Mastery of Cardiothoracic Surgery

Second Edition

Editors

Larry R. Kaiser, M.D.

The John Rhea Barton Professor and Chairman
Department of Surgery
University of Pennsylvania;
Surgeon-in-Chief,
University of Pennsylvania Health System
Philadelphia, Pennsylvania

Irving L. Kron, M.D.

William H. Muller Jr. Professor and Chairman, Department of Surgery
University of Virginia Health System
Charlottesville, Virginia

Thomas L. Spray, M.D.

Professor of Surgery, Department of Surgery
University of Pennsylvania School of Medicine;
Alice Langdon Warner Endowed Chair
Chief, Division of Cardiothoracic Surgery
The Children's Hospital of Philadelphia
Philadelphia, Pennsylvania

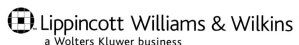

. Lippincott Williams & Wilkins
a Wolters Kluwer business

Philadelphia · Baltimore · New York · London
Buenos Aires · Hong Kong · Sydney · Tokyo

Acquisitions Editor: Brian Brown
Managing Editor: Julia Seto
Project Manager: Nicole Walz
Manufacturing Coordinator: Kathy Brown
Associate Marketing Director: Adam Glazer
Design Coordinator: Holly Reid McLaughlin
Cover Designer: Larry Didona
Production Service: Techbooks
Printer: Courier

Library of Congress Cataloging-in-Publication Data

Mastery of cardiothoracic surgery/[edited by] Larry R. Kaiser, Irving
   L. Kron, and Thomas L. Spray. — 2nd ed.
      p.   ; cm.
   Includes bibliographical references and index.
   ISBN 13: 978-078175-2-091
   ISBN 10: 0-7817-5209-4 (alk. paper)
   1. Heart—Surgery. 2. Chest—Surgery. I. Kaiser, Larry R. II.
   Kron,
Irving L. III. Spray, Thomas L.
      [DNLM: 1. Thoracic Diseases—surgery. 2. Cardiovascular Diseases—surgery.
      3. Thoracic Surgery—methods. WF 980 M423 2007]
RD598.M28 2007
617.4'12—dc22   2006026412

Care has been taken to confirm the accuracy of the information presented and to describe generally
accepted practices. However, the authors, editors, and publisher are not responsible for errors or omissions
or for any consequences from application of the information in this book and make no warranty, expressed
or implied, with respect to the currency, completeness, or accuracy of the contents of the publication.
Application of the information in a particular situation remains the professional responsibility of the
practitioner.

   The authors, editors, and publisher have exerted every effort to ensure that drug selection and dosage
set forth in this text are in accordance with current recommendations and practice at the time of
publication. However, in view of ongoing research, changes in government regulations, and the constant
flow of information relating to drug therapy and drug reactions, the reader is urged to check the package
insert for each drug for any change in indications and dosage and for added warnings and precautions.
This is particularly important when the recommended agent is a new or infrequently employed drug.

   Some drugs and medical devices presented in the publication have Food and Drug Administration
(FDA) clearance for limited use in restricted research settings. It is the responsibility of the health care
provider to ascertain the FDA status of each drug or device planned for use in their clinical practice.

   To purchase additional copies of this book, call our customer service department at
(800) 638-3030 or fax orders to (301) 223-2320. International customers should call (301) 223-2300.

   Visit Lippincott Williams & Wilkins on the Internet: at LWW.com. Lippincott Williams & Wilkins.
Customer service representatives are available from 8:30 am to 6 pm, EST.

10 9 8 7 6 5 4 3 2 1

To my dear Lindy, who can't figure out when I possibly can get any writing done. And to our children, Jon, Jeff, Garrett, Grace, Caroline, and the "little man," Daniel S. Kaiser.

—LRK

To my wife, Debbie, and our four terrific kids, Adam, Jason, Kristen, and Brian.

—ILK

To Melissa.

—TLS

Contents

Acknowledgments ix
Preface xi
Contributor xiii

Section I
General Thoracic Surgery

1. Endoscopy: Bronchoscopy and Esophagoscopy 1
   Joseph LoCicero III

2. Mediastinoscopy and Staging 11
   Mark Onaitis and David Harpole

3. Thoracic Incisions 26
   M. Blair Marshall

4. Right-Sided Pulmonary Resections 33
   Larry R. Kaiser

5. Left-Sided Pulmonary Resections 46
   Larry R. Kaiser

6. Pneumonectomy 53
   Robert Cerfolio

7. Bronchoplastic Procedures 64
   Anna Maria Ciccone, Federico Venuta, and Erino A. Rendina

8. Pulmonary Resections: Limited Resections
   and Segmentectomy 71
   Costanzo A. DiPerna and Douglas E. Wood

9. Tracheal Resection and Reconstruction 76
   Dean M. Donahue and Douglas J. Mathisen

10. Carinal Resection 82
    Dean M. Donahue

11. Video-Assisted Thorascopic Pulmonary
    Resections 88
    Allan Pickens and Robert J McKenna Jr.

12. Management of Pneumothorax and
    Bullous Disease 93
    Stephen D. Cassivi and Claude Deschamps

13. Thymectomy (Sternotomy) 100
    Francis C. Nichols and Victor F. Trastek

14. Thymectomy (Transcervical) 107
    Larry R. Kaiser

15. Resection of Posterior Mediastinal Lesions 113
    Brendon M. Stiles and Thomas M. Daniel

16. Antireflux Procedures 121
    Mark K. Ferguson

17. Transhiatal Esophagectomy 131
    Ahmad S. Ashrafi and R. Sudhir Sundaresan

18. Thoracic Approaches to Esophagectomy 139
    Alan G. Casson and H. Chrish Fernando

19. Minimally Invasive Esophageal Procedures 148
    Matthew J. Schuchert and James D. Luketich

20. Surgery for Achalasia and Other Motility
    Disorders 163
    Richard F. Heitmiller and Molly M. Buzdon

21. Esophageal Conduits and Palliative Procedures 174
    Wayne Hofstetter

22. Excision of Esophageal Diverticula 187
    Philip A. Rascoe and W. Roy Smythe

23. Lung Transplantation 194
    R. Duane Davis

24. Surgery for Emphysema 204
    Mark Ellis Ginsburg

25. Thoracic Outlet Syndromes 213
    Harold C. Urschel Jr. and Amit N. Patel

26. Chest Wall Resections 222
    John C. Kucharczuk and Larry R. Kaiser

27. The Diaphragm 228
    Christine L. Lau and Bryan F. Meyers

28. The Thoracic Duct and the Management
    of Chylothorax 244
    Bradley M. Rodgers

29. Pericardial Procedures 254
    John R. Roberts and Larry R. Kaiser

30. Surgical Management of Malignant
    Mesothelioma 262
    Joseph S. Friedberg and Shamus R. Carr

31. Mediastinal Lymph Node Dissection 271
    Ali Khoynezhad and Steven M. Keller

32. Surgical Management of Empyema: Tubes,
    Decortication, Open-Window Thoracostomy 280
    Mark S. Allen

33. Resection of Superior Sulcus Tumors 286
Christine Lau and G. A. Patterson

34. Surgery of Pulmonary Mycobacterial Disease 295
Marvin Pomerantz and John D. Mitchell

Section II
Adult Cardiac Surgery

Part A
General Considerations

35. Cardiopulmonary Bypass 305
Harry A. Wellons Jr. and Richard K. Zacour

36. Myocardial Protection 315
Constantine L. Athanasuleas and Gerald D. Buckberg

37. Database 326
Frederic Grover and Colleagues

38. Prevention of Neurologic Injury after Coronary
Artery Bypass 332
Christopher J. Barreiro and William A. Baumgartner

Part B
Acquired Valvular Heart Disease

39. Mitral Valve Repair 341
Lawrence H. Cohn

40. Mitral Valve Repair: Robotic Minimally Invasive 353
Alan P. Kypson, L. Wiley Nifong, and
W. Randolph Chitwood Jr.

41. Mitral Valve Repair: Ischemic 369
David H. Adams, Farzan Filsoufi, Lishan Aklog, and Sacha P.
Salzberg

42. Acquired Valvular Heart Disease: Mitral
Valve Replacement 378
Kwok L. Yun and D. Craig Miller

43. Reoperative Mitral Valve Replacement 391
G. Randall Green, Scott A. Buchanan, Reid W. Tribble, and
Curtis G. Tribble

44. Tricuspid Valve 403
Benjamin B. Peeler

45. Aortic Valve Replacement 410
David A. Fullerton

46. Aortic Valve Replacement: Ross Procedure 424
Ronald C. Elkins

Part C
Coronary Artery Disease

47. Coronary Artery Bypass Grafting Using
Cardiopulmonary Bypass 437
Robert S.D. Higgins and R. Anthony Perez-Tamayo

48. Coronary Artery Bypass: Hypothermic Ventricular
Fibrillation 449
Cary W. Akins

49. Off-Pump Coronary Artery Bypass Surgery 454
Howard K. Song and John D. Puskas

50. Robotic Coronary Artery Bypass Surgery 466
Saqib Masroor, L. Wiley Nifong, and
W. Randolph Chitwood Jr.

Part D
Surgery for Heart Failure

51. Left Ventricular Reconstruction 479
Constantine L. Athanasuleas and Gerald D. Buckberg

52. Mitral Valve Repair for Cardiomyopathy 494
Martin T. Spoor and Steven F. Bolling

53. Ventricular Assist 500
Nicholas C. Dang, Mehmet C. Oz, and Yoshifumi Naka

54. Surgery for Complications of
Myocardial Infarction 510
Mark F. Berry and Timothy J. Gardner

Part E
Thoracic Aortic Disease

55. Annuloaortic Ectasia 527
Tirone E. David

56. Aortic Dissection 534
Alberto Pochettino and Joseph E. Bavaria

57. Descending Thoracic and Thoracoabdominal
Aneurysms 545
John A. Kern and Irving L. Kron

58. Arch Aneurysms 556
Joseph S. Coselli, John Bozinovski, and Scott A. LeMaire

59. Acute Traumatic Aortic Transection 568
Daniel Martinez, Scott Johnson, O. L. Miller
and John Calhoon

Part F
Transplantation

60. Heart Transplantation 579
Christopher T. Salerno and Edward Verrier

61. Heart-Lung Transplantation 587
Bruce A. Reitz and Abdulaziz Alkhaldi

Part G
Arrhythmias

62. The Maze Procedure for the Surgical Treatment
of Atrial Fibrillation 599
John M. Stulak and Hartzell V. Schaff

63. Surgical Treatment of Atrial Fibrillation 606
A. Marc Gillinov

Part H
Other Cardiac

64. Cardiac Tumors 615
Himanshu J. Patel, Francis D. Pagani, and Richard L. Prager

65. Acute Pulmonary Embolus 621
    Thoralf M. Sundt

66. Chronic Pulmonary Thromboembolism
    and Pulmonary Thromboendarterectomy 626
    Michael M. Madani and Stuart W. Jamieson

Section III
Congenital Cardiac Surgery

67. Anatomy and Classification of Congenital
    Heart Disease 639
    Paul M. Weinberg

68. Echocardiographic Evaluation of Congenital
    Heart Disease 651
    Jack Rychik

69. Cardiac Magnetic Resonance Imaging 660
    Mark A. Fogel

70. Hemodynamic Assessment and Transcatheter
    Therapy for Congenital Heart Disease 679
    Nancy D. Bridges and Jonathan J. Rome

71. Palliative Operations for Congenital
    Heart Disease 693
    Carl L. Backer and Constantine Mavroudis

72. Anomalies of Systemic Venous Drainage 708
    Sanjiv K. Gandhi and Ralph D. Siewers

73. Patent Ductus Arteriosus 716
    Redmond P. Burke

74. Vascular Rings, Slings, and Other
    Arch Anomalies 722
    Erle H. Austin III and Minoo N. Kavarana

75. Atrial Septal Defects 739
    Richard D. Mainwaring and John J. Lamberti

76. Ventricular Septal Defects 750
    Christopher J. Knott-Craig

77. Aortopulmonary Window 759
    James S. Tweddell

78. Coarctation of the Aorta 768
    Irving Shen and Ross M. Ungerleider

79. Interrupted Aortic Arch Complex 779
    Richard G. Ohye, Takaaki Suzuki, Eric J. Devaney,
    and Edward L. Bove

80. Left Ventricular Outflow Tract Obstruction
    and Aortic Stenosis 789
    Flavian M. Lupinetti and Michael F. Teodori

81. Anomalies of the Sinuses of Valsalva and Aortico-Left
    Ventricular Tunnel 804
    Luca A. Vricella and Duke E. Cameron

82. Atrioventricular Canal Defects 811
    Martin J. Elliott, Mazyar Kanani, and Jeffrey P. Jacobs

83. Truncus Arteriosus 827
    Thomas L. Spray

84. Double-Outlet Ventricles 841
    Kirk R. Kanter

85. Transposition of the Great Arteries 855
    Thomas L. Spray

86. Congenitally Corrected Transposition of the
    Great Arteries 873
    Victor Bautista-Hernandez and Pedro J. del Nido

87. Pulmonary Stenosis and Pulmonary Atresia with
    Intact Septum 881
    Mark D. Plunkett and Hillel Laks

88. Pulmonary Atresia with Ventricular Septal Defect and
    Major Aortopulmonary Collaterals 895
    Malcolm J. MacDonald, V. Mohan Reddy, and Frank L.
    Hanley

89. Tetralogy of Fallot 907
    Robert D. B. Jaquiss

90. Cavopulmonary Shunts and the Hemi-Fontan
    Operation 916
    W. Steves Ring

91. Tricuspid Atresia/Single Ventricle and the
    Fontan Operation 925
    John E. Mayer Jr.

92. Hypoplastic Left Heart Syndrome 935
    Peter J. Gruber and Thomas L. Spray

93. Anomalies of Pulmonary Venous Return 947
    Benjamin B. Peeler, V. Seenu Reddy, and Irving L. Kron

94. Coronary Artery Anomalies in Children 959
    J. William Gaynor

95. Pediatric Heart Transplantation 973
    Charles B. Huddleston

96. Lung and Heart-Lung Transplantation
    in Children 985
    Thomas L. Spray

97. Ebstein's Malformation of the Tricuspid Valve
    in Children 998
    Brian L. Reemtsen and Vaughn A. Starnes

98. Mitral Valve Repair in Children 1008
    Christian Brizard

99. Aortic Valve Repair in Children 1017
    Mary Jane Barth, Chawki el-Zein, and Michel N. Ilbawi

100. Valve Replacement in Children/Ross Procedure ... 1024
     Ronald C. Elkins

101. Fontan Conversion/Arrhythmia Surgery 1035
     Constantine Mavroudis, Barbara J. Deal, and Carl L. Backer

Index   1043

Acknowledgments

First and foremost we would like to thank everyone who took time from their ever-busy schedules to revise, update, and in many cases, prepare new chapters for this book. Writing book chapters truly is a labor of love because there is little else to gain from textbook writing. Julia Seto at Lippincott Williams & Wilkins took on this project after it had begun, but has done a fantastic job of seeing the work to its conclusion. She was both cheerleader and coach, exhorting us on a regular basis to move ahead when it seemed as if we were stuck. Her pushing and prodding has ultimately paid off and for that we thank her.

Preface

When we set out to produce the first edition of the *Mastery* we were uncertain of the reception that it would receive from the cardiothoracic community. The book was modeled after the extremely successful *Mastery of Surgery* that appealed to a much larger demographic and the question remained whether there would be an audience for a *Mastery* dealing with a somewhat more limited subject. The fact that we have produced a second edition indicates the success with which the first edition was met, we are pleased to say. We set out to produce a book that fit into that narrow area between a comprehensive textbook and an atlas using recognized experts in their field for each chapter, and in the minds of many, we have succeeded. The editor's comments at the end of each chapter serve to put the information into context and, in some cases, even offer an opinion that differs from that expressed by the author of the chapter. Many people have commented on how much they have enjoyed these editorial comments and we have continued those in this edition.

We have completely revised this edition with a number of new chapters and some new authors. References have been updated and newer techniques have been added. We have maintained the original format of dividing the book into three sections, just as the specialty has defined itself. The book should prove extremely useful for the trainee in cardiothoracic surgery as well as for the experienced practitioner who may want to look up an infrequently performed procedure as a brief refresher. It is comprehensive enough both in scope and coverage to be useful, along with standard textbooks, in preparation for the in-training exam as well as for the written and oral board examinations. We feel that this book still serves as an excellent complement to the major textbooks in the field especially with regard to the performance of the actual surgical procedure. At a time when volumes of information are available online, it is not unreasonable to ask the question whether there is a future for the "hardcopy" textbook. We feel that the written work is alive and well and that practitioners want a book on the shelf to refer to when the need arises.

The field of cardiothoracic surgery currently finds itself at a crossroads. We have come to the realization that we are attracting fewer people to our chosen specialty for a number of reasons. A perception exists that the lifestyle of the cardiothoracic surgeon is not particularly desirable and this keeps some people away. There is a general view that few jobs are currently available in cardiac surgery and this may be dissuading some people from entering the field. Some individuals are attracted to general thoracic surgery as a career but are put off by the cardiac surgical requirements. Cardiothoracic surgery has resisted the urge to formally fragment the specialty by preserving a single certification board and there is no move afoot to change that. The specialty remains as one and our major professional organizations continue to support all areas of the field. Recent manpower surveys within the specialty show that the majority of practitioners do not limit their practice to one specific area but practice in at least two areas and the specialty must be cognizant of this as we continue to evolve new ways to educate surgeons. This is especially true in this era of work hour restrictions with the need to maximize the educational experience in the fewer hours that trainees are present. We need to find creative ways to continue to attract the most talented people to this great specialty of ours. It is our hope that the second edition of *Mastery of Cardiothoracic Surgery* will provide a concise, yet broad look at the specialty for the individual considering the field as his or her life's work.

Larry R. Kaiser, MD
Irving L. Kron, MD
Thomas L. Spray, MD

Contributors

David H. Adams, MD
Marie-Josèe and Henry R. Kravis Professor and Chairman
Department of Cardiothoracic Surgery
Mount Sinai School of Medicine
New York, New York

Cary W. Akins, MD
Clinical Professor
Department of Surgery
Harvard Medical School
Visiting Surgeon
Department of Surgery
Massachusetts General Hospital
Boston, Massachusetts

Lishan K. Aklog, MD
Chair
Cardiovascular Center
Heart and Lung Institute
Chief of Cardiovascular Surgery
St. Joseph's Hospital and Medical Center
Pheonix, Arizona

Mark S. Allen, MD
Professor of Surgery
Division of General Thoracic Surgery
Mayo Clinic
Chair, Division of General Thoracic Surgery
Department of Surgery
Mayo Clinic
Rochester, Minnesota

Abdulaziz Al-Khaldi, MBBS, MSC, FRCSC
Consultant
Department of Cardiac Surgery
King Abdulaziz Medical City
Riyadh, Saudia Arabia

Ahmad S. Ashrafi, MD, FRCS(C)
Fellow in Advanced Minimally Invasive Thoracic Surgery
Heart, Lung, and Esophageal Surgery Institute
University of Pittsburgh Medical Center
Pittsburgh, Pennsylvania

Constantine L. Athanasuleas, MD
Cardiac Surgeon
Department of Cardiothoracic Surgery
Norwood Clinic
Chief
Department of Cardiothoracic Surgery
Carraway Methodist Medical Center
Birmingham, Alabama

Erle H. Austin, III, MD
Professor
Division of Thoracic/Cardiovascular Surgery
University of Louisville
Rudd Heart and Lung Center
Louisville, Kentucky

Carl Lewis Backer, MD
Professor
Department of Surgery
Northwestern University Feinberg School of Medicine
A.C. Buehler Professor of Cardiovascular and Thoracic Surgery
Division of Cardiovascular Thoracic Surgery
Children's Memorial Hospital
Chicago, Illinois

Christopher Barriero, MD
Categorical General Surgery Resident
Department of Surgery
Johns Hopkins Hospital
Baltimore, Maryland

Mary Jane Barth, MD
Pediatric Cardiovascular Surgeon
The Heart Institute for Children
Christ Hospital Medical Center
Oak Lawn, Illinois

William A. Baumgartner, MD
Professor of Surgery
Department of Cardiac Surgery
Johns Hopkins University
Cardiac Surgeon-in-Charge
Johns Hopkins Hospital
Baltimore, Maryland

Victor Bautista-Hernandez, MD
Research Fellow
Department of Cardiac Surgery
Children's Hospital Boston
Boston, Massachusetts

Joseph E. Bavaria, MD
Professor
Department of Surgery
University of Pennsylvania
Vice Chief, Division of Cardiothoracic Surgery
Director, Thoracic Aortic Surgery Program
University of Pennsylvania Health System
Philadelphia, Pennsylvania

Mark F. Berry, MD
Resident, Cardiothoracic Surgery
Duke University
Formerly Chief Resident
Department of Surgery
Hospital of the University of Pennsylvania
Philadelphia, Pennsylvania

Steven F. Bolling, MD
Professor of Surgery
Section of Cardiac Surgery
University of Michigan
Ann Arbor, Michigan

Edward L. Bove, MD
Professor and Head
Section of Cardiac Surgery
Department of Surgery
University of Michigan
Ann Arbor, Michigan

John Bozinovski, MD, MSc, FRCSC
Assistant Professor
Division of Cardiothoracic Surgery
Baylor College of Medicine
Attending Surgeon
Cardiovascular Surgery Service
Texas Heart Institute at St. Luke's Episcopal Hospital
Houston, Texas

Nancy D. Bridges, MD
Chief, Clinical Transplant Section
Transplantation Immunobiology Branch
National Institute of Allergy and Infectious Diseases
National Institutes of Health
Bethesda, Maryland

Christian Pierre Brizard, MD
Associate Professor
Department of Pediatrics
The University of Melbourne
Director, Cardiac Surgery Unit
Royal Children's Hospital
Melbourne, Victoria, Australia

Scott A. Buchanan, MD
Attending Surgeon
Department of Cardiac Surgery
Maine Medical Center
Portland, Maine

Gerald Buckberg, MD
Distinguished Professor of Surgery
Department of Surgery
David Geffen School of Medicine at UCLA
Los Angeles, California

Redmond P. Burke, MD
Chief
Division of Cardiovascular Surgery
Miami Children's Hospital
Miami, Florida

Molly M. Buzdon, MD
Assistant Chief
Department of Surgery
Union Memorial Hospital
Baltimore, Maryland

John H. Calhoon, MD
Professor and Chief
Division of Thoracic Surgery
Department of Surgery
University of Texas Health Science Center at San Antonio
San Antonio, Texas

Duke E. Cameron, MD
Consultant
Department of Surgery
John Hopkins University Hospital
Baltimore, Maryland

Shamus R. Carr, MD
US Naval Hospital Gaum
Agana Heights, Gaum
Formerly Chief Resident, Surgery
University of Pennsylvania

Stephen D. Cassivi, MD, MSc, FRCSC, FACS
Associate Professor
Surgical Director of Lung Transplantation
Department of Surgery
Mayo Clinic College of Medicine
Consultant Surgeon
Division of General Thoracic Surgery
Mayo Clinic
Rochester, Minnesota

Alan Graham Casson, FRCSC
Professor
Department of Surgery
Dalhousie University
Chief, Division of Thoracic and Esophageal Surgery
Queen Elizabeth II Health Sciences Centre
Halifax, Nova Scotia, Canada

Robert James Cerfolio, MD, FACS, FCCP
Professor
Chief of Thoracic Surgery
Department of Surgery
University of Alabama at Birmingham
Birmingham, Alabama

W. Randolph Chitwood, Jr., MD, FACS, FRCS (Eng)
Professor
Division of Cardiothoracic and Vascular Surgery
Department of Surgery
Director, East Carolina Heart Institute
Brody School of Medicine at East Carolina University
Chief
Department of Surgery
Pitt County Memorial Hospital
Greenville, North Carolina

Anna Maria Ciccone, MD
Assistant Professor
Department of Thoracic Surgery
"La Sapienza" University of Rome
Staff Surgeon
Department of Thoracic Surgery
Ospedale Sant'Andrea
Rome, Italy

Lawrence H. Cohn, MD
Virginia and James Hubbard Professor of Cardiac Surgery
Harvard Medical School
Senior Surgeon
Division of Cardiac Surgery
Brigham and Women's Hospital
Boston, Massachusetts

Joseph S. Coselli, MD
Professor and Chief
Division of Cardiothoracic Surgery
Michael E. DeBakey Department of Surgery
Baylor College of Medicine
Chief, Adult Cardiac Surgery
Texas Heart Institute
Houston, Texas

Nicholas C. Dang, MD
Resident
Department of Surgery
Columbia University, College of Physicians and Surgeons
Resident
Department of Surgery
New York-Presbyterian Hospital, Columbia University Medical Center
New York, New York

Thomas M. Daniel, MD
Professor
Division of Thoracic and Cardiovascular Surgery
Department of Surgery
University of Virginia School of Medicine
Charlottesville, Virginia

Tirone E. David, MD
Professor
Department of Surgery
University of Toronto
Chief, Division of Cardiovascular Surgery
Toronto General Hospital
Toronto, Ontario, Canada

R. Duane Davis, Jr., MD
Professor
Department of Surgery
Duke University School of Medicine
Director of Transplantation
Duke University Medical Center
Durham, North Carolina

Barbara J. Deal, MD
Professor
Department of Pediatrics
Northwestern University
Feinberg School of Medicine
Chicago, Illinois

Pedro J. del Nido, MD
William E. Ladd Professor
Department of Surgery
Harvard Medical School
Chairman
Department of Cardiac Surgery
Children's Hospital of Boston
Boston, Massachusetts

Claude Deschamps, MD
Professor
Department of Surgery
Division of General Thoracic Surgery
Mayo Clinic College of Medicine
Chair, Department of Surgery
Mayo Clinic
Rochester, Minnesota

Eric J. Devaney, MD
Assistant Professor
Department of Surgery
University of Michigan Medical School
Ann Arbor, Michigan

Costanzo A. DiPerna, MD
Thoracic Surgery Resident
Department of Cardiothoracic Surgery
University of Washington
Seattle, Washington

Dean M. Donahue, MD
Assistant Professor Department of Surgery
Harvard Medical School
Assistant Surgeon
Massachusetts General Hospital
Boston, Massachusetts

Chawki el-Zein, MD
Pediatric Cardiovascular Surgeon
The Heart Institute for Children
Christ Hospital Medical Center
Oak Lawn, Illinois

Ronald C. Elkins, MD
Professor Emeritus
Department of Surgery
University of Oklahoma Health Sciences Center
Thoracic Surgeon
Department of Thoracic Surgery
Presbyterian Hospital
Oklahoma City, Oklahoma

Martin J. Elliot, MD, FRCS
Professor
Department of Cardiothoracic Surgery
University College London
Chairman of Cardiothoracic Services
The Great Ormond Street Hospital for Children NHS Trust
London, United Kingdom

Mark K. Ferguson, MD
Professor
Department of Surgery
University of Chicago
Head, Thoracic Surgery Service
University of Chicago Hospitals
Chicago, Illinois

Hiran Chrishantha Fernando, FRCS, FRCSEd
Associate Professor
Department of Cardiothoracic Surgery
Boston University School of Medicine
Director of Minimally Invasive Thoracic Surgery
Boston Medical Center
Boston, Massachusetts

Farzan Filsoufi, MD
Associate Professor
Department of Cardiothoracic Surgery
Mount Sinai School of Medicine
Associate Chief, Cardiac Surgery
Mount Sinai Medical Center
New York, New York

Mark A. Fogel MD, FAAP, FACC
Attending Cardiologist
Assistant Radiologist
Department of Cardiology
Children's Hospital of Philadelphia
Philadelphia, Pennsylvania

Joseph S. Friedberg, MD, FACS
Associate Professor
Department of Surgery
University of Pennsylvania
Chief, Division of Thoracic Surgery
Penn-Presbyterian Medical Center
Philadelphia, Pennsylvania

David A. Fullerton, MD
Professor
Department of Surgery
University of Colorado
Head, Cardiothoracic Surgery
University of Colorado Health Sciences Center
Denver, Colorado

Sanjiv K. Gandhi, MD
Associate Professor
Department of Surgery
Washington University
Pediatric Cardiac Surgeon
St. Louis Children's Hospital
St. Louis, Missouri

Timothy J. Gardner, MD
Clinical Professor
Department of Surgery
University of Pennsylvania
Philadelphia, Pennsylvania
Medical Director
Center for Heart and Vascular Health
Christiana Care Health System
Newark, Delaware

J. William Gaynor, MD
Associate Professor
Department of Surgery
University of Pennsylvania School of Medicine
Attending Surgeon
Children's Hospital of Philadelphia
Philadelphia, Pennsylvania

Marc Gillinov, MD
Surgeon
Department of Thoracic and Cardiovascular Surgery
Cleveland Clinic Foundation
Cleveland, Ohio

Mark Ellis Ginsburg, MD
Associate Clinical Professor
Department of Surgery
Columbia University
Associate Director
General Thoracic Surgery
New York-Presbyterian Hospital
New York, New York

G. Randall Green, MD
Physician
Department of Surgery
Rochester General Hospital
Rochester, New York

Frederick L. Grover, MD
Professor and Chair
Department of Surgery
University of Colorado
Director, Lung Transplantation
University of Colorado Health Sciences Center
Denver, Colorado

Peter J. Gruber, MD, PhD
Assistant Professor
Department of Surgery
University of Pennsylvania
Attending Surgeon
Children's Hospital of Pennsylvania
Philadelphia, Pennsylvania

Frank L. Hanley, MD
Professor
Department of Cardiothoracic Surgery
Stanford University School of Medicine
Chief, Pediatric Cardiothoracic Surgery
Lucille Packard Children's Hospital
Stanford, California

David H. Harpole, Jr., MD
Professor and Chief
Department of Surgery
Duke Medical Center
Durham, North Carolina

Richard F. Heitmiller, MD
Chief of Surgery
Department of Surgery
Union Memorial Hospital
Baltimore, Maryland

Robert A. D. Higgins, MD
Professor and Chairman
Department of Cardiovascular and Thoracic Surgery
Rush University
Director
Department of Cardiovascular and Thoracic Surgery
Rush University Medical Center
Chicago, Illinois

Wayne Hofstetter, MD
Assistant Professor
Department of Thoracic and Cardiovascular Surgery
The University of Texas MD Anderson Cancer Center
Houston, Texas

Charles B. Huddleston, MD
Professor
Department of Surgery
Washington University School of Medicine
Chief, Pediatric Cardiothoracic Surgery
St. Louis Children's Hospital
St. Louis, Missouri

Michel N. Ilbawi, MD
Director, Cardiovascular Surgery
The Heart Institute for Children
Christ Hospital Medical Center
Oak Lawn, Illinois

Jeffrey P. Jacobs, MD
Pediatric Cardiovascular Surgeon
All Children's Hospital
St. Petersburg, Florida

Stuart W. Jamieson, MB, FRCS, FACS
Distinguished Professor of Surgery
Chief of Cardiothoracic Surgery
University of California, San Diego
San Diego, California

Robert D. B. Jaquiss
Chief, Pediatric Cardiac Surgery
Arkansas Childrens Hospital
Professor of Surgery
University of Arkansas College of Medicine
Little Rock, Arkansas

Scott B. Johnson, MD
Associate Professor
Division of Thoracic Surgery
Department of Surgery
University of Texas Health Science Center
San Antonio, Texas

Larry R. Kaiser, MD
The John Rhea Barton Professor and Chairman
Department of Surgery
University of Pennsylvania
Surgeon-in-Chief
University of Pennsylvania Health System
Philadelphia, Pennsylvania

Mazyar Kanani, MRCS
British Heart Foundation Clinical Research Fellow
Institute of Child Health
London, United Kingdom

Kirk R. Kanter, MD
Professor
Department of Surgery
Emory University School of Medicine
Chief, Pediatric Cardiac Surgery
Children's Healthcare of Atlanta at Egleston
    Children's Hospital
Atlanta, Georgia

Minoo N. Kavarana, MD
Assistant Professor
University of Louisville
Louisville, Kentucky
Cardiovascular & Thoracic Surgeon
Marymount Hospital, London
London, Kentucky

Steven M. Keller, MD
Professor
Department of Cardiothoracic Surgery
Albert Einstein College of Medicine
Chief, Division of Thoracic Surgery
Montefiore Medical Center
Bronx, New York

John A. Kern, MD
Associate Professor
Division of Thoracic and Cardiovascular Surgery
Department of Surgery
University of Virginia Health System
Charlottesville, Virginia

Ali Khoynezhad, MD, Ph.D
Assistant Professor
Department of Cardiovascular and Thoracic Surgery
University of Nebraska Medical Center
Omaha, Nebraska

Christopher J. Knott-Craig, MD, FACS
Professor of Surgery
Division of Cardiothoracic Surgery
Oklahoma University
Chief, Pediatric Cardiothoracic Surgery
Children's Hospital of Oklahoma
Oklahoma City, Oklahoma

Irving Louis Kron, MD
William H. Muller, Jr. Professor and Chair
Department of Surgery
Chief, Division of Thoracic and Cardiovascular Surgery
University of Virginia Health System
Charlottesville, Virginia

John C. Kucharczuk, MD
Assistant Professor
Department of Surgery
University of Pennsylvania
Philadelphia, Pennsylvania

Alan P. Kypson, MD
Assistant Professor
Division of Cardiothoracic Surgery
Brody School of Medicine at East Carolina University
Attending Surgeon
Department of Surgery
Pitt County Memorial Hospital
Greenville, North Carolina

Hillel Laks, MD
Professor
Department of Surgery
Division of Cardiac Surgery
University of California, Los Angeles Geffen School of Medicine
Los Angeles, California

John J. Lamberti, MD
Professor of Surgery
Division of Cardiothoracic Surgery
University of California, San Diego
Director, Children's Heart Institute
Department of Cardiac Surgery
Children's Hospital, San Diego
San Diego, California

Christine L. Lau, MD
Assistant Professor
Department of Surgery
University of Michigan
Ann Arbor, Michigan

Scott A. LeMaire, MD
Associate Professor
Division of Cardiothoracic Surgery
Baylor College of Medicine
Attending Surgeon
Cardiovascular Surgery Service
Texas Heart Institute at St. Luke's Episcopal Hospital
Houston, Texas

Joseph LoCicero, III, MD
Director of Surgical Oncology
Maimonides Medical Center
Brooklyn, New York

James D. Luketich, MD
Sampson Family Endowed Professor of Surgery
Department of Surgery
University of Pittsburgh
Chief, Division of Thoracic and Foregut Surgery
Chief, Heart, Lung, and Esophageal Surgery Institute
University of Pittsburgh Medical Center
Pittsburgh, Pennsylvania

Flavian Mark Lupinetti, MD
Thoracic and Cardiovascular Surgeon
Department of Surgery
Casa Grande Regional Medical Center
Casa Grande, Arizona

Malcolm J. MacDonald, MD
Clinical Assistant Professor, Department of
    Cardiothoracic Surgery
Division of Pediatric Cardiac Surgery
Faek Cardiovascular Research Center
Stanford, California

Michael Mehrdad Madani, MD, FACS
Assistant Professor
Division of Cardiothoracic Surgery
Department of Surgery
University of California, San Diego
San Diego, California
Chief
Section of Cardiothoracic Surgery
San Diego Veterans Affairs Healthcare Systems
La Jolla, California

Richard D. Mainwaring, MD
Surgeon
Department of Pediatric Cardiovascular Surgery
Sutter Medical Center
Sacramento, California

M. Blair Marshall, MD
Associate Professor
Department of Surgery
Georgetown University
Chief
Division of Thoracic Surgery
Georgetown University Hospital
Washington, DC

Daniel Martinez, MD
Division of Thoracic Surgery
University of Texas Health Science Center
San Antonio, Texas

Saqib Masroor, MD, MHS
Director of Minimally Invasive Cardiac Surgery
Department of Surgery
Hackensack University Medical Center
Hackensack, New Jersey

Douglas J. Mathisen, MD
Hermes C. Grillo Professor of Thoracic Surgery
Harvard Medical School
Chief, General Thoracic Surgery
Massachusetts General Hospital
Boston, Massachusetts

Constantine Mavroudis, MD
Professor and Vice Chairman
Department of Surgery
Northwestern University Feinberg School of Medicine
Willis J. Potts Professor and Surgeon-in-Chief
Children's Memorial Hospital
Chicago, Illinois

John E. Mayer, Jr., MD
Professor
Department of Surgery
Harvard Medical School
Senior Associate
Department of Cardiac Surgery
Children's Hospital, Boston
Boston, Massachusetts

Robert J. McKenna, Jr., MD
Clinical Professor
Department of Thoracic Surgery
University of California, Los Angeles
Chief, Department of Thoracic Surgery
Cedars Sinai Medical Center
Los Angeles, California

Bryan F. Meyers, MD, MPH
Associate Professor
Department of Surgery
Washington University School of Medicine
Attending Physician
Barnes-Jewish Hospital
St. Louis, Missouri

D. Craig Miller, MD
Thelma and Henry Doelger Professor of Cardiovascular Surgery
Department of Cardiothoracic Surgery
Stanford University School of Medicine
Palo Alto, California

O.L. Miller, Jr., MD
Southeast Texas Heart and Lung Surgeons
Port Arthur, Texas

John D. Mitchell, MD
Associate Professor of Surgery
Department of Surgery
University of Colorado at Denver and Health Sciences Center
Chief, Section of General Thoracic Surgery
University of Colorado Hospital
Denver, Colorado

Yoshifumi Naka, MD, PhD
Herbert Irving Assistant Professor of Surgery
Department of Surgery
Columbia University, College of Physicians and Surgeons
Director, Cardiac Transplantation and Mechanical
    Circulatory Support Program
New York-Presbyterian Hosptial, Columbia University
    Medical Center
New York, New York

Francis C. Nichols, MD
Assistant Professor
Division of General Thoracic Surgery
Mayo Clinic College of Medicine
Consultant
Division of General Thoracic Surgery
Mayo Clinic
Rochester, Minnesota

L. Wiley Nifong, MD
Associate Professor of Surgery
Department of Cardiothoracic and Vascular Surgery
Brody School of Medicine at
    East Carolina University
Surgeon
Pitt County Memorial Hospital
Greenville, North Carolina

Richard G. Ohye, MD
Assistant Professor
Department of Surgery
University of Michigan Medical School
Ann Arbor, Michigan

Mark W. Onaitis, MD
Cardiothoracic Surgery Resident
Department of Surgery
Duke University Medical Center
Durham, North Carolina

Mehmet C. Oz, MD
Professor
Department of Surgery
Columbia University, College of Physicians and Surgeons
New York-Presbyterian Hospital, Columbia
    University Medical Center
New York, New York

Francis D. Pagani, MD, PhD
Associate Professor
Department of Surgery
University of Michigan
Director, Heart Transplant Program and Center for
    Circulatory Support
University of Michigan Medical Center
Ann Arbor, Michigan

Amit N. Patel, MD, MS
Assistant Professor of Surgery
University of Pittsburgh Medical School
Pittsburgh, Pennsylvania

Himanshu J. Patel, MD
Assistant Professor of Surgery
Section of Cardiac Surgery
University of Michigan Hospital
Chief, Section of Cardiac Surgery
Ann Arbor Veterans Hospital
Ann Arbor, Michigan

G. Alexander Patterson, MD
Evarts A. Graham Professor of Surgery
Chief, Division of Cardiothoracic Surgery
Washington University School of Medicine
Staff Surgeon
Barnes-Jewish Hospital
St. Louis, Missouri

Benjamin B. Peeler, MD
Assistant Professor
Department of Surgery
University of Virginia School of Medicine
Surgical Director
University of Virginia Hospital Children's Heart Center
Charlottesville, Virginia

R. Anthony Perez-Tamayo, MD, PhD
Assistant Professor
Department of Cardiovascular and Thoracic Surgery
Rush University Medical Center
Chief, Division of Cardiothoracic Surgery
Attending Cardiothoracic Surgeon
John Stroger Hospital of Cook County
Chicago, Illinois

Allan Pickens, MD
Assistant Professor
Section of Thoracic Surgery
Department of Surgery
University of Michigan
Ann Arbor, Michigan

Mark D. Plunkett, MD
Associate Professor
Department of Surgery
University of California, Los Angeles School of Medicine
Los Angeles, California

Alberto Pochettino, MD
Associate Professor
Department of Surgery
University of Pennsylvania
Philadelphia, Pennsylvania

Marvin Pomerantz, MD
Professor
Department of Surgery
University of Colorado at Denver and Health Sciences Center
University of Colorado Hospital
Denver, Colorado

Richard L. Prager, MD
Division Head, Professor of Surgery
Section of Cardiac Surgery
University of Michigan Hospital
Staff Surgeon
Section of Cardiac Surgery
Ann Arbor Veterans Hospital
Ann Arbor, Michigan

John D. Puskas, MD, MSc
Associate Professor and
Associate Chief of Cardiothoracic Surgery
Department of Surgery
Emory University School of Medicine
Chief of Cardiac Surgery
Emory Crawford Long Hospital
Atlanta, Georgia

Philip A. Rascoe, MD
Chief Resident
General Surgery
University of Texas Medical School of Houston
Houston, Texas

V. Seenu Reddy, MD, MBA
Assistant Professor Surgery
Department of Surgery
Director, Thoracic Aortic Surgery & Emerging Technology
Staff Surgeon, Santa Rosa Children's Hospital
Division of Thoracic Surgery
University of Texas Health Sciences Center at San Antonio
San Antonio, Texas

V. Mohan Reddy, MD
Associate Professor of Cardiothoracic Surgery
Chief, Division of Pediatric Cardiac Surgery
Lucile Packard Children's Hospital
Stanford University
Palo Alto, California

Brian L. Reemtsen, MD
Assistant Professor
Department of Cardiothoracic Surgery
University of Southern California School of Medicine
Surgeon
Children's Hospital Los Angeles
Los Angeles, California

Bruce A. Reitz, MD
Norman E. Shumway Professor of Cardiothoracic Surgery
Department of Cardiothoracic Surgery
Stanford University School of Medicine
Stanford, California

Erino A. Rendina, MD
Professor
Department of Thoracic Surgery
"La Sapienza" University of Rome
Chief Professor
Department of Thoracic Surgery
Ospedale Sant'Andrea
Rome, Italy

W. Steves Ring, MD
Professor and Chairman
Cardiovascular and Thoracic Surgery
University of Texas Southwestern Medical Center
Attending Surgeon
Pediatric Cardiothoracic Surgery
Children's Medical Center at Dallas
Dallas, Texas

John R. Roberts, MD
Sarah Cannon Cancer Center
Surgical Clinic
Nashville, Tennessee

Bradley M. Rodgers, MD
Professor
Departments of Surgery and Pediatrics
University of Virginia
Chief, Pediatric Surgery
University of Virginia Health System
Charlottesville, Virginia

Jonathan Jack Rome, MD
Associate Professor
Department of Pediatrics
University of Pennsylvania
Director, Cardiac Catheterization Laboratory
Departments of Cardiology and Pediatrics
Children's Hospital of Philadelphia
Philadelphia, Pennsylania

Jack Rychik, MD, FACC
Medical Director, Fetal Heart Program
Director, Echocardiography Laboratory
Attending Cardiologist
Department of Cardiology
Children's Hospital of Philadelphia
Philadelphia, Pennsylvania

Christopher T. Salerno, MD
Assistant Professor
Division of Cardiothoracic Surgery
University of Washington
Seattle, Washington

Sacha P. Salzberg, MD
Post-Doctoral Research Fellow
Department of Cardiothoracic Surgery
Mount Sinai Medical Center
New York, New York

Hartzell V. Schaff, MD
Stuart. W. Harrington Professor of Surgery
Chair, Division of Cardiovascular Surgery
Mayo Clinic College of Medicine
Rochester, Minnesota

Matthew J. Schuchert, MD
Assistant Professor of Surgery
Heart, Lung, and Esophageal Surgery Institue
University of Pittsburgh Medical Center
Pittsburgh, Pennsylvania

Irving Shen, MD
Chief
Department of Pediatric Cardiac Surgery
Inova Fairfax Hospital for Children
Falls Church, Virginia

Ralph D. Siewers, MD
Professor of Surgery (Retired)
Department of Surgery
University of Pittsburgh
Department of Cardiothoracic Surgery
Children's Hospital of Pittsburgh
Pittsburgh, Pennsylvania

W. Roy Smythe, MD
Chair
Department of Surgery
Texas A&M Health Science Center College of Medicine
Chief of Surgery
Scott & White Hospital
Temple, Texas

Howard K. Song, MD, PhD
Assistant Professor
Division of Cardiothoracic Surgery
Oregon Health and Science University
Portland, Oregon

Martinus Twyeffort Spoor, MD
Instructor
Section of Cardiac Surgery
University of Michigan
Attending Surgeon
Section of Cardiac Surgery
University of Michigan Hospitals
Ann Arbor, Michigan

Thomas L. Spray, MD
Alice Landon Warner Professor of Surgery
University of Pennsylvania
Chief
Division of Cardiothoracic Surgery
The Children's Hospital of Philadelphia
Philadelphia, Pennsylvania

Vaughn A. Starnes, MD
Hastings Professor and Chairman
Department of Cardiothoracic Surgery
Keck School of Medicine
University of Southern California
Los Angeles, California

Brendon M. Stiles, MD
Chief Resident
Department of Surgery
University of Virginia Health System
Charlottesville, Virginia

John M. Stulak, MD
Fellow in Cardiac and Thoracic Surgery
Division of Cardiovascular Surgery
Mayo Clinic
Rochester, Minnesota

R. Sudhir Sundaresan, MD
Professor
Department of Surgery
University of Ottawa
Head, Division of Thoracic Surgery
Ottawa Hospital- General Campus
Ottawa, Ontario, Canada

Thoralf M. Sundt, MD
Professor
Division of Cardiovascular Surgery
Department of Surgery
Mayo Clinic College of Medicine
Consultant
Department of Surgery
Mayo Clinic
Rochester, Minnesota

Takaaki Suzuki, MD, PhD
Assistant Professor
Department of Surgery
Keio University School of Medicine
Sinjuku-ku, Tokyo
Chief, Division of Cardiovascular Surgery
Tokyo Metropolitan Children's Hospital
Kiyose-shi, Tokyo
Japan

Michael F. Teodori, MD
Section Chief, Cardiothoracic Surgery
Phoenix Children's Hospital
Phoenix, Arizona

Victor F. Trastek, MD
Professor
Department of Surgery
Mayo Clinic College of Medicine
Scottsdale, Arizona

Curtis G. Tribble, MD
Professor and Chief
Division of Cardiothoracic Surgery
University of Florida College of Medicine
Gainsville Florida

Reid W. Tribble, MD
Carolina Cardiac Surgery Associates
Columbia, South Carolina

James S. Tweddell
Professor of Surgery and Pediatrics
Chief, Division of Cardiothoracic Surgery
Department of Surgery
Medical College of Wisconsin
Milwaukee, Wisconsin

Ross M. Ungerleider, MD
Professor
Head, Division of Cardiothoracic Surgery
Department of Surgery
Oregon Health and Sciences University
Portland, Oregon

Harold Clifton Urschel, Jr. MD
Professor
Department of Cardiovascular and Thoracic Surgery
University of Texas—Southwestern Medical School
Chair, Cardiovascular and Thoracic Surgical Research, Education,
     and Clinical Excellence
Baylor University Medical Center
Dallas, Texas

Federico Venuta, MD
Associate Professor
Department of Thoracic Surgery
"La Sapienza" University of Rome
Staff Surgeon
Department of Thoracic Surgery
Policlinico Umberto I
Rome, Italy

Edward Verrier, MD
Professor and Chief
Division of Cardiothoracic Surgery
University of Washington Medical Center
Seattle, Washington

Luca A. Vricella, MD
Chief of Pediatric Heart and Lung Transplantation
Assistant Director, Pediatric Cardiac Surgery
Assistant Professor of Surgery
Comprehensive Transplant Center
John Hopkins University Medical Center
Baltimore, Maryland

Paul M. Weinberg, MD
Professor
Departments of Pediatrics and Pathology, and Laboratory
    Medicine
Children's Hospital of Philadelphia, University of Pennsylvania
    School of Medicine
Senior Cardiologist and Consultant in Pathology
Division of Cardiology
Children's Hospital of Philadelphia
Philadelphia, Pennsylvania

Harry A. Wellons, MD
Professor of Surgery
Department of Thoracic and Cardiovascular Surgery
University of Virginia
Charlottesville, Virginia

Douglas E. Wood, MD
Endowed Chair in Lung Cancer Research
Professor and Chief
Division of General Thoracic Surgery
University of Washington
Seattle, Washington

Kwok L. Yun, MD
Assistant Chief
Department of Cardiac Surgery
Kaiser Permanente Los Angeles Medical Center
Los Angeles, California

Richard Zacour, CCP
Chief Perfusionist
Department of Thoracic-Cardiovascular Perfusion
University of Virginia Health System
Charlottesville, Virginia

I

General Thoracic Surgery

Endoscopy: Bronchoscopy and Esophagoscopy

Joseph LoCicero III

Bronchoscopy and esophagoscopy are integral techniques in the practice of thoracic surgery. Their use allows the surgeon not only to locate individual specific anatomic variations, but also to define abnormal endoluminal pathologic states. In addition, these techniques may be applied as therapeutic maneuvers in cases of foreign-body extraction, dilation of a stricture, or laser excision of obstructing tumors. Both the rigid and flexible techniques of bronchoscopy and esophagoscopy are important because each has distinct advantages (Table 1-1). Among the advantages of flexible endoscopy are that patients tolerate it well and are willing to undergo the procedure repeatedly. The procedure can be done under local anesthesia with minimal sedation, which allows patients to return to normal activity within a short period of time. Advantages of rigid endoscopy include the ability to obtain large biopsy specimens and to perform debridement easily and effectively. Suction attachments are larger and permit better, more effective clearing of debris. Rigid endoscopy is best for determining fixation or rigidity caused by scarring or cancer that might imply unresectability. In addition, rigid endoscopy is best for dilation and stent placement under direct vision. Appropriate application is based on the experience of the operator and the anticipated requirements.

Anatomic Considerations

Aerodigestive anatomy begins with the entry of air into the body via the nasopharynx and the oropharynx. Entry may be gained to the upper aerodigestive system through either the nose or the mouth. At the nares, there is a 3-mm to 4-mm opening below the lower turbinates, with direct access to the posterior pharynx. This entry is just medial to the pharyngeal tonsil and passes posterior to the soft palate. Entry through the mouth reaches the posterior pharynx beyond the soft palate. As the posterior portion of the tongue is passed, one reaches the vallecula. At this level, the epiglottis can be seen anterior to the aerodigestive tract. Immediately posterior to this structure, the vocal cords can be seen easily. They are attached anteriorly and move apart posteriorly. The vocal cords are bounded by the aryepiglottic fold and posteriorly by the corniculate tubercles. Just posterior to the tubercles is the entrance to the esophagus. Laterally, on both sides of the esophagus, are the pyriform recesses, which are often mistaken for the true esophagus but are false passages with a depth of 2 cm to 3 cm.

Tracheobronchial Tree

Past the vocal cords, the trachea consists of a series of C-shaped cartilaginous strips connected by angular ligaments and a membranous flexible portion posteriorly, which is adjacent to the esophagus. This extends for a distance of 10 cm to the tracheal bifurcation. The thoracic trachea is crossed anteriorly by the innominate vein. The innominate and carotid arteries lie along the anterolateral wall of the trachea. Beyond this, the arch of the aorta lies to the left of the trachea. Laterally, on the right side, the superior vena cava is in close proximity to the trachea. Lying posterolaterally are the right and left paratracheal lymph node chains. At the tracheal bifurcation, there is a sharp carina, which measures approximately 1.5 cm in diameter, dividing the distal trachea into the right and left mainstem bronchi, each of which is approximately 1 cm in diameter (Fig. 1-1). The first branch of the right mainstem bronchus is the right upper lobe, which usually branches within 1 cm of the carina (Fig. 1-2). This lobar branch takes off at a 90-degree angle to the right mainstem bronchus, extending laterally. Beyond the right upper lobe branch is the continuation of the principal bronchus, termed the bronchus intermedius. This extends for 2 cm before dividing into the distal branches. The right middle lobe orifice is directly anterior to and usually opposite the superior segmental bronchus of the lower lobe (Fig. 1-3). The remaining basilar bronchi are distal to this. The major vascular relationship on the right is the right main pulmonary artery, which crosses anteriorly to the right mainstem bronchus at its origin and extends down on the anterolateral surface of the bronchus.

The left mainstem bronchus extends for 3 cm from the tracheal bifurcation to the bifurcation of the upper and lower lobes (Fig. 1-4). This mainstem bronchus is longer than the right mainstem bronchus because it passes inferior to the aortic arch. In addition, the left pulmonary artery crosses the bronchus to lie on the posterolateral aspect of the mainstem bronchus and its divisions. The first branch is the left upper lobe bronchus, which takes off at a 110-degree angle from the left mainstem. The continuation of the left mainstem bronchus immediately becomes the lower lobe orifice.

The segmental anatomy of the right and left lung is shown in Fig. 1-5. The right upper lobe bronchus divides into three segmental bronchi, namely the apical, posterior, and anterior segments. The middle lobe divides into the medial and lateral segments. The lower lobe divides into the superior segment and four basal segments, including

Table 1-1   Advantages of Flexible and Rigid Endoscopy

Flexible endoscopy
    Well tolerated
    Requires only local anesthesia
    Minimal sedation required
    Patient acceptability
Rigid endoscopy
    Accepts larger forceps for biopsy/
      debridement
    Accepts larger suction tubes for
      high-volume use
    More helpful for evaluation of fixation/
      rigidity
    Better for dilation and stent
      placement

the anterior, medial, lateral, and posterior basal segments. Small anatomic variations occur with regularity. The variations most often seen are the relationships between the superior segment orifice and the orifice of the middle lobe. The usual anatomic position is branching directly opposite one another. However, one may be higher or lower than the other. Such variations may be important when planning resections of central lower lobe tumors. Another variation that occurs with less frequency is the presence of an apical bronchus. This is similar to the normal anatomy of pigs and sheep. The apical segment of the right upper lobe has its origin at the distal trachea separate from the right upper lobe orifice. This bronchus, which may have its origin as high as 2 cm from the tracheal bifurcation, is associated with its own bronchial artery and can lead

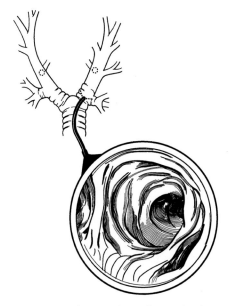

Figure 1-2. The view down the proximal right mainstem bronchus showing the origin of the right upper lobe bronchus. The close proximity of the upper lobe takeoff to the carina and the angle of its origin provide an anatomic landmark that can be used to determine orientation during bronchoscopy.

to confusion if it is not identified before an operative approach.

The segmental bronchi of the left lung are as follows. The left upper lobe bronchus divides into an upper division and a lower division. The upper division gives rise to the apicoposterior and anterior segments, the sum of which constitutes the upper lobe proper. The lower division is the lingula

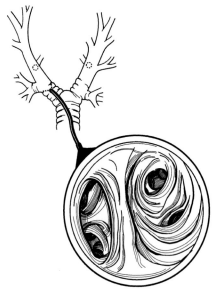

Figure 1-4. The left mainstem bronchus is significantly longer than the right and terminates at the bifurcation (or minor carina) into the upper lobe bronchus (composed of the upper lobe proper and lingular orifice) and the lower lobe bronchus.

and gives rise to the superior and inferior lingular segmental bronchi. Following the origin of the lower lobe bronchus, a large superior segmental bronchus is usually seen extending posteriorly. Within 1 cm of this bronchus, the airway divides into the anteromedial basal segment, the lateral basal segment, and the posterior basal segment. Anatomic variations of the left lung occur more rarely and are more often related to the subsegmental anatomy.

The Esophagus

By convention, the relationships of the esophagus are described with reference to the distance in centimeters from the incisors or front teeth. The cervical esophagus extends from 10 cm to 20 cm. This portion of the esophagus includes the cricopharyngeus. The major anatomic relationships are the membranous trachea anteriorly and the spine posteriorly. At 20 cm, the esophagus enters the chest and remains in intimate proximity to the membranous trachea anteriorly, the aorta laterally, and the spine posteriorly. The esophagus courses posterior to the left main bronchus as it passes inferior to the carina. The tracheal bifurcation occurs at approximately 25 cm from the incisors. At this point, the descending aorta remains at the posterior and left lateral portion of the esophagus throughout its

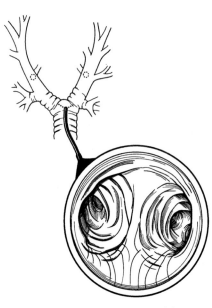

Figure 1-1. Bronchoscopic view of the trachea and carina.

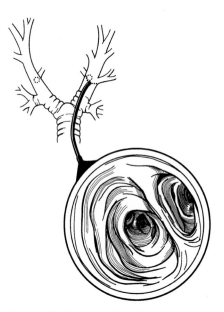

Figure 1-3. The view down the bronchus intermedius showing the middle lobe and lower lobe orifice.

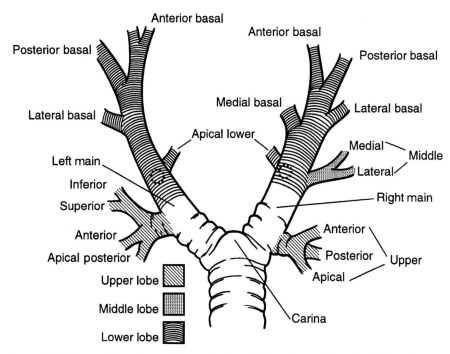

Figure 1-5. Segmental anatomy of the tracheobronchial tree in an orientation akin to that observed when performing bronchoscopy.

course in the chest. At 35 cm, the esophagus crosses the inferior pulmonary vein. At 40 cm from the incisors, the lower esophageal sphincter begins as the esophagus moves anteriorly and laterally to the left to enter the stomach. This relationship is the most variable. In short individuals, the sphincter may be at 38 cm, whereas in tall individuals, it may be at 45 cm. This relationship may also vary based on the timing of measurements. Measurements made during advancement of the scope tend to be longer than those made during retraction of the scope, particularly in patients with a sliding hiatal hernia.

Equipment

Standard equipment for any endoscopic examination includes a working instrument, a light source, suction, a forceps for biopsy, and irrigation solutions and a method to deliver them. Additional supplies that may need to be readily available include suction traps for specimen collection, endoscopic brushes, aspirating needles, and dilators. The size of the endoscope is determined as much by the purpose of the procedure as by the size of the patient. In general, diagnostic procedures are best performed with smaller instruments, whereas therapeutic procedures may require the largest scopes available.

Bronchoscopy

Flexible instruments for bronchoscopy should be small enough to allow ventilation around the scope by a spontaneously breathing patient. This is particularly important when used through an endotracheal tube. The standard-size scopes are 3.5 mm, with a 1.2-mm suction/biopsy port

(Fig. 1-6). This size requires an endotracheal tube of at least 8 mm. Most companies that manufacture endoscopy equipment make a smaller version that has a standard-size suction/biopsy channel. This allows the procedure to be performed through smaller endotracheal tubes. Accessories necessary during flexible endoscopy with an endotracheal tube include a bronchoscopy port adapter for the endotracheal tube. Additional supplies should include biopsy forceps, basket forceps for foreign-body extraction, disposable brushes, irrigation catheters, and biopsy/injection needles.

Rigid bronchoscopes provide a conduit for ventilation as well as for visualization and therefore should be as large as possible to permit adequate ventilation while manipulations are performed through the scope. The Jackson ventilating laser bronchoscope provides a separate port for ventilation that is out of the way of the operating port (Fig. 1-7). There are also separate ports for a flexible suction and laser fiber or flexible biopsy forceps. There is a removable eyepiece at the end of the scope that can be replaced by a cap fitted with a rubber tip, which allows placement of a telescope. The telescopes for viewing through a rigid scope may provide a 0-, 30-, or 90-degree viewing angle. The 30-degree angle is usually not necessary. The 0-degree angle allows wide visualization of the distal end of the scope and permits a view that would be seen with the naked eye. The 90-degree viewing angle is usually used to visualize the upper lobe on

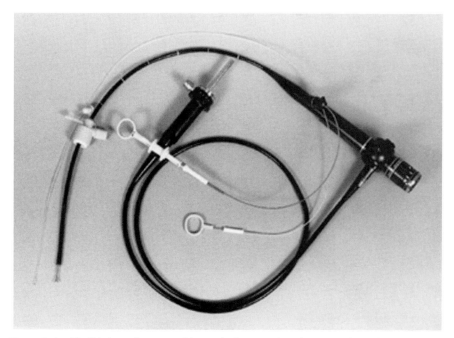

Figure 1-6. Flexible bronchoscope with standard accessories. Shown are the endotracheal tube ventilating adaptor, the biopsy forceps, and a disposable brush.

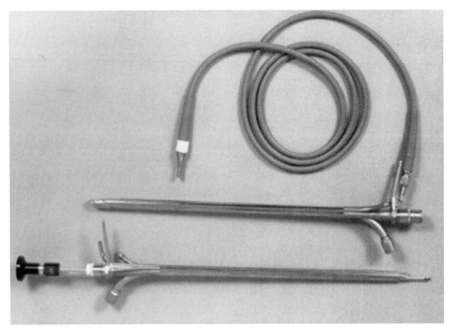

Figure 1-7. Jackson rigid ventilating laser bronchoscope. There is a side port for ventilation and a second port for placement of flexible tools. The light source is placed within the wall of the scope. The top scope demonstrates the eyepiece at the end, and the bottom scope demonstrates the telescope inserted through the special airtight adapter.

the right or the superior segmental orifices of the lower lobe.

Esophagoscopy

The flexible scopes for esophagoscopy are the standard upper endoscopy (gastroscopy) scopes, which come in standard and pediatric sizes. There is a variation of these scopes fitted with a white tip for laser use; however, this type of scope is rarely used. Accessories for esophagoscopy include biopsy forceps, a basket catheter for foreign-body and polyp removal, and cautery and needle catheters.

Rigid esophagoscopes are flatter than rigid bronchoscopes and have a more bulbous tip, are available in adult and pediatric sizes, and vary in length from 20 cm to 50 cm (Fig. 1-8). Accessories are similar to bronchoscopic accessories except that all of the instruments are longer. There is a special round esophagoscope that is 30 cm in length and is used for dilation under direct vision (Fig. 1-9). This scope can accept dilators up to and including 36 F (12 mm). The flatter esophagoscopes only permit dilators up to 20 F (6 mm) in size. Newer balloon dilators have a stem that allows the balloon to be inserted through an 8-F catheter, thus allowing more flexibility in use.

Direct dilators are most often used with the rigid endoscopes. This method of using Jackson dilators is rarely used today because

of the development of highly successful indirect dilators. Indirect dilators now come in two main styles: Savary, or wire-guided dilators, and Maloney, or unguided dilators (Fig. 1-10). A third style of inflatable dilator is available for both the esophagus and airway. The Savary-style dilators are passed over a guidewire, which is inserted under direct vision through a stricture or stenosis. Successive dilators are passed on the wire and removed to make room for the next dilator. Savary dilators come in sizes from 5 mm to 18 mm. The Maloney dilators look similar to the Savary dilators but do not have a hole to allow guided dilation. Maloney dilators once contained mercury but no longer

contain this potentially lethal substance. They are marked in centimeters to gauge depth of insertion. These measurements are shown both from the tip (American) and from the widest part (European) of the dilator. Maloney dilators come in sizes from 10 F to 60 F. The balloon dilators are available in two sizes that dilate to 15 mm and 20 mm, respectively.

Procedure

Basic principles for both bronchoscopy and esophagoscopy are similar. Flexible endoscopy is usually performed with the aid of a topical anesthetic often supplemented with intravenous sedation. Although rigid endoscopy can be performed with topical anesthesia, it is usually performed with the patient under general anesthesia. Preparation of the patient is similar in both cases. The American Society of Anesthesiology has published guidelines for conscious sedation (Table 1-2). Hospitals and many outpatient facilities require that the operators have specific privileges if they wish to use conscious sedation without the aid of an anesthesiologist or nurse anesthetist.

All patients should be monitored with an electrocardiogram, a noninvasive blood pressure monitor, and a pulse oximeter. A member of the team must be available to monitor and document these vital signs and notify the surgeon of any significant deviations. The patient should receive supplemental oxygen before, during, and after the procedure. The drug most often used for sedation is midazolam. This drug is usually given in 1-mg increments during administration of the local anesthetic. Midazolam is excellent because of its sedative and amnestic effects. Meperidine is a second agent given, particularly for more painful

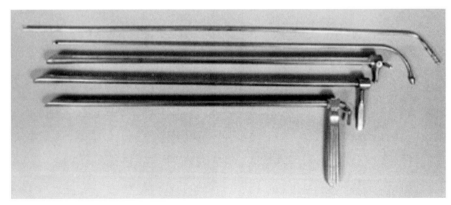

Figure 1-8. Standard Jackson esophagoscopes. Each varies slightly in the shape at the end, but in general they are flattened and shaped like the esophagus. Suctions have either an end hole or two side holes.

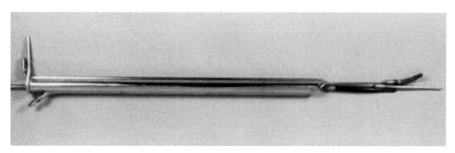

Figure 1-9. Dilating esophagoscope. This esophagoscope is round and will accept up to a 36-F dilator. Several varieties of Jackson rigid dilators are shown coming out of the end of the scope.

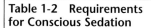

Table 1-2 Requirements for Conscious Sedation
Monitoring requirements
Electrocardiogram
Noninvasive blood pressure
Pulse oximetry
Documentation form
Supplemental oxygen
Intravenous access for sedation/drug administration
Assistant to deliver drugs and to monitor and document course
Monitored recovery

procedures such as dilation, rigid endoscopy, and stent placement. It is usually administered in 25-mg increments. After endoscopy under conscious sedation, the patient should be monitored for at least 1 hour. Administration of adequate local anesthesia is important for patients undergoing endoscopy under conscious sedation. For esophagoscopy, this is usually obtained with repeated administrations of tetracaine spray or viscous lidocaine gargle. A variety of methods can be used for bronchoscopy. These include lidocaine spray of the oral pharynx supplemented with lidocaine delivered to the vocal cords and trachea through the bronchoscope or via the cricothyroid membrane, inhaled nebulized lidocaine, and injection of lidocaine to produce superior laryngeal and transtracheal blocks. Nasal anesthesia for a transnasal approach is best done with 4% cocaine administered on swabs until effective anesthesia is achieved.

For general anesthesia, short-acting agents such as propofol are usually best. Dilation of the aerodigestive tract and rigid endoscopy are both highly stimulating and painful to the patient. This requires a deep plane of anesthesia for short periods of time. Agents best suited for this are intravenous thiopental (Pentothal) or propofol. These may be supplemented with total muscular paralysis with bolus doses of succinylcholine to give 45 to 60 seconds of complete relaxation. For bronchoscopy, the surgeon must be ready to intubate the trachea as soon as deep anesthesia has been reached. For rigid esophagoscopy, the airway should be intubated and the patient ventilated during the procedure. Even with the use of short-acting agents, emergence may be slow because of the deep plane required during stimulation. As soon as the endoscopic procedure is complete, the anesthesiologist should be notified so that emergence may begin.

Bronchoscopy

Flexible bronchoscopy is usually performed from the right side of the patient with the operator facing the head of the bed. The bronchoscope is held in the left hand, leaving the right hand to manipulate the scope or pass instrumentation down the biopsy/suction channel. The scope may be passed transnasally or orally, depending on the preference of the operator. The transnasal approach gives a more stable platform and a more direct approach to the larynx because of the fixation through the nares. The oral route requires flexion of the scope around the tongue and the epiglottis within a short distance and does not have a stable platform. With both techniques, there is complete visualization of the airway from the vocal cords down. Bronchoscopy through an endotracheal tube does not afford the opportunity to visualize the larynx or the upper trachea. All visualization of the airway is performed on the way in for the first time to observe any abnormalities undisturbed by potential scope trauma. Visualization is usually begun on the side opposite the area of suspected pathologic involvement and is usually performed in a sequential manner, with each segmental orifice being observed as described. Secretions may be collected in a trap, which should not be connected until the scope has passed the larynx. To prevent contamination by the oropharynx, the trap should be placed as close to the scope as possible, or the suction tubing from the scope to the trap should be changed at the time the trap is attached.

Rigid bronchoscopy is performed from the head of the bed. The patient's head should be placed on blankets or a "doughnut" to simulate an exaggerated sniffing position. This helps to straighten the route through the oropharynx into the trachea. A guard should be placed over the maxillary front teeth. The thumb and forefinger of the left hand are used as a fulcrum to stabilize the rigid endoscope, with the scope being moved by the right hand (Fig. 1-11). Even with a mouth guard in place, the teeth should never be used as a fulcrum, and care should be taken to avoid damage to the lips. The scope is passed beyond the tongue almost to the posterior pharynx (see Fig. 1-11, inset). The landmark is visualization of the epiglottis. The tip of the endoscope should then be used to elevate the epiglottis, and passing slightly inferior allows the vocal cords to be visualized. Passing the scope too far will elevate the entire larynx, and the operator will be looking at the cricopharyngeus. Once the vocal cords are visualized, the scope is rotated 90 degrees so as to make passage through the cords as atraumatic as possible. Visualization of the entire trachea is done by advancing the scope slowly using the thumb and forefinger

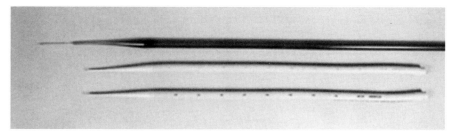

Figure 1-10. Flexible dilators. The Savary dilator **(top)** is a wire-guided dilator. The Maloney dilators are marked in centimeters to gauge depth of insertion in both American and European systems (see text).

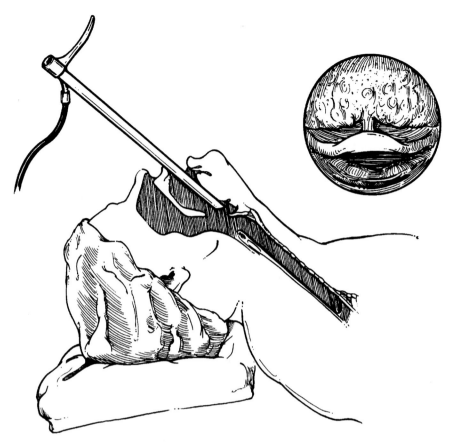

Figure 1-11. Patient positioning for rigid bronchoscopy. The inset shows the view once the bronchoscope is passed beyond the tongue into the posterior pharynx.

as a fulcrum. The right hand is used to stabilize the scope and to pass suction or biopsy forceps. An assistant should place the tip of the suction or the biopsy forceps into the bronchoscope so that the operator does not have to lose visualization. Once the carina is approached, the right or left mainstem may be intubated with the scope. This is done by rotating the patient's head in the opposite direction one wishes to go. For the right mainstem, the head is turned to the left; for the left mainstem, it is turned to the right. The lobar and segmental bronchi are identified as described. A 90-degree telescope is necessary to completely visualize the right upper lobe orifices.

After initial inspection, brushings, washings, and biopsy may be performed as indicated. In the case of an immunocompromised patient, a diagnostic bronchoscopy should include brushings of suspected infiltrates, bronchoalveolar lavage of a segment, and transbronchial lung biopsy. Brushing should be performed with a protected brush. These brushes come with a small plug at the end of the catheter that is pushed out when the brush is advanced. After brushing is performed, the brush should be re-

tracted back into the catheter and the entire catheter removed. Washings or lavage are best performed after brushing. Bronchoalveolar lavage is performed by wedging the scope into a subsegmental orifice so that the scope impacts the wall. Alternatively, there are balloon catheters that may be used for the same purpose. These occlude the segmental or subsegmental orifice completely. Lavage should be performed with sterile saline. One hundred milliliters is instilled in 25-ml increments. Each aliquot is retrieved using a syringe or gentle suction. A successful lavage retrieves 50% of the instilled solution. Transbronchial biopsies are performed by passing the biopsy forceps under direct vision beyond the subsegmental orifice. At this point, the forceps is opened and advanced until it meets resistance. A specimen is taken at this point. Several biopsy specimens should be obtained to ensure an adequate sample. An adequate sample includes respiratory epithelium and alveolar wall.

Another useful maneuver is a transbronchial needle biopsy of extrabronchial masses. This is performed with a Wang needle. There are several varieties of these needles, but all use the same basic principle. The

needle is in a sheath that is passed through the biopsy channel. It is advanced out of the catheter when it is in position. The length of the tubing is usually filled with saline beforehand to facilitate aspiration. The needle is advanced out of the catheter and through the wall of the trachea or bronchus into the mass or node to be biopsied. Several passes are made, and the needle is moved up and down during aspiration to increase the yield of the biopsy. The material obtained is placed on slides for cytologic interpretation. Some of the material also may be sent for culture.

Autofluorescence bronchoscopy is an approved modality used to evaluate the airway mucosa for malignant changes. If this modality is to be used, it should be performed first before the mucosa is damaged by suction or biopsy. A special autofluorescence bronchoscope (AF bronchoscope; Storz, Inc., Culver City, CA) is necessary. First, white-light bronchoscopy is performed to assess for gross abnormalities and to clear the airway of significant secretions. Next, the light source is changed to autofluorescence mode, which is ultraviolet light at 440 nm. Normal mucosa fluoresces green, mucus appears purple and mucosa from dysplasia to carcinoma appears pink. Biopsies can be better directed using this modality.

After completion of the procedure, the entire airway should be inspected for secretions or blood. These should be suctioned or lavaged away. Instillation of small amounts of a 1:10,000 solution of epinephrine is helpful in controlling slow continued hemorrhage. Blood pressure and pulse should be carefully monitored during this procedure because drugs are rapidly absorbed from the trachea. During recovery from the bronchoscopy, it is not necessary to obtain a chest roentgenogram as a routine. When a transbronchial biopsy is performed, a chest film should be obtained to assure that there is no pneumothorax.

Virtual bronchoscopy is under development. Like virtual colonoscopy, abnormalities discovered on radiologic evaluation need to be confirmed by visualization and biopsy.

Esophagoscopy

Both rigid and flexible esophagoscopy are performed through the mouth. For flexible esophagoscopy, the patient is usually placed in the left lateral decubitus position to allow oral secretions to drain out of the mouth easily during the procedure. The endoscopist stands facing the patient. The scope may be passed under direct vision posterior to the corniculate tubercles of the larynx into the esophagus. This permits visualization of the entire esophagus from its origin as the scope is advanced. An alternative method is to place the index and middle fingers in the mouth to move the tongue anteriorly, allowing the esophagus to open slightly. In this method, the scope is passed blindly through the upper esophageal sphincter. This makes placement of the scope within the esophagus easy with less potential for intubating the pyriform sinuses but does not permit initial visualization of the upper esophageal sphincter.

The upper esophageal sphincter is identified by seeing the mucosa flattened behind the larynx. As the scope is advanced, the opening gradually becomes larger, permitting the scope to pass. The upper esophageal sphincter is the first structure encountered as the scope is passed. At this point, a search should be made of the proximal esophagus to look for a possible lateral opening of a Zenker's diverticulum. After this, the scope should be slowly advanced through the thoracic esophagus and the mucosa observed. Intermittent air insufflation is helpful for visualization of the esophagus. It also helps in identifying areas of rigidity or fixation because these areas do not insufflate well. The scope is passed down to the lower esophageal sphincter, which should be at the same level as the diaphragm. The sphincter is usually closed, but it can be opened with small bursts of insufflation as the scope is passed into the stomach. Complete visualization of the esophagus includes observation of the undersurface of the lower esophageal sphincter by retroflexing the scope in the stomach to visualize the cardia. Most operators will continue the procedure by examining the stomach, the pylorus, and the first and second portions of the duodenum, although these are not integral parts of the esophagoscopic procedure. After examination and documentation of the level of any pathologic states, the scope is slowly removed and the esophagus reevaluated. Ideally, the operator should concentrate on the technical details of passing the instrument on insertion and evaluate any pathologic entities as the instrument is pulled back.

Rigid esophagoscopy is performed in a similar manner to rigid bronchoscopy. The patient should be intubated, although the procedure can be performed with the patient under local anesthesia with heavy sedation. The scope is held in the same manner as described for rigid bronchoscopy. The scope should be carefully advanced along the posterior pharynx, and once posterior to the larynx, the scope must be lifted using the thumb of the left hand as a fulcrum to visualize the cricopharyngeus. Once the cricopharyngeus is visualized, the scope is advanced carefully into the esophagus. Great care must be taken to avoid tearing the esophagus on the prominent C7 vertebral body. Rigid esophagoscopy is the most difficult endoscopic procedure to master and perform safely and carries the greatest risk to the patient. Rigid esophagoscopy cannot be performed in all individuals. Those individuals with significant arthritis who cannot extend the neck sufficiently cannot undergo esophagoscopy. In addition, some patients may have significant bony spurs on the spine, which may prevent the scope from advancing beyond that point. There is a high incidence of perforation when the operator persists in passing these bony spurs.

As with all endoscopy, photodocumentation is becoming widespread. Pictures help other practitioners to understand the nature of abnormalities. Photodocumentation makes follow-up much simpler because similar views of the abnormality or unusual finding may be compared over time. It is also a boon to education. All involved in the care of the patient may view live the proceedings. This is particularly important in critical care situations. The nursing staff rarely find out about the endobronchial or endoesophageal pathology. Visualization gives them a better appreciation for the situation and improves care. It also allows better teaching of technique when the surgeon in real time can direct the trainee through the procedure.

After endoscopic examination performed with topical anesthesia, the patient should not eat or drink until the oropharyngeal anesthesia has worn off. This usually takes about 30 minutes. The patient should not be released until he or she is able to drink without difficulty. No additional testing is necessary; however, if the patient complains of pain after esophagoscopy, this may be an indication of a perforation. A contrast study with dilute barium is best at defining any leak.

Conclusion

All trainees in thoracic surgery should master endoscopic examination of the upper aerodigestive tract, specifically bronchoscopy and esophagoscopy. The ability to pass a rigid bronchoscope rapidly can be a life-saving maneuver. The importance of the information to be gained by the surgeon performing the endoscopic examination before an open procedure cannot be overestimated.

SUGGESTED READING

Herth FJ, Ernst A, Becker HD. Autofluorescence bronchoscopy—A comparison of two systems (LIFE and D-Light). Respiration 2003;70:395.

Maniatis PN, Triantopoulou CC, Tsalafoutas IA, et al. Threshold selection in virtual bronchoscopy: Phantom study and clinical implications. Acta Radiol 2004;45:176.

Prakash UBS. *Bronchoscopy*. New York: Raven, 1994.

Shields TW, LoCicero J 3rd, Ponn RB. General Thoracic Surgery (5th ed). Philadelphia: Lippincott Williams & Wilkins, 2000.

Stradling P. Diagnostic Bronchoscopy: A Teaching Manual (6th ed). Edinburgh: Churchill Livingstone, 1991.

EDITOR'S COMMENTS

Dr. LoCicero makes several points that deserve amplification. First, the fact that the esophagus enters the mediastinum off the midline to the left so that it runs posterior to the left mainstem bronchus has great significance for proximal and midthoracic esophageal cancers. The assessment of airway involvement should include a close look at the proximal left mainstem bronchus. In addition, the endoscopist should be familiar with the relationship of the left and right main pulmonary arteries to their respective mainstem bronchi. It should be apparent to all that the location of the gastroesophageal junction mandates a left chest approach when that area needs to be approached from above.

Thoracic surgeons must become expert endoscopists. To some extent the ability to perform rigid endoscopy differentiates us from the majority of our medical counterparts and gives us a distinct advantage when performing therapeutic procedures, although the development of the interventional bronchoscopist has created a new threat in this regard. The familiarity with the anatomy gained by performing rigid endoscopy offers a new perspective when looking through a flexible endoscope. This further underscores the importance of teaching rigid endoscopy to thoracic surgical trainees, but unfortunately these techniques are in danger of becoming a lost art. Thoracic surgeons need to include rigid endoscopy as a component of the training program and must go out of their way to include rigid endoscopy as part of the procedure for any patient in whom an indication for its use exists. Often in the interest of time it is easy to overlook rigid endoscopic examination in the management of a patient who would otherwise be a candidate in favor of simply performing an examination with a flexible endoscope. The performance of rigid esophagoscopy seems to be especially rare in thoracic surgical programs. This procedure is the most difficult to master and is associated with the greatest risk to the patient. The ability to perform this procedure is a significant advantage when it comes to managing esophageal strictures, especially those related to anastomoses.

The surgeon always should perform his or her own bronchoscopic examination as part of any operative procedure despite the endoscopic procedure having been performed by the referring pulmonologist. The same holds true for esophagoscopy performed at the time of esophagectomy. It is difficult for me to even think of performing an open procedure if I have not seen the endoscopic findings. Yet, in the interest of time and the fear of offending one's medical colleagues, the endoscopic examination is often not repeated.

The complete thoracic surgeon should also be facile at performing therapeutic endoscopic procedures such as laser bronchoscopy, bronchial stent insertion, and the placement of endoesophageal prostheses despite the best efforts of our medical colleagues to take over these procedures.

L.R.K.

2

Mediastinoscopy and Staging

Mark Onaitis and David Harpole

Central to the staging algorithm for non–small cell lung cancer is accurate detection of the spread of tumors to mediastinal lymph nodes. Mediastinoscopy has assumed the most important role in the clinical staging of non–small cell lung cancer due to its ability to stage the mediastinum accurately. This chapter reviews mediastinoscopy and other modalities for mediastinal staging.

The Staging System

Classification of cancers according to primary tumor (T), lymph node (N), and metastatic (M) variables was introduced in the 1940s. The TNM system for lung cancer developed in 1985 is recognized internationally (Tables 2-1 and 2-2). Central to the system are the anatomy and nomenclature of the lymph node descriptors (Fig. 2-1). Four stages are defined. Stage I tumors are confined to the parenchyma and visceral pleura. Stage II tumors have metastasized to or directly invaded intrapleural (N1) but not mediastinal (N2) nodes. Stage III denotes extensive locoregional disease and is heterogeneous: IIIA is defined by ipsilateral mediastinal node metastases or direct invasion of potentially resectable structures; IIIB patients have involved scalene or contralateral thoracic nodes, malignant pleural effusion, or invasion of unresectable structures. Distant metastasis is the hallmark of stage IV.

Stage correlates with prognosis and guides treatment. Survival decreases significantly with advancing stage and specific descriptors within stages (Fig. 2-2). Operation usually is indicated in stages I and II. Complete resection in stage I yields a cure rate overwhelmingly superior to those with other therapies and is not enhanced by adjuvant regimens. Recent evidence seems to support a survival advantage for adjuvant therapy in resected stage II disease. Non-nodal stage IIIA (T3N0M0) tumors that can be resected en bloc are best treated surgically, with selective use of external and interstitial radiation. At the other end of the spectrum, stage IIIB and IV patients, with rare exceptions, do not benefit from surgical resection.

The role of surgical resection remains controversial in the large cohort of patients with nodal stage IIIA disease (T1–3N2M0). Five-year survival for clinical N2 disease treated by primary resection is <10%, in contrast to threefold superior results in pathologic N2 clinically staged as N0 or N1. Attempts to enhance survival by postresection adjuvant regimens have been disappointing, although several recent studies have shown improved survival with postoperative chemotherapy. Induction chemo(radio)therapy followed by operation in responders, in contrast, may be of benefit. Although there remains a small favorable N2 group (intranodal disease, single level, proximal station) who might be offered primary resection, initial treatment in most cases is nonsurgical. The primary issue in nodal evaluation therefore is not how to define "bulky" versus "resectable" N2 involvement, but rather how best to detect any clinical N2 disease in an accurate and cost-effective manner.

The Clinical Staging Process

Staging does not require all investigations in all cases. Evaluation is guided by history, physical examination, basic blood work, and findings on chest films and thoracic computed tomographic (CT) scans. Because the highest stage determines treatment, the conceptual sequence proceeds in the reverse order of the literal TNM descriptors—that is, from metastases to nodes to tumor. Documentation of M1 disease obviates the need for investigation of T and N; similarly, confirmation of N3 or N2 renders superfluous studies to define T or lower N variables beyond radiography. At all decision points, specific imaging and tissue sampling choices are influenced by available local expertise.

Distant Metastases

Early diagnosis of extrathoracic metastases may expedite treatment and avoid useless diagnostic procedures and potentially subjecting a patient to the risk of operation that would be of no long-term benefit. These considerations underlie two issues in metastatic staging: when to scan and when to biopsy scan abnormalities.

Metastases from primary bronchogenic carcinoma commonly are seen in lung, brain, bone, liver, and the adrenals. Upper abdominal CT scanning through the adrenals is performed as an extension of thoracic CT scanning because the additional temporal and monetary costs are minimal. The issue of multiorgan scanning therefore involves radionuclide bone scanning and cranial CT or magnetic resonance imaging (MRI) studies. Although some advocate brain scans (either MRI [preferable] or CT) in all cases, we consider the yield in truly asymptomatic patients with T1–2N0 insufficient to justify routine studies. In these cases, the negative predictive value of clinical screening is >90%. Furthermore, scan findings may be nonspecific. Bone scans are

11

Table 2-1   TNM Staging System for Lung Cancer

Stage	Description
Primary tumor	
TX	Tumor cannot be assessed, or is positive cytologically without demonstrable mass
T0	No evidence of primary
Tis	Carcinoma in situ
T1	Tumor of ≤3 cm surrounded by lung or visceral pleura and not invading proximal to a lobar bronchus
T2	Tumor >3 cm or involving visceral pleura or associated with atelectasis or obstructive pneumonitis extending to hilum but involving less than the entire lung. Proximal tumor at bronchoscopy must be >2 cm from carina
T3	Tumor of any size with extension into chest wall (including superior sulcus), diaphragm, mediastinal pleura, or pericardium, but not heart, great vessels, trachea, esophagus, or vertebral bodies, or tumor in main bronchus <2 cm from but not involving the carina
T4	Tumor of any size invading heart, mediastinum, great vessels, trachea, esophagus, vertebral bodies, or carina, or tumor associated with malignant pleural effusion
Lymph nodes	
N0	No metastasis to regional nodes
N1	Metastasis to ipsilateral peribronchial and/or hilar nodes. Includes direct extension (levels 10R–13)
N2	Metastasis to ipsilateral mediastinal and/or subcarinal nodes (levels 2, 4, 5, 6, 7, 8, 9, 10L)
N3	Metastasis to contralateral hilar and/or mediastinal nodes, or ipsilateral or contra-lateral scalene or supraclavicular nodes
Distant metastases	
M0	No distant metastasis detected
MI	Distant metastasis detected

Lung Cancer Stages			
Occult carcinoma	TX	N0	M0
Stage 0	Tis	N0	M0
Stage I	TI	N0	M0
	T2	N0	M0
Stage II	TI	NI	M0
	T2	NI	M0
Stage IIIA	T3	N0	M0
	T3	NI	M0
	TI-3	N2	M0
Stage IIIB	Any T	N3	M0
	T4	Any N	M0
Stage IV	Any T	Any N	MI

abnormal in 20% to 30% of older adults and may generate additional costly studies. Nonetheless, because the risk is low, the threshold for scans should be low and consider not only organ-specific findings, but also any harbinger of advanced disease, that is, nonspecific symptoms or signs (e.g., anemia, weight loss). Positron emission tomographic (PET) scans recently have become a significant part of the staging evaluation. A PET scan obviates the need for a separate radionuclide bone scan and may demonstrate occult metastatic disease in other sites. The radioactive fluorinated glucose moiety used in this study is trapped by malignant cells much more readily than in normal cells, and this study has been quite accurate in the diagnosis of the solitary pulmonary nodule but less so for distinguishing metastatic nodal disease. PET scanning has shown promise in identification of distant disease. The recent prospective trial from the American College of Surgeons Oncology Group (ACOSOG Z0050) revealed PET to be 83% sensitive and 90% disease specific. Of importance, the negative predictive value of PET was 99%. However, because the positive predictive value was only 36%, positive results should be confirmed pathologically if possible.

In most cases, diagnosis of metastasis is made by a synthesis of clinical and scan data. When uncertainty persists, a combination of plain radiography, conventional tomography or CT, MRI, and ultrasonography usually suffices. Guided fine-needle aspiration resolves most of the remaining dilemmas. For the thoracic surgeon, the rare case requiring open biopsy most often involves a rib lesion detected on a radionuclide scan. The major technical pitfall in rib biopsy lies in identifying the correct site because there is usually no palpable mass, and counting ribs is difficult except in very thin patients. Because skin markers are unreliable, preoperative localization is achieved with fluoroscopic or radionuclide guidance by injecting methylene blue directly into the periosteum. The aliquot is limited to one or two drops to avoid obscuring the surgical route by staining too much tissue. An aspirate is obtained before marking, and, if positive on immediate cytologic review, open biopsy is canceled.

Because adrenal adenomas occur in 2% to 9% of the population and adrenal metastases are common in lung cancer, adrenal masses are often identified by staging CT scans. A scenario of otherwise operable disease with treatment hinging on an adrenal mass, however, is uncommon. Because radiographic differentiation is fallible, percutaneous biopsy may be needed. If aspiration is nondiagnostic or not feasible, open biopsy can be done in a number of ways. Most common is adrenalectomy via an abdominal, flank, or posterior approach. Laparoscopy and thoracoscopy are options. We have had favorable experience with transpleural, transdiaphragmatic adrenalectomy for ipsilateral masses. With the patient in the thoracotomy position and intubated with a double-lumen tube, the costophrenic sulcus is entered after resection of 8 cm of posterior tenth rib. A diaphragmatic incision then provides access to the retroperitoneum, Gerota's fascia is opened, and the adrenal is resected or a biopsy specimen obtained. If only benign cells are found on frozen-section examination, lung resection is accomplished by a muscle-sparing thoracotomy under the same anesthetic and without repositioning.

Primary Tumor

Tumor size is determined radiographically, although central masses may be difficult to quantify because of adjacent structures and atelectasis. Size alone, however, is rarely

Stage 1A $\quad$ $T_1 N_0 M_0$

Stage 1B $\quad$ $T_2 N_0 M_0$

Stage II A $\quad$ $T_1 N_1 M_0$

$\quad$ II B $\quad$ $T_2 N_1 M_0$

$\qquad$ $T_3 N_0 M_0$

$\quad$ III A $\quad$ $T_1 N_2 M_0$

$\qquad$ $T_2 N_2 M_0$

$\qquad$ $T_3 N_1 M_0$

$\qquad$ $T_3 N_2$

$\quad$ III B $\quad$ T_4 any N M_0

$\qquad$ any T $N_3 M_0$

$\qquad$ any T any N M_1

VERIFY THE AUTHENTICITY OF THIS MULTI-TONE SECURITY DOCUMENT. BACKGROUND AREA CHANGES COLOR GRADUALLY FROM TOP TO BOTTOM.

ANTI-FRAUD PROTECTION - PATENTS 5,197,765; 5,340,159

SOUTHERN CALIFORNIA PERMANENTE MEDICAL GROUP

MV6962-00616

Patient Name	Medical Record	Phone No.	INITIAL As Applicable ☐ No Known Allergies
Address	Date of Birth	Gender ☐Male ☐Female	☐ Allergies List on Reverse (optional)

Rx Medication, Strength (Put Integer Left of Decimal) and Directions for Use ("Sig")	Initial Quantity	Initial Quantity	# of Refills or circle "No Refills"	Refill Quantity	Refill Quantity	Initial as Applicable
#1 ☐Do Not Substitute		☐1-24 ☐25-49 ☐50-74 ☐75-100 ☐101-150 ☐151 & over	"No Refills"		☐1-24 ☐25-49 ☐50-74 ☐75-100 ☐101-150 ☐151 & over	Worker's Comp.
#2 ☐Do Not Substitute		☐1-24 ☐25-49 ☐50-74 ☐75-100 ☐101-150 ☐151 & over	"No Refills"		☐1-24 ☐25-49 ☐50-74 ☐75-100 ☐101-150 ☐151 & over	Worker's Comp.
#3 ☐Do Not Substitute		☐1-24 ☐25-49 ☐50-74 ☐75-100 ☐101-150 ☐151 & over	"No Refills"		☐1-24 ☐25-49 ☐50-74 ☐75-100 ☐101-150 ☐151 & over	Worker's Comp.

NUMBER OF ITEMS PRESCRIBED: ***(All prescriptions void if number of items not noted.)*** ☐**Spanish Label**

Unless respective space is initialed, a Pharmacist may adjust "Sig" prn and dispense Pharmacy & Therapeutic Committee approved alternate. i.e., ________ Generic, ________ Pkg. Size / Qty., ________ Dosage Form/Strength or ________ Therapeutic Equivalent.

PAUL G. PERCH, M.D.
CARDIAC SURGERY • (323) 783-4595
1526 N EDGEMONT ST 3RD FL
LOS ANGELES, CA 90027
DEA NO. BP8257986 • CA LIC. NO. A82121

X ______________________________ DATE __________

KP Formulary Code _____ or initial _____ if NE Intended

RX-1252 (7-04)

HOLD AT AN ANGLE TO SEE THE MARK WHEN CHECKING AUTHENTICITY.

Table 2-2 Proposed Revisions to the TNM Staging for Lung Cancer

A revised lung cancer staging system has been accepted by the International Union Against Cancer. The aim of the revision is to further refine clinical prognostic stratification by separating some TNM categories and rearranging others and to include patterns of disease not previously addressed directly while simultaneously minimizing disruption and maintaining relevance of existing registries and databases. Prognostic accuracy by clinical stage is of paramount importance because it is likely that improvements in therapy will progress in small increments for the foreseeable future. The key features are as follows:

1. Division of stage I into two groups to reflect the significantly different implications of TI versus T2 in node-negative cases.
2. Division of stage II into two categories, similarly recognizing the impact of T1 versus T2, and also including T3N0 cancers, newly separating this subset from N2 disease because its biology and prognosis are different from cases with N2 nodal metastasis.
3. A first attempt to deal with the increasingly frequent dilemma of multiple lesions—T4 for lesions in the same lobe, M1 for those in separate lobes. We believe that the finding of multiple pulmonary sites of neoplasm represents a basic change in modem lung cancer presentation and warrants much attention in the future with respect to definitions as well as the implications of the number of lesions, refinements in histologic comparisons, unilaterality versus bilaterality, and appropriate treatment.

Proposed revised stages

Stage 0	Carcinoma in situ
Stage IA	T1 N0 M0
Stage IIA	T2 N0 M0
Stage IIB	T1 N1 M1
Stage IIIA	T2 N1 M0; T3 N0 M0
Stage IIIB	T4, any N, M0; any T, N3, M0
Stage IV	Any T; any M

Note: The authors gratefully acknowledge the support of Dr. Clifton F. Mountain for allowing us to include this information before its publication.

therapeutically determinative because T1 and T2 do not define different stages. Similarly, tumor site is defined by radiography. Bronchoscopy further confirms proximal bronchial or carinal locations, factors that independently affect stage (T3, T4). Determination of invasion, in contrast, may be difficult. In a minority of cases, radiographic signs are unequivocal—massive invasion, bone destruction, or vascular encasement. Diagnostic certainty is heightened by appropriate symptoms and signs such as pain, dysphagia, facial plethora, or hoarseness. Contiguity of central or peripheral tumors with adjacent structures, however, even with obliteration of fat planes, does not prove neoplastic transgression. Except in tumors of the superior sulcus, an MRI study adds little further information. If the area of potential invasion is resectable (T3), one may proceed to thoracotomy with preparations for chest wall or other extended resection. If the suspected involvement indicates unresectability (T4), confirmation is accomplished by mediastinoscopy, mediastinotomy, or thoracoscopy or may elude documentation short of thoracotomy.

Pleural effusions usually result from malignant pleural seeding but may rarely be parapneumonic or unrelated transudates.

Accordingly, fluid sampling is required when there are no other indicators of inoperability. The first step is thoracentesis with or without percutaneous pleural biopsy. Although repeat thoracentesis may produce positive results after a nondiagnostic aspirate, we generally perform thoracoscopy at this point and, depending on the findings, resect the tumor, insufflate talc for pleurodesis, or await the final result of histologic examination. Although the overall role of staging thoracoscopy remains to be determined, its usefulness for assessing pleural effusion is unquestioned.

The Lymph Nodes

Mediastinoscopy

Carlens and Pearson developed the technique of mediastinoscopy that is practiced today. The mediastinoscopes used today are modifications of the original instruments, with distal illumination, a beveled end, and a lateral slit for instrumentation. Standard mediastinoscopy allows assessment of the pretracheal and paratracheal, the subcarinal, and the tracheobronchial nodes (2R and L,

4R and L, 7, and 10R), as well as neoplastic invasion of the mediastinum or its airway and vascular components.

Mediastinoscopy is safely performed as an outpatient procedure because discomfort is minimal, most problems are apparent intraoperatively, and the usual patient is a resection candidate and fairly healthy. Because of the potential for hemorrhage, the venue is limited to hospital-based rather than free-standing facilities. A related issue is the timing of mediastinoscopy with respect to resection. Because frozen-section diagnosis is dependable and one may proceed to thoracotomy under the same anesthetic, practical considerations become determinative and include operating time, intensive care planning, epidural catheters, invasive monitoring, and patient preference. A one-stage inpatient approach is appropriate when there is a low expectation of finding positive nodes.

The ability of mediastinoscopy to detect malignant adenopathy in the superior mediastinum is well documented. Although by strict definition false positivity may result from biopsy of tumor rather than node, therapy is usually not affected. Because the lymphatic system is sampled rather than totally resected and some areas are beyond reach, there are inevitable false-negative results, but the rate is <10%. The negative predictive value of >90% translates into a high rate of curative resectability.

Indications

The need for mediastinal biopsy derives from the absence of a noninvasive modality that can be used to reliably differentiate benign from malignant nodes. The reported usefulness of CT scanning in staging the mediastinum varies widely (Table 2-3) and depends on size criteria, cell type, prevalence of N2 in the populations, and the method of histologic confirmation. Discrimination does not improve with MRI because there is much overlap of signal intensity. CT assessment relies mainly on size. The threshold for abnormality has been lowered over time to the currently accepted short-axis diameter of 1 cm. The result is greater sensitivity but lower specificity. Twenty percent to 40% of cases with radiographically apparent adenopathy are histologically benign, with hyperplasia caused by obstructive pneumonia or a preexisting process. This degree of discrepancy mandates that scan positivity be confirmed by tissue sampling. PET generated early excitement in staging the mediastinum, but more recent studies including

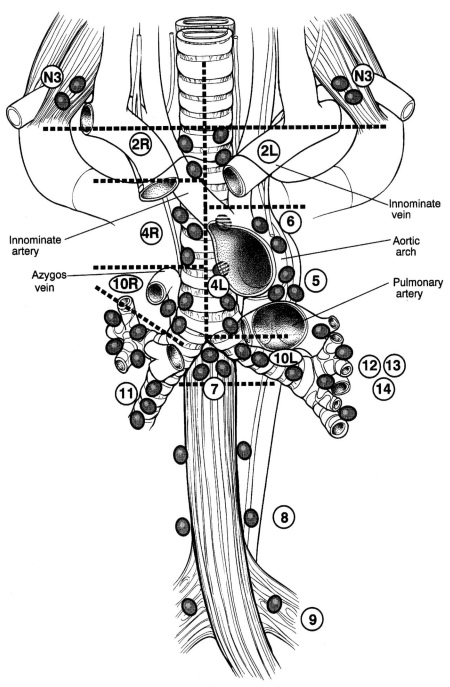

Figure 2-1. Lymph node map for TNM Staging of lung cancer.

constant negative predictive value of 90% or greater for modern CT technology. A recent randomized study comparing the rate of noncurative thoracotomy in routine (no CT scan) versus selective mediastinoscopy groups found a trend favoring the selective strategy by both clinical and cost criteria. We believe that it is reasonable to omit mediastinoscopy in most patients with peripheral tumors who have no radiographically apparent mediastinal or N1 adenopathy. The decision to bypass mediastinal invasive staging must be based on a high-quality, contrast-enhanced scan interpreted in collaboration with an experienced chest radiologist. Finally, at the extreme positive end of the radiographic spectrum, it is clinically safe to accept N2 staging without tissue in cases of massive, confluent mediastinal adenopathy or infiltration in a pattern not consistent with any benign process, especially if the PET scan also is positive.

In addition to staging, mediastinoscopy can often be used to diagnose lung cancer when other studies are unrevealing. In fact, patients with a lung mass, suggestive lymph nodes, and no evidence of metastases should undergo mediastinoscopy and bronchoscopy for diagnosis and staging at a single operation. In such cases, when mediastinoscopy is required and likely to produce a positive result, the practice of performing an initial transthoracic needle biopsy of the primary site or a diagnostic bronchoscopy is inefficient. Other causes of adenopathy in the upper mediastinum, such as lymphoma and sarcoidosis, as well as suitably located non-nodal masses, can be sampled by mediastinoscopy. Therapeutic applications include evacuation of bronchogenic cysts, abscess drainage, and the occasional resection of parathyroid adenoma. Variations of mediastinoscopy may be helpful in two other thoracic operations. Mediastinal lymph node dissection after induction therapy for lung cancer may be difficult because of fibrosis from tumor response and prior mediastinoscopy. Reopening the neck incision just before thoracotomy and blunt stripping of the pretracheal fascia may facilitate dissection from the pleural side. In transhiatal esophagectomy, passage of the mediastinoscope along the bluntly dissected upper esophagus may be helpful for clipping esophageal attachments and vessels.

the ACOSOG Z0050 trial reveal a sensitivity of 61% and a specificity of 84% for N2/N3 disease. The negative predictive value was 87%, and the authors concluded that mediastinoscopy still must be considered the gold standard. This is especially true if the PET scan is positive in the mediastinum. In this situation, because of the significant incidence of false positives, the mediastinal lymph nodes must be histologically documented to be positive. In contrast, surgeons are not of one mind regarding invasive staging in the absence of node enlargement. Proponents of routine mediastinoscopy cite the low accuracy of CT scanning and the high incidence of adenocarcinoma with its propensity for nodal metastases.

Others apply mediastinoscopy selectively. Indications include central tumors, known adenocarcinoma, the need for pneumonectomy, and superior sulcus cancers, but the most common criterion is adenopathy or suggested invasion on a CT scan. The selective approach is based on a fairly

Contraindications and Dangers

Anatomic conditions that preclude safe mediastinoscopy include huge cervical goiter, extensive calcification or aneurysm of the aortic arch or innominate artery, and

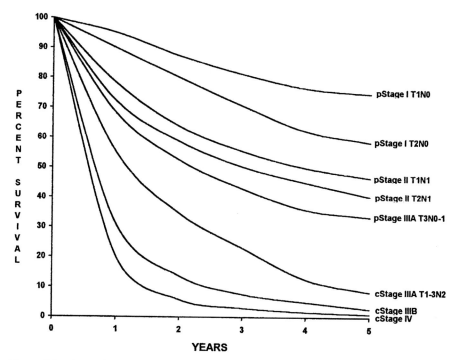

Figure 2-2. Approximate survival by stage and substage. Pathologic (p) early stages are contrasted to clinical (c) later stages to emphasize the importance of clinical staging. Stage IIIB survival also varies by N3 versus T4, and stage IV survival by intrapulmonary versus extrathoracic metastases.

difficult and may preclude multiple biopsies. Fortunately, a limited examination is adequate in most instances. The goal in superior vena cava syndrome is histologic diagnosis, and representative tissue often can be obtained in the high paratracheal region. Similarly, re-exploration is usually done to confirm residual or recurrent disease rather than to map all levels.

Surgical Technique

General anesthesia is required. The patient is positioned supine with the occiput at the very top of the operating table. The neck is moderately extended by an interscapular roll to draw the trachea from the mediastinum into the neck. The back of the operating table is elevated 20 to 30 degrees to decrease venous pressure but not enough to risk venous air embolism. The preparation includes the anterior chest for possible sternotomy, but this area is not shaved. The endotracheal tube exits the mouth on the anesthesiologist's side and is positioned as flat as possible (Fig. 2-3). If the tube protrudes anteriorly, it is subject to kinking and disconnection. Circulation to the right arm is monitored by a radial arterial cannula or pulse oximeter. A dampened waveform may indicate innominate artery compression and decreased right carotid perfusion. The degree and duration of compression should be minimized. Optical magnification is not required but can be achieved with an attachable swing-away lens. Alternatively, some surgeons find that loupes are helpful. Videomediastinoscopy is an option that provides both direct and monitor viewing. It aids teaching by obviating the inevitable shifts that occur when the scope is handed back and forth, thus ensuring that all observers are viewing the same structures. It cannot substitute, however, for the tactile experience of maneuvering the instrument.

A 3-cm to 4-cm transverse skin incision is centered between the anterior borders of the sternocleidomastoid muscles 1 cm above the sternoclavicular junctions and carried through the platysma (Fig. 2-4). The avascular space between the two layers of strap muscles is opened vertically. Palpation of the trachea aids in locating the narrow midline between the sternohyoid muscles. The deeper sternothyroid muscles are separated by a wide band of areolar tissue. The anterior wall of the trachea is now in view. If there is insufficient length of trachea caudad to the thyroid isthmus, this structure is retracted cranially. Rarely, the isthmus must be divided and its ends ligated or oversewn. The arteria thyroidea ima or a branch or branches

permanent tracheostomy after laryngectomy and radiation therapy. Although not contraindications, several other factors are signs of potential hazards. A carotid bruit, especially on the right, should prompt extra care to minimize neck extension and compression of the innominate artery. Prior sternotomy or cervical incision may render the search for the midline more difficult but does not affect the deeper dissection because the pretracheal fascia is intact. Previous mediastinoscopy, on the other hand, causes peritracheal fibrosis that extends into the mediastinum. Nonetheless, repeat mediastinoscopy can be safely accomplished in most cases. Particular care must be exercised

in separating the innominate artery from the trachea. Sharp dissection under direct vision is safer than the blunt approach used in first-time mediastinoscopy. The midline trachea–artery interface may sometimes be avoided by confining mediastinal entry to the left anterolateral aspect of the trachea. Mediastinoscopy can also be performed in the presence of obstruction of the superior vena cava. The most troublesome bleeding is from engorged superficial veins divided by the transverse skin incision rather than from the deeper veins, which are retracted laterally. It must be recognized, however, that mediastinoscopy in cases of superior vena caval obstruction or prior operation may be

Table 2-3 Correlation of Radiographic Studies and Mediastinoscopy with Pathologic Nodal Stages in Non-Small Cell Lung Cancer

	Computed Tomographic Scan[a]	Magnetic Resonance Imaging Scan	Chest Film	Mediastinoscopy
Sensitivity (%)	82 (60–96)	71	80	87
Specificity (%)	76 (52–96)	84	43	100
Accuracy (%)	81 (61–92)	83	57	95
Positive predictive value (%)	74 (32–97)	81	45	100
Negative predictive value (%)	91 (82–95)	84	79	93

[a]Range of values given in parentheses.

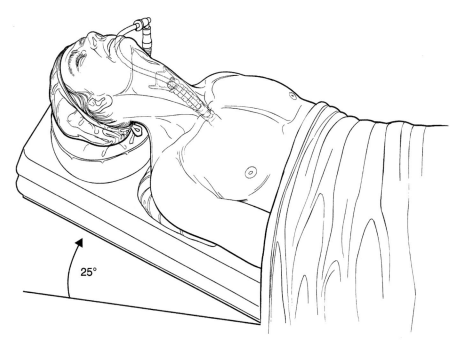

Figure 2-3. Patient position for mediastinoscopy. The neck is extended. The endotracheal tube is draped laterally to avoid the path of the mediastinoscope.

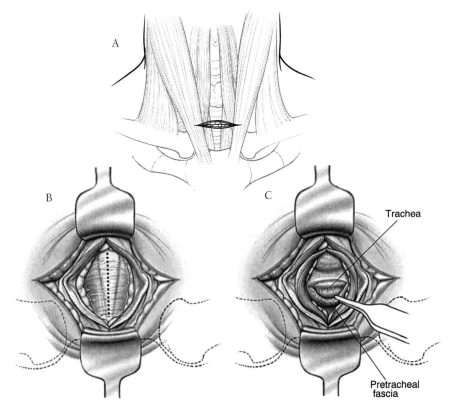

Figure 2-4. Cervical dissection. **(A)** Skin incision. **(B)** Vertical midline incision between the sternothyroid muscles after separation of the sternohyoids. **(C)** The pretracheal fascia is incised and elevated.

of the inferior thyroid vein must be ligated when these vessels cannot be retracted from the midline below the isthmus. It is essential to assess the area just above the sternal notch early in the dissection because cervical extension may draw the innominate artery up into the base of the neck where it can be injured by sharp dissection or cautery.

The pretracheal fascia is incised and elevated. A tunnel is created by insertion of the index finger for blunt dissection of the pretracheal space (Fig. 2-5). For purposes of palpation and later visualization, mediastinoscopy is a "tracheocentric" procedure: Anatomic orientation is defined at all times by the relationship to the trachea of the finger or the mediastinoscope. Tough fibrous bands between the trachea and fascia may be encountered proximally. Thereafter, gentle advancement and lateral sweeping clear the pretracheal and paratracheal spaces easily unless there is local fibrosis or malignant extranodal invasion. The dorsal aspect of the finger senses the tracheal rings in a stepladder fashion as one progresses distally. Dissection is carried to the full length of the finger and usually reaches a point 1 cm to 2 cm proximal to the carina. In short patients, the carina may be reached and is identified as a midline posterior depression. Simultaneously, the anteriorly directed volar surface of the finger palpates the innominate artery and the aortic arch more distally. Pressures within the superior vena cava and pulmonary artery are too low for these landmarks to be appreciated. During digital dissection, the surgeon formulates a mental map of the superior mediastinum by noting the presence of lymphadenopathy, mass, or invasion in relation to normal structures. Because the nodes are external to the pretracheal fascia, access requires penetration of the fascia within the mediastinum. This is usually accomplished digitally just beyond the innominate artery (Fig. 2-6). Enlarged nodes can then often be freed bluntly to a significant extent, which is a maneuver that facilitates subsequent endoscopic retrieval. Firm nodes in the upper right paratracheal area are particularly suitable because the finger can be hooked anteriorly around the innominate artery and blunt dissection performed against the chest wall.

The mediastinoscope is now introduced. As in all endoscopic procedures, the instrument is advanced only if it passes easily and there is a visible tunnel ahead. Passage is aided by blunt dissection with a metal or plastic suction-cautery apparatus. The "endodissectors" designed for laparoscopy also work well. After passage of the scope to the distal trachea, novice mediastinoscopists or vascular nature of the tissue in question, aspiration is carried out using a 20- or 22-gauge spinal needle and small syringe. Saline in the syringe, as opposed to a dry system, facilitates identification of small amounts of blood. In the rare case of a completely solidified mediastinum, when anatomic definition is impossible and biopsy hazardous, aspiration cytology or core tissue histology studies may have to suffice. In the majority of cases, however, it is possible to obtain substantial biopsy specimens. To prevent minor bleeding from obscuring the field, all target nodes are partially dissected before any biopsy specimens are taken. Node dissection through the scope is done bluntly, with the suction-cautery, endodissectors, or biopsy forceps (Fig. 2-9).

Once sufficiently freed, the node is grasped with a cupped laryngeal biopsy forceps, and traction is applied under direct vision. If the node cannot be extracted by gentle pulling and twisting, further dissection is carried out. It is occasionally possible and helpful to grasp the node and divide tethering attachments with a simultaneously introduced dissector or a second biopsy forceps. If further digital dissection seems helpful, the scope is withdrawn and the finger reintroduced. Alternating endoscopic and digital dissection can be repeated at multiple levels. Although removal of whole lymph nodes theoretically lessens the chance of tumor implantation and is aesthetically pleasing, it is not always feasible because of large size, friability, or adherence. In such instances, incisional biopsy specimens are taken with the laryngeal forceps. Particular care is taken when obtaining specimens near the tracheobronchial angles because of the proximity of the azygos vein and apical branch of the anterior trunk of the pulmonary artery on the right and the recurrent laryngeal nerve on the left.

The extent of biopsies depends on the clinical impression and operative findings. In lymphoma, sarcoidosis, or mediastinal mass, all that is needed is diagnostic tissue. For staging lung cancer, on the other hand, it is usually necessary to obtain specimens from more than one location. Samples are routinely taken from the high and low paratracheal regions, the subcarinal space, and the tracheobronchial angles (levels 2, 4, 7, and 10). If there is unequivocal extranodal tumor at a high station, lower levels need not be sampled because staging will not be altered. In general, however, the time taken for frozen-section confirmation is greater than the time and risk of taking more specimens. Routine biopsy of nodes contralateral to the

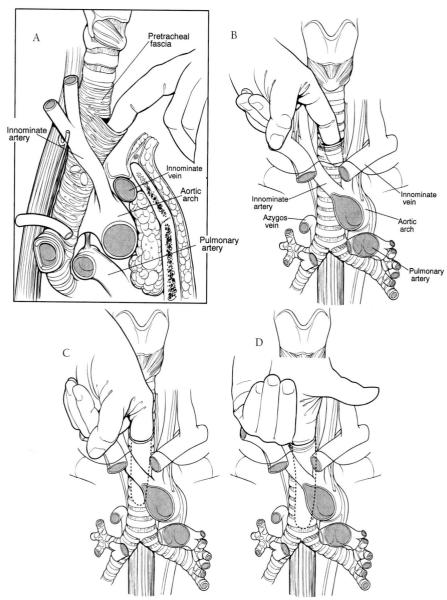

Figure 2-5. Development of the pretracheal tunnel and identification of landmarks and pathologic involvement. **(A, B)** Oblique and anterior views of a finger entering the pretracheal space and palpating the innominate artery. **(C)** Beyond and posterior to the innominate artery, palpating the trachea, artery, and nodes and enlarging the tunnel by lateral sweeping. **(D)** Fully inserted, palpating the arch, nodes, and sometimes the carina and proximal bronchi.

may be confused at not finding nodes despite visualizing the bifurcation. The problem is that the scope is within the pretracheal fascia, and its distal bevel, combined with the slope of the trachea from anterior to posterior as it descends through the mediastinum, angles the field of view directly onto the airway. The mediastinoscope must be withdrawn slightly and angled anteriorly to enter the extrafascial space previously created digitally or to indent the fascia so it can now be bluntly opened with the sucker (Fig. 2-7). The superior mediastinum is surveyed to confirm the findings of palpation by visualizing the pretracheal, paratracheal,

tracheobronchial, and subcarinal nodes, the azygos vein, the pulmonary artery, the proximal mainstem bronchi, and sometimes the bronchial take-off of the right upper lobe (Fig. 2-8). Nodes are identified by color and consistency and by reference to the map generated by palpation. Even to the experienced eye, however, the blue-gray hue of venous structures may simulate the appearance of an anthracotic node. Pulsations may be misleading by both their presence and absence because they may be transmitted to nonvascular structures and may be difficult to appreciate in the vena cava and azygos vein. If there is any doubt about the solid

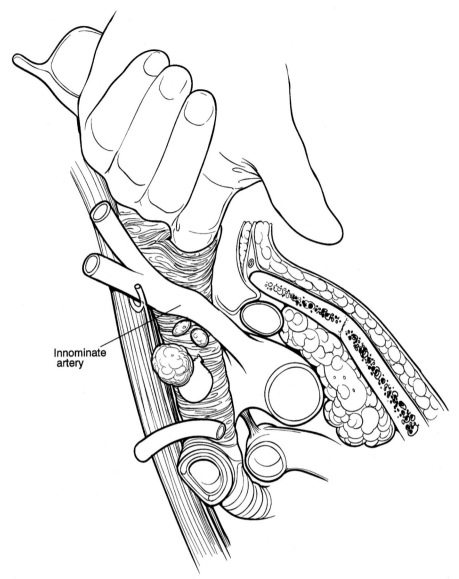

Innominate
artery

Figure 2-6. Oblique view of a finger piercing the pretracheal fascia to enter the node-containing space. Considerable blunt dissection of enlarged nodes can be accomplished.

primary tumor is essential in order not to understage IIIB (N3) cases as IIIA (N2). Labeling all specimens by numerical station is less subject to error than using their polysyllabic anatomic designations.

Bleeding is usually minor and requires no specific treatment. The mediastinoscope can perpetuate bleeding by keeping open the space beyond the scope, but it can also tamponade lateral bleeders. To assess hemostasis, the field therefore is observed as the scope is withdrawn slowly. Minor oozing can be stopped by packing the subcarinal or paratracheal spaces and withdrawing the mediastinoscope for a few minutes. This maneuver can be repeated as bleeding slows. Oxidized cellulose can be left in place for hemostasis and can also serve as a simple

quality control marker for comparing mediastinoscopy biopsy locations with the findings at later thoracotomy. If there is a visible small bleeding vessel, metal clips are placed with an applier designed for this purpose. Clipping is most useful for bronchial arteries in the subcarinal area. If cautery is used, it should be at low wattage and applied directly to raw node surface or small vessels to avoid arcing and thermal damage.

If there is concern about pleural or pulmonary puncture, the tunnel is filled with saline. Rapid disappearance of liquid may indicate a pleural rent; bubbling with inspiratory pressure suggests a parenchymal communication. If the leak is significant, a chest tube is placed. For closure, the strap muscles are reapproximated in the midline

with absorbable sutures. Ridge formation is lessened if the platysma is not closed separately. A subcuticular closure is used for the skin. Drainage is not necessary.

Variations

Extended cervical mediastinoscopy accesses the subaortic and anterior mediastinal nodes, areas beyond the reach of the standard pretracheal procedure. After clearing of the infraisthmic trachea or completion of standard mediastinoscopy, the space anterior to the aortic arch is opened by digitally piercing the fascia between the innominate and the left common carotid arteries. The innominate vein, separated from the operative area in standard mediastinoscopy by the arch arteries, now lies directly anterior to the tunnel. After normal and abnormal structures are palpated, the mediastinoscope is passed anterior to the aorta, and appropriate biopsy specimens are taken (Fig. 2-10). Direct invasion and mediastinal fixation can also be appreciated with the scope or the exploring finger. In *mediastinopleuroscopy*, the pleural space is intentionally entered. On the right, the pleura is opened posterior to the innominate artery, whereas on the left, entry is gained between the left common carotid and left subclavian arteries. In addition to pleural biopsy and fluid sampling, small lung biopsy specimens or larger, stapled wedge excisions can be obtained. However, the risk of seeding a clean mediastinum by transpleural biopsy of an upper lobe cancer or infection must be considered.

Postoperative Care

Patients are discharged after 2 to 3 hours of observation that includes standard postanesthesia vital signs, electrocardiographic monitoring, and pulse oximetry. Our unplanned admission rate is 1%. Chest radiographs are obtained only if there is known or suspected pleural entry, excessive bleeding, abnormal auscultation findings, or hypoxemia. Similarly, blood tests are done only when specifically indicated.

Complications

Mediastinoscopy is a low-risk procedure in experienced hands (Table 2-4). The mortality rate in large series ranges from 0.0% to 0.08%. Complications occur in up to 3% of cases, but are major in 0.5% or less. The most feared complication and the cause of most deaths is massive hemorrhage from damage to the aortic arch or its branches, the superior vena cava, the azygos vein, or the pulmonary artery. Lacerations of the innominate and jugular vein occur less commonly and are more easily

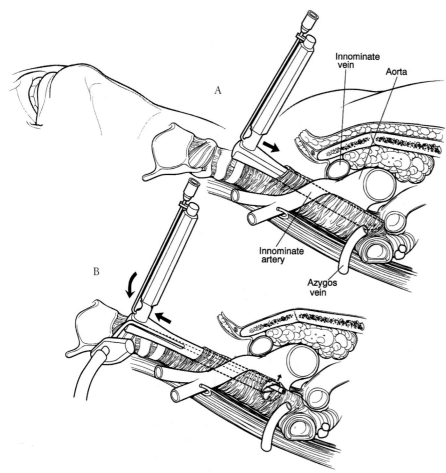

Innominate
vein

Aorta

A

Innominate
artery

Azygos
vein

B

Figure 2-7. **(A)** The passive angle of the mediastinoscope within the pretracheal fascia not previously opened digitally aims the bevel directly at the trachea. **(B)** The scope is angled anteriorly to tense fascia so it can be penetrated with a sucker. The innominate artery is subject to compression during this maneuver.

repaired. Injury to a bronchial artery may produce significant but not massive bleeding unless the vessel has been avulsed from the aorta. Although in some series surgical repair for hemorrhage was not required, it is inevitable that significant bleeding will occur on occasion. The incidence should not exceed 0.1%. If control cannot be achieved via the cervical incision, the mediastinum is packed while preparations are made for transfusion and operation. If there is a rent in the superior vena cava, lower extremity venous lines are placed. The decision to proceed with sternotomy or thoracotomy depends on the location of the vascular injury, the resectability of the tumor, and the patient's immediate status. Median sternotomy is generally preferable for innominate artery, aortic arch, and right pulmonary arterial injuries. Right thoracotomy is more useful for the more common azygous vein injury and for superior vena caval injury. In addition to provision of access for control of hemorrhage, a right thora-

cotomy allows resection of the right-sided tumor at the same setting. Surgical intervention may also be required for rare nonvascular injuries. Small tracheobronchial tears are treated by packing, but larger lacerations require direct or pedicled flap closure. Esophageal perforation, usually in the subcarinal region, may be detected and repaired early or may elude diagnosis until mediastinal sepsis complicates treatment. Recurrent nerve paralysis is infrequent, usually involves the left side, and is transient in one half of cases. Pneumothoraces are generally minor and not under tension because most result from pleural laceration rather than parenchymal injury. Treatment by observation, aspiration, or tube thoracostomy is dictated by the clinical situation. It has been suggested that stroke is a procedure-specific complication, especially of extended mediastinoscopy, and is caused by atherosclerotic embolization or cerebral hypoperfusion from arch or branch arterial compression. The incidence, however, is ex-

tremely low and probably not higher than expected with any operation and general anesthetic.

Alternative Procedures

In the absence of an accurate noninvasive modality, mediastinoscopy represents an ideal staging procedure because of its accuracy, safety, and minimal discomfort. In some instances, however, sufficient information can be obtained by other means. At bronchoscopy, enlarged paratracheal and subcarinal nodes can be sampled by transtracheal or transcarinal needle aspiration. Negative findings in an aspirate should not be considered definitive, and mediastinoscopy may follow later or at the same procedure. It is also essential to avoid false positivity from contamination of the aspirate by cells of the primary tumor (Fig. 2-11). Accordingly, we reserve this method for tumors located well distal to the carina and perform node aspiration before sampling the primary site. Aspiration replaces mediastinoscopy only when the situation requires diagnosis alone or confirmation of node positivity at a single level without concern about invasion or extracapsular extension. Endobronchial ultrasound is undergoing investigation as a means to stage and guide aspiration of suspicious nodes. Due to inability of the transducer to create a seal in the relatively large trachea, this modality may be more accurate for imaging hilar nodes, information that would not alter decision to proceed with thoracotomy. Others have evaluated endoscopic ultrasound (EUS)-guided fine-needle aspiration. Although sensitivity may approach 90%, the presence of air in the trachea makes imaging of levels 2 and 4 lymph nodes difficult. Thus, this modality may be useful for lower lobe tumors with their propensity to spread to level 7 before others. Transthoracic fine-needle aspiration may also be considered when limited information is required. In experienced hands, this procedure has a high yield. Because it is often unnecessary to traverse lung parenchyma, pneumothorax is less common than after lung biopsy. Although thoracoscopy may be valuable for left-sided adenopathy, we envision no advantage over mediastinoscopy in cases requiring right-sided and midline nodal investigation. Indeed, left paratracheal nodes are not reached by right thoracoscopy. When the situation calls for specific evaluation of posterior subcarinal or pulmonary ligament nodes or of tumor factors as well as nodes, thoracoscopy may be helpful.

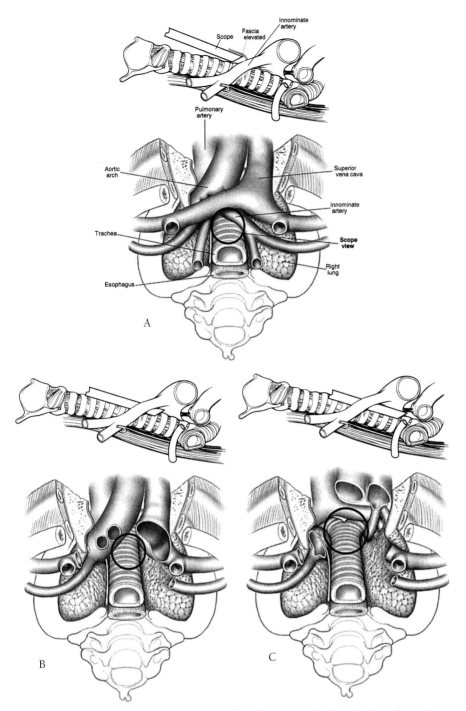

Figure 2-8. Craniocaudal (surgeon's orientation) and corresponding lateral views of superior mediastinal and adjacent structures at three levels. Circles outline potential views through the mediastinoscope at each level, depending on the anteroposterior and lateral angulation of the instrument. **(A)** Proximal tunnel. **(B)** Midtrachea. **(C)** Distal trachea and carina.

Indications

Cancer of the left upper lobe is the usual indication. The staging algorithm for tumors in this location differs from that for other sites because of the pattern of lymphatic metastases and because of unique surgical results in the presence of localized adenopathy. The left upper lobe drains not only to the subaortic and anterior mediastinal groups, but also to the ipsilateral paratracheal stations. A significant number of patients with left upper lobe tumors have metastases to the latter groups, involvement that presages the same poor surgical prognosis as in other clinical N2 cases. Resection of left upper lobe cancers with malignant but not bulky adenopathy confined to the subaortic window (level 5), in contrast, yields an approximate 30% 5-year survival, more than three times that of other clinical N2 cases. These considerations suggest that level 5 node biopsy need not be routine but should be used selectively when gross disease is suspected from the findings on CT scans. Mediastinoscopy, on the other hand, is frequently required for staging left upper lobe cancers. If one practices routine mediastinoscopy, the pattern of metastases from left upper lobe cancers dictates that these tumors not be excepted. When mediastinotomy is indicated by CT findings, it is preceded by mediastinoscopy. If right or left superior mediastinal nodes obtained via the mediastinoscope are positive for cancer, the invasive staging is complete, and other levels need not be sampled. If mediastinoscopy produces negative findings, the results of anterior mediastinotomy become determinative.

Like mediastinoscopy, anterior mediastinotomy may in some cases be the initial procedure for simultaneous diagnosis and nodal staging. The mediastinum, pulmonary vessels, and phrenic nerve can also be assessed for direct invasion. Mediastinotomy is frequently useful for obtaining tissue from anterior mediastinal tumors to secure a diagnosis, and occasionally hilar masses and upper lobe pulmonary lesions.

Contraindications and Dangers

Prior sternotomy is not an absolute contraindication but warrants caution. The procedure should generally not be performed, however, in the presence of a patent left internal mammary coronary bypass graft. To protect the graft in the event of a second sternotomy, most cardiac surgeons drape it laterally, often opening the pleura to do so. This places the artery anterior to the lung hilum, essentially along the course of the phrenic nerve, and subject to injury during node

Anterior Mediastinotomy

Anterior or parasternal mediastinotomy on the left allows assessment of areas inaccessible by standard mediastinoscopy: the subaortic and anterior mediastinal nodes as well as the proximal hilar structures. The left paratracheal and tracheobronchial nodes are obscured by the aortic arch, but contralateral level 4 and level 10 nodes are accessible by right mediastinotomy, as are the superior vena cava and superior right hilum. The upper lobes and pleura can also be exposed. Parasternal mediastinoscopy refers to the common practice of using a mediastinoscope through the anterior incision and does not denote a unique procedure.

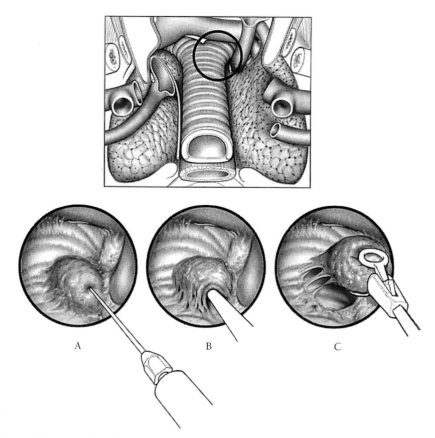

Figure 2-9. Node identification and dissection. **(A)** Aspiration to confirm nonvascular target. **(B)** Blunt dissection with a sucker. **(C)** A node grasped with forceps for further dissection and retrieval.

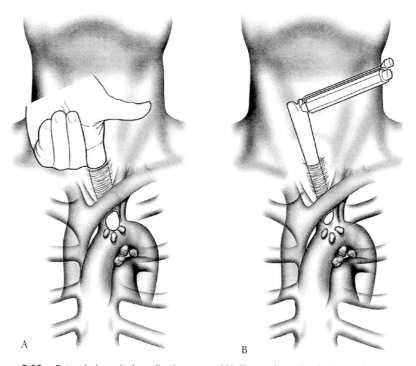

Figure 2-10. Extended cervical mediastinoscopy. **(A)** Finger dissection between the innominate and left carotid arteries. **(B)** The mediastinoscope in place for anterior mediastinal and aortopulmonary node biopsy.

biopsy. Although re-do mediastinoscopy has been shown to be safe, we are not aware of substantial similar experience for repeat mediastinotomy, have not performed such procedures, and consider reoperation in the absence of gross residual disease hazardous.

Surgical Technique

The patient is positioned supine and under general anesthesia. Selective lung ventilation via a double-lumen tube is not essential but may be helpful. A 6-cm to 8-cm transverse incision is made just lateral to the sternum at the second or third costal levels (Fig. 2-12). The fibers of the pectoralis muscle are split to expose the cartilage. The cartilage is resected from the sternochondral to the costochondral junction, and the mediastinum is entered through the posterior perichondrium. In some cases, adequate exposure is achieved through the intercostal space without removing the cartilage, but it is easier to remain extrapleural by removing the cartilage. The internal mammary artery and vein are retracted or ligated and divided. The mediastinal pleural reflection is separated bluntly from the posterior table of the sternum and retracted laterally staying extrapleural and taking care not to put a rent in the mediastinal pleura. Finger dissection opens the loose areolar tissue and extends inward until the aorta, pulmonary artery, and intervening space are identified and assessed for fixation, invasion, and adenopathy. During palpation, as in mediastinoscopy, the surgeon formulates a tactile map of normal and abnormal structures and can begin freeing nodes. Direct inspection confirms the nodal and vascular anatomy. The vagus and phrenic nerves can sometimes be identified along the aortic arch and the location of the recurrent laryngeal branch thereby inferred, but the phrenic nerve is usually not seen at the hilum unless the pleura is open.

Enlarged nodes are sampled directly by excisional or incisional biopsy. For smaller nodes, biopsy specimens are obtained through a mediastinoscope introduced through the costal incision. The techniques of dissection, identification, and hemostasis described for cervical mediastinoscopy apply here as well. In addition, anatomic definition may sometimes be clarified by opening the pleura and assessing the situation from both the mediastinal and pleural aspects. Some favor opening the pleura and obtaining specimens from the pleural side in all cases. Although the aortic arch is not amenable to retraction via mediastinotomy, on the right the vena cava can be retracted medially or dissection performed

Table 2-4   Complications of Mediastinoscopy

Death: ≤0.08%
Major complications: ≤0.5%
 Major hemorrhage
 Tracheobronchial laceration
 Esophageal perforation
 Recurrent nerve paralysis
 Phrenic nerve paralysis
 Thoracic duct injury
 Cerebrovascular accident
 Mediastinitis
 Venous air embolus
 Tumor implantation
Minor complications: ≤2.5%
 Pneumothorax
 Superficial wound infection
 Recurrent nerve paresis
 Minor bleeding
 Autonomic reflex bradycardia
 Mediastinal lymph node necrosis

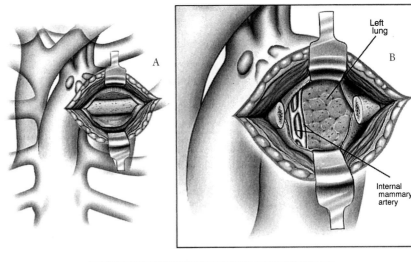

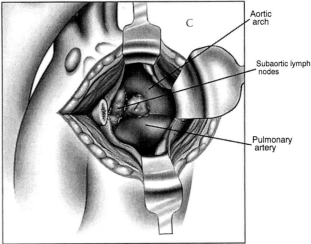

Figure 2-12.   Anterior mediastinotomy. **(A)** Incision over the second costal cartilage. **(B)** After resection of the costal cartilage. **(C)** View of enlarged subaortic nodes.

between the vena cava and the ascending aorta, depending on the target area. When mediastinotomy is done in conjunction with cervical mediastinoscopy, the neck incision is left open to allow bidigital palpation of the aortopulmonary region (Fig. 2-13). If needed, resection of a segment of osseous rib lateral to the excised costal cartilage provides substantial additional intrapleural exposure for pleural inspection, posterior hilar assessment, or generous stapled lung biopsy.

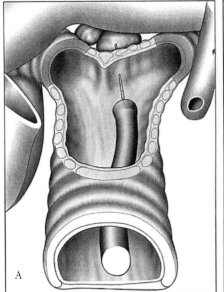

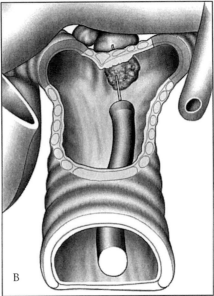

Figure 2-11.   Transcarinal aspiration of level 7 nodes. **(A)** Acceptable sample—the needle entering directly into nodes. **(B)** Contaminated sample—the needle traverses an endobronchial primary tumor.

Usually drainage is not needed. If the pleura was entered, a small tube is brought out through one edge of the wound. After closure, pleural air is evacuated by inflating the lungs to a pressure of 30 to 40 cm H_2O as the tube is withdrawn. If the lung was biopsied at operation, the tube is left in place and connected to suction, underwater seal, or a one-way flutter valve.

Complications

Because mediastinotomy is performed far less frequently than mediastinoscopy, there are no large series that assess the complication rate. Mortality should be exceedingly rare. Significant bleeding from injury to the aorta, the internal mammary vessels, the pulmonary artery, or the superior pulmonary vein is possible but uncommon. Diaphragmatic paralysis and hoarseness occur occasionally from damage to the phrenic or recurrent laryngeal nerves. Chylothorax has been reported. Pneumothorax can usually be handled conservatively. Tumor invasion of the incision is rare, but we have seen one

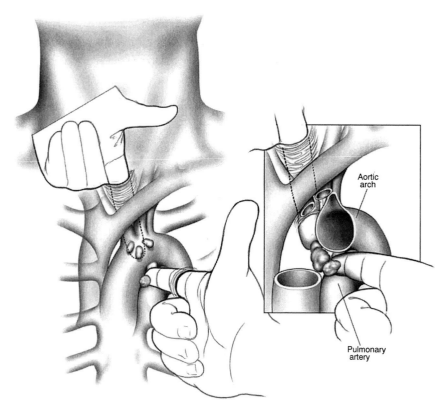

Aortic arch

Pulmonary artery

Figure 2-13. Bidigital palpation of the aortopulmonary region via cervical mediastinoscopy and left anterior mediastinotomy.

case each with lung cancer, germ cell tumor, and lymphoma.

Alternative Procedures

It is our bias that anterior mediastinotomy has important limitations for staging lung cancer. Discomfort is significant, and costal cartilage resection leaves a noticeable depression. Large masses that abut the anterior chest wall on CT scans can be biopsied without cartilage excision. In contrast, removal is generally required in patients with lung cancer because the area of interest is several centimeters from the incision. Tactile, direct visual, and endoscopic visual assessment are frequently suboptimal. The versatility of and the information gained by mediastinotomy are more impressive in theory than in practice. Massive adenopathy or gross tumor infiltration and fixation of major structures is easy to detect, but subtle involvement is difficult to appreciate. In contrast to mediastinoscopy for superior mediastinal exploration, we therefore often pursue alternatives to anterior mediastinotomy for assessing subaortic lymphadenopathy. Because biopsy is warranted only in the presence of node enlargement, transthoracic needle aspiration may be feasible. In some patients, thoracoscopy is valuable for left-sided nodal staging because it provides excellent access to the subaortic

area and can be done concomitant with negative findings on mediastinoscopic examination. When there is fixation of the lung to the mediastinum, however, thoracoscopic staging may require dissection of malignant adhesions and risk diffuse pleural implantation. We reserve thoracoscopy for cases with subaortic adenopathy separate from the primary site and without radiographically suggested lung fixation. Finally, extended mediastinoscopy can accomplish the goals of mediastinoscopy and mediastinotomy with the advantage of a single incision.

Scalene Biopsy

Scalene lymph node biopsy is an open procedure for sampling enlarged nodes in the scalene triangle, the low anterior cervical region superficial to the anterior scalene muscle. Scalene fat pad excision denotes resection of all the node-bearing areolar tissue in this region.

Indications

Before the introduction of mediastinoscopy, scalene biopsy was the mainstay of nodal staging in lung cancer. Routine biopsy was performed variously ipsilateral to the tumor, bilateral, or on the right for right-sided and left lower lobe tumors and on the left for left upper lobe cancers. The positivity

rate in the absence of palpable adenopathy varied from 3% to 20%, with central adenocarcinomas having the highest incidence. In the current era of CT scanning, the yield in patients without mediastinal node enlargement or an apical tumor is low, and routine biopsy is not warranted. Although the converse incidence—occult scalene metastases in clinical N2 disease—is unknown, it has been suggested that it may be as high as 10%. The question is important because studies of therapy for nodal IIIA cancer may be confounded by inclusion of an unsuspected cohort of IIIB cases (N3). Although one may speculate about a future resurrection of fat pad excision in N2 disease, scalene biopsy is limited to directed sampling of enlarged nodes. In contrast, in sarcoidosis, although surpassed by mediastinoscopy, the diagnostic yield of blind scalene biopsy is sufficiently high (75% to 90%) that the procedure may be substituted for mediastinoscopy when this disease is suspected, diagnosis is elusive by bronchoscopy or nonhistologic evidence, and general anesthesia must be avoided.

Contraindications and Dangers

Because poor healing, malignant wound seeding, and chylous fistula are prone to occur in cases with bulky adenopathy, extranodal tumor infiltration, and prior cervical radiation therapy, open biopsy should be avoided in this setting.

Percutaneous sampling is substituted for open biopsy when the nodes are sufficiently large and accessible. The procedure is performed in the office or clinic with a syringe and a 20-gauge needle for cytologic study or with a core biopsy device for histologic study. This approach is strongly recommended when the risk of lymphatic leak and poor healing is high.

Surgical Technique

Fat pad excision is described to highlight the anatomy (Fig. 2-14). In the presence of enlarged nodes, however, only abnormal tissue need be sampled by standard methods for incisional or excisional lymph node biopsy. Local anesthesia is adequate. The neck is extended and the head turned away from the operative side. A 4-cm incision centered between the heads of the sternocleidomastoid muscle and about 2 cm above the clavicle is deepened through the platysma. The two heads are retracted in opposite directions or the entire muscle is retracted medially. If needed, the clavicular head can be partly or totally transected near its insertion. The omohyoid is retracted cranially. The boundaries of the scalene triangle are

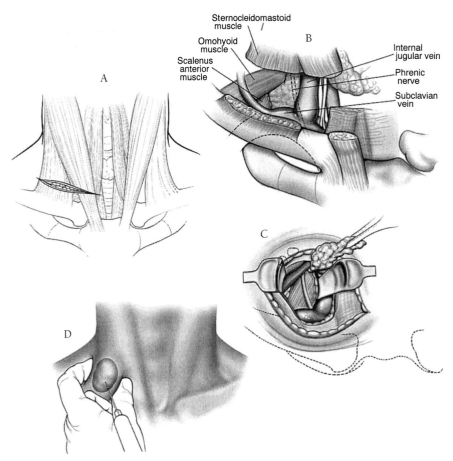

the jugular vein medially, the subclavian vein inferiorly, and the omohyoid muscle superolaterally. The anterior scalene muscle, with the phrenic nerve coursing along its surface, constitutes the deep margin of dissection. The fat pad is dissected from these structures from below upward. Visible lymphatic channels are clipped or ligated. The transverse cervical artery, arising from the subclavian and entering the fat pad inferiorly, may have to be ligated. On the left, the thoracic duct can often be seen near its entry into the superior aspect of the subclavian vein. If injured, it must be meticulously ligated. When fat pad excision is performed along with mediastinoscopy, the mediastinoscopy incision is extended 1 cm to the appropriate side, and a skin flap is developed. The fat pad can then be reached posterior to the sternal head of the sternocleidomastoid by retracting the muscle anteriorly or by transecting it at its insertion.

Complications

Mortality is negligible. Injury to the major veins should be rare. The jugular vein can be repaired easily, but a subclavian laceration may require clavicular resection. Phrenic nerve injury is prevented by avoiding the use of cautery deep to the fat pad. Pneumothorax may result from a rent in the pleural cupola or, less likely, puncture of the lung. Venous air embolism can occur, as in any cervical procedure.

Figure 2-14.   Scalene biopsy. **(A)** Skin incision over the sternocleidomastoid muscle. **(B)** Anatomy of the scalene triangle. **(C)** Resection of the fat pad, exposing the anterior scalene muscle and phrenic nerve. **(D)** Alternative—percutaneous needle aspiration of enlarged nodes.

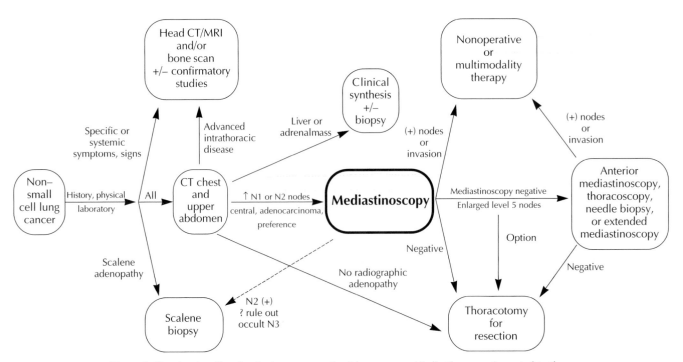

Figure 2-15.   An algorithm for staging non–small cell lung cancer. Mediastinoscopy is central to the clinical staging process. (CT, computed tomography; MRI, magnetic resonance imaging.)

Conclusion

Mastery of thoracic surgery is in large measure the cognitive and technical mastery of the process and procedures for staging lung cancer. Figure 2-15 presents a staging algorithm.

SUGGESTED READING

Barendregt WB, Deleu HWO, Joosten HJM, et al. The value of parasternal mediastinoscopy in staging bronchogenic carcinoma. Eur J Cardiothorac Surg 1995;9:655.

Canadian Lung Oncology Group. Investigation for mediastinal disease in patients with apparently operable lung cancer. Ann Thorac Surg 1995;60:1382.

Foster ED, Munro DD, Dobell ARC. Mediastinoscopy. A review of anatomical relationships and complications. Ann Thorac Surg 1972;13:273.

Ginsberg R, Rice TW, Goldberg M, et al. Extended cervical mediastinoscopy: A single staging procedure for bronchogenic carcinoma of the left upper lobe. J Thorac Cardiovasc Surg 1987;94:673.

Jepsen O. Mediastinoscopy: Bioptic Mediastinal Exploration by the Method of Carlens. Copenhagen: Munksgaard, 1966.

Mountain CF. A new international staging system for lung cancer. Chest 1986;89(Suppl):225S.

Pearson FG, DeLarue NC, Ilves R, et al. Significance of positive superior mediastinal nodes identified at mediastinoscopy in patients with resectable cancer of the lung. J Thorac Cardiovasc Surg 1982;83:1.

Puhakka HJ. Complications of mediastinoscopy. J Laryngol Otol 1989;103:312.

Shields T. The significance of ipsilateral mediastinal lymph node metastasis (N2 disease) in non–small cell carcinoma of the lung. J Thorac Cardiovasc Surg 1990;99:48.

Silvestri GA, Littenberg B, Colice GL. The clinical evaluation for detecting metastatic lung cancer. A meta-analysis. Am J Respir Crit Care Med 1995;152:225.

EDITOR'S COMMENTS

For a patient with lung cancer, mediastinoscopy is the definitive procedure for staging the superior mediastinal lymph nodes. Yet in a recent American College of Surgeons survey of 729 hospitals and >40,000 patients to determine patterns of surgical care provided patients with non–small cell lung cancer, mediastinoscopy was performed in only 27% of operated patients and a lymph node biopsy was performed in only 47% of those procedures (Little AG, Rusch VW, Bonner JA, et al. Patterns of surgical care of lung cancer patients. Ann Thorac Surg 2005;80:2051). This is simply amazing to me based on the amount of information that can be obtained from this procedure and the number of thoracotomies that could either be saved, if the mediastinoscopy were positive, or gained, if it were negative but expected to be positive. The reasons for this are somewhat baffling, although it may say something about the way we are educating thoracic surgeons. Mediastinoscopy is a difficult procedure to teach and a difficult procedure to do well even after the basics are learned. Thoracic surgical residencies seemingly are not providing adequate training in the performance of this procedure. This lack of mediastinoscopy also asks the question as to who is performing thoracic surgery. We know that thoracic surgical procedures are performed by general surgeons in many communities, surgeons who likely would have little if any training in the performance of mediastinoscopy.

With the mediastinoscope, it is possible to sample lymph nodes on both the right and left sides in the upper paratracheal (level 2), lower paratracheal (level 4), pretracheal (level 3), and subcarinal (level 7) locations. It is a common misconception that left paratracheal lymph nodes cannot be accessed by mediastinoscopy. Nodes on the left side are more difficult to find and tend to occur at a slightly higher location relative to the right side. While working on the left, great care must be taken to avoid injuring the left recurrent laryngeal nerve, which runs just lateral to where the paratracheal lymph nodes are located. This includes the careful and judicious use of electrocautery on the left side to avoid thermal injury to the nerve. It is actually easier to sample the left paratracheal lymph nodes at mediastinoscopy than at thoracotomy because of the limited access afforded to the tracheobronchial angle by the position of the aortic arch, and thus it may be preferable to perform mediastinoscopy routinely for left-sided procedures other than small T1 lesions. Certainly for left lower lobe lesions the threshold for performing mediastinoscopy should be low because of the prevalence of contralateral nodal disease with lesions in this location.

Extended cervical mediastinoscopy designed to allow the sampling of lymph nodes in the para-aortic (level 6) and subaortic (level 5) locations has never become a part of the practice of most thoracic surgeons. The procedure is difficult to perform, and the information provided really is of little use. If the findings on standard cervical mediastinoscopy are negative, even if the subaortic lymph nodes are found at thoracotomy to contain tumor, the prognosis still approximates that of N1 disease, as pointed out by Onaitis and Harpole. Isolated level 5 lymph node involvement is associated with the best prognosis of all N2 disease as long as the disease can be completely resected. If the question is one of resectability, the better procedure for assessing the subaortic window is parasternal mediastinotomy, in which the area may be palpated. This procedure may be performed through a tiny incision made at the left sternal border over the second costal cartilage. The cartilage is excised and the mediastinum entered by reflecting the pleural reflection laterally. The pleural space need not be entered in order to stage the para-aortic and subaortic lymph nodes. As pointed out by the authors, bidigital examination using both the parasternal and cervical mediastinoscopy incisions may provide valuable information regarding resectability for a central lesion located on the left side. Videothoracoscopy also provides excellent access to these nodal locations but requires placement of a double-lumen tube and single-lung ventilation and does not readily allow for palpation.

Accurate surgical staging recently has been brought to the fore because of the change in our thinking regarding postoperative adjuvant chemotherapy for completely resected stage Ib disease and greater. Most medical oncologists now recommend postoperative chemotherapy for these resected patients, recognizing that there seems to be a survival advantage in treated patients. This also places greater importance on the preoperative evaluation for distant disease. PET scanning has assumed an ever-increasing role in the noninvasive staging of lung cancer. A negative mediastinum on CT scan and PET means with almost 100% certainty that the mediastinal lymph nodes are not involved and mediastinoscopy is not indicated. The finding of PET-positive mediastinal nodes should be confirmed histologically with nodal tissue obtained via mediastinoscopy. Extranodal disease may also be assessed with PET. An enlarged adrenal gland seen on CT scan, if positive on PET, is fairly reliable evidence that metastatic disease is present. An enlarged adrenal gland should prompt further evaluation. Often an MRI scan will suffice to demonstrate that the enlargement is consistent with an adenoma. When MRI findings are equivocal, needle biopsy should be performed. If there is still a question, we favor laparoscopic adrenalectomy, a well-accepted procedure and certainly one that is performed more commonly and with less morbidity that the transdiaphragmatic approach favored by Onaitis and Harpole.

L.R.K.

3

Thoracic Incisions

M. Blair Marshall

The optimal approach to the thorax depends on a number of variables: (1) bony anatomy, (2) location and extent of the pathology, (3) location of the hilum, and (4) objectives of the procedure. Historically, the posterolateral thoracotomy has been the work horse for the majority of major thoracic procedures. With the movement toward minimally invasive procedures in both cardiac and general thoracic surgery, there has been renewed interest in additional approaches, such as the anterior thoracotomy and muscle-sparing incisions. These tailored approaches may favorably affect morbidity, operative time, postoperative pulmonary function, muscle strength, and postoperative pain. This chapter emphasizes the selective indications for these particular approaches and highlights the important technical details.

Posterolateral Thoracotomy

The posterolateral thoracotomy has been the most widely used approach for thoracic pathology. Although any pulmonary resection may be performed through this incision, which has led to its particular versatility, we no longer consider it the optimal approach for most resections.

As for most pulmonary procedures, a double-lumen endotracheal tube is placed and the patient is placed in the lateral decubitus position. A vacuum-type bean bag or other form of support keeps the patient from moving on the table. Pneumatic compression devices are used to prevent thromboembolic disease. The patient is positioned so that the hip overlies the point of flexion

in the table. Once the table is flexed, the abdomen is lengthened and traction opens the intercostal spaces slightly. In positioning, it is important to prep and drape widely, particularly along the posterior spine. One must be careful to avoid inadvertent injury to the arms and legs by using appropriate padding and support between the legs and around the elbows and wrists. The leg support is flexed toward the ceiling to provide additional support to the lower extremities.

The landmarks for this incision include the spine and the scapula. A gentle curve is drawn at the midpoint between the posterior angle of the scapula and spine to approximately one fingerbreadth below the tip of the scapula over to the anterior axillary line (Fig. 3-1). We tend not to use the full extent of this incision for most procedures to minimize tissue trauma and improve healing. Once the skin and subcutaneous tissues are divided, the latissimus dorsi is divided as well. Anteriorly, we routinely spare the serratus anterior muscle by freeing the fascial attachments to the chest wall and between the muscle and the latissimus dorsi muscle; this is done obliquely along the chest wall to avoiding division of the serratus fibers. Depending on the posterior extent of the incision, additional thoracic muscles such as the trapezius or rhomboids may need to be divided. This is particularly important when elevating the scapula off of the chest wall as in a chest wall resection or posterior approach to a Pancoast resection.

The scapula is elevated with a right-angled retractor, and the ribs are counted by manual palpation. Relying on the first rib can be misleading because the posterior first rib may be obscured. One can avoid errors by

using the insertion of the posterior scalene muscle onto the second rib as a reference.

A fifth-interspace thoracotomy incision is made by dividing the intercostal muscles directly above the superior margin of the sixth rib. This avoids injury to the neurovascular bundle that lies just inferior to the fifth rib in a slightly recessed groove. The division along the intercostal muscles extends fairly far beyond the limits of the skin incision to maximize rib separation. In patients with brittle ribs, excising a subperiosteal segment of the sixth rib at the costovertebral angle, so-called "shingling," can help to avoid rib fracture. A 1-cm segment is removed to prevent pain from periosteal friction following reapproximation. Resection of larger segments of rib is reserved for repeat thoracotomies. In this situation, entering the pleural space through the bed of the resected rib improves exposure for adhesiolysis of the pleural space. In approaching diaphragmatic pathology, the seventh or eighth intercostal space is suitable for optimal exposure.

Once the chest is entered, a Finochietto-type retractor is used to separate the ribs. For smaller incisions, smaller retractors provide adequate exposure. On completion of the procedure, a single modified thoracostomy tube usually provides adequate drainage. Additional drainage holes are cut in the tube, and it is tunneled transversely so as to lie in the diaphragmatic sulcus and course posterior to the apex of the chest; thus, it functions as both a basilar and an apical tube (Fig. 3-2). Large absorbable sutures are used to reapproximate the ribs. One must be careful not to overapproximate the ribs because this may contribute to postoperative pain. The remainder of the incision is closed meticulously in layers with absorbable sutures.

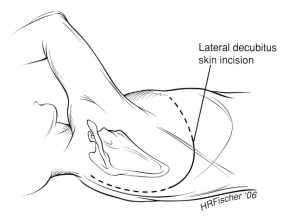

Figure 3-1. The patient in the lateral decubitus position. The scapular landmarks are defined, and the course of the skin incision is illustrated.

Axillary Thoracotomy (Muscle Sparing)

The axillary thoracotomy has replaced the posterolateral thoracotomy as my incision of choice for the majority of pulmonary resections. Because of the inherent limitations of exposure, it did not initially gain widespread use. Improved stapling devices and increased surgical experience have demonstrated its superiority. The advantages of this incision are several: (1) the major thoracic muscles are left intact, (2) there is increased ease and speed of both opening and closing the chest, (3) cosmesis is improved. The disadvantages are that if this incision is made small, it is difficult for two surgeons to have adequate simultaneous visibility. In addition, most posterior chest wall resections are more optimally suited for a posterolateral thoracotomy because elevating the muscles and scapula off of the chest wall facilitates the dissection. Some authors have suggested that complex resections, such as bronchial sleeve resections or pulmonary reconstructions, should not be performed through this approach, although we have not found this to be the case. We routinely perform complex procedures including lung transplantation and repeat thoracotomies through this incision.

The patient is positioned in the lateral decubitus position with a few adjustments. The elbow is rotated cephalad to open up the axilla. The body is rotated posterior so that more of the anterior and lateral chest is exposed. The skin incision for this approach may be oriented vertically or obliquely. We tend to use a vertical incision for open procedures and the oblique incision for video-assisted thoracic surgery (VATS) lobectomy. A 5-cm to 7-cm incision is made along the anterior axillary line aligned with the anterior superior iliac spine centered usually on the nipple in male patients or the fourth intercostal space (Fig. 3-3.) One should avoid placing this incision too far posterior because injury to the long thoracic nerve may occur. After the skin incision, the subcutaneous tissues are divided. The intercostal brachial nerve runs in the superior half of the incision and should be preserved if possible. Patients should be counseled preoperatively that they may have numbness in the area of distribution of this nerve. In addition, numbness along the lateral breast is common with this incision and eventually resolves.

After the subcutaneous tissues are divided, the pectoralis major muscle is undermined and the anterior border of the serratus anterior muscle is visualized. Often the pectoralis minor muscle must be reflected to see these anterior insertions of the serratus muscle. The serratus insertions must be mobilized off the chest wall by reflecting the costal attachments or split along the fifth interspace. Thus the insertions of the serratus anterior muscle are mobilized and reflected off of the fourth and fifth ribs. For pulmonary resections we use the fourth interspace, and for tracheal resections the third. Because this incision is anterior, one cannot rely on the posterior scalene muscle for counting ribs. The first rib is identified by palpating the tubercle. If one is unsure of the first rib, one can reach over the superior border and identify the thoracic outlet because there are no intercostals above the first rib.

The intercostal muscles along the appropriate space are divided as in a posterolateral thoracotomy. The intercostal incision is carried well beyond the limits of the skin incision almost to the level of the vertebral bodies. The incision in the intercostal space is kept away from the overlying chest wall muscles and is facilitated by progressive opening of the rib spreader, which provides countertraction. A pediatric Finochietto-type rib spreader is used to separate the ribs, and a Balfour is placed perpendicular to the rib spreader to retract the skin and subcutaneous tissues. The skin is quite pliable, and thus excellent exposure can be achieved through this relatively small skin incision because the intercostal incision essentially rivals or even exceeds that made with a posterolateral incision. At the completion of the procedure, a single chest tube is placed, pericostal sutures are placed to reapproximate the ribs, the insertions of the serratus anterior muscle are sewn to the pectoralis minor muscle anteriorly, and the rest of the closure proceeds as usual.

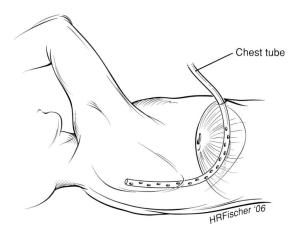

Figure 3-2. A single chest tube is modified with additional drainage holes and its course altered so that it functions as both basilar and apical drains.

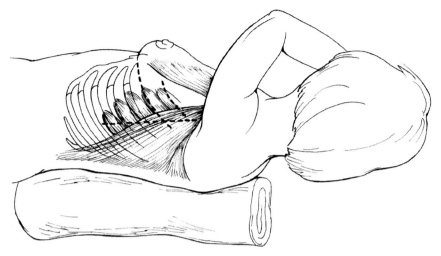

Figure 3-3. Axillary thoracotomy incisions: the vertical and oblique approaches are demonstrated.

Anterior Thoracotomy

With recent trends toward minimally invasive cardiac surgery, the anterior thoracotomy has regained popularity. Otherwise, it remains the incision of choice for open-lung biopsy and emergent thoracotomy. Open-lung biopsy, in contrast to a video procedure, may be the approach of choice in hypoxic, ventilated patients who require lung biopsy. These patients may not tolerate single-lung ventilation, and this procedure can be performed while both lungs are being ventilated by a single-lumen endotracheal tube.

The patient is positioned with a roll under the operative side. The ipsilateral arm is placed over the patient on an arm rest or alongside on a support. An incision is made from the anterior axillary line curving under the breast toward the sternum. The fourth or fifth intercostal space is entered. For an open-lung biopsy, we make a fairly limited incision, approximately 3 cm in size. For an emergency thoracotomy, the incision is obviously much larger and can be extended across the sternum to increase exposure as needed. (Fig. 3-4).

Median Sternotomy

The median sternotomy is mostly commonly used for cardiac surgical procedures but can be a useful tool in general thoracic surgery operations requiring access to both pleural spaces or resection of mediastinal disease.

The patient is placed supine with one or both arms tucked. A roll is placed behind the shoulders to extend the neck and expose the

sternal notch. The midline of the sternum is marked, and a knife divides the skin (Fig. 3-5). The subcutaneous layers are divided though the decussating fibers of the pectoralis major muscle, and the midline of the sternum is carefully marked with cautery. Palpating the intercostal spaces along the sternum allows one to accurately identify the midline. The interclavicular ligament is divided, and the retrosternal space is bluntly dissected. The xiphoid tip is dissected, and again the space posterior to this is developed. A reciprocating saw is used to divide the sternum. The bleeding periosteal edges are carefully cauterized. An appropriate sternal retractor is used to gradually spread the two sternal edges. Brachial plexus injuries may occur when the retractor is opened too quickly or widely.

After the procedure, one or two chest tubes are placed. Sternal wires are used to reapproximate the sternum. We place two in the manubrium and four around the sternal edges. The pectoralis fascia is closed over the

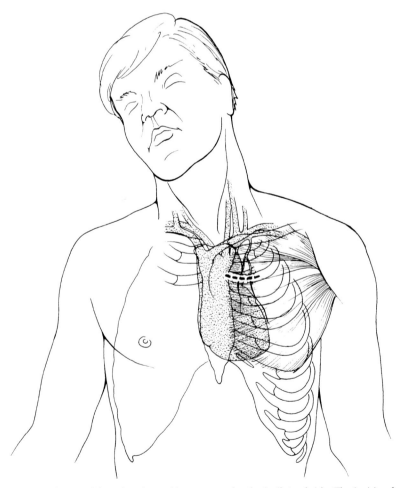

Figure 3-4. Patient positioned supine, with a support for the ipsilateral side. The incision for an anterior thoracotomy is illustrated. Depending on the purpose for this incision, the patient's position and the length of the incision can be modified.

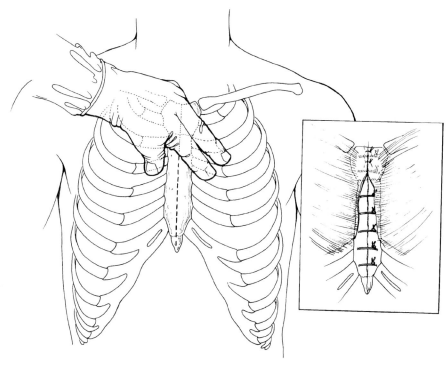

Figure 3-5. For the median sternotomy the patient is positioned supine and a roll is placed under the shoulders to optimize exposure of the sternal notch.

sternum, and the remainder of the wound is closed in layers. One should thoroughly irrigate the wound and carefully obliterate any potential spaces at the time of closure to attenuate the possibility of infection.

Bilateral Thoracosternotomy (Clamshell)

The bilateral thoracosternotomy had previously been the incision of choice for bilateral lung transplantation. Due to complications from poor healing of the transverse sternal division, most centers have abandoned this technique in transplant patients. However, it remains a very useful approach when wide access to both pleural spaces is required, as in selected patients with bilateral pulmonary metastases or those with large tumors of the anterior mediastinum, although admittedly it is used sparingly.

A transverse skin incision is made extending from one anterior axillary line along the inframammary crease to the other anterior axillary line (Fig. 3-6). The subcutaneous tissues are divided, and the fourth or fifth intercostal space is identified. The intercostal muscles along this space are divided, and the mammary vessels are identified and ligated prior to dividing the sternum. The

Lebsche knife is used to divide the sternum transversely. Rib spreaders usually are placed on both sides to allow for maximal exposure. After the procedure, paracostal sutures are placed and the sternum is reapproximated with wire.

Thoracosternotomy (Hemiclamshell)

The thoracosternotomy is a useful approach for large central pulmonary lesions and other special situations. Such tumors can interfere with one's access to the hilum, making the dissection and proximal control of the pulmonary artery difficult. With the thoracosternotomy, one can approach the dissection anteriorly and dissect the hilar vessels from within the pericardium without being blocked by a large tumor as occurs when trying to approach the hilum from a posterior approach. In addition, the brachiocephalic vessels are much more readily seen, exposed, and controlled through this anterior approach. This incision is extremely versatile, and we do not hesitate to use it for these special situations.

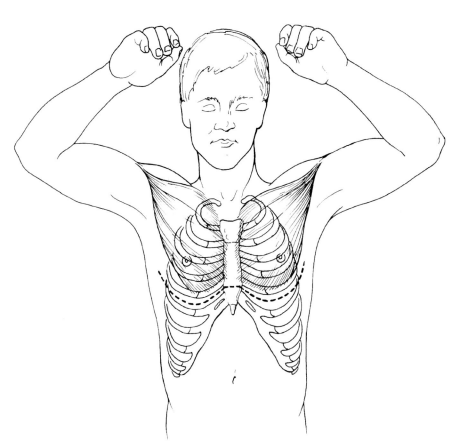

Figure 3-6. The clamshell incision is illustrated coursing along the inframammary creases and across the sternum.

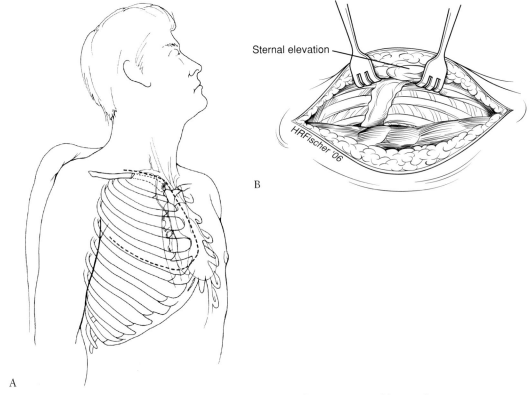

Sternal elevation

HRFischer '06

B

A

Figure 3-7. **(A)** The hemiclamshell incision incorporates the sternotomy with extension to a thoracotomy to increase the intrathoracic exposure. This incision can also be extended along the sternocleidomastoid when exposure of the brachiocephalic vessels is required. **(B)** A hemisternal retractor is used to elevate the sternum and increase the intrathoracic exposure.

The patient is positioned supine or with a small support elevating the ipsilateral chest. Both arms may be tucked, or the arm may be extended if additional exposure of the lateral chest is needed. The initial skin incision is an inframammary incision and opening of the fourth intercostal space to assess resectability and ensure that there is no diffuse pleural spread or other reason why the entire incision should not be made. The skin incision is then extended over to the sternum and up toward the sternal notch and then for a short distance along the anterior border of the ipsilateral sternocleidomastoid muscle (Fig. 3-7A). The subcutaneous tissues are divided through the decussating fibers of the pectoral muscles and then along the fourth intercostal space. Before dividing the sternum, the intercostal muscles in the fourth space are divided up to the mammary vessels. These are dissected, doubly ligated, and divided in advance. The sternal saw is used to perform a partial sternotomy curved out to the fourth interspace. A hemisternal retractor of the type used for harvesting the internal mammary artery is then placed and used to elevate the chest wall (Fig. 3-7B). One

should avoid excessive tension on the chest wall to prevent fracture along the costal margin.

Anterior Cervicothoracic Approach (Modified Thoracosternotomy)

For pathology at the level of the thoracic outlet or apex of the chest, a modified thoracosternotomy is used. This particular incision is used most commonly for apical intrathoracic pathology that may or may not involve resection of the apical chest wall.

A double-lumen tube is used. The patient is placed supine, with a soft support under the shoulders. The head is turned away from the side of pathology. An L-shaped skin incision is made along the anterior border of the ipsilateral sternocleidomastoid muscle to the sternal notch and then curving out below the clavicle going toward the deltopectoral groove (Fig. 3-8). Depending on the pathology, either the manubrium is divided and the cut carried out at the first or second intercostal space, or a portion

of the clavicle is either divided or excised (see later discussion). The sternal head of the sternocleidomastoid is reflected, and the interclavicular ligament is divided. The retrosternal space is freed with blunt dissection. The intercostal muscles are divided in either the first or second intercostal space, whichever is more suitable for the pathology. The mammary vessels are doubly ligated and divided. When working through the first intercostal space, we tend to address the mammary vessels after dividing the manubrium. This improves exposure of the vessels as they come through the outlet, avoiding inadvertent injury to the phrenic nerve. The Lebsche knife is used to divide the manubrium in an L-shaped fashion from the midline down to the appropriate intercostal space. A hemisternal retractor is used to elevate the chest wall and provide exposure.

To close this incision, the divided interspace is reapproximated with paracostal sutures and the manubrium is reapproximated with No. 5 stainless steel wires. The remainder of the wound is closed by reapproximating the muscle and fascia in the usual fashion.

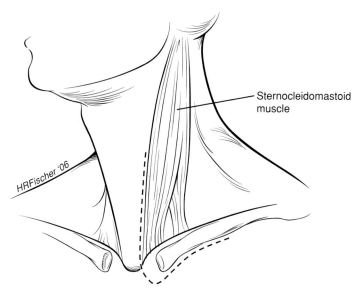

Figure 3-8. The L-shaped incision for a cervicothoracic approach. The incision begins along the border of the sternocleidomastoid muscle, proceeds to the sternal notch, and then curves out along the infraclavicular groove.

Transclavicular Approach (Modified Dartevelle)

If the pathology requires resection of apical chest wall and exposure of the brachiocephalic vessels and brachial plexus, we find this approach optimal. Again, an L-shaped skin incision is used and the border of the sternocleidomastoid is developed. The medial attachments of this muscle to the head of the clavicle and sternum are divided. The oscillating saw is used to divide the clavicle in an oblique fashion (Fig. 3-9), and a hemisternal retractor is used to elevate the clavicle and expose the supraclavicular fossa. Dividing the clavicle or excising the medial portion of the clavicle allows for easy access to the first rib, making resection of this rib considerably easier. Following ex-

amination of the subclavian fat pad and the vessels, the appropriate intercostal space below the level of the lesion, as identified on computed tomography or plain film, is entered. The extent of disease is evaluated, and the chest wall may be divided in the appropriate locations as identified by palpating the lesion. After all of the chest wall and intercostal attachments have been completely divided, the chest wall bloc with the attached underlying pulmonary parenchyma is dropped into the thorax though the defect. The pulmonary parenchymal resection may be completed without difficulty through this defect. On completion of the procedure, a chest tube is placed, and the chest wall is reconstructed with either Marlex mesh alone or with methyl methacrylate, depending on the size and location of the defect. Anterior defects should routinely be reconstructed with a rigid prosthesis to prevent a

"flail-like" physiology especially in the patient with borderline pulmonary function. The clavicle is reapproximated with two No. 5 sternal wires. The soft tissues are closed in layers. The patient's arm is maintained in a sling for 6 weeks.

Thoracoabdominal Incision

The thoracoabdominal incision provides wide exposure of the lower chest, retroperitoneum, and upper abdomen, especially the hiatus. It is common approach for the management of abdominal aortic aneurysms, occasional distal esophageal tumors, and anterior approach to the lower thoracic and lumbar spine.

The exact location of the skin incision varies in relation to the pathology. The chest portion of the incision may be over the sixth, seventh, or eighth intercostal space, and the abdominal portion may be either midline or paramedian in location (Fig. 3-10). The patient is positioned supine, usually with a small support extending from the hip to chest of the ipsilateral side. The arm can be supported at the patient's side, extended out at 90 degrees or suspended across the chest. The skin incision is made extending from the anterior axillary line, across the costal arch onto the abdomen. The costal arch and the intercostals are divided. The diaphragm can be divided radially from the chest wall to the hiatus or circumferentially leaving 3 cm to 4 cm along the chest wall for later reapproximation. One must be careful to avoid injury to the phrenic nerve. A rib spreader is placed to separate the ribs, or a self-retaining type of retractor that attaches to the operating table may be used to provide exposure in both the chest and abdomen.

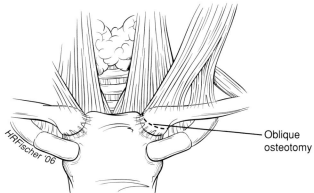

Figure 3-9. The oblique osteotomy through the head of the clavicle to allow for later reapproximation.

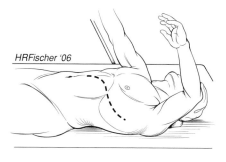

Figure 3-10. The thoracoabdominal incision courses over the costal margin down onto the abdomen in a paramedian or median location depending on the objectives of the procedure.

On completion of the procedure, a chest tube is placed. The diaphragm is closed with large nonabsorbable, interrupted sutures. We routinely excise the edges of the costal arch to prevent postoperative pain with rubbing reapproximation. Paracostal sutures are used to reapproximate the ribs, and the abdomen is closed in layers, again with large nonabsorbable sutures for the fascia.

SUGGESTED READING

Bains MS, Ginsberg RJ, Jones WG, et al. The clamshell incision: An improved approach to bilateral pulmonary and mediastinal tumor. Ann Thorac Surg 1994;58:30.

Fry WA. Thoracic incisions. Chest Surg Clin North Am 1995;5:177.

Heitmiller RF. Thoracic incisions. Ann Thorac Surg 1988;46:601.

Hennington MH, Ulicny Jr KS, Detterbeck FC. Vertical muscle-sparing thoracotomy. Ann Thorac Surg. 1994;57:759.

Korst RJ, Burt ME. Cervicothoracic tumors: Results of resection by the "hemi-clamshell" approach. J Thorac Cardiovasc Surg 1998;115: 286.

Nesbitt JC, Wind GG. Thoracic Surgical Oncology: Exposures and Techniques. Philadelphia: Lippincott Williams & Wilkins, 2003, Chapter 1.

Massimiano P, Ponn RB, Toole AL. Transaxillary thoracotomy revisited. Ann Thorac Surg 1988; 45:559.

EDITOR'S COMMENTS

Dr. Marshall has nicely summarized the basic, and not so basic, thoracic incisions. Most chest procedures may be accomplished through the standard posterolateral incision, but it is particularly important for the thoracic surgeon to be familiar with some of the nonstandard incisions for certain applications. With the advent of minimally invasive approaches to thoracic pathology it is thought by a number of authors that smaller incisions are associated with less postoperative pain, yet this assumption has never been convincingly proven. The so-called "utility" incision used for a VATS lobectomy may be the same size as the standard vertical axillary muscle-sparing incision, but it is the absence of rib spreading that may be the source of less postoperative pain in those patients who experience less pain. It has

been our experience, and that of many others, that despite the small incisions used in standard thoracoscopic procedures, patients do have significant postoperative pain simply because a hole has been made through the intercostal muscles. Limiting the degree of rib spreading for any open procedure to only that amount that is really needed for visualization will go a long way toward attenuating postoperative pain, that and the use of epidural analgesia or some other form of "local" pain control such as an extrapleural catheter for the administration of a local anesthetic.

Our routine incision of choice is the vertical axillary muscle-sparing incision that requires entry through the fourth intercostal space as opposed to the fifth interspace used for the standard posterolateral incision. The vertical axillary incision is an "anterior" incision, and thus opening the fifth space would put us down at the level of the hemidiaphragm. The intercostal incision is opened well beyond the confines of the skin incision taking care to preserve the overlying serratus anterior and latissimus dorsi muscles. Placing the rib spreader and gradually opening it as the intercostal incision is made provides needed countertraction to facilitate the completion of this incision. The only time this incision is absolutely contraindicated is when there is an expectation of the need for a chest wall resection. Women with large, pendulous breasts present a relative contraindication because the breast pulling on the healing incision has been associated with dehiscence and hypertrophic scar formation.

The cervicothoracic approach to the apex of the chest is the preferred one for dealing with apical pathology whether parenchymal or extraparenchymal such as apical nerve sheath tumors. When chest wall resection is not contemplated, the approach through the manubrium is ideal in that it preserves complete mobility of the ipsilateral upper extremity. If a chest wall resection is contemplated, then either the medial portion of the clavicle should be excised or an oblique osteotomy made in the head of the clavicle so as to allow unhindered access to the entire first rib. Once the clavicle is out of the way the first rib is readily approached and resected with excellent visualization and exposure so as to keep safe the subclavian vessels and brachial plexus. In my opinion this approach also is the preferred one for apical

lung, so-called Pancoast, tumors. I feel that the better exposure of the subclavian vessels and the brachial plexus adds a measure of safety to this approach not found with the standard extended posterolateral approach. It has been my impression that patients have less pain and functional disability with this approach as opposed to a large incision that extends up to the C7 vertebral body posteriorly and requires division of all chest wall musculature so that the scapula can be elevated off the chest wall. There is no question that resection of the medial clavicle results in some dysfunction of ipsilateral upper extremity range of motion, thus the modification as originally proposed by Dr. Marshall of the oblique clavicular osteotomy. The osteotomy should be closed with wires because plating has been associated with dehiscence of the closure. There are standard orthopedic plates made for clavicular fractures that likely would provide ideal fixation, but the application of these devices is somewhat complex and requires special expertise.

The thoracoabdominal incision has proven extremely useful in our practice for approaching the diaphragmatic hiatus in the setting of previous operations in this region. For instance, the failed fundoplication renders the approach to the hiatus particularly difficult through a midline incision alone. Being able to approach the esophagus from above, especially if the stomach has herniated through the chest, makes the thoracoabdominal approach ideal. I favor positioning the patient in full lateral decubitus for this incision and starting the skin incision lateral to the rectus muscle. The incision crosses the costal arch where the interspace is "straight," usually the seventh interspace. The diaphragm is taken down circumferentially leaving lateral attachments so as to facilitate closure. The edges of the diaphragm are marked to simplify the closure. Accurate closure of the intercostal space is critical to avoid overlap of the costal edges, a situation that patients find extremely uncomfortable. This incision should be the approach of choice to the re-do hiatus.

Surgeons should use an incision with which they are comfortable that provides the best exposure to the pathology at hand. Some of the "nonstandard" incisions should be mastered because these can simplify some very complex procedures.

L.R.K.

4

Right-Sided Pulmonary Resections

Larry R. Kaiser

General Introduction to Pulmonary Resections

Pulmonary resection is the operation that defines the thoracic surgeon. The specialty of thoracic surgery is relatively new, dating back less than 50 years, but it has really been defined during the last 30 years. Because of problems relating to positive-pressure ventilation in the patient with an open chest, the development of anatomic pulmonary resection moved slowly. The initial procedure, performed for a carcinoma of the lung, was a pneumonectomy carried out by mass ligation of the pulmonary hilum with subsequent suturing of individual hilar structures. During the first four decades of the twentieth century carcinoma of the lung was an uncommon disease, and most pulmonary resections were performed for inflammatory conditions or tuberculosis. Most lung cancers were treated by total removal of the lung when they were deemed operable, and this clearly was the operation thought to be required. Lesser resections were reserved for benign disease, mostly infectious problems. It took a number of years before surgeons recognized that a resection of less than an entire lung, though a more difficult operation, provided an acceptable alternative for the treatment for lung cancer, not unlike the recognition that less than a radical mastectomy could be done for breast cancer with comparable survival rates.

Recognizing that surgical excision is the optimal treatment for otherwise operable lung cancer, it is important that the appropriate procedure be performed. Lobectomy remains the definitive resection because it is an anatomic resection that assures removal of the regional lymph nodes that course along the lobar bronchus and thus provides

the best staging information and local control. Doing less than a lobectomy must be considered a compromise, although often it is tempting to consider a nonanatomic wedge excision for small primary tumors. Not only does a wedge excision not include the lobar bronchus, precluding evaluation of lobar lymph nodes, but also usually it provides only a minimal parenchymal margin and thus is accompanied by a significant incidence of local recurrence. The Lung Cancer Study Group (LCSG) addressed the question of lobectomy versus limited resection for T1N0 lesions (tumor <3 cm, negative lymph nodes) in a prospective, randomized trial. The initial analysis of the data demonstrated an increased incidence of local recurrence in the limited-resection group (>30% incidence) but failed to demonstrate a decrease in survival. The final analysis, however, revealed superior survival for patients in the lobectomy group. A number of other studies looked retrospectively at patients undergoing limited resection, which includes anatomic segmental resection, and demonstrated long-term survivors but the LCSG study stands as the only large randomized trial.

There are patients in whom lobectomy is not feasible and a lesser resection offers the best alternative, though admittedly a compromise. Patients in this category are those with borderline pulmonary function or those who have had previous pulmonary resections. Whenever possible the lesser resection should be an anatomic segmental resection, which by definition involves taking the appropriate segmental artery and vein as well as the segmental bronchus with its accompanying lymph nodes. Wedge resection, a nonanatomic form of resection in which the bronchovascular structures are not isolated and taken separately along with

regional lymph nodes, is another alternative, although it is not ideal for patients with primary lung cancers. With the advent of videothoracoscopic techniques and the simplicity of wedge resection via this approach, for a time there was renewed interest in utilizing this technique for T1N0 lung cancers. The American College of Surgeons Oncology Group (ACOSOG) has an ongoing study looking at limited resection combined with local implantation of radioactive seeds to assess whether there is a decreased incidence of local recurrence and whether this translates into a survival benefit. As it currently stands based on the LCSG data, wedge excision mostly should be avoided, and patients who are found to have a primary lung cancer should be offered the best possible procedure, which is, to the best of present knowledge, a lobectomy. Wedge resection, at best, is a compromise, and patients who otherwise can tolerate an anatomic resection are not well served by having a lesser procedure. This has become even more important as we are identifying more early-stage, small lung cancers picked up in patients who undergo screening spiral computed tomographic (CT) scans. These patients, despite having a small nodule, should be offered the procedure, lobectomy, that offers the best chance for cure based on present knowledge.

Prior to operation a decision must be made regarding which, if any, other studies should be carried out. The type and extent of the staging evaluation depend on a number of clinical factors. At minimum patients should have a recent chest radiograph and CT scan of the chest. Most, if not all, should have a recent set of pulmonary function studies including diffusion capacity. Positron emission tomographic (PET) scanning has become standard for the evaluation of a solitary pulmonary nodule, and there is convincing evidence of its usefulness in staging the mediastinum as well. The fluorinated glucose used for the PET scan is trapped preferentially in malignant cells as opposed to normal cells and thus show up as hot. Numerous studies have looked at the sensitivity and specificity of PET for both pulmonary nodules and mediastinal lymph nodes. A nodule that shows up positive on PET has a high (approaching 90%) likelihood of being malignant. A negative PET scan does not rule out malignancy because bronchioloalveolar carcinoma and carcinoid tumors do not readily take up the fluorinated glucose and thus have a significantly higher incidence of false-negative results. A solitary nodule that is negative on PET needs to be followed with serial CT scans and resected if growth is detected. In assessing mediastinal lymph nodes PET has a specificity of >90%, but the sensitivity is somewhat lower and approximates 80%. A CT scan without mediastinal lymph nodes >1.5 cm in size and a negative PET scan obviates the need for further mediastinal staging, whereas a PET-positive lymph node mandates the need for mediastinoscopy or needle aspiration of the suspicious node.

The decision to search for disseminated disease is a difficult one, and precise criteria for defining when an extent-of-disease work-up should be performed do not exist. A reasonable approach is to err on the side of performing a complete extent-of-disease evaluation if there is any reason at all to do so. Reasons would include any organ-specific or nonspecific signs or symptoms. Nonspecific signs include weight loss, easy fatigability, and anemia, and organ-specific signs includes bone pain, elevated liver enzymes, and localizing neurologic findings. If any of these findings is present, a complete staging evaluation should be obtained, not just the study pointed to by the organ-specific complaint. A PET scan obviates the need for a separate radionuclide bone scan, but magnetic resonance imaging (MRI) or (less likely) a CT scan of the brain is required for a complete extent-of-disease evaluation. Any patient with a past history of malignancy should have a search for distant disease, as should the patient who is at a higher risk for operation, such as an individual with multiple medical problems or borderline pulmonary function. In addition, any patient with locally advanced disease in whom the indications for operation are being extended (i.e., N2 disease) or the nonsmoker with a lung mass should have distant disease ruled out. The aim is to avoid subjecting a patient to the risk of an operation who then proceeds to manifest disseminated

disease within 1 year of operation, a finding that ideally should have been identified preoperatively.

An important aspect of the preoperative evaluation of a patient with lung cancer is the assessment of pulmonary function. Not all patients undergoing thoracotomy require pulmonary function testing, but the majority of patients with lung cancer also have some element of underlying lung disease as a result of the same risk factor that is associated with their cancer: cigarette smoking. Assessment of pulmonary function serves to identify both those patients at a significantly increased likelihood of postoperative morbidity and those patients who stand to benefit from preoperative manipulations designed to attenuate those risks. There is no single best test to evaluate pulmonary function in a patient who is slated to undergo pulmonary resection. Furthermore, there are no absolute values that contraindicate resection, although by using a combination of studies, it is at least possible to make a judgment as to which patients are at an increased risk for postoperative morbidity or mortality. Preoperative spirometry to measure flows and volumes should be performed. Important measurements include forced expiratory volume in 1 second (FEV$_1$), maximal voluntary ventilation (MVV), diffusing capacity, FEV$_1$/forced vital capacity (FVC) ratio, and the ratio of the residual volume (RV) to total lung capacity (TLC). An FEV$_1$ of <40% of predicted has been associated with increased postoperative morbidity and mortality. A reduced diffusing capacity has also been associated with postoperative morbidity. Any assessment of postoperative morbidity and mortality has to take into account the extent of the proposed resection. Often this is difficult to determine, and the experience of the surgeon is closely related to the likelihood of pneumonectomy. The surgeon operating on patients with compromised lung function should be experienced in the performance of segmental resections, sleeve resections, and nonanatomic resections, all techniques of lung preservation. Techniques of video-assisted thoracic surgery may also be of use in patients with limited pulmonary reserve who require pulmonary resection. There are a number of measures that can be instituted that are designed to attenuate the postoperative risk in these patients with compromised lung function. (Table 4-1) The sobering truth, however, is that it often comes down to a judgment on the part of the surgeon based on both objective and subjective factors that may be most important. There are some patients who just are not

Table 4-1   Measures to Decrease Postoperative Morbidity and Mortality of Patients Undergoing Thoracotomy for Lung Cancer

Preoperative
  Cessation of smoking
  Optimization of nutrition (ideal body weight ± 10%)
  Supervised plumonary rehabilitation with goals
  Appropriate inhalation bronchodilator therapy
  Control of secretions (when appropriate)
  Teaching techniques of using incentive spirometer, coughing, deep-breathing
Intraoperative
  Muscle-sparing incision, minimal rib spreading
  Video-assisted approach (when appropriate)
  Parenchyma-conserving operation (segmental resection, sleeve resection, wedge)
  Optimal bronchodilation
  Limited duration of anesthesia
  Control of secretions (bronchoscopy at conclusion of procedure)
  Conservative fluid management
  Avoidance of air leaks
Postoperative
  Thoracic epidural analgesia
  Proper use of incentive spirometry
  Early ambulation
  Aggressive secretion management (nasotracheal suctioning, bronchoscopy, minitracheostomy [infrequent])
  Experienced nursing staff

candidates for pulmonary resection for a variety of reasons that sometimes may be difficult to articulate.

Recent experience with lung volume reduction surgery in patients with severe end-stage emphysema has changed our thinking regarding operation for lung cancer in patients with compromised lung function. Nutritional assessment and therapy and a supervised program of pulmonary rehabilitation may further optimize borderline patients for pulmonary resection. Our tendency is to be quite aggressive in considering patients with pulmonary malignancies for resection. Rarely is a patient turned down for resection solely on the basis of his or her pulmonary function. At times the resections have to be somewhat creative, and there are a number of intraoperative factors that may contribute to a reduction in postoperative problems (Table 4-1). Patients with borderline lung function have to be strongly motivated toward resection. These patients are not the ones to be talked into an operation even if their other treatment options are limited; they really have to want it. The major morbidity and potential mortality in these patients occur in the early postoperative period, but one must also keep in mind the long-term sequelae of the resection of lung parenchyma in these individuals. Paradoxically there may be some improvement in lung function after pulmonary resection in these patients especially if the lung parenchyma removed receives a minimal amount of the pulmonary perfusion. A preoperative quantitative ventilation-perfusion lung scan is useful in assessing the significance of the loss of lung parenchyma. An estimate of the predicted postoperative FEV_1 may be obtained by subtracting the percentage removed by the proposed resection based on the percentage of perfusion received by that area of lung parenchyma. A residual FEV_1 of <800 ml has been associated with an increased risk of postoperative morbidity and mortality, but this is entirely dependent on what percentage of the predicted FEV_1 the 800 ml represents. For instance, in a 50-kg female and FEV_1 of 800 ml may represent a postresection FEV_1 of 60% of predicted or more. An algorithm for the preoperative assessment of risk in patients with lung cancer is presented in Fig. 4-1.

In addition to pulmonary function studies, an assessment of exercise capability for the patient with compromised lung function may be appropriate in some circumstances. This assessment may range from something as simple as having the patient climb one or two flights of stairs while monitoring oxygen saturation and pulse rate to formal exercise testing and calculation of maximal oxygen consumption (VO_2 max). One can be reasonably certain that a patient who can walk up two flights of stairs can tolerate a lobectomy. For truly borderline patients measurement of VO_2 max may be the deciding test.

A value of <15 ml/kg/min has been associated with significantly increased postoperative morbidity and mortality. Patients in this category should be scrutinized closely before one decides to proceed with resection. It is this type of patient who may do better with a limited resection such as a video-assisted wedge excision, a compromise to be sure, if the lesion is small and peripheral. It is highly unlikely that a patient with pulmonary compromise so marked could tolerate a pneumonectomy. Other parameters suggesting high risk include a pCO_2 of >45 torr and elevated pulmonary artery pressures.

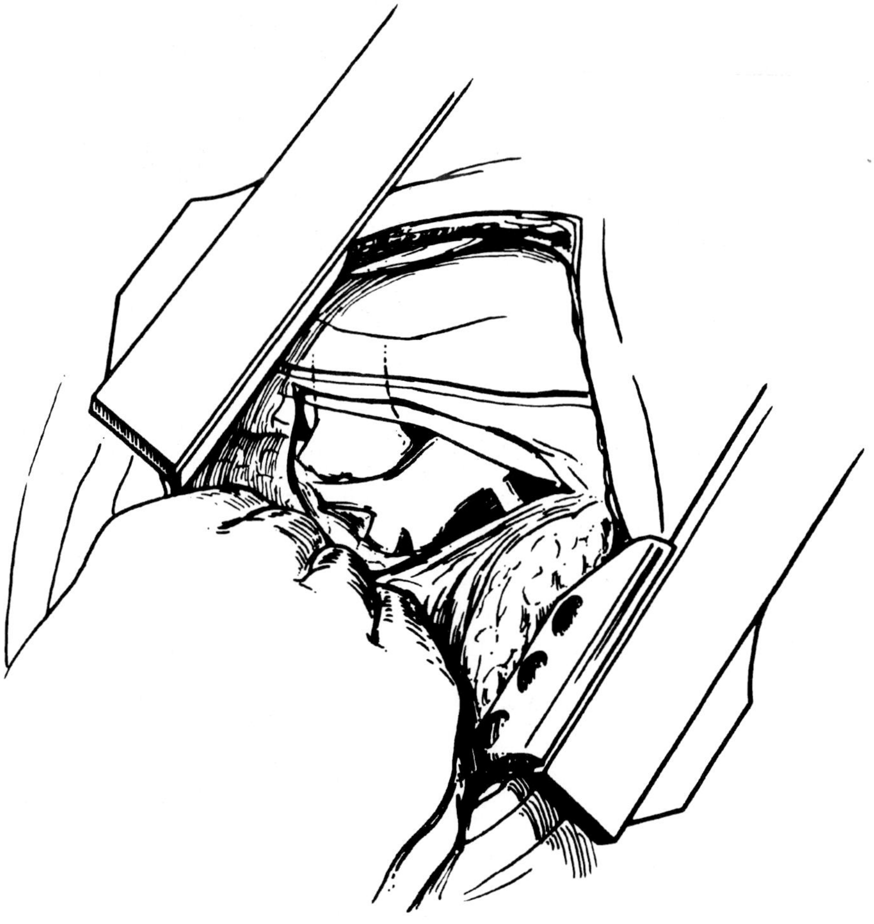

Some patients may undergo invasive staging prior to pulmonary resection. The decision to perform mediastinoscopy may be based on CT scan findings of enlarged mediastinal lymph nodes and the results of the PET scan. The criteria for defining "enlarged" vary, and the sensitivity and specificity of the technique vary depending on the size that is set. We perform mediastinoscopy when lymph nodes >1.5 cm in size are seen on the CT scan. Others perform mediastinoscopy on all patients prior to pulmonary resection recognizing that the majority of procedures will reveal only nodes without evidence of metastatic disease. Mediastinal lymph nodes that light up on PET scan mandate the need for mediastinoscopy unless there is such bulky adenopathy seen on CT scan that tissue confirmation would be redundant.

Whether mediastinoscopy is used selectively or routinely, the key point is accurate staging of the mediastinum in the patient with lung cancer. This mandates at a minimum mediastinal lymph node staging at thoracotomy or, preferably, complete lymph node dissection. The problem with lymph node staging alone is the issue of how lymph nodes are chosen to be sampled, a problem not present when a complete lymph node dissection is carried out. Mere palpation of a node or an assessment of nodal size will miss lymph nodes harboring intranodal or microscopic disease. It is not clear what percentage of nodal disease is missed with a staging procedure because of the variability in the selection of nodes to be sampled and the lack of a study in which nodes are first sampled followed by a complete lymph node dissection. From our experience 10% to 20% of resections where mediastinal lymph node disease is not suspected result in positive lymph nodes being identified by the pathologist. An operation without lymph node staging information must be considered incomplete. Accurate staging allows

Figure 4-1.   View of the right hilum as seen from the right side of the table. The hilar pleura has been incised, and the right main pulmonary artery and superior pulmonary vein are well seen. Note the middle lobe vein draining into the superior pulmonary vein. This vein must be preserved when performing a right upper lobectomy. The continuation of the artery distal to the apical-anterior trunk passes posterior to the superior pulmonary vein.

the surgeon to discuss prognosis realistically with the patient and allows the patient the opportunity to either participate in a trial of postoperative adjuvant therapy or be evaluated for treatment outside of a protocol setting. With three recent prospective, randomized clinical trials demonstrating improved survival of patients with completely resected N1 or N2 disease treated with postoperative adjuvant chemotherapy, the quality and completeness of the intraoperative staging has become even more important.

Despite the bias on the part of most physicians that postoperative radiation therapy is of value in resected patients who are found to have either N1 or N2 disease, there are no prospective data that demonstrate a survival advantage in patients so treated. One prospective, randomized trial of postoperative radiation therapy versus no further treatment for resected patients with squamous cell carcinoma demonstrated a significant reduction in local recurrence but absolutely no difference in survival. A randomized trial conducted by the collaborative efforts of the national cooperative cancer groups compared postoperative chemotherapy (cis-platinum, VP-16) and radiation therapy with radiation therapy alone. This trial required that patients either have mediastinoscopy performed or have a completely negative CT scan in addition to mandating what lymph nodes had to be sampled at the time of thoracotomy. The results of this trial showed no advantage for the combined radiation therapy and chemotherapy arm over radiation therapy alone and no significant difference when compared to historical controls. Interestingly, there did appear to be a survival advantage in the subgroup of patients who had mediastinal lymph node dissection as opposed to lymph node sampling only.

Long-term survival after pulmonary resection depends both on characteristics of the primary tumor (T stage) and presence or absence of lymph node disease (N stage). Table 4-2 summarizes survival data. Any analysis of survival is greatly dependent on how thoroughly the lymph nodes were staged, as discussed previously. These data, accumulated from studies performed by the Lung Cancer Study Group, are particularly enlightening because of the stringent requirement for nodal staging that was mandated for entering patients into these studies. Thus, when a patient was staged as N1 we can be assured that was an accurate staging evaluation because the mediastinal lymph nodes would have been sampled and found to be free of tumor.

Table 4-2 Five-Year Postoperative Survival by TNM Groups

Cancer Stage	Percentage Surviving with Squamous Cell Carcinoma	Percentage Surviving with Adeno-carcinoma
Stage I		
T1N0	83	69
T2N0	64	57
Stage II		
T1N1	75	52
T2N1	53	25
Stage IIIa		
T1–2N2	46	35
T3N0	37	21

Source: Data from Lung Cancer Study Group studies.

Introduction to Right-Sided Resections

There are a number of significant anatomic features relating to right-sided pulmonary resections that are unique to the right chest. The right main pulmonary artery is relatively long and courses posterior to the superior vena cava and across the carina. At times, this extra length of the artery is an advantage for some proximal lesions that in a similar location on the left side would not be resectable because of the short length of the left main pulmonary artery relative to the bifurcation. There has to be enough length of artery distal to the bifurcation to be able to place a clamp and divide and suture the artery so that the lesion can be removed. The distance between the carina and the origin of the right upper lobe bronchus usually is <2 cm, and the carina is readily mobilized from the right side. Access to the proximal left mainstem bronchus is significantly easier from the right side compared to the left side, where the aortic arch limits access to both the origin of the left main bronchus and the carina. Mobilization of the carina is not possible from the left chest, and even visualization of the carina from the left is difficult. Carinal resections, when indicated, are performed through a right thoracotomy or, at times, through a median sternotomy.

The superior mediastinum, the space accessed by the mediastinoscope, is well visualized from the right side. The area bounded by the azygous vein (inferior), the trachea (posterior), the subclavian vein (superior), and the superior vena cave (anterior) delineates this compartment, whose lymph node–bearing contents may be removed en bloc from the right side. No such access exists on the left side, where the left paratracheal nodes are relatively inaccessible because of the location of the aortic arch. As mentioned, with the access afforded to the carina from the right side it follows that the subcarinal space is readily dissected for lymph node removal.

On the right side the azygous vein is an important anatomic landmark. The vein courses from posterior to anterior across the main stem bronchus to drain into the superior vena cava. Just inferior to where it crosses the main bronchus is the origin of the upper lobe bronchus, a key anatomic feature. Rarely is it necessary to divide the azygous vein, but it may be taken with impunity if it is involved by tumor or limits access to the lymph node–bearing area.

In assessing resections from the right side, the upper lobectomy probably is the most straightforward resection, although the location of the posterior segmental arterial branch may, at times, be problematic. Right lower lobectomy is complicated by the location of the middle lobe artery and bronchus, and middle lobectomy is considered difficult, erroneously I might add, by some because of the minor fissure.

Surgical Technique

Right Upper Lobectomy

Right upper lobectomy is the prototypical pulmonary resection and is a good starting point for the trainee just starting out in pulmonary surgery. The long right main pulmonary artery with the apical-anterior branch and the discrete take-off of the upper lobe bronchus make this an ideal resection. The so-called "truncus anterior," the apical-anterior branch of the pulmonary artery, also facilitates segmental resections of the right upper lobe. Once this branch is divided the segmental bronchi are easily visualized.

A left endobronchial double-lumen tube is placed to allow for single-lung ventilation so that the right lung is collapsed for the lobar resection.

With the patient positioned on the left side (left lateral decubitus position) the chest is entered through either a standard posterolateral thoracotomy incision or one of the muscle-sparing incisions. The chest is accessed through the fifth intercostal space for the posterolateral incision or the fourth intercostal space for the more anterior muscle-sparing incision. The hilum and mediastinum are palpated to assess extent of involvement and determine resectability.

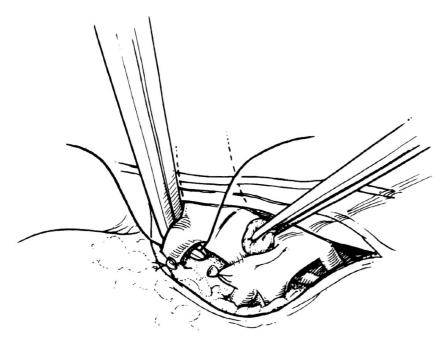

Figure 4-2.   At times the apical venous branch obscures the origin of the apical-anterior arterial trunk and must be divided prior to division of the arterial branch. Here the venous branch has been divided in preparation for division of the apical-anterior trunk. The right angle is around the arterial branch. The artery is divided between carefully placed 0 silk ligatures.

The lung is retracted posteriorly with the surgeon's left hand, and the hilar pleura anteriorly and superiorly is incised. The superior pulmonary vein is identified and dissected distally toward the lung parenchyma and proximally to the pericardial reflection. The vein is encircled with a finger once the appropriate plane of dissection is entered. Care must be taken to avoid injury to the pulmonary artery, which lies directly posterior to the superior pulmonary vein (Fig. 4-1). The middle lobe venous branch, which usually drains to the superior pulmonary vein, is identified and preserved. This vein almost always is a branch of the superior pulmonary vein but occasionally may be found entering the inferior pulmonary vein. Infrequently aberrant venous drainage on the right side, usually a small venous branch emptying directly into the vena cava, may be encountered. Lying just superior and posterior to the vein is the right main pulmonary artery. The artery is dissected circumferentially and followed proximally, where it is observed as it courses posterior to the superior vena cava. The artery is easily encircled with a finger once the appropriate plane of dissection is entered. Proximal control of the artery usually is established in this fashion if there is even a suggestion that the dissection may be difficult. It is not necessary to encircle the right main pulmonary artery in every case, but one cannot

be too safe in taking the extra precaution of having proximal control. After the artery is encircled an umbilical tape is passed and a Rumel tourniquet is placed. Should the artery be inadvertently entered it is a simple matter to snug down on the tourniquet and control the bleeding. The artery is dissected distally, and the apical-anterior arterial branch is identified (Fig. 4-2). This usually occurs as a common trunk, but the individual segmental branches may arise separately from the main artery with the branch to the anterior segment coming off the artery as the most proximal branch.

Dissecting out the pulmonary artery and its branches differs significantly from the manner in which other arteries are handled. Lacking a muscular coat, the main strength of the artery comes from the intima. Thus the artery is extremely fragile and must be handled with the utmost care. When dissecting the artery great care must be taken in using any "spreading" maneuver. Whereas in peripheral vascular surgery it is perfectly acceptable to dissect out an arterial branch by using the scissors to spread adjacent tissue, this move, if applied to a pulmonary arterial branch, can easily result in avulsion of the branch from the artery trunk. Likewise when attempting to use a right angle to encircle a branch of the pulmonary artery little or no force should be applied because one gets no tactile cues from this artery. An arte-

rial branch should be completely dissected free circumferentially prior to trying to pass a right-angled clamp. To do this the thin connective tissue overlying the artery is grasped with a forceps and lifted to allow a cut by the scissors. Once the correct plane on the artery is reached a closed, blunt-tipped scissors is used to gently push the artery away while continuing to hold the incised tissue. This rapidly creates the plane of dissection and frees up the adjacent arterial branch. If an attempt to pass a right angle is met with any resistance, further dissection should be performed rather than persisting with the right angle and potentially perforating the back wall of the arterial branch. A peanut dissector may also be used to dissect the pulmonary artery once the correct plane of dissection on the artery is encountered, but I do not favor use of this instrument.

Once the artery has been identified the dissection proceeds superiorly along the hilum to enter to the plane of the bronchus. The azygous vein is a significant landmark. This vein crosses the right mainstem bronchus just superior to the origin of the right upper lobe bronchus. The vein courses from posterior to anterior, and the bronchus lies medial to the vein. Once the artery is dissected away from the bronchus it is possible to encircle the upper lobe bronchus at this point if deemed necessary. At times it is advantageous to divide the bronchus first, especially if the primary tumor or lymph nodes involve the branches of the pulmonary artery.

The lung is retracted anteriorly by the assistant to reveal the posterior aspect of the hilum. Unlike the situation of operating in the abdomen, it quickly becomes clear when doing pulmonary surgery that the surgeon must be familiar with the anatomy and especially the relationships between structures from both an anterior and a posterior orientation. In the chest, the surgeon needs to think in three dimensions. To facilitate the performance of an upper lobectomy, dissection is begun by incising the overlying pleura in the bifurcation formed by the upper lobe bronchus and the bronchus intermedius (Fig. 4-3). This is one of the most significant moves of the entire procedure, and if understood greatly simplifies and speeds up the operation. Taking care to coagulate small bronchial vessels that are present in this "crotch," one incises the pleura. A lymph node is a constant finding in this location, and the dissection frees this node anteriorly away from the bifurcation. The upper lobe bronchus may be encircled at this point and taken, if desired (inset, Fig. 4-3). Just anterior to this lymph node,

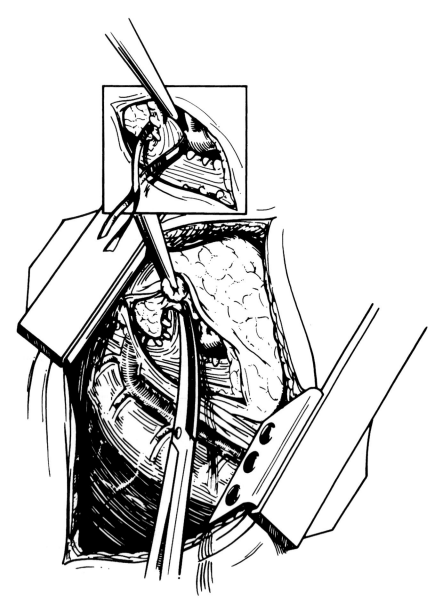

Figure 4-3. One of the most important concepts in pulmonary surgery is visualization of the anatomy in three dimensions. Much of the dissection may be done from behind or the posterior aspect of the hilum. Here the bifurcation between the bronchus intermedius and upper lobe bronchus is being dissected and the upper lobe bronchus skeletonized. There is the constant finding of a lymph node at this "crotch." Incision at the bifurcation and elevating the lymph node out of the area reveals the pulmonary artery within the fissure. **(Inset)** Once the bifurcation is dissected the bronchus may be encircled. Superiorly, if the artery has been dissected the bronchus may be taken at this point.

however, lies the branch of the pulmonary artery to the superior segment of the lower lobe, which is easily visualized from this posterior approach. Once this arterial branch is identified the posterior portion of the major fissure may be completed with a firing of the linear stapler (Fig. 4-4). The lower lobe superior segment arterial branch is the most posterior branch of the artery within the fissure, and the stapler may be safely passed just posterior to the branch. The pleura within the fissure needs to be in-

cised, and the appropriate location for placement of the stapler may be found by placing the forefinger in the "crotch" just dissected posteriorly and the thumb in the fissure. The fissure at the appropriate spot is quite thin and may be further thinned out by finger dissection of the parenchyma held between the thumb and forefinger. This move is safe because the location of the artery is known and it has been dissected free. It avoids extensive dissection in the fissure in a search for the pulmonary artery. Until the location

of the artery is known, firing a stapler across the fissure, as is commonly done, adds little; it really brings one no closer to the artery. Taking advantage of the anatomy posteriorly allows easy identification of the artery in the fissure without actually dissecting in the fissure and thus avoids air leaks. It is important to remember that the fissure, for that matter any fissure, is defined by the artery. Once the artery is identified and dissected in the correct plane the posterior portion of the major fissure is very simple to complete.

Alternatively the upper lobe bronchus may be encircled and divided at this point, which allows complete visualization of the artery from "behind" the fissure. This is the preferable move when there is nodal involvement in the fissure that makes dissection on the artery difficult. The arterial branch to the posterior segment of the upper lobe is adjacent (superior) to the superior segmental branch and occasionally may arise from this branch (Fig. 4-5). The arterial supply to the middle lobe usually arises just opposite the take-off of the superior segmental branch. There is usually one middle lobe arterial branch, but two branches are not uncommon.

Resectability must be assured prior to dividing any vascular structures. The ability to remove all disease, including mediastinal lymph node disease, if encountered, must be clear. It offers the patient no benefit to proceed with resection if gross disease will be left behind. There is no advantage to a palliative resection, only the disadvantage of the risk of the procedure. At times the surgeon must be prepared to be somewhat creative in completing a resection especially if the tumor involves the hilum of the lung and obscures the origin of the lobar vessels making individual dissection of these vessels impossible. Clamping the artery proximally allows the portion of the arterial wall containing the origin of the branches to be excised and the arterial wall either sutured primarily or patched with a piece of pericardium. Otherwise proximal involvement of the pulmonary artery may mandate pneumonectomy, but parenchymal conservation should always be considered if the cancer operation will not be compromised. Rarely should proximal tumor involvement or encasement of the right upper lobe bronchus in and of itself mandate pneumonectomy as long as the surgeon is facile with sleeve resection. The arterial branch to the anterior and apical segments is divided between ligatures, preferably silk because of the easy handling and tying features of this material. The ties must be placed so as to leave enough distance between them to allow the branch to be divided and leave a cuff of artery on each side. No upward traction should be exerted when tying because the artery may be easily disrupted at the origin of the segmental branch. Usually a single tie is placed on an arterial branch, but a suture ligature may also be placed adjacent to the proximal tie for added safety. To avoid any accidental pulling on a tie, each suture is cut after the knot is complete and prior to dividing the ligated arterial branch. Knowing how much force to exert when securing a knot on a pulmonary arterial branch is critical to avoiding injury to the vessel. Only enough force to feel the intima "crunch" should be applied and no more. The pulmonary artery is a low-pressure system, which does not mandate a huge amount of force to ligate a vessel. More force than is necessary may result in avulsion of the arterial branch. Alternatively a vascular stapler may be used to divide the apical-anterior arterial branch. Once this branch is divided the origin of the upper lobe bronchus is readily apparent. Lymph nodes lying along the bronchus are dissected upward to be removed with the specimen, a maneuver that completes the dissection around the bronchus.

The superior pulmonary vein either is divided with a vascular stapler or alternatively tied and suture ligated (Fig. 4-6). Alternatively a vascular clamp may be placed and the divided vein sutured with a horizontal mattress stitch, the clamp removed, and the suture run as a simple stitch anterior to the mattress stitch back to where it was begun. Once the vein is divided the continuation of the pulmonary artery is identified as it lies posterior to the vein. The middle lobe arterial branch is readily identified from the anterior aspect of the hilum, and, to facilitate division of the fissure and separation of the middle lobe from the upper lobe, the branch should be mobilized for a short distance. The arterial branch to the posterior segment of the upper lobe at times may be seen through this anterior exposure, or an additional anterior segmental branch may be identified. Once the artery is identified from this anterior approach and the middle lobe artery is seen, the minor fissure, which is usually incomplete, may be divided with an application of a linear stapler.

The posterior segmental branch of the artery is ligated and divided within the fissure. With the lung again retracted anteriorly the origin of the upper lobe bronchus is well seen, and a stapler is used to close the bronchus (Fig 4-7). The bronchus is taken as close as possible to its origin without compromising the lumen of the right main stem bronchus. The bronchus is divided and the

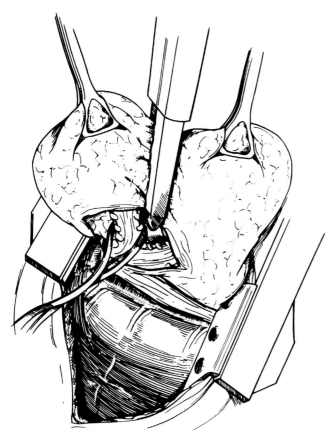

Figure 4-4.   Once the artery is identified and the branch to the superior segment of the lower lobe defined, the posterior aspect of the major fissure may be divided with a linear stapler. There are no arterial branches posterior to the superior segmental branch, thus allowing the fissure to be defined and divided. Here the stapler has been placed facilitated by the upper and lower lobes grasped with Duval lung clamps.

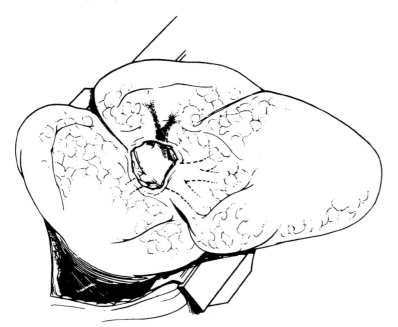

Figure 4-5.   View of the pulmonary artery from within the fissure showing the position of the arterial branch to the posterior segment of the upper lobe in relation to the middle lobe branch and the superior segmental branch. If the fissure is well developed, the overlying pleura may be incised and dissection carried down directly on the vessel. If the fissure is poorly developed, it is easier to divide the bronchus, identify and divide the posterior segmental branch, and then complete the fissure with several firings of the linear stapler.

upper lobe removed if the minor fissure has been divided. If the minor fissure remains, it is completed with a firing of the linear stapler. To obtain definitive staging information, a complete mediastinal lymph node dissection should be performed.

After division of the minor fissure and removal of the right upper lobe the middle lobe is left without tether because the oblique fissure usually is relatively complete. Postoperatively, this situation may predispose to torsion and infarction of the middle lobe. To prevent this very significant complication, the middle lobe is "reattached" to the lower lobe either by placing several absorbable sutures in a figure-of-eight fashion or by placing a row of staples between the two lobes. The middle lobe must be properly oriented prior to attaching it to the lower lobe.

There are several potential pitfalls to avoid when performing a right upper lobectomy. For the most part it is one of the most straightforward of the pulmonary resections, but problems may occur. The middle lobe vein must be identified and preserved when dividing the superior pulmonary vein. Once the superior pulmonary vein has been divided great care must be taken to avoid injury to the middle lobe artery especially when dividing the minor fissure. Traction exerted on the upper lobe while it is still attached to the middle lobe by the intact minor fissure may result in an avulsion injury to the middle lobe artery. As already mentioned, the right main bronchus may be narrowed if the upper lobe bronchus is taken with a stapler placed too close to its origin. This usually occurs when the lobe is retracted upward tenting the main stem bronchus prior to placing the stapler. If the main stem bronchus has been injured, it is best to proceed with sleeve resection and reanastomosis instead of trying to "repair" the damage. Waiting for a stricture to become symptomatic creates far more problems in the long run.

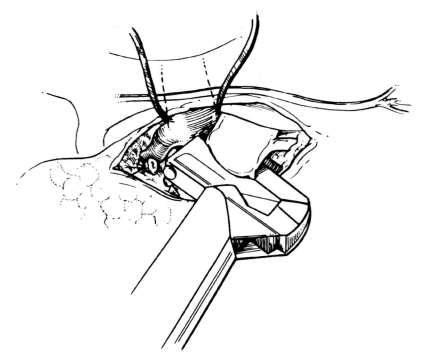

Figure 4-6.   Proximal control of the artery has been obtained by placing an umbilical tape around the artery. The superior pulmonary vein, with the middle lobe vein left intact, is divided between rows of vascular staples. Here the stapler is being applied to the vein.

Right Middle Lobectomy

Middle lobectomy is thought by many to be the most difficult lobectomy because of the problems presented by the fissures. This is an erroneous concept because it is possible to accomplish the bronchovascular dissection and division from an anterior approach if the fissures are problematic. The middle lobe is a common site for inflammatory disease and bronchiectasis. It is a common location for mycobacterial infections other than tuberculosis (MOTT).

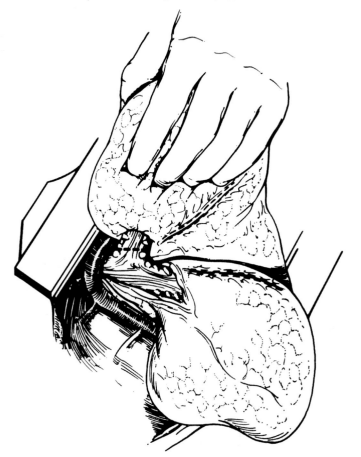

Figure 4-7.   The right upper lobe bronchus is divided as close to its origin as possible (*dashed line*). The point of division should not be so close that it compromises the lumen of the main bronchus or bronchus intermedius. It is safest to take the bronchus from this posterior approach because its origin is well seen.

The illustrations depict the view from the left side of the table, the ideal position from which to operate. If the major fissure is well developed and the pulmonary artery can be visualized easily within the fissure, the overlying pleura is incised. If the artery is not visible, the fissure overlying the artery must be divided to identify the artery. This creates air leaks and is generally messy and time consuming. To proceed with this "standard" approach, significant dissection in the fissure is required, and it is safest to gain proximal control of the pulmonary artery by incising the hilar pleura overlying the main pulmonary artery with the lung retracted posteriorly. Within the fissure the middle lobe arterial branch is identified as it originates from the pulmonary artery usually just opposite the branch to the superior segment of the lower lobe (Fig. 4-5). Most commonly there is a single arterial branch to the middle lobe, but occasionally two branches are identified. The arterial supply to the middle lobe is ligated with silk ligatures and divided. Once the arterial supply is divided the middle lobe bronchus may be seen lying deep to the artery and slightly inferior, as viewed from within the fissure. The bronchus is dissected back to its origin from the bronchus intermedius, stapled, and divided. Alternatively, the bronchus may be divided and closed with interrupted sutures of braided or monofilament absorbable material of size 3-0 or 4-0.

With the lung retracted posteriorly the anterior hilar pleura over the superior pulmonary vein is incised. The middle lobe venous branch or branches most commonly drain into the superior pulmonary vein but can drain into the inferior vein on rare occasions (Fig. 4-1). To ensure that a branch is coming from the middle lobe, the lobe may be grasped with a lung clamp and retracted laterally (upward toward the incision). This will avoid division of small branches coming from the upper lobe. The venous branch is then divided after ligating with silk ligatures and securing with a suture ligature.

Once the bronchovascular structures have been divided the minor fissure is completed with a firing of the linear stapler. The anterior portion of the major fissure likely is well developed and is easily completed and the lobe removed.

An alternative technique for middle lobectomy is also illustrated and is likely to be a more useful and versatile. This technique does not rely on the pulmonary artery being visible within the fissure and does not require extensive dissection in the fissure to identify the artery. The lung is retracted posteriorly. The hilar pleura overly-

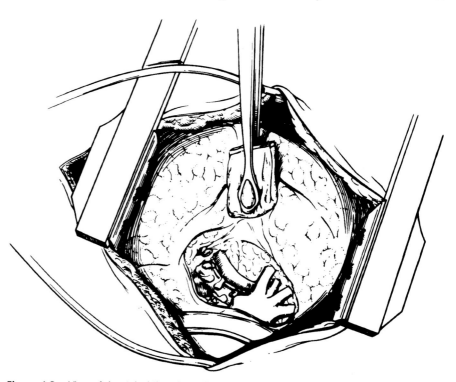

Figure 4-8. View of the right hilum from the left side of the table. The superior pulmonary vein has been dissected out and the middle lobe vein identified, ligated, and divided. The ligated stump of the middle lobe vein is seen. Immediately posterior to the vein lays the middle lobe bronchus. Usually the bronchus has to be divided to have optimal visualization of the middle lobe artery, but at times the artery is seen slightly superior and posterior to the bronchus. Division of the bronchus facilitates division of the artery and provides the exposure to assess whether there are other middle lobe arterial branches.

ing the superior pulmonary vein is incised and the middle lobe vein identified. The vein is ligated and divided, and the middle lobe bronchus lies immediately posterior and slightly superior to the vein (Fig. 4-8). The bronchus is surrounded by connective tissue, which is divided taking care to coagulate any bronchial arterial branches that are encountered. The bronchus should be followed back to its origin at the bronchus intermedius. The middle lobe arterial branch lies just posterior and slightly superior to the middle lobe bronchus but may not be visible prior to dividing the bronchus. The bronchus is encircled with a right-angled clamp staying close to the bronchial wall to avoid damage to the adjacent arterial branch (Fig. 4-9). The bronchus is divided with a scalpel using a right-angled clamp as a guide. The bronchial stump is closed with interrupted sutures. Alternatively, a stapler may be applied to close the middle lobe bronchus.

After division of the bronchus the middle lobe arterial branch is easily seen and is circumferentially mobilized (Fig. 4-10). The arterial branch or branches are ligated and divided. Once the bronchus, artery, and

vein are divided, the minor fissure as well as that portion of the oblique fissure in contact with the middle lobe are divided with several firings of the linear stapler and the lobe is removed. A mediastinal lymph node dissection is then completed to obtain the most accurate and complete staging information.

Despite the apparent simplicity of middle lobectomy as described there are several potential trouble spots. The middle lobe bronchus comes off the bronchus intermedius at essentially a right angle and is quite fragile and susceptible to injury. The origin of the middle lobe bronchus is not easily seen from the anterior approach, and the bronchus intermedius may be damaged when the middle lobe bronchus is taken with a stapler. The middle lobe arterial supply may also present problems if there is more than one branch. Sometimes the additional branch may be obscured and injured if its presence is not recognized. Care must also be taken when going around the middle lobe arterial branch from the anterior approach to avoid injuring the main pulmonary artery within the fissure.

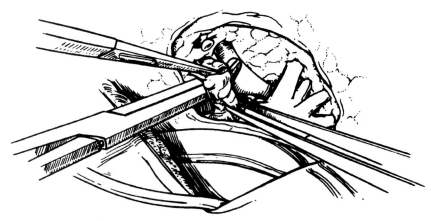

Figure 4-9. The middle lobe bronchus is encircled with a right-angled clamp and divided with a scalpel. It is important to identify the origin of the middle lobe bronchus to avoid damage to the bronchus intermedius. The bronchial stump is closed with interrupted absorbable sutures, or alternatively a stapler may be placed and the bronchus closed. Note the relationship of the middle lobe artery to the bronchus.

Right Lower Lobectomy

Because of the close proximity of the bronchovascular structures of the middle lobe, resection of the right lower lobe provides several unique challenges and is one of the more difficult lobectomies. Similar to the middle lobectomy, the pulmonary artery must be identified within the fissure to complete the resection, and in those cases where the fissure is poorly developed a direct attack through parenchyma often proves to

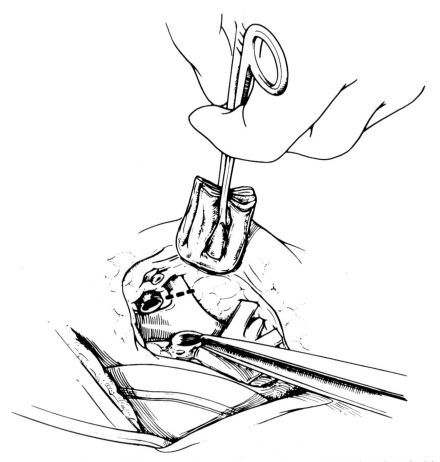

Figure 4-10. Following division of the middle lobe bronchus the arterial branch (or branches) is well seen and can be mobilized and divided (*dashed line*). Once the artery is taken the minor fissure is divided with a linear stapler, as is the anterior portion of the major fissure.

be quite challenging. The chest is entered through either a standard posterolateral thoracotomy incision (fifth intercostal space) or a vertical axillary muscle-sparing incision (fourth space). If disease is noted within the fissure or if the hilum is involved, it is best to obtain control of the proximal right main pulmonary artery. The hilar pleura is incised anteriorly and superiorly with the lung retracted in a posterior direction, and the proximal pulmonary artery is encircled just lateral to the superior vena cava.

If the fissure is reasonably well developed, the pleura overlying the pulmonary artery is incised and the dissection is carried down onto the plane of the artery (Fig. 4-11). The branch to the superior segment of the lower lobe is first identified, and the middle lobe arterial branch is most commonly found arising from the opposite aspect of the artery just across from the superior segmental origin. The dissection may be extended posteriorly along the superior aspect of the branch to the superior segment, which leads to the bifurcation of the upper lobe bronchus and bronchus intermedius. With the lung retracted anteriorly the pleura overlying this bifurcation posteriorly is incised, and a linear stapler encompassing the parenchyma within the fissure may be inserted from just above the superior segmental arterial branch through the area of the bifurcation. This move is possible because there are no vascular structures present posterior to the origin of the superior segmental arterial branch. On the superior aspect of the artery just opposite the superior segment, the posterior segmental branch, the so-called "recurrent" branch (posterior segmental), to the upper lobe arises and is easily visualized. Rarely this branch to the upper lobe may arise from the superior segment branch to the lower lobe, but this possibility should be kept in mind. The posterior aspect of the major fissure is then divided and completed.

The relationship of the superior segmental branch to the middle lobe arterial branch determines whether the lower lobe artery may be divided as a complete trunk or whether the superior segmental branch and basal trunk need to be taken separately. As illustrated in Fig. 4-11, the superior segmental branch must be taken separately to avoid damage to the middle lobe arterial supply. The dashed line indicates the position for division of the basal segmental trunk. This is usually a 1-cm to 2-cm trunk and should be double ligated with a suture ligature or closed with a vascular stapler and divided. The simplest stapling maneuver uses the endoscopic linear stapler with a vascular

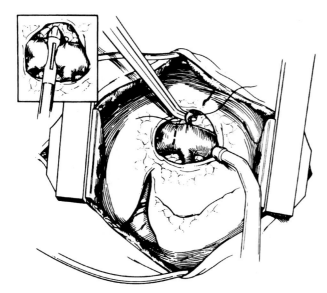

Figure 4-11. The pulmonary artery within the fissure has been identified and dissected. The position of the branch to the superior segment is such that it must be ligated and divided separately from the rest of the arterial supply to the lower lobe. The superior segmental branch is shown here being encircled by a right-angled clamp, and the point of division of the basal arterial trunk is marked (*dashed line*). Note the position of the superior segmental branch relative to the middle lobe artery. **(Inset)** The basal arterial trunk is shown being divided by the endoscopic vascular stapler, which both ligates and divides. The angle is usually ideal for placement of this stapler, which provides an extremely secure closure of three parallel rows of staples.

monofilament thread or doubly ligated prior to division. At the minimum, a tie and a suture ligature are placed to secure the vein. The anterior aspect of the major fissure is now easily completed with a firing of the linear stapler, which allows the lobe to be removed.

It is a common misconception that right lower lobectomy is difficult because of the necessity to identify the pulmonary artery within the fissure. If a "difficult" fissure is encountered, it is always best to obtain proximal control of the right main pulmonary artery as the initial maneuver. The artery may then be followed distally beyond the middle lobe branch, which leads up to the fissure and facilitates dissection of the fissure, minimizing air leaks. Alternatively, the artery may be identified posteriorly from within the "crotch" formed by the bronchus intermedius and the upper lobe bronchus and the posterior aspect of the fissure completed. Once the artery is identified further dissection within the fissure proceeds expeditiously. Rarely should it be necessary to dissect through the depths of the fissure to identify the artery.

cartridge for closure and division (inset, Fig. 4-11). The stapler may be placed obliquely to include the superior segment branch and avoid the middle lobe artery.

Dividing the pulmonary artery reveals the bronchus, which lies just deep (medial) to the artery. With the artery retracted superiorly the origin of the middle lobe bronchus may be visualized and the location for division of the lower lobe bronchus established (Fig. 4-12). The middle lobe artery lies superficial and superior to the middle lobe bronchus. Care must be taken to avoid compromising the origin of the middle lobe bronchus when stapling or dividing the lower lobe bronchus (Fig. 4-12, inset). The bronchus may be either closed with a stapler or divided with a scalpel and closed with interrupted absorbable sutures.

With the lung retracted toward the apex of the chest the inferior pulmonary ligament is divided up to the level of the inferior pulmonary vein (Fig. 4-13). An inferior pulmonary ligament lymph node (level 9) should be excised for staging purposes. The inferior pulmonary vein is dissected and encircled in preparation for division. A finger is passed around the vein after entering the appropriate dissection plane, and the vein is divided with a vascular stapler (Fig. 4-13, inset). Alternatively the vein may be clamped, divided, and sutured with a running

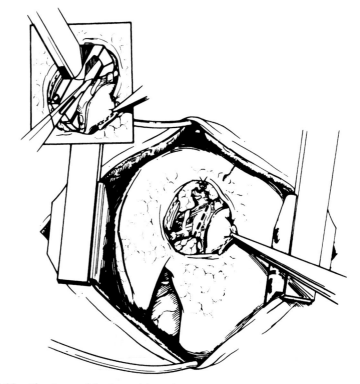

Figure 4-12. The stump of the lower lobe pulmonary artery is retracted superiorly to expose the lower lobe bronchus. The middle lobe bronchus, which comes off the bronchus intermedius at a 90-degree angle, must be identified and preserved. If a stapler is to be used, it must be placed in such an orientation as to avoid compromising the orifice of the middle lobe bronchus. The site of bronchial division is shown (*dashed line*). The bronchial division includes the bronchus to the superior segment as shown. Occasionally it is necessary to close and divide the superior segment bronchus separately. **(Inset)** A stapler is placed across the lower lobe bronchus distal to the origin of the middle lobe bronchus. Often the stapler has to be oriented in an oblique fashion to include the superior segment bronchus and avoid the middle lobe.

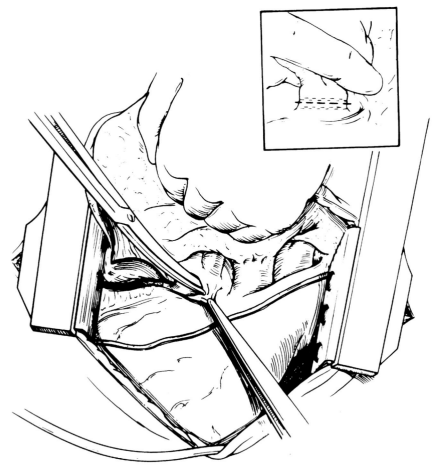

Figure 4-13. With the lung retracted superiorly the inferior pulmonary ligament is incised up to the level of the inferior pulmonary vein. The vein is shown being dissected by incising the overlying pleura. The vein may then be encircled with a finger and divided between rows of vascular staples or clamped, divided, and sutured closed. **(Inset)** The vein has been encircled and two rows of staples placed. The line of division is marked (*dashed line*). Often division of the vein precedes bronchial division, but there is no set order in which structures must be taken.

Bilobectomy

Occasionally, the location of a lesion will mandate removal of the middle and lower lobes, a procedure that can be accomplished en bloc because of the common origin of these lobes as the bronchus intermedius. A tumor originating in the bronchus intermedius usually requires removal of both lobes, but a lower lobe lesion that involves the external aspect of the lobar bronchus may also mandate taking the middle lobe. Where an indication exists for bilobectomy the vessels for each lobe are isolated and divided as described for each individual lobectomy. Once the pulmonary arterial branches have been divided the point of division of the bronchus becomes obvious; the bronchus should be divided above the origin of the middle lobe bronchus just distal to the upper lobe take-off (Fig. 4-14). Morbidity and mortality for bilobectomy exceed those for lobectomy alone, so this resection should

not be performed solely for ease or convenience. The middle lobe should never just be assumed to be expendable. The bronchial stump placed so close to the upper lobe bronchus may be at somewhat increased risk for breakdown compared to other bronchial closures.

Lesions within the bronchus intermedius often present additional problems for the surgeon. These tumors may invade the inferior pulmonary vein occasionally with proximal extension into the left atrium. Careful exploration is mandated to assess resectability before dividing any structures. Proximal involvement of the inferior pulmonary vein need not preclude resection if the vessel can be encircled or the extent of atrial involvement is not excessive. Some of these lesions may demand intrapericardial pneumonectomy because of the proximal involvement of the atrium. A sleeve resection of the main bronchus may also be performed if the proximal extent of the tumor involves

the bronchus at the level of the upper lobe bronchus. The right main bronchus may be divided proximal to the upper lobe origin and the upper lobe bronchus severed at its origin. The middle and lower lobes together with a portion of main bronchus are removed and the upper lobe anastomosed to the open end of the main bronchus.

Postoperative Mortality

Thirty-day mortality from pulmonary resections is approximately 4%. Lobectomies and lesser resections should have mortality between 1% and 2%, whereas pneumonectomies still carry a mortality of 6% to 7%. The mortality rate is directly proportional to increased age, associated diseases, and the extent of resection. Respiratory complications, not surprisingly, are the most common cause of postoperative mortality in patients undergoing pulmonary resection. Cardiac complications also account for a significant percentage of mortality, whereas technical problems such as hemorrhage, bronchopleural fistula, and empyema account for a small but significant percentage of complications leading to death.

Postoperative Morbidity

Approximately 30% of patients undergoing pulmonary resection will sustain a postoperative complication, of which approximately two thirds are minor and the other one third are nonfatal major complications. The most common complication is supraventricular arrhythmia, which occurs in up to 20% of patients, depending on how closely patients are monitored. Most of these respond to simple pharmacologic manipulation and rarely are hemodynamically significant at onset. With appropriate treatment, the rhythm reverts to sinus rhythm quickly, and patients may be taken off the antiarrhythmic drugs usually after 1 month. Other minor complications include postoperative air leaks lasting more than 7 days and atelectasis. Major nonfatal events most commonly are respiratory related with patients developing significant infiltrates and pneumonitis. A small percentage of patients require reintubation in the postoperative period for respiratory failure usually related to the development of an infiltrate. There are no definitive predictors for postoperative pulmonary complications, although significant risk factors for major complications include age >60 years, FEV_1 <2 liters, weight loss >10%, associated systemic disease, and extent of disease. Pulmonary complications can be minimized with meticulous attention to postoperative respiratory maneuvers

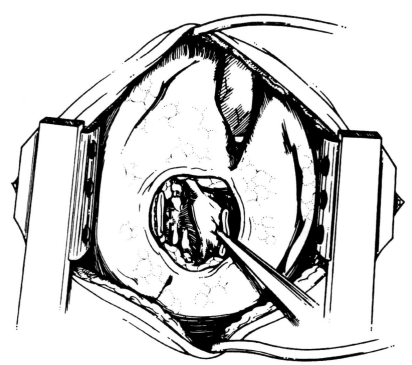

Figure 4-14.   To complete a bilobectomy, the pulmonary artery within the fissure is divided proximal to the middle lobe arterial origin, if possible. Often the middle lobe artery must be taken as a separate branch. The bronchus intermedius is then exposed by retracting the artery. The bronchus intermedius is divided proximal to the middle lobe origin and just distal to the take-off of the right upper lobe (*dashed line*). Surprisingly, the right upper lobe usually is adequate to fill the residual space, and space infection problems are unusual.

including chest physiotherapy and preoperative teaching.

Other complications of pulmonary resection include wound infections and disturbances in mental status especially in older patients. Notwithstanding our best efforts to avoid them, complications do occur. If recognized early, many can be treated without sequelae. Meticulous attention to detail in all phases of management—preoperative, intraoperative, and postoperative—goes a long way toward keeping problems to a minimum.

SUGGESTED READING

Deslauriers J, Ginsberg RJ, Piantadosi S, et al. Prospective assessment of 30-day operative morbidity for surgical resections in lung cancer. Chest 1994;106:329S.

Ginsberg RJ, Rubinstein LV. Randomized trial of lobectomy versus limited resection for T1 N0 non–small cell lung cancer. Lung Cancer Study Group. Ann Thorac Surg 1995;60:615.

Hatter J, Kohman LJ, Mosca RS, et al. Preoperative evaluation of stage I and stage II non–small cell lung cancer. Ann Thorac Surg 1994;58:1738.

Kawahara K, Akamine S, Tsuji H, et al. Bronchoplastic procedures for lung cancer: clinical study in 136 patients. World J Surg 1994;18:822.

Martini N, Kris MG, Flehinger BJ, et al. Preoperative chemotherapy for stage IIIa (N2) lung cancer: The Sloan-Kettering experience with 136 patients. Ann Thorac Surg 1993;55:1365.

Nakahara K, Fujii Y, Matsumura A, et al. Role of systematic mediastinal dissection in N2 non–small cell lung cancer patients. Ann Thorac Surg 1993;56:331.

Pierce RJ, Copland JM, Sharpe K, et al. Preoperative risk evaluation for lung cancer resection: Predicted postoperative product as a predictor of surgical mortality. Am J Respir Crit Care Med 1994;150:945.

Roth JA, Fossella F, Komaki R, et al. A randomized trial comparing perioperative chemotherapy and surgery with surgery alone in resectable stage IIIA non–small-cell lung cancer. J Natl Cancer Inst 1994;86:673.

Sugarbaker DJ, Strauss GM. Advances in surgical staging and therapy of non–small-cell lung cancer. Semin Oncol 1993;20:163.

Warren WH, Faber LP. Segmentectomy versus lobectomy in patients with stage I pulmonary carcinoma. Five-year survival and patterns of intrathoracic recurrence. J Thorac Cardiovasc Surg 1994;104:1087.

EDITOR'S COMMENTS

As noted by Dr. Kaiser, the preoperative evaluation of patients with lung cancer involves both radiographic and pulmonary physiologic testing. There should also be a low index of suspicion of performing a pharmacologic cardiac stress test if clinically indicated. In addition, whereas a preoperative histologic diagnosis of lung cancer is helpful, it is entirely appropriate to proceed to thoracotomy without a tissue diagnosis if the clinical history and radiographic appearance of the lesion strongly suggest a diagnosis of lung cancer. It is, however, prudent to have a histologic diagnosis of malignancy before performing a pneumonectomy.

What differentiates the casual from the expert thoracic surgeon is a thorough understanding of the corresponding lung's bronchovascular anatomy and the more common vascular anatomic variants. This permits the expert thoracic surgeon to move the case along and greatly increases the chances that the correct oncologic procedure can be done without the need to perform a pneumonectomy. As noted out by Dr. Kaiser, this point cannot be overemphasized. At the University of Virginia, we perform a pneumonectomy for lung cancer in fewer than 10% of our patients, preferring instead to perform sleeve resections and segmentectomies, with or without pulmonary artery resections and reconstruction. We prefer to use either autologous or bovine pericardium for extended pulmonary arterioplasties that cannot be closed primarily. It is also important to place a soft-tissue buffer (pericardial fat pad, pleura, etc.) between a bronchial suture or staple line and an overlying pulmonary arterioplasty to further minimize the remote possibility of a bronchovascular fistula.

An important point to emphasize with respect to the actual resection of either the right upper or lower lobe is the superiority of resecting the lobe using a fissure-less dissection. We rarely dissect in the fissure, and believe that inadvertent injury to the defining pulmonary arterial branches is more likely and that the incidence of postoperative air leaks is also greater. For instance, for upper lobe lesions, we routinely divide the superior pulmonary vein first, then the apico-anterior pulmonary branches, the upper lobe bronchus, and then the posterior ascending pulmonary artery branch. The minor and major fissures are then divided in continuity with serial applications of the stapler. Finally, when performing these identical right-sided resections using a video-assisted thoracic surgery (VATS) approach, the fissure-less dissection approach is even more expeditious and safe.

I.L.K.

5

Left-Sided Pulmonary Resections

Larry R. Kaiser

Left-sided resections have a number of unique features distinct from those carried out on the right. The aortic arch, in most cases, is a left-sided structure, and its position relative to the pulmonary artery and the left main bronchus is the major defining feature of resections on this side. Access to the proximal left main bronchus and carina is limited because of the aortic arch. Thus, the left paratracheal area, a lymph node–bearing area, is difficult to access at thoracotomy. There is no well-defined space or compartment where a lymph node dissection is carried out as on the right side. Lymph nodes are dissected from the aortopulmonary window and the subcarinal space and, at times, from the paratracheal area that can be accessed from the inferior aspect of the aortic arch.

Access to the most proximal aspect of the left main pulmonary artery may be gained by dividing the ligamentum arteriosum and then encircling the pulmonary artery. The left recurrent laryngeal nerve is highly vulnerable to injury because of its position in relation to the inferior surface of the aortic arch. This nerve originates from the vagus nerve as it crosses the arch and then "recurs" around the ligamentum arteriosum. Any dissection in the aortopulmonary window places the left recurrent laryngeal nerve at risk of injury. This is especially true if one attempts to excise the lymph nodes in the left tracheobronchial angle or paratracheal position.

The left main bronchus also varies significantly from the right. On the left there is a long segment of main stem bronchus prior to the bifurcation of the lobar bronchi as opposed to the right, where the right upper lobe bronchus originates within 1.5 cm to 2 cm of the carina. Upper or lower lobectomy with a sleeve resection of the main bronchus is certainly feasible on the left side, although these account for only a minority of these resections in any series.

The lingular segment is analogous to the middle lobe in that it has separate arterial and venous branches as well as a distinct bronchus. Lingular segmentectomy was one of the first segmental resections described, likely because of its well-defined, discrete bronchovascular anatomy.

Contralateral mediastinal lymph node involvement is much more common with left-sided lesions, particularly lesions of the left lower lobe. For that reason mediastinoscopy is critically important when assessing lesions of the left lower lobe.

Surgical Technique

Left Upper Lobectomy

Of the pulmonary resections the left upper lobectomy is, perhaps, the most technically challenging. The location of the pulmonary artery in relation to the aorta and the branching pattern of the left pulmonary artery contribute to the technical difficulties. There are a number of potential pitfalls that must be avoided to safely complete a left upper lobectomy. Lymphatics from the left upper lobe commonly drain to lymph nodes in the aortopulmonary window (level 5) or paraaortic location (level 6), and these lymph nodes must be removed to obtain complete staging information. Despite the classification of these nodal locations as mediastinal (N2), involvement of these lymph nodes

with tumor in the absence of other nodal disease is associated with a better prognosis than N2 disease in any other location. Survival with isolated involved level 5 or 6 lymph nodes approximates that of patients who have only N1 lymph node involvement (approximately 40% at 5 years) as long as a complete resection can be performed. As mentioned, access to the superior mediastinum is difficult from the left side because of the location of the aortic arch in relation to the left main bronchus and tracheobronchial angle. For this reason mediastinoscopy is extremely useful for left-sided lesions even without enlarged lymph nodes present on the CT scan because it allows accurate sampling of the paratracheal area in a manner that is significantly simpler and safer than trying to access this area during thoracotomy.

The left upper lobectomy is begun by incising the hilar pleura anteriorly and superiorly with the lobe retracted in the posterior direction. The pulmonary artery emerges from beneath the aortic arch and is located superior and posterolateral to the superior pulmonary vein. The apical segmental branch of the vein may cross the artery and partly obscure the apical-posterior segmental trunk of the pulmonary artery, necessitating division of the venous branch first (Fig. 5-1). The appropriate plane of dissection is entered on the pulmonary artery proximal to the take-off of the first branch, and careful circumferential dissection is carried out. The left main pulmonary artery is encircled with the index finger, and a blunt-tipped C-clamp is passed toward the encircled finger to pass an umbilical tape around the vessel. A Rumel tourniquet is placed but

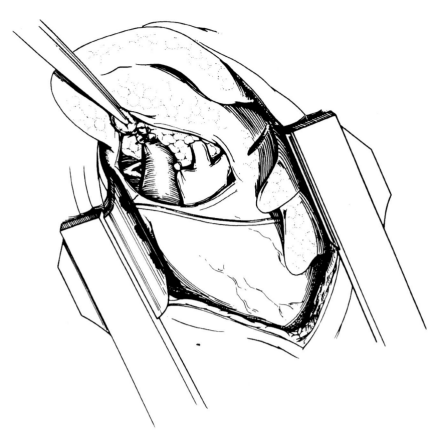

Figure 5-1.   View of the left pulmonary hilum from the right side of the table showing the pulmonary artery and vein. The line of division of the apical-posterior segmental branch of the artery is shown (*dashed line*). A venous branch partially obscuring the artery has been divided, and the ligated stump is shown.

not snared to allow the main pulmonary artery to be occluded if this should prove to be necessary. The superior pulmonary vein is dissected and encircled, taking care to include the lingular branch. The vein may be doubly ligated or stapled with a vascular stapler and divided. It is both safe and expeditious to employ vascular staplers to divide both pulmonary vessels, both venous and arterial branches. Parallel rows of staples are placed, and the vessel is divided. Alternatively, an endoscopic vascular stapler that cuts between parallel rows each with three layers of staples has also been used. Conversely, individual branches may be ligated with silk ligatures and divided. A suture ligature should be placed in addition to a single tie especially to secure venous branches.

The apical-posterior segmental branch of the pulmonary artery is a short, broad vessel that may be easily avulsed or torn if too much traction is applied when retracting the upper lobe (Fig. 5-1). This is a feared complication of left upper lobectomy, which may force a pneumonectomy depending on the extent of the injury to the artery following avulsion especially if

the tear extends proximally. If proximal control of the artery has not been secured, as discussed, this makes for a particularly disastrous complication. Trying to get around the left main pulmonary artery to place a clamp on the vessel is extremely difficult when at the same time it is necessary to staunch the hemorrhage from an injury to the artery. Often a significant amount of blood is lost during this maneuver. One should avoid the temptation to wildly try to place a clamp on the vessel. Without encircling the vessel this results in, at best, only partial occlusion and, at worse, further injury to the vessel. Proximal extension of a tear in this portion of the pulmonary artery may result in an irreversible situation with death due to exsanguination. If an injury to the main pulmonary artery occurs and proximal control has not been obtained, one should gently occlude the rent with a finger and assess the situation. Blood should be available in the room before further maneuvers are attempted. Additional help should be summoned if not already present. It is not feasible to try to suture the pulmonary artery without gaining proximal control.

Attempts to place sutures in the artery under these conditions may result in further injury to the artery because the torrential bleeding does not allow enough visualization to accurately place the sutures and the artery is easily torn. At this point, the pericardium should be opened to secure additional length of the artery, and the intrapericardial portion of the pulmonary artery should be encircled for proximal control while maintaining digital pressure on the arterial rent. It may be necessary to divide the ligamentum arteriosum to place a vascular clamp in proximally enough to allow for the artery to be repaired. Once proximal control is achieved the branch is completely divided if it has not been completely avulsed, and the artery is repaired with 5-0 or 6-0 monofilament, nonabsorbable sutures. Rather than frank avulsion of the apical-posterior arterial branch, a more common traction injury is a hematoma in the vessel from an intimal tear. The intima is what holds the pulmonary artery together structurally, so this has the potential to be a disastrous situation. Proximal control should be obtained and the vessel ligated preferably proximal to the intimal tear. Placing a ligature at the area of the tear may result in complete avulsion of the branch when the knot is placed. As noted, it is best to recognize that this arterial branch presents special problems, and the recognition of this should lead to great caution when retracting the left upper lobe because avoiding problems with the pulmonary artery is far better and simpler than having to repair the artery no matter how good the surgeon may think he or she is at fixing problem situations.

Dissection on the artery continues distally following the artery toward and into the fissure. The left main pulmonary artery resides in an Peribronchial location relative to the left main bronchus (Fig. 5-2). As the fissure is entered, the anterior segmental arterial branch to the upper lobe is encountered just proximal and opposite to the origin of the superior segmental branch to the lower lobe. Once the superior segmental branch is identified the posterior portion of the fissure may be completed with a stapler. The anterior segmental branch is divided between silk ligatures (Fig. 5-3), and the artery is followed further distally until the lingular branches are encountered. There may be a single lingular trunk or two separate branches. The lingular branches are ligated and divided, and the anterior portion of the fissure is completed with a firing of the linear stapler (Fig. 5-4). Alternatively, the fissure may be taken following division of the bronchus when it is all that remains holding the lobe in place.

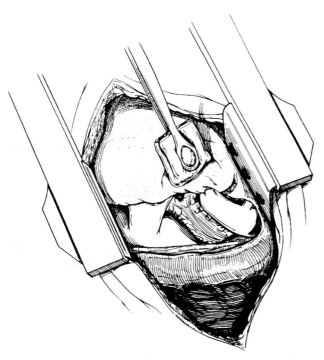

Figure 5-2. Relationship of the left main pulmonary artery to the left main bronchus seen from the posterior aspect. The main pulmonary artery lies in an epibronchial location. The inferior pulmonary vein is also seen from this posterior view.

Within the fissure the artery is bluntly reflected inferiorly away from the underlying bronchus, which is located medial (or deep) (Fig. 5-5). The bifurcation of the left main bronchus is visible at this point, and care should be taken to avoid damage to the lower lobe bronchus when the upper lobe bronchus is divided. The bronchus needs to be skeletonized and encircled prior to its division. Bronchial vessels should be either electrocoagulated or occluded with metal clips and divided, depending on their size. It should not be assumed that the stapler used to close the bronchus will occlude these vessels. Staplers used on the bronchus are not particularly hemostatic because of the size (3.5 mm or 4.8 mm) of the staples. To avoid postoperative bleeding from a bronchial artery, these vessels should be identified and ligated before dividing (or stapling) the bronchus.

Exposure of the left upper lobe bronchus is achieved both from the anterior aspect of the hilum and from within the fissure. Division of the superior pulmonary vein exposes the bronchus as seen when viewing the hilum from the anterior aspect. After division of the vein the bronchus may be further dissected with mobilization of peribronchial lymph nodes upward with the specimen. Incising the fibrous tissue on the plane of the bronchus at the level of the bifurcation also facilitates division of the anterior portion of the fissure. The thumb and first finger placed at the bifurcation may be used to thin out the parenchyma in this location so as to be able to divide the fissure by firing the linear stapler after placing it through the hole formed by the opposed thumb and forefinger. The upper lobe bronchus is stapled and divided as close as possible to the bifurcation (Fig. 5-5, inset). Alternatively, the bronchus may be divided with a scalpel (open technique) and closed with individual sutures of either a 3-0 or 4-0 monofilament or braided nonabsorbable material (Fig. 5-6). The bronchus is divided in an open fashion, that is, incised with a scalpel in the presence of endobronchial disease that may be close to the bronchial margin because the stapler, by virtue of its width, obscures what otherwise might be an adequate margin. The importance of a negative margin is obvious, and a frozen section of the bronchial margin should be obtained whenever an endobronchial lesion is present if not routinely for all but small peripheral lung cancers. The bronchial stump is checked under saline to assure that the closure is airtight. The anesthesiologist is asked to inflate the lung and hold a pressure of between 25 and 30 cm H_2O.

The inferior pulmonary ligament is incised, freeing up the lower lobe, which it tethers, although the value of this maneuver is questionable. The intent of incising the so-called inferior pulmonary ligament is to allow the lower lobe to more adequately fill the residual space following removal of the upper lobe. Lymph nodes in the para-aortic (level 6) and aortopulmonary window (level 5) locations are taken. The subcarinal

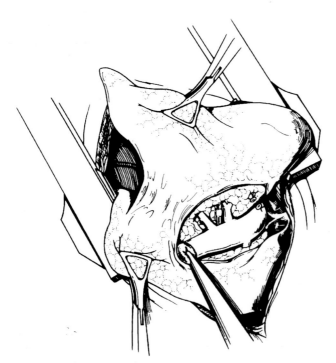

Figure 5-3. The anterior segmental branch of the pulmonary artery has been divided and the artery exposed in the fissure. Two lingular arterial branches are seen, as is the branch to the superior segment of the lower lobe.

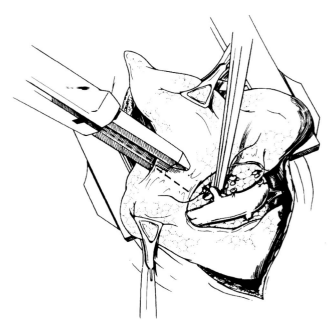

Figure 5-4. The anterior aspect of the fissure is taken with the linear stapler after the artery has been identified and dissected. A right-angled clamp is around a lingular arterial branch in preparation for ligation and division of the branch.

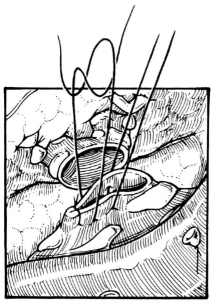

Figure 5-6. The bronchus has been divided with a scalpel and is being closed with sutures. The first suture should be placed at the midpoint of the closure, and all sutures should be placed before tying. The sutures should be evenly spaced and should be tied snugly but not so tight that they pull through the membranous bronchus, which is quite fragile. The bronchus is closed so that the membranous portion is apposed to the cartilaginous bronchus.

space is opened by incising the mediastinal pleura posteriorly and just inferior to the main bronchus. Small vagal branches going to the lung are divided between metal clips. The contents of the subcarinal space (level 7) are removed using blunt and sharp dissection along with the liberal use of metal clips. The left paratracheal and tracheobronchial angle lymph nodes are most easily sampled at mediastinoscopy, but if exposure of these nodal locations is required, it is obtained by dissecting inferior to the aortic arch heading medially. The pulmonary artery must be retracted inferiorly to permit this dissection, which is facilitated by dividing the ligamentum arteriosum (Fig. 5-7). On the left side there is not a well-defined packet of superior mediastinal lymph nodes that yields a nice clean dissection. The nodes must be removed individually. Great care must be taken to avoid the left recurrent laryngeal nerve, which courses around the ligamentum arteriosum. If the patient is hoarse in the postoperative period, the vocal cords should be examined with a laryngoscope to ensure that the left vocal cord is moving. If the left vocal cord is paralyzed, the patient's ability to cough and clear secretions in the postoperative period is markedly impaired, and aspiration with subsequent pneumonia becomes a significant risk.

A variation of the standard left upper lobectomy is a lingular-sparing upper lobectomy that is useful in patients with borderline lung function where the primary tumor is in the apical or posterior segment of the upper lobe. Lesions in the anterior segment sometimes are amenable to this approach as well. Basically, the dissection proceeds as for a standard left upper lobectomy, but the lingular branch of the superior pulmonary vein is preserved, as are the lingular arterial branches as they are identified in the fissure. The dissection on the bronchus is carried further distal than for standard upper lobectomy to identify the bifurcation between the upper lobe proper and the lingular bronchus. The lingular bronchus is spared as the stapler is applied to the upper lobe proper bronchus. The parenchyma is either "stripped," as described classically for segmentectomy, or divided with a stapler guided by the location of the remnants

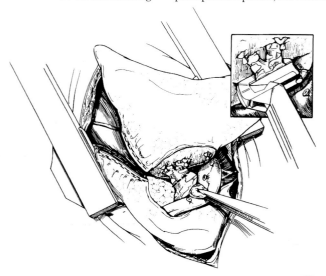

Figure 5-5. The pulmonary artery is retracted inferiorly to expose the origin of the left upper lobe bronchus. The point of division of the bronchus is shown (*dashed line*) just proximal to the bifurcation. The lingular bronchus and upper lobe proper are easily seen. **(Inset)** The stapler is applied to the bronchus proximal to the lingula and upper lobe proper bifurcation. This is done from within the fissure.

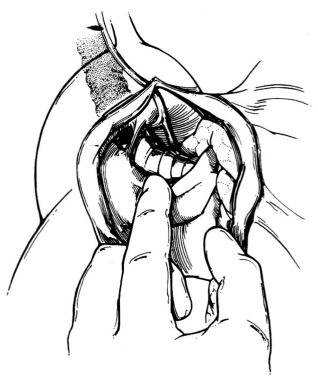

Figure 5-7. Exposure of the tracheobronchial angle is difficult from the left side because of the relationship of the left main bronchus to the aortic arch. To gain access to the tracheobronchial angle, the pulmonary artery must be retracted inferiorly. The ligamentum arteriosum is shown intact, but access to the left tracheobronchial angle is facilitated by dividing the ligamentum. The vagus nerve and the left recurrent laryngeal nerve are nicely demonstrated, showing how vulnerable the recurrent nerve is to injury during dissection in the aortopulmonary window.

with the mediastinoscope than at thoracotomy because of the location of the aortic arch relative to the left main bronchus.

The chest is entered through either a standard posterolateral thoracotomy incision (fifth intercostal space) or a muscle-sparing incision (fourth intercostal space). Even for lower lobectomy there is no advantage to being in a lower intercostal (sixth) space because the position of the hilar structures remains constant, although intuitively one would think that if the fifth space is used for upper lobectomy, the sixth must be appropriate for lower lobectomy. The pleural space is thoroughly explored to rule out visceral or parietal pleural spread of tumor, to assess lymph node involvement, to assess nodal disease within the fissure, and to establish whether left lower lobectomy is the procedure of choice. It is safest, especially for the less experienced operator, to gain proximal control of the left main pulmonary artery by starting the dissection with the upper lobe retracted posteriorly to allow access to the proximal pulmonary artery. The pleura overlying the pulmonary artery is incised anteriorly and superiorly, and dissection is carried down onto the artery. The appropriate plane is entered, and the artery is encircled, most safely, with the index finger, an umbilical tape is passed, and a Rumel

of the distal ends of the bronchovascular structures and the anterior segmental arterial branch.

Left Lower Lobectomy

In contrast to the left upper lobectomy, left lower lobectomy can be one of the easiest pulmonary resections and, like the right upper lobectomy, is an excellent resection for those just beginning their experience in pulmonary surgery. The anatomy is quite well defined, and there are only a few traps into which one might be led. Again the role that mediastinoscopy plays in lesions of the left side, particularly lower lobe lesions, must be emphasized. Carcinomas of the left lower lobe involve contralateral mediastinal lymph nodes more commonly than lesions in any other lobe because of the almost constant occurrence of lymphatics that cross the midline. For left lung lesions mediastinoscopy is the definitive invasive procedure for sampling right paratracheal lymph nodes, but it also provides access to the left paratracheal (level 2) and tracheobronchial angle (level 4) lymph nodes. The left-sided lymph nodes are actually easier to access

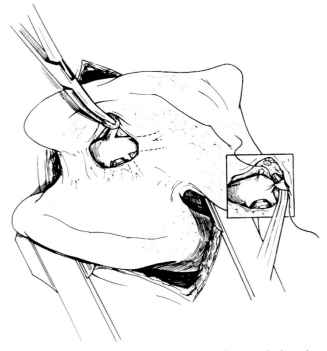

Figure 5-8. View of the left pulmonary artery in the fissure showing the branch to the superior segment to the lower lobe being exposed. Note the position of this branch relative to the anterior segmental branch (upper lobe) and lingular branch. Often the superior segment branch needs to be taken separately, but it may, at times, be able to be taken in combination with the basilar trunk. **(Inset)** The superior segment branch has been ligated and divided, and the basilar trunk is now being ligated.

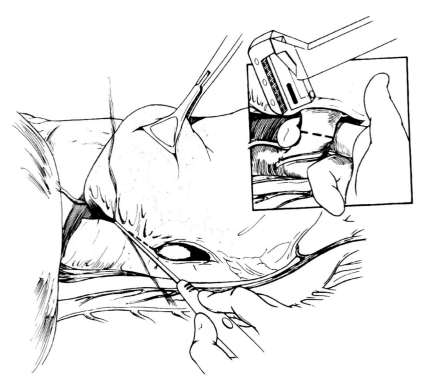

Figure 5-9. The inferior pulmonary ligament, a fibrofatty band tethering the lower lobe, is being incised with electrocautery as the lower lobe is elevated upward. The ligament is incised up to the level of the inferior pulmonary vein. **(Inset)** Once the inferior vein is dissected free it is encircled with a finger or clamp. A vascular stapler may be used to ligate the vein, or alternatively the vein may be doubly ligated or clamped, divided, and sutured closed.

trunk. Once the superior segmental branch of the artery is identified, the posterior aspect of the fissure may be completed by incising the pleura overlying the pulmonary artery posteriorly just before the artery enters the lung parenchyma. There are no branches coming off the inferior aspect of the artery posterior to the superior segment branch. This allows for placement of a linear stapler and completion of the fissure. Rarely should it be necessary to directly cut into lung parenchyma overlying the artery to complete a fissure. Likewise, the anterior aspect of the fissure may be completed with the linear stapler once the artery has been identified.

The inferior pulmonary ligament, a fibrofatty band tethering the lower lobe medially, is incised using electrocautery and divided up to the level of the inferior pulmonary vein (Fig. 5-9). The vein may be visualized from either the anterior or posterior aspect of the hilum and is encircled with a finger or right-angled clamp once the plane of dissection is entered. The vein is then ligated and divided with a vascular stapler (Fig. 5-9, inset) or clamped and sutured.

By retracting the proximal pulmonary artery stump superiorly one identifies the bronchus to the lower lobe (Fig. 5-10). The

tourniquet is placed but not cinched down. This establishes proximal control if needed, a maneuver that is much easier to carry out at this point than at a time of sudden hemorrhage if the pulmonary artery or one of its branches is entered inadvertently.

If the fissure is complete, that is, if the pulmonary artery is visible from within the fissure, dissection may begin in the fissure by incising the pleura overlying the pulmonary artery to enter the appropriate plane on the vessel (Fig. 5-8). Once this plane is reached dissection may proceed in both an anterior and a posterior direction along the artery. The superior segmental branch to the lower lobe is identified usually just opposite the anterior segmental branch of the artery to the upper lobe. This branch often needs to be divided separately depending on its location relative to the lingular branch (Fig. 5-8, inset). At times, the basal segmental trunk of the artery may be divided along with the superior segmental branch, but this is dependent on the superior segment branch coming off distal (i.e., inferior) to the take-off of the lingular branch. The artery to the lower lobe may be taken with a vascular stapler or doubly ligated. The linear endoscopic vascular stapler is ideally suited for ligation and division of the basal arterial

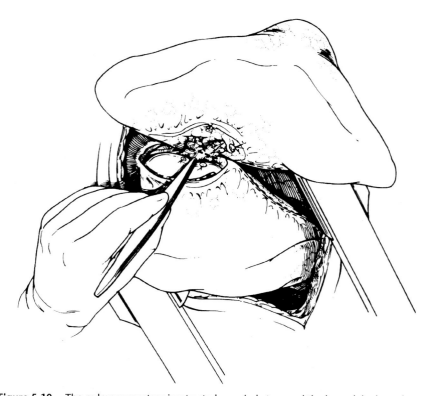

Figure 5-10. The pulmonary artery is retracted superiorly to reveal the lower lobe bronchus. The line of division (*dashed line*) is just proximal to the bifurcation between the superior segment bronchus and the basilar segmental bronchus. The line of division needs to be slightly oblique to encompass the origin of both of these. Most commonly the bronchus is closed with a stapler, but it may also be cut and sutured closed.

bifurcation of the left main bronchus will be seen with this maneuver, confirming its identity. Care must be taken to include the superior segmental bronchus with the division of the lower lobe bronchus. This may require division of the bronchus in a slightly oblique orientation, but this should be done as close as possible to the bifurcation. Identification of the lower lobe bronchus is also facilitated after division of the inferior pulmonary vein as the bronchus lies just posterior and superior to the vein. This identification may be helpful when there is lymph node involvement or tumor within the fissure making it difficult to approach the bronchus from that aspect.

A lymph node dissection is performed by taking the contents of the aortopulmonary window (level 5), the para-aortic location (level 6), and the subcarinal space (level 7). The subcarinal space is entered by retracting the lung anteriorly and incising the pleura just inferior to the left main bronchus posteriorly. Several vagal branches to the lung usually accompanied by small blood vessels are encountered that need to be clipped and divided. The contents of the subcarinal space are removed with the aid of metal clips placed on the small bronchial vessels. An inferior pulmonary ligament lymph node (level 9) is also taken. This is most often encountered as the inferior pulmonary ligament is incised and is usually found near the inferior pulmonary vein. These are the nodal levels not sampled by mediastinoscopy, and their excision completes the staging evaluation.

SUGGESTED READING

Graeber GM, Collins JJH, DeShong JL, et al. Are sutures better than staples for closing bronchi and pulmonary vessels? Ann Thorac Surg 1991;51:901.

Patterson GA, Piazza D, Pearson FG, et al. Significance of metastatic disease in subaortic lymph nodes. Ann Thorac Surg 1987;43:155.

EDITOR'S COMMENTS

This chapter nicely outlines the important technical caveats that are necessary when performing left upper or lower lobe pulmonary resection. Traction injuries to the anterior segmental branch to the upper lobe have appropriately earned this segmental branch the moniker "artery of sorrow." The intraoperative management of this complication is well described, and every thoracic surgeon should be familiar with the techniques described by Dr. Kaiser. Occasionally, the operator will notice a 2-mm to 3-mm subadventitial tear with or without a hematoma at the base of this artery. Although there is not immediate bleeding for this injury, any further retraction in a posterior-caudad direction is likely to convert that injury to the vessel into a surgical emergency. All traction on that lobe should immediately cease, and the injury should be inspected for expansion. If it remains stable, I have preferred to continue the upper lobectomy by dividing the superior pulmonary vein (if not done already) followed by the upper lobe bronchus from an anterior approach. The upper lobe bronchus can be easily identified just inferior and posterior to the lingular vein. Once divided, identification of pulmonary arterial branches within the fissure to the upper lobe can then be ligated and divided moving in an anterior-to-posterior direction. All these maneuvers can be done with little to no traction from the first assistant. The division of the upper lobe bronchus grants the operator increased flexibility in managing the bruised or injured anterior segmental artery because both proximal and distal pulmonary arterial control is now guaranteed. This "isolation maneuver" of the proximal pulmonary arterial segmental arteries is also very helpful when the proximal left pulmonary arterial branches are involved with tumor and either a pulmonary arterioplasty or formal pulmonary artery sleeve resection will be required to achieve an R_0 resection.

Although careful dissection of the station 5 and 6 lymph nodes should be done for accurate staging, it is not uncommon for there to be a pesky small bleeder in the aortopulmonary window after the dissection. The operator needs to resist any temptation to use cautery here and should also avoid clips unless the bleeding vessel is unequivocally identified. Gentle pressure with or without some topical hemostatic agents will stop almost all bleeding here and does not risk injury to the recurrent laryngeal nerve.

I.L.K.

6

Pneumonectomy

Robert Cerfolio

Pneumonectomy, defined as the removal of an entire lung, is technically one of the easiest and yet one of the riskiest operations performed in the chest. This risk is inherent to the final result of the procedure—having only one lung. Elective pneumonectomy when performed for non–small cell lung cancer (NSCLC) has an operative mortality that ranges from 3% to 12%. This is significantly higher than that for an elective coronary artery bypass grafting. Unlike other paired organs that are removed for malignancy, the lungs are unusual in the fact that a right-sided pneumonectomy has a significantly higher operative risk than one on the left. The indication for pneumonectomy affects the operative risk as well. When a pneumonectomy is performed for a destroyed lung from an inflammatory process such as tuberculosis, the reported operative mortality is higher and ranges from 3% to 30%, and the morbidity of this procedure has been quoted as high as 44%. In this chapter, I focus on pneumonectomy for NSCLC and do not discuss the specific issues and considerations of a pneumonectomy for mesothelioma, destroyed lung, or other less common clinical scenarios. Finally, because many regard a pneumonectomy as a disease in and of itself, thoracic surgeons should rarely go into an operation planning to do a pneumonectomy. More commonly, a pneumonectomy is done because there exists no other technical way to completely remove all of the cancer and achieve negative margins. Thus, pneumonectomy should most often be performed because a sleeve lobectomy will leave a positive margin for cancer. Finally, there are several different types of pneumonectomies. They will only be mentioned for completeness reasons; the description of most lies beyond the scope of this chapter.

Types of Pneumonectomies

There are several different types of pneumonectomy. These include a radical pneumonectomy, which is defined as the removal of the entire lung along with the ipsilateral pleura, hemidiaphragm, and hemipericardium. This type of operation is most commonly applied to patients with mesothelioma. Other types of pneumonectomy include completion pneumonectomy, which is removal of the entire remaining lung after a patient has had some other portion of that lung removed at a previous operation. There are also intrapericardial and extrapericardial pneumonectomies. The former is often performed for anatomic reasons such as for large central tumors. A carinal pneumonectomy refers to the removal of an entire lung and the carina as well. This requires an anastomosis between the remaining mainstem bronchus and the distal trachea. This chapter focuses on the surgical techniques of a standard pneumonectomy.

History

In 1895, Macewen performed the first multiple-stage pneumonectomy in a patient with tuberculosis and empyema. Until that time all previous attempts in humans had been unsuccessful. In 1910, Kummel performed the first pneumonectomy for lung cancer by clamping the pedicle and leaving the clamps in situ. Unfortunately, the effort was unsuccessful, and the patient died on postoperative day 6. In 1933, Graham and Singer, of St. Louis, reported the first successful removal of an entire lung for carcinoma. The operation was performed via

mass ligation of the hilar structures. However, the modern technique for pneumonectomy is attributed to Churchill. In 1930, he attempted removal of the entire lung for carcinoma. Initially he planned to mass ligate the hilum, but the tumor was very close to the hilum, necessitating individual ligation of the vessels and bronchus. Unfortunately, due to his failure to close the bronchus, the patient died 3 days later of bronchopneumonia. In 1933, Rienhoff, of Baltimore, was the first to perform a successful pneumonectomy for cancer. The patient's chest was closed postoperatively and he subsequently survived the hospitalization. Pneumonectomy then slowly became a well-established procedure thanks to these and other prominent pioneers in thoracic surgery. In fact, it became the only oncologically acceptable operation for lung cancer. Until the late 1950s and early 1960s, pneumonectomy was the standard operation for patients with lung cancer because the thinking was that only entire removal of the lung could possibly lead to cure. Subsequently, a number of studies were published that showed that lesser resections were better tolerated, offered similar survival, and had less morbidity and mortality.

Indications for Pneumonectomy

Before taking any patient to the operating room for a possible sleeve resection and/or what might turn out to be a pneumonectomy, one must carefully assess and clear the patient's pulmonary function and cardiovascular status. Often the inability to perform a lesser resection is discovered intraoperatively, so the preoperative evaluation should always include an assessment of the patient's ability to tolerate a pneumonectomy. This possibility should be discussed with the patient preoperatively. The thoracic surgeon and patient must weigh the risks and benefits of pneumonectomy, including increased morbidity and mortality and decreased exercise tolerance, against the benefit of potential cure and increased survival.

We perform a cardiac stress test and an echocardiogram on all patients. Reversible coronary artery disease is a contraindication to elective pneumonectomy; therefore a thorough evaluation of the patient's cardiac status must be undertaken. The patient should have areas of reversible myocardial ischemia revascularized and/or cardiologic clearance before elective pulmonary resection. On echocardiogram the presence of a patent foramen ovale should be known preoperatively, and significant valvular disease should be assessed and corrected if severe.

The starting pulmonary function and the extent of the planned resection help to guide the surgeon. There have been multiple studies listing lower limits of various pulmonary function study variables below which operative risks become prohibitive. These are guidelines only. Each decision must be made individually for each patient. The old teaching that the forced expiratory volume in 1 second (FEV_1) must be >800 ml after the completion of the pneumonectomy is obsolete. This old surgical dictum obviously does not take into account the size of the patient. An FEV_1 of 800 ml for a 4 foot 9 inch-tall, thin female is more than adequate. Thus, the percent predicted FEV_1 ($FEV_1\%$), which takes into account the various shapes and sizes that patients come in, is a much more precise measurement. The percent postoperative predicted ($popEV_1\%$) and percent postoperative predicted diffusion capacity of the lung for carbon monoxide ($popDLCO\%$) have been shown to be reliable predictors of postoperative morbidity and mortality. These values should be calculated with the aid of ventilation perfusion scans when patients have radiologic evidence of segmental, lobar or greater areas of atelectasis. Important studies have shown that when the $popFEV_1\%$ is <40% and the $popDLCO\%$ is <40% the operative risks are significantly increased. These values are guidelines, and each patient and each clinical situation is different. However, the presence of significant hypercapnea raises an important red flag. When the preoperative arterial blood gas, a mandatory test prior to possible pneumonectomy, shows a partial arterial carbon dioxide pressure of ≥48 mm Hg the operative risk becomes significant. However, the

surgeon and patient again must decide together in the clinic before surgery what will be done if a sleeve resection with parenchymal conservation is not technically feasible or if after the completion of a sleeve resection there is a positive margin that remains.

Finally, because a pneumonectomy is associated with a higher perioperative risk than a lobectomy, certain oncologic principles need to be considered. We believe that in general the presence of residual or recalcitrant N2 disease (after neoadjuvant therapy for biopsy-proven N2 disease) is an absolute contraindication for pneumonectomy (except in certain young patients with high $popFEV_1\%$ and $popDLCO\%$ or those who are having significant hemoptysis, etc.). After the decision has been made to perform a sleeve lobectomy or pneumonectomy the operation should follow certain principles and have a certain sequence.

The Surgical Procedure: Right-Sided Pneumonectomy

Despite the fact there have been vast improvements in the field of general thoracic surgery and anesthesia, a pneumonectomy done today is not much different from one done 30 years ago, except perhaps for the advent of stapling devices. After the careful preoperative staging with the use of integrated positron emission tomography (PET)/computed tomography (CT) scan and CT scan along with careful clearance of the cardiopulmonary system and the elimination of N2 disease via the use of mediastinoscopy, transesophageal ultrasound with fine-needle aspirate, and videoassisted thoracic surgery (VATS), a patient is finally prepared for pneumonectomy. Preoperative bronchoscopy is performed, and occasionally that alone can tell a surgeon that a pneumonectomy is required to achieve an R0 (negative margin) complete resection. If a lesion is attached (not into, but attached) to the right proximal bronchial wall and one is able to get distal to it with the bronchoscope and it continues as one contiguous lesion down into the bronchus intermedius and into the right lower lobe, then one must do a right pneumonectomy. One must be sure that it is not a tumor thrombus coming out of the right lower lobe bronchus but rather is adherent to the mainstem wall. Similarly, if a lesion is quite large and involves the main pulmonary artery on the right and courses distally involving branches of

the basilar pulmonary artery, a right pneumonectomy is required. Otherwise, in the vast majority of patients, a sleeve resection should be planned, and the decision to do a pneumonectomy is not made on preoperative bronchoscopy but rather on surgical exploration.

After the preoperative bronchoscopy the appropriate devices are placed: an epidural catheter (placed before induction of anesthesia), a double-lumen left endobronchial tube (placed by the surgeon if there is a large and/or bloody lesion in the proximal airway to avoid any blood from spilling into the soon-to-be-only lung), an arterial line, a central venous catheter, a warming blanket, and serial compression devices on the legs. The patient is turned onto the left lateral decubitus position with the right chest up, carefully padded, and secured to the table. There are several possible surgical approaches including a median sternotomy, vertical axillary thoracotomy, and so on, but we will focus on the most common approach for a pneumonectomy, the posterolateral thoracotomy. This can be performed in several ways as well, but we prefer cutting about half of the posterior aspect of the latissimus dorsi muscle, sparing all of the serratus anterior muscle and entering the chest over the uncut, unshingled, and unbroken sixth rib. We also strongly believe that an intercostal muscle flap should be harvested in any patient who is going to undergo a sleeve lobectomy or possible pneumonectomy (as shown in Fig. 6-1) for coverage of the bronchial stump or protection of the anastomosis. We have shown its usefulness in >400 patients. It should be harvested or mobilized with cautery dissection before the placement of a chest retractor. This provides a well-vascularized, soft, pliable muscle that is free of periosteum. It does not calcify over time when harvested in this manner. It can reach to buttress any bronchial stump or anastomosis, and it can help separate suture line between sleeved pulmonary artery and/or bronchus. The muscle can be interposed in between these structures to separate them. It should not be circumferentially wrapped around any anastomosis. It only takes 3 to 4 minutes to mobilize, and we have also shown in a prospective, randomized trial that it also decreases the pain of thoracotomy. If a sleeve resection is not performed, the muscle pedicle can then be tacked to the bronchial stump with the use of interrupted 3-0 double-armed Prolene sutures as shown in Fig. 6-2.

Once the retractor is placed, the chest is explored. The operation should be conducted like any other cancer operation. The

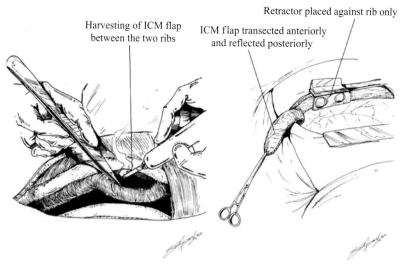

Harvesting of ICM flap
between the two ribs

ICM flap transected anteriorly
and reflected posteriorly

Retractor placed against rib only

Figure 6-1. Harvesting of an intercostal muscle (ICM) off of the inferior aspect of the sixth rib and carefully off of the top bottom part of the fifth rib using a cautery so it is devoid of periosteum.

chest is carefully inspected to rule out pleural effusions that could be consistent with T4 disease, metastatic nodules on the pleura or diaphragm that could represent M1 disease, or previously nonimaged pulmonary nodules. We prefer to remove all the mediastinal lymph nodes and perform a complete thoracic lymphadenectomy as opposed to just a sampling procedure. If any of the mediastinal lymph nodes look or feel suspicious or were imaged by CT and/or integrated fluorine-18 fluorodeoxyglucose (FDG)-PET-CT as suspicious and were not ruled out as harboring cancer prior to thoracotomy, frozen-section analysis should be performed. Once the decision has been made that resection is the appropriate option, the lung is retracted posterior and the anterior hilum is exposed. The overlying pleural is incised posterior to the phrenic

nerve. The superior pulmonary vein and the inferior pulmonary vein are dissected free. Lymph nodes from this area are removed, and the small veins that lead to the phrenic nerve are carefully coagulated so as not to injure the nerve. An intact phrenic nerve is best even if a pneumonectomy is performed because a paralyzed hemidiaphragm causes some degree of dysfunction to the contralateral diaphragm as well. In rare situations there is only one right pulmonary vein. This makes a sleeve resection more difficult if not impossible because the blood has to be baffled back into the left atrium. The inferior pulmonary ligament should have already been released during the inspection phase and to adequately remove the inferior ligament (level 9) and periesophageal (level 8) lymph nodes. The inferior pulmonary vein is then easily encircled with an index finger as shown in Fig. 6-3. If the subcarinal nodes have been completely removed, this move is somewhat easier because the finger is placed between the superior pulmonary vein and middle lobe vein and then comes around the vein and anterior to the right mainstem bronchus. We prefer placing a vessel loop around the vein. Dissection is then carried out anteriorly and more superiorly. Because a sleeve resection is usually attempted first, we often isolate the superior pulmonary vein next, depending on the size and location of the tumor, and usually remove the hilar and segmental lymph nodes. Very commonly, there is a large hilar lymph node that interdigitates between the superior aspect of the superior pulmonary vein and the main pulmonary artery just as it courses distally posterior to the superior vena cava. If one is able to completely remove this large node N1 node, the course of the distal main pulmonary artery becomes visible. This makes encircling the superior pulmonary vein safer and easier. The vein is carefully encircled around its posterior aspect so as not to injure the main pulmonary artery that runs just posterior to it. If the tumor is large, the pulmonary artery may have to be controlled first and encircled before the superior pulmonary vein. Sometimes, the pericardium may also have to be opened to do this. It should be opened away from the phrenic nerve, which must be visualized and spared. The advantage of opening the pericardium is that it allows central inspection of resectability and it makes proximal control of the vessels easier. However, it may increase the incidence of atrial fibrillation. A finger is then used to encircle the main pulmonary artery and the superior pulmonary vein, and once this is accomplished all the vasculature has been controlled. This entire

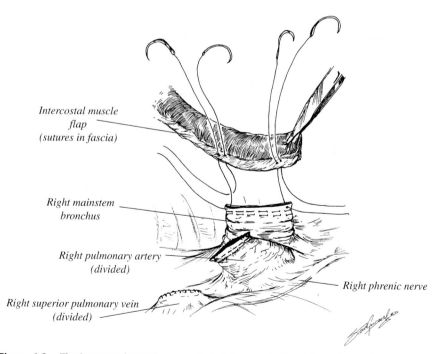

Intercostal muscle flap
(sutures in fascia)

Right mainstem bronchus

Right pulmonary artery
(divided)

Right superior pulmonary vein
(divided)

Right phrenic nerve

Figure 6-2. The intercostal muscle is parachuted down onto the right mainstem bronchi for coverage. Note the small bites on the bronchus that are taken distal to the staple line so as not to injure its blood supply. Note that the muscular aspect of the flap is brought down onto the right mainstem bronchus.

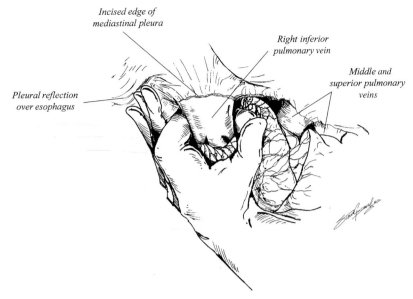

*Incised edge of
mediastinal pleura*

*Pleural reflection
over esophagus*

*Right inferior
pulmonary vein*

*Middle and
superior pulmonary
veins*

Figure 6-3.   A finger is placed around the right inferior pulmonary vein, and it is encircled.

process may only take 30 to 40 minutes, and if one knows early on that a pneumonectomy is needed, the entire operation often takes <1 hour.

The sequence of ligation of the hilar structures is highly dependent on the position of the lesion and the surgeon's preferences. Before taking any vessels, we have shown in a nonrandomized, but prospective trial that giving 250 mg of Solu-Medrol may help to prevent the complication of post-pneumonectomy pulmonary edema. Thus we recommend giving this 5 to 10 minutes before ligating the vessels. One should also test clamp the pulmonary artery for 1 to 2 minutes and ensure that the patient's hemodynamics tolerates the shunting of all of the pulmonary blood supply into the left lung. If the patient's blood pressure drops quickly and if the clamp or the fingers/hand used to clamp the pulmonary artery is not compressing the heart, this suggests that the patient will not tolerate a pneumonectomy. This move should be repeated several times, and if it continues to occur, the vessels should not be taken and the operation should be aborted. This is a very rare occurrence but is a final check of the patient's suitability for pneumonectomy. In this situation, despite the careful preoperative evaluation that suggested that the patient was a candidate for pneumonectomy, the procedure cannot be carried out.

There are few data that document the advantage or disadvantage of taking the vein prior to the artery. Kurusu reported an oncologic advantage in taking the vein before the artery because it may prevent the accidental dislodgement of cancer cells into

the systemic circulation during the manipulation and dissection of the tumor. Others believe that there is less blood lost in the removed lung when the vein is taken after the artery. There is no data to support these latter claims. The vessels can also be ligated in several different ways. We prefer to take the vein with a vascular stapler that staples and cuts simultaneously, but prefer to take the artery with a vascular stapler that staples only. The staplers disperse the closure of the vessel over its entire length as opposed to bunching it up into one suture ligature. Another method involves clamping the artery, cutting, and then oversewing the end with a running, nonabsorbable monofilament suture along its length. This obviously takes longer to do.

Once the vessels have been taken, the bronchus is the only remaining structure that is keeping the lung in vivo. We do not like to take the bronchus first on a right or left pneumonectomy as we often do on a right upper lobectomy because it is easier to provide a short stump if it is taken last. However, on the right side the bronchus can be taken before the vessels if needed. It can make the dissection easier for large anterior tumors that are too big to allow for anterior dissection of the hilar structures. It can be taken with a knife or a stapler (we use 4.8-cm-long staples) before the artery or veins are divided. If it is taken with a knife, one can visualize the trachea and ensure the position of the double-lumen tube. If it is taken with a stapler, one should ask the anesthesiologist to inflate and then deflate the balloon on the tracheal cuff side after closing the stapler but before firing the instrument

to ensure that it does not have the tracheal balloon of the double-lumen tube. Either way, a short stump is a crucial and mandatory part of a successful right pneumonectomy.

We divide the azygous vein first with a vascular stapler before stapling the right mainstem bronchus. One must ensure the central venous line is not in the azygous vein. It is usually very easy to see the blue tip of the central line in the superior vena cava or even in the azygous vein. In rare situations when an intercostal muscle is not available and if there is no pericardial fat pad, the azygous vein can be used as a form of bronchial coverage. This is accomplished by dividing the vein as far posteriorly as possible and then ligating the other end tied flush against the cava. The vein is cut as distally as possible, and this provides a long flap of a defunctionalized vein that can be split and used to cover the right mainstem bronchus. We frequently use this technique for a radical pneumonectomy for mesothelioma because the intercostal muscle is not useable because it may be contaminated with tumor cells. It is important to note that a pleural flap does not provide adequate coverage because it is paper thin and is often dead within 48 hours after surgery.

Once the vessels and the azygous have been ligated and divided the bronchus is taken last. The lung is retracted and pulled downward so the right mainstem bronchus is exposed. If all of the subcarinal lymph nodes have been removed and the large bronchial artery that comes from the undersurface of the carina to the subcarinal nodes has been clipped, the left mainstem bronchus is already exposed. A stapler is placed (more easily on the right than on the left because of the absence of the aortic arch on the right in most patients). It is placed so that it is flush against the trachea, and then the staples are fired. As described previously, one must ensure that there are no parts of the double-lumen tube in the staple line and that no suction catheters are within the bronchus before stapling and cutting. Although there is some literature about hand sewing the bronchus, there are no data that suggest that one technique is better than the other. We recommend the stapling technique. The specimen is then removed.

The bronchial margin should be sent for frozen-section analysis, as should the artery or vein margin if the tumor is close. The chest is then filled with warm water, not saline. We prefer the former because of the oncologic possibility that it may lyse tumor cells that are floating in the chest. In addition, it is easier to see through it than through saline, so it is easier to check the stump for a leak. The double-lumen tube should now be opened to both chests, and the stump should be tested. If any bronchial leaks are noted, interrupted sutures are placed under it in a vertical mattress fashion with knots opposite the pulmonary artery. It should be interrogated again until there is no stump leak. The intercostal muscle flap is then parachuted down to cover the entire bronchus (as shown in Fig. 6-2). The sutures that are placed in the bronchus should be small superficial bites so as not to injure the stump or its blood supply. The entire stump is covered. We have used this method to cover the bronchus after lobectomy and mainstem bronchus after pneumonectomy in >500 patients, including >100 who have had preoperative radiation, and have had only 2 bronchopleural fistulas.

We prefer placing a chest tube to monitor postoperative bleeding. The best way to handle the postpneumonectomized space has never been described. Some surgeons recommend aspirating the air with a syringe after the chest has been closed to set the mediastinum, just prior to leaving the operating room. Others recommend placing a chest tube and then rolling the patient on his or her back after the operation is completed and then removing it prior to going to the recovery room. We prefer leaving it in overnight on water-seal only to assess for postoperative bleeding. We attach it to a conventional pleural drainage system and place a sign on it that reads "NO SUCTION." This avoids errors postoperatively. A special "pneumonectomy" balanced drainage system is also available.

After a pneumonectomy the mediastinum shifts over time toward the operated side, and this shift can cause serious problems, specifically the rare postpneumonectomy syndrome, which is described later in this chapter. We believe that it is best to have the trachea just to the left of the midline after a right pneumonectomy because the remaining left lung will slowly displace the trachea toward the pneumonectomized right side over time.

The chest is closed after the placement of a chest tube using intracostal sutures to decrease pain as shown in Fig. 6-4.

The Surgical Procedure: Left-Sided Pneumonectomy

The oncologic and physiologic principles for a left pneumonectomy are the same

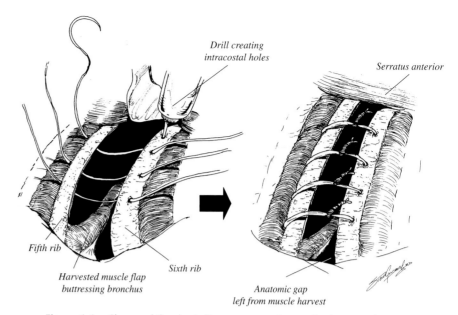

Figure 6-4. Closure of the chest after pneumonectomy using intracostal sutures.

as for one on the right. However, because the anatomy is different, some special considerations must be mentioned. The pulmonary artery on the left is shorter than that on the right. The ligamentum arteriosum tethers the left main pulmonary artery. This structure can be divided, but this technique, which is necessary for a left mainstem bronchial sleeve resection, is not needed for a standard left pneumonectomy. It should be avoided because the left recurrent laryngeal nerve is wrapped around this structure and may be injured when the ligamentum is divided. Because of the shorter pulmonary artery on the left, intrapericardial dissection is more commonly needed on the left than on the right. Because most patients with NSCLC are elderly smokers, many have had previous coronary artery bypass grafting. Care must be taken to avoid injuring the left internal mammary artery and the vein grafts when dividing adhesions to free up the lung before a left pulmonary resection, and in addition the distal aspect of the grafts must be avoided when entering the pericardial space.

After the decision has been made that a left pneumonectomy is indicated (the patient is mediastinal lymph node–negative, a sleeve resection is not possible, etc.) the dissection starts, as on the right, with the anterior hilar structures by incising the pleura reflection. The avascular plane between the pleural reflection and the pericardium is dissected, and the inferior and superior pulmonary veins are identified. Again, the phrenic nerve must be avoided. As described for the right side, the inferior pulmonary

ligament is released and the inferior pulmonary ligament lymph nodes are removed. The periesophageal and the subcarinal lymph nodes are also removed and assessed. If this is done, it is easy to get a finger between the inferior pulmonary vein and the left mainstem bronchus and encircle the inferior pulmonary vein with a vessel loop (as shown in Fig. 6-5). A finger can be used to get around the superior pulmonary vein as well, but before this is done, the edges of the vein must first be dissected free. Care must be taken when dissecting between the superior edge of the pulmonary vein and the inferior border of the left main pulmonary artery to avoid the anterior-apical trunk of the left pulmonary artery. In addition, the superior pulmonary vein lies superior in relation to the left mainstem bronchus. Large proximal endobronchial tumors with extraluminal disease can present a difficult problem when encircling the vein. Occasionally the bronchus can be taken first. However, on the left side especially, we prefer taking the bronchus last because it is much more difficult to achieve a short stump on the left than on the right. This is because the aortic arch obstructs access to the tracheobronchial angle. Once the superior pulmonary vein is encircled (as shown in Fig. 6-6), a loop is placed around it. The pulmonary artery is controlled just distal to the ligamentum arteriosum by dissecting its edges free. The index or middle finger can be placed around it, and the vessel is encircled. It should be test clamped and the patient's hemodynamics observed as described on the right side. Once all three vessels are encircled we favor

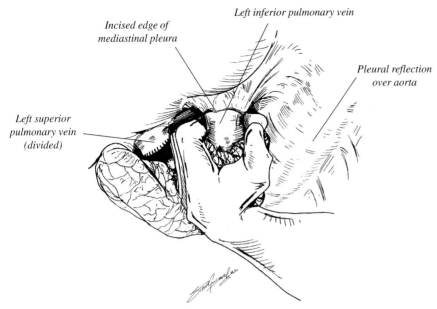

Figure 6-5. A finger is placed around the left inferior pulmonary vein, and it is encircled.

giving 250 mg of intravenous Solu-Medrol and test clamping the artery as described previously. The veins and artery are taken as described for the right side, leaving the left mainstem bronchus.

Probably the biggest difference between a right and a left pneumonectomy is the position and length of the bronchus. The mainstem bronchus is longer on the left than it is on the right. Because the vast majority of patients have a left-sided aorta, it is more difficult to achieve a short bronchial stump on the left than on the right. A short mainstem bronchial stump is a mandatory part of a pneumonectomy. It keeps the incidence of a bronchopleural fistula low by preventing the pooling of secretions. The best technique involves pulling the lung up and aggressively retracting it out of the chest. To do this, the pericardial reflection must be taken off of the left mainstem bronchus. Often there may be part of a subcarinal lymph node left that was not completely removed in the lymphadenectomy portion of the case. The remainder of that node should now be removed, and eventually the left mainstem

bronchus is visible. Care must be taken on the left side, as on the right, not to injure the opposite-side bronchus. The tracheal balloon of the double-lumen tube can distend the membranous part of the opposite mainstem bronchus, which is paper thin. This can be injured as the subcarinal node is swept off of the opposite mainstem bronchus. Once the entire left mainstem bronchus is seen and its junction with the trachea is visible a stapler (4.8-mm staples) is carefully slid under the aortic arch. The assistant must aggressively pull the lung out of the wound to provide the best access to the proximal left mainstem bronchus. The stapler is fired, the bronchus is cut, and the specimen is removed. As described for the right side, the bronchial margin should be checked on frozen section and the stump checked for a leak with a water submersion test. When taken properly the left mainstem bronchus will immediately retract well under the aortic arch. It should be difficult to see, and it should be covered by the surrounding mediastinal structures. This reduced exposure is probably a factor in the lower incidence of a bronchopleural fistula on the left compared to the right. We still recommend coverage with an intercostal muscle flap. To place these sutures in this short, retracted stump, one must retract the arch back carefully and avoid the pulmonary artery as well. Coverage is not as critical an issue on the left as on the right, but we prefer to cover the bronchi on both sides with an intercostal muscle flap. The chest is closed after the placement of a chest tube using intracostal sutures to decrease pain. Although the operation is often straightforward, the postoperative course can be difficult. Keys to successful outcomes include minimal amounts of intravenous fluid, strict aspiration precautions, and aggressive pulmonary and cardiophysiotherapy.

Management of Common Complications after Pneumonectomy

Vocal Cord Dysfunction

Because of their anatomic location around the aortic arch, the left vagus and recurrent laryngeal nerves can be invaded by intrathoracic malignant neoplasms. For the same reason these nerves can be injured or severed while isolating the hilum during lung resection or mediastinal lymph node dissection. However, this should rarely, if ever, occur. The right recurrent laryngeal nerve is also at risk during extensive mediastinal lymph

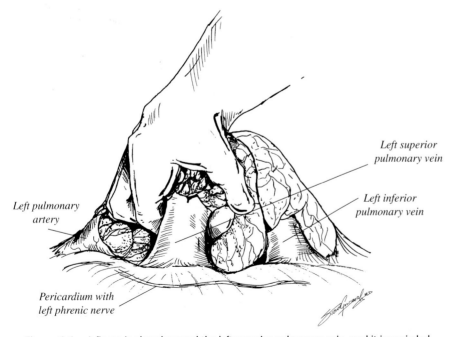

Figure 6-6. A finger is placed around the left superior pulmonary vein, and it is encircled.

node dissection up to the subclavian artery because of its close association with the right subclavian artery.

Vocal cord dysfunction has been reported to occur in about one third of patients after left lung resection and mediastinal lymph node dissection for cancer. The reported incidence rate of vocal cord paralysis after thoracic interventions is wide, ranging from 4% to 31% for postoperative recurrent laryngeal nerve paralysis after primary thoracic cancer surgery. However, surgical injury to the left or right recurrent nerve is extremely rare. There is also an increased morbidity because recurrent laryngeal nerve and vagus nerve injuries are associated with increased rate of reintubation, arrhythmias, and aspiration. Risk factors for recurrent nerve injury and vocal cord dysfunction include preoperative radiotherapy, left pneumonectomy, and pericardiotomy.

Mechanism of injury varies and can be caused by heat, stretch devascularization, or direct transection. Heat injuries usually result from using the electrocautery for hemostasis in the vicinity of the nerve. Stretching of the nerve causing neuropraxia occurs while dissecting out the hilum, especially when associated with a hilar tumor. The perineural vascular supply is delicate and can be injured easily during dissection. The anterior terminal branch of the recurrent laryngeal nerve, designated as the motor branch, is located laterally, a position that makes it particularly vulnerable to surgical wound or trauma.

Symptoms of recurrent laryngeal nerve injury on either side include hoarseness, aspiration, poor cough, and dysphagia. Diagnosis is made based on symptoms. When symptoms become apparent, a laryngeal examination should be done to confirm the diagnosis and prevent the consequences such as aspiration, bronchial obstruction, pneumonia, and reintubation. At laryngoscopy, recurrent laryngeal nerve paralysis results in location of the vocal fold in a nonmedian position and causes incomplete glottic closure. Treatment varies depending on the extent of injury. Patience is usually best because most injuries are not secondary to severing the nerve. The surgeon is usually aware if the nerve had to be cut to remove the tumor. If the nerve is intact, the edema will usually resolve in several weeks and the voice will return to normal. If the nerve has been severed, then medialization thyroplasty is indicated. If the nerve is preserved, then most clinicians would recommend waiting 6 months between the time of resection and medialization thyroplasty. During that time functional voice and swallowing therapy is

indicated. Occasionally these patients will regain function of their recurrent laryngeal nerve with no need for further therapy.

Arrhythmias

Arrhythmias after pulmonary resections continue to be a frustrating and common problem, with atrial arrhythmias most common. The incidence has been reported to range from 5% to as high as 40% after pneumonectomy depending on how closely the patients are monitored and how the condition is defined. Atrial fibrillation (AF) is by far the most common arrhythmia associated with pulmonary resection and has an incidence ranging from 10% to 20% after lobectomy to 40% after pneumonectomy. Supraventricular tachycardia (SVT) and ventricular tachycardia (VT) are much less frequent than AF. The incidence of SVT after pneumonectomy is reported to be between 13% and 26%. Most arrhythmias occur within the first 2 to 3 days after surgery and rarely after postoperative day 5. The incidence is higher if an intrapericardial dissection was required for resection of the tumor.

The etiology of these arrhythmias is poorly defined. Some studies have shown that an increase in right heart pressure and an increase in pulmonary vascular resistance predispose a patient to clinically significant arrhythmias. Factors that have been associated with postoperative arrhythmias after noncardiac thoracic surgery include hypoxia, intrapericardial dissection, pericardial manipulation, vagal irritation, pulmonary hypertension, older age, and preexisting cardiac or pulmonary disease. The prognostic significance of arrhythmias, especially AF, is difficult to determine because they are often associated with other, more serious cardiac or pulmonary complications. Studies have shown no differences in mortality between patients who develop AF not associated with other complications who were appropriately treated following noncardiac thoracic surgery than in those patients who maintain normal sinus rhythm. The fact remains that prevention of postoperative arrhythmia complications helps to decrease postoperative morbidity and reduce hospital costs and length of admissions as well as readmission rates.

The data suggest that prophylactic use of an antiarrhythmic drug perioperatively can decrease the incidence of AF in patients undergoing pneumonectomy. Historically, digoxin has been used to prevent and treat arrhythmias after noncardiac thoracic

surgery; however, there have been multiple randomized, controlled trials demonstrating minimal to no effect. Prophylactic betablocker administration has been shown in some studies to be effective in both prevention and treatment of postoperative AF, but its use after a pneumonectomy may not be best. Amiodarone has been proposed for prophylaxis and is currently used by many to treat AF and SVT. A prospective trial using intravenous amiodarone following pulmonary surgery to prevent SVT was halted due to the increased incidence of acute respiratory distress syndrome (ARDS) after pneumonectomy. There have been other studies, however, showing that prophylactic use of oral amiodarone resulted in a decrease in the incidence of SVT after pulmonary resection when compared to placebo with no reported increase in ARDS. Magnesium sulfate infusion postoperatively was shown in one randomized trial to be an effective agent in reducing the incidence of AF versus no treatment. The most commonly used drugs at this time for both prophylaxis and treatment of AF/SVT are calcium-channel blockers. We prefer a calcium-channel blocker, specifically diltiazem. Diltiazem has been shown in multiple studies to decrease the incidence of postoperative AF/SVT after pulmonary surgery when given both orally and intravenously. In a randomized, controlled trial by Amar it was shown that postoperative SVT occurred significantly less in the diltiazem-treated group versus the group given placebo. Specifically, a standard intravenous dose is given postoperatively on the day of surgery and subsequently converted to oral dosing on postoperative day 1. This regimen was shown to decrease the incidence of arrhythmias to 15% versus 25% in placebo patients, and another study had results of 14% versus 31% in those treated with digoxin. When a patient has any sign of an arrhythmia, underlying causes such as hypoxia, electrolyte abnormalities, and even silent myocardial ischemia must be ruled out. Symptomatic arrhythmias must be taken seriously and cardioverted when necessary. If the arrhythmia continues for >48 hours, the risks and benefits of anticoagulation and/or chemical or electrical conversion should be considered.

Postpneumonectomy Pulmonary Edema

Postpneumonectomy pulmonary edema (PPE) was first described by Gibbon in 1942 but not extensively covered in the literature until almost 40 years later. PPE is a dreaded complication that has no real consensus for its definition or prevention. It is reported to occur most often between 12 and 96 hours postoperatively and can be confused or occur in combination with any of the following: congestive heart failure, pulmonary thromboemboli or ARDS due to sepsis, pneumonia, and aspiration; all of these make PPE a diagnosis of exclusion. Most authors agree that to confirm a diagnosis, a patient must show progressive and refractory hypoxia, pulmonary edema on chest radiograph, and widened alveolar-to-arterial oxygen gradient after lung resection, usually pneumonectomy (but also reported after lobectomy and bilobectomy).

The incidence of this severe complication varies in the literature due to a lack of a consensus definition. Reported incidence of PPE after pneumonectomy is from 4% to 7% and after lobectomy 1% to 7%, but it may be as high as 12% to 15% according to authors who include mild cases. The reported mortality also varies but is uniformly high, ranging from 50% to 75% and even 100% in a few studies. Risk factors are variable but generally include perioperative transfusion (result of an immunologic reaction similar to transfusion-related lung injury, TRALI reaction), higher ventilation pressures intraoperatively, right pneumonectomy (reportedly a result of poor lymphatic drainage), perioperative fluid overload, older age, poor perioperative lung function, pre-existing cardiac disease, extensive lymphadenectomy, neoadjuvant therapy, and the hyperoxia, volotrauma, and hyperinflation associated with one-lung ventilation.

Histologic changes in PPE are almost identical to those that are well described in ARDS, prompting some authors to suggest that they are one and the same. Initially the endothelial integrity is lost with resulting extravasation and hemorrhage. Type I pneumocytes undergo necrosis, and platelet/fibrin microthrombi form. After about 5 days organization and repair begins with the proliferation of fibroblasts and type II pneumocytes. Also during this time squamous metaplasia of the epithelium begins, as well as hyaline membrane formation. Interstitial and alveolar fibrosis occurs at 10 days with widespread thrombotic, fibroproliferative, and obliterative changes occurring, as well as extensive remodeling of the pulmonary vascular bed. As the process continues past 14 days, collagen deposition dominates the remainder of the disease process through its course.

At times despite careful preoperative planning, intraoperative technique, and postoperative management, postpneumonectomy pulmonary edema occurs. When it does occur, treatment is at best difficult and resource consuming. The successful use of nitric oxide been reported. A precise mechanism, even with the knowledge of the histology, has never been clearly delineated, making prevention and prediction almost impossible. Treatment traditionally consists of fluid restriction, diuretics, and ventilator support. Similar to ARDS patients, PPE patients benefit from sedation and paralysis to improve oxygenation. Attempts should be made to keep peak airway pressures as low as possible using pressure-controlled ventilation and permissive hypercapnea. Positive end-expiratory pressure should also be used to keep the inspired oxygen concentration as low as possible.

The key to treatment is prevention. We described previously the use of Solu-Medrol before pulmonary artery clamping. This assumes that the steroid bolus helps to reduce the ongoing and subsequent inflammatory cascade caused by the manipulation of the lung and sudden shift in pulmonary blood flow. Although these data are very interesting, there have been no large prospective, randomized trials that either prove or disprove the utility of this intervention or elucidate potential complications.

Chylothorax

Chylothorax is a very uncommon complication after pneumonectomy. It is often avoidable with careful operative planning and intraoperative technique. It is an extremely difficult diagnosis to make after a pneumonectomy because one expects the pneumonectomized space to fill with fluid and one is reluctant to perform a thoracentesis after pneumonectomy for fear of iatrogenically infecting that space. The diagnosis should be considered when a patient returns with a significant mediastinal shift toward the nonoperated side instead of toward the pneumonectomized side. A thoracentesis will yield chylous (milky) fluid, and the diagnosis is confirmed by the presence of chylomicrons and a triglyceride content of ≥ 110 mg/dl, a lymphocyte count >90% of the total white blood cell count, and a total protein concentration approaching that of plasma. The medical history is usually not predictive. There are reports suggesting that a history of cirrhosis increases the risk secondary to the increased rate of flow in the lymphatics of the liver and the thoracic duct. Other risk factors have been identified including gross mediastinal lymph node disease, radical mediastinal lymphadenectomy, and pleural flap elevation along the thoracic aorta.

Chylothorax is often caused by leaking lymphatic ducts from dissection of lymph nodes that are malignant. However, even with complete thoracic lymphadenectomy, which we recommend, the incidence of chylothorax is very low. As opposed to esophageal resections, chylothorax after pulmonary resections, including pneumonectomy, is mainly due to injury to collaterals of the thoracic duct and is rarely due to injury to the main thoracic duct itself. Those patients with N2 disease, especially with extracapsular N2 disease, carry an increased risk of developing a chylothorax, likely due to the obstruction of lymphatic channels by metastatic disease. The mortality rate in the literature after iatrogenic/traumatic chylothoraces ranges from 4.5% to 10%.

Chylothoraces occur more often on the right side. This is explained both pathologically and anatomically. Bronchogenic carcinomas occur more often on the right side (ratio of 6:4), thus leading to more frequent mediastinal lymph node dissections on the right. Anatomically, the lymphatic drainage of the lungs predominates in the right chest for two reasons: (1) the right lung is larger and (2) the lymph flow to the right paratracheal nodes from the left lung is greater than the lymph flow from the right lung to the left paratracheal nodes.

Initial management of iatrogenic chylothorax following pulmonary resection is predominately conservative, using medium-chain triglyceride diets or occasionally total parenteral nutrition, as well as drainage via tube thoracostomy. There are a few nonsurgical treatments that have been reported for a chylothorax that does not close with conservative measures. Lymphangiography can be used for both diagnostic and anatomic detail. There are some studies that report spontaneous closure of the defect after the procedure due to the beneficial effects of the iodinated contrast on the laceration (if small). Percutaneous catheterization of the thoracic duct with embolization of the defect has also been reported. Pleuroperitoneal shunting has been used permitting reabsorption of the chyle by the peritoneum; this procedure makes documenting closure of the defect difficult, however, and is mainly reserved for postoperative pediatric patients and cases of nontraumatic malignant chylothoraces.

Surgical management is reserved for those patients who fail conservative measures. Prolonged drainage of a chylothorax leads to neutropenia and carries significant morbidity. Re-exploration via thoracotomy and pledgeted sutured ligation of the main duct with fibrin glue placement over the duct is best. The main duct can also be ligated via a laparotomy or laparoscopic approach. No matter what treatment is used, the thoracic surgeon must be aware of the potential for severe protein malnutrition, dehydration, and immune deficiency due to large losses of lymphatic constituents because the daily volume of the thoracic duct can approach 3 liters. Prompt treatment is necessary after diagnosis, and aggressive fluid and nutritional monitoring must be instituted. If conservative measures do not result in sealing of the leak within 5 to 7 days and if the output remains high (>800 mL/day), surgical ligation of the duct is best.

Pulmonary Embolism

Patients with malignant disease frequently suffer from coagulation abnormalities causing deep venous thrombosis and thromboembolic events despite normal routine clotting tests. The reduction in the cross-sectional area of the pulmonary arterial bed after lung resection may increase that risk. Patients who have had a pneumonectomy are at higher risk because they often suffer from more advanced-stage tumors, a higher reduction in cross-sectional area of the pulmonary arteries, and the potential for cross-embolization from the ipsilateral pulmonary artery stump when it has been left too long, predisposing it to thrombus formation.

Pulmonary thromboembolism (PTE) complicates as many as 30% of major general surgical procedures and is the cause of death in 3% of patients after orthopedic procedures. Up to 14% of thoracic surgical patients develop postoperative deep venous thrombosis, which is the most common source of PTE. The reported mortality rate is as high as 80% after pulmonary resection.

Several factors increase the risk for PTE after pneumonectomy, and they include age >50 years, patients who have been immobile before and after surgery, those with bronchogenic carcinoma, particularly adenocarcinoma cell type, large primary tumor, advanced stage, and the lack of prophylactic measures. Patients requiring pulmonary resection possess many of the traditional risk factors predisposing them to PTE and are theoretically likely to suffer more-severe symptoms. Because of the often vague and nonspecific nature of the symptoms, many patients remain undiagnosed after pneumonectomy. A high index of suspicion is needed. Symptoms are often attributed to

more common complications such as bronchospasm, atelectasis, pulmonary edema, and pulmonary insufficiency.

The diagnosis of a PTE can be made by several different modalities including ventilation-perfusion scanning, helical CT scan, and echocardiography. The gold standard is, of course, pulmonary angiography; however, this is often excluded secondary to the rapid clinical deterioration of these patients and the contrast load. Treatment of a clinically significant PTE varies depending on symptoms. Thrombolysis is recommended in cases of subtotal PTE with systemic or pulmonary artery catheter administration of thrombolytic agent. This obviously carries an increased risk of hemorrhagic complications. In cases of clinically significant PTE postoperatively, systemic anticoagulation is also advocated as a less risky alternative to thrombolysis with only limited success, mainly in patients with multiple small emboli.

Bronchopleural Fistula and Empyema

Postpneumonectomy bronchopleural fistula (BPF) is defined as a communication between the mainstem bronchial stump after a pneumonectomy and the ipsilateral pleural space. It is a life-threatening problem because infected material can be aspirated into the only remaining lung. It is by definition associated with a postpneumonectomy empyema. A postpneumonectomy empyema is defined as the presence of purulent material in the postpneumonectomy space and is usually but not always associated with a BPF. When it occurs within the first 6 months after a pneumonectomy there commonly is a BPF associated with it. Early recognition and aggressive treatment with reoperation are the keys to survival.

The overall incidence of BPF and empyema is greater after pneumonectomy than after lesser resections. After pneumonectomy for any reason, the incidence of BPF/empyema ranges from 2% to 16%. When stratified by disease state, the incidence rates for empyema and BPF after pneumonectomy for primary lung cancer are 5.8% and 4.1%, for metastatic disease 3.1% and <1%, and for benign disease 24% and 9.9%, respectively. When it occurs, BPF increases the mortality rate for pneumonectomy significantly, ranging from 30% to 50%. In the lung cancer literature one can also see an increasing incidence of BPF after pneumonectomy with the use of neoadjuvant treatments. Most data

indicate that there is also an increase in both cardiac and pulmonary complications and obviously increased hospital stay and costs after the occurrence of a BPF. Multiple studies have identified both local and systemic factors that are associated with the development of empyemas and/or BPF after pulmonary resections.

Local factors include the following:

1. Presence of carcinoma at the bronchial margin
2. Long bronchial stump
3. Disrupted bronchial blood supply
4. Technique of stump closure (controversial)
5. Pre-existing empyema
6. Extended resections
7. Preoperative radiation
8. Postoperative need for mechanical ventilation
9. Right versus left pneumonectomy

Systemic factors include the following:

1. Poor nutritional status
2. Diabetes
3. Sepsis
4. Preoperative chemotherapy
5. Underlying lung disease (including chronic infection and chronic obstructive pulmonary disease predicted by decreased predicted postoperative FEV_1 [$ppoFEV_1$] and ppoDLCO)
6. Preoperative immunosuppression (steroid therapy)
7. Older age (>70 years)
8. Postoperative sputum positive for AFB

Prevention of postpneumonectomy BPF and empyema centers on attention to careful intraoperative technique. One must limit the length of the bronchial stump, which will help to prevent pooling of secretions leading to increased risk of infection at the site of bronchial closure. Perioperative prophylactic antibiotics have a well-known benefit following general thoracic procedures. For patients with pre-existing infection/empyemas or the potential for significant pleural space contamination (destroyed lung or preoperative BPF) more specific culture-directed antibiotic regimens might be indicated. Method of closure of the bronchial stump remains controversial. There are a variety of studies that report the superiority of both hand-sewn and stapled closures. No matter what closure is chosen, most authors suggest bronchial stump reinforcement after pneumonectomy, especially in cases where breakdown is more likely (neoadjuvant therapy, presence of infection, and right-sided procedures). As described previously, we prefer an intercostal muscle flap. Other options are a pericardial fat pad, defunctionalized azygous flap, or, probably the worst choice, a pleural flap. The choice of tissue used for reinforcement varies among surgeons.

In cases where postpneumonectomy BPF or empyema is suspected, early diagnosis is paramount because the earlier it is diagnosed and treated, the better is the prognosis. Early empyemas without BPF are uncommon and are best managed by debridement of the space. When the space has been sterilized the space should then be filled with the debridement antibiotic solution (a Clagett procedure) and the tubes removed. Although management of postoperative BPF remains a problem, immediate drainage of the pleural space can be a lifesaving procedure because it may prevent aspiration of accumulated fluid into the contralateral lung. A variety of treatment strategies have been proposed for subsequent management. For small fistulas (<3 mm in size) with a short stump occasionally tube drainage alone is sufficient along with the injection of fibrin glue into the fistula. Sometimes these small fistulas close spontaneously, but that is very rare. In those cases where tube drainage does not result in closure of the small BPF, some authors advocate the use of videoscopic drainage and debridement combined with bronchoscopic closure using cauterization or metallic coils with the application of fibrin glue. For larger BPFs attempts at endoscopic closure are not recommended. Definitive surgery to close a postpneumonectomy BPF is quite involved, and therefore the patient's medical and nutritional status must be optimized, the postpneumonectomy space must be cleaned and healthy, the need for postoperative mechanical ventilation must be minimized, and there must be no evidence of recurrent carcinoma. A variety of procedures have been used for bronchial stump closure after development of a large (≥3 mm) BPF. The traditional, well-described procedure initially developed by Pairolero involved multiple debridements, the use of muscle flaps or omentum to plug the fistula, and finally closure via a Clagett procedure. Others have suggested a transsternal, transpericardial approach to the bronchial stump via the posterior pericardium and subsequent mobilization of the affected stump, reamputation, and a reinforced closure.

Postpneumonectomy Syndrome

Postpneumonectomy syndrome is an unusual complication occurring most often after right pneumonectomy. Resulting from an extreme shift and rotation of the mediastinum and contralateral lung into the empty pleural space, it produces symptomatic proximal airway obstruction and causes air trapping. The mainstem bronchus is stretched and compressed against the vertebral bodies, descending aorta, and/or remaining pulmonary artery branches. Patients present months to years after pneumonectomy with dyspnea, stridor, and recurrent pneumonias. Chest radiographs and computed tomography show an extreme shift of the mediastinal structures, and bronchoscopy reveals severe proximal airway obstruction and sometimes tracheomalacia. Other causes must be ruled out including recurrent malignancy, pulmonary hypertension, progression of underlying lung disease, pulmonary thromboembolism, and congestive heart failure.

Although it is impossible to predict, the syndrome is described mostly in children and young adults; however, there are occasional reports in the adult literature as well. Most surgeons attempt to prevent the acute shift of the mediastinum by avoiding chest tubes after pneumonectomy; if they are used, tubes are either clamped or left to water seal drainage only. To correct the shift when it does occur, the mediastinal structures must be shifted back to a more anatomic location. This can be done via anterior pericardiorrhapy, which anchors the pericardium to the parasternal chest wall, and by placing expandable saline-filled breast implants into the postpneumonectomy space, which is usually spared of adhesions, stabilizing the mediastinum. However, these techniques have fallen out of favor for fear of infecting the pneumonectomized space. Tracheomalacia after longstanding obstruction is an indicator of poor outcome. Treatment is often the placement of a silicone removable stent, which helps to keep the airway open.

SUGGESTED READING

Alexiou C, Beggs D, et al. Pneumonectomy for stage I (T1N0 and T2N0) nonsmall cell lung cancer has potent, adverse impact on survival. Ann Thorac Surg 2003;76:1023.

Algar FJ, Alvarez A, et al. Predicting pulmonary complications after pneumonectomy for lung cancer. Eur J Cardiothorac Surg 2003;23:201.

Balkanli K, Genc O, et al. Surgical management of bronchiectasis: Analysis and short-term results in 238 patients. Eur J Cardiothorac Surg 2003;2:699.

British Thoracic Society. Society of Cardiothoracic Surgeons of Great Britain and Ireland Working Party. BTS guidelines: Guidelines on the selection of patients with lung cancer for surgery. Thorax 2001;56:89.

Cerfolio RJ, Bryant AS, et al. Intraoperative Solu-Medrol helps prevent postpneumonectomy pulmonary edema. Ann Thorac Surg 2003;76:1029.

De Decker K, Jorens PG, Van Schil P. Cardiac complications after noncardiac thoracic surgery: an evidence-based current review. Ann Thorac Surg 2003;75:1340.

Deslauriers J, Gregoire J, et al. Sleeve lobectomy versus pneumonectomy for lung cancer: a comparative analysis of survival and sites of recurrences. Annals of Thoracic Surgery. 77(4):1152–56, Apr2004.

Foroulis CN, Kotoulas C, et al. Factors associated with cardiac rhythm disturbances in the early post-pneumonectomy period: A study on 259 pneumonectomies. Eur J Cardiothorac Surg 2003;23:384.

Fuentes PA. Pneumonectomy: A historical perspective and prospective insight. Eur J Cardiothorac Surg 2003;23:439.

Galetta D, Cesario A, et al. Enduring challenge in the treatment of nonsmall cell lung cancer with clinical stage IIIB: Results of a trimodality approach. Ann Thorac Surg 2003;76:1802.

Ghiribelli C, Voltolini L, et al. Survival after bronchoplastic lobectomy for nonsmall cell lung cancer compared with pneumonectomy according to nodal status. J Cardiovasc Surg 2002;43:103.

Kim YT, Kim HK, et al. Long-term outcomes and risk factor analysis after pneumonectomy for active and sequela forms of pulmonary tuberculosis. Eur J Cardiothorac Surg 2003;23:833.

Lardinois D, Horsch A, et al. Mediastinal reinforcement after induction therapy and pneumonectomy: Comparison of intercostals muscle versus diaphragm flaps. Eur J Cardiothorac Surg 2002;21:74.

Le Pimpec-Barthes F, D'Attellis N, et al. Chylothorax complicating pulmonary resection. Ann Thorac Surg 2002;73:1714.

Licker M, Spiliopoulos A, et al. Risk factors for early mortality and major complications following pneumonectomy for non–small cell carcinoma of the lung. Chest 2002;121:1890.

Okada M, Nishio W, et al. Evolution of surgical outcomes for nonsmall cell lung cancer: Time trends in 1,465 consecutive patients undergoing complete resection. Ann Thorac Surg 2004;77:1926.

Schneider B, Schickinger-Fischer B, et al. Concept for diagnosis and therapy of unilateral recurrent laryngeal nerve paralysis following thoracic surgery. Thorac Cardiovasc Surg 2003;51:327.

Thomas P, Doddoli C, et al. Stage I nonsmall cell lung cancer: A pragmatic approach to prognosis after complete resection. Ann Thorac Surg 2002;73:1065.

Watanabe S, Watanabe T, Urayama H. Endobronchial occlusion method of bronchopleural fistula with metallic coils and glue. Thorac Cardiovasc Surg 2003;51:106.

EDITOR'S COMMENTS

As the author correctly points out, pneumonectomy is a "disease" associated with multiple short- and long-term complications. Yet when a complete resection can be accomplished and pneumonectomy is the only alternative the benefits most frequently outweigh the risks. Patients who may potentially require pneumonectomy need to be assessed preoperatively to assure that they are candidates, as the author points out. Seemingly there are no "absolute" contraindications to pneumonectomy, only relative ones. I prefer not to perform pneumonectomy in most patients >70 years of age, yet occasionally this is necessary. The author feels that residual mediastinal lymph node disease after preoperative treatment is an absolute contraindication to pneumonectomy, yet we and others feel that if a complete resection can be achieved in a patient who is otherwise a candidate for pneumonectomy, then it should be done. A significant degree of hypercarbia, especially if associated with pulmonary hypertension, should preclude pneumonectomy.

As the author points out, pneumonectomy rarely should be planned preoperatively. There might be a strong suspicion that complete removal of the lung may be required, but we do everything possible to conserve lung parenchyma including bronchial sleeve resections as well as pulmonary artery resection with reconstruction. Pneumonectomy should be carried out when it is determined intraoperatively that parenchymal conservation is not feasible due to involvement of all lobes, proximal involvement of the pulmonary artery that precludes reconstruction, or inability to separate the veins mandating taking the veins at their confluence.

The author recommends a number of intraoperative maneuvers that are somewhat controversial and deserve some comment. The reason behind the use of a central venous catheter for resections where pneumonectomy is contemplated is not clear to me what information that can be gleaned from such a catheter is helpful during the resection. In addition, the recommendation for giving steroids before taking the pulmonary vessels has very little support in the literature and is not routinely done in most centers. That being said, there is probably little downside to giving it, and it might be helpful in preventing postpneumonectomy pulmonary edema. Buttressing the bronchial stump is something that many surgeons do, but there is little evidence that it truly is useful in preventing postoperative bronchial stump problems. I agree with the author that if one chooses to buttress the stump, either intercostal muscle or a pericardial fat pad pedicle is significantly better than a simple flap of pleura. The author recommends staple closure of the pneumonectomy stump, and I agree, and feel that the strength of the closure likely is better with the double or triple row of staples laid down by a mechanical device. The more important factor is keeping the bronchial stump as short as possible and as well vascularized as possible. We also leave a chest tube in a pneumonectomy space but would never leave this to a water-seal system. One significant cough could cause a shift of the mediastinum enough to impede venous return to a degree that could cause cardiac collapse. In addition, despite a sign to the contrary, it is too easy for someone to come along and assume that the tube should be hooked up to suction, which could cause immediate death. If one is to leave a tube in a pneumonectomy space, we strongly urge the use of a pneumonectomy balanced drainage system in the name of patient safety. The tube routinely is removed on the first postoperative morning but allows for the monitoring of blood loss within the pneumonectomy space during the immediate postoperative period.

Several postoperative issues discussed by the author also deserve mention. I take issue with the comment that vocal cord dysfunction should be expected in one third of patients undergoing left pneumonectomy. Even when it is found necessary to divide the ligamentum arteriosum, the recurrent nerve usually can be visualized and preserved. Vocal cord dysfunction should almost never occur unless the recurrent laryngeal nerve has been taken as part of the resection. The right recurrent nerve essentially should never be injured during a pulmonary resection because of its location where it recurs around the subclavian artery. Postoperative atrial arrhythmias occur in up to one third of patients, and there is no convincing evidence that this incidence can safely be decreased, although amiodarone shows promise in patients undergoing less than pneumonectomy. Treating prophylactically with calcium-channel blockers should keep the ventricular rate better controlled when the atrial arrhythmias occur but likely do not decrease the incidence of the complication. A postoperative chyle leak rarely, if ever, responds to medium chain triglycerides, and if conservative therapy is to be tried, it should be total parenteral nutrition. If after 7 days the chyle leak persists, ligation of the thoracic duct should be undertaken. This is most easily accomplished via a low right thoracotomy with ligation of the duct at the aortic hiatus where it enters the chest as a single trunk. Trying to identify the point of leakage usually is pointless and often fails. The diagnosis of a pulmonary embolus currently is made by spiral CT scan, and the use of pulmonary angiography for diagnosis has fallen by the wayside. Thrombolysis rarely is successful and is fraught with bleeding complications early after pneumonectomy. Systemic heparinization remains the treatment of choice in most centers. The presence of a postpneumonectomy empyema, whether accompanied by a bronchial fistula or not, requires treatment of the infected space first and foremost. This usually means an open-window thoracostomy for optimal drainage unless the fistula occurs very early in the postoperative course, in which case reoperation with reclosure of the bronchial stump is indicated. Dealing with an infected pneumonectomy space is a complex topic and is dealt with in another chapter. Transsternal closure of a bronchopleural fistula is reserved for complete bronchial dehiscence where enough bronchial stump remains for resection and reclosure. Despite the author's view, the postpneumonectomy syndrome, which occurs rarely, when symptomatic should be treated by the placement of tissue expanders in the pneumonectomy space with gradual inflation. No better treatment exists, and because this complication is seen many years after the resection space infection really is not an issue.

L.R.K.

7

Bronchoplastic Procedures

Anna Maria Ciccone, Federico Venuta, and Erino A. Rendina

History

The first sleeve lobectomy was performed by Price-Thomas in 1947 for an endobronchial adenoma. Five years later, Allison reported a sleeve lobectomy for carcinoma. It was Paulson and Shaw, however, who popularized sleeve resection with their 1955 paper, entitled "Bronchial anastomosis and bronchoplastic procedures in the interest of preservation of lung tissue." The use of their techniques allows the modern thoracic surgeon to perform parenchymal-sparing procedures on patients who would not tolerate a pneumonectomy. In the case of malignancy, sleeve resections are performed without compromise of oncologic principles.

Principles and Justification

Pneumonectomy is associated with an increased morbidity and mortality when compared to lobectomy and sleeve lobectomy. Thus, in our practice, we make every effort to avoid pneumonectomy. This includes complex bronchoplastic and bronchovascular reconstructions when required. The justification of this approach is simply that by avoiding pneumonectomy we avoid its attendant risks while providing an equivalent cancer operation. In addition, lung-sparing procedures allow us to offer curative operations to patients with poor pulmonary function who would otherwise not tolerate an operation.

Preoperative Assessment and Preparation

Our preoperative evaluation includes a complete history and physical examination. Special attention is focused on previous thoracic procedures and chest irradiation. Use of high-dose steroids or systemic illnesses that might interfere with bronchial anastomotic healing are noted. All patients have a chest x-ray, a chest computed axial tomography (CAT) scan, and pulmonary function testing with diffusion capacity. Patients with a diagnosis or suspicion of malignancy also have an extent-of-disease workup, which includes a bone scan and magnetic resonance imaging (MRI) of the brain when indicated.

We perform mediastinoscopy selectively in patients with malignant disease. Patients who have mediastinal adenopathy of >1.0 cm on CAT scan undergo mediastinoscopy before thoracotomy. If the mediastinoscopy is negative, we proceed with the thoracotomy. If the mediastinoscopy reveals ipsilateral N2 disease, patients are referred for preoperative chemo- or chemoradiation therapy and return later for resection. Those patients with contralateral N3 disease are referred for chemoradiation therapy and are not offered surgical resection.

Anesthesia

After induction of general anesthesia, all patients undergoing sleeve resection require bronchoscopy by the operating surgeon. This can be done with either a rigid or a flexible bronchoscope. Bronchoscopy allows visualization of the lesion and planning of the resection. After bronchoscopy it is important for the surgeon to have a complete discussion with the anesthesiologist regarding the operative plan. If a right-sided sleeve resection is contemplated, a left endobronchial double-lumen tube should be placed (Fig. 7-1). If a left-sided sleeve resection is contemplated, a right endobronchial tube is placed. For sleeve pneumonectomy or a carinal sleeve resection, a sterile anesthesia circuit is required to allow direct ventilation from the surgical field.

Operations

We have performed sleeve resections through standard posterolateral incisions, serratus-sparing posterolateral incisions, and lateral incision, which is quite satisfactory for exposure and dissection.

After entry into the chest, complete exploration is carried out to rule out metastatic disease to either the pleura or lung parenchyma and to assess resectability. On both the right and left side we begin our dissection in the anterior hilum and completely dissect out the main pulmonary artery. Special care must be taken on the left side to avoid damage to the short left main pulmonary artery and specifically the apical segmental arterial branch. If there is bulky disease or any difficulty is encountered with dissection, we do not hesitate

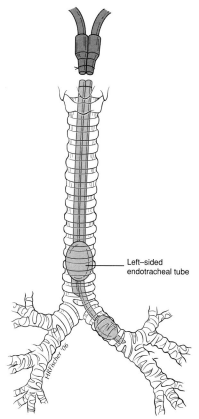

Figure 7-1. Left-sided endotracheal tube in place for right upper lobe sleeve.

to open the pericardium on either side to obtain proximal control. Next, we encircle the main pulmonary artery with an umbilical tape. The remaining steps are specific to the sleeve resection being performed and each will be described independently in what follows.

Right-Sided Resections
Right Upper Lobectomy Sleeve Resection: The Prototype Bronchoplastic Procedure

After proximal arterial control has been obtained, we continue our dissection superiorly and enter the plane of the right upper lobe bronchus (Fig. 7-2). The lung is retracted anteriorly, and we continue our dissection in the bifurcation between the right upper lobe bronchus and the bronchus intermedius. A "crotch" lymph node is a consistent finding in this location. This node is elevated away from the bifurcation to reveal the pulmonary arterial branch to the superior segment of the right lower lobe. Once this branch is identified, the posterior portion of the fissure is completed with a linear stapler. This approach avoids extensive parenchymal dissection in the fissure. The bronchus intermedius is encircled just distal to the right upper lobe take-off, and an umbilical tape is placed to aid in dividing the airway at the appropriate time. Up to this point we have not made any irreversible maneuvers. A complete inspection is carried out to ensure that all disease including nodal disease can be removed. Once complete resectability is confirmed we begin by ligating and dividing the pulmonary arterial branches to the right upper lobe. Likewise, the venous drainage is divided with a vascular stapler taking care to preserve the middle lobe venous drainage. The minor fissure is completed with a linear stapler. The mainstem bronchus is encircled at its origin, and an umbilical tape is placed. Before committing to the sleeve resection it is often productive to divide the right upper lobe bronchus at its origin to

see whether the tumor can be cleared with a negative bronchial resection margin. This is especially important with carcinoid tumors, in which the endobronchial component may be attached only at one point and the lesion simply pulled out leaving a clear bronchial margin. Once the bronchus has been opened the decision to proceed with sleeve resection may be made based on the findings either grossly or microscopically.

To begin the sleeve resection, we divide the mainstem bronchus with a No. 15 blade just proximal to the right upper lobe take-off. Likewise, the bronchus intermedius is divided just distal to the right upper lobe take-off (Fig. 7-3). For upper lobe sleeve resections these cuts must be perpendicular to the long axis of the airway and placed between cartilaginous rings so as to result in a clean cut. An angled division of the bronchus is to be avoided. The proximal and distal airway margins are cut from the specimen and the true margin inked by the surgeon. We personally take the margins to the pathologist so that the proper orientation can be demonstrated prior to frozen-section examination. Once the margins have been cleared, the reconstruction is started. Microscopic tumor present at a bronchial margin requires additional resection of the involved area or possibly pneumonectomy.

We perform the bronchial sleeve anastomosis in an interrupted fashion. The key to a successful bronchial sleeve anastomosis is a pneumostatic well-approximated, tension-free repair that accounts for any size discrepancy between ends by precise suture placement. We do not take a "tuck" in the proximal airway to make up

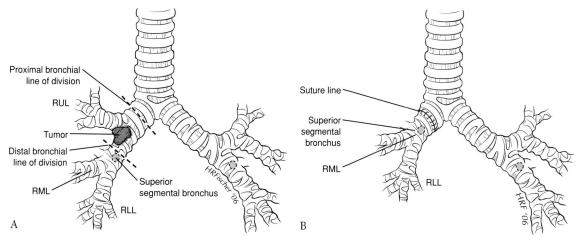

Figure 7-2. Tumor in right upper lobe bronchus requiring sleeve resection. (RLL = right lower lobe; RML = right middle lobe; RUL = right upper lobe.)

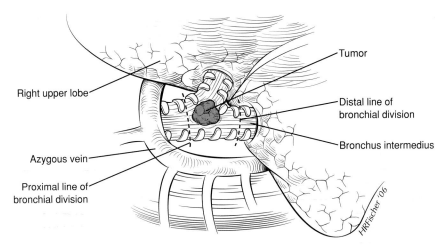

Right upper lobe

Tumor

Distal line of bronchial division

Bronchus intermedius

Azygous vein

Proximal line of bronchial division

HRFischer '06

Figure 7-3. Division of the right mainstem and bronchus intermedius during right upper lobe sleeve.

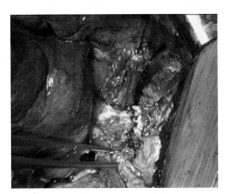

Figure 7-5. Pericardial fat wrapped around the anastomosis.

for a size discrepancy. Rather, we make up the size discrepancy along the entire circumference of the anastomosis by precise suture placement.

When performing an interrupted anastomosis, we use 4-0 oiled, absorbable, braided suture. The first suture is placed in an "outside-to-in" fashion at the junction of the cartilaginous and membranous bronchi. The suture is not tied, but is secured to a suture guide. Additional sutures are placed at 2-mm intervals to complete the first half of the cartilaginous anastomosis (Fig. 7-4). Once the midpoint of the cartilaginous bronchus is reached, we begin tying the sutures starting at the corner. The surgeon "crosses" the next suture in the series to relieve tension while the assistant ties. The cartilaginous anastomosis is completed from the midpoint down to the opposite corner in a similar fashion. The lung is retracted anteriorly to reveal the membranous portion of the bronchus. The membranous portion of the anastomosis is completed with interrupted sutures. The chest is filled with saline, and the anastomosis is tested to 20-cm water inflation pressure. Needle hole air leaks are ignored; however, air leaks between the cut edges of the bronchus, if small, are reinforced with simple interrupted sutures. A large area of leaking may require the entire anastomosis to be redone. We wrap all anastomoses with either a pleural flap or a pedicle of pericardial fat (Fig. 7-5).

We wrap most anastomoses with an intercostal muscle flap (Fig. 7-5), sometimes with an omental or pericardial flap. Although the reossification of the intercostal muscle flap can occur, it does not necessarily cause problems; in fact, the bronchus has very limited intrinsic motility and a stable caliber. If the intercostal muscle flap is loosely applied around the bronchus, even if some retraction occurs, there is no reason why the hardening caused by ossification should produce stenosis. When the sleeve resection is planned preoperatively, the intercostal pediole flap may be prepared before the insertion of the rib retractor to avoid crushing the intercostal vascular bundle, and is prepared at full thickness, encompassing a wide pleural flap. The flap is slid backward around the bronchial anastomosis, between it and the PA. The flap is then turned until its pleural side is in contact with the bronchial anastomosis, and the pleura is secured to the bronchus by interrupted sutures.

Middle Lobe Sleeve Resection

The middle lobe sleeve resection is an infrequently performed resection. After proximal arterial control, the middle lobe vein is identified, isolated, and divided (Fig. 7-6). The bronchus to the middle lobe lies immediately posterior to the middle lobe vein. The bronchus is followed back to its origin. A right-angled clamp is placed around the bronchus intermedius, and it is divided at a location proximal to the middle lobe orifice. The division is slightly angled. The distal division is also angled to preserve the orifice to the superior segment of the lower lobe. The pulmonary artery lies directly posterior and slightly superior to the bronchus, and care must be taken to avoid injury when dividing the bronchus. After division of the airway, the middle lobe arterial branch is easily visualized. The branch is ligated and divided. Next the minor fissure and anterior portion of the major fissure are completed with firings of a linear stapler.

After confirmation of negative margins, the airway anastomosis is performed. In an interrupted manner as described previously for the right upper lobectomy sleeve resection. Special considerations in performing a middle lobe sleeve resection must be given to the superior segmental orifice of the lower lobe. This orifice should not be narrowed or occluded when creating an anastomosis. Intercastal muscle flap is used to wrap the anastomosis and separate it from the pulmonary artery.

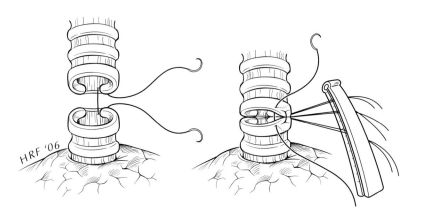

HRF '06

Figure 7-4. Interrupted anastomotic technique.

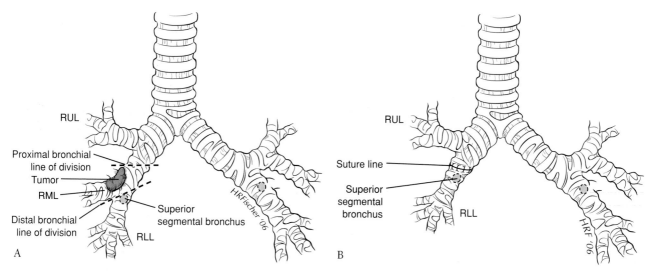

Figure 7-6. Middle lobe sleeve. Note that the bronchus transection is not perpendicular to the axis of the airway in order to preserve the superior segmental orifice to the lower lobe. (RLL = right lower lobe; RML = right middle lobe; RUL = right upper lobe.)

Bilobectomy Sleeve Resection

Bilobectomy sleeve resection is performed for an endobronchial lesion in the bronchus intermedius that extends up proximal to the upper lobe orifice (Fig. 7-7). The basic principles of proximal arterial control, microscopic negative margins, and a precise tension-free anastomosis apply. Here the right mainstem bronchus is divided just proximal to the right upper lobe take-off and the right upper lobe bronchus is divided at its origin. The right upper lobe bronchus is then anastomosed to the mainstem bronchus after removal of the middle and lower lobes, the so called "Y" sleeve. Due to the reorientation of the upper lobe bronchus after removal of the middle and lower lobes, special care must be taken to avoid torsion of the bronchus at the level of the anastomosis.

Left-Sided Resections

Left Upper Lobe Sleeve Resection

Proximal arterial control is obtained with care to avoid injury to the short apical-posterior segmental branch of the left pulmonary artery. We continue our dissection along the plane of the artery and identify the superior segmental branch to the lower lobe (Fig. 7-8). At this point, we complete the posterior fissure with a linear stapler. The anterior segmental artery is ligated and divided. The lingular branches of the pulmonary artery are identified, ligated, and divided. The lung is retracted posteriorly, and the upper lobe venous drainage is divided with a vascular stapler. The anterior portion of the fissure is completed with a linear stapler. The only remaining attachment to the specimen is the bronchus. The mainstem bronchus is encircled proximal to the bifurcation, and an umbilical tape placed to be used as a "handle." Two 2-0 silk stay sutures are placed in the proximal left mainstem and used for retraction. The mainstem bronchus is divided with a new No. 15 blade proximal to the bifurcation, and the left lower lobe bronchus is divided at its origin. The origin of the superior segmental

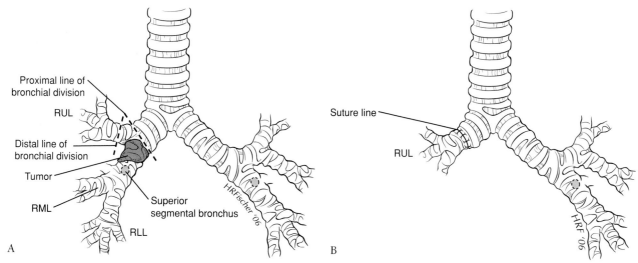

Figure 7-7. Bilobectomy sleeve. (RLL = right lower lobe; RML = right middle lobe; RUL = right upper lobe.)

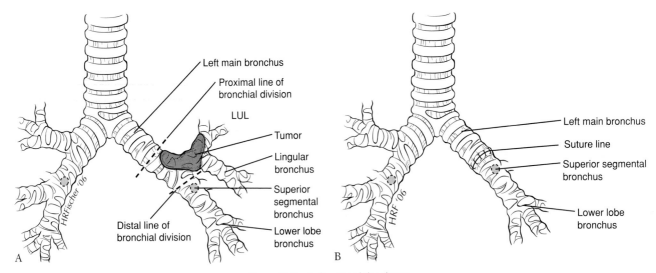

Figure 7-8. Left upper lobe sleeve.

bronchus can be quite close to the origin of the lower lobe bronchus, and the lobar division must leave the bronchus intact without separating the superior segmental bronchus. It is possible to take the superior segment, if necessary, to achieve a complete resection and sew the basal segments to the mainstem bronchus. The cuts across the bronchus should be perpendicular to the longitudinal axis of the airway and placed between cartilaginous rings. The margins are inked, and a frozen-section examination is performed. Once the margins are confirmed to be microscopically negative, the reconstruction is begun. We use an interrupted technique as described previously for the right upper lobe sleeve.

Because the left mainstem bronchus is long, extensive proximal resections can be performed. This can create a technically

challenging anastomosis because proximal exposure is obscured by the aortic arch. If required, the arch can be mobilized and carefully retracted to provide additional exposure. As greater amounts of proximal airway are removed, increased tension on the anastomosis is not a problem. Precise suture placement to account for size discrepancy between the lobar bronchus and the mainstem bronchus is particularly important. The inferior pulmonary ligament should be released.

Left Lower Lobectomy Sleeve Resection ("Y" Sleeve)

For lesions involving the left lower lobe orifice, with extension into the mainstem bronchus but sparing the upper lobe orifice, a lower lobectomy with sleeve resection

of the left upper lobe bronchus can be performed. The arterial and venous branches to the lower lobe are divided and the fissures are completed (Fig. 7-9). We dissect out and pass an umbilical tape around the left mainstem and left upper lobe bronchus. Two silk stay sutures are place in the mainstem bronchus and used for retraction. The left upper lobe bronchus is divided at its origin with a fresh No. 15 blade. It is important for the division to be perpendicular to the long axis of the airway. Next, the mainstem bronchus is divided proximal to the bifurcation and well beyond the extent of the tumor. The specimen is removed from the field, and frozen-section examination of the airway margins is performed. Once the margins are confirmed to be microscopically negative, the reconstruction is completed.

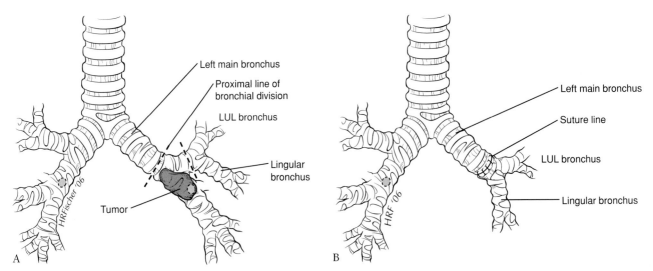

Figure 7-9. Left lower lobe sleeve.

The anastomosis is performed in an interrupted or running fashion as described previously for the right upper lobe sleeve resection. The lingular bronchus may arise quite proximally, and care must be taken when dividing the upper lobe bronchus to assure that the upper lobe bronchus remains intact. There is often a large size discrepancy between upper lobe bronchus and the mainstem. This requires precise placement of sutures so that the discrepancy is distributed over the entire circumference to the anastomosis.

Postoperative Care

After sleeve resection, the patient is extubated in the operating room. Postoperative pain relief is facilitated by a functioning thoracic epidural catheter. Pain control is re-evaluated periodically by the nursing staff and adjusted by the anesthesia pain service. The epidural catheter remains in place for the first 48 hours after surgery in the majority of patients, only in a few patients the epidural catheter remains in place until the chest tubes are removed. Atelectasis and subsequent pneumonia in the lung distal to the anastomosis must be avoided. This is accomplished by adequate pain relief and aggressive pulmonary toilet that may include frequent bronchoscopy, if necessary. We begin incentive spirometry as soon as the patient is awake and begin ambulation on postoperative day 1. The chest tube remains in place until there is no air leak, and the drainage is <200 ml/day. This usually occurs by postoperative day 3 to 5. The epidural is capped 12 hours after the chest tube is removed, and oral narcotics are started. If adequate pain relief is obtained on an oral regimen, the epidural catheter is removed. Awake flexible bronchoscopy should be performed before discharge to assess the integrity of the anastomosis.

Outcome

Major complications after sleeve resection include anastomotic dehiscence, empyema, and bronchovascular fistula. Fortunately, the incidence of these complications is low. We maintain a low threshold for bronchoscopy in the postoperative period. Persistent or evolving atelectasis in the lung distal to the bronchial anastomosis mandates bronchoscopy. A small partial anastomotic dehiscence (<30%) with a good pericardial fat wrap and no bronchopleural fistula can be treated conservatively, but consideration should be given to completion pneumonectomy based on the judgment of the surgeon. A complete dehiscence is caused either by anastomotic tension or more likely results from ischemia. This mandates reoperation and usually a completion pneumonectomy. An empyema can occur with or without a bronchopleural fistula. When it occurs without a bronchopleural fistula it is handled with drainage, antibiotics, and ablation of any residual space with muscle transposition. In this case it is likely related to preoperative postobstructive pneumonia. When empyema occurs with a bronchopleural fistula from the anastomosis a completion pneumonectomy is required, and management of the infected pneumonectomy space is problematic.

Bronchovascular fistula presents with massive hemoptysis. This occurs when there is an anastomotic breakdown with peribronchial abscess formation, which necessitates into the adjacent pulmonary artery. Under these circumstances, completion pneumonectomy is performed if this occurs in the hospital setting, which is unlikely because the time frame when this occurs usually approaches 3 weeks after operation. As expected, the mortality from this complication is very high.

The mortality rate for sleeve lobectomy is slightly higher than for routine lobectomy (3% to 5%). The most frequent respiratory complication is pneumonia, which can be minimized by aggressive postoperative pulmonary toilet and adequate pain control. Local recurrence rates after bronchoplastic procedures are low (<5%) and similar to that achieved by pneumonectomy as long as the resection margins are free of disease. This illustrates the importance of frozen-section examination of the bronchial margins before completing the airway anastomosis. Late bronchial anastomotic strictures occasionally occur and are related either to ischemia or a healed partial anastomotic dehiscence. These usually can be managed with dilation and, if indicated, bronchial stent placement.

REFERENCES

Deslauriers J, Gaulin P, Beaulieu M, et al. Long-term clinical and functional results of sleeve lobectomy for primary lung cancer. J Thorac Cardiovasc Surg 1986;92:871.

Ferguson MK, Lehman AG. Sleeve lobectomy or pneumonectomy: Optimal management strategy using decision analysis techniques. Ann Thorac Surg 2003;76:1782.

Gaissert HA, Mathisen DJ, Moncure AC, et al. Survival and function after sleeve lobectomy for lung cancer. J Thorac Cardiovasc Surg 1996;111:948.

Icard P, Regnard JF, Guibert L, et al. Survival and prognostic factors in patients undergoing parenchymal saving bronchoplastic operations for primary lung cancer: A series of 110 consecutive cases. Eur J Cardiothorac Surg 1999;15:426.

Newton JR Jr, Grillo HC, Mathisen DJ. Main bronchial sleeve resection with pulmonary conservation. Ann Thorac Surg 1991;52:1272.

Okada M, Yamagishi H, Satake H, et al. Survival related to lymph node involvement in lung cancer after sleeve lobectomy compared with pneumonectomy. J Thorac Cardiovasc Surg 2000;119:814.

Paulson DL, Shaw RR. Bronchial anastomosis and bronchoplastic procedures in the interest of preservation of lung tissue. J Thorac Surg 1955;29:238.

Price Thomas C. Conservative resection of the bronchial tree. J R Coll Surg Edin 1956;1:169.

Rendina EA, De Giacomo T, Venuta F, et al. Lung conservation techniques: Bronchial sleeve resection and reconstruction of the pulmonary artery. Semin Surg Oncol 2000;18:165.

Rendina EA, Venuta F, De Giacomo T, et al. Safety and efficacy of bronchovascular reconstruction after induction chemotherapy for lung cancer. J Thorac Cardiovasc Surg 1997;114:830.

Rendina EA, Venuta F, De Giacomo T, et al. Sleeve resection after induction therapy. Thorac Surg Clin 2004;14:191.

Suen HC, Meyers BF, Gutrie T, et al. Favorable results after sleeve lobectomy or bronchoplasty for bronchial malignancies. Ann Thorac Surg 1999;67:1557.

Tronc F, Gregoire J, Rouleau J, Deslauriers J. Long-term results of sleeve lobectomy for lung cancer. Eur J Cardiothorac Surg 2000;17: 550.

Van Schil PE, de la Rivière AB, Knaepen PJ, et al. Long-term survival after bronchial sleeve resection: Univariate and multivariate analysis. Ann Thorac Surg 1996;61:1087.

Vogt-Moykopf I, Fritz TH, Meyer G, et al. Bronchoplastic and angioplastic operations in bronchial carcinoma: long term results of a retrospective analysis from 1973 to 1983. Int Surg 1986;71:211.

EDITOR'S COMMENTS

Dr. Rendina and co-workers have beautifully described the full spectrum of sleeve resections including those that are rarely performed. The point here is that sleeve resections can be performed on any lobe in the interest of parenchymal preservation. When feasible, our choice always is to proceed with a lung conservation procedure instead of a pneumonectomy. Important technical points to keep in mind are the absolute necessity for a clean bronchial cut perpendicular to the long axis of the bronchus for both the proximal and distal ends. Precise suture approximation making up the size discrepancy is also key because the distal bronchus almost always is significantly smaller than the proximal bronchus. Although tempting, we avoid taking a "tuck" in the larger bronchus and prefer instead to make up any discrepancy with suture bites spaced evenly around the entire circumference of the anastomosis.

We also feel that it is important to wrap the anastomosis with a viable pedicle, and we prefer pericardial fat, which is attached both to itself and to the bronchus. Aggressive postoperative pulmonary toilet is key, and frequent therapeutic bronchoscopy may be required to clear secretions. Postoperative atelectasis of the reattached pulmonary parenchyma should prompt early bronchoscopy to assure patency of the anas-

tomosis as well as to clear any secretions. On the left side the superior segment of the lower lobe may be taken as part of a resection involving mainly the upper lobe and the basal segments sewn to the left mainstem bronchus. Depending on the size of the basal segmental orifice, there may be difficulties with secretion clearance as well as a fairly narrow lumen after the anastomosis. If there is any evidence of nonhealing, we err on the side of performing a completion pneumonectomy rather than wait to have major trouble with a bronchovascular fistula and its attendant high mortality.

The authors mention that anastomotic healing problems often stem from ischemia, but he does not comment on the role of mediastinal lymph node dissection in bronchial ischemia. It is my opinion that a complete lymph node dissection that completely

cleans out the subcarinal space may contribute to bronchial anastomotic ischemia, and it is my preference to perform lymph node sampling especially in this area. I am not aware of any studies that definitively show that the bronchus can be devascularized by a lymph node dissection, but intuitively it makes sense especially with a thorough clean-out of the subcarinal space with its rich bronchial blood supply.

Bronchial sleeve resection may need to be combined with pulmonary artery resection and reconstruction especially on the left side. We do not hesitate to perform such a double-sleeve resection if that is what is required to save pulmonary parenchyma. It is our preference, and that of many others, to preferentially perform sleeve resection even when the patient's underlying pulmonary function clearly indicates that the patient could tolerate pneumonectomy.

L.R.K.

8

Pulmonary Resections: Limited Resections and Segmentectomy

Costanzo A. DiPerna and Douglas E. Wood

Sublobar pulmonary resections encompass all pulmonary resections of less than an anatomic lobectomy. They are subdivided into two distinct categories: anatomic, otherwise known as segmentectomy; and nonanatomic, commonly referred to as a wedge resection. Segmental resections were originally considered for patients with segmental inflammatory disease, such as aspergilloma, tuberculosis, and bronchiectasis, but the indications have expanded to include metastatic disease to the lung as well as primary lung cancer in patients with poor pulmonary reserve.

It is easy to recommend sublobar resections for diagnostic procedures and benign disease, but it is a more complicated decision in malignant disease. For disease that is metastatic to the lung, segmentectomy or wedge resection is the procedure of choice if surgery is indicated and the anatomy is amenable to sublobar resection. There is no clear evidence that more radical resection results in better survival or lower recurrence, and frequently these patients require resection of more than a single site, usually dictating smaller individual resections.

The decision to choose a sublobar resection for primary lung cancer is complex and continues to evolve. The predominant indication is in patients with poor pulmonary reserve, yet this is ill defined and inconsistently applied. Traditional teaching has been that patients require a predicted postoperative forced expiratory volume in 1 second (FEV$_1$) of >0.8 to 1.0 liter/sec to have sufficient pulmonary reserve to tolerate surgery and have adequate short- and long-term functional capacity. However, two factors have modified these guidelines. First, improvements in surgery, anesthesia, postoperative pain management, and respiratory care have allowed successful thoracotomy and pulmonary resection even in patients with major comorbidity and/or with patients with a low preoperative FEV$_1$, even <0.5 liter/sec. Clearly these patients are at increased risk of pulmonary complications after pulmonary resection, but it is unusual that these risks are prohibitive. These patients also have relative contraindications to radiation or chemotherapy and may suffer similar or greater pulmonary complications or loss of function due to radiation when compared to surgery. In these patients with major comorbidity a discrete intervention like surgery is often better tolerated than the less immediate, but insidious and progressive consequences of radiation.

The second factor changing the indications for surgery results from the recent experience in lung volume reduction surgery, which paradoxically results in an increase in pulmonary function and exercise capacity when overinflated lung parenchyma is removed in selected emphysema patients. Patients with severe upper-lobe predominant emphysema, hyperinflation, and a tumor in the upper lobe may actually be well served by a lobectomy or a lung reduction style of wedge resection and have an improvement rather than a decrement in postoperative lung function.

The major factor that compels surgical consideration for lung cancer patients, even in those with major comorbidity, is that surgery provides the only meaningful opportunity for cure. This is probably not an important factor if a patient's anticipated life expectancy from their other disease(s) is <1 to 2 years, but for the majority of patients we should expend every effort to try to offer surgical therapy with curative intent. Standard lobectomy should be possible in the majority of patients with nonpulmonary comorbidity.

The Lung Cancer Study Group conducted a randomized trial that confirmed that lobectomy is the procedure of choice for patients with lung cancer, but segmentectomy and wedge resection are very reasonable compromise resections for those patients who are not able to tolerate a lobectomy. However, in the last few years several investigators have suggested that sublobar resections may have similar or equal outcomes to lobectomy in some patients. Lung cancer screening by low-dose spiral computed tomography (CT) has resulted in the identification of many small lung nodules, as well as nodules with an alveolar filling appearance rather than a solid appearance, known as a "ground glass opacities" (GGO). It is possible that the subcentimeter lung cancer may be adequately treated by wedge resection or segmentectomy, even in patients with adequate pulmonary reserve, but this has not been subjected to a prospective, randomized trial. The appearance of GGOs on screening CT scans has led to a renewed appreciation of the subset of lung cancer known as bronchioloalveolar carcinoma, which in its pure form is a noninvasive subset of adenocarcinoma that has little potential for lymphatic and hematogenous metastases. Yet bronchioloalveolar carcinoma (BAC) may spread within the airway resulting in a late parenchymal metastasis appropriate for further surgical resection. Ground glass opacities are frequently BAC and may be best treated by sublobar resections because they have a low malignant potential by traditional criteria, yet may need additional pulmonary resections in the future due to the natural history of BAC. However, it is important to differentiate pure BAC from invasive adenocarcinoma with BAC features. The former may be treated by sublobar resection, but the presence of invasive carcinoma should indicate the need for a lobectomy if possible.

There are anatomic considerations that influence appropriateness of sublobar resections as well. Although exceptions always exist, generally, segmentectomy and wedge resection is reserved for those patients with more peripheral and smaller tumors, a rough guideline being in the outer one third of the lung parenchyma and <3 cm in diameter, respectively. It is possible to consider limited resection for larger or more central tumors, but these will almost always require an anatomic segmentectomy to achieve adequate tumor margins. Another anatomic factor is the location of the tumor within the lung. A tumor that is close to or crosses an anatomic segment may require a bisegmentectomy or "cheating" into the adjacent segment with a staple line beyond the segmental boundary. Wedge resections are easiest (i.e., most successful) near acute lung edges, where it is possible to get adequate deep margins without encountering lung parenchyma that is too thick to staple. Therefore peripheral tumors at the lung apex, lung base, or adjacent to a fissure are most amenable to an effective wedge resection.

Segmental resections are based on the principle of following the lymphatic drainage and bronchial branches of the segments resected. This provides a theoretical, but unproven, advantage over nonanatomic wedge resection in the treatment of primary lung cancer. However, segmental resections are also the least common type of pulmonary resection performed and are technically more challenging than lobectomy or pneumonectomy. This frequently results in wedge resections being performed as a default sublobar resection when parenchymal preservation is desired, due to inexperience with the indications for segmentectomy and lack of confidence in the technical components of segmentectomy.

Wedge resection of the lung is performed for a wide variety of indications, including lung biopsy for interstitial or infiltrative processes, excisional biopsy of a lung nodule, and definitive resection of a primary lung cancer or metastatic disease. With the current variety of standard and endoscopic staplers, wedge resection has become extremely easy and reliable. As a result, however, wedge resection is at risk for being overutilized, the technical simplicity being a seductive attraction to the surgeon with little thoracic surgical training or experience. Most of these surgeons have little or no experience with segmentectomy and so frequently will prefer a wedge resection procedure when a segmentectomy, or even a lobectomy, would be preferred for anatomic or oncologic reasons.

There are clear theoretical reasons explaining why segmentectomy may be superior to wedge resection for primary lung cancer. A segmental resection results in more reproducible deep parenchymal margins because it extends the resection to the pulmonary hilum. Segmentectomy also incorporates the lymphatic drainage system and interlobar lymph nodes and so may result in both more thorough resection and better staging. Several studies have suggested decreased rates of local recurrence with segmentectomy, but no well-designed study comparing segmentectomy to wedge resection has been performed. However, it is quite possible that the appearance of better cancer outcomes after segmentectomy may be substantially biased because of inappropriate or inadequate wedge resections being performed by less experienced surgeons. It is reasonable to postulate that outcomes between wedge resection and segmentectomy for primary lung cancer may be similar as long as three principles are adhered to: (1) adequate sampling of N1 and N2 lymph nodes to exclude stage II and stage III disease, (2) an adequate 2-cm parenchymal margin around the tumor, and (3) restriction of lung cancer surgery to surgeons trained in thoracic surgical oncology and performing high-volume pulmonary resections in order to have the experience and expertise to select patients who truly require sublobar resection or who may benefit from segmentectomy rather than wedge resection.

Because sublobar resections are contraindicated in patients with nodal disease, careful preoperative and intraoperative lymph node staging should be performed. Positron emission tomography (PET) adds significant accuracy to the staging accomplished with chest CT, but still suffers from false-positive and false-negative results. Mediastinoscopy is indicated to confirm or exclude N2/3 nodal disease in cases of a positive PET scan. Our practice is to perform mediastinoscopy on every lung cancer patient during the same anesthetic as the planned pulmonary resection in order to detect all possible stage III patients prior to thoracotomy, but many would consider this optional for peripheral T1 N0 M0 tumors with a normal CT and PET in the hilum and mediastinum. At the time of thoracotomy representative N1 and N2 lymph nodes should be sampled because stage II/III patients require a lobectomy for there to be confidence of a complete resection.

Segmentectomy

Intimate knowledge of pulmonary anatomy and its variants is crucial in order to perform pulmonary segmentectomy. A complete bronchoscopic exam must be performed at the time of surgery. Identification of abnormal segmental anatomy will aid in the planning of surgery, and extrinsic segmental compression or presence of endoluminal tumor in the segmental orifice are contraindications to segmental resection. Those segments that are amenable to segmentectomy include the apical, anterior, and posterior segments of the right upper lobe and the superior segment and medial basilar segment of the right lower lobe. The middle lobe is rarely considered for segmentectomy because there is little gained from a sublobar resection with this small lobe. The left lung segments amenable to segmentectomy are the apicoposterior, anterior, and lingular segments of the left upper lobe and the superior and anteromedial basilar segments of the left lower lobe. The basilar segments may be resected as a unit on either side, sparing the respective superior segment, which can supply significant pulmonary function and help to fill the space of the lower hemithorax.

The initial steps of the operation involve assessment of the tumor size and location to determine the technical feasibility of segmentectomy and any evidence of pleural, mediastinal, or nodal involvement that precludes curative sublobar resection. The anterior and apical segment arteries are dissected at the medial and superior aspect of the pulmonary hilum, and the posterior, superior, and basilar segment arteries are found in the fissure (Fig. 8-1). After clearly identifying this segmental vessel, it is divided using standard technique. Dissection of the superior pulmonary vein from the hilum and extending into the lung parenchyma allows identification and division of the respective vein draining the upper lobe segments, although some surgeons prefer to divide the posterior segmental vein within the fissure. The separate superior segment vein and basilar segment

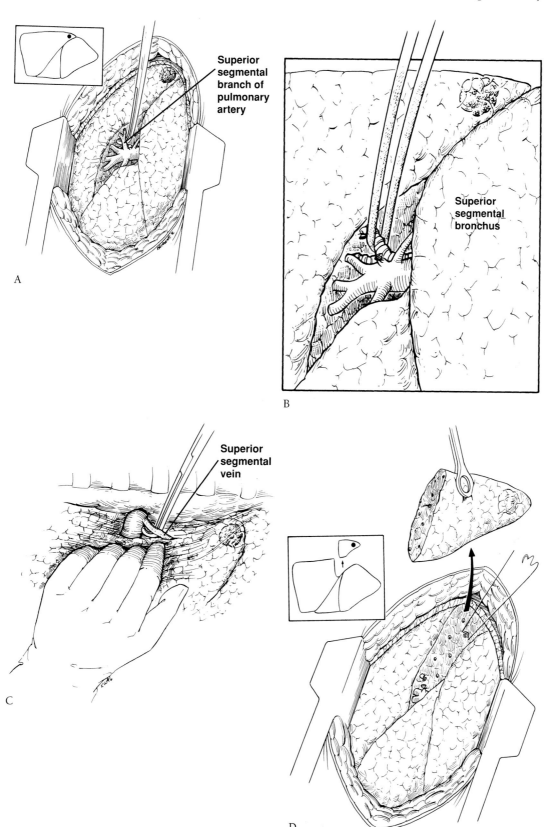

Figure 8-1. **(A)** With the fissure open, the pulmonary arterial branch to the superior segment is dissected out. Note the tumor at the apex of the right lower lobe. **(B)** The superior segmental branch of the pulmonary artery has been ligated, and the superior segmental bronchus is dissected out. **(C)** The lung is retracted medially, and the superior segmental branch of the inferior pulmonary vein is dissected out. **(D)** The intersegmental plane is opened, and the specimen is removed. Individual bronchioles and vessels can be ligated or cauterized.

confluence is readily identified after division of the pulmonary ligament and dissection of the inferior pulmonary vein, but identification of the medial basilar and anteromedial basilar vein is more difficult and requires following the basilar branches into the lung parenchyma. The posterior aspect of the fissure should be completed for posterior, apicoposterior, and superior segmentectomies, and the anterior fissure completed for the anterior, lingular, and basilar segments. No fissure division is necessary for the right apical segment. Lymph nodes encountered during vascular control and bronchial division should be resected and submitted to pathology to refine intraoperative tumor staging.

The segmental bronchus is identified deep to the divided pulmonary artery. Peribronchial lymph nodes are resected or reflected into the specimen to be resected, which facilitates encircling the airway and confirming that it is the true bronchus leading to the segment to be resected. The bronchus can be divided at its origin with a knife and oversewn with fine absorbable sutures, or alternatively can be divided using a stapler, and the stumped closed with reinforcing sutures.

The historical method of parenchymal division was accomplished by simultaneous traction on the divided segmental bronchus along with finger fracture blunt dissection along the intersegmental plane defined by the venous anatomy. This technique has the advantage of avoiding restriction of the adjacent segment by a staple line, as well as clear development of adequate margins, but it is tedious to oversew and cauterize the bleeding and air leak sites on the surface of the raw lung parenchyma, and prolonged air leak is a more common postoperative complication. Therefore, stapled division of the pulmonary parenchyma is almost universally employed because it is easy and fast, surgeons are more comfortable with the technique, and it minimizes the problems of postoperative air leak. To do this correctly, the surgeon must know the parenchymal extent of the segment very well. If there is any uncertainty, spending a few moments with a surgical atlas is a useful refresher. However, with the stapler it is perfectly acceptable to "cheat" into an adjacent segment if this will allow better resection of the tumor with a 2-cm margin. Retracting the nodule with one hand, fingers deep to the nodule on the underlying normal parenchyma while the other hand applies and fires the stapler can help to assure and maximize an adequate margin during stapling. The surgeon has to approximate the true margin, which is different in atelectatic versus inflated parenchyma, and recognize

that approximately 1 cm is removed by the pathologist (the staple line) before assessing the histologic margin.

Wedge Resection

The most common technique of nonanatomic pulmonary wedge resection uses the linear stapler, used for probably >95% of wedge resections. Stapling is readily available and effectively seals the lung parenchyma to minimize air leak. As mentioned, a stapled wedge resection is most amenable to lesions in the outer one third of the lung parenchyma and adjacent to an acute edge of lung at the fissure, apex, or base. These are rough guidelines, however, and deeper lesions can often be successfully wedged also, even if they do not fit the routine criteria for wedge resection. However, if a deep wedge resection removes a majority of the lobe or compromises the remaining lung parenchyma, the indications for sublobar resection should be re-examined and reconsideration given to formal lobectomy.

Although stapling is deceptively simple, there are a couple of important points to maximize success. First, margins are assured and maximized by the same strategy outlined in the segmentectomy section—manually lifting the nodule away from the underlying lung while applying and firing the stapler (Fig. 8-2). Second, one must carefully judge the thickness and pliability of the lung parenchyma to be stapled. Most areas of normal lung can be successfully incorporated and sealed with a 3.8-mm or 4.8-mm staple line, but some deep areas may be thicker and may not be amenable to a safe staple line. Other patients may have underlying interstitial lung disease or inflammation with thick and stiff lung. Attempts to force a stapled wedge resection in these cases may result in staple line dehiscence with serious bleeding and bronchial air leak. There are no gauges to guide the thickness of lung that can be successfully stapled, so this re-

quires surgical experience and judgment. If dehiscence does occur, it should be repaired with a running, absorbable monofilament suture, incorporating the faulty staple line, the edge of visceral pleura, and the raw lung parenchyma. We prefer a two-layer suture with a running horizontal mattress followed by a simple running suture.

The other major technique of wedge resection is cautery or laser excision, sometimes referred to as a "precision" resection or a Perelman procedure. This technique is excellent for a benign lesion, such as a hamartoma, particularly when the nodule is deeper and not presenting at a lung surface. In these cases the nodule can be essentially enucleated from the surrounding lung parenchyma with very minimal loss of normal lung tissue. The second indication for cautery excision is a metastatic nodule in the lung that is deeper in the lung parenchyma or near the pulmonary hilum. The technique of cautery excision may allow successful removal of the nodule with 1 cm to 2 cm of parenchymal margin with anatomy that would have otherwise required a lobectomy. The third indication is a nodule surrounded by thick or stiff lung that does not have the compliance to accept the compression of a staple line. Cautery resection is rarely performed for primary lung cancer, however, because, the margins are less than would normally be desired.

The technique of cautery excision is similar for the electrocautery and the Nd:YAG laser (Fig. 8-3). The desired boundary of the resection is marked on the visceral pleura with the lung partially inflated and then progressively deepened circumferentially

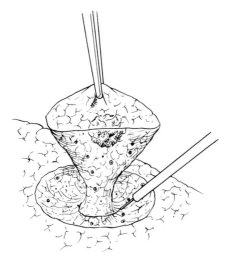

Figure 8-3. A deep-seated nodule is delivered up into the field, and a cone of lung is resected, using precision electrocautery.

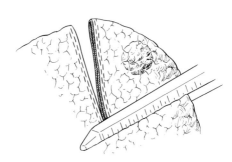

Figure 8-2. A wedge of lung is resected, using a linear stapler.

around the nodule with frequent examination of the margin. The excision is performed slowly to allow effective cauterization of the underlying parenchyma. When the resection is complete the raw lung parenchyma can be oversewn with a running two-layer closure as outlined, but the surface can also be left as a raw surface if it is superficial and hemostatic with a minimal air leak.

Video-assisted thoracic surgery (VATS), also known as thoracoscopy, can frequently be used in wedge resections, combining a minimally invasive approach to minimize recovery and morbidity. Much of the ability to palpate the lung is lost with VATS, however, making identification of the nodule more difficult and precluding a systematic bimanual palpation of the lung for other pathology. In these cases it is extremely important for the surgeon to have an ability to accurately interpret the two-dimensional CT images into a three-dimensional anatomic location to achieve a high yield of nodule identification. Then if one of the thoracoscopic ports can be placed near the nodule, it is possible to palpate the lung digitally through the port to help in localization. This technique is successful in nearly all cases of peripheral lung nodules. An alternative localizing strategy is for preoperative radiologic placement of a wire guide, but this adds to the time and complexity of the surgical procedure and should not be necessary with careful planning and minimally invasive palpation. VATS wedge resection does have a limitation of the technique, however. It is much more difficult to achieve the same degree of nodule retraction with direct tactile feedback, and so deep margins may be less reliable. On the other hand, this inability to hold the nodule can often result in the opposite effect, with overly large wedge resections performed to offset any uncertainty in the adequacy of the margin.

VATS is performed routinely for wedge resections, and is now also increasingly performed for standard lobectomy. However, the technical demands of a segmentectomy are still an indication for a thoracotomy at most, or all, thoracic surgery centers.

Conclusion

Sublobar pulmonary resections are an attractive option for benign or metastatic lung nodules, but wedge resection or segmentectomy may also be indicated in patients with primary lung cancer with poor pulmonary reserve, subcentimeter cancers, or small focal bronchioloalveolar carcinoma. Few surgeons are familiar with the technique of pulmonary segmentectomy. This is unfortunate because segmentectomy provides a useful option for patients with poor lung function and anatomy unfavorable to a wedge resection or those with primary lung cancer and the hope to accomplish a more anatomic resection. Patients undergoing sublobar resections should be carefully staged preoperatively and intraoperatively to exclude more advanced disease that is not appropriate for limited resection. Lobectomy is still the procedure of choice for non–small cell lung cancer, but sublobar resections are reasonable compromise resections that are superior to the alternatives of radiation and chemotherapy.

SUGGESTED READING

Bando T, Yamagihara K, Ohtake Y, et al. A new method of segmental resection for primary lung cancer: Intermediate results. Eur J Cardiothorac Surg 2002;21(5):894; discussion, 900.

Kodama K, Doi O, Higashiyama M, et al. Intentional limited resection for selected patients with T1 N0 M0 non–small-cell lung cancer: A single-institution study. J Thorac Cardiovasc Surg 1997;114:347.

Koike T, Yamato Y, Yoshiya K, et al. Intentional limited pulmonary resection for peripheral T1 N0 M0 small-sized lung cancer. J Thorac Cardiovasc Surg 2003;125:924.

Lung Cancer Study Group (prepared by Ginsberg RJ, Rubinstein LV). Randomized trial of lobectomy versus limited resection for T1 N0 non–small cell lung cancer. Ann Thorac Surg 1995;60:615.

Martin-Ucar AE, Nakas A, Pilling JE, et al. A case-matched study of anatomical segmentectomy versus lobectomy for stage I lung cancer in high-risk patients. Eur J Cardiothorac Surg 2005;27:675.

Okada M, Nishio W, Sakamoto T, et al. Effect of tumor size on prognosis in patients with non–small cell lung cancer: The role of segmentectomy as a type of lesser resection. J Thorac Cardiovasc Surg 2005;129:87.

Pastorino U, Valente M, Bedini V, et al. Limited resection for stage I lung cancer. Eur J Surg Oncol 1991;17:42.

Read RC, Yoder G, Schaeffer RC. Survival after conservative resection for T1 N0 M0 non–small cell lung cancer. Ann Thorac Surg 1990;49:391.

Warren WH, Faber LP. Segmentectomy versus lobectomy in patients with stage I pulmonary carcinoma: Five year survival and patterns of intrathoracic recurrence. J Thorac Cardiovasc Surg 1994;107:1087.

EDITOR'S COMMENTS

Given that the standard resection for primary lung cancer is an anatomic lobectomy, lesser resections represent a compromise, but in many instances may be the optimal approach. As DiPerna and Wood point out, for patients with compromised pulmonary function where a lobectomy may be contraindicated a segmental resection or nonanatomic wedge excision may suffice. One has to wonder, however, whether a patient who can tolerate a segmentectomy is really unable to tolerate lobectomy. This likely depends on the extent of the underlying lung disease and the distribution. If a lesion is present in a lower lobe in a patient where the lower lobe provides most of the functioning parenchyma, a superior segmentectomy sparing the basal segments may indeed be the procedure of choice.

The authors recommend that these resections be limited to thoracic surgeons trained in thoracic surgical oncology who perform a high volume of pulmonary resections. Although in principle I agree, in practice this might prove difficult. I also take issue with the authors who perform mediastinoscopy prior to every pulmonary resection. With the current generation of CAT scanners augmented by PET scanning it is hard to justify the performance of what must be called an unnecessary procedure in a patient without enlarged nodes on CT and a mediastinum that is negative on PET scan. The specificity of the combined modalities approximates 100%.

With regard to the technical details as described, I find that the segmental veins may best be taken after division of the segmental bronchus with the exception of the superior segmental vein. I agree with the authors that wedge excision is always less desirable than an anatomic resection, and one can expect that in up to one third of patients with primary lung cancers they will recur locally following a wedge excision. The procedure certainly is a compromise and should be used judiciously in patients with primary lung cancer.

L.R.K.

9

Tracheal Resection and Reconstruction

Dean M. Donahue and Douglas J. Mathisen

Anatomy

The adult trachea averages nearly 12 cm in length from the inferior border of the cricoid cartilage to the carina. There are 18 to 22 cartilaginous rings, with approximately two rings per centimeter. The only complete cartilaginous ring is the cricoid cartilage of the larynx. The first ring of the trachea is recessed into the broader ring of the cricoid.

The vocal cords are located in the middle of the larynx. The trachea begins 1.5 cm to 2.0 cm below the cords, with the initial portion of the subglottic airway located within the larynx. The posterior or membranous wall of the trachea is applied to the esophagus by an avascular plane of loose connective tissue. Laterally, connective tissue attachments allow vertical movement of the trachea with cervical motion. When the neck of a young person is hyperextended, more than one half of the trachea may be above the suprasternal notch. With the neck completely flexed forward, most of the trachea lowers into the mediastinum. With aging, the mobility of the trachea decreases.

The thyroid isthmus crosses the trachea anteriorly at the second or third ring. The thyroid is fixed to the trachea laterally by connective tissue and blood vessels. Below this, the innominate artery runs obliquely across the anterior wall of the trachea. The aortic arch runs over the anterolateral surface of the distal trachea and passes over the left main bronchus. The azygos vein arches over the right main bronchus at the tracheobronchial angle. The left recurrent laryngeal nerve runs in the tracheoesophageal groove along almost the entire length of the trachea. On the right, the nerve approaches the trachea superiorly, but ends in essentially the

same position. Both nerves enter the larynx medial to the inferior cornua of the thyroid cartilage.

The blood supply of the trachea is shared with the esophagus and the main bronchi. Supply to the upper trachea comes from the inferior thyroid artery and, to a lesser extent, the subclavian, supreme intercostal, internal thoracic, innominate, and superior and middle bronchial arteries. Many small lateral longitudinal anastomotic vessels exist. From these lateral anastomotic arcades, transverse vessels travel between the cartilaginous rings and feed the submucosa and the cartilages.

Understanding the vascular anatomy of the trachea is critical to a successful resection and reconstruction. The blood supply to the trachea comes mainly from end vessels and segments. It therefore becomes important not to devascularize the trachea circumferentially over more than a 1-cm to 2-cm length. Because these vessels enter the trachea laterally, it is safe to dissect along the entire pretracheal plane.

Etiology of Acquired Tracheal Lesions

The most common condition that requires tracheal resection and reconstruction is postintubation tracheal stenosis. Ischemia and necrosis of the tracheal mucosa can occur when a low-pressure cuff of an endotracheal tube is overinflated. A circumferential injury to the tracheal wall may then occur. If the erosion is deep enough, all layers of the trachea can be destroyed so that cicatricial repair creates a tight circumferential stenosis. It is important to emphasize the full-thickness nature of most postintubation

lesions. In our experience, full-thickness injuries are best treated by resection and reconstruction. They should not be treated by modalities aimed at the inner lining of the tracheal lumen (i.e., laser photoablation). The second means by which a postintubation stenosis can occur is at the site of a tracheostomy tube. Leverage from attached ventilatory equipment can erode part of the tracheal wall. These tend to be triangle-shaped lesions caused by contraction of the excessively eroded stoma during healing. The posterior walls of the trachea are usually intact. Endotracheal tubes can cause injury at the laryngeal level, even with short periods of intubation. Although most laryngeal injuries are the result of a cuff lesion, a tracheostomy that is placed too high on the trachea can result in subglottic injury.

Tracheal tumors, such as adenoid cystic carcinoma and squamous cell cancers, can be successfully treated with resection and reconstruction. These frequently require a lengthier resection than benign conditions. Idiopathic laryngotracheal stenosis is a condition almost exclusively seen in women. These are usually short lesions, but the laryngeal component adds to their complexity.

Tracheoesophageal fistulas are perhaps the most complex lesions. As a group they require the longest resections, and they have a higher incidence of requiring laryngeal release procedures to reduce tension on the anastomosis. The management of these lesions is beyond the scope of this chapter, but it should be stressed that definitive repair should be delayed in patients requiring positive-pressure ventilation until they can be weaned from ventilatory support. This is best accomplished by placing a tracheostomy tube with the balloon below the fistula to prevent soilage of the lung. A draining gastrostomy and a feeding jejunostomy are also placed. Single-stage repair is successful in 90% of patients.

Clinical Presentation

Clinically significant lesions manifest themselves as tracheal obstruction. The patient's symptoms progress from dyspnea on exertion to wheezing and ultimately to stridor. As the stenosis progresses, even small amounts of mucus may lead to severe obstruction at the level of the stenosis or tumor.

Diagnostic Studies

Radiographic studies of the trachea are useful in defining the presence and extent of a tracheal lesion. Lateral films of the neck with the chin raised demonstrate most lesions in the upper half of the trachea. If the patient has an existing tracheostomy stoma or tracheostomy scar, a radiopaque marker is placed on the skin to identify its relationship to the tracheal stenosis.

Tracheal tomograms are helpful in precisely measuring the extent of the lesion and the relative distance from the vocal cords and carina. The use of computed tomographic (CT) scanning is valuable in assessing the local extent of malignant tracheal pathologic involvement. CT scanning is of little value in assessing benign stenosis, with the exception of special cases such as goiter, compressive vascular lesions, or histoplasmosis.

In patients with a tracheostomy tube in place, the tube should be removed during radiographic examination to obtain the most useful information. This should be done under carefully supervised circumstances, and emergency equipment for immediate reinsertion should be available.

Bronchoscopy is mandatory in all patients with tracheal stenosis. Flexible bronchoscopy under local anesthesia is helpful in evaluating vocal cord function and the proximal extent of a stenotic lesion; however, no attempt should be made to pass the scope through the stenosis. This may precipitate respiratory distress, bleeding, increased secretions, or edema, requiring emergency tracheostomy. Bronchoscopy is best done in the operating room to allow for tracheal dilation with rigid bronchoscopes if airway compromise develops.

Indications for Surgery

Tracheal resection and reconstruction may be performed for a variety of indications. These indications can be divided into two groups: acquired and neoplastic.

Acquired lesions include stenosis from either intrinsic tracheal pathologic conditions (postintubation, inflammatory, idiopathic) or extrinsic compression (goiter, vascular rings, mediastinal masses). The treatment of a benign stenosis is based on the degree of symptomatic airway obstruction. Asymptomatic lesions may be followed closely with careful attention paid to the onset of dyspnea on exertion. Any lesion that produces enough symptoms to limit the activity of a patient should be considered for surgical correction. Traumatic injury to the airway may also require resection and reconstruction to debride the damaged portion of the trachea.

Benign tumors of the trachea can almost always be resected with primary end-to-end reconstruction as opposed to lateral resection with primary or patch closure, a procedure that is not our preferred method of treatment. Malignant lesions, either primary tracheal tumors or tracheal involvement by thyroid tumors, may also be treated with resection and reconstruction.

Treatment Options

Circumferential resection and reconstruction remains the best overall treatment strategy for symptomatic tracheal lesions. There are certain instances in which surgical management should be delayed. These include the presence of severe inflammation in the area of the planned resection or a patient on high-dose systemic corticosteroids. Repair in either of these instances may lead to restenosis. The initial management options in these situations include repeated dilations with a rigid bronchoscope and placement of a tracheostomy tube or T tube. If there is no existing stoma, the tube is placed directly through the stenotic lesion to avoid damaging uninvolved trachea. If there is a pre-existing stoma placed away from the site of stenosis, the stoma should be replaced with one through the stenosis to allow the old stoma area to heal. This may provide an additional length of trachea to be used for reconstruction. In other patients, reconstruction may not be advisable at all because of the length of stenosis. In these patients, a T tube may provide the best long-term management.

Surgical Technique

It is important to emphasize complete evaluation of the larynx before proceeding to tracheal reconstruction. If there is any question of vocal cord dysfunction, a fiberoptic evaluation of the larynx is performed preoperatively.

The surgical procedure begins with rigid bronchoscopic evaluation of the larynx and trachea. Bronchoscopes ranging in diameter from 3.5 mm to 9 mm should be available. If the tracheal lumen is <6 mm in diameter, the smaller instruments are serially passed through the stenosis to dilate this. This will prevent hypercarbia during the early part of the procedure until the trachea can be opened and ventilated across the field. Using the rigid bronchoscope, measurements should be carefully obtained beginning at the carina and defining the inferior border of the stenosis, the superior border of the stenosis, the cricoid cartilage, and the vocal cords. These measurements are useful in planning the resection and helpful in deciding if a release procedure should be used.

The degree of inflammation should also be evaluated because the presence of intense inflammation may require delaying definitive surgical correction. These patients can be temporarily managed by dilating the stenosis and inserting a fenestrated tracheostomy tube, or preferably a silicone rubber (Silastic) T tube.

Patients are positioned with the neck hyperextended with an inflatable thyroid bag beneath the scapula. The surgical field extends from the chin to below the sternum. Exposure is obtained through a collar incision (Fig. 9-1A). Although rarely needed, additional exposure can be obtained by partial upper sternotomy (Fig. 9-1B). The upper and lower flaps are elevated deep to the platysma from above the cricoid cartilage to the sternal notch. The strap muscles are separated along the midline. The thyroid isthmus is divided and suture ligated. The anterior surface of the trachea is cleared from the cricoid cartilage to the carina.

The area of stenosis is usually a full-thickness injury clearly visible on the outer surface of the trachea. Occasionally, the cartilaginous rings are not destroyed, and external identification of the stenosis may be difficult. In this case, the flexible bronchoscope is passed through the endotracheal tube, and the tube is pulled back above the stenosis. A 25-gauge needle is inserted into the trachea. Under direct vision through the bronchoscope, this needle is then positioned to determine the uppermost aspect of the stenosis. A fine suture is placed on the tracheal wall at this point, and the endotracheal tube is advanced.

Lateral dissection is then carried out along the entire extent of the stenosis and

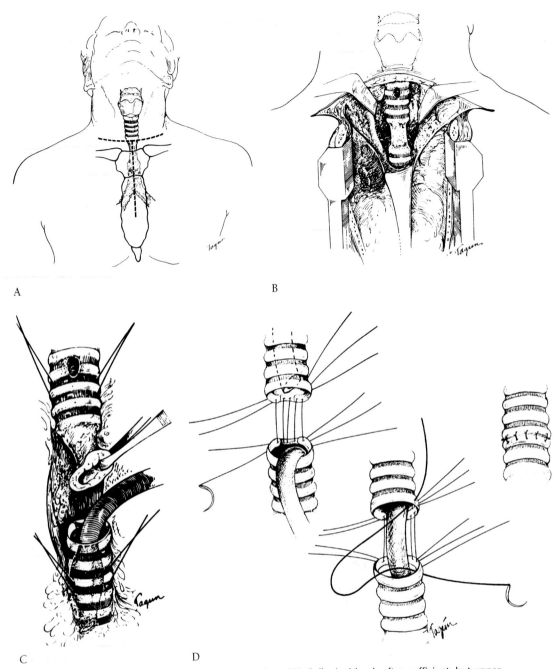

A

B

C

D

Figure 9-1.   Reconstruction of the upper trachea. **(A)** Collar incision is often sufficient, but upper median sternotomy improves access to the mediastinum. **(B)** Retraction of innominate vein and artery provides working space. **(C)** Division of the trachea and intubation across the operative field permit dissection of densely adherent lesion. **(D)** Posterolateral sutures are placed. The proximal airway is advanced and anterior sutures are placed. (Reprinted with permission from HC Grillo. Tracheal reconstruction: indications and techniques. Arch Otolaryngol 1972;96:31.)

for approximately 1 cm below the stenosis. No effort is made to visualize the recurrent laryngeal nerves. These will not be injured if the dissection is kept on the tracheal wall. Tiny blood vessels are carefully cauterized as they are encountered.

Dissection is then carried circumferentially to a point approximately 1 cm below the lower level of the stenosis. The trachea is then encircled with a Penrose drain for traction. It is important to emphasize that no more than 1 cm of normal trachea is dissected circumferentially below the area to be resected. This reduces the risk of devascularizing the portion of the trachea that is to be used for the reconstruction.

The trachea is then divided at the lower border of the stenosis. The divided trachea is intubated across the operative field with a flexible Tovell tube. Sterile corrugated tubing is then connected to the tube and passed out through the drapes to the anesthetist. The patient is ventilated while the stenotic segment is retracted upward with Allis forceps (Fig. 9-1C). The dissection continues close to the tracheal wall. A red rubber catheter is sutured to the endotracheal tube, which is then withdrawn upward through the vocal cords. The catheter will be used to guide the endotracheal tube back into the airway once the repair sutures are all placed. Traction sutures of 2-0 polyglactin 910 (Vicryl) are then placed on the lateral walls of each end of the trachea, 1 cm from the divided edge of the airway (Fig. 9-1C). Before the anastomosis is constructed, the patient's head is flexed. The traction sutures are then drawn together to ensure that approximation of the trachea can be accomplished without tension. The patient's neck is then allowed to re-extend, and the anastomosis is completed.

A 4-0 Vicryl suture is then placed in the midline posteriorly from outside the posterior membranous wall to inside the tracheal lumen in the upper tracheal end (Fig. 9-1D). This stitch is then passed from inside the membranous wall of the distal end of the trachea to outside. Each suture is placed approximately 3 mm from the cut edge of the trachea and passed through the full thickness of the tracheal wall. This posterior suture will be the last suture tied and is held by a hemostat at the upper end of the surgical field. The endotracheal tube is removed from the distal trachea intermittently to facilitate placement of the sutures. Interrupted 4-0 Vicryl sutures are then placed in a stepwise fashion toward the operator's side of the field. This is continued to the level of the lateral traction suture. Sutures are then placed from the initial midpoint posterior stitch, sewing away from the operator's side to the level of the lateral traction stitch on the opposite side of the field. Each of these sutures is clipped serially to the side of the drapes. The sutures for the anterior portion of the trachea are placed forehand, all anterior to the lateral traction sutures. These are all clipped serially to the drapes below the incision.

Once all anastomotic sutures have been placed, the endotracheal tube is advanced under direct vision into the distal trachea. The thyroid bag is deflated, and the patient's head is propped on folded blankets to maintain the neck in flexion. The lateral traction sutures on each side are then tied, thus drawing the ends of the trachea together. The anterior tracheal wall sutures are tied, followed by the posterior sutures (Fig. 9-1D). The trachea is rotated slightly by pulling on the lateral traction suture to facilitate tying of the posterior row of sutures. If possible, the thyroid isthmus is reapproximated anteriorly over the anastomosis. If there is concern regarding the postoperative airway, then a small silk suture is placed in an area of the trachea away from the anastomosis to mark a site for a possible future tracheostomy.

A small, closed suction drain is inserted through a stab wound lateral to the incision and placed in the pretracheal plane. The strap muscles are anatomically reconstructed and the platysma and skin closed with subcutaneous sutures. At the conclusion of the procedure, a guardian stitch is placed from the submental crease to the presternal skin. This will assist the patient in keeping the head in flexion.

Postoperative Management

All patients are allowed to wake up and are extubated while still in the operating room. This allows the surgeon to assess the airway and to be certain that the anastomosis is satisfactory. If the airway is not satisfactory, the patient is reintubated with a small endotracheal tube positioned below the anastomosis. Preferably this would be an uncuffed or a deflated cuffed tube. A postoperative tracheostomy is rarely needed. In our series, only 8% (71 of 901) of patients required one. This was typically due to laryngeal edema from a high anastomosis or vocal cord paralysis. Some of these tracheostomies were done routinely early in our experience with laryngotracheal reconstruction. We now find the routine use of tracheostomies in this patient population unnecessary. If a tracheostomy is necessary, it is placed through a small vertical incision away from the anastomosis. The anastomosis should then be covered with either mobilized thyroid isthmus or a pedicled strap muscle flap to separate it from the opened airway. Early in the postoperative course, the patients are observed for signs of tachypnea, dyspnea, or stridor. Oral intake is usually begun under close observation beginning with a thick liquid or soft solid diet. Thin liquids are avoided initially. If laryngeal reconstruction was performed or if there is hoarseness, oral intake is delayed to avoid aspiration. The surgical drains are managed based on their output, usually being removed on postoperative day 2. If there is concern regarding the airway, a flexible bronchoscopy may be done to evaluate the larynx and the anastomosis, as well as to clear any retained secretions. The guardian chin stitch is cut on the seventh postoperative day, and a flexible bronchoscopy is routinely performed to evaluate the repair.

The same principles apply to tracheal resection for tumor. The one exception is the need to identify the recurrent laryngeal nerves because of extraluminal neoplasm. Otherwise, the details of resection and reconstruction are the same as described for tracheal stenosis. It is important preoperatively to assess the extent of extratracheal involvement by tumor to accurately evaluate the feasibility of resection.

Results

In 2004, our group published a series of 901 patients undergoing a tracheal resection and reconstruction over a 28-year period. The patient characteristics of that series are listed in Table 9-1. The operative procedures performed are listed in Table 9-2, and the results of tracheal resection and reconstruction are listed in Table 9-3. Nearly 95% of patients had an intact airway without the need for tracheostomy or T tube. A permanent airway appliance was needed in 4.2% of patients. There were 11 deaths in the series.

Table 9-1 Tracheal Resection and Reconstruction: Patient Characteristics ($n = 901$)

Diagnosis (number of patients)	
Postintubation	589
Tumor	208
Idiopathic	83
Tracheoesophageal fistula	21
Age (years)	
Mean ± SD	47.4 ± 18.9
Range	4–86
Diabetes	10.7%
Preoperative steroids	7%
Obese (BMI >30 kg/m^2)	25.2%
Preoperative tracheostomy	30.6%
Reoperation	11.2%

BMI = body mass index; SD = standard deviation.

Table 9-2 Operative Procedures ($n = 901$)

Incisions	
Cervical	75%
Plus mediastinal	20%
Thoracotomy	5%
Length resected (cm)	
Mean ± SD	3.3 ± 1
Range	1–6.5
Laryngotracheal anastomosis	31.2%
Laryngeal release	9%
Postoperative tracheostomy	8%

SD = standard deviation.

Table 9-3 Tracheal Resection and Reconstruction: Results ($n = 901$)	
Complications	18.2%
Anastomotic complications	9%
Deaths	1.2%
Result	
Good	94.6%
Tracheostomy or T tube	4.2%

Anastomotic Complications

Complications following tracheal resection and reconstruction are infrequent. The most common and most serious complications are related to anastomotic healing. There were 81 anastomotic complications (9%) in our series of 901 patients undergoing tracheal resection and reconstruction between 1975 and 2003. These complications included separation of the suture line ($n = 37$), recurrent stenosis at the anastomosis ($n = 37$), and obstructing granulation tissue formation ($n = 7$). Treatment of these complications involved permanent T tube ($n = 20$), temporary T tube ($n = 16$), reoperation ($n = 16$), permanent tracheostomy ($n = 14$), temporary tracheostomy ($n = 7$), and repeated dilations ($n = 2$). After treatment, half of these patients had a good result and were without an airway appliance.

Multivariable analysis (Table 9-4) has shown that the most significant predictors for anastomotic complications were reoperation and diabetes. Other significant predictors were age ≤ 17, resection length ≥ 4 cm, the need for a laryngotracheal resection, and the presence of a preoperative tracheostomy. Early in our experience, the use of permanent braided suture led to the formation of granulation tissue in nearly one fourth of

Table 9-4 Multivariable Predictors of Anastomotic Complications		
Variable	Odds Ratio	p Value
Diabetes	3.32	0.002
Reoperation	3.03	0.002
Length of resection ≥ 4 cm	2.01	0.007
Age ≤ 17 years	2.26	0.03
Laryngotracheal resection	1.80	0.03
Preoperative tracheostomy	1.79	0.04

our patients. The majority of these complications could be addressed with bronchoscopic removal of the granulation tissue. In 1978, we began using braided absorbable polyglactin sutures. Since then, <2% of patients have developed significant granulation tissue at the anastomosis.

Other Complications

Laryngeal Dysfunction

Laryngeal dysfunction may result from injury to the recurrent laryngeal nerves during the dissection or from a high laryngotracheal anastomosis. In 5% of cases there were varying degrees of postoperative laryngeal dysfunction. Half of these patients had minor or temporary dysfunction that required no specific treatment. The remainder had more severe dysfunction requiring temporary or permanent tracheostomy or T tube. Two patients required gastrostomy tube feedings for persistent aspiration secondary to glottic dysfunction.

Laryngeal complications, mainly aspiration or vocal cord dysfunction, occurred in 4 of 9 patients undergoing thyrohyoid laryngeal release (44%) and in 8 of 40 (20%) undergoing suprahyoid release. In 8 patients, the combination of laryngotracheal resection plus laryngeal release resulted in a 50% complication rate. These complications included dysphagia in 3, with aspiration also in 1, malacia in 1, and partial or complete dehiscence in 3. Laryngeal function improved in 3 of the 4 patients with major complication, ultimately leading to a good result.

Hemorrhage

Since our institution's initial experience with this procedure in 1966, five patients bled from the innominate artery. Three of them died, two of whom had concomitant anastomotic separation. One patient was managed successfully with repair of the artery, and one was managed by division of the innominate artery.

Infection

Infectious complications developed in 6.8% of patients. These complications were evenly divided between wound infections and bronchitis or pneumonia. Half of the wound infections were minor infections that were treated with intravenous antibiotics only, but the remainder were more extensive sternal infections that required surgical debridement.

A majority of the patients with bronchitis or pneumonia required bedside bronchoscopic treatment and antibiotics. Three patients were managed with temporary tracheostomy and two with reintubation.

Deaths

Eleven perioperative deaths have occurred in the 901 patients operated on since 1975 (1.2%). Complications related to anastomotic dehiscence accounted for 6 deaths: 3 from acute airway obstruction, 2 from tracheoinnominate artery fistula, and 1 from mediastinitis. The 6 deaths unrelated to anastomotic complications were due to aspiration pneumonia ($n = 3$), pulmonary embolism ($n = 1$), and myocardial infarction ($n = 1$).

Conclusion

Postintubation stenosis is the most common indication for tracheal resection and reconstruction, and its causes have been well established. Prevention of these lesions is possible in most situations by use of large-volume, low-pressure cuffs and careful management of stomal tubes. However, we continue to see patients with these lesions, most likely caused by overinflation of plastic cuffs and traction on tracheostomy tubes.

Nonoperative treatments, including repeated dilation, local and systemic steroids, cryosurgery, fulguration, laser treatment, and prolonged or permanent stenting with T tubes and other stents, are only successful in carefully selected lesions. Failure rates with laser treatment range from 23% to 43% and reflect the fact that these lesions involve the full thickness of the tracheal wall.

Segmental tracheal resection remains the preferred definitive treatment for postintubation stenosis, as well as selected other tracheal lesions. In our series, good results were obtained in 94.6% of all resections, with failure in 4.2% and death in 1.2%. The increased failure rate mandates a continued cautious approach to laryngotracheal reconstruction. It must also be remembered that a permanent tracheal T tube may be the best solution for a patient with extensive tracheal damage where resection is questionable.

SUGGESTED READING

Gaissert H, Grillo HC, Mathisen DJ, et al. Temporary and permanent restoration of airway continuity with the tracheal T-tube. J Thorac Cardiovasc Surg 1994;107:600.

Grillo HC, Donahue DM, Mathisen DJ, et al. Postintubation tracheal stenosis: treatment and results. J Thorac Cardiovasc Surg 1995; 109:486.

Grillo HC, Mark EJ, Mathisen DJ, et al. Idiopathic laryngotracheal stenosis and its management. Ann Thorac Surg 1993;56:80.

Grillo HC, Mathisen DJ. Primary tracheal tumors: Treatment and results. Ann Thorac Surg 1990;49:69.

Grillo HC, Mathisen DJ, Wain JC. Laryngotracheal resection and reconstruction for subglottic stenosis. Ann Thorac Surg 1992;53:54.

Grillo HC, Suen HC, Mathisen DJ, et al. Resectional management of thyroid carcinoma invading the airway. Ann Thorac Surg 1992;54:3.

Wright CD, Grillo HC, Wain JC, et al. Anastomotic complications after tracheal resection: Prognostic factors and management. J Thorac Cardiovasc Surg 2004;128:731.

EDITOR'S COMMENTS

It is hard to add much in the way of commentary to the information provided by Drs. Donohue and Mathisen, given that the experience from the Massachusetts General Hospital (MGH) far exceeds that of any other place in the world. Homage must be paid to the pioneering contributions of the former leader of this group, Dr. Hermes Grillo, who single-handedly essentially defined the field of tracheal surgery. The material presented here primarily stems from his work and teachings. Fortunately in the current era of intensive care unit management ischemic tracheal strictures occur rarely, but this makes it difficult for an individual surgeon to acquire the expertise necessary to achieve the kind of results reported by the MGH group.

Technique, as stressed by the authors, and attention to detail are the hallmarks of tracheal surgery. To paraphrase Clem Hiebert, an MGH trainee and a superb surgeon, "tracheal surgery is either terribly simple or simply terrible." The ease with which one can devascularize the trachea with resultant anastomotic breakdown or stricture formation cannot be underestimated. As the authors point out, circumferential mobilization should be kept to a minimum because the blood supply is segmental and comes in laterally. Injury to one or both recurrent laryngeal nerves may occur if dissection veers away from the trachea, and the left nerve is especially vulnerable because one works in the tracheoesophageal groove to get around the trachea prior to dividing it. The initial division of the trachea should be done distal to the stricture or tumor and then the trachea retracted upward so as to facilitate dissection and separation of the involved segment off the esophagus. The proximal division then occurs once the trachea is separated away from the esophagus.

Airway management is key, and a sterile anesthesia circuit must be placed on the field before division of the airway. Periodic ventilation of the distal segment is interspersed with suture placement. Suture placement must be precise, and aligning the sutures properly so as to facilitate tying them is key. It is easy to get individual sutures twisted on one another making the completion of the anastomosis extremely difficult. Suture placement should be done with the neck extended but the sutures tied with the neck flexed to minimize tension on the suture line. The area in which experience and judgment comes into play is in deciding how much of the trachea can be resected and whether a release procedure should be performed. Thus the importance of the rigid bronchoscopy and the measurements relative to the carina and the vocal cords. This is crucial because laryngeal release procedures commonly are associated with swallowing dysfunction especially in older individuals. A stricture must be completely resected to achieve the best possible outcome, and tumors should be resected with negative margins. There is a tendency on the part of the inexperienced operator to be very conservative with the amount of trachea resected, thus leaving disease behind and doing the patient a disservice. This stems mainly from concerns on the part of the inexperienced operator regarding the ability to reconstruct the trachea without tension. The experienced tracheal surgeon recognizes that essentially half of the trachea may be resected and successfully reconstructed, but when one sees the distance between the two ends immediately following the resection it does give one pause and the beads of sweat begin to accumulate on the brow. This is especially true with tumors where extensive resections often are required and are made more complex by the presence of extraluminal disease. Rarely is a partial sternotomy required for proximal and mid-tracheal lesions. Subglottic stenoses require special consideration especially with regard to the cricoid cartilage and the technique for resecting a portion of the cricoid with preservation of the recurrent laryngeal nerves. Griff Pearson has contributed significantly to the techniques for these types of resections, which are somewhat more complex than a standard tracheal resection.

The chin stitch should be placed not so much to keep the chin on the chest as to serve as a reminder to the patient that neck extension should be avoided. As pointed out by the authors, the chin stitch should remain in place for 7 days.

Anastomotic dehiscence can be catastrophic and must be managed appropriately, usually with a T tube. It is this type of situation that requires the expertise of an operator experienced in tracheal surgery if these patients are to be salvaged. Here again the contributions of Dr. Grillo and the MGH group have defined the management techniques.

L.R.K.

10

Carinal Resection

Dean M. Donahue

Introduction

Resection of the carina may be performed with or without a pulmonary resection. It is an important option available to thoracic surgeons in the management of tumors of the central airways. Neoplasm accounts for approximately 90% of the indications for carinal resection and reconstruction. Benign or inflammatory conditions occasionally require this procedure to permanently relieve airway obstruction.

These aggressive procedures have several challenging issues that must be overcome, including patient selection, intraoperative anesthetic management, and reconstruction techniques. The location of the lesion determines the extent of resection required and the type of reconstruction that may be performed. The feasibility of central airway reconstruction guides the determination of resectability.

Patient Evaluation

As part of the preparation for carinal resection and reconstruction, the patient must undergo a standard medical evaluation. This includes examining cardiac and pulmonary comorbidities as well as other systemic illnesses and factors such as nutritional status. The initial patient evaluation is designed to identify risk factors that may be modified preoperatively, potentially improving the patient's postoperative course. Smoking cessation, improving the patient's nutritional status, and weaning corticosteroids are examples of risk modification before carinal surgery. Patients who previously underwent mediastinal irradiation represent an increased perioperative risk. There are several factors thought to contribute to this, including damage to the microvascular circulation at the anastomosis and reduced tissue pliability, which potentially increases anastomotic tension.

Evaluation of pulmonary function with static pulmonary function tests (PFTs), measurement of diffusion capacity, and quantitative ventilation and perfusion scan are useful in carinal surgery with pulmonary resection. It is critical if a sleeve pneumonectomy is being contemplated. The data from the quantitative perfusion scan can be used in conjunction with PFTs to calculate a predicted postoperative forced expiratory volume in 1 second (FEV_1). This is calculated as a percentage of the predicted value based on the patient's body surface area.

Computed tomography (CT) scans of the chest are mandatory for all patients before carinal surgery. For a malignant process, these scans can provide information on the extent of tumor within the airway, although this frequently underestimates the involvement. They can also visualize the tumor outside of the airway that is not appreciated by bronchoscopy. The size and location of mediastinal lymph nodes are identified, but a mediastinoscopy is recommended in all cases regardless of the nodal appearance. The CT scan should also be examined for the condition of the lung parenchyma, the presence of pneumonia, and any additional lesions within the lung. The presence of calcification within the coronary arteries may warrant further cardiac evaluation.

Patients undergoing carinal resection for a malignancy need a thorough metastatic evaluation. Given the increased risk of these resections, magnetic resonance imaging or contrast-enhanced CT scan of the brain is recommended in all patients. Positron emission tomography is helpful in evaluating regional and occult systemic disease. An abdominal CT scan is performed with special attention paid to the liver and adrenal glands.

Anesthesia

Positive-pressure ventilation increases the pressure on a freshly created airway anastomosis. Therefore, the goal of the anesthetic technique is to allow extubation at the completion of the surgical procedure. Short-acting or reversible agents facilitate this goal. When a pneumonectomy is planned, there must be judicious fluid administration, lower oxygen concentrations, and attention to airway pressures.

With resection of the carina, single-lung ventilation will be required. Unfortunately, standard double-lumen endotracheal tubes are impractical because they are difficult to reposition after the anastomosis has been constructed. Instead, an extra long (>31 cm), flexible single-lumen tube that is armored to avoid kinking is preferred. Because most central airway surgery is performed from the right chest, this tube is positioned in the left main bronchus using a bronchoscope.

Because the distal trachea and main bronchi will be opened, intubation of one main bronchus with a sterile apparatus across the operative field is required. Cross-field ventilation is then intermittently performed. There are brief periods when the tube is removed from the main bronchus to allow placement of anastomotic sutures. Frequent communication between the surgeon and anesthesia team is critical to maintain adequate gas exchange. For cases where oxygenation is difficult, jet catheters can be placed into the open bronchus to allow high-frequency ventilation. Once the sutures between the trachea and the main bronchus are completed, the endotracheal tube is advanced across the anastomosis for continued ventilation. If necessary, the second anastomosis reimplanting the remaining bronchus to the side of the airway can be constructed without interrupting ventilation.

Operative Technique

Intraoperative Evaluation

Bronchoscopy is the most effective way to evaluate the extent of airway involvement. This information is used to determine whether a reconstruction can be performed with acceptable anastomotic tension. As a general rule, the safe limit is 4 cm between the tracheal and left main bronchial margins. For bulky tumors, rigid bronchoscopy provides the added benefit of a core-out procedure. This technique allows debulking of the intraluminal tumor. If there is postobstructive pneumonia, this improves drainage before the planned resection.

Mediastinoscopy is recommended for all cases. A thorough lymph node evaluation, regardless of appearance on CT scanning, is required for accurate staging. If mediastinal lymph nodes are involved, resection may be considered after neoadjuvant therapy. Patients with contralateral or supraclavicular nodal (N3) disease are typically considered unresectable.

A mediastinoscopy will also open the anterior pretracheal plane along the length of the trachea. This facilitates tracheal mobility and reduces tension on the anastomosis. The mediastinoscopy is typically performed at the time of planned carinal resection. Performing this as a separate procedure will eventually lead to scar formation in the pretracheal plane, potentially reducing tracheal mobility.

Surgical Approaches

Due to the location of the aortic arch, exposure for most carinal resections is easier through a right posterolateral thoracotomy incision. This allows excellent exposure to the trachea, right bronchial tree, and much of the left main bronchus. Occasionally, the location of the lesion will require a left-sided thoracotomy. Exposure of the carina from this side is facilitated by mobilizing the left main pulmonary artery and the aortic arch (Fig. 10-1). One must be attentive to the location of the recurrent laryngeal nerve to prevent injury. Slings—usually umbilical tape or Penrose drains—are then passed around both the distal trachea and right main bronchus.

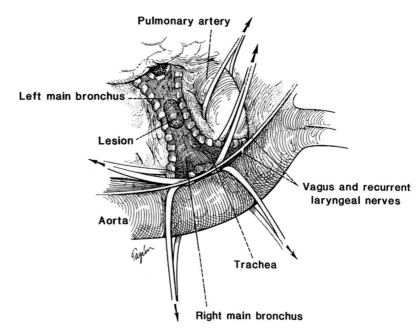

Figure 10-1. Exposure for left main bronchial resection. Note the tracheal, right main bronchial, pulmonary artery, and aortic retraction that provides improved exposure. (Reprinted with permission from Newton JR, Grillo HC, Mathisen DJ. Main bronchial sleeve resection with pulmonary conservation. Ann Thorac Surg 1991;52:1272.)

The carina can also be approached anteriorly, either through a median sternotomy or bilateral anterior ("clamshell") thoracotomy. The anterior and then the posterior pericardium is opened between the superior vena cava and ascending aorta. Mobilizing the brachial cephalic vessels in a cephalad direction and the right main pulmonary artery caudally provides exposure to the distal trachea and proximal main bronchi.

Resection of the Carina

If the operation is from the right chest, the azygous vein is divided to improve exposure of the carina. Occasionally a segment of the esophagus is encircled with a Penrose drain and retracted away from the airway. From the left side, the aortic arch is mobilized and encircled with two or three Penrose drains. This allows the arch to be lifted carefully away from the airway to improve exposure.

The carina and adjacent tissues are then dissected away from the surrounding structures. At this time the pretracheal plane should be reevaluated to ensure that it has been fully dissected up to the neck. Once it is fully mobilized, the airway resection may commence.

Typically, the left main bronchus is divided and lateral traction sutures are placed on each side. During this portion of the procedure, the bronchus is intubated as previously outlined. The trachea is then divided above the carina, and lateral traction sutures

are once again placed (Fig. 10-2). If any of the right lung is being preserved, the airway is divided at the appropriate level (i.e., the main bronchus or bronchus intermedius). Additional traction sutures can be placed in the right-sided bronchus. The mobility of the airway segments is then evaluated using the traction sutures. If tension is a concern, various release maneuvers may be performed.

Release Maneuvers

Avoiding anastomotic tension is another important principle in airway reconstruction. Factors such as the patient's age and the existence of scar tissue from prior surgery or radiation contribute to the intrinsic airway mobility. The simplest means of reducing tension is flexion of the neck. Slight cervical flexion can be maintained postoperatively with a guardian stitch between the chin and the presternal tissue.

An intrapericardial release is commonly performed. This will improve mobility of the main bronchi by 1 cm to 2 cm. The inferior pulmonary ligament is first divided, and a U-shaped pericardial incision is made around the inferior pulmonary vein. The raphe below the vein is then divided to complete this maneuver (Fig. 10-3).

A suprahyoid release does not usually improve mobility at the distal trachea. It may be used for more extensive resections that involve higher levels on the trachea.

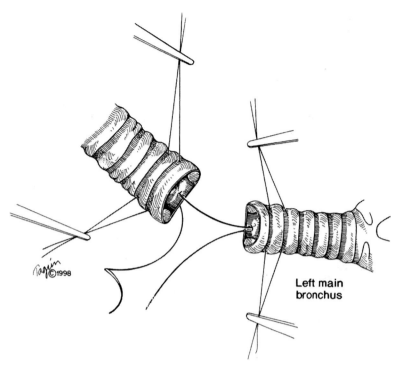

Left main bronchus

Figure 10-2. Technique of end-to-end anastomosis. (Reprinted with permission from Mitchell JD, Mathisen DJ, Wright CD, et al. Clinical experience with carinal resection. J Thorac Cardiovasc Surg 1999;117:39.)

Airway Reconstruction

Airway healing is facilitated by adequate blood supply on each side of the anastomosis. Most of the blood supply to the trachea comes from segmental vessels entering laterally. Mobilizing the pretracheal space improves mobility, but dissection laterally must be avoided to preserve these blood vessels. At the carina and main bronchi, the bronchial arteries provide most of the blood supply. These arteries include ante-rior branches arising from the subclavian artery, internal mammary artery, or coronary vessels. There are also posterior bronchial arteries from the aorta or intercostal arteries. The bronchial arteries create a plexus in the peribronchial areolar tissue.

Knowledge of the vascular anatomy allows one to understand one of the basic tenets of airway surgery: preservation of blood supply. The airway must be dissected circumferentially at the planned site of transection. To preserve collateral blood supply to the cut end, the extent of circumferential dissection is minimized to a length of approximately 3 mm to 4 mm from the end of the airway.

The first anastomosis is constructed between the trachea and the main bronchus in an end-to-end technique. This involves placing simple interrupted 4-0 Vicryl (polyglactin; Ethicon Inc., Somerville, NJ) sutures circumferentially. These are placed so that the knots will remain outside of the lumen. Once the sutures are in place, the endotracheal tube is advanced into the main bronchus. The traction sutures on either side of the anastomosis are then tied together to approximate the airways. If there is a size discrepancy, the bronchus can be allowed to intussuscept into the trachea. The individual anastomotic sutures are then tied down (Fig. 10-4).

If the location of the lesion allows any of the right lung to being preserved, an end-to-side anastomosis is constructed. The

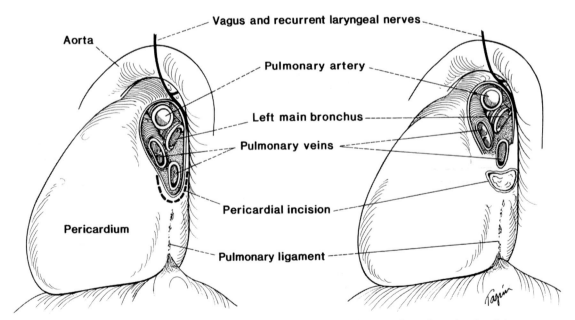

Vagus and recurrent laryngeal nerves
Aorta
Pulmonary artery
Left main bronchus
Pulmonary veins
Pericardial incision
Pericardium
Pulmonary ligament

Figure 10-3. The left-side intrapericardial hilar release technique showing the U-shaped pericardial incision allowing 1 cm to 2 cm of upward hilar mobility to facilitate the creation of a tension-free anastomosis. (Reprinted with permission from Newton JR, Grillo HC, Mathisen DJ. Main bronchial sleeve resection with pulmonary conservation. Ann Thorac Surg 1991;52:1272.)

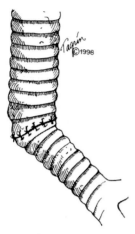

Figure 10-4. The trachea and contralateral bronchus are brought together in an end-to-end anastomosis. (Reprinted with permission from Mitchell JD, Mathisen DJ, Wright CD, et al. Clinical experience with carinal resection. J Thorac Cardiovasc Surg 1999; 117:39.)

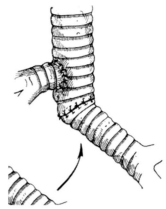

Figure 10-6. After end-to end anastomosis between the trachea and left mainstem bronchus, the bronchus intermedius is reimplanted into the trachea. (Reprinted with permission from Mitchell JD, Mathisen DJ, Wright CD, et al. Clinical experience with carinal resection. J Thorac Cardiovasc Surg 1999;117:39.)

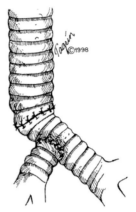

Figure 10-7. After end-to-end anastomosis between the trachea and left mainstem bronchus, the bronchus intermedius is reimplanted into the left mainstem. (Reprinted with permission from Mitchell JD, Mathisen DJ, Wright CD, et al. Clinical experience with carinal resection. J Thorac Cardiovasc Surg 1999;117:39.)

location of this anastomosis must be at least 1 cm away from the tracheobronchial anastomosis (Fig. 10-5). With a hilar release maneuver, the right bronchial anastomosis can usually be placed on the side of the trachea (Fig. 10-6). If there is still tension after release maneuvers have been performed, then the anastomosis should be placed on the side of the left main bronchus 1 cm beyond the

tracheal anastomosis (Fig. 10-7). In either location, the anastomosis should be placed along the lateral wall of the airway within the cartilaginous portion. The end-to-side anastomosis is constructed in a similar fashion with interrupted 4-0 Vicryl suture. Lateral traction sutures are occasionally omitted in favor of two 3-0 Vicryl sutures at each corner of the anastomosis.

Once all anastomoses have been completed they are tested for air leaks with controlled positive-pressure ventilation. They are then wrapped with a pedicled tissue flap. This is to provide additional blood supply to promote healing and to separate the suture line from the adjacent pulmonary arteries. A pericardial fat pad flap is preferred. If there are two anastomoses, the flap can be split distally to wrap around each one. A pleural flap may also be used in a patient at low risk for anastomotic complications. In high-risk cases, such as previous radiation therapy, a flap of omentum is strongly recommended.

Postoperative Care

Disruption of the normal mucociliary pathway created by an airway anastomosis results in abnormal secretion clearance. Adequate pain control with epidural or systemic analgesics optimizes a patient's ability to cough. Chest physiotherapy should be aggressively employed. If necessary, flexible bronchoscopy should be used to assist in pulmonary toilet.

Among the most frequent complications are atrial arrhythmias. These are frequently well tolerated and transient. Standard initial management includes rate control with β-blockers or calcium-channel blockers.

Within the first 3 days after a carinal pneumonectomy attention must be paid to the development of adult respiratory distress syndrome. This is characterized by tachypnea, hypoxia, and a ground-glass radiographic appearance in the remaining

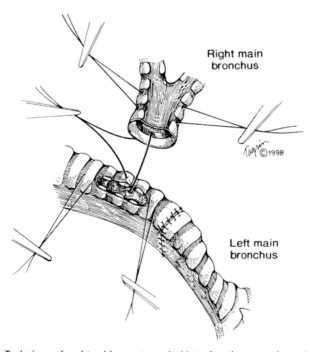

Right main bronchus

Left main bronchus

Figure 10-5. Technique of end-to-side anastomosis. Note that the created opening is entirely in cartilaginous wall to provide rigidity to the anastomosis. (Reprinted with permission from Mitchell JD, Mathisen DJ, Wright CD, et al. Clinical experience with carinal resection. J Thorac Cardiovasc Surg 1999;117:39.)

lung. The etiology for this condition is not known, but several factors have been implicated. Supportive measures, which are utilized as indicated, include ventilatory support, fluid restriction, and diuresis. The administration of inhaled nitric oxide has been reported to improve the clinical course of these patients, but no controlled studies have been performed.

Bronchoscopy is recommended to evaluate any concerns regarding airway integrity. It is routinely performed in all patients prior to discharge. Anastomotic complications occurring early in the postoperative course range from mild mucosal necrosis due to ischemia to anastomotic separation. An intact anastomotic wrap may prevent mediastinal contamination, and these patients may be successfully managed with a T tube extending beyond the anastomosis. If a bronchopleural fistula does develop, adequate drainage and antibiotic coverage must be established. A late anastomotic stenosis typically develops as a result of separation due to tension. Attempts can be made to dilate this stricture with rigid bronchoscopy.

Results

The complication rates in reported series of patients undergoing carinal resection and reconstruction range from 10% to 40%. The operative mortality in these same series is between 7% and 29%. As is the case with all lung cancer patients, the prognosis of tumors involving the central airways is related to the presence of lymph node metastasis. In a series of 60 carinal resections and reconstructions in patients with bronchogenic carcinoma performed at the Massachusetts General Hospital, there were 34 patients without lymph node metastasis. These patients had a 5-year survival of 51%. The 15 patients with N1 metastasis had a 32% 5-year survival of 32%. Patients with N2 or N3 disease ($n = 11$) had a 5-year survival of 12%.

Summary

Resection of the carina followed by airway reconstruction is a technically difficult endeavor carrying a high operative risk. Proper preoperative evaluation to identify reversible risk factors is helpful in improving outcome. Meticulous dissection is required with attention paid to the technical details of preserving blood supply and reducing tension on the anastomosis. The overall poor outcome of N2 disease in the presence of a carinal tumor mandates a thorough mediastinal lymph node evaluation. Maintaining adequate pulmonary toilet is critical to a successful recovery.

SUGGESTED READING

Dartevelle PG, Macchiarini P, Chapelier AR, et al. Tracheal sleeve pneumonectomy for bronchogenic carcinoma: Report of 55 cases [update]. Ann Thorac Surg 1995;60(6):1854.

Grillo HC. Carinal reconstruction. In: Grillo HC (ed). Surgery of the Trachea and Bronchi. Hamilton, Canada: BC Decker; 2004: 599.

Mitchell JD, Mathisen DJ, Wright CD, et al. Resection for bronchogenic carcinoma involving the carina: long-term results and effect of nodal status on outcome. J Thorac Cardiovasc Surg 2001;121:465.

Mitchell JD, Mathisen DJ, Wright CD, et al. Clinical experience with carinal resection. J Thorac Cardiovasc Surg 1999;117:39.

Porhanov VA, Poliakov IS, Selvaschuk AP, et al. Indications and results of sleeve carinal resection. Eur J Cardiothorac Surg 2002;22:685.

Roviaro GC, Varoli F, Romanelli A, et al. Complications of tracheal sleeve pneumonectomy: personal experience and overview of the literature. J Thorac Cardiovasc Surg 2001;121:234.

EDITOR'S COMMENTS

Donohue has provided a beautiful contribution on carinal resection, a procedure that his group and a few others have pioneered. The indications for these procedures are few, and only a small number of these operations are performed in any given year even in the busiest thoracic units.

Several key points made by Dr. Donohue deserve mention. All patients being considered for carinal resection should undergo mediastinoscopy at the time of the procedure both for staging purposes and to free up the anterior aspect of the trachea to facilitate the resection. Patients with N2 disease probably are not ideal candidates for this operation, which carries a significant operative mortality.

Most of these resections are approached from the right chest even if the lesion is in the left main bronchus. Alternatively the carina may be approached anteriorly via a median sternotomy. Approaching the carina from the anterior approach requires that the pericardium between the superior vena cava and the aorta be incised and that the right main pulmonary artery be mobilized away from the carina. This approach may be preferable for lesions involving the left main bronchus where a sleeve pneumonectomy is contemplated. The anastomosis between the right main bronchus and the distal trachea easily may be accomplished via this anterior approach, and the left lung may be removed, something that is not possible via a right thoracotomy. The key factor with carinal resection remains the reconstruction from the standpoints of both the blood supply and the tension that may be present after the construction of an anastomosis. This is especially important if much of the distal trachea must be resected. The factor that most limits reconstruction is the limited amount of mobilization that can be obtained from the left main bronchus because of the tethering effect of the aortic arch. This is particularly important during a right sleeve pneumonectomy if tumor extends up the distal trachea. The anastomosis between the distal trachea and the left main bronchus must be accomplished without tension and with preservation of the blood supply that is compromised by dissection in the subcarinal space. Circumferential dissection around the distal trachea must be confined to the level where the trachea is to be divided.

Several factors determine the type of reconstruction after carinal resection, but first and foremost is whether lung resection is required. If only the carina is to be resected, the major determinant of the reconstruction is the length of distal trachea resected. If minimal distal trachea is taken, a "neocarina" may be fashioned by anastomosing the left and right mainstem bronchi together at the medial wall followed by an anastomosis to the cut end to the distal trachea. If enough distal trachea has been taken to create tension with this type of reconstruction, then it may be necessary to anastomose the right main bronchus to the distal trachea and place the left main bronchus into the cartilaginous portion of the right main bronchus. Alternatively, if parenchymal resection is required, the major issues concern resection on the right side. If only the right main bronchus and upper lobe are resected, the bronchus intermedius should be anastomosed to the side of the left main bronchus that has been brought up and connected to the distal trachea. As Donohue points out, the end-to-side anastomosis between the bronchus intermedius and the left main bronchus should be placed on the cartilaginous portion of the bronchus without involvement of the membranous portion of the left main bronchus. This is relatively easily accomplished via a right thoracotomy. Ventilation during the time the airway is divided should be carried out with a sterile anesthesia circuit brought onto the operative field with an anode-type tube placed in the open bronchus periodically after short periods of apnea. In my opinion this type of setup is far easier to control than using jet ventilation and trying to keep the catheter in the airway.

Any surgeon contemplating a carinal resection should keep in mind that these procedures are associated with a significant postoperative mortality, usually from airway complications, but occasionally from post-pneumonectomy pulmonary edema if pneumonectomy has been carried out. Because so few of these resections are done, one should consider referring these procedures to colleagues who have performed more than just one or two of them or to institutions where specialized thoracic surgical units exist.

L.R.K.

11

Video-Assisted Thorascopic Pulmonary Resections

Allan Pickens and Robert J McKenna Jr.

Video-assisted thoracoscopic surgery (VATS) is an attractive alternate approach to conventional open surgery for selected patients. The tremendous success of laparoscopic procedures in the 1980s gave impetus to surgeons to apply this technology to the thoracic cavity. Modern VATS was made possible by improved endoscopic video systems and endoscopic staplers. The era of VATS is now long enough that there are enough data to determine how the results with VATS compare with those of open procedures for patients who need major pulmonary resections.

The first VATS lobectomy with anatomic hilar dissection was performed in 1992. The experience with VATS resections for patients with early stage bronchogenic carcinomas now is sufficiently large to show that the procedure, compared to conventional open thoracic procedures, can be performed safely and provide several benefits. Postoperative pain following VATS resections is significantly less, and patients return to full activity sooner. In addition, some studies document better preservation of pulmonary function. These attributes of VATS allow recruitment of older patients and patients with multiple comorbidities that would otherwise have made those patients unsuitable for conventional open thoracotomy. The momentum to perform minimally invasive pulmonary resections is growing in the field of general thoracic surgery.

The risk of bleeding during VATS and the difficulty of dealing with significant hemorrhage as well as the adequacy of VATS as a cancer operation remain sources of concern for some thoracic surgeons. Actually, dissection of vessels while looking at a monitor is a skill that can improve the accuracy of dissection with the enhanced illumination, magnification, and alternate views that

are provided by VATS. In a survey of 1,578 VATS lobectomies by MacKinlay, there was no intraoperative exsanguination, so that, although the theoretical risk of bleeding problems exists, it appears to be a rare occurrence and can be dealt with because experienced VATS surgeons know how to minimize the risk of bleeding and how to control the bleeding if it occurs. Bleeding may occur with both open and VATS procedures.

There are several oncologic issues regarding the use of VATS for cancer surgery. A cancer can recur in an incision after VATS resection. Placement of specimens in a bag for removal through a VATS incision, gentle handling of the tissue so as to not disseminate tumor cells, and copious irrigation of the hemithorax prior to closure significantly minimize the risk of incisional recurrence. Some critics have expressed concerns about the adequacy of VATS lobectomy as a cancer operation. Technically, VATS lobectomy should be the same anatomic operation with the same nodal sampling or complete nodal dissection as performed through a thoracotomy. As reported by Sagawa et al. in a prospective trial of systematic nodal dissection by VATS, the average number of nodes dissected by VATS is not significantly different from that by open thoracotomy. The true measure of any cancer operation is survival. Although some surgeons have reported exceptional survival after VATS lobectomy (e.g., Kaseda and Aoki reported 94% at 4 years), others have reported survival that is the same as reported with a thoracotomy for lung cancer (McKenna reported 72% at 5 years). It certainly appears that a VATS approach, at the very least, does not compromise survival for lung cancer patients.

Even the definition of a VATS lobectomy is controversial, in particular the length of

the utility incision, the need for rib spreading, the type of instruments (conventional or thoracoscopic), and the mode of operative visualization (by looking through the incision or at the monitor). Frankly, there does not need to be a consensus on these issues. The principal features of a lobectomy, whether open or closed, are an anatomic dissection with individual ligation of the pulmonary vessels and division of the lobar bronchus, prevention of tumor spread, and adequate assessment of lymph nodes. Each surgeon must evaluate his or her skills and resources to determine the subtle details that allow the safest, least traumatic, and most therapeutic operation for his or her patients.

Indications and Contraindications for Video-Assisted Thorascopic Surgery Pulmonary Resection

Wedge resections, segmentectomies, lobectomies, and pneumonectomies have all been performed using VATS. Wedge resections are not standard oncologic operations for lung cancer. VATS wedge resections for lung nodules are most commonly performed to determine a pathologic diagnosis. The local recurrence rate has been reported to be three times greater after wedge resection than after lobectomy for cancer. If the patient can physiologically tolerate the operation, a lung cancer should be resected via an anatomic procedure as dictated by oncologic principles. However, in patients with severely limited lung function or multiple risk factors,

Table 11-1   Relative Contraindications to Video-Assisted Thorascopic Surgery Pulmonary Resection
Intolerance of single-lung ventilation
Tumor size >5 cm
Anticipated sleeve resection
Hilar lymphadenopathy
Chest wall or mediastinal involvement
Neoadjuvant radiation therapy or chemotherapy

VATS wedge resection may be the only surgical option for treating small, peripheral lung cancer.

Although most pulmonary resections likely could be performed by VATS, fewer than 10% are currently performed with minimally invasive surgery. In 2003, McKenna and associates performed 89% of their 224 lobectomies using VATS (unpublished data). These resections were primarily for stage I lung cancer and occasionally for benign disease. The limitations were primarily the size of the tumor relative to the incisions, the safety of the vascular dissection, and the invasion of extrapulmonary structures. Table 11-1 lists relative contraindications for VATS lobectomy. Except for inability to tolerate single-lung ventilation, most limitations are due to anatomic considerations. If the tumor is >6 cm, the tumor limits the mobility of the lobe for dissection, and the ribs need to be spread to remove the lobe. For VATS lobectomy, the lobe is placed in a bag for removal from the chest. Pulling the bag through the intercostal space opens the space adequately for removal of tumors <5 cm without spreading the ribs. After preoperative treatment with chemotherapy, radiation therapy, or both, scar tissue destroys the normal planes of dissection. This makes the vascular dissection much more difficult, and often a muscle flap is used to reinforce the bronchial closure. Both benign and malignant pathologic lymph nodes attached to pulmonary vessels often require a thoracotomy for safe dissecting. Centrally located tumors need to be carefully evaluated to determine if the better procedure is a sleeve resection (vascular or bronchial) or a pneumonectomy. The assessment and performance of a sleeve resection usually requires a thoracotomy, although bronchial sleeve resections have been performed using VATS. The degree of chest wall or mediastinal involvement must be assessed to determine the advisability of resecting a tumor with VATS. Incomplete fissures are not a contraindication to a VATS lobec-tomy. Our approach is to dissect the vessels in the hilum first and complete the fissure after transection of the vessels and bronchus.

Preoperative Evaluation

The preoperative evaluation of patients undergoing VATS is similar to that of any patient undergoing a conventional open thoracic procedure. The surgeon should be familiar with the patient's history, physical exam, and recent studies. Knowledge of pulmonary function tests and their predictive value for the patient's postoperative pulmonary function is an integral part of the preoperative evaluation. Thoracoscopic procedures tend to be less stressful for the patient than posterolateral thoracotomy, and studies suggest that there may be fewer cardiopulmonary complications, such as atrial fibrillation or myocardial infarction; however, surgeons must always be cognizant of possible conversion to an open thoracotomy. Patients must be informed of the consequences of both VATS and open thoracotomy.

Operative Technique

VATS is neither simple nor uniform. Several variations exist due to evolving technology. Some surgeons express concern for the difficulty in teaching VATS techniques to residents, but this anxiety is tremendously reduced with experience. Absolute understanding of thoracic anatomy and video orientation is critical. Thoracoscopic examination is made difficult by paradoxical motion. Paradoxical motion is generated when the camera and instruments are facing each other. By turning the camera 180 degrees, one can restore a normal spatial relationship for the operator if needed.

Depending on the cardiopulmonary status of the patient and the expected duration of the operation, VATS can be performed using local, regional, or general anesthesia. Most VATS resections are performed with the patient under general anesthesia with controlled ventilation. Single-lung ventilation is used by most if the patient has sufficient pulmonary reserve. Double-lumen endotracheal tubes, endobronchial intubation, bronchial blockers, and specialized tubes with bronchial blockers capable of suction (Univent, Fugi Systems, Tokyo, Japan) can be used for lung isolation. Although some anesthesiologists use continuous positive airway pressure (CPAP) or intermittent ven-tilation of the lung to be operated on, this should rarely be necessary. Intra-operative hypoxemia, even in patients with very severe emphysema (forced expiratory volume in 1 second [FEV_1] <30%), is usually due to poor placement of the double-lumen endotracheal tube, and can be corrected by adjustment of the tube.

With the patient under single-lung general anesthesia, the patient is placed in full lateral decubitus position, as for a posterolateral thoracotomy. Care is taken to fully flex the patient to prevent the hip from obstructing movement of the thoracoscope and to maximize intercostal space (ICS). The surgeon stands on the anterior side of the patient, and the assistants stand on the posterior side of the patient. For preemptive analgesia, local anesthetic (0.5% bupivacaine with epinephrine) is injected into the ICS of the incision as well as one ICS above and one ICS below the incision. Care is taken to infiltrate the inferior border of ribs without injecting intravascularly. This provides a more effective intercostal nerve block, which reduces surgical stimulation and provides postoperative pain relief.

Incisions

The basic principle for thoracoscopic incisions involves triangulating the target tissue and inferior placement of the trocar for the camera. Alignment of the thoracoscope, pathology, and monitor is optimal. In general, the trocar and thoracoscope are placed in the eighth ICS in the midaxillary line on the right or the posterior axillary line on the left to avoid obstruction of vision by the pericardial fat pad. By placing the camera low in the chest, the best panoramic view of the thoracic cavity is achieved. The 30-degree lens allows much greater flexibility for the surgeon to see around structures in the hilum. This incision is placed anterior to a rib and angled superiorly toward the ICS to reduce irritation of the intercostal nerve. All other incisions are made directly into the middle of an ICS.

In the sixth ICS in the midclavicular line (as far anteriorly and inferiorly as possible), a 1-cm to 2-cm incision is made for ring forceps and staplers. Initially, a ring forceps manipulates the lung to allow for inspection of the pleura and exposure of the hilum to determine the proper position for the other incisions. Through this incision, the diaphragm can be depressed for visualization of the inferior pulmonary ligament.

The utility thoracotomy incision is a 2-cm to 4-cm incision from the anterior edge of the latissimus dorsi muscle to the anterior axillary line. It generally lies in the fourth ICS directly lateral to the superior pulmonary vein for an upper lobectomy or one ICS inferiorly for a middle or lower lobectomy. With gentle manipulation of the lung, most aspects of the lung can be directly palpated through this incision. Ribs are not spread, but a Weitlander retractor may be used to hold the soft tissues of the chest wall open for easier passage of instruments and to prevent the lung from expanding when intrathoracic suctioning causes a negative pressure in the chest. The hilar structures are easily accessible for dissection through this incision.

If needed, a posterior 1-cm to 2-cm incision in the sixth ICS at the auscultatory triangle allows additional manipulation of the lung for inspection. Inferior placement of this posterior incision improves the angle of the stapler for the superior pulmonary vein and assistance with a lower lobectomy. Slightly higher placement of the incision helps with paratracheal node dissection but makes the angle for the stapler on the pulmonary vein more difficult.

We do not recommend routine use of trocars, except for the thoracoscope. Ports make it difficult to use conventional thoracic instruments. Conventional instruments are familiar to surgeons and allow better tactile feedback. If there are any adhesions between the lung and the chest wall or mediastinum, they should be separated before starting the dissection. This mobilizes the lung for better palpation and visualization. By bringing the lung toward the palpating finger placed through different ports, most of the lung surface can be palpated. This is important because small nodules (<0.5 cm) can go undetected by thoracoscopic examination alone. Last, it is crucial to avoid torquing the instruments or thoracoscope onto the inferior surface of ribs because pressure on the intercostal nerves can cause significant postoperative neuralgia.

Wedge Resection

Wedge resections are the most commonly performed VATS pulmonary resection. Most wedge resections are done to obtain a pathologic diagnosis. Endoscopic staples are usually used for wedge resection of pulmonary nodules. Ring forceps through two incisions position the mass for the stapler. The stapler is often fired through both incisions to complete the resection. Alternatively, electrocautery can be used to resect the mass. Optimal function of the electrocautery requires good traction and counter traction. Smoke from the electrocautery can be prob-

lematic because suction causes expansion of the lung unless air can freely flow into the thoracic cavity through at least one incision. A Weitlander retractor provides good retraction of the soft tissue to allow ventilation. Following a wedge resection using electrocautery, the lung parenchyma must be sutured. We use 3-0 PDS suture and conventional needle holders through either incision to suture the lung. Wedge resection specimens should be placed in a bag for removal if malignancy is suspected. When treating primary lung cancer, the local recurrence following wedge resection is much higher, and such local recurrence is associated with a high rate of mortality due to cancer. If the wedge resection demonstrates a primary lung cancer, a formal lobectomy with lymphadenectomy is recommended.

Lobectomy

There are three types of VATS lobectomy described in the literature: video-assisted minithoracotomy, video-assisted simultaneously stapled lobectomy, and video-assisted non–rib-spreading lobectomy. We strongly believe that individual ligation of lobar vessels and bronchus, lymph node dissection, and avoidance of rib spreading are essential to VATS lobectomy. The surgical approach is planned according to the location of the lesion, yet the principles for dissection and division of the pulmonary vein, pulmonary artery, and bronchus are the same. Vessels in the hilum are dissected sharply through the utility thoracotomy incision with standard thoracotomy instruments, such as Metzenbaum scissors and Debakey forceps. Hilar lymph nodes are removed early as separate specimens to facilitate pathologic staging and passage of nonarticulating endoscopic staplers (EZ 35, Ethicon, Cincinnati, OH; Endo-GIA, US Surgical, New Brunswick, NJ). A braided, nonabsorbable 2-0 suture is frequently used to encircle vessels to identify the plane of dissection and provide traction. Appropriate traction is crucial in aligning the vessels and bronchus with the stapler. The fissure, bronchus, and pulmonary vessels >5 mm are transected with surgical staples. The 2.0-mm staples are used for the vessels, and the 4.8-mm staples are used for the fissure and bronchus. Articulation of the stapler is unnecessary when proper placement of incisions provides the correct angle for the stapler. The incisions that offer the best angle for stapling structures are shown in Table 11-2.

The fissure is usually completed after the vessels and bronchus are transected. One should not hesitate to complete the

Table 11-2 Recommended Incisions for Stapler Placement

Incision	Structure Stapled
Posterior incision	Superior pulmonary vein
	Upper lobe anterior trunk
	Middle lobe artery and vein
	Left upper lobe bronchus
Utility incision	Minor fissure
	Right upper lobe bronchus
Midclavicular incision	Inferior pulmonary vein
	Upper lobe anterior trunk
	Major fissure
	Additional left upper lobe arteries
	Lower lobe arteries
	Lower lobe bronchus

fissure earlier if this maneuver will provide better access to the vessels or bronchus. A largely fused fissure is not an absolute contraindication to VATS.

To minimize the risk of contaminating the incision with tumor, the resected lung specimen is placed in a bag for removal through the utility thoracotomy incision. The Lap Sac (Cook Urological, Spencer, IN) is a large, sturdy bag with the capacity to accommodate most pulmonary resections. The bag should be positioned in the apex of the thoracic cavity with the opening facing the camera. The entire lobe should be inside the bag before attempting removal. Removal of the bag containing the lobe is easier if the narrow part of the lobe is removed first and the bag opening is left open for decompression of air, but not blood.

Mediastinal node sampling or complete lymph node dissection can be performed by VATS. The lung is retracted posteriorly, and a ring forceps lifts the azygous vein for exposure of the tracheobronchial and pretracheal nodes. Standard thoracotomy instruments are used to perform the dissection through the utility thoracotomy incision. The pleura adjacent to the azygous vein is incised and the vein is retracted inferiorly. Paratracheal node dissection is easier if the azygous vein is transected, but this is not required. A ring forceps lifts the pleura and the paratracheal nodes as the plane is dissected along the superior vena cava, trachea, and pericardium over the ascending aorta, from the pulmonary artery inferiorly to the innominate vein superiorly. Anterior retraction of the lung provides exposure for the subcarinal node dissection, which begins at the inferior pulmonary vein and proceeds superiorly. The planes of dissection are the pericardium and main stem bronchi. Aortopulmonary window lymph nodes usually are resected before left upper lobectomy because it facilitates mobilization of the anterior trunk of the pulmonary artery and the superior pulmonary vein. Care must be taken to avoid injury to the vagus, recurrent laryngeal, and phrenic nerves. Based upon the lobe in which the cancer is located, surgeons customize their node dissections. Naruke's recommendations are as follows: right upper lobectomy (pretracheal #3 and lower paratracheal #4R); right middle lobectomy (retrotracheal #3 and subcarinal #7); right lower lobectomy (subcarinal #7); left upper lobectomy (aortopulmonary window #5 and para-aortic #6); left lower lobectomy (subcarinal #7). Nevertheless, a thorough assessment of lymph node involvement must be done in conjunction with any lobectomy.

Pneumectomy

VATS pneumonectomy can be performed safely using the same principles, but VATS pneumonectomies are rarely indicated because most tumors needing a pneumonectomy are either T3 or large hilar tumors. The technique is similar to that for an open pneumonectomy. The pulmonary veins, pulmonary artery, and main stem bronchus are dissected and divided sequentially using traditional instruments and staplers.

Outcomes

Morbidity and Mortality after Video-Assisted Thorascopic Surgery Pulmonary Resection

The morbidity and mortality following VATS resections is comparable to those for open resection. VATS wedge resection has a very low perioperative morbidity and mortality. Nonanatomic lung resections have been reported as safe with a morbidity of 9% and a mortality of 0.6%. The safety of VATS lobectomy continues to improve with advances in technology. In a review of multiple series, a morbidity rate of 10% to 21.9% after VATS lobectomy was reported. Prolonged air leak was the most frequent complication. The mortality was 0.6% (7 of 1,120 patients), but no deaths were due to massive hemorrhage. Conversion from VATS to open thoracotomy was necessary in 0.0% to 19.5% of the patients in the series. Overall, 119 of 1,120 VATS were converted to open thoracotomy (11.6%). Tumor characteristics, such as central location, vascular involvement, or unsuspected T3 lesions, were the most

common reasons for conversion. It is vital to understand that conversion from VATS to open thoracotomy is not a measure of defeat, but instead is the result of astute awareness of the need for wider exposure.

Reports indicate that patients have less pain following VATS lobectomy compared with lobectomy by open thoracotomy. Less muscle transection and lack of rib spreading are believed to contribute to the decreased pain. Less pain following VATS resection has been documented in several large case-controlled studies both by objective assessment of analgesic requirements and by subjective assessment of pain score. Consequently, better postoperative pulmonary function has been exhibited. When forced expiratory volume in 1 second (FEV_1) and forced vital capacity (FVC) values were measured preoperatively and at 3 months postoperatively, it was found that patients who underwent VATS lobectomy had better preservation of function than those who underwent a thoracotomy.

Survival

The success of a cancer operation is dictated by the long-term survival of the patients. The results from several studies on VATS major resections for stage I lung cancer show equivalent to or better survival, compared to survival after a thoracotomy for a lobectomy. A review of multiple studies reveals a mean survival of 90% with a mean follow-up of 34 months. Yim et al. reported a trend toward improved disease-free survival with VATS resection and suggested that less suppression of immunosurveillance was important to the survival benefit. The oncologic adequacy of VATS resection is vital because lung cancer patients who are candidates for VATS are in a potentially curable stage.

VATS pulmonary resections can be performed safely with several documented advantages compared to open thoracotomy resection. Benefits include smaller incisions, decreased postoperative pain, better preservation of pulmonary function, and earlier return to normal activities. These results are obtained without sacrificing oncologic principles of thoracic surgery. An anatomic resection and a thorough assessment of lymph node status are achieved with VATS. Most important, patient survival is equivalent, if not better, following VATS resection for lung cancer.

SUGGESTED READING

Demmy TL, Curtis JJ. Minimally invasive lobectomy directed toward frail and high risk patients: A case control study. Ann Thorac Surg 199;68:194.

Downey RJ, McCormack P, LoCicero J, et al. Dissemination of malignant tumors after video-assisted thoracic surgery: A report of twenty-one cases. J Thorac Cardiovasc Surg 1996;111:954.

Ginsberg R, Ruberstein L. Randomized trial of lobectomy versus limited resection for T1N0 non–small cell lung cancer. Ann Thorac Surg 1995;60:615.

Hermansson U, Konstantinov IE, Aren C. Video-assisted thoracic surgery lobectomy: The initial Swedish experience. Semin Thorac Cardiovasc Surg 1998;10:285.

Jaklitsch MT, DeCamp MM Jr, Liptay MJ, et al. Video-assisted thoracic surgery in elderly (a review of 307 cases). Chest 1996;110:751.

Kaseda S, Aoki T. Video-assisted thoracic surgical lobectomy in conjunction with lymphadenectomy for lung cancer. J Japan Surg Soc 2002;103:717.

Kaseda S, Aoki T, Hangai N, et al. Better pulmonary function with video-assisted thoracic surgery than with thoracotomy. Ann Thoracic Surg 2000;70:1644.

Kirby TJ, Rice TW. Thoracoscopic lobectomy. Ann Thorac Surg 1993;56:784.

McKenna RJ. Thoracoscopic evaluation and treatment of pulmonary disease. Surg Clin North Am 2000;80:223.

McKenna RJ, Fischel RJ, Wolf R, et al. Is VATS lobectomy an adequate cancer operation? Ann Thorac Surg 1998;66:1903.

Naruke T, Tsuchiya R, Kando H, et al. Lymph node sampling in lung cancer: How should it be done? Eur J Cardiothorac Surg 1999;16:517.

Roviaro G, Varoli F, Vergani C, et al. Video-assisted thoracoscopic surgery major pulmonary resections: The Italian experience. Semin Thorac Cardiovasc Surg 1998;313.

Sagawa M, Sato M, Sakurada A, et al. A prospective trial of systematic nodal dissection for lung cancer by video-assisted thoracic surgery: Can it be perfect? Ann Thorac Surg 2002;73:900.

Swanson SJ, Hasan FB. Video-assisted thoracic surgery resection for lung cancer. Surg Clin North Am 2002;82:211.

Walker WS. VATS lobectomy: The Edinbergh experience. Semin Thorac Cardiovasc Surg 1998;10:291.

Wilson WL, Lee TW, Lam SS, et al. Quality of life following lung cancer resection: Video-assisted thoracic surgery vs thoracotomy. Chest 2002;122:211.

Yim APC, Ko KM, Chau WS, et al. Video-assisted thoracoscopic anatomic lung resections: The initial Hong Kong experience. Chest 1996;109:13.

Yim APC, Wan S, Lee TW, et al. VATS lobectomy reduces cytokine responses compared with conventional surgery. Ann Thorac Surg 2000;70:243.

EDITOR'S COMMENTS

There is no doubt that pulmonary resection may be done via a thoracoscopic approach, although the correct terminology for most of the procedures would be "video assisted." As described by McKenna, a "utility" incision is employed through which standard instruments are used. The advantage is the lack of rib spreading, which is felt by many to be the major source of postoperative pain. As described in this chapter, resections done in this manner may be performed safely with results equal to those of a standard open cancer operation.

Does it take special skill to perform these resections? In my opinion, not really, just a willingness to take the extra time to perform the resection with the equivalent of one hand tied beyond one's back. The inability to use the hand is a disadvantage, but is not insurmountable, as a number of authors have shown. That the video-assisted operation is associated with less postoperative pain has not been conclusively documented, although with the advent of epidural analgesia postoperative pain has already been significantly attenuated with little if any morbidity. I remain impressed with how much pain patients have following a simple thoracoscopic procedure where no rib spreading has occurred but only a hole made through intercostals spaces. Fortunately chronic post-

thoracotomy pain is seen infrequently, and it is not known whether there is a lesser incidence of this after a video-assisted procedure.

One cannot argue that the video-assisted approach makes sense for a T1 lesion without associated lymphadenopathy and perhaps even for certain T2 lesions. Especially in the setting of resident teaching, for most cases I still prefer to gain proximal control of the main pulmonary artery, something that is not done with a video-assisted approach. Should a problem occur during a video-assisted procedure when stapling a pulmonary artery branch, I would submit that there will be a significant squeeze on the surgeon's coronary circulation until such time as the chest can be opened. These types of things rarely get written about. McKenna opines that video-assisted resections have allowed older patients and those with multiple comorbidities to have an operation, but I remain unconvinced that they would not do just as well with a muscle-sparing incision and a quick, well-monitored surgical procedure.

Surgeons for the most part should resist the temptation of doing a thoracoscopic

wedge resection for cancer thinking that they are doing the patient a favor by doing a less invasive procedure. A wedge resection for most malignant lesions is a compromise that brings with it a significant chance for local recurrence. If a surgeon is comfortable with a video-assisted anatomic resection, then by all means he or she should offer this to patients. In my experience, however, I have not seen patients clamoring for this procedure. Most people, when faced with a diagnosis of lung cancer, are motivated mainly to have their tumor removed in a fashion that will allow them the best chance of being "cured" of their disease. The number of days that their postoperative pain lasts usually is a fleeting memory when they look back with the feeling of being a survivor a few years later. The situation is not comparable, say, to radical prostatectomy, where a laparoscopic or robotic procedure offers a true functional advantage, at least in the short term. A lobectomy is a lobectomy whether performed looking directly at instruments or indirectly at a video monitor.

L.R.K.

12

Management of Pneumothorax and Bullous Disease

Stephen D. Cassivi and Claude Deschamps

The pleural space between the parietal pleura, lining the inside of the chest wall, and the visceral pleura, covering the outside surface of the lung, is a potential space during normal conditions. Pneumothorax is the presence of air in the pleural space and can be due to a number of causes. The etiology and volume of the pneumothorax and the resultant intrapleural pressure and condition of the underlying lung play a role in determining the clinical severity.

This chapter outlines the anatomy and basic physiology of the pleural space. The pathophysiology of the various etiologies of pneumothoraces is discussed, as are the diagnosis and management options. Special attention is directed to the particular condition of bullous disease.

Anatomy

The pleural space is lined by the visceral and parietal pleurae (Fig. 12-1). The visceral pleura is a thin layer (usually one cell thick) intimately covering the outer surface of the lung. It adheres to the underlying alveolar walls of the lung parenchyma via connective tissue made up of elastic fibers. There is therefore no true cleavage plane between the visceral pleura and the lung parenchyma that it envelops. The visceral pleura has no somatic innervation.

The parietal pleura is a more complex serous membrane. It lines the inside of the chest wall, diaphragm, and mediastinum and is attached to these by a fibrous and connective tissue layer known as the endothoracic fascia. It is the endothoracic fascia that is the dissection plane that allows the parietal pleura to be stripped off of the chest wall and other structures. It is thickest and most substantial along the chest wall, over-

lying the ribs, and thinnest as it covers the mediastinal structures and beneath the sternum. The parietal pleura is innervated by somatic, sympathetic, and parasympathetic nerve fibers via the intercostal nerves.

Physiology

The physiology of the pleural space is relatively straightforward, although dynamic. Functional residual capacity is the measure of lung volume with the patient at rest after normal exhalation. In this state, the elastic and retractive nature of the chest wall and lung pull the parietal and visceral pleurae away from one another, thus creating a negative intrapleural pressure usually in the range of -2 to -5 cm H_2O. During inspiration, the outward chest wall and diaphragmatic forces counteracting the normal elastic recoil of the lung parenchyma can create intrapleural pressures of -20 to -35 cm H_2O. Gravity also exerts an influence on this negative intrapleural pressure. In the upright position, the apex has a greater negative intrapleural pressure than the base of the lung in the region of the costophrenic sulci (0.25 cm H_2O/cm of height). This phenomenon may contribute to some degree to creating increased distention of alveoli in the apex and a greater predisposition to spontaneous pneumothoraces by rupture of apical blebs.

As a consequence of having more oxygen consumed than carbon dioxide produced during the respiratory cycle (respiratory quotient <1), there is a resultant partial pressure gradient between the gases in the venous blood and those of the arterial system and pleural space. This gradient, usually between 54 and 72 cm H_2O, ensures against spontaneous gas formation in the pleural

space as long as the intrapleural pressures do not become less than -72 cm H_2O. More practically, this also explains how pleural air, such as in the case of a pneumothorax, can be gradually reabsorbed by diffusion into the venous circulation.

Pleural gases can also be affected by barometric pressure. Whereas the relative proportions of gases do not change with variation in atmospheric pressure, there can be a significant change in the volume of these gases. Boyle's law states that at constant temperature, for a given mass of gas, pressure p multiplied by volume V is a constant:

$$pV = c$$

In more practical terms, the volume change in a gas is inversely proportional to the change in atmospheric pressure. This has a number of clinically significant consequences when considering pneumothoraces. First, although a person with a pneumothorax being transported by airplane is likely to be in a pressurized cabin, one can expect the barometric pressure to decrease, with a resultant proportional increase in the volume of their pneumothorax if there is not a path of egress for the intrapleural gas such as provided by a chest tube. Second, a clinician whose practice is located at a higher altitude (with lower atmospheric pressure) can expect a slower resolution of pneumothoraces by resorptive diffusion alone than that seen by a colleague practicing closer to sea level.

Etiology and Pathophysiology

Primary spontaneous pneumothorax is the most common cause of pneumothoraces and

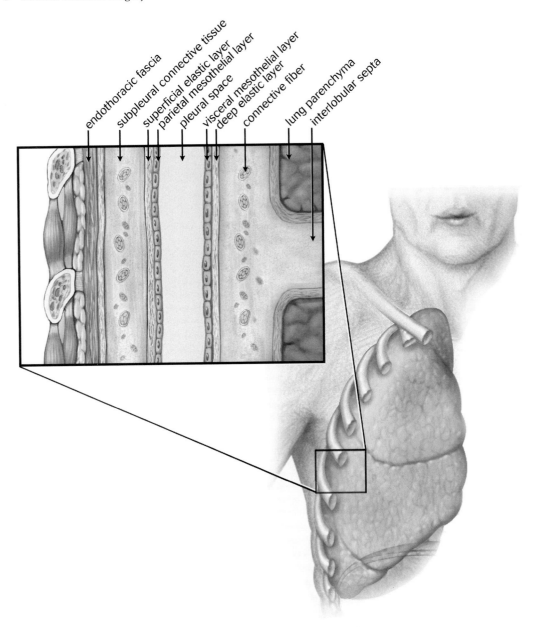

endothoracic fascia
subpleural connective tissue
superficial elastic layer
parietal mesothelial layer
pleural space
visceral mesothelial layer
deep elastic layer
connective fiber
lung parenchyma
interlobular septa

Figure 12-1. Anatomy of the pleural surfaces.

has an estimated overall incidence of 5 to 10 cases per 100,000 per year. It occurs predominantly in young, healthy men, with an incidence in this group as high as 1 in 500 per year, and is due in most cases to rupture of apical subpleural blebs in otherwise normal lungs (Fig. 12-2). The pathogenesis of these apical blebs is unclear, although it is postulated that higher transpulmonary pressures at the apex lead to greater alveolar distending pressures. The resultant rupture of alveoli traps air between the internal and external elastic membranes of the visceral pleura. It is noted that these types of pneumothoraces most often occur in tall, thin individuals, many of whom are smokers. The lifetime risk of developing a pneumothorax

in an otherwise healthy man is estimated at 0.1% whereas it is as high as 12% in one who is a smoker. There may also be an association with connective tissue disorders such as Marfan syndrome. A familial form of spontaneous pneumothorax has been described with autosomal dominant inheritance and incomplete penetrance.

Spontaneous pneumothorax can also occur as a result of underlying lung disease, in which case it is referred to as a secondary spontaneous pneumothorax. There are various pulmonary disease states leading to secondary pneumothoraces (Table 12-1). Most cases are related to bullous-type disease, with hyperinflation leading ultimately to rupture and subsequent pulmonary

parenchymal collapse. Diseases characterized by cystic lesions in the pulmonary parenchyma such as cystic fibrosis and lymphangioleiomyomatosis can also lead to spontaneous rupture and pneumothorax. Malignant pulmonary nodules, both primary and metastatic, usually located subpleurally, can rupture as they expand and result in a spontaneous pneumothorax.

Spontaneous pneumothoraces that occur and recur in relation to the menstrual cycle are referred to as catamenial pneumothoraces. These episodes occur within 72 hours before or after the onset of menstruation. Three distinct mechanisms have been proposed based on metastatic, hormonal, and anatomic models. The metastatic

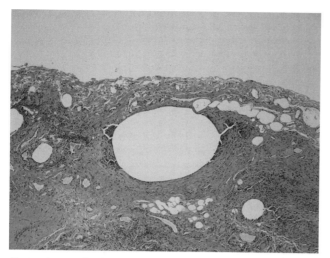

Figure 12-2.   Photomicrograph of apical resection for recurrent primary spontaneous pneumothoraces demonstrating subpleural bleb.

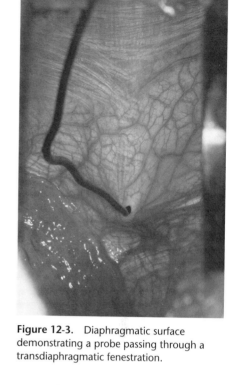

Figure 12-3.   Diaphragmatic surface demonstrating a probe passing through a transdiaphragmatic fenestration.

model hypothesizes migration of endometrial tissue via the peritoneal cavity through transdiaphragmatic lymphatic channels, via diaphragmatic fenestrations, or hematogenously into the pleural space. An alternative theory suggests that endometrial tissue may be deposited in the chest cavity during embryonal development. Endometrial deposits have been identified in the pleural space in 13% to 62.5% of these cases.

Hormonally regulated monthly sloughing of endometrial tissue is believed to result in pleural irritation, causing chest pain, and subpleural breaches, causing air leaks. The hormonal hypothesis suggests that high serum levels of prostaglandin F_2 at ovulation leads to vasospasm, associated ischemia with tissue injury, and alveolar rupture. The anatomic model for catamenial pneumothorax is based on the influx of

air into the pleural space from the peritoneal cavity via diaphragmatic fenestrations (Fig. 12-3).

Infectious diseases of the lung in their many forms may result in secondary spontaneous pneumothorax. This is most notable in the immunocompromised host such as individuals infected with the human immunodeficiency virus (HIV) and those with manifestations of acquired immunodeficiency syndrome. Pneumothorax occurs in 1% to 2% of hospitalized patients with HIV and is associated with 34% mortality. The most common etiologic agent in these cases is *Pneumocystis carinii*. Other virulent or opportunistic infections are also causally related to the occurrence of spontaneous pneumothoraces, including most recently severe acute respiratory syndrome (SARS).

Pneumothoraces may also be incited by iatrogenic or traumatic events. Penetration of the pleural space by a needle during a diagnostic or therapeutic procedure, whether deliberate or accidental, may result in a so-called acquired pneumothorax. This is usually due to a breach or laceration of the visceral pleura. This can occur during procedures such as transthoracic needle aspiration, central line placement in the neck, and thoracentesis. In the latter procedure, recent studies have shown that the incidence of iatrogenic pneumothorax can be significantly reduced by using ultrasound guidance.

Table 12-1 Etiologies of Pneumothorax	
Spontaneous	
Primary	
Rupture of subpleural bleb	
Secondary	
Bullous disease	Emphysema, chronic obstructive pulmonary disease (COPD), alpha-1 antitrypsin deficiency emphysema
Cystic disease	Cystic fibrosis, lymphangioleiomyomatosis
Malignancy	Primary lung cancer, lung metastases (especially osteogenic sarcoma), after chemotherapy
Catamenial	
Infectious	*Pneumocystis carinii* pneumonia, acquired immunodeficiency syndrome (AIDS), severe acute respiratory syndrome (SARS)
Eosinophilic granuloma	
Connective tissue disorders	Marfan syndrome
Acquired	
Iatrogenic	
Needle puncture	Transthoracic needle aspiration/biopsy, thoracentesis, central venous line placement
Transbronchial biopsy	
Laparoscopic surgery	
Traumatic	
Blunt	
Penetrating	
Barotrauma	Ventilator induced

Diagnosis

The most common presenting symptom of spontaneous pneumothorax is ipsilateral pleuritic chest pain of relatively sudden onset. Dyspnea may or may not be a prominent symptom and is usually proportional to the amount of lung collapse. Ipsilateral decreased breath sounds and hyper-resonance on percussion are usually noted. In the case of a tension pneumothorax there may also be deviation of the trachea to the contralateral side, tachycardia, hypotension, and diaphoresis. Although they are useful in suggesting the diagnosis of pneumothorax, clinical history and physical examination are not generally reliable in predicting the volume of underlying lung collapse.

Standard posteroanterior (PA) chest radiographs (CXR) remain the standard for diagnosis of spontaneous pneumothorax in the clinically stable patient. If the diagnosis is suspected but is not confirmed by a standard upright CXR taken on inspiration, a CXR taken either during expiration or in the lateral decubitus position may accentuate the pneumothorax and facilitate diagnosis. Computed tomography (CT) scans are the most sensitive and specific imaging modality for the diagnosis of pneumothoraces and can be especially useful in differentiating such a diagnosis from that of a large emphysematous bullae.

A large body of literature exists positing many methods of estimating the volume of the pneumothorax as a percentage of the pleural space volume. None of the methods has been universally accepted. CT scans are much more precise for such estimates because they take into account the nonuniform collapse that usually characterizes spontaneous pneumothoraces. However, the clinical usefulness of a precise measurement of pneumothorax size is debatable. Most often treatment decisions are made on the basis of a relative estimate of pneumothorax size, its evolution over time, and, more important, the clinical status of the patient.

Treatment

The most important factor to consider in the management of a patient with a pneumothorax is his or her clinical status. An unstable patient, whether due to the hemodynamic compromise of a tension pneumothorax or the respiratory compromise of a clinically significant simple pneumothorax, requires urgent treatment. This can be accomplished, in the case of a tension pneumothorax, by

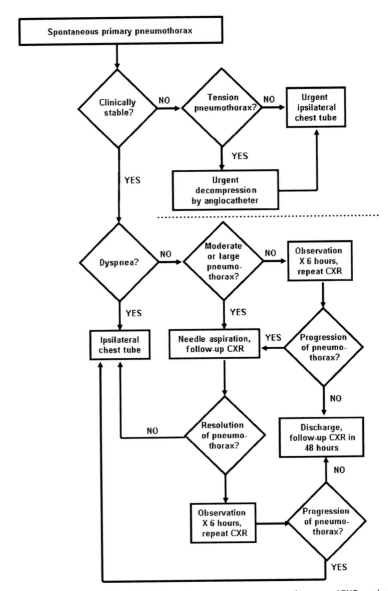

Figure 12-4. Algorithm for the treatment of spontaneous pneumothoraces. (CXR = chest x-ray.)

immediate insertion of a 14-gauge angio-catheter in the ipsilateral mid-clavicular line in the second interspace. This is followed by an expeditious insertion of an ipsilateral chest tube to evacuate the remaining air and re-expand the underlying lung.

There are a number of treatment options for patients with pneumothoraces, either primary or secondary (Table 12-2). In the clinically stable patient with a spontaneous pneumothorax, an evaluation should first be made of his or her level of dyspnea or breathlessness as well as the relative size of the pneumothorax (Fig. 12-4). In a patient with little or no breathing difficulties and a small pneumothorax (<20%), it is reasonable to observe the patient with a repeat CXR in approximately 6 hours. If the

Table 12-2 Treatment Options for Pneumothorax	
Observation	
Needle aspiration	
Chest tube	
Pleurodesis	
Thoracoscopy	With wedge resection
	With pleurodesis
	Mechanical
	Chemical
	With pleurectomy
Thoracotomy	With wedge resection
	With pleurodesis
	Mechanical
	Chemical
	With pleurectomy

pneumothorax has not progressed and the patient has not developed worsening symptoms, he or she can usually be observed further as an outpatient with return in 24 to 48 hours for reassessment by clinical exam and repeat CXR.

The rate of resolution of a spontaneous pneumothorax by reabsorption is between 1.25% and 1.8% per day. Using high concentrations of oxygen in the inspired gas in an effort to create a gradient of nitrogen favoring reabsorption of intrapleural gas has been shown to increase the resolution of pneumothoraces by up to four times the rate on room air. However, hospitalization for the sole purpose of providing high-flow oxygen in an effort to hasten the resolution of the pneumothorax is likely unnecessary and is not advocated.

In patients with few respiratory symptoms and moderate to large pneumothorax, there is growing evidence that a trial of needle aspiration may be warranted. The consensus guidelines from both the American College of Chest Physicians and the British Thoracic Society advocate an initial trial of needle aspiration in these cases. These recommendations are based on studies showing initial aspiration to be as effective as chest tube management in resolving pneumothoraces in patients with minimal symptoms. Recurrence rates were also equal in both groups. The most recent of these studies also shows that repeat attempts at needle aspiration after an initial failed attempt are of no use. In those instances a chest tube is warranted.

Needle aspiration of a pneumothorax can be accomplished by using the widely available disposable thoracentesis kits. Local anesthetic is used to numb the skin and subcutaneous tissues in the area of the second interspace in the ipsilateral midclavicular line. The small-bore catheter, loaded on the aspirating needle, is guided carefully into the pleural space just above the upper edge of the third rib. Suction on the syringe is applied as the needle is inserted, and once air is aspirated, the catheter can be advanced over the needle, which is ultimately withdrawn. With a syringe and three-way stopcock or one-way valve attached to the catheter, air is aspirated until no more can be evacuated. The catheter is then removed, and a postprocedure CXR is performed to assess adequacy of the aspiration. If the pneumothorax has resolved, a delayed CXR can be obtained at 6 hours to confirm resolution. The patient can then be followed as an outpatient and reassessed in 24 to 48 hours with a clinical exam and repeat CXR. If, however, on the initial postaspiration or the delayed

CXR there remains a moderate to large pneumothorax, insertion of a chest tube is warranted. Failure to resolve a pneumothorax after needle aspiration either on initial postaspiration or delayed chest films is likely due to a persistent air leak.

Chest tube drainage is usually advocated for large, asymptomatic or smaller, symptomatic pneumothoraces. The technique has been well described. Proper functioning of the tube requires deliberate directing of the tube in the desired position. For the most part, chest tubes are inserted in the anterior or mid-axillary line in the fourth or fifth interspace and should be guided posteriorly and cephalad. A tube positioned in this fashion will drain both air and fluid satisfactorily in the vast majority of cases. The usual pitfall of a tube placed anteriorly is that it will often find its way into the major fissure and cease to function adequately. Failure to adequately resolve a pneumothorax after chest tube insertion should be investigated with a view to ensuring correct positioning. If this is not clear by CXR, a CT scan should be obtained and in most cases will confirm proper or improper tube location.

Acquired pneumothoraces due to blunt, penetrating or ventilator trauma almost always require chest tube insertion as initial management. These injuries are usually more severe, and symptoms are not likely to resolve with mere observation or simple needle aspiration.

Most spontaneous primary pneumothoraces can be managed effectively by conservative measures: observation, needle aspiration, and/or chest tube drainage. The adjunctive use of chemical pleurodesis (talc, tetracycline, or other pleural sclerosant) is usually not necessary and is less effective than surgical alternatives discussed later in this chapter. Chemical pleurodesis should only be used in cases of treatment failure where the patient is either unwilling or unable to undergo surgical repair.

Operative Management of Pneumothoraces

Operative intervention for first occurrences of primary spontaneous pneumothorax is controversial because most resolve with conservative, nonoperative management, and a large number do not recur. However, recurrence of a primary spontaneous pneumothorax does occur, and the risk of recurrence within 4 years has been reported as high as 54%, with increased risk being

Table 12-3 Indications for Operative Intervention for Pneumothorax Treatment
Persistent air leak (>3–5 days) or failure of lung to fully re-expand with chest tube drainage
Hemopneumothorax
Recurrent ipsilateral pneumothorax
Bilateral spontaneous pneumothorax
First occurrence of contralateral pneumothorax
At-risk activities/professions (i.e., pilots, divers)
Poor access to medical treatment or follow-up

associated with smoking, increased height, male gender, and age >60 years. The risk of recurrence of a secondary pneumothorax is even higher and is associated with risk factors such as increasing age, pulmonary fibrosis, and emphysema.

The indications for operative intervention for the definitive treatment of pneumothorax are given in Table 12-3. The principle objectives of surgery in these cases are to resect the blebs or bullae and to obliterate the space to avoid further recurrences. The former can usually be accomplished by stapled wedge resection, and the latter can be approached by several means. Pleural space obliteration can be achieved by pleurodesis, either chemical or mechanical, or by parietal pleurectomy.

The findings at the time of surgery are variable. In the case of secondary pneumothorax, the underlying disease is the major determinant of surgical findings. In primary pneumothorax, the majority have blebs or bullae, usually located in the apex of the upper lobe and sometimes also in the superior segment of the lower lobe. The finding of abnormalities, however, is not universal. A classification of pleural findings has been suggested in which stage I refers to no discernible abnormalities, stage II refers to pleuropulmonary adhesions, stage III refers to blebs/bullae <2 cm, and stage IV refers to bullae >2 cm.

Open thoracotomy via a transaxillary or posterolateral incision is certainly possible with excellent effectiveness (recurrence rates <0.5%) and low morbidity (3% to 11%). In most cases in which surgical intervention is indicated, a thoracoscopic approach can also be used and tends to be the procedure of choice. A standard three-port approach is usually used with single-lung ventilation being obtained by way of a double-lumen endotracheal tube. The

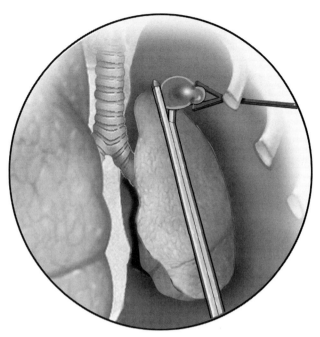

Figure 12-5. Wedge resection of apical blebs found at thoracoscopy.

deflated lung is examined, and if blebs are found, these are excised by stapled wedge resection (Fig. 12-5). This is followed by a procedure to obliterate the space by either pleurectomy or pleurodesis. Parietal pleurectomy appears to be the most effective way of achieving pleural symphysis and preventing further recurrences. Pleurectomy is usually accomplished in the apex and carried down to the level of the third or fourth rib or the azygous vein.

If no blebs are found (stage I), after a negative search for other pathology, pleurectomy is usually performed to obliterate the space. A recent retrospective review demonstrated reduced recurrences with the addition of an apical wedge resection. The addition of an apical staple line on the lung may encourage pleural adhesion and obliteration of the space when accompanying an apical parietal pleurectomy. This is our preferred approach as well.

Special Considerations

Bullous Disease

Whereas blebs are defined as small (<2cm) subpleural air collections contained within the visceral pleura, bullae are larger air pockets usually resulting from alveolar wall destruction. A practical classification system was developed to divide bullous disease into four groups (Table 12-4). Bullae can be associated with any form of emphysema.

Although the mechanism of secondary pneumothorax in bullous disease is for the most part similar to those with primary spontaneous pneumothoraces due to subpleural blebs, the underlying emphysema that usually accompanies the bullous disease accounts for the increased severity of the symptoms. These emphysematous patients often have such poor pulmonary reserve that symptoms of a pneumothorax can be quite marked and severe.

One of the more common problems encountered after chest tube placement is the development of a prolonged air leak. In an effort to avoid the increased morbidity and mortality of operative intervention in these patients, conservative management may be attempted with prolonged pleural drainage with or without chemical (talc) pleurodesis. Surgery is sometimes chosen or becomes necessary to definitively treat the persistent air leak. Bullectomy by stapled resection or ligation is the usual procedure used with

Table 12-4 Classification of Bullous Lung Disease		
Group	Number of Bullae	Underlying Lung Pathology
I	Single	Normal
II	Multiple	Normal
III	Multiple	Emphysema
IV	Multiple	Other lung diseases

From: De Vries WC, Wolfe WG. Surg Clin N Amer 1980;60:851–866.

concomitant parietal pleurectomy or mechanical/abrasive pleurodesis. When possible, this is preferably done by thoracoscopy to attempt to minimize postoperative respiratory complications due to the incisional pain of thoracotomy.

Another option in poor-risk patients unable to proceed to surgical resection is the Monaldi approach of intracavitary drainage. This was initially proposed as a treatment of tuberculous pulmonary abscesses and most recently advocated by Goldstraw and colleagues at the Royal Brompton Hospital. In this procedure, a small portion of rib overlying the bulla is excised subperiosteally. The pleurae and bulla are incised within a purse-string suture encompassing bulla wall and both parietal and visceral pleurae. A Foley catheter is inserted through this incision, and the purse-string suture is secured overtop of the Foley catheter balloon, which is within the bulla cavity. The catheter is connected to a usual chest drain suction device with underwater seal. This is supplemented by a talc pleurodesis of the bulla cavity and the intrapleural space.

Cystic Fibrosis

There is an approximate 10% incidence of pneumothorax in patients with cystic fibrosis. Due to the nature of their underlying lung disease, these patients may experience quite severe symptoms and sometimes fatal episodes. Conservative therapy with or without chest tube may be the initial treatment of choice for these patients. This alternative is usually undertaken in an effort to avoid pleurodesis in a patient who will subsequently undergo lung transplantation. It should be noted that pleurodesis, although it may increase the technical difficulty at the time of explanting the diseased lungs, does not in and of itself constitute an absolute contraindication to lung transplantation.

Catamenial Pneumothorax

There are many theories as to the etiology of catamenial pneumothorax, which is the most common manifestation of intrathoracic endometriosis. Diaphragmatic fenestrations are also encountered in these patients. These patients can often be treated thoracoscopically with wedge resection of visible endometrial implants and direct suture closure of diaphragmatic fenestrations with either mechanical pleurodesis or parietal pleurectomy. Nonsurgical options include hormonal suppression with gonadotropin-releasing hormone agonists such as leuprolide, oral contraceptives, and bilateral salpingo-oophorectomy.

In a prospective study, only 1 of 8 patients who underwent surgical repair of diaphragmatic defects suffered a recurrence during a mean follow-up period of 6.6 months (range 2 to 15 months). The retrospective analysis of 10 patients with catamenial pneumothorax revealed no recurrences during a mean follow-up of 33 months (range 12 to 48 months) in the 5 patients treated by diaphragmatic repair. These data suggest that surgical repair of diaphragmatic defects, often requiring only simple suture closure, is associated with an excellent therapeutic outcome.

SUGGESTED READING

Baumann MH, Strange C, Heffner JE, et al. Management of spontaneous pneumothorax: An American College of Chest Physicians Delphi consensus statement. Chest 2001;119:590.

Cassivi SD, Deschamps C. Chest tube insertion and management. In Albert RK, Spiro SG, Jett JR (eds), Clinical Respiratory Medicine, 2nd ed. Philadelphia: Elsevier Science, 2004: 175.

DeVries WC, Wolfe WG. The management of spontaneous pneumothorax and bullous emphysema. Surg Clin North Am 1980;60:851.

Flume PA. Pneumothorax in cystic fibrosis. Chest 2003;123:217.

Greenberg JA, Singhal S, Kaiser LR. Giant bullous lung disease: Evaluation, selection, techniques, and outcomes. Chest Surg Clin North Am 2003;13:631.

Henry M, Arnold T, Harvey J, Pleural Diseases Group SoCCBTS. BTS guidelines for the management of spontaneous pneumothorax. Thorax 2003;58(Suppl 2):ii39.

Jones PW, Moyers JP, Rogers JT, et al. Ultrasound-guided thoracentesis: Is it a safer method? Chest 2003;123:418.

Leo F, Pastorino U, Goldstraw P. Pleurectomy in primary pneumothorax: Is extensive pleurectomy necessary? J Cardiovasc Surg 2000;41:633.

Naunheim KS, Mack MJ, Hazelrigg SR, et al. Safety and efficacy of video-assisted thoracic surgical techniques for the treatment of spontaneous pneumothorax. J Thorac Cardiovasc Surg 1995;109:1198; discussion 1203.

Noppen M, Alexander P, Driesen P, et al. Manual aspiration versus chest tube drainage in first episodes of primary spontaneous pneumothorax: A multicenter, prospective, randomized pilot study. Am J Respir Crit Care Med 2002;165:1240.

Peikert T, Gillespie DJ, Cassivi SD. Catamenial pneumothorax. Mayo Clinic Proc 2005;80: 677.

Shah SS, Goldstraw P. Surgical treatment of bullous emphysema: Experience with the Brompton technique. Ann Thorac Surg 1994;58: 1452.

Tirnaksiz MB, Visbal, A.L., Deschamps C. Spontaneous pneumothorax and lung volume reduction surgery. In Bland KI (ed), The Practice of General Surgery, 10th ed. Philadelphia: W. B. Saunders, 2002: 881.

EDITOR'S COMMENTS

When we talk about spontaneous pneumothorax, it is necessary, as the authors point out, to distinguish primary spontaneous pneumothorax from secondary pneumothorax because the treatment and approach differ for the two entities. The usual patient who presents with a primary spontaneous pneumothorax is a young man commonly with a characteristic body habitus. These young men tend to be tall and thin and may have a family history of pneumothorax. The initial management needs to be individualized, but many of these cases can be managed with simple aspiration via the second intercostal space and a repeat chest radiograph to confirm the absence of a reaccumulation of air. Even if an air leak is suspected, initial management may consist of placing a small cannula connected to a Heimlich (one-way) valve and outpatient management. For a first primary spontaneous pneumothorax we proceed to operation only if the air leak lasts >48 hours or if the patient's occupation makes travel to remote areas likely. The chance of a recurrence approaches 30%, and thus there is a 70% chance that the patient will never have another pneumothorax. Either a recurrence on the ipsilateral side or a contralateral pneumothorax are indication for operation. If the second pneumothorax occurs on the contralateral side, consideration should be given to operation on both sides. The operation may be done thoracoscopically or open, but I prefer a "hybrid" operation that involves a small transaxillary incision with visualization afforded by placement of the videothoracoscope through the chest tube site. Graspers and a stapling device may be placed via the transaxillary incision because the interspace, usually the second, is quite wide. Apical bulla may be stapled and mechanical pleural abrasion, which is our preference, carried out. I tend to avoid apical pleurectomy because of the increased risk of bleeding, but this procedure may be readily carried out via the transaxillary incision.

Secondary spontaneous pneumothorax, usually occurring in the patient with significant emphysema and potentially bullous disease, requires a different approach than the one just discussed. Most of these patients are poor operative candidates, and conservative management with chest tube drainage often is the preferred approach. Thoracoscopic localization of the air leak often is difficult, and frequently the outcome of an operation is the creation of additional air leaks. If a residual space is present, the mobilization and transposition of a serratus anterior muscle flap into the space may be the treatment of choice, with the obliteration of the space likely to effect closure of the air leak. The approach to the patient with a secondary spontaneous pneumothorax must be individualized based on the patient's underlying clinical status and intrathoracic findings as demonstrated on a CT scan.

I would be remiss in not expanding on the issue of tension pneumothorax. The term tension pneumothorax often is misused based on a lack of understanding of the underlying physiology. The simple loss of the normal negative intrathoracic pressure leads to the entry of air into the hemithorax. This may or may not be accompanied by an ongoing parenchymal air leak. If the air leak is small, air accumulates in the pleural space and often in the soft tissue, that is, there is subcutaneous emphysema. A significant air leak usually caused by blunt or, more likely, penetrating trauma can lead to an accumulation of enough air in the chest that the mediastinum shifts and venous return to the heart is compromised. This is the definition of a "tension" pneumothorax. An air leak in a patient on positive-pressure ventilation frequently may be accompanied by tension physiology and requires emergent decompression of the pleural space with a needle placed in the second intercostal space followed by placement of a chest tube. It is the hemodynamic compromise that not only characterizes a tension pneumothorax but also threatens the patient's life, so emergent recognition and appropriate management is key.

L.R.K.

13

Thymectomy (Sternotomy)

Francis C. Nichols and Victor F. Trastek

The thymus gland continues to present challenges to thoracic surgeons. The thymus is the site of origin of benign and malignant neoplasms; it also is involved in cellular immunity and certain aspects of neuromuscular conduction. In 1939, Blalock and associates reported the successful resection in a young woman with myasthenia gravis (MG) of the thymus containing a cyst. After thymectomy, she slowly recovered from her neuromuscular disorder. In 1944, Blalock reported 20 cases of MG treated with transsternal thymectomy, and he noted similar clinical improvements particularly in young women with MG of short duration. Over time, numerous authors debated the role of thymectomy as treatment for MG. It has become clear that thymectomy improves the clinical outcome of patients with MG.

The surgical approaches for thymectomy include trans-sternal, transcervical, and video-assisted thoracic surgery (VATS), with there being proponents of each. The basic principles of thymic surgery should include exploration of the mediastinum, en bloc thymectomy including the cervical poles and adjacent mediastinal fat, protection of the phrenic nerves, and prevention of intrapleural dissemination. For patients with MG without thymoma, resection through a partial sternotomy remains our most common approach. In patients with thymoma, a full sternotomy is commonly used.

Surgical Anatomy

The thymus is a bilobed structure located in the anterior mediastinum overlying the pericardium and great vessels at the base of the heart (Fig. 13-1). The lobes are usually fused in the midline, giving the gland an H-shaped configuration. The upper horns extend into the neck and attach to the thyroid gland by the thyrothymic ligament. The lower horns are draped over the pericardium and attach to the pericardial fat pad. One or both lobes may occasionally lie posterior to the left innominate vein instead of anterior to it. Rare thymic locations include partial or complete failure of descent of one or both thymic lobes and aberrant islands of thymic tissue in the neck, mediastinum, pericardial fat, or within pulmonary parenchyma. In a small series of patients reported by Masaoka and colleagues in 1975, there was a 72% incidence of microscopic deposits of thymic tissue in the mediastinal fat tissue. Jaretzki and colleagues found thymic tissue in the neck, outside of the normal cervical extensions of the thymic lobes, in 32% of patients.

The arterial blood supply of the thymus is provided superiorly by small branches from the inferior thyroid arteries, laterally from the internal mammary arteries, and inferiorly from the pericardiophrenic branches. Venous drainage is predominantly via a single central vein or multiple branches emptying into the left innominate vein. Small veins accompanying the arteries may also partially account for the venous drainage.

The relation of the thymus to the phrenic nerve is critical because both nerves are intimately associated with the thymus as they pass from the chest into the neck at the thoracic inlet. The knowledge of this anatomy is crucial for a successful postoperative outcome because injury to the phrenic nerves can have dire respiratory consequences particularly in patients with MG.

The thymus gland in a newborn reaches a mean weight of 15 g, and grows until puberty, reaching a mean weight of 30 g to 40 g. Following puberty, a gradual process of thymic involution occurs continuing throughout adulthood, with the gland eventually decreasing to a weight of 5 g to 25 g. Ultimately, the thymus becomes almost totally replaced by fat.

Indications for Surgical Resection

Indications for thymectomy include MG, a thymic mass, or both. Approximately 10% to 15% of patients with MG will have an associated thymoma, whereas 30% or more of patients with thymoma will have MG. The indications for thymectomy in patients with MG at our institution include the following: young patients who have a short duration of symptoms, those who fail medical treatment, or those who cannot tolerate their medications. Patients with ocular symptoms alone or those with symptoms that are well controlled on medication are not usual candidates for thymectomy.

Preoperative Evaluation

Preoperative evaluation of a patient with MG requires a neurologic evaluation and computed tomographic scan (CT) of the chest with intravenous contrast enhancement to assess the thymus gland for a mass. Magnetic resonance imaging (MRI) may provide similar information, but the resolution of the CT scan exceeds that of MRI when assessing the contents of the anterior mediastinum. Although a diagnostic transthoracic needle aspirate (TTNA) can be helpful in patients with a thymic mass, we do not recommend it on a routine basis.

is performed. In a prospective study Seggia and associates found that plasmapheresis significantly improved respiratory function and muscle strength in myasthenic patients undergoing thymectomy.

Preoperative anesthetic medication is minimal, usually consisting of atropine and a mild sedative. Preoperative anticholinergic medications are avoided. On induction of anesthesia, we have found that the myasthenic patient does not pose any particular extra problems. Muscle relaxants are avoided, and deep anesthesia is maintained by an inhalation agent and short-acting narcotics.

Operative Technique

We recommend a partial sternal-splitting incision in patients requiring thymectomy for MG who do not have an associated thymic mass. This incision provides adequate visualization of the entire intrathoracic and cervical portion of the thymus gland. If a thymoma is unexpectedly found or exposure is not adequate, the incision can easily be extended into a full sternal-splitting incision. The goals of the operation include evaluation for a thymic mass, visualization and preservation of the phrenic nerves, and total thymectomy with resection of associated fatty tissue. We believe the partial sternal-splitting incision allows completion of these goals in a safe fashion and with a reasonable cosmetic result.

When a thymoma is present, full median sternotomy is commonly performed; however, if the tumor is very large or there is extension into the hilum of the lung, a clamshell incision may be useful (Fig. 13-2). Preoperatively, it can be difficult to determine whether a thymic mass is malignant. It is the surgeon's determination of invasive disease at the time of the operation that is the key finding in helping to resolve whether a thymoma is benign or malignant.

Partial Sternal-Splitting Incision

After induction of general endotracheal anesthesia using a single-lumen endotracheal tube, the patient is placed in the supine position and the neck, chest, and upper abdomen are prepared and draped.

The skin incision is started 1.5 cm below the sternal notch and extended down the midline of the sternum to the level of the fourth or fifth rib (Fig. 13-3). With cephaled skin retraction, the area below the sternal notch is dissected free so a finger can be

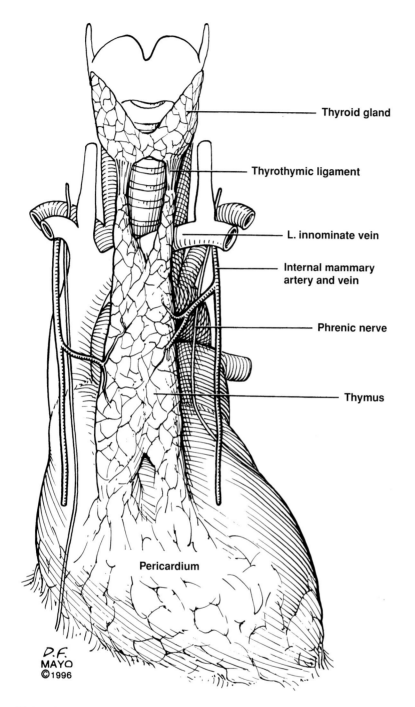

Thyroid gland

Thyrothymic ligament

L. innominate vein

Internal mammary artery and vein

Phrenic nerve

Thymus

Pericardium

D.F. MAYO ©1996

Figure 13-1. The thymus gland is located in the anterior mediastinum, overlying the pericardium and the great vessels of the heart. It is a bilobed structure with two upper and two lower horns. Arterial blood supply is predominantly from the internal mammary vessels laterally, whereas the venous drainage is central into the left (L.) innominate vein. Of key importance is the relationship of the thymus gland to both phrenic nerves, particularly in the middle portion of the gland.

Preoperative Preparation

We advocate the team approach in the care of the myasthenic patient undergoing thymectomy. This includes anesthesia, neurology, and the surgical team being involved preoperatively, operatively, and postoperatively. A patient undergoing thymectomy for MG must be in optimal condition and should be stabilized on a medical program. If this is not possible or the patient has a history of bulbar symptoms, preoperative plasmapheresis

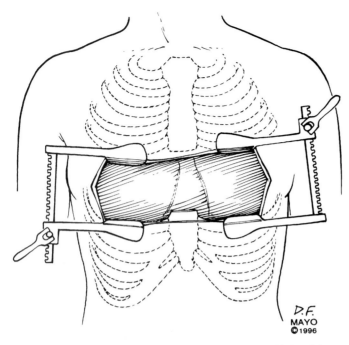

Figure 13-2. For resection of an extraordinarily large thymoma possibly involving one or both pulmonary hila, a bilateral thoracotomy or "clamshell" incision may be used.

placed under the sternum. The sternum is divided longitudinally in the center to the level of the fourth or fifth rib. As the sternum is spread with the retractor, one side will usually transversely split off at the interspace (Fig. 13-4). The overlying mediastinal pleurae are separated in the midline bringing the thymus and left innominate vein into view. Both pleural spaces are opened beginning inferiorly and then extended in a cephalad direction, with the surgeon making sure to identify and protect the phrenic

nerve on each side. The identification of the internal thoracic vein provides a landmark for the superior extent of the pleural opening as the phrenic nerve is in immediate proximity. Thorough exploration of the mediastinum, pleural spaces, and lungs is performed.

Thymectomy is begun by dissecting the middle of the right inferior horn off the pericardium. By using a right-angled clamp in a "walking technique," the inferior horn is dissected in a caudad direction well onto the pericardial fat pad until it can no longer be brought into view. The fat pad is then clamped, divided, and ligated with 2-0 silk. With one right-angled clamp still on the pericardial fat attached to the inferior horn, the right lobe is dissected off the pericardium in a cephalad direction. As the middle portion of the thymus is approached, the dissection is discontinued, and dissection of the right superior horn in the cervical area is begun (Fig. 13-5). This horn is freed circumferentially in its middle portion and, again, using the right-angled "walking technique," freed from its bed until the thyrothymic ligaments are identified. The horn is disconnected from the thyroid gland, and the ligament is ligated with 2-0 silk, leaving a right-angled clamp on the superior horn. With both the inferior and superior horns elevated by the respective right-angled clamps, a U-shaped incision 1 cm superior to the phrenic nerve is made in the mediastinal pleura. Using a right-angled clamp and blunt dissection technique, the middle portion of the right lobe and associated fatty tissue are pulled back from the area above the phrenic nerve up to the junction of the innominate vein and superior vena cava. The lateral vessels coming from the internal mammary are then carefully divided and ligated with 3-0 silk (Fig. 13-6). The thymus gland is then reflected further along the left innominate vein until the midline venous draining vessels are identified. The area of the phrenic nerve can be packed with gauze sponge. The cautery is not used in this area to avoid inadvertently injuring the phrenic nerve. This completes one half of the resection.

The same steps are carried out on the left side. However, the left side can be more difficult because the phrenic nerve tends to come closer, and there seems to be a greater amount of fatty tissue obscuring its view. Again, a blunt dissection technique in the critical area where the nerve runs close to the middle portion of the thymus gland helps to prevent injury to the nerve. Once all four horns have been successfully mobilized, the venous drainage is clamped, divided, and ligated with 3-0 silk (Fig. 13-7). We do not

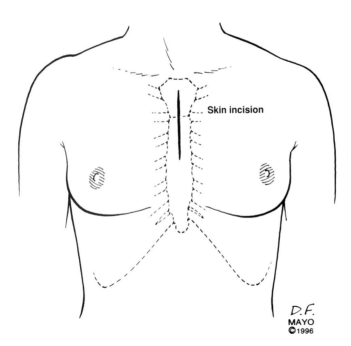

Figure 13-3. With the patient supine, the skin incision is begun 1.5 cm below the sternal notch, and is carried to the level of the fourth or fifth rib. This allows the incision to be well below the neck area and not visible when normal clothing is worn, providing for an acceptable cosmetic result.

use clips on the vein. If the extent of the thymus gland cannot be discerned during this dissection, separate margins are taken for frozen-section analysis to make sure no thymic tissue is left behind.

If the presence of a thymic mass is known ahead of time or if one is found at the time of dissection, careful evaluation of whether this mass is adherent or invading surrounding structures must be made by the surgeon. If present, the mass and associated structures should be resected en bloc and evaluated further in the frozen-section laboratory.

After thymectomy, hemostasis is meticulously obtained. We have found that postoperative bleeding can be increased in patients who have undergone preoperative plasmapheresis. A chest tube is placed below the right breast, through the chest wall, and across the pleural space and mediastinum, with the tip of the tube ultimately in the apex of the left chest (Fig. 13-8). The sternum is reapproximated with interrupted wire placing two or three wires in the manubrium and the remainder around the interspaces of the sternum. The remainder of the soft tissue closure is completed with multiple layers of absorbable suture including a subcuticular closure of the skin.

Full Median Sternotomy Incision

A single-lumen tube is usually used, although a double-lumen tube may be helpful if the mass is extraordinarily large. Large intravenous lines are placed. At exploration, the surgeon not only determines whether the thymic mass is invading surrounding structures, but also evaluates the lungs and pleura for metastases. If metastases are found, they should be resected, if possible, during the same procedure. Actual resection of the thymus gland proceeds in a manner similar to that described earlier. Involved adjacent structures should be resected en bloc with the thymic mass (Fig. 13-9). One phrenic nerve should always be spared. If total resection is not possible, debulking as much of the tumor as possible is worthwhile. Areas surrounding the resection should be clipped for further radiation therapy. Closure of the surgical incision is similar to that described previously.

Postoperative Recovery

After the operation is completed, the patient is taken to the recovery room, awakened, and evaluated frequently by the anesthesiologist. We strive for extubation in the

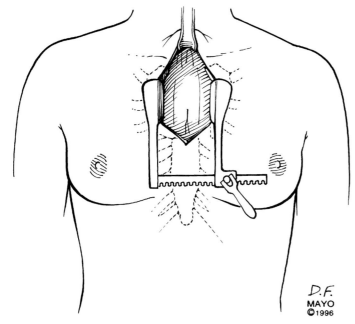

Figure 13-4. When the sternum is retracted, usually the third or fourth interspace will fracture transversely, allowing more than adequate exposure of the thymus gland in patients with myasthenia gravis and no associated mass. This fracture is easily repaired when the sternum is rewired. If necessary, the incision and partial sternal incision can always be lengthened. Both pleural spaces are entered inferiorly and opened cephalad to provide adequate exploration of the pleural spaces and lungs and full visualization of the phrenic nerve.

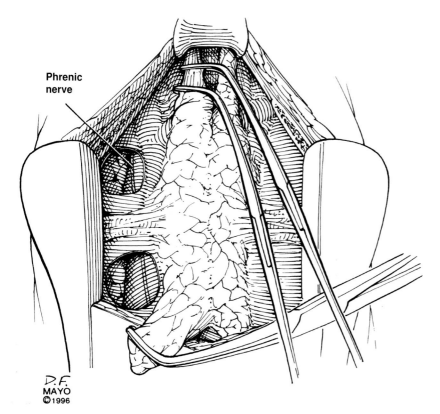

Figure 13-5. The dissection is begun on the right thymic lobe by freeing the inferior horn off the pericardium in a caudad direction by advancing the right-angled clamps in a "walking technique." This is continued well onto the pericardial fat pad, where it is then divided and ligated. The right-angled clamp is left on the pericardial fat attached to the inferior horn for retraction at a later time. The superior horn is then freed from the cervical area in a similar fashion by identifying and dividing the thyrothymic ligament.

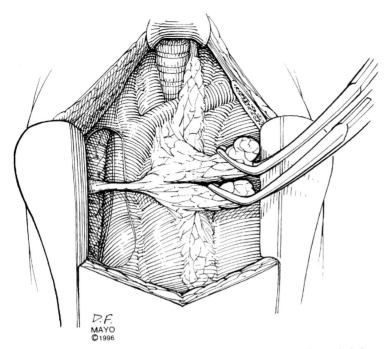

Figure 13-6. With both horns on the right side completely freed, the right-angled clamps are used to retract the horns medially to put tension on the vessels entering laterally from the internal mammary artery. This allows optimal visualization and protection of the phrenic nerve as these vessels are divided and ligated. The right lobe of the thymus and associated fatty tissue are then reflected medially. Use of cautery in this area should be avoided because it is possible to inadvertently injure the phrenic nerve.

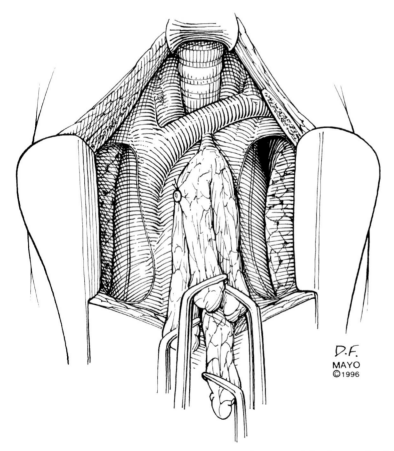

Figure 13-7. After the inferior and superior horns of the left portion of the thymus gland are mobilized, the venous drainage to the left innominate vein is ligated and divided.

recovery room if the respiratory effort and blood gas values are acceptable. It has been our experience that nearly all patients can be extubated in this manner. Patients are then transferred to the general thoracic surgical intermediate care area (ICA) or intensive care unit. Aggressive respiratory care and early ambulation for all thymectomy patients is important. Patients with MG are closely followed by both the surgical and neurology teams. Inspiratory-expiratory pressures and vital capacity are measured every 6 hours so that respiratory status can be evaluated. Anticholinesterase agents are restarted at the first sign of weakness. If the patient deteriorates from the respiratory standpoint, plasmapheresis is instituted. Occasionally, a patient may require reintubation. Once the patient is stable from the respiratory standpoint, he or she is transferred to routine surgical floor care, drains are removed, and the patient is discharged when recovery is complete.

Surgical Results

In 1987, Lewis and colleagues reported on 274 patients treated for thymoma at the Mayo Clinic, of whom 227 underwent total resection. The operative mortality in this group was 3.1%. Complications occurred in 89 patients (39.2%) and were more frequent in those who had preoperative MG or cardiovascular disease.

Since the advent of the team approach combined with aggressive preoperative and postoperative care, operative mortality has nearly been eliminated and morbidity is very low. We reviewed 364 patients seen at Mayo Clinic Rochester from 1982 through 2004 who underwent thymic resection. Of these, 241 (66.2%) had MG. A partial sternotomy was performed in 236 patients, full sternotomy in 126, and clamshell incision in 2. Two hundred thirty-six (98%) of the 241 patients with MG were extubated within the first few hours of the operation. The remaining 5 patients were extubated the following day. There was 1 operative death (0.27%) secondary to acute respiratory distress syndrome (ARDS). The average length of hospitalization was a mean of 4.8 days. Major complications occurred in 18 (4.9%) patients and included atelectasis in 10, atrial fibrillation in 4, respiratory failure requiring reintubation and bleeding in 3 each, and cylothorax in 1.

Improvement of the symptoms of MG after thymectomy can be variable. Buckingham and associates in 1976 reviewed 160 patients with MG and found that 33% of

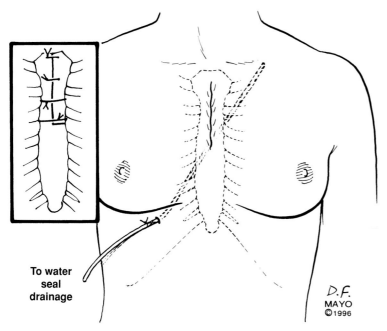

To water seal drainage

Figure 13-8. After hemostasis is achieved, a right chest tube is placed below the right breast, through the chest wall, and across the pleural space and mediastinum. The tip is placed in the apex of the left pleural space.

the 80 patients undergoing resection had complete remission when compared with a computer-assisted matched group of 80 patients treated medically, of whom only 8% had complete remission. There were 11 late deaths after thymectomy, but 34 late deaths in the medically treated group. In 1982, Olanow and associates reported on 47 consecutive patients, with a mean follow-up of 25.5 months, and found 83% of patients were free of generalized weakness and 61% were receiving no medications. In 1992, Kirschner stated what he believed to be realistic expectations of surgical treatment for MG, including remission in 20% to 25% of patients, with 10% to 20% being complete drug-free remissions, improvement in 35% to 50%, and no change in 10%. Only a few patients will do worse.

Survival for thymoma is based on stage of disease at the time of resection. Kondo and colleagues reported on the survival of 1,320 patients with thymic epithelial tumors from 115 Japanese institutes. The tumor was

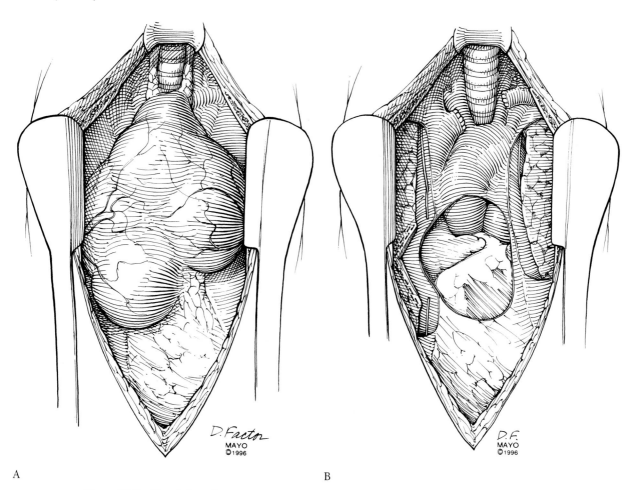

A   B

Figure 13-9. Via a full median sternotomy incision **(A)** the thymoma is evaluated and resection begun. **(B)** If the thymoma is invasive, total en bloc resection is carried out, including all associated involved structures, in this case lung, right phrenic nerve, portion of pericardium, and left innominate vein.

thymoma in 1,093 patients, thymic carcinoma in 186, and carcinoid in 41. Following total surgical resection the overall 5-year survival for stage I and II thymoma was 100% and 98%, respectively. For stages III, IVA, and IVB, 5-year survival was 88.7%, 70.6%, and 52.8% respectively. Of note, for patients with totally resected stage III and IV thymoma, 5-year survival was 92.9%. For thymic carcinoma, the 5-year survival rates for stage I plus II, III, and IV were 88.2%, 51.7%, and 37.6% respectively. Although adjuvant therapy is often recommended for patients with totally resected stage II, III, and IV thymomas and thymic carcinomas, Kondo and colleagues did not demonstrate such a benefit.

Conclusion

Thymectomy for MG without a thymic mass performed through a partial sternal-splitting incision provides excellent exposure and has minimal mortality and morbidity. Whether a more limited approach, such as video-assisted thoracic surgery (VATS) or cervical thymectomy, or a more aggressive approach, such as transcervical-trans-sternal maximal thymectomy, is more effective is difficult to prove. We believe that thorough preoperative evaluation, total thymectomy, and aggressive postoperative care using a team approach has helped to produce optimal postoperative results in patients undergoing thymectomy for MG. Although MG has in the past negatively influenced operative survival, this is no longer true.

Complete surgical resection remains the mainstay of therapy for early stage thymomas and perhaps after neoadjuvant chemotherapy for more advanced stage disease. A full median sternotomy incision provides excellent exposure with minimal mortality and morbidity in the majority of these patients.

SUGGESTED READING

Blalock A. Thymectomy in the treatment of myasthenia gravis: Report of twenty cases. J Thorac Surg 1944;13:316.

Blalock A, Mason MF, Morgan HJ, et al. Myasthenia gravis and tumors of the thymic region: Report of a case in which the tumor was removed. Ann Surg 1939;110:544.

Buckingham JM, Howard FM Jr, Bernatz PE, et al. The value of thymectomy in myasthenia gravis: A computer-assisted matched study. Ann Surg 1976;184:453.

Calhoun RF, Ritter JH, Guthrie TJ, et al. Results of transcervical thymectomy for myasthenia gravis in 100 consecutive patients. Ann Surg 1999;230:555.

Deeb ME, Brinster CJ, Kucharzuk J, et al. Expanded indications for transcervical thymectomy in the management of anterior mediastinal masses. Ann Thorac Surg 2001;72:208.

Jaretzki A. Thymectomy for myasthenia gravis: Analysis of controversies regarding techniques and results. Neurology 1997;48(Suppl 5):S52.

Jaretzki A, Penn AS, Younger DS, et al. Maximal thymectomy for myasthenia gravis: results. J Thorac Cardiovasc Surg 1988;95:747.

Kirschner PA. Myasthenia gravis and ther parathymic syndromes. In Benfield JR (ed), Chest Surgery Clinics of North America, Mediastinal Tumors. Philadelphia: Saunders, 1992;183.

Kondo K, Monden Y. Therapy for thymic epithelial tumors: A clinical study of 1,320 patients from Japan. Ann Thorac Surg 2003;76:878.

Lewis JE, Wick MR, Scheithauer BW, et al. Thymoma: A clinicopathologic review. Cancer 1987;60:2727.

Mack MJ, Landreneau RJ, Yim AP, et al. Results of video-assisted thymectomy in patients with myasthenia gravis. J Thorac Cardiovasc Surg 1996;112:1352.

Masaoka A, Nagaoka Y, Kotake Y, et al. Distribution of thymic tissue at the anterior mediastinum. J Thorac Cardiovasc Surg 1975;70:747.

Masaoka A, Yamakawa Y, Niwa H, et al. Extended thymectomy for myasthenia gravis patients: a 20-year review. Ann Thorac Surg 1996;62:853.

Nichols FC, Ercan S, Trastek VF. Standard thymectomy. In Shields TW, Locicero J, Ponn RB, et al. (eds), General Thoracic Surgery, 5th ed. Philadelphia: Lippincott Williams & Wilkins, 2005;2629.

Olanow CW, Wechsler AS, Roses AD. A prospective study of thymectomy and serum acetylcholine receptor antibodies in myasthenia gravis. Ann Surg 1982;196:113.

Patterson GA. Thymomas. Semin Thorac Cardiovasc Surg 1992;4:39.

Seggia JC, Abreu P, Takatani M. Plasmapheresis a preparatory method for thymectomy in myasthenia gravis. Arq Neuropsiquiatr 1995;53:411.

Stern LE, Nussbaum MS, Quinlan JG, et al. Long-term evaluation of extended thymectomy with anterior mediastinal dissection for myasthenia gravis. Surgery 2001;130:774.

Wright CD, Kessler KA. Surgical treatment of thymic tumors. Semin Thorac Cardiovasc Surg 2005;17:20.

EDITOR'S COMMENTS

Nichols and Trastek have nicely described their technique for thymectomy via median sternotomy. Their preferred approach is a partial sternotomy unless a thymoma is present, in which case they advocate a full median sternotomy. By their definition a partial sternotomy is carried down to the level of the fourth or fifth intercostal space, and it is not clear to me what advantage this offers over a full sternotomy. We and others have taken a more liberal approach with regard to indication for thymectomy in patients with myasthenia gravis (MG). The authors state that they do not currently offer thymectomy to those with ocular disease only or to those patients who are well controlled on their medication. They also note that their preference is for young patients or those who cannot tolerate the medication. Especially with a less invasive approach, such as the transcervical approach, the morbidity is so low that I see no reason why thymectomy should not be offered to every patient with MG. In our experience, as well as in the experience of several other groups, the outcome from transcervical thymectomy is equivalent to that achieved with an open approach, but it is important that results be stated in a clear fashion. Achieving a complete response is a continuous variable as more patients achieve this over time and thus is best expressed as the probability of achieving a complete response (Kaplan-Meier). This was the recommendation of a consensus panel convened by the Myasthenia Gravis Foundation, yet few authors have reported their data using this method. The authors' approach involves a significant amount of dissection around the phrenic nerves, yet in the review of their series they report no phrenic nerve injuries. Other large series that utilize the "maximal" thymectomy have all reported nerve injuries and an incidence of postoperative respiratory failure.

When dealing with thymomas it is critical to recognize, as the authors point out, the importance of performing a total thymectomy in addition to resecting the tumor. The authors refer to thymomas as "malignant," but it is probably preferable to refer to these lesions as either encapsulated or invasive because rarely do they behave like malignancies. It is also critically important to distinguish invasive thymoma from thymic carcinoma, an epithelial malignancy that is associated with a far worse prognosis.

L.R.K.

14

Thymectomy (Transcervical)

Larry R. Kaiser

Introduction

The classical and standard approach to thymectomy is via a median sternotomy. The preceding chapter discusses this approach in detail. There is no question that median sternotomy provides ideal exposure of the anterior mediastinum and thus makes removal of the thymus gland quite straightforward. It always struck me that this exposure was somewhat "maximal" for the removal of a fatty gland that just gets in the way of the cardiac surgeon prior to entering the pericardium. Papatestas, at Mt. Sinai Hospital in New York City, generated a large series of patients undergoing thymectomy via a cervical approach with results in patients with myasthenia gravis (MG) that were almost comparable to those achieved with median sternotomy. The idea of a cervical approach to the thymus gland was not original with Papatestas, but the large volume of patients with MG seen at Mt. Sinai prompted him to revive an approach that was less invasive for these patients, many of whom were not great candidates for a sternotomy with the attendant postoperative morbidity. It was really Joel Cooper, however, who popularized the transcervical approach to thymectomy by formalizing the procedure with the use of a specific retractor used for the procedure that allowed better visualization of the operative field. The operation performed by Papatestas relied on "blind" dissection of the gland within the mediastinum, but with Cooper's retractor the entire dissection is done under direct visualization, allowing the ability for a more complete thymectomy.

It is illustrative to contemplate that it was a surgeon, Alfred Blalock, who contributed as much as anyone to the recognition of the role of the thymus gland in the autoimmune disorder myasthenia gravis. In 1936 Blalock performed a thymectomy for a thymoma in a patient with MG, after which it was noted that the patient's symptoms improved remarkably. This was a seminal observation and one that easily could have been overlooked because the patient was operated on for removal of a neoplasm, a thymoma. It was not until years after this procedure that Blalock published the results of this case. He was able to make the leap in his thinking after the observation of improvement in myasthenic symptoms after thymectomy for thymoma excision, suggesting that thymectomy might be of benefit in myasthenic patients with thymoma. In 1941, building on this observation, he reported a series of 6 patients with MG who underwent thymectomy in the absence of a thymoma. This was an incredibly radical concept, that is, the removal of what otherwise appeared to be a normal gland in an attempt to improve symptoms from a neurologic disease that was poorly understood. In 1944 Blalock published a series of 20 patients with MG who underwent thymectomy. There were 4 deaths in the series, and the most favorable results with regard to symptom relief occurred in those patients whose symptoms had been present for 1 year or less.

It is important to recognize that thymectomy when a thymoma or other mass is not present in the anterior mediastinum most commonly is carried out in patients with MG in an attempt to improve the symptoms of the disease. Relatively few surgical operations are designed solely to result in a functional improvement, and those that are rarely, if ever, involve the removal of an organ to effect such improvement. Thus operation for MG may be unique in that removal of an organ, in this case the thymus gland, produces either complete or partial remission of the disease in up to 90% of patients. Despite the passage of 70 years since Blalock noted improvement in symptoms after removing the thymoma from the patient with MG, the relationship between the gland and the disease has not been fully elucidated. We do know that MG is a CD4+ T-cell–dependent autoimmune disease characterized by antibody-mediated skeletal muscle weakness and that the disease may be related to intrathymic expression of the neuromuscular type of acetylcholine (ACh) receptors. The thymus appears to be the site of autosensitization to the ACh receptor.

Thymectomy for MG is now a well-accepted procedure in the thoracic surgical community, although a number of controversies remain. Many neurologists remain hesitant to recommend thymectomy for patients with MG and feel that these patients present significant surgical risks and that many can be rendered symptom-free with medication. The mainstay of medical therapy for MG remains pyridostigmine (Mestinon), a cholinesterase inhibitor that is often accompanied by gastrointestinal (diarrhea, vomiting, mouth watering) and other side effects (blurred vision, increased sweating). Corticosteroids form the next line of therapy often used in addition to pyridostigmine. For nonresponders immune-suppressive agents such as azathioprine and cyclosporine have been used. For many patients, the opportunity to be relieved of their symptoms without the need for medication more than justifies an operative procedure especially if the procedure can be performed with minimal morbidity. The key to success from thymectomy in patients with MG has long been thought to be complete removal of the thymus gland, and it has been noted that thymic remnants may be found in aberrant locations. This is the major argument against any procedure other than a median sternotomy, the classic approach to thymectomy. Alfred Jaretzki described the "maximal" thymectomy, which involves a combined cervicothoracic approach and removes all mediastinal tissue from phrenic nerve to phrenic nerve as well as searches for aberrantly located gland. A similar approach has been taken by Greg Bulkley, who reported on 200 patients treated over a 30-year period. Although there were no early deaths, he reported a complication rate of >30% with a 6% incidence of respiratory failure. He noted that the maximal thymectomy was the greatest predictor of response in addition to no preoperative plasmapheresis and male gender.

The complete response rate increases over time; thus it must be considered as a continuous variable, and the best way to report these data is to use the Kaplan-Meier probability of achieving a complete response, a method employed by only a few investigators but one recommended by an expert working group. Transcervical thymectomy can achieve complete and total removal of the gland and may be performed as an outpatient procedure with minimal morbidity and no mortality. The long-term results are equivalent to those achieved by the trans-sternal approach as well as with the combined cervical/trans-sternal approach. Cooper reported on 100 consecutive transcervical thymectomies with 35% complete response at 5 years and 44% at 8 years. In a series of 78 patients we reported a 39.7% crude complete response rate and a Kaplan-Meier 5-year estimated probability of complete response of 43%. Despite these results, transcervical thymectomy is offered at only a few institutions because of the continued "belief" that the operation leads to less than complete removal of the gland and is unable to remove gland located aberrantly. Most surgeons who perform thymic surgery will see at most 5 to 10 patients per year with MG, thus making it difficult for them to develop the expertise necessary to perform the transcervical procedure. There is no question that a sternotomy is an easier operation for the surgeon but clearly not for the patient.

Preoperative Preparation

Patients with MG need to be individualized with regard to preoperative preparation. Most require nothing other than the usual preoperative laboratory work and perhaps cardiology clearance, based on their past history. The majority of patients with MG are young, although there is a second peak in incidence of the disease after age 50 years. Where the need for individualization comes into play is in the patient with severe symptoms especially bulbar or respiratory symptoms. All patients with MG should undergo measurement of their forced vital capacity (FVC). Those whose FVC is significantly reduced should be considered for either intravenous immunoglobulin treatment or plasmapheresis. I leave this decision up to the referring neurologist, but with the minimal morbidity that accompanies transcervical thymectomy I do not feel strongly about plasmapheresis even in the patient with a significant reduction in FVC. Because the sternum is not opened, the degree of respiratory embarrassment is negligible with the transcervical approach. Nonetheless in our experience approximately one fourth of patients undergo plasmapheresis before transcervical thymectomy. Usually this is accomplished with three exchanges done during the week prior to the thymectomy, most commonly as an outpatient procedure as long as the patient has reasonable venous access. Some patients require an inpatient stay for plasmapheresis. After plasmapheresis, patients experience an increase in strength for a variable period of time and usually report feeling quite good.

Technique of Transcervical Thymectomy

There are a number of anesthetic considerations in patients with MG, and an anesthesiologist experienced in the management of these patients is desirable. If muscle-relaxing agents are used, only small doses of nondepolarizing agents should be used, ideally only the short-acting drugs. The patient is placed on the operating table in the supine position with the head at the very upper edge of the table. The neck is maximally hyperextended using an inflatable bag behind the patient's shoulders or alternatively a rolled sheet. The head should be placed in a "doughnut" to keep it from moving. This operation is difficult under the best of situations but is particularly difficult in the patient whose neck can only be minimally extended. The amount of neck extension should be a consideration in the preoperative period in determining whether a patient is a candidate for the transcervical approach. Early in one's experience the transcervical operation should be avoided in the patient with minimal neck extension, but as one gains additional experience with the operation the "tricks" available become better known and these patients can be done transcervically.

It is important that the patient's head be at the very edge of the table, otherwise the reach required makes the procedure even more difficult. The arms are tucked at the side, and "toboggans" can be used to facilitate this. The arms need to be protected because the retractor will be placed on the table and the arms are at risk for a compression injury. The neck and anterior chest are prepped with povidone-iodine solution, and the draping should involve side drapes and a drape across the head that drops down to the floor. An ether screen cannot be used, and the anesthesiologist should be positioned to the side of the patient. The anesthesia tubing should be allowed to drop down and not be suspended on a "Christmas tree" that elevates the drapes. The procedure is conducted from the patient's head, and anything that elevates the draping impairs the operator's vision into the mediastinum. The skin incision is made just over the sternal notch and carried down through the platysma (Fig. 14-1). Making the incision even 1 cm or 2 cm superior to the notch leaves a bridge of skin that makes the mediastinal dissection more difficult. Once the incision is made through the platysma both superior and inferior subplatysmal flaps are raised. The superior flap should be carried up to just below the thyroid cartilage, and the inferior flap is carried below the suprasternal notch. Two Gelpi retractors are placed to separate the skin flaps.

The dissection is carried along the midline avascular plane separating the sternohyoid and sternothyroid muscles. The ligamentous attachment within the sternal notch must be incised and the substernal plane developed with the finger. With the assistant elevating the strap muscles the loose areolar tissue on the posterior aspect of the sternothyroid muscle is incised. The cervical portion of the gland appears salmon-pink, and it is the color and the presence of a thin fibrous capsule that distinguishes the gland from the surrounding cervical fat. This is more difficult than it sounds. The distinction of the gland from the cervical fat may be quite difficult, but hugging the posterior aspect of the strap muscle usually allows the operator to locate the gland. I usually identify the right lobe of the gland first because often it comes up higher in the neck than the left lobe. The gland is located anterior to

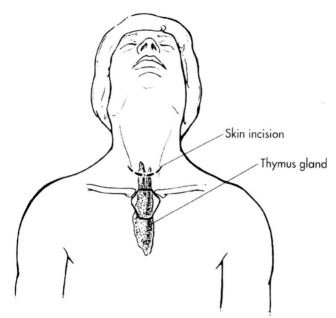

Figure 14-1. Transcervical thymectomy (TCT). (Reprinted with permission from LR Kaiser. Atlas of General Thoracic Surgery. St. Louis: Mosby, 1997.)

the inferior thyroid vein, and if the dissection is deep to the vein, the gland has been missed and the dissection needs to be more superficial.

Once the gland is located it must be freed up laterally and the inferior thyroid vein separated away. Occasionally there may be small venous branches from the gland draining into the inferior thyroid vein. These small branches should be clipped as the gland is followed superiorly. Not uncommonly, the gland can be followed up above the inferior aspect of the thyroid cartilage. The gland is gently pulled inferiorly as it is dissected superiorly until the superior aspect of the gland is reached. There will be a small vein that enters the superior aspect of the gland that must be clipped. The gland is then elevated and a right angle placed on the upper pole of the gland. A long silk tie is placed on the gland to be used as a "handle" to facilitate subsequent dissection (Fig. 14-2).

With the gland retracted anteriorly using the silk tie, it is sharply dissected away from surrounding soft tissue and elevated. The dissection is carried down toward the innominate vein. The opposite lobe of the gland is identified by following the elevated

lobe inferiorly. Again the avascular plane posterior to the strap muscles is incised to identify the opposite lobe. Again this lobe is followed to its termination superiorly and the vein is clipped and divided. A long silk suture to be used for traction is placed on this lobe as well. Hemostats are placed on both of the silk sutures to keep them separate. At this point a self-retaining retractor may be placed to separate the strap muscles to facilitate the dissection inferiorly. Both lobes are freed up down to the innominate vein. The surgeon now goes to the head of the table and sits on a stool on wheels. A headlight is mandatory for the successful completion of the mediastinal portion of this procedure. Some surgeons use magnifying loupes as well, usually with 2.5× magnification. Holding the lobes anteriorly and using peanut sponges on Kelly clamps, one bluntly frees the gland away from the innominate vein. As this is done, venous branches from the gland to the innominate vein will come into view. These branches will vary in size and location. Most commonly the gland passes anterior to the innominate vein, but in the rare patient one or both lobes of the gland may pass posterior to the vein. In that situation the lobes should be freed up until they can be passed underneath the vein and then brought away from the vein to identify the thymic venous branches. Smaller venous branches may be clipped before being divided while larger branches are ligated. The venous branches are isolated using the peanut sponges, and a right angle is then placed to grasp a silk ligature. With the assistant retracting the innominate vein superiorly using a peanut, the ligature is placed proximally on the thymic venous branch and tied (Fig. 14-3) The ligature is not cut but is used to apply countertraction as the distal ligature is placed and tied. The venous branch is then divided and the sutures cut. Commonly there are venous branches from the gland that drain laterally into the internal mammary vein. These must also be clipped and divided. Once all thymic venous branches are divided the gland may be freed away from the pericardium inferior to the innominate vein. From this point forward almost all of the dissection is done bluntly using ball sponges (tonsil sponges) placed on a ring forceps.

The anterior aspect of the gland is freed away from the sternum using the ball sponges (Fig. 14-4). The substernal plane has previously been exposed with the finger, and this makes placement of the ball sponges somewhat easier. Freeing the gland away from the sternum at this point may be done blindly with the ball sponges.

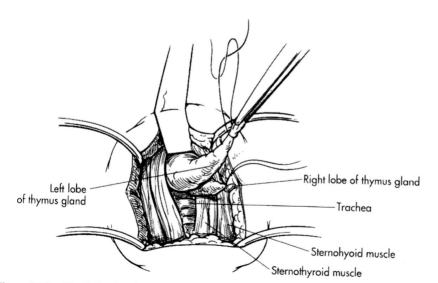

Figure 14-2. The tie is placed on the gland. (Reprinted with permission from LR Kaiser. Atlas of General Thoracic Surgery. St. Louis: Mosby, 1997.)

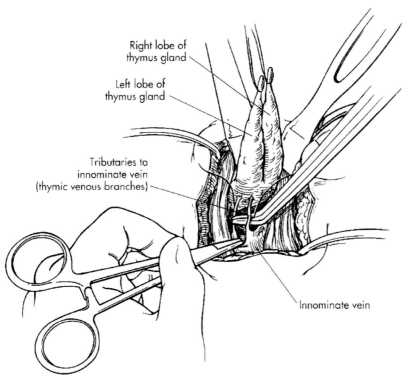

Figure 14-3. The ligature is placed proximally on the thymic venous branch and tied. (Reprinted with permission from LR Kaiser. Atlas of General Thoracic Surgery. St. Louis: Mosby, 1997.)

Elevating the gland anteriorly allows the ball sponges to free the gland away from the pericardium. The right lobe of the gland is pulled to the left with the ball, and lateral attachments that are easily visible are incised. The same is done for the left lobe of the gland.

Care should be taken to avoid any breach of the capsule of the gland, and the gland is retraced using the silk ligatures.

At this point the Cooper thymectomy retractor (Pilling Co., Fort Washington, PA) is placed. Clamps are applied over the drapes on each side of the table (Fig. 14-5). The side bars of the Polytract retractor (Pilling Co.) are placed through the clamps and adjusted to the appropriate height. The cross bar of the retractor is then put into place. The position of the retractor relative to the sternal notch is particularly important if the retractor is to remain in place. The arm of the retractor is placed into the sternal notch and placed through the connector on the cross bar. It is then lifted, usually with a significant amount of force, and locked in place. If the location of the retractor on the table is incorrect, the sternal portion of the retractor will not remain in place and the position of the side bars needs to be corrected. An alternative to the Cooper retractor, which is a custom piece, has been suggested. The Rultract retractor (Rultract Inc., Independence, OH), which is usually used for taking down the internal mammary artery, may also be used with an appropriate blade that fits into the sternal notch. This retractor may be more readily available than the Cooper retractor, and thus this procedure may become more accessible. Once the retractor is in place an Army-Navy retractor is placed on each side of the wound, each held in place by a Penrose drain tied around the retractor post on each side. The inflatable bag behind the shoulders is deflated to further improve visualization into the mediastinum. At this point the patient literally is being held up by the thymectomy retractor.

Attention is first directed to the right lobe of the gland, which is swept away from the right pleural reflection. The gland is easily distinguished from the fat of the pleural reflection. Care is taken to avoid entering the pleural space, but if it is entered, a red rubber catheter placed before closing is used to evacuate the hemithorax aided by a Valsalva maneuver. The tube is removed as the wound is closed. With the gland reflected anteriorly, using the silk sutures, it is separated completely from the pericardium to its inferior extent. This maneuver facilitates the sweeping of the gland away from each pleural reflection. After the right lobe is freed away from the pleural reflection it is brought over toward the left.

The left lobe is then swept away from the left pleural reflection. The left side always is more difficult than the right because of the tongue of gland that extends toward the aortopulmonary window. Freeing the gland away from the pleural reflection is done entirely bluntly with the use of the ball sponges. The phrenic nerves are vulnerable on each side especially near the sternal notch. Particularly on the left side as the gland is followed toward the

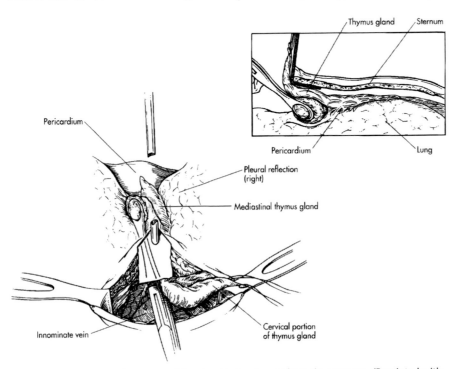

Figure 14-4. The anterior aspect of the gland is freed away from the sternum. (Reprinted with permission from LR Kaiser. Atlas of General Thoracic Surgery. St. Louis: Mosby, 1997.)

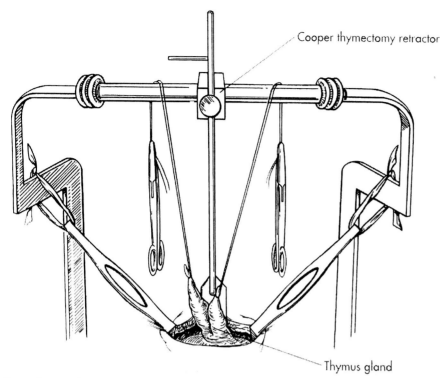

Cooper thymectomy retractor

Thymus gland

Figure 14-5. Clamps are applied over the drapes on each side of the table. (Reprinted with permission from LR Kaiser. Atlas of General Thoracic Surgery. St. Louis: Mosby, 1997.)

aortopulmonary window care must be taken to avoid traction on the phrenic nerve. Often the nerve is not seen, but its position must be assumed. No sharp dissection should be done in the vicinity of the nerve, especially near the apex of the chest, when the nerve is most anterior in location. Once the gland is freed away from each pleural reflection it is brought from inferior to superior. Some pericardial attachments may require sharp division, but these are easily seen. As the gland is brought above the innominate vein some attachments may remain. These should be clipped because often these are small thymic venous branches that had not been previously seen.

Once the gland is removed a thorough inspection should be made to ensure that there is no bleeding within the mediastinum. If one or both pleural spaces have been entered, a red rubber tube is placed into the pleural space, as mentioned previously. This is removed just as the closure is completed and a Valsalva maneuver is performed. The strap muscles are reapproximated, and the platysma is closed with absorbable suture. The skin is closed with a subcuticular suture. With a properly conducted anesthetic the patient is readily awakened and has adequate muscle strength to tolerate extubation. The patient is brought to the postanesthesia recovery area and allowed to fully awaken. A chest radiograph is obtained to ensure that no significant pneumothorax is present. Unless this is quite large and the patient is symptomatic, nothing needs to be done about a pneumothorax because there is no ongoing air leak. As soon as the patient is fully awake his or her usual medications are given by mouth. We plan to discharge the patient to home within a few hours of the operative procedure. Usually oral pain medication is required for the first 1 or 2 postoperative days.

Results

With >200 of these procedures performed, our mean operative time is a little greater than 1 hour. The mean length of stay is 0.5 day, with only the occasional patient staying overnight. We have no mortality, and no patient has remained intubated or required reintubation or an intensive care unit stay. We have noted 2 phrenic nerve injuries and 3 superficial wound infections. The mean preoperative Osserman grade was 2.55, and the mean postoperative grade was 1.07. Greater than 50% of the patients were either Osserman grade III or IV preoperatively. The crude complete response rate was 39.7% in the first 120 patients. The Kaplan-Meier probability of achieving a complete response

at 60 months is 43%. This compares with a Kaplan-Meier probability of approximately 50% with the maximal transcervical/transsternal thymectomy. A negative prognostic indicator was preoperative treatment with corticosteroids, and patients with thymomas had a higher likelihood of achieving a complete response than those with normal thymus or thymic hyperplasia.

Cooper noted a decrease in Osserman grade from 3.0 to 1.0 in 100 consecutive patients undergoing the procedure. Eighty-five percent of patients improved one or more Osserman grades, and 63% improved two or more grades. Thirty-five percent were in complete remission. Long-term follow-up of 52 patients followed for a mean of 8.4 ± 6.1 years showed a complete remission rate of 44.3% and a mean Osserman grade of 0.4.

Whatever approach is chosen, it is clear that thymectomy for MG provides an opportunity for complete remission of symptoms for a significant number of patients. In my opinion there is no reason why the operation should not at least be offered to every patient with MG including those with only ocular disease, especially if the operation can be done as an outpatient procedure via the transcervical approach. Only about 10% of patients will have no response to thymectomy. The challenge is getting the word out to the neurologists who care for these patients and making the case that an extirpative procedure can actually result in a functional improvement. Learning to perform transcervical thymectomy is challenging because the number of patients with MG seen by a given surgeon in one year usually is minimal. The operation is difficult to teach because of the limited visualization other than for the individual performing the procedure. This is one of those procedures where the little tricks are learned after doing a number of these procedures. For the surgeon who may do only two or three thymectomies per year it is doubtful that the transcervical procedure can be mastered, and either these patients should be sent to someone who does the transcervical operation or the trans-sternal approach should be offered.

SUGGESTED READING

Bulkley GB, Bass KN, Stephenson R, et al. Extended cervicomediastinal thymectomy in the integrated management of myasthenia gravis. Ann Surg 1997;226:324.

Calhoun RF, Ritter JH, Guthrie TJ, et al. Results of transcervical thymectomy for myasthenia gravis on 100 consecutive patients. Ann Surg 1999;230:555.

Jaretzki A, Barohn RJ, Ernstoff RM, et al. Myasthenia gravis: Recommendations for clinical research standards. Ann Thorac Surg 2000;70:327.

Jaretzki III A, Wolff M. "Maximal" thymectomy for myasthenia gravis. J Thorac Cardiovasc Surg 1988;96:711.

Kark AE, Papatestas AE. Some anatomic features of the transcervical approach for thymectomy. Mt Sinai J Med 1971;38:580.

Shrager JB, Deeb ME, Mick R, et al. Transcervical thymectomy for myasthenia gravis achieves results comparable to thymectomy by sternotomy. Ann Thorac Surg 2002;74:320.

EDITOR'S COMMENTS

Dr. Kaiser presents an elegant description of a transcervical thymectomy, and by virtue of the fact that he has done so many, he almost makes it seem as though it is an easy operation to do. It is not, and it should not be an operation performed by the casual general thoracic surgeon who only does one or two thymectomies per year. Most thoracic surgeons prefer a trans-sternal approach to the thymus gland, although there are an increasing number of surgeons who are managing small thymic tumors or patients with myasthenia gravis with thoracoscopic procedures.

There are several points made in this chapter that merit further emphasis. First, the results of transcervical thymectomies, in appropriately selected patients, are equivalent to the "larger," more invasive procedures described by Jaretski. Second, this operation is difficult to teach because of the limited visibility for any first or second assistant. Third, it takes some experience to correctly identify cervical fat or the beginning of the thymus gland. A common mistake is to proceed with the dissection more posteriorly than needed. As pointed out by the author, using the inferior thyroidal vein as an anatomic landmark to guide the depth of dissection is an important technical point and helps to keep the operator in the correct plane of dissection.

We have performed several of these procedures thoracoscopically through either a right-sided approach or a bilateral approach with the patient supine and arms elevated over the head much like the positioning for a double-lung transplant. Visualization is excellent, recovery is quick, and it is easier to teach to residents because of the thoracoscopic picture. Whatever approach is chosen, it is likely that referral of these patients for surgery will be facilitated with minimally invasive surgical approaches like the transcervical approach described by Dr. Kaiser.

D.R.J.

15

Resection of Posterior Mediastinal Lesions

Brendon M. Stiles and Thomas M. Daniel

Anatomists describe the posterior mediastinum as that part of the thorax behind the pericardium extending from the fourth thoracic vertebral body to the diaphragm. Anatomically, the division of the mediastinum into the superior, anterior, middle, and posterior compartments means that all components of the mediastinum above the fourth thoracic vertebral body belong to the superior compartment. Tumors of the anterior and posterior mediastinum, however, often extend to and can occupy the superior compartment, and most surgeons refer to only three divisions of the mediastinum: anterosuperior, middle, and posterior. The posterior mediastinum therefore contains all structures posterior to the pericardium and pericardial reflection and extends from the thoracic inlet to the diaphragm.

Within the posterior mediastinum are the thoracic aorta, thoracic duct, azygos and hemiazygos veins, esophagus, fibroareolar fatty tissue and lymph nodes, posterior intercostal veins, arteries and nerves, the vagus nerves and sympathetic chains, and widely scattered paraganglionic cells. Although posterior mediastinal tumors can arise from any of these structures, neurogenic tumors are by far the most common primary tumors of the posterior mediastinum and can arise from the sympathetic ganglia, paraganglia cells, intercostal nerves, or neural sheath cells (Fig. 15-1). In this chapter, we discuss the resection of posterior mediastinal neurogenic tumors. Although posterior mediastinal tumors can also be of esophageal, vascular, bone, lung, or lymphatic origin, these tumors are not specifically addressed in this chapter.

Posterior Mediastinal Neurogenic Tumors

The posterior mediastinum is relatively rich in neural tissue. Spinal nerves exit through the intervertebral foramina and immediately divide, sending one ramus laterally in the posterior mediastinum as the intercostal nerve. Another division of the spinal nerve root gives off branches to the sympathetic trunk, which runs along the posterior mediastinum on the rib heads. In most reported series, neurogenic tumors represent 55% to 60% or more of all posterior mediastinal masses. In addition, approximately 10% to 20% of posterior mediastinal neurogenic tumors have a spinal canal component. Based on the anatomic description of the spinal nerve roots and the intercostal nerves, it appears that neurogenic tumors arising in the region of the intervertebral foramen can grow in both directions along the involved nerve. These particular tumors are called dumbbell tumors and are usually composed of a larger, posterior mediastinal component and a smaller, intraspinal canal component connected by a narrow foraminal segment (Fig. 15-2). These tumors need to be accurately assessed preoperatively and mandate careful neurosurgical and thoracic surgical planning when resected. Failure to diagnose a dumbbell tumor preoperatively may lead to major complications intraoperatively while one is trying to resect the intrathoracic component of the tumor. Unknowingly cutting across the narrow foraminal tumor neck may result in tumor hemorrhage, which could cause spinal cord compression. In addition, the intercostal artery gives off a small branch artery that traverses the interverte-

bral foramen. Distorted anatomy due to the presence of a dumbbell tumor can lead to unexpected arterial bleeding that may be difficult to control. Significant cord compression from a resulting epidural hematoma is a disastrous complication.

Histologically, posterior mediastinal neurogenic tumors are classified based on the neural cell of origin. Tumors of nerve sheath origin comprise neurilemomas, benign and malignant schwannomas, benign neurofibromas, and malignant neurofibrosarcomas. Ganglionic tumors arising from the sympathetic chain are benign ganglioneuromas and malignant ganglioneuroblastomas. Tumors arising from the randomly scattered paraganglionic cells can be found anywhere in the mediastinum and include the relatively uncommon mediastinal pheochromocytomas and the nonchromaffin paragangliomas. Paragangliomas of the posterior mediastinum are usually found in the paravertebral sulcus and can be functional if they secrete hormones. Dumbbell tumors are usually benign tumors of nerve sheath origin (schwannoma, neurofibroma). The majority of all posterior mediastinal neurogenic tumors are benign.

Most posterior mediastinal tumors are first noted on a routine chest radiograph offered for other reasons. Patients tend to be asymptomatic. When symptoms are present, they are often caused by mechanical factors related to the size and location of the tumor. For example, back and chest pain may be present from involvement of ribs or intercostal nerves. Tumors involving the stellate ganglion and upper sympathetic trunk can cause Horner's syndrome or even compression of the brachial plexus with referred neurologic symptoms. Although dumbbell

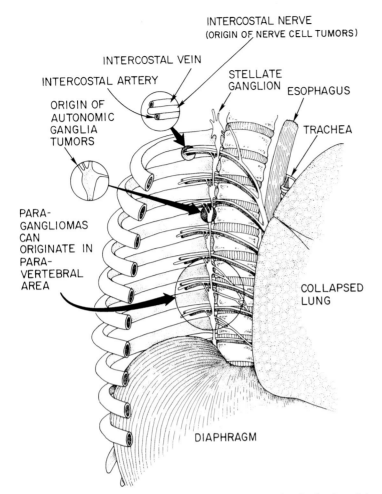

Figure 15-1. The anatomy of the posterior mediastinum showing the distribution of the common neurogenic tumors.

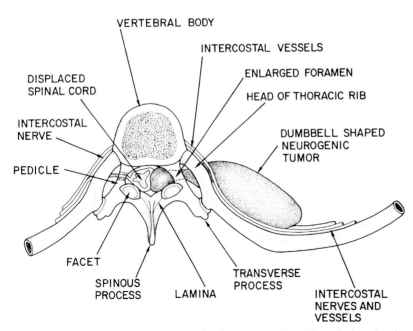

Figure 15-2. A neurogenic dumbbell tumor showing compression of the spinal cord, enlarged intervertebral foramen, and a large posterior mediastinal tumor component.

tumors at times can be surprisingly asymptomatic, the majority of these tumors will cause symptoms related to spinal cord or nerve root compression. Between 60% and 80% of patients with dumbbell tumors will have neurologic symptoms. Symptoms can also be caused by the production of hormones such as catecholamines from functional paragangliomas.

After the diagnosis of a posterior mediastinal tumor is made, further evaluation should begin with a computed tomographic (CT) scan. All patients with a posterior mediastinal tumor, even if asymptomatic, should be evaluated for the possibility of intraspinal extension. A CT scan can often aid in this distinction by showing an enlarged intervertebral foramen or the presence of an intraspinal canal mass. Often, further studies such as magnetic resonance imaging (MRI) or rarely a myelogram are needed to more accurately delineate the foraminal and intracanal anatomy. MRI scans are less invasive and are exceptionally accurate in making the diagnosis. Spinal angiography should be considered in select cases, particularly for lower thoracic posterior mediastinal tumors, in an attempt to identify the artery of Adamkiewicz. Loss of this artery may lead to spinal cord ischemia. Because fewer than 5% of posterior mediastinal tumors are malignant, an extensive search for metastatic disease is usually not warranted unless specific symptoms are present. Other lesions such as an anterior meningocele or a meningioma should be differentiated from true posterior mediastinal tumors based on preoperative imaging studies.

Tumors of the posterior mediastinum are often easily accessible to percutaneous biopsy techniques, but we believe that potentially resectable tumors should not be subjected to anything less than a complete excisional biopsy, assuming that the patient is a reasonable surgical candidate. Because the natural history of unresected tumors has not been well described, observation alone is controversial. Larger tumors for which more extensive resection may be necessary or tumors that are believed to be of questionable origin, such as sarcomas or metastatic lesions in patients with other primary tumors, may be sampled by percutaneous techniques. Dumbbell tumors can be assumed to be of neurogenic origin, and a preoperative tissue diagnosis is not needed because these tumors should always be resected.

Patients with the appropriate constellation of symptoms (hypertension, sweating, palpitations) and a posterior mediastinal mass should undergo appropriate hormonal screening and possibly metaiodobenzyl-guanidine (MIBG) scanning to further identify the source of a functioning tumor. Although rare, urinary catecholamine analysis may occasionally identify a patient with surgically correctable hypertension for a pheochromocytoma. Patients who are asymptomatic do not routinely need hormonal analysis. However, we recently evaluated an asymptomatic patient with a mediastinal paraganglioma that secreted dopamine. Although only 3% to 5% of posterior mediastinal neurogenic tumors are malignant, benign tumors may occasionally degenerate into their malignant counterparts, and the presence of malignancy may not be apparent on preoperative studies. In addition, asymptomatic tumors may continue to grow and ultimately produce troublesome symptoms.

The only patients in whom specialized preoperative management is indicated are those symptomatic patients with functioning paragangliomas or pheochromocytomas. These patients, if hypertensive, should receive 1 to 2 weeks of alpha-adrenergic receptor blockade and careful intravascular volume loading followed by beta-receptor blockade to control rebound tachycardia. All patients undergoing resection of a posterior mediastinal tumor should

be suitable candidates for thoracotomy because it may be required even for those patients undergoing attempted thoracoscopic tumor resection. Unless indicated by poor functional status, pulmonary function studies are not routinely necessary.

Surgical Principles

Patients with posterior mediastinal tumors without intraspinal extension can be managed in one of two ways. Well-circumscribed tumors <3 cm in maximum diameter without evidence of chest wall or bony invasion can be approached thoracoscopically. Improvements in video-assisted thoracoscopic surgical techniques (VATS) have led to reports of safe and successful resection of posterior mediastinal neurogenic tumors. Although no formal recommendations exist, we strongly believe that patients with posterior mediastinal tumors >3 cm in size or tumors that appear locally invasive should undergo posterolateral thoracotomy and open resection. In addition, any compromise in sound surgical technique should not be accepted when performing a thoracoscopic resection of a posterior mediastinal tumor. Patients should be prepared physically and psychologically to undergo a full thoraco-

tomy before any attempted thoracoscopic resection.

Patients with dumbbell tumors require special consideration and are probably best served by a single-stage operation performed through a combined neurosurgical and thoracic surgical approach. Occasionally these patients may require a true staged approach, with the neurosurgical component performed first, followed by resection of the thoracic component as discussed later in this chapter. Either an open or a thoracoscopic approach can be used to resect the thoracic component, with the decision based on the principles outlined earlier. With a true single-stage approach, however, the entire tumor can usually be resected either by performing a costotransversectomy or by extending the thoracic incision into a formal posterolateral thoracotomy as described later.

Surgical Technique

Thoracoscopic Resection

Single-lung ventilation is mandatory for thoracoscopic resection of a posterior mediastinal tumor, and accurate placement of a double-lumen endotracheal tube should be

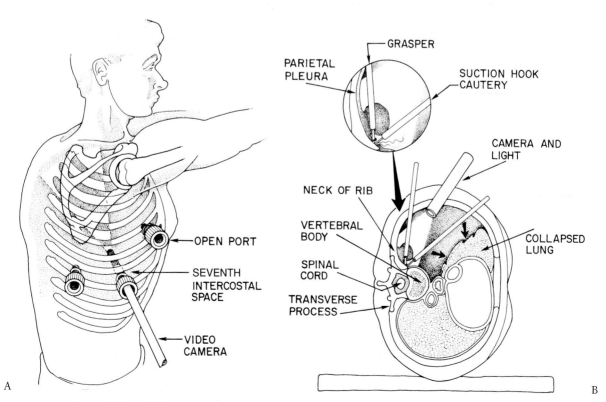

Figure 15-3. **(A)** Typical port placement for resection of an upper thoracic posterior mediastinal tumor. **(B)** Cross-sectional view of thoracoscopic posterior mediastinal tumor resection.

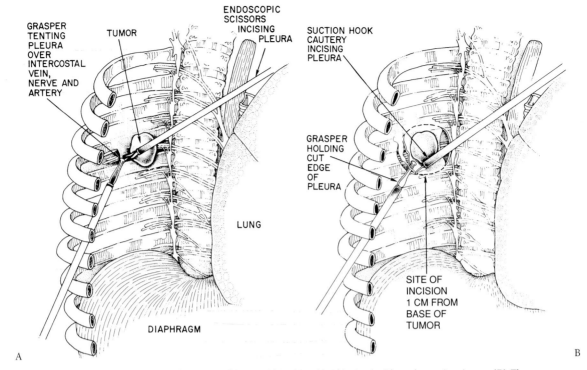

Figure 15-4. **(A)** The pleura near the tumor is grasped and incised with endoscopic scissors. **(B)** The suction-irrigating hook cautery device is used to open the pleura circumferentially around the tumor.

verified preoperatively by careful broncho-scopic examination. Patients are placed in full lateral decubitus position, and the skin is prepared widely to allow for a posterolateral thoracotomy should the exposure be needed or complications arise during the thoraco-scopic procedure. Trocar sites should be placed as far away from the tumor as possible to allow optimal visualization and working room within the rigid thorax. The camera port should be placed in the middle to an-terior axillary line in the seventh intercostal space for tumors of the upper half of the pos-terior mediastinum (Fig. 15-3A). The lung is collapsed, a 1.0- to 1.5-cm skin incision is made, and the pleural space is entered with a blunt Mayo scissors or Kelly clamp. A fin-ger is inserted into the chest to ensure that a patent pleural space is present, and a cam-era trocar is inserted. If pleural symphysis is found, the procedure is converted to an open thoracotomy. Other ports are inserted un-der direct thoracoscopic visualization. Ports should be placed higher on the chest for low posterior mediastinal tumors and lower on the chest for tumors located higher in the chest. Figure 15-3A depicts typical port placement for resection of a high posterior mediastinal tumor.

Rigid trocars are not needed for the work-ing ports because the instruments can be in-serted directly through the chest incisions.

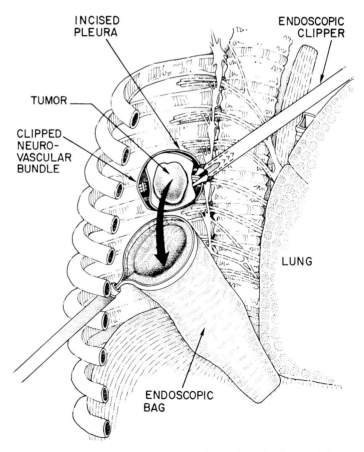

Figure 15-5. The neurovascular bundle is secured with endoscopic clips, and the tumor is dissected off the posterior chest wall and placed in an endoscopic bag for removal from the chest.

Generally, two or, if needed, three additional working ports are used in addition to the camera port (Fig. 15-3B). The pleura is grasped with endoscopic forceps approximately 1 cm from the tumor and incised with the hook cautery device or with endoscopic scissors (Fig. 15-4A). The pleura is incised completely around the tumor, with care taken to stay 1 cm to 2 cm away from the tumor to ensure adequate margins (Fig. 15-4B). The tumor is mobilized until it is tethered only by the neurovascular bundle from which it is seen to arise. The neurovascular bundle is carefully dissected free with the hook cautery device and is secured proximal and distal to the tumor with the endoscopic clip applier (Fig. 15-5). The vascular bundle is doubly clipped to ensure hemostasis. The tumor is then carefully dissected completely free from the posterior chest wall and is placed in an endoscopy bag and is removed through one of the working trocar sites (Fig. 15-5). The skin incision through which the tumor is delivered may need to be enlarged to allow removal of the entire tumor. The tumor should be delivered through the chest wall in a bag to avoid any potential seeding of the trocar site by a malignant tumor. This is a rare occurrence but is being reported with increasing frequency after other thoracoscopic and laparoscopic tumor resections. After hemostasis is obtained, a single chest tube is placed through the anterior trocar site and directed posteriorly toward the apex. The camera trocar is removed, and the remaining trocar sites are closed with subcuticular absorbable sutures. Larger incisions may require muscle closure. The trocar sites may be infiltrated with 0.2% ropivacaine with epinephrine for postoperative analgesia, and the chest tube is removed on the first or second day.

Posterolateral Thoracotomy for Resection of Larger Tumors

A double-lumen endotracheal tube is placed to allow for single-lung ventilation during the procedure. The patient is placed in a lateral decubitus position and the chest is prepped widely. A standard posterolateral thoracotomy skin incision is made two fingerbreadths below the tip of the scapula. The body of the latissimus dorsi muscle is divided. The serratus is seen originating from the scapula and is mobilized down to its insertion on the lower ribs. The scapula is retracted, and the ribs are counted. Depending on the location of the tumor, either the fifth or sixth intercostal space is entered. The intercostal incision is made on the superior surface of the rib. Again depending

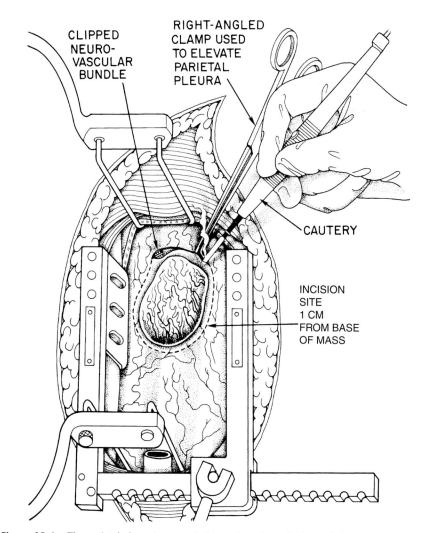

Figure 15-6. The parietal pleura is opened at least 1 cm from the base of the tumor, and the intercostal neurovascular bundle is secured with vascular clips.

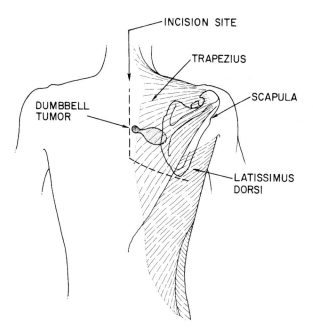

Figure 15-7. Incision for single-stage resection of a dumbbell neurogenic tumor.

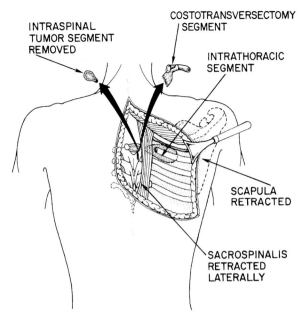

INTRASPINAL
TUMOR SEGMENT
REMOVED

COSTOTRANSVERSECTOMY
SEGMENT

INTRATHORACIC
SEGMENT

SCAPULA
RETRACTED

SACROSPINALIS
RETRACTED
LATERALLY

Figure 15-8. A hemilaminectomy and foraminectomy allow exposure and possible resection of the intraspinal component of the tumor. A costotransversectomy is often adequate for resection of the intrathoracic component.

Resection of Neurogenic Dumbbell Tumors

Various methods for resection of dumbbell neurogenic tumors of the posterior mediastinum have been described. Grillo in 1983 was one of the first to strongly endorse a "single-stage" approach for resection of neurogenic dumbbell tumors, and since then others have followed his lead. However, the single-stage approach as described in the literature includes a variety of combined neurosurgical and thoracic approaches and incisions. These are often single stage only in the sense that two separate operations are performed under a single session of anesthesia. We believe that when possible, a true single-stage approach should be used. At our center, the single-stage approach involves both the neurosurgeon and thoracic surgeon working through the same incision with the patient in the prone position using a costotransversectomy or extension to a posterolateral thoracotomy. The tumor is approached posteriorly through a midline incision, which is curved slightly laterally on the side of the tumor. Most tumors can be completely excised through this approach; however, on occasion a true two-stage approach may be preferred or required owing to a lengthy or complicated neurosurgical

on the location of the tumor, a rib above or below is transected or "notched." This enhances exposure by allowing greater rib retraction. For resection of a posterior mediastinal neurogenic tumor, we find it unnecessary to resect a rib. Further exposure can be achieved by taking the serratus muscle off its insertion on the lower ribs anteriorly. A muscle-sparing incision can also be used, depending on the size of the tumor. After the pleura is entered, a rib spreader is used to spread the ribs, and a Balfour retractor is positioned perpendicular to the rib spreader to retract the serratus anteriorly. The lung is collapsed and gently retracted anteriorly, and the pleura over the tumor is opened with a surgical margin of 1 cm to 2 cm (Fig. 15-6). The pleura is reflected circumferentially, and the tumor is mobilized on its neurovascular bundle. The neurovascular bundle is clipped proximal and distal to the tumor, and the tumor is removed.

The chest is closed after a single chest tube is positioned through a separate stab wound. Large absorbable pericostal sutures are used to reapproximate the ribs. The edges of the mobilized serratus muscle are tacked down with running absorbable sutures. The latissimus is reapproximated. Scarpa's fascia is closed with a running absorbable suture, and the skin is closed with subcuticular sutures. An epidural catheter is placed before the operation begins in all patients undergoing a thoracotomy. This aids greatly in postoperative pain control and

usually remains in place 2 to 3 days. Aggressive pulmonary toilet and early ambulation are encouraged to prevent atelectasis and pneumonia. The chest tube is generally removed on the first or second day.

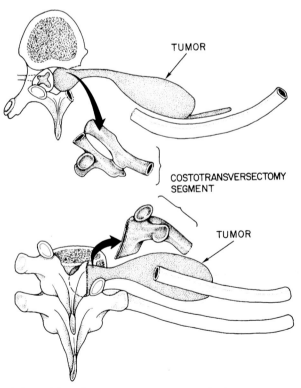

TUMOR

COSTOTRANSVERSECTOMY
SEGMENT

TUMOR

Figure 15-9. Artist's rendition of a costotransversectomy and subsequent exposure of a dumbbell tumor.

resection of a large intraspinal tumor component. In such cases, the neurosurgical resection is generally performed first through a posterior midline incision and a hemilaminectomy and foraminectomy at the appropriate level or levels, and the intraspinal component of the tumor is completely resected. After this, the patient is repositioned into the lateral decubitus position, and the intrathoracic mediastinal component of the tumor is resected either thoracoscopically or through an open thoracotomy using the principles and techniques described previously. The thoracotomy should follow the neurosurgical resection to allow decompression of the spinal cord.

Single-Stage Approach

The first step of the single-stage approach is performed by the neurosurgical team. The thoracic surgeon should, however, be present to ensure an optimal incision and exposure for the subsequent intrathoracic part of the procedure. After the safe induction of anesthesia, the patient is placed prone, and all pressure points are carefully padded. Other surgeons have described a single-stage operation with the patient in a semilateral prone position, thereby facilitating extension of the incision should a formal posterolateral thoracotomy be required. The chest and back must be prepared widely to allow the neurosurgeon access to the midline of the back while still enabling exposure of the posterolateral chest. A midline incision is made over the spinous processes and should extend well above and below the tumor. The inferior aspect of the incision is curved laterally below the scapula if a thoracotomy is planned as shown in Fig. 15-7. The deep fascia of the back is sharply dissected off the spinous processes, and the trapezius is identified. The trapezius and rhomboid muscles are elevated off the spinous processes, and the resulting myocutaneous flap is reflected laterally. The paraspinal muscle mass is then mobilized for the length of the incision and is retracted laterally. A hemilaminectomy and foraminectomy is performed at the appropriate level, and the intraspinal portion of the tumor is neurosurgically resected or fully exposed (Fig. 15-8). Excessive traction on the tumor should be avoided. The paraspinal musculature is then retracted medially, and the intrathoracic portion of the tumor is exposed through the same incision by retracting the scapula and myocutaneous flap laterally. The rib overlying the bulk of the tumor is resected subperiosteally along with the accompanying transverse process.

This costotransversectomy is often adequate to expose enough of the intrathoracic portion of the tumor to allow full mobilization and subsequent resection (Figs. 15-8, 15-9). A rib spreader may be used to gently retract the ribs to enhance exposure. Because of its site of origin, the tumor can often be resected without entering the pleura, and some surgeons strongly endorse a total extrapleural resection. If densely adherent, however, the pleura should be resected with the tumor. The appropriate neurovascular bundle is secured with clips or ties, and the tumor is removed. For larger dumbbell tumors that cannot be resected through a costotransversectomy alone, the incision is extended laterally, a posterolateral thoracotomy is done, the ribs are spread further, and the tumor is resected through this extended incision (Fig. 15-10). The intercostal musculature and periosteum of the resected rib are closed, a chest tube is placed if the pleura was entered, and the deep fascia of the back is reapproximated with absorbable sutures. If extensive myocutaneous flaps have been fashioned, a subcutaneous drain is placed. The chest tube and drain are removed when drainage decreases, usually after 2 to 3 days.

Surgical Considerations for Resection of Dumbbell Tumors

We make every attempt to resect dumbbell tumors using a true single-stage approach with a costotransversectomy or very limited posterolateral thoracotomy. This approach does require a costotransversectomy,

however, and some surgeons believe this results in some degree of instability of the already laminectomized spine. A separate thoracotomy or thoracoscopic resection of the intrathoracic component of the tumor could avoid a costotransversectomy altogether and perhaps yield a more stable postoperative spine. However, postoperative pain is likely to be more troublesome after a thoracotomy, and disability, if a muscle-sparing thoracotomy is not used, may be greater. If a single-level laminectomy is performed and the rib resection is limited during the costotransversectomy, we believe spinal integrity is not a major issue, and postoperative pain is more easily managed than after extension to a full thoracotomy. If the intrathoracic component of the tumor is small, the optimal situation may be to resect the intraspinal component first through a hemilaminectomy and foraminectomy and avoid any resection of the posterior ribs and transverse processes and resect the intrathoracic portion of the tumor through the thoracoscope as shown in Figs. 15-3 through 15-5.

We consider the following algorithm appropriate for the resection of posterior mediastinal neurogenic dumbbell tumors. Tumors with an intrathoracic component that is <2 cm to 3 cm can be considered for thoracoscopic resection after the intraspinal component is resected first through a posterior midline incision over the spinous process. The incisions are smaller, pain is minimized, ribs are not resected or spread, and a costotransversectomy is avoided. Dumbbell tumors with an intrathoracic component of >2 cm to 3 cm but <6 cm should be resected

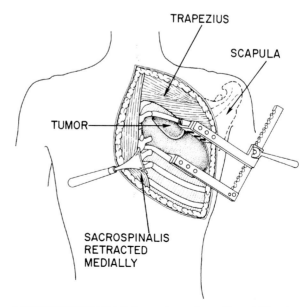

TRAPEZIUS

SCAPULA

TUMOR

SACROSPINALIS
RETRACTED
MEDIALLY

Figure 15-10. A posterolateral thoracotomy can be performed for additional exposure for resection of larger dumbbell tumors.

in one stage using a single posterior approach and a costotransversectomy. In this situation, thoracoscopy is not indicated because of the size of the tumor, but a full thoracotomy is avoided, pain is limited, and functional recovery is excellent. Patients with posterior mediastinal dumbbell tumors >6 cm or that cannot be resected through a costotransversectomy or patients requiring multilevel laminectomies may need to undergo extension of the incision to a posterolateral thoracotomy for resection of the intrathoracic component of the tumor.

Postoperative Considerations

Intensive care monitoring is generally not required for most patients undergoing resection of posterior mediastinal neurogenic tumors. Older patients or patients with poor pulmonary function undergoing a formal thoracotomy probably should be observed for 24 hours in a step-down unit; most other patients can be managed on a surgical floor. Early ambulation and aggressive pulmonary toilet with active incentive spirometry are mandatory to help prevent atelectasis and subsequent pneumonia. Diet is rapidly advanced, and chest tubes and drains are usually removed within the first 2 to 3 days. Patients undergoing thoracoscopic resection are usually ready for discharge by the third or fourth postoperative day. Specific complications are rare after resection of these tumors, with the most disastrous being a spinal neurologic catastrophe after resection of a dumbbell tumor.

Posterior mediastinal neurogenic tumors are rare enough that most surgeons will see only a few of them during their surgical career. Even large tertiary-care referral centers average only two or three such cases per year. When resecting these rare tumors, the thoracic surgeon must be able to tailor the operation to fit the clinical situation, and surgeons in other disciplines, specifically neurosurgery, should be consulted when indicated. In addition, only techniques and procedures with which the surgeon is familiar should be used when resecting a posterior mediastinal tumor.

SUGGESTED READING

Grillo HC, Ojemann RG, Scannell JO, et al. Combined approach to "dumbbell" intrathoracic and intraspinal neurogenic tumors. Ann Thorac Surg 1983;36:402.

Konno S, Yabuki S, Kinoshita T, et al. Combined laminectomy and thoracoscopic resection of dumbbell type thoracic cord tumor. Spine 2001;26:130.

Landreneau RJ, Dowling RD, Ferson PF. Thoracoscopic resection of a posterior mediastinal neurogenic tumor. Chest 1992;102:1288.

Naunheim KS. Video thoracoscopy for masses of the posterior mediastinum. Ann Thorac Surg 1993;56:657.

O'Reilly G, Jackowski A, Weiner G, et al. Lateral parascapular extrapleural approach for single-stage excision of dumbbell neurofibroma. Br J Neurosurg 1994;8:347.

Osada H, Aoki H, Yokote K, et al. Dumbbell neurogenic tumor of the mediastinum: A report of three cases undergoing single-staged complete removal without thoracotomy. Jpn J Surg 1991;21:224.

Ricci C, Rendina EA, Venuta F, et al. Diagnostic imaging and surgical treatment of dumbbell tumors of the mediastinum. Ann Thorac Surg 1990;50:586.

Saito A, Yagi N, Miura K, et al. Videothoracoscopic resection of a posterior mediastinal tumor. Surg Laparosc Endosc 1995;5:142.

Shadmehr MB, Gaissert HA, Wain JC, et al. The surgical approach to "dumbbell tumors" of the mediastinum. Ann Thorac Surg 2003;76:1650.

EDITORIAL COMMENTS

Posterior mediastinal lesions usually are picked up as incidental findings on a chest radiograph. As pointed out by the authors, the majority of these are benign, and malignant posterior mediastinal tumors in adults are extremely rare. Though often talked about, malignant degeneration of benign neurogenic tumors is even more uncommon. The question commonly arises as to whether a small, asymptomatic posterior mediastinal tumor without intraspinal extension simply can be followed. If a needle biopsy confirms the presence of a neurogenic tumor, it is my opinion, shared by a number of others, that these lesions can be followed because many grow very slowly, if at all, and likely will never cause symptoms. The late Bob Ginsberg favored this approach and recognized that it is very hard to make an asymptomatic patient better. I was particularly intrigued by the authors' one-stage approach to the so-called dumbbell lesions. This represents a very attractive alternative to two incisions, allows for complete removal of the lesion, and likely causes less postoperative pain. If the procedure can be performed without entering the pleura, even the need for a chest tube is obviated. It is my preference to resect these rare dumbbell tumors in collaboration with the neurosurgeons via a single incision with the patient prone, avoiding a separate thoracotomy incision. It is particularly important to recognize the intraspinal component preoperatively so that the appropriate team can be put into place. If there is any question of involvement within the canal, an MRI scan should be done to assess this. Routine CT scanning will not show involvement within the canal.

For those lesions where tumor in the canal is not demonstrated, the importance of complete resection must be underscored. A thoracoscopic approach cannot compromise the completeness of the resection despite how tempting it may be to accomplish resection with minimally invasive techniques. Just as the authors describe, the pleura should be incised circumferentially around the lesion and then the mass dissected away from the vertebral body and surrounding structures. Care must be taken at the foraminal level to assure that the tumor has not invaded the foramen yet remains outside of the canal. If there is any question of foraminal involvement, the neurosurgeon should be consulted, and a formal foraminotomy may be necessary to make sure that all tumor is resected. Avulsion of the tumor at this level may result in a cerebrospinal fluid leak from a dural tear. Neurogenic tumors occurring at the apex of the chest may also be problematic from an exposure viewpoint, especially larger lesions. Patients with lesions in this location should be informed of the possibility of a Horner's syndrome subsequent to the operation.

L.R.K.

16

Antireflux Procedures

Mark K. Ferguson

Although peptic esophageal injury was first described in the early twentieth century, it was not until the late 1940s that the relationship between gastroesophageal reflux and abnormalities of the anatomy and function of the lower esophageal high-pressure zone were recognized. In the 1950s and 1960s, Nissen and Belsey separately introduced surgical procedures that were designed to limit gastroesophageal reflux. The use of these procedures antedated by decades the thorough understanding of mechanisms that promote gastroesophageal reflux disease, which necessitated the introduction of techniques for evaluating esophageal motility and acid exposure. Indeed, although our knowledge of esophageal physiology has increased greatly, our understanding of the factors that promote acid reflux disease is incomplete.

Surgical therapy for gastroesophageal reflux disease has been in a process of evolution since its introduction. The development of pharmacologic agents that inhibit gastric acid production and the introduction of potent prokinetic drugs have changed the frequency with which surgical therapy is used for this condition. Since the early 1990s, the development of laparoscopic techniques for fundoplication has altered further the surgical approach to gastroesophageal reflux disease. This progress has made both the selection of candidates for antireflux surgery and the choice of approach to such patients increasingly complex. This chapter provides an overview of the approach to selecting patients and operations for managing gastroesophageal reflux disease.

Indications

Gastroesophageal reflux is a common condition that affects >80% of the population to varying degrees. When the frequency or severity of the symptoms is greater than the expected norm for the population, the condition is referred to as *gastroesophageal reflux disease* (GERD). Patients who suffer from GERD require therapy, usually consisting of lifestyle modifications and, in some instances, pharmacologic management. Lifestyle changes include weight loss for patients who are overweight, avoidance of food intake for several hours before retiring for the night, elimination of foods and medications that promote lower esophageal sphincter dysfunction, cessation of smoking, and elevation of the head of the bed. Medications that are typically used for GERD of mild to moderate severity include antacids and cytoprotective agents. Patients at the far end of the GERD spectrum require intensive medical therapy for symptoms that include severe heartburn, frequent regurgitation, dysphagia caused by dysmotility or peptic stricture formation, oropharyngeal complications, and pulmonary complications. Medications that are commonly used under these circumstances include high-dose histamine H_2-receptor blockers (cimetidine, ranitidine, famotidine, nizatidine, ethintidine, roxatidine) and H^+/K^+ adenosine triphosphatase (proton pump) inhibitors (omeprazole, pantoprazole, rabeprazole, lansoprazole).

Patients who continue to have symptoms despite optimal medical therapy are candidates for surgical intervention. In addition, some patients are unable to comply with medical therapy for emotional, psychiatric, or financial reasons. Some of these patients may also be appropriately considered for surgical intervention. Complications of GERD such as esophageal stricture are relative indications for surgery. The combination of intensive acid suppression therapy and esophageal dilation is successful in relieving dysphagia in approximately 75% of patients with a peptic esophageal stricture. Between 20% and 30% of patients require only a single dilation, whereas most of the remaining patients need additional dilations over an interval of 1 to 2 years. The risk of complications is low, making acid suppression and dilation the best initial therapy for most patients with a reflux-induced stricture. Other relative indications for surgery include the presence of pulmonary complications, such as asthma and chronic cough, substantial symptoms or severe esophagitis in young patients, and, rarely, bleeding from erosive esophagitis. Pulmonary symptoms typically respond poorly to medical therapy and also constitute a relative indication for antireflux surgery. In younger patients with severe manifestations of GERD, surgical therapy is a less expensive and more effective intermediate-term treatment than medical therapy. The success rate of fundoplication surgery diminishes over time, so that patients are not guaranteed permanent relief of symptoms if they experience initial success after their operations. This must be kept in mind when making a recommendation for fundoplication surgery.

One of the most controversial issues regarding selection of patients for fundoplication is whether successful fundoplication surgery materially influences the development and/or subsequent behavior of Barrett's esophagus. No randomized trial has demonstrated a reduced incidence of the development of Barrett's esophagus in response to fundoplication; regression of the extent of Barrett's esophagus and a reduced rate of progression to dysplasia or invasive cancer similarly have not been demonstrated. However, there is an increasing amount of uncontrolled data that suggest that Barrett's esophagus is less likely to pose problems after antireflux surgery than after medical management.

Principles of Antireflux Surgery

After an accurate diagnosis is established and proper indications for surgery are confirmed, an operative strategy must be selected. Factors of importance in this selection include the type of wrap used, the operative approach, and whether other, associated procedures are necessary. The importance of adaptability in operations for GERD cannot be overemphasized; a single surgical approach will not suffice for all patients. Most operations for uncomplicated reflux are performed laparoscopically; since the early 1990s this approach has largely supplanted the open abdominal approach. Both laparoscopic and open approaches provides access to other intra-abdominal pathologic conditions if present, avoid the need for a chest tube (which is necessary in thoracic approaches), and are less painful than open thoracic approaches. Laparoscopy permits a smaller incision, reducing the risk of postoperative incision hernia, and provides for earlier discharge from the hospital and return to work than open laparotomy. Obesity is only a relative contraindication to either of the abdominal approaches. The transthoracic approach is indicated for patients who have severe peptic strictures, particularly when they are associated with esophageal shortening, for patients with other intrathoracic pathologic conditions, and for some patients who require reoperation for recurrent GERD. A relative contraindication to the transthoracic approach is the presence of severe respiratory insufficiency. The availability of continuous epidural analgesia, smaller access incisions, and improved techniques of pulmonary toilet have eliminated most of the drawbacks that previously made the transthoracic approach less than optimal.

Operations that successfully prevent reflux must adhere to several basic principles of antireflux surgery. Esophageal mobilization is necessary to restore an adequate intra-abdominal segment of esophagus, the length of which is inversely correlated with the amount of residual postoperative reflux. The acuteness of the angle of His is restored by a gastric wrap, whether partial or complete, providing a mechanical advantage to the sling and clasp fibers that normally constitute the lower esophageal high-pressure zone. The gastric wrap also calibrates the esophageal orifice at the junction of the esophagus and stomach. This abrupt change in luminal diameter brings into play the law of LaPlace, making the intragastric surface tension greater than the intraesophageal surface tension, promoting an increase in the resting tension of the lower esophageal high-pressure zone. Finally, the size of the hiatal orifice is calibrated by approximating the crural fibers, which helps to prevent herniation of the repair.

Selection of the type of gastric wrap to use is a matter of individual training and experience. Complete wraps, such as the Nissen fundoplication, provide better long-term control of reflux symptoms than do partial wraps but cause more early postoperative dysphagia and are associated with the development of the "gas-bloat" syndrome in a small number of patients. Because long-term control of reflux is likely to be better after a total fundoplication, this operation is used in most patients with GERD. Partial wraps, such as the Belsey, Toupet, and Hill techniques, are almost as effective as complete wraps in controlling reflux symptoms and are not associated with a high incidence of postoperative dysphagia or the inability to eructate. These wraps produce a lower resting pressure in the distal esophageal sphincter postoperatively and are useful in the management of patients with substantial esophageal dysmotility. Such wraps, especially the Hill, are also useful for patients who have had partial gastric resection, in whom the creation of a total fundoplication is not possible.

Patient Preparation

Patients are maintained on intensive acid suppression therapy to minimize the degree of esophagitis present at the time of operation. Patients with peptic stricture are dilated preoperatively to ensure that the stricture can be successfully dilated; failure of preoperative dilations suggests that a patient should be prepared for possible resection and reconstruction rather than simple antireflux surgery. If pulmonary symptoms are present preoperatively, treatment, including bronchodilators and pulmonary toilet, is optimized before surgery. There is little need for a formal bowel preparation (as is customary before colon surgery), although the use of a clear liquid diet and cathartics to cleanse the colon often facilitates the conduct of an operation. The patient takes nothing by mouth the night before surgery and can be admitted to the hospital on the day of surgery. Intravenous perioperative antibiotics are usually not necessary because fundoplication surgery is classified as a clean, uncontaminated operation.

Operative Techniques

Laparoscopic Fundoplication

The patient is anesthetized and positioned either in a modified lithotomy position (surgeon stands between patient's legs) or supine (surgeon stands to patient's right). The operating table is placed in steep reverse Trendelenburg position. The first assistant stands on the patient's left and the camera operator stands on the right side of the table when the patient is in lithotomy position or opposite the surgeon when the patient is supine. After peritoneal insufflation is achieved with CO_2 to a pressure of 15 cm H_2O, a camera port is placed in a supraumbilical location and retracting/operating ports are placed near the right and left costal margins (Fig. 16-1). Most of the operation is performed using a 30-degree telescope.

The left lobe of the liver is mobilized and displaced with a retractor anteriorly and to the patient's right using either a right lateral subcostal port or a subxiphoid port. The stomach is grasped with an atraumatic clamp placed through a left subcostal port and is retracted to the patient's left. The

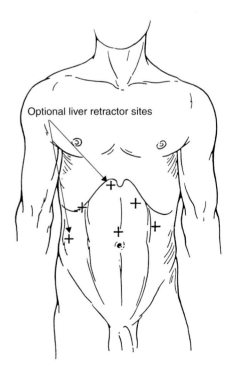

Optional liver retractor sites

Figure 16-1. The sites for access port placement for laparoscopic fundoplication surgery.

gastrohepatic omentum is divided above the level of the nerve of Latarjet, and the right crus is identified and dissected proximally until the anterior limit of the esophageal hiatus is reached. The esophagus lies medial to this crus and is bluntly mobilized from its bed into the mediastinum, with the surgeon taking care to keep the anterior vagus nerve intact on the wall of the esophagus. The peritoneum on the anterior surface of the esophagus is divided using electrocautery or ultrasound shears.

The stomach is regrasped by the first assistant and is retracted down and to the patient's right to reveal the short gastric vessels. It is usually necessary to divide several of these to the level of the fundic tip using an ultrasound shears to achieve sufficient proximal mobilization of the stomach to permit performance of the wrap without tension. The posterior gastric attachments to the diaphragm are mobilized to enable the development of a window posterior to the esophagus and stomach. The left crus is identified and the esophagus is dissected from it. The esophagus is encircled with a Penrose drain, the ends of which are clipped to facilitate grasping, and is retracted to the patient's left. The esophagus is mobilized bluntly posteriorly to reveal the posterior vagus branch, which is carefully preserved. The dissection of the esophagus is complete when the esophagogastric junction lies comfortably in the abdomen and a large window posterior to the esophagus and esophagogastric junction has been developed.

The esophagus is retracted superiorly and to the patient's left. Large interrupted nonabsorbable sutures are placed in the crura to close the hiatus to a normal caliber. The surgeon's judgment and experience provide guidance on how tightly the crural fibers should be approximated. Normally two or three such sutures are required. The gastric fat pad is removed with electrocautery to expose the esophagogastric junction anteriorly.

The gastric fundus is grasped with an atraumatic clamp passed behind the esophagus and is drawn to the patient's right (Fig. 16-2). While the fundus is held in place, a large bougie is passed orally by an assistant into the stomach. A second atraumatic grasper is used to draw a portion of the stomach up across the esophagogastric junction to meet the tip of the gastric fundus that has been wrapped around the esophagus posteriorly. The adequacy of tissue volume and mobilization is assessed using the "shoeshine" maneuver with a grasper on each portion of the fundus to be used in the wrap. Interrupted nonabsorbable fun-

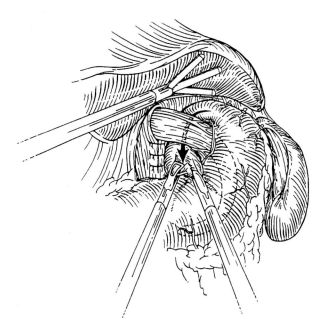

Figure 16-2. The stomach is brought posteriorly around the esophagus, and a large bougie is passed across the esophagogastric junction.

doplication sutures are placed through the lateral fundus, through the muscularis of the esophagus, and through the wrapped portion of the fundus (Fig. 16-3). The wrap is performed around the esophagus, making sure the most inferior suture is placed above the esophagogastric junction. Three sutures spaced 1 cm apart produce a 2-cm fundoplication. Some authors recommend use of pledgets to prevent sutures from eroding through the stomach. The stitches are tied and cut as soon as they are placed to avoid having redundant suture material in

the field while the subsequent stitches are placed. The bougie is removed. The port sites are inspected and are closed in a standard fashion.

Transabdominal Total Fundoplication (Nissen)

The patient is anesthetized and is placed supine. No special intravenous or intra-arterial monitoring is required. The abdomen is accessed through a midline or a subcostal incision. The left lobe of the liver

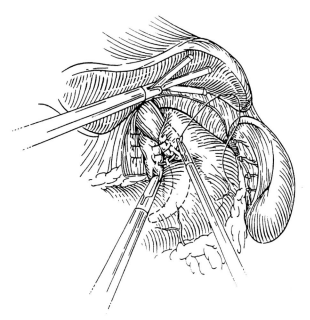

Figure 16-3. Three stitches are placed to complete the laparoscopic Nissen fundoplication.

is mobilized and retracted to the right and anteriorly. The abdominal esophagus is dissected and encircled with a small rubber drain for use in retraction. The distal thoracic esophagus is mobilized using a combination of sharp and blunt dissection, ensuring that an adequate length of esophagus is available to permit the performance of a wrap that will rest within the abdomen without tension. Care is taken not to enter either pleural cavity. Both vagus nerves are preserved and will be included within the fundoplication wrap. Several short gastric vessels are divided, extending to the proximal gastric fundus, and the proximal portion of the gastric fundus is dissected from any attachments to the retroperitoneum and inferior surface of the diaphragm. The gastric fat pad is dissected to expose the esophagogastric junction and is excised. It is useful to mark the level of the esophagogastric junction with a single hemoclip to enable its identification on plain postoperative radiographs (this, of course, is not feasible if vascular clips are used for other parts of the procedure). After the esophagus is retracted to the patient's left, the crura are approximated with large interrupted nonabsorbable sutures to close the hiatus sufficiently so that only the tip of a finger can pass comfortably into the mediastinum (Fig. 16-4).

A large bougie (56 to 60 F) is passed transorally by an assistant into the stomach. The surgeon grasps the gastric fundus with the right hand and passes it posteriorly around the esophagus, grasping it to the right of the esophagus with an atraumatic bowel clamp.

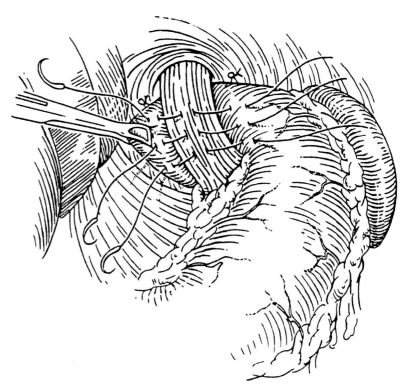

Figure 16-5.   After the tip of the gastric fundus is brought posteriorly around the esophagus, sutures are placed from the stomach, through the esophagus, and through the gastric fundus to complete the Nissen fundoplication.

A point high on the stomach is selected and is brought anterior to the esophagus to meet the posterior portion of the wrap slightly to the right of the esophageal midline. A so-called "shoeshine" maneuver is used to ensure adequate mobility of the segments of the gastric fundus and body to permit performance of a tension-free fundoplication. Interrupted nonabsorbable sutures are placed between the stomach to the left of the esophagus and through the gastric fundus that has been passed posteriorly and to the right of the esophagus, taking a deep bite of the muscular wall of the esophagus in between. Three stitches are placed approximately 1 cm apart to create a 2-cm wrap (Fig. 16-5). The sutures are tied with the bougie in place. Some surgeons use pledgets to reinforce the repair, which theoretically carry the risk of erosion into the stomach or esophagus and could potentiate an infection if contamination developed. It is not necessary to anchor the repair to the diaphragm to prevent herniation because adequate mobilization and proper crural approximation almost completely eliminate this risk. After removing the bougie, the surgeon tests the wrap, which should permit passage of one finger within it alongside the esophagus. The abdomen is closed in a standard fashion.

Transabdominal Partial Fundoplication

Partial fundoplications can be performed using open or laparoscopic approaches. The

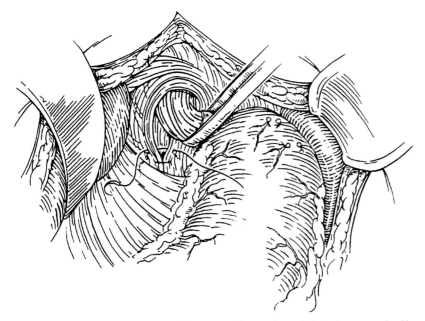

Figure 16-4.   Crural stitches are placed to narrow the esophageal hiatus to a normal caliber before performing a fundoplication.

partial fundoplications that are currently in use are the posterior (Toupet, Lind), the anterior (Dor, Thal), and the Hill gastropexy with a combined partial anterior and posterior fundoplication. This chapter describes only the Toupet technique, which is the most commonly used partial fundoplication that is performed transabdominally for treating GERD.

The initial steps in performing the posterior partial fundoplication (Toupet) are similar to those for performing a total fundoplication. The abdominal esophagus is mobilized circumferentially taking care not to injure the vagus nerves. It is sometimes useful to divide a few of the proximal short gastric vessels, but removal of the gastric fat pad is not necessary. The crura are dissected free of surrounding tissue. The tip of the gastric fundus is brought posteriorly around the esophagus as for a total fundoplication (Fig. 16-6). Using three or four interrupted nonabsorbable sutures, the surgeon sutures the anterior aspect of the wrapped portion of the stomach to the right lateral wall of the esophagus just anterior to the anterior vagus nerve. The posterior aspect of the wrap is sutured to the right crus. The gastric fundus is sutured to the left side of the esophagus just anterior to the posterior vagus nerve, and the stomach is also sutured to the left crus. This completes a 180- to 210-degree posterior wrap (Fig. 16-7).

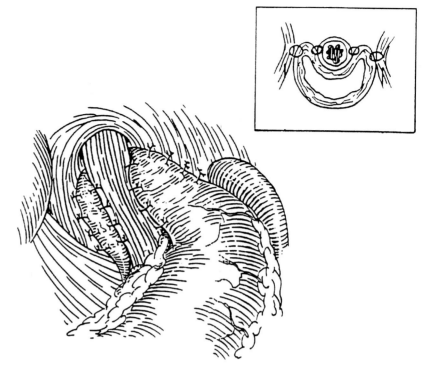

Figure 16-7. Two rows of sutures are place on the stomach to complete a Toupet fundoplication, one to the esophagus, the other to the left crus.

Transthoracic Total Fundoplication (Nissen)

The anesthesiologist places a double-lumen tube or bronchial blocker to permit single-lung ventilation. The patient is placed in the right lateral decubitus position with the left side up. A lateral thoracotomy is performed in the seventh interspace, preserving the serratus anterior muscle. A 1-cm segment of the eighth rib may be taken posteriorly deep to the level of the paraspinous muscles to allow greater rib spreading without causing a fracture. The distal esophagus is mobilized to the level of the inferior pulmonary vein taking care not to enter the right pleural space. The vagus nerves are preserved and are left on the esophagus. The phrenoesophageal membrane is divided near its insertion on the esophagus to enable entry into the peritoneal cavity through the esophageal hiatus. The esophagogastric junction is mobilized circumferentially. This requires division of retroperitoneal tissues, including an inconstant communicating artery between the left gastric and inferior phrenic arteries (Belsey's artery). When the crura and the left lobe of the liver are exposed, the hiatal dissection is complete. The proximal stomach is pulled into the chest. The gastric fat pad is excised to permit apposition of the gastric serosa to the esophagus. A hemoclip is used to mark the level of the esophagogastric junction so that it can be identified on plain radiographs postoperatively. Several short gastric vessels are divided to provide adequate mobilization of the stomach.

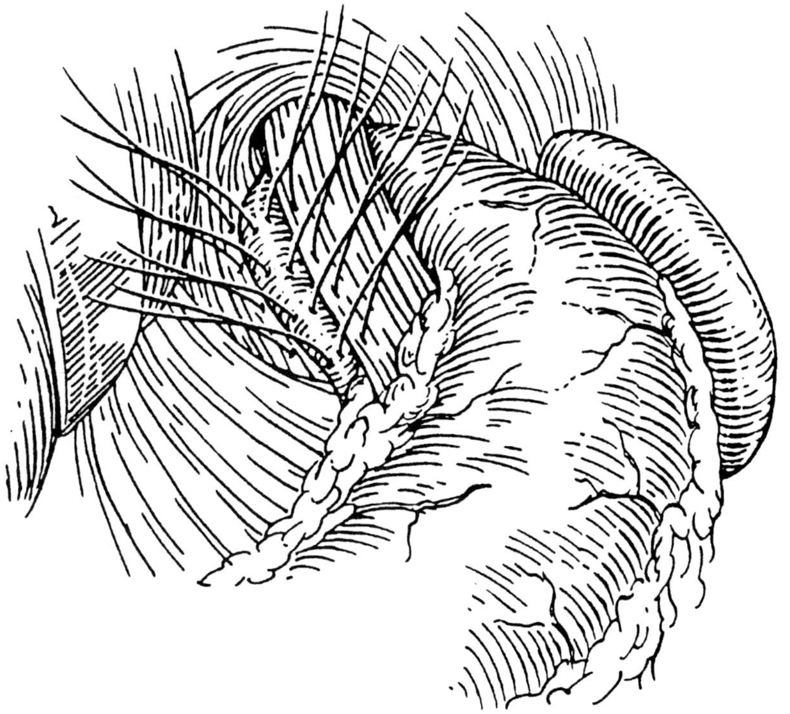

Figure 16-6. A Toupet fundoplication requires two initial rows of sutures, one from the wrapped fundus to the esophagus, the other from the wrapped fundus to the right crus.

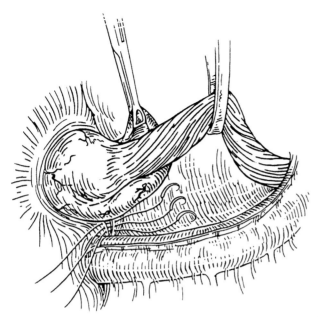

Figure 16-8. All transthoracic fundoplications are preceded by placement of crural stitches, which are left untied until the fundoplication wrap is completed. The fundus of the stomach is brought posterior to the esophagus in preparation for a Nissen fundoplication.

Interrupted nonabsorbable sutures are placed in the crura for future hiatal repair. The first suture is placed at the initial decussation of the crural fibers, and subsequent stitches are placed cephalad at 1-cm intervals until an adequate closure of the hiatus is possible. This usually requires three or four sutures. The stitches are left untied until the fundoplication wrap is completed. A large (56 to 60 F) bougie is placed orally by an assistant so that it traverses the esophagogastric junction. The tip of the gastric fundus is grasped in the surgeon's left hand and is brought posteriorly around the esophagus, where it is held with an atraumatic clamp (Fig. 16-8). A portion of the stomach high on the body is pulled across the esophagus to meet the wrapped portion of the fundus. Three interrupted sutures are placed through the stomach to the left of the esophagus, through the muscularis of the esophagus, and again through the gastric fundus lying to the right of the esophagus. These are spaced at 1-cm intervals to create a 2-cm wrap (Fig. 16-9). After the fundoplication sutures are tied, the bougie is removed, and the wrap is reduced below the diaphragm, where it should rest without tension. The crural stitches are tied to calibrate the esophageal hiatus, leaving enough room to allow the tip of one finger to be admitted easily alongside the esophagus. A nasogastric tube is placed by an assistant, and the chest is closed after an intercostal drain is placed.

Transthoracic Partial Fundoplication (Belsey Mark IV)

The initial portions of the operation are performed in a manner similar to that described for the transthoracic total fundoplication, although it is usually not necessary to divide any of the short gastric vessels. Crural sutures are placed but are left untied. The partial fundoplication wrap is begun by placing mattress sutures of interrupted nonabsorbable material through the stomach 1 cm distal to the esophagogastric junction and through the esophagus 1 cm proximal to the junction (Fig. 16-10). Three sutures make up the first layer: one just anterior to the anterior vagus nerve, one just anterior to the posterior vagus nerve, and one midway between these two. After these sutures are tied, a second row of mattress sutures is placed. These are first passed through the diaphragm, close to the margin of the central tendon. They then are placed through the stomach and esophagus in a mattress fashion, encompassing an additional 1 cm of stomach distal to and 1 cm of esophagus proximal to the previous sutures, and finally are brought through the diaphragm again (Fig. 16-11). The wrap is reduced below the diaphragm, where it should rest without tension. The second row of sutures is then tied to create a 240- to 270-degree wrap that is anchored underneath the diaphragm (Fig. 16-12). The crural sutures are tied to calibrate the esophageal hiatus, leaving sufficient room to admit the tip of one finger posteriorly alongside the esophagus. A nasogastric tube is placed, and the chest is closed after an intercostal drainage catheter is inserted.

Gastroplasty and Fundoplication

Gastroplasty (Collis gastroplasty) and fundoplication was originally described for use in patients who suffered from esophageal shortening caused by peptic stricture with severe contraction fibrosis. It was designed to create a tube from the lesser gastric curvature tissues with a diameter similar to that

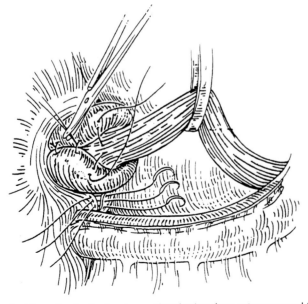

Figure 16-9. The Nissen fundoplication is completed using three sutures spaced 1 cm apart, extending from the stomach, through the esophagus, to the wrapped fundic tip.

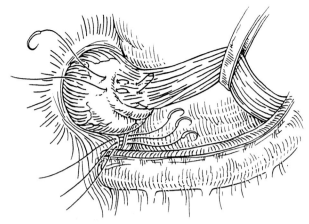

Figure 16-10. A Belsey fundoplication is begun by mobilization of the upper stomach into the chest. The initial row of three mattress sutures incorporates 1 cm of stomach and 1 cm of esophagus and is evenly spaced between the vagus nerves.

of the esophagus that would permit the creation of an intra-abdominal fundoplication around this "neoesophagus" without placing tension on the repair. This technique eliminates the necessity for performing an intrathoracic fundoplication, which exposes the patient unnecessarily to the risks of gastric perforation and strangulation, and enables preservation of the esophagus when resection would be the only remaining viable option. Recent reports suggest that the operation can be used (in a "cut" or "uncut" fashion) for the routine treatment of GERD, even in the absence of esophageal shortening.

The operation is performed through an open transthoracic approach for patients who have clinically apparent esophageal shortening. The esophagus is mobilized from its bed as described previously, with the exception that the mobilization is extended to the level of the aortic arch to maximize esophageal length. The phrenoesophageal membrane is divided, the hiatus is dissected circumferentially, and the stomach is mobilized. The gastric fat pad is removed, and several short gastric vessels are divided. Interrupted nonabsorbable stitches are placed in the crura but are not tied. If it is determined at this point that a standard, tension-free intra-abdominal fundoplication cannot be created, a lengthening procedure is performed.

If there is a peptic esophageal stricture, the esophagus is dilated under direct vision. A large (56 to 60 F) bougie is passed by an assistant orally into the stomach. A linear cutting stapler is placed adjacent to

the dilator beginning at the esophagogastric junction and extending inferiorly, parallel to the lesser curvature (Fig. 16-13). The stapler is fired, creating a staple line 5 cm in length and preserving all of the gastric fundus. The staple line is oversewn (Fig. 16-14). In some situations, surgeons prefer to use an uncut gastroplasty, which uses only a staple line and does not expose the patient to the small risk of opening the stomach. The gastric fundus then is used to create either a partial or a total fundoplication around the "neoesophagus" using techniques identical to those described previously (Fig. 16-15). After the fundoplication is completed, it is reduced into the abdomen and the crural sutures are tied.

In some patients an open abdominal or laparoscopic approach is used for fundoplication, and the need for esophageal lengthening isn't discovered until during the operation. Esophageal lengthening can be achieved by using a linear stapler as described previously during an open abdominal antireflux operation. If the operation is being performed laparoscopically and gastroplasty is necessary, the stapler can be introduced through a thoracoscopy port and directed through the esophageal hiatus under direct vision from the laparoscope or using a thoracoscope. Alternatively, a window is created using a circular stapler positioned adjacent to the bougie lying against the lesser gastric curvature. A linear cutting stapler is inserted through this window and is fired parallel to the bougie in a cephalad direction, completing the gastroplasty. The fundoplication is then completed around the "neoesophagus."

Postoperative Care

The stomach is drained with a nasogastric tube during the early postoperative period in patients who undergo open fundoplication. The need for gastric decompression after laparoscopic fundoplication is less well defined, and nasogastric drainage often is avoided unless there is evidence of gastric stasis or if a gastroplasty has been performed. Oral intake commences when bowel activity is evident, usually on the third or fourth postoperative day after open repair and on the day of surgery or the first postoperative day after laparoscopic repair. A liquid diet is often appropriate for the first several days after oral intake has begun. Patients may have dysphagia to solids during the first several weeks after repair, especially after total fundoplication. Typically, reassurance and time are all that is necessary in

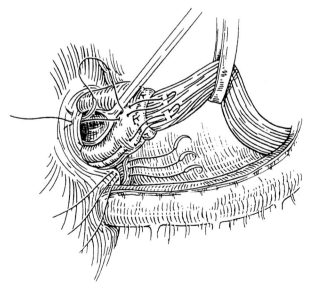

Figure 16-11. A second row of sutures for the Belsey fundoplication is placed 1 cm from the first, and incorporates the diaphragm at the beginning and end.

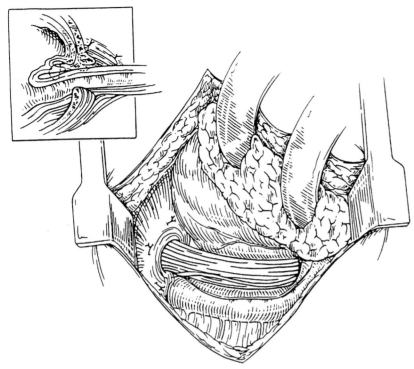

Figure 16-12. The completed fundoplication showing the wrap anchored below the diaphragm by the second row of sutures.

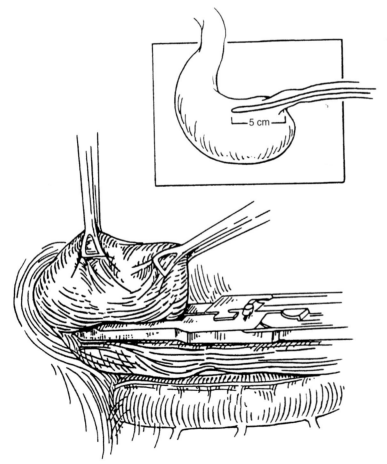

Figure 16-13. A Collis gastroplasty is created by firing a stapler parallel to the lesser gastric curvature, snugly placed against a bougie that has been positioned across the esophagogastric junction.

the management of this short-term problem. It is often useful to maintain patients with esophagitis on acid suppression medication for several weeks postoperatively until the esophageal inflammation has subsided.

Surgical Complications

Serious complications are rare after fundoplication surgery. Gastric perforation, esophageal leak, and acute development of gastric herniation through the dissected hiatus occur in <1% of patients. The management of these problems is urgent reoperation and repair of the defect. The outcome in patients who are diagnosed and treated expeditiously is good.

The most common early complication of fundoplication surgery is dysphagia. It is diagnosed more often in patients who have total fundoplication than in those with partial fundoplication, which is likely an effect of the tightness of the wrap. Dysphagia often is more common in patients undergoing transthoracic than transabdominal fundoplication, probably because of the additional mobilization that is performed in the former group of patients. If dysphagia is persistent or severe, it is possible that underlying esophageal motility problems are present or that a technical complication occurred during the operation. Anatomic problems that cause severe postoperative dysphagia usually are evident radiographically, and include a wrap that is too tight or too long, paraesophageal hernia, slipped fundoplication, and herniation of the fundoplication wrap into the chest. In patients in whom severe motility problems are suspected, prokinetic agents may be of some therapeutic benefit.

One complication that appears to be unique to total fundoplications is the "gas bloat" syndrome. It is characterized by the inability to belch or vomit and by postprandial fullness. The etiology of this problem is multifactorial and is likely related to vagal nerve injury, an overly tight fundoplication, delayed gastric emptying, or chronic swallowing of air. Most patients experience considerable improvement over time and require no specific therapy. In patients with persistent symptoms, an evaluation should include esophageal manometry, endoscopy, barium contrast study of the esophagus and stomach, esophageal pH monitoring, and a gastric emptying scan. Findings of a high resting pressure in the lower esophageal sphincter combined with radiographic and endoscopic evidence for a tight wrap are usually an indication for reoperation to take down the fundoplication and create a looser

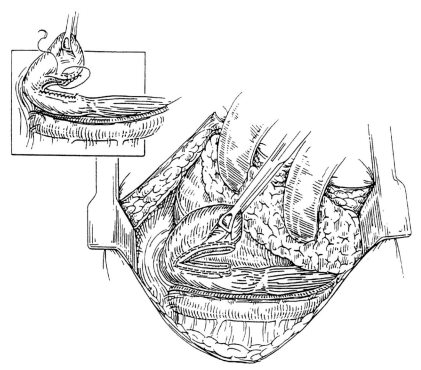

Figure 16-14. The staple line of the gastroplasty is oversewn, creating an extended esophagogastric tube and enlarging the gastric fundus.

is not necessarily an indication for reoperation. The antireflux mechanism remains intact, and most patients have recurrent but easily controlled symptoms. Telescoping of the stomach through a total fundoplication, or the "slipped Nissen" syndrome, is more problematic. Affected patients typically have a hiatal hernia, and acid-producing mucosa is trapped above the wrap, resulting in dysphagia and prolonged exposure of the esophagus to gastric acid. Reoperation is usually necessary for such patients.

Results of Surgery

The results of surgery for GERD are related to the severity of symptoms, the degree of esophageal and gastric dysfunction, and the amount of anatomic deformity present before the operation. The outcome is also directly related to the experience and skill of the surgeon. Between 85% and 90% of patients with normal esophageal motility and without esophageal stricture experience good or excellent results. The type of fundoplication created, whether total or partial, appears to have little influence on the ultimate results of the operation. Similarly, there are no data that demonstrate the superiority of the transthoracic, open transabdominal, or laparoscopic approaches in the management of patients with uncomplicated GERD. The initial advantages for the laparoscopic approach are potentially substantial and include cost savings as a result of decreased hospitalization time and earlier return to work as well as decreased pain. There are no follow-up data on these patients extending beyond 5 years, however, and the durability of these repairs has yet to be demonstrated. Standard fundoplication operations in the management of esophageal stricture are successful in 75% to 80% of patients, whereas gastroplasty and fundoplication for such patients is successful in about 85% of cases. Long-term follow-up suggests that results continue to worsen over time, such that an early (5-year) success rate of 90% evolves into a success rate of only 75% after 15 years.

wrap. Most chronic problems, however, are related to delayed gastric emptying. Therapy with prokinetic agents should be considered initially, whereas balloon dilation of the pylorus is indicated if there is gastric outlet obstruction resulting from scarring or vagal nerve dysfunction.

Other complications of fundoplication are gastric ulceration and technical failures.

The latter can be classified as either breakdown of the repair, slippage of the wrap into the chest, or telescoping of the stomach through a total fundoplication wrap. Fundoplication breakdown occurs more often with partial than with total fundoplication because the esophageal tissues do not hold sutures well. The slippage of an intact wrap into the chest, usually a total fundoplication,

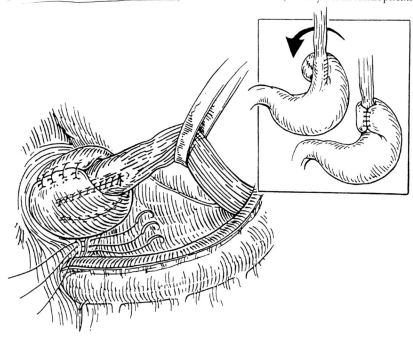

Figure 16-15. A partial or total (shown) fundoplication is performed after completing the gastroplasty.

SUGGESTED READING

Campos MD, Peters JH, DeMeester TR, et al. Multivariate analysis of factors predicting outcomes after laparoscopic Nissen fundoplication. J Gastrointest Surg 1999;3:292.

Chrysos E, Tsiaoussis J, Zoras OJ, et al. Laparoscopic surgery for gastroesophageal reflux disease in patients with impaired peristalsis: total or partial fundoplication? J Am Coll Surg 2003;197:8.

Fernando JC, Luketich JD, Christie NA, et al. Outcomes of laparoscopic Toupet compared to laparoscopic Nissen fundoplication. Surg Endosc 2002;16:905.

Flum DR, Koepsell T, Heagerty P, et al. The nationwide frequency of major adverse outcomes in antireflux surgery and the role of surgeon experience, 1992–1997. J Am Coll Surg 2002;195:611.

Oelschlager BK, Barreca M, Chang L, et al. Clinical and pathologic response of Barrett's esophagus to laparoscopic antireflux surgery. Ann Surg 2003;238:458.

Oleynikov D, Eubanks TR, Oelschlager BK, et al. Total fundoplication is the operation of choice for patients with gastroesophageal reflux and defective peristalsis. Surg Endosc 2002;16:909.

Pera M, Deschamps C, Taillefer R, et al. Uncut Collis-Nissen gastroplasty: Early functional results. Ann Thorac Surg 1995;60:915.

Peters JH, Heimbucher J, Kauer WK, et al. Clinical and physiologic comparison of laparoscopic and open Nissen fundoplication. J Am Coll Surg 1995;180:385.

EDITOR'S COMMENTS

Dr. Ferguson has provided a very clear and lucid discussion of antireflux procedures. There is no question that the laparoscopic Nissen fundoplication has become the procedure of choice for most patients. As Schuchert and Luketich point out in Chapter 19, the surgeon must be aware of the foreshortened esophagus and be prepared to deal with it lest the wrap be under tension, an excellent predictor of failure. Unfortunately, many thoracic surgical programs are not providing the cardiothoracic residents experience with laparoscopic fundoplication because the procedure has been ceded to the gastrointestinal surgeons or the "minimally invasive" surgical specialist who performs the "advanced" laparoscopic procedures. This may not be as undesirable as it would seem on first glance. It is incumbent on the thoracic surgeon with a particular interest in esophageal disease to seek out the additional training required to be proficient in these procedures. At several institutions divisions of thoracic surgery are being reincarnated as divisions of thoracic and foregut surgery to reflect the interest and expertise in diseases of the esophagus. This was an idea first proposed by DeMeester, whose disciples have gone on to form their own units in other institutions.

The decision as to whether to do a partial wrap as opposed to a total 360-degree wrap needs to be carefully considered if the patient has evidence of a motility disorder. As Dr. Ferguson points out, the total wrap is associated with better symptom relief from reflux but is associated with early dysphagia and occasionally with the "gas bloat" syndrome. The patient with disordered motility, such as the amotile esophagus seen in achalasia, may not tolerate a 360-degree wrap well. Dr. Ferguson points out the principles that need to be considered in doing an antireflux procedure, and if these are followed carefully, selected patients should have significant and durable relief of their reflux symptoms. Results are significantly poorer following a re-do procedure, and thus the experience of the surgeon is of great importance. There seems to be a tendency toward more failures following laparoscopic procedures perhaps because of the failure to recognize esophageal shortening. Many of these surgeons are capable of performing the re-do procedure laparoscopically as well, which never ceases to amaze me.

L.R.K.

17

Transhiatal Esophagectomy

Ahmad S. Ashrafi and R. Sudhir Sundaresan

Introduction

Esophageal resection continues to pose a significant challenge to the thoracic surgeon. Although malignancy is the most common indication for removing the esophagus, end-stage benign diseases of the esophagus do occasionally require resection. Esophageal cancer is a very aggressive malignancy that affects patients in the middle and older age group. Esophagectomy offers the only chance for cure and the best palliation. The goal of surgical resection should therefore be to maximize chance of cure and to minimize morbidity and mortality. The factors influencing the approach to the operation are many, and include the level and size of the tumor and the potential for adherence of the esophagus or tumor to surrounding mediastinal structures. Although Denk was the first surgeon to describe transhiatal esophagectomy in 1913, it was Orringer and Sloan who reintroduced and popularized it in 1978. Transhiatal esophagectomy (THE) is a safe procedure, and its greatest advantage is the avoidance of a thoracotomy. Furthermore, the esophagogastric anastomosis is placed in the neck, thereby reducing the high morbidity and mortality associated with an intrathoracic anastomotic leak. THE can be utilized to resect both benign and malignant lesions of the proximal, middle, and distal one thirds of the esophagus. This operation is ideally suited for resection of lower esophageal cancers (below the inferior pulmonary vein level) and proximal cancers in patients undergoing total pharyngolaryngoesophagectomy with gastric pull-up to the hypopharynx. Contraindications for THE include bulky middle-third tumors, situations in which there is increased risk of airway, aortic, or azygous vein injury during mediastinal dissection. In addition, if the patient has undergone prior esophageal surgery, the surgeon should have a lower threshold to convert to a transthoracic approach in order to deal with the mediastinal fibrosis safely. In this chapter, we describe *transhiatal esophagectomy*. Surgical technique is the main focus, but we also discuss pertinent preoperative and postoperative issues that maximize a successful outcome.

Preoperative Assessment and Preparation

All patients evaluated for THE require a complete history and physical examination. Preoperative workup must include basic blood work, barium swallow, upper endoscopy, and pulmonary function tests. A computed tomographic (CT) scan of the chest, abdomen, and pelvis is necessary for staging esophageal cancer, but it also provides vital anatomic information. An aberrant subclavian artery (passing posterior to the esophagus) increases the risk of vascular injury during transhiatal dissection and should prompt the surgeon to consider an alternate approach. All patients are assessed in a pre-admission unit by an anesthesiologist and a physiotherapist. Some patients may be sent for further cardiopulmonary assessment if deemed necessary by the anesthesiologist. If the patient has had a previous partial gastric resection, insertion of a gastrostomy tube, or previous gastric disease that might preclude using a gastric tube as the replacement conduit, an alternate conduit (typically colon) must be prepared. Preoperative assessment of the colon entails mesenteric angiography and either a colonoscopy or barium enema to rule out vascular or other colonic pathology. The patient should undergo a bowel prep preoperatively.

Operative Technique

All radiographic studies should be displayed in the operating room before starting. A thoracic epidural catheter is placed for postoperative pain relief. Prophylactic antibiotic is administered after induction of anesthesia. Full monitoring capacity, including two large-bore intravenous (IV) lines, a radial artery line, and a Foley catheter, is implemented. General anesthesia is administered using an uncut single-lumen endotracheal tube. If a central venous line is required, a right-sided subclavian or internal jugular approach should be used. Antiembolic stockings and sequential compression devices are applied. The patient is positioned supine with an inflatable bag placed beneath the shoulders to extend the neck. The patient's arms are securely padded and tucked at the sides, and the head is turned slightly toward the right (Fig. 17-1). A wide sterile field is prepared and draped from the mandibles to the suprapubic hairline, extending laterally to the midaxillary lines. Use of a headlight by the surgeon will maximize operative field illumination, especially while conducting mediastinal dissection.

Abdominal Phase

A small upper midline laparotomy incision is made to initially explore the abdomen and rule out intra-abdominal spread of tumor. The full incision is then created and

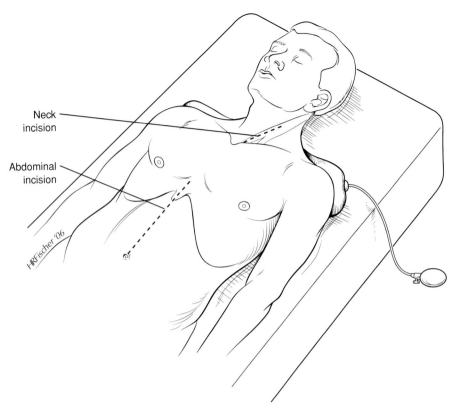

Figure 17-1. The patient is positioned supine with the neck extended and turned slightly to the right and with the arms at the sides. Laparotomy and neck incisions are indicated.

Neck
incision

Abdominal
incision

HRFischer '06

making the ligation and division of the short gastric vessels a relatively easy task. All of these vessels are divided between ligatures until the upper greater curve and fundus are completely free.

The greater curvature of the stomach is then reflected superiorly, and the left gastric pedicle is identified. All of the fatty tissue and contained lymph nodes are carefully mobilized toward the stomach. The left gastric pedicle is divided using one or two firings of the endovascular stapling instrument, staying nearly flush with the upper border of the pancreas.

Transhiatal dissection of the esophagus is then performed. The operating table is tipped into Trendelenburg position. The Penrose drain around the terminal esophagus is used to retract the esophagogastric junction caudally and alternating to the left and then to the right. A long, curved sponge forcep is used to provide countertraction away from the esophagus. A malleable retractor is also used to gently retract the pericardium anterosuperiorly. The surgeon uses the headlight to provide maximal visualization and illumination of the thoracic esophagus. These maneuvers allow the esophagus to be mobilized by blunt and cautery dissection under direct vision to the level of the carina.

Cervical Phase

An 8-cm oblique incision is made along the anterior border of the left sternocleidomastoid muscle, starting at the level of the cricoid cartilage and ending with a "hockeystick" extension in the suprasternal notch (Fig. 17-1). After division of the platysma, the avascular plane deep to the sternocleidomastoid muscle is entered, mobilizing it laterally. The omohyoid muscle is divided using electrocautery. The fascia along the lateral border of the strap muscles is divided vertically, exposing the contents of the carotid sheath, the airway, and the thyroid gland. The larynx, trachea, and esophagus are retracted medially. The left recurrent laryngeal nerve must be identified in the tracheoesophageal groove and protected at all times. Of note, one should use fingers rather than metal retractors to retract the structures medially and laterally, as described. The middle thyroid vein and the inferior thyroid artery are divided between ligatures. The adventitial surface of the esophagus is dissected circumferentially, allowing it to be encircled with a Penrose drain and gently retracted cranially. Using blunt finger dissection, the esophagus can now be safely mobilized caudally. Sponge sticks are used

spans the xiphoid process to the umbilicus. Excision of the xiphoid process facilitates maximal visualization of the upper abdomen (Fig. 17-1). A table-mounted retractor is positioned to allow upward and lateral retraction of the costal arches and lateral retraction of the abdominal wall (Fig. 17-2). The falciform and round ligaments are divided with cautery. The triangular ligament is divided using electrocautery paying careful attention to the hepatic vein, and the left lobe of the liver is folded to the right using a malleable retractor blade. The pars lucida in the lesser omentum over the caudate lobe of the liver is divided, and this is extended up to the right crus. The gastroesophageal junction is dissected free of the crura and encircled using a Penrose drain. The inferior phrenic vein is ligated and divided. The hiatus is generously enlarged by notching the crural sling anteriorly with cautery. The peritoneal reflection from the left crus to the upper fundus is divided.

The lesser sac is entered through the avascular plane in the greater omentum. This is perhaps one of the most crucial parts of the operation, and it is important to handle the stomach with care. Using a gauze sponge to hold the stomach will minimize the direct pressure applied on the stomach

as it is being mobilized. As this mobilization of the omentum is being carried out, a distance of approximately 2 cm should be kept beyond the gastroepiploic vascular arcade on the greater curve. This will reduce the chance of injuring the vascular pedicle as it is being developed. This sequential division and ligation of vessels along the greater curvature is taken toward the right beyond the pylorus. Kocherization of the duodenum is performed using cautery and Metzenbaum scissors. We prefer performing a pyloroplasty as a drainage procedure: Two stay sutures are applied transversely on the pylorus, identifying the corners of the pyloroplasty. A 2-cm to 3-cm longitudinal entry is made using the electrocautery. The pyloroplasty is closed transversely with the use of several interrupted, nonabsorbable, full-thickness sutures,. Recall that the duodenal mucosa is fixed, whereas the gastric mucosa is very mobile, so care is taken with the gastric bites to include the serosa and the mucosa.

The greater omentum is then mobilized in identical fashion toward the left, to the lower pole of the spleen, revealing the left gastroepiploic and short gastric vessels. One or two sponges are placed posterior to the spleen to rotate it anteriorly and medially,

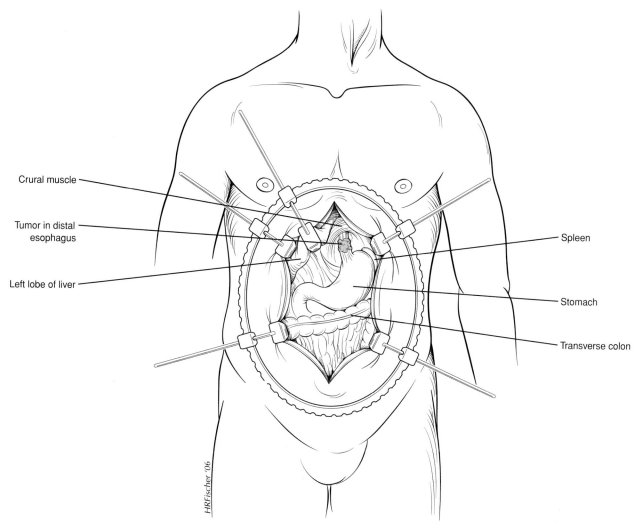

Crural muscle

Tumor in distal
esophagus

Left lobe of liver

Spleen

Stomach

Transverse colon

HRFischer '06

Figure 17-2. Use of a table-mounted retractor with maximal upward pull on the costal arches and lateral abdominal wall is essential to optimize exposure of the hiatus and upper stomach.

on the adventitia of the esophagus to free it to the level of the carina. Attention must be paid to surrounding structures, including the left recurrent laryngeal nerve in the tracheoesophageal groove, the membranous airway, the azygos venous arch, and the arch of the aorta.

The next phase of the operation completes the esophageal dissection from the mediastinum. The anesthesiologist is warned that manual dissection and division of the last few attachments around the midesophagus, conducted through the hiatus from the abdomen, may lead to transient cardiac compression and hypotension. This is the only part of the operation that is done using "blind" blunt dissection (Fig. 17-3). Preemptive increasing of preload may help to reduce the resultant hypotension. After complete dissection of the esophagus, it is partially delivered out of the cervical incision, and using a GIA stapler, it is divided

with at least 5 cm extra distally. This extra length is kept until the conduit is delivered to the neck and one is certain that adequate length is available for a tension-free anastomosis. A long umbilical tape is stapled to the upper margin of the distal esophagus. Once this is passed into the abdomen, the tape traverses the entire mediastinum. The mediastinum is inspected, blood is evacuated, and the mediastinum is packed. Both pleura are also inspected to determine whether a chest tube is needed to drain the pleural space at the time of closure.

The first step in preparing the conduit is to clean off the serosa at the mid-lesser curvature and ligate and divide the contained right gastric vessels. Using a GIA stapler, the lesser curve is divided parallel to the greater curve starting at the fundus. Once again, the stomach must be handled with utmost care; using a gauze sponge to hold the stomach will minimize the direct trauma. Typically,

four separate firings of the 75-cm linear cutting stapler will be needed (Fig. 17-4). The lesser-curve staple line on the gastric conduit is oversewn with a continuous 4-0 PDS Lembert suture.

The conduit is then appropriately oriented with the greater curvature in the left lateral position, and it is placed in a laparoscopic camera bag tied to the umbilical tape. One hand can be used to push the conduit from the abdomen through the hiatus into the mediastinum while the second hand exerts upward traction on the tape to gently pull the conduit upward (Fig. 17-5). Once again all effort must be given to maintaining proper orientation and avoiding torsion of the conduit. Once the fundus is delivered to the neck, the tip of the conduit is grasped through the cervical incision using a Babcock clamp. The orientation of the stomach is checked. The greater curvature should be to the patient's left and the staple line to the

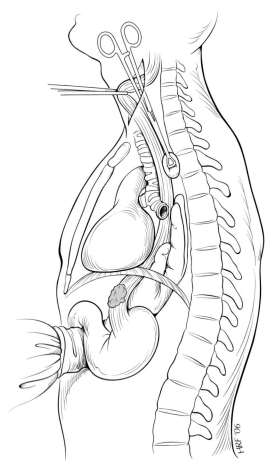

Figure 17-3. The only part of the operation that requires "blind/blunt" mobilization is the careful manual freeing of the last few attachments to the esophagus around the carina.

patient's right. The stomach must also be inspected from the abdomen to make sure it has not been twisted 360 degrees.

The esophagus is then assessed to determine the site of anastomosis. We start with a circular (transverse) myotomy and divide the esophageal mucosa at the distal end of the myotomy. This allows for a nice mucosal rosette, and the true margin of the esophagus is sent to the pathologist for frozen section. The anastomosis is hand-sewn in two layers using a continuous 4-0 PDS suture for each. To begin, we use two stay sutures identifying the corners of the esophagus by applying the suture through the muscle only and 180 degrees apart. The anastomosis is performed in an end-to-side fashion, away from the gastric tip, along the upper greater curvature. An outer posterior layer is started using the double-armed suture, half-way between the stay sutures. A seromuscular bite is taken on the stomach and sutured to the esophageal muscle layer (Fig. 17-6A). After the posterior outer layer is completed, an oblique gastrotomy is performed using electrocautery, roughly matching the size of the esophageal mucosal tube. The inner layer is sutured in a similar running fashion, with a double-armed suture starting in the middle and working out to each corner. This inner layer incorporates the esophageal mucosa to the full thickness of the stomach (Fig. 17-6B). Before completing the anterior inner layer, the anesthesiologist is asked to advance the nasogastric tube across the anastomosis. Once the tip is verified to lie just below the diaphragm, the tube is securely taped to the patient's nose. The anastomosis is completed by finishing the anterior inner layer and continuing with the previous sutures to finish the outer layer. In our experience, this anastomotic technique has proven effective as well as expedient. It has become our preferred approach for all esophagoenteric anastomoses, regardless of neck or chest position. The esophageal anastomosis is then reduced into the upper mediastinum below the thoracic inlet. We do not place "tacking" sutures in the prevertebral fascia because this can potentially lead to major neurologic and septic complications, such as epidural abscess or osteomyelitis. This is especially more likely if the anastomosis leaks. A Penrose drain is placed alongside the anastomosis and brought out through the lower end of the skin incision. The neck is closed in layers using absorbable sutures in the platysma and staples in the skin. The drain is secured to the skin with a suture.

The mediastinum, pleura, and peritoneal cavity, including the pyloroplasty site, are inspected, and a feeding jejunostomy is inserted 20 cm to 30 cm from the ligament of Treitz, using the Witzel technique. The jejunum is secured to the abdominal wall over a 10-cm to 12-cm length to avoid volvulus around the jejunostomy site, and the feeding tube is secured to the skin. Sponge, needle, and instrument counts are checked for accuracy, and the abdomen is closed with a running No. 1 PDS suture; skin is closed

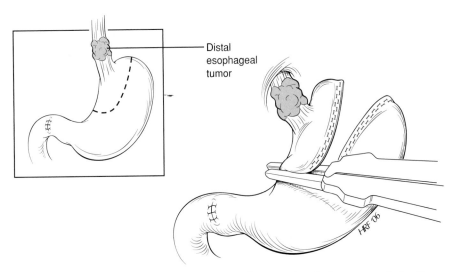

Distal esophageal tumor

Figure 17-4. It is essential to preserve the fundus when resecting the lesser curve during the preparation of the gastric conduit.

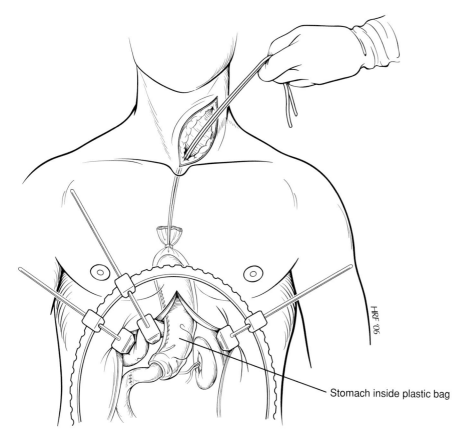

Stomach inside plastic bag

Figure 17-5. Gentle upward pull on the umbilical tape is all that is required to transpose the conduit to the neck because friction between the plastic bag and the gastric serosa will facilitate cephalad movement.

with staples. Wounds are cleansed and appropriate dressings are applied. The patient is transferred to the post–anesthetic care unit (PACU) or the intensive care unit (ICU) with monitors and kept intubated if deemed necessary by the anesthetist.

Intraoperative Complications

In addition to intraoperative complications associated with any laparotomy or neck exploration, certain complications specific to THE merit separate discussion.

During mobilization of the stomach, the right gastroepiploic artery is at risk of injury. Although rare, this occurrence seriously jeopardizes the blood supply of the conduit and renders it unsafe for use. Intraoperative consultation for a microvascular repair of the artery may be appropriate for a minimal (tangential) injury, but this is probably not advisable. A safer alternative is to use the colon, which can be done immediately if the bowel has been prepared. If not, the

operation is best abandoned and the patient brought back to the operating room after adequate preparation. Microvascular anastomosis in the neck has been reported as an unusual means of restoring perfusion to the conduit.

Pneumothorax can arise during the mediastinal dissection. Once recognized, it is managed by insertion of a 28-F chest tube through the operative field.

Traction injuries to the aorta or azygous vein occur rarely during the mediastinal dissection and require immediate thoracotomy. The mediastinum should be packed, the anesthetist should be notified, and blood must be called for immediately. Azygos vein injury is managed through a right anterior thoracotomy. Thoracic aortic injury is extremely rare and potentially lethal. In spite of making an urgent left thoracotomy, the exposure of the injury is difficult, and the magnitude of the hemorrhage can lead to exsanguination before satisfactory exposure and control are achieved. Attempts should be made to pack the mediastinum and control the bleeding before performing the thoracotomy. Extra expert help should immedi-

ately be called to the operating room in the event of such a complication.

The final potential complication involves injury to the membranous airway. If this occurs, the anesthesiologist is asked to advance the uncut endotracheal tube distally into the airway. The esophagectomy is then completed, after which the injury is repaired. For high tracheal injuries, repair can generally be accomplished from the neck; lower tracheal injury is repaired via a right posterolateral thoracotomy.

Postoperative Care

The epidural infusion is started immediately upon arrival of the patient in the ICU or PACU. An electrocardiogram (ECG), chest radiograph, arterial blood gas, and basic blood work are obtained. The initial intravenous fluids consist of crystalloid resuscitation. Urine output is measured hourly, and the heart rate, heart rhythm, blood pressure, and arterial oxygen saturation are monitored continuously. Adequate pain control facilitates immediate extubation and allows the patient to breathe and cough effectively to clear secretions and prevent atelectasis. Prophylactic antibiotic is continued for 24 hours. Deep vein thrombosis (DVT) prophylaxis is given in the form of subcutaneous heparin or low-molecular-weight (LMW) heparin, combined with a sequential compression device. The nasogastric tube and jejunostomy tube are irrigated every 4 hours to maintain patency.

The head of the bed is kept at 30 to 45 degrees, and the patient is maintained on an H_2 antagonist or a proton-pump inhibitor. A dedicated physiotherapist who has seen the patient preoperatively assesses the patient on postoperative day 1, and the patient is ambulated. Jejunostomy tube feeds are started on postoperative day 1 at 20 ml/hr and kept at this rate. The intravenous regimen is converted to a maintenance fluid and rate. The nasogastric tube is left in place until a thin barium swallow on postoperative day 5 shows a patent anastomosis without leak. The nasogastric tube is then removed, and the patient is allowed to slowly progress with oral intake. A dietician assesses the patient for recommendations and education. The jejunostomy feeds are stopped before discharging the patient, although the tube is kept in place and removed during a subsequent postoperative visit. If adjuvant treatment is required or the patient is not taking sufficient oral nutrition, the feeding tube may be used for a longer period, even at home.

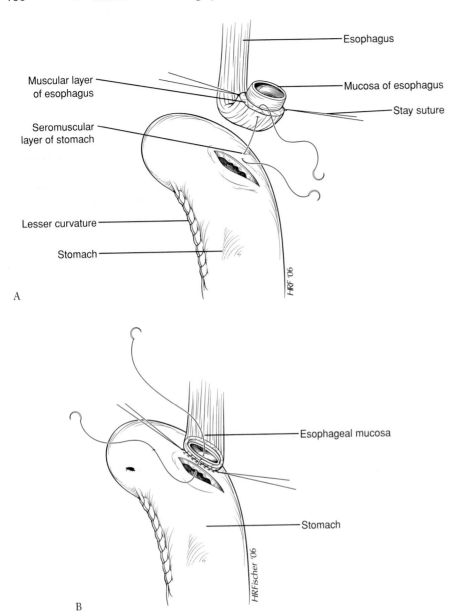

Esophagus

Muscular layer
of esophagus

Mucosa of esophagus

Stay suture

Seromuscular
layer of stomach

Lesser curvature

Stomach

HRF '06

A

Esophageal mucosa

Stomach

HRFischer '06

B

Figure 17-6. **(A)** The esophagogastric anastomosis is performed in two layers with continuous 4-0 monofilament suture for each. The outer layer is being constructed by approximating the esophageal muscle to the seromuscular layer of the stomach. **(B)** Completion of the outer posterior layer will set up apposition of the esophageal and gastric mucosal tubes. The inner layer approximates the esophageal mucosa to the full thickness of the stomach.

Postoperative Complications

In addition to the usual postoperative complications associated with any major operation (such as myocardial infarction, DVT, pulmonary embolism, cardiac arrhythmias, etc.), certain complications of THE merit consideration (Table 17-1).

Left recurrent laryngeal nerve injury is infrequent (<10%) and results from direct injury to the nerve usually during the cervical phase of the operation. The patient is

Table 17-1   Complications of Transhiatal Esophagectomy
Recurrent laryngeal nerve injury
Pneumonia
Anastomotic stricture
Anastomotic leak
Gastric tip necrosis
Cervical vertebral osteomyelitis
Epidural abscess
Tracheoesophageal fistula
Chylothorax

noted to be hoarse postoperatively. However, the consequence of this injury is far more serious, in that the inability to protect the airway with a closed glottis can lead to aspiration, which can lead to life-threatening pulmonary sepsis. Patients will need education by a speech pathologist and a dietician to swallow safely and minimize the risk of aspiration. Patients should be followed carefully thereafter. For the minority who do not demonstrate spontaneous recovery or accommodation within 4 to 6 months, referral to an ear, nose, and throat surgeon for vocal cord medialization is appropriate.

Intraoperative injury to the thoracic duct can lead to chylothorax. A high suspicion of a chyle leak should exist if the patient rapidly develops a pleural effusion (usually right sided) or, if a chest tube has been placed intraoperatively, there is an excessive amount (>1,000 mL/day) of drainage that turns "milky" when the patient starts on a regular diet. Chylothorax should be suspected and confirmed by analysis of the pleural fluid. This complication is initially managed conservatively by instituting parenteral nutrition and stopping oral intake and tube feeds. However, transection injuries of the duct rarely respond to these measures, and thus reoperation is usually necessary. Surgical correction consists of a low right thoracotomy and mass ligation of the tissue between the azygous vein and aorta on the vertebral body, which will include the thoracic duct.

Anastomotic leak must be suspected in any patient with fever and redness in the neck incision. After fluid resuscitation, broad-spectrum IV antibiotics, and a septic workup, the neck wound must be opened immediately at the bedside. The wound is cultured, and a chest x-ray is obtained to assess the mediastinum and pleural spaces. The patient is started on twice- to thrice-daily dressing changes. We prefer to obtain a CT scan of the neck and chest with oral contrast to rule out mediastinal or pleural collections as well as to quantify the anastomotic leak. If the patient does not show prompt clinical improvement, gastric tip necrosis must be suspected and ruled out by an urgent upper endoscopy. The endoscopy must be performed very carefully to minimize trauma to a relatively fresh anastomosis. If the upper stomach is found to have sloughed, the patient will need urgent reoperation, consisting of neck exploration, creation of cervical esophagostomy, and resection of the necrotic stomach. The abdomen must also be reopened to reduce the viable stomach and create a gastrostomy. The patient subsequently must undergo delayed reconstruction with a substernal colon interposition.

Results of Transhiatal Esophagectomy

There is ongoing debate as to whether THE is as safe and as oncologically adequate an operation as transthoracic esophagectomy (TTE). Several single-institution studies and meta-analyses have analyzed these questions. Collective results of four randomized trials including 258 patients showed a cumulative operative mortality of 6.7% for TTE and 4% for THE. Two large series comparing THE and TTE showed a higher mortality for TTE (9.2%, 9.5%) than THE (5.7%, 6.3%); however, the differences were not statistically significant. Although mortality rates are comparable, virtually all studies have demonstrated a higher anastomotic leak rate for the cervical anastomosis in THE (13.6%, 16%) as compared to intrathoracic anastomosis (7.2%, 10%). These data highlight the fact that cervical anastomotic leaks are infrequently associated with mediastinitis or uncontrolled sepsis, the usual cause of mortality in esophagectomy patients. Finally, the 5-year survival was similar for patients undergoing TTE (23%, 26%) and THE (21.7%, 24%).

Rentz and colleagues conducted a 10-year prospective analysis of 945 patients in 105 hospitals. These authors demonstrated no significant difference in postoperative morbidity and mortality between THE and TTE.

Despite ongoing debate about THE and TTE, in the hands of an experienced and careful surgeon, both operations provide satisfactory results. Surgeons must be familiar with both approaches and carefully select the best approach for the individual patient.

Summary

Transhiatal esophagectomy has existed since the beginning of the twentieth century, and after a long dormant phase was repopularized by Orringer and Sloan in 1978. The operation can be used to resect the entire esophagus for both benign and malignant diseases. Methodical and careful execution of the procedure is necessary to maximize success and minimize serious complications. Inexperience or inexpert conduct of the surgery can lead to devastating intraoperative difficulties and potential for serious postoperative morbidity.

SUGGESTED READING

Bolton JS, Teng S. Transthoracic or transhiatal esophagectomy for cancer of the esophagus—Does it matter? Surg Oncol Clin North Am 2002;11:365.

Denk W. Zur radikaloperation des oesophaguskarzinoms. Zentralbl-Chir 1913;40:1065.

Orringer MB, Sloan H. Esopagectomy without thoracotomy. J Thorac Cardiovasc Surg 1978;76:643.

Orringer MB, Marshall B, Iannettoni MD. Transhiatal esophagectomy for treatment of benign and malignant esophageal disease. World J Surg 2001;25:196.

Petsikas D, Shamji FM. Revascularization of the ischemic gastric tube using the left internal thoracic artery. Ann Thorac Surg 1996;62:568.

Rentz J, Bull D, Harpole D, et al. Transthoracic versus transhiatal esophagectomy: A prospective study of 945 patients. J Thorac Cardiovasc Surg 2003;125:1114.

Valji AM, Maziak DE, Allen MW, et al. The stomach as a microvascularly augmented flap for esophageal replacement. Ann Thorac Surg 2000;69:1593.

EDITOR'S COMMENTS

It has been conclusively shown that morbidity and mortality associated with certain operations are linked to the volume of cases performed by the individual surgeon and in some cases to the number of cases done in a given institution. Esophagectomy is one of those procedures in which the outcome clearly is dependent on the volume done by the surgeon, that is, the surgeon who does a "large" volume of esophageal resections has results that demonstrate lower morbidity and mortality than the surgeon who does only the occasional esophagectomy. That being said, it is incumbent on the surgeon who performs esophageal resection to be expert at a variety of operations because one operation is not indicated for every patient who needs surgery. Transhiatal esophagectomy should be one of the operations used, and, in my opinion, the most frequent operation used, but clearly there are times when a thoracotomy is indicated. A bulky mid-esophageal lesion in which the most difficult part of the dissection will be in the area most difficult to assess via a transhiatal approach mostly mandates thoracotomy, although some surgeons disagree with this.

The key to the transhiatal approach, as the authors point out, is the completion of most of the mediastinal dissection under direct vision, as opposed to a "blind" or "blunt" approach. With the patient in a Trendelenburg position, an appropriate retractor placed in the hiatus, and headlight illumination, the portion of the dissection up to the carina is carried out under direct vision. It is difficult, if not impossible, to stay out of one or both pleural spaces, and I favor placing a chest tube into an opened pleural space at the conclusion of the procedure because one can be almost assured that an effusion will accumulate if this is not done. The tube(s) may be removed as the drainage decreases over the first few postoperative days.

The authors recommend the routine performance of a drainage procedure because bilateral truncal vagotomy is a consequence of the esophageal resection. There are many who feel that a drainage procedure is not necessary and may be avoided. My preference is to do a pyloromyotomy and thus avoid another mucosal suture line.

Bringing the gastric remnant through the posterior mediastinum up to the neck can be problematic, as the authors mention. The use of the camera bag has been well established and provides an excellent vehicle to accomplish this. The stomach should be marked with a line to assure that twisting has not occurred during the transit up to the neck.

There are a number of issues relating to the esophagogastric anastomosis that deserve mention. The authors prefer a two-layer closure and use this routinely. This anastomosis is associated with a significant postoperative stricture rate that will require dilation. Over the last few years we have adopted the technique, first proposed by Orringer, of using the linear staple to construct the anastomosis with suture closure of the "hood," the open portion through which the stapler was placed. This results in a large anastomosis that is associated with a significantly lower rate of leakage and a lower incidence of stricture formation. Perhaps it is the sheer size of the anastomosis that results in the lower leakage rate.

Finally, with regard to intraoperative complications, recurrent laryngeal nerve injury is a significant complication that should rarely occur with appropriate technique. The nerve must be visualized in the neck and protected from retraction or other injury. It must be recognized that the nerve may also be injured during the mediastinal dissection when a portion is done "blindly" at or above the carina. Care should be taken to stay close to the esophagus during this part of the resection. Injury to the thoracic duct must be treated aggressively once it is recognized in the postoperative period. Total parenteral nutrition should be instituted, but if there is not a significant decrease in the amount of drainage and if the leak has not sealed within 7 days, the duct should be ligated via a low right thoracotomy with mass ligation of the tissue along the spine between the azygous vein and the aorta at the level of the aortic hiatus. No attempt should be made to "find" the leak; ligation of the duct not only is preferable, but is far easier.

Despite the best of intentions and even in experienced hands, esophageal resection is associated with a morbidity rate of close to 40%, with the most common complications being pulmonary related. Aggressive pulmonary toilet should be the norm, and overall postoperative care should be conducted in units accustomed to taking care of these patients if morbidity is to be minimized.

L.R.K.

18

Thoracic Approaches to Esophagectomy

Alan G. Casson and H. Chrish Fernando

In selected patients, esophagectomy may be required to treat either malignant or benign esophageal disease. Examples of the latter include end-stage achalasia or motor disorders, recurrent stricture secondary to chronic gastroesophageal reflux or lye ingestion, and esophageal trauma and perforation. Esophageal resection may also be indicated for patients with premalignant Barrett epithelium with high-grade dysplasia. However, in current clinical practice, esophageal cancer is the most frequent indication for esophagectomy, which offers the potential for cure and improved quality of life. Several techniques of esophagectomy are described, including the popular transhiatal approach discussed in the preceding chapter. This chapter focuses on current thoracic techniques, including the role of evolving minimally invasive approaches that incorporate thoracoscopic esophageal dissection.

Although the incidence of esophageal cancer in North America and Europe is relatively low, recent epidemiologic studies reported a steady rise in incidence for adenocarcinomas of the lower esophagus and esophagogastric junction. The reasons underlying this changing pattern of disease are unknown, although several lifestyle risk factors, including tobacco and alcohol consumption, obesity, and dietary factors, have been proposed. The recent identification of molecular markers associated with Barrett metaplasia-dysplasia-adenocarcinoma progression may provide further insight into the molecular pathogenesis of this disease. Despite recent advances in, and increasing clinical utilization of, neoadjuvant and adjuvant therapy, the prognosis for invasive esophageal cancer remains generally poor. Because several modalities are available for treating esophageal cancer, patients initially may be evaluated and managed by a variety of medical specialists. It is important that the thoracic surgeon appreciate the indications, limitations, and potential complications of all therapeutic options to effectively manage patients with this disease. However, it is likely that surgery will continue to play a key role in the treatment of esophageal cancer in the foreseeable future.

Early attempts at potentially curative surgical excision of esophageal cancer were often associated with high operative mortality rates. This led to divergent opinions regarding the goal of surgical treatment of this disease with respect to "palliative" or "curative" resection. Although recent reports indicate that an operative mortality of <5% should be routinely achieved, esophageal resection is still associated with relatively high morbidity, even in high-volume units. The surgeon treating esophageal cancer therefore not only must be skilled at the technical aspects of esophageal resection and reconstruction, but also must use sound judgment in preoperative evaluation and be meticulous in the postoperative management of these patients. Although a complete resection of a localized esophageal tumor offers the best hope of long-term survival, a single-stage operation with immediate reconstruction of the upper gastrointestinal tract will restore swallowing expediently and improve quality of life. Because there is no single accepted approach to esophagectomy, the choice of operation for carcinoma of the esophagus often depends on several factors, including the site of the tumor, the general condition of the patient, and the experience or preference of the surgeon, rather than on sound oncologic principles alone.

Preoperative Evaluation

A thorough history is obtained and a physical examination is performed to evaluate symptoms related to the local effects of the primary tumor, possible metastatic sites, and the general physiologic status of the patient. A contrast esophagram and esophagogastroscopic examination are frequently obtained early in the investigation of esophageal disease, and these investigations should be regarded as complementary. A barium swallow study (upper gastrointestinal series) is performed initially to define foregut anatomy, the anatomic site and extent of the primary tumor, and the degree of esophageal obstruction before esophageal instrumentation. Esophagogastroscopy permits direct visualization of the primary tumor, and biopsy specimens should be taken to confirm the diagnosis of malignancy and establish the histologic subtype. Esophagogastroscopy also is useful in assessing the stomach for reconstruction of the upper gastrointestinal tract and in excluding coexisting gastric disease. If the patient is unable to swallow, the obstructing tumor also should be dilated to palliate dysphagia while further investigation or definitive treatment is planned.

For many solid tumors, accurate staging is frequently the most reliable predictor of survival and underlies treatment strategies. TNM staging systems require evaluation of the primary tumor (T), regional lymph nodes (N), and distant metastases (M). A totally satisfactory staging system has not been developed for esophageal cancer. There are many reasons for this, including the relative inaccessibility of the esophagus for accurate preoperative tumor staging; inconsistent correlation between preoperative and operative findings; uncertainty as to the etiology and staging of adenocarcinoma at the esophagogastric junction; advanced tumor stage at diagnosis (T3, T4, N1, M1); and lack of agreement as to which nodal stations represent regional and distant disease. Lymph node mapping, based on a numeric system and precise anatomic boundaries for each nodal station, is under evaluation for staging esophageal cancer.

In clinical practice, computed tomographic (CT) scanning of the chest is the most frequent noninvasive radiologic investigation for staging the primary esophageal tumor, regional lymph nodes, and distant visceral metastases. Whereas magnetic resonance imaging (MRI) appears to offer little advantage over CT scanning for staging intrathoracic locoregional disease, this technology continues to evolve, and it is anticipated that the staging accuracy of MRI will continue to improve. Endoscopic ultrasound (EUS) has been used with increasing frequency in several centers to image the esophageal wall and periesophageal lymph nodes for staging nonobstructing esophageal tumors. Although a few studies have reported EUS to be more accurate than CT scanning, this promising technique warrants further prospective evaluation and at present should be considered complementary to conventional CT scanning for locoregional (T, N) staging of esophageal cancer. Over the last decade, positron emission tomography (PET) has been used with increasing frequency to stage locoregional and distant disease and to determine response to induction therapy.

Although a detailed description of all techniques used to stage esophageal cancer is beyond the scope of this chapter, bronchoscopy should also be performed on all patients in whom the tumor is in close proximity to the airway (at or above the level of the carina) to exclude involvement of an airway by the tumor. There has also been interest in using minimally invasive, video-assisted laparoscopic and thoracoscopic techniques to stage esophageal cancers in a manner similar to the use of mediastinoscopy to stage lung cancer. Although this approach may well improve the accuracy of preoperative staging, additional clinical studies are warranted to evaluate this strategy for staging esophageal cancer.

Before the operation, a careful evaluation of cardiac and pulmonary function is essential, especially if the thoracotomy is planned. Because a majority of patients with esophageal cancer are cigarette smokers, poor pulmonary function may be improved (often significantly) preoperatively by cessation of smoking and chest physiotherapy. Patients with obstructing esophageal tumors may have radiographic evidence of aspiration pneumonia, which should be treated by esophageal dilation, chest physiotherapy, and antibiotics after the possible presence of a tracheobronchial fistula has been excluded. Oral hygiene should be improved whenever possible. Hepatic and renal function should be evaluated biochemically, especially in patients with a history of alcohol intake. The value of preoperative enteral or parenteral nutrition, either short term or long term, in an attempt to minimize weight loss is uncertain. However, dehydration and anemia should be corrected by the intravenous administration of fluids or transfusion of blood products before general anesthesia.

The evaluation of patients with benign esophageal disease for esophagectomy is done on an individual basis and depends on the underlying disorder and efficacy of previous treatment. In addition to a barium swallow study and esophagogastroscopy to define foregut anatomy, esophageal function studies (manometry, 24-hour ambulatory pH monitoring) are often necessary to complete the preoperative assessment in these patients.

Indications for the Thoracic Approach

The thoracic approach for esophagectomy is preferred in the following situations:

1. For an extended or radical en bloc resection incorporating any (or part) of the following mediastinal structures: the thoracic esophagus and its surrounding connective tissue, pleura, regional lymph nodes, pericardium, azygos vein, thoracic duct, and diaphragmatic crura.
2. For tumors adjacent to the airway or mediastinal vascular structures in cases in which preoperative staging has not conclusively defined the interface between tumor and normal tissues.
3. For benign esophageal disease, such as lye or peptic stricture, that may be associated with dense periesophageal reaction and fibrosis.
4. When mediastinal fibrosis after previous radical mediastinal radiation therapy or esophageal perforation is suspected.
5. In the uncommon situation in which (a) technical limitations with the esophageal substitute suggest that an intrathoracic anastomosis will be necessary or (b) the patient has associated pulmonary disease that requires a lung biopsy.

It should be remembered that these situations are relative rather than absolute indications for thoracotomy. Contraindications to thoracotomy, such as poor pulmonary function, general medical status, and so forth, should also be considered when planning surgery. Indications for a minimally invasive approach are evolving.

Principles of Transthoracic Esophageal Resection and Reconstruction

Immediately before the operation, a mechanical bowel preparation is performed. This is done regardless of the planned esophageal substitute because occasionally it will be necessary to use colon. Prophylactic antibiotics are administered intravenously, and an epidural catheter is placed before induction of general anesthesia. If the surgeon has not performed an esophagogastroscopic examination (or bronchoscopy for a proximal tumor), it is essential to do so at this time. A double-lumen endotracheal tube or bronchial blocker is placed to isolate the appropriate lung and to facilitate exposure of the mediastinum during thoracotomy.

Because preoperative staging of esophageal cancer is not completely reliable, the surgeon must not only assess the resectability of the primary tumor, but also assess potential sites of metastatic disease in the chest. Suspected metastases should be biopsied, and an intraoperative frozen-section examination performed in consultation with the pathologist. In general, the finding of distant metastatic disease would preclude esophagectomy. The sequence of assessment of (1) resectability of the primary tumor, (2) metastases, and (3) the esophageal substitute may vary somewhat. A laparotomy may be performed initially to exclude intraabdominal metastases and to assess and mobilize the conduit for reconstruction, followed by a thoracotomy and esophageal resection. This sequence is appropriate for the Ivor Lewis (laparotomy/right thoracotomy) approach. Similarly, when a left thoracoabdominal approach is used, the abdomen may be explored initially by performing the abdominal part of the incision and subsequently extending the incision posteriorly to gain access to the left chest. If a three-hole approach (right thoracotomy/laparotomy/neck) is planned, the right thoracotomy may be performed initially to evaluate and mobilize the primary tumor. The esophagus remains in situ while the patient is positioned supine, and the laparotomy is performed next to exclude abdominal disease and prepare the conduit for transposition to the neck. The mobilized esophagus is then removed through the abdominal and neck incisions.

With appropriate technique, the full length of the intrathoracic esophagus can be dissected using either a right or left thoracotomy. Although no clinical trials have directly compared right and left thoracic approaches, operative mortality and outcome appear comparable. Because the aortic arch may limit the exposure of middle-third or upper-third tumors, left thoracic or thoracoabdominal approaches have generally been advocated for tumors of the lower one third of the esophagus or at the esophagogastric junction. A right thoracotomy has traditionally been used for middle-third tumors, but recently this approach has been used with increasing frequency for lower-third lesions. Indeed, a right thoracotomy or video-assisted thoracic surgical (VATS) approach will permit excellent exposure of the intrathoracic esophagus at any level. Transsternal approaches are used infrequently for esophageal resection, although a partial upper sternotomy will provide suitable exposure of upper-third thoracic esophageal cancers. Further exposure may be obtained by adding a lateral anterior thoracotomy incision to the sternotomy.

The extent of esophageal resection remains controversial. Autopsy studies demonstrated that longitudinal spread of carcinoma to the proximal esophagus along submucosal lymphatics diminishes with distance from the primary tumor. However, even at 10 cm, microscopic tumor will be found in up to 3% of cases. Therefore, to ensure an adequate proximal margin, it would appear that a total thoracic esophagectomy, with an anastomosis in the neck, would be preferable to a subtotal or partial esophagectomy. Few studies have evaluated the extent of submucosal spread of tumor distally to the lower esophagus and stomach. For primary esophageal cancers at or adjacent to the esophagogastric junction, it is important to resect a sufficient amount of lesser curvature of the stomach to ensure a negative distal resection margin. Generally, 4 cm to 6 cm of the lesser curve, with lesser omentum and its corresponding four to six vascular arcades, will be sufficient. However, this should be confirmed histologically. The extent of dissection required

to achieve adequate lateral (radial) margins is unknown. An en bloc resection of tumor, periesophageal connective tissue, pleura, regional lymph nodes, and involved adjacent structures would seem appropriate but is reported to have increased morbidity. It is unclear whether survival is improved with more-radical en bloc procedures. Similarly, the value of an extended lymphadenectomy is also unknown because the majority of patients with lymph node metastases are likely to have systemic (occult) disease at the time of resection.

A single-stage procedure, with immediate reconstruction of the upper gastrointestinal tract, restores swallowing and improves quality of life. Although stomach, colon, and jejunum have been used successfully to replace the esophagus at any level, the stomach is preferred for several practical reasons. This organ has an excellent blood supply and, after mobilization, easily reaches the neck, where a single anastomosis is performed. To ensure adequate mobilization of the stomach, a Kocher maneuver is performed routinely. Further length may be obtained by constructing a gastric tube rather than the whole stomach. Although it is controversial, a pyloromyotomy may be performed in an attempt to ensure that gastric emptying is not delayed. Satisfactory functional results are generally reported after gastric transposition, even long term in patients with benign disease.

The stomach, or other conduit, is most frequently positioned in the posterior mediastinal (orthotopic) location. Occasionally it is necessary to use a substernal, subcutaneous, or transthoracic route. If the substernal route is used, the thoracic inlet should be enlarged by resecting the medial portion of the clavicle, the first rib, and part of the manubrium to prevent obstruction at the thoracic inlet. Theoretically, substernal interposition protects the gastric mucosa should postoperative radiation therapy be administered to the esophageal bed. However, the most direct route is through the posterior mediastinum. Use of a sterile plastic sleeve to deliver the conduit to the neck has been particularly helpful because this avoids rotation of the conduit, damage to its vascular supply, and serosal tears. If orthotopic placement of the substitute is planned after a transthoracic resection, displacement or volvulus of the transposed conduit into the pleural space has been reported to occur postoperatively. Techniques to "mediastinalize" the conduit after thoracotomy have been described and include, where possible, reapproximation of mediastinal pleura, preservation of the azygos vein, suture of

lung to the posterior mediastinum, and effective decompression of the interposed organ throughout the early postoperative period (Fig. 18-1).

After a total thoracic esophagectomy, the transposed conduit is anastomosed to the remaining cervical esophagus in the neck. Anastomotic technique varies widely among surgeons and ranges from entirely hand-sewn anastomoses, using absorbable or nonabsorbable sutures in an interrupted or running manner, to use of mechanical stapling devices. Although mechanical stapling techniques are effective at reducing operative time and leak rates, they require just as much technical precision as a hand-sewn anastomosis. Regardless of anatomic site (intrathoracic, cervical) or technique used, the following principles apply to any gastrointestinal anastomosis. Accurate mucosal apposition, no tension, and a good blood supply are essential to achieve excellent immediate and long-term functional results. Metal clips may be applied adjacent to the anastomosis to aid radiographic localization postoperatively. A nasogastric tube is placed carefully across the anastomosis to decompress the stomach postoperatively. A feeding jejunostomy is placed before the abdomen is closed. A large catheter is preferred and is secured without compromising the lumen of the jejunum. Enteral feeding may be started within 24 hours.

Although some surgeons advocate using colon as the primary esophageal substitute, it is most commonly used as an alternative when the stomach is unsuitable for use because of previous gastrectomy, involvement with tumor, or inadequate length. If a colonic interposition is planned, it is important to exclude intrinsic colonic disease. Because the blood supply to the colon is generally more tenuous than that to the stomach, it is helpful, but not essential, to define colonic vascular anatomy by preoperative angiography. The final assessment of its blood supply, however, is made by the surgeon at operation. Extreme care also must be taken to avoid compromising the arterial and venous blood supply during mobilization. Isoperistaltic segments of left colon, based on the left colic artery, or transverse colon, based on the left or middle colic artery, are the preferred substitutes. Although sufficient length may be obtained using any part of the colon, it is important to avoid redundancy, which may result in poor transit and impaired function postoperatively. The major objection to using colon routinely is that three anastomoses are required, consequently increasing operative time and potential morbidity. Limited

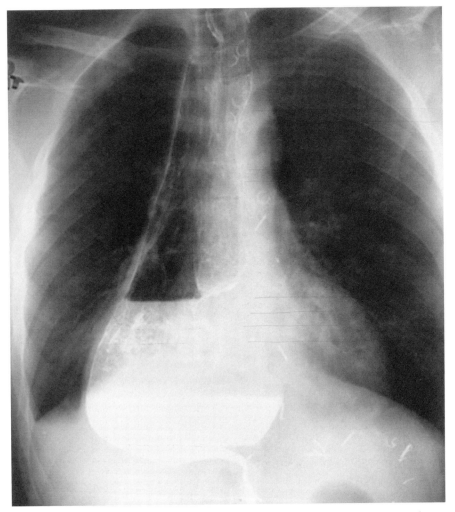

Figure 18-1. The barium swallow study of a patient referred with recurrent aspiration and dysphagia after esophagectomy and gastric interposition. A gastric drainage procedure had not been performed at the time of this procedure. This study illustrates a dilated intrathoracic stomach with displacement into the right chest secondary to gastric outlet obstruction. Attempts at balloon dilation were unsuccessful, and a pyloroplasty was required to improve gastric emptying.

mobility and an unpredictable blood supply have restricted use of jejunum in replacement of the lower esophagus, generally below the level of the inferior pulmonary vein. Free jejunal interposition, using microvascular application, has seen increasing application as an alternative to gastric pull-up for reconstruction of the cervical esophagus after resection of hypopharyngeal tumors.

The principles just summarized are also applicable for benign esophageal disease. Although the extent of resection is limited to resection of the diseased tubular esophagus, mediastinal dissection may be difficult in the presence of dense periesophageal fibrosis resulting from severe reflux or previous esophageal perforation. Few studies have critically evaluated long-term function of

esophageal substitutes. Although colonic replacement was widely thought to be preferable for benign disease, a properly constructed interposed stomach is an extremely durable substitute with quite satisfactory long-term function.

Surgical Technique

Although surgical techniques for esophageal resection and reconstruction vary considerably, the following sections summarize key technical components of commonly used thoracic approaches. Several steps of each operation, such as gastric mobilization, are common to each approach, and therefore are discussed only in the first section.

Right Thoracotomy/ Laparotomy

In 1946, Ivor Lewis proposed a two-stage approach, comprising an initial laparotomy with mobilization of the stomach followed 10 to 15 days later by a right thoracotomy, esophagectomy, and esophagogastric anastomosis. This combined approach evolved as a single-stage procedure, typically for middle-third or lower-third esophageal tumors. Although it is used widely, the disadvantages of this approach are that only a subtotal esophagectomy is performed and the esophagogastric anastomosis is intrathoracic.

With the patient supine, a laparotomy is performed first, to explore the abdomen and mobilize the stomach, which is the preferred substitute. Dissection at the hiatus is facilitated by ensuring the midline abdominal incision is taken up to the xiphoid and by using an "upper-hand" self-retaining retractor to elevate the lower sternum and left costal margin. The left triangular ligament is divided, and the now-mobile left lobe of the liver is retracted using the malleable blade attachment. The abdominal esophagus is dissected circumferentially, and the crura are defined. The lower esophagus is mobilized transhiatally under direct vision. Depending on the location of the primary tumor, an assessment is made as to its resectability. If the hiatus appears to be small, it may be enlarged by dividing the left crus laterally with electrocautery.

The stomach is mobilized as follows. The lesser sac is entered through the greater omentum, several centimeters away from the greater curvature, taking care not to compromise the right gastroepiploic artery. In the presence of adhesions or a fused lesser sac, the correct plane of dissection may be identified by first dividing the lesser omentum and gently elevating the stomach from above. The greater curvature of the stomach is mobilized by clamping, cutting, and ligating omental branches of the right gastroepiploic artery distally toward the pylorus and proximally toward the fundus. At a variable distance along the greater curve, the short gastric vessels will be identified. Careful dissection may identify anastomotic vessels between several short gastric vessels and the right gastroepiploic artery, and these should be preserved if possible to ensure additional vascularization of the greater curve of the stomach. Occasionally, it is necessary to dissect into the splenic hilum to preserve these anastomoses. The short gastric vessels are dissected individually in the gastrosplenic ligament and are ligated and

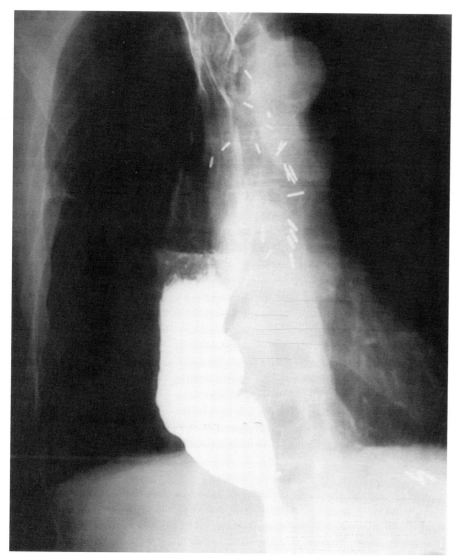

Figure 18-2. A barium swallow study illustrating the anatomy of an interposed stomach 8 years after esophagectomy for cancer. After transthoracic resection, the interposed stomach tends to be displaced into the right chest, especially if not "mediastinalized." In this case, displacement was minimal (compare with Fig. 18-1), and the patient swallowed normally.

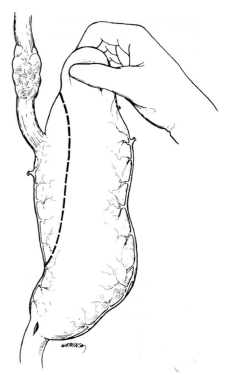

Figure 18-3. Construction of a gastric tube. The extent of resection of the lesser curve of the stomach is illustrated by the broken line, which incorporates four to six vascular arcades with associated lesser omentum. Additional length of stomach is obtained by several applications of a mechanical stapler from distal to proximal. The suture line is oversewn. A pyloromyotomy is also illustrated.

divided. The left gastric artery and vein are dissected to their origin by elevating the stomach and sweeping any associated lymph nodes toward the lesser curve. These vessels are suture-ligated individually. The lesser curve of the stomach is mobilized, incorporating the lesser omentum and four to six vascular arcades, a minimum of 5 cm, distal to the esophagogastric junction. The right gastric artery is preserved if possible. A suture is placed on the anterior wall of the stomach to ensure correct orientation when delivered into the chest. A Kocher maneuver, pyloromyotomy, and placement of a feeding jejunostomy are performed before the abdominal incision is closed.

The patient is then repositioned for a right posterolateral thoracotomy. The chest is entered through the fifth or sixth interspace, depending on the location of the tumor and body stature. The lung is excluded and retracted anteriorly to expose the mediastinum. The tumor is mobilized (Fig.18-2), although the extent of mediastinal dissection may vary. An en bloc dissection of the esophagus incorporating all tumor and involved structures necessary to ensure negative lateral margins is the goal. The esophagus is transected as high in the chest as possible to achieve a negative proximal resection margin. The mobilized stomach is delivered into the chest through the hiatus. It is essential to ensure that the stomach is correctly orientated and that the hiatus is an appropriate size to prevent gastric outlet obstruction (too tight) or herniation of abdominal viscera in to the chest (too loose). The lesser curve of the stomach, incorporating the esophagogastric junction, associated nodal tissue, and-lesser omemtum, is excised using a mechanical stapling device, and the staple line is oversewn. To maximize the length of the gastric tube, the stapler should be applied to the lesser curve from distal to proximal, with the apex of the fundus held with some degree of tension (Fig. 18-3). The stomach is anastomosed to the transected esophagus by hand (Fig. 18-4) or using a mechanical stapler (Fig.18-5). It is important to ensure that the interposed conduit remains in the posterior mediastinum because a redundant intrathoracic conduit will tend to prolapse in to the right chest. As discussed earlier, several techniques are described to "mediastinalize" the conduit.

Right Thoracotomy/ Laparotomy/Cervical Incision

The three-hole approach, comprising a right thoracotomy, laparotomy, and cervical

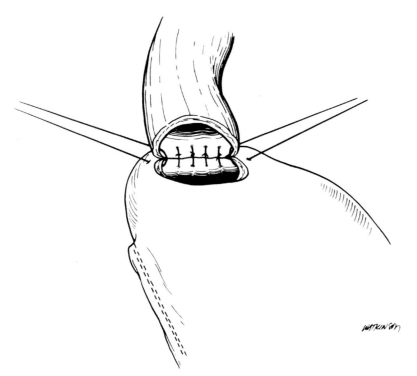

WATKINSON

Figure 18-4. Illustration of a hand-sewn esophagogastrostomy in which a single layer of interrupted absorbable sutures is used. This technique is used for neck anastomoses.

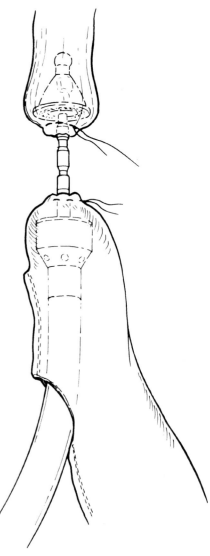

Figure 18-5. Illustration of the use of a mechanical stapler for esophagogastrostomy. The esophagus should be dilated carefully to accept the largest anvil without splitting the mucosa. A running monofilament suture secures the esophagus and stomach while the instrument is approximated and fired. The site of entry for the stapler on the stomach is closed by application of an additional mechanical stapler. All staple lines are oversewn.

incision, is the preferred transthoracic approach for benign and malignant esophageal disease. This operation is suitable for resection of esophageal cancer at any level of the thoracic esophagus, with the further advantage that the anastomosis is in the neck. There are several variations of this approach, related to the thoracotomy and sequence of incisions (Fig. 18-6). A full posterolateral thoracotomy may be performed as the initial step, which may be especially helpful if a difficult technical resection for cancer at or above the level of the carina is anticipated. After the thoracic esophagus is mobilized, the thoracotomy incision is closed and the patient repositioned supine for the laparotomy and neck dissection. An alternative is to perform the laparotomy and neck incisions first, with the patient supine. The conduit is then transposed substernally and anastomosed to the esophagus in the neck. After the abdominal and neck incisions are closed, the patient is repositioned for a right posterolateral thoracotomy, and a total thoracic esophagectomy is performed. A further modification of the three-hole approach is to perform right anterior thoracotomy, laparotomy, and neck incision synchronously. The patient is positioned supine with the right chest elevated slightly. A right anterior thoracotomy is performed through the fourth intercostal space. Exposure of the thoracic esophagus is generally satisfactory

using this anterior approach, provided that the right lung is collapsed by use of a double-lumen endotracheal tube. Use of a bronchial blocker is less helpful because it tends to dislodge as the lung is retracted. A laparotomy and neck dissection to mobilize the conduit and cervical esophagus, respectively, are performed without repositioning the patient. Use of two surgical teams further reduces operative time.

The cervical esophagus is approached through an incision along the anterior border of the left sternocleidomastoid muscle. The omohyoid and strap muscles are divided using electrocautery. Ligation of the middle thyroid vein and inferior thyroid artery facilitate the dissection. The left recurrent laryngeal nerve is identified in the tracheoesophageal groove, and care is taken not to damage this structure. The anterior wall of the esophagus is dissected from the posterior membranous trachea under direct vision. This is facilitated by gentle finger retraction of the trachea and left lobe of the thyroid. Dissection is continued posterolaterally to the anterior longitudinal ligament of the spine, from which the posterior esophageal wall is elevated. The esophagus is encircled, with the surgeon taking care not to incorporate the right recurrent laryngeal nerve during this maneuver. The mobilized cervical esophagus is then dissected under direct vision into the superior mediastinum until the

mobilized thoracic esophagus is identified. After transaction, the conduit is transposed to the neck and anastomosed to the cervical esophagus.

Left Thoracotomy

Left transthoracic approaches were initially developed to resect cancers of the lower one third of the esophagus or at the esophagogastric junction (Fig. 18-7). With appropriate technique, the full length of the

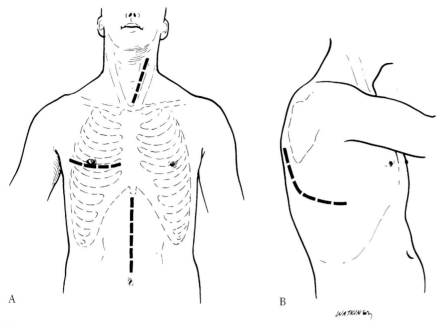

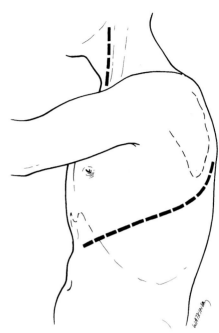

Figure 18-6. Right thoracotomy incisions for esophagectomy. **(A)** A right anterior thoracotomy may be performed synchronously with laparotomy and neck incisions with the patient supine. **(B)** Alternatively, a full right posterolateral thoracotomy may be used and the patient repositioned.

Figure 18-8. A left thoracotomy may be extended anteriorly across the costal margin as a thoracoabdominal incision or posteriorly to facilitate exposure at or above the aortic arch. If a total thoracic esophagectomy is performed, the interposed stomach is anastomosed in the left neck.

thoracic esophagus may be mobilized through a left posterolateral thoracotomy. However, the aortic arch may limit the en bloc dissection of more proximally situated tumors and may influence placement of the anastomosis. Although the abdomen can be explored and the stomach mobilized entirely through the diaphragm, it is generally more expedient to extend the incision across the costal margin in to the left upper quadrant of the abdomen.

Left Thoracoabdominal Approach

Because a left thoracoabdominal incision allows excellent exposure of the upper abdomen, it is particularly useful for primary esophageal cancers involving the esophagogastric junction. If sufficient stomach is available for reconstruction, it may be anastomosed to the transected esophagus in the chest, either below or above the aortic arch. Because a total thoracic esophagectomy is preferred for primary esophageal cancers, this approach may be modified to include a left neck incision and cervical anastomosis (Fig. 18-8). The left thoracoabdominal incision is also useful for resection of adenocarcinomas of the esophagogastric junction (cardia), subcardia gastric and fundic cancers, when a total gastrectomy including the lower esophagus (extended gastrectomy) is planned. In this situation, reconstruction is done using jejunum in a Roux-en-Y manner, with an intrathoracic anastomosis.

The patient is placed in a right lateral decubitus position. The left chest, abdomen and neck are exposed, and the left arm is free-draped. The abdominal part of the incision is made obliquely in the left upper quadrant of the abdomen from the mid-line to the left costal margin. The abdomen is explored first. The incision is extended across the costal margin as the lateral component of a left posterolateral thoracotomy incision. The chest is generally entered through the sixth interspace; the exact interspace may vary among patients. Should further

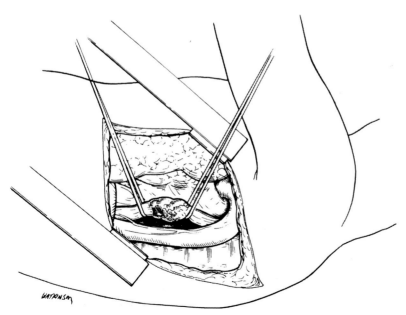

Figure 18-7. Esophageal mobilization using a left thoracotomy. Although typically used for lower esophageal tumors, with appropriate technique the full length of the thoracic esophagus can be mobilized using this approach.

exposure of the upper esophagus be necessary, the incision is extended upward between the scapula and vertebrae as the posterior component of the posterolateral thoracotomy. The diaphragm is divided circumferentially; care is taken to ensure that a sufficient cuff remains on the chest wall for reconstruction, and colored sutures are used to aid orientation. The principles of esophageal dissection and reconstruction are similar to those for other thoracic approaches. If the esophagus is mobilized above the aortic arch, care is taken to avoid injury to the thoracic duct, the posterior membranous trachea and bronchus, the left vagus, and its recurrent laryngeal nerve. The cervical esophagus is mobilized in the left neck, transected, and anastomosed to the transposed stomach as described. During closure of the thoracoabdominal incision, the diaphragm is carefully reconstructed with nonabsorbable, interrupted or running sutures. The costal cartilage may be reapproximated with interrupted, heavy, nonabsorbable monofilament sutures or a portion resected.

Minimally Invasive Approaches to Esophagectomy

Minimally invasive surgical techniques are increasingly used for the staging and treatment of esophageal cancer. Rapid advances in technology over the last decade have facilitated the development of video-assisted laparoscopic, transhiatal, and thoracoscopic approaches for esophageal resection and for gastric mobilization for reconstruction. It is important that the indications for surgery and the principles of esophageal resection are not compromised when considering a minimally invasive approach. The issue of outcomes becomes even more critical when considering a minimally invasive esophagectomy (MIE). The learning curve and the potential for disaster are great after MIE. On the other hand, the potential for lower mortality, lower morbidity, and reduced pain is attractive to patients. Ideally, if MIE is performed, this should be restricted to high-volume centers where there is also significant expertise with minimally invasive techniques.

A number of operative approaches have been referred to as MIE. Most are hybrid approaches that combine a minimally invasive procedure in one body cavity with an open procedure in another. The first completely minimally invasive approach to esophagec-tomy was described by Depaula from Brazil. He used a laparoscopic transhiatal approach, primarily for patients with end-stage achalasia. Swanstrom subsequently reported the first North American experience using the same technique in nine patients. Most of the tumors in his series were early-stage cancers or high-grade dysplasia.

There are some disadvantages with the laparoscopic transhiatal approach. Dissection of the mediastinal esophagus is tedious via a completely laparoscopic approach, and the effectiveness of lymph node dissection is compromised, making this more suitable for small patients with early-stage cancers or high-grade dysplasia. For this reason, Luketich et al. modified the approach by Depaula to include thoracoscopy. The key components of this operation are (1) right VATS to mobilize the entire thoracic esophagus, (2) laparoscopic creation of a gastric conduit, laparoscopic jejunostomy, and in most cases a laparoscopic pyloroplasty, and (3) cervical anastomosis. This approach, which is described in greater detail in another chapter, can be applied to a greater number of patients than the laparoscopic transhiatal technique.

Although no randomized data comparing MIE to open esophagectomy are available, preliminary reports are encouraging. Table 18-1 compares published outcomes after MIE and open esophagectomy. The results after MIE are as good if not better than some of the open series, demonstrating the feasibility of this approach, at least in a single-center setting. The Eastern Cooperative Oncology Group and the Cancer and Leukemia Oncology Group are evaluating the feasibility of MIE using the thoracoscopic/laparoscopic approach in a multicenter setting. If this procedure is indeed found to be feasible, further studies will need to compare MIE to open esophagectomy in a randomized setting.

Minimally invasive approaches to esophageal disease are discussed in detail in the following chapter.

Postoperative Management

Careful attention to postoperative management and an awareness of specific complications related to esophagectomy are essential in minimizing the morbidity associated with this procedure. With excellent epidural analgesia, most patients are extubated immediately in the operating room. Occasionally a short period of mechanical ventilation (<12 hours) may be required, especially if operating time is prolonged, with subsequent extubation when fully awake, pain-free, and able to maintain an airway. Prolonged intubation and ventilation are unnecessary and should be avoided. All patients are subject to chest physiotherapy and are ambulated early to further reduce potential respiratory complications. Pleural drains are removed as soon as possible provided there is no air leak and drainage is minimal, but mediastinal drains placed adjacent to an intrathoracic anastomosis should be left in place until integrity of the anastomosis is confirmed radiographically. Enteral feeding is usually started within 24 hours postoperatively through the feeding jejunostomy. The volume and concentration of the

Table 18-1 Comparison of outcomes for minimally invasive and open esophagectomy

	Luketich et al. (2003)	Nguyen (2003)	Orringer (1999)	Bailey (2003)	Rizk (2004)	Atkins (2004)
Number of patients	222	46	1,085	1,777	510	379
Approach	MIE	MIE	Open	Open	Open	Open
Mortality (%)	1.4	4.3	4	9.8	6.2	5.8
Leak rate (%)	11.7	4.3	13	NA	21	14
Pneumonia (%)	7.7	2.2	2	21.4	NR	15.8
Length of stay (days)	7	8	10[a]	NA	23[b] 11[c]	10

[a]Median not reported, 53% discharged by 10 days.
[b]Patients with technical complications.
[c]Patients without technical complications.
MIE = minimally invasive esophagectomy; NA = not available
Sources of data: Atkins 2004; Bailey 2003; Luketich JD, Alvelo-Rivera M, Buenaventura PO, et al. Minimally invasive esophagectomy: Outcomes in 222 patients. Ann Surg 2003;238:486; Nguyen 2003; Orringer 1999; Rizk 2004.

formula are titrated and advanced in a step-wise manner to avoid abdominal distention. If the patient develops signs of sepsis at any stage during the postoperative course, investigations are initiated immediately to determine the cause. In addition to the usual sites of postoperative infection, the following should be carefully evaluated: the anastomosis and conduit, the pleural spaces, and the subphrenic and subhepatic spaces. Suction is applied to the nasogastric tube to decompress the transposed conduit. A contrast study, initially with water-soluble contrast followed by dilute barium, is obtained on the fifth to seventh postoperative day. If no anastomotic leak is seen and satisfactory gastric emptying is demonstrated, the nasogastric tube is removed and the patient is started on clear liquids by mouth. At the time of discharge from the hospital, the patient should be able to manage several small meals of solid food daily. The patient is discharged with the feeding tube clamped; this is removed at the first postoperative follow-up visit, generally 3 weeks later.

SUGGESTED READING

Casson AG, Darnton SJ, Subramanian S, et al. What is the optimal distal resection margin for esophageal carcinoma. Ann Thorac Surg 2000;69:205.

Casson AG, Rusch VW, Ginsberg RJ, et al. Lymph node mapping of esophageal cancer. Ann Thoracic Surg 1994;58:1569.

Casson AG, van Lanschot JJB. Improving outcomes after esophagectomy: The impact of operative volume. J Surg Oncol 2005;92:262.

DePaula AI, Hashiba K, Ferreira EA, et al. Laparoscopic transhiatal esophagectomy. Surg Laparosc Endosc 1995;5:1.

Griffin SM, Shaw IH, Dresner SM. Early complications after Ivor Lewis subtotal esophagectomy with two-field lymphadenectomy: Risk factors and management. J Am Coll Surg 2002;194:285.

Hulscher JBF, van Sandick JW, de Boer AGEM, et al. Extended transthoracic resection compared with limited transhiatal resection for adenocarcinoma of the esophagus. N Engl J Med 2002;347:1662.

Koh P, Turnbull G, Attia E, et al. Functional assessment of the cervical esophagus after gastric transposition and cervical esophagogastrostomy. Eur J Cardiothorac Surg 2004;25:480.

Korst RJ, Rusch VW, Venkatraman E, et al. Proposed revision of the staging classification for esophageal cancer. J Thorac Cardiovasc Surg 1998;115:660.

Krasna MJ, Jiao X, Sonett JR, et al. Thoracoscopic and laparoscopic lymph node staging in esophageal cancer: Do clinicopathologic factors affect outcome? Ann Thoracic Surg 2002;73:1710.

Luketich JD, Alvelo-Rivera M, Buenaventura PO, et al. Minimally invasive esophagectomy: Outcomes in 222 patients. Ann Surg 2003;238:486.

Swanson SJ, Batriel HF, Bueno R, et al. Transthoracic esophagectomy with radical mediastinal and abdominal lymph node dissection and cervical esophagogastrostomy for esophageal carcinoma. Ann Thorac Surg 2001;72:1918.

Swanstrom LL, Hansen P. Laparoscopic total esophagectomy. Arch Surg 1997;132:943.

Urschel JD, Blewett CJ, Bennett WF, et al. Hand-sewn or stapled esophagogastric anastomosis after esophagectomy for cancer: Meta-analysis of randomized controlled trials. Dis Esoph 2001;14:212.

Visbal AL, Allen MS, Miller DL, et al. Ivor Lewis esophagogastrectomy for esophageal cancer. Ann Thorac Surg 2001;71:1803.

Wallace MB, Nietert PJ, Earle C, et al. An analysis of multiple staging management strategies for carcinoma of the esophagus: Computed tomography, endoscopic ultrasound, positron emission tomography, and thoracoscopy/laparoscopy. Ann Thorac Surg 2002;74:1026.

EDITOR'S COMMENTS

This chapter nicely complements the preceding chapter by pointing out similarities between the two approaches, differences in indication, and potential pitfalls and morbidity. What strikes home in both chapters is the importance of doing a total esophagectomy and recognizing that esophageal carcinoma, especially adenocarcinoma, may occur at multiple levels. In addition, the functional result achieved with a total esophagectomy and gastric transposition exceeds that attained with a partial esophagectomy. It does not make sense to perform an operation for an adenocarcinoma of the distal esophagus, with or without Barrett's mucosa, that leaves esophagus behind, and thus, the continued opportunity for reflux of gastric contents.

Several technical aspects described by the authors deserve comment. The standard "3-hole" esophagectomy, as described, utilizes an anterior thoracotomy with the patient supine with the right side slightly elevated. Thus, an anterior thoracotomy is being used to resect a posterior structure which is not an ideal situation. In my opinion, it is preferable to utilize a posterolateral thoracotomy when one feels that a thoracotomy is indicated. This requires the patient to be in full lateral decubitus position; a position and an incision that facilitates dissection of this posterior mediastinal structure. For bulky mid-esophageal lesions, it is preferable to start with the right thoracotomy, assure that the tumor is resectable, and completely mobilize the esophagus in the chest. Following chest closure, the patient is positioned supine and a laparotomy and neck incisions are made as they were for the transhiatal approach, except that the mediastinal portion has already been completed. The gastric remnant is brought up through the posterior mediastinum and an anastomosis constructed in the left neck. The authors do not express a preference for one anastomotic technique over another, but each surgeon should establish a technique that they feel comfortable and confident with.

The left thoracoabdominal incision has great utility for distal lesions, but in particular, for situations in which previous operations in the hiatus have been carried out. Such is the case for a patient with a failed Nissen fundoplication whom now requires esophagectomy. The patient should be in the full right lateral decubitus position, and the abdominal portion of the incision need not extend beyond the lateral border of the rectus muscle. Full access to the abdomen may be gained by this approach, but it is difficult to mobilize the duodenum or perform a gastric emptying procedure via this approach. However, the access provided to the re-do hilum is simply superb and outweighs any disadvantages. Closure of the costal margin is key to avoid the uncomfortable situation of overlapping edges that will certainly cause patients to complain.

Once again, this chapter serves to point out the importance of the ability to utilize one of a number of approaches to esophagectomy depending on the individual clinical situation encountered.

L.R.K.

19

Minimally Invasive Esophageal Procedures

Matthew J. Schuchert and James D. Luketich

Introduction

With the widespread development of minimally invasive surgical techniques and instrumentation, the last decade has witnessed a revolution in the video-assisted surgical approach to diseases of the esophagus. The continued challenge for the minimally invasive surgeon is to maintain the fundamental principles of esophageal surgery that have been established with decades of open experience while avoiding ill-advised shortcuts. The more complex the esophageal intervention, the more likely we are to see difficulty in reproducing the key technical steps of any given minimally invasive procedure. Although in most cases it is not the intent of the surgeon to perform a less than perfect operation, he or she may be prodded by reports from other centers, as well as by patient and referring physician opinions seeking good results from small incisions. Therefore, as we evolve toward a less invasive culture and embrace new technologies, it is important to continue to critically interpret and publish our results while adopting a thoughtful attitude toward accomplishing the best outcomes possible.

This chapter summarizes the role of minimally invasive surgery in the treatment of acquired shortening of the esophagus, giant paraesophageal hernias, and esophageal cancer. Although laparoscopic fundoplication represents one of the cornerstones of minimally invasive esophageal surgery, this topic is discussed in detail in Chapter 16 on antireflux procedures. Similarly, other advanced minimally invasive esophageal techniques, including myotomy with fundoplication for esophageal motility disorders, diverticulectomy, advanced endoscopic modalities, and palliative esophageal

procedures, are covered elsewhere in this book. The discussion of minimally invasive approaches highlighted in this chapter includes some of the published operative and short-term results, as well as a comparison to the comparable open procedures. In some cases, we report early results of minimally invasive procedures that are not yet comparable to our prior open experience. In some instances, this represents the effect of the learning curve, and in other cases may truly represent areas that have not yet achieved uniformly equal results compared to open surgical approaches. Long-term results for the majority of these procedures are either absent or only now becoming available. Very complex procedures such as the laparoscopic Collis gastroplasty, laparoscopic giant paraesophageal hernia repair, and minimally invasive esophagectomy are routinely being performed in only a limited number of specialized centers. Prospective trials will ultimately be required to objectively identify the benefits and limitations of these minimally invasive approaches.

Laparoscopic Collis Gastroplasty

Acquired Shortening of the Esophagus

Acquired shortening of the esophagus is a known sequela of complicated gastroesophageal reflux disease; however, the frequency and degree of its existence are controversial in the surgical community, although it is so clear in some cases that it is difficult to deny its existence (Fig. 19-1). However, in other cases it may be quite subtle, and arguably can be overcome in

a number of these instances by extensive esophageal dissection. We have noted it more commonly in the setting of ulcerative esophagitis, peptic strictures, and paraesophageal herniation and after failed antireflux operations. The proposed mechanism is the development of reflux-induced transmural inflammation leading to repeated cycles of injury and repair over time, which ultimately results in scarring and contraction of the esophagus and cephalad displacement of the gastroesophageal (GE) junction (Fig. 19-1). Such shortening can reduce or eliminate the ability to achieve adequate esophageal mobilization and length during fundoplication, contributing to a higher incidence of wrap slippage and failure.

The overall incidence of acquired shortening of the esophagus is unknown, and some authors question its very existence. In a review of the open and laparoscopic literature, the frequency of esophageal shortening ranges widely, from 60% to 0% in some laparoscopic series. Its prevalence is perhaps greatest in the setting of giant paraesophageal herniation, where the GE junction is chronically displaced within the mediastinum in as many as 77% to 100% of patients. Objective results on esophageal length have been measured between the manometrically defined upper and lower esophageal sphincters. In normal patients, or in those with a simple hiatal hernia, this length is approximately 20 cm; in the setting of giant paraesophageal hernias it is only 15 cm.

Unrecognized esophageal shortening is potentially a major contributor in the development of recurrent herniation, which is the most common cause of fundoplication failure. It is also a primary explanation for a "slipped" Nissen fundoplication. In many such instances the initial repair

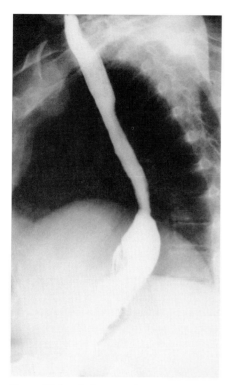

Figure 19-1. Barium esophagram demonstrating acquired shortening of the esophagus.

is constructed around proximal tubularized stomach rather than the terminal esophagus. Although there is no ideal method of firmly establishing the presence of a shortened esophagus, the combination of radiographic studies (barium swallow) and endoscopic findings will alert the surgeon to situations in which esophageal shortening is likely. Large hiatal hernias (>5 cm) that fail to reduce during barium roentgenography, as well as esophageal strictures, are most likely associated with esophageal shortening. Adequate intraoperative assessment of the location of the true gastroesophageal junction requires complete dissection of the esophagogastric fat pad overlying the junction. Many surgeons do not routinely do this. It should also be kept in mind that the presence of pneumoperitoneum elevates the diaphragm, which could provide the false impression that an adequate length of intra-abdominal esophagus is present. Similarly, downward retraction via a Penrose drain looped around the GE junction, as well as the downward pressure produced by the presence of a bougie, can provide the illusion of an additional 2 cm to 3 cm of intra-abdominal length.

When a shortened esophagus is encountered, maximal mobilization of the distal esophagus should be performed. This may be accomplished most readily via an open

thoracotomy where direct access to the entire intrathoracic esophagus may lend itself well to lengthy mobilization. In any case, if a tension-free 2-cm to 3-cm segment of intra-abdominal esophagus cannot be obtained with esophageal dissection, then an esophageal-lengthening procedure should be considered.

Many treatment options have been proposed for the management of esophageal shortening, including esophagopexy, esophagectomy, transthoracic fundoplication, and lengthening procedures. Hill has long recommended an esophagogastropexy (Hill procedure) as a treatment for all patients with gastroesophageal reflux disease (GERD), including those with esophageal shortening. Although the reported results are excellent, this approach has failed to obtain widespread acceptance due to its perceived complexity. On occasion, total esophagectomy with gastric pull-up or a transthoracic approach may be the best option for a severely damaged, dysfunctional esophagus. However, these approaches are typically reserved for extremely severe or recalcitrant cases. A circular esophagomyotomy to promote esophageal length in the setting of fundoplication has been used by some surgeons. This method has failed to achieve clinical acceptance because of its technical difficulty, perceived patient risk, and compromise of distal esophageal motility.

Originally described by J. L. Collis in 1957, the Collis gastroplasty creates a tube of neo-esophagus using the gastric cardia and fundus, allowing reduction of the GE junction below the diaphragm and recreation of the angle of His. This neo-esophagus remains in an intra-abdominal location without tension, promoting the reconstructing of a physiologic antireflux barrier. However, a Collis gastroplasty alone does not consistently achieve control of reflux without an associated wrap. Pearson and colleagues were the first to describe a transthoracic Collis-Belsey combination for patients with a shortened esophagus, highlighting the importance of restoring the GE junction to an intra-abdominal position without undue tension. The transthoracic approach allows complete mobilization of the esophagus and efficient repair of the diaphragmatic hiatal defect while providing adequate exposure of the proximal stomach for fundoplication. The long-term control of reflux may be problematic with a Collis-Belsey procedure, and a transthoracic Collis-Nissen procedure may provide an alternative. The Collis-Belsey and Collis-Nissen procedures have traditionally been performed through the chest

due to the difficulty in achieving complete esophageal mobilization as well assessing proximal esophageal tension through an abdominal incision. A Collis-Nissen procedure using gastrointestinal stapling devices has gradually become the preferred approach for esophageal lengthening while avoiding the attendant complications of thoracotomy. With the advent of laparoscopy, the traditional transabdominal and transthoracic approaches, have, in our opinion, been supplanted by minimally invasive techniques. If an adequate length of tension-free intra-abdominal esophagus cannot be obtained with extensive mobilization, additional intra-abdominal esophageal length can be attained with a Collis or wedge gastroplasty in conjunction with a Nissen fundoplication. Similar to the open approach, the goal of a laparoscopic gastroplasty is to create a 2-cm to 3-cm segment of intra-abdominal neo-esophagus only if the native esophagus fails to achieve this goal after extensive mobilization. The exact length of the Collis segment is dependent on where the true GE junction lies after complete mobilization; in some cases it may be very short.

A careful preoperative assessment is performed to identify those patients at risk for esophageal shortening. Patients with a long history of GERD or those who develop recurrent symptoms after a failed antireflux operation are at high risk for esophageal shortening. Barium esophagography will identify patients with large hiatal or giant paraesophageal hernias as well as those with strictures, all of which suggest the likelihood of a shortened esophagus. Esophagoscopy typically reveals esophagitis (possibly Barrett's), strictures, and displacement of the GE junction not uncommonly >5 cm above the diaphragmatic hiatus. Manometry frequently documents a hypotensive lower esophageal sphincter with variable degrees of esophageal motility dysmotility.

Technique: Laparoscopic Collis Gastroplasty

The anesthetized patient is placed in a comfortable supine position. We recommend routinely performing on-table upper endoscopy to gain detailed information regarding the endoluminal appearance of the esophagus and stomach, the presence and extent of ulcers, strictures, Barrett's esophagus, and/or hiatal hernia. Care is taken to minimize insufflation so as not to overdistend the stomach and small bowel. A urinary catheter is inserted to decompress the bladder. Subcutaneous heparin is

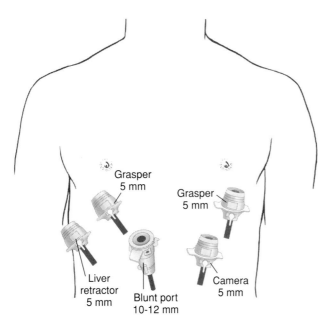

Figure 19-2. Standard port placement for laparoscopic Nissen fundoplication with Collis gastroplasty.

administered, and inflatable compression stockings are worn on the lower extremities for perioperative deep venous thrombosis prophylaxis. Many surgeons prefer either the lithotomy or "inverted-Y" position. We favor the standard supine position, with the surgeon standing to the patient's right and the first assistant standing to the patient's left. The patient is placed in a steep reverse-Trendelenburg position. Video monitors are positioned on either side of the head of the table. Access to the abdomen is achieved via a direct cut-down technique or with a Veress needle. With a closed (Veress) technique, a 2-mm skin incision is made at the umbilicus or just inferior to the left costal margin. A Veress needle is then inserted into the abdominal cavity. Two pops should be heard as the needle penetrates the fascial layers. Before insufflation, the needle position should be confirmed with the drop test. We prefer to perform a direct, open cut-down approach to minimize the risk of inadvertent injury to the abdominal contents. This approach is particularly useful in patients with prior abdominal surgery, who may have adhesions and distorted anatomy.

Our preferred port placement is demonstrated in Fig. 19-2. We begin with placement of a 10-mm blunt port through the right rectus muscle via direct cut-down technique, at a level near the midpoint between the umbilicus and the xiphoid. This port may be positioned superiorly in the setting of larger hiatal hernias, where extensive mediastinal dissection is anticipated. Care is taken to preserve the rectus musculature, gently spreading with blunt retractors rather than dividing with electrocautery. This simple step will help to minimize delayed portsite hernias. After insufflation with carbon dioxide to a pressure of 15 mm Hg, a 5-mm 30-degree camera is used for visualization. A 5-mm port is then placed in the mid-clavicular line just inferior to the left costal margin. A second 5-mm port is placed through the left rectus, three to four fingerbreadths to the left of the initial 10-mm port. A third 5-mm port is placed along the right costal margin toward the right shoulder. A liver retractor is then introduced through a 5-mm port positioned just inferior to the right costal margin in the mid-axillary line (Fig. 19-2). Attachment to a table-mounted mechanical arm facilitates liver retraction. The patient is then placed into steep reverse-Trendelenburg (Fowler) position, allowing gravity to assist in the displacement of the bowel and stomach from the diaphragm. A toothed, noncrushing atraumatic grasper (Snowden-Pencer, Tucker, Georgia) is used in the surgeon's left hand, and the harmonic scalpel (Ultracision, Inc., US Surgical, or similar) is used in the right hand. The 30-degree laparoscopic camera is positioned in the assistant's left hand to provide enhanced visualization of the retrogastric and retroesophageal structures. The gastrohepatic omentum is then opened, and the caudate lobe of the liver is exposed. An aberrant left hepatic artery branch arising from the left gastric artery may be present in up to 25% of patients, and should be avoided if possible, although many are small and can be divided with little consequence. The right crus is exposed, and care is taken to preserve the peritoneal lining over both crura. The phrenoesophageal ligament is divided with the autosonic shears or harmonic scalpel along its anterior border, care being taken to identify and preserve the anterior vagus nerve. The GE junction and distal esophagus are circumferentially mobilized, frequently as high as the level of the camera. The esophageal fat pad is then carefully reflected to the right of the esophagus, with care being taken to identify and preserve the nearby anterior vagus nerve. If the GE junction does not remain below the diaphragmatic hiatus with an adequate segment of tension-free intra-abdominal esophagus (ideally 2 cm to 3 cm), a Collis gastroplasty is performed prior to fundoplication. An esophageal bougie is placed into the stomach and is aligned along the lesser curvature (Fig. 19-3A). The diameter of the bougie is determined by the patient's history, size, and esophageal manometry results. Assuming adequate motility, a 54-F bougie is typically employed. A large, tapered needle attached to a No. 2 paracostal Vicryl suture is straightened and secured to the point of a 21 mm EEA stapler anvil. At a level corresponding to the desired point of esophageal lengthening, the needle is then passed anteriorly through the stomach immediately adjacent to the bougie (Fig. 19-3B). The needle serves as a guide for the passage of the anvil, which is carefully pulled through the posterior and anterior stomach walls, respectively. It is important to maintain outward and downward traction on the gastric fundus during this maneuver to optimize positioning of the anvil. Electrocautery can be employed sparingly to assist in passage of the anvil tip. The EEA stapler is then inserted through the right paramedian 10-mm port and is attached to the anvil. The EEA stapler is fired, creating a circular defect in the stomach wall (Fig. 19-4). The Endo GIA II stapler (U.S. Surgical Corp., Norwalk, CT) is then deployed in a cephalad direction, positioned snugly against the bougie, allowing the creation of the desired length of tension-free, intra-abdominal neo-esophagus (Fig. 19-5). The staple line is carefully inspected for leaks by direct visualization and endoscopic insufflation. The neo-esophagus is then wrapped by the mobilized gastric fundus, achieving a 2-cm to 3-cm floppy Collis-Nissen fundoplication

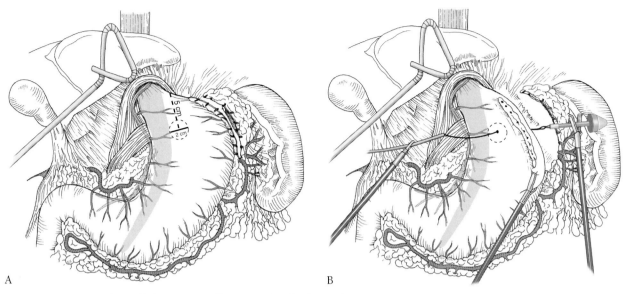

Figure 19-3.   Position of bougie **(A)** and delivery of EEA anvil **(B)** during Collis gastroplasty.

(Fig. 19-6). The bougie is then removed, and a nasogastric tube is inserted under direct visualization. The crura are then reapproximated posteriorly as described for Nissen fundoplication.

The nasogastric tube is typically removed on postoperative day 1, and a barium swallow is performed to rule out leak and/or obstruction. If the barium study demonstrates good passage of contrast without leakage, the patients are started on clear liquids. Patients are usually discharged to home on postoperative day 1 or 2 after receiving nutritional counseling.

Results

Decades of experience with open fundoplications have identified several key principles essential for successful surgical outcomes in the treatment of chronic GERD. Among the most important include thorough preoperative testing, routine division of the short gastric vessels, closure of the crura, and the creation of a tension-free fundoplication while maintaining 2 cm to 3 cm of intra-abdominal esophagus. The defining feature of a tension-free hiatal hernia repair is the recognition and proper treat-

ment of an intrinsically shortened esophagus. Failure to recognize or treat a shortened esophagus can lead to hiatal disruption and wrap slippage, accounting for up to one third of surgical failures after open or laparoscopic fundoplication. Excellent long-term results have been achieved in patients undergoing open surgery for complicated gastroesophageal reflux disease when the Collis gastroplasty is performed with a partial or complete fundoplication. More recently, minimally invasive techniques have been developed that duplicate the open results, with >90% control of reflux symptoms. A potential advantage of a thoracoscopic as opposed to laparoscopic approach is that the stapler can be angled through the chest and placed flush against the esophageal bougie prior to firing, closely approximating the orientation of the open procedure. The disadvantage of this approach is the requirement for thoracic incisions, which produce increased pain, decreased postoperative respiratory function, and the requirement for chest tube drainage.

The EEA/GIA technique (as outlined here) done via laparoscopy obviates the need for thoracoscopy or thoracotomy. In the largest series of laparoscopic Collis-Nissen fundoplications to date, we reported on 50 consecutive patients who underwent Collis-Nissen antireflux surgery at the University of Pittsburgh. Subjective follow-up results were good to excellent in 96% of patients. There were no mortalities, and the median hospital stay was 3 days. Complications of the laparoscopic Collis procedure included dysphagia, staple-line leaks, and pneumothorax. In this series, five (10%)

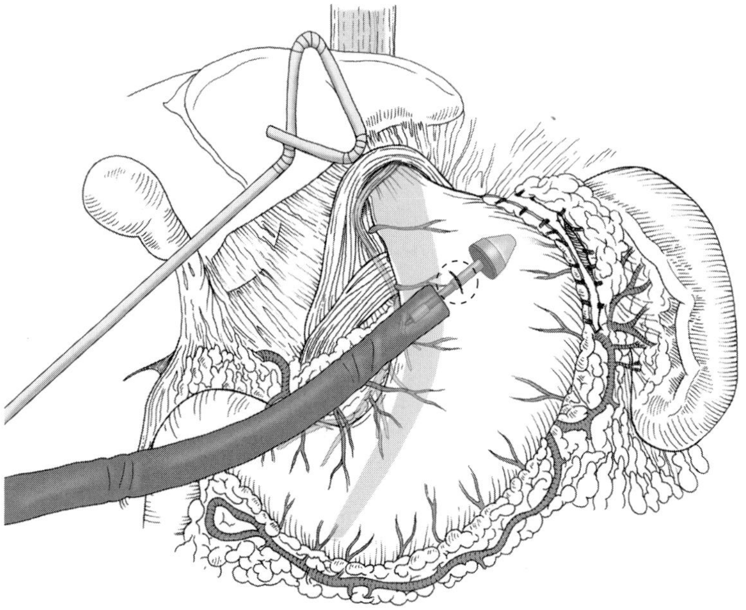

Figure 19-4.   Creation of circular gastric staple line with a 21-mm EEA stapler.

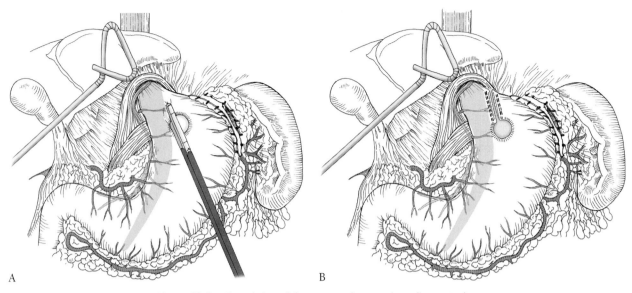

Figure 19-5. Completion of the neo-esophagus using a linear stapler.

intraoperative complications occurred: one vagus nerve injury and four pneumothoraces. There were four (8%) major postoperative complications (two pulmonary emboli (PEs) and two staple-line leaks). The control of reflux symptoms and the low complication rate compare favorably with published open series.

Several preoperative clinical features have been identified that have been found to independently predict the need for a Collis gastroplasty. These include the presence of a stricture, paraesophageal hernia, or Barrett's

esophagus and the need for re-do antireflux surgery; all are independently associated with the need for gastroplasty. Theoretical concerns regarding the complications of Collis gastroplasty have been raised. Staple-line leaks have been reported, although their incidence is <2% in both the open and larger laparoscopic series. A second concern arises from the potential for impaired esophageal motility of the neo-esophageal segment. This immotile segment may be at risk for dilation and may play a role in the development of postoperative dysphagia, al-

though this theoretical relationship has not been clearly established in the open or laparoscopic literature. An additional concern is the disposition of a segment of gastric mucosa proximal to the newly created high-pressure zone.

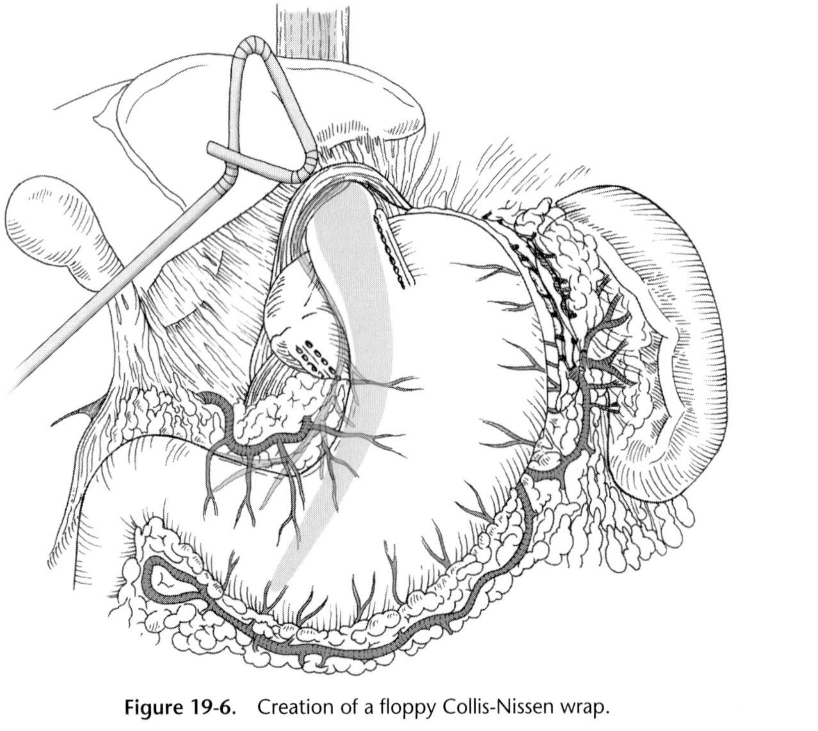

Several authors advocate an extended mediastinal dissection as an alternative to gastroplasty in the treatment of patients with esophageal shortening, claiming that in the majority of instances meticulous esophageal mobilization provides adequate intra-abdominal length for a tension-free fundoplication. In certain hands, overall outcome and failure rates may be equivalent to those achieved with a Collis gastroplasty.

Laparoscopic antireflux procedures have become increasing popular and prevalent and are being performed by an ever-increasing number of practitioners. This will undoubtedly increase the number of patients with a short esophagus who are referred for surgical treatment. The Collis-Nissen procedure has an established excellent long-term success rate for this complex problem. With the development and refinement of laparoscopic Collis techniques, conversion to a laparotomy or a thoracotomy when a short esophagus is encountered is no longer necessary. Although the creation of a Collis segment can be viewed as a compromise in the surgical correction of hiatal hernias and refractory GERD, the addition of a laparoscopic Collis gastroplasty during Nissen fundoplication provides an important tool for the management of patients with acquired shortening of the esophagus, allowing the creation of a tension-free

Figure 19-6. Creation of a floppy Collis-Nissen wrap.

intra-abdominal segment of neo-esophagus that may enhance the results of fundoplication.

Giant Paraesophageal Hernia Repair

Paraesophageal hernias represent a subtype of hiatal hernia. The most common form of hiatal hernia is the simple or sliding (type I) hiatal hernia (95%), in which the GE junction migrates above the diaphragmatic hiatus, frequently associated with incompetence of the lower esophageal sphincter. The remaining forms of hiatal hernia can be classified as paraesophageal hernias (5%). Type II paraesophageal hernias are characterized by the position of the GE junction below the diaphragm, with a portion of the fundus and greater curvature migrating through a hiatal defect alongside the esophagus. This type of hernia is rare, with a reported prevalence of only 3% among all paraesophageal hernias. In type III paraesophageal hernias, both the GE junction and the fundus protrude through a hiatal defect (Fig. 19-7). Type IV hernias are defined by herniation of the entire stomach, omentum, and/or transverse colon into the mediastinum. The characteristic anatomic defects of paraesophageal hernias include enlargement of the diaphragmatic hiatus and abnormal laxity of the gastrosplenic and gastrocolic ligaments, allowing migration of the stomach (and other abdominal contents) into the chest. Giant

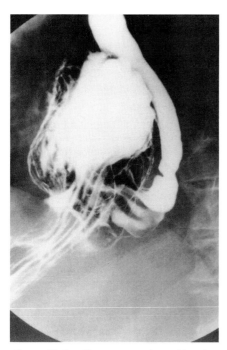

Figure 19-7. Giant paraesophageal hernia.

paraesophageal hernias are defined by the presence of greater than one third of the stomach within the chest.

The incidence of paraesophageal hernias is unknown. It is estimated that they make up 3% to 15% of all hiatal hernias, producing an estimated incidence of 15 to 45 per 100,000 individuals within the general population. Symptoms of paraesophageal hernia frequently include those found in GERD (e.g., heartburn, regurgitation, etc.). Chest pain (especially postprandial) is a common finding and is frequently mistaken for anginal symptoms. Postprandial distress, nausea, bloating, and anemia are also commonly encountered. A relatively asymptomatic but insidious symptom is occult gastrointestinal bleeding. Anemia is reported in 20% to 30% of patients with paraesophageal hernias in published series, but the rate of blood loss is slow and rarely is associated with hemodynamic compromise. A significant fraction of patients with paraesophageal hernia are asymptomatic or complain of only minor symptoms. The exact proportion of such patients is difficult to estimate for obvious reasons. Interestingly, it has been estimated that up to 89% of patients denying symptoms will actually describe some symptoms when questioned carefully.

Symptoms can be progressive, however, and can result in catastrophic complications with nonsurgical management. Mortality from strangulation may be greater than 50%, depending on the patient's age and the delay in diagnosis. This has led many to argue that symptomatology is not a reliable predictor of who might progress to acute complications, and that elective surgery should be performed on most patients with a giant paraesophageal hernia, in particular those with organoaxial rotation diagnosed on barium esophagram. Prompt elective repair is thus recommended after diagnosis to avoid the development of such complications. When the repair is performed electively, excellent control of symptoms (>90%) and a death rate of <1% to 2% can be achieved.

Despite the foregoing observations, the beliefs held by surgeons are still largely based on small patient series and anecdotal case reports. There is little doubt that patients presenting with obstructive symptoms, bleeding, or both should undergo elective hernia repair. However, surgical correction of asymptomatic or minimally symptomatic paraesophageal hernias is controversial. Recent studies suggest that asymptomatic patients have an 85% annual probability of remaining asymptomatic. This implies that about 1 in 6 patients will develop new symptoms, which can then be

treated with elective repair. The probability that a patient's initial presentation would require an emergency operation has been estimated to be only 1% per year. Although mortality of an emergency operation has been reported as high as 50%, a pooled analysis of the largest series demonstrated an aggregate operative mortality rate of 17%. In a larger analysis of a nationwide database, the mortality rate for emergency operation for paraesophageal hernia ($n = 1,035$) in 1997 was only 5.4%. Thus, for a 65-year-old asymptomatic patient, who has an 18% lifetime risk of developing life-threatening symptoms (1% per year) requiring emergency surgery (5.4% mortality), the overall lifetime risk of death with observation is approximately 1%, comparable to the expected 1% to 2% mortality of elective repair. Decision-analysis models have failed to demonstrate a gain in quality-adjusted life expectancy with elective laparoscopic repair of asymptomatic paraesophageal hernias when compared with watchful waiting.

When symptoms arise, the only effective treatment of paraesophageal hernias is surgical repair. The surgical technique involves reduction of the herniated contents back into the abdomen, excision of the hernia sac, and closure of the hiatal defect. These procedures can be performed transthoracically, transabdominally, or laparoscopically. In extremely high-risk patients with minimal symptoms, an anterior gastropexy can be performed to help prevent the development of incarceration or organoaxial volvulus. In the absence of reflux symptoms, the need to perform an antireflux procedure is debatable. However, up to 60% of patients with type III hernias have also been shown to have hypotensive lower esophageal sphincter (LES) pressures and abnormal 24-hour pH monitoring studies. Such findings support the routine performance of an antireflux procedure with paraesophageal hernia repair. The use of partial (Dor, Toupet) or complete (Nissen) wraps has been reported, each with good results. The choice of wrap is determined by the individual patient's underlying anatomy, symptom complex, and esophageal motility and surgeon preference.

Traditionally, repair of a giant paraesophageal hernia (GPEH) has been performed through an open laparotomy or thoracotomy. Increasingly, repair of GPEH is being performed using minimally invasive techniques. Preoperative assessment includes a barium esophagram that ordinarily establishes the diagnosis (Fig. 19-7). Upper endoscopy allows assessment of the gastric anatomy as well as the extent of mucosal injury. Esophageal manometry and 24-hour

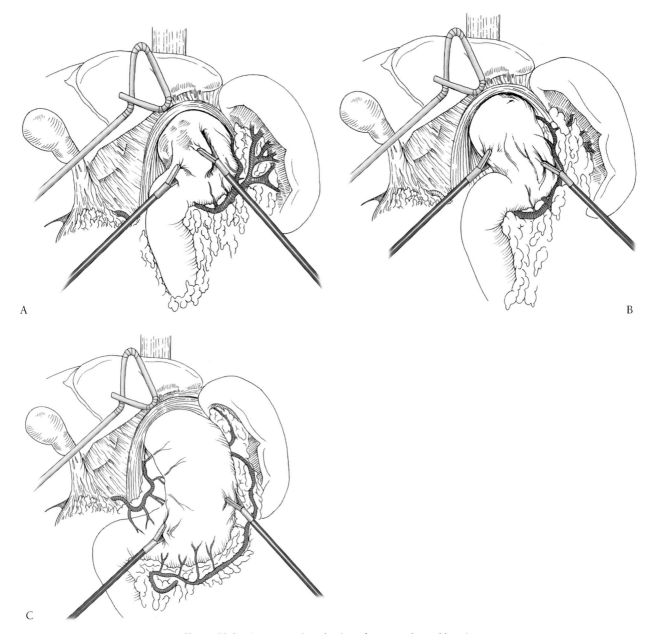

Figure 19-8. Laparoscopic reduction of paraesophageal hernia.

pH studies are not routinely performed because the degree of anatomic distortion frequently interferes with the reliable performance of these studies.

Technique: Giant Paraesophageal Hernia Repair

Standard laparoscopic port placement is used as shown in Fig. 19-2. The abdominal port incisions can be shifted slightly cephalad in the case of a giant paraesophageal hernia to facilitate ease of mediastinal dissection. The left lateral segment of the liver is retracted anteriorly with a 5-mm flexible retractor (Snowden Pencer, Genzyme, Tucker,

GA) and secured to a stationary holding device (Mediflex, Islanda, NY). After exposure, the herniated stomach is reduced back into the abdomen using atraumatic graspers (Snowden Pencer) in a hand-over-hand fashion (Fig. 19-8). Dissection is begun by inverting the mediastinal hernia sac and pulling it back into the abdomen. The crural reflection of the sac is then incised, and the flimsy mediastinal attachments to the sac are carefully taken down by the ultrasonic shears (Fig. 19-9). Care is taken to identify and preserve the proximal anterior and posterior vagus nerves during this portion of the dissection. Similarly, the adjacent pleura must be identified and swept later-

ally away from the plane of dissection. The surgeon and the anesthesiologist must communicate closely during this portion of the procedure because changes in blood pressure or inspiratory pressures may indicate the development of a tension pneumothorax, which can be readily treated by placement of a pigtail catheter or a chest tube. The complete dissection and reduction of the hernia sac is a critical component of successful surgery for giant paraesophageal hernias. The gastrohepatic ligament is then divided just medial to the lesser curvature of the stomach using the harmonic scalpel (Ethicon, Cincinnati, OH) or the ultrasonic shears (U.S. Surgical Corp, Norwalk, CT).

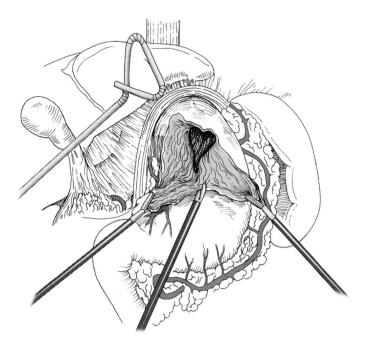

Figure 19-9.   Excision of paraesophageal hernia sac.

The right crus of the diaphragm is subsequently exposed. The dissection is carried anteriorly over the surface of the esophagus, with care being taken to identify and preserve the anterior vagus nerve. Inferior traction on the gastric fundus and epiphrenic fat pad is then performed to allow exposure of the anterior portion of the left crus. A retrogastric/retroesophageal window is then created to expose the posterior portion

of the left crus. At this point, division of the short gastric vessels is performed.

Careful identification of the gastroesophageal junction after fat pad excision frequently reveals a shortened esophagus in the setting of a GPEH. The esophageal fat pad is carefully and completely mobilized medially, sweeping the anterior vagus to the right of the esophagus (Fig. 19-10). The distal esophagus is then mobilized at the level of

the diaphragmatic hiatus circumferentially to determine whether esophageal shortening is present. The surgeon then assesses for tension by pulling on the stomach caudally once the gastroesophageal junction has been mobilized. If the GE junction does not remain below the diaphragmatic hiatus with an adequate segment of tension-free intra-abdominal esophagus (ideally 2 cm to 3 cm), a Collis gastroplasty is then performed prior to fundoplication (see the prior discussion of the Collis gastroplasty). Care is taken to cover the point of overlap of the EEA circular staple line and the Endo GIA II staple line with the gastric wrap because this represents the weak point of the neo-esophageal staple line. The crura are reapproximated posteriorly to complete the surgical procedure as outlined previously. In most cases the crura are approximated primarily without excess tension. In unusual cases of an excessively large defect, a patch of Gore-Tex (W. L. Gore, Flagstaff, AZ) or Surgisis (Cook, West Lafayette, IN) is used to reinforce the closure. A gastrostomy or a gastropexy is not routinely performed, although this technique can be useful after hernia reduction in patients unfit for the definitive conventional repair. Before closing, endoscopy is routinely performed with intraluminal insufflation to rule out esophageal or gastric leaks. A nasogastric tube is placed under laparoscopic guidance. After surgery, the nasogastric tube is typically removed on postoperative day 1, and a barium swallow is obtained to evaluate the repair and verify the absence of a leak. If no leak is present, clear liquids are started. If a clear liquid diet is tolerated, the patient is usually discharged to home on postoperative day 2. Advancement to a soft diet occurs over the subsequent 1 to 2 weeks.

Results

Although laparoscopic Nissen fundoplication has become a well-established procedure in the treatment of GERD, laparoscopic management of giant paraesophageal hernias is somewhat controversial. Although early studies of laparoscopic repair of GPEH were promising, concerns have arisen about the safety and efficacy of a minimally invasive approach in handling this complex problem. Dahlberg reported the Mayo clinic experience in 37 patients undergoing laparoscopic repair of GPEH. Successful repair was accomplished laparoscopically in 35 of the 37 patients. Intraoperative complications included two splenic injuries and one crural tear. Postoperatively, there were two cases of esophageal leak and one

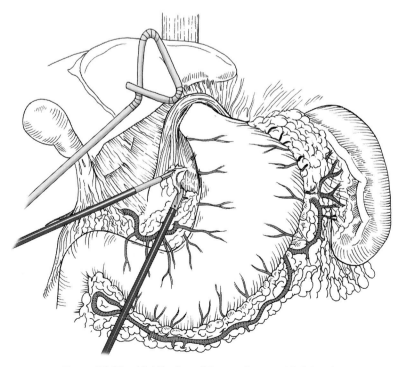

Figure 19-10.   Mobilization of the esophagogastric fat pad.

small-bowel obstruction at a port site. Mortality was 5.4%. In short-term follow-up, 4 of 37 patients (12.9%) developed recurrent paraesophageal herniation. It was concluded that laparoscopic repair of giant paraesophageal hernia is a technically challenging operation associated with significant morbidity and mortality. Similar results were obtained in a series of 60 patients by Weichman. In this series, reoperation for recurrent herniation occurred in 5.5% of patients, with an associated 1.9% mortality. This study also concluded that laparoscopic repair of GPEH is a technically challenging procedure, but that with increasing experience and technical refinements, results could approximate those of the open approach.

As experience with advanced laparoscopic techniques has developed, improved results after laparoscopic repair of giant paraesophageal hernias have been noted.

We reported on the outcome of 100 consecutive laparoscopic repairs of giant PEH from July 1995 to February 2000. The median surgical time was 3.67 hours (range 2.0 to 11.5 hours). The median length of stay was 2 days. Complete sac removal and crural repair was performed in all patients. The crural repair was primary in 96 patients; 4 had a mesh repair. All but 1 of the patients underwent an antireflux procedure. There were 72 Nissen procedures and 27 Collis-Nissen fundoplications. There were 3 conversions to open procedures (2 cases of severe adhesions, and inability to reduce the stomach safely in 1 patient). Intraoperative complications included pneumothorax requiring a chest tube ($n = 4$), esophageal perforation ($n = 5$), and gastric perforation ($n = 3$). The perforations were small and easily repaired laparoscopically. The 30-day mortality was zero. In a separate report, we demonstrated that laparoscopic repair of moderately sized and giant paraesophageal hernias resulted in less blood loss, shorter intensive care unit stays, faster recovery from ileus, and shorter length of hospital stay when compared with patients undergoing open repair.

In the largest series reported to date, we updated the University of Pittsburgh experience in the laparoscopic repair of 203 consecutive giant paraesophageal hernias. Median follow-up was 18 months. The most common symptoms included heartburn (47%), dysphagia (35%), epigastric pain (26%), and vomiting (23%). Laparoscopic procedures included 69 Nissens, 112 Collis-Nissens, and 19 other procedures. Only 3 patients were converted to open

nonurgently secondary to adhesions. Median length of stay was 3 days. Complications (minor or major) occurred in 57 of 203 patients (28%). There were 6 postoperative esophageal leaks (3%) and only 1 death. Five patients (2.5%) required reoperation for recurrent hiatal hernia. Good to excellent results were obtained in 92% of patients based on postoperative questionnaire. The mean postoperative GERD Health-Related Quality-of-Life score was 2.4 (scale 0 to 45; 0 = no symptoms, 45 = worst).

As the experience with antireflux surgery in the setting of GPEH has increased, we have come to recognize the important role of esophageal shortening in this condition. As described earlier, 75% to 90% of patients with true GPEH will have a GE junction located well above the diaphragmatic hiatus. In addition, proper assessment of esophageal length can be tricky because there is a tendency to overestimate the intra-abdominal length of the esophagus because of the diaphragmatic elevation caused by the pneumoperitoneum as well as the downward traction that is applied to the stomach. On the basis of such results, an esophageal-lengthening procedure should be strongly considered during the repair of GPEH. As such, the rate of Collis gastroplasties has tripled from 27 per 100, as reported in our initial series, to 86 per 103. In total, 113 patients (56%) received a Collis gastroplasty in the University of Pittsburgh series.

In addition to esophageal lengthening, proper reconstruction of the hiatal defect is also critical to the long-term success of the repair. In the majority of patients the crura can be approximated primarily without undue tension. In most open series, however, a recurrence rate of up to 10% can be seen. The radiographic recurrence rate has been reported to be higher using a laparoscopic approach, ranging from 23% to 42%. Crural breakdown and wrap migration has been implicated in up to two thirds of these failures. Failure rates are particularly prominent when the hiatal defect exceeds 5 cm. The crura may be quite attenuated and not hold sutures well. Faced with this situation, the surgeon has several options. One possibility is the use of a relaxing incision in the diaphragm that reduces the tension at the level of the hiatus. The relaxing incision is then closed with a polytetrafluoroethylene patch. This approach serves to reduce tension during approximation of the hiatus. The second approach, advocated by several authors, is mesh cruroplasty. Mesh may be used to buttress the crural muscle so that sutures do not tear through or to actually serve as a patch to achieve closure of the

hiatus. Several authors have reported that the use of mesh lowers recurrence when compared with nonmesh techniques. Longer-term analysis will be necessary to determine the overall efficacy of this approach.

In summary, laparoscopic repair of GPEH is feasible, safe, and effective in centers with extensive experience in minimally invasive esophageal surgery. The laparoscopic approach should adhere to the principles established in open series: complete stomach reduction, complete hernia sac excision, careful assessment for esophageal shortening, and crural repair. Liberal use of the Collis gastroplasty may reduce the incidence of recurrent herniation and improve long-term functional results. Long-term follow-up will be necessary to confirm the durability of these laparoscopic techniques.

Minimally Invasive Esophagectomy

Minimally invasive esophagectomy (MIE) is a complex and technically challenging procedure that is performed in only a few medical centers worldwide. Open esophagectomy approaches (e.g., transhiatal, Ivor Lewis) remain the standard approach in most medical centers. These operations, however, are associated with significant morbidity and mortality rates (in the range of 6% to 7%) even in experienced centers.

The earliest descriptions of MIE involved a combination of open surgery with either thoracoscopy or laparoscopy. There have been multiple subsequent reports of esophagectomy for cancer performed by thoracoscopy and open laparotomy. These studies demonstrated the feasibility of thoracoscopic-assisted esophagectomy, but the overall benefit was not well established.

The most popular minimally invasive approaches to esophageal resection are hybrid approaches that combine elements of thoracoscopy or laparoscopy with open techniques. The most widely practiced variant is the "thoracoscopic esophagectomy," which utilizes thoracoscopy to achieve esophageal mobilization in combination with standard laparotomy and cervical incisions for the completion of the esophagectomy. Other approaches include "lap-assisted esophagectomy," in which laparoscopy is used for mobilization and preparation of the gastric tube, as well as "hand-assisted laparoscopic transhiatal esophagectomy," which introduces a hand port to assist with mediastinal mobilization during transhiatal esophagectomy (THE). Most recently, robotic video-assisted thoracoscopic surgery/laparotomy approaches have been developed using the da Vinci operating robot.

Totally minimally invasive esophagectomy (total MIE) techniques have been developed using thoracoscopy and/or laparoscopy exclusively. The most popular totally minimally invasive approaches to esophagectomy are the Ivor Lewis and three-hole MIE (see later discussion). Which minimally invasive approach is best remains to be determined. Until further randomized data become available, the chosen approach should be based on tumor and patient characteristics, as well as the surgeon's personal preference and expertise.

The first totally laparoscopic esophagectomy at the University of Pittsburgh was performed in 1996. This initial approach has evolved into one combining thoracoscopy and laparoscopy for several reasons. Laparoscopic esophageal mobilization can be tedious and cumbersome via the completely laparoscopic approach. In addition, visualization of paraesophageal structures (such as the inferior pulmonary vein and the mainstem bronchi) and the performance of mediastinal lymph node dissection can be very limited when using an exclusively transabdominal approach. In the first 77 patients at the University of Pittsburgh undergoing MIE, a combined thoracoscopic/laparoscopic approach was used in the majority, achieving a median length of hospital stay of 7 days and a stage-specific survival similar to or better than open surgery results. The authors have performed MIE on >500 patients with high-grade dysplasia or cancer. When MIE is compared to open approaches, a shorter hospital stay, less morbidity, and similar operative times are noted. In some centers, a complete thoracoscopic/laparoscopic approach is not feasible or preferred, and the use of hand-assisted techniques in the approach to esophagectomy has been explored. Though offering some potential advantage in cases in which organ integrity is important, a hand inserted near the esophageal hiatus or into the mediastinum frequently obscures the view and is generally unnecessary during MIE.

MIE should be performed by surgeons who have extensive experience in minimally invasive esophageal surgery. Patients must be deemed fit for operation and must have resectable lesions as characterized by endoscopic ultrasound and/or computed tomography (CT). During the early portion of the learning curve, surgeons should consider performing surgery in patients who have high-grade dysplasia, small tumors, a favorable body habitus, and minimal or no prior abdominal or thoracic surgery. As experience increases, we have found that previous abdominal or thoracic surgery and preoperative chemoradiation are not contraindications to a minimally invasive approach for either staging or resection of esophageal cancer.

Technique: Minimally Invasive Esophagectomy

The thoracoscopic/laparoscopic esophagectomy performed at the University of Pittsburgh will be highlighted here.

The procedure is begun with an on-table esophagogastroduodenoscopy (EGD) to assess the tumor's location, as well as the suitability of the gastric conduit for reconstruction. If the EGD, endoscopic ultrasound (EUS) or CT scan findings suggest gastric extension, T4 local invasion, or possible metastases, we perform a staging laparoscopy, a thoracoscopy, or both. The patient is intubated with a double-lumen tube to permit single-lung ventilation and is placed in the left lateral decubitus position. With the right lung collapsed, four thoracoscopic ports are introduced (Fig. 19-11). The camera port (30 degrees, 10 mm) is placed at the seventh-eighth intercostal space slightly anterior to the midaxillary line. A 5-mm port is placed at the eighth or ninth intercostals space 2 cm posterior to the posterior axillary line for the ultrasonic coagulating shears (U.S. Surgical Corp., Norwalk, CT). A 10-mm port is then placed in the anterior axillary line at the level of the fourth intercostal space and is used for placement of a fan retractor to assist with anteromedial lung reflection and exposure of the esophageal bed. The last 5-mm port is placed posterior to the tip of the scapula. In most cases, a retracting suture (0-Surgidac; U.S. Surgical Corp.,

Norwalk, CT), is placed in the central tendon of the diaphragm and brought out of the inferior anterior chest wall through a 1-mm skin nick using the Endo-Close device (U.S. Surgical Corp., Norwalk, CT). This traction suture allows downward retraction on the diaphragm without the need for providing manual retraction and provides excellent exposure of the distal esophagus at the level of the diaphragm.

Next, the inferior pulmonary ligament is divided. The mediastinal pleura overlying the esophagus is divided, and the entire thoracic esophagus is exposed. The authors generally choose a plane distant to the tumor while dissecting circumferentially around the esophagus. Encircling the esophagus with a Penrose drain facilitates traction and exposure (Fig. 19-12). The azygos vein is then isolated and divided using the Endo GIA stapler with a vascular load. Care is taken to preserve the pleura above the azygos vein. We believe that this pleural layer helps to maintain the gastric tube in a mediastinal location, and it may also help to seal the plane around the gastric tube near the thoracic inlet, thereby minimizing the extension of a cervical leak downward into the chest. Circumferential mobilization of the esophagus is then performed (including the surrounding lymph nodes, periesophageal tissue, and fat) from the level of the diaphragm to the thoracic inlet, following the plane along the pericardium and aorta as well as the contralateral mediastinal pleura, up to (but not including) the thoracic duct and azygos vein laterally. We do not routinely dissect out the recurrent laryngeal lymph nodes or perform a cervical lymph node dissection. Aortoesophageal vessels are sequentially ligated and divided with the Autoclip and Autosonic shears (U.S. Surgical Corp., Norwalk, CT). Deployment of clips during this dissection (especially laterally) minimizes the risks of bleeding and thoracic duct leak. By this technique, the thoracoscopic part of this procedure can be

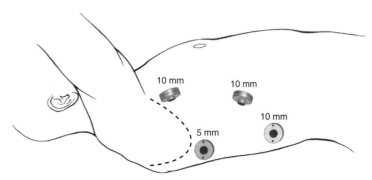

Figure 19-11. Thoracoscopic port placement for minimally invasive esophagectomy.

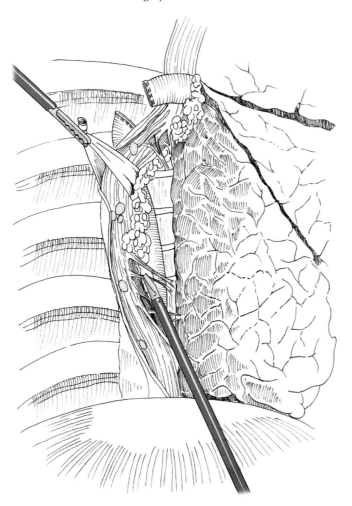

Figure 19-12. Thoracic esophageal mobilization.

performed within 1 to 2 hours in most cases. The intercostal nerves are then blocked with 1 to 2 cc of bupivacaine (0.5%) in dilute epinephrine for control of immediate postoperative pain. A single 28-F chest tube is then inserted in the camera port, the lung is reinflated, and the port sites are closed.

The patient is then turned into the supine position. Access to the abdomen is obtained through a standard five-port technique, essentially identical to that described for laparoscopic Nissen fundoplication (Fig. 19-2). The anterior incisions are typically made 2 cm to 3 cm lower to facilitate gastric mobilizations, pyloroplasty, and J-tube insertion. The left lateral segment of the liver is retracted anteriorly to expose the esophageal hiatus using a liver retractor (Diamond-Flex; Snowden-Pencer, Tucker, GA), which is secured into position with a self-retaining system (Mediflex; Velmed, Wexford, PA). The abdominal dissection is initiated with division of the gastrohepatic ligament, allowing exposure of the right crus of the diaphragm. At this stage of the operation, we avoid dividing the phre-

noesophageal membrane because early entry into the mediastinum may lead to loss of pneumoperitoneum into the chest cavity and difficulties with exposure. The dissection is then carried over the anterior surface of the esophagus, with care being taken to identify and preserve the anterior vagus trunk. The diaphragmatic attachments of the spleen are taken down at the level of the left crus, which allows the spleen to fall away, greatly facilitating the retroesophageal and left crural portions of the dissection. The short gastric vessels are then divided with the ultrasonic coagulating shears. The dissection continues along the greater curvature of the stomach, preserving the right gastroepiploic vessels. The stomach is then folded over and reflected superiorly allowing dissection of the undersurface of the stomach and extraction of celiac and gastric vessel lymph nodes. The left gastric artery and vein are then exposed and divided using the Endo GIA vascular stapler.

After complete gastric mobilization, a pyloroplasty is then performed using ultrasonic shears and is closed transversely

with the Endostitch device (2-0; U.S. Surgical Corp., Norwalk, CT) (Fig. 19-13). The lesser curve fat and nodes are dissected en bloc with the stomach. Care is taken to preserve the right gastric vessels. A gastric tube is then constructed using the Endo GIA II 3.5- or 4.8-mm stapler (Fig. 19-14). There is some variability in the construction of the gastric tube based on the characteristics of the resected lesion. Variable portions of the stomach may need to be resected as part of the specimen, and a narrow tube may need to be created. If gastric extension is found to be significant, then an adequate margin is ensured and a chest anastomosis can be performed. For most patients operated on, gastric involvement has been minimal. We prefer a tube measuring 5 cm to 6 cm in diameter. Extreme caution must be exercised during gastric tube mobilization and stapling to avoid trauma. The gastric tube is attached to the esophagogastric specimen using two 2-0 Endostitch sutures. Marking sutures are also placed on the anterior surface of the proximal gastric tube to aid in the prevention of twisting as the tube is brought up into the neck (Fig. 19-15).

We routinely place a laparoscopic jejunostomy feeding tube during minimally invasive esophagectomy. In most cases, an additional 10-mm port is inserted in the right lower quadrant to facilitate suturing of the jejunum to the anterior abdominal wall. The colon is retracted cephalad, and the ligament of Treitz is identified. The jejunum is then followed distally 25 cm to 50 cm and is tacked to the left anterior abdominal wall with an Endostitch. A needle jejunostomy feeding catheter kit (Compat Biosystems, Minneapolis, MN) is placed percutaneously into the peritoneal cavity under direct laparoscopic vision and is directed into the isolated loop of jejunum. A guide wire is advanced, and the catheter is threaded over the guide wire. The puncture site is then sealed with three tacking sutures positioned circumferentially. A small amount of air is injected into the lumen to confirm appropriate positioning of the catheter. If there is any concern regarding the intraluminal position of the J-tube, an on-table Gastrografin injection can be performed.

The phrenoesophageal membrane is then divided to complete the esophageal mobilization. If necessary, the right and left crura can be divided with the ultrasonic shears to widen the hiatus, allowing passage of the specimen into the chest. This maneuver can help to minimize diaphragmatic compression of the gastric conduit, which is a potential cause of delayed gastric emptying postoperatively. A 4-cm to 6-cm

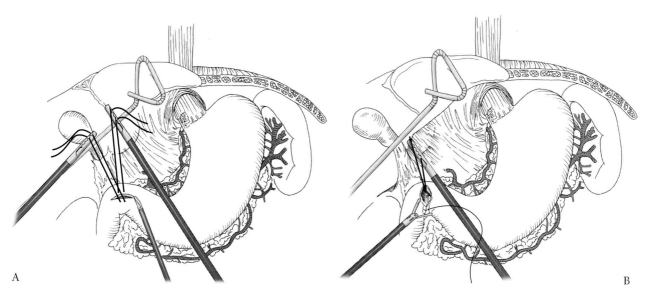

Figure 19-13. Laparoscopic pyloroplasty.

horizontal left neck incision is then made two fingerbreadths above the sternal notch (Fig. 19-16). The cervical esophagus is mobilized and exposed. A finger or sponge stick is used to retract the thyroid and avoid retraction on the recurrent laryngeal nerve. The dissection is carried distally until the thoracic dissection plane is encountered. The esophagus is divided 1 cm to 2 cm below the cricopharyngeus, and the esophagogastric specimen is carefully pulled out of the wound while the laparoscopic assistant carefully delivers the specimen and gastric tube in proper alignment into the mediastinum (Fig. 19-16). The specimen is sent to pathology for frozen section analysis of the surgical

margins. An anastomosis is then performed between the esophagus and gastric tube using a hand-sewn, end-side EEA or side-side technique with an Endo GIA II stapler (Fig. 19-17). We prefer the 25-mm EEA stapler. We prefer a very high anastomosis to ensure adequate resection of any tumor or Barrett's involvement, as well as to enable anastomotic leak drainage through the neck incision. A nasogastric tube is passed through the anastomosis distally into the gastric tube for postoperative decompression. Any redundant gastric conduit is then pulled back into the abdomen under direct visualization. The gastric tube is then tacked to the diaphragm to prevent herniation of

abdominal contents into the chest, using the Endostitch. Care is taken to avoid injury to the gastric vessels. The abdominal instrumentation is withdrawn, and the ports are closed. The skin of the neck is loosely approximated with staples. The completed reconstruction is shown in Fig. 19-17.

Results

In the initial 222 cases at the University of Pittsburgh, there were 186 (84%) men and 36 (26%) women. The median age was 66.5 years (range 39 to 89 years). Preoperative indications included carcinoma (79%) and high-grade dysplasia (21%). Neoadjuvant

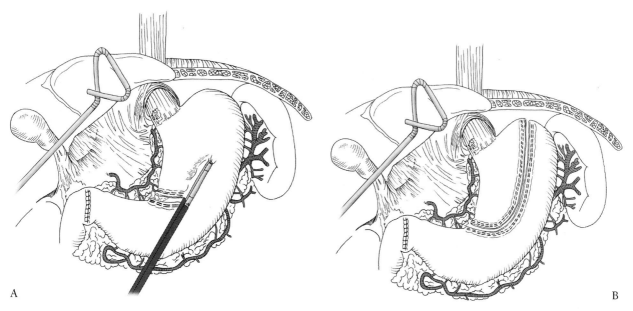

Figure 19-14. Creation of the gastric tube.

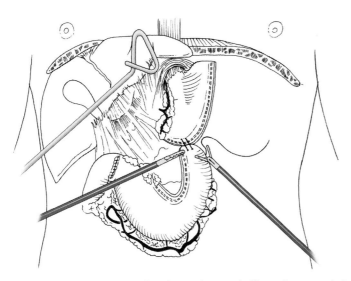

Figure 19-15. The gastric tube is sutured to the specimen to facilitate alignment during pull-up.

chemotherapy was used in 35% of patients and radiation in 16%. Prior to MIE, esophageal stents were inserted in 6% of patients and feeding tubes (G- or J-tubes) in 3%, with previous open abdominal surgery having been performed in 25% of the patients. The majority of cases can be completed using a minimally invasive approach, with open conversion ranging between 0% and 29% in reported series. Reasons for

conversion include dense pleural adhesions, bleeding from esophageal and intercostals vessels, and difficulty with an intrathoracic anastomosis. Open thoracotomy is occasionally necessary in the setting of locally advanced tumors. In the initial 222 cases performed at this institution, minithoracotomy was liberally performed in 8 of the first 15 patients, with only 4 additional thoracotomies used in the next 207 cases. We have subsequently discovered that thoracoscopy permits full esophageal and lymph node dissection. Conversion to open laparotomy was performed in 4 patients due to dense abdominal adhesions. Overall MIE was successfully completed in 206 patients (93%), with a 30-day operative mortality of 1.4% ($n = 3$). The reason for this trend is not established, although lower rates of respiratory and wound-related complications are evident when compared with the open procedure, which in turn may account for the lower mortality.

The most frequent minor complication was atrial fibrillation (12%), followed by pleural effusion (6%), which was treated with bedside thoracentesis or pigtail catheter drainage. Major complications occurred in 32% of patients. The most common major complication was anastomotic leak (12%). Most anastomotic leaks were localized to the neck and were managed conservatively. Pneumonia was the second most common major complication, occurring in 8% of patients. Vocal cord palsy (4%), chylothorax (3%), and gastric tip necrosis (3%) were rare, but serious, complications. Early Teflon or Gelfoam injection of the vocal cords in the setting of recurrent laryngeal nerve palsy improves swallowing function and lowers the risk of aspiration. These results compare very favorably with both open and minimally invasive series.

When compared to open esophagectomy, the minimally invasive approach resulted in similar operative time, less blood loss, and shorter intensive care stays. The incidence of respiratory complications (pneumonia, pulmonary embolism, respiratory failure) seems to be similar between the two approaches.

The early results of MIE compare favorably to those of many open series. In a recent analysis of esophagectomy outcomes in the national Medicare claims database published by Birkmeyer, high-volume hospitals were found to have the least mortality (8.1%). By comparison, 30-day operative mortality after MIE in our series was 1.3%, with a median hospital stay of 7 days. The low incidences of pneumonia (8%) and acute respiratory distress syndrome (5%)

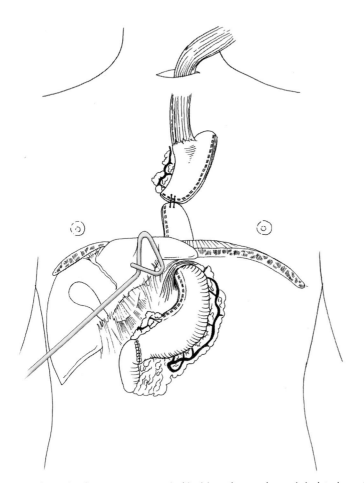

Figure 19-16. Through a low transverse cervical incision, the esophagus is isolated proximally and divided and the esophagogastric specimen is pulled out of the wound.

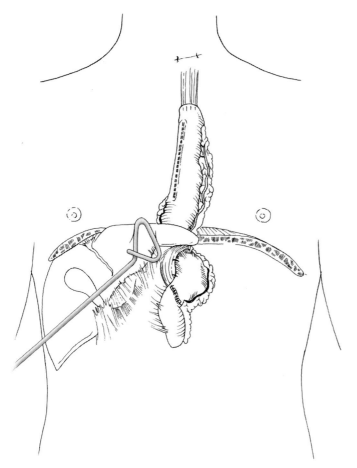

Figure 19-17. Completed cervical anastomosis.

suggest an advantage for the minimally invasive approach. Prospective, randomized studies will be required to more accurately delineate the possible survival advantage afforded by MIE compared to open techniques.

Quality-of-life subjective assessments were found to be similar to preoperative values and population norms. In our series of 222 patients, the mean postoperative dysphagia score was 1.4 on a scale from 1 (no dysphagia) to 5 (severe dysphagia). Because reflux can be an issue after esophagectomy, heartburn severity was measured using the Health-Related Quality of Life Index (HRQOL). The mean heartburn score was 4.6 (on a scale from 0 to 45), which represents a normal (no reflux) score. SF36 Health Survey scores were also measured and were not significantly different from to age-matched normal values during follow-up.

Minimally invasive esophagectomy is technically demanding with a steep learning curve. Operative times have been shown to decrease from 7 to 8 hours down to 4 to 5 hours after performing 20 operations. Therapeutic outcomes compare quite favor-

ably (and in many instances superiorly) to most open series. Such encouraging results will serve to broaden the applicability of this technique to higher-risk patient groups such as the elderly. Prospective studies will be required to determine whether postoperative pain, recovery time, and cost are improved. A Phase II Intergroup Study (E2202) is being developed to evaluate the clinical and oncologic results of MIE for cancer compared with traditional open surgery. Until these results are available, the optimal surgical approach for each patient should be decided based on surgical experience, tumor characteristics, and patient preference.

SUGGESTED READING

Fernando HC, Christie NA, Luketich JD. Thoracoscopic and laparoscopic esophagectomy. Semin Thorac Cardiovasc Surg 2000;12:195.

Glasgow RE, Swanstrom LL. Hand-assisted gastroesophageal surgery. Sem Laparosc Surg 2001;8:135.

Lal DR, Pellegrini CA, Oelschlager BA. Laparoscopic repair of paraesophageal hernia. Surg Clin North Am 2005;85:105.

Luketich JD, Alvelo-Rivera M, Buenaventura PO, et al. Minimally invasive esophagec-

tomy: Outcomes in 222 patients. Ann Surg 2003;238:486.

Luketich JD, Grondin SC, Pearson FG. Minimally invasive approaches to acquired shortening of the esophagus: Laparoscopic Collis-Nissen gastroplasty. Sem Thorac Cardiovasc Surg 2000;12:173.

Luketich JD, Schauer PR, Christie NA, et al. Minimally invasive esophagectomy. Ann Thorac Surg 2000;70:906.

Nguyen NT, Gelfand D, Stevens CM, et al. Current status of minimally-invasive esophagectomy. Minerva Chir 2004;59:437.

Pierre AF, Luketich JD. Technique and role of minimally invasive esophagectomy for premalignant and malignant diseases of the esophagus. Surg Oncol Clin North Am 2002;11:337.

Pierre AF, Luketich JD, Fernando HC, et al. Results of laparoscopic repair of giant paraesophageal hernias: 200 consecutive patients. Ann Thorac Surg 2002;74:1909.

Schuchert MJ, Luketich JD, Fernando HC. Complications of minimally-inavsive esophagectomy. Semin Thorac Cardiovasc Surg 2004;16:133.

Stylopoulos N, Gazelle GS, Rattner DW. Paraesophageal hernias: Operation or observation?. Ann Surg 2002;236:492.

Stylopoulos N, Rattner DW. Paraesophageal hernias: When to operate. Adv Surg 2003;37:213.

EDITOR'S COMMENTS

The authors provide an excellent discussion of foreshortening of the esophagus, a distinct clinical entity whose presence continues to be debated by some. It is inconceivable that the long-term consequences of gastroesophageal reflux and subsequent scarring would not result in transmural involvement with shortening. Trying to pull the scarred foreshortened distal esophagus into the peritoneal cavity and then completing a wrap under tension is bound to fail. Luketich and colleagues have greatly added to our knowledge regarding this entity, and their proposed solution of a Collis gastroplasty combined with a 360-degree wrap seems to be the procedure of choice. The fact that this may be done exclusively via a laparoscopic approach is a great technical advance and avoids the added morbidity and especially pain of going into the chest. They touch on the learning curve and point out that these procedures should only be performed by those with significant advanced laparoscopic skills. The problem remains that in certain areas of the country relatively few patients are referred for antireflux surgery, and it may be difficult for many surgeons to acquire the requisite experience with minimally invasive esophageal procedures to overcome the learning curve.

The cases needed to traverse the learning curve ideally should be acquired in a relatively short period of time for the operator to truly be able to capitalize on the learning gleaned from each procedure. It probably is not beneficial to think that acquiring 10 or 20 cases over a 3-year period is going to lead to proficiency in performing a given procedure.

The issues involving minimally invasive esophagectomy for cancer are complex. Esophageal cancer occurs with considerably less frequency than, for instance, colon cancer, so that a prospective, randomized trial of the minimally invasive approach versus the standard open approach would take many years to complete. Nonetheless, it was just such a trial that was felt to be necessary before recommending laparoscopic colectomy as an equivalent cancer operation. The relatively small number of esophageal cancers also makes it problematic to get over the learning curve. Very few places do 20 esophageal procedures per year, and in those that do, not all are for esophageal cancer. One only needs to look at the paucity of esophageal cases, especially resections, reported by candidates applying for certification to the American Board of Thoracic Surgery to see that these types of cases rarely are concentrated in any one institution. The authors report a complication rate of 32%, and they are the best in the world, or certainly the most experienced, in performing the operation. A leak rate of 12% can hardly be justified in light of recent reports where the leak rate is considerably lower, and should be. There seem to be few advantages to the minimally invasive approach. Length of stay does not change nor should it because the healing of an anastomosis is not hastened just because the operation has been done with a small incision. In my mind transhiatal esophagectomy truly represents a minimally invasive approach in that the chest is not entered at all, even with small incisions. If the argument is that more lymph nodes can be taken with a thoracoscopic mobilization of the esophagus, then the logical conclusion to this is that all patients should have radical esophagectomy as espoused by Skinner, in which even more nodes and surrounding fatty areolar tissue can be taken. The facts seem to support very little if any difference in survival between the transhiatal approach and other approaches. The minimally invasive approach may very well find a home for those patients with Barrett's mucosa and high-grade dysplasia in whom the operation is being done for the prevention of invasive malignancy. For that matter, I'm not sure, based on current results, that it is imperative that every surgeon performing esophageal resections needs to be proficient with minimally invasive approaches, and it may be best that these procedures be performed by surgeons like Luketich who have made it their life's work. Surgeons simply need to be willing to refer patients who would benefit from a minimally invasive operation to the Luketiches of the world, perhaps the hardest thing for most of us. That being said, it's hard not to stand in awe of someone who has already amassed over 500 minimally invasive esophagectomies in his personal series, putting him in a class by himself.

L.R.K.

Surgery for Achalasia and Other Motility Disorders

Richard F. Heitmiller and Molly M. Buzdon

The surgical techniques available for the management of esophageal motility disorders are limited and have not changed significantly since their inception. They include esophagomyotomy to relieve sphincteric obstruction or muscle-induced pain secondary to esophageal spasm, partial or complete fundoplication to control reflux, combined esophagomyotomy and fundoplication, and esophageal resection and replacement for patients in whom the esophageal disease is thought to be irreparable. Whenever possible, concomitant esophageal pathologic conditions such as diverticula are repaired at the same time. Since the previous edition of this book there has been a dramatic change in the incisional approach to performing these corrective surgeries from predominantly open *thoracotomy* techniques to minimally invasive *laparoscopy* methods. This change has altered surgical methods, the background and training of the surgeon who performs the surgery, and even, for some motility disorders, the indications for surgery to first-line treatment from treatment reserved for patients who fail nonoperative therapy. This chapter discusses the achalasia, vigorous achalasia, diffuse esophageal spasm (DES), hyperperistalsis (supersqueeze esophagus), and scleroderma. A section is devoted to one of the most common esophageal motility disorders—reflux-related dysmotility. The full scope of antireflux surgery, however, is discussed in another chapter.

Achalasia

Definition

Achalasia is a motility disorder characterized by failure of the lower esophageal sphincter (LES) to relax with a swallow and absent or ineffective peristalsis of the esophageal body. The name *achalasia* is attributed to Sir Cooper Perry and is derived from the Greek root *chalan,* which means "to loosen." The name therefore underscores the LES dysfunction, which is the most important component of this disorder.

Incidence

Achalasia is an uncommon disorder and occurs with an incidence of 1 to 6 patients per 100,000 population. Between 2% and 14% of patients being evaluated for symptomatic esophageal disease are found to have achalasia. It occurs equally in men and women, and in whites more often than in blacks, and has a peak incidence in the third decade of life.

Etiology

It is well documented that achalasia is a degenerative nerve process that exclusively involves the esophagus. The neural abnormality has two components: (1) loss of ganglion cells in the myenteric plexus, which mediate peristalsis; and (2) interruption of inhibitory vagal nerve innervation, which mediates LES relaxation. A number of causes have been proposed for the degenerative neural process including congenital, postinfectious (viral, parasitic, etc.), and toxic causes. In fact, there appear to be a number of ways to produce the same degenerative nerve process that results in the clinical disease achalasia. Therefore, achalasia represents a single acquired disease process with multiple possible inciting causes.

Symptoms and Diagnosis

Dysphagia and regurgitation are the most common symptoms. Regurgitation becomes increasingly prominent with increasing esophageal diameter. Chest pain from esophageal spasm is associated with the variant "vigorous achalasia," which is discussed later in this chapter. Historically, the diagnosis was made by failure to demonstrate, by esophagoscopic examination or passage of bougies, a fixed mechanical lesion in a patient with dysphagia and distal esophageal obstruction. Currently, esophageal manometry is the most definitive way to diagnose achalasia because it is a manometrically defined disorder. A contrast-enhanced esophagogram demonstrates a dilated esophagus that ends in a tapered end ("bird's beak") at the LES and that empties slowly. A barium-enhanced esophagogram is reported to have a diagnostic accuracy of 85% in patients with achalasia. If achalasia is suspected on contrast-enhanced esophagogram, esophagoscopy is recommended to rule out an occult malignancy presenting as pseudoachalasia. Radionuclide studies to document bolus transit time through the esophagus are best used to document the effects of therapeutic interventions, not for primary diagnosis.

Treatment

Principles

There is no cure for achalasia. Treatment is palliative. Treatment principles are the same regardless of the treatment method used. They include the following:

1. Relieve the obstructing symptoms caused by the nonrelaxing LES.
2. Prevent gastrointestinal reflux (GER) caused by weakening of the LES; GER can be especially severe for patients whose

163

esophagus cannot effectively clear the re-fluxed material.

3. Achieve results that are long lasting.

Treatment Options

Treatment options include the nonopera-tive options of medications, pneumostatic dilation, botulinum toxin (Botox) injection, open or minimally invasive esophagomy-otomy with or without fundoplication, and esophageal resection and replacement.

Nonsurgical Treatment Options

The focus of this text is on surgical treat-ment options and techniques. However, operation is only one of many treatment options designed to palliate the patient with achalasia over a lifetime of follow-up. In fact, the majority of patients are treated with more than one treatment method. Therefore, nonoperative treatment options will be briefly discussed in this chapter. A number of medications have been tried to pharmacologically relax the LES. Nifedipine is generally thought to be the most effective of these medications. Even so, it has limited efficacy and potentially significant side effects, and thus it is indicated for patients with mild symptoms or as adjunctive therapy. Pneumatic dilation is a technique in which the LES is forcibly stretched (and torn) by means of a large angioplasty-type balloon that is fluoroscopically positioned across the LES in an attempt to perform an "endoscopic myotomy."

Pasricha and colleagues pioneered the use of the nerve toxin botulinum toxin as a means of managing patients with achalasia. The toxin is administered endoscopically by four-quadrant injection of the LES using a sclerotherapy-type needle. The rationale was to use this agent to block the uninhibited resting LES tone and therefore improve esophageal emptying. Subsequent clinical studies performed at Johns Hopkins Medical Institutions have confirmed the safety of Botox therapy and demonstrated clinical results that are comparable with those of pneumatic dilation. The therapy has the added advantage of being an outpatient procedure. Results have been most favorable in older patients and for patients with vigorous achalasia. The therapeutic response lasts 8 to 14 months, after which it must be repeated.

Surgical Treatment Options

The surgical treatment options of (1) esophagomyotomy with or without fundo-plication using minimally invasive or open techniques and (2) esophageal resection are discussed in detail in the surgical technique section.

Indications for Surgery

Advances in laparoscopic esophagomy-otomy techniques have dramatically shifted the risk/benefit balance in favor of early surgical therapy, especially in otherwise healthy patients. There is no cure for achalasia, and treatment is projected to last throughout a patient's lifetime. Because the average age of presentation for achalasia is 40 years, it is important not to run out of treatment options too quickly. Historically, open surgical methods have been effective at relieving symptoms. However, if surgery was ineffective or later failed, it was thought that there were no good remaining treatment options and that, speaking metaphorically, management bridges had been burned. Laparoscopic surgical methods yield favorable results similar to open methods and are associated with low morbidity, mortality, length of stay, and cost. In contrast to open methods, however, initial laparoscopic surgery does not prevent nonoperative treatment options, repeat laparoscopic surgery, or open surgery.

Whereas some physicians still feel that surgery, using any methods, is indicated only after nonoperative methods have been exhausted, there is a clear shift in practice plans toward early consideration of laparoscopic myotomy for patients with achalasia. These recommendations for early laparoscopic surgery stand only if the surgeon is specifically trained in and experienced with laparoscopic esophagomyotomy techniques.

Surgical Technique

Laparoscopic Esophagomyotomy

The patient is placed in modified lithotomy, reverse Trendelenburg position. Sequential compression devices are placed on the legs to diminish the risk of deep venous thrombosis. A Foley catheter and an orogastric tube are placed preoperatively. A 5-mm incision is made in the midline at one third of the distance from the umbilicus to the xiphoid process. A Veress needle is inserted, and the abdomen is brought to 15 mm Hg of pressure. Four additional 5-mm trocars are placed. Two are located in the mid-clavicular line below the costal margin and two others are placed lateral to the rectus muscle on the right and left sides, approximately 3 cm superior to the umbilicus (Fig. 20-1). A 5-mm liver retractor is used to retract the left lateral segment of the liver to expose the gastroesophageal (GE) junction. The dissection begins along the greater curvature, ligating the short gastric arteries with the ultrasonic dissector. The peritoneum overlying the left crus is opened sharply, and the esophagus is carefully identified and dissected free from the left crus. The gastrohepatic ligament is opened, and the right crus is then exposed. Starting at the most inferior aspect of the right crus, the peritoneum is divided, and blunt dissection is performed to free the esophagus from the crus. The phrenoesophageal ligament is divided. The anterior vagus runs on the anterior left portion of the esophagus, and the myotomy should be performed to the right of the vagus nerve. The fat pad at the gastroesophageal junction is excised. The fibers of the muscularis externa are scored with the back of the hook cautery (Fig. 20-2). We begin at the base of the esophagus and use a 5-mm dissector in the left hand to distract the esophageal muscle fibers. The hook cautery is placed in the right hand, and the muscle fibers are carefully divided with electrocautery. The myotomy is extended up

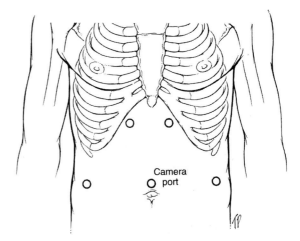

Figure 20-1. Trocar port positions. Five 5-mm trocars are used. The supraumbilical, midline port is used for the videocamera and the right lateral port is used for liver retraction.

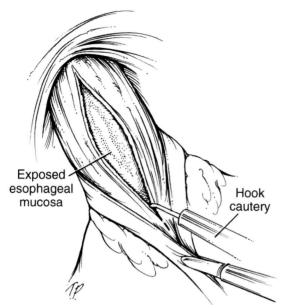

Figure 20-2. Laparoscopic myotomy. Downward retraction on the esophagogastric junction using a Penrose drain optimizes exposure to the lower esophagus and esophagogastric junction. A hook cautery is used to create the myotomy, which extends 5 cm onto the esophagus and 2 cm onto the stomach.

approximately 6 cm along the esophagus. The myotomy must also extend down at least 2 cm past the GE junction onto the stomach. While performing the myotomy, we prefer to place a manometry catheter and perform intraoperative manometry to assess the results of the fundoplication. After an adequate myotomy is performed, the manometry catheter is slowly withdrawn into the esophagus to ensure that no further high-pressure zone exists. Usually, the distal extent of the myotomy onto the stomach needs to be extended, as determined by manometry values. In patients treated with botulinum toxin, the dissection of the mucosa from the muscularis propria becomes more challenging. If an inadvertent perforation of the esophagus or stomach occurs, figure-of-eight suture closure is used to close the defect. We prefer to perform an anterior (Dor) fundoplication in all patients to prevent postoperative reflux. In the event of a perforation of the esophagus or stomach, the Dor fundoplication will also provide added coverage (Fig. 20-3).

Thoracoscopic Esophagomyotomy

In this era of cost containment, the possibility of performing esophagomyotomy using minimally invasive techniques is particularly competitive with nonsurgical methods. Experience with videothoracoscopic esophagomyotomy has not included an added antireflux procedure. General double-lumen endotracheal anesthesia is required, and patients are positioned as for a left thoracotomy. Patients sign a consent for a thoracotomy approach should the need arise. There are several trocar placement strategies that have been reported, but they have in common video camera port placement in the fourth, fifth, or sixth interspace posterior to the posterior axillary line so that the esophagus is viewed in a "downward" fashion; two working ports (anterior and posterior to the line of the esophagus); and one or two ports for lung and diaphragm retraction, respectively (Fig. 20-4). The often-dilated esophagus is not encircled, which would be difficult and potentially dangerous. Instead, the distal esophagus is identified and "retracted" toward the surgeon by means of intraoperative flexible esophagoscopy. With the use of endoscopic scissors or a hook cautery, a longitudinal esophagomyotomy is performed that extends approximately 0.5 cm onto the stomach (Fig. 20-4, inset). The esophageal hiatus is undisturbed. A single chest drain is placed through an inferior port incision, the lung re-expanded, and the trocar incisions closed. Postoperative nasogastric drainage is not routine, an early contrast swallow is obtained, oral feedings are resumed, and the patient is discharged after 3 to 4 days.

Modified Heller Myotomy

Esophagomyotomy plus an antireflux procedure is termed a *modified Heller myotomy*. The rationale for combining these procedures is based on the recognition that it is difficult to determine how far to extend the myotomy onto the stomach (even more so because achalasia is an infrequent indication for surgery), but a transthoracic antireflux repair is a common procedure that most thoracic surgeons perform with confidence. Extending the myotomy well onto the stomach minimizes the likelihood of persistent LES obstruction, and the fundoplication is effective at minimizing gastroesophageal reflux, which invariably results from an extended myotomy. As a result, it is my preference to perform a modified Heller myotomy if surgery is indicated for achalasia.

General anesthesia with a double-lumen endotracheal tube is required. Special attention must be directed toward protecting

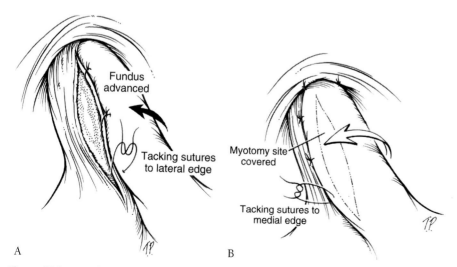

Figure 20-3. Dor fundoplication. An anterior partial fundoplication covers the myotomy site and is secured in place with six sutures: three to the left muscle edge (placed first) and three to the right muscle edge, as shown.

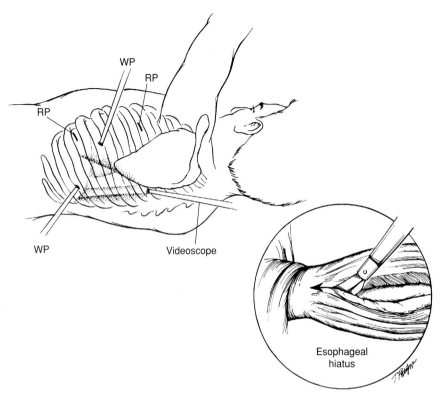

Figure 20-4. Videothoracoscopic esophagomyotomy requires thoracotomy positioning, a port for the videoscope, two working ports (*WP*), and two ports (*RP*) for retracting the diaphragm and lung, respectively. **(Inset)** Videothoracoscopic esophagomyotomy. The myotomy is carried just to the stomach.

the aorta, by palpating it, grasping it with a long Babcock clamp, and subsequently dissecting it, or by following the right (anterior with the patient in the thoracotomy position) limb around medially. The peritoneum is opened anteriorly. One has to avoid being too far anterior and extraperitoneal or being too close to the GE junction and dissecting into the gastric wall. Once the peritoneum is opened, a clear space is attained that can be digitally probed for confirmation. The GE junction is identified and delivered into the chest through the hiatus. The GE junction fat pad is split in the midline and each half, along with the anterior vagal branches, is reflected medially and laterally. The hiatus is narrowed by interrupted nonabsorbable sutures in the crus, which displace the esophagus anteriorly. These are placed but not tied. A longitudinal myotomy is performed using Metzenbaum scissors (see Fig. 20-5). Initially the thickened muscle is split in one site until the esophageal mucosa is identified. The myotomy is then continued (Fig. 20-6A) in this extramucosal plane distally onto the stomach for 1.0 cm to 1.5 cm and proximally onto the dilated portion of esophagus, where its muscle mass thins, for a total myotomy length of approximately 10 cm. The cut muscle edge is sharply dissected off

against aspiration on induction because of the potential for retained food and fluid within the esophagus. A nasogastric tube is inserted after induction. Patients are positioned in the right lateral decubitus position and a sixth, seventh, or eighth intercostal space approach through a left lateral thoracotomy is used (Fig. 20-5, inset). The specific interspace should be individually selected to provide direct exposure of the lower esophagus, the gastroesophageal (GE) junction, and hiatus. For most patients a 10- to 12-cm incision is all that is necessary for exposure. The left lung is deflated, the inferior pulmonary ligament is divided, and the lung is gently retracted cephalad and medially. The esophagus is encircled with a 0.25-in. Penrose drain (Fig. 20-5). Care must be taken to avoid perforating the esophagus while encircling it because of its wider diameter and to include and protect both vagal trunks with the mobilization. Proximal mobilization of the esophagus is usually not necessary because the esophagus is elongated as well as widened. The esophageal hiatus is delineated beginning with the right (anterior) limb, followed by the left limb. The left limb can be identified posterior to the esophagus, medial to

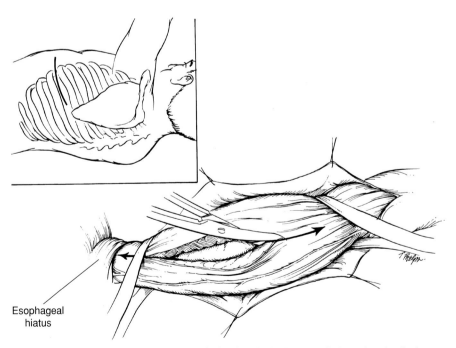

Figure 20-5. After the esophagus is encircled with 0.25-in. Penrose drains, a longitudinal myotomy is performed with scissors. **(Inset)** Operative positioning. An incision in the left sixth, seventh, or eighth interspace is used.

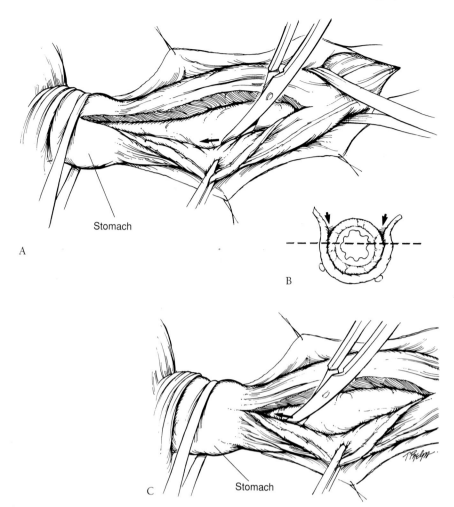

A

B

C

Stomach

Stomach

Figure 20-6. There are two main esophagomyotomy techniques. One extends the myotomy 1.0 cm to 1.5 cm onto the stomach **(A)**, and the other carries the myotomy just to the stomach **(C)**. Regardless of the technique used, the cut muscular edges are dissected off the anterior aspect of the mucosa **(B)** to prevent reapproximation.

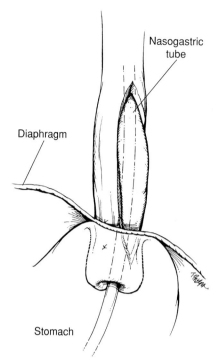

Nasogastric tube

Diaphragm

Stomach

Figure 20-8. The completed modified Heller esophagomyotomy (myotomy plus fundoplication).

Heller Myotomy

Not all authors agree that an esophagomyotomy needs to be modified with the addition of an antireflux procedure. Ellis and coworkers have long advocated limited, early esophagomyotomy before the development of significant esophageal distention. The procedure involves double-lumen endotracheal anesthesia, the same care to avoid aspiration, and a left thoracotomy

the anterior half of the esophageal diameter to minimize the chance for reapproximation of the sphincter muscle (Fig. 20-6B). A "two-stitch" Belsey-type partial fundoplication is performed (Fig. 20-7). A double-armed suture of nonabsorbable braided material is ideal for this. The fundoplication, in addition to its antireflux effect, assists to hold the cut muscle edges apart. Once the GE junction and partial fundoplication are reduced through the hiatus into the abdomen, the sutures in the crus are tied (Fig. 20-8). The hiatus should be tightened so that it just accommodates the tip of a finger alongside the esophagus (with the nasogastric tube in place). The pleural space is irrigated and is drained with a single chest tube, and the thoracotomy is closed in layers.

Postoperatively, the nasogastric tube is removed on day 3, and oral feedings are advanced after gastrointestinal peristalsis returns.

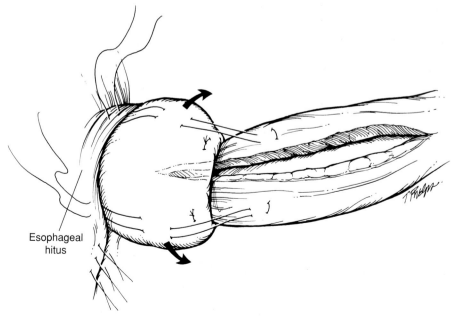

Esophageal hitus

Figure 20-7. A two-stitch fundal wrap.

approach. The ipsilateral lung is deflated and retracted to expose the distal esophagus, which is encircled. This procedure differs from the modified Heller approach in that the hiatus is not disturbed, the longitudinal esophagomyotomy extends just onto the stomach (1 cm or less), and the overall length of the myotomy is shorter (approximately 7 cm) (Fig. 20-6C). The cut muscle edges are reflected off the mucosa to prevent later reapproximation with healing (Fig. 20-6B). Closure and postoperative care are similar to those described for a modified Heller myotomy.

Esophageal Resection and Replacement

Esophageal resection and replacement should be considered for patients who have failed to respond to a technically proper esophagomyotomy and patients whose esophagus is so markedly dilated and elongated that standard surgical or nonsurgical techniques to relieve LES obstruction would be technically difficult and result in anticipated persistent poor esophageal emptying. The ideal surgical approach resects all dilated, aperistaltic, intrathoracic esophagus; is suitable for patients in whom there has been previous esophageal surgery; minimizes the possibility of esophageal injury with mediastinal spillage; replaces the esophagus as for benign disease; and is safe. A three-incision technique with gastric pull-up and cervical esophagogastric anastomosis accomplishes these goals (Fig. 20-9, incision A, B, C).

General double-lumen endotracheal anesthesia is used, and a nasogastric tube is inserted. Patients are placed in the left lateral decubitus position, and a right lateral thoracotomy incision is made. A lengthy incision is not required. A fifth or sixth interspace approach is used, and the ipsilateral lung is deflated and retracted medially. The azygos vein is doubly ligated and divided, and the mediastinal pleura is incised over the esophagus. The esophagus is encircled with a 0.25-in. Penrose drain at the level of the carina. Again, care must be taken not to injure the often-dilated esophagus during this maneuver, and this is usually an area away from adhesions and where exposure is particularly good. With the esophagus encircled, its mediastinal attachments are divided from chest apex to hiatus. Generous use of the electrocautery is recommended. There is little chance of injury to mediastinal structures as the esophagus is being progressively lifted up out of the mediastinum (Fig. 20-10A).

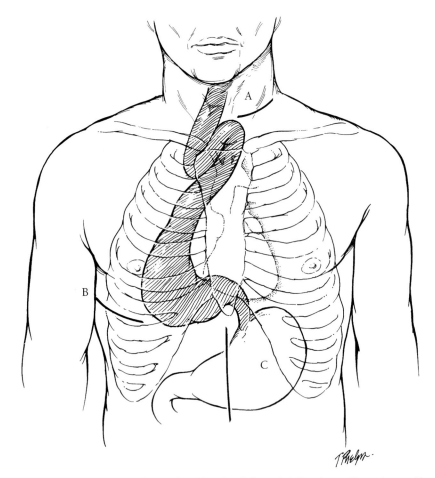

Figure 20-9. An achalasia patient with a dilated and distended ("end-stage") esophagus. The incisions used with a three-incision (A, B, C) esophagectomy.

The cautery should not be used near the apex of the chest to avoid injuring the right recurrent laryngeal nerve. If there is concern over possible injury to the thoracic duct, it may be ligated low in the chest. A single chest tube is placed inferiorly, the lung is expanded, and the thoracotomy is closed in layers. The patient is returned to the supine position and reintubated with a single-lumen endotracheal tube, and the neck is extended as for a transhiatal esophagectomy (THE). The remainder of the procedure is identical to a THE approach except that the intrathoracic and lower cervical esophageal dissection has already been accomplished. Modified left collar and midline abdominal incisions are made, and the stomach is mobilized with preservation of the right gastroepiploic and, if possible, the right gastric artery as well. The stomach is divided parallel to the cardia with a GIA stapler. The staple line is oversewn with 4-0 polypropylene (Prolene). The esophagus and cardia are withdrawn out through the cervical incision, and the stomach is pulled into the neck, setting up the cervical

anastomosis using a technique described by Stone and Heitmiller (Fig. 20-10B,C; Fig. 20-11). We prefer a two-layered inverting 4-0 silk anastomotic method, but this can be varied according to the surgeon's preference. Incisions are closed in layers. A jejunostomy is performed using a technique that permits postoperative percutaneous replacement if needed. Postoperatively, the nasogastric tube is removed on postoperative day 5, a videoesophagogram is performed on postoperative day 6, and oral intake is resumed thereafter if no leak, significant obstruction, or aspiration was seen on the esophagogram.

Surgical Results

The results are virtually identical and excellent regardless of which surgical approach is used for esophagomyotomy or whether an antireflux procedure is added. Reported operative mortality, success in relieving dysphagia, and associated GER are 0% to 2%, 87% to 93%, and 7% to 11%, respectively. Arain and colleagues recently demonstrated that achalasia patients with a high

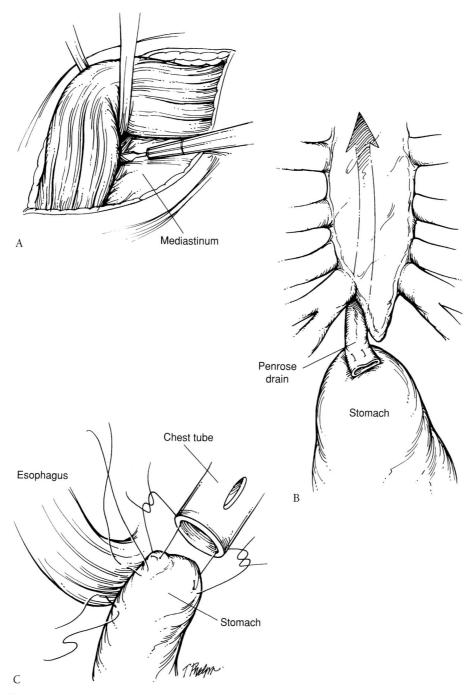

Figure 20-10.   The three-incision esophagectomy technique. The esophagus is dissected from the mediastinum under direct vision **(A)**. After the stomach is mobilized, it is drawn up into the neck with the fundus as the leading point **(B)**, and a cervical end-to-side esophagogastric anastomosis is fashioned **(C)**.

resting LES pressure were more likely to have relief of dysphagia following myotomy. Douard and colleagues documented comparable safety and effective outcomes for laparoscopic versus open myotomy methods. The laparoscopic approach resulted in a shorter length of hospital stay. Kesler and colleagues reported similar findings when comparing thoracoscopic myotomy

to open thoracotomy outcomes. Both approaches yielded excellent relief of dysphagia; however, the thoracoscopic approach resulted in less postoperative narcotic use and shorter hospital stay and recovery times. Studies do not indicate any significant differences in outcomes whether a fundoplication is performed or not. Frantzides and colleagues successfully performed laparo-

scopic esophagomyotomy with "floppy" Nissen fundoplication with excellent results and a low incidence (4%) of postoperative dysphagia.

Gockel and colleagues demonstrated that Heller myotomy may be performed successfully after prior failed pneumostatic dilation (PD). However, the success rate with surgery fell dramatically with the number of

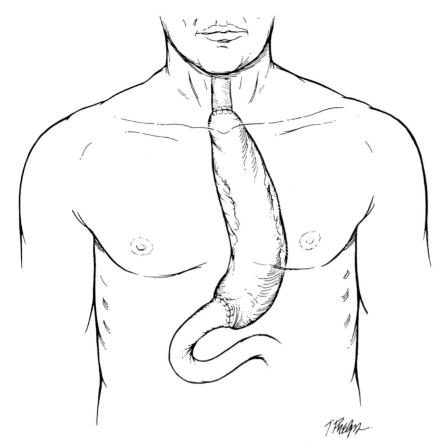

Figure 20-11. The completed gastric pull-up.

region is not identified, a long myotomy is performed to the level of the aortic arch (Fig. 20-12). An antireflux procedure may be added depending on the surgeon's practice for managing standard achalasia. Postoperative patient care is identical to that described for achalasia.

Diffuse Esophageal Spasm

Definition

Diffuse esophageal spasm (DES) is an esophageal motility disorder that is very specifically defined. DES is characterized by simultaneous, repetitive, high-pressure muscular contractions that result in chest pain from elevated esophageal wall tension and dysphagia from disordered peristalsis with segmentation. At least 10% to 20% of wet swallows must exhibit these high-pressure contractions, and there must be evidence for normal peristalsis during swallows without DES. This differentiates DES from (vigorous) achalasia.

Incidence and Etiology

DES is a rare clinical entity that has been reported to occur in only a small percentage of patients who are being evaluated for known esophageal symptoms. The cause is unknown. Patients with DES have markedly hypertrophic esophageal musculature that is hypersensitive to stretch (e.g., as with swallowed food or fluid bolus). It is unclear

prior PDs performed. As a result, the authors concluded that young patients may benefit from early referral for primary surgical therapy. Similar findings have been reported with Botox injection therapy prior to surgery, which suggests that Botox should be reserved for patients who are not candidates for surgery or to treat symptoms as a bridge to surgery.

Orringer and Stirling reported 1 operative death in 26 patients (3.8%) who underwent THE for achalasia.

Vigorous Achalasia

In some patients with achalasia, esophageal spasm-type pain is especially prominent, and this entity is termed *vigorous achalasia*. Esophageal manometry in these patients shows frequent high-amplitude, nonperistaltic contractions in response to a swallow. The LES demonstrates little or no relaxation. The etiology for this achalasia variant is unknown.

Treatment options are similar to those described for patients with achalasia. Transthoracic (including thoracoscopic) surgical therapy is directed at relieving LES obstruction *and* esophageal spasm by means

of esophagomyotomy. For vigorous achalasia, the myotomy needs to be extended proximally to include the region of high-amplitude, nonperistaltic waves noted on preoperative manometry. If a specific

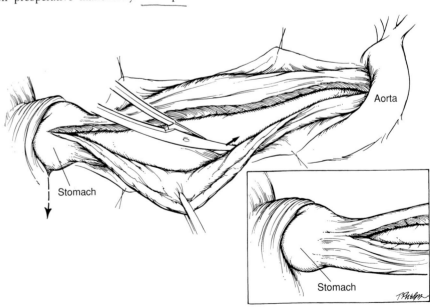

Figure 20-12. The technique of long esophagomyotomy. As with achalasia, there are two variations in technique, depending on whether or not the myotomy extends onto the stomach **(Inset)**.

whether these changes are the cause or the consequence of this disorder.

Diagnosis

The diagnosis is best made by esophageal manometry demonstrating repetitive, simultaneous nonperistaltic contractions of abnormally high pressure. High-pressure contractions must be present in at least 10% to 20% of wet swallows, and the presence of some normal peristaltic activity must be identified. Notably, LES pressure and function are normal in 70% of patients. Findings on contrast-enhanced swallow studies that are classic for DES include a corkscrew appearance, with holdup of contrast within the esophagus as a result of "segmentation." Axial hiatal hernia and esophageal diverticula are associated lesions found in patients with DES.

Treatment

Treatment strategies for patients with DES are directed at preventing the characteristic high-amplitude muscular contractions, muscular hypersensitivity, or both.

Nonoperative therapy includes medications, pneumatic dilation, and endoscopic botulinum toxin injection. Nitrates, especially sublingual nitroglycerin, and nifedipine are the most widely used medications. Pneumatic dilation or botulinum toxin injection may be considered for patients in whom esophageal manometry demonstrates a localized process. In most patients, however, the disease process diffusely involves the esophageal body.

Indications for surgery include failure of nonoperative therapy to relieve spasm-related pain or dysphagia or to manage DES in patients in whom there are associated pathologic conditions, such as a diverticulum, that requires surgical correction.

Surgical Technique

A long esophagomyotomy is the procedure of choice. The term "long" implies extending the myotomy from the hiatus to at least the level of the aortic arch. There is some controversy over whether the myotomy should be extended across the LES and whether to add an antireflux procedure. In the majority of patients, the LES is normal. For these patients, a long myotomy alone is sufficient. If the LES is abnormal or if there is uncertainty regarding LES function, the myotomy should include the LES and a partial fundoplication added. The optimal length of myotomy has also been questioned because of the favorable results using laparoscopic methods.

Laparoscopy

Champion and colleagues described laparoscopic esophagomyotomy with posterior partial fundoplication for diffuse esophageal spasm with relief of dysphagia and chest pain. There has not been widespread experience with these techniques because the mainstay of therapy has been nonoperative in the majority of cases.

Thoracoscopic Long Myotomy

A double-lumen endotracheal tube is used. Patients are positioned on the right side as for a left thoracotomy. The same trocar strategy is used as for patients with achalasia (Fig. 20-4). The only difference is that the esophagomyotomy should be extended proximally to the level of the aortic arch in patients with DES.

Long Myotomy Alone

Double-lumen endotracheal intubation is used, and a nasogastric tube is inserted. The patient is placed in the right lateral decubitus position, and a lateral thoracotomy at the left seventh interspace is used. The ipsilateral lung is deflated, the inferior pulmonary ligament is divided, and the lung is retracted cephalad and medially. The esophagus is encircled midway between the inferior pulmonary vein and the esophageal hiatus with a 0.25-in. Penrose drain. The vagal trunks are included and preserved. A long esophagomyotomy is performed from the hiatus to the level of the aortic arch, dividing the thickened esophageal musculature (Fig. 20-12, inset). In my experience, the myotomy is most easily and safely performed with Metzenbaum scissors. Another technique that has been described is to expose the mucosa at one point; develop the extramucosal plane with a right-angled clamp; and then divide the overlying muscle with scissors, knife, or electrocautery. When the myotomy is complete, the exposed esophageal mucosa is partially "degloved" by dissecting the cut muscle edges off one half of the diameter of the esophagus (Fig. 20-6B). The exposed mucosa is inspected to be sure there are no perforations. Some prefer to fill the chest with irrigation fluid and to gently insufflate air into the esophagus to make sure the exposed mucosa is intact. A single chest tube is placed inferiorly, the lung is re-expanded, and the thoracotomy is closed in layers. The nasogastric tube may be removed early in the postoperative course, and liquids are resumed once there is return of gastrointestinal function. The diet is advanced as tolerated.

Long Myotomy Including the Lower Esophageal Sphincter and Partial Fundoplication

The procedure for long myotomy including LES and partial fundoplication is identical to that described previously except that the hiatus is opened, the myotomy is extended across the LES onto the stomach, and a two-stitch partial fundoplication is added exactly as described for patients with vigorous achalasia (Fig. 20-12).

Surgical Results

The results from surgery are limited because of the small number of DES cases. Henderson and colleagues treated 34 DES patients with long myotomy with fundoplication and followed them for at least 5 years. Thirty-two (88%) patients reported long-term relief of dysphagia and pain, and 94% reported an overall good quality of life. Eypasch and colleagues reported similar, favorable outcomes regardless of whether myotomy was used or esophagectomy. In both groups, 90% of patients stated that they would have the operation again. Champion and colleagues demonstrated similar favorable outcomes when they compared thoracoscopic and laparoscopic myotomy for patients with a wide range of esophageal motility disorders including DES. They documented a lower incidence of dysphagia and chest pain with laparoscopy compared to thoracoscopic methods.

High-Amplitude Peristaltic Contraction

Definition

High-amplitude peristaltic contraction (HAPC) is a motility disorder characterized by persistent high-amplitude esophageal contractions, most commonly of the distal esophagus, which results in sharp, episodic chest pain. This disorder is also referred to as "nutcracker" or supersqueeze esophagus. Unlike DES, the contractions in HAPC are peristaltic and coordinated, and therefore dysphagia is uncommon (approximately 10% of patients).

Incidence and Etiology

HAPC is uncommon and its etiology is unknown.

Diagnosis

Clinically, patients present with episodic, sharp, noncardiac chest pain. HAPC is the most common esophageal motility disorder for patients who present with noncardiac chest pain. Dysphagia is uncommon because the high-amplitude contractions are propagated. Contrast esophagogram and endoscopy may be normal. Manometry shows intermittent high-amplitude esophageal contractions two standard deviations above normal. LES findings are inconsistent.

Therapy

The goal of therapy is to reduce the incidence and amplitude of the abnormal muscular contractions. Medical therapy using diltiazem has been shown to reduce chest pain associated with this disorder. There are no data to support pneumatic or static bougienage. There is limited but favorable experience with myotomy and partial fundoplication using techniques that have already been described. The fact that HAPC most commonly involves the lower esophagus makes it accessible to laparoscopic myotomy with or without fundoplication. The same laparoscopic approach as described for the treatment of achalasia would apply.

Scleroderma

Definition and Etiology

Scleroderma, or progressive systemic sclerosis, is a collagen vascular disease characterized by calcinosis, Raynaud's phenomenon, esophageal dysmotility, sclerodactyly, and telangiectasia (CREST). It is the most common collagen vascular disease affecting esophageal function, with reported esophageal involvement in 50% to 80% of patients. The etiology is unknown. Histopathologic findings include smooth muscle atrophy affecting the distal two thirds of the esophagus, deposition of collagen in connective tissue, and subintimal arteriolar fibrosis. The result is an atonic esophagus with poor or absent LES tone and significant gastroesophageal reflux, often with peptic stricture formation.

Diagnosis

In all patients with scleroderma, the possibility of esophageal involvement should be suspected and gastroesophageal reflux aggressively treated. A contrast-enhanced esophagogram demonstrates an atonic ("lead pipe") esophagus with reflux. There is often an associated hiatal hernia. Manometry demonstrates ineffective, low-amplitude

peristaltic contractions involving the distal two thirds of the esophagus. LES tone is diminished or absent.

Treatment

Treatment goals are aggressive gastroesophageal reflux therapy and management of any reflux-related sequelae such as peptic strictures. Nonsurgical therapy for the esophageal component of scleroderma includes aggressive antireflux therapy and bougie dilation of esophageal strictures. Proton-pump inhibitors have markedly improved medical antireflux therapy. Surgical therapy is reserved for a very small subset of patients who fail medical antireflux therapy and whose systemic disease justifies consideration of surgery. Antireflux surgery is covered separately in this text. However, two points specifically related to patients with scleroderma are noted. The first is that partial fundoplication (Fig. 20-13A) is favored over complete fundoplication. In my experience, for scleroderma and other esophageal motility disorders, complete fundoplication is too often associated with obstructive symptoms to justify its use. The second point is that the operative approach should be designed to permit esophageal lengthening (Fig. 20-13B), such as a Collis–Belsey procedure, because esophageal connective tissue fibrosis may result in esophageal shortening.

Surgical Results

The number of reported series and patients who require surgery for scleroderma-related GER is small. The following points, however, are uniformly raised in these series. Antireflux surgery, by whatever method, can be performed safely. There does not appear to be an increase in procedural morbidity and mortality as a result of the scleroderma. The operating surgeon must be prepared to perform an esophageal lengthening (Collis) procedure. Series report a need for an adjunctive Collis lengthening procedure in 8% to 21% of cases. A complete fundoplication may be used to control reflux without creating severe obstructing symptoms. Finally, the recurrence rate of symptomatic GER is high. All of these results are from earlier series using open surgical techniques. Whether laparoscopic methods and earlier surgical intervention to control GER in scleroderma patients will favorably affect these outcomes has yet to be determined.

Gastroesophageal Reflux–Related Motility Disorders

The most common motility abnormality, GER-related esophageal motility changes, is generally not included with the motility disorders covered in this chapter. How-

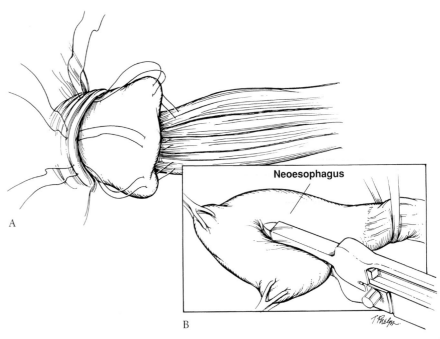

Figure 20-13. For the few patients with scleroderma who require surgical intervention, surgical options include **(A)** a partial fundoplication and **(B)** esophageal "lengthening" with partial fundoplication.

ever, because they are highly prevalent, clearly defined, and potentially surgically treated, a few comments will be made here. A detailed account of antireflux surgery is covered in another chapter. The motility abnormality associated with GER in the majority of cases has now been termed ineffective esophageal motility (IEM). This is defined as distal esophageal amplitudes of <30 mm Hg or nontransmitted contractions greater ≥30%. Ho and coworkers reported that 49% of patients with GER met criteria for IEM. GER-related motility changes include a decrease in LES strength that leads to a cycle of increasing reflux. Reduction in the amplitude of lower esophageal peristaltic contractions, simultaneous contractions, and repetitive segmental contractions have also been identified. The result of these three changes is a less effective esophageal clearance of refluxed material that also leads to increasing symptoms and damage. The simultaneous contractions are similar in nature but generally of higher amplitude than those seen in idiopathic DES. Finally, an increase in upper esophageal sphincter (UES) tone has been identified. There appears to be a direct correlation between the severity of documented GER (by pH-probe studies) and the prevalence of GER-related esophageal motility disorders. Treatment of GER-related motility disorders involves antireflux therapy. Medical therapy is well defined and will not be covered here; antireflux surgery is covered in another chapter. Effective antireflux therapy appears to reverse the pretreatment motility abnormalities in the majority of cases. The procedure does not need to be tailored for the patient's preoperative motility because similar results are seen after Nissen fundoplication in patients with normal or ineffective esophageal motility.

SUGGESTED READING

Arain MA, Peters JH, Tamhankar AP, et al. Preoperative lower esophageal sphincter pressure affects outcome of laparoscopic esophageal myotomy for achalasia. J Gastrointest Surg 2004;8(3):328.

Beckingham IJ, Cariem AK, Bornman PC, et al. Oesophageal dysmotility is not associated with poor outcome after laparoscopic Nissen fundoplication. Br J Surg 1998; 85(9): 1290.

Booth M, Stratford J, Dehn T. Preoperative esophageal body motility does not influence the outcome of laparoscopic Nissen fundoplication for gastroesophageal reflux disease. Dis Esophagus 2002;15:57.

Champion JK, Delisle N, Hunt T. Laparoscopic esophagomyotomy with posterior partial fundoplication for primary esophageal motility disorders. Surg Endosc 2000;14(8):746.

Champion JK, Delisle N, Hunt T. Comparison of thoracoscopic and laparoscopic esophagomyotomy with fundoplication for primary esophageal motility disorders. Eur J Cardiothorac Surg 1999;16(Suppl 1):S34.

Douard R, Gaudric M, Chaussade S, et al. Functional results after laparoscopic Heller myotomy for achalasia: A comparative study to open surgery. Surgery 2004;136:16.

Eypasch EP, DeMeester TR, Klingman RR, et al. Physiologic assessment and surgical management of diffuse esophageal spasm. J Thorac Cardiovasc Surg 1992;104(4):859.

Frantzides CT, Moore RE, Carlson MA, et al. Minimally invasive surgery for achalasia: A 10-year experience. J Gastrintest Surg 2004;8(1):18.

Gockel I, Junginger T, Bernhard G, et al. Heller myotomy for failed pneumostatic dilation in achalasia: how effective is it?. Ann Surg 2004;239(3):371.

Henderson RD, Ryder D, Marryatt G. Extended esophageal myotomy and short total fundoplication hernia repair in diffuse esophageal spasm: Five-year review in 34 patients. Ann Thorac Surg 1987;43(1):25.

Ho SC, Chang CS, Wu CY, et al. Ineffective esophageal motility is a primary motility disorder in gastroesophageal reflux disease. Dig Dis Sci 2002;47(3):652.

Kesler KA, Tarvin SE, Brooks JA, et al: Thoracoscopy-assisted Heller myotomy for the treatment of achalasia: Results of a minimally invasive technique. Ann Thorac Surg 2004;77(2):385.

Orringer MB, Stirling MC. Esophageal resection for achalasia: Indications and results. Ann Thorac Surg 1989;47:340.

Pasricha PJ, Ravich WJ, Hendrix TR, et al. Intrasphincteric botulinum toxin for the treatment of achalasia. N Engl J Med 1995;332:774.

Pellegrini C, Wetter LA, Patti M, et al. Thoracoscopic esophagomyotomy. Ann Surg 1992;216:291.

Stone CD, Heitmiller RF. Simplified, standardized technique for cervical esophagogastric anastomosis. Ann Thorac Surg 1994;58:259.

EDITOR'S COMMENTS

As I pointed out in the previous edition, motility disorders are, for the most part, infrequently seen by thoracic surgeons; with the advent of minimally invasive procedures, however, more of these patients are coming to surgical attention. These problems present a significant therapeutic challenge over and above the usual extirpative procedures that surgeons perform more commonly. An improvement in function characterizes a successful outcome, which for achalasia is manifest by relief of dysphagia and food sticking. Laparoscopic Heller myotomy has become the procedure of choice for patients with achalasia, and the procedure not only results in excellent outcomes in most cases, but also has been embraced by gastroenterologists, who seem to be referring their patients in record numbers. Most of the procedures being performed add a fundoplication of some sort and thus fall under the classification of a modified Heller myotomy, as the authors point out. In my opinion the laparoscopic approach is superior to the thoracoscopic approach, and the question is whether thoracic surgeons will continue to see these patients. Most thoracic surgical programs are not heavily focused on laparoscopic procedures, yet after completion of a general surgery residency most trainees are well educated in laparoscopic techniques. As gastrointestinal surgery continues to define itself as a subspecialty, it is likely that most of these cases will be sent to them unless a particular interest is shown by a thoracic surgeon who defines himself or herself as an esophageal surgeon. We should be teaching these techniques in our thoracic residencies, and it remains to be seen whether we will be able to do this.

For patients who have failed to respond to a properly performed antireflux procedure where the esophagus is "burned out," resection is the treatment of choice. Depending on past procedures, these can be challenging operations. The authors discuss approaching these with a three-hole procedure starting off in the right chest. We have found that a left thoracoabdominal incision that crosses the costal arch in the seventh or eighth intercostal space provides ideal exposure to the hiatus for patients who have had extensive work performed previously in this location. The dissection at the hiatus via laparotomy with the patient supine, as they suggest, may be quite difficult. After the thoracoabdominal mobilization an anastomosis is constructed in either the chest or the neck.

Surgeons should be aware that functional results from myotomy for the other motility disorders described may not approach those seen for achalasia. This is especially true for patients with diffuse esophageal spasm and nutcracker esophagus. Great care should be taken properly to select patients for operation after a manometric diagnosis of one of these more unusual disorders.

L.R.K.

21

Esophageal Conduits and Palliative Procedures

Wayne Hofstetter

Esophageal Replacement Conduits

There are several different options for re-establishing gastrointestinal continuity after esophageal resection, and there has been a significant amount of debate regarding the operative results and postoperative function of each conduit. The decision on which to choose—stomach (whole or partial), jejunum, or large bowel—depends on appropriateness, organ availability, and surgeon preference and experience. Each option has benefits and drawbacks, and no conduit has proven the equal of the native esophagus; options are weighed according to individual patient requirements. Actual "proof" of superiority for any individual conduit is lacking, and there are conflicting experiences documented in the literature for every type of reconstruction.

This chapter describes the technical aspects of the most frequently performed esophageal replacement procedures with the addition of the potential advantages, disadvantages and indications for each. Any surgeon who has interest in esophageal disease will find that it is necessary to be familiar with all of the options for replacement in order to devise an esophageal replacement plan for each individual patient. One must also look beyond the technical feasibility of re-establishing continuity when individualizing a treatment plan and take into account the long-term implications of each conduit option.

Gastric Pull-up Procedures

A gastric pull-up procedure is the most common conduit choice for re-establishing gastrointestinal continuity after subtotal esophagectomy. The technique of gastric mobilization will be covered in other chapters; therefore I will focus on some operative details and consider the advantages and disadvantages of the whole or tubularized gastric conduit.

Gastric mobilization is accomplished effectively via midline or subcostal laparotomy, laparoscopy, or thoracoabdominal incisions. The main concern of any approach is to accomplish adequate margins if there is a malignancy, preserve critical mucosal blood supply, and successfully re-establish patency of the foregut. The stomach normally receives a redundant blood supply from the right and left gastric arteries, the right gastroepiploic artery, the short gastric, and pancreaticogastric arteries. Branches of the phrenic artery supply the fundus and gastroesophageal junction as well. The mobilized stomach is supplied by the right gastric and right gastroepiploic arteries, sacrificing the other vascular supply to allow the stomach sufficient freedom to reach high into the chest or neck (Figs. 21-1 and 21-2). Whereas an esophagogastric anastomosis in the chest has relatively abundant blood supply from these vessels, arterial and venous blood supply to the tip of the mobilized fundus for an anastomosis in the neck is maintained by submucosal vessels fed from the epiploic arcade. Care must be taken to preserve the gastroduodenal and right gastroepiploic artery arcades when mobilizing the greater curvature and gastrocolic ligament, allowing extra attention around the anatomic area of the splenic tip. At this point, the artery may have some variability that can ultimately affect the outcome of an anastomosis. Rarely does a true left gastroepiploic artery exist to form a straight anastomosis with the right. The right gastroepiploic artery usually terminates two

thirds of the way up the greater curve, at which point the short gastric vessels begin, although in some patients it appears to terminate earlier. Careful attention while dissecting in this watershed area can often reveal that a potentially early termination of the right gastroepiploic artery is actually supplemented by a salvageable arcade within the gastrocolic ligament, which can be preserved by careful dissection and maintain crucial blood supply to the relatively avascular tip of the mobilized stomach.

Vagal-Sparing Gastric Pull-up

The vagal-sparing esophagectomy was devised by Merendino and later modified by Akiyama in an attempt to minimize the side effects from sacrificing the vagus nerves, and because it is a limited oncologic procedure it is appropriate only when esophagectomy is required for high-grade dysplasia, limited intramucosal lesions, or selected benign conditions. Collard later described a further modification that would allow the stomach to be used as a conduit while preserving the distal gastric innervation (Fig. 21-3).

Preservation of the vagal branches to the antrum and pylorus of the stomach requires distinct differences in the technique of mobilization. Dissection begins at the phrenoesophageal ligament where the distal esophagus and vagus nerves are identified. In the same manner in which a proximal, highly selective vagotomy is performed, the esophageal fat-pad and gastrohepatic ligament along with vessels and nerves are dissected off of the lesser curvature right on the esophageal and gastric wall from the esophagus down to the level of the angularis incisura of the stomach. The esophagus is encircled with a Penrose drain, leaving the vagal trunks outside the drain. On the greater curvature, dissection proceeds as a

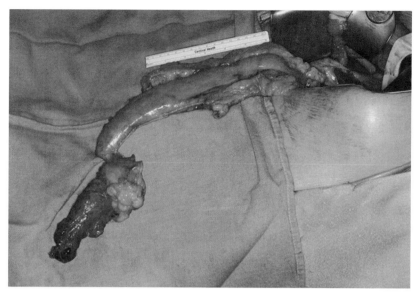

Figure 21-1. Mobilized gastric conduit. Note the termination of the right gastroepiploic artery two thirds of the way up the greater curvature of the stomach.

normal gastric pull-up, but care must be taken when mobilizing high and posterior on the stomach to avoid injury to the posterior vagal trunk. The result is a fully mobilized stomach with intact vagal innervation to the pylorus.

Removal of the esophagus is accomplished by transhiatal dissection directly on the wall of the lower esophagus and mediastinal stripping of the upper esophagus. In patients with favorable anatomy and proper positioning the surgeon can dissect nearly to the carina under direct visualization. Attention is turned to the neck. A left cervicotomy is performed, and the proximal esophagus is mobilized with care to avoid injury to the recurrent laryngeal nerves. Mobilization is performed on the esophageal wall with delicate finger dissection, separating the vagus and recurrent laryngeal nerves from the esophagus. The esophagus is transected proximally at this point, allowing for a margin if there is metaplasia or dysplasia and leaving enough length to perform a cervical anastomosis below the cricopharyngeus. Distally the transection is performed on the proximal stomach allowing for appropriate margins and gastric length. The esophagus is then "stripped" through the mediastinum using a large vein stripper passed up the lumen of the esophagus and tied stoutly to the full thickness of the proximal cut end. Hemostasis is obtained, and the posterior mediastinum is carefully dilated with a Foley catheter (30-cc balloon) that is sequentially passed through the cavity. This allows the mobilized stomach to be passed up the mediastinum without undue traction. Anastomosis in the neck re-establishes continuity.

Advantages and Disadvantages

By far, the most significant advantages of the gastric pull-up procedure are the ease of operation and sturdiness of the conduit. A pull-up procedure requires only one anastomosis, and it is uncommon (<1%) to lose an entire conduit secondary to ischemia. Anastomotic leak occurs in approximately 3% to 20% of cases when the anastomosis is performed in the neck and less often in cases with a thoracic anastomosis (3% to 10%). Mortality at large centers averages approximately 4% and stricture rate is approximately 10% to 20%. Patients return to eating relatively normal meals in a short period of time after the procedure and are usually not chronically dependent on enteral or parenteral supplementation. Most patients who want to return to work do so, and long-term function in terms of quality of life is generally good, although it is often considered to be somewhat less than normal. Avoiding potential early complications following a gastric pull-up can be accomplished by taking into account issues

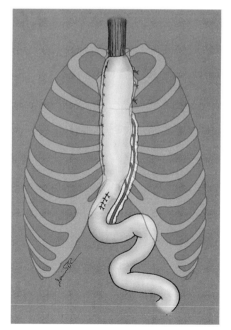

Figure 21-2. Gastric interposition. (Reprinted with permission of David Rice, MD; copyright David Rice, MD.)

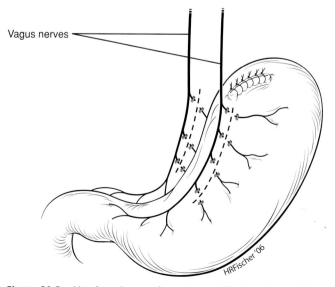

Vagus nerves

Figure 21-3. Vagal-sparing esophagectomy with colon interposition.

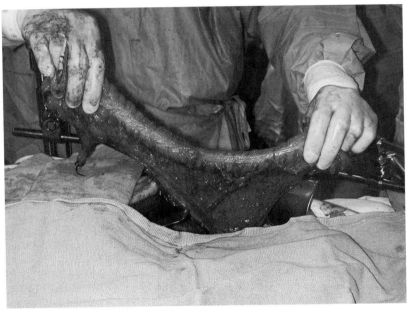

Figure 21-4. Vagal-sparing gastric mobilization.

procedure has led to innovation and development of alternative options for esophageal replacement.

Colon Interposition

The colon provides an excellent option for esophageal replacement in experienced hands. Some surgeons prefer this option for younger patients with a long life expectancy even when the stomach is available. A subtotal or total esophagectomy with partial or complete gastrectomy can be reconstructed with a left or right colon graft. Either of these potential conduits involves the use of some to most of the transverse colon, which receives its blood supply when interposed from marginal arteries and the arc of Riolan (left colon) (Fig. 21-4). Transposition of the colon graft is typically based on the ascending branch of the left colic artery (left colon) or the middle colic vessels (right colon). Our preference is to use an isoperistaltic left colon when possible because it has a thicker wall and better size match to the esophagus. If the right colon must be used, we advocate excluding the cecum.

Preparation

Any patient who is likely to need colon for esophageal reconstruction should undergo endoscopic evaluation prior to surgery to assess for synchronous primary tumors, widespread diverticular disease, or vascular lesions. Angiography is usually not necessary prior to a routine interposition in a patient with a naïve abdomen. Evaluation with magnetic resonance (MR) or computer tomographic (CT) angiography is appropriate in patients suspected of having resection of colon or colonic vessels or of having vascular embarrassment secondary to peripheral vascular disease or central vascular disease. In some situations, invasive angiography may be necessary. Oral hygiene is important, and septic teeth or significant periodontal disease should be addressed prior to surgery. Transposing an unprepared colon is associated with a high morbidity, and therefore a complete bowel cleansing regimen prior to surgery is warranted. Advising the patient to stay on liquid diet for 2 days before surgery will make the preparation better and easier. Although some surgeons advocate preoperative selective gut decontamination for 24 hours before surgery with oral antibiotics, there is no direct evidence that this prevents complicated outcomes, and there are incidences of toxicity from the oral agents themselves.

of conduit length, diameter, and arterial anatomy. Whereas a stomach can be tubularized to reach above the cricopharyngeus muscle, the optimal pull-up is anastomosed below the cricoid, has at least a 4-cm width all the way to the tip, and has the right gastroepiploic artery reaching two thirds of the way up the greater curvature.

Major late drawbacks of the gastric pull-up procedure are dumping (5% to 25% long term), dysphagia, early satiety, regurgitation, and duodenal gastric reflux, the later issue being a concern for patients who have a long life expectancy. We are now seeing more patients who are surviving 5 years or more beyond esophagectomy. Multiple studies have found that many patients who originally presented with benign disease or high-grade dysplasia or were fortunate enough to have been cured of their malignancies are having difficulty with recurrent metaplasia, dysplasia, and even cancers within the esophageal remnant. Several studies have investigated the issue of recurrent metaplasia with gastric-pull up. Most are in agreement that a high percentage of patients who are followed after surgery and are carefully assessed will have evidence of bile reflux. A significant proportion of patients surviving beyond 3 years will have recurrent Barrett's metaplasia, and upward of 80% of patients with an intrathoracic anastomosis will manifest reflux and subsequent esophagitis.

Other drawbacks are early satiety. Almost all patients lose some body weight after gastric pull-up, although many will approach their ideal body weight and stabilize. Approximately 30% of gastric pull-up patients struggle with early satiety in the long term and must eat small meals throughout the day to maintain their weight. Upward of 30% of patients after gastric pull-up complain of difficulty maintaining weight despite these maneuvers and are dependent on oral nutritional supplements. Overall, nutritional issues are understudied in postesophagectomy patients, and a better understanding of postresectional metabolism would aid in the overall care of this cohort of patients.

Aspiration is frequently a complaint of gastric pull-up patients. Although most can return to lying flat with some precautions such as avoiding late and large meals prior to sleeping, many patients must sleep in a semirecumbent position to avoid nocturnal aspiration. Patients should also be counseled regarding positional regurgitation. Younger patients whose occupations require a head-down position should be counseled of the potential for chronic regurgitation and encouraged to make a vocational change. Alternatively, it may also be appropriate to consider choosing another type of conduit in these situations.

To summarize, the gastric conduit provides a reliable form of reconstruction and is the most commonly used procedure, and there is a large international experience with this in its various forms. The fact that it may be unavailable or inappropriate in an individual patient and that there are concerns regarding the side effects with the

Procedure

I will describe the procedure for a left colon interposition. Differences for the right colon are significant in that the pedicle for a left colon interposition is based on the left colic vessels, whereas the right colon is based on the middle colic vessels. The operation can proceed as a transhiatal or three-field esophagectomy placing the proximal anastomosis in the neck via a left anterior neck incision.

The abdomen is entered, and the left and right colon are mobilized taking down both the hepatic and splenic flexures. The omentum is mobilized away from the colon. Special care must be taken while mobilizing the transverse colon and the gastrocolonic ligament not to injure the transverse mesocolon and inadvertently disrupt important vasculature. Once the colon has been mobilized, the mesocolon is transilluminated to visually assess the vasculature. The mesocolon is opened on either side of the middle colic vessel; the optimal anatomy for a left colon interposition is a single trunk at the middle colic artery, which will ensure arterial arcade anastomosis in the transverse colon. To determine the length of the colon necessary for interposition, an umbilical tape measured from 5 cm below the xiphoid to the jaw angle will provide enough colon length for a posterior mediastinal interposition. If a retrosternal route is necessary, measure to the earlobe; one can trim excess or dusky-looking ends before performing the anastomoses.

Returning to the colon, the ascending and descending branches of the left colic artery are identified and the mesocolon between these is opened. Before making any incisions in the colon one must check for viability in the proposed length of graft. The vasculature of the segment is isolated based on the proposed blood supply (ascending branch for left, middle colic for right) by placing bulldog clamps on the marginal vessels on either side of the graft and the major vasculature that will be sacrificed. To transpose the left colon, the patient must have adequate vascular anatomy. The inferior mesenteric artery, arc of Riolan, marginal artery, and middle colic artery must be assessed and found to be patent to achieve a functioning interposition. The isolated segment is temporarily left, and attention is turned elsewhere in the operation. The graft is reassessed, and it should be confirmed by palpation and visualization that the segment remains viable, has a pulse, and is not engorged (purple) due to venous hypertension. A Doppler can

be useful to confirm adequate isolation of the segments but should not be relied on for viability. When ready for the graft, the middle colic artery is ligated at its origin from the superior mesenteric artery. The length of the colon interposition that is necessary (measure three times, cut once) is reconfirmed, and the bowel is divided approximately 1 cm away from the feeding vessels of the marginal arteries. The mobilization of the mesocolon is completed. The colon is placed in an isoperistaltic position taking note of the tension-free position in which the colon and mesocolon will need to be placed in the mediastinum. Several authors have placed emphasis on positioning the colonic segment in an isoperistaltic orientation, and this is our practice as well. Based on existing motility data for patients with colon interpositions, however, the colon interposition may be a passive conduit playing little to no role in the bolus transit within the conduit. The hiatus is opened to ensure that no mesocolon entrapment has occurred because the graft will course through the crus. The graft is passed through the lesser sac in a retrogastric position and then through the mediastinum by placing the colon in a camera or bowel bag. Care must be taken to avoid twists in the graft throughout the mediastinal course. In cases in which a retrosternal route is chosen, the hemimanubrium and ipsilateral clavicular head are removed to assure adequate room for the conduit. Adequate venous circulation is as critical as arterial blood supply. Pressure on the mesocolon and/or the colon at the thoracic inlet or outlet can impede venous return and jeopardize the anastomosis, function of the interposed colon, and overall outcome of the operation.

Once it is delivered into the neck the blood supply of the proximal bowel is assessed. The staple line is cut off of the colon sharply, the mucosa is visualized, and there should be bleeding from the submucosa. This should be brisk and bright. Any redundant colon or dusky ends are trimmed off. Mobilization of the mesocolon away from the end of the graft is minimized to avoid inducing ischemia at the anastomosis, with just enough being dissected away to facilitate the anastomosis. The esophagocolonic anastomosis is completed with an absorbable suture. The nasogastric tube is threaded into the colon under direct visualization before completing the anastomosis. The mediastinum and neck are drained with a closed suction drainage system. Any intrathoracic redundancy of the colon is removed with gentle traction, and the colon is tacked at the hiatus to avoid future redundancy, torsion, or abdominal

content herniation. The cologastric anastomosis is completed on the posterior side of the stomach allowing no more than 10 cm of intra-abdominal colon to function as a positive-pressure, antireflux zone. With the exception of vagal-sparing colon interpositions, the stomach should be partially resected whether involved with malignancy or not. We recommend one-half to two-thirds gastrectomy in vagotomized patients to avoid gastric-stasis issues. (When performing a vagal-sparing esophagectomy with a colon interposition the anastomosis is placed at the fundus and most of the stomach reservoir can be preserved.) (Fig. 21-5) The colocolonic anastomosis is then performed. Care must be taken to avoid ischemia at the colocolonic anastomosis as well. The dusky ends must be trimmed, and adequate blood supply to the remaining colon must be confirmed. Closure of the mesenteric defect should take place on top of the interposition. Pyloric drainage and feeding jejunostomy complete the procedure.

Results

In experienced centers colon interposition achieves good short- and long-term results. There are several potential advantages with use of the colon compared to a gastric reconstruction. A longer segment of esophagus can be resected, even up to the pharynx, with less worry of conduit ischemia. In cancer cases involving the gastroesophageal junction the surgeon can perform a more robust gastric resection to achieve negative margins. Colon interposition provides a reflux barrier from the stomach to the esophagus that will minimize the incidence of recurrent metaplasia and perhaps cancer. Although peptic colitis is described, colonic mucosa has some resistance to acid and bile compared to the esophagus. Using colon can preserve at least some of the reservoir function provided by the stomach, allowing the stomach to be a stomach. Long-term function may be superior to gastric transposition. Some authors report lower anastomotic stricture rates in colon when compared to stomach, and when strictures do occur they may be more easily dilatable. In experienced hands leak, morbidity, and from mortality are not significantly different what is found with gastric transposition, as described by several authors.

However, there are drawbacks to using the colon as a conduit. Most would agree that there is an increased complexity in a colonic reconstruction as it requires three anastomoses, significantly longer operating room time, and the need for bowel

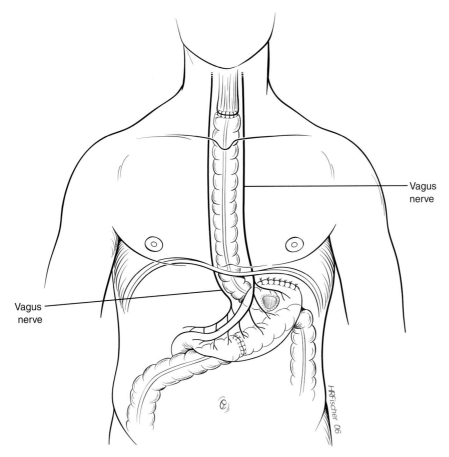

Figure 21-5. Mobilized left colon for interposition.

small bowel conduits are used preferentially for esophageal reconstruction in patients with limited options and as a "final-effort" reconstruction after discontinuity procedures.

Course of Operation
Critical factors that affect the overall short- and long-term function of the small bowel pedicle graft are as follows:

1. Lack of redundancy.
2. Straight course.
3. Adequate jejunal arcade vessels.
4. Adequate cervical or mammary vessels and for microvascular reconstruction.

In the abdomen, the jejunum is mobilized to the ligament of Treitz. The vascular arcade pattern of the bowel is assessed by transillumination of the mesentery. This conduit requires a normal-type vascular arcade with several main branches off of the superior mesenteric artery (SMA) feeding the jejunum in continuous arcades (Fig. 21-6) rather than a single, dominant-type vessel branching sending multiple small discontinuous arcades to the bowel. The superior mesenteric artery is exposed at the base of the mesentery and ligated, and the branches that supply the loops of jejunum required for interposition are divided. The first vascular arcade at the ligament is spared, and generally the next three to four branches must be taken for adequate length (Figs. 21-7 and 21-8). This provides enough jejunum to reconstruct gaps of up to 40 cm to 50 cm in length. Straightening the curve out of the small bowel by opening the normally foreshortened small bowel mesentery is important and results in better functional performance of the flap. If necessary, the most distal arcade vessels can be divided at the arch, leaving that arch intact for microvascular anastomosis to the neck or internal thoracic vessels (Fig. 21-9). The "supercharged" portion of the flap will provide blood supply to the upper one third of the conduit. The distal arcade within the small bowel mesentery is left intact as a pedicle off of the SMA to supply the lower two thirds of the conduit. The conduit is passed retrocolic, retrogastric, and then preferably in the posterior mediastinum to the neck (Fig. 21-10). An optional retrosternal course is employed when the esophageal bed is not available. This route often requires a hemi-manubrectomy and resection of the ipsilateral clavicular head to avoid pressure on the microvascular anastomosis. Transpleural and subcutaneous routes are infrequently used and are associated with a significantly increased incidence of emptying problems.

preparation. Conduit ischemia is more common in the colon compared to the stomach (historical data, not randomized), and as a result several authors have investigated the use of cervical arterial augmentation via microvascular anastomosis or a "super-charged" colonic interposition. Venous insufficiency can affect the survival or function of the graft and may present early or late, from 1 to 2 months out. In the long term, reoperation is necessary for dysfunction caused by redundancy or dilation and stasis in up to 30% of patients.

Jejunal Interposition

Alternatives to colon or gastric reconstruction may, by necessity, need to be sought for long-segment or segmental reconstructions of the esophagus. Small bowel lends itself to reconstruction of any required length and position of esophageal replacement. It is abundant and readily available without preparation and is resistant to acid and bile. Although previously considered a conduit that was only appropriate as a short-segment

pedicled interposition or a short cervical free-flap, it is now being applied to reconstruction of long segments spanning the entire length of the esophagus as well.

Long-Segment Reconstruction
Roux described the first known long-segment jejunal interposition, performed in 1907. Subsequent to this, several adept surgeons applied this technique but noted a 22% incidence of gangrene in the interposed segment. It was therefore thought that reconstruction with a long-segment jejunal interposition after total esophagectomy was not a feasible option, and the procedure was abandoned. In 1946, William Longmire treated a patient for a long-segment esophageal defect who had limited reconstruction options. Combining his experiences in plastic and thoracic surgery, he added cervical microvascular augmentation to facilitate Roux's reconstruction. The procedure was successful but did not gain popularity until the most recent decade. There are several experienced centers where

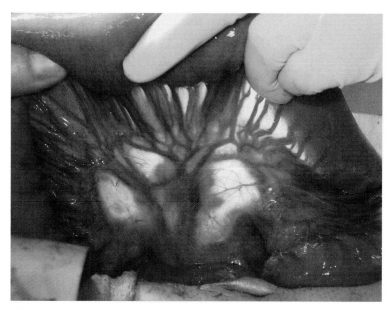

Figure 21-6.   Transillumination of normal branching within jejunal mesentery.

Back in the abdomen, the jejunogastric anastomosis is performed high up on the posterior wall of the stomach to avoid a saddle bag deformity and poor gastric emptying. Some residual reservoir is preferential to a complete gastrectomy if possible, the caveat being that a vagotomized whole stomach may also lead to slow emptying. Side-to-side jejunojejunal anastomosis completes continuity. If a previous gastrectomy had been performed, then intestinal continuity is accomplished via a Roux-en Y jejunojejunostomy. Figure 21-11 illustrates the straight course and excellent size match that can be attained with a jejunal interposition.

Advantages

By using microvascular techniques longer gaps can reliably be bridged with a low incidence of flap loss. From our unpublished series of patients with previous discontinuity, only 2 of 26 (8%) long-segment supercharged pedicled jejunal flaps were lost. One was secondary to excessive tension placed on the graft at the time of transposition in the mediastinum. The intimal flap that was created was recognized immediately, and an alternate conduit was chosen. The second was lost in a patient who had poor venous circulation in the flap but a patent venous and arterial anastomosis. Review of long-term function shows excellent results; patients tend to maintain weight, they are able to return to work including occupations that require bending at the waist, eating is rated as good to excellent in 85% of patients, and risks of gastroesophageal reflux seen in gastric pull-up procedures are avoided.

Patients undergoing long-segment jejunal interposition are usually at increased risk of complications secondary to previous surgery, discontinuity procedures, or the need for extensive gastric resection as well as esophagectomy. Disadvantages to the procedure include a higher cervical anastomotic leak rate, prolonged operating room time, and the need for three bowel and two microvascular anastomoses. Morbidity is generally higher with these procedures than with gastric pull-up, although this issue has never been directly evaluated. Stricture is an uncommon occurrence even after cervical leaks because the blood supply to the neck anastomosis tends to be brisk. Redundancy, dilation, and stasis within the conduit can be seen as late complications but are felt to occur less frequently than with colon interpositions. Long-term follow-up of a significant number of these patients is lacking.

Care must be taken while passing the conduit into the chest and neck to avoid tearing arcades or creating intimal flaps within the delicate blood supply of the jejunum. Microvascular anastomoses are performed at the cervical or internal mammary vessels. An esophagojejunal anastomosis is completed in the neck by interrupted absorbable suture in a single layer. Forgetting to pass the nasogastric tube before completing the anastomosis can prove to be an unfortunate memory lapse; blind application of the tube can easily lead to a perforation in the mid-portion of the flap within the thorax, where it can go unrecognized at the time of surgery. One should consider placing a gastric tube rather than performing a blind passage. An indicator flap representing 2 cm to 3 cm of the terminal portion of the jejunal flap is separated at the bowel wall but left intact to the vascular arcade and mesentery. At the completion of the cervical portion of the case, this portion of the small bowel is left outside the wound to monitor the microvascular anastomosis by periodically assessing bowel color, motility, and Doppler signal.

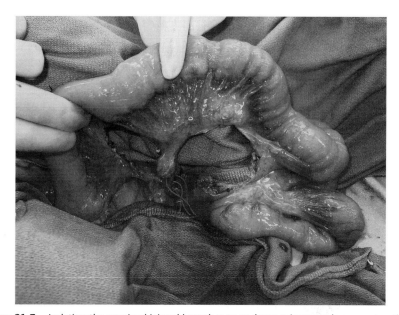

Figure 21-7.   Isolating the proximal jejunal branches to undergo microvascular reconstruction in the neck.

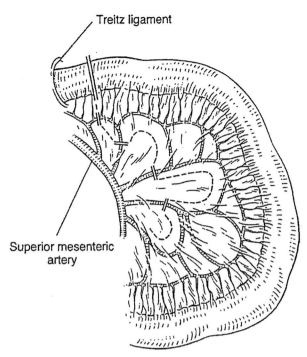

Figure 21-8. Normal jejunal branching pattern and preparation for long-segment jejunal interposition. (Reprinted with permission from Omura K, Kanehira E, Ohtake H. Reconstruction of the thoracic esophagus using Jejunal pedicle with vascular anastomoses. J Surgical Oncol. 75;3:217–219.)

Distal Segmental Esophagectomy (Merendino Procedure)

It is evident that many of the persistent side effects of esophagectomy are due to vagotomy and the loss of reservoir function that the stomach provides. An effort to reduce the long-term sequelae of esophageal resection in patients with excellent prognosis has produced a recent resurgence in interest for the distal segmental esophageal resection. Patients with short-segment Barrett's esophagus with high-grade dysplasia, esophageal cancer strictly limited to the mucosa, or benign pathology where distal esophagectomy is indicated may be considered for vagal-sparing procedures. Merendino originally described this as a surgical solution to cases of peptic stricture where he performed a distal esophagectomy via a vagal-sparing technique and re-established continuity by interposition with a portion of pedicled jejunum. A transverse or left colon graft can be used in this position as well. The interposition of small or large bowel is preferable to pulling the stomach part-way up into the chest because exclusion of the lower esophageal sphincter and subsequent low-thoracic esophagogastric anastomosis is a severe reflux-generating operation and is not recommended.

Procedure

The harvest is similar to the procedure described for long-segment jejunal flap, except that the length that is required is far shorter and there is no need for revascularization. Usually one arcade of bowel length is sufficient to bridge the segmental defect. The bowel with its mesentery is easily interposed in a retrogastric position with minimal mobilization. The esophagojejunal anastomosis is completed in the chest from a transhiatal position and is facilitated by end-to-end anastomosis (EEA) staplers. Small bowel and jejunogastric anastomoses complete continuity of the gastrointestinal tract. Allowing some length (5 cm to 10 cm) of the interposed bowel to reside in the abdomen can cut down on reflux of gastric contents. Care must be taken not to allow redundancy, however, because this will lead to stasis and poor function. Repair of the mesentery must not impinge on the feeding pedicle of the interposed segment.

Advantages and Disadvantages

Advantages include proximal esophageal preservation for preserved swallowing, vagal sparing to decrease dumping and the infrequent dysmotility syndrome, and preservation of the gastric reservoir to combat early satiety.

There are specific disadvantages to this procedure. Gastric emptying can be delayed in the early postoperative period. Conduit redundancy or dilation may require later remedial operations. Marginal ulceration has been described as a late complication to jejunal interposition; therefore we recommend acid reduction as a lifelong therapy. The procedure requires three anastomoses. Due to the loss of the lower esophageal

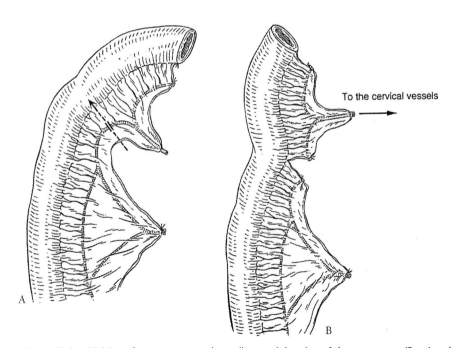

Figure 21-9. Division of uppermost arcade to allow straightening of the mesentery. (Reprinted with permission from Omura K, Kanehira E, Ohtake H. Reconstruction of the thoracic esophagus using Jejunal pedicle with vascular anastomoses. J Surgical Oncol. 75;3:217–219.)

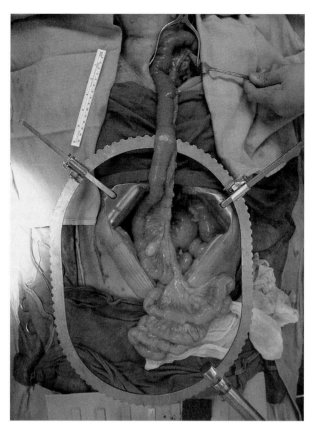

Figure 21-10.   Long-segment jejunal interposition.

sphincter and close proximity of the esophagus to the stomach, this is somewhat of a reflux-generating surgery. Positive pressure in the abdomen forces gastric contents into the interposed segment and even into the native esophagus, which resides in a negative-pressure thoracic environment. To combat this, some authors have advocated a technique in which the proximal portion of the conduit is wrapped around the esophagus similar to a partial fundoplication. Others have described a distal anastomotic intus-susception to fashion a valve at the jejunal-gastric anastomosis.

Short-Segment Small Bowel Transposition

Segmental cervical esophageal defects are also commonly repaired with a free jejunal flap transposed into the neck. The loop of small bowel is harvested just as a pedicled graft, but is then removed as a flap and can be revascularized by microvascular technique to the cervical vessels. Results from these procedures are generally very good.

Pyloric Drainage Procedure

The addition of a drainage procedure to the vagotomized stomach has been traditionally added due to early experience with a whole vagotomized stomach for ulcer disease that resulted in a significant number of patients with secondary gastric stasis, and this procedure is generally our practice as well. Recently, however, the need for a drainage procedure in a partially resected, vagotomized stomach has been questioned. Several physiologic gastric emptying studies have shown that patients undergoing esophagectomy with formation of a tubularized stomach pull-up have accelerated gastric emptying with or without a drainage procedure. Subsequently some surgeons have advocated a "selective approach," electing not to perform a pyloric drainage operation and reserving an endoscopic dilation or drainage procedure for the 10% to 20% of patients who will manifest persistent gastric stasis in the postoperative period. Drainage procedures are not routinely performed in patients who have undergone vagal-sparing procedures, and it is felt that this contributes to the decreased incidence of dumping postoperatively.

Conduit Position

Many retrospective and descriptive studies have been published covering the topic of conduit complications and function in regard to position of the reconstruction within the mediastinum. In general, all studies lack sufficient evidence or homogeneity among various patient populations to make a definitive recommendation. Most surgeons would agree that the posterior mediastinal position is a shorter route, requiring less conduit length and therefore potentially reducing ischemia, stricture, and leak rate. Conduit emptying may be better when

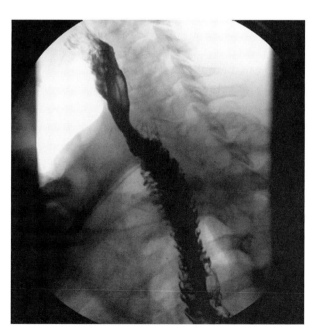

Figure 21-11.   Postoperative barium swallow status after jejunal interposition. Note the size match and straight course.

placed in the posterior mediastinum as well. In contrast, there are single-institution, retrospective studies that show good function with the conduit in the retrosternal or posterior mediastinal position. Given this, most surgeons use the posterior mediastinal route as a preferred pathway, reserving the retrosternal pull-ups for patients who have circumstances that preclude the use of the posterior mediastinum. Disadvantages to the retrosternal route include the frequent need for hemimanubrial resection with subsequent arm and shoulder sequelae, the possibility of a higher leak rate, sternal osteomyelitis, and slower emptying. In contrast, the retrosternal route may be preferable in re-do patients, in those with advanced tumors where there is a risk of local regrowth and conduit dysfunction, in cases where postoperative radiation is needed (R2 resection), or in cases where a tracheoesophageal fistula was taken down.

Palliation

The natural history of esophageal cancer is such that the majority of patients who contract the disease will manifest symptoms that seriously affect their quality of life. Many patients present with significantly advanced disease and are never considered for curative procedures. Other patients, although presenting with only locally advanced disease, may not be candidates for surgery or aggressive medical therapy due to comorbidity or poor performance status. Palliative treatment is appropriate in symptomatic patients, which manifests as malignant dysphagia in 70% of patients presenting with locally advanced esophageal cancer. Other common symptoms presenting for palliation include bleeding, fistula, perforation, pain, and malnutrition.

The various treatment modalities for palliation of advanced esophageal cancer include operation (bypass, feeding tubes), radiation (external beam, brachytherapy), systemic therapies (chemotherapy), local ablative therapies, and dilation and stenting. Most of these types of procedures can be complementary to one another, and a combination of modalities will often provide the most effective palliation. When choosing among the treatment options for palliation one must consider the location of the tumor, the specific symptoms requiring palliation, the potential side effects of any proposed therapy, and the patient's comorbidity and performance status. We encourage an open discussion with patients before embarking on any course of palliative treatment.

Surgical

Given the available endoluminal treatment modalities and results of nonprocedural palliative procedures such as chemotherapy and radiation, there is no role for the strictly palliative esophagectomy. Patients with symptomatic but inoperable locally advanced esophageal neoplasms and those presenting with metastatic disease are best treated with nonoperative modalities because many of these patients have a life expectancy of <1 year. There are, however, several indications for surgical palliation of symptoms related to esophageal cancer.

Frequently, heavy tumor burden pushes a patient into a catabolic state, and many patients with already low reserve have a limited ability to maintain adequate nutrition even after other palliative procedures have been successfully performed. Despite having a patent esophagus, patients may not be capable of maintaining their weight. Because of this, we recommend early administration of adjunctive nutritional support. A minilaparotomy or laparoscopic feeding jejunostomy can provide rapid and effective nutritional palliation. Similarly, gastric feeding tubes may be used and may have the added advantage of a gastric reservoir that will often allow for more convenient bolus feedings rather than pump dependence (Most would avoid a gastric tube, however, if the patient is potentially resectable or if the tumor involves stomach for reasons of pain, satiety, and tube-site tumor metastases).

The patient that presents with a perforated esophageal cancer may require esophagectomy and/or esophageal diversion to control sepsis and ongoing mediastinal soiling. Although covered esophageal and tracheal stents have proven to be fairly effective palliation for rupture, leaks, and fistulas as well. although bleeding tumors were also traditionally treated with palliative surgery, current endoscopic ablative therapies are capable of treating this with good results while minimizing morbidity.

Overall, surgical palliation is limited to uncontrolled fistulae or ruptures, uncontrollable bleeding, or adjunctive nutritional support. Given the efficacy of other nonoperative palliation efforts, esophageal resection performed strictly for dysphagia is generally of historical interest.

Chemotherapy and Radiation

Esophageal cancers are responsive to both chemotherapy and combined chemoradiotherapy. Current protocols are aimed at preserving swallowing function and prolonging life in patients with advanced disease. Platinum-based regimens have proven to be the most active cytoreductive agents for treating dysphagia caused by squamous cell or adenocarcinomas, with overall response rates as high as 90%. Toxicity may be significant, however, and therefore this regimen is not routinely employed for palliation, although it does exemplify the potential of this modality for palliation of dysphasia.

Overall, chemotherapy with or without the addition of radiation can be an effective cytoreduction agent that will result in significant improvement in swallowing function and other side effects seen in advanced esophageal cancers. However, due to toxicity these modalities should be chosen only for patients with sufficient physiologic reserve to tolerate the treatment. Endoluminal therapies used in combination with systemic and/or radiation treatment may enhance the palliative results and improve a patient's quality of life.

Brachytherapy

Endoluminal radiation therapy has been reported to palliate malignant dysphagia in approximately 50% to 90% of patients receiving treatment. There are still major concerns with toxicity, however, and debate regarding the overall dose and fractionation continues in the radiotherapy literature. Low-dose-rate intraluminal radiotherapy may be more easily tolerated with fewer complications but takes longer to achieve palliation. High-dose-rate brachytherapy (HDR-ILRT) (12 Gy to 20 Gy given in one or two fractions) seems to have emerged as the dose delivery of choice. With 15 Gy of HDR-ILRT given in one or two fractions a significant number of patients can expect significant palliation of dysphasia. Stent placement may result in a higher number of complications than HDR-ILRT without a significant improvement in dysphagia or improved quality of life.

In summary, brachytherapy is an option for palliative treatment of esophageal lesions, but concern regarding esophageal fistulas, especially those associated with lesions in the mid-upper esophagus, may limit the efficacy of this treatment modality.

Endoscopic Endoluminal Palliative Procedures

There is a wide array of endoscopic treatment modalities used for the palliation of symptomatic malignant esophageal neoplasms. Recent technologies that are easily administered and have high efficacy rates have, for the most part, replaced the older methods of caustic injections and several methods of thermal ablation. The mechanical methods that are now commonly employed are endoluminal ablative therapies or dilation therapy. Either can be used in conjunction with endoluminal stenting. Ablative therapies, such as laser ablation, photodynamic therapy (PDT), and brachytherapy, can be used independently or in conjunction with other therapies such as chemotherapy, radiotherapy, and dilation and stenting.

Ablative Therapies

Ablation therapies are effective at producing rapid palliation in the majority of patients with malignant dysphagia or bleeding. Generally, they are best suited for lesions located in the distal esophagus, gastroesophageal junction (GEJ), or very proximal esophagus. Although lesions in the proximal and mid-esophagus are amenable to ablative therapies, they are at higher risk for complication such as tracheoesophageal fistula. There are several modern endoscopic ablative modalities that are routinely employed.

Photodynamic Therapy. Photodynamic therapy (PDT) is appropriate for patients with symptomatic malignant dysphasia or bleeding from a primary or recurrent esophageal cancer and is reapplicable in cases that have recurred from tumor regrowth. This modality is well suited for lesions in the middle, distal, or very proximal esophagus and is capable of accomplishing some degree of palliation in 85% to 100% of patients in which it is attempted.

PDT is accomplished by exposing the tumor to a specific wavelength of light after the patient is administered an intravenous injection of a hematoporphyrin, a photosensitizer that will concentrate in cellular membranes and then ultimately on intracellular organelles. Malignant tissue is believed to selectively retain these compounds at a higher concentration than normal tissue, making them particularly susceptible to this form of therapy. On the second postinjection day, the tumor is endoscopically exposed to infrared light at 630 nm wavelength. Once exposed, the tumor undergoes necrosis mediated by oxygen free-radical cell death. PDT also selectively affects capillary beds, which can lead to additional tumor destruction by avascular necrosis. Two days after the initial treatment the necrotic tumor is debrided with an endoscope and then re-treated with light exposure. Because the degree of tumor necrosis is generally proportional to the amount of light exposure, carefully planning the overall tumor dose prior to therapy is necessary to minimize the risk of perforation and maximize efficacy. Patients with

very bulky tumors are difficult to adequately treat, and some authors advocate placing the probe directly into the tumor (interstitial exposure) for better results. Likewise, totally obstructing lesions may require initial treatment with laser ablation and/or guidewire placement followed by dilation to obtain adequate access to perform PDT. Complications are infrequent and can range from mild to quite severe. Temporary chest pain, odynophagia, and pleural effusion may occur frequently as a result of treatment and are not necessarily related to more ominous complications. Tumor necrosis can lead to full-thickness tissue loss and potential perforation. Because the amount of necrosis directly correlates to tumor light dose, overexposure increases the risk of perforation, which occurs in approximately 2% of treated patients.

Tracheoesophageal fistula has been reported in 5% to 30% of patients. Although PDT is well suited for lesions in the GEJ or the distal or very proximal esophagus, it is believed that proximal to mid-esophageal lesions, although amenable, may have a higher fistula rate, and therefore, other modalities such as a Celestin or Montgomery salivary tube, could be considered.

Treatment-related esophageal stricture rate is reported in up to 11% for esophageal PDT overall. However, it is less common in patients who have received PDT strictly for palliation because the depth of the treatment is usually less than a full-thickness burn. Many patients also suffer from relapse of dysphasia from tumor regrowth, and therefore stricture is not likely to be as commonly reported. To combat the formation of post-treatment stricture, photodynamic therapy is often combined with the liberal use of esophageal dilation, which may decrease the incidence of this complication.

Patients are vulnerable to sunlight and even bright, indoor light for a period of time after PDT. Cutaneous photosensitivity, or "lightburn," occurs in approximately 5% to 20% of patients who undergo this therapy despite precautions. Because the photosensitizer is administered intravenously, the porphimer will concentrate even on normal cell membranes in sufficient quantities to cause damage to any area of skin that is inadvertently exposed to light for a prolonged duration. Often, incidental light overexposure results in mild, reversible skin irritation, but extensive burns have been described. For this reason, patients must arrive to their initial intravenous injection completely protected against sun and bright indoor light, including eye protection, and must remain so for a period of 4 to 6 weeks

as the photosynthesizer is metabolized. Sunblocks are not effective at preventing this complication because these block ultraviolet but not infrared light. "Photobleaching," a process of allowing limited exposure to light, hastens the metabolism of the porphimer and can decrease the incidence of light-related complications and allow patients to return to normal light exposure sooner. Other cutaneous complications that are reported with some frequency are erythema multiforme from drug-related toxicity and herpes zoster infection.

Esophagitis is a fairly infrequent complication occurring in approximately 2% of patients after PDT. The usual etiology is *Candida* infection.

Mortality is generally quoted as 0% to 2% for palliative photodynamic therapy.

Duration of Efficacy. A significant proportion of surviving patients will represent within 60 to 90 days, with recurrence of malignant dysphasia requiring further treatment. In cases that recur, PDT can be reapplied, or other palliative procedures may be performed such as the use of a self-expanding metal stent, laser ablation, dilation, or a combination of these.

Laser Ablation. Thermal ablation with a neodymium:yittrium-aluminum-garnet (Nd:YAG) laser has the benefit of ease of applicability and rapid relief of dysphasia. It is performed by delivering pulsed or continuous laser energy via a fiberoptic catheter advanced through an endoscope allowing for direct visualization of the tumor during ablation. When employed as a single modality for palliation it is ideally suited for patients with short-segment, partially obstructing tumors of the esophagus. Most patients will require multiple treatment sessions (three or more) to gain relief from dysphagia, and the sessions are time consuming. However, some authors advocate performing Nd:YAG ablation even on large, obstructing lesions as the solitary modality in a single treatment session and report that essentially all patients improved after therapy. These results were obtained using a retrograde ablation technique and usually required dilation before ablation to allow the endoscope to pass through the tumor. This method has an associated 10% incidence of perforation. Patients with large, obstructing tumors may also benefit from Nd:YAG ablation to gain initial access to the lumen when other methods such as PDT or stenting are being planned.

The major advantage of this modality is that patients may obtain rapid relief of dysphagia without the potential negative impact on quality of life caused by PDT secondary to light sensitivity. Disadvantages of laser ablation are the frequent need for multiple applications to clear tumor burden and a relatively short duration of palliation (30 to 60 days on average) especially when laser ablation is not combined with other palliative procedures such as stenting. Other disadvantages are the incidence of perforation (8%), tracheoesophageal fistula (1% to 6%), and mortality (1% to 5%). Clinicians should be aware of a risk of fire when performing laser ablation in an area that has previously been stented.

When thermal ablation is compared with expandable metal stents it has been noted that both methods resulted in a decrease in dysphagia scores in most patients, although there was no difference between the methods. Stents may be necessary after laser ablation as a bail-out due to recurrent malignant stenosis or immediately after thermal ablation secondary to adverse events (perforation or fistula). Cost and hospital admissions were found to be twice as high for thermal ablation compared to expandable metal stents. Duration of efficacy seems to favor thermal ablation.

Stents

Esophageal stents used as a single modality or in conjunction with ablative therapies provide effective and rapid palliation of malignant dysphasia. They are also frequently used in cases of fistula, rupture, or contained spontaneous malignant perforations. Unlike ablative therapy, which is mainly limited to endoluminal disease, stenting is suitable for use when extrinsic lesions are causing compression of the esophagus as well as when exophytic tumors cause luminal narrowing. Proximal esophageal lesions are also prone to fistulize to the trachea or cause stridor from external tracheal compression; placement of a self-expanding metal stent (SEMS) in the *trachea* has proven to be very valuable in these cases.

There are multiple stents approved by the Food and Drug Administration, and decisions on which to choose should depend on the type and location of lesion to be palliated. Lesions causing intrinsic or extrinsic compression can be palliated with expanding metal stents, which are available in covered (Fig. 21-12) or uncovered varieties. They tend to have high radial forces, and although they are good for rapid relief of dysphagia, they have the disadvantage of increased patient discomfort compared to other modalities. Another option for this type of lesion is a Nitinol stent (Fig. 21-13),

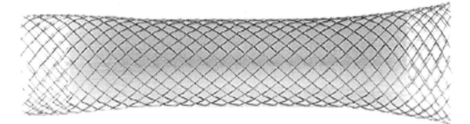

Figure 21-12.   Coated self-expandable metal stent. (Courtesy, Boston Scientific, Natick, MA.)

which is generally softer and better tolerated than traditional metal stents but tends to expand more slowly and the covered version has a slightly higher incidence of migration. Palliation of an esophageal leak or fistula calls for using covered stents. There are newer, removable plastic stents (Polyflex, Boston Scientific, Natick, MA) that are fully covered and may be a promising technology for all types of lesions in most areas of the esophagus and airway.

When considering location, middle to distal lesions are suited to treatment with SEMS, but placement at or above the cricopharyngeus muscle is undesirable because patients tolerate expanding stents in this area poorly. Lesions in this area are more amenable to flexible plastic stents such as a Celestin tube or alternative palliative therapies. Very distal and GEJ tumors can be effectively palliated with stents; however, clinicians and patients should be aware that the incidence of symptomatic reflux and regurgitation is very high in these cases because the distal end of the stent hangs free in the gastric lumen.

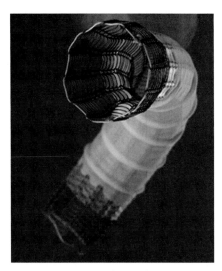

Figure 21-13.   Coated Nitinol self-expandable metal stent with proximal flare. (Ultraflex Stent, courtesy, Boston Scientific, Natick, MA.)

Technique. Stents are placed by an endoscopic approach in a sedated or completely anesthetized patient with an applicator (Fig. 21-14). Fluoroscopic guidance (Fig. 21-15) can be very helpful or critical in some cases. A precise assessment and measurements of the stenosed area are critical in judging the length and width of the stent to be deployed. In general, stents with a smaller lumen will lead to ongoing or continued dysphasia, more frequent food bolus obstruction, and shorter duration of dysphasia relief as regrowth of tumor obstructs the lumen. Alternatively, choosing too large a lumen (overstenting) will result in more patient discomfort from radial forces and incomplete deployment of the stent that can then lead to food and secretion deposition and early blockage. We generally choose a diameter between 17 mm and 20 mm. Length must be estimated such that an uncovered proximal portion of the stent anchors within normal esophageal wall (Fig. 21-16) and the stent traverses the entire length of the stricture. Distal anchoring is possible in mid-esophageal lesions, but it is common to have the distal end of the stent project into the gastric lumen for more-distal lesions. Generally, a stent that is 4 cm longer than the lesion would appropriately allow 2 cm on either end for anchoring.

If no lumen is present on endoscopy, gentle probing with a guide-wire under fluoroscopic guidance can often establish the pathway to the lumen. Once established, a pre-stent dilation performed by balloon or Savary-type dilators will allow one to adequately assess the malignant stricture and choose an appropriate stent. Other modalities for establishing a proper working lumen are Nd:YAG laser ablation or PDT. A gently inflated transendoscopic balloon dilator will help to deploy the stent and place it in optimal positioning.

Results. Care must be taken to avoid major or potentially disastrous complications. Overzealous expansion of a mid-esophageal lesion can compress proximal or distal

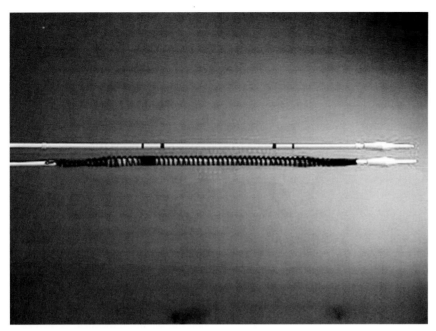

Figure 21-14. Self-expandable metal stent application system. (Courtesy, Boston Scientific, Natick, MA.)

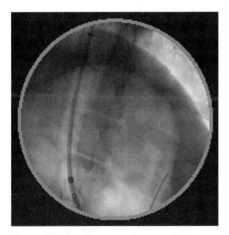

Figure 21-15. Fluoroscopic control of stent placement. (Courtesy, Boston Scientific, Natick, MA.)

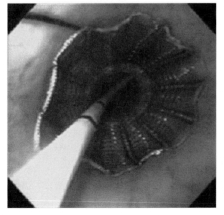

Figure 21-16. Self-expandable metal stent placed with proximal flange in normal esophageal wall for anchoring. (Courtesy, Boston Scientific, Natick, MA.)

airways. Likewise, aggressive dilation can result in a ruptured esophagus and/or fistula formation. Overall, stent placement is associated with a 5% perforation rate. Other potential complications include bolus obstruction, migration, mortality, and eventual recurrent malignant stenosis due to tumor overgrowth. Uncovered stents migrate less often (2% vs. 10% to12% for covered stents), but recurrence due to overgrowth and the need for further therapy due to recurrence of dysphagia are more common with this type of stent. Covered stents migrate more often, but have a longer duration of palliation. Covered stents are also ideal for nonsurgical palliation of esophageal fistulas.

Summary

In summary, there are multiple methods for palliating symptoms from esophageal cancer that are effective and rapid. Although there have been multiple studies comparing the efficacy the modalities, there is no single dominant therapy. Individualizing treatment to a patient is most likely to produce significant durable palliation and should be done so with a minimum amount of discomfort.

SUGGESTED READING

Akiyama H, Tsurumaru M, Ono Y, et al. Esophagectomy without thoracotomy with vagal preservation. J Am Coll Surgeons 1994;178; 83.

Barkley C, Orringer MB, Iannettoni MD, et al.

Challenges in reversing esophageal discontinuity operations. Ann Thorac Surg, 2003; 76:989.

Christie NA, Buenaventura PO, Fernando HC, et al. Results of expandable metal stents for malignant esophageal obstruction in 100 patients: Short-term and long-term follow-up. Ann Thorac Surg 2001;71:1797.

Collard JM, Romagnoli R, Goncette L, et al. Whole stomach with antro-pyloric nerve preservation as an esophageal substitute: An original technique. Dis Esophagus 2004;17:164.

Dallal HJ, Smith GD, Grieve DC, et al. A randomized trial of thermal ablative therapy versus expandable metal stents in the palliative treatment of patients with esophageal carcinoma. Gastrointest Endosc 2001;54:549.

DeMeester TR, Zaninotto G, Johansson KE. Selective therapeutic approach to cancer of the lower esophagus and cardia. J Thorac Cardiovasc Surg 1988;95:42.

Dresner SM, Griffin SM, Wayman J, et al. Human model of duodenogastro-oesophageal reflux in the development of Barrett's metaplasia. Br J Surg 2003;90:1120.

Gaspar LE, Winter K, Kocha WI, et al. Swallowing function and weight change observed in a phase I/II study of external-beam radiation, brachytherapy and concurrent chemotherapy in localized cancer of the esophagus (RTOG 9207). Cancer J 2001;7:388.

Gerzic ZB. Modification of the Merendino procedure. Dis Esophagus 1997;10:270.

Harvey JA, Bessell JR, Beller E, et al. Chemoradiation therapy is effective for the palliative treatment of malignant dysphagia. Dis Esophagus 2004;17:260.

Holscher AH, Voit H, Buttermann G, et al. Function of the intrathoracic stomach as esophageal replacement. World J Surg 1988; 12:835.

Homs MY, Eijkenboom WM, Coen VL, et al. High dose rate brachytherapy for the palliation of malignant dysphagia. Radiother Oncol 2003;66:327.

Homs MY, Steyerberg EW, Eijkenboom WM, et al. Single-dose brachytherapy versus metal stent placement for the palliation of dysphagia from oesophageal cancer: Multicentre randomised trial. Lancet 2004: 364:1497.

Ilson DH, Forastiere A, Arquette M, et al. A phase II trial of paclitaxel and cisplatin in patients with advanced carcinoma of the esophagus. Cancer J 2000;6:316.

Ilson DH, Saltz L, Enzinger P, et al. Phase II trial of weekly irinotecan plus cisplatin in advanced esophageal cancer. J Clin Oncol, 1999;17:3270.

Isolauri J, Koskinen MO, Markkula H. Radionuclide transit in patients with colon interposition. J Thorac Cardiovasc Surg 1987;94:521.

Kolh P, Honore P, Degauque C, Gielen, et al. Early stage results after oesophageal resection for malignancy—Colon interposition vs. gastric pull-up. Eur J Cardiothorac Surg 2000;18:293.

Lightdale CJ, Heier SK, Marcon NE, et al. Photodynamic therapy with porfimer sodium versus thermal ablation therapy with Nd:YAG laser for palliation of esophageal cancer: A multi-center randomized trial. Gastrointest Endosc 1995;42:507.

Litle VR, Luketich JD, Christie NA, et al. Photodynamic therapy as palliation for esophageal cancer: Experience in 215 patients. Ann Thorac Surg, 2003;76:1687.

Longmire WP. A modification of the Roux technique for antethoracic esophageal reconstruction. Surgery 1947;22:94.

Lord RV, Wickramasinghe K, Johansson JJ, et al. Cardiac mucosa in the remnant esophagus after esophagectomy is an acquired epithelium with Barrett's-like features. Surgery 2004;136:633.

Merendino KA, Dillard DH. The concept of sphincter substitution by an interposed jejunal segment for anatomic and physiologic abnormalities at the esophagogastric junction; with special reference to reflux esophagitis, cardiospasm and esophageal varices. Ann Surg 1955;142:486.

Mitty RD, Cave DR, Birkett DH. One-stage retrograde approach to Nd:YAG laser palliation of esophageal carcinoma. Endoscopy, 1996;28:350.

Moghissi K, Dixon K. Photodynamic therapy (PDT) in esophageal cancer: A surgical view of its indications based on 14 years experience. Technol Cancer Res Treat, 2003;2:319.

Monga A, Kumar D, Jain SK. Laser palliation of esophageal carcinoma. J Assoc Physicians India 2002;50:1017.

Nash CL, Gerdes H. Methods of palliation of esophageal and gastric cancer. Surg Oncol Clin North Am 2002;11:459.

O'Riordan JM, Tucker ON, Byrne PJ, et al. Factors influencing the development of Barrett's epithelium in the esophageal remnant postesophagectomy. Am J Gastroenterol 2004;99:205.

Roux C. A new operation for intractable obstruction of the esophagus (L'oesophago-jejuno-gastrosiose, nouvelle operation pour retrecissement infranchissable de l'oesophage). Sem Med 1907;27:34.

Schroder W, Gutschow CA, Holscher AH. Limited resection for early esophageal cancer? Langenbecks Arch Surg 2003;388:88.

Sharma V, Mahantshetty U, Dinshaw KA, et al. Palliation of advanced/recurrent esophageal carcinoma with high-dose-rate brachytherapy. Int J Radiation Oncol Biol Phys 2002;52:310.

Shibuya S, Fukudo S, Shineha R, et al. High incidence of reflux esophagitis observed by routine endoscopic examination after gastric pull-up esophagectomy. World J Surg 2003;27:580.

Stein HJ, Feith M, Siewert JR. Cancer of the esophagogastric junction. Surg Oncol 2000;9:35.

Urschel JD. Does the interponat affect outcome after esophagectomy for cancer? Dis Esophagus, 2001;14:124.

Urschel JD, Blewett CJ, Young JE, et al. Pyloric drainage (pyloroplasty) or no drainage in gastric reconstruction after esophagectomy: A meta-analysis of randomized controlled trials. Dig Surg 2002;19:160.

Vakil N, Morris AI, Marcon N, et al. A prospective, randomized, controlled trial of covered expandable metal stents in the palliation of malignant esophageal obstruction at the gastroesophageal junction. Am J Gastroenterol 2001;96:1791.

EDITOR'S COMMENTS

One size clearly does not fit all when it comes to esophageal surgery. Anyone attempting to pursue esophageal surgery, whether for malignant or benign disease, needs to have a variety of techniques, both extirpative and reconstructive, at the ready and be facile with all of these approaches. The surgeon who is equipped with only one esophageal operation does his or her patients a disservice. Dr. Hofstetter provides an excellent description of each type of reconstruction. Our preference for most indications is the gastric transposition, basing the gastric remnant on the right gastroepiploic vessel. As the author points out, there are indications for the use of colon and jejunum, but these are unusual. We have been quite satisfied with the "hybrid" anastomosis most recently championed by Orringer, which uses a linear stapler with one blade placed through a small gastrotomy and the other in the esophageal lumen. This leaves a small "hood' that must be sutured closed. We have found that leaks rarely occur with this technique, perhaps because of the sheer size of the anastomotic lumen. This anastomosis may be completed in either the chest or the neck. Functional results with this technique have been excellent, with a reduced incidence of patients requiring postoperative dilation. The transhiatal approach with a total esophagectomy and gastric transposition is, in our opinion, the preferred operation for Barrett's esophagus with high-grade dysplasia as well as for invasive adenocarcinoma. Lesions in the mid-esophagus, especially bulky lesions, usually require a thoracotomy, particularly if they are located close to the carina, the so-called "no-man's land" for the transhiatal approach. A total esophagectomy with a cervical anastomosis bringing the gastric remnant through the posterior mediastinum is still the preferred approach.

Colon interposition introduces another level of complexity to an esophageal resection but is the conduit of choice if the gastric remnant is not available. Having to complete three anastomoses clearly increases the risk and potential morbidity of the operation, and the blood supply to the interposed colon is quite a bit more tenuous than that supplying the gastric remnant. In the postoperative period after colon interposition the slightest downturn in the patient's condition should prompt endoscopic evaluation of the interposed segment to assure viability. If not dealt with promptly, a dead colon segment is associated with significant mortality.

We have had limited experience with the long jejunal segment. The occasional patient has required a composite reconstruction using colon and a jejunal segment. The idea of "supercharging" either a jejunal or colon graft is an excellent one, but this should be done with a plastic surgery colleague experienced in microvascular techniques. Usually a short segment of jejunum is used as a free graft vascularized via a microvascular vein and arterial hook-up in the neck.

I was intrigued by the thought that a drainage procedure should rarely be required after esophagectomy where the vagi are taken as routinely occurs. I have always performed a pyloromyotomy, believing that this adds little if any morbidity to the procedure and prevents the need to go back to do an emptying procedure even on an occasional basis. All it takes is one stomach that doesn't empty to convince oneself that an emptying procedure is probably not a bad idea, especially a pyloromyotomy.

L.R.K.

22

Excision of Esophageal Diverticula

Philip A. Rascoe and W. Roy Smythe

Diverticula of the esophagus are uncommon disorders that are usually classified according to their location (cervical, thoracic, or epiphrenic), their pathogenesis (pulsion or traction), and their morphology (true or false).

The great majority of esophageal diverticula are acquired lesions that occur predominantly in elderly adults. Pulsion, or false, diverticula are the most commonly encountered type of esophageal diverticula. These localized outpouchings lack a muscular coat, and their wall is formed entirely by mucosa and submucosa. Almost all are the result of a functional obstruction to the advancing peristaltic wave, usually caused by an abnormal upper or lower esophageal sphincter. Occasionally, impedance to peristaltic progression may be the result of peptic strictures or localized motility disorders such as spasm. Pulsion diverticula thus occur most commonly at the level of the cricopharyngeus where there is a weak area of the crossing muscle fibers in Killian's triangle or the distal 10 cm of the thoracic esophagus between the inferior pulmonary vein and the diaphragm (epiphrenic location); however, they may also occur within the midthoracic esophagus.

True, or traction, diverticula are usually seen in the middle one third of the thoracic esophagus in a peribronchial location. These diverticula are the result of paraesophageal granulomatous mediastinal lymphadenitis secondary to disorders such as tuberculosis or histoplasmosis. The ensuing desmoplastic reaction tents the full thickness of the esophageal wall, producing a conical, wide-mouthed true diverticulum. They most frequently project to the right because subcarinal lymph nodes in this area are closely associated with the right anterior wall of the esophagus. These outpouchings are rarely seen in the Western world and are usually of little or no clinical significance except in rare instances when ongoing mediastinal inflammation results in a fistulous communication with the airway or other intrathoracic structures.

Zenker's Diverticulum

The British surgeon Abraham Ludlow is credited with the original description of a pharyngoesophageal diverticulum from an autopsy specimen that remains on display at the Royal Infirmary Pathology Museum in Glasgow, Scotland. Almost a century later, the German pathologist Zenker provided a complete clinical and pathologic description of 34 cases. The pathogenesis of this lesion was first suggested in 1926 by Jackson, who proposed that the tonically contracting upper esophageal sphincter (UES) impeded the progress of the swallowed bolus. A localized increase in intraluminal pressure forces the mucosa to herniate through the posterior midline of the inferior pharyngeal constrictor in the anatomically bare area (Killian's triangle) between the oblique fibers of the thyropharyngeus and the horizontal fibers of the cricopharyngeus. The diverticulum deviates away from the rigid vertebrae and usually presents on the left side. The exact nature of this cricopharyngeal motor dysfunction remains unclear, but most commonly an incomplete or incoordinated opening of the UES is present.

Clinical Presentation

Zenker's diverticulum is primarily a condition of the elderly and is twice as common in men. Dysphagia for solid food and regurgitation of undigested food are the most common symptoms and are typically present. Halitosis, noisy swallowing or "gurgling" after deglutition, and globus sensation are also common. Aspiration may also result from this condition, and it may manifest as a mild nocturnal cough, morning hoarseness, or new adult bronchospasm caused by repeated laryngeal penetration and irritation and, on rare occasion, present as chronic lower respiratory tract infection or even lung abscess. Despite the association among hiatal hernia, gastroesophageal reflux, and Zenker's diverticulum, only a few patients present with severe heartburn and rarely do they require surgical correction of their reflux.

Diagnosis

A barium esophagogram using a lateral or oblique projection usually demonstrates the diverticulum, which can be large and may protrude well into the superior mediastinum (Fig. 22-1). Esophageal manometry adds little information and should not be routinely performed. Endoscopy can be considered, but often adds little to the diagnosis. Perforation of the diverticulum can result from aggressive endoscopic examination because the flexible endoscope often enters the diverticulum rather than the true esophageal lumen. Malignant change is possible but is exceedingly rare in these diverticula, with squamous cell carcinoma having been reported in no more than 0.5% of patients. If diverticulopexy or endoscopic management is planned, the diverticulum should be palpated to rule out a nodular density in the wall, and a preoperative endoscopic examination should be considered to evaluate the interior of the sac because there will be no pathologic specimen.

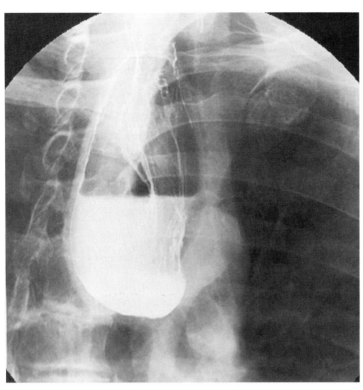

Figure 22-1. Barium esophagram demonstrating a large Zenker's diverticulum.

Treatment

Once a diagnosis is made, treatment is suggested because these diverticula will often enlarge over time and can lead to the more bothersome complications such as aspiration. The gold standard for the surgical treatment of Zenker's diverticulum is cricopharyngeal myotomy combined with either diverticulectomy or diverticulopexy via an open transcervical approach. However, advances in instrumentation for minimally invasive surgery now allow for the management of Zenker's diverticula via a transoral endoscopic creation of a stapled esophagodiverticulostomy in many patients. This procedure creates a cricopharyngeal myotomy while bringing together the lumina of the pouch and esophagus. Carefully selected patients may be offered endoscopic management with the caveat that conversion to an open procedure may be necessary should the minimally invasive approach prove technically unfeasible intraoperatively.

Preoperative Management

Endoscopic management is not the preferred procedure in some patients due to anatomic constraints. Difficulty in placing the diverticuloscope may be encountered in patients with retrognathia, limited jaw mobility, prominent incisors, or rigid cervical kyphosis that limits neck extension. In addition, the size of the diverticulum on barium esophagogram should be assessed because small diverticula (<2 cm) are generally not amenable to stapling. A small pouch limits access of the stapler head and prohibits adequate length of myotomy. Diverticula >6 cm should also be managed with an open approach because endoscopic stapling results in a large pharyngeal cavity that does not empty completely. This information is helpful in preoperative discussions with the patient concerning the likelihood of conversion to an open procedure. All patients should be prepared and give consent for an open procedure in the event that endoscopic instrumentation proves unfeasible or a complication is encountered. Patients are instructed to limit their diet to clear liquids the day before surgery.

Although many cervical operative procedures are now performed under local anesthesia, a general endotracheal anesthetic is suggested for this procedure, along with the usual preincision antibiotic prophylaxis.

Endoscopic Surgical Technique

After induction of general anesthesia, a shoulder roll is placed to achieve neck extension in the standard position for rigid esophagoscopy. An upper jaw dental guard is placed. Direct endoscopy is performed using a lighted suspension laryngoscope. The esophageal lumen, diverticular lumen, and their common wall are visualized. The distal blades are opened slightly to enter the esophagus anteriorly and the diverticular lumen posteriorly. The distal blades of the scope are opened, keeping the common wall between the esophagus and diverticulum centered in the scope's aperture. The proximal scope is then widened, and the laryngoscope is attached to a suspension system to allow for bimanual instrumentation during the stapling procedure. A 0-degree bronchoscope telescope attached to an endoscopic camera is then inserted laterally through the laryngoscope. The pouch is examined to exclude malignancy and to assess the depth of the pouch and length of the septum. A 30-mm linear stapler is then introduced through the laryngoscope, and its jaws are positioned on the common wall with the longer end containing the staple cartilage within the esophageal lumen. The position of the jaws is confirmed using the telescope. If the position of the jaws is in question, the stapler is opened and the device reapplied. If necessary, traction sutures can be placed laterally in the common wall using an Endosuture device and used to help pull the common wall into the jaws of the stapler. If proper positioning of the stapler cannot be confirmed before firing, the minimally invasive approach cannot safely be performed and should be abandoned in favor of an open procedure. Once proper position is confirmed, the stapler is fired and removed. The stapler divides the common wall, including the cricopharyngeus muscle, between the diverticulum and esophagus and closes the wound edges with a triple row of staples on each side. The divided edges of the septum should retract laterally revealing an open esophageal lumen. The cut edges should be inspected to ensure hemostasis. Should a significant septum and diverticular sac still be present, a second stapler application should be performed in a similar fashion. Once the septum is completely divided and hemostasis is confirmed, the procedure is terminated. Patients are offered a liquid diet the following day, and if fluids are tolerated, they are advanced to a soft diet and discharged on the second postoperative day. All patients should have a chest x-ray postoperatively to exclude air in the retropharyngeal space or mediastinum.

Open Surgical Technique

After general anesthesia is induced, a shoulder roll is placed and the neck is extended with the head turned slightly to the right. An incision is made along the anterior border of the left sternocleidomastoid muscle down to near the suprasternal notch. The subcutaneous tissue and platysma are subsequently divided. A superficial cervical cutaneous nerve is present in the upper one third of the field and should be protected if possible to prevent postoperative dysesthesia of the submandibular skin. The incision is deepened through the cervical fascia medial to the sternocleidomastoid muscle. The fascia overlying the omohyoid muscle is incised, and the muscle is divided. The prethyroid muscles are retracted medially to reveal the thyroid gland, the jugular vein, and the carotid artery. The middle thyroid vein is ligated and divided, and the larynx is retracted medially. The inferior thyroid artery is ligated and divided as laterally as possible to protect the recurrent laryngeal nerve, which is located immediately beneath its branches in the tracheoesophageal groove behind the thyroid. The thyroid and cricoid cartilage are rotated medially while retracting the carotid sheath and its contents laterally, and the use of manual retraction is preferred to self-retaining devices to prevent a traction or direct compression injury to the recurrent laryngeal nerve. With the use of blunt dissection, the prevertebral fascial plane is entered posterior to the esophagus and diverticulum, and further rotation of the larynx then everts the lateral posterior pharyngoesophageal junction. The diverticulum can usually be visualized adherent within its filmy attachments to the posterior aspect of the cervical esophagus at or below the level of the cricoid cartilage. The adventitial tissues are gently dissected in the posterior midline to free up the pouch. The tip of the diverticulum is grasped with an atraumatic Babcock or similar type of clamp and is dissected away from the esophagus using a combination of sharp and blunt dissection (Fig. 22-2). The sac is elevated until its neck is clearly defined, and this may require some additional sharp dissection from the known surface of the diverticular sac toward the investing muscle fibers and scar tissue, if present. Once the neck is displayed, a cricopharyngeal myotomy is created starting at the inferior border of the diverticulum on the left posterolateral or posterior aspect of the esophagus. The muscle is separated from the underlying submucosa bluntly using a small right-angled clamp. The myotomy should be extended inferiorly for approximately 3 cm (Fig. 22-3). The submucosa will bulge between the edges of the sectioned muscle. With the myotomy completed, small diverticula (<1 cm) will often

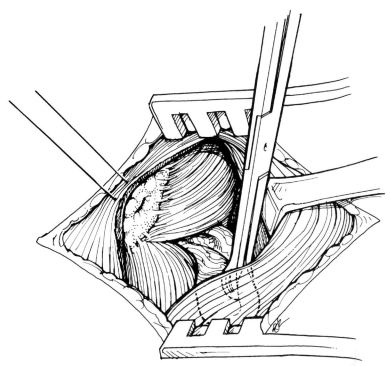

Figure 22-2.   Exposure of Zenker's diverticulum. The sac is grasped with an atraumatic clamp and dissected away from the esophagus.

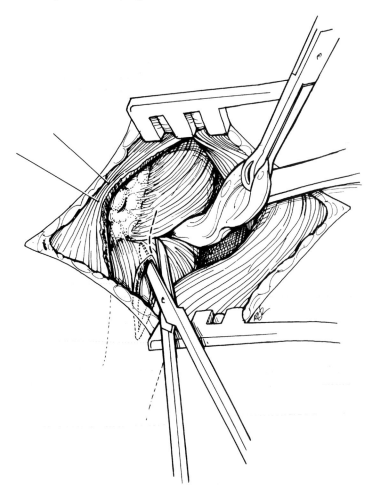

Figure 22-3.   The esophageal muscle is incised from 2 cm to 3 cm below the diverticulum and extended toward the cricopharyngeus.

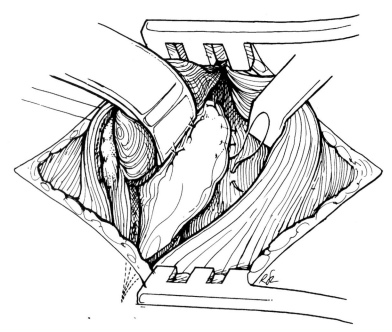

Figure 22-4.   Once the myotomy is completed, the diverticulum should be resected or sutured superiorly to the prevertebral fascia.

disappear when released into the bulging submucosa, and thus myotomy alone is sufficient. Those that do not spontaneously resolve should be further treated with either diverticulopexy or excision. Diverticula <5 cm in length are amenable to diverticulopexy, which is a simpler and faster procedure that does not require opening the esophageal lumen. After myotomy, the tip of the diverticulum may be suspended either to the posterior wall of the pharynx or to the prevertebral fascia with two to four simple 3-0 silk sutures (Fig. 22-4). Care should be taken not to transfix the sac to avoid any contamination of the surgical field. Diverticula >5 cm are too large to be suspended and should usually be resected. After myotomy, a large bougie (40 F or larger, depending on patient size) is inserted into the cervical esophagus to prevent an excessive mucosal resection. If possible, a linear stapling device is applied transversally across the neck of the sac, and the sac is transected distal to the staple line. In the rare cases in which a stapler cannot be applied, the sac may be resected and the defect repaired using interrupted sutures. Care must be taken here to not remove an excessive amount of submucosa with the resection. It is better to have more than needed because tissue can be gathered into the suture line to make the lumen an appropriate size. Before closure, a nasogastric tube is passed into the proximal esophagus, and the mucosal integrity is tested by air insufflation by placing saline in the incision and compressing the distal

esophagus below the nasogastric tube with a tonsil sponge on a ring forceps. The nasogastric tube is subsequently removed, and after hemostasis is ensured, the wound is closed in two layers without drainage. If the ends of the omohyoid are large enough, they may be reapproximated using a figure-of-eight suture technique. Patients are allowed a clear liquid diet the morning after surgery and advanced to a soft diet the following day in most cases. Most patients are discharged on the second or third postoperative day. A postoperative barium swallow is not routinely required before discharge. When at home, a soft diet may be suggested for the first week following surgery.

Surgical Results

There have been no randomized, controlled trials comparing the different open surgical approaches, nor have there been randomized studies comparing endoscopic stapled esophagodiverticulostomy with open surgical techniques. Several case series describing endoscopic techniques have reported satisfactory outcomes in at least 90% of patients, with both morbidity and recurrence rates <10%. These figures closely approximate those reported in series of open surgical techniques. Complications are similar after both techniques and most commonly include hemorrhage, transient vocal cord paralysis, and perforation resulting in mediastinitis. Reported advantages of the minimally invasive approach include

shorter anesthetic time, earlier resumption of normal diet, and shorter hospital stay. The endoscopic stapling technique is an effective procedure that is likely to find increasing application. However, follow-up data regarding recurrences are limited to 2 years. Therefore, conventional open techniques should be considered gold standard therapy at present.

Thoracic Diverticula

Diverticula of the thoracic esophagus are relatively uncommon and typically account for <30% of all esophageal diverticula. As stated earlier, their classification according to location or pathogenesis is probably unnecessary because midesophageal traction diverticula are now a rarity in the Western hemisphere. Almost all thoracic esophageal diverticula are associated with and perhaps caused by an esophageal motor disorder, most commonly achalasia, diffuse esophageal spasm, hypertensive lower esophageal sphincter, and nonspecific motor disorders. Using cinefluorography and manometry, Cross et al. concluded that in 150 patients with esophageal disorders, esophageal diverticula were the result of excessive intraluminal pressures. This segmental increase in pressure, caused by increased esophageal tone or a delay in sphincteric opening, acts on weakened areas of the esophagus and results in outpouching of the mucosa.

Clinical Presentation

Most patients are >60 years of age, and many are asymptomatic or have only minimal and often vague symptoms. There is usually no correlation between diverticular size and the presence of symptoms. Many vague symptoms may be attributable to the underlying motility disorder rather than the diverticulum. Symptoms include dysphagia, postural regurgitation, belching, retrosternal pain, heartburn, and epigastric pain. As in pharyngoesophageal diverticula, pulmonary symptoms are often present but underestimated. These symptoms range from mild nocturnal cough to life-threatening massive aspiration.

Diagnosis

The diagnosis is suggested by a posterior mediastinal air-fluid level on chest roentgenogram and is almost always confirmed by a barium esophagogram. The presence of an associated hiatal hernia or carcinoma within the diverticulum (both uncommon occurrences) can be assessed by endoscopic examination, which should be performed in every case. Esophageal manometry is not essential for the diagnosis but may help to define the nature and the extent of the underlying motor disorder. Manometry may require directed passage of the catheter beyond the diverticulum if difficulty is encountered.

Indications for Surgery

Most would agree that surgical intervention is necessary in symptomatic patients, those with large diverticula, and those with established complications such as bronchopulmonary infection (Fig. 22-5). The indication for surgery in asymptomatic or minimally symptomatic patients is less clearly defined by the literature, and yearly surveillance for patients with an asymptomatic thoracic esophageal diverticulum is often the most prudent option.

The basic elements of the operation are resection of the diverticulum and a myotomy to alleviate the underlying motor disorder. Although some authors advocate that a myotomy be done only if a documented underlying motor disorder is present, this is a hazardous proposition because it risks the integrity of the diverticulectomy staple line in the postoperative period and a possible recurrence of the diverticulum later. Another point of controversy is the length of the myotomy. Although a limited myotomy may be satisfactory in many situations, a long myotomy from the level of the aortic arch down to the first 1 cm to 2 cm of the stomach adds little to the duration of the operation and essentially eliminates the need for reoperation. Naturally, once the cardia is mobilized, a nonobstructive type of antireflux repair must be added to avoid the almost certainly ensuing gastroesophageal reflux, which the aperistaltic esophagus cannot adequately clear.

Surgical Procedure

All patients receive a preoperative dose of ampicillin/sulbactam, and this antibiotic is continued for 24 hours postoperatively. Patients with large diverticula should have the contents of the sac evacuated by a large tube preoperatively. Rapid sequence induction of general anesthesia is necessary to secure rapid control and protection of the airway against aspiration.

Notwithstanding that most diverticula project into the right side of the chest, the preferred approach is through a left thoracotomy, which permits excellent exposure of the lower half of the thoracic esophagus, the diverticulum, and the cardia should an antireflux repair be necessary. The patient is placed in the right lateral decubitus position, and the left chest is entered through the sixth intercostal space. The use of a double-lumen endotracheal tube with deflation of the left lung greatly improves the exposure. The mediastinal pleura is incised over the esophagus, the incision extending from the aortic arch to the esophageal hiatus. The esophagus is mobilized at some distance away from the diverticulum and encircled proximally and distally with Penrose drains including both vagus nerves (Fig. 22-6). The sac is freed from the surrounding mediastinal structures with blunt and sharp dissection. Occasionally, the sac is firmly adherent to the right lung or the right mainstem bronchus (in midesophageal diverticula), and upward traction on the esophagus allows a careful dissection of the sac from those attachments.

The sac may be invested in an inflammatory rind of tissue, and this must be carefully removed to expose the submucosal wall. The neck of the diverticulum is sharply dissected from the surrounding esophageal muscle and residual scar if present, and the submucosal layer should be separated from the surrounding overlying muscle at its margins so that the true neck is obvious for later division. The vagus nerves may be very adherent to the sac, and can be embedded in the inflammatory tissue surrounding it. Care must be taken not to injure the nerves during this part of the procedure.

Dissection then proceeds caudally to mobilize the gastric cardia. The phrenoesophageal membrane is sharply divided, and the hiatus is manually dilated. The mobilization of the cardia is completed by dividing the posterior attachments between the two vagi and entering the lesser sac, followed by complete excision of the fat pad just superior to the cardia in this region. The posterior attachments here may harbor an enlarged arterial branch emanating from the left gastric artery, and failure to recognize this can result in hemorrhage.

At this time, a 44-F or larger bougie is placed by the anesthesiologist with manual guidance by the surgeon past the diverticular opening. The diverticulum is then brought into view by grasping its fundus with an atraumatic clamp and rotating the diverticulum and the esophagus anteriorly and then to the left (Fig. 22-7). If possible, a diverticulectomy is now performed by excising the sac about 5 mm from its neck using a linear stapling device. If this is not possible due to the size of the neck or necrosis at its junction at the esophageal wall, it can be sharply excised after placement of stay sutures on the cranial and caudal extents of the neck. This can then be repaired using interrupted 3-0 absorbable sutures. A nasogastric tube is passed, and the stapled closure is tested for leak by air insufflation under water with distal esophageal compression. The muscle layer is then approximated over the mucosal closure with interrupted 3-0 silk sutures (Fig. 22-8). On occasion, the muscular layer may be too edematous

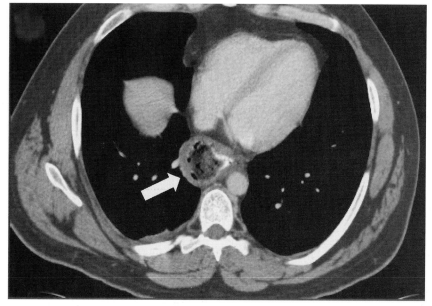

Figure 22-5. Large epiphrenic pulsion diverticulum associated with pain and intermittent regurgitation of undigested food.

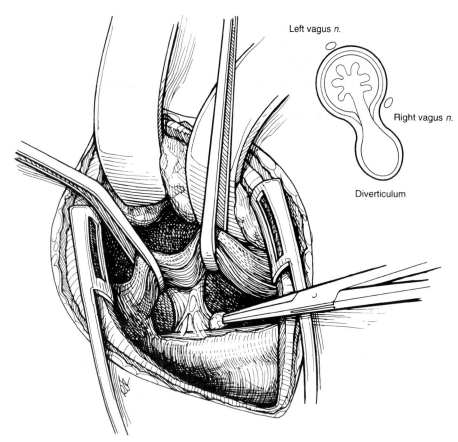

Figure 22-6. Mobilization of the esophagus for thoracic diverticulum. Penrose drains are used to encircle the esophagus proximal and distal to the diverticulum, including vagus nerves. (n. = nerve.)

or attenuated for a good second-layer closure. If this is the case, an intercostal muscle flap may be mobilized and approximated to the linear repair using interrupted small silk sutures on the muscular margins. If this is necessary, placing it around the esophagus posteriorly and then onto the left anterior surface will facilitate comfortable position

when the esophagus is rotated back to the right. A long myotomy is then performed on the left lateral aspect of the esophagus 180 degrees from the excised diverticulum. The muscle is divided at least 2 cm proximal to the diverticular repair, and if feasible from just below the aortic arch and carried across the gastroesophageal junction onto

the stomach for approximately 1 cm. The edge of muscle is gently dissected off the underlying mucosa for several millimeters on either side to preclude premature healing of the myotomy. A nonobstructive antireflux repair should then be performed to prevent reflux sequelae. The repair of choice is the Belsey Mark IV partial fundoplication, with sutures placed on either side of the myotomy in the muscular layer. Once the second layer of sutures is placed, the cardia is gently repositioned into the abdomen and the second layer of sutures is tied. The crura are reapproximated with large nonabsorbable suture so that it will accommodate the tip of the operator's index finger, and the nasogastric tube is advanced into the stomach.

Minimally invasive treatment of thoracic esophageal diverticula has been performed, but the laparoscopic approach should not be used for those diverticula that are positioned higher near the inferior pulmonary vein. When this approach is feasible, a Dorr fundoplication is the preferred procedure after resection of the diverticulum and myotomy. Thoracoscopic approaches have also been reported, and the components of the operation are no different from the open procedure described previously, with the caveat that very large diverticuli may be difficult to dissect and rotate into the field adequately. These minimally invasive techniques are attractive, although the relatively rare nature of these lesions as symptomatic or very large lesions at presentation has precluded systematic study of this approach.

Surgical Complications and Postoperative Care

Retention of the nasogastric tube is encouraged for 3 to 4 days, at which time a barium esophagram is performed to rule out leak at the repair or myotomy or mechanical obstruction. If no leak is present, a clear liquid diet is begun and is rapidly advanced to a soft mechanical diet with discharge typical on the sixth or seventh postoperative day. Although success rates are very high, there has been moderate morbidity reported and a mortality of up to 9% in some series, substantiating the recommendation that small or asymptomatic diverticula should be observed. Causes of death are more frequently mediastinitis as a result of esophageal leakage and aspiration pneumonia. Morbidity and mortality are obviously negatively influenced by the advanced age of many candidates.

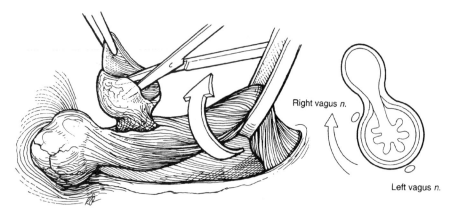

Figure 22-7. The esophagus is rotated to the left and anteriorly to expose the diverticulum, which is most often located on the right side. (n. = nerve.)

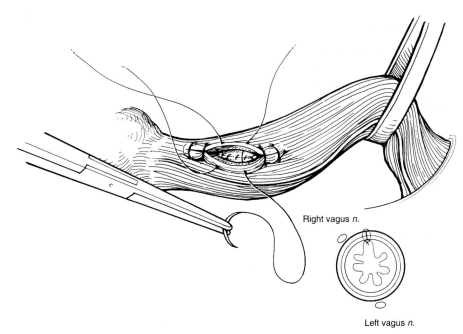

Right vagus *n.*

Left vagus *n.*

Figure 22-8. After removal of the diverticulum, the mucosal and muscular layers are closed with interrupted sutures. The closure may be tested for leak by air insufflation and distal occlusion. (n. = nerve.)

SUGGESTED READING

Adams J, Sheppard B, Andersen P, et al. Zenker's diverticulostomy with cricopharyngeal myotomy: The endoscopic approach. Surg Endosc 2001;15:34.

Allen MS. Treatment of epiphrenic diverticula. Semin Thorac Cardiovasc Surg 1999;11:358.

Aly A, Devitt PG, Jamieson GG. Evolution of surgical treatment for pharyngeal pouch. Br J Surg 2004;91:657.

Bremner CG. Zenker diverticulum. Arch Surg 1998;133:1131.

Rice TW, Baker ME. Midthoracic esophageal diverticula. Semin Thorac Cardiovasc Surg 1999;11:352.

Sen P, Bhattacharyya AK. Endoscopic stapling of pharyngeal pouch. J Laryngol Otol 2004; 118:601.

Sideris L, Chen LQ, Ferraro P, et al. The treatment of Zenker's diverticula: A review. Semin Thorac Cardiovasc Surg 1999;11:337.

White PS, Mountain RE. Endoscopic treatment for Zenker's diverticulum. Semin Laparosc Surg 1999;6:177.

EDITOR'S COMMENTS

By far the most common diverticulum of the esophagus is the pharyngoesophageal, or Zenker's, diverticulum, which, as the authors point out, is not a true diverticulum because it is a mucosal protrusion, not a true full-thickness outpouching of the esophagus. Most commonly these patients present with difficulty swallowing, noisy swallowing, and often signs and symptoms of aspiration, especially at night. Many of these patients are elderly, and many are told they are not operative candidates because of the risk. It is safe to say that the risk is minimal, and it is likely that there is far greater risk to the patient by allowing the diverticulum to remain, especially if the patient has signs of aspiration. If the patient is felt to be at significant risk for general anesthesia, the procedure may be carried out under local anesthesia.

It has been and remains our preference to approach a Zenker's diverticulum via the open technique. This involves an incision along the anterior border of the left sternocleidomastoid muscle with dissection down to the prevertebral fascia. The left side is used even if the diverticulum protrudes to the right because the esophagus is easily mobilized and the left recurrent nerve is less at risk than the right. The myotomy is begun at the base of the diverticulum and carried well down onto the esophagus taking care to incise both the longitudinal and circular muscle fibers. For all but the largest diverticula I prefer to perform a diverticulopexy, excluding the diverticulum from the flow of material in the esophagus but avoiding a mucosal entry. If a diverticulectomy is to be carried out, a large (50 F) bougie is placed to avoid tenting of the mucosa and excessive excision that could lead to a stenosis. A staple line is placed across the diverticulum, and the patient is not fed for several days. A contrast study assures integrity of the staple line before feeding.

As described by the authors, an endoscopic approach to the treatment of Zenker's diverticulum has been described. An instrument specifically for this purpose, the Weerda diverticuloscope, should be used for proper visualization of the diverticulum and endoscopic stapler placement. One blade of the stapler must be in the esophageal lumen and the other in the lumen of the diverticulum for the procedure to be successful. This accomplishes obliteration of the "party wall" between the diverticulum and the lumen of the esophagus and accomplishes a myotomy. The long-term results of this procedure have not been well established.

It is critical to recognize that any esophageal diverticulum or pseudodiverticulum represents the manifestation of a motor disorder of the esophagus, which underscores the importance of a complete myotomy. The myotomy is especially important if the diverticulum has been excised to assure the integrity of the staple line. The terms "pulsion" and "traction" diverticula rarely are used in present-day nomenclature. Even the so-called epiphrenic diverticula are manifestations of a motor disorder, and when operation is indicated a myotomy must also be performed. Patients with an epiphrenic diverticulum also are subject to aspiration, but many, if not most, patients with these diverticula do not require operation. Most are asymptomatic and merely represent curiosities on plain chest radiographs or barium contrast studies. The mere presence of a large epiphrenic diverticulum is not an indication for operation, especially because these must be approached via a thoracotomy.

L.R.K.

23

Lung Transplantation

R. Duane Davis

After the initial report of human lung transplantation by Dr. James Hardy in 1963 at the University of Mississippi, numerous subsequent attempts failed until the first successful transplant by Dr. Joel Cooper at the University of Toronto in 1983. In the succeeding years, lung transplantation has become a viable and effective treatment for patients with end-stage lung disease and has been performed in >20,000 recipients worldwide. Progress has been made in surgical techniques, donor lung preservation, lung reperfusion protocols, perioperative care, and long-term medical management of this challenging patient population. These refinements in care are reflected in survival improvements. One-year survival reported by the Organ Procurement and Transplantation Network (OPTN) has improved from 74% in 1994 to 84% in 2004. Similar improvements in survival have occurred in the experience in the Duke Lung Transplant Program (Fig. 23-1A). In the most recent 3-year cohort, 30-day, 1-year, and 2-year survival have been 98%, 92%, and 81%, respectively. Death early after transplant is commonly related to a primary graft dysfunction (PGD) that is usually caused by ischemia-reperfusion injury. PGD rates have substantially decreased with better lung preservation and controlled reperfusion strategies. Early post-transplant recipient survival and lung allograft survival now approximate rates seen with other solid-organ transplants; however, longer-term survival continues to be suboptimal, with 5- and 10- year survival in registry data of 45% and 25%, respectively. Late deaths are most frequently related to chronic allograft dysfunction, the causes of which are related to both immunologic and nonimmunologic factors. The control of these factors with better immunosuppressive regimens and by minimizing nonimmunologic injury such as with the use of surgical fundoplication to limit gastroesophageal reflux–related aspiration into the tracheobronchial tree appears to be improving long-term survival.

Indications for Lung Transplantation

Lung transplantation has been successfully applied as a treatment for patients with a number of different end-stage lung diseases. Although specific listing criteria and indications have been widely reported, lung transplantation is typically performed in patients (1) with a limited life expectancy secondary to lung failure, estimated to be 6 to 12 months, (2) with the capability of tolerating and following the complicated post-transplant medical regimen, and (3) without comorbidities that would significantly affect post-transplant survival and quality of life, such as concurrent/recent malignancy, extrathoracic infection, or significant dysfunction/failure of other organs. In select patients, concomitant other organ transplant or reparative cardiac procedures can be performed with acceptable results.

The choice to perform a single versus a bilateral, sequential lung transplant depends on recipient characteristics and balancing the value of increasing the number of recipients transplanted by performing two single-lung transplants (SLT) from a single donor with the benefit of improved long-term survival as seen in bilateral lung transplants (BLT). Although the majority of patients with nonseptic lung disease, such as chronic obstructive pulmonary disorders (COPD), idiopathic pulmonary fibrosis (IPF), and primary pulmonary hyperten-

sion, can safely undergo single-lung transplant, patients with septic lung disease, such as bronchiectasis from either cystic fibrosis (CF) or non-CF, require bilateral lung transplantation to prevent infectious complications emanating from the residual native lung. Because of the numerous complications arising from the native lung such as infection, hyperinflation of emphysematous lung, malignancy, and a 25% absolute difference in survival at 7 years (Fig. 23-1B), the practice at the Duke Lung Transplant Program has been to perform bilateral, sequential lung transplants in all patients. This chapter describes the steps in procuring, preparing, and transplanting lungs in a bilateral, sequential fashion. These techniques also are used when only one lung is being transplanted.

Donor Lung Retrieval

The improved outcomes have led to an increased number of recipients waiting for transplant. In the United States, approximately 4,000 patients are listed waiting for lung transplant. Annually, approximately 1,100 lung transplants are performed, whereas 450 deaths occur on the waiting list. The shortage of organs is not unique as compared to other organs, but there are a number of differences. Of organs commonly transplanted, the lungs are the most sensitive to exogenous damage. Events prior to brain injury, such as smoking, and events associated with brain injury, such as aspiration, mechanical ventilation, or neurogenic pulmonary edema, may compromise the suitability of the donor lungs for transplantation. However, there is a wide variety of opinions regarding what is a suitable lung for transplantation. In the United States,

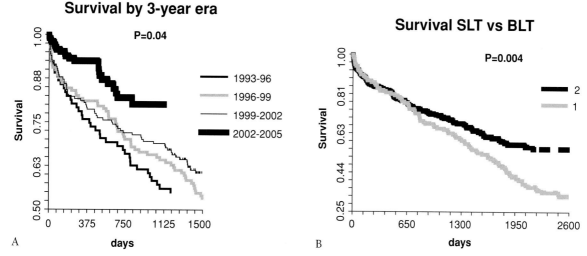

Figure 23-1. Actuarial survival for lung transplant recipients of the Duke Lung Transplant Program **(A)** for the four consecutive 3-year intervals from 1993 to 2005 and **(B)** for patients receiving single (1) as compared to bilateral (2) transplants. Survival has significantly improved with each subsequent time period and for patients receiving bilateral transplants.

there has been a gradual increase in the percentage of organ donors (to 17%) in which lungs were retrieved. However, this number is substantially less than the best-performing regions in the United States as well as in Australia, where the utilization is 40% to 50%. Moreover, survival rates in the recipients from these regions exceed registry data. Aggressive donor management with hormonal replacement, particularly with respect to corticosteroid administration, appropriate ventilatory settings with alveolar recruitment measures, suitable fluid management and vasoactive drug administration, aspiration prevention, and use of bronchoscopic suctioning have been shown to increase the yields of donor lungs. In addition, aggressive evaluation and placement strategies also are factors in increasing donor lung yield.

The donor lungs must (1) be ABO compatible with the recipient, (2) have no unacceptable HLA antigens if the recipient has anti-HLA antibodies, which can be determined by prospective cross-match or virtual cross-match, (3) not transmit diseases such as hepatitis B or C infection, HIV infection, or malignancies, (4) be size compatible, and (5) be able to function physiologically to immediately sustain cardiopulmonary function in the recipient. With respect to disease transmission, donors who test as serologic positives for hepatitis B, hepatitis C, or HIV or have non–central nervous system, non-skin malignancy (excluding melanoma) are not used except in extraordinary circumstances. One exception is that donors with positive hepatitis core antibody but negative

surface antigen serologies can be used with very low rates of disease transmission.

Donor evaluation includes obtaining a thorough medical history for the potential donor. Specific donor criteria depend on the transplant center, but in general, the focus is on the donor's blood type, size, age, smoking habits, pulmonary diseases, thoracic procedures, and mode of death. Additional information that should be provided at the time of a donor offer includes radiographic findings, arterial blood gas, ventilator settings, peak airway pressures, endotracheal tube size, and bronchoscopic findings. In older donors with substantial smoking history, obtaining a high-resolution chest computed tomography scan can greatly assist in evaluating the lung parenchyma and better assess the presence of emphysema, lung nodules, and interstitial lung disease that would be contraindications to the use of the lungs. Corticosteroids (methylprednisolone 1,000 mg) should be administered to the donor, and ventilatory settings should be optimized. Underventilation and inappropriate use of positive end-expiratory pressure (PEEP) are common, and optimization can improve the donor arterial blood gas results. The most recent chest radiograph is examined for pathology and can be used to help with sizing of the organs. Atelectasis does not preclude transplantation; however, clear consolidation would prevent the use of the organs, unless the area could be easily excised or the contralateral lung were to be utilized. This differentiation is rarely possible without direct visualization and palpation of the organs. Atelectasis is the most common

reversible cause of low donor ratios of arterial oxygen partial pressure (PaO_2) to fraction concentration of oxygen in the inspired air (FiO_2). On-site evaluation of prospective donors greatly increases the number of lungs retrieved. In the absence of poor airway compliance (elevated peak airway pressure in the absence of a small endotracheal tube or morbid obesity) or combined abnormalities such as an older donor with extensive tobacco exposure and marginal arterial blood gases, we attempt to evaluate all donors.

Size matching of the donor and the recipient is initially based on height. Matching within 4 inches between donor and recipient is usually without consequence. However, recipients with obstructive lung disease will have larger-than-normal thoracic cavities, and larger donors are preferred. Recipients with restrictive lung disease, on the other hand, will have smaller-than-normal thoracic cavities, and smaller donors are preferred. Comparison of chest measurements, both vertical and horizontal dimensions, between donor and recipient from the chest x-ray provides additional information regarding sizing. It is important to account for size reformatting with digitized films. Although significant size differences between donor lung size and recipient thoracic volume can be managed successfully in the operating room, appropriate size matching before committing to the transplant procedure is optimal.

Fiberoptic bronchoscopy is performed to evaluate for evidence of airway inflammation, intraluminal pathology, and anatomy, as well as to remove secretions from the airways. Although it is common to encounter some purulent secretions, this is not a contraindication to organ utilization unless the secretions do not clear or they recur after being suctioned clear. Donor airway cultures and Gram stains are useful for determining recipient antibiotic administration.

Donor lung procurement is usually performed in the context of cardiac and hepatic organ procurement. The following donor procurement procedure can be used in all circumstances. Exposure of the thoracic and abdominal organs is through a median sternotomy with an extension of the incision in the midline to the pubis. The pericardium is opened in the midline with wide extensions laterally at the level of the diaphragm inferiorly. Pericardial stay sutures are placed for exposure. Both pleural spaces are opened widely, extending from the diaphragm inferiorly to the mammary pedicles superiorly. Adhesions are divided with the electrocautery. Manual examination of both lungs is performed serially to assess the general appearance, nodules, atelectasis, consolidation, edema, and compliance. Suspicious findings should be excised and sent for pathologic analysis to rule out malignancy. The elastic recoil of the lungs is then determined by inflating the lungs with bagged breaths and allowing the lungs to deflate independently by temporarily disconnecting the endotracheal tube from the ventilator. Lungs with adequate compliance should rapidly deflate after disconnection from the ventilator. During this phase of the evaluation, an aggressive alveolar recruitment is performed. In conjunction with the anesthesiologist, the lungs are hand ventilated to expand any atelectatic areas. An arterial blood gas is obtained following these maneuvers. We use a minimum PaO_2 of 300 mm Hg on an FiO_2 of 1.0 and PEEP of 5 cm H_2O as criteria for suitability. Additional information can be obtained and nonpulmonary shunt causes of impaired oxygenation can be identified by individually sampling from the four pulmonary veins. The expected PaO_2 should be >400 mm Hg from the veins draining appropriately functioning regions. This approach can identify areas of lung inappropriate for transplantation. Not infrequently, contused segments or areas of consolidation can be resected by wedge resection, lobectomy, or the use of only one lung. These resections are ideally done as a "back table" procedure after the procurement. Similarly, when the donor lung is oversized for the recipient chest cavity, lung resection can be performed, again, preferably as a back table procedure. In these situations, our preference is to perform a

middle lobectomy on the right and a lingulectomy on the left, with a curvilinear wedge resection from the anteroapical section of either upper lobe. When even greater oversizing occurs, implanting only the lower lobe may be optimal.

Once the decision is made that the donor lung(s) are suitable for procurement and this is communicated to the implanting surgical team, preparation for surgical procurement begins by mobilizing the great vessels. Using primarily cautery dissection, one dissects the ascending aorta from the pulmonary artery (PA) and the superior vena cava (SVC). The SVC is mobilized by cautery dissection from the innominate vein to the right atrial juncture. This dissection is continued on to the heart to develop Waterston's (interatrial) groove. By fully mobilizing the SVC and adequately developing the interatrial groove, one can minimize the two most common sites of procurement injury: (1) injury to the right pulmonary artery posterior to the SVC often at the level of the right PA trunk bifurcation and (2) an inadequate anterior right-sided left atrial cuff. The inferior vena cava (IVC) can usually be mobilized quickly with finger dissection. Commonly, temporary hemodynamic instability occurs, but this can be lessened by placing the donor in Trendelenburg position before these maneuvers. The IVC should be well exposed below and above the diaphragm to ensure adequate tissue for abdominal and cardiac transplant teams.

The trachea is located by incising the posterior pericardium after gently retracting the SVC laterally and the aorta medially. An umbilical tape can be used to encircle the trachea after the plane is developed manually. Once all procuring teams are ready to cannulate, the donor is fully heparinized (250 units/kg). The ascending aorta is cannulated for standard antegrade cardioplegia. The cannula is secured using a 4-0 Prolene mattress or purse-string suture and a Rummel tourniquet. Placement of the PA cannula occurs in a similar fashion as the aortic cannula with placement comfortably distal to the pulmonary valve but adequately proximal to ensure equal perfusion through both pulmonary arteries. Care should be taken to ensure that the bent tip of the curved cannula is directed toward the bifurcation of the PA. After placement of the cannulae, a 500-μg bolus dose of prostaglandin E_1 (prostacyclin) is administered directly into the pulmonary trunk, near the pulmonary cannula. Immediately after infusion of the prostacyclin, the SVC is ligated doubly or occluded using a vascular clamp and the IVC is divided allowing decompression of the right heart. The

aorta is cross-clamped, and the cardioplegia solution is infused through the aortic cannula. Even if the heart is not to be procured, aortic cross-clamping should be performed to prevent bronchial artery flow. The IVC should be divided above the pericardial reflection to provide adequate cuff for both the liver and heart implantations. Left heart decompression is achieved by performing a large left atrial appendage incision. Once this incision is created, perfusion of the lungs through the PA catheter is initiated with either of Perfadex or Celsior preservation solutions (extracellular-based solutions). The height of the solution bag above the PA cannula should not be more than 30 inches. Approximately 3 liters of perfusate (35 to 50 mL/kg) is flushed through the PA (antegrade flushing of the lungs). On commencement of perfusate flow, the thoracic cavity should be bathed in iced saline solution. The procuring surgeon then assesses biventricular filling by directly palpating the heart. Exsanguination and subsequent flow of clear fluid from the left atrial appendage should be observed because it usually indicates successful antegrade flushing of the preservation solution throughout the pulmonary vasculature. Ventilation of the donor lungs should continue during preservation solution administration. To optimize visibility for the subsequent organ removal, the abdominal IVC should be vented inferiorly and not into the chest.

After adequate infusion of the appropriate preservation solutions into the aorta and the PA, removal of the heart is performed. It is paramount that adequate tissue for implanting be achieved for both the heart and lung allografts. The heart is retracted to the right, and a left atriotomy is initiated midway between the coronary sinus and the left pulmonary veins. The interatrial groove on the right is further developed to ensure adequate atrial cuff size. The initial atriotomy is extended inferiorly and superiorly using scissors while being mindful of the left pulmonary veins. The surgeon on the left side of the table typically has the optimal view of the right pulmonary vein orifices and should finish creating the atrial cuff while directly visualizing these orifices. Enough cuff width should be available for the left atrial anastomosis. The SVC is divided between the silk ligatures; alternatively, by using a vascular clamp one can maximize the length of SVC taken by repositioning the clamp distally at this time. The main PA is transected at the bifurcation and the aorta is divided proximal to the cross-clamp. As with the SVC, the vascular clamp may be moved distally to maximize the length of the aorta. The heart is removed from the field.

After the heart is passed off the table, retrograde flushing of the lungs is performed through each large pulmonary vein orifice. Adequate retrograde perfusion can be determined when the perfusate eluting from the PA becomes clear. Usually this requires approximately 1 to 2 liters of the preservation solution (250 mL to 500 mL of solution for each of the four pulmonary veins). Removal of the remaining thoracic contents ensues by dividing the inferior pulmonary ligaments and posterior attachments. The trachea is mobilized by blunt dissection to at least three cartilaginous rings proximal to the carina. Before stapling the trachea, the anesthesia team ventilates the lungs with several bagged breaths. The endotracheal tube is pulled proximally, the lungs are allowed to deflate to approximately two thirds of vital capacity, and the trachea is stapled with the TA-30 stapler two to three rings above the carina. A second row of staples is immediately placed proximally, and the trachea is divided between the two staple lines with a scalpel or scissors. Overexpansion of the lungs is avoided to prevent alveolar stretch injury and subsequent allograft failure.

Heavy scissors can now be used to swiftly divide the remaining posterior mediastinal tissue inferiorly and superiorly in the plane anterior to the esophagus, completely freeing the lungs for removal. Alternatively, the esophagus can be divided after removal of the nasogastric tube proximally and distally with a GIA stapler. The remaining dissection then occurs between the esophagus and the spine with subsequent removal of the lungs en bloc with the esophagus. At this point, they can be bagged together for travel; if the right and the left lungs are going to separate institutions, they require division at the procurement hospital. Our preference is to perform back table dissection at the implanting hospital when possible because of better lighting and equipment.

The lungs are divided by incising the posterior pericardium, the left atrium midway between the two sets of veins, and the main PA at its bifurcation (Fig. 23-2). When lungs are traveling to separate institutions, the left bronchus can be transected between staples just distal to the carina to maintain its inflation pressure for transport. On arrival to the transplanting institution, the grafts are prepared for implantation. This primarily involves dividing the main bronchus for each lung either one or two rings proximal to the upper lobe take-off. Because of the reliance of the bronchus and airways

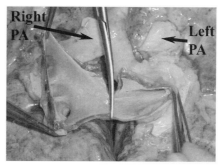

Figure 23-2. Preparation for implantation of the lungs for separate single-lung or sequential bilateral lung transplantation requires division of the donor lungs by incising the posterior pericardium, the left atrium between the two sets of veins, and the main pulmonary artery (PA) at its bifurcation. It is important to remove pericardial attachments from the vascular cuffs to prevent later anastomotic complications.

on collateral perfusion from the PA, the length of the bronchus is kept to a minimum. Care should be taken to minimize dissection along the length of the bronchus. The pulmonary arteries are inspected for the presence of pulmonary emboli. If present, they are removed with forceps, and retrograde flushing through the pulmonary veins is repeated until the perfusate clears. All structures are inspected for injuries. Reconstruction of vascular injuries or inadequate cuff lengths is best achieved on the back table before initiating implantation. Direct repair is usually possible, but autologous tissue from the explanted lungs, allograft tissue from the donor, and pericardium from the recipient can be used to repair injuries. The arteries and atrial cuff should also be evaluated for residual pericardial attachments, and these should be removed at this time. If retained, they may lead to kinking and blood flow occlusion after the anastomosis is completed. Samples of donor bronchus for microbiologic testing can also be taken at this time.

Recipient Procedure

Anesthetic Considerations

Suitable large-bore intravenous access is required for potential large-volume fluid administration. All recipients have a radial artery catheter and a pulmonary artery catheter placed via an internal jugular vein. We also routinely place a femoral arterial catheter because of the frequent poor functioning of the radial arterial line, particularly with clamshell incisions. Patients

are intubated with a double-lumen endotracheal tube with the tip placed into the left bronchus. Confirmation of tube placement is made by fiberoptic bronchoscopic visualization. In small recipients in which a 37-F or greater double-lumen tube cannot be placed, single-lumen intubation is done with the plan to perform the majority of the procedure on cardiopulmonary bypass. Whereas others have used single-lumen tubes using bronchial blockers to isolate the left lung and advancement of the tube into the left bronchus to isolate the right, we prefer to use cardiopulmonary bypass to avoid airway complications such as tube occlusion from inspissated mucous. When performing single-lung transplant, it is preferable to transplant the side that has a normal pleural space and the worst function as determined by quantitative perfusion. All transplants are done with the availability of cardiopulmonary bypass for the transplant procedure and extracorporeal membrane oxygenation (ECMO) for post-transplant support if necessary. During the procedure, minimal fluids, particularly crystalloid solutions, are administered, and inotropic agents (epinephrine) are used liberally to maintain appropriate hemodynamics. Communication by the surgeons to the anesthesiologists before retracting on cardiovascular structures that will cause hemodynamic compromise greatly aids in the appropriate administration of boluses of vasoactive agents to prevent hemodynamic compromise. Maintenance of an appropriate red blood cell volume and clotting factors throughout the procedure is paramount. This is especially important in patients with substantial bleeding and those with pulmonary hypertension and passive hepatic congestion. We routinely use transesophageal echocardiography (TEE) to monitor cardiac function and filling, as well as to interrogate the left atrial anastomoses.

Positioning of the Patient and Skin Incision

For left single-lung transplants, the recipient is placed in a right lateral decubitus position, with access to the left groin for possible femoral vein cannulation. The procedure is performed through a standard fifth-intercostal-space posterolateral thoracotomy. Muscle-sparing thoracotomy can be used, particularly for patients with COPD. Right single-lung transplants can either be performed through a standard fifth-intercostal-space posterolateral thoracotomy or, preferably, through a

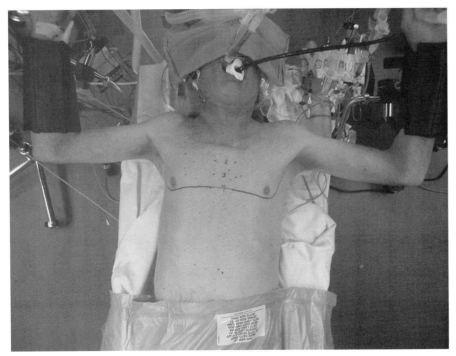

Figure 23-3. Positioning and incision utilized for the clamshell incision. The patient is placed in a supine position with the arms lifted anteriorly and abducted. The forearms are rested on cushioned support as the arms are flexed slightly at the level of the elbow. A warming blanket is placed to cover the lower body below the level of the umbilicus. For a male patient the incision is performed at the level of the fourth intercostal space.

fourth-intercostal-space anterolateral thoracotomy. Access for cardiopulmonary bypass cannulation can be achieved most easily in the chest, and the groins are not exposed. For patients undergoing a bilateral lung transplant, we use a bilateral fourth-intercostal-space anterotrans-sternal thoracotomy (clamshell) incision (Fig. 23-3). The patient is placed in a supine position, and both arms are lifted anteriorly and abducted. The forearms are rested on cushioned support as the arms are flexed slightly at the level of the elbow. A warming blanket or device is routinely used and is positioned from the umbilicus down for right and bilateral transplants and from the thigh down for left lung transplants. It is imperative that the patient's chest and upper abdomen are prepped widely. For a female patient, the skin incision is made at or below the infra-mammary crease, and the chest is opened through the fourth intercostals space after a breast flap is developed and retracted superiorly on each side. After ligating the internal mammary pedicles, we routinely divide the sternum transversely. Although we have had a low incidence of sternal complications, other groups have reported more sternal wound problems and preferentially perform the procedure without division of the sternum through separate bilateral an-

terolateral thoracotomies. At this point, it is important to divide the mediastinal pleura superiorly to the level of the mammary vein and inferiorly to the level of the pericardium with cautery. The pericardium should remain intact at this point but may be opened if the use of cardiopulmonary bypass is anticipated. Before widely opening the retractors, the intercostal muscles in the fourth intercostal space (ICS) are divided in the lateral and posterior direction to maximize the overall exposure with the clamshell incision. The overlying muscles (e.g., latissimus dorsi and serratus anterior) are relatively spared laterally. Adhesions are routinely encountered and are particularly prevalent in patients with cystic fibrosis, previous pneumothoraces, or previous pulmonary resections. The adhesions located along the chest wall, diaphragm, and to the mediastinum well anterior to the phrenic nerve should be divided using electrocautery. Dissection of mediastinal adhesions in the area of the phrenic nerve should be done sharply and with great caution. After lung reduction surgery or previous lobectomies, adhesions to the mediastinum may be such that the phrenic nerve cannot be identified. In these circumstances, it is often prudent to divide the overlying lung tissue using a GIA stapler and to leave a small amount of residual lung

to prevent phrenic nerve injury. This usually is accomplished after all other aspects of the pneumonectomy have been performed. Frequently, this is the most time-consuming portion of the operation.

In recipients with small chest cavities such as most patients with IPF, a figure-of-eight traction suture (0-silk) is placed into the fibrous dome of the diaphragm, and this suture is brought out of the chest using a crochet hook passed through a 14-gauge angiocatheter placed in the most inferolateral aspect of the pleural cavity. The diaphragm is retracted inferiorly while pulling down with the suture, and the suture is secured external to the chest wall with a small clamp. To aid in the exposure of the left hilum, a heavy silk retraction stitch is placed inferiorly on the pericardium, posterior to the phrenic nerve and anterior to the inferior pulmonary vein. The silk suture is passed through a heavy-duty Rummel tourniquet fashioned from a red rubber Robinson catheter, which allows the heart to be safely retracted upward and to the right to provide improved exposure during further dissection of the hilar structures and implantation of the donor lung. For bilateral lung transplants, we routinely mobilize (but do not divide) both hilar structures completely before initiating the recipient pneumonectomy. Which pneumonectomy is done first depends on several factors listed in the relative order of importance: (1) normal chest cavity size and configuration, (2) donor lung quality (a donor lung with contusion, consolidation, or procurement injury is done second), (3) worst native lung function (this side should preferentially be done first), and (4) the degree of technical difficulty for each side (more technically difficult side, usually the left, should be done first, which shortens the period in which only one transplanted lung is being perfused).

The recipient pneumonectomy differs from conventional pneumonectomies in that intrapericardial dissection is always done, division of the pulmonary artery is done at or beyond the take-off of the branch vessels, and the bronchus is divided immediately proximal to the upper lobe orifice. The use of the Endo GIA stapler facilitates the ligation and division of the pulmonary arteries and the pulmonary veins. After the lung is removed, the pericardium around the hilar structures is circumferentially incised. Development of Waterson's groove on the right side and division of attachments from the roof of the left atrium to the pulmonary artery and the posterior left atrial wall and pericardium facilitate subsequent left atrial clamp placement

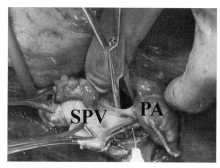

Figure 23-4. Division of the attachments between the left pulmonary artery (PA) and superior pulmonary vein (SPV) and left atrium is initiated laterally and continued medially. Completing the mobilization of the roof of the left atrium from the right side greatly assists in the placement of vascular clamps on the left atrium and subsequent anastomoses.

(Fig. 23-4). The pulmonary arteries are mobilized proximally. On the right side, this requires division of attachments anteriorly to the SVC. On the left side, attention to avoiding recurrent laryngeal nerve injury is paramount. Particularly in the anterosuperior portion of the left PA, the use of electrocautery is avoided. It is important to establish hemostasis, especially in the posterior mediastinum, before initiating lung implantation. Particularly in patients with cystic fibrosis and sarcoidosis, bleeding from lymph nodes can be problematic. Wide extirpation of these lymph node groups with clip ligation of the bronchial artery and other source vessels provides excellent hemostasis, improves exposure, and can assist in preventing vascular anastomotic complications. The vagus nerve located posterior and lateral to the right-sided lymph node group should be identified and protected.

In patients undergoing bilateral lung transplantation, once hemostasis and adequate lengths of PA, left atrium, and bronchus are achieved, two sets of figure-of-eight No. 1 Maxon pericostal sutures are placed in the posterior and lateral aspect of the thoracotomy wound in preparation for closure of the chest at this point of the operation because of the excellent exposure obtained while the lung is out of the pleural cavity. Similarly, posterior pleural drainage tubes are placed in the costovertebral gutter. We use a 36-F right-angled chest tube and a 24-F flexible Blake drain. A smaller-caliber suction catheter placed into this chest tube and connected to suction device then facilitates the drainage of blood and fluid throughout the case. A flexible drainage tube can also be placed at this time in the axillary space, between the rib cage and the

latissimus muscle; in female patients, the tip of this catheter can later be guided into the submammary space near the end of the operation.

Cardiopulmonary Bypass

Most lung transplants can be performed safely and efficiently without the use of cardiopulmonary bypass (CPB). However, CPB should be used whenever recipient hemodynamics, poor systemic perfusion, or technical factors dictate. We use CPB on a planned basis for patients (1) with severe pulmonary hypertension, although occasionally some patients have been treated without bypass by use of nitric oxide and inotropic support, (2) requiring intracardiac procedures such as atrial septal defect (ASD) or ventricular septal defect (VSD) closure or valve repair, (3) with a small recipient airway, (4) who are large relative to the donor lung, to avoid full cardiac output through a small vascular bed, and (5) with fragile left atrial tissue or inadequate donor left atrial cuff, to allow the anastomoses to be performed without clamps using either cardioplegic arrest or fibrillatory arrest. Particularly for patients with pulmonary hypertension and presumed passive hepatic congestion, the bypass circuit is primed with fresh-frozen plasma to mitigate peritransplant coagulopathy. For right and bilateral lung transplants, cannulation is performed in the chest using the right atrial appendage for placement of a 120-degree double-stage cannula for venous return and ascending aorta cannulation for arterial return. For left lung transplants, femoral venous cannulation is performed with a long Bio-Medicus venous cannula (15 F to 23 F) for venous return and descending aorta cannulation for arterial return. Frequently, the femoral venous cannulation is difficult in the decubitus position. In urgent situations venous return can be achieved by cannulating the left pulmonary artery, which allows more time to achieve femoral venous access. Alternatively, we have been able to access the right atrial appendage after initiation of CPB. Although CPB can be performed at any point in the operation as needed, our preference is to perform as much of the dissection including a pneumonectomy before initiating bypass. When CPB is used, we perform both pneumonectomies and full mobilization of all bronchus, pulmonary arteries, and left atrial cuffs before initiating any portion of the implant procedure.

Lung Implantation

There is little difference between the implantation of the left and the right lung. Usually,

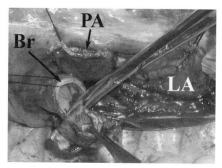

Figure 23-5. The bronchus (Br) is divided anteriorly with a scalpel and a retraction suture is placed anteriorly to aid in the positioning of the bronchus for the subsequent anastomosis. Shown is division of the membranous bronchus. The excised recipient bronchus is sent for culture studies. (LA = left atrial; PA = pulmonary artery.)

the left lung implantation is slightly more difficult when performing a bilateral lung transplant because the heart and left atrial appendage impede the exposure for the left atrial anastomosis. Heparin is administered through a central vein (100 U/kg) with a goal activated clotting time (ACT) of approximately 300 seconds.

The mainstem bronchus is cut with a scalpel just proximal to the takeoff of the upper lobe bronchus. After the cartilaginous portion of the bronchus is divided with a blade, a retraction stitch is placed anteriorly to secure control over the bronchus. The remainder of the bronchial wall (posterior, membranous portion) is then divided with a pair of sharp scissors (Fig. 23-5). The recipient bronchus is now ready for anastomosis, and any secretions within the lumen are aspirated. Confirmation of endotracheal tube location is performed. The pleural space, bronchus, and endotracheal lumen are irrigated with an antibiotic solution. After the antibiotic solution is aspirated, iced laparotomy sponges are placed posteriorly in the pleural cavity, and the donor lung is orthotopically positioned in the pleural cavity. The recipient bronchus and donor bronchus are aligned, and the bronchial anastomosis is performed with a 4-0 PDS suture in a running fashion. The posterior, membranous portion of the bronchial anastomosis is performed first, starting from one corner of the membranocartilaginous junctions (Fig. 23-6). The anterior, cartilaginous portion of the bronchus is anastomosed similarly using the running technique. Usually one bronchus is clearly larger, most commonly the recipient. By placing a transition stitch from the outside of the smaller bronchus into the inside of the larger

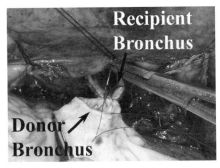

Figure 23-6. The bronchial anastomosis is created using a running suture of 4-0 absorbable monofilament starting from the membranous-cartilaginous junction. The membranous portion is performed in an end-to-end manner.

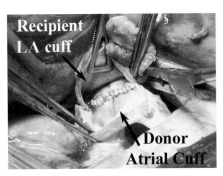

Figure 23-8. The left atrial (LA) anastomosis is created using a running 5-0 polypropylene suture. Retraction of the anterior LA cuff by the assisting surgeon greatly assists exposure, particularly on the left side. Emphasis is placed on creating an intima-to-intima approximation without incorporating muscular tissue.

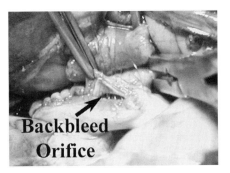

Figure 23-9. The lungs are de-aired through the anteriormost aspect of the left atrial anastomosis. Following partial removal of the pulmonary artery clamp and full removal of the left atrial clamp, the anastomosis is secured and tied.

bronchus, an intussusception is created. The orientation of the anatomy is preserved with membranous-to-membranous and cartilaginous-to-cartilaginous apposition with approximately a one-ring intussusception. After the bronchial anastomosis is completed, it is evaluated for an air leak under water while the anesthesiologist manually inflates the donor lung with room air.

After completing the bronchial anastomosis, the already stapled recipient PA is occluded proximally with a Satinsky vascular clamp, and the staple line is trimmed away. The donor PA is similarly trimmed to an appropriate length. Care must be taken not to leave the donor or recipient PA too long to avoid kinking after the anastomosis is made. The recipient PA and the donor PA are aligned in preparation for the anastomosis, which is begun in one corner with a 6-0 Prolene suture in a running fashion (Fig. 23-7). On the left side, identifying the anterior and apical lobar branches of

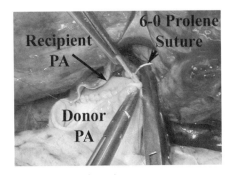

Figure 23-7. The pulmonary artery anastomosis is performed in an end-to-end manner using a running 6-0 polypropylene suture. Frequently, a substantial size discrepancy exists that can be addressed by elongating the distensible smaller pulmonary artery (PA) and taking numerous bites.

the donor facilitates proper alignment. Assessment of the PA anastomosis is done by placing a second vascular clamp (e.g., Harken II) distal to the anastomosis and subsequently removing the previously placed Satinsky clamp from the recipient PA.

Placement of the left atrial clamp is assisted by retracting the stapled superior and inferior pulmonary vein stumps laterally with Pennington clamps. A large Satinsky vascular clamp is placed on the body of the left atrium. The staple lines are excised, and the orifices of the superior pulmonary vein and inferior pulmonary vein are connected, creating a large, recipient left atrial cuff. Placing a Pennington clamp on the anterior portion of the atrial cuff and retracting superiorly and medially greatly improves exposure, particularly on the left side (Fig. 23-8). Exposure for the left-sided anastomosis often requires substantial retraction of the heart. This can be facilitated by retraction of the previously placed pericardial stitch and by manual retraction. During this period, placement of the patient into Trendelenburg position and bolus administration of inotropic agents may be necessary. Occasionally, widely opening the pericardium to allow the heart to herniate anteriorly and to the right may be necessary to provide exposure and suitable hemodynamics. An endothelial-to-endothelial anastomosis is created using a running suture of 5-0 Prolene suture with a concerted effort to include the intimal layer and exclude the muscular tissue. Once the posterior portion of the anastomosis is completed, an intravenous bolus of methylprednisolone (500 mg) and mannitol (25 gm) is given.

Reperfusion

With the last few throws of the 5-0 Prolene suture left loose anteriorly (Fig. 23-9), the vascular clamp on the PA is partially released to allow blood to flow into the newly implanted lung through the right PA anastomosis in order to remove air from within the pulmonary vasculature. Immediately before the 5-0 Prolene suture is tied, the Satinsky clamp on the recipient left atrium is released to force out any residual air. Reperfusion is carefully controlled to minimize the risk of primary graft dysfunction (PGD). Controlled, low-pressure perfusion of the lung is achieved by gradually releasing the PA clamp over 10 to 15 minutes. Ventilation with room air is initiated by hand and then by mechanical ventilation. Pressure control mode of ventilation is preferred with 5 cm to 8 cm of PEEP, distending pressure of 16 cm to 22 cm, and minimal FiO_2—preferably <30%. During this reperfusion period, hemostasis of the donor lung tissue is achieved. At the time of full release of the pulmonary artery clamp, the pulmonary artery pressures should be normal. Use of nitric oxide and loop diuretics is initiated if pulmonary artery pressures are elevated or if poor systemic oxygenation is present. An anterior 28-F pleural tube is placed on each side.

When implantation occurs on CPB, as previously mentioned, both pneumonectomies are performed, posterior thoracotomy sutures and pleural drains are placed, and both lungs are implanted before reperfusion. The first lung that is implanted is packed in ice slush during implantation of the second lung. Methylprednisolone (1 g) and mannitol (50 g) are administrated before reperfusion. While the lungs are ventilated with room air, gradual reperfusion is initiated starting at 5 to 10 mm Hg mean PA pressure and increasing by 5 mm Hg every 5 minutes until normal systemic pressures are achieved. Reperfusion of the lungs with oxygenated, hypocarbic blood may be especially advantageous to maximize pulmonary vascular recruitment and parenchymal recovery.

In patients undergoing double-lung transplants without CPB, once appropriate hemodynamics and oxygenation are confirmed after reperfusion of the first transplanted lung, the remaining native lung is removed. Implantation proceeds in a similar fashion as for the first lung. The performance initially of bilateral dissection and mobilization greatly reduces the duration of time for which the entire systemic blood flow passes through only one transplanted lung, which also appears to minimize the development of PGD.

For single–lung transplants, closure of the posterolateral thoracotomy is conventional with large-bore chest tubes placed in the anterior and posterior pleural space. For bilateral transplants performed using a clamshell incision, the anterior aspect of the clamshell opening is approximated with three sets of No. 5 wires, one simple set in the midline of the sternum and one set of figure-of-eight on each side of the midline with the lateral aspect placed lateral to the mammary pedicle. The remainder of the clamshell opening is reapproximated with a series of No. 1 Maxon sutures in a figure-of-eight fashion. As described earlier, the Maxon sutures on the lateralmost aspect of the clamshell opening were placed while the native lungs were either deflated or removed. If not already done, a Blake drain into each of the axillary space is placed. The pectoral fascial layer, the subcutaneous layer, the subdermal layer, and the skin are then approximated.

Chest tubes are placed to suction, except in circumstances in which the recipient pleural space is substantially larger than the donor lung size. In these situations, chest tubes are left to water seal to prevent overdistension of the lung allograft, stretch injury, and severe pulmonary graft dysfunction. This situation can be identified by marked differences in tidal volumes between when the pleural tubes are on and off suction.

After dressings are applied, the double-lumen endotracheal tube is removed and a large single-lumen endotracheal tube is placed. Fiberoptic bronchoscopy is performed to (1) assess the adequacy of the anastomosis, (2) clear secretions, (3) assess for the development of PGD as manifested by severe pulmonary edema, and (4) evaluate for torsion or malrotation of the allograft manifest by abnormal, crescent-shaped distal airways.

Primary Graft Dysfunction

By using extracellular-based pulmonary perfusion solutions, adding retrograde pulmonary perfusion to lung preservation, minimizing the oxygen exposure at the time of reperfusion, controlling the initial pressure and flow through the lung allograft, and using oxygen free-radical scavengers, the incidence of severe primary graft dysfunction (PGD) has decreased from 15% to 25% to as little as 5%. However, development of severe allograft dysfunction as demonstrated by marked hypoxia, pulmonary edema, elevated pulmonary artery pressures, and poor compliance requires immediate investigation for reversible causes. It is especially important that anastomotic or mechanical causes, especially venous out-flow problems, are identified and corrected immediately. With respect to venous out-flow obstruction, correction later than 4 to 6 hours will be unlikely to achieve reasonable allograft recovery. Interrogation of the anastomoses includes visual inspection to assess for torsion or kinking; TEE to assess for turbulent or absent pulmonary vein flow, left atrial anastomotic quality, and presence of intraluminal clot; and direct measurement of pressures across the anastomosis. Cardiac etiologies can usually be identified by TEE including left-sided valvular abnormalities, left ventricular failure, intracardiac shunts, and tamponade. We routinely obtain a quantitative perfusion scan within the first hours after the transplant, with lobar or greater perfusion defects necessitating further assessment, most preferably by operative exploration. Asymmetric pulmonary edema and crescent-shaped airways on bronchoscopic evaluation may be indicative of mechanical problems. PGD can be caused by humoral lung injury from circulating antidonor antibodies. These antibodies are identified by donor–recipient

---

Table 23-1   Duke University Immunosuppression Protocol

Preoperative
FK506: 0.04 mg/kg PO on admission
Azathioprine: 2 mg/kg IV on induction of anesthesia

Intraoperative
Solu-Medrol: 500 mg IV before reperfusion of each transplant lung if bilateral; 500 mg IV before reperfusion of single transplanted lung.
Basiliximab (Simulect): 20 mg IV after induction of anesthesia.

Postoperative
FK506: 0.04 mg/kg given sublingually every 12 hrs; *for patients who will also receive voriconazole or itraconazole postoperatively, reduce dose to 0.02 mg/kg;* adjust to achieve a trough level of 10–15 ng/mL; switch to PO when gastrointestinal motility is restored; if creatinine >1.5, target FK506 level is 8–12 ng/mL.
Azathioprine: 2 mg/kg IV or PO daily to maintain white blood cell count >4,000. Steroids: Solu-Medrol 125 mg IV every 12 hrs for 48 hrs, then prednisone 20 mg PO daily
Basiliximab (Simulect): 20 mg IV on postoperative day 4.

Maintenance
FK506: Every-12-hr dosing adjusted to maintain trough FK506 levels: months 0–6, 10–15 ng/mL; >6 months, 8–12 ng/mL; lower level may be required if patient develops significant renal insufficiency.
Azathioprine: 2 mg/kg/d PO adjusted to maintain white blood cell count >4,000.
Prednisone: months 0–3, 20 mg/d; months 4–6, 15 mg/d; months >6, 10 mg/d.

Treatment of rejection

Minimal or mild rejection episodes (ISHLT grade 1 or 2): Solu-Medrol 500 mg IV daily for three doses followed by oral prednisone taper starting at 60 mg and decreasing by 5 mg/d until original dose is reached.

Moderate (ISHLT grade 3) or steroid-resistant rejection: RATG (Thymoglobulin) 1.5 mg/kg IV for three doses; premedicate with Solu-Medrol 40 mg IV, diphenhydramine 50 mg IV, and acetaminophen 650 mg PO 30 min before each dose.

ISHLT = International Society for Heart and Lung Transplantation; IV = intravenous; PO = oral; RATG = rabbit antithymocyte globulin.

cross-matching. Treatment is multimodal, including plasmapheresis, column absorption, intravenous immunoglobulin, and anti–B cell therapies such as anti-CD20 (rituximab).

Severe PGD causes or significantly contributes to the majority of early post-transplant deaths. Unless reversible causes could be identified, treatment has been supportive with optimization of ventilator parameters, inotropic support, and nitric oxide. We have shifted to a strategy of early institution of venovenous (V-V) ECMO when recipients develop severe pulmonary edema or require $FiO_2 > 60\%$. Venovenous cannulation typically is instituted via the right femoral vein with a venous catheter (Bio-Medicus) and the left internal jugular vein with a pediatric arterial cannula (Medtronic, Minneapolis, MN). Cannulae are placed percutaneously using a modified Seldinger technique over a guidewire following serial dilations. The circuit consists of a hyaluron-based, heparin-coated $\frac{3}{8}$-inch tubing (GISH Biomedical, Inc., Rancho Santa Margarita, CA) with a Jostra Quadrox hollow fiber membrane oxygenator and Jostra Rotaflow pump (MAQUET CardiopulmonaryAG, Hirrlingen, Germany). The optimal placement of circuit inflow and outflow ports is determined by the level of recirculation noted in the system. ECMO flows are approximately 2.5 to 3.5 liters/min with a sweep gas flow adjusted to maintain the partial pressure of carbon dioxide around 30 mm Hg so as to maximize pulmonary vasodilation. During V-V ECMO support, a protective ventilatory strategy is used including low-oxygen, low-pressure ventilation. Weaning from V-V ECMO involves discontinuing membrane gas flow and increasing ventilatory parameters as needed. No increase in anticoagulation is required for V-V ECMO weaning. With the use of this strategy, all patients have been weaned from ECMO, usually after 3 to 5 days of support, because pulmonary vascular resistance decreases following institution of ECMO and pulmonary capillary leak usually resolves more quickly (often within 24 hours). The 30-day survival in patients requiring V-V ECMO at our institution is approximately 90%.

Principles of Postoperative Care

Although an extensive discussion of postoperative care is beyond the scope of this text, a few principles are important. Optimal pain control, especially for bilateral trans-plant recipients, is achieved with an epidural analgesia. Most patients with good allograft function should be extubated within 24 hours of the transplant and can be discharged from the hospital within 10 days of the transplant. Although the optimal immunosuppressant regimen is not known, most programs use a triple-drug regimen including a calcineurin inhibitor (cyclosporine, tacrolimus), an antiproliferative agent (Imuran, mycophenolate mofetil), and corticosteroids. Induction therapy using an anti-CD25 agent (basiliximab, daclizumab) or an immune cell–depleting agent, either a polyclonal anti–T cell agent (Thymoglobulin, ATGAM) or, most recently, anti-CD52 (Campath), is used in approximately 50% of lung transplant recipients. Although acute rejection occurs commonly after lung transplant with 40% to 60% of patients having at least one episode of rejection in the first 6 months, it is an uncommon cause of early mortality. Mortality early after lung transplant is most commonly secondary to poor allograft function, infection, and neurologic and cardiac events. The immunosuppression and infection prophylaxis protocols used by the Duke Lung Transplant Program are outlined in Tables 23-1 and 23-2.

A factor that appears to be related to lung allograft injury and is underestimated in its frequency is that of aspiration injury. In addition to the infrequent classic massive aspiration pneumonitis, repetitive injury secondary to microaspiration appears to occur commonly. Factors that increase the risk of aspiration include the high prevalence of gastroesophageal reflux in patients with end-stage lung disease, particularly in those patients with IPF and cystic fibrosis.

Table 23-2   Duke University Infection Prophylaxis

Bacterial
Standard regimen[a]:
Ceftazidime: 2 g IV preoperatively on induction per anesthesia, then 1 g IV every 8 hrs for 7–10 d or until invasive lines are out (adjust doses for renal insufficiency)
Vancomycin: 1g IV preoperatively on induction per anesthesia, then 1 g IV every 12 hrs for 7–10 d or until invasive lines are out (adjust doses for renal insufficiency)

CMV/HSV/EBV[b,c,d]
Donor negative/recipient negative: leukoreduced PRBCs only; if HSV-negative, no prophylaxis; if HSV-positive, acyclovir 200 mg PO thrice daily for 12 wks
Donor positive/recipient negative: ganciclovir 5 mg/kg IV every 12 hrs for 4 wks followed by ganciclovir 5 mg/kg IV daily for 10 wks, followed by Valcyte 450 mg PO daily indefinitely.
Donor negative/recipient positive OR donor positive/recipient positive: ganciclovir 5 mg/kg IV every 12 hrs for 2 wks followed by ganciclovir 5 mg/kg IV daily for 2 wks

Pneumocystis carinii: Septra DS, one PO every Monday, Wednesday, Friday starting 1 wk postoperatively, continuing indefinitely; if sulfa allergy: dapsone 50 mg PO daily OR aerosolized pentamidine 300 mg every month continuing indefinitely.

Fungal: Nystatin suspension 5 cc swish and swallow daily for oral Candida prophylaxis; continue for 6 mos; inhaled amphotericin B 50 mg daily for 4 d, then weekly while hospitalized immediately post-transplant (dose to be reduced to 25 mg once patient is extubated)

***Toxoplasmosis gondii* (use only for donor positive/recipient negative):** Septra DS, one daily starting 1 wk postoperatively (also covers *P. carinii* prophylaxis); if sulfa allergy: pyrimethamine (Daraprim) 50 mg PO daily and folinic acid (leucovorin) 10 mg PO daily for 6 mos (use in addition to pentamidine for *P. carinii* prophylaxis); if patient is intolerant of daily pyrimethamine, use dapsone 50 mg daily and pyrimethamine 50 mg weekly and folinic acid 10 mg weekly

---

CMV = cytomegalovirus; EBV = Epstein-Barr virus; HSV = herpes simplex virus; IV = intravenous; PO = oral; PRBC = packed red blood cells.
[a]The standard regimen should be amended as indicated to include the following: (1) coverage for any other known preoperative pathogens in the recipient; this is particularly indicated for recipients with cystic fibrosis, bronchiectasis, and other septic lung diseases; (2) coverage for any additional organisms identified from donor bronchial washings; OR if first bronchoalveolar lavage (BAL) cultures are negative at 72 hrs postoperatively, change IV antibiotics to Levaquin or moxifloxacin 500 mg PO daily for 7 d.
[b]Use Valcyte 450 mg PO twice daily for the duration of the above protocols as long as patient is tolerating POs, has good PO intake, normal gastrointestinal function, white blood cell count >5,000, and creatinine <1.5.
[c]For all EBV-negative recipients: ganciclovir 5 mg/kg IV every 12 hrs for 4 wks, followed by Valcyte 450 mg PO daily indefinitely.
[d]Patients receiving rabbit antithymocyte globulin (RATG; Thymoglobulin) therapy treated with ganciclovir at a dose of 5 mg/kg IV every 12 hrs (or appropriate treatment dose based on renal function) for 3 weeks for CMV prophylaxis.

Gastroesophageal reflux is even more common and of greater severity after lung transplant because of issues related to both the medication regimen and, more important, to vagal nerve injury. Vagal nerve injury also contributes to gastroparesis, which can exacerbate the amount of esophageal reflux. In addition, abnormal oropharyngeal swallowing appears to occur in many patients often as a result of left recurrent laryngeal nerve injury. We routinely assess all patients for gastroesophageal reflux both before and early after lung transplant as well as perform an endoscopic swallow evaluation after transplant and before initiating oral intake. In patients with severe reflux, surgical fundoplication is performed early after the lung transplant, often during the transplant admission. Patients who fail their swallow evaluation receive nutritional support via intestinal and not gastric tubes (i.e., gastrojejunal tube or nasojejunal tube) until their oropharyngeal function normalizes. In patients with vocal cord paralysis or paraparesis, vocal cord medialization is performed.

Bronchoscopic examination is performed frequently in the early post-transplant period. It is applied, often in conjunction with obtaining transbronchial biopsies, to investigate new infiltrates, fevers, or allograft dysfunction as manifest by worsening oxygenation, hypercapnia, and decreased spirometric values. Although pulmonary embolism is uncommon after transplant, the potentially devastating consequence of pulmonary infarction because of the lack of bronchial artery inflow requires a high degree of vigilance with respect to diagnosis and treatment. Surgical embolectomy of large pulmonary emboli is often indicated.

Conclusions

Tremendous progress has occurred in lung transplantation over the last two decades. One-year patient and allograft survival now is comparable to those of liver and cardiac transplantation. As with all solid-organ transplantations, the shortage of available donor organs and the development of chronic allograft injury are the primary limitations to a greater applicability to the treatment of end-stage lung diseases. Although development of alternative organ sources through xenotransplantation, lung organogenesis, and non–heart beating donors will greatly affect the future number of lung transplants performed, there appears to be a substantial number of suitable organs, especially the lungs, that would become available if the majority of donors were evaluated appropriately. With a better understanding of the causes of lung allograft injury and ongoing work toward developing immunologic tolerance, improved long-term outcome is achievable.

SUGGESTED READING

Cantu III E, Appel III JZ, Hartwig MG, et al. Early fundoplication prevents chronic allograft dysfunction in patients with gastroesophageal reflux disease. Ann Thorac Surg 2004;78:1142.

de Perrot M, Snell G, Babcock W, et al. Strategies to optimize the use of currently available lung donors. J Heart Lung Transplant 2004; 23:1127.

Patel VJ, Messier RH, Davis RD. Clinical outcome following coronary artery revascularization and lung transplantation. Ann Thorac Surg 2003;75:372.

EDITOR'S COMMENTS

Davis and his colleagues at Duke have contributed greatly to improvements in lung transplantation in recent years. Perhaps no other procedure is so dependent on rigorous attention to even the most minute detail. The Duke group recommends bilateral sequential lung transplant for all patients, even those in whom a single lung would suffice, based on improved long-term survival for patients receiving two lungs. It is difficult to argue with this rationale, except to point out that the number of potential recipients waiting for transplant far exceeds the supply of donor lungs, so for most programs it makes sense to use a single lung in certain recipients.

Because of problems with sternal wound healing after the transverse sternotomy used with the bilateral thoracosternotomy incision, many groups have gone to using bilateral anterior thoracotomies, accepting the poorer exposure. Davis points out that they have not had problems with sternal wound healing, and there is no question that the exposure afforded by division of the sternum significantly facilitates both the removal of the native lungs and implantation of the donor lungs. Secure wire closure of the transverse sternotomy should promote healing and decrease the incidence of wound problems.

The aggressive use of venovenous extracorporeal membrane oxygenation is novel, but it is hard to argue with a 30-day 90% survival. The key here is the early institution of the ECMO support, as the Duke group espouses, if there is significant graft dysfunction. The other strategies mentioned to attenuate the incidence of primary graft dysfunction should be adopted by all institutions based on the outstanding results reported here.

The recognition that occult gastroesophageal reflux may contribute to lung allograft infection and injury is particularly important. We have long known that swallowing dysfunction accompanies pneumonectomy, and it also has been recognized in those undergoing lung transplantation. What is newly recognized is the significant incidence of gastroesophageal reflux and aspiration. I applaud not only the author's aggressive use of medical antireflux management, but also the early use of surgical fundoplication in these patients. A number of patients have undergone fundoplication during the post-transplant hospitalization.

All groups performing lung transplantation would be wise to adopt many of the protocols put into use by the Duke group.

L.R.K.

24

Surgery for Emphysema

Mark Ellis Ginsburg

Introduction

Emphysema is characterized by "an abnormal permanent enlargement of airspaces distal to the terminal bronchioles, accompanied by destruction of their walls without obvious fibrosis." This pathologic process proceeds relentlessly, leading to breathlessness, reduced exercise capacity, respiratory failure, and, ultimately, death. Surgical therapy is designed to address the physiologic derangements imposed by this process in an attempt to palliate symptoms and, in very select cases, improve survival.

Emphysema has always presented a formidable therapeutic challenge for thoracic surgeons. Encountered both as a primary disease and as a comorbidity, it has long challenged the surgeon's skills and innovation. The rediscovery and refinement of lung volume reduction surgery (LVRS) by Dr. Joel Cooper and colleagues in 1994 was a powerful impetus toward developing new techniques and a better understanding of the natural history and pathophysiology of this disease. Once seen as an untreatable and progressive illness with little hope of improvement, it has now become a target of new therapeutic interventions and hope.

This chapter deals with lung volume reduction surgery and its techniques, but it should be appreciated that broad advances are being made in understanding the physiology, pharmacology, and radiology of emphysema. The future has never been more optimistic for this unfortunate group of patients.

History

Over the course of the last century a number of well-intentioned but poorly conceived procedures have attempted to address the mechanical and physiologic derangements of the emphysematous lung. Surgical techniques to accommodate the hyperinflated lung by enlarging the chest cavity included costochondrectomy and transverse sternotomy. Paravertebral thoracoplasty attempted to reduce pulmonary hyperinflation. These procedures fell far short of their goals, and, not achieving any objective benefit, were quickly abandoned. The valid observation that the typical flattening of the diaphragm seen in advanced emphysema was associated with limited ventilation led to misconceived attempts to restore diaphragmatic contour by phrenicectomy, pneumoperitoneum, and abdominal belts. Parietal pleurectomy was used to address reduced parenchymal perfusion, with the hope of promoting collateral circulation from the chest wall. Pulmonary denervation attempted to reduce bronchospasm and secretions but was also of no benefit.

Despite the foregoing, there have been some notable successes in the surgical efforts to treat emphysema. Giant bullectomy did result in demonstrable and durable improvement but proved useful in only a limited and specifically defined group of patients. Otto Brantigan first conceptualized the idea of pulmonary remodeling to alter the compliance and function of the diseased lung. His concept was that the elastic recoil holding open small airways was lost due to hyperinflation, and that reducing the size of the lung would improve expiratory airflow. He applied this concept of lung reduction using multiple wedge resection but was unable to provide convincing evidence of effectiveness and applicability. Lung transplantation has proven successful for emphysema, but again it remedies only a narrow spectrum of patients. Laser bullectomy, popularized by Wakabayashu in the early 1990s, triggered renewed interest in the disease but was neither efficacious nor safe.

The reintroduction of lung volume reduction for emphysema by Cooper and colleagues and the subsequent data provided by the National Emphysema Treatment Trial have shown that a large number of emphysema patients can benefit by surgical treatment.

Pathophysiology of Emphysema

The most widely accepted hypothesis for the pathogenesis of emphysema is that an imbalance in the proteinase–antiproteinase system leads to a net excess of proteolytic activity in the lung. This imbalance results from either an excess of proteinase activity by external irritants or a reduction in antiproteinase activity due to a genetic predisposition. These enzymatic processes result in a degradation of the elastin and collagen matrix and ultimately destruction of lung tissue and loss of elastic recoil. Physiologically, this damage leads to a limitation of airflow, alterations in pulmonary mechanics, abnormalities in gas exchange, and changes in pulmonary hemodynamics. The clinical consequences are dyspnea, reduced exercise capacity, recurrent pulmonary infections, and finally respiratory failure. More recent evidence suggests far more complex interactions of injuries involving metalloproteinases, tumor necrosis factor, polymorphonuclear cells, CD4 cells, CD8 cells, and macrophages. Work by Hogg and colleagues showed that recurrent injury and remodeling of terminal bronchioles results in irreversible airway obstruction. They postulated that this process is driven by colonization and repeated infections and is mediated by an adaptive immune response.

The reduction in expiratory airflow measured by spirometry is evident by a decrease in the ratio of the forced expiratory volume in 1 second (FEV_1) to the forced vital capacity (FVC) and an absolute decrease in FEV_1 itself. Hyperinflation, a primary characteristic of emphysema, is a direct result of the loss of elastic recoil and acts as a compensatory mechanism by which increasing lung static volumes creates decreases in air flow resistance at the level of the most distal bronchi. This phenomenon is in contrast to asthma and chronic bronchitis, in which inflammatory airway disease leads primarily to an increase in airway resistance but minimal hyperinflation. Distinguishing between these two varieties of obstructive lung disease is critical to patient selection for operation for emphysema.

In response to hyperinflation, the diaphragm flattens and the chest wall increases in size. Progressive diaphragmatic flattening leads to a reduction in muscle fiber length, decreased inspiratory force generation, decreased surface apposition, and reduction in transpulmonary pressure. When extreme, diaphragmatic contraction can lead to a reduction of the chest cavity during inspiration. All these changes place the chest wall and accessory muscles at a mechanical disadvantage during ventilation compared to normal individuals and result in an increased work of breathing.

Classically, emphysema is characterized by fairly well preserved gas exchange. There is a reduction in diffusing capacity due to loss of alveolar surface area, but marked hypoxemia is uncommon except in end-stage disease. There is a marked ventilation-perfusion (V/Q), with ventilation going to already high V/Q areas (dead-space ventilation).

The hemodynamic effects of emphysema are not well documented. There appear to be increases in pulmonary vascular resistance, pulmonary artery systolic pressure, and pulmonary capillary wedge pressure at rest and a limitation of cardiac output with exercise. The causes of pulmonary hypertension are multifactorial and include vasoconstriction, loss of pulmonary capillary bed, and thickening of the pulmonary arteries due to remodeling. Hyperinflation during exercise may limit cardiac filling, resulting in reduced cardiac output. These alterations result in further limitation in peripheral O_2 delivery during exertion.

Selection of Patients for Surgical Therapy

Patient selection for operative intervention is limited by a relative lack of clinical experience and long-term data. Initial screening should include a comprehensive history and physical examination, pulmonary function tests, chest x-ray, and computed tomography scan of the chest. It is important to establish the diagnosis of emphysema with hyperinflation, the distribution of disease, and the degree of disability prior to proceeding to a costly and intrusive workup. Many patients can be excluded from further consideration based on this limited screening. The major indications and contraindications for LVRS are outlined in Tables 24-1 and 24-2.

A thorough history should be elicited for the degree of disability from emphysema per se, the rate of progression of symptoms, the frequency of hospitalizations, and the amount and quality of daily sputum production. The physical examination should make note of the breathing pattern at rest and during exercise, especially the contribution of the accessory muscles, signs of reactive airway disease, and the degree of physical deconditioning.

Those patients who have disability felt to be severe enough to warrant further consideration for surgical intervention, who have emphysema with little evidence of reactive airway disease or chronic bronchitis, and who meet the general criteria for LVRS should then undergo an extensive evaluation that includes cardiac testing, comorbid disease assessment, exercise capacity, and

quality-of-life metrics (Table 24-3). At this point, a frank discussion of the goals for surgical therapy and the limitations of this approach should be undertaken. Other options should be explored including refining medical therapy, pulmonary rehabilitation, and, if appropriate, lung transplantation.

Distinguishing emphysema from chronic bronchitis or reactive airway disease is critical for identifying those patients most likely to benefit from LVRS. Although most patients have some element of inflammatory airway disease, the closer the patient is to pure emphysema, the classical "pink puffer,"

Table 24-2 Relative Contraindications to Lung Volume Reduction Surgery

Computer tomography evidence of significant bronchiectasis

Partial arterial pressure of CO_2 $\geq$60 mm Hg

Pulmonary artery systolic pressure $\geq$45 mm Hg, mean pulmonary arterial pressure $\geq$35 mm Hg

Prior lobectomy ipsilateral to targeted disease

Significant systemic illness or malignancy expected to compromise survival

Significant pleural or interstitial lung disease

Chronic bronchitis or asthma

Cardiac disease precluding major thoracic surgery

Use of $\geq$20 mg of prednisone daily, or equivalent steroid, intractable to weaning

Oxygen requirements at rest exceeding 6 liters/min to keep O_2 saturation $\geq$90%

Six-minute walk distance $\leq$140 m post-rehabilitation

Psychosocial instability

Ventilator dependence

Active nicotine abuse

Body mass index $\geq$31.1 kg/m2 in men and $\geq$32.3 kg/m2 in women

---

Table 24-1 Relative Indications for Lung Volume Reduction Surgery

History and physical exam consistent with emphysema

FEV_1 $\geq$15% or $\leq$40% of predicted

TLC $\geq$100% of predicted

Residual volume $\geq$150% of predicted

Room air PaO_2 $\geq$45 mm Hg

Room air $PaCO_2$ $\leq$55 mm Hg

Nonsmoker for >6 months

Computed tomography evidence of severe emphysema

Acceptable cardiac risk for surgery

Ability to comply with a pulmonary rehabilitation program

FEV_1 = forced expiratory volume in 1 second; $PaCO_2$ = partial arterial carbon dioxide pressure; PaO_2 = partial arterial oxygen pressure; TLC = total lung capacity.

Table 24-3 Preoperative Evaluation

Complete history and physical examination

Serum cotinine level

Alpha-1 antitrypsin level

High-resolution inspiratory and expiratory computed tomography scan of the chest

Perfusion lung scan

Transthoracic echocardiogram with assessment of pulmonary artery pressure

Dobutamine radionuclide stress test

Spirometry, pre- and post-bronchodilator

Lung volumes by plethysmography

Cardiopulmonary exercise test

Six minute walk

Room air ABG

the more likely LVRS will be beneficial and appropriate. Evidence of reactive airway disease includes significant dependence on steroid therapy, inspiratory or expiratory wheezing, and a lack of hyperinflation on chest x-ray. Such patients may have similar physiologic profiles to emphysema patients but tend to have a greater spirometric bronchodilator response. Patients with significant daily sputum production or computed tomography scan evidence of bronchiectasis are also poor candidates for LVRS and should be excluded from surgical consideration.

Heterogeneity of disease and upper lobe predominance have repeatedly been shown to correlate favorably with improved outcomes after LVRS. The computed tomographic scan and the perfusion lung scan are particularly helpful in determining the degree of heterogeneity and, therefore, potential target areas for resection. It is important to review the posterior-anterior, lateral, and oblique views of the perfusion scan when assessing the pattern of disease.

The chest radiograph, computed tomographic scan, and lung volumes assessed by plethysmography are all helpful in assessing the degree of hyperinflation. Whereas lung volume measurements alone have not consistently correlated with improvement after surgery, the lack of hyperinflation is an important negative predictor, implying significant reactive airways disease as opposed to emphysema.

Evidence of an indeterminate pulmonary nodule or proven lung cancer deserves special mention. Prior to the reintroduction of LVRS, most patients with severe emphysema were excluded from consideration for resection because of inadequate pulmonary function. The lessons of LVRS have demonstrated that many such patients with this confluence of pathology can now undergo surgical resection, in some cases accomplishing both curative cancer surgery and improvements in pulmonary function. These patients require individual evaluation and planning based on the location of the tumor and the geography of their emphysema, but they should no longer be summarily excluded from surgical consideration based solely on pulmonary function testing.

Cardiac assessment should include measurement of pulmonary pressures and assessment of coronary artery disease. Patients should undergo echocardiography to assess right-sided pressures and dobutamine stress testing for coronary artery evaluation. Suggestion of significant disease mandates cardiac catheterization. Scharf et al. demonstrated that in patients with emphysema assessed for the National Emphysema Treatment Trial (NETT), significant pulmonary hypertension (pulmonary artery systolic pressure >45 mm Hg, mean pulmonary arterial pressure >35 mm Hg) was relatively uncommon. Coronary artery disease was more common but rarely excluded patients from surgery. Given the common primary risk factor of smoking, it may be that most patients with either severe coronary disease or significant pulmonary hypertension have already been naturally deselected because of death or advanced deconditioning.

Less often considered but of great importance are other comorbidities such as depression and osteoporosis. Aggressive assessment and treatment are important both for perioperative consideration as well as long-term outcomes. Untreated depression affects motivation during pulmonary rehabilitation and decreases later quality-of-life improvement after surgery. Untreated osteoporosis can lead to painful fractures and chronic pain syndromes, negating any pulmonary function benefits from the surgical procedure.

The timing of palliative surgery with respect to a long and chronic illness is always difficult. There is little available data suggesting when in the course of emphysema surgical intervention is optimal. It is noteworthy, however, that patients randomized to medical therapy in the NETT had a mortality of 0.11 deaths per person-year. Clearly, many patients pass through a window of opportunity during which LVRS is reasonable therapy. Ultimately, further progression of disease leads to ineligibility due to further loss of functional lung tissue, progressive deconditioning, or death.

Preoperative Preparation

Preoperative preparation consists of two broad areas: physical reconditioning and optimizing medical therapy. Almost all patients suffer from deconditioning and obtain substantial benefit from pulmonary rehabilitation. Pulmonary rehabilitation has been shown to improve exercise tolerance, decrease dyspnea, and improve quality of life. It has not been shown to change pulmonary function. We require a period of physical reconditioning in a formal pulmonary rehabilitation program that is familiar with our clinical goals and experienced in the management of pulmonary patients. Other, nonpulmonary-oriented programs are usually inadequate. The plateau in functional improvement is often reached within 6 to 10 weeks, but individual assessment is necessary.

All patients are evaluated for optimization of medical therapy, especially bronchodilator and steroid therapy. Most patients can been weaned from steroids or reduced to a minimal dose. Failure to achieve this goal should raise suspicions of a significant component of reactive airway disease rendering the patient a poor candidate for LVRS. In addition, evaluation and treatment of osteoporosis, depression, and anxiety disorders are important. Finally, we require a prolonged period of abstinence from nicotine products. This must be supported by laboratory evidence including serum cotinine levels.

Because LVRS is elective, surgery should be deferred until the maximum benefit has been obtained from preoperative therapy.

Surgical Techniques
Choice of Approach and Selection of Target Areas

The selection of target areas and the surgical approach go hand in hand. Initial assessment of potential areas for resection is made on review of the high-resolution computed tomography scan of the chest and the perfusion scan. The computed tomographic scan performed during inspiration and expiration can further refine areas of air trapping.

The choice of approach is largely surgeon dependent based on his or her comfort level with the technique. Posterior pleural disease and left lower lobe pathology are difficult to access from a median sternotomy. Unilateral procedures can be performed using either a video-assisted thoracoscopic approach or open thoracotomy. Bilateral video-assisted thoracic surgery is an excellent technique for LVRS but requires excellent minimally invasive skills. The assessment of lung size, the identification and management of air leaks, and the creation of pleural tents can be difficult using a video-assisted approach.

Bilateral Trans-Sternal Lung Volume Reduction Surgery

Our preferred approach for most patients is a median sternotomy (Fig. 24-1). This approach provides excellent bilateral exposure and is remarkably well tolerated by most patients. A thoracic epidural catheter is placed and tested prior to induction of general anesthesia. Narcotics are avoided because of the risk of hypercarbia and the often

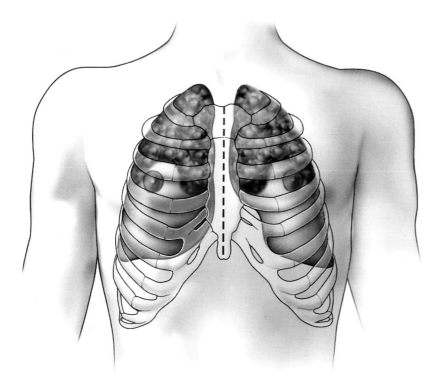

Figure 24-1. A median sternotomy provides excellent exposure for bilateral lung volume reduction surgery.

The entire lung must be fully mobilized to allow the lung to reposition in the hemithorax and avoid pleural space problems. The inferior pulmonary ligament is divided, with care taken to avoid a traction injury to the phrenic nerve during exposure. We avoid grasping any lung tissue that is not destined for resection because of its inherent fragile nature. A large sponge stick is very useful for retraction. Adhesions must be carefully divided, and if this proves difficult, extrapleural mobilization is a useful technique. Recalcitrant adhesions in the area of the phrenic nerve can be managed by stapling off a small area of lung tissue, leaving it attached to the nerve. Placing laparotomy sponges behind the lung or floating the lung in warm saline can improve the exposure by bringing the lung into better position.

Once the lung has been mobilized and the areas of lung parenchyma identified for resection, stapling is performed using Endo-GIA staplers (United States Surgical Corp., Norwalk, CT) reinforced with either bovine pericardium (Peristrips, Biovascular, Minneapolis, MN; Instat, Johnson and Johnson, Brunswick, NJ) or Gore-Tex strips (Core-guard, W. L. Gore, Flagstaff, AZ). GIA staplers are used for thicker lung tissue. Stapling begins anteriorly (Fig. 24-3) and proceeds toward the posterior lung, gently using the resected area to elevate the remaining lobe (Fig. 24-4). Care must be taken to avoid resecting too deep into the lobe or near hilar structures. Sizing, that is, determining how much parenchyma to resect, is critical, but optimal size guidelines remain elusive. Over-resection will result in pleural space problems and air leaks, under-resection in potentially inadequate therapeutic effectiveness. We try to size the inflated lung to fill the hemithorax from diaphragm to apex with the diaphragm in the normal anatomic position.

slow and prolonged emergence from anesthesia. After general endotracheal anesthesia has been induced, flexible bronchoscopy is performed though a single-lumen endotracheal tube. This step allows assessment, culture, and clearance of secretions as well as evaluation for central endobronchial malignancies, which can occasionally be found in this high-risk patient group. The patient is then reintubated with a double-lumen endotracheal tube. A median sternotomy is performed and a Bugge retractor (Pilling, Fort Washington, PA) is placed to elevate the sternal table (Fig. 24-2). We perform lung reduction initially on the side with the least perfusion. The pleura is opened posterior to the sternum from the diaphragmatic surface to just below the internal mammary vein. Care must be taken not to open the pleura too cephalad in order to avoid injuring the phrenic nerve. The lung is initially examined in the ventilated state, and ventilation is then interrupted to the operative lung. We use pressure-controlled ventilation to the contralateral lung to avoid barotrauma. As deflation of the operative lung occurs, visual inspection allows the surgeon to identify the areas of lung that become atelectatic first. Absorptive atelectasis occurs fastest in the least severe areas of emphysema. After a few minutes, perfusion differences are evident, with the best-perfused areas

desaturating the fastest. Finally, limited reinflation allows the surgeon to distinguish the areas of lung parenchyma with the greatest compliance. These observations, together with the computed tomography scan of the chest and the perfusion lung scan, provide the surgeon with the information necessary to determine the target areas of lung most amenable to resection.

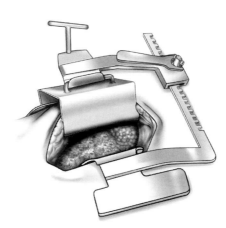

Figure 24-2. The sternum is elevated using a Bugge retractor. The pleura is opened just posterior to the sternum from the diaphragm to the mammary vessels. Care must be taken not to incise too cephalad to avoid injury to the phrenic nerve. Ventilation to the operative lung is interrupted allowing visual inspection of deflation.

Once unilateral resection is complete, the lung is gently inflated, holding manual pressure on all suture lines. Airway pressure is kept to the minimum necessary to achieve reinflation. Air leaks are assessed by filling the hemithorax with warm saline, and every reasonable attempt is made to minimize or eliminate them using additional reinforced staple or suture lines or biologic glue, as necessary. Contralateral resection is then performed in a similar fashion. Two chest tubes are placed in each hemithorax, with care taken to position them for optimal apical and basilar drainage. When necessary, a pleural tent can be performed to aid in obliterating excess apical space. Pleurodesis is not routinely performed but is not unreasonable.

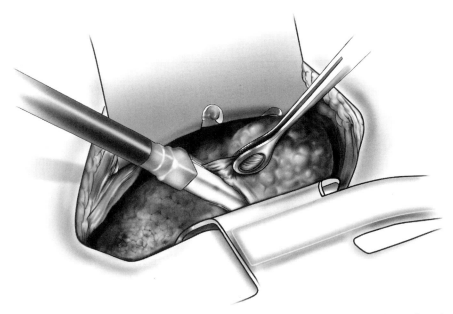

Figure 24-3. The targeted lung tissue is grasped anteriorly and an Endo-GIA stapler reinforced with bovine pericardium is used to start the resection.

Before extubation, secretions are vigorously cleared and bronchodilators are instituted. It is important that patients are pain free, alert, and not significantly hypercarbic at the time of extubation. The chest tubes are initially placed to water seal, and chest x-rays are checked frequently. If a large pneumothorax develops, minimal suction on the chest tubes will be necessary.

Video-Assisted Bilateral Thoracoscopic Lung Volume Reduction Surgery

Careful positioning and planning is critical to this technique. We position the patient supine with the arms above the head and well padded on an ether screen (Fig. 24-5). The patient is secured to the operating table,

and the chest is prepped widely. The anesthetic technique and intraoperative ventilatory management are similar to those described for trans-sternal LVRS. Three ports are used as illustrated in Fig. 24-6. The most inferior port for the camera is located in the sixth intercostal space in the anterior axillary line. The stapling port is placed in the fourth intercostal space in the mid-clavicular line. The instrument port used is placed in the third intercostal space in the mid-axillary line. The inferior pulmonary ligament is divided with electrocautery, and adhesions are dissected with great care to avoid air leaks. Extrapleural dissection is used when adhesions are difficult. The lung is grasped anteriorly, and an Endo-GIA stapler is placed through the anterior port, stapling the lung from inferiorly toward the apex (Fig. 24-7). The stapling is continued around the apex of the lung toward the posterior aspect of the lobe. Again, care is taken not to staple too close to the hilum or to over-resect. Calibrating the correct lung size is more difficult to assess using this technique. When resection is complete, the chest cavity is partially filled with warm saline, and the lung is gently inflated at low pressures to assess for air leaks. Anterior and posterior chest tubes are positioned, and attention is directed to the contralateral hemithorax. Extubation is performed in a manner similar to the trans-sternal approach.

Unilateral Procedures

There are a number of situations in which a unilateral procedure is preferred over a bilateral approach. These indications include selective cases of pulmonary nodules or malignancies requiring major resection, severe contralateral pleural disease, prior lobectomy, and primary ipsilateral disease. In these cases we individualize the surgical approach, but in most cases we use a video-assisted thoracoscopic technique or a limited thoracotomy.

Postoperative Care

LVRS patients require particular diligence in postoperative care due to their limited tolerance for untoward events. Successful outcomes after LVRS require a dedicated team of surgeons, pulmonologists, anesthesiologists, respiratory therapists, physiotherapists, and nurses experienced in the management of advanced lung disease. A well-coordinated, multidisciplinary team approach provides the best outcomes, anticipating the unique consequences and potential complications of this procedure.

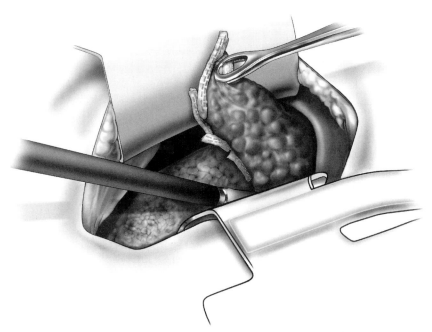

Figure 24-4. The resection is continued apically and posteriorly using gentle traction to expose the posterior aspect of the lung. Filling the hemithorax with warm saline allows the lung to float toward the surgeon, which improves visibility.

Routine extubation occurs at the completion of surgery and reduces the risk of barotrauma, which may result in difficult-to-manage air leaks. Successful extubation and effective pulmonary toilet require excellent pain management. Pain control is achieved initially by epidural administration of local anesthetics until the partial pressure of CO_2 has normalized and the patient is alert. Narcotics are then slowly added, titrated to avoid oversedation and hypoventilation. Patients are mobilized early postoperatively, and aggressive pulmonary toilet is instituted using incentive spirometry, coughing, deep breathing, and nasotracheal suctioning. Hypotension induced by epidural anesthesia is best treated with fluids because vasoconstrictors have been associated with mesenteric ischemia in some patients.

The chest tubes are maintained on water seal unless an increasing pneumothorax ensues, in which case low wall suction at 10 cm H_2O is employed. Pleural drainage is continued for 3 to 5 days. If an air leak persists, a Heimlich valve is connected to the chest tubes, and chest x-rays are closely followed for the next 24 hours. Patients can be discharged with a Heimlich valve if the lung remains stable for 48 hours. It has been our experience that the need for reoperation for uncontrolled air leaks is rare.

Bronchodilator therapy is reinstituted immediately postoperatively. Steroids are avoided unless there is evidence of reactive airway disease, worsening secretions, or respiratory failure. If secretions are not being adequately cleared with less invasive methods, bronchoscopy should be employed liberally. Antibiotics are begun preoperatively and continued postoperatively as needed. We send an intraoperative and daily sputum sample for culture and Gram stain to guide antibiotic therapy, as needed.

Some patients will require reintubation, often for reversible events. If the patient shows signs of respiratory failure despite adequate control of pain, bronchospasm, and secretions, intubation should be done electively instead of allowing a failing patient to decline precipitously. These patients should be rested for several days and the precipitating event treated prior to extubation. Tracheostomy and mobilization is recommended if early re-extubation cannot be accomplished.

Results of Surgery

Since the initial report by Cooper et al., there have been numerous case series and small randomized trials reporting the results of

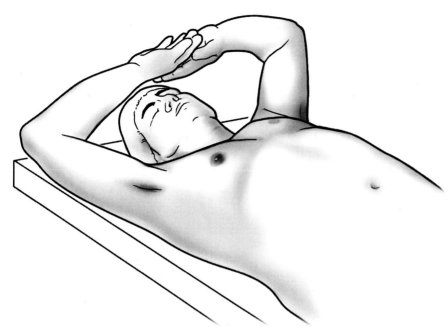

Figure 24-5. For bilateral lung volume reduction through a video-assisted thoracoscopic approach the patient is positioned supine with the arms placed above the head supported on a well-padded ether screen.

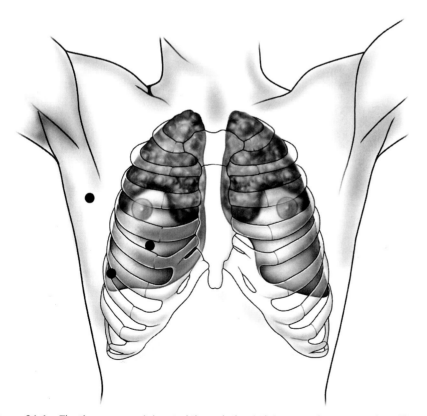

Figure 24-6. The thoracoscope is inserted through the sixth intercostal space anterior axillary line. An empty sponge stick clamp is placed through the third intercostal space mid-axillary line and is used to grasp the lung. The stapling device is placed through the fourth intercostal space mid-clavicular line, and the resection begins anteriorly toward the apex.

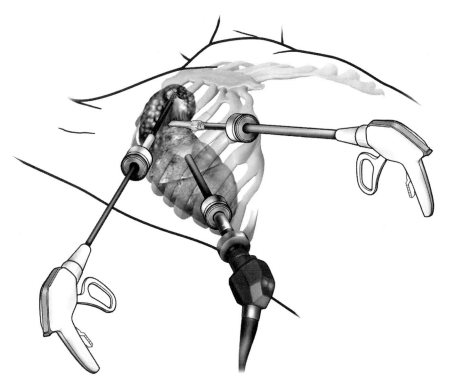

Figure 24-7. The resection is continued around the apex in a manner similar to the trans-sternal approach.

LVRS performed by a variety of approaches and techniques. These studies have consistently shown that LVRS results in improvement in FEV_1, respiratory muscle function, exercise capacity, and dyspnea. Postoperative mortality has ranged from 5% to 15%. Morbidity has been significant and includes prolonged air leaks, respiratory failure, myocardial infarction, pneumonia, and stroke.

Long-term results are limited. Yusen et al., reported on the first 200 patients undergoing LVRS at Washington University followed for a mean of 3.7 years. Dyspnea scores were improved in 81% at 6 months, 52% at 3 years, and 40% at 5 years after surgery. Improvements in physical functioning assessed by SF-36 testing were evident in 93% of patients at 6 months, 78% of patients at 3 years, and 69% of patients at 5 years. They concluded that patients undergoing LVRS achieved a substantial benefit over medical therapy and that this benefit persisted for at least 5 years. These improvements appear to be separable from the effects of medical therapy and pulmonary rehabilitation and to be nonlinearly related to pulmonary function changes.

The National Emphysema Treatment Trial was the largest prospective, randomized study to establish the validity of lung volume reduction surgery for the treatment of emphysema. This trial, funded by the

Centers for Medicare and Medicaid Services and the Agency for Healthcare Research and Quality and administered by the National Heart, Lung, and Blood Institute, was conducted at 17 U.S. academic medical centers over a 7-year period. It compared maximal medical therapy including pulmonary rehabilitation to bilateral lung volume reduction surgery in 1,218 patients followed for a mean of 2 years. This trial identified characteristics of five subgroups of patients that demonstrated either a benefit or harm from LVRS. Although limited in scope and design, this trial is now the basis for patient selection and prediction of outcomes guiding clinicians.

The five subgroups identified in the NETT were based on baseline exercise capacity, diffusing capacity for carbon monoxide (DLCO), architecture of disease, and FEV_1 (Table 24-1). Two of the five subgroups exhibited deleterious effects from LVRS, and three subgroups showed improvement. Only one group showed a survival advantage with LVRS. These results are summarized in Table 24-4.

The analysis showed that patients with upper lobe predominant emphysema and low baseline exercise capacity achieved a significant benefit in survival, exercise capacity, and quality-of-life indices. Patients with non–upper lobe predominant emphysema and low baseline exercise capacity only achieved a benefit in quality of life and exercise capacity. Patients with non–upper lobe predominant emphysema and low exercise capacity achieved a benefit only in quality of life.

Patients with an $FEV_1 \leq 20\%$ of predicted and either homogeneous distribution of emphysema or a DLCO $\leq 20\%$ of predicted who underwent LVRS had a significantly increased mortality with surgery. Survivors had a small but clinically insignificant benefit in quality of life and exercise capacity. Likewise, patients with non–upper lobe predominant emphysema and a high baseline exercise capacity also suffered increased mortality with surgery, without a significant clinical benefit.

Studies comparing median sternotomy to bilateral video-assisted thoracoscopic surgery have consistently failed to show any meaningful differences with respect to survival or functional improvement between the two approaches. In the NETT, functional outcomes were not significantly different between patients undergoing median sternotomy or video-assisted thoracoscopy. However, patients undergoing video-assisted thoracoscopic surgery were living

Table 24-4 Primary Results of the National Emphysema Treatment Trial	
Subgroup	**Outcome from LVRS**
$FEV_1 \leq 20\%$ and DLCO $\leq 20\%$ or homogeneous disease	Decrease survival
Upper lobe predominant disease/low exercise capacity[a]	Increased survival
	Increased exercise capacity
	Decreased symptoms
Upper lobe predominant disease/high exercise capacity	Increased exercise capacity
	Decreased symptoms
Non–upper lobe predominant disease/low exercise capacity	Decreased symptoms
Non–upper lobe predominant disease/high exercise capacity	Decreased survival

[a]Low baseline exercise capacity <25 W for women and <40 W for men.
DLCO = diffusing capacity for carbon monoxide; FEV_1 = forced expiratory volume in 1 second; LVRS = lung volume reduction surgery.

independently sooner, and overall costs were less than after median sternotomy.

There is ample evidence that bilateral lung volume reduction results in greater functional improvement than unilateral volume reduction. However, unilateral procedures for patients who have lung tumors, isolated unilateral pleural disease, prior lobectomy, or unilateral emphysema have shown good results. How much contralateral effect occurs is unknown and is probably minimal given the lack of significant lung–lung interaction. Post-transplant lung volume reduction of the native lung has also been shown to be of benefit, but it is unclear whether the benefit is related to effects in the transplant or native lung.

The application of lung volume reduction techniques to patients with lung nodules or proven lung cancers has opened surgical therapy to a group of patients previously felt to have inadequate lung function to allow resection. Each case requires individual consideration and surgical design, but lesions both in areas of severe emphysema as well as in less diseased areas of lung but amenable to limited resection can now be approached. Combining lung volume reduction with tumor resection has been shown to be feasible, but no long-term studies of efficacy are available.

Future Directions

The National Emphysema Treatment Trial provided incontrovertible evidence that remodeling the lung can improve pulmonary function. Much work remains to further define the optimal timing and technique of surgery. The NETT contains a trove of unmined data yet to be analyzed. Especially intriguing is the opportunity to perform digital analysis of the extensive radiologic studies performed on this well-studied group of patients.

New technologies are being investigated that hold the possibility of achieving a lung volume reduction effect or, at the least, improving the efficiency of ventilation through a bronchoscopic approach. These include endoscopically placed one-way valves and other devices. Early studies suggest that these techniques are safe and achieve improvements similar to that of surgical lung volume reduction by redirection of ventilation, amelioration of dynamic hyperinflation, and, in some cases, atelectasis as well. Whether these technologies will translate into a meaningful clinical benefit remains to be established.

A unique opportunity exists for clinicians interested in the treatment of emphysema. The excitement that has swirled around lung volume reduction surgery has stimulated new lines of investigation and opened the opportunity to new discoveries and treatment strategies. In this context, lung volume reduction surgery should be viewed as only the beginning of a new era in the surgical treatment of emphysema.

SUGGESTED READING

Cooper JD. Technique to reduce air leaks after resection of emphysematous lung. Ann Thorac Surg 1994;57:1038.

Cooper JD, Trulock EP, Triantrafilou AN, et al. Bilateral pneumonectomy (volume reduction) for chronic obstructive pulmonary disease. J Thorac Cardiovasc Surg 1995;109:106.

Hogg JC, Chu F, Utokaparch S, et al. The nature of small-airway obstruction in chronic obstructive pulmonary disease. N Engl J Med 2004;350:2645.

Martinez FJ, de Oca MM, Whyte RI, et al. Lung volume reduction improves dyspnea, dynamic hyperinflation, and respiratory muscle function. Am J Respir Crit Care Med 1997;55:1984.

McKenna RJ Jr, Brenner M, Fischel RJ, et al. Should lung volume reduction surgery for emphysema be unilateral or bilateral? J Thoracic Cardiovasc Surg 1996;112:1331.

McKenna RJ Jr, Fischel RJ, Brenner M, et al. Use of the Heimlich valve to shorten hospital stay after lung reduction surgery for emphysema. Ann Thorac Surg 1996;61:1115.

National Emphysema Treatment Trial Research Group. A randomized trial comparing lung volume reduction surgery with medical therapy for severe emphysema. N Engl J Med 2003;348:2059.

Pauwels RA, Buist AS, Calverley PM, et al. Global strategy for the diagnosis, management, and prevention of chronic obstructive pulmonary disease: NHLBI/WHO Global Initiative for Chronic Obstructive Pulmonary Disease (GOLD) Workshop summary. Am J Respir Crit Care Med 2001;163:1256.

Wisser W, Tshernko E, Wanke T, et al. Functional improvements in ventilatory mechanics after lung volume reduction surgery for homogeneous emphysema. Eur J Cardiothorac Surg 1997;12:525.

Yusen RD, Lefrak SS, Gierada DS, et al. A prospective evaluation of lung volume reduction surgery in 200 consecutive patients. Chest 2003;123:975.

EDITOR'S COMMENTS

There has been considerable interest in surgery for emphysema since Joel Cooper first reintroduced the idea of lung volume reduction surgery in 1994. After his initial report many of these procedures were performed, often with poor outcomes and high mortality, approaching 30% in some institutions. Criteria for selecting patients for operation varied greatly, as did the technique for operation. Recognizing the potential for a huge expenditure, the Center for Medicare and Medicaid Services (CMS) stopped paying for lung volume reduction surgery but ultimately agreed to pay for the procedure as part of a clinical trial sponsored by the National Heart, Lung, and Blood Institute (NHLBI). Seventeen centers ultimately participated in the study, which failed to accrue anywhere near the number of patients initially predicted but did demonstrate a survival advantage for one particular group of emphysema sufferers. Currently CMS will pay for the procedure done in approved centers that follow the criteria established to select candidates for operation. Despite the positive results of the NETT, the number of patients referred for lung volume reduction surgery is miniscule. It seems that the pulmonary medicine community has become disillusioned with the procedure and discourages patients from seeking the operation. Optimal medical management includes pulmonary rehabilitation, which does improve exercise capability and overall well-being. However, no medical therapy has been shown to improve survival or the quality of life as measured by a variety of tools the way that lung volume reduction surgery can in selected patients.

The knowledge gained from operating on these patients with severe emphysema has had a definite effect on patients with borderline pulmonary function who present with lung cancer. Whereas previously many of these patients were denied operation because they were felt to have too little reserve to undergo resection, we now operate on most of them. Depending on the location of the tumor, resection may accomplish an element of volume reduction in some of these overinflated lungs, thus improving overall lung function, even though only a unilateral procedure is performed. On occasion a resection accompanied by a contralateral lung volume reduction procedure is performed that results in an improvement of the patient's pulmonary function as well as resection of the tumor. Rarely are patients turned down for operation based strictly on pulmonary function numbers without consideration of a number of other factors including the location of the tumor, location of the most severe emphysema (in particular, whether the disease is heterogeneous), nutritional status, and motivation.

There are some technical features of the lung volume reduction procedure that bear mentioning. The amount of lung to resect generally approximates 20% to 30% of the volume on each side, but precise measurements or ways to calculate the amount of lung to resect do not exist. The operator has to rely on individual experience to best judge how much parenchyma to resect. Too little, and the patient will not benefit from the procedure and will have been subjected to all of the risk nonetheless. Too much, and the patient may suffer from the loss of an excessive amount of gas-exchanging parenchyma, thus the importance of heterogeneous disease. For the most part this operation is not for the patient with homogeneous disease without distinct target areas, with the occasional exception. Injury to the phrenic nerve must be avoided. The nerve is easily injured if, in trying to maximize exposure, the pleural reflection is opened too far superiorly where the nerve is quite anterior. The incision into the pleural reflection must stop inferior to the internal thoracic vein. Whether buttressing staple lines with prosthetic material aids in preventing or attenuating air leaks remains an open question, although several studies have shown no advantage. Many of the parenchymal leaks occur just adjacent to the buttress material as the lung is reinflated. I have tended to buttress staple lines on open procedures but not on thoracoscopic procedures, and it has been my impression that there are not significant differences in rate or duration of air leaks. Pain control in the postoperative period is crucial, and the epidural must be functioning properly or it should be replaced. Control of pain allows the patient to actively participate in mobilizing secretions. If the patient is unable to effective cough, I opt for placement of a "mini-trach" via the cricothyroid membrane for secretion management. I err on the side of placing this early in the course if there is any suggestion of secretion retention.

Despite the seeming ease of the surgical procedure, these patients present significant challenges in the postoperative period, and lung volume reduction surgery probably should be limited to centers with significant experience in dealing with patients with advanced lung disease. These do not have to be centers where lung transplantation is performed, but likely there is some advantage to that, and with the number of procedures being done, this probably is feasible. On the other hand, any center that can demonstrate expertise in the care of patients with end-stage emphysema should be able to seek approval to perform the procedure. Lung volume reduction surgery can provide selected patients with significant improvement in their quality of life and perhaps lengthen their life.

L.R.K.

25

Thoracic Outlet Syndromes

Harold C. Urschel Jr. and Amit N. Patel

Thoracic outlet syndromes involve compression of one or more of the major anatomic structures passing through the thoracic outlet (i.e., the space between the spine and shoulder under the clavicle). These include the upper and lower brachial plexus and peripheral nerves, the sympathetic nervous system with branches along the artery, and the axillary subclavian artery and vein. In addition to a careful history and physical examination, the diagnosis of vascular or nerve compression is specific and must be objectively documented. Although standard objective vascular tests are well recognized, accurate ulnar and median nerve conduction velocity tests are more difficult to perform. To assess the effects of treatment, either conservative or surgical, in either primary or recurrent thoracic outlet syndromes, it is absolutely essential for the nerve conduction velocity measurements to be reliable and reproducible because of the subjectivity inherent in the assessment of pain. Stellate ganglion block may predict the efficacy of dorsal sympathectomy in many cases.

Most nerve compression syndromes are mild and chronic and can be treated effectively with conservative targeted physiotherapy. The more severe sensory or motor deficits secondary to brachial plexus or peripheral nerve compression; peripheral vascular responses mediated by the sympathetic nervous system, including chest pain, arterial insufficiency, arterial emboli, or occlusion; and venous obstruction present greater challenges and frequently require surgical management.

Indications for Surgical Therapy

Indications for surgery include the failure of conservative measures to attenuate the symptoms caused by nerve compression after a 3-month period and the presence of prolonged conduction velocities in the ulnar or median nerve. Other surgical indications include (1) the presence of atypical chest pain unrelieved by conservative management (not related to coronary artery, esophageal, or pulmonary pathologic conditions), (2) the presence of hypersympathetic activity, (3) the narrowing or occlusion of the axillary subclavian artery with or without peripheral emboli, and (4) thrombosis of the axillary subclavian vein (Paget-Schroetter syndrome, effort thrombosis).

For nerve compression, the preferred initial surgical approach is the transaxillary approach for first-rib resection, with decompression of the axillary subclavian artery and vein as well as the brachial plexus. In contrast to the supraclavicular approach, the transaxillary approach allows the first rib to be removed, the scalene muscles divided and resected if necessary, and the outlet decompressed with minimal risk to the critical neurovascular structures that lie away from the first rib. It is particularly important to remove the rib completely to minimize recurrence of the symptom complex as a result of regeneration of bone or fibrocartilage from an incompletely removed "stump" or rib remnant. To remove the first rib completely using a supraclavicular approach,

the brachial plexus and neurovascular structures must be retracted, which is a situation that results in a higher complication rate.

For recurrent thoracic outlet syndrome after either primary transaxillary or supraclavicular operations, the posterior "thoracoplasty" operation provides a safer approach and better access for removing bone remnants and scar from the brachial plexus and subclavian vessels and allows a dorsal sympathectomy to be performed for causalgia and reflex sympathetic dystrophy (sympathetic-maintained pain syndrome).

For arterial reconstruction, the combined supraclavicular-infraclavicular approach is often used when bypass grafts are necessary for either occlusion or aneurysm. For venous occlusion (Paget-Schroetter syndrome), the ideal management combines clot lysis with administration of urokinase through a catheter followed by prompt decompression of the thoracic outlet by transaxillary resection of the first rib. Prolonged delay of clot lysis markedly increases morbidity, and failure to perform prompt first-rib resection and thoracic outlet decompression leads to extremely high rates of recurrence. Compression and sympathetic nerve hyperactivity not relieved by medical therapy should be treated by dorsal sympathectomy usually performed in conjunction with resection of the first rib through the same exposure.

Surgical Principles

Thoracic outlet decompression surgery generally involves (1) removal of the first rib,

213

(2) decompression of the axillary subclavian vein and artery, (3) division of the costoclavicular ligament, (4) resection of the anterior and middle scalene muscles from the first rib up into the neck to prevent reattachment to Sibson's fascia, and (5) neurolysis of the C7, C8, and T1 nerve roots as well as the middle and lower trunks of the brachial plexus. This is performed under magnification provided by the thoracoscope, which is an excellent light source and a superior teaching tool.

The surgical approach should be tailored to the individual patient, and the surgeon should be familiar with all approaches. We prefer the transaxillary approach for primary decompression and a posterior thoracotomy for reoperation for recurrent symptoms. Sympathectomy may be added to this procedure for reflex sympathetic dystrophy (sympathetic-maintained pain syndrome), Raynaud's phenomenon or disease, or other "causalgia-like" symptoms.

Dorsal sympathectomy, with or without resection of the first rib, may be performed from the transaxillary, supraclavicular, or posterior approaches. Stellate ganglion blocks may be used to evaluate the effectiveness of the procedure to relieve symptoms. Although some surgeons cauterize the dorsal sympathetic ganglion through the thoracoscope, primarily for hyperhidrosis, we consider it important to resect the ganglia and obtain frozen-section pathologic evidence of "ganglion cells." Resection of the T2 and T3 ganglia with the incorporated sympathetic chain will relieve most symptoms (in 90% of patients). Adding the T1 ganglia increases it to almost 100% (by adding the nerve of Kuntz). For Raynaud's disease, it is usually necessary to produce a Horner's syndrome by taking the entire stellate ganglion (C7, C8, and T1) to relieve the symptoms.

Surgical Technique

Transaxillary First-Rib Resection (with Dorsal Sympathectomy)

A double-lumen tube is used to collapse the lung on the side to be treated, minimizing the chance for an unplanned pneumothorax. A lighted right-angled breast retractor and a narrow Deaver retractor are used for optimal exposure. The video thoracoscope is used both as a light source and to provide magnification and facilitate teaching. The patient is placed in the lateral decubitus position with an axillary roll under the "down"

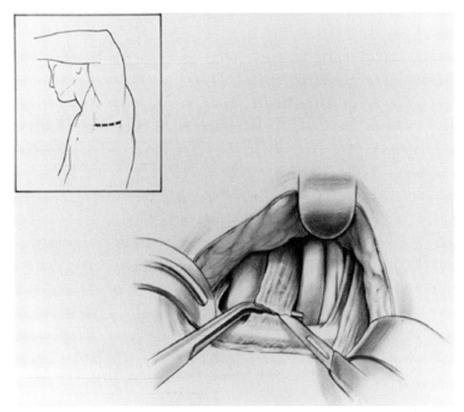

Figure 25-1.   Division of the insertion of the anterior scalene muscle off the first rib. A right-angled clamp is used to protect the neurovascular bundle. **(Inset)** Location of the skin incision at the hairline of the axilla extending from the pectoralis major to the latissimus dorsi muscle. (Adapted from HC Urschel Jr, JD Cooper. Atlas of Thoracic Surgery. New York: Churchill Livingstone, 1995.)

side. The arm on the "up" side is wrapped and elevated over a traction apparatus with a 1-pound weight. A special arm holder is used to hold the arm at 90 degrees from the chest wall; hyperabduction or hyperextension of the shoulder is avoided. Care is taken to relax the arm every 2 minutes or as often as necessary. The arm, axilla, and chest wall are prepared and draped.

A transverse incision is made below the axillary hairline, between the pectoralis major muscle anteriorly and the latissimus dorsi muscle posteriorly (Fig. 25-1, inset). The incision is carried directly down to the chest wall without angling it up toward the first rib. When the chest wall is encountered, the dissection is carried superiorly to the first rib, and the intercostal brachial nerve that exits between the first and second ribs is identified. It is preserved by retracting it anteriorly or posteriorly. (Dividing this nerve produces 6 months to 1 year of numbness on the inner surface of the upper arm.) The first rib is dissected subperiosteally with a Paulson periosteal elevator, and the anterior scalene muscle is identified. A right-angled clamp is placed behind the muscle, with the surgeon taking care not to injure the sub-

clavian artery or vein. The anterior scalene muscle is divided near its insertion on the first rib (this avoids injury to the phrenic nerve, which courses away from the muscle at the level of the first rib) (Fig. 25-1).

After the anterior scalene muscle is divided, the rib is dissected free in a subperiosteal plane and separated from the pleural apex. A triangular piece of the rib is removed in the avascular area. The vertex of this triangle is at the scalenus tubercle. The anterior section of rib is removed by dividing the costoclavicular ligament and resecting the rib back to the costicartilage of the sternum (Fig. 25-2).

The posterior part of the rib is freed up back to the transverse process, where it is divided with a pair of rib shears. Any rib remaining posteriorly may be taken with an Urschel-Leksell rongeur. Care is taken to avoid injury to the C8 and T1 nerve roots as the middle scalene muscle is freed off the rib (Fig. 25-3).

After the transverse process is visualized, the head and neck of the rib are removed with an Urschel reinforced pituitary rongeur (Fig. 25-4). It is necessary to completely remove the head and neck of the rib so as to

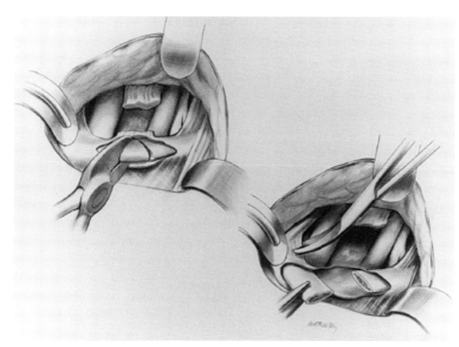

Figure 25-2. After division of the anterior scalene muscle, a wedge of bone is excised from the middle portion of the rib **(left)**, which allows the anterior aspect of the rib to be grasped **(right)** and dissected anteriorly toward the sternum. (Adapted from HC Urschel Jr, JD Cooper. Atlas of Thoracic Surgery. New York: Churchill Livingstone, 1995.)

minimize regeneration. Care is taken not to injure the T1 nerve root inferiorly or the C8 nerve root superior to the first rib at the level of the neural foramina. After the first rib is completely removed, a neurolysis of the C7, C8, and T1 nerve roots as well as the middle and lower trunks of the brachial plexus is performed. A video thoracoscope may be used for this purpose because of its magnification and light. The middle and anterior scalene muscles are resected up into the neck so that they will not attach to Sibson's fascia or the pleura. Fibrous bands are removed from the axillary-subclavian artery

and vein. Great care is taken to maintain hemostasis.

If a dorsal sympathectomy is indicated for an upper-extremity pain syndrome such as reflex sympathetic dystrophy, it is performed through the same incision. After the rib has been removed, the pleura and lung are retracted inferiorly with a sponge stick, the plane of separation being below the T1 nerve root. The stellate ganglion and dorsal sympathetic chain are identified (Fig. 25-5).

Clips are placed on each of the gray and white rami communicans to the intercostal nerves. The ganglion is sharply divided so that the T1, or the lower one third, is removed (Fig. 25-6). The chain is resected, with the T1, T2, and T3 ganglia removed, and a clip is placed across the chain inferiorly. Electrocautery is used to control bleeding and also to scarify the area. Frozen-section studies are obtained to ensure that ganglion cells are present. A 20-F chest tube is placed through a separate stab wound inferior to the axilla if the pleura has been opened. After the wound is irrigated with antibiotic solution, corticosteroid (Depo-Medrol) is injected over the area of neurolysis. The wound is closed in layers with a 3-0 polyglactin 910 (Vicryl) suture used for the skin.

Posterior Thoracotomy First-Rib Resection (with Dorsal Sympathectomy) for Recurrent Thoracic Outlet Syndrome

Although posterior thoracotomy first-rib resection (with dorsal sympathectomy) may be used for primary large first-rib or cervical rib resection, it is usually used for reoperations. The transaxillary or supraclavicular route is preferred for the initial procedure. Reoperation for recurrent compression incorporates a dorsal sympathectomy for causalgia-like symptoms, sympathetic-maintained pain syndrome, or Raynaud's phenomenon.

The patient is placed in the lateral decubitus position with the arm placed as for a thoracotomy. An incision approximately 6 cm in length is made with the midpoint at the angle of the scapula and located between the scapula and spinous processes (Fig. 25-7, inset). This is carried through the skin and subcutaneous tissue down to the trapezius muscle. The trapezius and rhomboid muscles are split (Fig. 25-7).

The posterior superior serratus muscle is divided and the first rib stump identified

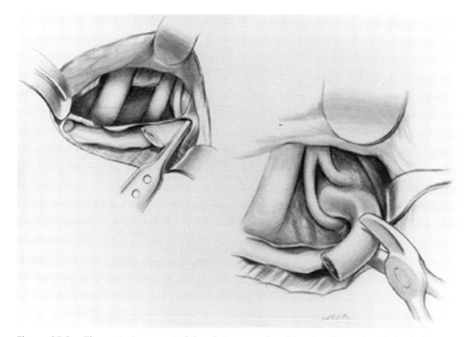

Figure 25-3. The posterior aspect of the rib is grasped and freed up in a subperiosteal plane heading posterior toward the transverse process **(left)**. The neck of the first rib sits between the C8 and T1 nerve roots, and care must be taken to avoid injury to these roots **(right)**. (Adapted from HC Urschel Jr, JD Cooper. Atlas of Thoracic Surgery. New York: Churchill Livingstone, 1995.)

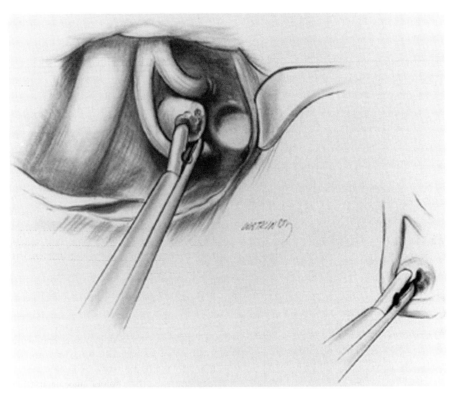

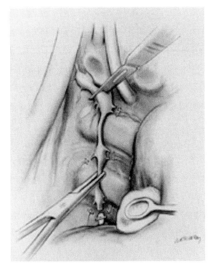

Figure 25-6. The sympathetic chain is divided at the inferior aspect of the superior cervical or stellate ganglion. Branches are clipped and cut as shown. The T1, T2, and T3 ganglia are removed. (Adapted from HC Urschel Jr, JD Cooper. Atlas of Thoracic Surgery. New York: Churchill Livingstone, 1995.)

Figure 25-4. The head and neck of the first rib are removed in a piecemeal fashion with the Urschel rongeur to avoid injury to the C8 and T1 nerve roots. The rib must be removed in its entirety for the best chance of a successful outcome. The most common reason for reoperation is the presence of residual posterior rib. (Adapted from HC Urschel Jr, JD Cooper. Atlas of Thoracic Surgery. New York: Churchill Livingstone, 1995.)

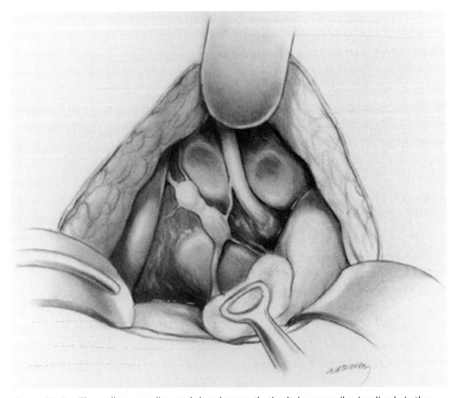

Figure 25-5. The stellate ganglion and dorsal sympathetic chain are easily visualized via the transaxillary approach. (Adapted from HC Urschel Jr, JD Cooper. Atlas of Thoracic Surgery. New York: Churchill Livingstone, 1995.)

medially. Electrocautery is used to expose the first-rib remnant and to incise the periosteum (Fig. 25-8, panel 1). A periosteal elevator is used to remove the stump (Fig. 25-8, panel 2). The head and neck of the rib often will be found intact, having been left at the first operation. Rib shears are used to divide the rib, and an Urschel-Leksell reinforced pituitary rongeur is used to remove the head and neck of the rib (Fig. 25-8, panels 3, 4). The T1 nerve root is identified inferior to the first rib remnant (Fig. 25-8, panel 5).

After the T1 nerve root is identified, neurolysis is carried out using a right-angled clamp, a knife, and special microscissors (Fig. 25-9). A stimulator may be helpful if extensive scarring is present. The neurolysis is extended up to the C7 and C8 roots and onto the lower cord of the brachial plexus. All the scar is removed as far forward as necessary so that the roots as well as the upper, middle, and lower cords of the brachial plexus lie free. Care is taken to avoid injury to the long thoracic nerve or any other brachial plexus branch.

The second rib is dissected free, and electrocautery is used to open the periosteum. A 2-cm section of the rib is resected posteriorly, medial to the sacrospinalis muscle, to perform the sympathectomy (Fig. 25-10).

After the head and neck of the second rib are excised, the sympathetic chain is identified on the vertebral body. The stellate ganglion lies in an almost transverse

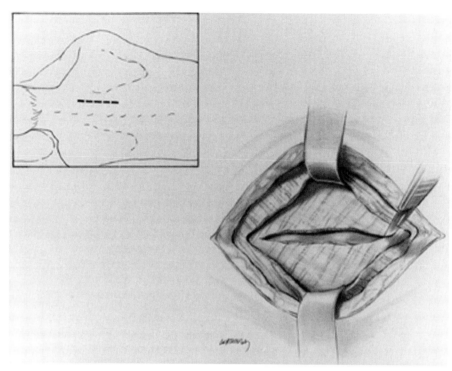

Figure 25-7. The incision for a posterior approach for resection of the first rib, which is usually reserved for use in reoperative procedures. **(Inset)** The location of the posterior incision for resection of the first rib. (Adapted from HC Urschel Jr, JD Cooper. Atlas of Thoracic Surgery. New York: Churchill Livingstone, 1995.)

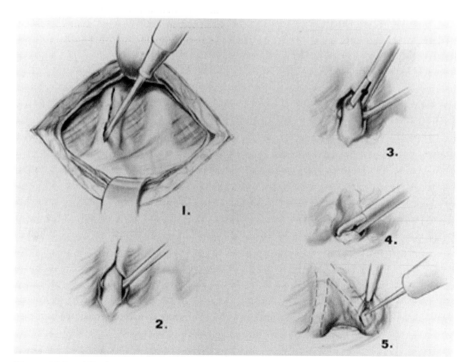

Figure 25-8. **(1)** The periosteum overlying the posterior first rib is incised with electrocautery. **(2)** The rib is mobilized and encircled in the subperiosteal plane to facilitate excision. **(3)** Rib shears are used to divide the rib and rongeurs are used to remove the rib in pieces. **(4)** Rongeurs are used to remove the head and neck of the rib so as to leave no posterior remnants. **(5)** The C8 and T1 nerve roots are identified by their location in relation to the neck of the first rib. (Adapted from HC Urschel Jr, JD Cooper. Atlas of Thoracic Surgery. New York: Churchill Livingstone, 1995.)

orientation rather than a vertical position (Fig. 25-11).

The lower one third of the stellate ganglion (T1) is sharply divided, and the gray and white rami communicans are clipped and divided (Fig. 25-12). The T1 and T2 segments and ganglia are removed along with the sympathetic chain; clips are used on all of the branches. Electrocautery is used to effect hemostasis and to char the area so regeneration of the sympathetic chain is discouraged. The wound is closed in layers with sutures placed in a figure-eight fashion in each of the muscle layers. A large, round Jackson-Pratt drain is placed in the area of neurolysis through a separate stab wound several centimeters below the inferior part of the incision.

Transthoracic Dorsal Sympathectomy

The patient is placed in the lateral decubitus position. The arm may be placed in a traction-pulley system with a 1-pound weight, or an arm holder may be used. A double-lumen endotracheal tube is used so that the ipsilateral lung may be collapsed. A transverse incision is made at the inferior border of the axillary hairline extending between the pectoralis muscle anteriorly and the latissimus dorsi posteriorly. It is extended down to the chest wall. The second interspace is identified, and the intercostal muscle is opened between the second and third ribs.

The pleura is entered, and the lung is collapsed and retracted. The sympathetic chain is identified lying over the neck of the ribs through the parietal pleura, and the pleura is incised.

The dorsal sympathetic chain and its branches, including the gray and white rami communicans to the intercostal nerves, are clipped and divided. The T1, T2, and T3 ganglia are removed with the sympathetic chain. The lower one third of the stellate ganglion is resected sharply (T1). Frozen section studies of the ganglia are obtained to document that ganglion cells are present. A chest tube is placed through a separate stab wound and the lung inflated.

Venous Thrombosis of the Axillary-Subclavian Vein (Paget-Schroetter Syndrome)

Effort thrombosis of the axillary-subclavian vein (Paget-Schroetter syndrome, PSS) is

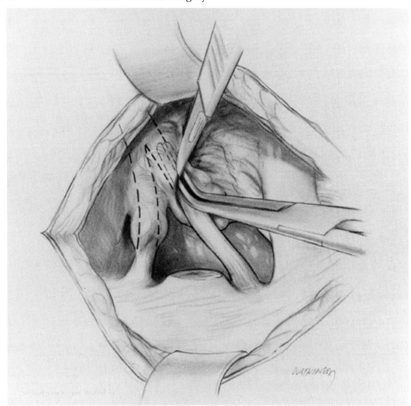

Figure 25-9. After the nerve roots are identified, a neurolysis is carried out to free up the nerves from any scar tissue or fibrous bands that may be encasing them. It is thought by many that the neurolysis is the most important aspect of the procedure. (Adapted from HC Urschel Jr, JD Cooper. Atlas of Thoracic Surgery. New York: Churchill Livingstone, 1995.)

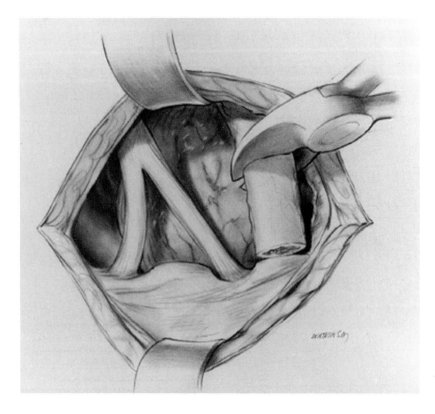

Figure 25-10. To improve exposure of the sympathetic chain through this posterior approach, a 2-cm section of the posterior second rib is removed. (Adapted from HC Urschel Jr, JD Cooper. Atlas of Thoracic Surgery. New York: Churchill Livingstone, 1995.)

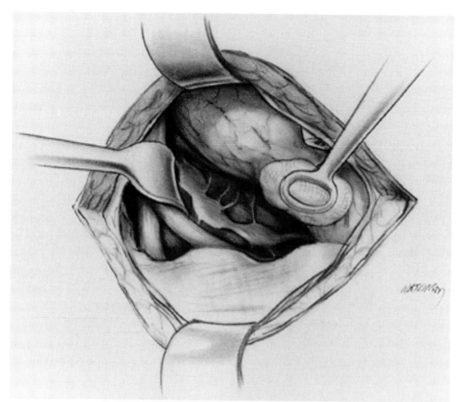

Figure 25-11. The dorsal sympathetic chain is exposed, and the stellate ganglion, which lies almost in a transverse orientation, is identified. (Adapted from HC Urschel Jr, JD Cooper. Atlas of Thoracic Surgery. New York: Churchill Livingstone, 1995.)

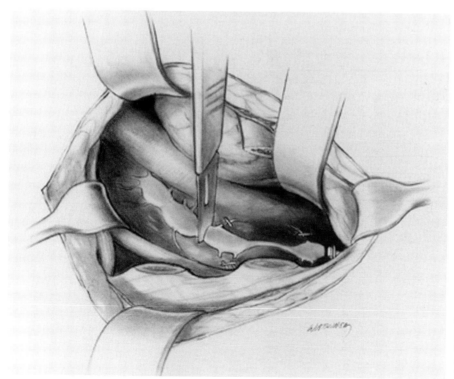

Figure 25-12. The dorsal sympathetic chain is divided at the level of T1. Clips are placed on branches, which are then divided. (Adapted from HC Urschel Jr, JD Cooper. Atlas of Thoracic Surgery. New York: Churchill Livingstone, 1995.)

secondary to compression in the thoracic outlet.

Most patients demonstrate congenital lateral insertion of the costoclavicular ligament (medial to the axillary-subclavian vein.) With enlargement of the scalenus anticus muscle lateral to the vein, dehydration or coagulopathy, the vein occludes, producing acute swelling of the arm and, without proper treatment, often long-term morbidity.

The treatment of choice is a prompt diagnosis clinically, by venous Doppler and venography, and immediate thrombolytic therapy followed by prompt transaxillary first-rib resection and neurovascular decompression. No long-term anticoagulants are necessary. Because the compression is external to the vein, pericutaneous transvenous angioplasty or stents are contraindicated.

Results and Complications

Transaxillary first-rib resection results in at least 90% immediate relief of symptoms in the classic syndrome. The recurrence rate is approximately 12% to 15%, depending on the individual, the "hyperscarring" or keloid formation, or failure to remove the rib completely. Upper brachial plexus compression (median nerve) occurs less frequently, but transaxillary first-rib resection alone is as effective as the combined supraclavicular and transaxillary approaches. Recurrent neurologic symptoms generally can be treated medically unless a rib remnant or regenerated fibrocartilage is present. Again, indications for reoperation depend on persistent symptoms, failure of physiotherapy, and prolonged conduction velocities in the ulnar or median nerve.

Arterial or venous syndromes rarely recur if they are properly treated initially. Often, the opposite limb is at risk and should be assessed before the onset of symptoms if an operation has been required on one side.

Nerve injury from the supraclavicular approach is reported in 5% of patients and involves the brachial plexus or its branches, the peripheral nerves, the phrenic nerve, or long thoracic nerves. With the transaxillary approach, nerve injury occurs in <1% of cases. In cases of arterial insufficiency, amputation is occasionally required if early, expeditious management is unsuccessful. Chronic venous obstruction produces arm edema and often the postphlebitic syndrome. Phlegmasia cerulea dolens may

result if acute severe venous obstruction is not relieved.

Conclusion

Upper-extremity pain syndromes present a significant challenge to the surgeon from both a diagnostic and a therapeutic standpoint. A trial of medical therapy, usually a targeted physical therapy regimen, should be completed before a surgical approach is even contemplated. Patient selection is critically important to achieve optimal results. Not all patients who fail conservative management are good candidates, and desperation is never a very good indication.

Acknowledgment

We thank Rachel Montano for her dedication and commitment to the completion of this chapter.

SUGGESTED READING

Cheng SWK, Stoney RJ. Supraclavicular reoperation for neurogenic thoracic outlet syndrome. J Vasc Surg 1994;19:565.

Mackinnon SE, Patterson GA, Urschel HC Jr. Thoracic Outlet Syndromes. In Pearson FG, Deslauriers J, Ginsberg RJ, et al. (eds), Thoracic Surgery. New York: Churchill Livingstone, 1995.

Urschel HC Jr. Dorsal sympathectomy and management of thoracic outlet syndrome with VATS. Ann Thorac Surg 1993;56:717.

Urschel HC Jr, Cooper JD. Atlas of Thoracic Surgery. New York: Churchill Livingstone, 1995.

Urschel HC Jr, Patel AN. Paget Schroetter syndrome therapy: Failure of intravenous stents. Ann Thorac Surg 2003;75:1693.

Urschel HC Jr, Razzuk MA. Current concepts: Management of the thoracic outlet syndrome. N Engl J Med 1972;286:1140.

Urschel HC Jr, Razzuk MA. The failed operation for thoracic outlet syndrome: The difficulty of diagnosis and management. Ann Thorac Surg 1986;42:523.

Urschel HC Jr, Razzuk MA. Thoracic Outlet Syndrome. In Sabiston DC Jr, Spencer FC (eds), Gibbon's Surgery of the Chest (6th ed). Philadelphia: Saunders, 1995.

Urschel HC Jr, Razzuk MA. Upper plexus thoracic outlet syndrome: Optimal therapy. Ann Thorac Surg 1997;63:935.

Urschel HC Jr, Razzuk MA. Neurovascular decompression in the thoracic outlet: Changing management over 50 years. Ann Thorac Surg 1998;228:609.

Urschel HC Jr, Razzuk, MA. Paget-Schroetter syndrome: What is the best management? Ann Thorac Surg 2000;69:1663.

Urschel HC Jr, Razzuk MA, Hyland JW, et al. Thoracic outlet syndrome masquerading as

coronary artery disease. Ann Thorac Surg 1973;16:239.

EDITOR'S COMMENTS

Dr. Urschel is one of the most experienced surgeons in the world when it comes to dealing with thoracic outlet syndrome. This includes his tremendous experience in dealing with recurrent symptoms following thoracic outlet decompression. That being said, most thoracic surgeons go the other way when faced with a patient with an upper-extremity pain syndrome. Vascular surgeons have picked up many of these patients, and it is not unusual to see the occasional vascular surgeon "specializing" in the treatment of thoracic outlet syndrome. The difficulty with thoracic outlet syndrome resides not in the surgical procedure but in making the diagnosis and deciding who should be operated on and when. It remains the opinion of many experts, including neurologists, that there are no characteristic, consistent, or reproducible objective findings that allow one to make a diagnosis of thoracic outlet syndrome. This, combined with the psychiatric overlay that often accompanies the syndrome, the frequency of litigation related to this problem, and the issue of work-related disability causes many surgeons to avoid dealing with these patients altogether. Other than the presence of a cervical rib, there is no anatomic abnormality that can be visualized on imaging studies, including both computed tomography and magnetic resonance imaging. Specifically this is the case when dealing with the patient with an upper-extremity pain syndrome as opposed to the patient with vascular or Paget-Schroetter syndrome. Results for patients treated for vascular compression are far more satisfying than those achieved for the much more common "neurogenic" compression patients. It has been my experience that patients with upper-extremity pain rarely are satisfied long term after operation. Often the early results are striking, but following a short interval these patients usually re-present with additional complaints. It is almost as if they have a "need" to have the pain syndrome. Relief of one set of symptoms usually is replaced by another.

The authors do not mention the need for a neurosurgeon or hand surgeon interested in peripheral nerve disease, but a combined approach with one of these specialists may be beneficial. The neurolysis of the brachial plexus may be more important than previously realized, and these specialists are more adept at dealing with these large nerves than most thoracic surgeons. The question comes up as to how to deal with a cervical rib. If the cervical rib is to be resected, this probably should be done through a supraclavicular approach, which puts the neurovascular structures at greater risk. I base my approach on the size of the cervical rib. A large cervical rib probably should be resected via the supraclavicular approach, whereas a diminutive cervical rib can be best dealt with by a transaxillary resection of the first rib, which removes the adhesive bands that attach to the cervical rib but does not resect the actual accessory rib.

The video thoracoscope probably adds little to the transaxillary approach to the first rib especially if a lighted right-angled breast retractor is used. A special set of first-rib instruments with grooved and nongrooved Overholt periosteal elevators, special retractors, and angled and straight first-rib cutters is mandatory for a safe transaxillary first-rib resection. The key to the procedure is proper positioning of the upper extremity, which, in my opinion, needs to be held, not simply suspended with a weight, by an assistant who can move the arm at various times during the procedure to obtain the best exposure. The arm is prepped and covered with a stockinette to facilitate this. Despite the appropriate equipment and arm positioning, getting the posterior aspect of the rib remains difficult. The rib is divided and the anterior portion removed first. Then the posterior aspect of the rib is excised, but getting exposure of the transverse process is not easy. Use of the rongeur, as the authors point out, allows the surgeon to get the most posterior portion of the rib. There remains considerable doubt as to whether it is necessary to remove every last bit of the posterior aspect of the first rib to effect relief of the compression. This raises the question of whether there is ever an indication for a "re-do" procedure, and this clearly remains controversial.

L.R.K.

26

Chest Wall Resections

John C. Kucharczuk and Larry R. Kaiser

Introduction

Indications for chest wall resection are broad and varied. They include resection of both primary and secondary chest wall lesions. Primary chest wall lesions are those that arise within the normal constituents of the chest wall including skin, connective tissue, muscle, bone, and cartilage. These can be either benign or malignant. They are relatively uncommon, and resection is often warranted for diagnosis and treatment. Secondary chest wall masses are caused by invasion from a process originating in contiguous organs such as the lung or breast. Lung cancer with chest wall invasion is the most common indication for chest wall resection. In these cases, chest wall resection is performed in stage-appropriate candidates as part of an en bloc resection for attempt at cure.

The three basic tenets of chest wall resection are (1) resection of all disease with wide margins, (2) provision of healthy soft tissue coverage, and (3) preservation of respiratory mechanics. The intent of this chapter is to review the indication and techniques of chest wall resection with reconstruction from the simple to the complex. The discussion focuses on the proper selection of reconstructive techniques from "off the self" synthetic material to complex soft tissue transfers.

Preoperative Evaluation

Patients being considered for chest wall resection undergo a complete medical evaluation. Special attention is focused on any past medical or surgical history that will affect the approach for resection and the choices for reconstruction or influence wound heal-

ing. These factors include previous chest procedures, a history of radiation, evidence of active infection, and immunosuppression. All patients have radiographic imaging including a chest radiograph and computed tomography (CT) scan of the chest. For patients with a primary chest wall lesion magnetic resonance imaging may be helpful in delineating the local extent of disease, but as a general rule it cannot distinguish between benign and malignant masses. Patients with underlying lung cancer and contiguous chest wall invasion undergo a complete extent of disease workup to rule out metastatic disease, and if negative, they are considered for resection. If partial vertebral body resection is entertained or there is concern regarding involvement at the level of the neural foramen, preoperative neurosurgical consultation is obtained. Likewise, the need for transfer of large volumes of soft tissue for coverage or unfamiliarity with the available techniques for complex tissue transfer should prompt consultation with an experienced reconstructive surgeon.

Operative Planning: Optimizing the Approach

In selecting the appropriate incision it is imperative that the surgeon be thoughtful, flexible, and experienced. The optimal surgical approach allows for assessment of the extent of disease without violation of the lesion. Lateral chest wall lesions are generally approached through posterolateral incisions. If there is a planned need for soft tissue transfer, the latissimus dorsi and serratus anterior muscles are mobilized but not divided before entering the pleural cavity. If

there is no need for tissue transfer, we generally divide the latissimus dorsi muscle but spare the serratus anterior in case it should be needed in the future. The pleural cavity is entered either an interspace below the lesion or at a site anterior to the lesion. The lesion is palpated to determine the extent of resection required. Primary chest wall lesions usually do not invade the lung, and pulmonary resection usually is not required. In cases of lung cancer with contiguous chest wall involvement the chest wall resection is performed as shown in an en bloc fashion. Attempts to develop an extrapleural plane or strip the tumor off the chest wall should be avoided because it risks violation of the tumor with contamination of the pleural cavity and consequently high rates of recurrence. Once the chest wall resection is complete, the chest wall bloc remains attached to the underlying pulmonary parenchyma and the pulmonary resection is performed. We do not attempt to separate the chest wall bloc from the underlying lung.

Lesions involving the apex of the chest can be approached via the traditional Shaw-Paulson technique. This approach uses a long posterolateral incision carried up to the C7 vertebral body, elevation of the scapula off the chest wall after division of the trapezius and the rhomboids, and chest wall resection from a posterior approach. These lesions may be more effectively managed through the anterior cervicothoracic approach described by Dartevelle and subsequently modified by others. Anterior chest wall lesions are often best approached with the patient supine and an anterior incision over the location of the lesion.

Regardless of the surgical approach chosen, the basic tenets of chest wall resection, which include a wide margin of excision, en bloc anatomic resection with the attached

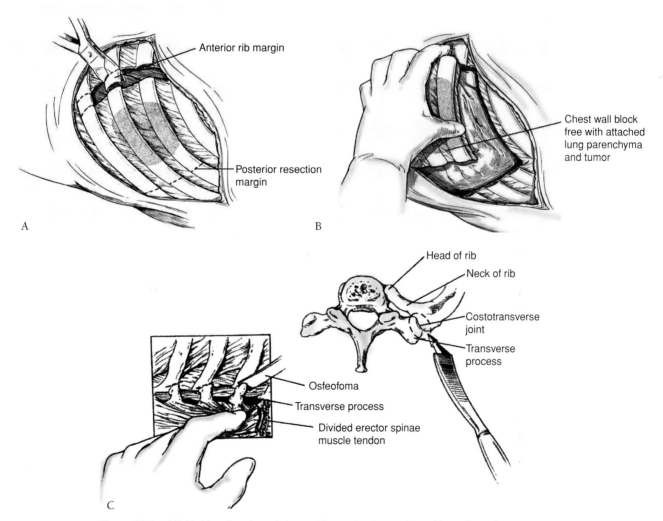

lung parenchyma, and appropriate reconstruction of the chest wall defect when required, must be fulfilled.

Technique of Chest Wall Resection

A suspicion that the chest wall may be involved often occurs because the patient presents with pain associated and a peripheral lesion seen abutting the chest wall on CT scan. In general, it is not possible reliably to differentiate chest wall invasion from simple abutment merely by looking at the CT scan. A posterolateral incision is made, and the latissimus dorsi muscle and serratus anterior muscles are either divided or mobi-

lized if they are needed for pedicled muscle flaps. The chest usually is entered via the fifth intercostal space and exploration carried out. If the lesion involves the fifth rib, the entry into the hemithorax should be either anterior or posterior to the presumed area of involvement. Before initiating the chest wall resection, palpation of the hilum and mediastinum should be carried out to ensure resectability. It serves little purpose to take down the chest wall block only to find locally advanced disease or diffuse pleural disease that precludes resection. The combination of mediastinal lymph node positivity and chest wall involvement portends a poor outcome. If there is any suspicion of nodal involvement, mediastinoscopy must be carried out before chest exploration. A positive mediastinum usually precludes chest wall

resection outside of a protocol setting, although some surgeons proceed with resection after neoadjuvant chemotherapy. Most studies have shown essentially no 5-year survivors with chest wall involvement and positive mediastinal lymph nodes.

Once it has been determined that the tumor is resectable, the chest wall resection is begun. Depending on the location, the scapula may need to be mobilized off the chest wall, and this requires division of the trapezius and rhomboid muscles. At least a portion of one rib above and one rib below the lesion should be resected. The extent of resection is determined by the intrathoracic exploration. The anterior portion of the resection is done first by determining the appropriate rib and incising the periosteum several centimeters anterior to the lesion.

Figure 26-1. **(A)** En bloc chest lateral chest wall resection in a patient with a primary lung cancer. The anterior line of resection is far away from the primary site of invasion, and small, 1-cm portions of the anterior ribs are removed and labeled as margins. **(B)** The completed chest wall resection; at this juncture the entire chest wall bloc is allowed to fall into the pleural cavity and the pulmonary resection is performed through the chest wall defect. **(C)** Disarticulation of the posterior rib from the transverse process with an osteotome. (Reprinted with permission from LR Kaiser. Atlas of General Thoracic Surgery. St. Louis: Mosby, 1997.)

A wide excision should be performed to ensure negative margins. We prefer to take a 1-cm piece of rib and submit this separately at each level as the anterior resection margin (Fig. 26-1A). This move creates a small amount of space for ligation of the intercostal bundle at each level. Starting at the inferior extent of the resection and working superiorly, the anterior margin is taken at each level with the pleura excised as the resection proceeds. The intercostal muscles at the inferior and superior extent of the resection are divided along with the pleura, and the posterior portions of the involved ribs are divided. There is no need to take a separate posterior margin at each level; this margin will be marked on the en bloc resection specimen. Depending on the location of the lesion, the posterior rib division may be either through the rib as demonstrated in Fig. 26-1B or may require disarticulation of the rib from the respective transverse process of the spine as shown in Fig. 26-1C. If there is any doubt, the rib should be disarticulated, and at times even the transverse process may need to be resected. As always, the intent is to have a negative resection margin. As always the intent is to have a negative resection margin; anything less (i.e., a positive margin) is associated with a poor long-term survival.

If the posterior portion of the ribs simply is divided, this is done in a subperiosteal fashion with ligation of the intercostal bundle. The bundle at each level has already been ligated and divided anteriorly, and thus only a single ligature at each level is required. If disarticulation from the transverse process is required, the intercostal bundle must be ligated at the level of the neural foramen. To disarticulate the ribs from the transverse process, the paraspinous ligament must be reflected away from the spine down to the level of the transverse process with the use of the electrocautery because there are numerous perforating vessels that must be controlled. Once down to the transverse process, the rib is pulled anteriorly as the cautery incises the cartilaginous junction between the neck of the rib and the transverse process of the spine. The correct location has been identified when the cartilage appears to "melt" with the application of the cautery and the rib neck begins to separate slightly. Once through this cartilaginous symphysis, a curved osteotome is inserted between the neck of the rib (Fig. 1C, inset) and the transverse process and, with the transverse process as a fulcrum, is rocked forward disarticulating the neck of the rib from the transverse process and the head of the rib from the vertebral

body. This is facilitated by having incised the overlying pleura from within the chest. The osteotome is directed anteriorly toward the vertebral body and thus away from the spinal canal, so there is no chance of injuring the spinal cord. The force is directed upward away from the vertebral body so as to lift the head of the rib. The rib should be gently disarticulated so as to not avulse the intercostal nerve because the dural sheath may be torn with a resultant cerebrospinal fluid leak. Once the rib has been disarticulated enough to see the intercostal nerve exiting the neural foramen, the nerve and intercostal vessels should be ligated and divided. It is not uncommon to experience some bleeding from the foramen because there are multiple small venous channels that may be avulsed. Only bipolar cautery should be used at the foraminal level to staunch any bleeding so as to prevent any thermal injury to the spinal cord. The foramen should NOT be packed with Surgicel or gel foam to control bleeding; these materials can expand within the foramen leading to spinal cord compression with neurologic consequences.

Once the posterior ribs have either been divided or disarticulated the chest wall bloc remains attached to the underlying lung parenchyma, and if the tumor is a primary lung, once the chest wall bloc has been entirely separated it is left attached to the underlying lung parenchyma. The appropriate anatomic pulmonary resection (lobectomy or, at times, segmentectomy) is performed. A complete mediastinal lymph node dissection should be part of the procedure even if a mediastinoscopy has been done so that accurate staging information is obtained. If

the lesiona is a primary chest wall tumor, the specimen is removed and the reconstruction is begun.

Removal of the first rib requires some special techniques and expertise. One must be intimately familiar with the relationship of the brachial plexus and subclavian vessels to the first rib to avoid injuring any of these structures. Special first-rib instruments are necessary for safe first-rib resection. These include special angled first-rib periosteal elevators either with a groove or not, rongeurs, and angled rib cutters. If first-rib resection is required, the scalene muscles that insert on the rib must be detached. The posterior scalene inserts on the second rib, so this will have already been taken. The middle scalene inserts on the first rib between the subclavian vein and artery and should be reflected with the periosteal elevator following cautery incision of the periosteum. The anterior scalene should be incised and reflected off the rib. The inferior aspect of the rib is freed up with the use of a grooved elevator. A Matson elevator is placed under the rib to expose the medial aspect of the rib so as to protect the nerves and vessels. Once the medial aspect of the rib is cleared, a first-rib cutter is used to cut the anterior aspect of the rib. If the first rib needs to be disarticulated from the transverse process, care must be taken to identify the C8 and T1 nerve roots that combine to form the lower cord of the brachial plexus. These nerve roots may be identified by visualizing the head of the first rib, which is located immediately between these two structures. If the roots are not identified as they exit their respective foramina, the lower cord of the plexus may be inadvertently divided if the operator

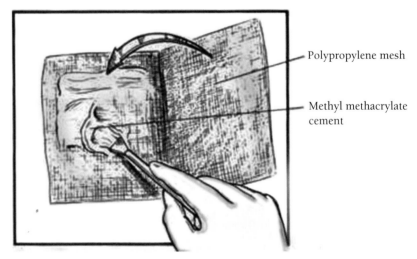

Figure 26-2. Creation of a polypropylene mesh/methylmethacrylate "sandwich" to be used as an inset prosthesis for lateral chest wall reconstruction. (Reprinted with permission from LR Kaiser. Atlas of General Thoracic Surgery. St. Louis: Mosby, 1997.)

mistakenly thinks that this is the T1 nerve root. The T1 root may be taken as part of the resection if it is involved, but division of the C8 root leaves a nonfunctional hand. The degree of disability that occurs after division of the T1 nerve root usually is minimal to at most moderate.

Synthetic Material Choices

The synthetic materials available for chest wall reconstruction are polypropylene mesh and polytetrafluoroethylene (PTFE) patches. Both have been used in large series of patients and appear to have equivalent outcomes. Polypropylene is significantly less expensive and can be reinforced with methylmethacrylate to create a rigid prosthesis that can be contoured to the chest wall. This may provide a better cosmetic result. Figure 26-2 shows the creation of a mesh/methylmethacrylate "sandwich" for chest wall reconstruction. Regardless of the material selected for reconstruction, it is inset into the defect with interrupted, nonabsorbable suture. We use No. 1 polypropylene sutures placed through the cut edges of the lateral ribs and around the uncut superior and inferior ribs as shown in Fig. 26-3. A small drill facilitates placement of suture through the cut ribs. If no superior rib remains for fixation, the prosthesis is secured on the remaining three sides with room at the apex to avoid erosion into the structure of the thoracic inlet. The synthetic material is covered with healthy soft tissue. Usually this simply requires closure of the cut muscle edges over the prosthesis followed by soft tissue closure. In cases where there has been significant soft tissue or muscle resection, complex soft tissue transfer is required.

Reconstruction of the chest wall defect is not required if a posterior resection has been done and the entire defect is covered by the scapula. If the fifth rib has been taken, however, the tip of the scapula has a tendency to be trapped underneath the sixth rib, a situation that is very uncomfortable for the patient. Thus if the fifth rib has been taken posteriorly, chest wall reconstruction with a patch of polypropylene mesh should be undertaken to prevent entrapment of the scapular tip. Rigid fixation is not required in this location. Other posterior or posterolateral chest wall defects should be reconstructed either with polypropylene mesh alone or with mesh and methylmethacrylate. Anterior chest wall defects usually require a

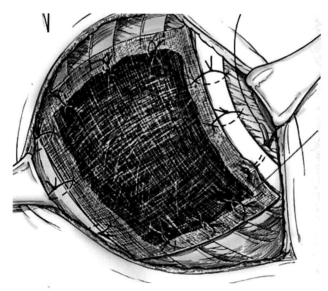

Figure 26-3. Chest wall prosthesis inset with interrupted nonabsorbable sutures. (Reprinted with permission from LR Kaiser. Atlas of General Thoracic Surgery. St. Louis: Mosby, 1997.)

rigid prosthesis to prevent respiratory embarrassment due to altered chest wall dynamics in the early postoperative period. This is especially important in the patient with borderline pulmonary function, where the "flail chest" physiology created by the chest wall defect often is enough to mandate mechanical ventilation without rigid fixation of the chest wall.

Tissue Transfer Options

The major muscles of the chest wall provide a good source of autologous tissue for soft tissue coverage of large chest wall defects. They may be utilized to cover prosthetic material in cases where significant soft tissue has been removed or alone without underlying prosthetic reconstruction in cases of infection. The rectus abduminus and omentum can also be transferred from the abdomen to the chest to provide coverage.

Table 26-1 lists the tissue available to transfer to the chest along with the blood supply of each flap. Preservation of the neurovascular bundle of a pedicle flap is critical to its success and is an absolute requirement.

Figure 26-4 illustrates the anatomic features of each pedicle flap used in the chest. Anterior chest wall coverage is best provided by pectoralis major advancement flaps. A pedicle rectus abdominals flap or omental flap with skin graft may also be utilized. Lateral defects are best addressed with pedicle serratus and/or latissimus flaps. If a composite flap (skin, soft tissue, and muscle) cannot be used, muscle alone can be transferred and a split-thickness skin graft can be applied.

Sternal Resections

Primary sternal tumors are rare, and when they occur they almost always are chondrosarcomas arising from the body of the

Table 26-1 Pedicled Flaps Available as Either Simple Muscle or Composite Tissue Transfers for Chest Wall Reconstruction[a]

Muscle	Arterial Supply	Use in Chest Wall Reconstruction
Latissimus dorsi	Thoracodorsal	Anterior and lateral chest wall
Pectoralis major	Thoracoacromial	Anterior and midline chest wall
Serratus anterior	Lateral thoracic	Lateral chest wall
Rectus abdominis	Superior epigastric	Anterior and midline chest wall
Omentum	Gastroepiploic	Midline chest wall

[a]The neurovascular bundle that must be preserved in each flap is listed. These transfer flaps as well as a variety of others can also be used as "free flaps" with use of microsurgical techniques to establish arterial inflow and venous drainage in complex cases.

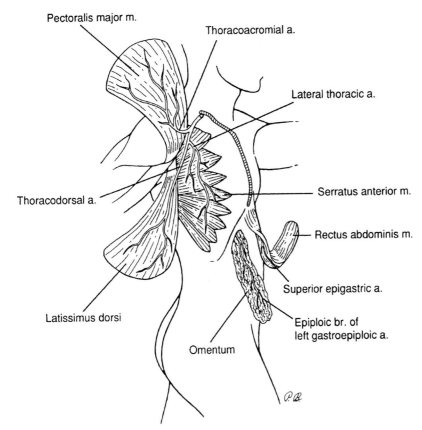

Figure 26-4. Pedicle muscle flaps available for reconstruction of chest wall and sternal defects. (a. = artery; m. = muscle.)

sternum. These tend to be low-grade lesions, and the best opportunity for cure is total sternectomy to achieve negative margins and immediate reconstruction with prosthetic material. The likelihood of cure and propensity for recurrence with sarcomas are related to the tumor's histologic grade.

Defects created by partial sternectomy may be small and reconstructed with simple pectoralis advancement flaps without the need for prosthetic material. Total sternectomy results in significant soft tissue and structural loss. It usually requires complex reconstruction. This is especially true if the sternum is being resected for recurrent breast cancer after excision and radiation therapy.

Technique for Sternal Resection

A vertical midline incision is made over the sternum, and skin flaps may need to be raised, depending on the size of the lesion. The pectoralis muscles are reflected laterally unless muscle is involved, in which case it is left with the sternum to be resected. The sternal notch is dissected and the retrosternal plane is developed. Inferiorly the xiphoid process is excised and the retrosternal plane entered from this aspect as well. The pleural reflections are swept laterally. The costal cartilage at each level is divided after removal of the perichondrium. The posterior perichondrium is incised to separate it from the sternum. This is facilitated by the use of a bone hook to elevate the sternum.

Often the manubrium can be preserved with total removal of the body of the sternum. If this is the case, the body of the sternum is disarticulated from the manubrium. If resection of the manubrium is required to achieve a complete resection, the clavicular heads are disarticulated and the first costal cartilage on each side incised. This allows complete removal of the sternum. Reconstruction is carried out with a polypropylene mesh/methylmethacrylate "sandwich," which is fitted into the defect and contoured appropriately. The prosthesis is inset with monofilament nonabsorbable suture placed through the cut rib edges and clavicular heads.

Figure 26-5 illustrates an intended total sternectomy for a primary sternal lesion. The reconstruction is completed as shown in Fig. 26-6A. The omentum has been transferred to cover the mediastinum; a mesh/methylmethacrylate prosthesis is covered by bilateral pectoralis major turnovers. If the skin is not removed as part of the resection, it is closed over drains to complete the

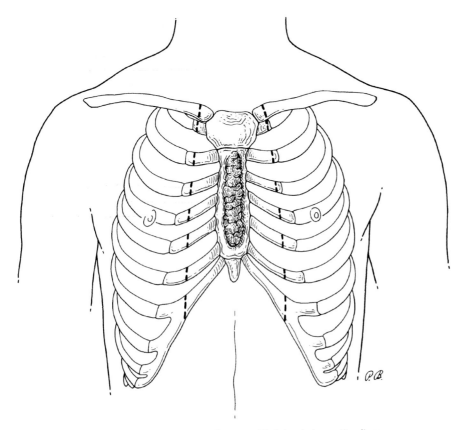

Figure 26-5. Primary sternal tumor with intended resection lines.

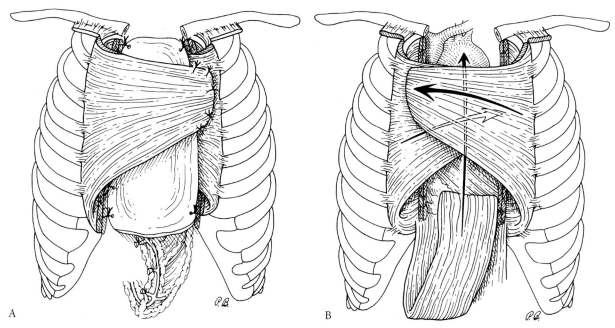

A   B

Figure 26-6. **(A)** Reconstruction of sternal resection with omental transfer to cover the mediastinum followed by bilateral pectoralis muscle turnover flaps to cover a polypropylene mesh methylmethacrylate prosthesis. If soft tissue and skin coverage is also needed, the prosthesis can be completely covered by a rectus flap as shown **(B)** and the reconstruction completed with a skin graft.

reconstruction. If significant skin and soft tissue has been resected, the prosthesis can be completely covered with the addition of a rectus abdominus flap (Fig. 26-6B) and a split-thickness skin graft applied.

Conclusion

Primary and secondary lesions of the chest wall and sternum can be resected in appropriate patients with good clinical outcomes. Taking on these cases requires proper preoperative planning and a working knowledge of a variety of reconstructive techniques.

SUGGESTED READING

Arnold PG, Pairolero PC. Chest wall reconstruction: An account of 500 consecutive patients. Plast Reconstr Surg 1996;98:804.

Burt M. Primary malignant tumors of the chest wall. The Memorial Sloan-Kettering Cancer Center Experience. Chest Surg Clin North Am 1994;4:137.

Chapelier AR, Missanna MC, Couturaus B, et al. Sternal resections and reconstruction for primary malignant tumors. Ann Thorac Surg 2004;77:1001.

EDITOR'S COMMENTS

Dr. Kaiser presents an elegant description of a transcervical thymectomy and because he has done so many, he makes it seem like an easy operation to do. It is not and should not be an operation performed by the casual general thoracic surgeon who only does one or two thymectomies per year. Most thoracic surgeons prefer a transsternal approach to thymus gland, although there are an increasing number of surgeons who are managing small thymic tumors or patients with myasthenia gravis with thoracoscopic procedures.

There are several points made in this chapter that merit further emphasis. First, the results of transcervical thymectomies, in appropriately selected patients, are equivalent to the "larger", more invasive procedures described by Jaretski. Second, this operation is difficult to teach secondary to the limited visibility for any first or second assistant. Third, it takes some experience to correctly identify cervical fat or the beginning of the thymus gland. A common mistake is to proceed with the dissection more posteriorly than needed. As pointed out by the author, using the inferior thyroidal vein as an anatomic landmark to guide the depth of dissection is an important technical point and helps keep the operator in the correct plane of dissection.

We have performed several of these procedures thoracoscopically through either a right-sided approach or through a bilateral approach with the patient supine and their arms elevated over their head, much like the positioning for a double lung transplant. Visualization is excellent, recovery is quick, and it is easier to teach to residents because of the thoracoscopic picture. Whatever approach is chosen, it is likely that referral of these patients for surgery will be facilitated with minimally invasive surgical approaches like the transcervical approach described by Dr. Kaiser.

David R. Jones and I.L.K.

27

The Diaphragm

Christine L. Lau and Bryan F. Meyers

Introduction

The diaphragm is a dome-shaped, musculoaponeurotic structure separating the thoracic and peritoneal cavities. It is from this anatomic function that it derives its name (Greek *dia* [in between] and *phragma* [fence]). This constantly active striated muscle increases the volume of the thoracic cavity with contraction and reduces thoracic volume on relaxation. These volume changes in turn result in cyclical changes in intrathoracic pressure with the movement of air into and out of the lungs. Voluntary or involuntary sustained contraction of the diaphragm assists in increasing abdominal pressure to assist in defecation or vomiting.

The embryologic development of the diaphragm begins between the eighth and tenth weeks of intrauterine life. The anterior and pericardial portions are formed from the septum transversum, which originates between the heart and the liver. The posterolateral portion of the diaphragm is formed by the fusion of the dorsal mesentery and the receding wolffian body and pleuroperitoneal membrane. The muscle of the diaphragm is formed from the invasion of these membranous structures by two muscle masses that originate from the cervical myotomes and migrate caudally with the septum transversum.

The multiplicity of origins and the complexity of development may explain the number and variety of congenital diaphragmatic defects that occur. Defects occurring before membranous fusion result in defects without a sac, whereas defects occurring after membrane fusion as a result of incomplete muscle invasion will have a pleuroperitoneal hernia sac.

Anatomy

Any operation or incision involving the diaphragm requires a thorough knowledge of its anatomy. The diaphragm consists of a peripheral muscular zone that inserts into a central aponeurotic tendon. The peripheral portion of the diaphragm originates circumferentially from four points: sternum, ribs, anterior muscular, and posterior muscular. The sternal origin consists of two short slips of muscle that arise from each side of the xiphoid, extending superiorly and posteriorly to insert in the central tendon (Fig. 27-1). The costal origin consists of muscle bundles arising from the inner aspect of the lower six costal cartilages. These muscle bundles interdigitate with the muscle bundles from the transversus abdominis muscle, and they insert into the anterior and lateral portions of the central tendon. The posterior portion of the diaphragm arises from the medial and lateral arcuate ligaments (Fig. 27-2). The medial ligament is the thickened anterior portion of the psoas fascia, which extends from the body of L2 to the tip of the transverse process of L1. The lateral ligament is a thickening of the anterior fascia of the quadratus lumborum muscle and extends from the tip of the transverse process of L1 to the lower border of the twelfth rib. The diaphragmatic crura are posterior bundles of muscle that arise inferiorly from the sides and bodies of the lumbar vertebrae and intervertebral discs. The right crus arises from L1 to L3 and the left crus from L1 to L2. As the muscle fibers ascend, the medial fibers of both muscles decussate in front of the descending aorta. The fibers on the right continue to ascend and encircle the esophagus before inserting into the central tendon. The aorta penetrates the

diaphragm at T12, and the esophagus penetrates it at T10. The slips of muscle that make up the diaphragm coalesce centrally as they insert in the trifoliate (three-leafed) central tendon. The three leaves are the left, right, and pericardial. The right tendon is perforated by the vena cava approximately 1 in. to the right of the midline at T8.

The phrenic nerves provide both sensory and motor function (Fig. 27-2). The right phrenic nerve penetrates the diaphragm just lateral to the caval foramen, and the left penetrates just lateral to the left heart border. Each nerve divides into roughly four trunks: an anterolateral trunk, a posterolateral trunk, a sternal trunk, and a crural trunk. After giving off the sternal trunks, each nerve penetrates the diaphragm and courses immediately below the peritoneal lining on the inferior surface of the muscle and therefore cannot be seen from the chest.

The arterial blood supply to the diaphragm comes from the left and right phrenic arteries arising from the abdominal aorta near the aortic hiatus (Fig. 27-3). They bifurcate posteriorly near the dome and course along the margin of the central tendon. A large anterior branch runs anteriorly and superiorly and merges with the pericardiophrenic artery. A smaller, posterior branch of the phrenic artery courses laterally and posteriorly along the dorsal, lumbar, and costal origins of the diaphragm and merges with the intercostal vessels. Additional blood supply comes from the musculophrenic and pericardiophrenic branches of the internal mammary artery and the intercostal arteries. Venous drainage is via the right and left inferior phrenic veins, which run near the artery and drain medially into the inferior vena cava. The arterial and the

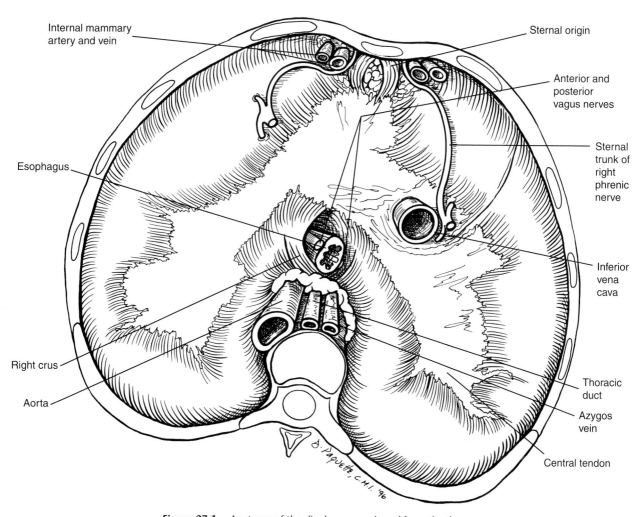

Figure 27-1. Anatomy of the diaphragm as viewed from the thorax.

Labels in figure:
Internal mammary artery and vein
Sternal origin
Anterior and posterior vagus nerves
Esophagus
Sternal trunk of right phrenic nerve
Inferior vena cava
Right crus
Aorta
Thoracic duct
Azygos vein
Central tendon

venous drainage are best visualized from the abdominal side of the diaphragm.

Incisions

Incisions in the diaphragm are commonly made to provide exposure during a variety of thoracic or abdominal operations. Knowledge of the distribution of phrenic innervation allows the surgeon to preserve diaphragm function in most cases. The relationship between the phrenic nerve and common diaphragmatic incisions is shown in Fig. 27-4. Generally, the best incision is made circumferentially approximately 2 cm from the muscle's lateral origin. This incision can be made from either pleural space or as a lateral extension of a thoracoabdominal incision. As an incision is made along the diaphragm peripherally, the index and middle fingers are kept against the chest wall above and below the diaphragm. This keeps

the incision the proper distance from the chest wall and protects unseen viscera from injury. There is little risk of significant injury to either the phrenic artery or phrenic nerve in this location. An incision extending into the crura may injure the terminal portion of the crural nerve or the posterior branch of the phrenic nerve, but these injuries are of little significance. Closure of this circumferential incision results in minimal additional impairment of respiratory function compared to thoracotomy or laparotomy alone.

Occasionally, shorter incisions in the central tendon can provide additional limited exposure of an underlying structure such as the splenic hilum or short gastrics during a fundoplication. Small diaphragmatic arterial vessels may be cut and easily controlled with a figure-of-eight suture. These central incisions should not extend too far medially to avoid cutting the posterior branch of the phrenic nerve. A mid-

line incision may also be made safely in the diaphragm, whether anteriorly or posteriorly. The only significant structure crossing the midline is the left inferior phrenic vein, which must be ligated. In Merendino's classic paper on incisions, two other incisions were described as safe: a paracardiac incision medial to the phrenic nerve and a posterior radial incision at the level of the esophageal hiatus.

Repair of the Injured or Incised Diaphragm

Various techniques may be used to close or repair the diaphragm. Simple incisions through the central tendon are easily repaired with a nonabsorbable 0 suture (Fig. 27-5A). We prefer a running horizontal mattress suture that everts the cut edge. The everted edge can then be oversewn by

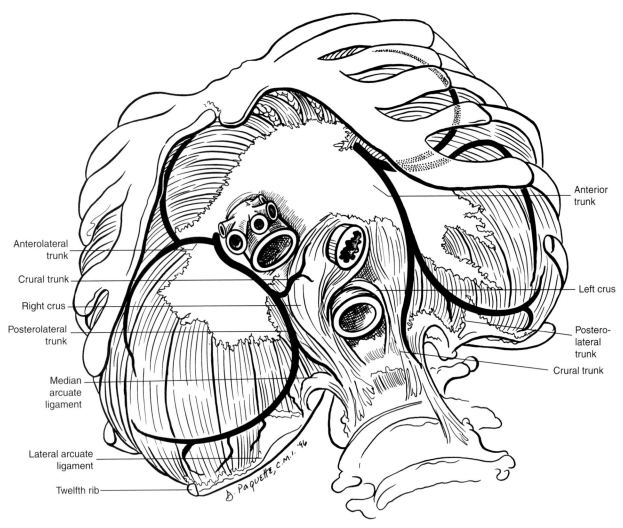

Figure 27-2. Anatomy of the diaphragm with the branches of the phrenic nerve as viewed from the abdomen. The sternal branch of the phrenic nerve is seen in Fig. 27-1.

continuing the suture back in over-and-over fashion above the first suture. For repair of incisions or defects through the muscular portion of the diaphragm, we prefer interrupted horizontal mattress sutures of a nonabsorbable 0 material (Fig. 27-5B). We utilize this suture technique to close peripheral incisions in the diaphragm. Small penetrating wounds can be closed easily with simple interrupted sutures. When we encounter ragged, torn, or thinned-out diaphragmatic muscle, however, we buttress our horizontal mattress sutures with polytetrafluoroethylene (Teflon) pledgets. The resection of primary tumors of the diaphragm or tumors of the lung, pleura, or chest wall that invade the diaphragm may leave a defect that cannot be closed primarily. Reconstruction should re-establish separation of the thoracic and abdominal viscera and maximize the restoration of pulmonary function. Various materials accomplish these goals in-

cluding polypropylene mesh, woven polytetrafluoroethylene (PTFE) patch, bovine pericardium, Surgisis (Cook Surgical), and polyester (Dacron) patch. The material is sutured to the muscular portions of the diaphragm with interrupted horizontal mattress sutures. A running suture may be used to approximate the material to the central tendon. When the defect is large and significant immobility of the reconstructed diaphragm is anticipated, it is important that the repaired leaf be relatively taut to prevent paradoxical movement and to maintain vital capacity. This is discussed in more detail in the section on diaphragmatic paralysis. When peripheral defects are present, it is sometimes possible to reattach the diaphragm to the chest wall at a higher level to maintain function. To accomplish this, we utilize interlocking horizontal mattress sutures and bring them out through the chest wall.

Anterior Retrosternal Diaphragmatic Hernia of Morgagni

The retrosternal diaphragmatic hernia described by Morgagni in 1769 makes up <2% of reported diaphragmatic defects (Fig. 27-6). The hernia occurs between the xiphoid process of the sternum and costochondral attachments of the diaphragm where the internal mammary vessels pass through the diaphragm to become the epigastric vessels. It results from a failure of muscle tissue to spread over the area. This potential space is covered by pericardium on the left side, and so more hernias occur on the right. The hernia usually has a sac, unless the sac has ruptured in prenatal life. This rare hernia may be found in childhood but is more likely to be present in adults. The symptoms vary, and they may be only

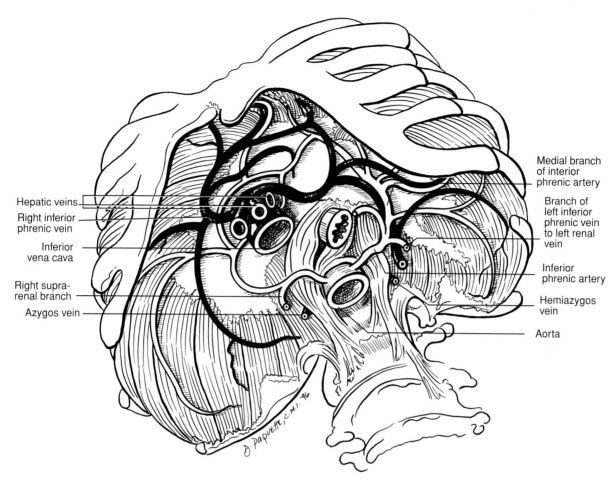

Hepatic veins

Right inferior phrenic vein

Inferior vena cava

Right supra-renal branch

Azygos vein

Medial branch of interior phrenic artery

Branch of left inferior phrenic vein to left renal vein

Inferior phrenic artery

Hemiazygos vein

Aorta

Figure 27-3. Abdominal view of the diaphragm showing the arterial supply and venous drainage.

vague fullness and cramping to obstructive in nature. There seems to be a larger percentage of female patients, and obese patients are more symptomatic. The hernia frequently presents as an incidental abnormal finding on chest x-ray films. The film may show a mass or even a fluid level. The viscera in the sac usually include one or more of the following: colon, omentum, stomach, and small bowel. An upper gastrointestinal series or barium enema can characterize abdominal contents in the sac. Computed tomographic scanning is particularly useful and has a reported 100% sensitivity for diagnosis.

Patients should have 24 hours of clear liquids before surgery. Antibiotics should be given before the surgical incision. The repair is best done through an abdominal approach. A midline or subcostal incision will allow for excellent visualization of the hernia and its contents. Recently, laparoscopic repair of these hernias has been increasingly used. After the abdomen is entered, the contents of the sac can be reduced with gentle traction. If necessary, a catheter can be in-

troduced into the sac to equalize pressure. In the rare case of incarceration, the skin incision can be extended across the costochondral arch into the intercostal space to allow bimanual manipulation to reduce the hernia into the abdomen. The sac margins are identified, and the sac is resected. When there is a complete rim of diaphragm muscle around the hernia defect, it can be closed with heavy, braided permanent suture placed in horizontal mattress fashion (Fig. 27-7A). A second running layer of sutures should be placed between the mattress sutures after they have been tied. When a complete rim of muscle is absent anteriorly, the free crescent edge of the unattached diaphragm is sutured to the costal margin with heavy, braided mattress sutures (Fig. 27-7B). When the wound is closed, if the pleura has been entered, air can be removed by sucking it out with a catheter before the last suture is placed or by inserting an intercostal tube and placing it to water seal drainage.

If a previously unsuspected hernia is discovered during a thoracotomy, the hernia

should be repaired (Fig. 27-7C). The hernia is reduced and the sac resected. Two rows of permanent braided sutures are placed in mattress fashion, one at the edge of the defect and one another 2 cm proximal to the edge. The sutures are brought out through the chest wall and tied, bringing a 2-cm area of diaphragmatic surface in contact with the chest wall. A postoperative chest film is taken to evaluate lung expansion.

Posterolateral Diaphragmatic Hernia of Bochdalek

Bochdalek described a congenital posterolateral defect in the diaphragm (Fig. 27-6). Failure of the pleuroperitoneal canal to close at the eighth week of gestation allows the foregut to herniate into the chest as it returns to the abdominal cavity. The herniated gut occupying the pleural cavity can lead to a failure of the lung bud to mature. The resultant pulmonary hypoplasia is the

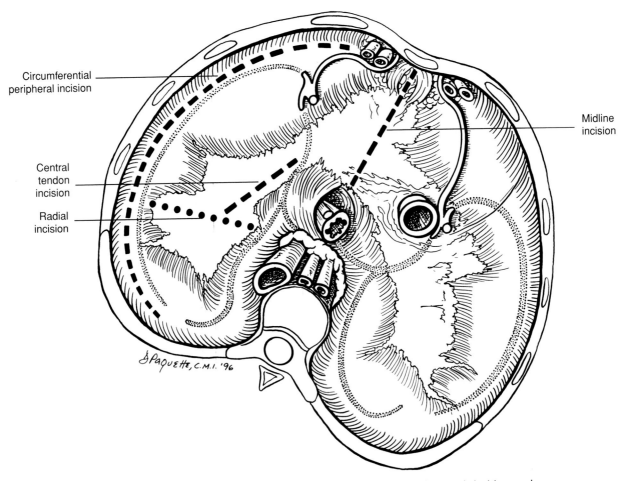

Circumferential peripheral incision

Central tendon incision

Radial incision

Midline incision

SPAQUETTE, C.M.I. '96

Figure 27-4.   Thoracic view of the diaphragm showing the common diaphragmatic incisions and their relationship to the branches of the phrenic nerve.

main cause of morbidity and mortality associated with this disease, which occurs in 1 of 4,000 births. In 1953, Gross reported a series of 63 infants who underwent repair of the defect with an operative mortality of 12%. With the advent of early diagnosis through the use of prenatal ultrasound, many smaller infants with additional comorbidities are considered for repair. Despite the early diagnosis and advanced intensive care available to these sick children, the operative mortality approaches 50%.

The diagnosis can be made by prenatal ultrasound and is obvious later when a radiograph shows intestinal contents in the chest. Symptomatic hernias are more common on the left side. Other anomalies of the central nervous system, genitourinary tract, and cardiovascular systems should be investigated.

Perioperative management is just as important as the surgical repair. A nasogastric tube prevents air from getting into the herniated bowel and thus prevents further pulmonary compromise. Blood gases need to

be monitored and assisted ventilation introduced if necessary. Common sense would suggest rapid surgical correction—reduce the hernia and close the defect. In reality, surgery may worsen the clinical status. With the infant sedated or paralyzed, mechanical ventilation can often regulate satisfactory gas exchange without surgery. Infants who do not respond appropriately to maximum treatment may be placed on extracorporeal membrane oxygenation (ECMO). There is neither solid data nor empirical consensus as to whether the repair should proceed while the infant is on ECMO or be delayed until after decannulation. The preference at our center is to wait until the child has been removed from ECMO in order to reduce the bleeding complications. The final word on the timing of operation has not been established, but it is clear that emergency surgery is not necessary.

The repair begins with a subcostal transverse incision, leaving 2 cm to 3 cm between the incision and the costal margin. A self-retaining retractor affords excellent vi-

sualization. The viscera can be seen entering the defect and should be gently reduced. A vein retractor beneath the anterior lip of the defect and a catheter in the sac to equalize the air pressure can assist in the task. A hernia sac, present in 20% of cases, should be sought out and resected. The ipsilateral lung will be seen, and care should be taken to avoid hyperinflation. A chest tube can be placed at this time. The posterior lip of the defect should be identified. It appears above the adrenal gland and should be freed sufficiently to enhance closure of the defect. The anterior and posterior edges are approximated with 2-0 sutures of nonabsorbable braided synthetic material placed in horizontal mattress fashion. A large defect, however, will need to be closed with a prosthesis (Fig. 27-8). A Gore-Tex patch cut larger than the defect is fashioned. It is sutured in place with nonabsorbable monofilament sutures tied over Teflon pledgets. If no posterior rim is found, the sutures can be placed around the rib or deep into the intercostal muscles. Pedicled abdominal wall muscle flaps

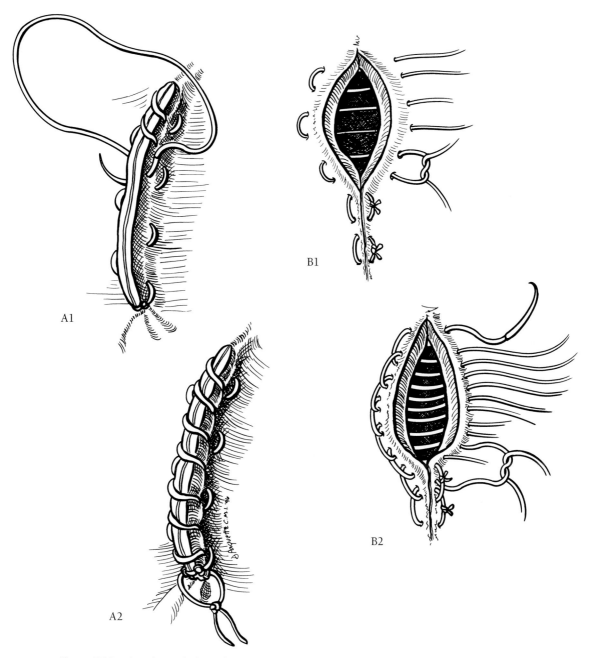

A1

B1

A2

B2

Figure 27-5. Suturing techniques for repair of the diaphragm. **(A1, A2)** Repair of the central tendon. **(B1, B2)** Repair of diaphragmatic muscle with simple or interlocking interrupted horizontal mattress sutures.

to repair the defect do not appear to be as efficacious as the prosthesis.

After the diaphragm is repaired, the bowel needs to be returned to the abdomen. It may be necessary to develop a ventral hernia by just closing the skin or to construct a silo to accommodate the viscera without tension. The hernia or pouch can be closed over the next several days.

Postoperative care may be very difficult. The chest tube is placed to an underwater seal with no suction. Alternatively, balanced thoracic drainage tubes can be used to prevent further lung injury. The lungs are at risk of rupture. Barotrauma with a pneumothorax may develop in either lung. Minor changes in ventilation can precipitate intense pulmonary vasoconstriction. Generalized capillary leakage is present in the first 48 hours. Cardiomyopathy and renal failure are constant threats if severe hypoxia was present during early resuscitation.

Mortality is higher in neonates requiring rapid treatment in the first 6 to 24 hours of life. Chronic bronchopulmonary dysplasia, mental retardation, and neurologic defects are not uncommon after extraordinary methods are initially successful. The case fatality rate remains above 50%. Attempts have been made to correct the defect in utero, to obstruct the fetal trachea to cause pulmonary hypertrophy, and even to perform lung transplantation. The final

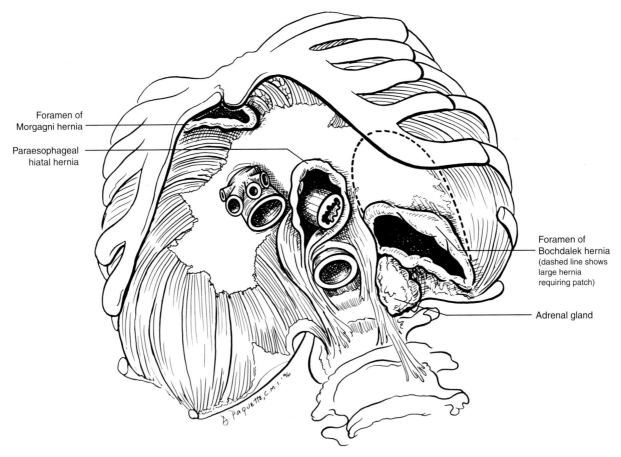

Foramen of
Morgagni hernia

Paraesophageal
hiatal hernia

Foramen of
Bochdalek hernia
(dashed line shows
large hernia
requiring patch)

Adrenal gland

Figure 27-6. Abdominal view of the diaphragm showing the location of the common hernias.

answer for this intriguing problem remains a surgical puzzle.

Hiatal Hernia

The type I, or sliding, hiatal hernia is discussed in Chapter 16. The type II hernia is the uncommon paraesophageal hernia that begins with a focal weakening in the phrenico-esophageal membrane anterior and lateral to the esophagus (Fig. 27-6). In the type II hernia, the gastric cardia and distal esophagus remain below the diaphragm. As the phrenico-esophageal membrane weakens, the gastric fundus protrudes through a defect and gradually obtains a higher and higher position within the chest. As it ascends, it rotates along the axis of the lesser gastric curvature, which is fixed by the duodenum, left gastric artery, and esophagogastric junction. The fundus and the antrum ascend into the chest, leaving the cardia and pylorus below the diaphragm in the abdomen (Fig. 27-9A). This produces the mechanical effect of obstruction at the level of the diaphragm and the classic ap-

pearance on barium swallow studies of the upside-down stomach. The type III hernia is a combination of type I and type II, and a type IV hernia is a generalized enlargement of the hiatus with the presence of other viscera besides the stomach in the chest.

Significant controversy surrounds paraesophageal hernias. Many believe that the type II hernia is rare and that most paraesophageal hernias are type III with a supradiaphragmatic esophageal sphincter. Figure 27-9B shows a radiograph illustrating a type III hernia. Many believe that an antireflux procedure should be a part of the repair in all patients regardless of symptoms, whereas others believe that it should be reserved for patients with demonstrated reflux. Many believe that the presence of a parahiatal hernia is an indication for operation, and recently others have shown that this may not be necessary with an absence of symptoms. Finally, the hernia may be repaired via the thorax or the abdomen, and each approach has its proponents and detractors.

Most patients complain of postprandial discomfort but a few complain of dysphagia. Substernal fullness or pressure is common

and may be partially relieved by belching or regurgitation. Symptoms of reflux may or may not be present. When gastric volvulus or obstruction occurs, patients may present in extreme distress with severe nausea, epigastric pain, and an inability to regurgitate or vomit. The patient may not be able to swallow his or her saliva. These patients require emergency surgery to prevent strangulation and infarction, which carry a high mortality.

In patients without prior abdominal surgery a laparoscopic approach to repair of paraesophageal hernias may be considered. One potential cause of recurrence when approached laparoscopically is failure to treat acquired esophageal shortening. For this reason when we approach these laparoscopically we do not hesitate to perform a Collis gastroplasty when <2 cm of esophagus is intra-abdominal after full mobilization. To facilitate the gastroplasty, we place the patient positioned on a 30-degree incline (right side up) at the time of the operation and perform the Collis procedure by making a thoracoscopic incision for an endoscopic gastrointestinal anastomosis (GIA) stapler.

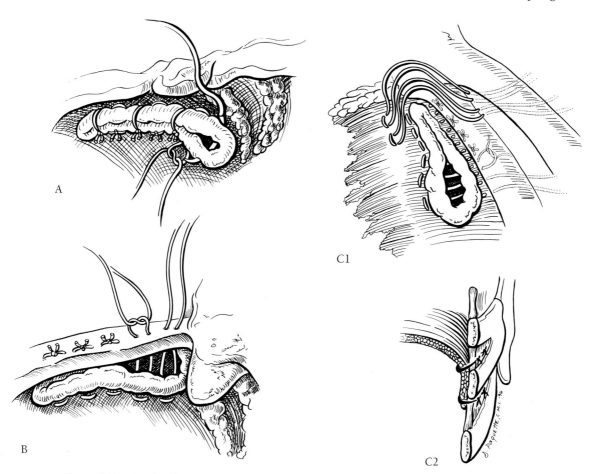

Figure 27-7.   Repair of hernia of Morgagni. **(A)** Abdominal approach when an anterior rim of muscle is present. **(B)** Abdominal approach when an anterior rim of muscle is absent. **(C1, C2)** Thoracic approach: anterior and lateral views. Note how the diaphragm is buttressed against the chest wall for a firm closure.

For the open approach, we prefer the thoracic approach using a left seventh interspace incision with shingling of the eighth rib posteriorly. This allows wide separation of the ribs and avoids entrapment of the intercostal nerve at the site of the fracture. The vagus nerves are identified and are encircled with vessel loops, with every effort to avoid injuring them. The hernia sac is dissected free from the thoracic cavity and resected. Often the sac extends well into the right chest. The crura are identified and their edge freed up. If the esophagus appears shortened, we perform a Collis gastroplasty. A Belsey-Mark IV fundoplication is performed in the chest, and the wrap is reduced below the diaphragm (Chapter 16). In our opinion, the incidence of reflux after surgery without an antireflux operation is sufficiently high (approximately 15%) as to warrant fundoplication. We prefer the Belsey to the Nissen procedure when a Collis gastroplasty is required because we found a high incidence of dysphagia when we performed the Collis-Nissen procedure. The crura are

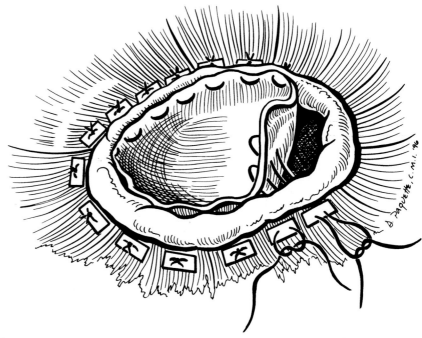

Figure 27-8.   Repair of a large hernia of Bochdalek with a Gore-Tex patch. The interrupted mattress sutures are buttressed with Teflon pledgets.

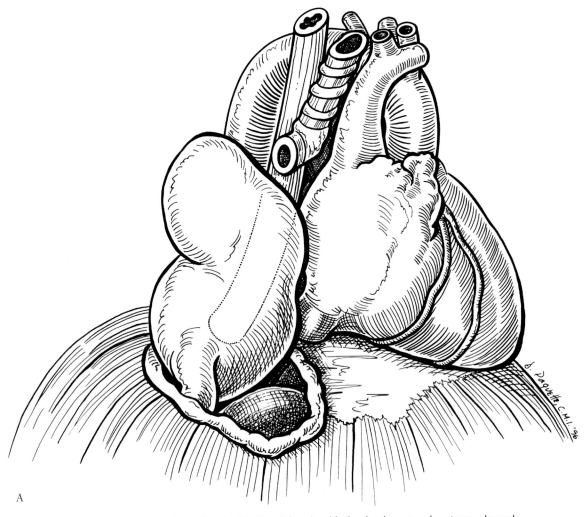

A

Figure 27-9. Paraesophageal hernia. **(A)** Type II hernia with the duodenum and gastroesophageal junction anchored below the diaphragm. **(B)** Type III hernia with migration of the gastroesophageal junction and duodenum into the chest. (*Continued*)

approximated with interrupted nonabsorbable 0 sutures 1 cm to 2 cm from the margin. Approximately five sutures are used. Once the last suture is tied, one should be able to pass a little finger beside the esophagus with an indwelling nasogastric tube. If the hiatus is too large after the last suture is placed, an additional suture may be placed in the crura anterior to the esophagus. Gastric stasis may be more prolonged than after a type I repair.

Diaphragmatic Paralysis

Diaphragmatic paralysis or paresis is most often seen after cardiac procedures. Openheart procedures and reoperations have a higher incidence. Most often the paralysis is temporary. In infants, direct injury is most common, whereas in adults, the injury is most often attributed to hypothermia and almost always occurs on the left side. The overall incidence of injury has been reported as approximately 2%. Direct invasion of the phrenic nerve by tumors of the lung or mediastinum are common causes of phrenic nerve paralysis, and these are usually identified on a computed tomography (CT) scan of the chest. Direct injury to the nerve during a noncardiac thoracic or cervical operation may or may not be associated with transection. Traction on the nerve, pressure from a retractor, or the use of cautery near the nerve may cause paralysis or paresis. Severe trauma associated with sudden deceleration or blast may produce phrenic nerve injury, and it is also seen occasionally in neuromuscular disorders, after a difficult birth, or after viral, bacterial, syphilitic, or tuberculous infection. In many cases the cause remains elusive.

In the young child or infant, life-threatening respiratory insufficiency may develop after diaphragmatic paralysis. This has been attributed to three factors. The intercostal muscles are weak and do not allow a significant increase in intrathoracic dimensions. The mediastinum is extremely mobile and shifts excessively away from the paralyzed side on inspiration, limiting lung expansion. Finally, the tendency toward recumbency allows the abdominal viscera to exert undue force in an upward direction.

In an adult, unilateral diaphragmatic paralysis produces little respiratory dysfunction in a majority of patients. An early reduction of 20% to 30% in vital capacity and total lung capacity frequently returns to normal after 6 months. In the supine position, however, vital capacity and expiratory flow rates remain diminished. It has been reported that the majority of patients whose major symptoms were cough or chest pain improved on follow-up, whereas two thirds of patients whose principal symptom was dyspnea on

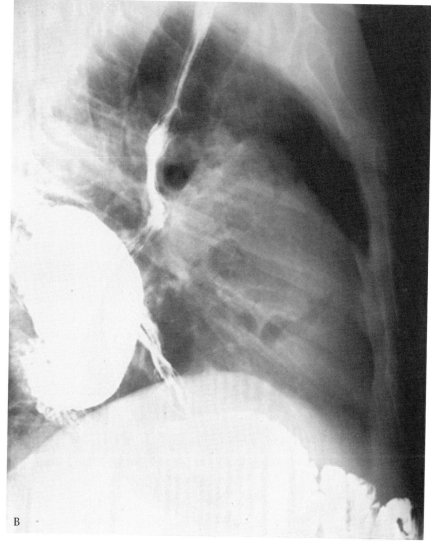

Figure 27-9.   (*Continued*)

exertion remained unchanged or got worse. In the rare patient with bilateral paralysis, excessive accessory muscle movement may be seen but is associated with marked reductions in vital capacity and flow rates.

Normal diaphragm motion is easily evaluated fluoroscopically, and the so-called "sniff test" can provoke and uncover abnormal paradoxical motion during vigorous inspiration. Recently, cine-magnetic resonance imaging (MRI) has been used in equivocal cases to evaluate degrees of diaphragmatic paresis.

In an infant or young child, early assessment of phrenic nerve function at the bedside has been useful in ventilated patients. Diaphragmatic plication for unilateral paralysis has been used in infants and children as well as adults to improve respiratory function. In infants and children <18 months of age, the timing for intervention has generally varied from 1 to 8 weeks. More recently,

several authors have recommended early intervention within 2 weeks of diagnosis. In patients treated with early plication, both the duration of intubation and the intensive care unit stay have been reduced. In children >18 months of age, plication has generally not been necessary. Additional support for early plication lies in the demonstration that plication does not interfere with the return of normal diaphragmatic function. In these patients, we recommend the technique originally described by Schwartz and Fuller in 1978. The diaphragm is plicated centrally with interrupted 3-0 horizontal mattress sutures buttressed with Teflon pledgets and spaced approximately 0.5 cm apart. The sutures are spaced in the diaphragm so as to avoid the main branches of the phrenic nerve and are placed only in muscle. The diaphragm is grasped with forceps between the branches of the nerve, and each arm of the suture is passed through the muscle,

avoiding the peritoneum below. Enough diaphragm has to be included in each pleat to make the diaphragm moderately taut. In a rare case when repeated plications have failed, fixation of the diaphragm with a prosthetic material may be required.

In an adult, plication should be entertained only when the timing or nature of injury precludes regeneration of the phrenic nerve, and when significant symptoms merit the additional surgery. This time period is generally 1 year. An occasional patient with postsurgical diaphragmatic paralysis and significant underlying lung disease may not have sufficient ventilatory reserve to compensate for the paralysis and may benefit from early plication. Plication changes the configuration of the diaphragm, allowing vital capacity and lung capacity to increase, and increases the ability of the diaphragm to act as a pressure generator by making it relatively taut. Furthermore, the observed improvement in the forced vital capacity and forced vital capacity at 1 second, total lung capacity, residual volume, diffusing capacity, and partial arterial oxygen pressure after plication may continue to improve for up to 1 year. The improvement in symptoms after plication appears to be durable.

To plicate the diaphragm in adults, we recommend thoracotomy through the eighth intercostal space. The phrenic nerve is stimulated directly just above its entrance into the diaphragm to confirm paralysis. The lateral and posterior portions of the diaphragm are gathered on themselves in pleats with interrupted horizontal mattress sutures buttressed with Teflon pledgets (Fig. 27-10A, B). A double-armed 0 nonabsorbable suture is used. The pleats are oriented circumferentially beginning at the peripheral margin of the diaphragm and extending medially to or into the central tendon. It takes approximately 10 to 20 sutures at 1-cm intervals to accomplish the goals of reducing the diaphragm to the position of peak inspiration and making it taut. Patients generally tolerate the procedure well, and patients plicated in the postsurgical setting may wean rapidly from mechanical ventilation.

Eventration

Eventration of the diaphragm is a congenital defect acquired during fetal life. It is characterized by a failure of muscle to develop in the otherwise membranous structure of the septum transversum. It is frequently associated with spinal and chest wall anomalies, hypoplasia or aplasia of the

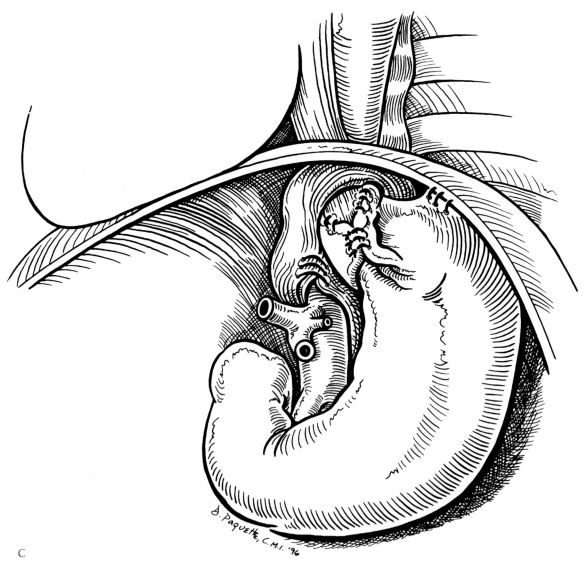

C

Figure 27-9. (*Continued*)

lung, extrapulmonary sequestration, and visceral transposition. Severe cardiorespiratory symptoms in a newborn or neonate are usually caused by hypoplasia of the lung on the involved side. The major challenge in these patients is respiratory support including extracorporeal membrane oxygenation. Immediate repair is required, generally via the thoracic approach. The thinned diaphragm is incised near its costal attachment, stretched out, and reattached with horizontal mattress sutures. Another defect frequently associated with pulmonary hypoplasia is the presence of an accessory diaphragm. A CT scan is frequently necessary to make this diagnosis, and these should be excised.

Recently repair of diaphragmatic eventration has been described using a video-assisted-thoracoscopic technique. A dual-lumen tube is placed, and the patient is placed in the lateral decubitus position. A 10-mm camera port is placed in the fifth intercostal space in the posteroaxillary line and second 5-mm port is placed anteriorly on the mammary line in the fifth intercostal space. A 5-cm minithoracotomy is made in the ninth or tenth intercostal space on the posterior axillary line. Two superimposed series of transverse back-and-forth sutures are used. The first suture invaginates the eventration, and the second row allows the desired tension on the diaphragm. The technique is shown in Figure 27-10C. Modifications of this technique have been proposed that avoid the minithoracotomy by the insertion of two 5-mm ports in the eighth and ninth intercostal spaces.

Diaphragmatic Pacing

Diaphragmatic pacing may be beneficial in two groups of patients: those with central alveolar hypoventilation (Ondine's curse) and those with high cervical cord injuries (quadriplegics). Although diaphragmatic pacing has occasionally been used in two other groups, patients with chronic obstructive pulmonary disease (COPD) and patients with intractable hiccups, its value in these patients is much less well defined. Patients with injury to the diaphragm or phrenic nerve do not respond to diaphragmatic pacing.

Patients with central alveolar hypoventilation (CAH) have a diminished response of the receptors in the medulla to

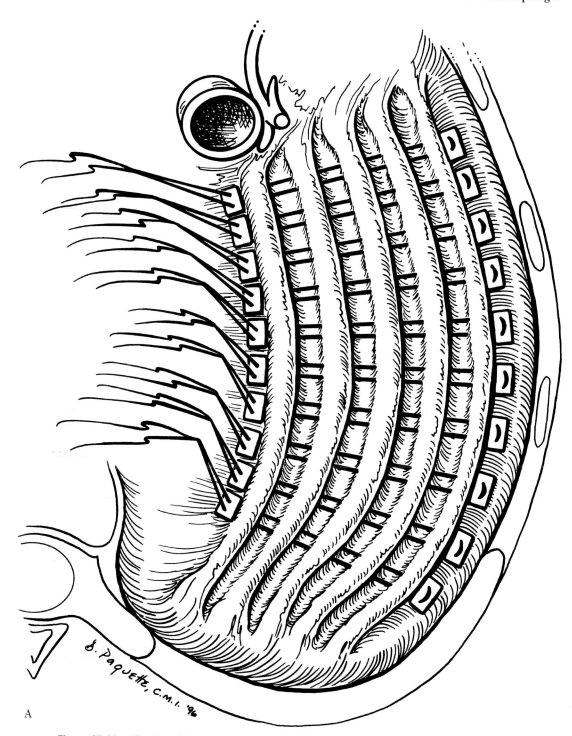

A

Figure 27-10. Plication of the right diaphragm in an adult. **(A)** Sutures buttressed with Teflon pledgets extend anteriorly to the level of the vena cava. **(B)** Plicated diaphragm. **(C)** Repair of diaphragmatic eventration using a video-assisted-thoracoscopic technique to plicate the diaphragm. (ICS = intercostal space.) (Reprinted with permission from Mouroux J, Padovani B, Poirier C, et al. Technique for the repair of diaphragmatic eventration. Ann Thorac Surg 1996;62:905–907.) (*Continued*)

hypercarbia and hypoxia. The normal increase in ventilation with hypercarbia or hypoxia is blunted or absent in patients with CAH. Although this response is abnormal at daytime as well as at night, when the patient is awake he or she can make a conscious effort to breathe. When sleeping however, the conscious effort is lacking. It is important to differentiate CAH from obstructive sleep apnea, which occurs only while sleeping and is secondary to an anatomic obstruction. The differentiation between the two is important because treatment is markedly different for obstructive sleep apnea (weight loss, positive-pressure ventilation support, and in severe cases uvulopalatopharyngoplasty) compared to CAH (diaphragm pacing).

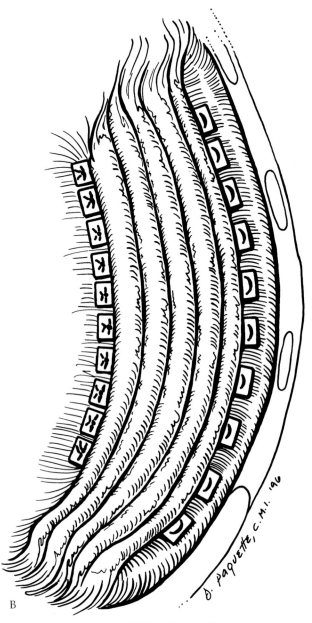

Figure 27-10.   (*Continued*)

Cervical spinal cord injury can occur in patients secondary to motor vehicle accidents, sports-related injures, or falls. High cervical spine injuries (those above C3) are most amenable to phrenic nerve pacing because the phrenic nerve is intact. When the injury involves the nerve roots at C3–5, less benefit is obtained because of the lack of contribution from the involved roots. Injuries below C5 do not affect the phrenic nerve, and such patients do not benefit from phrenic nerve pacing.

Patients with severe COPD become accustomed to chronic hypercarbia and rely on hypoxic drive to ventilate. When supplemental oxygen is required they may lose their hypoxic drive and hypoventilate. Phrenic nerve pacing, although theoretically useful in this setting, is rarely used. Pacing has been reported for patients with intractable hiccups, but many patients find pacing uncomfortable and discontinue it voluntarily.

Pacing the diaphragm is accomplished by placing an electrode in contact with the phrenic nerve. Most commonly this is performed via a limited anterior thoracotomy in the second or third interspace, although a cervical approach or thoracoscopic approach can be useful as well. The phrenic nerve must be handled with care to prevent accidental injury that would preclude successful pacing. Muscle relaxants should be avoided to allow awareness of irritation and stimulation of the nerve. Use of perioperative antibiotics and sterile technique is imperative. The electrode is placed flat against the mediastinum and underneath the phrenic with the other end connected to a receiver unit in a subcutaneous pocket. In the functioning system, the receiver unit communicates through the skin with an external pacemaker. Usually one side is done at a time and the implantation for the other side is performed a few weeks later.

Trauma

Injuries to the diaphragm may be apparent immediately after trauma or may present late. This is true of injuries that occur after penetrating or blunt trauma. Penetrating injuries are 5 to 10 times more common than blunt injuries and occur randomly on both sides of the chest. They usually measure from 1 cm to 4 cm in length and generally may be repaired with simple sutures. Most penetrating wounds that affect the diaphragm occur below the level of the nipple, and any injury below that level should be suspected of involving the diaphragm. Most knife wounds to the chest occur with a downward motion, whereas most wounds to the abdomen occur with an upward motion. In general, knife wounds are more common in the chest and bullet wounds are more common in the abdomen. In the case of an abdominal wound, surgical exploration is usually undertaken and diaphragmatic injury must be excluded at some time during the procedure to prevent the late herniation through the defect. Laparoscopic evaluation and repair of the diaphragm have recently been recommended in cases of penetrating injury. When injury is to the chest, a diaphragmatic injury may be missed because not all patients are explored. These patients need to be followed carefully.

Blunt trauma may result in rupture of the diaphragm. The left side is affected about 20 times more commonly than the right, and in most cases rupture is secondary to a motor vehicle collision. The laceration usually varies from 10 cm to 15 cm in length and may occur any place in the diaphragm. Different series have claimed that the posterolateral, anterolateral, or pericardial areas are more commonly affected. The transmission of force through the abdominal viscera is the most commonly accepted explanation for the cause of these tears, and the attenuation of that force by the liver explains the left predominance. One third of

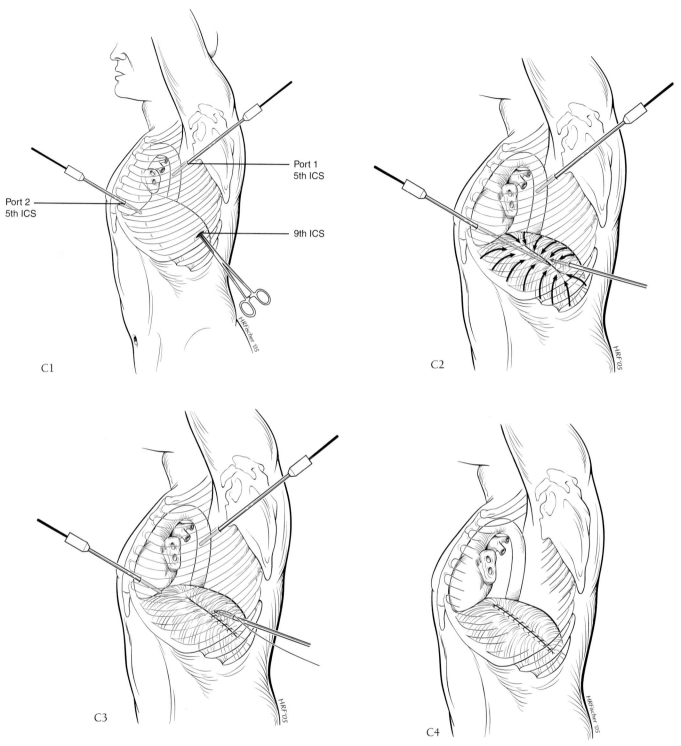

Figure 27-10.   (*Continued*)

the cases of blunt diaphragmatic rupture, however, occur after thoracic injury, and the association between diaphragmatic injury and acute aortic dissection has been recognized. Up to 5% of patients with significant blunt trauma will have diaphragmatic injury. Most often, the diaphragmatic injury is of secondary importance to some other

catastrophic injury. However, rupture of the diaphragm can occur without signs of external injury in children because of the increased compliance of the thoracic cage. The approach to these injuries dictates the approach to the diaphragm. Most often, acute left-sided injury is best explored through the abdomen, whereas right-sided injuries or in-

juries that become manifest later are best explored through the chest.

Only 50% of patients with blunt rupture will demonstrate herniation of abdominal viscera on presentation. The stomach, spleen, colon, and small intestine herniate most commonly in this order. Most patients, however, will demonstrate some abnormality on chest x-ray films, usually a pneumothorax, hemothorax, or elevation of the diaphragm. A high index of suspicion is the single most important factor in making the diagnosis. Although the chest x-ray film is an important diagnostic test, several views may be required to establish the diagnosis. Passing a nasogastric tube and distending the stomach with air or creating a pneumoperitoneum is sometimes helpful. An upper gastrointestinal series, barium enema, or intravenous pyelogram may be useful with left-sided injuries, and a liver scan, liver-lung scan, or angiogram may be diagnostic on the right. We have found that CT of the chest and abdomen with oral and intravenous contrast is most helpful in screening patients with significant trauma, and this may uncover a defect.

Diaphragmatic injuries that are missed may present late as diaphragmatic hernias. They commonly present as acute emergencies with intestinal obstruction or acute abdominal pain with or without chest pain or dyspnea. Other patients will present with nonspecific upper abdominal complaints.

The eighth or ninth interspaces are used to approach the diaphragm in cases of delayed presentation. The hernia is identified, and the abdominal viscera are freed from any adhesions that may have developed. Once the abdominal viscera have been returned to the abdomen, most defects can be closed primarily as previously described. Occasionally, a defect will require reconstruction with a patch.

Tumors

Primary tumors of the diaphragm are rare. Most are of mesenchymal origin, and the remainder (approximately 10%) are of neural origin. A majority are benign, and most of these consist of cystic lesions such as bronchial, mesothelial, or teratogenous cysts. If cysts are excluded, the majority of mesenchymal tumors are malignant, and the prognosis is poor with or without resection. The most common malignant tumor is the fibrosarcoma. On the other hand, the majority of neural tumors are benign. All tumors should be excised when feasible for diagnosis and treatment. Involvement of the diaphragm by tumors arising in adjacent structures is far more common. Tumors of the lung, pleura, chest wall, mediastinum, liver, stomach, and esophagus may all extend directly into the diaphragm. When appropriate, an en bloc resection of the primary tumor and involved diaphragm can be undertaken. Isolated metastases to the di-

aphragm do occur and, if they represent a sole site of metastasis, may be resected.

Benign tumors are generally asymptomatic and are most commonly an incidental finding on chest x-ray or CT studies. Symptoms generally are nonspecific and include lower chest pain, cough, dyspnea, and the feeling of central or subcostal fullness. Clubbing or hypertrophic pulmonary osteoarthropathy has been associated with more than one half of the neurogenic tumors reported.

A CT scan is the best imaging modality for tumors of the diaphragm. When liver involvement is suspected, angiography may be helpful. Occasionally MRI will clarify findings obscured on the CT scan.

Malignant tumors should be resected with a wide margin of normal tissue without regard to the extent of the defect. An entire leaf can be removed without undue physiologic derangement. Complex resections involving the removal of large areas of the diaphragm and adjacent chest wall have been reported for primary tumors of the lung or chest wall. Prosthetic material can be used to repair these defects. If additional soft tissue coverage is needed, a variety of muscle flaps may be rotated to cover the defects and, when necessary, free grafts with microvascular anastomoses can be constructed. It is important to take into account the degree

of diaphragmatic function lost in resection. If a large area is removed, it is important to position the repaired diaphragm near the position of full inspiration to maintain adequate vital capacity and avoid paradox.

Porous-Diaphragm Syndromes

Porous-diaphragm syndromes are a diverse group of diseases that share a common etiology: a defect in the diaphragm that allows for the transphrenic migration of substances (fluid, gases, tissue, or exudates) from the peritoneal cavity into the pleural spaces. The most common site of the diaphragmatic defect is in the tendinous part of diaphragm. These defects may be congenital but more often are acquired, and for various reasons (the peritoneal circulation, the piston effect of the liver) the thoracic involvement is seen more commonly on the right side.

Meigs syndrome (fibroma or fibroma-like benign ovarian tumor, ascites, pleural effusion, usually right sided, and cure of ascites and hydrothorax by removal of the ovarian tumor) appears to be the quintessential example of porous-diaphragm syndrome despite the fact that diaphragmatic defects have never been proven to occur in this syndrome. Surgical removal of the ovarian

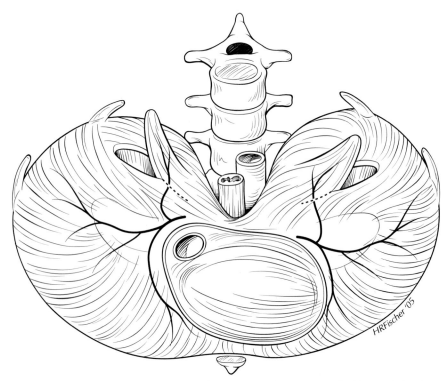

Figure 27-11. Technique for harvesting a diaphragmatic flap. (Reprinted with permission from TC Mineo, V Ambrogi. The diaphragmatic flap: A multiuse material in thoracic surgery. J Thorac Cardiovasc Surg 1999;118:1084.)

tumor treats the syndrome, and therefore unless a chest tube is required for the hydrothorax, it is uncommonly seen by the thoracic surgeon.

Catamenial pneumothorax is another example of a porous-diaphragm syndrome. This syndrome presents as spontaneous pneumothorax, usually right sided, occurring with the onset of menses. Endometriosis implants along the diaphragm and undergoes cyclical necrosis associated with hormone fluctuations, causing perforations in the diaphragm. The air causing the pneumothorax is presumed to travel retrograde through the fallopian tubes. Treatment involves closure of the diaphragm defect and medical control of the endometriosis. Thoracotomy, thoracoscopy, or pleurodesis is routinely employed to fix the diaphragm defect.

Diaphragmatic Flap

Although it is infrequently used, the diaphragmatic pedicled flap can provide excellent protection of bronchial stumps as well as vascularized coverage of bronchopleural fistulas and esophageal leaks. The flaps blood supply is provided by the phrenic artery. The technique for harvesting is shown in Figure 27-11. The harvesting technique can be aided by introducing a light source into the abdomen through the initial phrenotomy to transilluminate and protect the phrenic artery branches. In addition, this maneuver prevents inadvertent injury to abdominal organs. Division of the diaphragm starts on the posterior margin to protect the

origin of the phrenic artery. To ensure a vital flap, the width of the base should be about one fourth of the entire length. The flap can be marked with radiopaque clips if radiation therapy is to be used in the adjuvant setting. The defect created in the diaphragm by the flap is then closed with interrupted heavy silk.

SUGGESTED READING

Merendino KA, Johnson RJ, Skinner HH, et al. The intradiaphragmatic distribution of the phrenic nerve with particular reference to the placement of diaphragmatic incisions and controlled segmental paralysis. Surgery 1956;39:189.

Skandalkis JE, Gray SW, Ricketts RR. The Diaphragm. In Skandalkis JE, Gray SW, Ricketts RR (eds), Embryology for Surgeons. The Embryological Bases for Treatment of Congenital Anomalies (2nd ed). Baltimore: Williams & Wilkins, 1994;491.

The Diaphragm. Chest Surg Clin North Am 1998;8(2). Moores, DWO, ed.

EDITOR'S COMMENTS

We rarely think about surgical problems related to the diaphragm other than hernias. Primary tumors of the diaphragm are exceedingly rare, and we can excise an entire hemidiaphragm or portion thereof in the course of a resection for either lung cancer that directly invades or during an extrapleural pneumonectomy for mesothelioma. The authors have nicely summarized significant issues involved with reconstruction of the hemidiaphragm. A more vexing problem involves diaphragm paralysis. First, a firm diagnosis must be made and a fluoroscopy preformed—a sniff test usually is the best way to accomplish this. Significant paradoxical motion must be seen in order to establish the diagnosis, because passive movement of a paralyzed diaphragm may occur simply with excursion of the contralateral hemidiaphragm. Distinguishing a paralyzed diaphragm from a chronic diaphragmatic hernia or eventration may also cause difficulties. We have found that a contrast study may be helpful, but perhaps a more useful study is the coronal reconstruction of the MRI scan.

Diaphragm placation clearly has a place in the management of diaphragm paralysis in selected patients. As the authors point out, because many of the symptoms these patients manifest may disappear, there should be a period of observation, but the patient with significant paradoxical motion and persistent dyspnea may benefit greatly from this procedure. A great amount of care must be taken when the paralysis is on the right side, because the liver exerts considerable tension on the repair leading to dehiscence if the repair is not buttressed. Consideration should be given to the use of prosthetic material to buttress a repair of the right hemidiaphragm lest the repair dehisce with the first episode of significant coughing.

Readers should carefully study the excellent anatomic description provided by the authors, as this will aid in any manipulations on the part of the surgeon.

L.R.K.

28

The Thoracic Duct and the
Management of Chylothorax

Bradley M. Rodgers

Chylothorax is the abnormal accumulation of fluid from the lymphatic system within the pleural space. Chyle is composed mainly of the lymphatic drainage from the intestine, but also includes lymph from the lungs, liver, abdominal wall, and the extremities. The amount of lymph originating from the extremities as a component of chyle is negligible under normal circumstances. Chylothorax may be either congenital or acquired (Table 28-1). Congenital chylothorax is thought to occur either secondary to disruption of the thoracic duct during delivery or to congenital anatomic abnormalities of the duct, such as atresias. Acquired chylothorax can arise from multiple causes. Disruption of the thoracic duct most commonly occurs after blunt thoracic trauma. Occasionally the duct is injured in penetrating thoracic trauma, although the posterior location of the duct makes this form of injury quite uncommon. The thoracic duct may be lacerated during placement of left subclavian venous catheter. The most common cause of traumatic injury to the duct or its tributaries, however, occurs during thoracic operations. Chylothorax has been estimated to occur after 0.25% to 0.50% of all intrathoracic operations. Chylothorax has been described after nearly every form of thoracic surgical procedure but appears to be more common after cardiac procedures requiring considerable mediastinal dissection at the base of the heart or after esophagectomy.

Mediastinal neoplasms are responsible for the majority of chylothoraces that develop spontaneously in adult patients. Most of these are secondary to obstruction of lymphatic pathways from mediastinal lymphomas. Infections are an uncommon cause of chylothorax in the United States, but tuberculous lymphadenitis is a more common cause in many other countries. Miscellaneous causes for chylothorax include thrombosis of the subclavian vein or superior vena cava, usually secondary to long-dwelling intravenous catheters, child abuse, and pulmonary lymphangiomatosis (Table 28-1).

Anatomy

The thoracic duct is the largest lymphatic channel in the body. It conveys the majority of the lymph within the body into the circulatory system. The duct arises embryologically as paired channels with numerous crossing anastomoses. In most instances, the paired structures fuse to form a singular vascular channel with the right duct persisting in the lower thorax and the left persisting in the upper chest (Fig. 28-1). Although up to 50% of individuals may have anomalous patterns of thoracic duct anatomy, in its most classic anatomic position the duct arises from the cisterna chyli anterior to the first or second lumbar vertebral body. The duct runs cephalad from the cisterna along the right side of the aorta and enters the chest through the aortic hiatus. The duct ascends in the right thorax, medial to the azygos vein and posterior to the esophagus. At the level of the fourth or fifth thoracic vertebra, the duct crosses anterior to the vertebral body and behind the esophagus to become a left-sided structure, dorsal to the aortic arch. The duct passes through the thoracic inlet posterior and to the left of the esophagus and forms an arch that rises 3 cm to 4 cm above the clavicle to the level of the sixth or seventh cervical vertebrae. It crosses anterior to the subclavian artery and the thyrocervical trunk as it extends laterally and terminates by opening into the angle of the junction of the left subclavian and the internal jugular veins (Fig. 28-2). A bicuspid valve at the lymphaticovenous junction prevents the reflux of blood into the duct at this junction. The duct is 3 mm to 5 mm in diameter at its origin in an adult, but its caliber diminishes in the midthorax to dilate again just proximal to its venous termination. The duct receives numerous lymphatic tributaries from the thoracic wall as it ascends through the chest, and there are multiple lymphaticovenous anastomoses between the duct and the azygos and intercostal veins.

Riquet described two major thoracic duct tributaries from the heart. The right efferent trunk primarily drains lymph from the right ventricle and ascends between the aorta and pulmonary artery, connecting to the thoracic duct high in the left chest. The left efferent trunk drains lymph primarily from the left ventricle and ascends behind the pulmonary artery, usually connecting with the azygous vein in the right chest. Injury to the right efferent trunk may account for many cases of chylothorax or chylopericardium after cardiac surgery.

Although this represents the most common anatomic configuration of the duct, there are numerous variations that may be of considerable surgical significance. The most common variation in anatomy is a duplicate duct, occasionally at the lower thoracic, but more commonly at the cervical level. The

Table 28-1 Etiology of Chylothorax
Congenital
Traumatic
Ductal anomalies
Acquired
Traumatic
Surgical
Blunt trauma
Penetrating trauma
Child abuse
Nontraumatic
Malignant
Inflammatory
Idiopathic

level at which the duct crosses the vertebral column may also be variable.

Physiology

There are multiple valves throughout the length of the thoracic duct, particularly in the cephalic end, that ensure unidirectional flow. The wall of the thoracic duct contains smooth muscle cells with an intrinsic contraction interval of 10 to 15 seconds. Movement of chyle through the thoracic duct is modulated primarily by the intrinsic contraction of the duct wall and the pressure gradient between the abdomen and thorax. The rate of lymph formation from the intestine and liver also affects the rate of flow through the duct. Flow through the thoracic duct varies between 0.38 and 3.9 mL/min.

The function of the thoracic duct is to transport ingested fat and lymphatic fluid from the abdominal viscera and lower body into the venous circulation. Approximately 60% to 70% of all ingested fat is absorbed by the intestinal lymphatics and transported by the thoracic duct. Fatty acids containing <10 carbon atoms are absorbed directly into the portal venous system, whereas larger fats are formed into chylomicrons and transported into the lymphatics. The thoracic duct also is the main pathway for return of extravascular plasma proteins and lymphocytes to the vascular space. Prolonged loss of thoracic duct lymph can lead to fat and protein malnutrition as well as to immunocompromise secondary to loss of T lymphocytes.

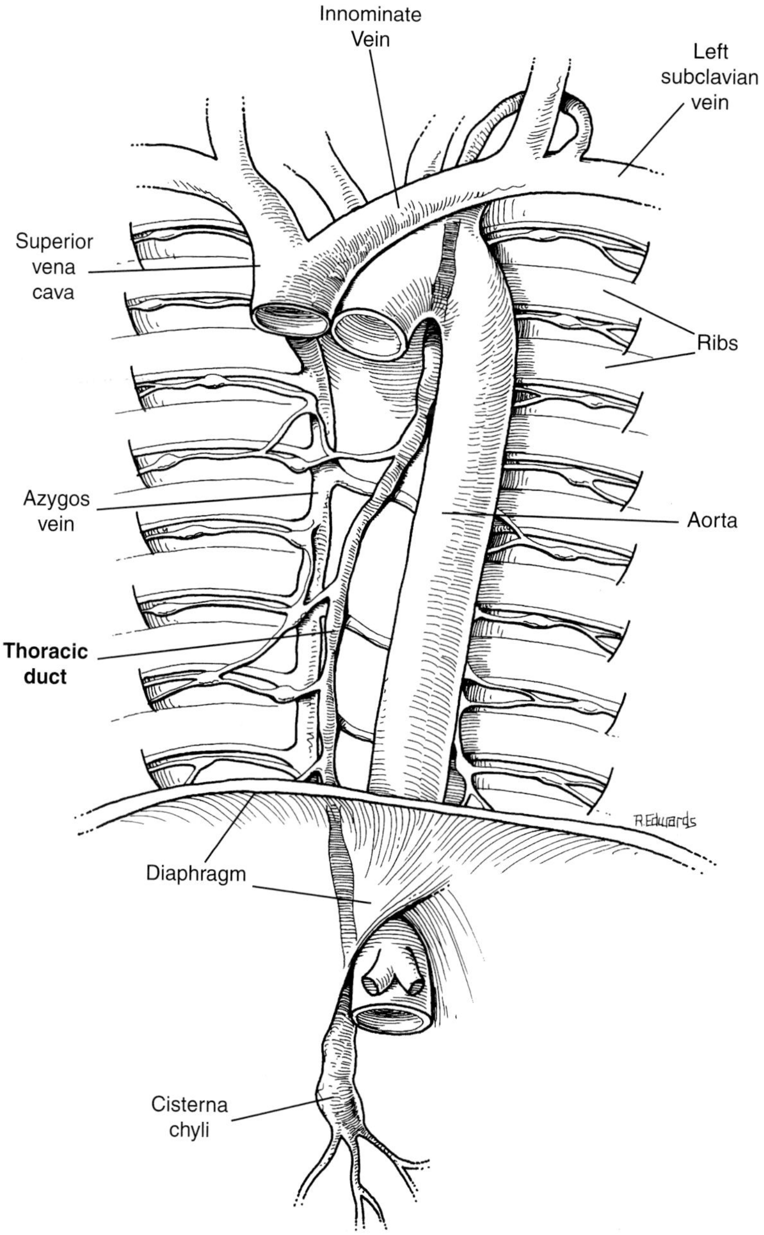

Diagnosis

The diagnosis of chylothorax is suspected with the development of a pleural effusion in certain high-risk clinical settings, such as after esophagectomy. The diagnosis is confirmed by examination of the pleural fluid obtained by thoracentesis. In an individual consuming a normal diet, the diagnosis is usually quite evident, with a milky appearance to the fluid. Often, however, the patient has not received normal fats enterally before the development of the chylothorax, and the fluid in this clinical setting has the appearance of serum. Chemical analysis of the fluid reveals elevated triglyceride and total protein levels (Table 28-2). Cell counts reveal a marked predominance of lymphocytes, with numbers ranging from 400 to 7,000 per milliliter. Chronic pleural effusions secondary to tumors or infections may occasionally appear milky because of the accumulation of cholesterol in the fluid. This so-called pseudochylothorax can be differentiated from true chylothorax by determination of the triglyceride level in the effusion. Most chylous effusions have a cholesterol/triglyceride ratio of <1, whereas nonchylous effusions have a ratio of >1. Pleural fluid with a triglyceride level of >110 mg/dL has a 99% chance of being chyle. If the triglyceride level is <50 mg/dL, the probability of a chylous effusion is only 5%.

The thoracic duct may be visualized by standard lymphangiograms or by nuclear scintigraphy. Often these studies will

Figure 28-1. The most common anatomic pattern of the thoracic duct. The duct enters the chest as a right-sided structure and crosses to the left chest at the fourth thoracic vertebra.

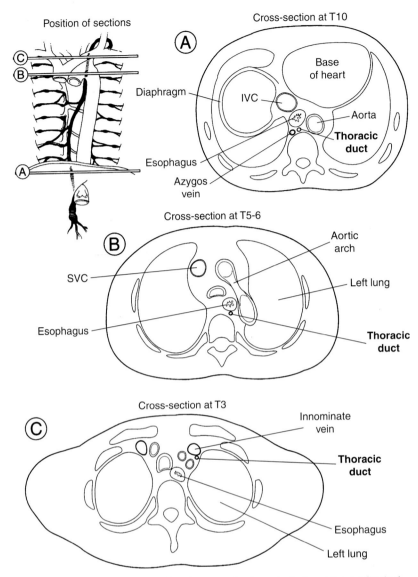

Figure 28-2. The anatomic relationships between the thoracic duct and the mediastinal structures at various levels in the chest. (IVC = inferior vena cava; SVC = superior vena cava.)

Table 28-2 Composition of Chyle	
pH	7.4–7.8
Specific gravity	1.012–1.025
Lymphocytes	400–7,000/dL
Culture	Sterile
Fat globules	Staining with Sudan red
Total protein	2.2–5.9 g/dL
Albumin	1.2–4.2 g/dL
Globulin	1.1–3.6 g/dL
Fibrinogen	16–24 g/dL
Total fat	0.4–6.0 g/dL
Triglycerides	>plasma
Cholesterol	65–220 mg/dL
Electrolytes	= plasma
Glucose	48–200 mg/dL
Cholesterol/triglyceride ratio	<1

demonstrate the anatomy of the duct and the level of the lymphatic leakage. They are rarely helpful, however, in the management of these patients and should not be considered a routine part of their evaluation.

Clinical Presentation

Chylothorax primarily causes symptoms of respiratory insufficiency as the volume of the effusion gradually increases. Most cases of chylothorax are slow in their progression, and symptoms do not occur for several days to several weeks after the initial injury to the duct. Rapid accumulation of chyle with production of severe respiratory symptoms is uncommon but is occasionally encountered after complete transection of the duct by traumatic or surgical injury. Chyle it-

self is bacteriostatic, probably because of its high fatty acid content, and symptoms of pleural infection are uncommon. Patients with longstanding chylothorax with loss of significant volumes of chyle often become hypoproteinemic. These patients also often develop lymphopenia from the loss of T lymphocytes in the chyle and may become relatively immunocompromised. In fact, malnutrition and infection account for the majority of deaths after the development of a chylothorax.

Management

Control of chylothorax is thought to occur with the formation of pleural adhesions in the region of the chylous leak, thus preventing flow of lymph from the thoracic duct or its branches. The management of patients with confirmed chylothorax therefore begins with attempts to completely drain the lymphatic fluid from the chest. In some cases, this may be accomplished by thoracentesis, whereas in most patients, with more rapid fluid accumulation, a tube thoracostomy is required. Measures are then instituted to reduce total thoracic duct lymphatic flow, initially using an oral diet containing fats primarily in the form of medium-chain triglycerides, which are absorbed directly into the portal venous system. Patients in whom significant lymphatic flow persists may require total elimination of enteral nutrition, with the institution of intravenous alimentation.

Recently, several clinical reports have suggested that the use of somatostatin or its longer-acting synthetic analogue octreotide may stop persistent chylous accumulation. The effect of somatostatin on thoracic duct flow is probably secondary to its reduction of splanchnic blood flow and its reduction of intestinal fat absorption, reducing chylomicron synthesis. Somatostatin has generally been administered as an intravenous infusion, using 250 μg/hr in adults and 3.5 to 10 μg/kg/hr in children. The dose may be increased in stepwise fashion to maximal response. Octreotide has generally been administered subcutaneously at doses of 100 μg twice or thrice daily for adults and 10 to 40 μg/kg per day in children (Table 28-3). Children and diabetic adults should be monitored for hyperglycemia or hypoglycemia, and adults are occasionally noted to have cardiac arrhythmias. The safety profile of these drugs, however, appears excellent, and they should be used early in patients with persistent chylous effusions to attempt to avoid protein and fat loss.

Table 28-3 Somatostatin/Octreotide Dore

Somatostatin	
Adult	250 μg/hr IV
Child	3.5–7.0 μg/kg/hr IV
Octreotide	
Adult	100 μg twice to thrice daily SC
Child	10–40 μg/kg/day SC

IV = intravenous; SC = subcutaneous.

The length of time that it is reasonable to persist with conservative therapy is somewhat controversial and depends on the cause of the chylothorax and the volume of lymphatic loss. Some authors suggest surgical intervention in cases of traumatic chylothorax when the daily loss of chyle exceeds 1,500 mL in adults or 100 mL per year of age in children for a 5-day period, when the output of chyle has not diminished over a 14-day period, or when nutritional complications appear imminent. Review of our clinical experience suggested that surgical intervention was highly effective and seemed warranted if the chylothorax had not responded after a maximum of 5 to 7 days of medical therapy in both adults and children.

The mortality for patients with chylothorax was approximately 50% until Lampson described mediastinal ligation of the thoracic duct in 1948. This procedure remains the most commonly used operation for persistent chylothorax, although several alternative procedures have been developed in recent years. In patients with unilateral chylous effusions, the chest should be opened on the ipsilateral side, whereas in cases of bilateral effusion, the right chest should be chosen initially. Many authors recommend instillation of 100 mL to 200 mL of olive oil or cream into the stomach several hours before the operation to increase the fat content of the thoracic lymph and make the area of leakage from the duct itself more easily identifiable. After the induction of general anesthesia with orotracheal intubation, the patient is placed in a full lateral decubitus position. A posterolateral thoracotomy is performed, and the chest is entered through the seventh or eighth intercostal space. If the chylothorax has developed after a previous thoracotomy, the original incision is opened. The mediastinal tissues are examined carefully for evidence of chylous leak. If such an area is identified, this region should be obliterated with nonabsorbable sutures, occasionally using polytetrafluoroethylene

(Teflon) pledgets to compress larger areas of tissue. Whether or not a specific area of leakage is identified and controlled, the main thoracic duct should be ligated as it enters the chest through the aortic hiatus. To accomplish this, the esophagus is encircled and retracted anteriorly, and the tissues between the azygos vein and the descending aorta just cephalad to the aortic hiatus are ligated with nonabsorbable sutures (Fig. 28-3). In most cases, the actual thoracic duct may be identified in this area and ligation performed, whereas in other cases mass ligature of the tissues in this area is accomplished, without direct identification of the duct itself. The chest is closed in layers with a single large chest tube connected to a water seal. A retropleural approach to the thoracic duct has been described. The patient is placed under general anesthesia and positioned prone, and a segment of the right posterior eighth rib is resected after the periosteum is stripped. The posterior mediastinal pleura is dissected bluntly from the chest wall in this region, and the thoracic duct is identified medial to the azygos vein. The duct is obliterated with nonabsorbable suture material, and the incision is closed in layers without drainage.

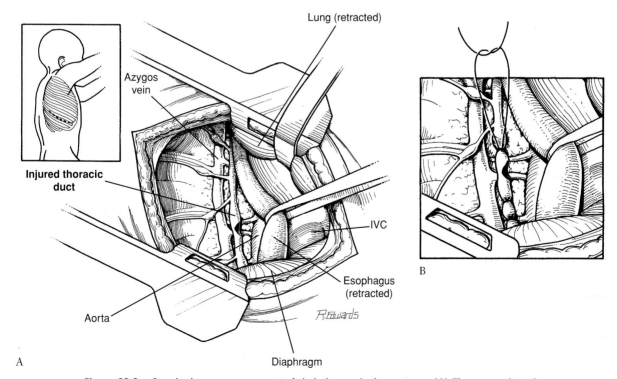

A

B

Lung (retracted)

Azygos vein

IVC

Esophagus (retracted)

R. Edwards

Aorta

Diaphragm

Injured thoracic duct

Figure 28-3. Standard open management of chylothorax via thoracotomy. **(A)** The approach to the thoracic duct through a right posterolateral thoracotomy incision. The duct is exposed by anterior retraction of the esophagus. **(B)** The duct is ligated with nonabsorbable suture material as it enters the chest. **(Inset)** Thoracotomy incision (over the seventh or eighth intercostal space). (IVC = inferior vena cava.)

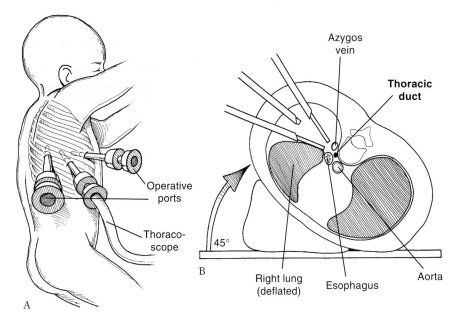

Figure 28-4.   The thoracoscopic approach to the thoracic duct and placement of thoracoscopic instruments. **(A)** The patient is placed in an exaggerated lateral decubitus position to expose the posterior mediastinal structures. **(B)** The thoracic duct is identified behind the esophagus, between the aorta and azygos vein.

Patients in whom the source of the chylothorax is suspected to be relatively localized, such as patients developing a chylous effusion after blunt or penetrating thoracic trauma, may benefit by thoracoscopic control of the lymphatic leak. Although the procedure may be performed under local anesthesia in these patients, the use of general anesthesia with unilateral ventilation greatly enhances the exposure of the mediastinum. The patient is placed in a full lateral decubitus position or rolled slightly forward to facilitate exposure of the posterior mediastinum. The initial trocar for the thoracoscope is placed in the sixth intercostal space in the midaxillary line. A second trocar is placed posteriorly in the same or adjacent interspace (Fig. 28-4). The residual pleural lymph is aspirated, and the pleura overlying the posterior mediastinum is carefully examined from the level of the inferior pulmonary ligament to the innominate vein. In some cases, a defect in the parietal pleura will be discovered with lymphatic leakage through this region. We have preferred to use metallic clips on this tissue to obliterate the leak, although others have used direct suture ligation (Fig. 28-5). After the pleural leak is controlled in this region, the entire area is flooded with fibrin glue to form a seal over the parietal pleura. In most cases, the inferior pulmonary ligament is then divided with the electrocautery, and the thoracic duct is clipped or ligated at the level

of the aortic hiatus. A single chest tube is placed through one of the trocar tracks while the other trocar sites are closed with subcuticular sutures.

If the origin of the chylous effusion is suspected to be more diffuse, such as in those patients who have undergone thoracic surgery or in patients with lymphangiomatosis or superior vena cava (SVC) thrombosis, placement of a pleuroperitoneal shunt may be the best treatment strategy. In choosing to use a pleuroperitoneal shunt, the surgeon must decide between an internalized system, which is completely buried under the skin, and an exteriorized system, which leaves the pumping chamber exposed. The internalized system has the advantage of not requiring any maintenance of the catheter entrance or exit sites, but it does require a responsible patient or parent who is willing to compress the chamber as frequently as necessary in spite of some potential discomfort. The exteriorized system has proven quite helpful in small infants who may not tolerate chest wall compression well and has advantages in obese patients in whom the internalized chamber may be difficult to localize. This system facilitates control of high-volume chylous leaks that require frequent pump compression. The disadvantage of the exteriorized system is the need for cleaning and dressing the catheter exit sites and the potential for infection through these sites.

Both the internalized and externalized systems may be placed under local anesthesia, although the use of general anesthesia facilitates the procedure. It is helpful in placing either of these systems to have some residual chyle within the chest at the time of the operation. This allows the surgeon to test the patency of the shunt system. If a chest tube is already in place, it may be clamped the night before the procedure to allow accumulation. The patient is placed in the supine position with the affected chest elevated 30 to 45 degrees with a wedge. The entire chest and abdomen of the affected side are prepared and draped. The pleuroperitoneal shunt system is placed on the body surface to determine the optimal position of the shunt and the incisions. It is helpful to

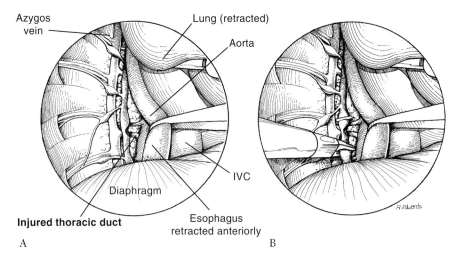

Figure 28-5.   Thoracoscopic management of chylothorax. The thoracic duct is exposed behind the esophagus **(A)** and occluded with metallic clips just above the level of the diaphragm **(B)**. (IVC = inferior vena cava.)

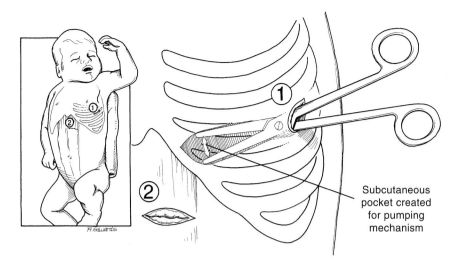

Figure 28-6. Placement of an internalized pleuroperitoneal shunt. The patient's hemithorax is elevated slightly, and short incisions are placed over the eighth intercostal space in the posterior axillary line and the anterior rectus sheath. A generous subcutaneous pocket for the pumping chamber is developed from the thoracic incision. (1 = incision for pleural end of shunt; 2 = incision for peritoneal end of shunt.)

mark the incisions with a skin pencil at this time. The pumping chamber for the internalized system should be placed in a subcutaneous pocket overlying the lower ribs of the anterolateral chest wall. The pleural catheter should be directed as far posteriorly as possible to allow optimal dependent drainage. A 2-cm skin incision is made just caudad to the proposed intercostal entrance of the pleural catheter. A generous subcutaneous pocket is dissected caudad from this area over the lower ribs. A 2-cm transverse incision is made overlying the anterior rectus sheath midway between the umbilicus and the xiphoid process (Fig. 28-6). The anterior rectus sheath is divided transversely, and the fibers of the rectus muscle are separated to expose the posterior rectus sheath and peritoneum. Two concentric purse-string sutures of 4-0 polypropylene (Prolene) are placed in the posterior rectus sheath. The pleuroperitoneal shunt system is filled with sterile saline by compressing the pumping chamber while the entire system is under fluid. Careful attention must be paid to orienting the pumping chamber in the proper direction because there are two unidirectional valves within the chamber. The pleural catheter is trimmed to appropriate length and placed across the intercostal space in tangential fashion. This is the most critical portion of the operation, and care must be taken not to kink the catheter as it crosses the chest wall. A long clamp is then passed from the lower incision to the upper incision, through the subcutaneous pocket, and the distal catheter and pumping cham-

ber are drawn into the pocket by traction (Fig. 28-7). The pumping chamber must be seated well within the pocket to ensure that neither of the incisions is directly over the compression chamber. Patency of the system is confirmed by repeatedly compressing the pumping chamber and observing for free flow of chyle through the distal tubing (Fig. 28-8). The peritoneal catheter is trimmed to appropriate length, and the posterior rectus fascia and peritoneum are opened within the purse-string sutures and the catheter passed

into the abdominal cavity. Both purse strings are tied securely around the catheter. The patency of the system is checked once again by repeatedly compressing the pumping chamber to ensure free flow of fluid. The two incisions are closed with subcutaneous and subcuticular absorbable sutures.

Planning for an exteriorized system starts as for the internalized system. The shunt is placed on the body surface to determine the best position for the incisions. Subcutaneous tunnels of approximately 6 cm to 10 cm in length are made for proximal and distal tubing. A 1-cm incision is made overlying the interspace through which the thoracic catheter will be placed, and a 2-cm incision is made overlying the anterior rectus sheath just above the level of the umbilicus. The thoracic catheter is drawn through the subcutaneous tunnel by passing a clamp in a caudad direction from the interspace incision. The Teflon cuff surrounding the catheter is placed at the level of the thoracic insertion (Fig. 28-9). The abdominal catheter is drawn through the subcutaneous tunnel by passing a clamp cranially from the rectus incision, and the cuff is positioned to lie at the level of the peritoneum. Two concentric purse-string sutures are placed through the posterior rectus fascia and peritoneum, as for the insertion of the internalized system, and the peritoneal catheter is inserted (Fig. 28-10). The two purse-string sutures are tied, and each is sutured to the Teflon cuff of the abdominal catheter. The thoracic cuff is not sutured to the thoracic fascia. The incisions are closed in layers

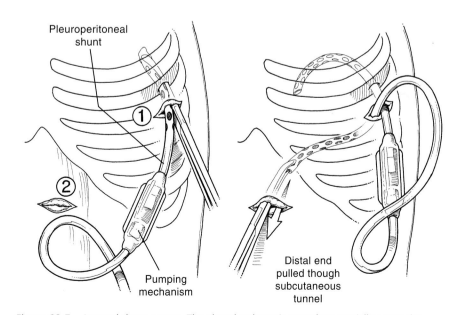

Figure 28-7. Internal shunt system. The pleural catheter is passed tangentially across the intercostal muscle into the pleural space. The distal catheter and pumping chamber are advanced by a clamp inserted through the abdominal incision.

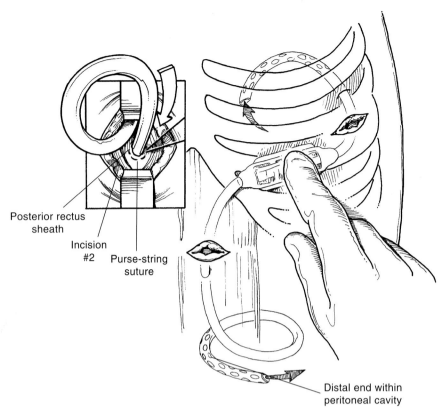

Figure 28-8. Internal shunt system in position. The peritoneal catheter is placed through two concentric purse-string sutures in the posterior rectus sheath and peritoneum. Patency of the system is confirmed by repeated compression of the pumping chamber. (Dark arrows indicate direction of flow.)

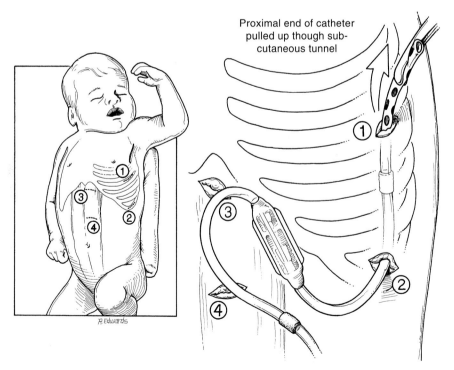

Figure 28-9. Placement of an externalized pleuroperitoneal shunt. Long subcutaneous tunnels are developed for the pleural and peritoneal catheters. (Numbers indicate incision sites.)

after the system is tested by compressing the exteriorized pumping chamber (Fig. 28-11). The catheters are sutured to the skin at the exit sites, and sterile dressings are applied.

Postoperatively a schedule of pump compression is established that will allow complete evacuation of chyle from the thorax. An estimate of the frequency of compression necessary can be made by identifying the preoperative volume of lymphatic leakage and estimating that each compression of the chamber pumps approximately 2 mL of chyle from the chest to the abdomen. Usually the patients are asked to compress the chamber for a certain number of times, four times a day. With the exteriorized chamber, the patient can easily tell when the chest is empty because the chamber will not fill with chyle after compression.

When the flow of lymph through the pleuroperitoneal shunt has diminished to a minimum, the patient is instructed not to pump the chamber for an interval of 2 weeks, after which a chest radiograph is obtained to be certain that there is no reaccumulation of fluid. If the chest is dry, the shunt is removed by simply withdrawing the pleural catheter. The abdominal catheter is dissected out, and the entrance through the posterior rectus fascia is closed with interrupted absorbable sutures to prevent visceral herniation.

Recently, successful occlusion of the thoracic duct using percutaneous puncture and catheterization through the cisterna chyli has been reported by several interventional radiologists. These procedures may be performed under local anesthesia with intravenous sedation. The duct is occluded with microcoils and fibrin glue. The success of these procedures suggests that they should be considered early in patients with substantial chyle losses. They may have special utility for debilitated patients.

The results of all of these invasive procedures for chylothorax are excellent. Sporadic case reports suggest that thoracic duct ligation is successful in controlling the chylous leak in approximately 85% of patients. Murphy indicated that pleuroperitoneal shunts are successful in 100% of patients with chylothorax after cardiac surgery and in 75% of patients with chylothorax secondary to caval obstruction. The success of thoracoscopic control of chylothorax appears comparable to that of these other procedures. Percutaneous techniques appear to be successful in approximately 70% of patients. Occasionally, a patient with diffuse lymphatic leak, such as a patient with caval obstruction or lymphangiomatosis, will fail to respond to these procedures. In these

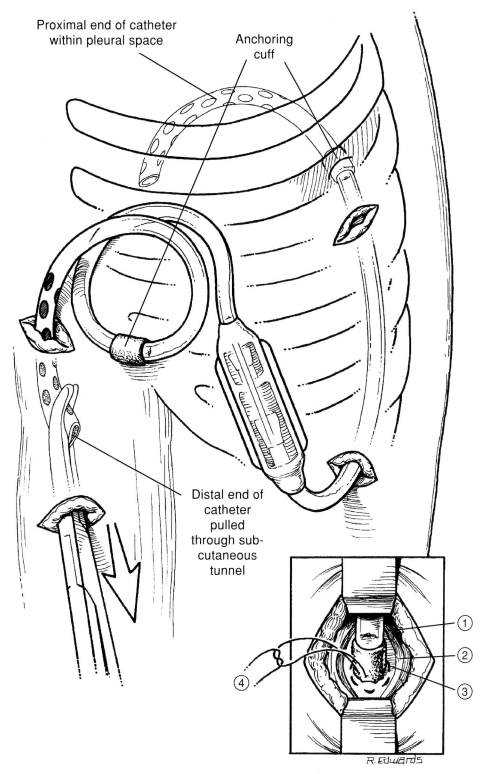

Proximal end of catheter within pleural space

Anchoring cuff

Distal end of catheter pulled through sub-cutaneous tunnel

R. Edwards

Figure 28-10. The catheters are placed with the polyethylene terephthalate (Dacron) cuffs at the level of the intercostal muscle and the posterior rectus sheath. **(Inset)** Purse-string suture pulled up through cuff.

patients a pleurodesis on the affected side will virtually always control the chylous leak. This may be performed by thoracoscopy, using either pleural abrasion or talc pleurodesis, or by an open pleurectomy.

It is important to recognize that the development of chylothorax is not a benign condition. Treatment should be prompt and aggressive to minimize loss of protein, fats, and lymphocytes. The effusion must be drained, and the patient should be placed on a medium-chain triglyceride diet or total parenteral nutrition immediately. Somatostatin or octreotide should be instituted in those patients with drainage persisting

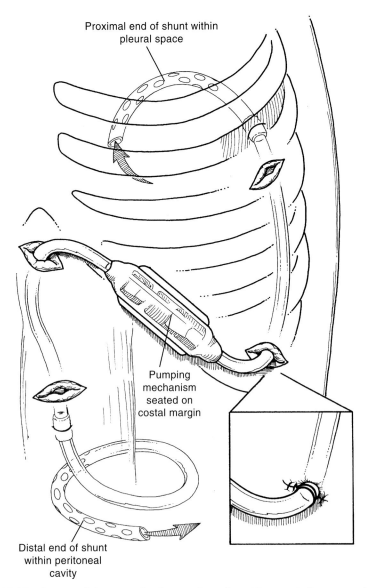

Proximal end of shunt within
pleural space

Pumping
mechanism
seated on
costal margin

Distal end of shunt
within peritoneal
cavity

Figure 28-11. Patency of the externalized system is confirmed by repeatedly compressing the pumping chamber. The catheters are secured at the skin exit site. **(Inset)** Securing suture wrapped around shunt tube.

for more than 3 days, and surgical therapy should be contemplated for effusions lasting 7 to 10 days. The choice of surgical procedure for the treatment of refractory chylothorax is determined by the experience of the surgeon and the cause of the chylothorax. Patients with direct injury to the duct from blunt or penetrating chest trauma may be the best candidates for posterolateral thoracotomy and direct control of the chylous leak as well as ligation of the main trunk of the thoracic duct. Patients with chylothorax arising secondary to thoracic surgical procedures in whom re-exploration may be difficult or prohibitively stressful may be excellent candidates for placement of a pleuroperitoneal shunt or percutaneous techniques, which may be performed under

local anesthesia. Patients with long-standing and loculated chylothorax may benefit from thoracoscopic control, which enables the surgeon to disrupt the multiple loculations within the pleural space while controlling the leak of chyle.

SUGGESTED READING

Al-Zubairy SA, Al-Jazairi AS. Octreotide as a therapeutic option for management of chylothorax. Ann Pharmac 2003;37:679.

Cerfolio RJ, Allen MS, Deschamps C, et al. Postoperative chylothorax. J Thorac Cardiovasc Surg 1996;112:1361.

Cope C, Kaiser LR. Management of unremitting chylothorax by percutaneous embolization and blockage of retroperitoneal lymphatic

vessels in 42 patients. J Vasc Interv Radiol 2002;13:1139.

Graham DD, McGahren ED, Tribble CG, et al. Use of video-assisted thoracic surgery in the treatment of chylothorax. Ann Thorac Surg: 1994;57:1507.

Johnstone DW, Feins RH. Chylothorax. Chest Surg Clin North Am 1994;4:617.

Lampson RS. Traumatic chylothorax. J Thorac Surg 1948;17:778.

Milsom JW, Kron IL, Rheuban KS, et al. Chylothorax: An assessment of current surgical management. J Thorac Cardiovasc Surg 1985;89:221.

Murphy MC, Newman BM, Rodgers BM. Pleuroperitoneal shunts in the management of persistent chylothorax. Ann Thorac Surg 1989;48:195.

Riquet M, Le Pimpec Barthes F, Souilamas R, et al. Thoracic duct tributaries from intrathoracic organs. Ann Thorac Surg. 2002;73:892.

EDITOR'S COMMENTS

And I thought I knew a lot about chylothorax. Rodgers has written an absolutely superb chapter that should be mandatory reading for all thoracic surgical residents as well as practicing cardiothoracic surgeons. I'm including even those surgeons who limit their practice to adult cardiac surgery because chylothorax rears its ugly head on occasion following cardiac surgical procedures, as Dr. Rodgers points out. I would bet that the majority of surgeons are not aware of the location where the thoracic duct is most vulnerable during a cardiac procedure, but by being aware of the right efferent trunk's location they may be able to avoid a problem. I would submit that it is far easier to avoid a problem with the thoracic duct than to fix a problem with the duct, not to mention the morbidity that results from a chyle leak. Should a chylothorax occur, however, the surgeon should be familiar with the problem and the potential solutions because time is of the essence.

I have not had any personal experience with somatostatin or octreotide in managing chylothorax, but other than the expense, either of these agents might be tried early in the course of a chylothorax especially if the patient is draining less than 500 mL/day. Having waited too long to ligate the thoracic duct on at least one patient, I now wait no longer than 7 days to carry out this procedure if the leak does not stop with conservative measures. The morbidity of hypoalbuminemia and immunosuppression in an early postoperative patient is simply too great to take any chances. We have been the major proponents of percutaneous techniques for sealing the duct. My colleague in interventional radiology and one of the true pioneers of the field, Stan Cope, described a technique of direct puncture of the cisterna chyli, threading of a small catheter into the thoracic duct, and then placing of platinum coils and fibrin glue to obliterate the duct. The success of this procedure is limited only by the ability to puncture the cisterna chyli. Previous upper abdominal procedures may distort the anatomy to the extent that direct puncture cannot be accomplished. The cisterna must be visualized with contrast, and to do this requires a lymphangiogram, truly almost a lost art. If we are able to "light up" the cisterna and successfully puncture it, the duct may be obliterated with sealing of the leak 100% of the time. Unfortunately the cisterna can only be punctured successfully approximately 70%

of the time in the best of hands. Whether the average interventional radiologist can master this procedure remains to be determined. It is my impression that use of this technique is not widespread because it is difficult to master a technique where, fortunately, the case numbers are low.

The standard approach to ligating the duct remains a low right thoracotomy with ligation of the duct near the aortic hiatus where it remains as a single trunk. Failure of this approach usually means that the duct was ligated too high in the chest, thus leaving a branch, or branches, patent. The thoracoscopic approach may be useful, although it is not easy, and the incidence of failure may be slightly higher than that achieved with an open procedure. For a left-sided effusion the duct may be approached via a left thoracotomy, as Dr. Rodgers points out. Lig-

ation of the duct for a chylothorax caused by diffuse obstruction of mediastinal lymphatics by tumor, usually lymphoma, tends to have a significantly greater failure rate, and resolution of the effusion usually is accomplished by treatment of the malignancy. It is in these situations that the pleuroperitoneal shunt may be of more help than simple ligation of the duct. Especially in those patients with higher output, rarely have we been successful simply by trying to effect pleurodesis.

The bottom line to all of this: Act quickly and decisively in managing an iatrogenic chylothorax. We recommend not waiting any longer than 7 days before proceeding with ligation or obliteration of the thoracic duct if the leak has persisted despite total parenteral nutrition.

L.R.K.

29

Pericardial Procedures

John R. Roberts and Larry R. Kaiser

Introduction

Operations for diseases of the pericardium are uncommon but can be critical for patients who require diagnostic or therapeutic intervention to resolve physiologically significant effusions or constriction. An understanding of the anatomic and physiologic dynamics of the pericardium and the consequences of interrelated diseases is key to management.

Anatomy of the Pericardium

The pericardium, like the pleura, consists of two mesothelial layers, one closely adherent to the myocardium and the second separated from the heart by a variable amount of fluid. The visceral pericardium is synonymous with the epicardium and is usually a monocellular serosal layer. The parietal pericardium, or the pericardial sac, is the better-known structure and is a tough, fibrous structure separated from the visceral pericardium by pericardial fluid, normally 15 mL to 50 mL of plasma ultrafiltrate. The visceral and parietal pericardium fuse over the great vessels and pulmonary veins.

The parietal pericardium attaches to the ascending aorta superiorly. It then extends across the superior vena cava and courses down over the right superior and inferior pulmonary veins to encircle the inferior vena cava. On the left side, the parietal pericardium extends inferiorly from the arch of the aorta down across the left pulmonary artery and then encircles the left ventricle. It then merges with the right side of the pericardium and fuses with the diaphragm inferiorly. Posteriorly the pericardium attaches to the left atrium. Two major recesses exist within the pericardial space: the transverse sinus and the oblique sinus. The transverse sinus is located posterior to the proximal ascending aorta and the pulmonary artery and anterior to the atria and superior vena cava. The oblique sinus lies inferior to the transverse sinus, between the right and the left pulmonary veins, and medial to the inferior vena cava.

Pericardial Effusions

Etiology

Tumors that commonly metastasize to the pericardium include breast and lung malignancies. Both are common, and these malignancies account for the majority of patients who require surgical pericardial drainage. Primary (or contiguous) pericardial malignancies include lymphomas, leukemias, thymomas, malignant mesotheliomas, teratomas, angiosarcomas, and rhabdomyosarcomas. Debulking of tumor that invades the pericardial space is seldom beneficial, although drainage procedures can be helpful if other reasonably effective adjunctive therapy is available, as is the case for breast cancer, for instance. Most pericardial effusions result from advanced and incurable malignant processes, and so drainage techniques must be relatively painless and require only short hospital stays.

Physiology of Pericardial Tamponade

The parietal pericardium is tough and noncompliant but can enlarge to accommodate slowly accumulating fluid. Rapid fluid accumulation, however, overwhelms the ability of the pericardium to distend and increases the pressure within the pericardial space. In these circumstances, the pericardium is less able to distend than the right atrium and right ventricle. This increased pressure compromises the diastolic filling of the heart and thus limits the stroke volume. For this reason, patients with hemodynamically significant pericardial effusions can increase cardiac output only by increasing heart rate or by increasing intravascular volume.

Pericardia tamponade is the accumulation of fluid within the pericardial space such that increased intrapericardial pressure diminishes diastolic filling of the heart and therefore stroke volume and cardiac output. Pericardial pressure does not relate linearly to volume of pericardial fluid. Acute accumulation of small amounts of fluid may be sufficient to cause tamponade. A large pericardial effusion can accumulate without hemodynamic significance if it develops over a significant period of time. Exceeding the elastic limit of the pericardium raises the intrapericardial pressure dramatically. Pericardial effusion therefore is an anatomic diagnosis, whereas tamponade is a physiologic one.

Diagnosis of Cardiac Tamponade

Making the diagnosis of a pericardial effusion is the first step in its treatment. Symptoms of increasing dyspnea, weakness, and substernal pressure may indicate accumulation of pericardial fluid. Signs of cardiac tamponade include increasing pulse rate, decreasing pulse pressure, paradoxical pulse, and distended neck veins. Transthoracic echocardiography reveals an inspiratory increase in right ventricular diastolic diameter and a reciprocal decrease in left ventricular dimensions in normal patients.

As cardiac tamponade develops, cardiac output decreases secondary to decreased stroke volume. The first defense is tachycardia. A more chronic decrease in cardiac output prompts secretion of mineralocorticoids and an increase in intravascular blood volume that supports cardiac preload and thus improves filling.

Although the left side of the heart has greater intracardiac pressures than the right side of the heart, cardiac tamponade typically results in relative filling of the right heart at the expense of the left heart. Echocardiography can demonstrate that early cardiac tamponade results in compression of the right atrium and further compression of the right atrial wall during systole. As the intrapericardial pressure increases, progressive leftward shift of the interventricular septum increasingly compromises the ability of the left ventricle to fill and thus diminishes the stroke volume of the heart. Echocardiography-guided drainage can demonstrate improved function as the drainage is performed.

Pericardial Procedures for Treating Effusions

Pericardiocentesis

Pericardiocentesis is a diagnostic and therapeutic procedure performed through a subxiphoid or transthoracic approach. Local anesthesia is usually adequate. For the subxiphoid approach, the area between the xiphoid process and the left costal margin is anesthetized. A needle is inserted between the two structures and directed toward the left shoulder; aspiration is performed as the needle is slowly advanced. Attaching the needle to a precordial electrocardiographic lead may help to identify contact with the myocardium. If air is encountered, the needle is withdrawn and reinserted more medially. If blood is withdrawn, 5 mL is placed on a gauze sheet and observed for clot formation. Defibrinated pericardial blood does not clot. At this point, a Seldinger technique is used: A wire is passed through the needle, and a drainage catheter is passed over the wire. The remaining pericardial effusion can then be withdrawn.

Performance of pericardiocentesis through the fourth intercostal space traverses a shorter distance to reach the pericardial space. After palpation of the fourth rib, local anesthesia is infiltrated at least one fingerbreadth lateral to the sternal edge to avoid injury to the internal mammary artery. The needle tip should be directed toward the right shoulder; aspiration is performed as the needle is advanced. As described, aspiration of air requires redirecting the needle more medially, whereas aspirated blood should be placed on a gauze sheet and observed for clot formation. Aspiration of pericardial fluid allows placement of an intravenous catheter by way of the Seldinger technique, as described.

Anatomic landmarks, echocardiographic guidance, or fluoroscopic guidance aids in the performance of these techniques. Placement of the catheter allows drainage of the pericardial fluid, thus converting an urgent, dangerous surgical drainage procedure into a safe, elective one. For many patients, simple drainage of the fluid will be sufficient to treat their pericardial effusion. If the fluid recurs, particularly a malignant effusion, sclerosis with doxycycline (usually 1,000 mg injected intrapericardially daily until drainage decreases) or sterile talc helps to prevent recurrent pericardial effusions. Ultrasound-guided pericardioplasty, in which a catheter is placed into the pericardial space and used to create and dilate an opening in the pericardium, has been described and allows drainage of fluid into the pleural space. The long-term patency of these windows is unknown. Long-lasting surgical approaches involve formation of a pericardial window by a subxiphoid approach, a left thoracoscopic approach, or a right thoracoscopic approach.

Subxiphoid Pericardial Window

Subxiphoid pericardial windows are most frequently performed with the patient under general anesthesia, although significantly compromised patients may require drainage under local anesthesia. When general anesthesia is used, patients with cardiac tamponade commonly lose their sympathetic tone and require inotropic and chronotropic support to maintain their blood pressure. When the procedure is performed on an awake patient, local anesthesia is infiltrated in the midline area, on both sides of the xiphoid process and around the xiphoid process extending inferiorly approximately 4 cm to 5 cm. The operation is performed through a 4-cm to 6-cm longitudinal midline incision beginning at the xiphisternal junction and extended inferiorly (Fig. 29-1A, inset). Subcutaneous fat is divided to identify the linea alba that is divided in the midline. Typically the xiphoid process is removed (Fig. 29-1A). Portions of the left and right costal arches may also be resected if needed for exposure but this is rarely required.

The diaphragm and peritoneal fat are swept inferiorly until the pericardium is identified (Fig. 29-1B). The pericardium is grasped and nicked anteriorly to allow some fluid to escape. This creates additional space to allow resection of a piece of pericardium at least 2 cm in diameter and larger if possible (Fig. 29-1B, inset). The peritoneum can be opened for a short distance and allows a direct opening for drainage of pericardial fluid into the peritoneal cavity, but this is not necessary for the procedure to be effective. If drainage into the peritoneum is desired, the resected specimen includes a small portion of the anterior diaphragmatic pericardium. Fluid obtained is then sent for culture and cytologic examination. The piece of pericardium is sent for culture as well as histologic examination.

After evacuation of all fluid, a finger is placed into the pericardial space and swept inferiorly and bilaterally to break up any loculations. If the peritoneum is not opened, a right-angled chest tube is placed through stab incisions on either side of the midline incision and positioned into the inferior aspect of the pericardium (Fig. 29-1C). The wound is closed by reapproximating the linea alba and fascia. The remainder of the wound is closed in typical fashion using interrupted nonabsorbable sutures for the midline fascia and absorbable sutures for the subcutaneous tissue and the skin. The chest tube in the pericardial sac is placed to suction. If drainage of the fluid is performed intraperitoneally, the patient usually can leave the hospital soon because no chest tubes are in place. Adhesions eventually obliterate the window between the pericardium and peritoneum. However, the communication between the pericardium and peritoneum typically provides excellent drainage of the pericardium to provide at least short-term palliation. If chest tubes are placed, they remain until the combined drainage for 24 hours is <100 mL. They are then removed at the bedside. Large amounts of persistent drainage can be treated with doxycycline or tetracycline sclerosis as described for percutaneous drainage. The procedure is straightforward and without significant morbidity (Table 29-1) as long as the diagnosis is correct. Patients with severely compromised cardiac function who have not been percutaneously drained should not undergo general anesthesia for the procedure because loss of sympathetic tone may result in severe hypotension. These patients should undergo a subxiphoid pericardial window using local anesthesia and sedation.

Clinically significant, loculated effusions may occur as a consequence of isolated or

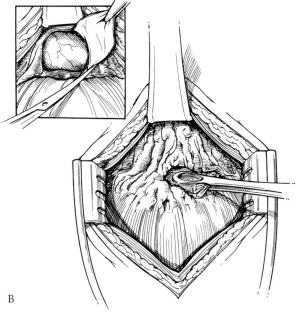

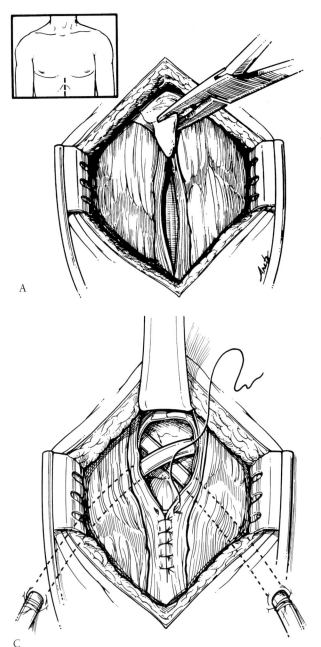

Figure 29-1. Subxiphoid pericardial window. **(A)** The subcutaneous tissue is divided with cautery, and the linea alba is divided in the midline to expose the xiphoid process. It is then resected at the junction with the sternum. **(Inset)** A subxiphoid incision should begin just superior to the xiphisternal junction and extend 5 cm to 6 cm inferior to it in the midline. **(B)** A sponge stick is used to sweep away the preperitoneal fat while a retractor elevates the sternum anteriorly. The pericardium is identified just posterior to the sternum and superior to the diaphragm. **(Inset)** After a nick is made in the pericardium, a 2-cm² area is resected. A finger is swept within the pericardium to break up loculations. The pericardial edges are then sutured to extrapericardial tissues to keep the window open. **(C)** The pericardial space is drained with two chest tubes, either two right-angled tubes positioned inferiorly just over the diaphragm or a single straight tube positioned anteriorly and a right-angled tube positioned inferiorly.

diffuse pericardial adhesions. This situation highlights the importance of assuring complete pericardial evacuation. If there is uncertainty of complete removal of fluid and adhesions, intraoperative transesophageal echocardiography should be performed.

Table 29-1   Pitfalls of Subxiphoid Pericardial Window

Putting hemodynamically compromised patients under general anesthesia

Injuring the heart while opening the pericardium secondary to pericardial adhesions or loculated fluid

Failing to completely drain loculated fluid

Thoracoscopic Pericardial Window

Thoracoscopic pericardial window can be performed from either side of the chest and functions by providing pleural surfaces to absorb excess pericardial fluid. Access ports are required as for any thoracoscopic procedure—typically three are necessary (Fig. 29-2A). The first port is placed in the sixth or seventh interspace in the anterior axillary line. The second and third ports are placed more posteriorly in the posterior axillary line, at approximately the eighth and fifth interspaces (Fig. 29-2A). The inferior pulmonary ligament is divided with the cautery. On the left side, the phrenic

nerve is carefully identified along its course from the hilum down to the diaphragm. It lies in the middle portion of the pericardium (Fig. 29-2B). To avoid phrenic nerve injury, pericardial windows are performed both anterior and posterior to the nerve. The pericardium is grasped with an instrument placed through the anterior port. After the pericardium is retracted laterally away from the heart, endoscopic scissors are used to nick the pericardium. A pulsatile rush of bloody pericardial fluid that mimics frank blood can raise fears that the heart has been injured. In most instances, however, this is not the case, and a generous pericardial resection of 3 cm² to 4 cm² can be resected (Fig. 29-2B).

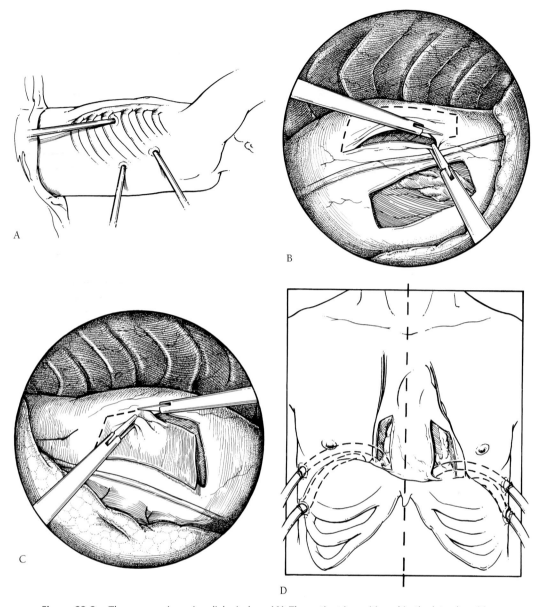

Figure 29-2. Thoracoscopic pericardial window. **(A)** The patient is positioned in the lateral position with an axillary roll under the down axilla and the upper arm appropriately supported. Three ports are usually necessary; the positions of these ports may be adjusted to the patient's habitus. The patient depicted has one port in the anterior axillary line at the seventh intercostal space. This port is typically used to grasp the pericardium. Two additional ports for viewing and operating are placed in the posterior axillary line at the fifth and eighth intercostal spaces. **(B)** The view from the left chest reveals the phrenic nerve running in the approximate middle of the pericardium. Windows anterior and posterior to the nerve are depicted. **(C)** On the right side it is usually possible to make a single window anterior to the nerve. **(D)** Chest tubes are placed in usual position in the anterior axillary line. One right-angled tube can be positioned within the pericardium.

The second window can then be performed anterior to the phrenic nerve in similar fashion. The inside of the pericardial space is examined with a sponge stick placed transpleurally into the pericardium to break up loculations (Fig. 29-2C). A right-angled chest tube placed through the pleural space into the posterior pericardial window drains the pericardial space. A second right-angled chest tube serves to drain the pleural space (Fig. 29-2D).

Thoracoscopic windows on the right side are performed similarly with identical port positioning (Fig. 29-2A). Again, a grasping port is located in the anterior axillary line at the sixth or seventh interspace. The operating ports are positioned in the posterior axillary line at approximately the fifth and eighth intercostal spaces. The right phrenic nerve runs close to the hilar blood vessels, relatively more posteriorly on the surface of the right pericardium. A single larger window anterior to the right phrenic nerve effectively drains the pericardial space (Fig. 29-2C). Again, the pericardium is grasped with an instrument placed in the anterior port while the thoracoscope and

Table 29-2 Pitfalls of Thoracoscopic Pericardial Windows

Choosing the wrong chest
Injury to the lung
Injury to the phrenic nerve
Inadequate window formation
Injury to the heart

Table 29-3 Causes of Constrictive Pericarditis

Cause	Incidence
Idiopathic	~75%
After an episode of acute pericarditis	10%–15%
Tuberculous pericarditis	3%
Mediastinal irradiation	Rare
Rheumatoid disease	Rare
Sarcoidosis	Rare
Trauma/hemopericardium	Rare
Cardiac surgery	1%–4%

operating instruments project through the posterior ports. A significant piece of pericardium, 3 cm to 4 cm in diameter, is resected (Fig. 29-2C). Drainage of pericardial fluid and clearing of pericardial loculations proceed as described. The pericardial and pleural spaces are drained with two right-angled chest tubes (Fig. 29-2D).

Thoracoscopic pericardial window formation is straightforward for surgeons trained in thoracoscopic techniques. Possible pitfalls are rare (Table 29-2). When the surgeon is deciding on which side of the chest to make the window, certain factors in the patient's history should be taken into consideration. A coexistent pleural effusion, pleural thickening, prior chest irradiation, and a previous thoracotomy can prevent or preclude a satisfactory procedure. Performing a thoracoscopic window on the same side as a previously existing primary tumor with malignant pleural effusion allows simultaneous drainage of the pleural effusion and pleurodesis. A history of therapeutic chest irradiation should prompt careful consideration. Whereas mediastinal irradiation does not affect the formation of pericardial windows, primary tumor irradiation may result in pleural fibrosis and obliteration of the pleural space. Attempts to place windows in these pleural spaces will likely result in pulmonary parenchymal injury, be technically tedious, and unlikely to yield long-term drainage of the pericardial space. In general, thoracoscopic pericardial windows are best placed in the chest opposite the tumor. Preoperative chest radiographs and computed tomographic (CT) scans help to identify pleural or intrathoracic disease that can direct management plans or determine the optimal side on which to perform the procedure. Pleural thickening suggests pleural inflammation, pleural tumor, or pleural fusion, any of which may cause failure of subsequent pericardial windows.

Cardiac injury is very rare but can result when dense adhesions bind the pericardium to the myocardium. A fluid-filled pericardium should tent laterally when grasped—if not, the initial opening in the pericardium should be made elsewhere. Formation of even a small opening allows careful dissection of the pericardium away from the heart and subsequent resection.

Pericardiectomy

Although pericardiectomy can be used to treat pericardial effusions that recur despite pericardial windows, more typically it is used to treat chronic constrictive pericarditis. In most cases, the cause of chronic constrictive pericarditis remains unknown, even after therapy for the process (Table 29-3). Furthermore, the clinical syndrome of chronic constrictive pericarditis may develop years after the original insult.

Diagnosis

Initial signs and symptoms are vague and nonspecific. Fatigue with moderate dyspnea on exertion and neck vein distention may be the first indicators. Hepatomegaly and ascites develop, with or without peripheral edema in the later stages. Breathlessness occurs only with exertion. Although significant fluid overload results in ascites and peripheral edema, the lungs are protected such that orthopnea and paroxysmal nocturnal dyspnea are rare.

With mild early disease, the clinical findings are limited to elevated jugular venous pressure, mild peripheral edema, and slight hepatomegaly. Progressive severity of constriction results in worsening peripheral edema, ascites, and pleural effusions. Patients with severe disease often develop supraventricular tachyarrhythmias and a reduction in pulse pressure. Pulsus paradoxus is to be expected in patients still in sinus rhythm. Rapid ventricular filling in early diastole results in a loud, early, third heart sound—a pericardial knock. The electrocardiogram commonly demonstrates nonspecific abnormal findings. Most patients will have diffuse nonspecific ST-segment and T-wave changes. Approximately one half of

patients with documented constrictive pericarditis will have low QRS voltages; one third will present with an atrial arrhythmia.

Chest radiographs may be unremarkable, although some series have shown pericardial calcification in up to 40% of patients. Although computed tomographic (CT) scans may reveal pericardial thickening, it may not be possible to differentiate between pericardial thickening and pericardial fluid. Nuclear magnetic resonance imaging allows for more accurate determination of pericardial thickening and can also measure various chamber sizes, demonstrating the characteristic right atrial dilation and right ventricular narrowing.

At catheterization, chronic constrictive pericarditis is characterized by an equal elevation of end-diastolic pressures in the right atrium, pulmonary artery, and left atrium, so-called equalization of pressures. The right intraventricular pressure tracings demonstrate an early diastolic fall and subsequent rapid rise to an elevated plateau ("the square root sign"). Left ventricular tracings may or may not be similar. In contrast, mean right atrial pressure fails to decrease normally during inspiration or may rise slightly. Equivocal hemodynamic findings can sometimes be resolved by the rapid intravenous infusion of 1,000 mL of normal saline during catheterization. This maneuver will evoke diagnostic features of occult chronic constrictive pericardial disease (including striking elevations of filling pressures, development of typical pressure pulse characteristics, and loss of respiratory variation of right atrial pressure). Even so, the differentiation between constrictive pericarditis and restrictive cardiomyopathy can be difficult, requiring a limited anterior thoracotomy or thoracoscopic exploration and pericardial biopsy. If the surgical diagnosis is chronic constrictive pericarditis, the incisions can be extended and a pericardiectomy performed. If the pericardium is normal, a diagnosis of restrictive cardiomyopathy is confirmed and the minor procedure terminated. If a recurrent pericardial effusion is identified, an extended pericardial window can be performed with a relatively minor incision.

Technique of Pericardiectomy

Two approaches for pericardiectomy are in common use and have essentially equivalent results. The approach by median sternotomy is somewhat more efficacious for complete pericardiectomy of the right ventricle and great veins, whereas an anterolateral thoracotomy allows complete release of the left ventricle. Patients should be monitored

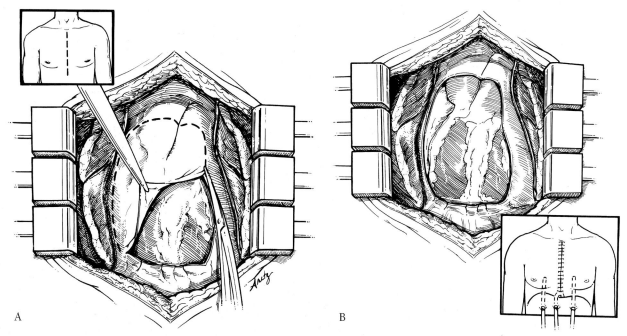

Figure 29-3. Pericardiectomy via median sternotomy. **(A)** The resection is usually begun at the diaphragmatic junction and carried to both phrenic nerves and to the aorta and pulmonary arteries above. The complete extent of the resection is not shown to depict the phrenic nerves. Typically, the phrenic nerves are difficult to see because they are quite posterior at this level. **(Inset)** A typical median sternotomy incision from the sternal notch to just below the xiphoid process is depicted. If aesthetic considerations are strong, the superior extent of the incision can be limited to as much as 5 cm below the sternal notch with only mild compromise of the operative field. **(B)** A completed resection goes to both phrenic nerves and frees the right atrium, aorta, and pulmonary artery. **(Inset)** The space is usually drained with three tubes and can be expected to be productive for several days after the procedure.

by placing a radial artery catheter and a central venous catheter. Even slightly compromised patients will require a pulmonary artery catheter to monitor right heart pressures.

Median Sternotomy

The patient is positioned supine, and a median sternotomy is performed in the usual manner (Fig. 29-3A, inset). After the sternum is split, the pleurae are opened bilaterally, and the phrenic nerves are identified (Fig. 29-3A). These nerves are positioned anteriorly in the superior mediastinum and track close to the pulmonary hila before entering the diaphragm posteriorly. Usually, the phrenic nerves are not visible without retracting the lungs—in the illustration, the nerves are depicted more anteriorly than is their typical position to demonstrate the appropriate extent of resection. The ultimate goal of the procedure is to resect the anterior pericardium between the phrenic nerves and to free the remainder of the cardiac surfaces within the posterior pericardium.

The greatest danger of the procedure is damage to the myocardium, coronary arteries, or phrenic nerves. Limited, loculated

pericardial spaces, even in patients with chronic constrictive pericarditis, can usually be identified just above the diaphragm and at the origins of the major vessels. The operation is started with transverse incisions in these areas to identify a pericardial space and to begin creating a pericardial flap or peel. Loculated fluid or frank pus may be encountered at this time and are sent for culture.

Care is taken to avoid injuring a coronary artery while the flap is created. Small islands of pericardium are left if necessary to avoid injury to coronary vessels or to the atrioventricular grooves, as long as no constricting bands remain to compromise the outcome of the procedure. The flap is then used as a retractor to dissect superiorly, laterally, inferiorly, and posteriorly to gradually free the myocardium from the peel. Calcified plaques or bars may be encountered and require piecemeal removal with bone cutting instruments. Calcified deposits imbedded deeply in myocardium are left in situ.

The left ventricle ideally should be freed of the constrictive pericardium first to avoid potentially catastrophic right ventricular failure. If the pericardium over the right

ventricle is resected first, this allows simultaneous increases in preload (by allowing complete diastolic filling of the right ventricle) and afterload (maintaining high "downstream" pressures by failing to free up the left ventricle). This risks causing right ventricular dilation and failure. The anterior pericardium is resected between the phrenic nerves. Posteriorly it is usually not necessary to remove the pericardium because the heart can be adequately mobilized and released with complete dissection from the constricting pericardium (Fig. 29-3B). With some difficulty, however, the pericardium posterior to the phrenic nerves can be resected via median sternotomy. If this is necessary, the patient is placed on cardiopulmonary bypass to allow better mobilization of the heart. The pericardial peel is then dissected away from the heart. The phrenic nerve is identified, and, with the heart decompressed, the pericardium is divided 1 cm posterior to the nerve under direct vision. A finger within the pericardium and posterior to the phrenic nerve can lift it into view. Thus freed, the phrenic nerve is retracted medially, and further pericardial resection is performed as necessary.

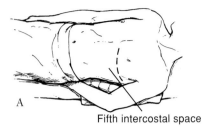

A
Fifth intercostal space

Figure 29-4. Pericardiectomy via anterolateral thoracotomy. **(A)** The patient is positioned at approximately 45 degrees, with the left hand tucked beneath the left buttock. A submammary incision begins just lateral to the sternum and curves posteriorly to overlie the fifth rib and enter the fourth or fifth intercostal space. **(B)** The phrenic nerve is identified and, with its accompanying fat and vessels, dissected free of the pericardium. An island of pericardium is harvested along with the nerve if necessary to avoid injury. **(C)** The pericardium is carefully dissected away from the myocardium to avoid injury.

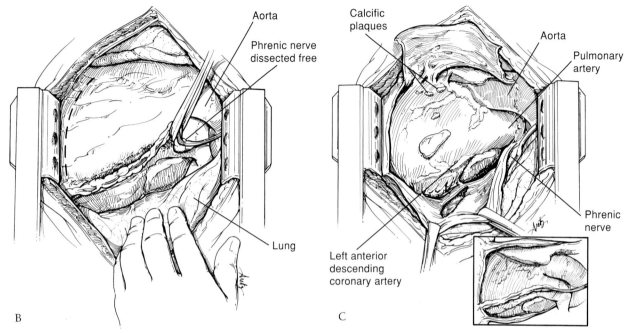

B   C

Occasionally, resecting the pericardium will reveal a thickened, constricting epicardium or visceral pericardium. This structure must then be resected or scored in such a manner as to allow normal cardiac filling; otherwise the procedure will fail to relieve symptoms. Ultrasonic dissectors can assist in this aspect of the procedure. Care is taken to remove localized constricting bands in the atrioventricular groove and at the origins of the great veins. The mediastinum is then drained anteriorly and posteriorly (Fig. 29-3B, inset). Large pleural effusions are drained before closure. Massive ascites should be drained if the quantity is such that respiration will be compromised.

Left Anterior Thoracotomy

The classic approach for pericardiectomy is by left anterolateral thoracotomy. A submammary incision and entry into the chest via the fourth or fifth intercostal space gives good access to the left ventricle and left atrium and allows for easy preservation of the left phrenic nerve. Access to the right ventricle, atrium, and great veins is not straightforward and may require dividing the sternum. Furthermore, conventional

intrathoracic cardiopulmonary bypass may not be possible from this approach; therefore, both groins should be prepared and draped to allow femorofemoral bypass if needed.

The patient is positioned supine with the left hand beneath the buttocks and the torso angled to 45 degrees (Fig. 29-4A). A submammary anterolateral thoracotomy is directed posteriorly to overlie the fifth rib. The pectoralis major muscle is divided anteriorly, and the chest is entered through the fourth or fifth interspace. Disconnecting the fifth costal cartilage from the sternum improves exposure. Often the internal mammary vessels must be divided. The inferior pulmonary ligament is divided, and the lung is retracted superiorly. The phrenic nerve is identified along its course from the hilum to the diaphragm. The nerve is preserved with its accompanying vessels and fat. If necessary, a tongue of pericardium is harvested along with the phrenic nerve to preserve it (Fig. 29-4B). The pericardium is opened, with care taken to avoid damage to the myocardium. Again, limited pericardial spaces with loculated fluid are often found above the diaphragm and at the origin of

the great vessels; incisions are best made in these areas. A flap is then created and used as a handle to gradually dissect the pericardium away from the myocardium. The inferior edge of the resection is placed at the junction of the diaphragm and pericardium. The superior extent of the resection extends almost to the cephalad pericardial line along the pulmonary artery and aorta (Fig. 29-4C). The dissection is carried to the right, deep to the thymus and prepericardial fat, to the atrioventricular groove. The resection on the left side extends posterior to the position of the phrenic nerve to the left atrium, including freeing the left atrium. Mediastinal and pleural tubes are placed in routine fashion.

Pericardiectomy via Thoracosternotomy or Bilateral Thoracotomy

Thoracosternotomy or bilateral thoracotomy approaches may be used for extensive pericardiectomies. They have been uncommonly applied because of relatively greater morbidity associated with this incision.

Table 29-4 Potential Pitfalls of Pericardiectomy via Median Sternotomy
Right ventricular failure
Myocardial failure
Phrenic nerve injury
Coronary artery injury
Incomplete epicardial decortication

Pitfalls

These procedures are technically demanding and tedious. Potential technical pitfalls include myocardial injury, phrenic nerve injury, and coronary artery injury (Table 29-4). Direct myocardial injury from cardiopulmonary bypass or cardiac overdistension (as a result of release of the chronic constriction) can contribute to ventricular failure. Cardiac failure is not uncommon and can be avoided by invasive cardiac monitoring, aggressive pharmacologic support, and early intervention with intra-aortic balloon pump counterpulsation. Specific right ventricular dilation and failure can result when the right ventricle is freed from its pericardial constraints before the left ventricle is freed. This allows increased right ventricular filling in the setting of persistently increased right ventricular afterload, resulting in acute right ventricular dilation and failure. This acute right ventricular failure can sometimes be treated by manually compressing the right ventricle to prevent dilation and urgently putting the patient on cardiopulmonary bypass. It is best prevented, however, by first performing pericardiectomy over the left ventricle.

SUGGESTED READING

Fitzpatrick DP, Wyso EM, Bosher LH, et al. Restoration of normal intracardiac pressures after extensive pericardiectomy for constrictive pericarditis. Circulation 1962;25:484.

Mack MJ, Aronoff RJ, Acuff TE, et al. Present role of thoracoscopy in the diagnosis and treatment of diseases of the chest. Ann Thorac Surg 1992;54:403.

McCaughan C, Schaff HV, Piehler JM, et al. Early and late results of pericardiectomy for constrictive pericarditis. J Thorac Cardiovasc Surg 1985;89:340.

Naunheim KS, Kesler KA, Fiore AC, et al. Pericardial drainage: Subxiphoid vs. transthoracic approach. Eur J Cardiothorac Surg 1991;5:99.

Quale JM, Lipschik GY, Heurich AE. Management of tuberculous pericarditis. Ann Surg 1987;43:653.

Reinmuller R, Gurgan M, Erdmann E, et al. CT and MR evaluation of pericardial constriction: A new diagnostic and therapeutic concept. J Thorac Imag 1993;8:108.

Seifert FC, Miller DC, Oesterle SN, et al. Surgical treatment of constrictive pericarditis: Analysis of outcome and diagnostic error. Circulation 1985;72(Suppl II):II-264.

Shepherd FA, Morgan C, Evans WK, et al. Medical management of malignant pericardial effusion by tetracycline sclerosis. Am J Cardiol 1987;60:1161.

EDITOR'S COMMENTS

Drainage of a pericardial effusion is a common problem faced by thoracic surgeons. Pericardiocentesis may be all that is required if fluid only provides adequate diagnostic material. Most commonly, however, the pericardium requires definitive drainage and ideally something to prevent a recurrence of the effusion. The subxiphoid approach is the most direct and technically simple procedure and is our choice for most indications. It may be performed using local anesthesia with the patient awake if there is a concern about the induction of general anesthesia. It is far simpler than the video-assisted thoracic surgery (VATS) approach, which requires placing an endobronchial tube, positioning the patient, and making intercostal incisions. A larger piece of pericardium may be taken via a VATS approach than through the subxiphoid approach, but there is reason to believe that a pericardial window is successful at preventing the reaccumulation of fluid because it promotes the formation of pericardial symphysis and thus obliteration of the potential space. There is no fistula created either between the pericardium and the peritoneum or the pericardium and pleura that lasts for any significant period of time, and the success of the procedure is not dependent on the creation of such a fistula.

After a subxiphoid drainage procedure to promote sclerosis, we leave a tube connected to suction drainage in the pericardial space for at least 5 days after the procedure. This is especially important after drainage of a malignant effusion.

The indications for VATS pericardial drainage remain controversial. The presence of a significant pleural effusion as well as pericardial effusion makes a VATS procedure advantageous because both are accessible. Given a choice, I prefer to perform a VATS pericardial drainage procedure from the right side because there is more room available in which to work and a greater area of pericardium is visible, which facilitates excision.

The diagnosis of constrictive pericarditis remains elusive. The clinician must have a high index of suspicion to make this diagnosis. The distinction between constriction and restrictive cardiomyopathy is difficult, and it often comes down to the surgical procedure to allow one to make the definitive call. Obviously pericardiectomy is not going to be of help in restrictive cardiomyopathy. For those cases of constrictive pericarditis it is imperative that a complete pericardiectomy be performed even if this requires cardiopulmonary bypass. These are tedious and not particularly interesting procedures, yet the outcome can be quite gratifying. Despite what was pointed out in this chapter, the importance of completing the left side first is somewhat controversial, and many surgeons do not hesitate to release the right side as the first step.

L.R.K.

30

Surgical Management of Malignant Mesothelioma

Joseph S. Friedberg and Shamus R. Carr

Although it is the most common primary tumor of the pleura, malignant pleural mesothelioma is a very rare cancer. In contrast to non–small cell lung cancer, which accounts for close to 200,000 cases each year in the United States, there are only several thousand cases of mesothelioma. The tumor is most commonly linked to asbestos exposure and occurs several decades after exposure. Despite the relatively recent mandates to protect the public from asbestos, it is expected that the incidence of mesothelioma will continue to increase for the foreseeable future. In addition, there is some research indicating a potential relationship between the SV40 virus and mesothelioma. Millions of doses of vaccine, specifically polio vaccine, that were administered in the late 1950s and early 1960s were tainted with this virus, and there is some concern that this also could lead to an increase in the incidence of mesothelioma, but this remains controversial.

The natural history of malignant pleural mesothelioma (MPM), which is almost always unilateral, is inexorable local progression with encasement of the lung and invasion of the chest wall, diaphragm, and mediastinum. The majority of patients succumb to the disease less than 1 year from the time of diagnosis. Although the disease has a reputation for being a purely localized tumor, at least half of patients have occult metastases at the time of their death. The clinical manifestations of metastases have become more common as investigators have developed aggressive multimodal approaches that may extend survival and control the local tumor.

Patients commonly present with dyspnea secondary to a pleural effusion. Other presenting symptoms, such as weight loss or pain from chest wall invasion, are even more ominous and tend to reflect more advanced disease. Radiographic studies may reveal only the pleural effusion and no other detectable disease. Unless a history of asbestos exposure is obtained, the diagnosis may initially elude a clinician not familiar with this rare cancer. Thoracentesis is usually the first attempt at diagnosis, but it is frequently fruitless. Depending on the interpreting cytologist, thoracentesis may be nondiagnostic in nearly half of cases. The recurrent nature of an undiagnosed effusion or an initial visit with a clinician experienced with mesothelioma should lead to referral to a thoracic surgeon.

A diagnosis and palliation of the effusion are best accomplished thoracoscopically. All of this can be performed through a single 10-mm incision. If the patient is potentially a candidate for an aggressive treatment protocol, then the surgeon involved in that protocol should be involved in the planning of the thoracoscopy for a number of reasons. Mesothelioma is a tumor with a propensity to seed and grow in surgical sites, mandating excision of the biopsy site at the time of the major resection. As a result, it is important to limit the size of the biopsy site and place it in a location where it can be excised without compromising future incision closure. What, if any, maneuvers are made to palliate an effusion is the other decision that should be deferred to the surgeon who will be heading the multimodality team treating the patient.

The modalities that have been used to treat mesothelioma include systemic therapy (chemotherapy, immunotherapy), radiation, photodynamic therapy (PDT) intraoperative hyperthermic chemotherapy lavage, and gene therapy. The treatments for MPM that have met with the greatest measure of success are those that use aggressive surgery for debulking gross disease and use other modalities in an effort to treat the residual microscopic disease, usually postoperative radiation, intraoperative PDT, or intraoperative hyperthermic chemotherapy lavage. Any of these treatment strategies may also be combined with systemic treatment. Protocols that employ hemithoracic radiation therapy require a pneumonectomy because of the dose-limiting toxicity imposed by radiation pneumonitis if there is lung in the radiation field. Protocols that use intraoperative PDT or intraoperative chemotherapeutic lavage may offer the possibility of a lung-sparing procedure.

The decision to offer a patient an aggressive treatment protocol is predicated on their predicted ability to tolerate the surgery and the absence of any metastatic disease (Table 30-1). Our standard radiographic evaluation includes a positron emission tomography (PET) scan to rule out bone metastases or other unsuspected metastatic disease, magnetic resonance imaging (MRI) of the brain, and a chest/upper abdominal computed tomography (CT) scan. Our medical evaluation includes a cardiology evaluation, pulmonary function tests, and, if there is any suspicion of arterial disease, carotid noninvasive studies. A quantitative ventilation-perfusion study can be very helpful if the patient's pulmonary function tests are borderline and a pneumonectomy is planned. It is common for patients with gross pleural disease to have only minimal function in the lung to be removed. The role for invasive staging studies is controversial. We perform a laparoscopy with peritoneal lavage for cytologic analysis. We have found occult abdominal disease by this technique and have not proceeded with any aggressive interventions. Some groups use laparoscopy to look for transdiaphragmatic transgression

Table 30-1 Eligibility Criteria for Extrapleural Pneumonectomy
Medical clearance
Cardiac evaluation
Pulmonary function tests
Ventilation-perfusion scan, quantitated in thirds
Radiographic staging
Magnetic resonance imaging of the brain
Computed tomography of the chest/abdomen with contrast
Positron emission tomography scan
Invasive staging
Bronchoscopy
Esophagogastroduodenoscopy
Staging laparoscopy
Mediastinoscopy

of the tumor, whereas others rely on MRI or reconstructed CTs for this purpose. It has been our experience that even MRI can give false-positive or false-negative results with respect to actual invasion into the abdomen. Mediastinoscopy is another area of controversy. In one of our trials using intraoperative PDT we found that involvement of mediastinal lymph nodes did not appear to correlate with outcome, and we have not been performing mediastinoscopy when planning this type of treatment. At this time, a safe guideline would be to perform mediastinoscopy before embarking on any multimodal protocol in which the mediastinal lymph nodes have been shown to have prognostic significance.

If a patient is not a candidate for an aggressive protocol or does not wish to proceed after a candid discussion of the expected risks and benefits, then a referral should be made to an oncologist with experience in treating mesothelioma. Although recent positive results with pemetrexed (Alimta) have slightly altered the natural history of this disease with a slight prolongation of survival, it is common for patients to encounter clinicians with a very nihilistic view and to not be offered any treatment options.

There is a TNM staging system for mesothelioma, but other staging systems also exist. This is likely a reflection of the limited number of patients being treated and the numerous different treatment combinations being employed. Some staging systems, such as the Brigham Staging System, are very accurate when employed with the treatment combination on which it was based but may not be accurate with a different treatment schema. It should be noted, however, that no staging system takes into account whether the tumor is of the epithelial, mixed, or sarcomatous subtype. The fact that the mixed and especially the sarcomatous cell types portend a worse prognosis is one of the few things on which most of the investigators studying this disease agree.

OPERATIVE TECHNIQUES

Diagnosis, Palliation of Pleural Effusion, and Invasive Staging

Sometimes a diagnosis is established on the basis of fluid cytology from a thoracente-sis or a closed pleural biopsy. Commonly, however, a surgical biopsy is required. This is best accomplished using a thoracoscopic technique that should be performed through a single 10-mm incision (Fig. 30-1). After medical clearance the patient is brought to the operating room. Once general anesthesia is induced, bronchoscopy is performed. On one occasion, we discovered a contralateral endobronchial metastasis that served as a contraindication for any aggressive treatment options. In the setting of a large effusion or bulky pleural disease, the expected appearance of the airway is extrinsic compression. If there is a significant amount of secretions in the airway, the surgeon should plan on performing a completion therapeutic bronchoscopy at the conclusion of the operation to maximize lung expansion.

Diagnosis and Palliation for Patients Presenting with Effusion

Once the patient is turned, the position of the double-lumen tube or bronchial blocker is confirmed and the lung on the operative side is isolated. After the patient is prepped and positioned in the appropriate lateral decubitus position, a potential thoracotomy incision is drawn on the chest wall. We excise the seventh rib when planning aggressive surgery, and we draw an S-shaped thoracotomy incision that allows for such an entry. Starting in the anterior axillary line and working forward as necessary, the chest is sounded with a 25-gauge needle, along the potential future incision line, until fluid

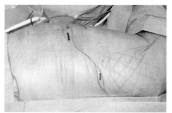

Planned incision

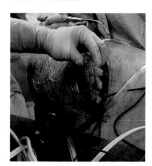

Excising biopsy sites

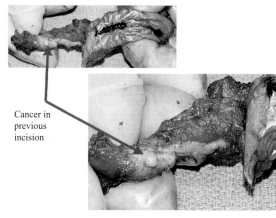

Cancer in previous incision

Figure 30-1. Pleural biopsy.

is encountered. This sample is saved for microbiology stains and cultures if there is any chance that the effusion is secondary to an infectious process. Once a safe site for entry is determined, a local cutaneous and intercostal block is performed with a long-acting local anesthetic, and a 10-mm incision is then created. The chest is then entered through this incision, and fluid is aspirated to allow visualization. The fluid is collected for cytologic evaluation in the event that lesional tissue is not confirmed on the pleural biopsies. When this is required, we send an entire suction canister of pleural effusion.

A 5-mm, 30-degree thoracoscope is then introduced, and the hemithorax is inspected. Remaining fluid is then aspirated, and a mediastinoscopy biopsy forceps is introduced into the chest through the same incision. The 30-degree angle allows the surgeon to maneuver the scope and the biopsy forceps without interference. The earliest-stage cases of mesothelioma may reveal only injected appearing pleura, in which case extensive parietal pleural biopsies are performed. More-advanced stages reveal nodular lesions that eventually coalesce into plaques coating the chest wall and lung, diaphragm, and mediastinum. It is important to never violate the visceral pleura, or a persistent air leak can result. All biopsies should be taken from the parietal pleura. Biopsy specimens need to be sent to the pathologist for frozen-section analysis, and "lesional tissue" needs to be confirmed along with a sufficient quantity of specimen for the pathologist to use for immunohistochemical analysis to be able to render a final diagnosis. Although most diagnoses are made on the basis of morphology and the immunohistochemical profile, some institutions may still run electron microscopy, which may require special handling of the specimen.

If the patient is scheduled for a definitive procedure in the near future, then placement of a chest tube without pleurodesis may be appropriate. If the patient is likely to have any significant interval between biopsy and further intervention, then palliation of the effusion should be considered. Again, planning of the palliation should be coordinated with the surgeon who will be performing the definitive procedure. If the lung expands and there is no contraindication, then it is our bias to perform an intraoperative talc pleurodesis. If the lung does not expand, then placement of a long-term cuffed, Silastic, valved pleural catheter for external drainage can provide good palliation.

Diagnosis for a Patient Presenting with a Pleural Rind

If a patient has a thick pleural rind, then the diagnosis can be obtained without entering the pleural space. Based on the CT scan, a spot along a potential future thoracotomy incision is selected where there appears to be significant pleural tumor thickness. Under general anesthesia, the area is infiltrated with local anesthetic. Depending on the thickness of the soft tissue between the skin and the target, the incision can be as small as 1 cm or may need to extend to 3 cm to 4 cm. The soft tissue is incised, and the dissection is carried into the underlying interspace, where a hard, white mass is encountered. Specimens are harvested using a scalpel or a biopsy forceps. Great care needs to be taken to avoid full-thickness penetration of the tumor and violation of the underlying visceral pleura. Again, it is imperative to confirm the presence of lesional tissue. It would be the exception to have a free pleural space in the presence of bulky pleural disease and the absence of an effusion, so there is unlikely to be a role for videothoracoscopy in these cases. If additional tissue is required, it is best to harvest tumor along the interspace rather than risk deeper biopsies that may enter the lung. Once the pathologist has confirmed the presence of lesional tissue and a sufficient quantity of specimen to establish a diagnosis, the procedure is terminated. The incision is irrigated with sterile water or saline. With the incision filled with liquid, the area is observed during several breaths to ensure that the fluid does not drain into the chest. This would indicate the presence of pleural patency and may require placement of a chest tube. The anesthesia team is then requested to deliver a prolonged inspiration, and the site is inspected for bubbles to assess for an air leak. If it appears that the lung has been entered, a soft drainage tube should be placed in the bed of the incision and treated like a chest tube. If there are no bubbles and the fluid level is static, then the incision can be closed in layers without any drainage.

Invasive Staging Studies

Given that there is no standard of care for the treatment of mesothelioma, it behooves the surgeon to be as certain as possible that a patient stands to benefit from an aggressive operation. With very rare exceptions, there is no role for surgery alone for this disease, and there is certainly no role for aggressive surgery in the setting of metastatic mesothelioma. At a minimum, the patient should undergo a radiographic staging workup. We also complement these studies with an outpatient procedure that includes a bronchoscopy, laparoscopy, and, in select cases, an upper endoscopy. The role of the laparoscopy is to rule out diaphragmatic transgression and/or peritoneal metastases. On several occasions, occult peritoneal metastases were uncovered with cytologic analysis of a saline peritoneal lavage. In addition, we have discovered both false-positive and false-negative readings on the radiographic interpretation of diaphragmatic invasion. We use mediastinal lymph node sampling if the patient is to undergo a prescribed treatment plan in which the paratracheal nodal status has been previously demonstrated to confer significant prognostic information, the nodal disease is more suggestive of distant metastases (like a suspicious aortopulmonary node in the setting of a right-sided tumor), or the patient is enrolling in a protocol that mandates mediastinoscopy.

If the patient is not excluded from further treatment on the basis of the bronchoscopy or upper endoscopy, the patient is prepped in the supine position for the laparoscopy. A small incision is made, and the abdomen is entered through a 5-mm periumbilical port using the surgeon's preferred technique. We use a 30-degree laparoscope to facilitate visualization of the entire peritoneal cavity and especially the diaphragm. After it is confirmed that there was no injury on entry, a second 5-mm subcostal port is placed on the side of the tumor. At this point, the entire peritoneal cavity is explored. The subcostal port is used to provide sufficient visualization of the undersurface of the diaphragm. Any suspicious areas are biopsied. The abdomen is then lavaged with 1 liter of sterile saline, and the fluid is collected for cytologic analysis. We have always considered any peritoneal disease as a contraindication to proceeding with a chest procedure, especially extrapleural pneumonectomy.

Debulking with "Curative Intent" as Part of a Multimodal Approach

Introduction

If the patient is a suitable candidate for an aggressive multimodal approach from an oncologic and medical perspective, then the surgeon needs to consider the operative approach. The goal of any debulking procedure should be to leave the patient with no visible or palpable disease. The surgical options for debulking are limited by the planned adjuvant strategy. Specifically, if hemithorax radiation is planned, then the lung must be removed to avoid the toxicity of extensive radiation pneumonitis. If other local adjuvants, like PDT or pleural lavage, are planned, then the option of saving the lung may be feasible. If a lung-sparing procedure is planned, then it will be critical for the surgeon to ensure that the lung is fully expanded at the conclusion of the procedure because debulking the lung most commonly requires stripping the entire visceral pleura from the underlying parenchyma. This results in a colossal air leak that will seal in several days if the lung fully expands. If there is a residual space from incomplete decortication or from pulmonary resection, the surgeon runs the risk of creating a persistent air leak.

Successful treatment combinations are likely to alter the natural history of mesothelioma with regard to both life expectancy and disease behavior. For years mesothelioma had a reputation of being a purely local malignancy. This perception likely was due to the fact that the vast majority of patients succumbed before there was any evidence of disease outside of the affected hemithorax. With a successful multimodal approach, patients are likely to live longer than without treatment, and there is a high likelihood that disease will recur in distant locations, with or without local recurrence. It is the pattern of recurrences reported in surgical series, particularly in the abdomen, that biased physicians toward attempting to maintain natural barriers whenever possible. That is, with a "classic" extrapleural pneumonectomy, there is en bloc resection of the lung, bony hemithoracic parietal pleura, and the ipsilateral diaphragm and pericardium. When pneumonectomy is planned, our approach is the same, except that the diaphragm and pericardium are stripped of all visible or palpable disease. Some tumors leave the surgeon with no option but to resect these structures, but frequently it is possible to strip the tumor from the pericardium and leave partial thickness of the diaphragm.

Positioning and Incision

In addition to the standard preparation for a procedure of this extent, it is critical to confirm that any special equipment and/or personnel are available. Examples of such items are an argon beam coagulator for chest wall cautery and prosthetic patches for pericardial and/or diaphragm reconstruction. For cases in which we perform intraoperative PDT, for instance, we also test our tunable dye laser, filter the overhead lights and surgical headlights, and coordinate the case with technicians who operate the light-measuring dosimetry system.

Before the patient is positioned, a nasogastric tube should be placed because this facilitates identification of the esophagus and can also be left in place if one chooses to leave the patient intubated at the conclusion of the operation. The patient is then positioned in the appropriate lateral decubitus position and draped in a manner that allows extension of the incision to the costal margin. All previous incisions should be marked and, if possible, incorporated into and excised with the thoracotomy incision to avoid the complication of mesothelioma growing in biopsy sites. The previous incisions are incorporated as ellipses. The cutaneous ellipse is grasped in one hand and the deep portion is palpated. If the biopsy track is palpable, then it is traced, with a margin, into the interspace and can be amputated at the pleural level or left en bloc to be removed with the main specimen. If there is no palpable abnormality, then the ellipse is taken as a full-thickness skin and subcutaneous fat specimen down to muscle.

There is a premium on minimizing trauma to the chest wall musculature with multiple excisions, particularly if the patient is going to have a pneumonectomy and require a watertight closure of the chest wall. Occasionally patients may have had biopsies through one or several incisions that cannot be incorporated into any reasonable incision or that would require a degree of re-excisions that may compromise chest closure. If there is high suspicion of tumor growth in the biopsy sites, then they need to be excised. If not, then preoperative consultation with a radiation oncologist for consideration of biopsy-site irradiation should be obtained if adjuvant radiation has not already been incorporated as part of the multimodal strategy.

Once the patient is positioned and prepped, a limited thoracotomy incision is created and the seventh rib is identified (Fig. 30-2). The incision is then extended, overlying the rib, to within several centimeters of the costal margin. This anteroinferior extension of the incision is very helpful in providing exposure to the diaphragmatic sulci, commonly the most difficult areas to debulk and reconstruct. The latissimus muscle is divided under the incision, but the serratus muscle is mobilized to the level of the rib insertions. Occasionally the muscle can be spared if adequate exposure can be obtained by retracting the muscle anteriorly. Otherwise the muscle is divided at the level of the rib insertions, leaving enough soft tissue to reattach it. In addition to better preserving muscle function, having the serratus intact under the incision provides a measure

of overlapping coverage and facilitates a watertight closure.

The seventh rib is then excised in a subperiosteal fashion. At this point it is our practice to vary the next step depending on whether a pneumonectomy or lung-sparing procedure will be performed. The goal of our surgical procedures is to leave the patient with no remaining visible or palpable disease. We do not plan, a priori, to resect the pericardium and diaphragm. It is our intention to preserve these natural barriers if it is possible to debulk these structures as completely as the bony hemithorax is debulked by developing the extrapleural plane. Commonly, the pericardial barrier can be preserved. The diaphragm is much more difficult and frequently requires partial or full-thickness resection. If a significant portion of the diaphragm is preserved, then we make an extra effort to preserve the phrenic nerve, which commonly can be stripped of any detectable disease and be left in continuity.

Lung-Sparing Procedure

Tumor can be removed, even with bulky disease, in the majority of patients. In developing this technique we explored different sequences for tumor resection and found that first debulking the lung and subsequently debulking the parietal pleural surfaces worked best. The reason for this is twofold. First, there seems to be less blood loss if the parietal pleural surface is not oozing for the duration of the lung debulking. Second, having the tumor tethered to the borders of the hemithoracic facilitates separation from the lung.

Although occasionally the visceral pleura can be separated from the tumor, the majority of cases require resection of the visceral pleura and result in a complete denuding of the lung, even within the fissures. To accomplish this, it is easiest to use a split ventilation technique. In this technique, the operative lung is kept on positive end-expiratory pressure (5 cm to 40 cm of water) during the majority of the decortication. This is accomplished by having the anesthesiologist maintain normal ventilation of the nonoperative lung and running nitrogen or room air through a positive end-expiratory pressure (PEEP) valve to the operative lung. The amount of positive pressure can be adjusted as required and provides the much-needed counter traction to separate the tumor from the lung parenchyma.

The first order of business is to identify the lung surface once the seventh rib is resected. With the anesthesiologist maintaining 10 cm of positive pressure on the lung, a fresh scalpel is used to incise along

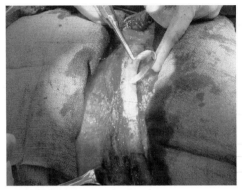

Resecting seventh rib

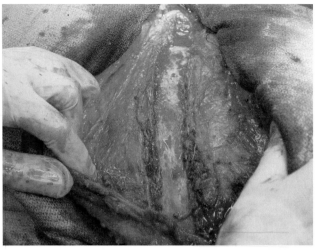

Bed of seventh rib through which extrapleural plane is entered and developed

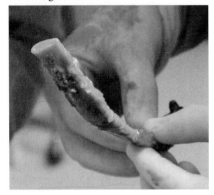

Seventh rib

Figure 30-2.   Incision with retractors.

a broad distance in the middle of the seventh rib bed. As this incision is carefully deepened by cell layers, it may be possible to determine the border between tumor and visceral pleura, in which case that plane should be developed. Commonly, the visceral pleura is not distinguishable as more than a pigmented layer as the deepest portion of the tumor, and the first indication that the visceral pleura has be violated is the leakage of air. This plane is then developed using whatever dissection technique seems to be working the best: sharp dissection, blunt dissection, or electrocautery. Anesthetic gas flow will need to be turned up to accommodate the resulting air leak, which can be massive. This continuous positive pressure on the operative lung greatly facilitates separation of the tumor from the lung, and it should be varied as needed to accomplish this task (Fig. 30-3). The tumor will dive into the fissures, and these areas also need to be resected. Great caution must be adopted at the base of these dissections as the pulmonary artery is approached. Occasionally, the pulmonary artery within the fissure will need to be skeletonized. If the artery is actually encased in tumor, then a lung-sparing procedure is not feasible. This situation should be evident on the preoperative CT scan.

Once the lung is completely debulked, it is deflated. The bleeding from the parenchymal surface usually stops at this point. Any areas of active bleeding are cauterized with a bipolar cautery. Attention is then focused on the parietal pleura. The plane is developed by working under the cephalad surface of the eighth rib with a broad-tipped scissors or a rounded dissector. Once the plane is sufficiently opened with instruments, the surgeon introduces a finger and subsequently a hand to further develop the plane. A characteristic feel to the cleavage plane will be appreciated if the surgeon is separating tumor from the chest wall at the correct level. Before working too caudally, the plane is developed posteriorly and anteriorly such that it can be extended to undermine the area under the sixth rib. The goal is to undermine enough space such that the chest retractor can be placed under the ribs, providing better exposure. An argon beam cautery is very useful for maintaining hemostasis when the parietal pleura is separated from the bony hemithorax. This dissection commonly results in a large surface area with diffuse oozing that is best controlled with surface cautery using the argon beam. If this device is not available, a standard cautery can be used if it is set to a level high enough to allow arcing of the current rather than re-

quiring contact, which will rapidly result in bothersome tip charring.

Although there is no absolute order in which the parietal pleura is separated, it is generally best to first start working posteriorly (Fig. 30-4). On the right side, the surgeon is looking for the azygous vein. If the surgeon is in the correct plane, the azygous vein will remain down on the mediastinum but will be completely skeletonized as the tumor is elevated. If the azygous vein or its tributaries are not seen in the expected location, then the surgeon is likely in a plane that is too deep and is elevating the veins with the tumor. The posterior intercostals should then be identified and traced anteriorly to identify the correct plane. Posteriorly, on the right side, the surgeon must be cognizant of the esophagus, which can be readily identified before it is well visualized, by palpating the nasogastric tube. The azygous vein will lead to the caval junction, which must not be disrupted. Once the plane over the cava is identified, then the apex can be liberated by following the cava and phrenic nerve medially and extending the cephalad chest wall dissection. The separation of the tumor occasionally requires sharp dissection or cautery, but it is best to perform as much as possible using blunt digital dissection because this elevates tumor in continuity

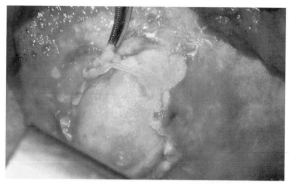

Stripping tumor off lung

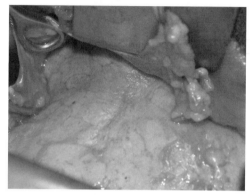

Lung with tumor elevated from surface

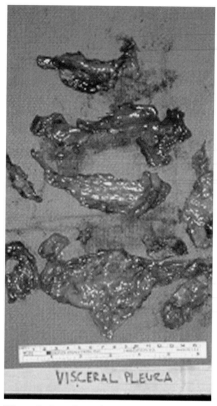

VISCERAL PLEURA

Visceral pleural specimen

Figure 30-3.   Visceral pleural debulking with anesthesia positive-pressure setup.

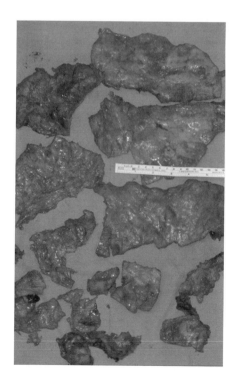

Figure 30-4.   Parietal pleurectomy. A 15-cm ruler is shown for size reference.

and avoids leaving tumor deposits in the cavity.

A similar strategy is used on the left side, except that the key posterior structure is the descending aorta. There is commonly a sulcus between the posterior aspect of the aorta and the chest wall. It is easy to stray behind the aorta, which may result in avulsion of intercostals vessels, so once this edge is identified, it is important to work the plane anteriorly over the medial surface of the aorta. The descending aorta is then used as a guide to the arch and, subsequently, the left subclavian artery to liberate the apex as on the right side, taking care to avoid damage to the vagus nerve as it courses across the aortic arch.

On both sides the dissection is extended caudally until the soft muscular fibers of the diaphragm are encountered. At this point the tumor has been separated from the bony hemithorax. The next area to be liberated is the pericardium. This surface is usually approached from the cephalad dissection, but occasionally there is an easy cleavage plane that allows the surgeon to swing around the anterior recess and onto the pericardium. In either case, the phrenic nerve should be identified, looped if necessary, and stripped

of tumor. The pericardial fat is resected with the tumor and leads to the appropriate plane on the fibrous pericardium. If the tumor does not elevate off the fibrous pericardium with the same "feel" as the separation from the chest wall, then wall can be entered and portions of the fibrous pericardium can be removed with the tumor, leaving the serous pericardium intact. The pericardium tends to be a very robust barrier, but if the tumor is involving the serous layer, it will need to be removed. In the setting in which we perform intraoperative PDT, we debulk the pericardium and wait until after PDT to resect the invaded portion of pericardium to avoid direct illumination of the heart. If the patient is not undergoing an intraoperative adjuvant requiring shielding of the heart, then the pericardium can be resected at this time. On the left side, special care must be taken to protect the recurrent laryngeal nerve and to also identify and preserve the phrenic nerve, which is slightly less obvious than on the right, where it lies on the superior vena cava.

As the mediastinal dissection is developed posteriorly, it will eventually connect with the hilar dissection from the lung liberation. At this point, all that remains is the tumor on the diaphragm. As opposed to the pericardium, it is much more difficult to separate the parietal pleura from the diaphragm. This can be a tedious dissection, but if the diaphragm can be debulked, it can avoid a prosthetic reconstruction. Commonly, this area requires sharp scissor dissection, but if there is not deep diaphragmatic invasion, the majority of the muscle can be spared. If the muscle is involved, then it is separated from the peritoneum, which is spared. Any violation of the peritoneum is immediately closed with absorbable suture to avoid possible abdominal seeding. If there is a thin layer of tumor, a CO_2 laser may be helpful. Special care must be taken at the site of phrenic penetration of the diaphragm.

Although many of the mediastinal lymph nodes are removed in the course of the parietal pleurectomy, any additional lymph nodes should be removed at this point. Again, special care needs to be taken in the aortopulmonary window to avoid injury to the recurrent laryngeal nerve. In addition to the lymph nodes routinely harvested as part of lung cancer operations, the surgeon needs to be attentive to less common stations like internal mammary nodes.

Once the mediastinal lymphadenectomy is complete, hemostasis is achieved, and any intraoperative adjuvant treatment is complete, then it is time to focus on closure. Before closure, on right-sided operations, the thoracic duct should be ligated. It is common to actually see the duct, and it should be ligated at the level of the aortic hiatus. If the visceral pleura has been removed, then the surgeon can anticipate a formidable air leak. This can be of a magnitude that overwhelms the flow rate of the anesthesia machine if the chest tubes are placed to suction prior to extubation. It is essential that the lung is fully decorticated to allow full expansion and that the chest is well drained. Straight chest tubes are placed anteriorly and posteriorly to the apex, both with additional drainage holes cut in the tubes to access the lower chest. A rongeur is helpful for making extra holes in the chest tubes. A right-angle tube is also placed along the diaphragm into the posterior costophrenic recess. Once the patient is extubated, the tubes are placed to -20 cm of suction, and the massive air leaks are tolerated because there is a premium on keeping the lung fully expanded and the chest evacuated of hematoma. If the lung is not fully expanded, then the suction should be increased to achieve this. Having all three chest tubes connected to separate collection devices allows the surgeon to assess leaks and drainage in a more useful manner. If the tubes are still leaking after 2 days, then the

suction can be decreased as long as the lung remains fully inflated. Once on waterseal, the leaks tend to stop quickly. Tubes can then be removed per routine criteria. Despite the enormity of the initial leaks, persistent air leaks are extremely rare events.

Extrapleural Pneumonectomy

The technique for mobilizing the pleural envelope for an extrapleural pneumonectomy is similar to that described for the parietal pleurectomy. If the pericardium can be spared, then the artery, veins, and bronchus can be exposed and divided once the pleural envelope is reflected back onto the hilum. If the pericardium needs to be sacrificed, then it is simpler to isolate and divide the vessels intrapericardially.

Extrapleural pneumonectomy for bulky tumors requires a siege mentality. The specimen can be quite bulky and minimally compressible. This results in very little working room and minimal visibility, making the dissection difficult. These cases require an intimate knowledge of the anatomy and a "feel" for the correct plane of separation. It is still our preference to save the diaphragm debulking for last, but some of these tumors may require the lung to be fully mobilized to have enough mobility of the specimen to access the hilar structures. The airway is divided flush with the carina to avoid pooling of secretions in the stump and potential fistula formation. In addition to a lymphadenectomy, the thoracic duct is ligated at the level of the aortic hiatus on the right side. There is usually a portion of pericardial fat remaining that can be crafted into a pedicle graft to buttress the bronchial stump using absorbable sutures. Reconstructions, if necessary, are performed, and a single 28-F chest tube is placed low and posterior in the hemithorax, attached to a balanced drainage collection system.

Reconstruction

Pericardial reconstruction is performed with a Gore-Tex (W. L. Gore & Associates, Flagstaff, AZ) pericardial patch. The patch is sewn in with nonabsorbable monofilament sutures (Fig. 30-5). It is fenestrated to avoid tamponade. The challenge in fashioning the reconstruction is not to make the patch too constrictive. Bearing in mind that the mediastinum is weighted away from the operative chest when the patient is in lateral decubitus position, the surgeon must build redundancy into the pericardial repair. This is particularly important on the right side, where it is easy to constrict the inferior vena cava. The opening for the cava should admit one to two fingers, and the

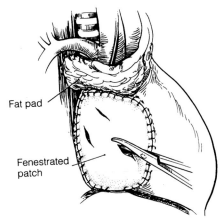

Figure 30-5. Pericardial fat pad/pericardial patch. (Reprinted with permission from D Sugarbaker. Extrapleural Pneumonectomy in the Setting of a Multimodality Approach to Malignant Mesothelioma. Chest. 1993; 1035:4.)

patch should be loose enough to admit several fingers over the heart. Even with these precautions, the patient should be observed for dramatic hemodynamic changes at the conclusion of the procedure when being turned from the lateral decubitus to the supine position. As always, the instruments and the room should be maintained in a sterile condition until the patient leaves the room. If there are hypotensive changes consistent with pericardial constriction or venous inflow obstruction, the patient should be immediately turned back to the lateral decubitus position. If the hemodynamic compromise resolves when the mediastinum is neighed, then consideration should be given to patch revision.

If the diaphragmatic musculature has been preserved along with the phrenic nerve, then it may not be necessary to sew in a patch. It is preferable to avoid placing prosthetics in the hemithorax. Although infections are rare, they become an even more formidable problem with artificial material in the chest. If only a small portion of the diaphragm has been removed, then it can be primarily reconstructed. If the diaphragm has been resected in its entirety or to the point at which it lacks integrity and will compromise breathing mechanics with paradoxical motion, then it should be reconstructed. Reconstruction of the diaphragm is performed with a 20 × 30 cm × 2-mm-thick Gore-Tex soft tissue patch. The patch is anchored to the previous diaphragm insertions (Fig. 30-6). It can also be anchored around ribs. The patch is sewn in with heavy monofilament, nonabsorbable suture. If the anchoring tissue is stout, a running suture

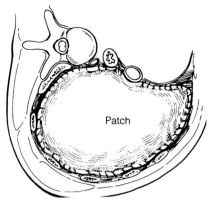

Figure 30-6. Diaphragm reconstruction/peritoneal patch. (Reprinted with permission from D Sugarbaker. Extrapleural Pneumonectomy in the Setting of a Multimodality Approach to Malignant Mesothelioma. Chest. 1993;1035:4.)

can be used. If there is any concern that some of the bites may pull through, an interrupted technique is used. Depending on the expertise of the radiation oncologist and the facility capabilities, the elevation of viscera, particularly the liver, into the hemithorax may represent a dose-restricting obstacle. It is always good to sew in the patch as low and as taut as possible to both stabilize breathing mechanics and move the abdominal viscera out of the radiation field.

Closure of the pneumonectomy space needs to be meticulous. The goal is to make the closure as watertight as possible to avoid developing a seroma that is actually an extension of the pleural fluid that is contained only by the skin. This is a tentative situation in which a wound infection can lead to empyema, which is potentially catastrophic, especially with prosthetic patches in the chest. Multiple layers of absorbable sutures are used for the closure, and the skin edges are approximated perfectly to decrease the chances of a wound infection.

Depending on the surgeon's routine and the available postoperative support, it is usually best to extubate the patient in the operating room to avoid positive pressure on the bronchial stump. Another option is to change the double-lumen endotracheal tube to a single-lumen tube and leave the patient intubated overnight. When this option is selected, the patient is maintained on a short-acting sedative, like propofol, and ventilated on a pressure-limited ventilation mode using the minimal pressures necessary to maintain adequate gas exchange. Unless oxygenation is an issue, PEEP does not need to be used. The patient can then be bronchoscoped the following morning and secretions cleared and then extubated after

sedation is held and pain control is assured. If the patient had a pericardial reconstruction, it is prudent to maintain a supine posture and allow for only minimal rolling for the first day. Otherwise, having the patient up and ambulating immediately is critical for pulmonary toilet.

Postoperative management of the pleural space is different for the extrapleural pneumonectomy patient than for the standard pneumonectomy patient. Very rapid filling of the hemithorax can occur and may result in tension hydrothorax if the tube is removed too soon. The trend of the drainage is important, and the tube can be safely removed when the output is decreasing and the drainage is several hundred milliliters per day. Although controversial, it is our practice to maintain patients on antibiotics until the chest tube is removed and to instill a very small volume of broad-spectrum antibiotics into the chest cavity just before tube removal. Otherwise, the postoperative care of the extrapleural pneumonectomy patient is similar to that of other pneumonectomy patients: adequate pain control, early and frequent ambulation, pulmonary toilet, and maintenance of a relative state of dehydration until the threat of postpneumonectomy pulmonary edema has passed.

SUGGESTED READING

Barbanti-Brodano G, Sabbioni S, Martini F, et al. Simian virus 40 infection in humans and association with human diseases: Results and hypotheses. Virology 2004;318(1):1.

Friedberg JS, Mick R, Stevenson J, et al. A phase I study of Foscan-mediated photodynamic therapy and surgery in patients with mesothelioma. Ann Thorac Surg 2003;75(3):952.

Grondin SC, Sugarbaker DJ. Pleuropneumonectomy in the treatment of malignant pleural mesothelioma. Chest 1999;116(6 Suppl):450S.

Hahn SM, Smith R, Friedberg JS. Photodynamic therapy for mesothelioma. Curr Treat Options Oncol 2001;2:375.

Rodriguez E., Baas P, Friedberg JS. Innovative therapies: Photodynamic therapy. Thorac Surg Clin 14(4):557.

Sugarbaker DJ, Mentzer SJ, DeCamp M, et al. Extrapleural pneumonectomy in the setting of a multimodality approach to malignant mesothelioma. Chest 1993;103(4 Suppl):377S.

EDITOR'S COMMENTS

The surgical management of this disease remains controversial, and many surgeons and oncologists are content to offer palliative

treatment only. Because most of the symptoms relate to the pleural effusion, effective palliation usually involves removal of the fluid and creation of pleural symphysis either with insufflated talc or instilled doxycycline. The bulk of the tumor that often is present may preclude successful pleurodesis, and the occasional patient is treated with a palliative debulking to effect pleurodesis. Friedberg and others have taken a much more aggressive approach to the treatment of this disease based mainly on the concept that the disease remains limited to the pleural space at least during the early phase. Thus a local approach may prove to be effective in this disease, whereas it would not even be reasonable for tumors.

What Friedberg did not discuss in detail are the criteria for selection of patients for an aggressive approach. Most others and we have limited extrapleural pneumonectomy to patients younger than the age of 60 or 65 years who have excellent performance status as well as reasonably preserved pulmonary function. Obviously they must have pulmonary function that will allow them to tolerate pneumonectomy, but the required excision of the hemidiaphragm introduces another "twist" to the operation over and above a standard pneumonectomy. A quantitative perfusion lung scan demonstrating that most of the perfusion is going to the lung that will remain is also a helpful finding. Based on the work of Sugarbaker and colleagues, extrapleural pneumonectomy also should be reserved for those patients with the purely epithelial type of mesothelioma for whom, it is felt, based on preoperative imaging, the disease may be completely removed. The long-term survivors after this extensive operative procedure are those in whom there is no lymph node involvement, who are able to have a complete resection with negative margins, and whose tumor is purely the epithelial type. Mixed-type or sarcomatous tumors do poorly following resection, and the risk of an extrapleural pneumonectomy likely is not justified in patients with these types of tumors. Overall mortality from extrapleural pneumonectomy may approach 10% depending on how rigorous the selection process is.

Friedberg argues that he favors preservation of the "natural barriers," the hemidiaphragm and pericardium, whenever possible so as to prevent the spread of tumor. It is extremely difficult to remove tumor burden from the hemidiaphragm such that all tumor is completely removed, and often to accomplish this requires resection of the hemidiaphragm. If tumor can be removed along with muscular diaphragm preferentially the underlying peritoneum should be left, but replacement with prosthetic material is still desirable to obtain the best closure and prevent migration of abdominal viscera into the empty pleural space, especially on the left side. Often tumor may be stripped off the pericardium leaving the pericardial membrane intact.

Lung-sparing procedures for mesothelioma also remain highly controversial, and it is highly likely that tumor remains behind, thus mandating the addition of some form of adjuvant treatment. Friedberg has been a proponent of photodynamic ther-

apy, and it remains to be seen whether the outcome is better with this modality. Others have used intracavitary chemotherapy whether at normothermia or with heating of the chemical agent. Postoperative radiation given with sophisticated treatment planning to protect the lung has also been used in some centers after a lung-conserving procedure.

The postoperative care of these patients is key, as Friedberg points out. Too rapid filling of the pneumonectomy space needs to be dealt with by drainage of the space. For patients in whom the lung has been spared, management of the huge postoperative air

leak by avoiding any residual space is critically important. A space infection in one of these patients is a disastrous complication. Potential morbidity from the photodynamic therapy must also be looked for closely.

There is much room for improvement in the outcome of the patient with malignant pleural mesothelioma. Aggressive approaches have had an overall impact on survival only in carefully selected patients. There have been some minimal advances in systemic therapy of this disease, and approaches with gene therapy also have been encouraging.

L.R.K.

31

Mediastinal Lymph Node Dissection

Ali Khoynezhad and Steven M. Keller

The thorough dissection of mediastinal lymph nodes constitutes an integral portion of an appropriately performed operation for lung cancer. Just as it is the responsibility of the surgeon to note the extent of the primary tumor and accomplish its complete removal, so too the surgeon must examine the intrathoracic lymph nodes and assure the histologic determination of the presence or absence of tumor. Accurate intraoperative staging of lung cancer provides important prognostic information that permits the physician to make more cogent recommendations regarding the need for additional therapy. Furthermore, only through the standardization of the technique of mediastinal lymph node dissection, the acceptance of definitions regarding the precise anatomic location of lymph node levels, and agreement on their N category can the results of treatment reported by different investigators be properly interpreted.

Since the first anatomic resection for lung cancer performed by Evarts Graham in 1933, surgeons have recognized the ubiquitous occurrence of identifiable lymph nodes in constant peribronchial and mediastinal locations. During the ensuing decades, numerous authors proposed labeling the sites in a variety of manners using competing nomenclatures. Currently, the Mountain lymph node map and definitions are the internationally accepted standard.

Intrathoracic Lymphatic Anatomy

The classic description of the mediastinal lymphatics was given in *Anatomie des Lymphatiques de l'Homme* by Rouvière . Meticulous post mortem dissection was combined with dye injection of lymphatics to identify common drainage paths. However, it was only recently that the patterns of intrapulmonary and mediastinal lymphatic drainage in living human subjects was described.

A dynamic in vivo investigation of drainage of the normal human intrathoracic lymphatics was conducted by Hata using ^{99m}Tc-labeled colloid injected into the submucosa of each segmental bronchus under bronchoscopic guidance. The resulting lymphoscintigrams were compared with the patient's chest x-ray to determine the anatomic drainage patterns. The results of 192 studies performed in 179 patients are presented in Fig. 31-1. The apical and posterior segments of the right upper lobe drained into the ipsilateral scalene nodes via the hilar nodes, tracheobronchial angle nodes, and upper paratracheal lymph nodes. Drainage from the anterior segment of the right upper lobe was varied. Approximately 50% of patients demonstrated flow similar to that in the other upper lobe segments. The remainder of drainage from the anterior segment of the right upper lobe was either via the subcarinal lymph nodes or into the anterior mediastinal lymph nodes. The former continued to the right scalene nodes via the pretracheal and paratracheal nodes (there was rare flow to the left paratracheal nodes). The latter proceeded along the left innominate vein and the left anterior mediastinal nodes and into the left scalene nodes.

The middle lobe and superior segment of the lower lobe shared similar patterns, with drainage to the ipsilateral scalene nodes via the two paths just described. However, a minority of patients demonstrated flow from the middle lobe to the left scalene nodes through the subcarinal and left paratracheal nodes. The basal segments of the lower lobes reached the subcarinal nodes via the hilar nodes. Further drainage reached the right scalene nodes by way of the right paratracheal lymph nodes.

Lymphatic flow from the left lung proved to be highly variable. However, a number of common patterns were discernible. The apical posterior segment of the left upper lobe drained primarily via the subcarinal lymph nodes and then either along the left vagus nerve to the left scalene nodes or along the recurrent laryngeal to the mediastinal lymph nodes. The anterior and lingular segments drained along the phrenic nerve through the para-aortic nodes to the ipsilateral scalene lymph nodes. Lymph from the basilar segments flowed via the subcarinal nodes to the pretracheal and contralateral paratracheal lymphatics to the right scalene nodes. Some flow along the ipsilateral paratracheal region with drainage to high mediastinal lymph nodes was demonstrated. Drainage from the superior segment was least constant and occurred via all paths.

Patterns of Intrathoracic Lymphatic Metastases

Borrie detailed the intrapulmonary patterns of lymphatic metastases in the resected specimens of 42 patients with right lung cancers and 50 patients with left lung cancers. He demonstrated the common occurrence of metastases from all lobes of the right lung to the lymph nodes found along the bronchus intermedius between the origins of the upper and middle lobe bronchi. Similarly, he determined that tumors from both the left upper and lower lobes commonly metastasized to those lymph nodes located between the origins of the lobar bronchi. These lymph nodes have become

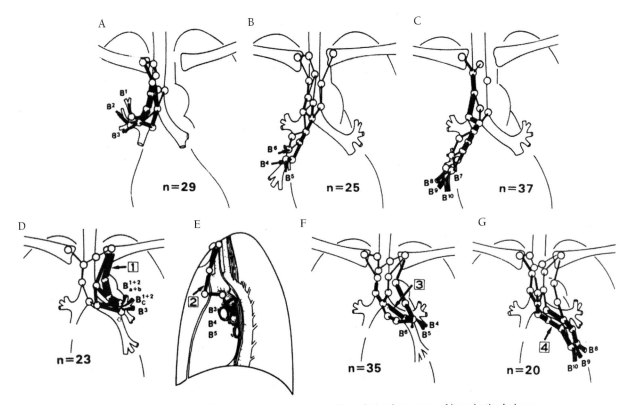

Figure 31-1. The width of each arrow corresponds to the relative frequency of lymphatic drainage. **(A)** Apical and dorsal segments of the right upper lobe. **(B)** Middle lobe and superior segment of the lower lobe. **(C)** Basal segments of the lower lobe. **(D–G)** Four routes of drainage were identified from the left lung: **(D)** through the subaortic lymph nodes and then proximally along either the vagus nerve to the scalene nodes or along the recurrent laryngeal nerve to the mediastinal nodes; **(E)** by way of the phrenic nerve to the scalene nodes; **(F)** along the mainstem bronchus to the paratracheal nodes; **(G)** under the mainstem bronchus to the subcarinal lymph nodes. (Reprinted with permission from E Hata, K Hayakawa, H Miyamoto, R Hayashida. Rationale for extended lymphadenectomy for lung cancer. Theor Surg 1990;5:19.)

known as the lymphatic sumps of Borrie. The mediastinal lymph nodes were not studied.

Nohl-Oser confirmed the findings of Borrie regarding the lymphatic sumps and made the supplementary observation that although it is common for lower lobe tumors to spread cephalad to these sumps, upper lobe tumors rarely metastasize caudal to these lymph nodes. In addition, Nohl-Oser summarized the pattern of regional metastases determined by mediastinoscopy, scalene node biopsy, or thoracotomy in 359 patients with lung cancer and mediastinal and scalene node metastases. Among the 152 patients with right upper lobe tumors, subcarinal, contralateral mediastinal, and contralateral scalene node spread was uncommon (<5%). Ipsilateral mediastinal lymph nodes represented the most common metastatic site (75%). In contrast, among the 104 patients with tumors originating in the left upper lobe, metastases occurred more frequently to the contralateral

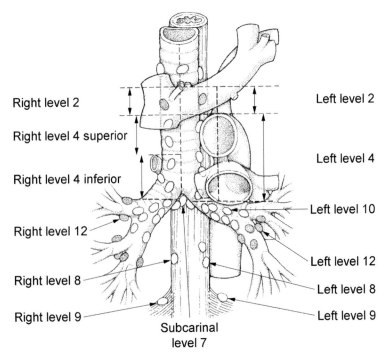

Figure 31-2. Graphic representation of current lymph node definitions. (Courtesy of Steven M. Keller, MD.)

mediastinal (13%) and scalene lymph nodes (10%). Tumors originating within the right lower lobe were rarely found in the contralateral mediastinal or scalene nodes (7%). The subcarinal (22%) and ipsilateral mediastinal (36%) regions were the common metastatic sites. Contralateral scalene node (14%) and contralateral mediastinal (25%) metastases were, however, prominent features of left lower lobe tumors.

Asamura described the intrathoracic lymph node metastatic patterns of 166 patients with biopsy-proven N2 non–small cell lung cancer. Tumors in all lobes appeared to metastasize to the mediastinum by way of the interlobar and hilar nodes. Right upper lobe tumors most commonly spread to the lower pretracheal nodes (74%). Metastases to the subcarinal nodes were much less frequent (13%). Right middle lobe tumors involved the subcarinal nodes most frequently (88%), followed by the lower pretracheal nodes (75%). Right lower lobe tumors metastasized to the ipsilateral paratracheal nodes as well as the upper and lower pretracheal nodes (76%) and, less frequently, to the subcarinal nodes (58%). Left upper lobe tumors, collectively, spread most commonly to the aortopulmonary window (59%) and para-aortic nodes (32%). Subcarinal nodes were less frequently involved (21%) but were the most common site for tumors of the lingular segment. Left lower lobe tumors most commonly metastasized to the subcarinal nodes (58%). Superior mediastinal or aortic nodes were also involved quite frequently (58%).

Kotoulas reviewed the lymph node metastatic patterns of 557 patients who underwent pulmonary resection and lymph node dissection. The results are summarized in Table 31-1 and are in general agreement with the findings of Nohl-Oser and Asamura. In addition, centrally located tumors from all lobes were more likely to metastasize to the subcarinal nodes than peripherally located tumors. This may explain the unexpected findings of Watanabe, who found frequent metastasis from the right upper lobe to the subcarinal nodes.

Although anatomic considerations would predict a regular and orderly sequence of metastases beginning in the intrapulmonary lymph nodes and progressing to the mediastinal and finally to the scalene lymph nodes, this pattern is frequently not observed. From among 216 patients with proven mediastinal lymph node metastases, Keller documented the absence of intrapulmonary lymph node metastases in 71 (33%) patients. Right upper lobe tumors "skipped" commonly to the ipsilateral

Table 31-1 Pattern of Intrathoracic Metastases in Patients with N2 Lymph Node Involvement[a]

Primary Location	n	N2 Nodal Levels								
		1	2	3	4	5	6	7	8	9
Right upper lobe	17	1	2	9	13			1	1	
Right middle lobe	2				1			1		
Right lower lobe	12	1	1		1			5	7	2
Right central	23		5	10	12			13	4	2
Left upper lobe	19		2	5		16	1	1	1	1
Left lower lobe	9			1	1			4	4	2
Left central	41		2	10		20	11	16	2	1

[a]Central tumors are not classified into a particular lobe and thus are considered separately.
Right upper lobe tumors tended to metastasize to the right paratracheal and lower pretracheal nodes. Right and left lower lobe tumors predominantly metastasized to the lower mediastinal and subcarinal nodes. Left upper lobe tumors spread to the aortopulmonary window, pretracheal, and left paratracheal nodes. Centrally located tumors on both sides frequently involved the subcarinal nodes.
Reprinted with permission from CS Kotoulas, CN Foroulis, K Kostikas, et al. Involvement of lymphatic metastatic spread in non–small cell lung cancer according to the primary location. Lung Cancer 2004;44: 183.

paratracheal lymph nodes, whereas left upper lobe tumors frequently metastasized to the aortopulmonary window lymph nodes. Skip metastases originating from tumors of either lower lobe were generally found in the subcarinal region.

Lymph Node Dissection

Definitions

Since Cahan first described mediastinal lymph node dissection after pulmonary resection numerous techniques for assessing the intrathoracic lymph nodes have been detailed. These range from simple biopsy of abnormal-appearing lymph nodes to radical resection of all mediastinal and supraclavicular lymphatic tissue. Discordant claims have been made regarding the accuracy of these techniques in identifying mediastinal lymph node metastases and their effect on patient survival.

The lack of uniform terminology has compounded the difficulty in assessing the efficacy of these techniques. The term *sampling* should be used when only those lymph nodes that were obviously abnormal to visual or tactile inspection were removed. *Systematic sampling* refers to routine biopsy of lymph nodes at levels specified by the author. *Complete mediastinal lymph node dissection* indicates that all ipsilateral lymph node–containing tissue was routinely removed at those levels indicated by the investigators. *Radical lymph node dissection* refers to resection of all ipsilateral mediastinal lymph nodes at those levels indicated by

the investigators as well as contralateral mediastinal or supraclavicular nodal tissue.

Comparison of Sampling, Systematic Sampling, and Complete Mediastinal Lymph Node Dissection

Accuracy

Gaer compared intraoperative visual evaluation of lymph nodes with pathologic examination. Based on inspection and palpation of the lymph nodes after dissection, the surgeon recorded his impression regarding the presence or absence of metastatic tumor in 95 consecutive patients with non–small cell lung cancer who underwent pulmonary resection and mediastinal lymph node dissection. Two hundred and eighty-seven nodal levels were removed (Table 31-2). Sensitivity was 71% and the positive predictive value was 64%. If tactile inspection of the nodal levels through unopened mediastinal pleura had been performed, the intraoperative appraisal would have presumably been even less accurate.

The need for routine intraoperative systematic lymph node sampling was further demonstrated by Graham, who reported the results of systematic sampling of right levels 2 to 4 and 7 to 10 or left levels 4 to 10 in 240 patients with clinical T1–3N0 non–small cell lung cancer. Mediastinoscopy was performed before thoracotomy if the computed tomography scan demonstrated mediastinoscope-accessible lymph nodes >1.5 cm. No patient with documented N2

Table 31-2 Intraoperative Assessment of Lymph Nodes

Assessment	Number of Node Stations	Number of Patients
True negative	238	88
True positive	25	16
False positive	14	11
False negative	10	9
Total number of resections	95	

Accuracy, 91.6%. Predictive value: positive, 25/(25 + 14) = 64.1%; negative, 238/(238 + 10) = 96.0%.
Reprinted with permission from JAR Gaer, P Goldstraw. Intraoperative assessment of nodal staging at thoracotomy for carcinoma of the bronchus. Eur J Cardiothorac Surg 1990;4:207.

disease underwent thoracotomy. Mediastinal lymph node metastases were demonstrated in 20% of patients, the majority of whom had T1 or T2 tumors.

A number of investigators have evaluated the extent of mediastinal biopsy necessary to obtain accurate staging information. Izbicki conducted a randomized, prospective trial containing 182 patients comparing systematic lymph node sampling to complete mediastinal lymph node dissection. The number of N2-positive levels was greater in the patients who had full lymph node dissections, although the percentage of patients found to have N1 or N2 disease was not significantly different between the two study arms. Keller compared the staging of 387 patients who had been accrued to a phase III adjuvant therapy trial, 187 of whom underwent systematic sampling and 186 complete lymph node dissection. N2 disease was demonstrated in 60% and 59%, respectively. Among the 222 patients with N2 metastases, multiple levels of N2 disease were documented in 30% of patients who had complete node dissection and 12% of patients who underwent systematic sampling. Thus, it appears that systematic lymph node sampling is as accurate as mediastinal lymph node dissection for staging non–small cell lung cancer but will identify fewer levels of N2 disease.

Techniques of Mediastinal Lymph Node Dissection

General Considerations

Mediastinal lymph node dissection can be accomplished either before pulmonary resection or after removal of the lung parenchyma. If documentation of nodal metastases will alter the nature of the operative procedure, lymph node dissection should be performed before pulmonary resection. A complete node dissection can be comfortably accomplished via a posterolateral thoracotomy or a vertical muscle-sparing incision. It is difficult to gain access to many of the nodal levels via sternotomy. Use of a double-lumen endotracheal tube greatly facilitates the node dissection. Clips are preferred for hemostasis in close vicinity to the lymph nodes because cautery may destroy their architecture. The operative procedure is lengthened 20 to 30 minutes.

If the resected specimens are not correctly labeled, even the most detailed lymph node dissection will provide little information. To ensure that each level is reported separately and that levels are not lumped together as "mediastinal lymph nodes," each level must be sent from the operating room as a discrete specimen. During a right thoracotomy, levels 4, 10, 7, 8, and 9 are routinely removed. Levels 5 or 6, 7, 8, and 9 are resected during a left thoracotomy.

Right Hemithorax

The superior mediastinum, encompassed by the trachea, superior vena cava, and azygos vein, is exposed by retracting the lung inferiorly (Fig. 31-3). The phrenic nerve is identified on the lateral border of the superior vena cava. The vagus nerve traverses the superior mediastinum and is usually visible through the unopened mediastinal pleura. The mediastinal pleura cephalad to the azygos vein (between the trachea and superior vena cava) is grasped with a forceps and incised to the level of the innominate artery. The pleural edge over the trachea is retracted, and, with the use of a peanut sponge rolled tightly on a clamp, the mediastinal fat pad is dissected from the anterolateral tracheal surface (Fig. 31-4). Traction is placed on the pleural edge over the superior vena cava, and the mediastinal fat pad is gently dissected from the junction of the superior vena cava and azygos vein to the level of the innominate artery. A small vein draining from the mediastinal fat pad directly into the superior vena cava is frequently present.

The mediastinal fat pad is removed from the superior vena cava anteriorly to the trachea posteriorly, and from the cephalad border of the azygos vein inferiorly to the caudal border of the innominate artery superiorly. Nonmagnetic clips (to avoid artifacts on future computed tomographic scans) are used liberally. Right level 2 lymph nodes are located between the cephalic border of the aortic arch and the cephalic border of the innominate vein. Lymph nodes distal to the aortic arch and proximal to the azygos vein are labeled right level 4 superior (Fig. 31-5).

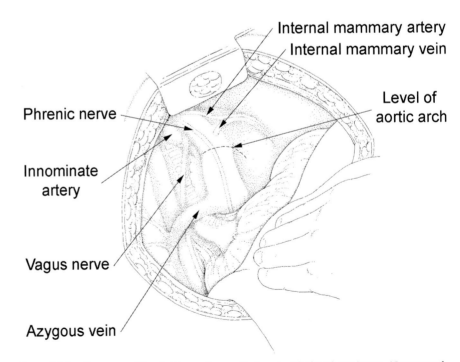

Figure 31-3. Exposure of the right superior mediastinum with the pleura intact. (Courtesy of Steven M. Keller, MD.)

Internal mammary artery
Internal mammary vein
Level of aortic arch
Phrenic nerve
Innominate artery
Vagus nerve
Azygous vein

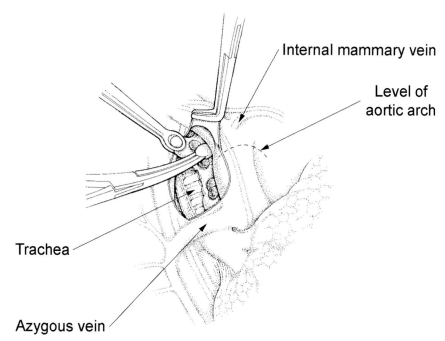

Figure 31-4. Dissection of the right level 2 lymph nodes. Because the aortic arch is not visible from the right hemithorax, the juncture of the internal mammary vein and the superior vena cava can be used as a surrogate marker to distinguish level 2 and level 4 superior lymph nodes. (Courtesy of Steven M. Keller, MD.)

A vein retractor is used to elevate the azygos vein, and the lymph nodes located between its cephalic border and the origin of the right upper lobe bronchus are removed (Fig. 31-6). During dissection of these level 4 inferior lymph nodes, care must be taken not to injure the pulmonary artery. Dissection between the esophagus and membranous portion of the trachea will reveal level 3 posterior nodes. Level 3 anterior lymph nodes are found anterior and medial to the superior vena cava at the insertion of the azygos vein.

Right level 10 lymph nodes are located along the anterior border of the bronchus intermedius distal to the pleural reflection (Fig. 31-7). Level 11, interlobar, lymph nodes are found in the sump of Borrie and are exposed by retracting the pulmonary artery anteriorly. Level 12 nodes are adjacent to the distal lobar bronchus and are removed with the specimen (Fig. 31-8).

The level 7 subcarinal region is exposed by retracting the lung anteriorly (Fig. 31-9). The mediastinal pleura is opened, and the edge overlying the esophagus is grasped with a right-angled clamp. The esophagus is retracted posteriorly, and the subcarinal lymph node packet is grasped with a ring clamp and elevated from the pericardium. Before transection, the attachments to the right and left main-stem bronchi are clipped. Blood vessels course along the anterior border of the trachea and enter the subcarinal lymph nodes from the region of the carina. These arteries and veins must be identified and controlled before transection.

The inferior pulmonary ligament contains the easily visualized level 9 lymph nodes, which are grasped with a ring forceps and removed with cautery or clips. Paraesophageal, level 8, lymph nodes are not always present.

Left Hemithorax

The aortopulmonary (levels 5 and 6) and subcarinal (level 7) lymph nodes are exposed by incising the pleura in a cephalad direction midway between and parallel to the vagus and phrenic nerves (Fig. 31-10). The ligamentum arteriosum is not usually seen, but it is readily palpated. The pleural edge closest to the phrenic nerve is grasped, and the lymph node–containing fat pad anterior to the ligamentum arteriosum is removed. Dissection of the level 6 lymph nodes is best accomplished with blunt instruments. The location of the phrenic nerve must be constantly known to avoid iatrogenic diaphragm paralysis. Level 5 lymph nodes are located posterior to the ligamentum arteriosum and are exposed with blunt dissection. Although it is rare, vocal cord paralysis is a potential complication. To avoid electrical injury to the nearby nerves, vessels should be controlled with clips or ties.

The level 7 subcarinal lymph nodes are approached with the lung retracted anteriorly (Fig. 31-11). The left main-stem bronchus is identified, and the pleura is opened anterior and parallel to the aorta. The lymph nodes are grasped with a ring clamp, and clips are liberally applied before removal of the nodal packet. The arterial vessel that commonly enters the lymph nodes from the anterior border of the trachea at the level of the carina must be

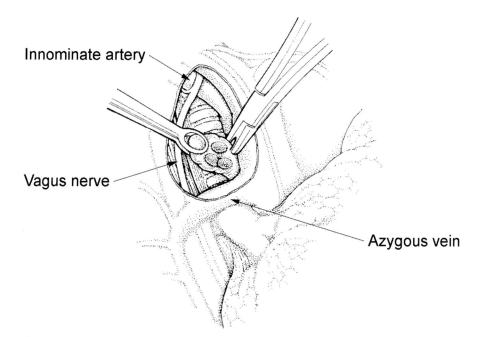

Figure 31-5. Dissection of right level 4 superior lymph nodes. (Courtesy of Steven M. Keller, MD.)

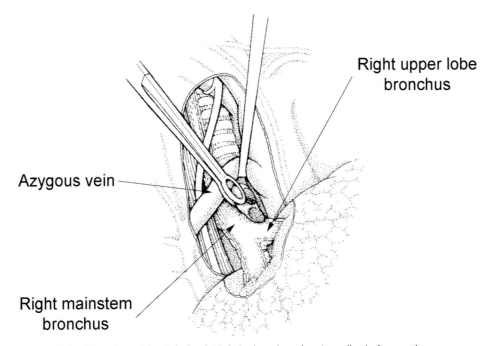

Figure 31-6.   Dissection of the right level 4 inferior lymph nodes. A small vein frequently seen draining into the superior vena cava must be ligated. (Courtesy of Steven M. Keller, MD.)

identified and clipped to avoid postoperative hemorrhage.

Level 11 interlobar lymph nodes are best visualized with the lung retracted anteriorly. The interlobar pulmonary artery must be avoided when clips or cautery are utilized. Level 12 lymph nodes are located along the distal lobar bronchus near its junction with the mainstem bronchus and are removed with the specimen (Fig. 31-12). Level 9, pulmonary ligament lymph nodes are identified within this structure and removed with cautery or clips. The esophagus courses posteriorly, and injury must be avoided.

Other Techniques

Those surgeons who believe that more extensive mediastinal lymph node dissections provide superior staging or lead to improved survival have devised more radical operations. The description given by Izbicki is representative. During a right thoracotomy, a mediastinotomy is performed along the superior vena cava, from the azygos vein to the thoracic inlet. All soft tissue in the superior mediastinum is removed, baring the right subclavian artery, right recurrent laryngeal nerve, and ascending aorta. In addition, the mediastinal tissue anterior to the superior vena cava is included in the dissection. A thymectomy is accomplished, and the right and left brachiocephalic veins, phrenic nerve, and ascending aorta are skeletonized. The thoracic duct is identified and ligated at the level of the carina. Dissection in the left hemithorax includes ligation and division of the ligamentum arteriosum, permitting anterior mobilization of the aortic arch and removal of lymph nodes from left levels 2 and 4.

Virtually all investigators who advocate radical lymphadenectomy believe that a right thoracotomy suffices to provide access to the necessary ipsilateral lymph nodes, although some recommend removal of the supraclavicular lymph nodes if the highest mediastinal lymph nodes are found to contain tumor. However, many of these same surgeons contend that a left thoracotomy does not allow sufficient exposure for resection of the requisite left mediastinal lymph nodes. Therefore, they approach left upper lobe tumors via a median sternotomy. The pericardium between the superior vena cava

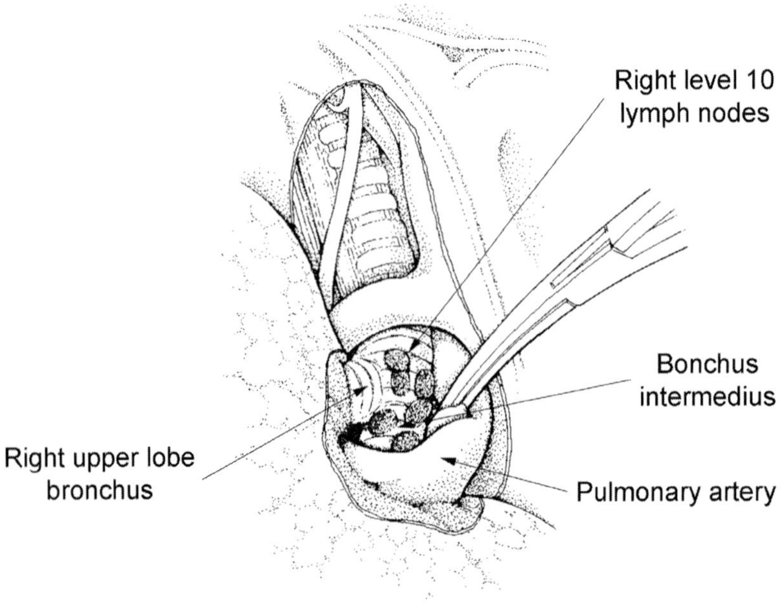

Figure 31-7.   Exposure of the level 10 lymph nodes is accomplished by retracting the pulmonary artery anteriorly. (Courtesy of Steven M. Keller, MD.)

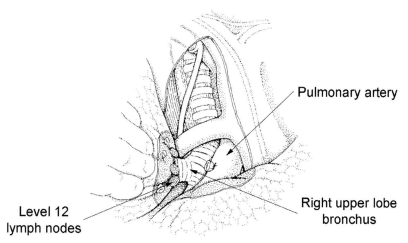

Figure 31-8. Dissection of the right level 12 lymph nodes. Cautery is used rather than clips to avoid interference with the application of a stapling device. (Courtesy of Steven M. Keller, MD.)

and ascending aorta is opened, and the former structure is retracted to the right and the latter to the left. This permits resection of the primary tumor, exenteration of the anterior mediastinum, and removal of pretracheal, bilateral paratracheal, subcarinal, aortopulmonary window, and bilateral tracheobronchial angle lymph nodes. Left upper lobe tumors not resectable via a sternotomy and all left lower lobe tumors are first approached via a standard thoracotomy. After completion of the procedure, the incision is closed and a sternotomy performed.

Morbidity

Perhaps the reason most cited by surgeons for not performing a thorough mediastinal lymph node dissection is a perceived substantial increase in operative morbidity. A retrospective analysis of 199 consecutive patients on whom the author performed a pulmonary resection and mediastinal lymph node dissection revealed 2 reoperations for bleeding and 2 inadvertent recurrent laryngeal nerve injuries. Both episodes of hemorrhage were caused by an unsecured blood vessel that led to the subcarinal lymph nodes.

In a retrospective analysis, Bollen found no significant difference in the median operative blood loss among patients who had undergone complete mediastinal lymph node sampling, systematic sampling, and no lymph node biopsy. However, he did demonstrate an increase in the absolute volume of chest tube drainage after complete node dissection or systematic sampling when compared to no lymph node biopsy. In addition, 5% of patients who underwent complete lymph node dissection suffered recurrent nerve injury and 3% developed a chylothorax. A prospective, randomized trial comparing complete lymph node dissection to systematic sampling demonstrated no difference in intraoperative blood loss, reoperations, or length of hospitalization.

Survival

Several studies have reported a survival benefit for patients who underwent mediastinal lymph node dissection when compared to those who underwent systematic sampling. Izbicki demonstrated that mediastinal lymph node dissection improved survival ($p = .058$) and prolonged disease-free survival ($p = .037$) in patients with pN1 or limited (single-node) pN2 disease. The mediastinal lymph node samples of 100 of the 169 patients entered in this prospective trial were retrospectively examined with immunohistochemical techniques using the Ber-Ep4 antibody to determine the presence or absence of tumor not seen by routine histology. Micrometastases were detected in an additional 23% of patients. When all 100 patients were analyzed as a group, no survival advantage was demonstrated for patients who had undergone complete mediastinal lymph node dissection when compared to those who underwent systematic sampling. However, those patients whose lymph nodes were negative for micrometastases by immunohistochemistry had a significantly

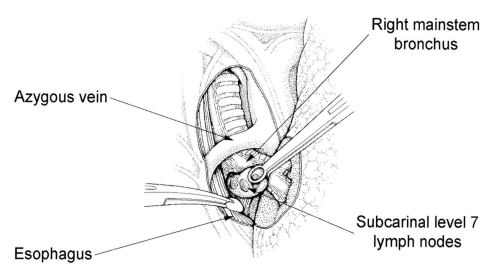

Figure 31-9. Dissection of the level 7 lymph nodes from the right hemithorax. The esophagus and membranous portion of the mainstem bronchi must not be injured. (Courtesy of Steven M. Keller, MD.)

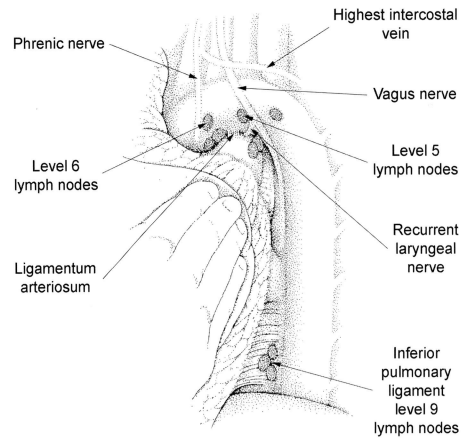

Phrenic nerve

Highest intercostal vein

Vagus nerve

Level 5 lymph nodes

Recurrent laryngeal nerve

Level 6 lymph nodes

Ligamentum arteriosum

Inferior pulmonary ligament level 9 lymph nodes

Figure 31-10. Exposure of the level 5, level 6, and left level 9 lymph nodes. Exposure of the left level 2 and level 4 lymph nodes would require mobilization of the aortic arch. (Courtesy of Steven M. Keller, MD.)

improved survival if they had undergone complete mediastinal lymph node dissection rather than systematic sampling.

In a prospective, nonrandomized trial of 373 patients with stage II and IIIA disease, Keller found that complete mediastinal lymph node dissection conferred a survival advantage compared to systematic sampling (median survival 57.5 vs. 29.2 months, $p = .004$) in patients with tumors of the right lung. Wu conducted a prospective, randomized trial of 532 patients with stage I–stage IIIA non–small cell lung cancer who underwent pulmonary resection and were randomized to either complete mediastinal lymph node dissection or systematic sampling. The 5-year overall survival was 48% in the mediastinal lymph node dissection group and 37% in the systematic sampling group ($p = .0001$). A survival benefit in patients who underwent mediastinal lymph node dissection was also seen when patients were compared according to disease stage ($p = .0104$, $p = .028$, and $p = .024$ for stages I, II, and IIIA, respectively). In addition, mediastinal lymph node dissection reduced the rate of local recurrence and distant metastasis. A meta-analysis containing 997 patients in four trials that compared complete mediastinal lymph node dissection and systematic sampling yielded a statistically significant survival advantage for those patients who had undergone complete mediastinal lymph node dissection ($p = .002$). The odds ratio for death was decreased by 0.33 in patients who underwent complete mediastinal lymph node dissection when compared to those who underwent systematic sampling.

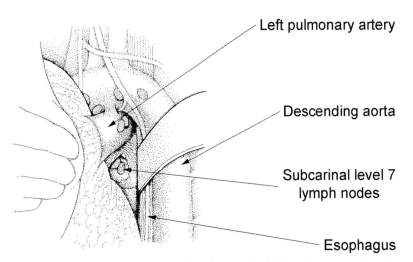

Left pulmonary artery

Descending aorta

Subcarinal level 7 lymph nodes

Esophagus

Figure 31-11. Exposure of the level 7 lymph nodes from the left hemithorax. A malleable retractor is used to retract the aorta and esophagus posteriorly. (Courtesy of Steven M. Keller, MD.)

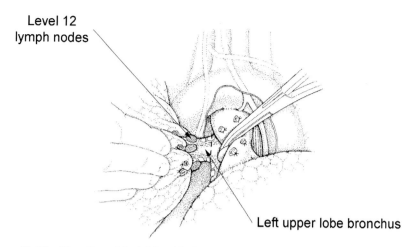

Level 12
lymph nodes

Left upper lobe bronchus

Figure 31-12.   Dissection of the left level 12 lymph nodes. (Courtesy of Steven M. Keller, MD.)

Why should complete mediastinal lymph node dissection influence survival? It is likely that the spectrum of non–small cell lung cancer includes a cohort of patients with metastatic disease that is truly limited to the regional lymph nodes. These are the patients who will benefit from aggressive resection of the intrathoracic lymph nodes.

A multicenter phase III trial, stratified by pathologic stage and with sufficient patients to permit detection of a clinically important survival difference, is the only means by which a definitive result will be obtained. The American College of Surgeons–Oncology Group has completed a prospective, randomized trial of 1,000 patients (protocol Z0030) to further study diagnostic and survival differences between systematic sampling and complete mediastinal lymph node dissection.

SUGGESTED READING

Asamura H, Nakayama H, Kondo H, et al. Lobe-specific extent of systemic lymph node dissection for non–small cell lung carcinomas according to a retrospective study of metastasis and prognosis. J Thorac Cardiovasc Surg 1999;117:1102.

Bollen ECM, van Duin CJ, Theunissen PHMH, et al. Mediastinal lymph node dissection in resected lung cancer: Morbidity and accuracy of staging. Ann Thorac Surg 1993;55:961.

Graham ANJ, Chan KJM, Pastorino U, Goldstraw P. Systematic nodal dissection in the intrathoracic staging of patients with non–small cell lung cancer. J Thorac Cardiovasc Surg 1999;117:246.

Izbicki JR, Passlick B, Pantel K, et al. Ef-fectiveness of radical systematic mediastinal lymphadenectomy in patients with resectable non–small cell lung cancer. Ann Surg 1998;227:138.

Izbicki JR, Thetter O, Habekost M, et al. Radical systematic mediastinal lymphadenectomy in non–small cell lung cancer: A randomized controlled trial. Br J Surg 1994;81:229.

Keller SM, Adak S, Wagner H, Johnson DH. Mediastinal lymph node dissection improves survival in patients with stages II and IIIa non–small cell lung cancer. Ann Thorac Surg 2000;70:58.

Mountain CF. Revisions in the system for staging lung cancer. Chest 1997;111:1710.

Naruke T, Suemasu K, Ishikawa S. Lymph node mapping and curability at various levels of metastasis in resected lung cancer. J Thorac Cardiovasc Surg 1978;76:832.

Nohl-Oser HC. An investigation of the anatomy of the lymphatic drainage of the lungs. Ann R Coll Surg Engl 1972;51:157.

Sugi K, Nawata K, Fujita, et al. Systematic lymph node dissection for clinically diagnosed peripheral non–small-cell lung cancer less than 2 cm in diameter. World J Surg 1998;22:290.

Wu Y, Huang Z, Wang S, et al. A randomized trial of systematic nodal dissection in resectable non–small cell lung cancer. Lung Cancer 2002;36:1.

EDITOR'S COMMENTS

The authors provide a very thorough historical perspective, data review, and technical description of mediastinal lymph node dissection. At this point it is safe to say that a patient who undergoes a pulmonary resection without a mediastinal lymph node dissection has received an incomplete operation. Not only is the information provided by the mediastinal lymph nodes of great prognostic significance, but, as the authors point out, it may also have therapeutic implications. Considering that a mediastinal lymph node dissection adds only 15 to 20 minutes to a standard pulmonary resection and may be accomplished with little, if any, morbidity, there is no reason not to do it. This has become even more important with recent reports showing a survival advantage for completely resected patients with stage IB and greater disease who receive postoperative adjuvant chemotherapy. This reinforces the significance of knowing the status of the mediastinal lymph nodes.

The authors also point out that there is increased chest tube drainage after mediastinal lymph node dissection and up to 3% of patients may have a chylothorax. Care must be taken to use metal clips when performing a node dissection. It is likely that chylothorax is caused by an aberrant branch of the thoracic duct that is not clipped. Most of these will stop with watchful waiting, but when the output is >500 mL/day for >7 days a procedure should be done to stop the chyle leak because of the excessive loss of lymphocytes and protein.

It is particularly important for the surgeon to properly label lymph nodes as they are removed. Ideally the nodes should be described by their numerical level. For those surgeons not intimately familiar with the lymph node map, a copy of the map should hang in the operating room to be referred to for proper labeling. Specimens should go to the pathologist labeled with the lymph node station. They should then be reported according to station such that there is no confusion regardless of who reads the pathology report.

The occasional author has considered the possibility of sentinel lymph node sampling for lung cancers, but this has not caught on primarily because of the ease of performing a complete mediastinal node dissection with no additional morbidity. There is no additional incision to be made because the nodes are taken via the same incision. There is no particular morbidity in opening the mediastinal pleura. Thus there really is nothing to be gained even if a sentinel node could be identified.

All surgeons operating on lung cancer should be familiar with the technique of mediastinal lymph node dissection. A number of years ago Keller prepared a video of the operative technique, which is still available.

L.R.K.

Surgical Management of Empyema: Tubes, Decortication, Open-Window Thoracostomy

Mark S. Allen

Introduction

An empyema, or empyema thoracis, is a collection of purulent material in the pleural space. The management and presentation varies considerably by managing physician, geographic location, and economic resources. In the United Kingdom, up to 40% of patients with an empyema come to surgery after failed catheter drainage, and "overall 20% of patients with empyema die." In third world countries, the usual organisms that cause an empyema differ greatly from what is seen in the developed world. Management varies from simple open drainage to complex interventional radiologic drainage with expensive fibrinolytics. This chapter reviews the surgical treatment of empyema thoracis, concentrating on closed-tube drainage, decortication, and open-window thoracostomy.

The first mention of an empyema is attributed to Hippocrates. He described the natural history of empyema by stating, "In pleuritic afflictions when the disease is not purged off in 14 days, it usually results in an empyema." The "surgical" management was as follows: "prepare a warm bath, set him on a stool, which is not wobbly ... listen to see on which side a noise is heard; and right at this place, preferably on the left, make an incision, then it produces death more rarely." The method of open drainage described by Hippocrates has remained in use for more than 2,000 years. Trousseau, in 1843, described the use of thoracentesis and drainage. Several years after Trousseau's introduction of thoracentesis, Hewett described closed pleural drainage. A major advance in treatment outcome occurred as a

result of the report of Graham and Bell as part of the U.S. Army Corps Empyema Commission in 1918. Before their report, open drainage was the standard treatment for all empyema that developed during World War I. The mortality rate was a staggering 30% to 70%. Through careful analysis of the patient population, they deduced that the treatment should follow several principles. There was drainage, but with careful avoidance of an open pneumothorax. They further described the concepts of early sterilization and obliteration of the cavity and the importance of nutrition in these patients. With adoption of these simple principles the mortality fell to 10% to 15%. In 1945, Tillet described the use of fibrinolytics, and in 1972, Clagett published a paper describing closure of the pleural cavity by filling it with antibiotic solution. More recently, Pairolero as well as Miller have expanded the understanding of the use of muscle flaps to treat difficult empyemas.

When treating a patient with a suspected empyema, there are several decisions to make to determine the best management. Initially, almost any patient with an effusion associated with sepsis or pneumonic illness should have a diagnostic pleural fluid sampling. If fluid cannot be obtained, then the use of computed tomography or ultrasound can help to localize the area to be sampled. Patients with frank pus or cloudy fluid should have a chest tube placed immediately. Even a delay of 12 to 24 hours can allow the fluid to thicken so that a decortication will be required. Similarly, when bacteria are seen on Gram stains of the pleural effusion, a chest tube should be inserted. Occasionally, culture and parapneumonic effu-

sion secondary to *Pneumococcus* may resolve with antibiotics alone, but the possibility of a mixed infection must be considered. Patients with a pH <7.2 should also have a chest tube placed. Other conditions or reasons to place a chest tube include large effusion, loculated (either by computed tomographic scan or ultrasound) effusion, and a patient not responding clinically to antibiotic therapy (Fig. 32-1).

Chest tubes can usually be placed at the bedside using mild sedation and infiltration of local anesthetic. The pleural space will usually be acidic, and thus adequate analgesia will be more difficult. Nevertheless, it should be possible to place a chest tube with minimal discomfort when properly performed. The tube should be placed into the pleural fluid collection and located to promote dependent drainage, but not so that the patient has to lie on the tube.

There have been no clinical trials comparing the efficacy of traditional large-bore (32- to 36-F) chest tubes versus the thin (10- to 14-F) tubes placed radiographically. Most papers in the literature report good results with either type tube (Fig. 32-2). Similarly, there is no consensus on the best way to manage the chest tube. Small-bore tubes usually need intermittent irrigation with 10 to 30 mL of normal saline solution via a three-way stopcock. Irrigation is usually not performed with large-bore tubes, because in practice it is more difficult to maintain negative intrapleural pressure and irrigate the tubes. Repeated irrigation may introduce bacteria into the pleural space, but this has also not been studied. Chest tubes are usually placed to 20 cm H_2O suction and kept in place until the drainage has fallen to

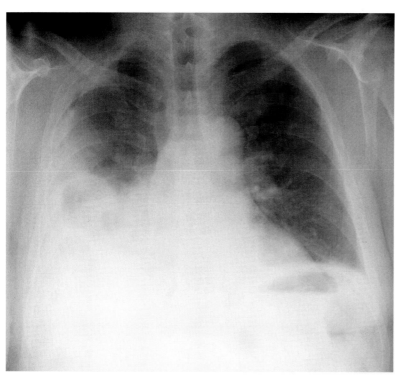

Figure 32-1. Chest roentgenogram demonstrating a large right pleura effusion that requires at least a chest tube for complete drainage.

<300 mL/24 hours, but again, there is no scientific data to support either of these "standard" practices. If the lung fully expands to fill the pleural space, the empyema will usually not recur after closed chest tube drainage alone.

Streptokinase

Instillation of intrapleural fibrinolytic therapy to break up loculations and to improve the drainage of an empyema has been in use since approximately 1949.

Although initial use was associated with numerous problems, including allergic reactions and leukocytosis, newer agents have rekindled interest in the use of intrapleural fibrinolytic drugs to improve pleural drainage. There are four small randomized trials, the largest of which included 128 adult patients who were randomized to receive either intrapleural urokinase, streptokinase, or controlled flushes. The patients who received the urokinase or streptokinase did have increased fluid drainage, but it is unclear whether the instillation of these medications reduced the morbidity, mortality, or need for surgical intervention. There is a larger randomized trial ongoing in the United Kingdom by the Medical Research Council and the British Thoracic Society. It is hoped that this will yield some insight into whether these techniques are valuable because their use is variable and based on anecdotal evidence.

Complications associated with the intrapleural fibrinolytics include allergic reactions and fever; however, it is difficult to determine whether the reactions are secondary to the primary illness or are from the introduction of the fibrinolytics. There is also the theoretical possibility that these agents may cause a systemic response, thus interfering with later fibrinolytic therapy that is given systemically for a myocardial infarction or as therapy for other emboli that may develop in the body. For streptokinase the recommended dosage is 250,000 IU daily or 250,000 IU every 12 hours for 3 days; for urokinase, it is 100,000 IU once daily for 3 days. The concept is to improve the drainage via the chest tube and reduce the need for surgery. These medications are most often used in children or in older adults in whom there would be a high risk of numerous comorbidities with surgical intervention.

Other intrapleural agents include streptodornase-alpha 1 DNAse. The concept behind this type of therapy is that the DNAse would liquefy some of the viscous material in the pleural space and improve the drainage. Again, clinical trials will be necessary to assess whether these are effective.

When chest tube drainage is ineffective, surgical intervention is required. Typically,

operation is indicated when there is persistent sepsis or a persistent pleural collection that is multiloculated (Fig. 32-3). Other considerations include whether there is a question of malignancy, whether there is a large amount of foreign material in the chest cavity, and whether the patient is immunosuppressed. Bronchoscopy should be performed in most patients who have an empyema because of the possibility of bronchial obstruction, which could be the etiologic factor leading to the empyema. Although this has never been randomly studied, in one British chest physician's series of 119 patients, 40% underwent bronchoscopy, usually to exclude a cancer that was causing the empyema. Tumor was found in <4% of the total sample. However, even though the number is small, the complication rate from the bronchoscopy was extremely low, and thus it would seem to be indicated in patients with an empyema.

The goal of the surgical procedure is to remove the infected material and the fibrinous material to allow the lung to expand so that the parietal and visceral pleura are in apposition. This is accomplished by a decortication. The first successful description of a decortication was by Fowler in 1893. The procedure had also been described by a French surgeon, DeLormae, but the patient died after the procedure. Decortication is most often done through a thoracotomy incision to allow wide access to the pleural cavity and to allow débridement of all the pleural material, as well as the thick rind that has been deposited on the parietal and visceral pleurae. Recently, decortication has been described using a video-assisted thoracoscopic (VATS) approach; however, with the minimally invasive technique, it is difficult and quite time consuming to remove sufficient quantity of the pleural thickening to affect an adequate re-expansion of the lung. The purpose of removing the thickened peel over the surface of the lung is so that it can re-expand and the pleural surfaces can be reopposed, eliminating the potential space that harbors bacteria. If the decortication proves to be technically impossible, such that when the visceral pleura is removed, the lung is torn, or an adequate plane cannot be found, it is possible to perform incisions into the visceral pleura, either in a parallel fashion or in a checkerboard fashion, to allow the lung to re-expand. This was first described by Ransohoff in 1900.

At the time of decortication, the fibrinopurulent material removed should be sent for culture and for pathologic examination to rule out pleural malignancy. At the completion of the procedure, the chest cavity

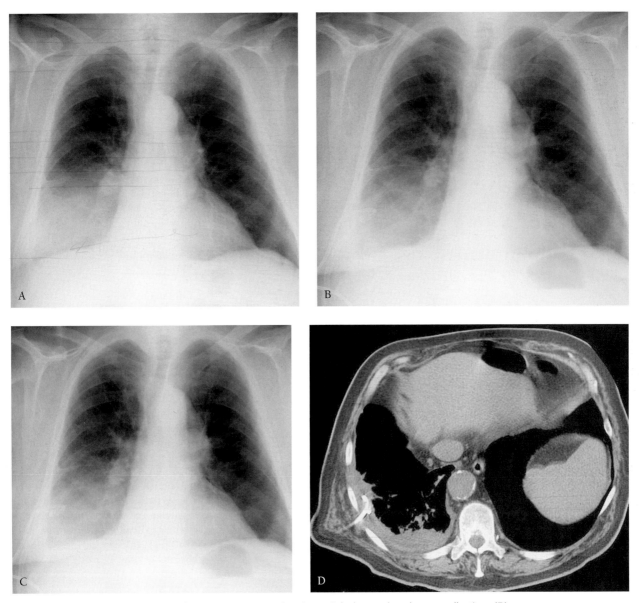

Figure 32-2. **(A)** Chest roentgenogram showing a right lower pleural space collection. **(B)** Computed tomography of the patient in panel A, demonstrating a empyema of the right chest. **(C)** Chest roentgenogram of the patient in panels A and B after placement of a pigtail catheter via computed tomography guidance. **(D)** Computed tomography of the patient showing the pigtail catheter in the nearly completely drained empyema.

should be irrigated with copious quantities of saline solution. Any large air leaks should be repaired with sutures. Smaller peripheral air leaks will usually seal very quickly after surgery. Large-bore chest tubes should be carefully placed in the posterior, anterior, and inferior pleural space and connected to suction immediately to continue to drain the pleural cavity in the postoperative period. Once the drainage has decreased to an acceptable level, usually <300 mL/chest tube/day, and if there is no air leak, the chest tubes can be removed. Success rates with an open decortication are extremely high.

A reason for failure is incomplete decortication, leaving a residual space. Certainly, just removing the purulent material and not removing the rind on top of the lung is a setup for failure and almost certainly will result in another operation (Fig. 32-4).

In some patients, a thoracotomy under general anesthesia is prohibitively risky, and they therefore are not candidates for a decortication. In this very small subset, it is possible to treat the patient with an old-fashioned method by either prolonged chest tube drainage or a thoracotomy and open drainage. As was shown in the

1918 Army Empyema Commission led by Graham and Bell, the mortality rate from empyema dropped significantly when a rib resection and wide surgical drainage was performed after there was complete fusion between the parietal and visceral pleura. Performing a rib resection or open drainage early in an empyema will lead to lung collapse and will be fatal >50% of patients. Long-term chest drainage can be performed by placing a chest tube and initially connecting it to closed suction drainage. This will allow the bulk of the infected material to drain. Once a significant period has gone by,

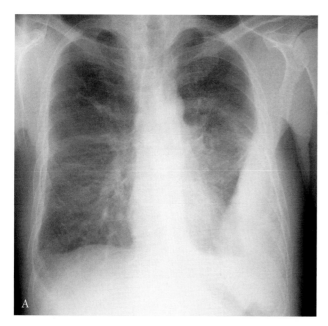

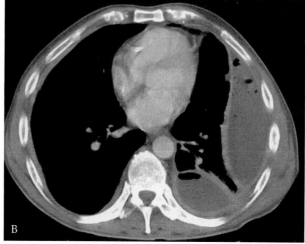

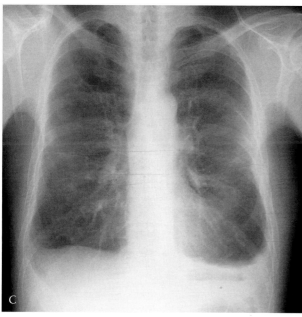

Figure 32-3. **(A)** Chest roentgenogram of a multiloculated empyema that requires decortication. **(B)** Computed tomographic picture of the multiloculated empyema. **(C)** Chest roentgenogram of the patient 1 month after undergoing a decortication via left thoracotomy.

usually 1 to 2 weeks, the chest tube can be converted to open drainage and a chest x-ray obtained to make sure that the lung does not collapse. If it does not collapse, the chest tube can be shortened and allowed to drain into a gauze sponge. This chest tube is then withdrawn from the chest cavity 2 cm to 4 cm every other week while the residual space closes and heals by secondary intention. Obviously this is not a very cosmetic or socially acceptable method of therapy for most patients; however, it is an option when patients are too ill to undergo general anesthesia or have a small to moderate-sized fixed space. This usually results in excellent apposition of the pleural space, although it is quite

inconvenient for the patients because they require frequent trips back to the doctor's office for management of the chest tube.

Another option, as derived from Eloesser's initial description, is to perform a rib resection and create a flap of skin and subcutaneous tissue that keeps the hole open, a procedure known as an open-window thoracostomy. Initially described by Leo Eloesser (1881–1976) in an article in *Surgery Gynecology and Obstetrics* in 1935, this flap was to be a one-way valve for patients with tuberculous empyema. The flap was not adequately described in the initial reference, so it is unclear how Eloesser was able to provide exit of air

from the chest cavity with no collapse of the lung. The subsequent development of antituberculous drugs and antibiotics made the Eloesser flap an obsolete, and the operation rarely needs to be used. There are times, however, when chronically ill patients require open dependent drainage, and this can be performed once there has been pleural synthesis by resecting one or more ribs from the dependent portion of the pleural cavity to be drained. The skin is sutured to the thickened pleural rind to keep the drainage site open (Fig. 32-4). This cavity can then be irrigated daily by the patient, and dressing sponges can be applied. Often, this is a chronic cavity and

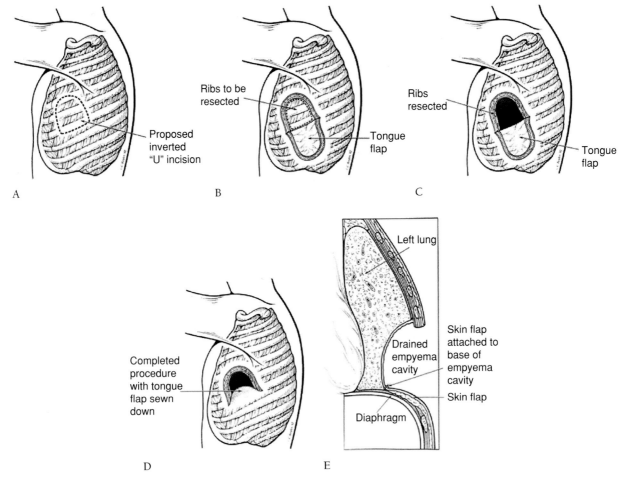

Figure 32-4. **(A)** Site of skin incision for an open drainage procedure. **(B)** Skin flap for open drainage of empyema. **(C)** The chest cavity has been opened by removal of a few ribs. **(D)** Skin is sewn to the lining of the pleural cavity. **(E)** Cutaway view of the completed open pleural flap. The lung must be completely adherent to the pleura before this technique can be used.

will remain open for the rest of the patient's life. Rarely will the cavity heal by secondary intention and close spontaneously. In either event, this is a very disabling procedure and should rarely be used except for the most extreme circumstances.

In summary, empyema should be treated by closed-chest drainage. This is usually successful when therapy is instituted early. When closed drainage is unsuccessful, an open decortication should be done. The goal is to remove all the purulent material and allow the lung to expand so the parietal and visceral pleurae can come together. When patients are too ill to tolerate an operation, a small window can be made after sufficient time has allowed the pleural surfaces to fuse, so the lung will not collapse from this open pneumothorax.

SUGGESTED READING

Deschamps C. Management of post pneumonectomy empyema and bronchopleural fistula. Chest Surg Clin North Am 1996;6: 519.

Ferguson AD, Prescott RJ, Selkon JB, et al. Empyema Subcommittee of the Research Committee of the British Thoracic Society. The clinical course and management of thoracic empyema. Q J Med 1996;89:285.

Hurvitz RJ, Tucker BL. The Eloesser flap: Past and present. J Thorac Cardiovasc Surg 1986; 92:958.

Katariya K, Thurer RJ. Surgical management of empyema. Clin Chest Med 1998;19: 395.

Light RW, Nguyen T, Mulligan ME, et al. The in vitro efficacy of varidase versus streptokinase or urokinase for liquefying thick purulent exudative material from loculated empyema. Lung 2000;178:13.

Merriam MA, Cronan JJ, Dorfman GS, et al. Radiographically guided percutaneous catheter drainage of pleural fluid collections. AJR 1988; 151:1113.

Miller JI. The history of surgery of empyema, thoracoplasty, Eloesser flap and muscle flap transposition. Chest Surg Clin North Am 2000; 10:45.

Miller KS, Sahn SA. Chest tubes. Indications, technique, management and complications. Chest 1987;91:258.

Munnell ER. Thoracic drainage. Ann Thorac Surg 1997;63:1497.

Poe RH, Marin MG, Israel RH, et al. Utility of pleural fluid analysis in predicting tube thoracostomy/decortication in parapneumonic effusions. Chest 1991;100:963.

Silverman SG, Mueller PR, Sainic S, et al. Thoracic empyema: Management with image-guided catheter drainage. Radiology 1988;169:5.

Simpson G, Roomes D, Heron M. Effects of streptokinase and deoxyribonuclease on viscosity of human surgical and empyema pus. Chest 2000;117:1728.

Somers J, Falser LP. Historical development in the management of empyema. Chest Surg Clin North Am 1996;6:403.

Staves J, van Sonnenberg E, Casola G, et al. Percutaneous drainage of infected and noninfected thoracic fluid collections. Journal Thorac Imaging 1987;2:80.

Ulmer JL, Choplin RH, Reed JC, et al. Image-guided catheter drainage of the infected pleural space. J Thorac Imaging 1991;6:65.

Wescott JL. Percutaneous catheter drainage of pleural effusion and empyema. Am J Radiol 1985;144:1189.

EDITOR'S COMMENTS

The management of empyema, despite being elucidated in detail by Graham in 1918 and by many others since, remains poorly understood by most. As pointed out by Dr. Allen, an early empyema, usually postpneumonic in origin, usually can be successfully managed by tube drainage alone. If there is no residual space following drainage of the infected fluid, simple chest tube drainage and removal of the tube when the drainage diminishes usually suffices. When chest tube drainage fails to completely drain the space, the situation becomes somewhat more complex, and measured surgical judgment is required. Incomplete drainage, if noted early, often will respond to videothoracoscopic debridement of the fibrinous material with complete re-expansion of the lung and obliteration of any residual space. It is the residual space that is the enemy of the thoracic surgeon. A persistent space remains a nidus of infection and must be obliterated. If the space is small and contained, it might suffice to place an empyema tube, usually through the bed of a resected rib. The tube is managed by open drainage and slowly advanced out over a period of weeks.

As Allen mentions, in place of a tube, an open-window thoracostomy may be constructed, but it needs to be placed in a dependent area so as to effect maximal drainage and must be large. This type of procedure most commonly is employed for a postpneumonectomy empyema with or without a bronchial stump leak. The location of the open window is particularly important and should be placed fairly far posterior so that the hemidiaphragm does not interfere with drainage. The Eloesser flap, as originally described, rarely is used because the simple suturing of the skin to the thickened pleura suffices to keep the window open.

Formal decortication is required when a significant amount of parenchyma is encased in a fibrous peel, the result of a pleural space infection. To allow the lung to reexpand, the visceral pleural peel must be removed. This requires precise entry into a decortication plane that leaves the visceral pleura intact. There is an element of timing involved because if decortication is attempted too early before the peel has "matured," defining a plane becomes extremely difficult. One should wait several weeks, if possible, before attempting definitive decortication. The ideal procedure includes a parietal pleurectomy with a decortication because pleural symphysis usually has occurred. Once the parietal pleura is taken down, a scalpel is used to cut through the parietal pleural peel and down into the decortication plane. This is facilitated by keeping the lung inflated and, at times, having the anesthesiologist perform a Valsalva maneuver, which acts as a counter traction when trying to define the appropriate plane in which to begin the dissection. Once the appropriate decortication plane is entered, traction is applied to the peel with counter traction applied to the lung surface. Often this traction–counter traction maneuver suffices to facilitate blunt dissection off the visceral pleura. Areas that are most difficult are the fissure and along the diaphragm. The peel should be cut as the decortication proceeds so as to not have to work in a hole.

At times the decortication can be quite tedious with numerous entries made into the visceral pleura. These usually close readily in the postoperative period. When the peel is appropriately mature, the decortication can be quite satisfying. The aim is to allow for complete expansion of the lung to obliterate any residual space. I often leave the patient intubated overnight following decortication to allow the positive-pressure ventilation to act as an "inner" stent to keep the lung expanded, because there is a tendency for it to collapse. Suction applied to the pleural drainage tubes also allows the decorticated parenchyma to remain expanded. Adequate pain relief, usually in the form of thoracic epidural narcotic, must be provided so as to facilitate cough and the clearing of secretions. Bronchoscopy should be used liberally in the postoperative period if the patient experiences problems in clearing secretions. Chest radiographs must be followed closely in the postoperative period.

Complete drainage of the infected fluid and fibrinous debris and obliteration of any residual space are the two hallmarks of the management of empyema. If the lung fails to expand to fill the space, the transposition of muscle, usually serratus anterior or latissiumus dorsi, usually serves this purpose. Thoracoplasty, the excision of ribs to allow the chest wall to drop into a residual space, was the method originally described during the tuberculosis era to fill spaces. Occasionally, this technique may be used to obliterate a space if muscle is either not available or inadequate to fill a space. Muscle transposition largely has supplanted the deforming procedure of thoracoplasty to fill residual spaces.

L.R.K.

33

Resection of Superior Sulcus Tumors

Christine Lau and G. A. Patterson

Superior sulcus tumors are understood to be primary bronchogenic cancers located at the apex of the lung with chest wall involvement. These lesions can present with pain in the nerve distribution of the eighth cervical and first and second thoracic nerve roots. In addition, Horner syndrome may be present as a result of invasion of the stellate ganglion. Such patients have the classic presentation described by Pancoast-Tobias syndrome. Patients with C8–T1 nerve root involvement may also present with typical neurologic findings of the "ulnar hand." However, the majority of patients with superior sulcus tumors present with nondescript but persistent shoulder or upper chest pain. Posteroanterior and lateral chest x-ray may demonstrate nothing more than apical pleural thickening. Computed tomography (CT) and magnetic resonance imaging (MRI) usually depict the lesion clearly.

Anatomic Considerations

The insertion of the anterior, middle, and posterior scalenus muscles on the first and second ribs, respectively, divides the thoracic inlet into three compartments (Fig. 33-1). The anterior compartment contains the platysma and sternocleidomastoid muscles, the external and anterior jugular veins, the inferior belly of the omohyoid muscle, the subclavian and internal jugular veins and their major branches, and the scalene fat pad. The middle compartment includes the anterior scalene muscle with the phrenic nerve lying on its anterior aspect, the subclavian artery with its primary branches except the posterior scapular

artery, the trunks of the brachial plexus, and the middle scalene muscle. Finally, the posterior compartment, which lies posterior to the middle scalene muscle, includes the long thoracic and external branch of the spinal accessory nerves, the posterior scapular artery, the sympathetic chain and stellate ganglion, vertebral bodies, intervertebral foramina, and intercostal nerves.

Clinical Considerations

The anatomic location and extension of the superior sulcus tumor determine the presenting symptoms and signs. Anterior apical tumors generally present with chest wall or shoulder pain. Hand or arm swelling suggests subclavian vein invasion on the left or brachiocephalic invasion on the right. The phrenic nerve may be involved as it crosses the scalenus anticus muscle. These anterior lesions usually do not involve the brachial plexus.

Tumors invading the middle compartment of the thoracic inlet may present with signs and symptoms related to compression or infiltration of the middle and lower trunks of the brachial plexus, which manifest clinically as pain radiating to the shoulder and upper extremity. Often these tumors spread along the fibers of the middle scalene muscle.

Posterior tumors usually present with all the signs and symptoms of the Pancoast-Tobias syndrome and are usually located in the costovertebral groove, involving the nerve roots of C8 and T1, the posterior aspect of the subclavian and vertebral arteries, the sympathetic chain, the stellate ganglion, and prevertebral muscles. These tumors have a propensity to spread along the nerve roots up to the spinal canal through

the intervertebral foramina. In addition, vertebral bodies may be involved by direct extension.

Diagnostic Considerations

Unfortunately, the diagnosis of superior sulcus tumor is often made late because symptoms are not specific, neurologic findings are sometimes absent, and routine imaging of the chest and shoulder are often not revealing. Often symptoms are mistakenly attributed to arthritis or other inflammatory conditions of the shoulder or cervical spine. The radiologic findings can be subtle because these lesions are often hidden behind the first rib and clavicle. Posteroanterior and lateral chest x-ray have little role in evaluation of the superior sulcus tumor. Superb imaging of the lesion and its local extension can be obtained using modern computerized tomographic techniques. High-resolution images with three-dimensional volume averaging allow precise location of extent of the tumor, nerve involvement, and spinal invasion. Specific nerve root or vascular invasion is better assessed by magnetic resonance imaging. The easiest way to obtain tissue diagnosis is by fine-needle aspiration biopsy. Transbronchial biopsy may be considered, but these lesions are so peripheral that this option is rarely useful. If there is a suspicion of extensive pleural invasion or pleural metastases, video assisted thoracic exploration may be utilized for diagnostic purposes. All patients should undergo a thorough search for hematogenous metastases. Positron emission tomography (PET) imaging should be a routine part of the evaluation to assess both regional lymph node

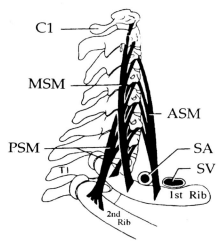

Figure 33-1. The insertion of the anterior scalenus muscle (ASM), middle scalenus muscle (MSM), and posterior scalenus muscle (PSM) on the first two ribs divides the thoracic inlet into anterior, middle, and posterior compartments. (SV = subclavian vein; SA = subclavian artery.)

involvement as well as distant metastatic disease. Because these are T3 lesions, we employ mediastinoscopy and supraclavicular lymph node biopsy in every patient. Patients with N2 or N3 nodal involvement are not candidates for resection. The initial investigation of the potentially operable patient also includes preoperative cardiopul-

monary functional tests and other investigations required for any major pulmonary resection.

Indications

Determination of specific root involvement is important. T1 invasion may be evident only from pain and paresthesia in the medial aspect of the upper arm. C8 invasion will be associated with loss of strength in intrinsic muscles, lack of thumb opposition, and numbness in the small finger and medial half of the ring finger. These observations can be confirmed by electromyography, but clinical examination is usually sufficient. Phrenic nerve invasion is detected by elevation and immobility of the ipsilateral diaphragm. Vascular invasion is usually apparent by good-quality contrast CT scans, but additional information can be obtained by magnetic resonance imaging. If vascular invasion is suspected, arteriography may be helpful, and Doppler ultrasound will demonstrate associated cerebrovascular arthrosclerotic changes, which might affect the decision regarding operability. Radiologic determination of vascular and nerve root invasion is sometimes equivocal. Apposition of the tumor to major structures does not confirm invasion or preclude surgical exploration to determine resectability (Fig. 33-2).

Spinal invasion or extradural extension is often evident on CT scans, but occasionally MRI is necessary to rule out subtle spinal involvement.

These investigations are not merely academic. Extent of disease and, therefore, likelihood of complete resection must be determined preoperatively. Loss of the T1 nerve root is inconsequential, but resection of T1 and C8 will leave a severely impaired "ulnar hand," which the patient may not accept. Subclavian vein or arterial invasion is not a specific contraindication to resection. The vein can be resected without reconstruction. Arterial resection will require primary reconstruction or interposition grafting. Vascular invasion describes a T4 lesion and predicts a decreased long-term survival. Limited involvement of the vertebra, for example, transverse process, partial vertebral body involvement, is not a contraindication to resection. In fact, these resections can be conducted with only local resection of the affected bone through tumor-free margins. Patients with more extensive single or double vertebral involvement may be candidates for complete resection. Recent advances in techniques of vertebral resection and spinal stabilization make such resection feasible. Limited experience with such resections has been reported from a small number of experienced centers, and early results are encouraging.

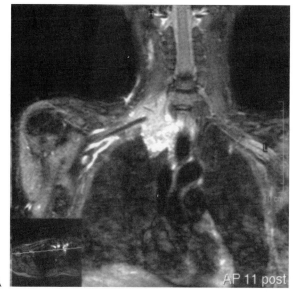
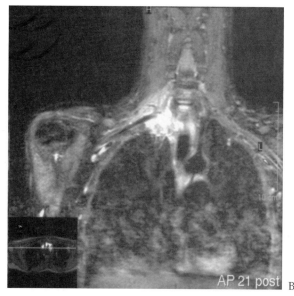

Figure 33-2. **(A)** Preinduction MRI of a patient with a right superior sulcus tumor highly suspicious for involvement of subclavian vessels. **(B)** Postinduction (chemoradiation) MRI of the same patient still suspicious for vascular invasion. The patient was explored initially through a supraclavicular approach. The vessels were found to be uninvolved, and a complete resection was performed using a standard Shaw-Paulson approach.

Absolute contraindications to resection include N2 or N3 disease, extensive vascular invasion, brachial plexus involvement more extensive than C8 and T1, and multiple-level vertebral involvement with extension into the spinal canal.

After the 1924 and 1932 magnum opuses of Henry K. Pancoast describing the tumors of the thoracic apex, the entity was considered incurable until the report of Chardack and MacCallum in 1956 and the description of Shaw and Paulson in 1961. Radiation therapy given preoperatively over a 20-day period at a dose of 30 Gy to 45 Gy had been the standard approach since the Shaw and Paulson report. In recent years, demonstration of tumor response following induction chemoradiation gave rise to an interest in its application in patients with superior sulcus tumors. A recent multicenter trial by Rusch and colleagues demonstrated that cisplatin and etoposide and 45 Gy of radiation improved the rate of complete resection, pathologic complete response, local recurrence, and intermediate-term survival compared to historical controls treated only with induction radiotherapy. For this reason and because of the success of combined-modality therapy in stage IIIA lung cancer, induction chemoradiation has become the standard of care for superior sulcus tumors in most centers. Recently, Krasna and colleagues argued that induction therapy should include higher doses of radiation.

Perioperative Patient Management

Preoperative preparation is as for any major pulmonary resection. A double-lumen endotracheal tube or bronchial blocking catheter for left-sided lesions is helpful. Standard monitoring lines include an arterial line in the contralateral radial artery. Two venous lines should be placed to allow for rapid volume expansion as needed.

Operative Technique

Different operative approaches are necessary depending upon the location of the primary tumor. The surgeon must be familiar with these various approaches. The goal of the operation is en bloc resection of the upper lobe along with involved ribs and other structures including transverse processes, the lower roots of the brachial plexus, the stellate ganglion, and the upper dorsal sympathetic chain.

There are three approaches most commonly employed for these lesions. The posterior approach described by Shaw and Paulson is ideal for lesions situated posteriorly. The anterior cervicothoracic approach described by Dartevelle is ideal for management of anterior lesions. The hemiclamshell approach is less commonly employed, but is useful for anterior or posterior lesions.

We believe that whatever approach is selected, an initial cervical exploration is warranted. This is particularly true when a posterolateral Shaw-Paulson resection is anticipated. With the patient supine, shoulders elevated, neck extended, and head turned to the contralateral side, a transverse incision is made immediately above the clavicle. The platysma muscle is divided, as is the clavicular head of the sternomastoid muscle. The supraclavicular fat pad is excised and submitted for frozen-section examination to rule out N3 disease in supraclavicular lymph nodes. The phrenic nerve is elevated away from the scalenus anticus muscle, which is then divided. This exposes the subclavian artery and the lower roots of the brachial plexus. Anterior displacement of the brachial plexus exposes the scalenus medius muscle, which is then divided, taking care to preserve the long thoracic nerve. By mobilizing and inspecting these structures through a small cervical incision, tumor extent can be assessed and judgments made regarding the possibility of subsequent complete resection before exposing the patient to the morbidity of a major posterior thoracotomy and rib resection. In addition, this anterior superior mobilization facilitates subsequent dissection and resection through the posterolateral thoracotomy.

Posterolateral Approach (Shaw-Paulson)

The patient is placed in the lateral decubitus position, leaning slightly forward. The upper arm is loosely supported by folded sheets and is free to move as the scapula is elevated. The skin preparation is carried out from the base of the skull (included are the spinal processes above C7) and down to the iliac crest and to the midline posteriorly and anteriorly.

Incision

A limited posterolateral incision is made, dividing the latissimus muscle, and entry is made into the chest through the fourth or fifth interspace. The pleural space and hilum are examined to exclude the presence of metastatic disease. This initial exploration also permits assessment regarding anterior

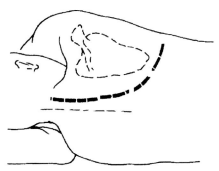

Figure 33-3. The posterolateral thoracotomy incision. The pleural cavity is entered through a limited posterolateral thoracotomy, and resectability is determined. If the lesion is deemed resectable, the incision is extended posteriorly to the level of the C7 spine.

(several centimeters away from the lesion) and inferior (one rib and one interspace) margins of resection.

Subsequently the incision is extended superiorly between the spinous processes and the medial border of the scapula to the level of the seventh cervical vertebra (Fig. 33-3). The trapezius muscle is divided along the full length of the incision. The rhomboid muscles from superior to inferior are then divided in the line of the incision. The rhomboid muscles insert into the medial border of the scapula. Care should be taken to avoid injury to the dorsal scapular nerve and the satellite scapular artery, which run down the medial border of the scapula. The division of the rhomboid muscles elevates the medial border of the scapula from the chest wall.

A large Finochietto retractor is then placed with its lower blade in the interspace incision and the upper blade on the tip of the scapula. Opening the retractor elevates the scapula off the chest wall and exposes the subscapular musculature. These muscles are then divided with cautery up to the level of the first rib.

Chest Wall Resection

The chest wall resection is completed first, allowing the lung to be completely mobilized and permitting a safer subsequent pulmonary resection. All involved chest wall should be resected en bloc. Extrapleural dissection without rib excision risks incomplete resection and local recurrence. The lowermost rib to be preserved is identified, and an interspace incision is made along its superior border, extending from the anterior margin of resection to the transverse process posteriorly. The division of the ribs is started anteriorly. Intercostal muscles are divided with electrocautery.

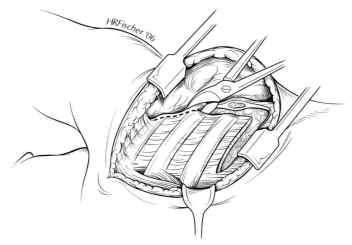

Figure 33-4. Using rib shears, the ribs are divided anteriorly in succession from inferior to superior after the neurovascular bundle is ligated or clipped. (Adapted from HC Urschel, JD Cooper [eds], Atlas of Thoracic Surgery. New York: Churchill Livingstone, 1995;185, Fig. D.)

Using rib shears, the ribs are divided anteriorly in succession from inferior to superior (Fig. 33-4). Traction on the previously divided anterior margins of the involved ribs exposes the anterior aspect of the first rib. For posterior tumors, the anterior aspect of the first rib can easily be encircled and divided with angled rib shears. The anterior and middle scalene muscles, previously divided from above, are exposed. The posterior scalene muscle is divided where it crosses the lateral border of the first rib. The superior margin of the first rib is then exposed by careful superior mobilization of the subclavian vein, artery, and inferior aspect of

the brachial plexus. At this point the operation is continued posteriorly.

The erector spinae muscle is incised along its anterior border and retracted posteriorly from the first rib to the lowermost resected rib. This exposes the angle of the invaded ribs and transverse processes. Hemostasis can be obtained by packing the space between muscles and bony structures. If there is no radiologic evidence of rib or spinal invasion, the transverse processes can be left intact. The costotransverse process joint is opened, and the heads of the ribs are disarticulated by placing a periosteal elevator in the joint and levering forward (Fig. 33-5). This elevates the head of the rib from the spine. If rib invasion is present, leaving the transverse processes compromises the margin of resection. Therefore, the transverse processes (Fig. 33-6) and (if rib heads are involved) lateral cortex of the vertebra are amputated using an osteotome (Fig. 33-7). With completion of the bony

resection at each level, the intercostal bundle is ligated and divided. Occasionally, significant venous hemorrhage is encountered from the orifice of the intervertebral foramen. Loose packing with hemostatic material can be used, taking care to avoid excessive pressure, which can result in migration of material into the spinal canal or occlusion of the anterior spinal artery. This posterior portion of the resection is continued superiorly until the angle of the first rib is reached.

Dissection of the Brachial Plexus

At this point, the first thoracic nerve (T1) below and the eighth cervical nerve (C8) above the neck of the first rib are visualized. The head of the first rib is then disarticulated from the spine. Usually, the T1 nerve is involved as it crosses the first rib. The nerve root is ligated or clipped and divided as it emerges from the intervertebral foramen. If the eighth cervical nerve is not involved, every effort should be made to protect it (Fig. 33-8). If the tumor also involves the eighth cervical nerve, the nerve root can be divided at the intervertebral foramen and the lower trunk of the brachial plexus divided lateral to the area of invasion. The nerve roots are ligated or clipped to prevent cerebrospinal fluid (CSF) leak. If a CSF leak is noted, the foramen should be covered with a pedicled flap of erecta spinae muscle in an effort to help seal the leak.

Dissection of Subclavian Vessels

Dissection of the subclavian artery can usually be carried out in a subadventitial plane (Fig. 33-9). Branches such as the internal mammary artery and the thyrocervical trunk are ligated and transected as necessary. If the subclavian artery is invaded, it should be cross-clamped (after adequate systemic heparinization, e.g., 0.5 mg/kg) proximal and distal to the involved segment and revascularized either by an

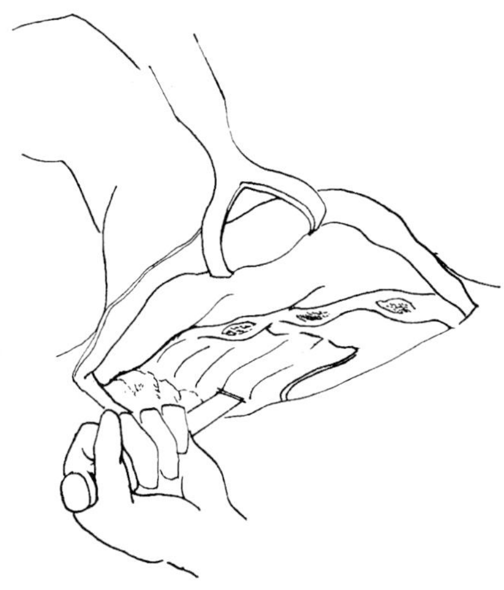

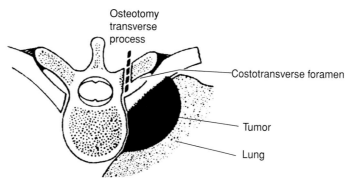

Figure 33-5. The rib may be disarticulated from the transverse process in the costotransverse angle if the parietal pleura and not the ribs or vertebrae are invaded by the tumor.

Figure 33-6. The osteotomy is performed at the level of the transverse process if the tumor erodes the rib posteriorly.

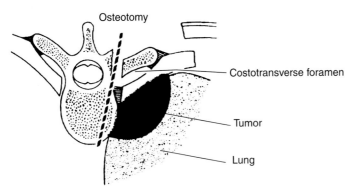

Figure 33-7. If the tumor is fixed to the paravertebral fascia, a partial excision of the vertebral body can be done as illustrated here.

end-to-end anastomosis or by interposing a polytetrafluoroethylene (PTFE) graft (6 mm or 8 mm). If the subclavian vein is involved or occluded by tumor, the segment of vein should be excised and the proximal and distal ends suture ligated. No attempt should be made to bypass the excised segment of vein. Management of the subclavian vessels can be difficult through the posterior approach, particularly if the tumor extends medially. In this circumstance it is sometimes necessary to resect a segment of the anterior scalene muscle and phrenic nerve.

Vertebral Body Resection

Limited invasion of the body of the vertebra mandates vertebrectomy for complete resection. Recent advances in spinal instrumentation allow complete resection of tumors involving vertebral bodies or neural foramina (Fig. 33-10). This is a reasonable strategy for limited vertebral invasion (one or two vertebral bodies) without extension into the spinal canal. For more extensive spinal invasion, there is no justification for resection.

For en bloc resection of the involved vertebrae with the chest wall and lobe, a transcervical as well as a posterior midline approach is used, or alternatively a cervicothoracic transmanubrial approach plus a midline posterior incision can be used. The anterior incision is used to assess resectability. Tumor-bearing structures are removed with lateral division of the involved nerve roots, ribs, and partial midline division of the vertebrae. A standard lobectomy is performed leaving the lobe in place. After this, the posterior midline approach is used for unilateral laminectomies, nerve root division within the spinal canal, and midline vertebral body division. After the resection is complete, spinal stabilization is performed.

Pulmonary Resection

The chest wall specimen is still attached to the upper lobe. Anatomic upper lobectomy is the preferred parenchymal resection even if the lesion is small. The lobectomy is performed through the defect created by the

chest wall resection or through the original exploratory intercostal incision (Fig. 33-11). Complete mediastinal node dissection or, at the minimum, nodal sampling is mandatory.

Postresection chest drainage is accomplished through two separate chest tubes, one of which must be placed at the apex of the pleural space. For chest wall resections down to the fourth rib, the scapula covers the chest wall defect, and therefore prosthetic reconstruction is not necessary. Muscle, subcutaneous tissue, and skin closure is accomplished in standard fashion.

Tatsamura recently proposed an approach for apical lung tumors that invade the thoracic inlet in which an incision is started at the level of the spinous process of the second or third thoracic vertebra, continued downward along the paravertebral line around the tip of the scapula, and continued upward to above the nipple level, following the axillary line up to the level of the sternoclavicular joint (Fig. 33-12). The management of the thoracic inlet through this incision is the same as for the Shaw-Paulson and anterior approaches.

Anterior Approaches

Transclavicular Approach

This approach is ideally suited for anterior lesions. The patient is placed in the supine position with the shoulders elevated, the neck hyperextended, and the head turned away from the involved side. The operative field extends from the mastoid down to the xiphoid process and from the midaxillary line laterally to the hemiclavicular line.

An L-shaped incision is made that includes an oblique pre-sternocleidomastoid

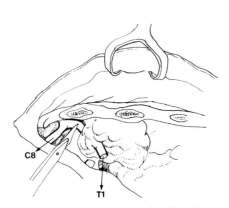

Figure 33-8. Division of the first thoracic nerve root (T1) as it emerges from the intervertebral foramen and before its fusion with the eighth cervical root (C8).

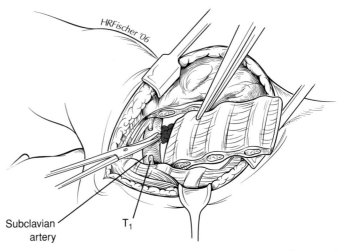

Figure 33-9. Dissection of the subclavian artery from the tumor can usually be carried out in a subadventitial plane. (Adapted from HC Urschel, JD Cooper [eds], Atlas of Thoracic Surgery. New York: Churchill Livingstone, 1995;187, Fig. H.)

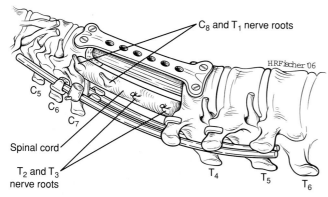

Figure 33-10. Multilevel thoracic vertebrectomy and laminectomy, reconstruction with methylmethacrylate, placement of anterior locking plate and screw construct, and posterior fixation with hooks and rods. (Reprinted with permission from S Gandhi, GL Walsh, R Komaki, et al. A multidisciplinary surgical approach to superior sulcus tumors with vertebral invasion. Ann Thorac Surg 1999;68:1778.)

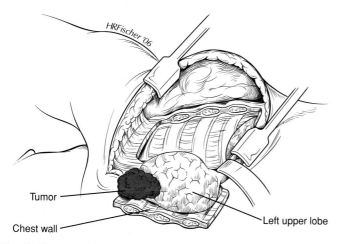

Figure 33-11. En bloc removal of the chest wall and lobe. (Adapted from HC Urschel, JD Cooper [eds], Atlas of Thoracic Surgery. New York: Churchill Livingstone, 1995;188, Fig. I.)

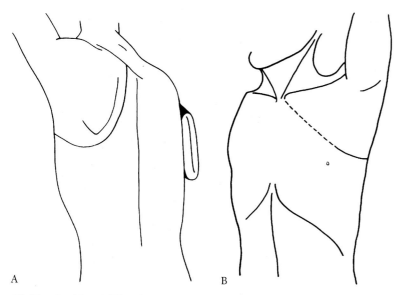

Figure 33-12. Semidorsal **(A)** and semiventral view **(B)** of the incision. (Reprinted with permission from T Tatsamura, H Sato, A Mori, et al. A new surgical approach to apical segment lung diseases, including carcinomas and inflammatory diseases. J Thorac Cardiovasc Surg 1994;107:32.)

incision extended horizontally below the clavicle and lateral to the deltopectoral groove (Fig. 33-13). By raising a subplatysmal flap laterally, one can resect the supraclavicular fat pad and rule out supraclavicular N3 disease. The sternocleidomastoid muscle is freed up inferiorly from the clavicle and manubrium to create a myocutaneous flap, which is then reflected back to yield a full exposure of the neck and the thoracic inlet. Superior mediastinal invasion is assessed by inserting a finger along the lateral aspect of the tracheoesophageal groove. Extension of the tumor into the thoracic inlet is carefully assessed. Resection through this approach requires visualization of the thoracic inlet immediately posterior to the medial clavicle. Dartevelle and colleagues described resection of the medial clavicle. However, medial clavicular resection can result in significant morbidity and limitation of shoulder motion postoperatively. A number of authors have described techniques that preserve the sternoclavicular joint and elevate the entire clavicle from medial to lateral. After resection is complete, the clavicle-sternal unit is rigidly fixed back to the sternum.

Dissection of the Subclavian Vein. Division of the internal, external, and anterior jugular veins makes visualization of the venous confluence at the origin of the innominate vein easier. On the left side, the thoracic duct should be identified, ligated, and divided. Division of the internal jugular vein improves exposure of the subclavian vein. If the subclavian vein is involved, it should be resected after proximal and distal control have been achieved. The phrenic nerve is evaluated and preserved whenever possible. The anterior scalene muscle is then divided either at its insertion on the scalene tubercle of the first rib or well away from the tumor (Fig. 33-14). If the tumor has invaded the superior aspect of this muscle, the muscle should be divided at the insertion on the anterior tubercle of the transverse processes of C3 through C6.

Dissection of the Subclavian Artery. As for the posterior approach, the subclavian artery is mobilized by dividing branches as necessary. The vertebral artery is sacrificed only if involved and provided that no significant extracranial occlusive disease was detected on preoperative Doppler ultrasound examination. Usually the artery can be dissected away from the tumor. If invaded, the artery should be resected and reconstructed as for the posterior approach (Fig. 33-15).

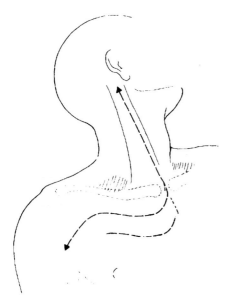

Figure 33-13. Right transcervical incision. The patient is placed in the supine position with the neck hyperextended and the head turned away from the involved side. An L-shaped skin incision is made from the angle of the mandible down to the sternal notch. This is extended horizontally under the internal half of the clavicle and prolonged into the deltopectoral groove or into the bed of the second/third intercostal space, as indicated by the extension of the lesion.

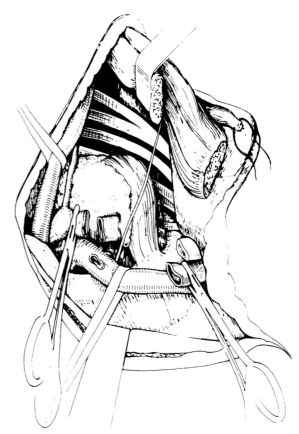

Figure 33-15. The subclavian artery is divided after proximal and distal control is achieved.

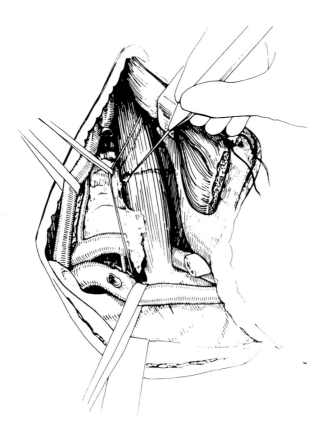

Figure 33-14. After division of the insertion of the anterior scalenus muscle on the scalene tubercle of the first rib, the subclavian artery is exposed. If the phrenic nerve is not invaded it must be preserved.

Dissection of Brachial Plexus. The middle scalene muscle is divided above its insertion on the first rib or higher as indicated by the extension of the tumor. Depending on the extent of the tumor, especially if there is invasion of the middle compartment of the thoracic inlet, the muscle may have to be taken by dividing the attachments to the posterior tubercles of the transverse processes of the second through seventh cervical vertebrae. The nerve roots of C8 and T1 are then easily identified and dissected distally until they coalesce to form the lower trunk of the brachial plexus. Thereafter, the prevertebral muscles are detached along with the dorsal sympathetic chain and stellate ganglion from the anterior surface of the vertebral bodies of C7 and T1. This permits visualization of the intervertebral foramina. The T1 nerve root, if involved, is divided proximal to the tumor at the level of the T1 intervertebral foramen. Although the tumor may extend well superior into the brachial plexus, neurolysis is usually achieved without division of any nerve roots above T1. Damage to the lateral and long thoracic nerves should be avoided to prevent a winged scapula.

Chest Wall Resection. The skeletal chest wall is divided anteriorly. For true anterior lesions, this may require resection of the lateral border of the sternum down to the lowest rib of resection. For lesions more lateral in location, the costal cartilage can be divided from the sternum. The intercostal space is divided laterally and posteriorly well beyond the margins of tumor involvement. The resected ribs are then divided or disarticulated from the spine through tumor-free margins.

Pulmonary Resection. This creates a chest wall defect through which an anatomic upper lobe en bloc resection can be performed. The anterior superior exposure mandates resection from anterior to posterior, that is, on the right division of the superior vein, arterial branches, and bronchus; on the left, superior vein, upper lobe bronchus, and arterial branches. It is rarely necessary to reposition the patient after closure of the anterior wound and complete the lobectomy through a standard posterolateral thoracotomy. However, it is very difficult, if not impossible, to visualize the inferior pulmonary ligament and divide it safely through this anterior superior defect without videothoracoscopic equipment.

Chest Wall Closure. If the medial clavicle is resected, the sternomastoid muscle is fixed to the upper edge of the sternum. An anterior skeletal chest wall prosthesis is advised if the second rib and mandatory if the third rib is included in the resection. Marlex methylmethacrylate, Gore-Tex, and Prolene mesh are useful substitutes. Standard closure and chest drainage is employed.

Hemiclamshell or Trap-Door Incision

The hemiclamshell or trap door incision combines a partial sternotomy and anterior thoracotomy (Fig. 33-16). The patient is positioned supine, usually with the ipsilateral operative side elevated.

Our preference is to begin the procedure with an incision in the inframammary crease and enter the chest through the third intercostal space. An assessment of operability and judgments regarding resectability are then performed. The incision is then extended superiorly through the upper sternum extending along the anterior border of the sternomastoid muscle. The internal mammary arteries are ligated and divided. A retractor or sternal hook is then placed, elevating the chest wall superolaterally. This allows exposure of the upper half of the superior mediastinum and the apex of the thoracic cavity. The superior vena cava and

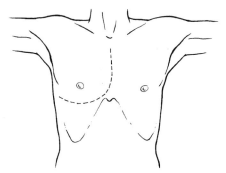

Figure 33-16. The hemiclamshell incision, made with the patient lying supine. (Reprinted with permission from MS Bains, RJ Ginsberg, WG Jones, et al. The clamshell incision: An improved approach to bilateral pulmonary and mediastinal tumors. Ann Thorac Surg 1994;58:30.)

ipsilateral innominate vein are then dissected laterally until the subclavian vein is exposed. The medial clavicle is removed for better exposure of the subclavian vessels and brachial plexus. The involved ribs are divided at the costochondral or costosternal junctions, and the appropriate intercostal space is entered below visible tumor. The posterolateral aspects of the involved ribs are then divided, and the specimen is released within the chest cavity superiorly, remaining attached to the apical fascia. The dissection and management of the subclavian vein, artery, and brachial plexus are similar to those described for the transclavicular approach, and a lobectomy is completed.

Masaoka Incision

The Masaoka incision involves an upper median sternotomy combined with an incision in the anterior fourth intercostal space below and a transverse cervical incision at the base of the neck superiorly (Fig. 33-17). Dissection then proceeds as described.

Surgical Complications and Postoperative Care

The potential complications that may occur after resection of apical lung tumors are similar to those for any major pulmonary resection. There are several complications unique to these resections. A CSF leak, if noted intraoperatively, must be sealed. This may require neurosurgical consultation, foraminotomy, and direct dural repair. If identified postoperatively by clear fluid drainage from chest tubes, aggressive management including re-exploration should be undertaken.

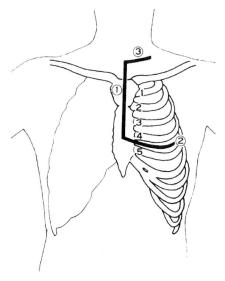

Figure 33-17. The Masaoka approach includes a proximal median sternotomy (1) extending to the fourth anterior intercostal space below (2) and the base of the invaded neck above (3, transverse collar incision). (Reprinted with permission from A Masaoka, Y Ito, T Yasumitsu. Anterior approach for tumors of the superior sulcus. J Thorac Cardiovasc Surg 1979;78:413.)

Consequences of a persistent CSF leak such as subarachnoid or ventricular air embolism and meningitis warrant aggressive management.

The possibility of Horner syndrome and nerve deficits secondary to division of nerve roots should be discussed with the patient preoperatively. Resection of the lower trunk of the brachial plexus (C8 and T1) results in an atrophic paralysis of the forearm and intrinsic muscles of the hand (Klumpke-Déjérine syndrome). This can be a disabling situation for the patient. Hemothorax may occur as the result of chest wall resection along with the difficulty and risks of securing small veins at the level of the intervertebral foramina. Chylothorax is also a possible complication and can be avoided by individual ligation of the thoracic duct and its branches. If chylothorax is identified and persists, aggressive management including thoracic duct ligation is mandatory. If the subclavian vein has been resected, the ipsilateral forearm should be elevated to facilitate venous drainage and minimize edema. The radial pulse must be monitored to assess patency of the revascularized subclavian artery.

Conclusions

Tumors of the superior sulcus are challenging lung cancers to treat because of their close association and often involvement of surrounding structures (brachial plexus, subclavian vessels, or spine). A multimodality approach consisting of induction chemoradiation followed by surgery is the standard for patients deemed preoperatively to have resectable disease. As for any lung cancer resection, negative resection margins have been shown to significantly improve survival. Complete resection is essential. The choice of incision is important. Anterior approaches have allowed complete resections of anterior apical lesions involving the subclavian vessels. Newer techniques of spine resection and stabilization enable complete resection in patients with posterior tumors with vertebral involvement.

SUGGESTED READING

Bains MS, Ginsberg RJ, Jones WG, et al. The clamshell incision: An improved approach to bilateral pulmonary and mediastinal tumors. Ann Thorac Surg 1994;58:30.

Chardack WM, MacCallum JD. Pancoast tumor. Five year survival without recurrence or metastasis following radical resection and postoperative radiation. J Thorac Cardiovasc Surg 1956;31:535.

Dartevelle P, Chapelier A, Macchiarini P. Anterior transcervical approach for radical resection of lung tumors invading the thoracic inlet. J Thorac Cardiovasc Surg 1993;105:1025.

Detterbeck FC. Changes in the treatment of Pancoast tumors. Ann Thorac Surg 2003;75:1990.

Fadel E, Missenard G, Chapelier A, et al. En bloc resection of non–small cell lung cancer invading the thoracic inlet and intervertebral foramina. J Thorac Cardiovasc Surg 2002;123:676.

Gandhi S, Walsh GL, Komaki R, et al. A multidisciplinary surgical approach to superior sulcus tumors with vertebral invasion. Ann Thorac Surg 1999;68:1778.

Grunenwald DH, Mazel C, Girard P, et al. Radical en bloc resection for lung cancer invading the spine. J Thorac Cardiovasc Surg 2002;123:271.

Grunenwald D, Spaggiari L. Transmanubrial osteomuscular sparing approach for apical chest tumors. Ann Thorac Surg 1997;63:563.

Masaoka A, Ito Y, Yasumitsu T. Anterior approach for tumors of the superior sulcus. J Thorac Cardiovasc Surg 1979;78:413.

Pancoast HK. Importance of careful roentgen-ray investigations of apical chest tumors. JAMA 1924;83:1407.

Pancoast HK. Superior sulcus tumors. JAMA 1932;99:1391.

Rusch VW, Giroux DJ, Kraut MJ, et al. Induction chemoradiation and surgical resection for non–small cell lung carcinomas of the superior sulcus: Initial results of Southwest Oncology Group Trial 9416 (Intergroup Trial 0160). J. Thorac Cardiovasc Surg 2001;121:472.

Shaw RR, Paulson DL, Kee JL, Jr. Treatment of the superior sulcus tumor by irradiation followed by resection. Ann Surg 1961;154:29.

Suntharalingam M, Sonett JR, Hass ML, et al. The use of concurrent chemotherapy with high-dose radiation before surgical resection in patients presenting with apical sulcus tumors. Cancer J 2000;6:365.

Tatsamura T, Sato H, Mori A, et al. A new surgical approach to apical segment lung diseases, including carcinomas and inflammatory diseases. J Thorac Cardiovasc Surg 1994;107:32.

EDITOR'S COMMENTS

Can anybody point out the superior sulcus to me? I've never been able to identify this as an anatomic structure, yet the term has persisted. Perhaps it would be better to label these as "apical lung tumors" and recognize that not all apical lung tumors are so-called Pancoast tumors. The important distinction involves the recognition of those apical lung tumors that involve structures in the thoracic inlet so that preoperative chemoradiotherapy can be given, because this regimen has been shown in a large intergroup trial to be associated with improved survival when compared to historical controls. This preoperative regimen has now become the standard of care for these lesions, supplanting the time-honored, but poorly tested, radiation therapy alone given in 30-Gy fractions over a 10-day period. Preoperative radiation therapy had been given for these lesions since the initial description by Shaw and Paulson despite a lack of data demonstrating efficacy.

Diagnosis of these lesions can be difficult, and patients often have been followed for many months with shoulder pain attributed to musculoskeletal problems before a chest radiograph and chest CT scan are obtained. The apex of the lung is a difficult area on the chest radiograph, and this area accounts for a large percentage of lesions missed by radiologists. Persistent shoulder pain in a smoker without a specific inciting cause should be looked at with great suspicion and a chest radiograph and CT scan obtained early. Apical lung lesions are the one area where MRI scans, and especially the coronal reconstructions, have added to our diagnostic capabilities and enhanced our operative planning expertise. MRI provides a significant improvement in our ability to see the brachial plexus as well as the brachiocephalic vessels and at least get a sense of whether there is invasion of these structures.

I agree with the authors' recommendation of sampling the supraclavicular fat pad prior to proceeding with resection, even when this area is not clinically suspicious. PET scanning may point to this area, but because of the close proximity with the primary tumor, it may not be possible to distinguish nodal disease. My preference is to perform a bronchoscopy and mediastinoscopy with supraclavicular fat pad biopsy as a separate procedure before initiating preoperative chemoradiotherapy, because if N2 or N3 disease is present, the "curative" radiation therapy course will differ from that given as a preoperative regimen.

As opposed to the authors, it is my feeling that the anterior cervicothoracic approach through an L-shaped incision along the anterior border of the sternocleidomastoid is the preferred approach for all apical lung tumors including posterior ones. One should keep in mind that the distance between anterior and posterior at the thoracic inlet is only a few centimeters. The anterior approach offers significantly improved access to the brachiocephalic vessels and the brachial plexus and still allows for complete chest wall excision and potentially vertebral body resection. Either the medial portion of the clavicle may be excised or, as we prefer, an oblique osteotomy can be made through the clavicular head and subsequently wired back in place to minimize upper extremity dysfunction. As opposed to the posterior approach, where the rib is disarticulated from the transverse process and then levered off the vertebral body, from the anterior approach the head of the rib is taken first and the neck subsequently separated away from the transverse process. We reserve the hemiclamshell incision for very large upper lobe lesions involving the thoracic inlet, feeling that the cervicothoracic approach works well in most instances. The anatomic pulmonary resection can always be accomplished through the anterior incision.

With respect to some of the smaller technical details, we use bipolar cautery if bleeding is encountered at the level of the neural foramina and avoid any packing with hemostatic material. CSF leaks should be assiduously avoided by careful ligation of the neurovascular bundle prior to division. If a leak is detected, a neurosurgery colleague should be consulted, preferably to directly repair the dural rent and not just "pack" the area. If there is a question of a CSF leak postoperatively, a skull film should be obtained to see whether air is present in the ventricles. With a CSF leak the patient usually will have a headache. Once a leak is demonstrated, a neurosurgeon should be involved. Conservative management involves placing a spinal drain, but as the authors point out, optimal treatment involves taking the patient back to the operating room for a direct dural repair.

L.R.K.

34

Surgery of Pulmonary Mycobacterial Disease

Marvin Pomerantz and John D. Mitchell

Pulmonary mycobacterial infections present a major problem for the thoracic surgeon. Infection with *Mycobacterium tuberculosis* (MTB), a virulent organism, can destroy previously normal lung. The development of resistant organisms, and particularly those resistant to rifampin and isoniazid (multidrug-resistant tuberculosis, MDRTB), represent a major health hazard. MTB and MDRTB are both transmitted by airborne droplets from person to person.

Worldwide there are 3 million deaths from tuberculosis (TB) yearly, and currently approximately 2 billion people harbor the TB organism, although they do not have the active disease. In the United States there were 14,871 cases of tuberculosis in 2003.

There are other mycobacterial infections that are *not* transmitted from person to person, are more indolent, and usually infect previously diseased lung tissue. These organisms as a group have gone through a series of name changes; originally called atypical mycobacteria, then non-*tuberculosis Mycobacterium* (NTM), then *Mycobacterium* other than *tuberculosis* (MOTT), and now environmental *Mycobacterium* (EM). The last-named term seems most appropriate because these mycobacteria are found in the environment, are inhaled, and usually settle in abnormal lung tissue. The most common EM infection is with the *Mycobacterium avian* complex (MAC). This includes infection with *M. avian* and *M. intracellularae*, which are similar infections and hard to distinguish from each other.

Other EM infections include those with *M. chelonae, abscessus, fortiutum, Kansasii, xenopi,* and *malmoense* and a number of other less common organisms.

The incidence and recognition of EM infections is increasing. Each of these infec-

tions has specific drug sensitivities and may also develop resistance. The rapid growers such as *M. abscessus* and *M. chelonae* are difficult to treat medically because there are few antibiotics to which these organisms are sensitive.

As noted earlier, characteristically, EM infections are less virulent and more indolent than infections with MTB and tend to invade hosts with abnormalities of their underlying lung. Once these organisms have established a foothold of infection in the pulmonary parenchyma, they frequently become resistant to available drug therapy and should be treated surgically earlier than is currently the practice.

Diagnostic Considerations and Indications for Surgery

Diagnosis of mycobacterial infection is made by smear and culture. On smears, the acid-fast organisms of MTB and EM appear the same, and therefore the subsequent culture and sensitivity data are critical for appropriate identification. On smears, however, some estimate of the infectious load can be made, and the smear can be used as a rapid method of following the patient's response to treatment. Historically, the field of thoracic surgery was born with surgery for tuberculosis. In the 1960s, however, rifampin was introduced, and this, along with isoniazid, has markedly decreased the need for surgical treatment of tuberculosis. Unfortunately, because of immigration patterns and increases in the numbers of immunocompromised individuals, homeless persons, and crowded prison populations, a ready source for transmission of these organisms has been reestablished.

Standard indications for surgical treatment of tuberculosis include massive hemoptysis (>600 mL in 24 hours), bronchopleural fistula, bronchostenosis, the question of malignancy, and re-expansion of a significantly trapped lung. Currently in the United States, however, the most common indication for operative intervention in tuberculosis is the presence of a multidrug-resistant organism (MDRTB). This means that a specific culture has identified lack of sensitivity to isoniazid, rifampin, and usually several other of the antituberculosis drugs. In surgical cases associated with the presence of organisms in the patient's sputum, there is usually a localized cavity, a destroyed lobe, or a destroyed lung. These findings are usually evident on standard radiographs. However, they are more accurately identified on computed tomographic (CT) scans of the thorax. Preoperative risk assessment involves pulmonary function testing, ventilation-perfusion scanning, and room-air arterial blood gas analysis in addition to routine laboratory evaluation and resting electrocardiogram in patients older than 40 years. Patients who demonstrate no evidence of severe cardiopulmonary limitation by history and physical examination are surgical candidates if the following criteria are met. First, the predicted postoperative forced expiratory volume in 1 second (FEV$_1$) must be >800 mL and preferably >1 liter. Second, there is no evidence on preoperative workup of pulmonary hypertension, specifically a pulmonary artery diastolic pressure of >20 mm Hg or elevated pulmonary vascular resistance. Patterns of disease include localized cavitary disease in the upper lung field, destroyed lobe or destroyed lung, and localized disease in the lingula or the middle lobe, which we have observed in a subgroup of EM patients. In

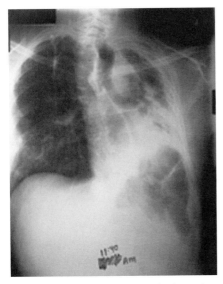

Figure 34-1. A chest radiograph of a patient with a destroyed left lung secondary to multidrug-resistant tuberculosis.

cases of MTB and MDRTB, there appears to be a pattern of selective left lung destruction in that the presentation with total lung destruction is seen twice as often on the left as it is on the right side (Fig. 34-1). In EM patients, this predilection for left lung destruction does not exist. With lobar involvement or cavitary disease, the right upper lobe is the most common region of involvement in both patients with MTB and MDRTB and

patients with EM infections (Fig. 34-2). Patients with EM infections tend to be older than those with MTB, more often are female, and in the United States usually are white. Patients with MTB and MDRTB are younger and are distributed throughout all racial groups.

Perioperative Management

All patients who are considered to be surgical candidates should be placed on culture-specific multidrug regimens for approximately 3 months before surgery. Typically, treated cases of localized tuberculosis that are drug susceptible should respond to a regimen of isoniazid and rifampin for 6 months and pyrazinamide for 2 months. This regimen should result in negative sputum findings usually within 3 months. If sputum positivity remains, the patient likely has MDRTB. The persistence of localized disease in this setting is an indication for surgical resection. Some patients, however, may require resection earlier. Patients who have drug-resistant organisms and a poor response to medical therapy, who have progression of disease on medical therapy, or who have the onset of other tuberculosis-related complications such as massive hemoptysis or bronchopleural fistula should be operated on more urgently.

EM patients responding poorly to medical therapy may need to be referred for surgical intervention sooner than is the current practice. The timing of surgical intervention is extremely important. All of these ground rules have been laid over many years in the medical treatment of tuberculosis. A thoracic surgeon should be involved in the planning of treatment and be aware that it might be necessary to altering the timing of surgery.

Another important factor in perioperative management is the nutritional resuscitation of these often cachectic, nutritionally depleted patients. This can be extremely difficult because of the catabolic wasting nature of the disease. We have found that several interventions are extremely helpful in this regard. It is often necessary to establish a secondary source of alimentation. Frequently these patients are unable to orally ingest a sufficiently large caloric load, and therefore, there should be supplementation via feeding tubes. If need be, parenteral nutrition is used to supplement the enteral route. For the stimulation of appetite, megestrol acetate (Megace) has been used along with human growth hormones and anabolic steroids. The goal in nutritional resuscitation is to achieve an albumin level of >3.0 g/dL and an anabolic state. All patients are preoperatively instructed in incentive spirometry, use of the acapella valve, coughing, and deep breathing.

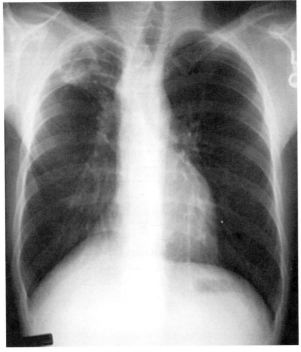

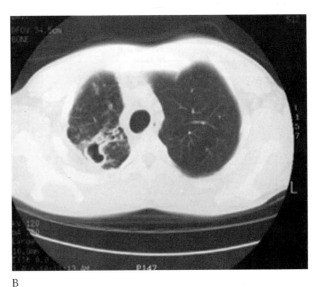

Figure 34-2. **(A)** A chest radiograph of a patient with cavitary disease of the right upper lobe secondary to multidrug-resistant tuberculosis. **(B)** A computed tomographic scan of the same patient.

Operative Technique

After the induction of anesthesia, patients are intubated, and a fiberoptic bronchoscope is used to inspect the bronchial anatomy. Critical information at this stage is the presence or absence of copious secretions and the occasional presence of tuberculous bronchitis at the proposed site of bronchial division, which poses a significant hazard to bronchial healing and would either mitigate against proceeding or require a change in the planned level of resection. After bronchoscopy is completed, the single-lumen tube is replaced with a double-lumen endobronchial tube placed into the left main bronchus with bronchoscopic verification. Patients with limited pulmonary or cardiac reserve should have a pulmonary artery catheter inserted. Inhalational anesthesia is used and is supplemented by epidural narcotic for perioperative infusion or an intrathecal dose of narcotic. Subsequently, the patient is placed in a full lateral thoracotomy position. Because of the length of these procedures, careful attention to appropriate positioning and padding of pressure points is essential.

The approach is through a standard posterolateral thoracotomy. Patients with bronchopleural cutaneous fistulas or previously created Eloesser flaps have these openings incorporated into the incision if they are in the appropriate location. The usual approach is through the fifth intercostal space. Patients with extensive disease usually have a contracted hemithorax; therefore, rib resection is often necessary for adequate exposure. The serratus muscle is preserved, being retracted anteriorly, and the latissimus muscle is elevated and preserved if it is to be used as a muscle flap to cover the bronchial stump. Subsequently, the appropriate plane of dissection is entered. Mycobacterial infections usually produce extensive adhesions between the visceral and parietal pleurae. Dissection, therefore, often must be done extrapleurally. This is especially true with cavitary disease, a completely destroyed lung, or when a completion pneumonectomy is being undertaken. In this situation, several points of dissection must be accomplished with care to avoid injury to mediastinal and intrathoracic structures. Specifically, when dissecting posteriorly and approaching the esophagus and the azygos vein, care must be taken to avoid injury to these structures. Similarly, in the apex of the chest, the subclavian vessels must be carefully avoided when approaching them bluntly through the extrapleural plane. Finally, in the anterior

region and around the heart, care must be taken to avoid injury to the mammary artery and the heart itself. In addition, injury can occur to the recurrent laryngeal nerves during blunt mobilization in the extrapleural plane.

In mycobacterial surgery, muscle flaps are frequently used. Indications for the use of a muscle flap include a positive sputum for mycobacteria at the time of surgery, the presence of a bronchopleural fistula, hemithorax polymicrobial contamination, and the anticipation of a residual postoperative space after lobectomy. The muscle flap of choice is the latissimus dorsi. This muscle is freed from its extensive origin on the lower thoracic, lumbar, and sacral spine, and the posterior iliac crest to its insertion on the intertubercular groove of the humerus (Fig. 34-3). The thoracodorsal artery, which is the blood supply to the latissimus dorsi muscle, must be preserved during the dissection toward the insertion site. After complete mobilization of latissimus dorsi, the inferior portion is divided with electrocautery to complete the mobilization. Subsequently, if necessary, a 2- to 3-cm portion of the anterior second or third rib is exposed and removed with care to avoid the intercostal vessels (Fig. 34-4). After resection is

completed, the latissimus dorsi muscle is passed into the hemithorax through the space defined by removal of this piece of rib and is sutured to the bronchial stump and hilar area with the remaining latissimus muscle used to fill as much space as possible and as needed (Figs. 34-5 and 34-6). In some patients with a thin latissimus muscle, it can be passed through the intercostal space without rib resection. Use of serratus anterior muscle is discouraged because it introduces the morbidity of a winged scapula, which frequently interferes with healing of the posterior aspect of the thoracotomy wound in these usually thin patients. In cases in which the latissimus dorsi muscle is not available, because it has been divided during a previous thoracotomy, a pedicle of gastrocolic omentum based on the right gastroepiploic artery is harvested. The omentum may be harvested with the patient supine before positioning in the lateral decubitus position. The omentum is our bronchial stump coverage of choice in patients with EM infections who require a right pneumonectomy because of the high incidence of bronchial stump dehiscence in these patients. It is theorized that the highly vascular omentum may promote healing in these situations. We also prefer to use the omentum after

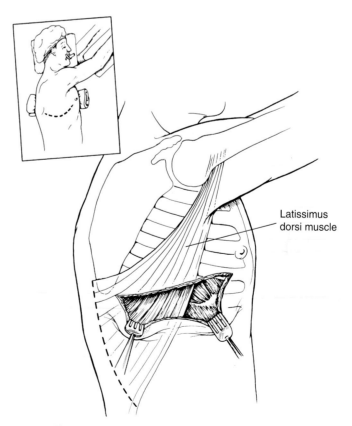

Figure 34-3. Outline of the latissimus dorsi muscle.

Latissimus dorsi muscle

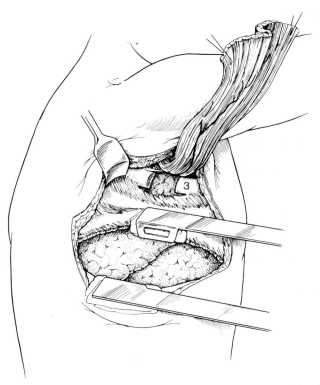

Figure 34-4. Mobilized latissimus dorsi muscle with resection of a portion of the third rib.

pneumonectomy in cases of massive intrathoracic contamination from tuberculosis or polymicrobial superinfection.

Usually the most difficult portion of the operation is the pleural and extrapleural dissection to free the lung from the thoracic cavity along its entire circumference. However, the hilum often is free of dense adhesive scarring and can be approached readily when performing a pneumonectomy. In

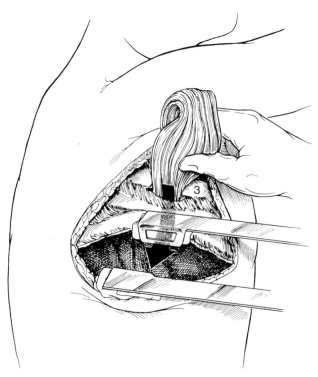

Figure 34-5. The latissimus muscle being passed into the chest.

some cases of completion pneumonectomy in patients who have had prior resections for tuberculosis or EM infections, the hilum may be encased by dense adhesions. This may necessitate an intrapericardial approach to the pulmonary vessels such that safe proximal control of these vessels is achieved. During a right upper lobectomy for tuberculosis in which the fissure is extremely adherent and dissection of the branch vessels in the fissure is difficult, it is often easier to resect the right upper lobe from a posterior approach, dividing the bronchus to the lobe before arterial division.

After the resection is completed, the pleural cavity is irrigated copiously with warm saline solution containing antibiotic. Because of the general poor nutritional status of these patients, wound closure demands strict attention to detail. Multiple pericostal sutures are placed. Muscle layers are approximated with absorbable braided suture (size 0), the subcutaneous tissue is approximated with 2-0 suture, and the skin is closed with a running subcuticular absorbable suture. Before emergence from anesthesia, all patients should again undergo bronchoscopy specifically to remove secretions that may have accumulated during the procedure, which may contaminate the uninfected bronchial orifices.

As with other major thoracic surgical procedures, aggressive postoperative respiratory care is mandatory. It is essential for patients undergoing resections for mycobacterial infections to have precise fluid replacement intraoperatively and postoperatively. These procedures are longer and more laborious than routine lobectomy or pneumonectomy for cancer. Therefore, it is possible for patients to receive too much fluid intraoperatively or perioperatively. This may be a particularly dangerous situation because the onset of postresection pulmonary edema in these infected patients is a highly morbid complication. All lobectomy patients older than age 50 years receive prophylactic digoxin, as do all pneumonectomy patients older than age 40 years. The digoxin is discontinued either at discharge or after 6 weeks in the absence of arrhythmias or signs of left ventricular failure. In the presence of arrhythmias or heart failure, the digoxin is continued for 3 months, and the patient is re-evaluated at that time. Some surgeons prefer the use of beta-blockers and/or calcium-channel blockers rather than digoxin. Hard data are difficult to come by regarding the best drugs to use postoperatively.

In 2001, we reported on 172 patients with MDRTB undergoing 180 pulmonary

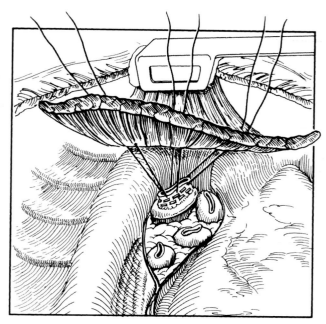

Figure 34-6. The latissimus muscle being sutured to the right mainstem bronchus after a pneumonectomy.

resections. Operative mortality was 3.3% and late mortality was 6.8%. Only 2% of the patients remained sputum positive postoperatively compared to 50% preoperatively. In 2004, Chan et al. reviewed the same group of patients and compared the results to a previous series treated at the National Jewish Medical and Research Center without surgery. Statistical improvement was found for the series treated with surgery (plus medical therapy) and among older patients treated with fluoroquinolones.

In 2003, Iseman et al. extensively reviewed the current status of patients infected with EM. The increasing patient population with EM infections makes this report important not only for medical doctors, but also for surgeons.

Surgical Complications and Postoperative Care

Mortality after resection in patients with mycobacterial disease should be <5%. Morbidity, however, is common, with bronchopleural fistula the most serious complication. Factors that predispose to fistula formation are the presence of mycobacteria in the sputum at the time of surgery, previous chest irradiation, extensive polymicrobial superinfection, and a previous thoracotomy. Furthermore, bronchial stump dehiscence after pneumonectomy is more common on the right side in the setting of EM infections

than in resections for tuberculosis. If this occurs initially, drainage of the hemithorax must be achieved to control infection and limit spillage to the remaining lung. Patients with limited pulmonary reserve and airway embarrassment from a large bronchopleural fistula often need intubation of the left mainstem bronchus when the right stump has dehisced. Patients must then be evaluated for the presence of ongoing infection and treated appropriately. Usually, the stump dehiscence occurs late (>6 weeks) after the resection, making the success of closing the stump in an immediate trip back to the operating room unlikely. An Eloesser procedure may be required, and after this procedure, the hemithorax can be packed with gauze lightly soaked in half-strength diluted sodium hypochlorite solution (Dakin's solution). This both controls the bronchopleural fistula and treats the infection until definitive closure can be done.

After the space infection is controlled, the bronchopleural fistula may be closed in several ways if the fistula does not close with drainage alone. Further resection can be carried out if less than a pneumonectomy was done, or the stump can be closed by a variety of methods if a pneumonectomy was performed. The bronchus can be approached through a trans-sternal approach between the aorta and the superior vena cava and division of the posterior pericardium. With this approach, the distal bronchus must be separated from the new staple or suture line and preferably removed. In such a

reoperation for bronchial dehiscence, it is preferable to cover the bronchial stump with a viable flap. The first choice for coverage is the omentum. Muscle transposition is another possibility if enough muscle tissue is available. Thoracoplasty is reserved for failure of all these techniques, although its use in combination with muscle flap transposition may be useful in certain cases.

Other complications after resection that can occur postoperatively include empyema without bronchopleural fistula, recurrent laryngeal nerve injury, wound infections, postpneumonectomy pulmonary edema, and bleeding, which occurs more commonly in this patient population because of the extensive adhesions in the hemithorax. Postpneumonectomy pulmonary edema usually occurs 2 to 5 days postoperatively and carries a mortality of >50%. Accordingly, it is recommended that fluid administration be limited to <1,500 mL/day for the first 5 postoperative days. Strict attention should be paid to intake and output, and nutritional supplementation should be given in the early postoperative period. The treatment of postoperative empyema without fistula is similar to that carried out when a fistula is present. After pneumonectomy and after initial tube drainage, an open-window thoracostomy (Eloesser) is performed, packing is carried out for 4 to 6 weeks, antibiotics are instilled, and the window is closed (Clagett procedure). This time course represents the ideal; many of these patients require prolonged drainage via the open-window thoracostomy.

Conclusion

In summary, surgery for tuberculosis in the United States is primarily for MDRTB associated with cavity formation, with destroyed lung, and with or without positive sputum. Similar indications are used when evaluating patients with EM infections. EM patients also have a more relapsing chronic type of disease, and after right pneumonectomy there is a high incidence of bronchopleural fistula. The complications after surgery in these patients are higher when there is positive sputum, a previous thoracotomy, chest irradiation, or polymicrobial contamination, and the patient's nutritional status is borderline. When there is localized disease, surgery for MDRTB produces a better cure rate when combined with adequate antibiotic therapy for up to 2 years than if the MDRTB is treated with antibiotics alone. It is recommended that in MDRTB and EM patients, muscle and omental flaps be used liberally for the reasons noted. It is important to use nutritional supplementation in these patients, and it is recommended that surgery be performed early in the course of the disease in many EM patients, before they develop more advanced disease, which makes resection more complex and is associated with a higher incidence of complications.

SUGGESTED READING

Bates JH, Nardell E. Institutional control measures for tuberculosis in the era of multiple drug resistance. Chest 1995;108:690.

Brown JM, Pomerantz M. Extrapleural pneumonectomy for tuberculosis. Chest Surg Clin North Am 1995;5:289.

Chan ED, Laurel V, Strand MJ, et al. Treatment and outcome analysis of 205 patients with multi-drug-resistant tuberculosis. Am J Respir Crit Care Med 2004;169:1103.

Dye C, et al. Global burden of tuberculosis estimated incidence prevalence and mortality by country. JAMA 1999;282:677.

Iseman MD, DeGroote M. Environmental Mycobacterium (EM) Infections. In Gorbach SL, Bartlett JG, Blacklow NR (eds), Infectious Diseases (3rd ed). Philadelphia: Lippincott Williams & Wilkins, 2003.

Iseman MD, et al. Pectus excavatum and scoliosis: Thoracic anomalies associated with pulmonary disease due to M. avian complex. Am Rev Respir Disease 1991;144:914.

Pomerantz BJ, Cleveland JC, Olson HK, et al. Pulmonary resection for multi-drug resistant tuberculosis. J Thoracic Cardiovasc Surg 2001;121:448.

Pomerantz M. Surgery for pulmonary infections with Mycobacterium other than tuberculosis (MOTT). Chest Surg Clin North Am 1993; 3:737.

Pomerantz M, et al. Resection of the right middle lobe and lingua for mycobacterial infections. Ann Thoracic Surg 1996;62:990.

Pomerantz M, Madsen L, Goble M, et al. Surgical management of resistant mycobacterial tuberculosis and other mycobacterial pulmonary infections. Ann Thorac Surg 1991;52:1108.

Reichman LB. Time bomb: The global epidemic of multi-drug resistant tuberculosis. New York: McGraw-Hill,2002.

Treasure RL, Seaworth BJ. Current role of surgery in Mycobacterium tuberculosis. Ann Thorac Surg 1995;59:1405.

EDITOR'S COMMENTS

To reiterate what I stated in the last edition, there is no one with more experience in dealing with these difficult problems than Dr. Pomerantz, and all of us can greatly benefit from his wisdom and experience. For most thoracic surgeons, mycobacterial disease represents only the occasional case, which in the mind of most is a good thing, I presume. However, when confronted with a patient with MDRTB who has indications for operation, the points Drs. Pomerantz and Mitchell make are extremely important. First, they update us on terminology. Just a couple of years ago we referred to the cause of non-tuberculous mycobacterial infections as MOTT, or Mycobacterium other than tuberculosis. Now the more appropriate term is EM, or environmental Mycobacterium, which more appropriately takes into account their source of origin.

Surgeons undertaking these cases should be forewarned that they usually are difficult and time consuming, and several points should be underscored. Patients should be on drug therapy before operation, although the time course of treatment varies and there is no well-established time for the duration of such therapy. Nutritional repletion is of the utmost importance, and we usually place either a percutaneous endoscopic gastrostomy tube or jejunostomy tube for a prolonged period of enteral feeding. Timing of the operation is also important, and the authors make the point that earlier, rather than later, operative intervention is preferred. The use of muscle flaps greatly adds to these procedures, and the authors are very clear as to why the latissiumus dorsi muscle is preferred to the serratus anterior muscle. A pedicle of gastrocolic omentum also finds great utility, and this may be harvested with the patient in the lateral decubitus position, which avoids the need to change position, as the authors recommend. The omentum is brought into the chest via a substernal route, and then directed through the pleural reflection into the appropriate pleural space. Use of the omentum can be combined with a muscle flap as well.

Because of the difficulty of the resection, we strongly recommend gaining proximal control of the pulmonary artery before attempting a lobectomy in these patients. This may involve intrapericardial dissection of the artery to safely accomplish this, depending on the extent of adhesions and fibrosis at the hilum. Especially on the right side, pericardium should not be excised, if at all possible, so that primary closure of the pericardium can be accomplished, avoiding the need for prosthetic material in a chest where infection is a distinct possibility.

The authors recommend prophylactic digoxin for these patients, especially those undergoing pneumonectomy. Attempts at prophylaxis of postoperative arrhythmias mostly have proven ineffective, with the exception of rate control when atrial arrhythmias occur. Digoxin in most centers is not the drug of choice; we prefer a beta-blocker or amiodarone.

I predict that this chapter will frequently be consulted by those who are faced with the occasional pulmonary resection in this group of patients.

L.R.K.

II

Adult Cardiac Surgery

A

General Considerations

35

Cardiopulmonary Bypass

Harry A. Wellons, Jr. and Richard K. Zacour

Cardiopulmonary bypass is a remarkably flexible tool when properly used by the surgical team, including the cardiac surgeon, anesthesiologist, and perfusionist. All three must be experienced and knowledgeable in their understanding of the physiology of cardiopulmonary bypass, its risks and limitations, and the potential injuries that may result from its misuse.

A written protocol for the use of cardiopulmonary bypass is established for the treatment of each major category of acquired and congenital cardiovascular disease. Standardization is important for efficiency and safety. These protocols are developed collaboratively, and any deviation from a protocol should be based on the needs of the individual patient and agreed to by all three team members.

If the surgeon is to realize the full advantage of cardiopulmonary bypass, he or she must have knowledge of the perfusion circuit in use at that institution. This includes priming solutions, speed and ability to vary perfusate temperature, maximum and minimum flow rates, and available cannula sizes.

There must be prior agreement among surgeon, anesthesiologist, and perfusionist on the chain of command and the sphere of responsibility of each member in the operating theater as well as concise, professional, and open communication.

Developing a Plan

Before each procedure, the surgeon must develop a plan for conducting the operation, especially the use of cardiopulmonary bypass. Although it is unnecessary for the perfusionist or the anesthesiologist to know the technical surgical details, it is critical that he or she understands the planned incisions, methods of cannulating the heart and great vessels, the systemic and myocardial temperatures desired, the possible need for low flow or circulatory arrest, and any anticipated pathologic or anatomic variations that may require alterations in the plan. The site of placement of a monitoring line may be controlled by the procedure such as use a radial artery as a graft.

It is advantageous for the surgeon to think through the entire operation before arriving in the operating room. This intellectual exercise begins by considering the critical elements of the operative procedure, which will determine the anatomic exposure required. For example, repair or replacement of the mitral valve requires maximum exposure of the right lateral part of the heart and the interarterial groove; although neither the ventricles nor the left side of the heart need to be elevated, they must be able to collapse into the left chest. On the other hand, aortic valve replacement can usually be performed with simple aortic cannulation and minimal manipulation or dissection of the ventricles. In general, coronary bypass requires exposure of all surfaces of the ventricles. Adequate exposure will be achieved by dissecting and freeing the cardiac structures from the pericardium, appropriately suspending the pericardium, and selecting and placing cannulas for perfusion and decompression of the heart. The operative plan will include the steps for myocardial protection and an estimate of the myocardial and systemic temperatures required for the specific operation.

Finally, there should be a mental review of "what if...," including potential anatomic variants and potential catastrophic events. Examples of anatomic variants might include mitral regurgitation with a heavily calcified posterior mitral annulus requiring a longer and more complex operation with additional steps to protect the myocardium, a persistent left superior vena cava accompanying an atrial septal defect, or a tetralogy of Fallot with a variant coronary artery crossing the right ventricular outflow tract. Potential catastrophic events should be reviewed frequently because they occur suddenly, and all members of the surgical team must be prepared to deal with them rapidly and precisely. Catastrophic events during reoperative surgery are obvious and include unexpected right ventriculotomy or aortotomy before cardiopulmonary bypass. Other catastrophic events include ventricular fibrillation before the heart has been exposed or rupture of the ascending aorta as the pericardium is opened in a patient with a type I dissecting aneurysm.

Preparation

From the time the patient arrives in the operating room, a member of the surgical team should be present. The anesthesiologist is responsible for induction of anesthesia, endotracheal intubation, and the placement or insertion of most monitoring devices. Only under extreme circumstances should a patient undergo induction of anesthesia before an adequate peripheral intravenous line and a stable electrocardiographic display have been established. In patients who are hemodynamically unstable, direct arterial pressure measurement should be established and a pulmonary artery catheter inserted before the induction of anesthesia.

Positioning the Patient

After all monitoring lines have been placed, the patient is positioned and pressure points padded to prevent pressure necrosis. All monitoring cables and lines are secured to prevent displacement or disconnection during the operation. Exposure will be through a median sternotomy in the majority of operations, which requires that the sternum be parallel to the operating room floor and the patient's arms placed at his or her side to avoid brachial plexus injury. This is achieved by placing a padded roll beneath the patient's shoulders and a padded ring under the head. In the occasional case in which a right anterior thoracotomy may be desired, the right chest is elevated 30 degrees with the patient's right arm at the side.

Skin Preparation and Draping

After the patient is positioned properly and all monitoring devices are secured, a protective screen is placed at the head of the table to support the sterile drapes. This is positioned to allow easy exposure of the entire operative field without interfering with the movements of the surgeon and first assistant. The neck, chest, abdomen, and both groins (and, for coronary artery bypass, both lower extremities) are treated with a two-solution preparation, and drapes are placed around the operative fields. For every open-heart operation, it is prudent to prepare and drape the groins to permit rapid institution of cardiopulmonary bypass before the sternum is opened, should it become necessary, or to permit insertion of additional monitoring lines or an intra-aortic balloon.

The height of the operating room table is adjusted so the surgeon's wrists are 1 cm to 3 cm below the elbows while operating. The assistants adjust their position and elevation to accommodate the surgeon. The operating room lights are positioned slightly above and behind the surgeon's left side if he or she is right-handed. The pump and cell-saving equipment are brought into position and the pump lines are passed to the field. The pump lines are located such that the operative field and the surgeons are unhampered, and the lines should be secured in a standard manner so that even excessive force cannot displace them. Inexperienced members of the team are instructed not to touch or compress the lines.

Incisions

The selection of the incision site for exposure and cannulation of the heart is based on considerations of safety, exposure, and cosmesis. Anatomic and pathologic variations, such as a large ascending aortic aneurysm pressing against the sternum or severe pectus excavatum in which the entire heart is displaced to the left chest, may require careful planning to avoid catastrophe. Obviously, variations in the incision to achieve cosmesis must not compromise safety or adequate exposure.

The pericardium is opened in the midline from its reflection on the aorta down to the diaphragm. The pericardium is released from the diaphragm with a transverse incision, with care being taken to avoid entering the pleural space. At this point, consideration is given to the specific exposure that will be required for the operation. Heavy silk sutures are placed in the cut edges of the pericardium and tied to the presternal fascia on the ipsilateral side of the incision to elevate and stabilize the appropriate cardiovascular structures.

Cannulation

The pericardial reflections on the aorta are freed to allow identification of the origin of the innominate artery. The cannulation site will be just proximal to the innominate artery and slightly to the left of the midline. In adults, two opposing purse-string sutures are used. The diameter of the area of the aorta enclosed by the inner purse-string suture should be 1 1/3 times the outer diameter of the tip of the cannula. The purse-string sutures for adults are double-armed, 3-0 monofilament polypropylene with a single polytetrafluoroethylene (Teflon) felt pledget. Each needle takes three bites of aorta, penetrating to the media but not the lumen of the aorta. The first double-armed suture is placed from left to right, and the needles are left clamped in their needle holders. The second suture is placed from right to left, and after the third bite of the aorta, each arm is passed through the Teflon felt of the opposite suture (Fig. 35-1). The two needles from the other purse string are now passed through the opposite felt pledget. The needles are cut, and the sutures drawn through tubing to form a "tourniquet." In children weighing <30 kg, a single circular purse-string suture of 4-0 polypropylene without felt pledgets is placed in the ascending aorta just proximal to the innominate artery. The diameter of this single circular purse-string suture is 1 1/3 times the external diameter of the tip of the arterial cannula

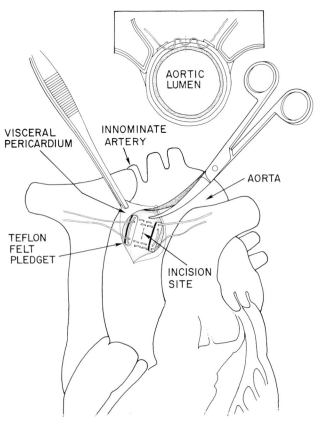

Figure 35-1.   Preparing an adult ascending aorta for cannulation.

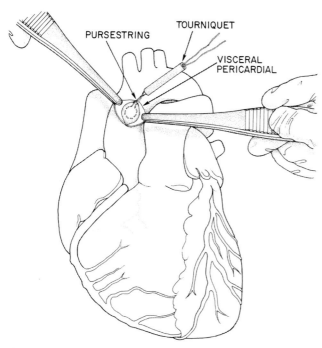

Figure 35-2. Preparing an infant or pediatric aorta for cannulation.

(Fig. 35-2). If the vena cavae are to be cannulated separately, the purse-string suture for the inferior cannula is placed first. This is a simple circular purse-string suture placed laterally and just above the inferior vena cava. The diameter should be 1 1/3 times the diameter of the tip of the venous cannula to be used. This purse-string suture will be placed laterally in the crista terminalis, and the needle should not enter the lumen of the atrium. The purse-string suture for the superior vena caval cannula is most easily placed in the atrial appendage using the same principles and dimensions.

At this point, the surgeon prepares to inject heparin into the right atrium through the purse-string suture in the atrial appendage. Before injection, it is important to draw back the plunger and observe blood entering the syringe. The standard heparin dose will vary among practices and needs; however 300 units per kilogram of patient body weight is satisfactory for most patients. However, heparin activity is patient specific and may vary if underlying coagulation defects are present.

Confirmation of systemic anticoagulation is achieved by performing an activated clotting time (ACT). This test measures heparin activity, which plays a more significant role in anticoagulation management than heparin concentration. Whereas the normal baseline ACT is between 86 and 147 seconds, the optimal range for cardiopulmonary bypass has not been defined.

We prefer to maintain ACTs between 400 and 600 seconds because ACTs of <180 seconds are dangerous and ACTs of >600 seconds are unnecessary (Table 35-1).

While awaiting circulation of the heparin and retrograde cardioplegia is planned, a smaller purse-string suture of 4-0 polypropylene is placed slightly anteriorly and inferiorly in the right atrium for the retrograde cardioplegia cannula. The inter-arterial groove on the right side of the heart

Table 35-1 Anticoagulation Management Protocol

Add 4 U of beef lung heparin per milliliter of the pump prime to the cardiopulmonary bypass circuit.

The surgeon injects 300 U of beef lung heparin per kilogram of patient body weight into the right atrium.

An uncontaminated whole-blood sample is drawn 3–5 mins after heparin injection for an activated clotting time (ACT) measurement.

The ACT must be >2.5 times the baseline ACT before initiating cardiopulmonary bypass, and must be maintained at >480 secs during cardiopulmonary bypass.

The ACT should be monitored every 20 mins during normothermic cardiopulmonary bypass, every 30 mins during hypothermic cardiopulmonary bypass, and more frequently if the patient shows heparin resistance.

is dissected in the area of the superior pulmonary vein. A 3-0 polypropylene purse-string suture is then placed at the junction of the right superior pulmonary vein and left atrium for insertion of a vent to decompress the left ventricle.

When an adequate activated clotting time is confirmed, the anesthesiologist lowers the blood pressure to facilitate aortic cannulation. With scissors and forceps, the visceral pericardium is cleared from the area of the aorta enclosed by the purse-string sutures, clearly exposing the aortic adventitia (Fig. 35-3). In adults, cannulation of the aorta is accomplished by the following sequence: A No. 15 scalpel is passed into the aorta within the inner purse string while the cannula is held in the other hand, with the tip pressing against the aorta immediately adjacent to the scalpel. The scalpel is then advanced to create an incision parallel to the flow of the blood, the length of which equals the diameter of the cannula, and the cannula is insinuated into the aorta as the knife is withdrawn. The incision must be the diameter of the cannula to avoid the need for mechanical dilation, which can result in tearing of the aortic wall. The cannula must be inserted into the incision perpendicular to the flow of blood to ensure direct entry of its tip into the lumen of the aorta without dissection or fraying of the intima. As soon as 2 mm to 5 mm of cannula has entered the aorta, the angle of insertion is changed to be parallel with the flow of blood, and the cannula is advanced to the full length to be inserted. When using a soft-tipped cannula, the length of cannula inserted must be 25% to 30% longer than the diameter of the aorta to prevent the tip from migrating proximally into the ascending aorta; however care must be taken to avoid passage of the cannula into an arch vessel (Fig. 35-4).

As soon as the cannula is in place, the tourniquets on the purse-string sutures are drawn tight. With a longer soft-tipped cannula, the tip should lie on the inner curve of the aortic arch and extend only slightly beyond the pericardial reflection. This can be confirmed by gentle palpation of the inner curve of the aorta where it exits the pericardium. The cannula is secured by a heavy silk tie incorporating the cannula and the proximal tourniquet, de-aired, and attached to the arterial pump line.

In infants and young children, the aorta is cannulated with a wire-wound, thin-walled cannula (Fig. 35-5). The aorta within the purse string is cleared of its visceral pericardium to expose the aortic adventitia, and the assistant, using two fine-tipped forceps, grasps the visceral pericardium on each side

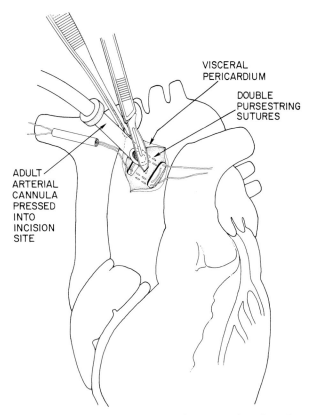

Figure 35-3. Incision of an adult ascending aorta and insertion of a soft aortic cannula.

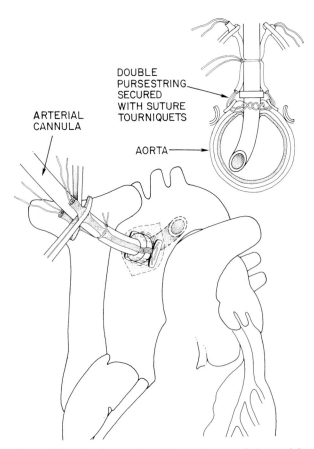

Figure 35-4. The final position of the aortic cannula in an adult.

of the purse string. The surgeon, using a scalpel with a No. 11 blade, makes an incision equal in length to the diameter of the cannula. As the scalpel is withdrawn, the assistant presses the cut edges of the aorta together to prevent bleeding. When the surgeon is ready, the forceps are parted, and the aorta is raised to give counterpressure as the surgeon inserts the cannula, entering the aorta at a right angle to the direction of blood flow and tilting the external cannula inferiorly as he or she advances it the equivalent of 1 1/3 times the aortic diameter (Fig. 35-6). The position of the cannula is confirmed by palpation to be sure it has not entered the innominate artery and that the tip lies on the inner curve of the aortic arch just distal to the pericardial reflection. The purse-string suture is drawn tight in its tourniquet and secured to the cannula with a heavy ligature. After the aortic cannula has been de-aired and connected to the arterial pump line, it is secured to the drapes to avoid undue tension.

When both venae cavae are to be cannulated, the inferior cannula is inserted first. The assistant places traction on the right atrium, anteriorly and medially, to expose the inferior purse-string suture. The surgeon, using a No. 15 scalpel blade, makes an incision within the purse string by inserting the scalpel inferiorly and drawing it superiorly. The scalpel is withdrawn and inserted a second time at a right angle to the previous incision to produce a cruciate opening (Fig.35-7). The cannula is now easily inserted and guided laterally and posteriorly to avoid the Eustachian valve and hepatic veins. This cannula should be positioned so that the side holes will be no more than 1 cm distal to an occluding caval tourniquet. Cannulation of the superior vena cava or insertion of a single cannula is performed through the atrial appendage, the tip of which is incised, and the trabeculations within the appendage divided (Fig. 35-8). If both venae cavae are cannulated, the superior cannula is positioned with its side holes above the caval-occluding tourniquet. If a single, two-stage venous cannula is used, it is inserted through the purse-string suture, and the first stage is guided into the inferior vena cava. The cannulas are secured to their tourniquets in the same way as for the arterial cannula (Fig. 35-9).

In infants and young children, venous cannulation is performed by modifying commercially available thin-walled, wire-wound cannulas. For double caval cannulation, the unwired portion of the tip is trimmed to provide two proximal side holes and an oblique bevel. Insertion techniques

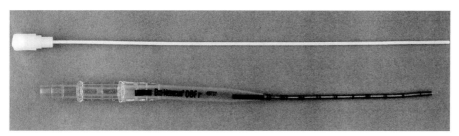

Figure 35-5. A wire-wound pediatric aortic cannula and obturator. This is an 8-F cannula. Because of the thin wall, it will permit flow rates of 800 mL/min and is adequate for patients weighing as much as 5.0 kg.

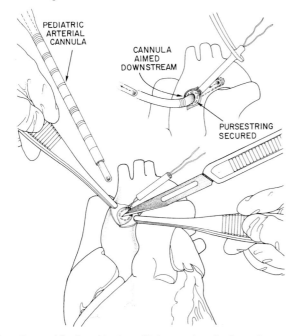

Figure 35-6. Insertion and final positioning of infant and pediatric aortic cannulas.

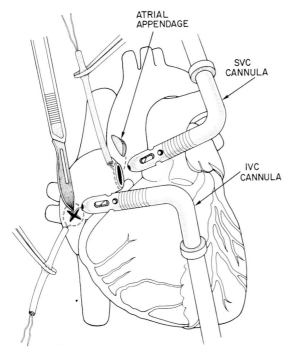

Figure 35-7. Double venous cannulation. (IVC = inferior vena caval; SVC = superior vena caval.)

are similar to those for adults (Fig. 35-10). When a single venous cannula is to be used in infants, it is modified to leave four side holes and is inserted so that only the tip lies in the orifices of the inferior vena cava to provide free drainage of the right atrium. A retrograde cardioplegia cannula is more easily inserted after placement of the venous cannulas but before cardiopulmonary bypass is instituted. The previously placed anterior mid-right atrial purse string is exposed and an appropriate incision made. The cannula should have a slight curve, and the surgeon places a palpating finger just beneath the inferior vena cava to facilitate insertion. The cannula is secured to its tourniquet, the pressure-measuring line is connected to the document an appropriate waveform, and the cannula is de-aired.

If a left ventricular vent is needed, it is inserted before cardiopulmonary bypass. The anesthesiologist performs a Valsalva maneuver to elevate the left atrial pressure. An incision is made in the purse-string suture at the juncture of the right superior pulmonary vein and left atrium, and the fluid-filled cannula is immediately inserted. The cannula should have a curve that forms nearly a right angle and should be aimed with its tip hugging the anterior atrial surface and directed toward the left ventricular apex. Except in mitral stenosis, it will pass immediately into the left ventricle in its appropriate position, which can be confirmed by signs of pulsatility within the cannula or by a palpating hand in the oblique sinus.

When antegrade cardioplegia is used, a small purse-string suture is placed in the proximal ascending aorta, and the cannula is inserted and secured. All pump lines are inspected for security and placement (Fig. 35-11). All clamps are removed from the arterial lines and cannulae unless two venous cannulae are used, in which case one cannula remains clamped until cardiopulmonary bypass is instituted. This is because frequently there is a small amount of air in the venous lines, and if both are unclamped, differential pressure between the inferior and superior vena cava would permit air embolus.

Alternate Arterial Cannulation

In some cases where cannulation in the aortic arch may not be feasible, such as aortic dissection of the ascending aorta and aortic arch or large aneurysms involving the arch, it may be necessary to place a graft on

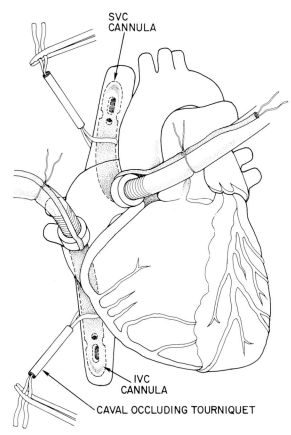

Figure 35-8. The final position for double cannulation. Note that the side holes must be distal to the vena caval tourniquets. (IVC = inferior vena caval; SVC = superior vena caval.)

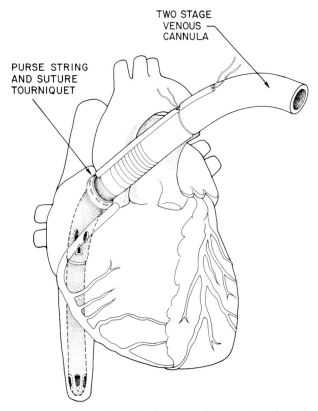

Figure 35-9. Single venous cannulation. The "two-stage" construction places drainage ports in the right atrium and the inferior vena cava.

the right axillary artery through which the arterial line may be connected or to consider retrograde cannulation of a femoral artery.

The axillary artery is exposed through a short infraclavicular incision. The underlying pectoralis muscle is divided and the axillary artery is mobilized with care to avoid injury to the adjacent brachial plexus. A segment of the artery is isolated between vascular clamps, and an 8-mm longitudinal incision is made in the vessel. A short 8-mm graft is sewn into place with a running 5-0 polypropylene suture. The arterial cannula is then inserted into the graft and fixed into place with a heavy silk ligature. After bypass is discontinued and the patient is stable, the arterial cannula is removed and the graft transected, leaving a small cuff that is closed with a running suture.

For femoral cannulation, an incision is made just below the inguinal ligament, and the common femoral artery is mobilized. The superficial femoral and profunda femoris arteries are encircled at their origin for distal control. For proximal control and to fix the cannula in place, an umbilical tape is passed around the femoral artery and drawn through a tourniquet. After a proximal vascular clamp is applied, a transverse arteriotomy is made, through which an appropriate-sized cannula is inserted in a retrograde manner. The tourniquet is tightened just enough to achieve hemostasis and secured to the cannula with a heavy silk ligature. On completion of cardiopulmonary bypass the cannula is removed and the arteriotomy closed with a 5-0 or 6-0 polypropylene suture.

Cardiopulmonary Bypass Circuit

The basic principle of cardiopulmonary bypass management is to minimize the patient's metabolic adaptation to a nonphysiologic state, a state of "controlled shock." To accomplish this, the perfusionist must meticulously prepare the extracorporeal circuit and manage the dynamic characteristics of cardiopulmonary bypass (Fig. 35-12).

The circuit design and the selection of the arterial and venous cannulas are based on the calculated blood flow rate necessary to provide hemodynamic support and gas exchange (Table 35-2). The arterial cannula tip is the narrowest component of the extracorporeal circuit and creates high-resistance, high-pressure gradients and turbulence. The cannulas are described by either French size or diameter in millimeters (mm), which reflects only the external dimensions, not

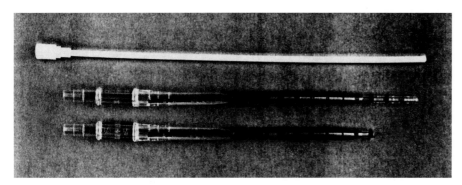

Figure 35-10. A thin-walled venous cannula for infants and children. The tip of the cannula is removed from the lower cannula so that only two side holes remain distal to the wire reinforcement.

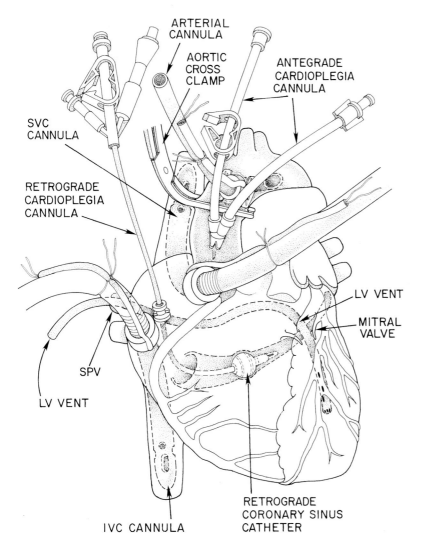

ARTERIAL CANNULA

AORTIC CROSS CLAMP

ANTEGRADE CARDIOPLEGIA CANNULA

SVC CANNULA

RETROGRADE CARDIOPLEGIA CANNULA

LV VENT

MITRAL VALVE

SPV

LV VENT

RETROGRADE CORONARY SINUS CATHETER

IVC CANNULA

Figure 35-11. Completed cannulation for total cardiopulmonary bypass. The left ventricular venting catheter has been inserted adjacent to the right superior pulmonary vein (SPV). The retrograde cardioplegia catheter is in the coronary sinus. The antegrade cardioplegia catheter is in the ascending aorta proximal to the aortic occluding clamp. (IVC = inferior vena caval; LV = left ventricle; SVC = superior vena caval.)

the internal diameter or performance characteristics. Although flow characteristics and pressure drops can be calculated for straight tubing, cannula performance characteristics discredit these calculations because of varying lengths, the presence of side holes, curves, or irregular diameters. These factors, along with ratio of internal diameter to external diameter (ID/OD), need to be considered when selecting a cannula. A pressure gradient across an arterial cannula should not exceed 100 mm Hg at full flow.

The performance characteristics of venous cannula are even more vital than those of the arterial cannula because blood flow through the extracorporeal circuit depends on the venous return, which may be either passive or "assisted." Although passive venous return is the more traditional method, and is dependent on gravity, the height of the operating table above the venous reservoir, and large-bore tubing, "assisted" venous return is achieved by applying a vacuum to the venous line or reservoir.

"Assisted" venous return provides some advantages over the traditional venous drainage, such as permitting smaller venous cannula, tubing, and incisions and lowering the priming volume; however it also offers a disadvantage, a potential increase in gaseous microemboli if the vacuum is too great and the reservoir volume is too low to allow proper dissociation. Because of this concern, we limit the amount of vacuum to less than −60 mm Hg and prefer to maintain a venous reservoir volume at or greater than 1,000 mL. Regardless of which method is utilized, venous return will be reduced if the side ports of an oversized venous cannula are obstructed by an overstretched vein, or if the internal diameter of the venous cannula is too small to accommodate the expected blood flow, overdistention of the right heart or flooding of the operative field will occur. A proper venous cannula will have a pressure gradient of <30 mm Hg, and will not allow an excessive negative pressure to develop (the ideal venous pressure should be at or slightly above 0 mm Hg). The patient's size determines the design of the extracorporeal circuit and the priming volume (Tables 35-3 and 35-4).

The degree of hemodilution may be calculated before bypass is initiated, and if the expected priming volume would cause an "unacceptable" anemia, packed red blood cells may be added to the extracorporeal circuit (Table 35-5):

Hemodilutional hematocrit (hct) (%) =

$$\frac{\text{Patient blood volume} \times \text{wt (kg)} \times \text{hct (\%)}}{[\text{Patient blood volume} \times \text{wt (kg)}] + \text{priming volume (mL)}}$$

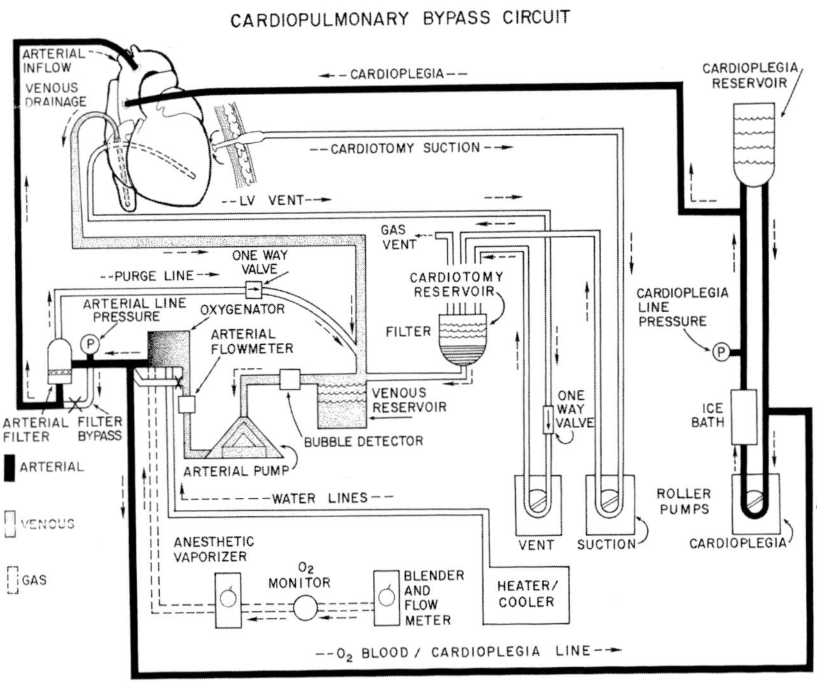

Figure 35-12. Example of a complete cardiopulmonary bypass circuit. (LV = left ventricle; P = pressure transducer.)

Hemodilution provides an advantageous effect for perfusion by decreasing viscosity and augmenting blood flow. One deleterious side effect of hemodilution is the reduction of oncotic pressure, which results in tissue edema. There is an inverse relationship between tissue edema and colloid oncotic pressure, and when albumin or mannitol is added to the extracorporeal circuit to obtain an oncotic pressure of 16 mm Hg, extracellular fluid accumulation is reduced. Although blood flow reflects the interaction of many influences, hemodilution aids to negate those inherent effects by diminishing blood's viscosity and resistance to flow and promotes increased microcirculatory flow and tissue perfusion.

Hypothermia also influences blood rheology and vascular geometry. A decrease in temperature provokes direct vasoconstriction and increases viscosity, creating sludging and stasis at the capillary level, and a reduced blood flow. These effects are counteracted by hemodilution.

Is there an "acceptable" degree of hemodilution? It is common to see hematocrits of 18% to 21% during cardiopulmonary bypass, and even extreme hemodilutional hematocrits of <15% are well tolerated when used for circulatory arrest cases or for patients who are Jehovah's Witnesses. A general rule of thumb is that the hematocrit in percent should not exceed the desired level of hypothermia in degrees Celsius.

Instituting Cardiopulmonary Bypass and Decompressing the Left Heart

Cardiopulmonary bypass is begun at the instruction of the surgeon. Visual inspection of the field, monitors, and bypass lines as the perfusionist initiates cardiopulmonary bypass will provide an immediate assessment of the conversion. After confirming the surgeon's instruction, the perfusionist initiates cardiopulmonary bypass by releasing the arterial line clamp and slowly transfusing the patient with the volume. The arterial blood flow of the extracorporeal circuit should be free-flowing and exhibit a reasonable extracorporeal line pressure. A sudden spike in the extracorporeal line pressure may indicate an occluded arterial line, a malpositioned aortic cannula, or an aortic dissection. Should this occur, cardiopulmonary bypass is terminated immediately and the cause identified and corrected.

As soon as it is obvious that arterial flow is unobstructed, the perfusionist releases the venous clamp, diverting the patient's venous blood into the cardiopulmonary bypass circuit. The right heart should be decompressed and the central venous pressure should be <5 mm Hg. A high central venous pressure and poor venous drainage at the initiation of cardiopulmonary bypass may indicate a malpositioned venous cannula, a kinked venous line, an "air-lock," venous cannulas that are too large or too small, an inappropriate height between the operating table and the venous reservoir, an inappropriate amount of vacuum, or a vacuum leak.

During this transition period of 1 to 2 minutes, the perfusionist gradually increases the rate of arterial flow, the ventricles receive less blood, and the pulsatile arterial waveform diminishes and becomes "flat-lined." Once total bypass is achieved, a continued pulsatile arterial waveform signifies that the left ventricle is receiving unwanted blood from aortic insufficiency, excessive bronchial venous return, or incomplete drainage of the systemic venous return.

An acute, transient state of systemic arterial hypotension, resulting from hemodilution and vasoactive substance release, is common on the initiation of cardiopulmonary bypass. Treatment with alpha-agonists is usually not necessary to overcome this acute state because the mean arterial pressure will generally increase with the initiation of systemic cooling (due to its induced vasoconstriction) and increased levels of endogenous catecholamines and angiotensin.

The arterial pressure during total cardiopulmonary bypass is a mean or "flat-line" pressure unless an artificial means is used to general pulsatile flow. The mean pressure should be viewed as an index of the relationship among blood flow, volume, and arteriolar resistance and not as a measure of perfusion adequacy. Although the subject

	1. Blood Flow Rate (BFR; in liter/		**2. Blood Flow Rate**
Age (yrs)	**min per m² from Body Surface Area (BSA, in m²)**	**Body Weight (kg)**	**(in mL/min per kg) from from Body Weight (in kg)**
0–2	BSA × 2.6	0–5	150
2–4	BSA × 2.5	6–10	125
4–6	BSA × 2.4	11–15	100
6–9	BSA × 2.3	16–25	90
>9	BSA × 2.2	>25	70

Table 35-2   Two Methods for Calculating "Full" Blood Flow Rates

Table 35-3	Required Inside Tubing Diameter for Different Patient Weights		
Patient Weight (kg)	Arterial Line (in.)	Venous Line (in.)	Vacuum-Assisted Venous Line (in.)
<8	1/4	1/4	1/4
8–17	1/4	3/8	3/8
17–50	3/8	3/8	3/8
>50	3/8	1/2	3/8

Removal of Air from the Heart

of much debate, an "acceptable" mean arterial pressure ranges from 35 to 90 mm Hg. However, in the presence of known coronary artery stenosis or ventricular hypertrophy, a perfusion pressure of 60 to 80 mm Hg should be maintained. In general, if the systemic vascular resistance index and mixed venous blood gases are normal, the resultant mean arterial pressure is "acceptable."

In patients with severe aortic regurgitation, the surgeon should be ready to cross-clamp the ascending aorta if ventricular fibrillation occurs. If the heart continues to beat, the left atrium should not be entered until the aorta has been cross-clamped to prevent embolization of air to the brain. In children and infants with congenital heart disease, the right heart should not be opened until the aorta is cross-clamped or ventricular fibrillation has occurred. However, decompression of the left ventricle is best achieved in infants and small children by tightening the vena cava tapes, opening the right atrium, and passing a small suction line through the patent foramen ovale into the left ventricle. If the foramen is not patent, a small stab wound will permit this approach.

The perfusionist can begin cooling the perfusate to induce hyperthermia once full flow and adequate decompression are established. The primary advantage of hypothermic cardiopulmonary bypass is the reduced metabolic rate and oxygen consumption; although not linear, this approximates 5% to 7% per degree Celsius. In addition, hypothermia sustains intracellular reservoirs of high-energy phosphates (essential for cellular integrity), and preserves high intracellular pH and electrochemical neutrality (a constant OH^-/H^+ ratio). As a result of these associated interactions, hypothermic patients can survive periods of circulatory arrest of up to 1 hour without suffering from the effects of anoxia (Table 35-6).

Hypothermia may be induced by surface cooling using cooling blankets and ice packs applied directly to the patient or by core cooling with cold perfusate from the extracorporeal circuit. Because tissues and organs have varying blood flows, systemic cooling is not a uniform process. To minimize this, we combine the two methods, maintain high perfusion flow rates of 2.2 to 2.5 liters/min/per m^2, and limit the rate of the cooling to <1 degree Celsius per minute until the desired temperature is reached. Thereafter, perfusion flow rates are adjusted to maintain "normal" mixed venous blood gases. Bladder and nasopharyngeal temperatures are monitored to ensure uniform temperatures.

Systemic rewarming is instituted by gradually increasing the perfusate temperature. Rewarming is slower than cooling because of the maximum permissible temperature gradient of 10 degrees Celsius between perfusate and nasopharyngeal temperatures, the maximum allowable blood temperature of 42°C, and the reduced thermal exchange as the temperature gradient between the patient and perfusate narrows. During this state, the warming blanket is set to 40°C, the perfusion flow rates are increased to 2.5 to 3.0 liters/min/per m^2, and, pressure permitting, pharmacologic vasodilation is used. When the bladder temperature reaches 32°C, the patient begins to vasodilate spontaneously and the pharmacologic vasodilator may be terminated.

With the aorta cross-clamped, the patient is placed in a 30-degree head-down position, the caval tourniquets are loosened, and the perfusionist restricts venous return to the pump. The right heart begins to fill, and the anesthesiologist ventilates the lungs. The heart is gently massaged while the vent in the left ventricle continues drain. The antegrade cardioplegic cannula is placed on suction, and, as more blood is massaged through the left heart, some air appears in the cardioplegic cannula. After all air appears to have been evacuated, the balloon of the retrograde cardioplegic cannula is deflated, pump flow is reduced to one half of calculated flow, arterial pressure is reduced to 50 mm Hg, and the aortic cross-clamp is removed while suction is maintained on the antegrade cardioplegic cannula. Transesophageal echocardiography is used to determine whether there is residual air within the heart. If there is, the operating table is rocked from side to side, the left atrial appendage is inverted, and gentle massage of the heart is continued. The heart is defibrillated when all air has been evacuated. Venous return is restricted intermittently to allow the heart to eject. Suction on the intracardiac vent is discontinued, and suction is maintained on the aortic cardioplegic/vent cannula as the heart continues to eject. When echocardiography confirms that the left heart is free of air, the operating table is restored to a level position and the aortic cardioplegic/vent cannula and the retrograde cardioplegic cannula are removed.

Appropriate postoperative monitoring lines are inserted, and, if indicated, temporary pacing wires are sutured to the right ventricle and the right atrium. Rewarming is continued until the nasopharyngeal temperature is 37°C and the bladder temperature is >36°C; this usually takes 3 to 5 minutes per 1°C increase.

Termination of cardiopulmonary bypass is performed gradually, with constant communication among surgeon, perfusionist, and anesthesiologist. Because the heart cannot generate a cardiac output until the central blood volume is restored, the perfusionist progressively occludes the venous return line, translocating blood volume from the venous reservoir into the patient's vascular system. The patient is now on "partial" cardiopulmonary bypass, with blood flowing through the heart and pulmonary circulation. When the blood volume in the heart reaches an adequate level, the aortic

Table 35-4	Priming Volume per Length of Tubing of Given Diameter	
Tubing Diameter (in.)	Priming Volume (mL/ft)
3/16	5.00
1/4	9.65
3/8	21.71
1/2	38.61

Table 35-5	Patient Blood Volume
Age	Blood Volume (mL/kg)
Premature	100
Newborns	90
1–12 mos	80–85
1–10 yrs	75–80
Adult	70–75

Table 35-6   Definition of Levels of Hypothermia and Approximate "Safe" Circulatory Arrest Times

Hypothermia Level	Patient Temperature (°C)	Circulatory Arrest Times (mins)
Mild	37–32	5–10
Moderate	32–28	10–15
Deep	28–18	15–60
Profound	>18	60–90

valve begins to open with each heart beat, and a measurable cardiac output will be observed. The translocation of volume is continued until the arterial systolic pressure reaches 100 mm Hg. The perfusionist then terminates cardiopulmonary bypass by completely occluding the venous and arterial lines. Thereafter, the perfusionist transfuses volume to the patient to maintain a systolic blood pressure of 100 mm Hg unless the heart becomes distended.

If the heart does not function effectively when cardiopulmonary bypass is terminated, bypass is reinstituted to prevent overdistention or hypoxia. If the heart functions appropriately with hemodynamic stability, decannulation can begin. If two venous cannulas were used, the inferior venacaval cannula is removed, and the purse-string suture is tied. The superior cannula is removed, and the tourniquet is drawn tight. A few minutes is allowed to confirm hemodynamic stability and adequate cardiac function. Transesophageal echocardiography will confirm that the repair is complete and myocardial function is adequate. Two chest tubes are inserted: a flat chest tube behind the heart in the oblique sinus (in infants this is performed using a flat, 10-mm–wide Jackson-Pratt catheter cut to the appropriate length) and a round chest tube is placed in the anterior mediastinum. If the pleural envelopes are opened, the anterior mediastinal tube is omitted and a round tube is placed in each pleural space entered. When it is time to reverse the heparin with protamine, all pump suctions are turned off, and the anesthesiologist is instructed to administer one third of the total calculated dose of protamine. Under no circumstances should shed blood be returned to the extracorporeal circuit once protamine is introduced into the patient's circulation. If there has been no hemodynamic instability from this dose of protamine after 5 minutes, the arterial cannula is removed from the aorta. In adult patients with two purse-string sutures, both are removed from their tourniquets. The surgeon supports the arterial line while the assistant places the first overhand throw in the purse-string suture on his or her side. When the arterial cannula is removed, the first purse-string is tied and held in position for hemostasis. The surgeon takes the purse-string on his or her side and ties this firmly. The assistant then completes tying the other purse-string suture. Once all protamine has been administered and the patient is stable, the purse-string suture on the right atrial appendage is tied and, if necessary, reinforced with a second suture. Thereafter, final hemostasis and surgical closure of the wound are performed according to protocol.

Acknowledgment

We thank our mentor and friend, Dr. Stan Nolan, because the original chapter as the basic description has not changed appreciably and represents the current practice at our institution.

SUGGESTED READING

Castaneda AR, Jonas RA, Mayer JE Jr, et al. (eds). Cardiac Surgery of the Neonate and Infant. Philadelphia: Saunders, 1994.

Castheely PA, Bregman D (eds). Cardiopulmonary Bypass: Physiology, Related Complications, and Pharmacology: Mount Kisco, NY: Futura, 1991.

Gravlee GP, Davis RF, Utley JR (eds). Cardiopulmonary Bypass—Principles and Practice. Philadelphia: Lippincott Williams & Wilkins, 2000; Chs 3–7.

Kaplan JA. Cardiac Anesthesia (3rd ed). Philadelphia: Saunders, 1993.

Kirklin JW, Barratt-Bowes BG (eds). Cardiac Surgery (3rd ed). Philadelphia: Churchill Livingstone, 2003.

Mora CT (ed). Cardiopulmonary Bypass—Principles and Techniques of Extracorporeal Circulation. New York: Springer-Verlag, 1995.

Reed CC, Kurusz MA, Lawrence AE Jr (eds). Safety and Techniques in Perfusion. Stafford, TX: Quali-Med, 1988.

Thys DM (ed). Textbook of Cardiothoracic Anesthesiology. New York: McGraw-Hill, 2001.

EDITOR'S COMMENTS

The authors carefully analyzed the techniques of cardiopulmonary bypass and focused on those uses at the University of Virginia. All cardiac surgeons must know this subject thoroughly. There are many variations in how cardiopulmonary bypass is provided. One's team must have a consistent approach. The versatile surgeon must have multiple alternative cannulation techniques, particularly in the face of a calcified ascending aorta or in terms of complex reoperative surgery. Percutaneous femoral cannulation approaches have been important to us for minimally invasive operations or in situations or some reoperations. Another technique that I think should become more available is the technique taught to us by the Cleveland Clinic, which is the use of suction venous drainage. There seems to be little if any more morbidity associated with it. It also provides for truly excellent drainage and avoids air locks.

I.L.K.

36

Myocardial Protection

Constantine L. Athanasuleas and Gerald D. Buckberg

This chapter reviews current concepts regarding myocardial protection during cardiac procedures. We provide the rationale of our strategy and describe the methodology of our approach in detail.

The strategies available for myocardial protection have led to adversarial positions regarding warm versus cold blood cardioplegia, antegrade versus retrograde delivery, and intermittent versus continuous perfusion. This creates confusion and deprives the patient of the benefits of each method. Cardioplegia markedly reduces oxygen demand in the arrested heart and must be delivered in sufficient quantity to all regions to match this low demand (Fig. 36-1). This has led to the use of antegrade and adjunct retrograde delivery, cold methods to reduce demands allowing bloodless visualization, and warm perfusion for resuscitation.

Our "integrated method" is a strategy of myocardial protection that combines the advantages of different concepts. It allows the operation to be conducted without interruptions. This method (1) provides unimpaired vision, (2) avoids unnecessary ischemia and cardioplegia overdose, and (3) permits aortic unclamping and discontinuation of bypass shortly after cardiac repair.

Electromechanical activity during cardiac arrest raises oxygen demand during ischemia. Hypothermia is a crucial component of myocardial protection because it reduces electromechanical activity (Fig. 36-1). Blood cardioplegia is now preferred by most surgeons because of its versatility. It maintains oncotic pressure, is a natural buffering agent, has advantageous rheologic properties, and is a free-radical scavenger. Blood cardioplegia also limits reperfusion injury and reverses ischemia/reperfusion changes in the acutely ischemic myocardium. These beneficial features may not be possible with crystalloid cardioplegia.

Noncardioplegia methods have been applied in special situations. For example, when a severely calcified aorta is encountered, the preferred technique is deep hypothermic arrest (approximately 20°C) without aortic clamping. Saphenous vein or arterial conduits can be attached to the innominate or mammary artery.

Cold Blood Cardioplegia

Cold blood cardioplegia allows complete myocardial recovery after 4 hours of ischemia in normal hearts. Normal preoperative function, however, is rare. Hypothermia lowers myocardial oxygen demand and ischemic damage when coronary flow is interrupted in the course of the revascularization procedure, provided the cardioplegic perfusate is distributed adequately with reinfusions. Hypothermia alone, however, does not avoid injury in chronically "energy-depleted" (ischemic) hearts (Fig. 36-2). Furthermore, hypothermic crystalloid cardioplegia adds some disadvantages, such as shifting the oxyhemoglobin association curve leftward, retarding Na^+/K^+ adenosine triphosphatase to produce edema, and activation of platelets, leukocytes and complement. Blood cardioplegia consists of four parts of blood to one part of crystalloid solution. This limits the hemodilution seen with crystalloid cardioplegia during repeated infusions.

Warm Blood Cardioplegia

Warm blood cardioplegia (37°C) given initially (induction) limits reperfusion damage in ischemic hearts. It enhances metabolic repair by channeling aerobic adenosine triphosphate production to reparative processes. Other cardioplegic components, citrate phosphate dextrose (CPD) and buffers (THAM [tromethamine; tris-hydroxymethyl aminomethane]), limit calcium influx and acidosis. Clinical studies confirm our experimental findings and show that warm blood cardioplegia ("hot shot") after ischemia improves recovery. Warm cardioplegic induction and reperfusion solutions are augmented with the amino acids glutamate and aspartate to replenish key Krebs-cycle intermediates depleted by ischemia. These additions enhance the reparative processes after a period of myocardial ischemia (Fig. 36-2B).

Warm (37°C) cardioplegia may also be used after aortic unclamping to restore rhythm and improve hemodynamics in the unstable patient following cardiac surgery. When used for impaired hemodynamics, the left ventricle is vented to reduce demands, and antegrade flow is given for 10 to 20 minutes. We have observed marked rhythm and hemodynamic improvement after witnessed cardiac arrest of up to 120 minutes with this approach.

Multidose Cardioplegia

Multidose cardioplegia infusions are used because noncoronary collateral flow from mediastinal collaterals displaces cardioplegia with warmer systemic blood. Topical hypothermia slows rewarming but may cause pulmonary complications (phrenic palsy) without supplementing the cardioprotective effects. Multidose cardioplegic reinfusions with buffers and low ionized calcium

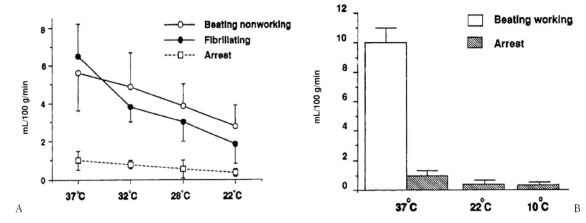

Figure 36-1. **(A)** Left ventricular oxygen requirements of beating nonworking, fibrillating, and arrested hearts from 37°C to 22°C. Note the lowest requirements during arrest. **(B)** The left ventricular oxygen requirements of a beating working and an arrested heart at 37°C, 22°C, and 10°C. Note in panel A the low oxygen demands of arrest and in panel B the negligible change between 22°C and 10°C as the heart rewarms from collateral flow. Panel B shows higher demands than panel A if electromechanical activity recurs when systemic perfusate washes out the cardioplegic solution

may limit reperfusion damage. Delivery at 10- to 20-minute intervals maintains arrest and restores substrates depleted during ischemia. Intraoperatively, adequate distribution of cardioplegia is noted as the dark blood that returns into the aorta during retrograde cardioplegia becomes red 1 to 2 minutes after infusion. Hyperosmolarity counteracts edema and may enhance myocardial compliance postoperatively.

Antegrade/Retrograde Perfusion: Alternating or Simultaneous?

A cardioplegic perfusate is effective only if it is well distributed. Adding retrograde perfusion improves subendocardial perfusion, avoids ostial cannulation during aortic valve procedures, limits removals

of retractors during mitral procedures, and permits flushing of air and atheroma during coronary reoperations. Transatrial coronary sinus cannulation allows safe and rapid retroperfusion into the coronary sinus and is used by the majority of surgeons worldwide. Experimentally, right ventricular nutritive flow appears limited, but hypothermia lowers oxygen demand. Clinical studies show that switching from

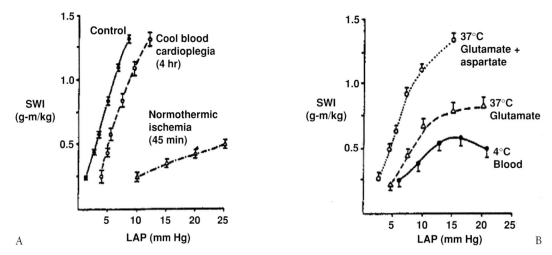

Figure 36-2. **(A)** Left ventricular function in normal hearts subjected to 4 hours of aortic clamping with cardioplegia with blood every 20 minutes compared with depressed function after 45 minutes of normothermic arrest without cardioplegia. The type of protection is more important than the duration of aortic clamping. **(B)** Left ventricular function when jeopardized hearts undergoing 45 minutes of normothermic ischemia are subjected to 2 more hours of aortic clamping. Note (1) no further improvement when only cold cardioplegic perfusate is given over the 45-minute arrest period and (2) progressively increased recovery when the cardioplegic solution is supplemented with warm glutamate and aspartate during induction of cardioplegia and reperfusion with intermittent cold doses of blood every 20 minutes of supplemental aortic clamping. These data suggest the value of amino acid enrichment in jeopardized hearts. (LAP = left atrial pressure; SWI = stroke work index.)

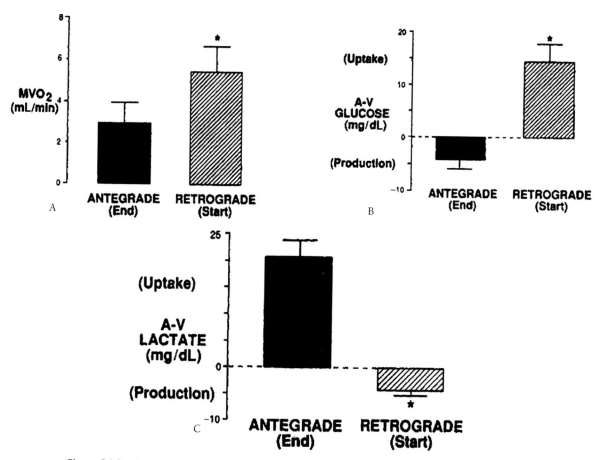

Figure 36-3. Myocardial metabolic changes in coronary patients when administration of the cardioplegic induction solution is converted from antegrade to retrograde. Note the increase in myocardial oxygen uptake (MVO2), glucose uptake, and lactate production, suggesting different areas of perfusion by the antegrade and retrograde methods of delivery. This implies an advantage to both methods. (A-V = arteriovenous.)

antegrade to retrograde perfusion increases oxygen uptake and lactate washout, indicating that each mode perfuses different areas. Therefore, both antegrade and retrograde perfusion are required (Fig. 36-3).

The limitations of antegrade and retrograde delivery were first overcome by *alternating* between antegrade and retrograde perfusion, but recent studies show that combined benefits are possible by *simultaneous* delivery of retrograde cardioplegia via the coronary sinus and antegrade cardioplegia via direct ostial or vein graft infusion. Myocardial venous hypertension is prevented by drainage through the Thebesian veins. Studies document the safety of simultaneous vein graft and coronary sinus perfusion, especially in high-risk patients.

Intermittent/Continuous Infusion

Continuous cardioplegic perfusion has been advocated to avoid ischemia by antegrade or retrograde delivery, but adequate protection may not be achieved at usual flow rates, and vision becomes obscured during infusion. A quiet/dry field requires "intentional" ischemia by intermittently stopping the flow of cardioplegic solution. Intermittent replenishment restores hypothermia, flushes accumulated metabolites, and counteracts acidosis and edema. Initially, the heart is arrested with high-dose potassium (20 mEq/liter) blood cardioplegia (Table 36-1), and multidose low-dose cold potassium (8 to 10 mEq/liter) blood cardioplegia (Table 36-2) is used for intermittent doses. Reinfusions are delivered even if no electromechanical activity occurs. Such reinfusions are retrograde in mitral procedures, and via the right coronary ostia each 15 minutes in aortic procedures during simultaneous retrograde perfusion. Initially, continuous retrograde perfusion with cold noncardioplegic blood (approximately 10°C) may be an adjunct when vision is not a problem (e.g., during proximal grafting of graphs to the aorta). A noncardioplegic

blood solution (approximately 10°C) that contains CPD, THAM, magnesium, and mannitol (Table 36-3) is used when vision is not a problem. Cold blood with a hematocrit of approximately 20% is infused at a pressure of <35 mm Hg. However, intermittent cardioplegic infusion is given at least every 15 minutes to prevent electromechanical activity. At the completion of the cardiac procedure, all hearts receive a dose of warm cardioplegia ("hot shot"), administered first antegrade and then retrograde. This is followed by a continuous infusion of warm blood into the aortic root while the cross-clamp is still in place at a flow of 300 to 350 mL/min and with pressure ≤80 mm Hg. The aortic clamp is released within 5 minutes after adequate contractility is observed.

Single Period of Aortic Clamping

Coronary bypass grafting is the most common cardiac operation, and the risk of

Table 36-1   Warm Blood Cardioplegia Solution

Cardioplegia Additive	Volume Added (mL)	Component Modified	Concentration Delivered[a]
Potassium chloride (2 mEq/mL)	15	Potassium ion	16–20 mEq/liter
Tromethamine (0.3 mole/liter)	225	pH	pH 7.5–7.7
Citrate-phosphate-dextrose	225	Calcium ion	0.2–0.4 mmol/liter
Aspartate, glutamate	250	Substrate	13 mmol/liter each
50% Dextrose in water	40	Glucose	<400 mg/dL
5% Dextrose in water	200	Osmolarity	380–400 mOsm

[a]When mixed in a 4:1 ratio with blood.

intraoperative cerebral atheroemboli is increased among elderly patients undergoing revascularization. Atheroemboli are more likely after repeated aortic tangential clamping for proximal anastomoses. The use of single aortic cross-clamping has been avoided by some because of a concern that this method extends the ischemic time. There is evidence that morbidity and cost are reduced despite a longer aortic clamp time when the aforementioned protective strategies are employed. These findings contradict the axiom that there is a constant battle against the clock when the aorta is clamped. The extent of cardiac damage is related to *how* the heart is protected rather than *how long* the clamp is in place. Blood cardioplegia provides sufficient cardiac nourishment during aortic clamping to contradict the belief that aortic clamping and the period of ischemia are synonymous.

Clinical Applications

Loop showed the advantages of blood cardioplegia in a report from the Cleveland Clinic on more than 3,300 patients. The method of myocardial management we

use incorporates warm/cold blood cardioplegia, antegrade/retrograde delivery, and blood/cardioplegic perfusate during a single period of aortic clamping for all procedures.

Cannulas and Devices for Delivering and Monitoring Antegrade/Retrograde and Simultaneous Antegrade/Retrograde Cardioplegia

All operations include use of a cardioplegic heat exchanger for cold and warm perfusion (Fig. 36-4), cannulas for antegrade and retrograde delivery, and a monitoring-infusion system. The system we use is shown in Fig. 36-5. The three controls are placed in a triangle for ready access:

1. A stopcock, which switches between antegrade and retrograde infusion. Attached to these infusion lines are smaller ones that measure infusion pressures.
2. A flow clamp to activate the aortic vent.
3. A flow clamp on the tubing attached to the retrograde infusion line, which controls infusion of cardioplegia through the vein graft or through a handheld infusion catheter placed into the coronary

ostia during aortic valve procedures (Fig. 36-5). Additional lines can be attached to either the antegrade or retrograde lines (Fig. 36-6).

Antegrade Cannula

An antegrade cannula is placed high in the right ascending aorta. This site is not used as a proximal graft site. A 3-0 mattress suture with a tourniquet is used to secure the cannula and is tied at the end of the procedure. The cannula contains a pressure line and vent port to suction air and blood between infusions. After commencement of cardiopulmonary bypass the heart should empty, as indicated by collapse of the pulmonary artery, indicating good systemic venous drainage. The aorta is clamped, and antegrade cardioplegia is delivered for 2 minutes at a rate of 200 mL/m with pressure flow to exceed 70 mm Hg. Flow rate is decreased if this pressure is exceeded. It is increased by 50 to 75 mL/m if hypertrophy is present. Additional antegrade cardioplegia is delivered through saphenous vein graft introducers or into the aortic root after a proximal vein graft anastomosis is completed. In uncomplicated coronary operations we do distal/proximal anastomoses in sequence, although tangential clamping is used in many centers. All proximal grafts may also be done last while the aorta is vented. The vent is clamped after flow is initiated to exclude trapped air in the antegrade cannula. During proximal grafting, low active suction through a "pop-off" valve (approximately 175 mm Hg) or gravity keeps aortic flow to just below the suture line to avoid collapsing the aorta and drawing air into it. Cold continuous blood is concomitantly infused retrograde at a rate of 150 mL/min and is suctioned out of the ascending aorta. The antegrade catheter is intentionally placed slightly below the anterior surface of the aorta to avoid having blood in the field of the anastomosis.

Retrograde Cannula

Transatrial approaches permit coronary sinus cannulation without right heart isolation. Cannulation is performed after venous cannulation and takes 10 to 15 seconds. We use a malleable stylet and self-inflating balloon cannula and introduce it anterior to the two-stage venous cannula. A low atrial incision with a 3-0 mattress suture is first placed. We retract the atrioventricular groove superiorly and to the left to reduce intra-atrial redundancy and avoid intraoperative displacement. The suture is secured through a tourniquet.

Table 36-2   Cold Multidose Blood Cardioplegia Solution

Cardioplegia Additive	Volume Added (mL)	Component Modified	Concentration Delivered[a]
Potassium chloride (2 mEq/mL)	10	Potassium ion	8–10 mEq/liter
Tromethamine (0.3 mole/liter)	200	pH	pH 7.6–7.8
Citrate-phosphate-dextrose	50	Calcium ion	0.5–0.6 mmol/liter
5% Dextrose in water 1/4 isotonic saline solution	550	Osmolarity	340–360 mOsm

[a]When mixed in a 4:1 ratio with blood.

Table 36-3 Modified Cold Blood Maintenance Solution

Solution Additive	Volume Added (mL)	Component Modified	Concentration Delivered[a]
Tromethamine (0.3 mole/liter)	50	pH	pH 7.5–7.6
Citrate-phosphate-dextrose	50	Calcium ion	0.5–0.6 mmol/liter
Magnesium chloride (2 mEq/mL)	10	Magnesium ion	4–6 mg/liter
5% Dextrose in water 1/4 isotonic saline solution	1,000	Osmolarity, glucose	340–360 mOsm
Mannitol (25%)	50	Osmolarity, oxygen radical scavenger	340–360 mOsm

[a]When mixed in a 4:1 ratio with blood.

The cannula can be placed from the left side of the table by the assistant, who directs the device at a 45-degree angle from the orifice of the coronary sinus to a position beneath the left atrial appendage (Fig. 36-7). Placement from the right side of the table is done by directing the stylet toward the left atrial appendage (Fig. 36-8). Placing the index finger at the junction of the inferior vena cava and right atrium allows the cannula tip to be palpated, guides entrance, and veri-fies correct placement. The cannula should always enter the coronary sinus easily. The cannula is advanced until it meets resistance within the coronary sinus, usually adjacent to the left atrial appendage. The tip of the cannula is easily felt (Fig. 36-9). If the cannula tip is in the posterior descending vein, it should be reinserted (Fig. 36-10). In "re-do" surgery, the retrograde cannula is placed without palpation. Position is confirmed when dark blood appears. Retroperfusion

for induction during coronary reoperations limits embolization and allows debris to be flushed out from cut grafts. Its position is checked after bypass is started and the heart arrested.

Cannulation on partial bypass is done with the right atrium slightly distended to keep the coronary ostium open. Failure to intubate the coronary sinus is rare (1% to 2%) and indicates a fenestrated Thebesian valve or a flap over the ostium. A finger placed through a small atriotomy incision sometimes allows direct cannula advancement. Alternatively, bicaval cannulation can be used. The right atrium is opened with a small incision and cannulation is performed directly after the flap is retracted or the Thebesian valve is opened. If the right atrium is open, a purse-string suture around the coronary sinus prevents reflux.

During retrograde infusions, the posterior descending vein fills readily with oxygenated blood, which confirms an extensive myocardial venovenous collateral network. The cannula is withdrawn slightly if there is failure to fill the posterior descending vein or if there is no egress of blood from the right coronary ostium or open right artery during aortic or coronary operations. This blue blood signifies nutritive flow despite some shunting into the right atrium with self-inflating balloons. The blood becomes red, which reflects adequate perfusion. This is especially important if normothermic continuous cardioplegia is delivered. When delivering simultaneous antegrade flow through vein grafts and retrograde flow into the coronary sinus, the retrograde pressure is measured and does not increase because of Thebesian vein drainage.

Coronary Sinus Injury

The coronary sinus can be injured due to forceful cannulation or continued administration of cardioplegia when coronary sinus pressure exceeds 50 to 60 mm Hg. This can occur while the heart is elevated during circumflex artery grafting. The perfusionist notes high pressure, then low pressure as a consequence of acute perforation, or the surgeon sees red blood accumulation within the pericardial well during infusions. Perforation can be repaired directly with 6-0 sutures or with pericardial pledgets if the tear site is not distinct. Coronary sinus rupture from balloon overinflation can also be repaired by suturing a pericardial patch over the disrupted region to the adjacent cardiac surface. Hematomas can sometimes be

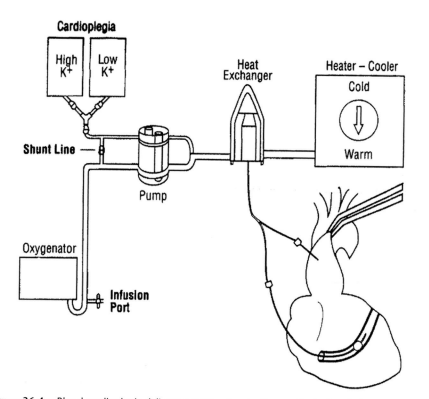

Figure 36-4. Blood cardioplegic delivery system, whereby the cardioplegic solution contains high-dose and low-dose potassium bottles. These are mixed 4:1 with blood from the oxygenator. The shunt line allows delivery of terminal regular blood through the roller head of the pump after the warm reperfusate is given.

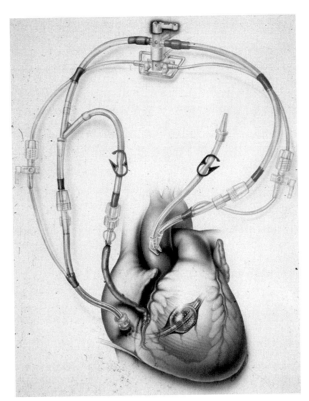

Figure 36-5.   Tubing use for antegrade, retrograde, and vein perfusion connected to the retrograde arm. Note the stopcock that allows simultaneous delivery of cardioplegic perfusate and monitoring of arterial or coronary sinus pressure. The arm is connected to the retrograde limb, allowing simultaneous retrograde/antegrade perfusion down the vein graft or right coronary ostium during aortic valve replacement.

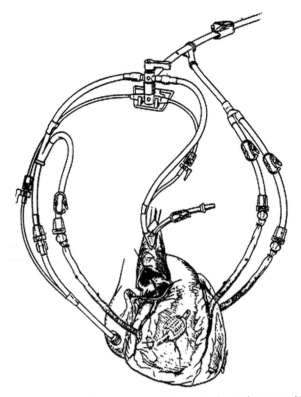

Figure 36-6.   Cardioplegia setup for coronary grafting and valve replacement. Note that the organization allows for simultaneous perfusion of the grafts and the coronary sinus when cardioplegic perfusate is given. The separation of the vein graft limbs does not allow crossing the field during work on the aorta.

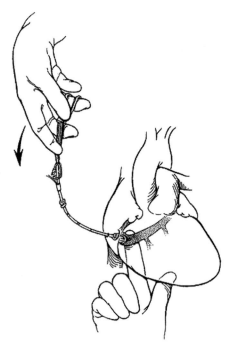

Figure 36-7.   Method for introducing the retrograde cannula from the left side of the operating table. Note the direct course at 45 degrees from the coronary sinus to the junction of the coronary sinus and the left atrium.

left unattended because low venous pressure allows self-containment after heparin reversal.

Monitoring Pressure

Measuring infusion pressure avoids edema and endothelial damage. It also detects aortic insufficiency produced by distortion of the noncoronary aortic cusp by the venous cannula or clinically insignificant regurgitation. Repositioning an adherent venous cannula away from the noncoronary cusp or compression of the right ventricular outflow tract with a sponge stick will compress the septum against the posterior left ventricle and limit this problem. During retrograde infusion, measurement of pressure verifies correct placement of the coronary sinus cannula.

Antegrade Pressure

Blood cardioplegia is given over time to ensure maximal oxygen delivery, and measured aortic pressures during induction range from 60 to 80 mm Hg at flow rates of 200 to 250 mL/m. Failure to arrest means inadequate systemic venous drainage (full pulmonary artery), incomplete aortic clamping or aortic insufficiency, delivery of a low-potassium dose, or nonocclusion of the

During the final warm cardioplegia infusion, the aortic root pressure should not exceed 50 mm Hg to avoid endothelial dysfunction.

Retrograde Pressure

Coronary sinus pressure ranges from 20 to 40 mm Hg at an infusion rate of 200 to 250 mL/m. A coronary sinus pressure of >50 mm Hg means improper positioning or cardiac retraction that kinks the venous system. This is treated by reducing flow rate immediately, repositioning the catheter, and resuming flow. Textured balloons should not be moved during infusion because of coronary sinus wall traction and possible injury. Coronary sinus pressure of <20 mm Hg implies that the balloon is not inflated or not occluding the coronary sinus. The cannula tip and balloon should then be palpated and repositioned. Added maneuvers to improve retroperfusion include compressing the junction of the coronary sinus and right atrium (Fig. 36-11) and placing a snared suture around the coronary sinus,

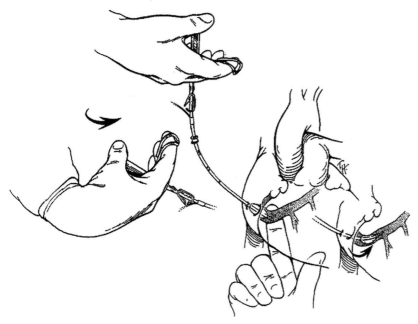

Figure 36-8. Method for introducing the retrograde cannula from the right side of the table. Note that the cannula is rotated anteriorly and toward the left shoulder to follow the course of the coronary sinus. Using force without rotation from the right side after the cannula is introduced may injure the coronary sinus.

cardioplegic line at the pump head. Treatment includes improving venous drainage, replacing the aortic clamp, checking the pump, and repeating the cardioplegic solution dose. An aortic pressure of <30 mm

Hg means antegrade flow is insufficient, and only retrograde infusion should be used. High aortic pressure (>100 mm Hg) occurs with extensive coronary disease, and antegrade distribution is unpredictable.

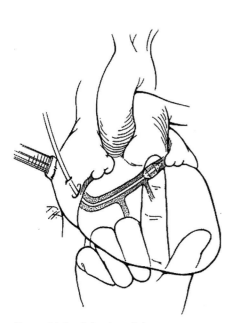

Figure 36-9. Palpation of the coronary sinus cannula for position. Note the posterior position of the cannula and the ability to feel the cannula tip. If only the body of the cannula is felt at this time, the cannula should be withdrawn slightly; otherwise, it will be wedged, and high pressures will be recorded.

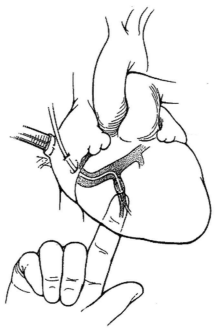

Figure 36-10. Palpation of the cannula tip without deep palpation. This means the cannula is in the posterior descending vein and it should be withdrawn and repositioned so that it can be palpated far posteriorly, as in Fig. 36-9.

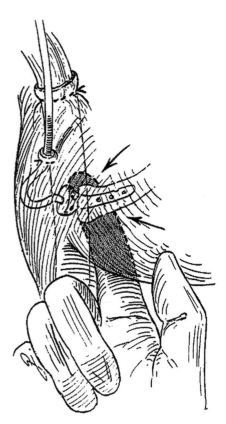

Figure 36-11. Method of compressing the coronary sinus at the junction of the right atrium and inferior vena cava if the cannula retracts intraoperatively but remains in the coronary sinus. This restores coronary sinus pressure, but reinsertion of the cannula is preferable to this transient intervention.

thus fixing it in place and preventing regurgitation of cardioplegia into the atrium. Other causes of low pressure are (1) persistent left superior vena cava, (2) failure of balloon inflation, and (3) rare left atrial unroofing of the coronary sinus noted during mitral procedures. The presence of a left superior vena cava is usually determined before cardiopulmonary bypass, and the vessel is occluded with a tourniquet only if an intact innominate vein is present. If the innominate vein is absent, only antegrade cardioplegia is used, to avoid myocardial underperfusion.

Measuring Pressure in the Cardioplegic Delivery System and the Vascular System Receiving the Cardioplegic Solution

Measuring pressure in the cardioplegia delivery system allows detection of inadvertent line occlusion by clamping or kinking. However, using the delivery system pressure to estimate aortic or coronary sinus pressure is inaccurate as shown in Fig. 36-12. The only exception is in aortic operations, when the right coronary ostium is directly perfused. The infusion line pressure allows an approximation of the vascular pressure.

Delivery and Monitoring of Antegrade/Retrograde Cardioplegic Perfusion or Simultaneous Antegrade/ Retrograde Cardioplegic Perfusion

A monitoring infusion set allows rapid switching from antegrade to retrograde perfusion with corresponding monitoring of aortic and coronary sinus pressures. The side arm attached to the retrograde line permits the following benefits during retroperfusion:

1. Simultaneous antegrade/retrograde delivery of solution (e.g., antegrade via the distally attached saphenous graft, or antegrade via the right coronary ostium [in aortic procedures] with *simultaneous* coronary sinus delivery).
2. Testing for distal suture line leaks.
3. De-airing of the graft as the suture line is secured during retrograde infusion.
4. Identifying graft twisting.
5. Allowing length measurement of the distended graft before aortic anastomosis.

Cardioplegic Solutions

Two important features of blood cardioplegia must be kept in mind: (1) Blood optimizes the rate of aerobic metabolism and (2) oxygen uptake occurs over time, so that infusion duration is more important than dose. Delivery at a fixed pressure for too short a time (especially with warm infusions) deprives the myocardium of the benefits of a full dose. The setup, therefore, provides two controls for the perfusionist (Fig. 36-4): (1) flow clamps to alternate between high-dose and low-dose potassium cardioplegic solutions for induction, maintenance, and reperfusion and (2) flow clamps to activate a shunt line to give a terminal noncardioplegic blood infusion. In addition, the cardioplegic solutions are delivered through an "inline" white blood cell filter to add leukodepletion to the cardioprotective strategy.

The following guidelines are used for flow rates in normal hearts and are increased by 50 to 100 mL/min for hypertrophied hearts (Table 36-4). Many formulations with various additives are used with excellent results. We use the high-dose potassium (20 mEq/L) solution that contains components described previously. It arrests the heart promptly during either warm or cold induction and remains available if electromechanical activity recurs. Enrichment with amino acids (glutamate/aspartate) is useful in high-risk patients (Table 36-1), those with low output, ischemia, or hypertrophy. It is switched to the low-dose, nonenriched potassium solution immediately after arrest with cold induction to limit hyperkalemia. The low-dose potassium (8 to 10 mEq/L) solution (Table 36-2) is used for maintenance doses during cold cardioplegic infusions and does not contain amino acids. The cold noncardioplegic solution in Table 36-4 is used between cardioplegic doses instead of cold blood. At the completion of all cardiac repairs, all patients receive a terminal warm, substrate-enriched cardioplegic perfusate ("hot shot") for 3 to 5 minutes followed by noncardioplegic warm normal blood with the aorta clamped. The same solution as in Table 36-1 is used, but the solution dose of KCl is reduced to 10 mEq to yield a KCl concentration of 8 to 10 mEq/L in the warm blood cardioplegic reperfusate. During infusion of the warm reperfusate, it is not uncommon to observe a mild degree of transient hypotension due to vasodilation.

Normocalcemic blood from the extracorporeal circuit is added to the cardioplegia

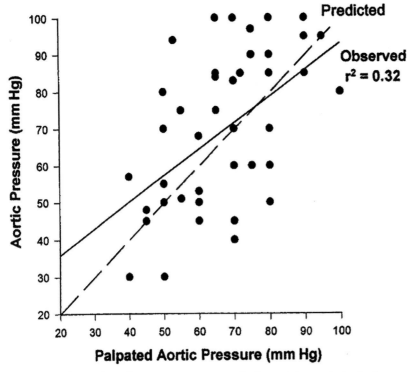

Figure 36-12.   Comparison of pressure measurements in the aorta by surgical palpation (*abscissa*) and measured aortic pressure (*ordinate*). Note the marked discrepancy between the estimated and measured pressures.

Table 36-4 Delivery of Cardioplegic Perfusate

Induction	Antegrade Perfusion	Retrograde Perfusion
Cold	300 mL/min × 2 mins	200 mL/min × 2 mins
Warm	300 mL/min until arrest, then 150 mL/min × 2.5 mins	150 mL/min × 2.5 mins
Maintenance	200 mL/min × 1 min	200 mL/min × 1 min
Reperfusion	150 mL/min × 2 mins	150 mL/min × 2 mins
Noncardioplegic blood	200 mL/min	200 mL/min

solution. In adult patients, we use citrated solutions (CPD); therefore, calcium should be added to the cardiopulmonary bypass circuit primed with noncalcemic solutions. This avoids unintentional hypocalcemia, which can damage the membranes of the sarcolemma. In pediatric patients, systemic hypocalcemia occurs when the pump is primed with citrated blood. Consequently, no calcium is added until the end of the procedure, when the calcium concentration is normalized before bypass is stopped.

Coronary Bypass Procedure

During coronary bypass the body is kept at 33°C to 34°C. The heart is arrested with high-potassium *cold* blood cardioplegia in elective low-risk operations with good ventricular function. For simplicity, one uses this solution, which contains the amino acid additives, rather than prepares another solution without these. Alternatively, this same high-potassium enriched *warm* blood cardioplegia ("warm induction") is used initially to arrest the heart in cases where acute ischemia is present or in cases of severely depressed systolic function. The administration of substrates in this situation has been proven to aid in the recovery of function after surgical repair. After the warm induction, low-potassium cold blood cardioplegia is infused into the aortic root and retrograde into the coronary sinus. Intermittent low-potassium cold blood cardioplegia is used during the course of the grafting (Table 36-4). The ventricle is palpated because cardiac distortion or aortic insufficiency (low aortic root pressure) may harmfully distend the ventricle. Similarly, retraction of the heart during retrograde delivery raises coronary sinus pressure by kinking the venous system. If pressure exceeds 50 mm Hg, flow is reduced.

Following cardioplegic arrest, all anastomoses are constructed in a dry operative field using distal/proximal grafting in sequence. The right coronary graft is constructed first because retrograde nutritive perfusion is limited. Retrograde perfusion (200 mL/min for 1 minute) is started after the last suture is placed in the first distal anastomosis with the suture line patulous to allow de-airing of the coronary artery with blood. The flow clamp connected to the graft is opened to evacuate air from the graft and to provide simultaneous graft antegrade and whole-heart retrograde cardioplegic perfusion while the suture is tied.

The vent is closed to distend the aortic root. Determination of the graft length is facilitated by holding the distended vein or arterial graft adjacent to the pericardium opposite either the pulmonary artery or the superior vena cava. During proximal grafting of vein to the aorta, retrograde cold noncardioplegic blood is infused at 200 mL/m. The cold solution maintains arrest, limits potassium overdosing, and contains CPD, THAM, magnesium, and mannitol, and thereby prevents resumption of low-level electromechanical activity. The aorta is vented during proximal grafting, which allows good visualization. Cardioplegia is then switched to the antegrade mode. Air is evacuated from the aortic root as the proximal suture line is secured. Air is also evacuated from the grafts during antegrade cardioplegia infusion with a 27-gauge needle.

Newly constructed grafts perfuse the heart after each proximal connection. The next distal graft is then constructed in a dry operative field while the heart is vented. The sequence is repeated for each distal and proximal anastomosis, leaving one proximal graft to be connected to the aorta after the final distal left internal mammary artery (LIMA) anastomosis is constructed. Systemic rewarming is started while the LIMA anastomosis is begun, and the perfusionist switches to a warm cardioplegic solution for the last dose.

After the LIMA is inserted into the anterior descending artery, antegrade warm cardioplegia is delivered for 2 minutes at a flow rate of 150 mL/min, followed by retrograde warm cardioplegia, also at a flow rate of 150 mL/min. During this retrograde infusion, the last proximal vein graft is sewn to the aorta. After the infusion of cardioplegia, the perfusionist delivers warm blood at a flow rate of 250 to 300 mL/min until the proximal grafting is complete. The heart usually begins to contract, and systolic compression of the capillary bed raises coronary sinus pressures but is of no concern. Clamps on all grafts are removed just before the proximal suture line is secured. Antegrade flow is started to de-air the aortic root, as before, and the grafts are de-aired to prevent air embolus.

In combined valve/coronary procedures, distal grafts are first placed. The valve is then replaced or repaired. Every 15 to 20 minutes, maintenance cold blood is delivered through the unattached vein grafts and simultaneously into the coronary sinus. All proximal anastomoses are then performed last with the aorta still cross-clamped. The proximal right graft is sewn last to maximize right ventricular perfusion. The warm (3 to 5 minutes) cardioplegic reperfusion is started at the end of the next-to-the-last proximal anastomosis. The perfusionist then delivers 37°C blood in a retrograde manner, and the aorta is vented gently while the final right graft is sewn to the aorta. By this point the high-potassium cardioplegia is washed out, and the heart begins to contract slowly.

The stopcock is switched to antegrade infusion, and warm blood is then infused into the aortic root with the cross-clamp in place at a flow of 250 to 300 mL/m. Mean aortic root pressure is kept at about 75 mm Hg, and flow is reduced as needed to prevent hypertension. The heart resumes vigorous contractility within a couple of minutes. The aortic clamp is then released, and the aorta is vented as the heart is filled. Cardiopulmonary bypass in then discontinued.

Evolving Myocardial Infarction

The procedure is modified in patients with acute evolving myocardial infarction. The left ventricle is vented via the right superior pulmonary vein to minimize myocardial oxygen demands. A final enriched *regional* perfusate is delivered into the vein graft attached to the infarct-related artery at 50 mL/min (≤50 mm Hg pressure) for 20 minutes. Sometimes this can be done via a vein side branch to optimize prolonged warm reperfusion during proximal grafting (Fig. 36-13). The proximal grafts are

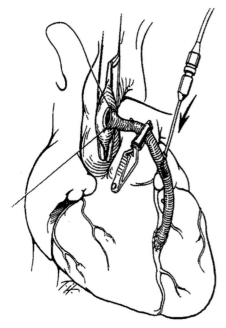

Figure 36-13. Method of performing tangential grafting in a patient who has acute ischemia from the catheterization laboratory or a naturally occurring infarction. Note that a tangential clamp is used for proximal anastomosis. Consequently, the 20-minute warm perfusate is infused down the graft if the side branch is available, and pressure is monitored by the perfusionist from the blood cardioplegia delivery system in this instance. Simultaneously, the proximal anastomosis is constructed because of the bulldog clamp on the graft.

constructed with tangential aortic clamping as the heart is beating. Bypass is continued for 30 more minutes to allow recovery of the newly revascularized infarcted myocardium. We have observed significant return of regional contractility despite more than 6 hours of ischemia. The details and outcome of this technique have been previously described.

Repeat Cardiac Surgery

The integrated cardioplegia method described earlier has been found to be particularly useful in repeat operations. In coronary bypass operations, a generally accepted rule is that old grafts should be left undisturbed. This "no-touch" technique prevents embolization of friable atherosclerotic debris into the distal vasculature.

After sternotomy, only the aorta and the right atrium are dissected free of surrounding adhesions. After cannulation and institution of cardiopulmonary bypass, the retrograde cannula is inserted. The aorta is

clamped, and induction cardioplegia is administered into the aortic root to arrest the heart. Retrograde cardioplegia follows with monitoring of the septal temperature to assure adequacy of distribution. The aorta is vented to decompress the heart, and only then is the heart freed of surrounding pericardial adhesions. This avoids compression of old vein grafts and embolization. The added time of ischemia is only about 10 minutes, and the hemodynamics are not compromised by avoiding mobilization by dissection of the beating heart before arrest. Distal and proximal grafts are constructed in sequence as with all coronary operations. The single aortic cross-clamping technique avoids compression of old grafts and ischemia that can be induced by the side biting method, in which graft flow is temporarily interrupted.

Clinical outcomes with this method in repeat coronary bypass grafting have demonstrated no increased mortality, even in patients with markedly reduced systolic function preoperatively.

Myocardial Protection during Aortic Root Replacement

The myocardium must be carefully protected during extensive and long operations on the aortic root, as encountered with ascending aortic aneurysm or dissection. Here the coronary ostia are often isolated for reimplantation into a graft. Intermittent cardioplegia can be administered directly into these unattached ostia, but care must be taken to avoid injury, particularly if operation is indicated because of dissection. An approach we have found useful is to graft the right coronary artery with saphenous vein. The proximal right coronary artery is temporarily occluded with a Silastic vascular loop. Cardioplegia can then be administered intermittently antegrade via the right coronary artery and simultaneously retrograde into the coronary sinus. This permits maximal distribution throughout the myocardium and does not interfere with the operation. The aortic root and ascending aorta can be repaired with ease in a dry field. After the root has been reconstructed and the ostia reimplanted into the graft, the saphenous vein graft is ligated at the anastomosis to the right coronary artery, either with a running suture or with a large hemoclip. The extra 5 minutes needed to execute this protective method assures global myo-

cardial protection and avoids injury to the friable coronary ostia.

Ventricular Restoration

An alternate approach is used in rebuilding the ventricular chamber in congestive heart failure patients undergoing ventricular restoration. These patients are in the highest risk category and normally undergo coronary grafting, and approximately 25% need mitral valve repair. Both coronary artery bypass grafting (CABG) and mitral repair are accomplished with the integrated method, and then the aortic clamp is removed to reconstruct the spherical left ventricular chamber into an oblique shape. The method of protection is the "beating open" technique. Competence of the aortic valve together with ventricular venting via the left superior pulmonary vein avoids ventricular filling during repair.

Aortic perfusion pressure is kept at >75 mm Hg because both experimentally and clinically, this higher pressure improves subendocardial perfusion: An improvement in the force of twisting is usually observed when perfusion pressure is increased. Restoration, with continuous perfusion, is *always* done *after* coronary grafting is completed to take advantage of the improved flow provided by the CABG procedure. Ventricular palpation with the beating method is very useful in the thick-walled akinetic heart, in which visual distinction between scar and viable muscle is difficult, especially if there is trabecular scar, or in the early phases after infarction when there is no evidence of scarring. Other advantages include (1) limiting ischemia by allowing ongoing coronary perfusion in severely dilated hearts during early learning curve, when the time period of restoration may be prolonged, (2) continuous perfusion to repay the "ischemic debt" after prolonged aortic clamping with cardioplegic protection was needed during the CABG and mitral repair phases of the procedure, and (3) more rapid discontinuation of bypass as the reperfused heart undergoes a long period of nutritive flow during restoration. Consequently, the beating method offsets the interval of "resting the heart" by prolonging the end of the procedure.

Determination of preoperative aortic insufficiency by ventriculogram or intraoperatively by echo is critical because only a small amount (i.e., 500 mL/min) will obscure the field. We normally use the beating technique but make some changes. If aortic regurgitation is anticipated, the aortic clamp is left

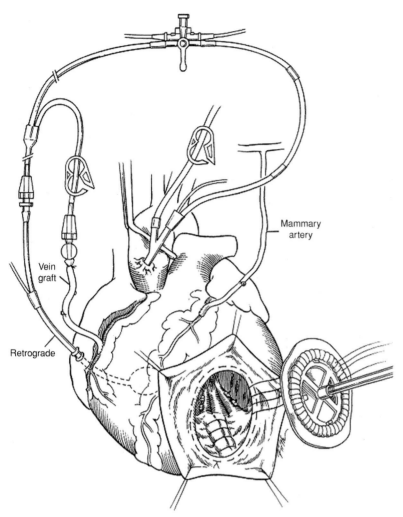

Figure 36-14.   Beating heart myocardial protection during systemic vascular resistance in a patient with aortic insufficiency. Note the clamped aorta, with perfusion via the internal mammary artery, vein grafts, and retrograde via the coronary sinus. This method is used with either anterior or inferior repairs.

in place; proximal grafts are perfused via a Y connector rather than connected to the aorta, the internal mammary artery graft is opened, and retrograde normal blood perfusion is delivered to the beating heart during repair as shown in Fig. 36-14.

Conclusion

Integrated myocardial management as described here is useful in all adult cardiac procedures by allowing them to proceed smoothly and more rapidly than usual because there is no interruption or delay for infusion of cardioplegic perfusate or noncardioplegic blood. The duration of cardiopulmonary bypass is actually shortened while one simultaneously takes advantage of the benefits of different methods. Ongoing studies will likely lead to the incorpo-

ration of additional cardioprotective methods such as preconditioning agents, white blood cell filters, oxygen radical scavengers, endothelium-enhancing agents, and molecular factors that will further improve the safety of ischemic intervals and limit reperfusion damage.

SUGGESTED READING

Ali IS, Al-Nowaiser O, Deslauriers R, et al. Continuous normothermic blood cardioplegia. Semin Thorac Cardiovasc Surg 1993;5:141.

Allen BS, Buckberg GD, Fontan F, et al. Superiority of controlled surgical reperfusion vs. PTCA in acute coronary occlusion. J Thorac Cardiovasc Surg 1993;105:864.

Allen BS, Buckberg GD. Myocardial Protection Management during Adult Cardiac Opera-

tions. In Baue AE, Geha AS, Hammond GL, et al. (eds), Glenn's Thoracic and Cardiovascular Surgery. Norwalk, CT: Appleton & Lange, 1995;1653.

Buckberg GD. Antegrade/retrograde blood cardioplegia to ensure cardioplegic distribution: operative techniques and objectives. J Card Surg 1989;4:216.

Calafiore AM, Teodori G, Mezzetti A. Intermittent antegrade warm blood cardioplegia. Ann Thorac Surg 1995;59:398.

Flameng W. Intermittent ischemia. Semin Thorac Cardiovasc Surg 1993;5:107.

Guyton RA. Oxygenated crystalloid cardioplegia. Semin Thorac Cardiovasc Surg 1993;5:114.

Ihnken K, Morita K, Buckberg GD, et al. The safety of simultaneous arterial and coronary sinus perfusion: Experimental background and initial clinical results. J Card Surg 1994;9:15.

Kirklin JW, Digerness SB, Fontan FM, et al. Controlled aortic root reperfusion in cardiac surgery. Semin Thorac Cardiovasc Surg 1993;5:134.

Kronon MT, Allen BS, Halldorsson A, et al. Delivery of a non-potassium modified maintenance solution to enhance myocardial protection in stressed neonatal hearts: a new approach. J Thorac Cardiovasc Surg 2002;123:119.

Loop FD, Higgins TL, Panda R, et al. Myocardial protection during cardiac operations. J Thorac Cardiovasc Surg 1992;104:608.

Teoh KH, Christakis GT, Weisel RD, et al. Accelerated myocardial metabolic recovery with terminal warm blood cardioplegia. J Thorac Cardiovasc Surg 1986;91:888.

EDITOR'S COMMENTS

The authors have presented a thorough review of myocardial protection. Dr. Buckberg has developed many of the methodologies that we use to this day and clearly has made myocardial protection safe and practical. There is no one unique technique of myocardial protection. If we questioned 10 experts in cardiac surgery, we would hear 10 different myocardial protection strategies. However, the individual surgeon must have a consistent approach. It must be known by the perfusionist, the nurses, and the surgeon's colleagues. The techniques must be flexible to allow for intraoperative conversions or to deal with specific clinical situations. However, even the best techniques of myocardial protection do not make up for a normally perfused heart. No matter what technique is used, time is of the essence, and this must always be considered by the operating surgeon.

I.L.K.

37

Database

Frederic Grover and Colleagues

Quality improvement endeavors within the field of cardiac surgical care have made substantial progress over the last 30 years. A key aspect that has promoted improvement in the processes and structures of cardiac surgical care is the development of multi-institutional databases to monitor outcomes following cardiothoracic surgery. Databases offer several inherent advantages to surgical practice. Combined with statistical analyses, complete and high-quality databases offer an assessment of the interactive effects of multiple risk factors on outcome, which is a complex and difficult task without the assistance of statistical prediction models.

The majority of these databases in cardiac surgery initially began with relatively crude measures of unadjusted operative (30 day) mortality as their primary outcome criteria. Since the mid-1990s, there has been a progressive increase in the level of sophistication in the databases. For example, risk models can be constructed from a list of preoperative variables, and these models can be used to predict the likelihood of adverse outcomes. Whereas database outcomes initially focused on mortality, more recent efforts seek to define risk-adjusted outcomes such as morbidity and efficiency outcomes such as length of stay. Databases offer the opportunity for both feedback and information exchange to facilitate the comparison of institutions and provide data to local clinical care teams to assess performance and coordinate future improvement strategies. This exchange offers the potential to further improve the processes, structures, and outcomes of care in cardiac surgery.

Historical Considerations

Local databases have been used by many institutions for more than 30 years. For example, hospital-based databases have been used by Duke University, the Cleveland Clinic, the Mayo Clinic, and others to monitor volume and mortality statistics within their institutions. The first large, multi-institutional monitoring of cardiac surgery outcomes began in the Department of Veterans Affairs (VA) with the establishment of the Cardiac Surgery Consultants Committee (CSCC) in 1972. Under a congressional mandate, the VA semiannual reports were combined with ongoing surveillance work toward the goal of assuring the quality of cardiac surgical care in the VA system. Until 1988, the CSCC used unadjusted mortality and volume as the main parameters to judge outcomes. Takaro and colleagues analyzed the VA experience from 1975 to 1984 and noted that the annual volume of cardiopulmonary bypass surgery rose from 3,000 to more than 6,400 procedures. Correspondingly, the observed mortality rate for coronary artery bypass procedures dropped from 4.7% to 3.6%. They noted that patient-related comorbidities accounted for most of the operative mortality, but advances in surgical and medical techniques also may have played an important role in this mortality rate reduction.

On March 12, 1986, the Department of Health and Human Services Health Care Financing Administration (HCFA) released to the public raw mortality data for coronary artery bypass grafting (CABG). This report actually listed hospitals that had mortality rates for Medicare patients under-

going CABG that were in excess of predicted mortality rates. Although these data were originally to be used for state peer review organizations as a quality improvement tool, HCFA was forced to release these data through the Freedom of Information Act. These mortality rates were unfortunately not risk-adjusted for clinical patient risk factors. In addition, diagnostic categories were grouped together without comprehensive clinical patient-specific risk adjustments related to severity of disease and comorbidity present. Furthermore, the public release of these data prompted widespread concern that non–risk-adjusted mortality could not offer an accurate reflection of the caseload mix within an individual program. Without appropriate patient-specific clinical risk stratification, accurate comparison of cardiac surgery outcomes between programs was widely perceived to be not useful for patient care, program management, or policy decisions. This action by HCFA served as a strong stimulus for the Society of Thoracic Surgeons (STS) to initiate its own cardiac surgical database with risk-adjusted methods.

In 1987, the VA Cardiac Surgery Advisory Group, now called the VA Cardiac Surgery Consultants Committee, was also concerned with the use of unadjusted operative mortality and volume as major quality indicators for the approximately 45 VA cardiac surgery programs. Using the logistic regression method approach developed by the Collaborative Study in Coronary Artery Surgery, Drs. Hammermeister and Grover initiated a multivariate discriminate analysis of the clinical and angiographic predictors of operative mortality. The VA developed a risk model for coronary artery bypass and valve replacement operations. The method included capturing data on all cardiac surgery procedures performed using a single-page data sheet (originally of 52 data elements) including patient-specific clinical risk factors, cardiac catheterization assessment data, operative details, and a set of both mortality and major morbidity outcome variables. These initial efforts proved successful in the attempt to "level the playing field" by accounting for the individual patient risk factors that could play a role in determining outcomes after cardiac surgical procedures. Based on these early events, two large national databases, the STS National Adult Cardiac Surgery Database and the VA Cardiac Surgery Database, emerged in a complementary and synergistic manner to provide routine reports of cardiac surgical practices for their use in their own local quality improvement endeavors. Similarly, large regional databases also evolved including (but not limited to) the Northern New England Cardiovascular Study Group (NNE) and the New York State databases.

Database Construction

The factors that may account for observed differences in outcomes include differences in significant risk factors among patients, random variation, and differences in the processes and structures of care. A conceptual model that was clinically relevant was built to evaluate the patient demographic factors, socioeconomic factors, severity of cardiac disease, comorbidities, and patient lifestyle/health behaviors that may influence the outcomes of cardiac surgical procedures adversely. Risk factors are assessed as close to the time frame of the cardiac surgical procedure as possible to most accurately and reliably evaluate the patient's inherent characteristics.

Random variation may be accounted for by using appropriate statistical techniques. Therefore, the purpose of risk stratification is to attempt to account for patient-specific characteristics for a given procedure performed that influence patient outcomes. This examination of risk-adjusted outcomes provides an indirect surrogate metric with which to begin studying the differences in the quality of care.

Virtually all of the databases in current use attempt to provide predictive risk stratification. Surgeons must, however, be aware of the limitations and factors pertaining to the design, construction, and management of a particular database if it is to be optimally utilized. Of primary importance are the completeness, accuracy, reliability, timeliness, sensitivity to change, and integrity of the data entered. "Garbage in = garbage out" is operative in considering any analysis of a database. Ideally, all patients receiving a cardiac surgical procedure should be entered for analysis and outcomes validated appropriately. For any given patient record, the data submitted must also be internally consistent. For example, patients entered into the database as needing emergent operations should have firm clinical data supporting the need for such a classification. Both intrafield and interfield edit checks may be used to evaluate discrepancies and updates performed appropriately. Finally, standardized definitions (with training for the data capture team) are important for all data elements captured. Common inconsistencies in application of definitions have been demonstrated for patient-related outcomes, such as perioperative morbidities, where the use of different diagnostic test assessments routinely are not consistently performed (e.g., the assessment of perioperative myocardial infarction varies due to the routine assessment of clinical pathology laboratory tests versus clinical lab tests performed based on clinical suspicion of a perioperative myocardial infarction having occurred). Surgeons should be aware of important aspects of the management/ operation of any given database, including the following:

1. Which outcomes are examined, and are definitions for the measured variables standardized? Mortality, for example, is the most widely used outcome because of its importance and because it is readily available from hospital records. Such a dichotomous variable would seem relatively standard. However, some databases measure in-hospital mortality, whereas others track 30-day mortality after CABG (including both in-hospital deaths and deaths that occur within 30 days postsurgery). Other important variables include the occurrence of other major complications (infection, stroke, prolonged ventilation, renal failure, etc.), cost, and length of hospital stay. These other measures constitute important outcomes but are more difficult to measure because complications may be not uniformly recorded across sites in the medical record. Standardized definitions for these major morbid events as perioperative complica-

tions exist and are rigorously defined by both the STS and VA cardiac databases.

2. What is the intent of the data analysis? The database may be designed to provide a predicted outcome for a given patient or to compare surgeon-specific or program-specific outcomes. In addition, outcomes analysis may be used to drive national policy decisions or managed care accreditation. Discussions have been initiated about also using risk-adjusted outcomes for physician profiling and credentialing.

3. How are the data collected? Input for databases may be gathered in a retrospective, concurrent, or prospective manner. Depending on the database, data acquisition may be mandatory (VA database) or voluntary (STS database). Data acquisition and entry may be collected by members of the patient care team or by independent data collectors. For example, in the VA database, data are collected by nurse investigators who are independent of the surgical team. It is believed that independent collection of such data may result in more thorough and unbiased reporting (e.g., self-reporting for complications may not be consistent uniformly across surgeons).

4. How are the missing data treated? Any large database will have incomplete data elements. This happens more commonly in databases in which data are entered retrospectively. If the outcome of interest is missing, then the records with missing outcome data must be discarded because no reasonable method exists that is well accepted to input outcomes. For all other non-outcome variables, a variety of statistical techniques are used. Occasionally, there are enough missing data elements within any record to justify dropping this specific case. Other common imputation techniques derive a value to be inserted for the missing variable based on values for other patients. For example, serum creatinine is often missing as a variable in the STS database, and in analyses of these data, one may either insert an indicator variable for "missing" or substitute a normal value of 1.0 for missing values. In addition, many more imputation techniques exist that trade off statistical rigor with clinically reasonable estimates (e.g., within-range estimates). As the completeness rates for cardiac surgery databases increase, however, the need for complex imputation techniques has begun to diminish.

5. What is the patient population from which the data are derived? Multicenter databases receive data from centers of different sizes and surgical volumes. This factor may introduce institutional bias into the database and weight it toward those programs entering the largest numbers of patients. Databases may include data from diverse surgical programs. For example, the STS database receives data from surgical programs of such diversity as large and small community practices, university-based training programs, and military hospitals. Alternatively, databases may receive data from relatively uniform patient populations. The VA database, for example, includes data for patients only undergoing surgery in VA medical centers. Different statistical techniques can be used to account for provider-specific fixed and random effects. The key is to check that any difference that one wishes to compare is not adjusted for one that is accounted for in the analysis.

How did the predictive model perform that was generated from the database? Construction of a predictive model typically involves several steps. First, a conceptual model that is clinically relevant is used to list the variables (risk factors) that are thought to be associated with a particular outcome in study (e.g., mortality). In context of the literature in the field, these clinical models are constructed by a panel of experts. After these risk factors have been predetermined, they must be rigorously and accurately defined to standardize the data collection. After all database completeness, accuracy, and reliability verifications (including any data record updates required), one may then perform a univariate and multivariate analyses for a specific outcome for a procedure for a selected population of patients to determine which of the chosen risk factors are statistically associated with patient outcome. The outcome rates for patients with a given risk factor are compared with the outcome rates for patients without the risk factor. The number of patients required for such an analysis varies based on the nature and frequency of the outcome studied, the number of patient risk variables planned for evaluation, and the preferred statistical approach planned. Based on the rule that in logistic regression analysis there should be no more than 1 risk factor assessed per 10 to15 adverse events, if one uses approximately 7 to 10 risk variables, >2,000 cases are required to develop a logistic regression model for CABG-only procedure, assuming an average mortality rate of <3%.

After univariate analyses have been performed, a multivariable predictive model is generated. In the majority of the cardiac surgical literature, the endpoints analyzed have been risk-adjusted mortality or presence/absence of major morbidity. For a dichotomous endpoint, the analytical technique originally used by the STS to generate a predictive equation was initially based on Bayesian theory to address the inherent challenges in a voluntary database related to missing data. However, the STS switched to multivariate logistic regression in 1997 when the data record completeness and quality improved such that the performance of the logistic regression approach was evaluated to be more rigorous than the prior approach. For dichotomous endpoints, moreover, the NNE, VA, and New York State databases all use multivariate logistic regression.

Multivariate logistic regression is a statistical technique that evaluates the likelihood of a specific event based on model building within a pre-established set of events. Often, large databases are partitioned into "learning" and "testing" datasets, with records proportionally stratified for dichotomous variables to assure adequate subgroup representation between groups. Other sampling techniques include (but are not limited to) boot-strapping techniques (a database resampling strategy). Logistic regression models can be used for either explanation (to understand associations between risk factors and outcomes) or prediction (to estimate risk for new and different populations). To apply the logistic regression equation for prediction purposes, risk factors are normally entered into the mathematical equation for a given patient. Thus, the logistic regression equation can yield the statistical probability of the dichotomous outcome of interest for such a patient.

Finally, the statistical modeling performance must be assessed. The accuracy of a predictive model is not an insignificant problem. The "predictive power" of the model describes the relationship of the predicted outcome to the observed outcome. It is the predictive validity that interests most surgeons. The c-statistic is commonly used to evaluate the predictive model's ability to discriminate between the occurrence and nonoccurrence of a dichotomous outcome. The c-statistic is based on the area under the receiver operating characteristic (ROC) curve. The ROC graphically relates the true-positive rate (sensitivity) and the false-positive rate (1 − specificity). For example, a c-statistic of 0.5 represents a useless test because a positive result would have an equal likelihood of being a true positive

or a false positive, indicating a benefit that is no greater than a random-chance guess. Graphically, a model with good discrimination generally is seen to pass near the upper left corner of the ROC plot; this point describes a high true-positive rate and a low false-positive rate.

Another key metric for model performance related to logistic regression is the model's calibration. Calibrating the model describes how well the model performs over the range of risk estimates generated in comparison to the observed outcome rate. Models may work well for high- or low-risk situations but not uniformly work well for all ranges of risk. A common metric used to assess model performance related to calibration is the Hosmer-Lemeshow test for "goodness of fit."

Current Adult Cardiac Surgery Databases

New York State Database

In response to the HCFA release of cardiac surgery data, New York State organized a Cardiac Surgery Advisory Committee, which was charged with investigating issues related to quality assurance for cardiovascular disease. This group developed a patient-specific cardiac surgical report form. This form reported demographic data, surgical procedures, admission and discharge dates, and information on risk factors, complications, and discharge status. Data forms are completed at each surgical program and forwarded to the Department of Health for analysis. Data reporting is mandatory. The patient variables captured are listed in Table 37-1.

The first report on these data was published in 1990 and described hospital mortality rates for 28 hospitals, 4 of which had significantly higher than expected mortality rates. The overall statewide mortality rate for cardiac surgery was 4.87%. Site reviews of the hospitals with excess mortality confirmed that significant quality-of-care issues existed in them.

Subsequently, in 1991, *Newsday* sought access to surgeon-specific mortality rates. The New York State Department of Health was concerned about the possibility of misleading the public because the volume of cases performed by each surgeon was quite smaller than the volume used to calculate hospital mortality rates. However, *Newsday* filed a successful lawsuit against the New York State Department of Health using the Freedom of Information Law to force release of surgeon-specific information for 1989

Table 37-1 Adult Preoperative Risk Factors: New York State Database

Age
Race
Gender
Payer
Reoperation (cardiac or great-vessel procedure performed during any previous admission)
Ejection fraction
Previous myocardial infarction
Morbid obesity (1.5 times ideal weight)
Hypertension history (requiring therapy)
Preoperative intra-aortic balloon pump
Dialysis dependence
Disasters (acute structural defect, renal failure, cardiogenic shock, gunshot)
Intractable congestive heart failure (CHF)
New York Heart Association functional class IV; symptoms of CHF at rest
Diabetes requiring medication
Greater than 90% narrowing of left main trunk
Percutaneous transluminal coronary angioplasty "crash"
Cardiac catheterization "crash"
Unstable angina
Chronic obstructive pulmonary disease resulting in functional disability, hospitalization, or forced expiratory volume in 1 second <75% predicted; or requiring bronchodilator therapy
Type of operation (coronary artery bypass graft, valve, coronary artery bypass graft plus valve, other)

From Hannan EL, Kilburn HK Jr, O'Donnell JF, et al. Adult open heart surgery in New York State. JAMA 1990;264:2768.

through 1990. Thus, in December 1992, surgeon risk-adjusted mortality rates for the 3-year period 1989 through 1991 for surgeons who performed at least 200 isolated CABG operations in the time period were publicly reported. Subsequent publications from the New York State Database continue to show improvement in risk-adjusted CABG mortality using this quality improvement platform. The New York State Database remains active and continues to identify significant independent risk factors for cardiac surgery in New York State.

Northern New England Cardiovascular Disease Study Group

The Northern New England Cardiovascular Disease Study Group was organized in 1987. This group comprises representatives from six institutions performing cardiac surgery in the northeast: Eastern Maine Medical Center, Maine Medical Center, Optima Health Care and Dartmouth-Hitchcock Medical Center in New Hampshire, Fletcher-Allen Health Care in Vermont, and Beth-Israel Deaconess Medical Center in Boston. This group of institutions voluntarily reports outcomes on cardiac surgical patients. At last report, more than 60,000 patients had been registered with this database, and the group contributes roughly 8,000 cases annually. This database was originally founded as a regional prospective study to examine whether the observed differences in outcomes following CAB in this region were solely the consequence of differences in patient case mix. The initial report from this database in 1991 evaluated 3,055 patients undergoing isolated coronary artery bypass grafting operations. This study noted that crude, unadjusted mortality rates provided insufficient data to gauge performance. Although the study documented a range for in-hospital mortality from 3.1% to 6.3%, these regional data also suggested that differences in observed in-hospital mortality rate could not be explained solely by differential patient case mix. Rather, the data suggested that differences in isolated CAB outcomes may have resulted from unmeasured differences in care.

This group then explored a regional strategy to learn "best practices" from each other. This strategy employed four components: regular feedback of outcomes data, efforts to determine causes of mortality, structured round-robin visits between organizations, and determinations of cause-specific mortality. This innovative sharing of information resulted in a subsequent reduction in the CAB mortality rate for the region by 24% over an 18-month period despite a higher-risk population being operated on during this period. Furthermore, the group identified low cardiac output as the most common mode of death after isolated CAB. The NNE cardiovascular group continues to explore regional efforts to prevent, recognize, and treat low cardiac output in the perioperative period.

Veterans Administration Database

The Cardiac Surgery Consultants Committee was organized under a congressional mandate to review the surgical results of the 43 VA medical centers performing cardiac surgery since 1972. In 1987, the committee acknowledged the limitations of using raw mortality data to determine whether the appropriate level of surgical care was being delivered. This group sought and received authorization and funding from the VA to initiate a study concerning the incorporation of patient risk factors for the assessment of cardiac surgical results. Since 1991, data entry has been performed by independent nurse investigators who work within each reporting VA medical center. These nurses are independent of the surgical team, and data entry from each surgical program is mandatory. Data are submitted for 6-month periods. The VA database now has enrolled data from several thousand patients.

The patient risk factors recorded are shown in Table 37-2. Data are entered at each individual site by the nurse investigators, and these data are then centrally processed. The expected mortality rate for each cardiac surgery program is computed by

Table 37-2 Coronary Artery Bypass Graft (CABG) Mortality Model: Veterans Administration Cardiac Surgery Database

Risk Variables	Odds Ratio
Age, odds ratio for 10-yr increments	1.5
Gender	
Male	Reference
Female	2.6
Chronic obstructive pulmonary disease	1.3
Vascular disease	
Peripheral	1.4
Cerebrovascular	1.3
Creatine level (mg/dL)	
<1.5	Reference
1.5–3.0	1.6
>3.0	2.6
Prior heart surgery	2.1
Prior myocardial infarction	
None	Reference
>7 days preoperatively	1.2
<7 days preoperatively	2.1
Preoperative intra-aortic balloon pump use	1.7
Cardiomegaly	1.5
Resting ST depression	1.4
New York Heart Association functional class	
I	Reference
II	1.5
III	1.5
IV	2.3
Canadian Cardiovascular Society class (angina)	
I	Reference
II	1.0
III	1.0
IV	1.4

calculating the expected probability of 30-day mortality for each patient and then averaging the probabilities for all patients having cardiac surgery at the given hospital. A ratio of the observed mortality rate to the expected mortality rate is then calculated. This information is reviewed by the VA Cardiac Surgery Consultants Committee semiannually. The blinded results of each VA cardiac surgical program are provided to the individual programs every 6 months. In the VA cardiac surgery database, only program-specific data are available, and not patient-specific nor surgeon-specific data.

Within the VA system, the risk-adjusted surgical results are used for two purposes: (1) as measures to prompt oversight review by the Cardiac Surgery Consultants Committee of the individual cardiac surgical programs and (2) as feedback to individual programs to provide comparison data with the other VA cardiac surgical programs such that continuous quality assurance may be sought.

Society of Thoracic Surgeons Adult Cardiac Surgery Database

In 1989, the STS similarly developed a voluntary risk-adjusted database in an effort to help members to assess the quality of care in their individual practices and affiliated hospitals. The goal of this database was to establish accurate data with analysis by sophisticated risk-adjustment techniques. An objective of the STS was to counterbalance the release of unadjusted and misleading mortality data compiled by other organizations and agencies. Data for more than 2 million cardiac surgical patients have been entered into the STS database, and a significant reduction in mortality for CAB and valve procedures has been demonstrated. The variables that are significant predictors of operative mortality following CAB are listed in Table 37-3.

The STS database is the largest repository of cardiac surgery data in existence. Thus, it provides a rich resource for scientific articles regarding the effect of new technologies and outcomes for cardiac surgical procedures. A prime example involves the effect of off-pump coronary artery bypass grafting on morbidity/mortality after coronary artery bypass grafting. Analysis of the STS database revealed a 20% risk reduction for mortality in the STS database for patients operated on with an off-pump versus an on-pump approach. Because they are observational, retrospective data, conclusions based on them must be interpreted

Table 37-3 The 1996 Coronary Artery Bypass Graft–Only Risk Model: Society of Thoracic Surgeons	
Variable	Odds Ratio
Age (in 10-yr increments)	1.64
Female gender	1.157
Nonwhite	1.249
Ejection fraction	0.988
Diabetes mellitus	1.188
Renal failure	1.533
Serum creatinine level (if renal failure present)	1.080
Dialysis dependence (if renal failure present)	1.381
Pulmonary hypertension	1.185
Cerebrovascular accident timing	1.198
Chronic obstructive pulmonary disease	1.296
Peripheral vascular disease	1.487
Cerebrovascular disease	1.244
Acute evolving, extending myocardial infarction	1.282
Myocardial infarction timing	1.117
Cardiogenic shock	2.211
Use of diuretics	1.112
Hemodynamic instability	1.747
Triple-vessel disease	1.155
Left main artery disease >50%	1.119
Preoperative intra-aortic balloon pump	1.480
Status	
Urgent or emergent	1.189
Emergent salvage	3.654
First reoperation	2.738
Multiple reoperations	4.282
Arrhythmias	1.099
Body surface area	0.488
Obesity	1.242
New York Heart Association functional class IV	1.098
Use of steroids	1.214
Congestive heart failure	1.191
Percutaneous transluminal coronary angioplasty within 6 hrs of surgery	1.332
Angiographic accident with hemodynamic instability	1.203
Use of digitalis	1.168
Use of intravenous nitrates	1.088

cautiously. However, these data have been successfully used to argue compellingly for a randomized, controlled trial to study off-pump CAB in the VA system. Such an investigation is underway and is to be concluded by 2007.

Society of Thoracic Surgeons Congenital Cardiac Surgery and General Thoracic Surgery Databases

Based on the successful implementation of its adult cardiac surgery database, the STS initiated two other databases: a congenital cardiac surgery database and a general thoracic surgery database. The congenital

cardiac surgery database now has 22 participating sites with accrual of 25,000 patient records. This database has developed a data dictionary with complete descriptions of the definitions for the multiple variations of congenital defects. This database is still in its development phase, but seeks to integrate the Aristotle Score into its report. In a similar fashion, the General Thoracic Surgery Database has 46 participating sites with roughly 5,000 patient data entries reported. With the development of commercially available software in 2004, data will soon be transferred to the Duke Clinical Research Institute for analysis. Data will then be returned in the form of annual or semi-annual reports to participating sites so that they may compare their outcomes with the national cohort.

Challenges and Future Directions of Databases

The Health Insurance Probability and Accountability Act of 1996 (HIPPA) provided a major challenge for multi-institutional databases. Because these databases are necessary components of quality improvement programs, some form of patient identifier will be necessary to provide longitudinal follow-up. Furthermore, to improve the efficiency and ease of prompt data analysis and feedback of such data, the use of the Internet will be desirable. The STS is in the process of incorporating patient consent for encrypted core data collection and transmission of patient data for quality improvement and longitudinal follow-up. However, the patient consent process may lead to some patients refusing participation. This refusal could bias data and have a negative effect on the accuracy and reliability of data for use in quality improvement.

Another challenge is maintaining and verifying the high quality of data submitted. New York State audits data, as does the NNE group. The VA has the added advantage of having several parallel databases that can be used to verify the accuracy of the national cardiac surgery database. Since the STS has paired with the Duke Clinical Research Institute (DCRI) as its repository and analytical site for its data, the DCRI has instituted various software checks for completeness of data. In addition, outliers of various risk factors and outcome variables automatically trigger data software checks in the STS database. The STS continues to provide a major effort in the education of data managers and surgeons with regard to definition of risk variables and the importance of data completeness and quality. Finally, the STS developed high and low thresholds for mortality and morbidity. Reported values outside these limits generate a query to the local group.

Efforts to improve the quality and monitor outcomes in cardiac surgery progressed throughout the last decade. Consumer groups, purchasers of health care, and patients demand access to the highest quality of care in cardiac surgery. The implementation of these databases has allowed for the appropriate use of outcomes data in cardiac surgery. These databases have proven enormously useful in providing feedback to surgeons and hospitals performing cardiac surgery. A future direction for adult cardiac surgery databases would include sharing demographic variables with the American College of Cardiology database such that center-specific cardiac care outcomes would be reflected. Cardiothoracic surgeons should be proud of their efforts to lead the rest of the health care system in understanding and defining the need for risk-adjusted quality measures of care and outcomes. Clearly the STS, the VA, and others have positively affected health care delivery in the twenty-first century via the development of these sophisticated databases.

Summary

Clinicians should use risk-adjusted outcome information only as a screening tool to evaluate where to further investigate for possible quality-of-care challenges and opportunities for improvement. Risk-adjusted outcomes may play an important role in patient–clinician discussions related to the informed consent process, clinical decisions related to comparing alternative therapies for a patient with prespecified risk profile, initiating local quality assessment and improvement discussions related to care provided, comparison of provider performance for further investigation, and enhancing national policy discussions. The key point is that risk-adjusted outcomes information alone is insufficient, but can be used to start an interactive dialogue with others toward the goal of improving patient cardiac surgical care.

SUGGESTED READING

Cleveland JC Jr, Shroyer AL, Chen A, et al. Off-pump coronary artery bypass grafting significantly decreases risk-adjusted mortality and morbidity. Ann Thorac Surg 2001;72: 1282.

Grover FL, Cleveland JC Jr, Shroyer LW. Quality improvement in cardiac care. Arch Surg 2002;137:28.

Hannan EL, Kilburn HK Jr, O'Donnell JF, et al. Adult open heart surgery in New York State. JAMA 1990;264:2768.

Hannan EL, Kilburn Jr HK, Racz M, et al. Improving the outcomes of coronary artery bypass surgery in New York State. JAMA 1994;271:761.

Kennedy JW, Kaiser GC, Fisher LD, et al. Multivariate discriminant analysis of the clinical and angiographic predictors of operative mortality from the Collaborative Study in Coronary Artery Surgery (CASS). J Thorac Cardiovasc Surg 1980;80:876.

Nugent WC. Innovative uses of a cardiovascular database. Ann Thorac Surg 1999;68:359.

O'Conner GT, Plume SK, Olmstead EM, et al. A regional prospective study of in-hospital mortality associated with coronary artery bypass grafting. JAMA 1991;266:803.

Takaro T, Ankeney JL, Laning RC, et al. Quality control for cardiac surgery in the Veterans Administration. Ann Thorac Surg 1986;42:37.

EDITOR'S COMMENTS

The use of databases has taken on increasing importance. Individual surgeons are judged by results, and in many states the results are available for public access. In addition, many insurance companies plan reimbursement based on data results. Our group is entering into contracts with insurance companies that will give us a premium if our results, including specific quality indicators, are in the top quartile.

In addition, the maintenance of competence initiative from the American Board of Thoracic Surgery will require the use of a database to prove that one is attending to one's own data and is making quality improvements based on them. I can't imagine one would be able to perform cardiac surgery in the future without the use of a database. Therefore, appreciating the developments cited in this chapter and appropriately interpreting one's own data will be critical to careers in cardiac surgery.

I.L.K.

38

Prevention of Neurologic Injury After Coronary Artery Bypass

Christopher J. Barreiro and William A. Baumgartner

Introduction

Coronary artery bypass (CAB) surgery has been proven to increase long-term survival compared to medical therapy for patients with significant coronary artery disease. Operative mortality continues to decline with improvements in anesthesia, surgical technique, and myocardial preservation. Despite these improvements, neurologic injury continues to be a significant risk for patients undergoing CAB. Aside from being a leading cause of morbidity in these patients, neurologic sequelae also result in escalating medical costs in the form of increased length of hospital stay and subsequent rehabilitation.

The spectrum of neurologic injury ranges from frank stroke, which is seen in up to 6% of patients undergoing CAB, to much more prevalent, subtle neurocognitive changes. These include mild deficits in memory, attention, concentration, and language. The three main etiologic factors involved are atherosclerotic emboli, cerebral hypoperfusion, and generalized perioperative inflammation. Identifying both the mechanism of injury and potential modifiable risk factors for unfavorable neurologic outcomes is a very active area of research, and many potential neuroprotective strategies have emerged.

Preoperative predictors of neurologic sequelae after cardiac surgery include advanced age, prior neurologic events, hypertension, diabetes, and peripheral vascular disease. These risk factors identify individuals with widespread cerebrovascular disease, impaired cerebral blood flow, or increased susceptibility to thromboembolic events. Studies have also identified intraoperative predictors for perioperative neurologic events. These independent risk factors include the presence of significant aortic arch atherosclerosis, longer duration of cardiopulmonary bypass (CPB), and CAB with concomitant carotid endarterectomy. The preoperative recognition and assessment of risk factors is an important step in reducing the morbidity and mortality associated with perioperative strokes.

Mechanism of Neurologic Injury

Neurocognitive deficits have been reported to occur in up to 60% to 70% of patients undergoing cardiac surgery. The development of potential therapeutic strategies is dependent on our understanding of the mechanism of neuronal cell injury following cardiac surgery. "Glutamate excitotoxicity" is a major mechanism of neuronal injury. Glutamate is the major excitatory amino acid neurotransmitter in the central nervous system (CNS) and can lead to neuronal hyperactivity and death during periods of metabolic stress such as hypoxia or ischemia (Fig. 38-1). Glutamate initiates a cascade of events via binding to an N-methyl-D-aspartate (NMDA) receptor, ultimately resulting in neuronal necrosis or apoptosis. Histologically, the areas of the brain most significantly affected are those in which NMDA receptors are prominent: the hippocampus, cerebellum, and basal ganglia. Pharmacologic blockade of this receptor was also shown to provide some degree of neurologic protection in animal models, thus validating this mechanism of injury.

Nitric oxide (NO) is a ubiquitous molecule also found to act as a neurotoxin. Induction of neuronal nitric oxide synthase (nNOS) via a hypoxic/ischemic insult leads to widespread NO production in the brain. NO and its metabolite peroxynitrite have toxic effects on the neuronal mitochondria, resulting in free radical proliferation and DNA fragmentation (Fig. 38-2). Mitochondrial energy failure is considered to play a central role in neuronal cell death. Investigations using a canine model of hypothermic circulatory arrest (HCA) showed that inhibition of nNOS results in decreased NO production and superior neurologic function compared to untreated HCA canines. These studies demonstrated that pharmacologic intervention at specific points in the injury cascade may potentially mitigate the neurologic deficits that can result from cardiac surgery.

Cerebral Protection Techniques

Minimizing the Systemic Inflammatory State

Cardiopulmonary bypass is associated with an intense inflammatory response due to contact of blood with the artificial bypass surfaces, conversion to laminar, nonpulsatile flow, and leukocyte and endothelial cell activation following ischemia/reperfusion. The systemic inflammatory response is characterized by activation of the complement, fibrinolytic, and

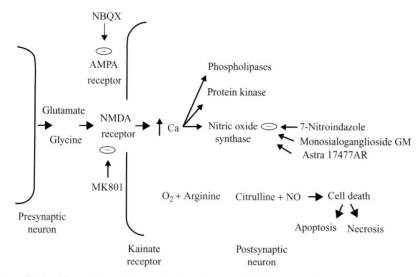

Figure 38-1.   The excitotoxicity mechanism of neuronal cell injury and points of intervention. (AMPA = α-amino-3-hydroxy-5-methylisoyazole-4-propionic acid; NMDA = N-methyl-D-aspartate.). (Reprinted with permission from WA Baumgartner. Neurologic injury after cardiopulmonary bypass surgery. J Neurosurg Anesthesiol 2004;16:102.)

cytokine cascades. Complement activation occurs immediately after the blood comes into contact with the foreign surfaces of the bypass circuit. This leads to increased inflammatory cytokine production and leukocyte activation. The leukocyte–endothelial cell interactions result in microvascular occlusion and end-organ ischemia. This inflammatory response is the suspected mechanism underlying the global cerebral edema seen on post-CPB magnetic resonance imaging.

Many therapeutic strategies have been used in an attempt to mitigate the CPB-induced inflammation. These include both pharmacologic and mechanical therapeutic modalities. Corticosteroids have been shown to reduce CPB-induced inflammation by decreasing complement activation and levels of circulating cytokines. However, the use of steroids remains controversial due to the theoretical risks of increased postoperative infections and delayed wound healing. The serine protease inhibitors such as aprotinin are another group of pharmacologic agents under investigation. Previous studies showed them to reduce the inflammatory response post-CPB and to decrease the postoperative stroke risk. Mechanical strategies to reduce the release of proinflammatory cytokines include leukocyte and hemoconcentration filters, which essentially wash the cells before returning them to the bypass circuit. However, significant clinical bene-

fit has not been shown in human studies. In an attempt to increase the biocompatibility of CPB, heparin-coated circuits have been shown to reduce complement activation, proinflammatory cytokine levels, and neutrophil adhesion. A prospective, randomized trial of heparin-coated circuits even demonstrated a significant improvement in postoperative neuropsychometric tests as compared to conventional circuits.

Maintenance of Cerebral Perfusion

Cerebral autoregulation maintains a constant cerebral blood flow (CBF) over a wide range of systemic arterial pressures (50 to 120 mm Hg). Below 50 mm Hg, cerebral oxygen delivery (CDo_2) becomes pressure dependent. This can be compensated for by an increase in cerebral oxygen extraction. Therefore, CDo_2 remains relatively constant even at systemic pressures as low as 30 mm Hg during moderate hypothermia. However, because of the common comorbidities of our patient population, including hypertension, diabetes, and cerebrovascular disease, the ischemic tolerance and autoregulatory capacity of the brain is altered. For this reason, higher minimal perfusion pressures may be required to support adequate cerebral oxygenation. With this in mind, flow rates during CPB are adjusted to preserve end-organ and cerebral perfusion above an ischemic threshold. However, the watershed areas of the brain still remain at greatest risk for neurologic sequelae. A prospective, randomized trial of 248 elective CAB patients showed that those maintained at lower perfusion pressures (50 to 60 mm Hg) had significantly higher mortality and stroke rates than those maintained at a higher perfusion pressure (80 to 100 mm Hg). This study demonstrated that maintaining patients on CPB at a higher perfusion pressure was technically safe and effectively improved outcomes after cardiac surgery. The current perfusion practices, which err on the side of higher perfusion pressures, result in excellent outcomes in the vast majority of patients, and there is little evidence to suggest that altering these practices will have a positive influence on CBF.

Embolization Reduction

There are three main types of embolic phenomena encountered during cardiac surgery that may result in postoperative neurologic dysfunction: particulate, gaseous, and lipid embolization. Perhaps the most significant of these is the particulate emboli resulting from atheromatous debris present in

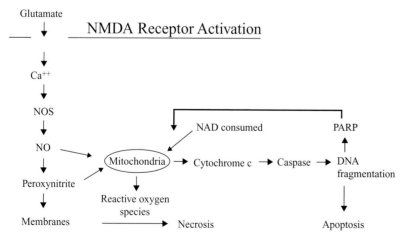

Figure 38-2.   The role of the mitochondria in neuronal cell injury. (NAD = nicotinamide adenine dinucleotide; NMDA = N-methyl-D-aspartate; NOS = nitric oxide synthase; PARP = poly ADP-ribose polymerase. (Reprinted with permission from WA Baumgartner. Neurologic injury after cardiopulmonary bypass surgery. J Neurosurg Anesthesiol 2004;16:102.)

the diseased aorta and great vessels. The platelet-fibrin aggregates and debris generated by the CPB circuit itself also have a causative role. To limit particulate embolization, surgical manipulation of the heart and great vessels must be minimized and care should be taken in the placement of cannulae and clamps on atherosclerotic vessels. In addition to intraoperative palpation, transesophageal echocardiography (TEE) and epiaortic ultrasonography are commonly used to assess the degree of aortic atherosclerosis and to identify more favorable areas for cannulation and clamping. In a recent study, patients undergoing epiaortic scanning showed a lower incidence of cognitive dysfunction than patients evaluated only with aortic palpation.

Cross-clamping of the atherosclerotic aorta can result in dislodging of plaque material and cerebral embolization. A number of recent studies evaluated the use of a single-clamp technique (SCT) versus a double-clamp technique (DCT) for cerebral protection during CAB. In the DCT, the cross-clamp is removed before the proximal aortic anastomoses, which are then performed using a partial occluding clamp. This technique reduces overall CPB and myocardial ischemic time but results in increased aortic manipulation and risk of embolization. A retrospective study of 189 SCT versus 272 DCT patients showed DCT to be an independent risk factor for neurologic injury on multivariate analysis. A recent prospective trial randomized 268 patients undergoing CAB to either SCT or DCT. The DCT group included 2 patients (1.5%) with a postoperative stroke and 2 patients (1.5%) with postoperative confusion. The SCT patients demonstrated improved cerebral protection, with no postoperative neurologic complications, and no adverse effect on myocardial protection or postoperative outcome.

Novel alternatives have also evolved to decrease aortic manipulation and subsequent embolic risk. Endovascular balloon occlusion of the ascending aorta has been described as one method for avoiding the potential injury caused by cross-clamping of the aorta. Intra-aortic filtration systems (Embol-X; Embol-X Inc., Mountain View, CA) have also been developed for deployment before cross-clamp release in an effort to reduce the embolic burden. A large, randomized trial of >1,200 patients demonstrated the filtration system to be both safe and effective with a filter embolic capture rate of 96.8%. However, postoperative event rates including mortality, stroke, transient ischemic attack, and renal insufficiency

showed no significant differences between the control and filter arms of the study. Aortic manipulation/clamping can also be minimized with the use of automated aortic connectors for the construction of sutureless proximal saphenous vein graft–aortic anastomoses. Again, a recent prospective trial of 77 primary CAB patients randomized to either the automated anastomotic device or conventional handsewn anastomosis demonstrated no significant differences in neurocognitive deficits, stroke, or mortality.

Cerebral air embolization is another potential source of postoperative neurologic dysfunction. Air can be entrained into the heart from the surgical field. However, this is more of an issue with open-chambered procedures such as valve surgeries than with routine CAB surgery. Flooding the surgical field with CO_2 is one method used to lessen the embolic load. The CPB circuit can introduce air into the patient, but this is theoretically avoided by the venous reservoir design and arterial line filter. The number of perfusionist interventions, defined as the administration of drugs or the injection of blood into the venous reservoir, has also been correlated with the incidence of air microemboli. A prospective study of 83 CAB patients demonstrated that those with increased perfusionist interventions, and therefore increased gaseous microemboli, had significantly worse performance on neurocognitive testing. This study further implicates the CPB circuit as a potential source of clinically significant microemboli. TEE is routinely used to assess the amount of intracardiac air and can assist in de-airing procedures.

Fat embolization into the cerebral circulation is a common occurrence due to aspiration of mediastinal and cardiac fat into the cardiotomy suction and CPB circuit. This lipid material is often small and deformable, and so is easily passed through arterial line filters. Lipid emboli in the cerebral circulation are an extremely common occurrence in post–cardiac surgery patients, as determined at autopsy. These emboli are associated with an upregulation of inflammatory cytokines in the brain, which may result in the systemic inflammatory response seen in some patients. Therefore, the current practice at our institution is to avoid the use of cardiotomy suction to prevent the return of lipid debris to the pump. Cell-saver or blood-salvage devices, however, can decrease the amount of particulate or lipid debris returned to the CPB circuit. The main drawback to these devices is the washing away of platelet and coagulation factors that

also occurs. The overall significance of lipid embolization is not entirely known, but may contribute to the postoperative delirium and cognitive dysfunction that can be seen early after CAB surgery.

Temperature Management

The issue of hypothermic versus normothermic CPB has been a topic of debate. The potential benefit of hypothermic CPB is a decreased cerebral metabolic rate, which has been shown to decrease the neuronal injury associated with ischemia. Mild hypothermia also allows for lower flow rates, which can lower the risk of embolization. This risk, however, is greatest during aortic cannulation, cross-clamping and unclamping, and onset of CPB. Unfortunately, the brain remains normothermic during these critical time periods due to the timing of hypothermia after the onset of CPB. In addition, hypothermia requires rewarming, which lengthens CPB and overall operative time. The rewarming process itself also has the potential to cause moderate hyperthermia if performed too rapidly, which has been associated with worsened neurologic outcomes. It is therefore important that during the rewarming phase the bladder temperature does not exceed 37°C to 37.5°C. Studies examining the effect of hypothermic versus normothermic CPB have yielded conflicting results. Some studies suggest a decreased stroke rate and improved neuropsychologic outcomes associated with hypothermic CPB, whereas others report no difference in neurologic complications. Overall, common practice is to induce a mild state of hypothermia (30°C to 32°C), which is generally protective of all organs during CPB.

Acid–Base Management

The increased solubility of carbon dioxide in blood at lower temperatures has resulted in two different methods of acid–base management during hypothermic CPB. The pH-stat management technique uses a temperature-corrected arterial blood gas and maintains the pH at 7.40. This technique can result in a loss of cerebral autoregulation and an increased risk of neurologic injury. The α stat management technique, however, does not use temperature-corrected arterial blood gases and therefore maintains the autoregulation of CBF. Studies comparing these two management strategies have had varied results. Some animal studies have advocated the use of the pH-stat method due to improved functional outcomes and less severe neuronal injury. However, other studies report a higher incidence of postoperative neurologic dysfunction in patients treated with the pH-stat method. This may be due to increased CBF associated with the loss of autoregulation, which can lead to an increased delivery of microemboli. Despite conflicting opinions, the majority of adult practices today utilize the α stat management technique.

Pharmacologic Intervention

Many different pharmacologic agents have been explored for their potential neuroprotective effects in both experimental and clinical models. However, there are no approved therapies for the prevention of CAB-associated neurologic events. Various anesthetic agents have been used in conjunction with electroencephalography in an effort to suppress cerebral oxygen metabolism. Anti-inflammatory agents have been tried to prevent the adverse inflammatory sequelae of cerebral ischemia. However, the limited success with these agents may not be caused by any direct neuroprotective effect, but rather by an indirect effect on cerebral emboli. As the mechanism of injury is further elucidated, the potential targets for intervention continue to increase. Our understanding of glutamate excitotoxicity with increased nitric oxide production and neuronal cell death has led to the rational exploration of glutamate-receptor blockers and nitric oxide synthase inhibitors. These agents have shown beneficial neurologic effects in our laboratory canine model of circulatory arrest. HCA is considered to carry the greatest risk of neurologic injury and is therefore a useful model for pharmacologic investigations.

The inhibition of mitochondrial energy failure is another strategy for preventing the ischemia-induced neuronal injury in our canine HCA model. Ischemic preconditioning (IPC) is a paradoxical form of protection against lethal ischemia by exposure to brief episodes of conditioning ischemia before primary insult. Although initially described in cardiac myocytes, a similar mechanism was also found in neurons and may provide mitochondrial protection. One potential mechanism of IPC relies on the opening of ATP-dependent K^+ channels on the inner mitochondrial membrane. This effect can be achieved pharmacologically by using a variety of different agents. Diazoxide, an antihypertensive medication no longer in clinical use, is one such ATP-dependent K^+-channel agonist. Pretreatment with diazoxide before neurologic insult has been

correlated with improved functional outcomes and histopathology. This has been further substantiated by the antagonistic effect of glibenclamide, an ATP-dependent, K^+-channel antagonist. In the current age of rational drug design, further successes in pharmacologic neuroprotection are inevitable as our mechanistic understanding continues to improve.

Hematocrit Management on Cardiopulmonary Bypass

Hemodilutional anemia has been used during hypothermic CPB to reduce blood viscosity to allow maintenance of baseline CBF. This technique is believed to reduce the risks of adverse outcomes due to arterial hypertension such as aortic dissection and collateral blood flow to the coronary arteries during cross-clamping of the aorta. Although a goal hematocrit level of approximately 21% is common practice, multiple studies have questioned the appropriateness of this technique. In a review of >6,900 coronary artery bypass grafting patients by DeFoe and colleagues, patients were categorized based on their lowest hematocrit on CPB. The data showed a trend toward increasing risk of death for patients with a hematocrit of <23%, and patients with a hematocrit of <19% had mortality rates approximately twice as high as those with a values of $\geq$25%. There was no difference in perioperative stroke rates. In a randomized trial of 147 infants, Jonas and colleagues randomly assigned patients to a lower-hematocrit strategy (21.5%) or a higher-hematocrit strategy (27.8%) during hypothermic CPB. The lower-hematocrit group had worse perioperative outcomes with significantly lower scores on the Psychomotor Development Index at 1 year of age. Further randomized studies are necessary to refine the optimum hematocrit level during hypothermic CPB to improve outcomes of cardiac surgery.

Glucose Control

Disruption of cerebral energy metabolism plays a causative role in the neurologic injury that occurs following cerebral ischemia. Episodes of brain ischemia initiate anaerobic glycolysis with resultant intracellular lactic acidosis, which is toxic to the cell. An increase in blood glucose concentration at the time of ischemia provides more substrate for anaerobic metabolism with worsening of the acidosis. Studies show that hyperglycemia at the onset of cerebral ischemia worsens postischemic neurologic function and histopathologic injury. In a primate

model of complete cerebral ischemia, animals receiving a glucose infusion immediately before ischemic insult had significantly worse neurologic function at 96 hours than control animals receiving a crystalloid infusion. CPB can potentially result in both global and local cerebral ischemia through hypoperfusion and microembolization. The appropriate intraoperative management of hyperglycemia and its affects after cardiac surgery remain controversial, and conflicting studies are found in the literature. In a prospective study of 171 infants undergoing cardiac surgery at Boston Children's Hospital, intraoperative hyperglycemia was not associated with neurodevelopmental outcomes at 1, 4, and 8 years. However, because postoperative infections have been demonstrated to be reduced in patients with tight glucose control, most practices are using this approach.

Intraoperative Cerebral Monitoring

Intraoperative neurophysiologic monitoring has been shown to reduce the incidence of neurologic complications after CPB. Some of the different modalities available include near-infrared cerebral oximetry, jugular bulb oximetry, EEG, somatosensory-evoked potentials (SEP), and transcranial Doppler (TCD) ultrasound. These multi-modality strategies can help detect cerebral hypoperfusion and dysoxygenation, which are major causative factors for brain injury during cardiac surgery. Cerebral oximetry is a simple method of measuring cerebral oxygenation. The level of cerebral oxygenated hemoglobin has been shown to correlate with high-energy phosphates and can predict histologic brain injury in an animal model. In addition, near-infrared spectroscopy can be used to obtain transcranial measurements of cerebral venous oxygen saturation (CVOS). CVOS remains remarkably stable, and any significant change reflects a marked imbalance between oxygen delivery and consumption. Jugular bulb oximetry provides similar information regarding oxygen imbalance. However, it is slightly more invasive due to the need for jugular vein cannulation. EEG and somatosensory-evoked potential monitoring have also been used as measures of cerebral metabolic activity. EEG silence and the disappearance of somatosensory-evoked potentials can be used as markers of adequate cerebral protection and can potentially shorten the cooling period during CPB. These two techniques, however, are more commonly used for patients undergoing hypothermic circulatory arrest. TCD ultrasound can detect sudden changes in either blood flow or vascular resistance, as well as aid in the identification of embolic phenomena. In addition to detecting abnormalities, these neurodiagnostic modalities can be used to make adjustments in perfusion, oxygenation, or anesthetic administration. When used effectively, this has been shown to shorten hospital stay and, decrease costs and, most important, neurologic complications.

Off-Pump Coronary Artery Bypass

With the development of cardiac immobilization techniques that allow complete revascularization of the beating heart, off-pump CAB (OPCAB) has increased in popularity. CPB is associated with an intense inflammatory response secondary to the conversion to laminar flow, blood contact with the artificial bypass surface, cold cardiac ischemia, and reperfusion. In addition, other CPB related factors such as hemodilution and aortic cross-clamping play a significant role in postoperative neurologic dysfunction. OPCAB has the potential advantage of avoiding the inflammatory response and micro-/macroemboli that may result from the CPB circuit and manipulation of the atheromatous aorta. Some retrospective studies suggest a decreased stroke rate with OPCAB. However, other studies fail to demonstrate significant neurologic benefit over routine CPB surgery. A prospective, randomized study evaluated cognitive dysfunction in 281 patients undergoing OPCAB and found a reduction in cognitive decline in the early postoperative period. However, no difference was detected in cognitive function between the groups at 1-year follow-up. Although OPCAB may offer some theoretical advantages, its ability to reduce the risk of neurologic complications is unclear and will only be determined through further clinical investigations.

Assessing Neurologic Injury

Neuropsychologic Testing

Traditional studies in the area of post–cardiac surgery neurologic outcomes focused on clinically obvious neurologic and psychologic dysfunction such as stroke, disorientation, and depression. However, with the introduction of neuropsychometric testing much more subtle injury patterns can be detected. This testing typically includes measures of language, memory, attention, concentration, and psychomotor performance. In a prospective study of 127 patients undergoing CAB surgery, patients were given a battery of cognitive tests preoperatively and 1 month and 1 year postoperatively. This study established that the incidence of cognitive decline varies among the different domains of cortical function tested. More important, however, these patients must be followed longitudinally because initial deficits may eventually show either improvement or further decline. A more recent prospective study from our institution looked at the longitudinal neuropsychologic performance of CAB patients versus nonsurgical controls with coronary artery disease. The results of cognitive testing at 3 months and 1 year after baseline examination were comparable between the two groups. This suggests that the cognitive decline during the early postoperative period after CAB may be transient and reversible. Therefore, any long-term cognitive dysfunction may be related to age and other comorbidities, as opposed to CPB exposure. Through the use of an objective measure of neurologic injury, the underlying etiology of neuropsychologic deficits can be identified and alleviated. However, no such gold standard exists. With further research into neurobehavioral assessment techniques, it will be possible to evaluate the effectiveness of surgical and pharmacologic strategies for mitigating neurologic injury after CAB surgery.

Molecular Markers

Various proteins released by the injured brain have been used to measure cerebral injury. Neuronal, glial, and endothelial cells of the CNS elaborate these substances in response to ischemia/reperfusion injury. Assaying for these biochemical markers provides a relatively noninvasive way of measuring the degree of injury. If these assays can demonstrate a direct correlation with clinical outcomes, this can provide a simpler way of assessing postoperative cognitive dysfunction. Brain-specific creatine phosphokinase (CPK-BB) is one such biochemical marker. Increased blood levels were found in 98% of 421 CPB patients in a study conducted at the Cleveland Clinic. However, there was no correlation between CPK-BB concentrations and neurologic dysfunction. A more recently investigated protein is $S100\beta$, which normally promotes axonal growth, glial proliferation, and neuronal differentiation. This protein is released by injured glial cells and also demonstrates increased blood concentration after cardiac surgery. It has been shown to correlate with intraoperative cerebral microemboli quantified with transcranial Doppler sonography. More important, a significant correlation could also be made with neuropsychologic deficits assessed at 6 months post–cardiac surgery in a small study of 16 patients. Similar studies have been conducted with various other biochemical markers. Although none are used routinely yet, a reliable, noninvasive biochemical test for detecting subtle neurocognitive deficits would provide a great benefit to the postoperative care of CAB patients.

Magnetic Resonance Imaging

Magnetic resonance imaging (MRI) has demonstrated cerebral edema as early as 1 hour after CAB surgery. This is often clinically insignificant and resolves by 1 week. Diffusion-weighted MRI can also help to differentiate acute from chronic brain ischemia; however, it has been difficult to correlate the presence of lesions on MRI with clinical cognitive dysfunction. Magnetic resonance spectroscopy (MRS) is another useful adjunct, which may have better predictive value for cognitive dysfunction. We have used MRS in our laboratory canine HCA model, which has allowed us to detect and quantify subcellular metabolic changes within the brain after HCA. The most significant finding on MRS was a decline in the ratio of N-acetyl-aspartate to choline (NAA:Cho) 24 hours post-HCA, which is a known marker of neuronal mitochondrial dysfunction. MRS also provided a way of assessing the efficacy of different pharmacologic agents. Pretreatment with diazoxide limited neurologic injury versus controls, which was reflected in a preserved NAA:Cho ratio. These results could be correlated with the degree of clinical neurologic injury observed. Similarly, MRI/MRS and neurocognitive testing were performed serially during the pre- and postoperative period in a clinical study of 35 CAB patients. Transient changes were detected in the ratio of NAA to creatinine (NAA:Cr), with the degree of decline closely correlating with deterioration in neurocognitive function, increased patient age, and longer CPB times. Normalization of the NAA:Cr ratio also accompanied the recovery of neurocognitive performance over time. These studies clearly demonstrate that MRS may offer an early, noninvasive means of assessing neurologic injury and the effectiveness of neuroprotective agents.

Conclusion

Neurocognitive dysfunction remains a significant complication after CAB surgery. This is especially true given the continual improvements in surgical and anesthetic techniques that allow us to operate on older and sicker patients today. Therefore, it is important that the individual risk profile of each patient be taken into consideration. The various neuroprotective strategies available to the cardiac surgeon continue to expand. Pharmacologic neuroprotection is an attractive option for preventing neurologic injury and therefore is a very active area of research. Although we have had success in some laboratory and small clinical studies, no single agent is available for routine use in CAB patients. However, as our mechanistic understanding of the neurologic injury associated with cardiac surgery continues to improve, we will be better equipped to develop further neuroprotective agents in the future.

SUGGESTED READING

Baumgartner WA, Walinsky PL, Salazar JD, et al. Assessing the impact of cerebral injury after cardiac surgery: Will determining this mechanism reduce this injury? Ann Thorac Surg 1999;67:1871.

Bucerius J, Gummert JF, Borger MA, et al. Stroke after cardiac surgery: A risk factor analysis of 16,184 consecutive adult patients. Ann Thorac Surg 2003;75:472.

Hammon JW, Stump DA, Butterworth JB. Approaches to reduce neurologic complications during cardiac surgery. Semin Thorac Cardiovasc Surg 2001;13:184.

Mahanna EP, Blumenthal JA, White WD, et al. Defining neuropsychological dysfunction after coronary artery bypass grafting. Ann Thorac Surg 1996;61:1342.

Roach GW, Kanchuger M, Mangano CM, et al. Adverse cerebral outcomes after coronary bypass surgery. N Engl J Med 1996;335:1857.

Van Dijk D, Jansen EW, Hijman R, et al. Cognitive outcome after off-pump and on-pump coronary artery bypass graft surgery: a randomized trial. JAMA 2002;287:1405.

EDITOR'S COMMENTS

Drs. Barreiro and Baumgartner have given an excellent overview on prevention of neurologic injury after cardiac surgery. Their group has done a great deal of investigation into this injury. They have clearly separated strokes from neurocognitive deficits. The mechanisms of both are obviously different. The difficulty for the practicing surgeon is to determine what is theoretical and what is real. We know for sure that one should not manipulate an atherosclerotic aorta. Surgery should either be done off pump or with alternative cannulation techniques. In addition, there are patients in whom the atherosclerotic aorta is not diagnosed preoperatively. Certainly, minimizing aortic manipulation such as by using a single cross-clamp has at least theoretical advantages.

The difficulty is in knowing when to use other modalities. For example, there is evidence that patients with low hematocrit have worse outcomes than those with higher hematocrit. However, there are no data, at least in adults, on whether transfusing these patients improves their outcomes. We know there is a downside to transfusion as well, and that is why this continues to be a dilemma in our practice. We have taken the stance that blood-reducing transfusion is better, but we still do not know what to do with the truly high-risk patient.

Finally, the question of what to do about the cerebral oximetry. We have begun to use this in our practice. I am not sure that minor changes need to be manipulated, but certainly major ones need to be dealt with. We do not have enough information yet to know the right approach here. Neurologic injury is probably the most important source of morbidity after cardiac surgery and remains a major topic of interest for us.

I.L.K.

B

Acquired Valvular Heart Disease

39

Mitral Valve Repair

Lawrence H. Cohn

Introduction

Reparative procedures for pathologic conditions of the mitral valve have become standard surgical therapy for mitral regurgitation in the current era. The evolution of surgical techniques over the last 20 years has led to definitive and reproducible operative procedures that ensure long-lasting, competent valves. When first introduced, many of these procedures were thought to be too complex, or the pathology too esoteric, to achieve repair. The long-term results of these operations, as well as the development of minimally invasive techniques permitting surgical intervention through smaller, less traumatic incisions, have shown otherwise. Once new and unfamiliar approaches to mitral valve pathology, these complex reparative valve procedures have become the standard of care in many valve centers.

This chapter delineates techniques and surgical concepts related to four classes of mitral valve pathology: (1) the floppy myxomatous mitral valve, (2) ischemic mitral regurgitation, (3) valves affected by endocarditis, and (4) the rheumatic mitral valve. Basic elements of the pathoanatomy and indications for mitral valve repair or replacement are reviewed, followed by a detailed description of surgical techniques and selected long-term results from the large patient series of mitral valve repair at Brigham and Women's Hospital.

Development of Techniques of Mitral Valve Repair

Mitral valve repair is associated with the first successful heart operation, performed by Elliott Carr Cutler in 1923 at the Peter Bent Brigham Hospital (the Peter Bent Brigham Hospital, founded in 1912, was renamed Brigham and Women's Hospital after it merged with the Robert Breck Brigham Hospital and the Boston Hospital for Women in 1980). His patient was a 12-year-old girl with severe rheumatic mitral stenosis. In his laboratory, Cutler had been investigating instruments and operative techniques for the treatment of mitral stenosis resulting from rheumatic heart disease, a scourge of the first half of the twentieth century before antibiotics were available. He had devised a technique *to create* moderate mitral regurgitation, thereby opening the flow of blood from the left atrium to the left ventricle. His first case was referred before development of the instrument, then known as a cardiovalvulotome, was complete. Improvising, he used a neurosurgical tenotomy knife to perform a transventricular commissurotomy via a median sternotomy on the noncalcified commissures of his young patient to open up the stenosed mitral valve. The patient survived the operation and lived for four more years. Isolated successes with this operation were rare until after World War II, when Harken in Boston and Bailey in Philadelphia independently began to perform large-scale closed mitral commissurotomies using the finger fracture method. Their large-scale success stimulated surgeons worldwide to begin using these techniques to relieve mitral stenosis. Until the 1970s, closed mitral commissurotomy was probably the most widely performed heart operation in the world.

Although pathologic mitral regurgitation was recognized early on and some attempts were made at surgical repair, few innovative procedures were performed until the development of the heart-lung machine for open-heart surgery in the early 1950s, which permitted surgeons to perform open mitral commissurotomy. In the late 1950s and early 1960s, several suture annuloplasty techniques were developed to relieve mitral regurgitation with moderate success. Probably most successful was the technique developed by Harold Kay in Los Angeles, who obliterated the commissures using a sequence of mattress sutures, which helped to relieve the mitral regurgitation. Circumferential suture of the annulus, a technique developed by both Paneth and DeVega, also aided in these attempts. Unfortunately, the recurrence rate with suture techniques was relatively high, and true success in mitigating mitral regurgitation awaited the advent of prosthetic mitral valve replacement devices, most notably the Starr-Edwards ball valve in 1961. These devices yielded far more predictable and reproducible results for the treatment of mitral regurgitation. In the early 1960s, Dwight McGoon proposed a reparative technique that involved resecting only those sections of the mitral valve with ruptured chordae, rationalizing that smaller resections would prevent overall distortion of the valve. This was a successful operation and similar to techniques used in current practice, but because of the reproducibility and ease of prosthetic mitral valve replacement, it was largely ignored at that time.

The inherent limitation of the early techniques used for mitral valve replacement was that surgeons of that era believed that it was necessary to cut all of the papillary muscle and chordal attachments to ensure an anatomically secure valve replacement. Late cases of severe ventricular decompensation from cardiomyopathy began to emerge, particularly in patients with severe mitral regurgitation. Many surgeons retreated from operations involving severe mitral regurgitation because of the false perception that the "pop-off valve" of the left atrium was no longer available and the stress on the ventricle would be far too great. This concept was popularized by John Kirklin in 1971, but later proved to be erroneous when laboratory data documented the importance of the interaction between the papillary muscle and chordal leaflet.

The late 1970s heralded a new development that stimulated the use of mitral valve reconstructive surgery for mitral regurgitation. This development was based on the use of a prosthetic suture annuloplasty ring to stabilize the annulus, which enabled mitral valve reconstructive operations to be reproduced by surgeons worldwide. The work of Alain Carpentier and Carlos Duran, who used these prosthetic rings to refashion and remodel the mitral valve annulus, was seminal to this effort. In addition to describing a series of reparative techniques for abnormalities of the mitral leaflets, Dr. Carpentier outlined the basic principles of repair in a formative lecture presented to the American Association for Thoracic Surgery in 1983. Techniques of mitral valve repair soon began to proliferate, including resection of the anterior and posterior leaflets, leaflet advancement, patching of leaflets, transposition of chords, and so forth. Both Duran and Carpentier wrote several papers outlining the long-term effects of mitral valve repair in the degenerative myxomatous valve, as well as the rheumatic valve, indicating long-term successful repair. A number of surgeons have subsequently developed rings of different caliber, consistency, and shape, but the basic principles remain faithful to the initial tenet outlined by Carpentier and Duran, namely that remodeling the mitral annulus with an annuloplasty ring is an important adjunct to the success of mitral valve repair.

Principles of Mitral Valve Repair

The principles of mitral valve repair have evolved from experience with all four underlying etiologies of mitral regurgitation: rheumatic, endocarditic, ischemic, and myxomatous mitral valve disease. Regardless of etiology, the principles are the same: create apposition of the anterior and posterior leaflets at systole, increase valve mobility, prevent valve stenosis, reduce annular dilation, and remodel the annulus. In addition, in patients with mitral regurgitation caused by endocarditis, a principal goal is

to eradicate all of the infection, yet preserve enough of the valve to achieve a functional result after reconstruction.

Principles and Techniques of Repair of the Myxomatous Floppy Mitral Valve

Repair techniques for the myxomatous floppy mitral valve have been in use for about thirty years. The original papers of Carpentier and Duran did a great deal to advance the surgical theory and science of this important area of mitral valve disease, primarily because of the use of remodeling annuloplasty rings as discussed above. The following principles of floppy mitral valve repair are now commonly accepted:

1. Equal apposition of the posterior and anterior leaflets at systole.
2. Reduced height of the posterior leaflet such that the prolapsing segment found in the posterior leaflet is obliterated or reduced, causing the overall height of the leaflet to be considerably shortened.
3. Stabilization of the anterior leaflet by repairing or replacing the ruptured chords present in affected segments, or shortening very elongated chords.
4. Remodeling of the annulus, which is invariably distorted, distended, and eccentric, using an annuloplasty ring, either a full encircling ring or a partial "C" ring.

Many techniques have been developed to achieve these four basic principles of repairing the floppy myxomatous mitral valve. The highlights of these various approaches are summarized below, with emphasis on the author's personal preference. Conventional terminology used to describe the normal partitions of the posterior and anterior mitral valve leaflets first outlined by Duran are depicted in Fig. 39-1A. The surgical anatomy of the mitral valve and surrounding structures is illustrated in Fig. 39-1B.

Apposition of the anterior and posterior leaflet at systole is fundamental to providing a long-lasting repair of the mitral valve with complete elimination of mitral regurgitation. This optimal level can be predetermined by the so-called Carpentier reference point in unaffected areas of the posterior leaflet in comparison with the anterior leaflet, denoting the areas where alterations may have to be made in the height of either leaflet. Once this has been determined, the first obligation is to reduce the height of the posterior leaflet so that it will serve as a "doorstop" for the anterior leaflet, which has the greatest area.

In approximately 80% of cases of floppy mitral valve syndrome, the middle section of the posterior leaflet (P2) is severely prolapsed, with either markedly elongated and stretched chordae or actual rupture of the chordae as shown in Fig. 39-2A. To repair this defect, the middle (or P2) section is usually resected to reduce the height of the posterior leaflet, thus eliminating the mitral regurgitation. Several techniques are available. My preference is to perform a limited resection of the affected segment of the posterior leaflet, removing the minimal number of adjacent chordae and only as much of the supporting structure of the posterior leaflet as necessary. To accomplish this, a silk suture is placed at the middle of the offending segment to be resected. With a straight surgical scissors, the area is excised in a trapezoidal shape, with the narrowest portion of the trapezoid at the annulus, thus ensuring the maximum preservation of adjacent chordae as depicted in Fig. 39-2B.

After removing this section, the remaining parts of the posterior mitral leaflet (PML) must be brought together. There are two ways to proceed. The first was popularized by Duran and attempts to bring the two areas together by imbricating the annulus back into the left atrium. This simple approach can be very effective when small sections of the PML are resected. The drawback to this technique is that it may actually distort the annulus. Once the two annular anchor stitches are brought together, a running stitch is used to run up and back to the atrium to close the imbricated annulus, and then a running Prolene stitch is used from the tip of the preserved leaflets back down toward the annulus, and the two stitches are tied together.

The second, more common approach, and my personal preference, is the leaflet advancement technique. With this technique, one incorporates the excess tissue from the remaining segments of the posterior leaflet, bringing the remaining segments together, and in the process preserving as many of the support chordae as possible. As shown in Figs. 39-2C and 39-2D, one can simply fold over parts of the remaining elongated posterior leaflet toward both commissures and proceed with a gradual reattachment of the two remaining leaflet segments to the annulus by advancing the remaining leaflet tissue in the space of the annular tissue vacated by the resected segment of P2. This is a personal technique modified from Carpentier's technique discussed later. The running 4-0 monofilament suture is then brought back toward the center, and with our technique, the two advancement sutures that

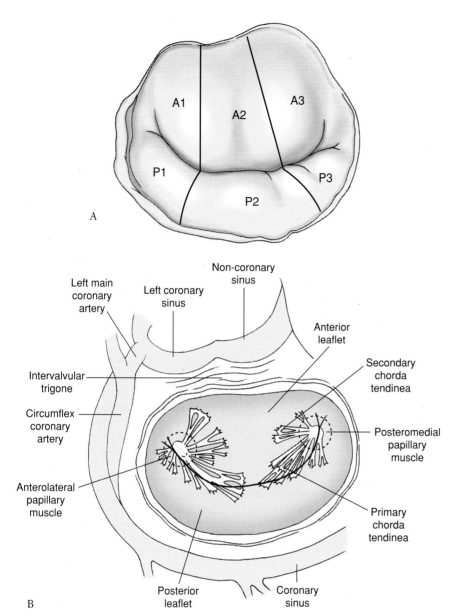

A

B

Figure 39-1.   (A) Anterior and posterior segments of the mitral valve. This figure illustrates the normal partitions of the anterior and posterior leaflets of the mitral valve as first described by Duran. In the figure, the leaflets appear in closed position obscuring the valve orifice. This conventional terminology, which is used to describe and measure optimal points of repair, divides each leaflet into three segments. (Reprinted with permission from NT Kouchoukos, EH Blackstone, DB Doty, et al. Kirklin/Barratt-Boyes Cardiac Surgery: Morphology, Diagnostic Criteria, Natural History, Techniques, Results, and Indications. Philadelphia: Churchill Livingstone, 2003:21.) **(B)** Surgical anatomy of the mitral valve. Thorough familiarity with the surgical anatomy of the mitral valve is key to avoiding injury to the coronary vasculature and other surrounding structures during reparative procedures. (Reprinted with permission from AM Gillinov, DM Cosgrove III. Mitral valve repair. In: LH Cohn, LH Edmunds Jr, eds. Cardiac Surgery in the Adult, 2nd ed. New York: McGraw-Hill, 2003:934.)

approximate the two leaflets at the annulus are left untied (Fig. 39-2D).

After both segments have been approximated at the annulus with the two running 4-0 sutures held on tension, we close and suture the segments of the residual, now reduced posterior leaflet using a single suture of 4-0 Prolene begun at the leading edge of the leaflet. The two segments of Prolene are tied at this point with four knots, and then each of these lengths of suture is run down toward the annulus, suturing the leaflet edges together and tying a knot with the adjacent advancement suture previously left untied (Fig. 39-2E). This is done twice as an over-and-over double layer to prevent any chance of dehiscence. I developed this technique several years ago because of the flexibility it affords and the reduction in time over the use of simple sutures or mattress sutures. The technique allows remodeling of the tissue, which can be easily adjusted to the residual tissue and height of the leaflet. We do not use pledgets of any kind at any time on mitral valve leaflets because they tend to produce scarring or provide a site for potential thrombus and eventual thrombolization. Once the posterior leaflet is repaired, reshaped, and refashioned, it is tested for competency. In my experience, even without a supporting ring or other alteration, the competency of the valve is reasonably secure in about 90% of cases in which this repair has been used. However, despite the apparent integrity of the repair at this point, because of the risk of annular distortion that will eventually lead to mitral valve leakage, we know from experience that the long-term competency of the valve is enhanced with placement of an annuloplasty ring.

The more classic leaflet advancement technique is depicted in Fig. 39-3 and details the procedure as it is performed in extreme cases of Barlow syndrome, where all of the segments of the PML are diseased. As shown in Fig. 39-3C, the dotted line of the leaflet is actually cut off the annulus almost back to the commissure on both sides. A running monofilament suture is then used to put the leaflet back onto the annulus. At the same time, the leaflet is advanced slightly, so that by the time the two parts of the leaflet are brought together, they are touching and an easy approximation is accomplished (Fig. 39-3D,E). The height of the leaflet is also significantly lowered when the running suture is carried out. This is particularly important in patients with Barlow syndrome, in which the height of the entire posterior leaflet may be quite high. Care must be taken not to sever any chordae while performing this maneuver, and all the chordae are pushed toward the lumen so that the leaflet may be dissected off the annulus without chordal injury.

Placing the annuloplasty ring is the final step of the basic mitral valve repair technique. The ring ensures a reproducible result, the most important aspect of any good operation. Sizing, placement, and fixation of the ring are keys to remodeling the annulus of the floppy valve. There are many different types of annuloplasty rings: full rings, partial C-rings, totally flexible rings, totally rigid rings, and so forth. In my experience, the

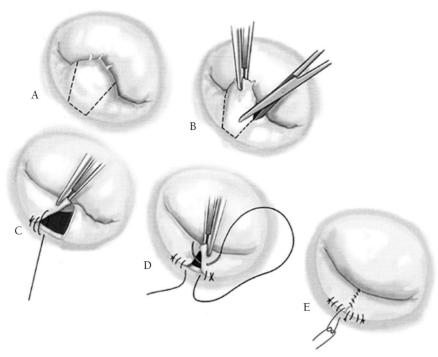

Figure 39-2.   Repair of the myxomatous floppy mitral valve using the leaflet advancement technique. This figure depicts a valve with ruptured chordae underlying the middle segment (P2) of the posterior leaflet.

most important aspect of ring selection is to find a size and shape that accomplishes the physiologic purpose of stabilizing the area between the trigone of the anterior leaflet of the mitral valve, which is the underside of the noncoronary leaflet of the aortic valve. It has long been held that the intertrigonal distance, as shown in Fig. 39-4, does not dilate, and therefore it is quite reasonable to use a partial or C-ring in this repair. Recent information has cast some doubt on this theory, but practically speaking, there is still relatively little movement of the intertrigonal area. I have found a C-type ring, such as the Cosgrove ring (Cosgrove-Edwards Annuloplasty System, Edwards LifeSciences Corporation, Irvine, CA), Medtronic Future ring (CG Future Annuloplasty System, Medtronic, Inc., Minneapolis, MN), or the partial Duran ring (Medtronic Duran Flexible Annuloplasty System, Medtronic), to be quite acceptable as long as the major principles of application are observed.

We place U stitches in the ends of the C-ring in the trigonal area well above the extra commissure as shown in Fig. 39-4A. It is important not only to stabilize the intertrigonal area, but also to use wide mattress sutures across both commissures where there is intercommissural cinching by the stitches that are used to implant the ring. Rings can be implanted by running sutures, but most commonly, deep intraventricular annular mattress sutures are placed and are the strong points of repair. For example, one of these sutures placed in the area of the commissure tends to flatten and narrow the commissure, another aid to preventing dilation. As shown in Fig. 39-4B, 9 to 11 sutures usually are sufficient to completely encircle even the most dilated annular ring. It is important to take wide bites, taking care that the needle passes into the ventricle at the annular level and out again, thus ensuring a secure fixation. The sizing of the ring, irrespective of type, can be accomplished by two methods. The first is to evaluate the intertrigonal distance between the two sutures placed in the expanse of the trigonal area. The second and perhaps more relevant method is to evaluate the height of the anterior leaflet. This approximation can be made by means of intraoperative transesophageal echocardiography before opening the heart. With myxomatous valve disease, this measurement is made using the sizer set provided by the manufacturer. In general, for patients with myxomatous valve disease, it is better to upsize the ring than downsize because this minimizes the possibility of developing systolic anterior motion (SAM) of the mitral valve. We believe that the height of the anterior leaflet is the key measurement and use it more commonly than the intertrigonal dis-

tance. Once the ring has been properly sized, it is fixated by placing the mattress sutures in a sequential fashion into the ring and tying the suture. The valve is tested, and if the repair is satisfactory, there should be minimal mitral regurgitation, even with high-volume saline infusion. The left atrium is closed with a 3-0 monofilament suture.

Variations on a Theme

There are numerous variations to this simple approach to mitral valve repair. In most cases, the critical element is shortening the height of the posterior leaflet, even with bileaflet prolapse, and relatively little needs to be done to the anterior leaflet. Occasionally, commissuroplasty is useful and is discussed later in the section on anterior leaflet pathology (Fig. 39-5). Other minor variations in technique for the posterior leaflet include the finding of natural clefts in the posterior annulus. These clefts may be accentuated when the leaflet advancement procedure is being performed. In this event, a mattress suture of 4-0 Prolene may be required to put together the two areas of the valve leaflet surrounding the cleft. Another variation includes the use of Gore-Tex chordae in the posterior leaflet to avoid abridging the distance of the annulus in any way. This method is possible when the leaflet itself is not severely compromised by myxomatous disease or if the ruptured chordae are bridged at a fairly narrow distance. In other cases, there may be only very short segments of valve that need to be resected. This technique can be effected by removing a narrow triangular wedge of tissue containing only one or two isolated chordal ruptures. This is sometimes seen with ischemic mitral regurgitation, which may permit this type of limited resection. The ring is then placed in the usual fashion. In addition, in cases of limited resection with a high PML, a "folding plasty" of sections of the resected PML may be done as shown in Fig. 39-6. With this technique, the leading edge of the elongated PML is tacked to the underside of the leaflet at the annulus, decreasing the height by 50%.

A problem occasionally encountered in repair of the PML is subannular calcification associated with severe myxomatous degeneration. This finding usually occurs in elderly patients with long-standing disease. Elderly patients benefit greatly by mitral valve repair, and in our series, we have found that the risk is equal to that of the younger age group. Considerable judgment must be exercised in removing annular calcifications, and a more conservative approach is recommended. In certain instances, when the annulus is not affected and the calcification is subannular, the calcification can be partially resected if it is not entirely circumferential to the PML. A technique developed by Carpentier involving radical resection of the entire block of calcium is useful when dealing with an extensive calcification requiring a large tissue resection. In this procedure, the atrium is separated from the ventricle. The calcium is removed en bloc, and then the atrium and ventricle are precisely reapproximated after the calcium has been removed. In most instances, however, we have found subtotal excision of calcium to be very precise and usually quite satisfactory for leaflet coaptation, leaflet advancement, and placement of annuloplasty rings of adequate size. On a rare occasion, we encounter a patient with massive calcification involving the entire annulus and leaflet, with ruptured chordae in the middle posterior leaflet, in whom replacement is considered extremely hazardous. In select individuals, the repair may still be carried out without placement of the annuloplasty ring because there is already a rigid ring of calcium in place around the entire posterior mitral leaflet preventing further annular dilatation. This rare circumstance is generally seen only in elderly patients.

Systolic Anterior Motion

Systolic anterior motion (SAM) is a problem that was seen much more frequently in years past with rigid encircling rings, when the height of the posterior leaflet was inadequately reduced. SAM signifies an obstruction of the left ventricular outflow tract formed by a very large anterior leaflet and the ventricular septum. In many instances, patients with floppy valves are protected from this problem by the existence of certain chords that prevent SAM. These chords are usually preserved during mitral valve repair procedures, and the chance of SAM is small. In cases where there is a potential for SAM to occur, for example, in patients who have an extremely large, redundant anterior mitral valve leaflet and the posterior leaflet has not been reduced sufficiently, other alternatives must be considered. First and foremost, one may have to re-resect and relower the posterior leaflet. Other methods for fixing the anterior mitral leaflet may be necessary, as discussed in the next section. Upsizing the annuloplasty ring prophylactically is an important consideration in cases of Barlow degeneration.

Anterior Leaflet Pathology

Most experienced mitral valve repair surgeons concur that if one sufficiently reduces

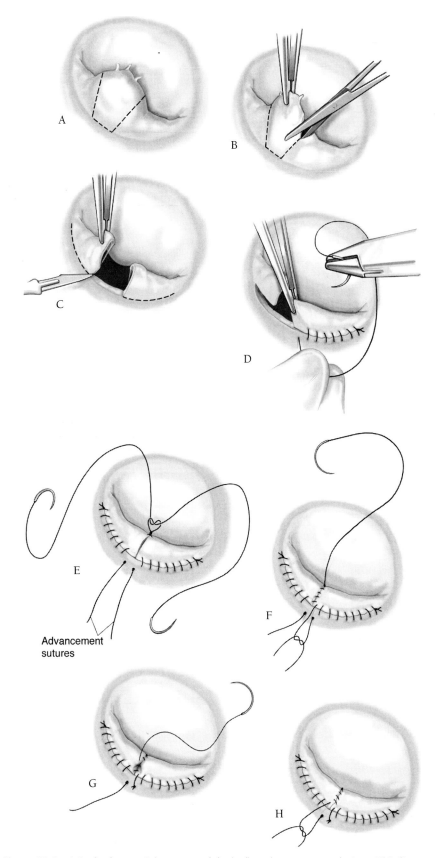

Figure 39-3. Mitral valve repair by means of the leaflet advancement technique. This figure illustrates the classic leaflet advancement technique in an extreme case of Barlow syndrome.

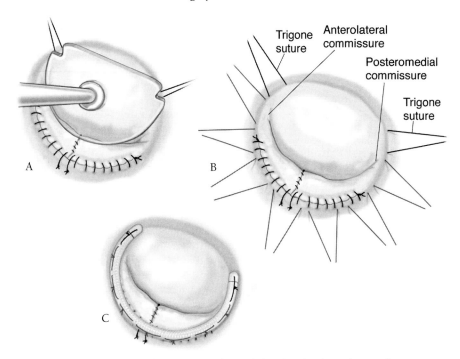

Figure 39-4.   Stabilization of the intertrigonal area. **(A)** A ring sizer is used to mark suture placement within the intertrigonal space. Nine to 11 sutures are generally sufficient to encircle even the most dilated annular ring. **(B)** Generally speaking, the intertrigonal space is not prone to dilation, which makes either a full encircling or partial C-ring suitable for repair. **(C)** U stitches are placed at the ends of the partial C-ring well in the trigonal area.

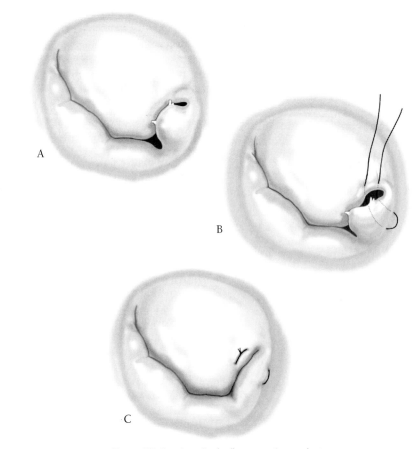

Figure 39-5.   Anterior leaflet commissuroplasty.

the height of the posterior leaflet, adequately upsizes the annuloplasty ring, and performs an appropriate annuloplasty ring suture placement, it is relatively unusual to have to fix the anterior leaflet by further surgical means. Nevertheless, there are a few techniques that the reparative surgeon needs to master to provide satisfactory repair in the face of major anterior leaflet pathology. First is the circumstance in which the anterior leaflet, particularly at A2, is severely elongated by a number of chords or chords in this area are ruptured. Burying the chordae in a trench of papillary muscle, which lowers the AML, was one of the first techniques used to reduce the height of the anterior mitral leaflet. The cleft in the mitral papillary muscle was then sutured shut, fixing the lowered chordae in place (Fig. 39-7). This was an original technique developed by Carpentier, but it was shown later by Cosgrove and associates to be associated with a high incidence of recurrent rupture of the chordae because the scissoring motion of the papillary muscles sometimes caused erosion and chordal rupture.

When it is absolutely required to lower the height of the anterior leaflet, it is now more common to use artificial chordae made of Gore-Tex suture. Several different techniques for achieving this effect have been popularized. Mattress sutures of 5-0 Prolene are placed in the papillary muscle adjacent to the area of leaflet that needs to be lowered, and several loops of suture may be used to connect the papillary muscle to the edge of the anterior leaflet in the affected area. The object is to prevent the anterior leaflet from prolapsing beyond the posterior leaflet. The sutures are carefully tied on the anterior leaflet. These techniques have been in use for at least 10 years and have been judged to be quite safe, reproducible, and adequate for reducing anterior leaflet prolapse without difficulty. Gore-Tex suture may also be used for PML pathology as shown in Fig. 39-8.

Another technique, first popularized by Duran, is the "flip-over" technique (Fig. 39-9). The surgeon incises an uninvolved segment of the posterior leaflet with its attached normal chordae of normal length immediately across from the affected area in the AML. This healthy PML segment is "flipped over" onto the anterior leaflet and attached along with its normal chordae to the anterior leaflet. Thus the attachments of the anterior leaflet to the normal papillary muscle are maintained, but the height of the anterior leaflet is lowered to the level already known to be normal for the PML. In my opinion, the only disadvantage of this procedure is

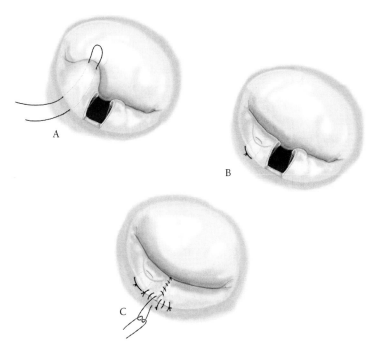

Figure 39-6. Folding plasty technique. Used in cases of limited resection with a high posterior mitral leaflet.

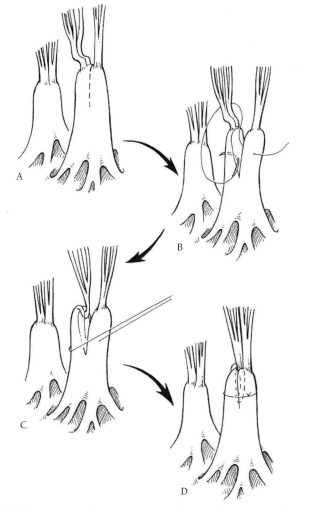

Figure 39-7. Technique of chordal shortening. (Reprinted with permission from DD Muehrcke, DM Cosgrove. Mitral valvuloplasty. In: LH Edmunds Jr, ed. Cardiac Surgery in the Adult. New York, McGraw-Hill, 1997:1006.)

the necessity of incising an uninvolved area of the posterior leaflet, which, with other means to accomplish the same effect, could be avoided.

Finally, a technique that has been recently discussed is the edge-to-edge repair, also known as the Alfieri technique (Fig. 39-10). This technique is appropriate when all other attempts to reduce SAM in a reconstructed large myxomatous valve have failed. The edge-to-edge suture technique makes a figure-of-eight orifice of the mitral valve, and in my opinion, should only be used in those patients with large myxomatous valves when the possibility of stenosis of the valve is extremely unlikely. We have used this technique on a number of occasions when SAM seemed inevitable or developed despite our best efforts and in the presence of compromised left ventricular function with ruptured anterior leaflet chordae only, when we felt a rapid and efficacious operation was necessary. For example, we used this repair in a 50-year-old man who presented with an ejection fraction of 10% and six ruptured chordae in the middle segment of the anterior leaflet. This patient had New York Heart Association (NYHA) class IV symptoms. A rapid operation was essential. Therefore, we performed a left atrial exposure and an edge-to-edge repair at the site of the six ruptured chordae in the anterior leaflet at A2 to P2 and placed a 36-mm Cosgrove ring. The cross-clamp time was 30 minutes. The patient tolerated the procedure well, and his left ventricular ejection fraction increased to about 20% within 6 weeks of the procedure, with the patient well on the way to remodeling his ventricle. Thus, an alternative technique can be used in an adjunctive way where anterior leaflet pathology is very difficult or a very rapid operation is essential in a critically ill patient.

Other techniques for shortening or reducing the height of the AML are the triangular resection technique (Fig. 39-11) and the AML shortening technique of Duran (Fig. 39-12). These techniques may correct SAM but are somewhat more unpredictable in terms of resecting the AML. I concur with Carpentier on this point, that in terms of AML resection, as little as possible is the most desirable approach.

Repair of the Ischemic Mitral Valve

Mitral valve repair in the setting of ischemic heart disease is an area of confusion, debate, indecision, and much controversy. Questions central to this issue concern what type of repair technique should be used and what degree of regurgitation should be

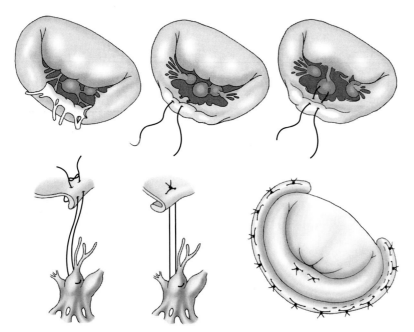

Figure 39-8. Technique for chordal replacement in the posterior mitral leaflet using expanded polytetrafluoroethylene (ePTFE) suture. (Reprinted with permission from JJ Nigro, DS Schwartz, RD Bart et al. Neochordal repair of the posterior mitral leaflet. J Thorac Cardiovasc Surg 2004;127:440.)

repaired. In ischemic mitral regurgitation, the pathology of the mitral valve is secondary to ischemia of the myocardium, which is, in turn, secondary to obstruction of the coronary artery circulation. Mitral valve ischemia is a disease of the left ventricle caused by segmental wall motion abnormalities or diffuse global hypokinesia and dilation. Dilation of the left ventricle produces a dilated annulus, which causes the mitral leaflets to separate, thus producing regurgitation in the face of a

structurally normal leaflet and subchordal mechanism.

Patient selection is another area of debate. Many, including the Emory group (Atlanta, GA), believe that most cases of ischemic mitral regurgitation can be ameliorated by a complete coronary artery bypass graft (CABG) operation. Those of the Brigham camp hold that the ordinary CABG procedure is not sufficient, particularly when there is persistent mitral regurgitation, that is, not just limited to the ischemic

episodes. In my opinion, chronic mitral regurgitation secondary to moderate to moderately severe ischemia should be repaired. The decision to repair should be made well in advance of the surgical procedure, not intraoperatively when the hemodynamic load is altered because of general anesthesia. These patients usually have some element of congestive symptoms to support this approach. Once the decision has been made and the coronary bypass completed, attention is turned to the left atrium.

Carpentier provided the definitive summary of the three classes of ischemic mitral regurgitation (types I, II, and III). Clearly, ruptured papillary muscle secondary to myocardial infarction constitutes an additional form of ischemic mitral regurgitation, but it is rare and difficult to repair because the wall to which the papillary muscle must be reattached is considerably weakened from the ischemia. This gives rise to some concern about postoperative recurrence. Because these patients are also among the most ill as a result of pulmonary edema, a very conservative surgical approach is warranted; and valve replacement in this circumstance is commonly preferred.

Some surgeons question whether a complete ring versus a C-ring is an important element of this repair, but the necessity of downsizing is well established to bring the anterior and posterior leaflets and annular attachments closer together. The concept that there is a "cure" for ischemic mitral regurgitation is relatively uncertain because the etiology of the disease is commonly the left ventricle, and the left ventricle may continue to dilate after surgery, as would be observed in a diffuse cardiomyopathy. The papillary muscles continue to be drawn down, and hence the leaflets may continue to show signs of leakage postoperatively if the dilation continues.

Dr. Irving Kron suggested an alternative operation, which involves tacking the papillary muscles back to the annulus. This technique may be of some benefit in those cases where it is anticipated that the papillary muscles will continue to stretch downward and outward. This relatively new technique has not been evaluated over the long term.

Dr. Robert Levine, of the Massachusetts General Hospital, proposed actually cutting the chordae in certain patients with ischemic mitral regurgitation. Dr. Levine believes that this approach may enhance coaptation of the leaflets because of the so-called restrictive nature of the valve lesions. Bolling and others championed the use of a very small, downsized ring to maintain control over the annular dilation as noted previously. This

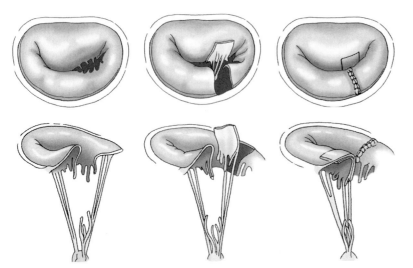

Figure 39-9. "Flip-over" technique. In this technique developed by Duran, a small portion of the posterior leaflet with attached viable chordae is excised and transferred (flipped over) to support a portion of the anterior leaflet with ruptured chordae. (Reprinted with permission from AM Gillinov, DM Cosgrove III. Mitral valve repair. In: LH Cohn, LH Edmunds Jr, eds. Cardiac Surgery in the Adult, 2nd ed. New York: McGraw-Hill, 2003:940.)

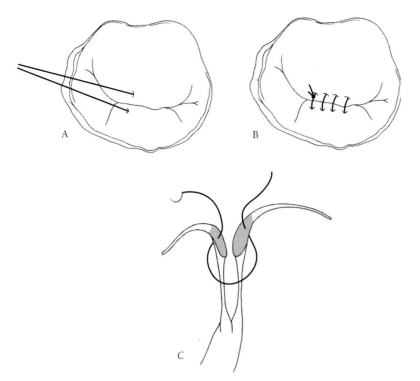

Figure 39-10.   The double-orifice technique. **(A)** A central stitch is used to check the symmetry of the orifice. **(B)** Running suture is placed along the free edge of the leaflets. **(C)** Deep bites are taken the rough zone of the leaflets to avoid tearing by the suture. (Reprinted with permission from F Maisano, JJ Schreuder, M Oppizzi. The double-orifice technique as a standardized approach to treat mitral regurgitation due to severe myxomatous disease. Surgical technique. Eur J Cardiothorac Surg 2000;17:201.)

technique adds little to the operative time (15 to 20 minutes for placement of a ring) and greatly improves the patient's hemodynamics. Overall the risks of operations for ischemic mitral regurgitation have decreased considerably from the 1980s, when operative mortality for repair or replacement procedures for ischemic mitral regurgitation with CABG ranged from approximately 10% to 12%, to present values ranging from 3% to 3.5%.

Device manufacturers have attempted to simulate these surgical treatments with new experimental percutaneous devices. These devices aim to reduce, if not totally obliterate, ischemic mitral regurgitation by various means including coronary sinus stenting, pushing the posterior leaflet up toward the anterior leaflet, or simulating the edge-to-edge repair Alfieri process. All of these devices are awaiting clinical trial and Food and Drug Administration approval.

Debate continues on the efficacy of mitral valve repair for moderate to moderately severe ischemic mitral regurgitation. It is clear, however, that the pathophysiologic state of the left ventricle is the determinant of early and late mortality, not necessarily the operation, whether repair or replacement is being performed. Clearly, rapid placement of the annuloplasty ring with preservation of the papillary muscles and chordae is the ideal approach and a trend to which most surgeons now ascribe.

Endocarditis of the Mitral Valve

The principles of repair for an infected mitral valve are the same as the surgical precepts for treating infection in any part of the body. All infected material must be removed and placement of prosthetic material into any potentially infected area should be assiduously avoided. This presents a dual challenge to the surgeon, who must not only eradicate the infection while leaving sufficient material to make a functional mitral valve, but also remodel the annulus with a suitable annuloplasty ring yet avoid placing any prosthetic material in an infected area. A variety of ingenious approaches have been performed over the years. A conventional leaflet closure accomplished with the leaflet advancement procedure is carried out using monofilament sutures. Local treatment with iodine solution is recommended. Although there is no scientific evidence to support its use, it is reasonable to treat severe local infection empirically with antiseptic therapy. Endocarditis that has encroached on the mitral valve may require triangular resection or possibly eradication using the flip-over technique from the posterior leaflet to the anterior leaflet to support the anterior leaflet with new chordae. With extensive infection, particularly in the posterior annulus, the entire leaflet may have to be removed. In this instance, the annular infection is debrided, and an autologous pericardial lining may be needed to line the annulus before it is reattached to the posterior leaflet. The valve repair is subsequently performed on top of the autologous pericardium. If the region is infected with a benign organism, such as *Streptococcus*, and there is adherent vegetation but the valve itself is not infected, simply excising the vegetation with a narrow leaflet resection using Prolene suture in a nondilated annulus may be all that is

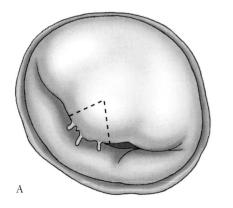

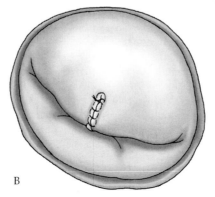

Figure 39-11.   Triangular resection of the anterior mitral leaflet. The technique of triangular resection for an isolated segmental prolapse of the anterior mitral leaflet. (Reprinted with permission from R Fasol, E Joubert-Hubner. Triangular resection of the anterior leaflet for repair of the mitral valve. Ann Thorac Surg 2001;71:381.)

**AML Redundancy – AML Shortening
(Resection with basal chords re-implantation**

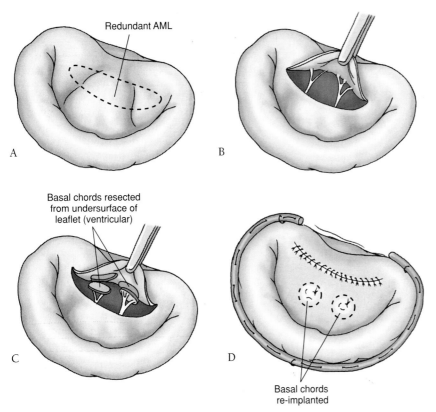

Figure 39-12. Duran's technique for anterior leaflet shortening. To reduce height, the base of the anterior mitral leaflet (AML) body is excised. The incision closest to the AML base is straight, and the other incision is curved along the free edge contour of the AML. Note that after excision, the "stay" basal chords are reimplanted into the ventricular aspect of the AML. (Reprinted with permission from CMG Duran. Surgical techniques for the repair of anterior mitral leaflet prolapse. J Card Surg 1999;14;471.)

required. In this case a prosthetic ring may not be needed. In cases in which there is severe destruction of the entire annulus with massive sepsis, the valve may have to be completely removed, debrided of infection, and the annulus relined with pericardium around the entire circumference, or the valve may have to be completely replaced with a prosthetic device. There have been attempts to use homograft mitral valves or pulmonic valves, but the long-term results are somewhat uncertain.

Repair of the Rheumatic Mitral Valve

Treatment of rheumatic mitral valve disease was the first consistent operation performed by cardiac surgeons. As mentioned in the introduction to this chapter, the first successful repair of a stenotic mitral valve secondary to rheumatic heart disease was performed in a 12-year-old girl at the Peter Bent Brigham Hospital in 1923 by Elliott Cutler. After World War II, Harken and Bailey began a large series of closed mitral commissurotomies, actually fracturing the stenotic mitral valve by inserting a finger or instrument through the valve. Throughout the 1950s and 1960s the closed mitral commissurotomy was a huge operation for treating mitral valve stenosis in patients with rheumatic heart disease. In the late 1970s, after cardiopulmonary bypass was well established, most surgeons converted to the open mitral commissurotomy. With the advent of balloon valve dilation for mitral stenosis and the decline in rheumatic valve disease in Western countries, operations for rheumatic mitral stenosis decreased. Nevertheless, even though balloon valve dilation is the most common treatment for rheumatic mitral stenosis in the current era, patients with rheumatic heart disease will come to

surgery with severe rheumatic mitral regurgitation and contraindications for balloon treatment. The technique of open mitral commissurotomy repair is illustrated in Fig. 39-13. Mitral regurgitation is associated with mitral stenosis. The hemodynamic situation is alleviated by the commissurotomy, after which the valve leaflets may become more flexible and demonstrate considerably better coaptation. In addition, incision into some of the fused chordae and papillary muscles below the valve may aid flexibility of the mitral valve leaflet, permitting better coaptation. Severe calcification is probably a contraindication to repair, and valve replacement will be required. Another contraindication to repair is an inadequate length of the subvalvar chordae, which diminishes flexibility and leaflet coaptation. If there is fusion of chordae and papillary muscle, repair is hopeless, and valve replacement is the only alternative.

Once the commissurotomy is completed, the chordae are more flexible and the leaflets perhaps even thinned by the removal of some of the rheumatic fibrosis. An annuloplasty ring is still implanted. This was the type of patient included in Carpentier's first group of mitral valve repairs and thus formed the concept of remodeling annuloplasty. As noted in many previous series, the longevity of the repair of the rheumatic valve is much more problematic than the degenerative or myxomatous valve, and the instance of the reoperation has been significantly higher in this group over the years. It is extremely safe, and in the properly selected patients provides excellent long-term results and freedom from reoperation that may last many years.

Mitral Valve Re-Repair

Re-repair of the myxomatous mitral valve after a failed repair may be accomplished in a small number of cases. In our total experience of almost 2,000 valve repairs, 0.7% had comprised mitral valve repairs. Analysis of these cases reveals four important causes of valve failure: (1) rupture of another chord in the mitral valve unrelated to the previous repair, (2) failure to lower the height of the posterior leaflet, (3) failure to adequately lower the anterior leaflet to the height of the posterior leaflet, and (4) failure to use an annuloplasty ring or using a ring that is too small. The latter is probably the most important factor leading to mitral valve re-repair. In many of our re-repair cases, the valve originally repaired was large and undersized rings were

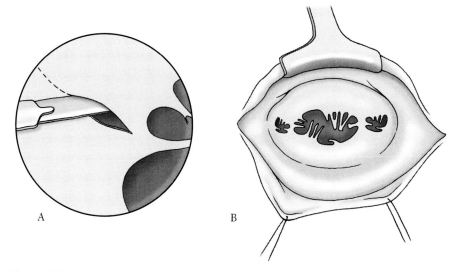

Figure 39-13. An open mitral commissurotomy performed using the triple-orifice technique. **(A)** The leaflets of the mitral valve are sharply separated at the anterior commissure after first enlarging the central orifice. **(B)** Completed commissurotomy with enlarged central orifice. (Reprinted with permission from BL Aaron, RR Lower. Advantages of open mitral commissurotomy using a triple-orifice technique. Ann Thorac Surg 1975;19:654.)

used in making the initial repair. Dehiscence with hemolysis can occur. In a previously reported work from our series that documented the validity of the use of mitral valve rings, we found that not using a ring led to a five-times greater incidence of valve repair failure. For these re-repair procedures, the rings are simply removed, the necessary reparative steps are carried out, and the patient is fitted with a larger ring providing significant reduction of recurrent mitral regurgitation.

Summary

Surgical experience over the last three decades culminating in a series of recent reports regarding the long-term results with mitral valve surgery have coalesced our conceptual thinking about the best approach to mitral valve disease. The role of reparative techniques is clearly supported over prosthetic or bioprosthetic valve replacement. A variety of surgical techniques have been developed to address the four principal etiologies of the diseased mitral valve: myxomatous degeneration, ischemia, endocarditis, and rheumatic mitral valve disease. With these procedures, the normal ventricular physiology, for the most part, is maintained and anticoagulation can be avoided. Most recently, in cases of chronic and paroxysmal atrial fibrillation, the Maze operation, using radiofrequency or other techniques,

has been increasingly used to manage ventricular physiology.

It is also noteworthy that many of these mitral valve repair techniques are amenable to minimally invasive surgical methods, including use of the lower ministernotomy and right thoracotomy (thoracoscopic or robotic), which are associated with decreased morbidity and mortality. The accessibility of the mitral valve and the wide variety of successful techniques supported by 30 years of surgical experience support current practice favoring repair over replacement.

SUGGESTED READING

Bolling S. Mitral valve reconstruction in the patient with heart failure. Heart Fail Rev 2001; 6:177.

Carpentier A, Pellerin M, Fuzellier JF, et al. Extensive calcification of the mitral valve annulus: Pathology and surgical management. J Thorac Cardiovasc Surg 1996;111:718.

Cohn L, Rizzo R, Adams D, et al. The effects of pathophysiology on the surgical treatment of ischemic mitral regurgitation: Operative and late risk of repair versus replacement. Eur J Cardiothoracic Surg 1995;9:568.

Duran C. Surgical techniques for the repair of the anterior mitral leaflet prolapse. J Card Surg 1999;14:471.

Duran C, Pekar F. Techniques for ensuring the correct length of new mitral chords. J Heart Valve Dis 2003;12:156.

Frater R, Vetter H, Zussa C, et al. Chordal replacement in mitral valve repair. Circulation 1990;82(Suppl IV):IV-125.

Greelish J, Cohn L, Leacche M, et al. Surgery for acquired cardiovascular disease. Minimally invasive mitral valve repair suggests earlier operations for mitral valve disease. J Thorac Cardiovasc Surg 2003;126:365–71; discussion, 371–3.

Grossi E, Sharony R, Colvin S. Mitral valve in ischemic versus idiopathic dilated cardiomyopathy. J Thorac Cardiovasc Surg 2003; 26:922.

Kron I, Green G, Cope J. Surgical relocation of the posterior papillary muscle in chronic ischemic mitral regurgitation. Ann Thorac Surg 2002;74:600.

Maisano F, Schreuder J, Oppizzi M, et al. The double-orifice technique as a standardized approach to treat mitral regurgitation due to severe myxomatous disease: Surgical technique. Eur J Cardiothorac Surg 2000;17: 201.

Mihaljevic T, Paul S, Leacche M, et al. Tailored surgical therapy for acute native mitral valve endocarditis. J Heart Valve Dis 2004;13: 210.

Nifong L, Chu V, Bailey M, et al. Robotic mitral valve repair: Experience with the da Vinci system. Ann Thorac Surg 2003;75:438.

EDITOR'S COMMENTS

Dr. Cohn presents a complete description of mitral valve repair. I've seen him do mitral valve repairs, and he is an excellent technician and one of the leaders in mitral valve surgery. I agree completely with the principles he espouses. I would like to repeat the most important ones, which are apposition of the posterior and anterior leaflets, reduction of the height of the posterior leaflet in myxomatous disease, and finally remodeling of the annulus with a ring. These techniques are the most critical. The rest have a certain amount of flexibility. We have some minor differences with some of the other techniques Dr. Cohn describes. Rather than quadrangular resections, we tend to do triangular resections of the posterior leaflet at the suggestion of the Mayo Clinic group. This has worked surprisingly well and has reduced our need for sliding "plasties." We have used artificial cords for the anterior leaflet, but I have also done some limited triangular resections as well with surprisingly good results. We were hesitant at one time to do this because of Carpentier's teaching, but we have noted that this has worked and, at least in our minds, may be a little simpler to do than using artificial chords.

We agreed with Cohn that the trench technique of reducing chordal length may result in reduced long-term results. Finally, we agree completely with Dr. Cohn's approach to ischemic mitral disease. This is a disease of the muscle and annulus in chronic situations that is usually not fixed with coronary bypass alone. The degree of ischemic mitral regurgitation decreases with dropping of the blood pressure during general anesthesia. We agree completely that the decision to repair should be made preoperatively, not in the operating room. Finally, Dr. Cohn describes many good bailouts. He suggests the Alfieri stitch as a bailout for SAM. I have not used this yet, but I will keep it in the back of my mind.

I.L.K.

40

Mitral Valve Repair: Robotic Minimally Invasive

Alan P. Kypson, L. Wiley Nifong, and W. Randolph Chitwood, Jr.

Introduction

In the 1950s, Bailey, Harken, Davila, and Glover made early attempts to repair mitral valves. These methods usually related to epicardial reduction of the mitral annulus or reduction of a regurgitant orifice by "plugging" with cone-shaped prosthesis. In the 1960s, Kay, Woller, and Reed developed intra-cardiac suture annuloplasties to reduce the posterior mitral annulus, improving leaflet coaptation. McGoon in 1960 performed the first repairs for ruptured chordae tendineae, and Austin in 1965 first replaced a mitral valve for a papillary muscle rupture. The advent of mechanical valves impeded the progress of mitral valve repair surgery until the early 1970s, when Carpentier and Duran pioneered novel reconstructive techniques. Despite mitral valve repair successes in Europe, skepticism pervaded the United States until Carpentier in 1983 showed excellent long-term repair results. These results were based on his elucidation of the functional anatomy in insufficient mitral valves and the development of reproducible repair methods. By the late 1980s, numerous reports from other centers were being published validating the long-term durability of repairs, freedom from anticoagulation, and decreased mortality compared with mitral replacements.

Traditionally, mitral valve surgery has been performed through a median sternotomy, which provides generous operative exposure and global cardiac access. However, during the last decade, improvements in instruments and endoscopes, as well as patient demand, resulted in a substantial increase in minimally invasive general and subspecialty surgical procedures. Endovascular port-access technology first allowed

a less invasive surgical approach to mitral valve surgery, avoiding a median sternotomy. Advances in closed-chest cardiopulmonary bypass and myocardial protection, as well as intracardiac visualization, instrumentation, and robotic telemanipulation, have hastened the shift toward efficient and safe minimally endoscopic cardiac surgery. Today, mitral valve surgery done through small incisions using robotic or endoscopic assistance has become standard practice for an increasing number of cardiac surgeons.

Robotic Technology

Computer-assisted, or robotic, cardiac surgery has been developed to facilitate surgeons' hand motions in limited operating spaces. These devices offer advantages of improved access, magnified vision, and stabilized instrument implementation. Six degrees of freedom are required to allow any free orientation in space. Thus, standard endoscopic instruments with only four degrees of freedom reduce dexterity significantly. When working through a fixed entry point or fulcrum, such as a trocar, the operator must reverse hand motions. At the same time, instrument shaft shear, or resistive drag, induces higher forces needed to manipulate the operating tips, leading to hand muscle fatigue. In addition, human motor skills deteriorate with visual–motor incompatibility, which is associated commonly with endoscopic surgery. Computer-enhanced instrumentation systems can overcome these and other limitations. These systems provide simultaneous tele- and micromanipulation of tissues in working small spaces. The surgeon operates from a console, immersed in a three-dimensional operative field.

Through a computer interface, his or her motions are reproduced in scaled proportion through "micro-wrist" instruments that are mounted on robotic arms inserted through the chest wall. These instruments emulate human XYZ-axis wrist activity throughout a full seven degrees of freedom.

There are two types of computer-enhanced surgical systems in use. These can be classified according to the tasks they help to perform. The first group functions as an assisting tool that simply holds and positions instruments during surgery. The Automated Endoscopic System for Optimal Positioning (AESOP; Intuitive Surgical, Inc., Mountain View, CA) guides an endoscope through voice-activated control. Voice commands order the robot to hold a specific camera position or reorient it to a specific operative field, providing a clear and steady view without camera tremor. Surgical telemanipulators, the second group, were invented to facilitate remote fine instrument tip manipulations guided by three-dimensional endoscopic vision. Through a computer interface, the surgeon's hand motions are emulated in scaled proportion through "micro-wrist" instruments that are mounted on robotic arms. These instruments reproduce human wrist activity exactly throughout seven full degrees of freedom. Tremor filtering and motion scaling are translated into enhanced dexterity in confined operating spaces, such as the left atrium in a near closed chest. The da Vinci system (Intuitive Surgical, Inc., Mountain View, CA) is the telemanipulation system used most commonly for mitral valve surgery.

The da Vinci system comprises a surgeon console, an instrument cart, and a visioning platform (Fig. 40-1). The console is removed physically from the patient and allows the surgeon to sit comfortably, resting his or her

353

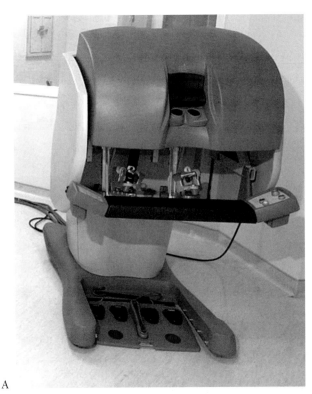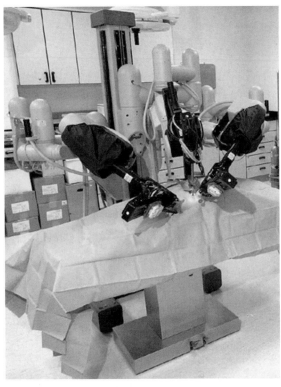

A   B

Figure 40-1. The da Vinci robotic telemanipulation system. **(A)** The operative console at which the surgeon is seated. **(B)** The instrument cart with two instrument arms and a camera arm that stands next to the operating room table.

arms ergonomically with head positioning in a three-dimensional vision array. Digital images are translated to analog natural depth perception with high-power magnification (10×). Analog surgeon hand motions are registered through sensors in digital memory banks. Concurrently, these data are transferred to an instrument cart, which converts them into synchronous surgical executions in the "end-effector" instruments. Every analog finger movement, along with inherent human tremor at 8 to 10 Hz/sec, is converted to binary digital data, which are smoothed and filtered to increase micro-instrument precision. A clutching mechanism allows constant readjustment of surgeon hand positions to maintain an optimal ergonomic attitude with respect to the visual field.

Evolution of Minimally Invasive Mitral Valve Surgery

Initially, minimally invasive mitral valve surgery was based on modifications of previously used incisions and performed under direct vision. Minimal-access incisions

provided adequate direct-vision mitral valve exposure, and surgeons showed that mitral valve operations could be done as safely and precisely as through a larger incision. Large series showed that surgical mortality (1% to 3%) and morbidity were comparable to those of conventional mitral surgery. One study reported 25 patients operated using a parasternal approach with no hospital mortality or repair failures, although follow-up was less than 1 year. A different study reported 43 minimally invasive mitral operations done with few complications, with improved patient satisfaction, and with solid economic benefits. Clearly, by employing familiar approaches and relying on direct vision, the initial steps in minimally invasive mitral surgery became less daunting.

With experience acquired, a shift from direct vision to video assistance occurred, and operations began to be performed using secondary vision. In 1996, Carpentier performed the first video-assisted mitral valve repair through a right minithoracotomy using ventricular fibrillation. In 1997, Chitwood described the first mitral valve replacement using videoscopic vision. The operation was done using a 6-cm right anterior minithoracotomy, peripheral cardiopulmonary bypass, a percutaneous

transthoracic aortic cross-clamp, and retrograde cardioplegia. In 1998, Mohr reported the Leipzig experience of 51 minimally invasive mitral operations done using port-access technology, a 4-cm incision, and three-dimensional videoscopy. In these patients, video technology was helpful for replacements and simple repair operations; however, complex reconstructions were still approached under direct vision. Concurrently, our group at East Carolina University reported 31 patients operated on using video assistance with a two-dimensional 5-mm camera. Complex repairs, including quadrangular resections, sliding valvuloplasties, and chordal replacements, were done with no major complications and a mortality of <1%.

In 1997 Mohr used the term "solo mitral surgery" to connote the first use of AESOP to perform endoscopic mitral surgery, bringing cardiac surgery into the robotic age. This technology enabled the use of even smaller incisions with better valvular and subvalvular visualization. In June 1998, our group performed a completely video-directed mitral operation using AESOP and a Vista three-dimensional camera (Vista Cardiothoracic Systems, Inc., Westborough, MA) with a head-mounted video display. The combination of three-dimensional visualization, robotic camera control, and instrument-tip articulation was the next essential step needed to enable totally endoscopic mitral operations.

Innovations in computer-assisted telemanipulation occurred rapidly in the mid 1990s. In 1998, Carpentier performed the first truly endoscopic mitral valve repair using an early prototype of the da Vinci surgical system. Within a week, Mohr performed five mitral repairs with the same device. In May 2000, our group performed the first complete mitral valve repair in North America using the da Vinci system. In that operation, a large P_2 trapezoidal resection was done with the defect closed using multiple interrupted sutures, followed by implantation of an annuloplasty band. The same year Grossi and colleagues did a partial mitral valve repair using the Zeus system (Intuitive Surgical, Inc., Mountain View, CA). Lange and associates in Munich were the first to perform a totally endoscopic mitral valve repair using only 1-cm ports and da Vinci. Although we still use a 4-cm incision for assistant access, robotic technology has progressed to a point where totally endoscopic mitral procedures are the routine operation of choice for patients having isolated mitral valve pathology.

Patient Selection

All patients with isolated degenerative mitral valve disease are now being considered for a robotic mitral repair. Complex mitral disease is tackled readily with the techniques described here. Contraindications include a prior right thoracotomy and circumferential annular calcification (Table 40-1). Moderate annular calcification alone does not preclude patients from undergoing a minimally

Table 40-1 Robotic Mitral Surgery Exclusion Criteria

Previous right thoracotomy
Renal failure
Liver dysfunction
Bleeding disorders
Pulmonary hypertension (pulmonary artery systolic blood pressure >60 torr)
Significant aortic or tricuspid valve disease
Coronary artery disease requiring surgery
Recent myocardial ischemia (<30 days)
Recent stroke (<30 days)
Severely calcified mitral valve annulus
Body mass index >35 kg/m^2

invasive approach. However, extensive "bar" calcification remains for us a contraindication to this approach.

Patients with poor lung function undergo pulmonary testing to ascertain whether they will tolerate single-lung ventilation. Should they not be able to tolerate isolated lung ventilation, then cardiopulmonary bypass is instituted earlier for intrathoracic preparation. The preoperative transesophageal echocardiogram remains the gold standard for perioperative planning. It is important to correlate the dynamic echo anatomy with both the Carpentier functional class and the intraoperative pathology. In patients older than age 40 years or with a strong family history or symptoms of coronary disease angiography is done preoperatively.

Robotic Mitral Valve Surgery

Anesthesia and Monitoring

To provide single-lung ventilation, either a dual-lumen endotracheal tube or a bronchial blocker is used. Hemodynamic monitoring is done with a radial arterial line and a flow-directed pulmonary artery catheter. For superior vena caval drainage, the right jugular vein is cannulated percutaneously with a 17-F thin-walled Biomedicus (Medtronic, Inc., Minneapolis, MN) cannula using the Seldinger guidewire technique. Transesophageal echocardiography (TEE) is used to evaluate cannula placement, annular size and quality, the leaflet coaptation plane, leaflet length, and the subvalvular mitral apparatus. The intensity and direction of regurgitant jets help to determine the significance of leaflet pathology. The transgastric view is very helpful for determining exactly which mitral segments need correction. Currently, we select the annuloplasty band size based on TEE measurements of anterior leaflet length, annular diameter, and septal thickness. Simplicity and reproducibility remain our watchwords. To gain optimal intracardiac access for placement of the robotic arms and camera, patient-side surgeon comfort and direct vision are most important. Loupes with long focal length (3.5×) are most helpful for peering through the 4-cm incision when preparing for either a video-assisted or a da Vinci repair. In the latter operation, the surgeon sits comfortably at the console while the table-side surgeon passes and retrieves sutures, needles, and tissue specimens through the working port.

Operative Techniques and Technology

For either da Vinci or AESOP operation, the patients are prepared the same with the right side elevated 30 degrees on a roll, and the arms secured by their side. A 4-cm minithoracotomy incision is made in the submammary fold in the anterior axillary line. The pectoralis muscle is spared, and the fourth intercostal space is entered after right lung deflation. Pericardial exposure is obtained without rib resection or division, and a soft-tissue retractor (Cardiovations, Inc., Somerville, NJ) is inserted to displace the skin, fat, and muscle layers, leaving an oval space between the ribs. To prepare the internal operative field, a 4-cm retractor (Estech, Inc., Danville, CA) is placed temporarily through the soft-tissue retractor. If the right hemidiaphragm obstructs the operative approach, a retraction suture is placed in the central tendon, pulled through the chest wall using a "crochet hook" instrument, and then secured for retraction. The pericardium is opened 2 cm anterior to the phrenic nerve and extended to both the inferior vena caval (IVC) and aortic reflections. Transthoracic pericardial retraction sutures should be placed near the superior vena caval reflection and the atrio-IVC juncture to distract the posterior (dorsal) pericardial edge laterally. To minimize intracardiac air retention, a 14-G catheter, placed through the chest wall, is used for continuous carbon dioxide insufflation (2 to 3 liters/min). If the da Vinci system is used, instrument arm trocars are placed through the third and fifth intercostal spaces and sighted to be in direct line with the mitral annulus (Fig. 40-2). It is important to maintain at least 8 to 10 cm between these arms to avoid intracardiac instrument collisions.

For cardiopulmonary cannulation, an oblique 2-cm right-groin incision is made and superficial purse-string sutures are placed in both the femoral artery and vein. Then, coaxial dilators are introduced over a guidewire. Under TEE guidance, a 22- to 25-F venous cannula (Cardiovations, Inc., Somerville, NJ) is positioned in the central right atrium. This cannula is not suture-anchored, because intraoperative manipulation may be needed to provide optimal venous return. By the same method, the femoral artery is cannulated with either a 17-F or a 19-F Biomedicus arterial cannula. Patients are cooled to 28°C with the use of (kinetic-assisted) suction venous drainage. The ascending aortic antegrade cardioplegia/vent catheter is placed just distal to the right coronary ostium. This position allows

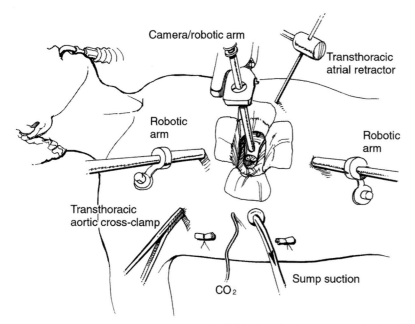

Figure 40-2. Robotic mitral valve repair: operative field. The robotic camera arm is placed into the center of the 4-cm incision. Both robotic arms are placed through the chest wall in a triangular fashion at least 5 cm to 7 cm apart to avoid any instrument arm conflicts. A soft-tissue retractor holds the incision open for the passing of suture and tissue. The transthoracic aortic cross-clamp is placed in the midaxillary line, low enough so that there is no conflict with the left robotic arm. The transthoracic atrial retractor is placed just off the lateral edge of the sternum, avoiding the internal mammary artery.

Table 40-3 Aesop Mitral Procedures (N = 303)	
Valve replacements	88 (29%)
Mitral valve repairs	215 (71%)
Ring annuloplasty	88 (40.9%)
Quadrangular/trapezoidal/ triangular resection	64 (29.8%)
Resection plus sliding annuloplasty	10 (4.7%)
Chordal replacements/ transfers	45 (20.9%)
Alfieri	16 (7.4%)
Concomitant procedures	42 (13.9%)
Closure of patent foramen ovale	6 (14.3%)
Ablation	26 (61.9%)
Atrial septal defect	2 (4.8%)
Tricuspid	2 (4.8%)
Miscellaneous	6 (14.3%)

deployment of the transthoracic clamp without crowding the cardioplegia/vent catheter. Retrograde coronary sinus catheters can also be placed across the right atrial wall and positioned using the TEE.

The interatrial (Waterston's, Sondergaard's) groove is dissected minimally and the oblique sinus is opened behind the IVC. To occlude the aorta, a 4-mm transthoracic aortic clamp (Scanlan, Inc., Minneapolis, MN) is placed through the second interspace in the midaxilla with the posterior clamp fixed-tine directed through the transverse sinus, passing posterior (dorsal) to the ascending aorta. Care must be taken to avoid injury to the right pulmonary artery, the left atrial appendage, or the left main coronary artery. After the clamp is applied, the heart is arrested with antegrade and/or retrograde cold blood cardioplegia.

A short atriotomy is made medial to the right superior pulmonary vein with extension toward the superior vena cava (SVC) and inferiorly behind the IVC. The arm of a percutaneous left atrial retractor is positioned just lateral to the sternal edge and medial to the incision, avoiding internal mammary vessel injury (Fig. 40-2). The retractor blade is inserted into the left atriotomy and attached to the arm. A ventral retractor blade elevates the interatrial sep-

tum to provide optimal mitral valve exposure. A left inferior pulmonary vein sump scavenges residual left atrial blood. The da Vinci instrument arms are then passed and positioned through trocars into the left atrium and the three-dimensional endoscope is positioned through the incision. Valve function is studied by the use of cold saline injections. The table-side surgeon exchanges the various microtipped

Table 40-2 Robotic Mitral Procedures (N = 114)	
Valve replacements	2 (1.8%)
Valve repairs	112 (98.2%)
Ring annuloplasty	21 (18.4%)
Posterior leaflet resection	47 (41.2%)
Quadrangular/trapezoidal resection plus sliding annuloplasty	32 (28.1%)
Posterior/anterior cleft repair	4 (3.5%)
Chordal replacements (Gore-Tex)	11 (9.6%)
Chordal transfer	23 (20.2%)
Alfieri	8 (7.0%)
Concomitant procedures	29 (25.4%)
Closure of patent foramen ovale	10 (34.5%)
Mini maze	19 (65.5%)

instruments. Standard reconstructive methods have been used in all of our da Vinci mitral valve repairs (Table 40-2) as well as in our AESOP-assisted patients (Table 40-3). We are comfortable in performing leaflet resections, sliding plasties, chordal transfers, chordal replacements, and annuloplasties. Currently, even Barlow's bileaflet disease does not escape our robotic repairs.

Mitral Valve Disease and Repair Techniques

Degenerative Mitral Disease

At our center, robotic instruments are used daily to repair degenerative (myxomatous) mitral valves. Classic features of this disease include leaflet prolapse and annular dilation. Carpentier's functional classification of mitral insufficiency is based on leaflet motion characteristics. Insufficiency with normal leaflet motion is type 1, with exaggerated (prolapse) leaflet motion is type 2, and with restricted leaflet motion is type 3. Most commonly, robotic mitral repairs are amenable to type 1 and 2 pathologies. Chordae tendineae may be thinned, elongated, and/or ruptured. Posterior (P_2) chordal rupture and/or elongation with a dilated annulus are the most common problem we repair. In the past, only symptomatic patients with 3+ or 4+ mitral regurgitation and ruptured/elongated posterior leaflet chords were referred for surgery. With the advent of safe, effective, minimally invasive, and robotic mitral surgery, more asymptomatic patients with moderate to severe regurgitation are being referred earlier. This is especially true for patients who already have some left ventricular impairment or dilation. There is clear evidence that patients with a chordal rupture and a flail leaflet segment should be repaired to enhance longevity. In asymptomatic patients, these newer indications are predicated on preventing ventricular dysfunction, left atrial dilation, and the development of atrial fibrillation.

Posterior Leaflet Prolapse

As mentioned, posterior leaflet prolapse/flail occurs most commonly. Robotic microscissors and tissue forceps are used for leaflet resections. Robotic needle holders should never be used to grasp delicate leaflet and chordal tissues. Posterior leaflet prolapse is treated by either quadrangular or trapezoidal resection of the diseased chordal leaflet segment (Fig. 40-3). We try to limit the length of the annular gap, especially in patients who do not require a sliding leaflet

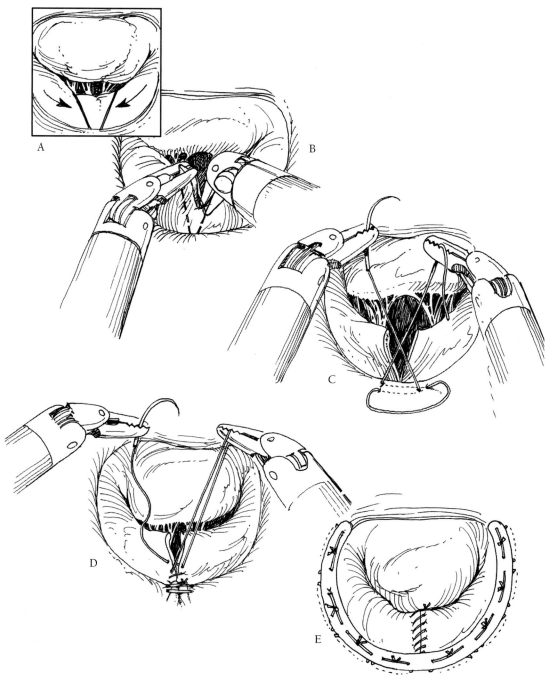

Figure 40-3. Robotic posterior leaflet resection. **(A, B)** A trapezoidal incision is created in P$_2$ with robotic scissors. **(C)** Figure-of-eight annular compression sutures (2-0 Ti-Cron) are placed. **(D)** The leading edges of the remaining P$_2$ leaflet are then brought together using interrupted or continuous 5-0 Cardionyl sutures. **(E)** A band annuloplasty is performed using interrupted 2-0 Ti-Cron sutures.

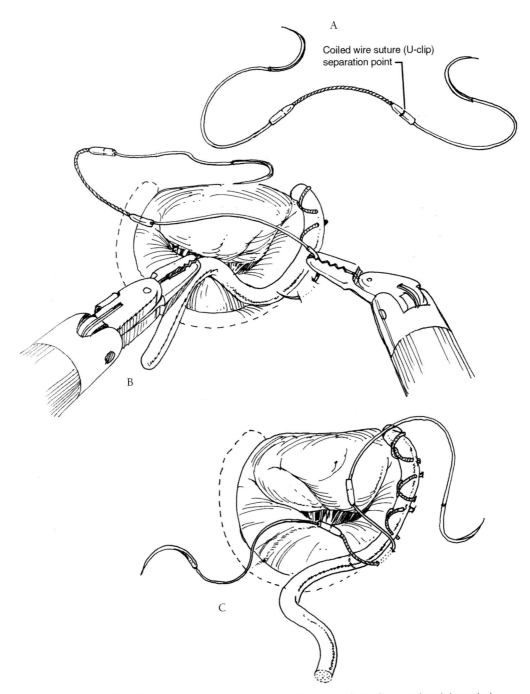

Figure 40-4.   (A) Nitinol U-clip used in robotic mitral valve repair. These clips are placed through the annulus **(B, C)** like conventional sutures, with each arm then placed through the annuloplasty band **(D, E, F)**. The locking mechanism, which deploys the clip, is released using robotic needle holders **(G)**. Nitinol retains a preformed shape **(H, I)** securing the annuloplasty band tightly against the tissue. The U-clip arms are carefully laid over the annuloplasty band to secure it firmly. (*continued*)

plasty to reduce the posterior leaflet height. The narrow annular defect is then closed robotically with 2-0 Ti-Cron figure-of-eight sutures. Residual leaflet edges are reapproximated with 4-0 or 5-0 Cardionyl interrupted sutures. In robotic operations, we have used the Cosgrove annuloplasty band, which is placed between each fibrous trigone using either 2-0 Ti-Cron sutures or special mitral repair U-clips that are deployed via a release mechanism (Coalescent Inc., Sunnyvale, CA) (Fig. 40-4).

When one is concerned about systolic anterior motion (SAM) of the anterior leaflet, a sliding leaflet repair is indicated and can be performed with the da Vinci system. Postrepair SAM can develop in patients with excess posterior leaflet tissue (posterior height >1.5 cm), a long anterior leaflet (>34 mm), left ventricular outflow-track septal hypertrophy, and in the presence of an acute angle between the planes of the aortic and mitral valve annuli. Moreover, SAM can be caused by an undersized

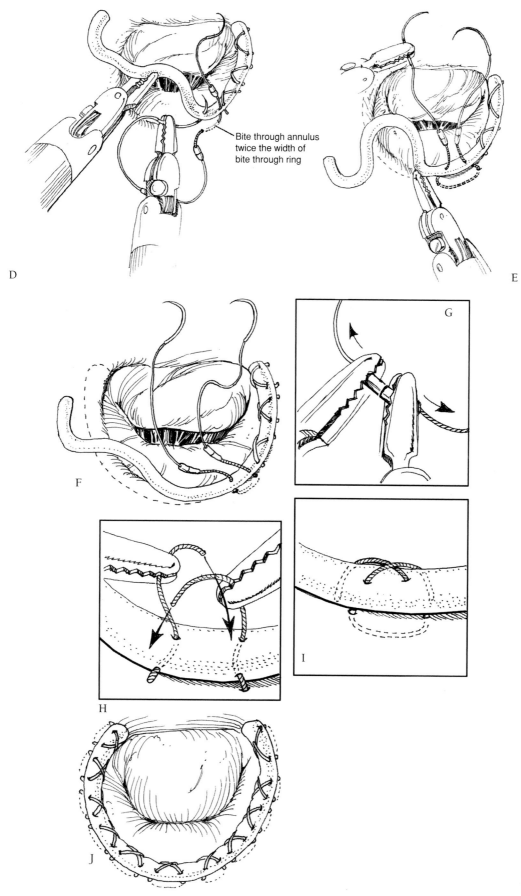

Bite through annulus twice the width of bite through ring

D

E

F

G

H

I

J

Figure 40-4.   (*Continued*)

annuloplasty ring or band. It is not true that SAM cannot develop when a flexible ring or intertrigonal band is used. The potential for SAM is created when a mitral reconstruction forces the middle or basal anterior leaflet to coapt with the tip of the posterior leaflet. During systole the ante-rior leaflet tip moves toward the septum, where outflow-jet "lift" increases unphys-iologic leaflet movement toward the out-flow septum. This displacement can open the mitral coaptation point, causing signif-icant regurgitation, even in a "saline test"-competent valve. It makes sense that ven-tricular hypertrophy and inotropic drugs can decrease the leaflet-septum space, in-creasing SAM and the outflow gradient.

The purpose of the *sliding leaflet repair* (Fig. 40-5) is to reduce the height of the posterior leaflet, which moves the anterior leaflet coaptation point more posterior and

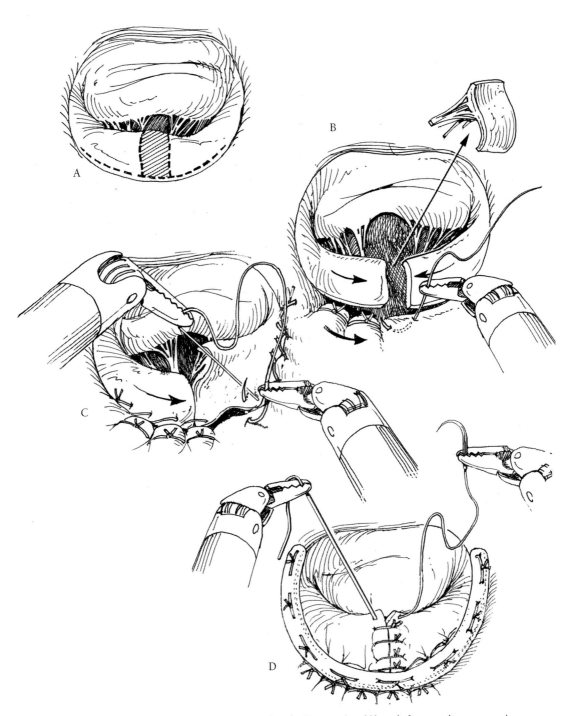

Figure 40-5. A robotic sliding leaflet repair. After the P$_2$ resection **(A)** and after annular compression sutures are placed to reduce tension on the repair **(B)**, a running suture sliding plasty is performed using 4-0 Cardionyl sutures from both the right and left trigones toward the middle of the annulus **(C)**. These sutures are then tied together, and the valve undergoes final repair with an interrupted 5-0 Cardionyl leaflet repair with subsequent annuloplasty band placement **(D)**.

away from the ventricular septum. After a quadrangular resection, the posterior leaflet is detached from the annulus on either side of the resection. Multiple annular compression sutures are used to reduce the gap symmetrically. Then the leaflet remnant is advanced along the annulus using a running 4-0 Cardionyl suture. Often both portions must be advanced centrally, much like closing barn doors. Leaflet edges are then reapproximated as described, and an annuloplasty completes the repair.

Anterior Leaflet Prolapse

A variety of techniques have been used to repair mitral anterior leaflet prolapse. The most common methods include *chordal transfers* and *prosthetic chord replacements*.

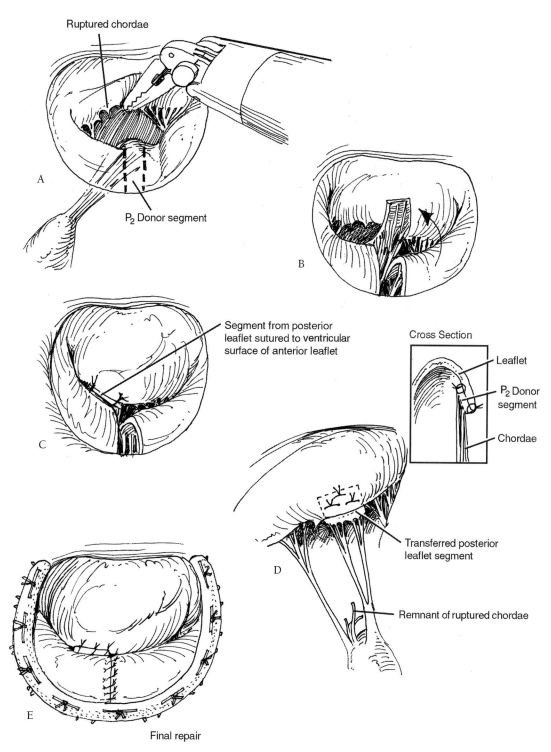

Figure 40-6.   A robotic posterior chordal transfer for anterior leaflet prolapse secondary to a ruptured A_1 chord. A portion of P_2 is resected **(A, B)**, transferred, and sewn to the ventricular edge of A_2 with interrupted 5-0 Cardionyl suture **(C, D)**. A ring annuloplasty is then placed **(E)**.

Using the da Vinci system, we prefer to reduce the anterior leaflet to the coapting plane by transferring either marginal or large basal chords. The three-dimensional high-magnification camera and microscissors allow us to detach anterior leaflet basal chords and transfer them directly to the flail edge of the leaflet. Moreover, primary chordae from the posterior leaflet can be transposed to the unsupported region of the anterior leaflet. Many prolapsing or flail posterior leaflet segments still have some good, thick chords remaining, and these can be transferred anteriorly with a patch of leaflet for anchorage.

Generally, by swinging either basal (secondary) anterior leaflet or residual posterior leaflet primary chords to the anterior leaflet edge, the radial movement geometrically reduces the anterior leaflet prolapse. The defect in the posterior leaflet is repaired as described for a standard quadrangular resection (Fig. 40-6). For significant anterior leaflet prolapse, multiple chords must be transferred with the saline test used to confirm appropriate edge reduction. Because of the lack of tremor, visioning systems, microinstruments, and improved access, it is much easier to transfer chords using the

da Vinci system than using conventional instruments and direct vision through a sternotomy.

Our second choice for reduction of anterior leaflet prolapse is chordal replacement using polytetrafluoroethylene (PTFE, Gore-Tex). With the da Vinci surgical system, papillary muscle access is magnificent. A short (16-cm) double-armed 4-0 Gore-Tex suture is passed in a figure-of-eight fashion through the papillary muscle fibrous head. Thereafter, the needles are passed through the leaflet edge at the rupture/prolapse site. Then the same suture is looped around the

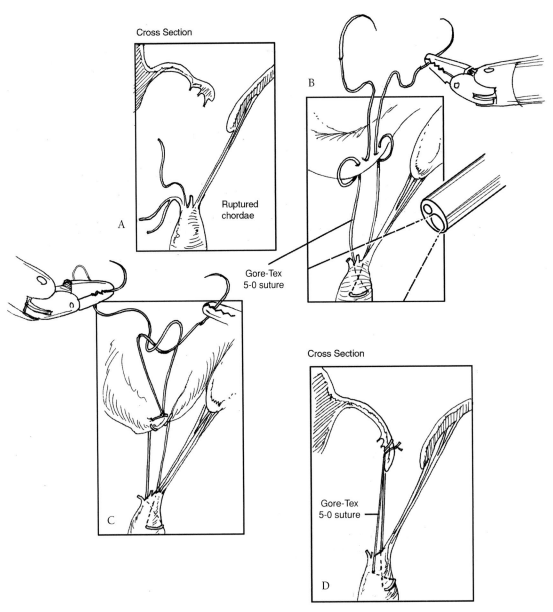

Figure 40-7.   Use of Gore-Tex neochords to correct an anterior leaflet prolapse resulting from ruptured chordae **(A)**. A 4-0 Gore-Tex is passed in "criss-cross" fashion through a viable papillary muscle head, and sutures are passed through the edge of the leaflet and looped to repenetrate the leaflet **(B)**. The suture is then tied while we perform the saline test and remeasure chordal lengths to ensure perfect leaflet coaptation **(C, D)**.

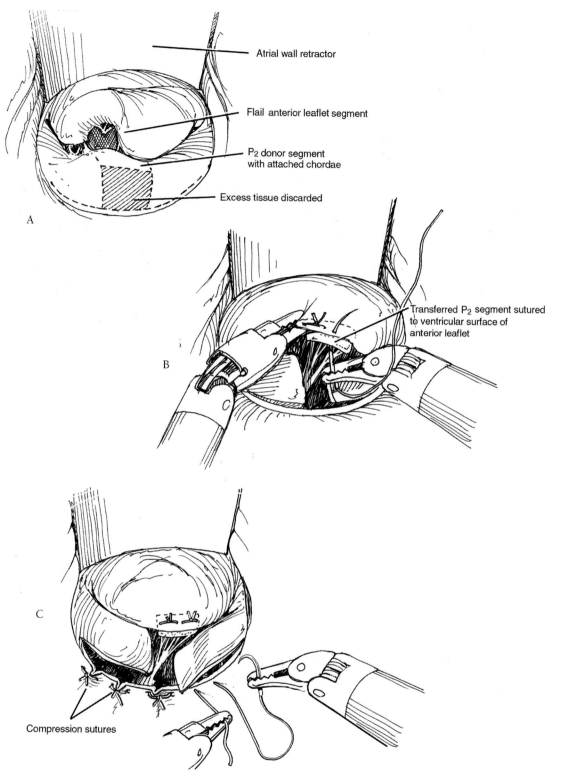

Atrial wall retractor

Flail anterior leaflet segment

P2 donor segment
with attached chordae

Excess tissue discarded

A

Transferred P2 segment sutured
to ventricular surface of
anterior leaflet

B

C

Compression sutures

Figure 40-8. Robotic repair of a Barlow valve. A segment of P_2 is resected and transferred to the ventricular surface of A_2 **(A, B)** using 5-0 Cardionyl suture for fixation. Compression sutures (2-0 Ti-Cron) are placed in the annulus and tied **(C)**. Then, a running sliding annuloplasty with 4-0 Cardionyl is often performed to approximate P_1 and P_2 segments **(D)**. Annuloplasty-band insertion completes the repair **(E)**. (*continued*)

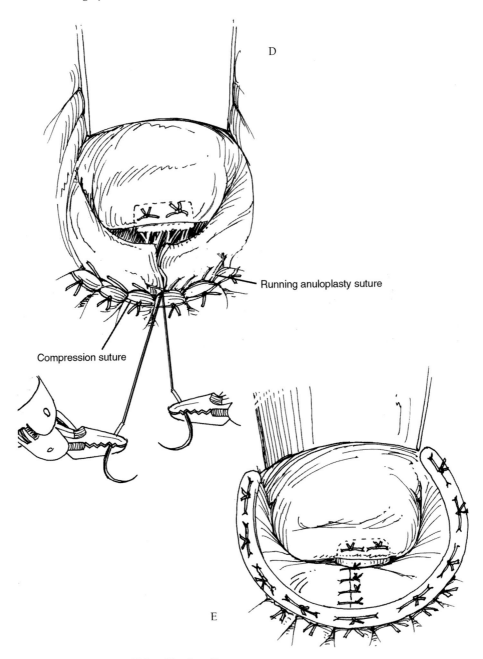

Figure 40-8. (*Continued*)

coapting edge and back through the leaflet, creating a "locking loop" (Fig. 40-7). The second chord is placed in similar fashion, with a gap between it and the first of 3 mm. After chordal length adjustment and before the two chords are tied by telemanipulation, saline testing is done robotically to assure optimal neochordal length and leaflet coaptation.

In all of our mitral valve repairs, we have abandoned Carpentier's method of chordal shortening by tucking an elongated chord into a papillary trench. Simpler methods have been very satisfactory, and reports of late chordal ruptures with the trench

method have shifted our focus from correction at the papillary end to that at the leaflet end. Robotic methods lend themselves better to the methods described here, and we have had no late ruptures in chordal transfers or replacements. In severe Barlow's bileaflet disease we generally transfer a long strip of chord-bearing posterior leaflet (usually P_2) to prolapsing segments of A_1–A_3. Then the resected part of the posterior leaflet is closed using the reducing sliding plasty, and commissural prolapse is corrected with the edge-to-edge method. Of course, a properly sized annuloplasty is done to complete the robotic repair (Fig. 40-8).

Annuloplasty

Annular dilation is present in most patients with degenerative mitral disease. An annuloplasty is performed in conjunction with all repairs to restore the native geometry, reduce the annular size, prevent further dilation, and reinforce the repair. Reducing the anterior–posterior annular diameter increases the leaflet coaptation surface. Annuloplasty support prostheses are either flexible or rigid and surround the mitral annulus either completely or incompletely. The latter notion suggests that the mitral-aortic curtain or central fibrous body, between the trigones, is nonmuscular and does not dilate. The Cosgrove-Edwards annuloplasty band is anchored at each trigone and for the more muscular intervening annulus both reduces and remodels. An ideal prosthesis should be flexible, soft, and easy to handle using robotic instruments. To date no complete ring satisfies these requirements, and the Cosgrove-Edwards band has served our repairs well, because the major etiology has been from degenerative causes and not ischemia.

Short (14-cm) double-armed 2-0 sutures are unavailable and, therefore, the band is attached using the single-arm method shown (Fig. 40-9). Initially, sutures are placed into each fibrous trigone to aid in exposure. In addition, we have detached the band from the template to manipulate it in the small interatrial space. This is not optimal, because nonlinear placement of sutures or variations in spacing can cause kinking of the band and annular asymmetry. The band is first anchored to the right fibrous trigone, and suture placement proceeds clockwise. The last two sutures at the anterior commissure and left fibrous trigone are placed before tying either. Care must be taken in this region to avoid the aortic root and the circumflex coronary artery. Good anchoring bites can be obtained here but the needle must remain perpendicular to the annulus and not tangential to the aorta or circumflex region. The camera in the da Vinci system allows precise placement of deep bites in the annulus. In the most recent 60 patients, we used double-armed nitinol U-clips successfully to anchor the band. In our experimental studies we have seen adequate annular compression, ease of placement, and band security. Moreover, we have found that our band implantation times have decreased significantly compared with the suture technique described.

When using the video-assisted method and AESOP, we use long instruments and traditional suturing methods. The surgeon must adjust the needle angles extracorporeally to correctly execute each intra-atrial maneuver. Sutures are arranged extracorporeally in guides radially placed around the

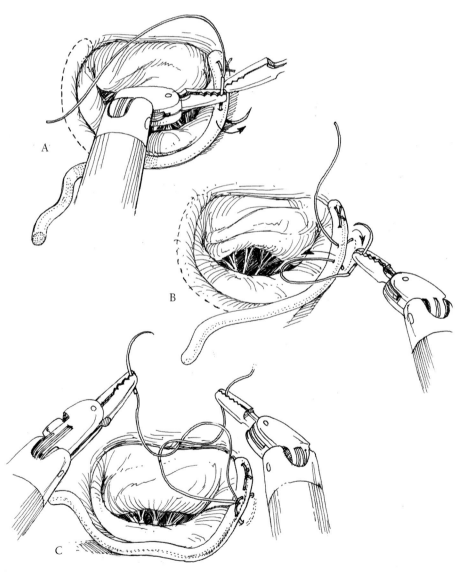

Figure 40-9.   Robotic suture placement for a mitral band annuloplasty. Twelve-centimeter 2-0 Ti-Cron sutures are placed and tied serially. With the use of a robotic needle holder, this single arm suture is placed first through the band **(A)** and then through the annulus **(B)** and back through the band. Six knots generally will secure the band tightly with the proper amount of annular compression **(C)**.

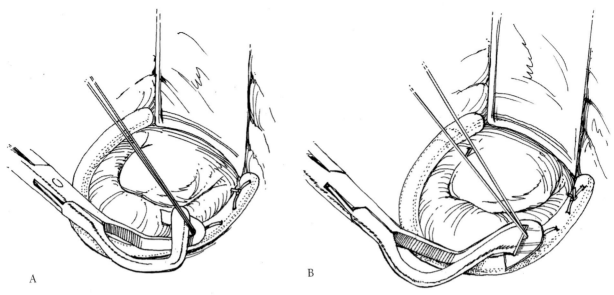

A   B

Figure 40-10.   The Chitwood extracorporeal knot-tier (pusher). This device has an offset to ensure visualization during tying through 4-cm incisions. Two half-hitches are placed to avoid "air-knots," and then square knots are placed to approximate the band tightly against the annulus. This instrument also has a scissor component that allows the surgeon to cut the suture without having to change instruments.

incision. Sutures are tied using a specialized device (Fig. 40-10).

Clinical Outcomes

We have performed nearly 400 mitral repairs using video assistance with AESOP. Furthermore, we have performed nearly 150 robotic mitral valve repairs with the da Vinci system. Our training program has trained over 200 surgeons in mitral repair surgery using the da Vinci system, and many of them are already successfully doing repairs.

AESOP Video-Assisted Mitral Valve Repairs

We began to use AESOP in 1999, and our first published series showed no operative mortality and 0.9% 30-day mortality in 72 patients. In comparison, our 30-day mortality for 100 serial conventional mitral patients was 2.2%. Two robot-assisted patients required conversion to a sternotomy secondary to bleeding. There were no aortic clamp injuries or retrograde dissections. When the 72 robot-assisted cases were compared to 55 patients who were manually assisted, perfusion times were found to have fallen significantly (172 to 143 minutes). Concurrently, cross-clamp times fell from 128 minutes with human assistance to 90 minutes in the AESOP-assisted group.

Clearly, AESOP camera stabilization and voice control enhanced surgeon freedom and decreased camera-cleaning events, both of which helped to reduce operative times. The average length of stay was 4.6 days, and 67% of patients required no blood transfusions. In the AESOP group, 1 patient had a failed repair.

More recently, we reviewed our first 300 patients operated using AESOP. Of these, 70% were mitral repairs, with cross-clamp and perfusion times averaging 98 and 138 minutes, respectively. The operative and 30-day mortalities were 0.3% and 3.0%, respectively. Complex repairs were done in most of these patients, and 2.5% were reoperated on for valve-related failures. For this larger group 4% had significant bleeding, requiring re-exploration, but only 24% received blood products. The overall hospital length of stay was 5 days. Trends seen in this larger group have persisted in additional mitral repair operations with video assistance and AESOP. Our continued experience has shown this approach to be safe and effective, with operative results that are similar to traditional methods. Patient satisfaction and recovery have been excellent. Other groups have published similar results using AESOP minimally invasive mitral surgery. Reichenspurner showed similar operative times and no 30-day mortality in 20 patients. Later, Trehan showed in 120 patients that operative times were comparable to ours. They

had a 0.5% operative mortality with no reoperations.

da Vinci Robotic Mitral Valve Repairs

In the year 2000, in the first Food and Drug Administration (FDA) safety and efficacy trial of robotic mitral valve repair, quadrangular leaflet resections, leaflet sliding plasties, chord transfers, PTFE chord replacements, reduction annuloplasties, and annuloplasty band insertions were performed at East Carolina University in 20 patients. These first cardiac arrest times were long times at 150 minutes, but were only 52 minutes for leaflet repairs. Moreover, it took an additional 42 minutes to anchor the Cosgrove-Edwards annuloplasty bands (mean 7.5 sutures). The operative times were long, but the results were good, and there were no device-related and few procedure-related complications. The average postoperative stay was 4 days (3 to 7 days). At 3-month follow-up, echocardiographies revealed nothing more than trace mitral regurgitation. All patients returned to normal activity by 1 month after surgery.

A subsequent multicenter, phase II FDA trial studied 112 da Vinci patients operated on in 10 U.S. centers. Again, repairs included quadrangular resections, sliding plasties, edge-to-edge approximations, and both chordal transfers and replacements. Leaflet repair and annuloplasty times fell to 37 and 39 minutes, respectively, compared to the phase I trial. Aortic cross-clamp and cardiopulmonary bypass times averaged 2.1 and 2.8 hours, respectively. There was little difference in operative times among centers. At 1-month follow-up, transthoracic echocardiography revealed 9 patients (8.0%) had greater than or equal to grade 2 mitral regurgitation, and 6 (5.4%) of these had reoperations. Although the reoperative rate was disturbing, the failed repairs were distributed across the group evenly and some centers had performed fewer than 10 robotic operations. There were no deaths, strokes, or device-related complications. This study demonstrated that multiple surgical teams could perform robotic mitral valve surgery safely early in the development of this technique, albeit with a learning curve with regard to operative times and repair results. The device was FDA approved in November 2002 for use in the United States based on these two studies.

Learning curve data from our first 38 da Vinci mitral repairs were encouraging. Patients were evaluated in two cohorts: Early ($N = 19$) and Late ($N = 19$). Operative times were measured starting after the robot was positioned to begin the repair. Total robotic operating times decreased from 1.9 to 1.5 hours ($p = .002$), respectively, between Early and Late groups. Concomitantly, leaflet repair times fell from 1.0 to 0.6 hours ($p = .004$), respectively. Both cross-clamp and bypass times decreased significantly with experience as well. Total length of stay was 3.8 ± 0.6 days, with no difference between the two groups. Of all patients in the study, 84% demonstrated three grades or greater reduction in mitral regurgitation at follow-up. There were no device-related complications or operative deaths.

We have completed nearly 150 robotic mitral valve repairs with the da Vinci system. There has been 1 operative death from a protamine reaction but no device-related complications. In the entire series there have been 2 late deaths, and we have reoperated on 3 patients for valve repair failures. However, even at the 100th case we continued to see improvement in operative time. No doubt this is related to the use of U-clips for annuloplasties, improved robot setup and deployment times, closer team working relations, and surgeon experience. However, there are parts of this operation that can only be improved by new technology and not just experience. For example, the robotic knot-tying times did not change significantly with

experience from the first 25 patients, averaging 1.8 minutes, to the next 25 patients, averaging 1.56 minutes ($p = $ N.S.). Thus, as we found in using the U-clips, new methods for retraction and exposure as well as visioning must be developed. Moreover, instrument arm sizes must be reduced and a greater variety of end-effector tips developed before we truly see the robotic era in mitral surgery.

Limitations/Future Directions

Despite rapid procedural advances, our early clinical experience with computer-enhanced mitral surgery has defined many of the technological limitations. Force or haptic feedback is absent in these devices; however, new strain sensors may soon allow for more control of force applied at the robotic end-effector. Thus far, we have been able to overcome the limitations of "touchless" surgery by relying on "ocular tactility." That is, with a high degree of visual acuity and magnification we can sense when knots are tight, bands are approximated closely to tissues, and calcifications are present. Nevertheless, the addition of haptic feedback will provide more latitude with these devices. As shown, conventional suture and knot tying add significant time to each procedure. Technological advances, such as the use of nitinol U-clips, have begun to decrease operative times significantly. For example, in a series of animal experiments, both average suture versus clip placement times and knot-tying versus clip deployment times decreased significantly when using U-clips. During implantation of experimental mitral annuloplasty bands, clip deployment was greater than 3.5 times faster than sutures. Pathologic review showed excellent clip and band incorporation at 3 and 6 months, and there was no discernible echocardiographic stenosis or regurgitation. Recently, 5-mm arms with finer instrument tips have been developed for da Vinci (Fig. 40-11).

We have examined learning curves both experimentally and clinically that are associated with robotic mitral valve repairs. A retrospective review of the first 80 mitral valve repairs using the da Vinci system suggested that learning curves can be flattened. To study these curves, we divided the group of 80 patients into eight equal groups of 10 chronological cohorts. Valve resection, repair, suture placement, knot-tying, total robotic, cross-clamp, and bypass times were analyzed in the first 5 cohorts of 10 patients. All showed significant reductions from the first group compared to the most recent operations (Table 40-4). As expected, we proved that intraoperative robotic mitral repair surgery times decreased as more procedures were performed. Interestingly, the learning curve was most evident through the first 20 operations, but there were incremental improvements thereafter. With further refinements and development of adjunctive technologies, computer-enhanced cardiac surgery should evolve, and promises to be beneficial for many patients. Future surgical imaging and positioning systems may allow us to do these repairs using 1-cm ports alone and perhaps even inside the beating heart under echo guidance.

Conclusions

A renaissance in cardiac surgery has begun, and robotic technology is providing benefits to cardiac surgeons and their patients. With improved optics and instrumentation, incisions are smaller, and simulated three-dimensional vision enhances surgeon hand–eye coordination. The placement of wristlike articulations at the end of the instruments moves the pivoting action to the plane of the mitral annulus. This improves dexterity in tight spaces and allows ambidextrous suture placement. Furthermore, the robotic system may have potential as an educational tool. In the near future, surgical vision and training systems may be able to model most surgical

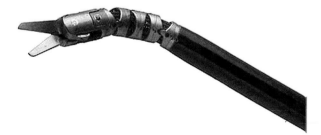

Figure 40-11. View of 5-mm robotic arms currently under development. These are more flexible and occupy less work space, which results in fewer instrument arm conflicts. These new arms should allow more ergonomic control by the surgeon when operating in close spaces.

Table 40-4   Intraoperative Times for the First 50 Robotic Mitral Valve Repairs

	RST[a]	RPT[a]	SPT[a]	KTT[a]	TRT[b]	CCT[b]	CPB[b]
First 10	8.8 ± 2.5	54.9 ± 2.8	2.7 ± 0.27	1.9 ± 0.11	2.1 ± 0.15	2.7 ± 0.07	3.4 ± 0.10
Second 10	5.6 ± 1.0	52.2 ± 8.2	1.9 ± 0.11	1.7 ± 0.09	2.0 ± 0.50	2.7 ± 0.16	3.4 ± 0.17
Third 10	4.7 ± 0.8	38.1 ± 5.4	1.5 ± 0.08	1.5 ± 0.08	1.5 ± 0.33	2.1 ± 0.13	2.7 ± 0.14
Fourth 10	2.9 ± 0.4	29.1 ± 2.9	1.5 ± 0.09	1.5 ± 0.08	1.5 ± 0.17	2.1 ± 0.10	2.7 ± 0.15
Fifth 10	2.6 ± 0.6	27.8 ± 3.1	1.3 ± 0.09	1.5 ± 0.07	1.4 ± 0.17	2.0 ± 0.09	2.5 ± 0.13
p	0.005	0.001	0.001	0.001	0.001	0.001	0.001

[a]Minutes (mean ± standard error of the mean).
[b]Hours (mean ± standard error of the mean).
RST = valve resection time; RPT = valve repair time; SPT = individual suture placement time; KTT = knot-tying time, TRT = total robotic time; CCT = cross-clamp time; CPB = cardiopulmonary bypass time.

procedures through immersive technology. Thus, a surgeon may be able to simulate, practice, and perform the operation based strictly on a patient's preoperative imaging data.

This new science is a trek and not a destination. In this era of outcomes-based medicine, surgical scientists must continue to evaluate robotics and all new technology critically. Despite enthusiasm, caution cannot be overemphasized. Surgeons must proceed carefully, because indices of operative safety, speed of recovery, level of discomfort, procedural cost, and long-term operative quality remain poorly defined. Traditional valve operations still enjoy long-term success with ever-decreasing morbidity and mortality, and remain our measure for comparison. However, robotically assisted mitral valve surgery has developed to become a safe and successful modality that surely will be modified as technological advances occur in all surgical disciplines.

SUGGESTED READING

Carpentier A. Cardiac valve surgery—The "French correction." J Thorac Cardiovasc Surg 1983;86:323.

Carpentier A, Loulmet D, Aupecle B, et al. Computer assisted open-heart surgery. First case operated on with success. C R Acad Sci II 1998;321:437.

Chitwood WR Jr, Nifong LW, Elbeery JE, et al. Robotic mitral valve repair: Trapezoidal resection and prosthetic annuloplasty with the da Vinci surgical system. J Thorac Cardiovasc Surg 2000;120:1171.

Chitwood WR Jr, Wixon CL, Elbeery JR, et al. Video-assisted minimally invasive mitral valve surgery. J Thorac Cardiovasc Surg 1997;114:773,.

Cosgrove DM, Chavez AM, Lytle BW, et al. Results of mitral valve reconstruction. Circulation 1986;74:182.

Felger JE, Chitwood WR Jr, Nifong LW, et al. Evolution of mitral valve surgery: Toward a totally endoscopic approach. Ann Thorac Surg 2001;72:1203.

Gorman PJ, Meir AH, Krummel TH. Simulation and virtual reality in surgical education: Real or unreal. Arch Surg 1999;134:1203.

Meir AH, Rawn CL, Krummel TM. Virtual reality: Surgical application—Challenge for the new millennium. J Am Coll Surg 2001;192:372.

Mohr FW, Falk V, Diegeler A, et al. Minimally invasive port-access mitral valve surgery. J Thorac Cardiovasc Surg 1998;115:567.

Mohr FW, Falk V, Diegeler A, et al. Computer-enhanced "robotic" cardiac surgery: Experience in 148 patients. J Thorac Cardiovasc Surg 2001;121:842.

Nifong LW, Chitwood WR Jr, Argenziano M, et al. Robotic mitral valve surgery: A United States multi-center trial. J Thorac Cardiovasc Surg 2005;129:1395.

Nifong LW, Chu VR, Bailey BM, et al. Robotic mitral valve repair: Experience with the da Vinci system. Ann Thorac Surg 2003;75:438.

Sand ME, Naftel DC, Blackstone EH, et al. A comparison of repair and replacement for mitral valve incompetence. J Thorac Cardiovasc Surg 1987;94:208.

EDITOR'S COMMENTS

Chitwood's group at East Carolina University has been the standard bearer for robotic mitral valve surgery. They analyzed these procedures in this well-written chapter and clearly demonstrated excellent results and reductions in time. Whether we agree or not, patients prefer small incisions, and the use of the robot has allowed many surgeons to perform excellent mitral valve repairs through small incisions. Clearly, the major issue with the robot is the learning curve and the lack of sense of feel. The advantages are the excellent utilization, the loss of tremor, and the ability to manipulate in small spaces. I am still not sure where robotic mitral valve surgery fits in, but it is clearly an advancing field. This excellent analysis by the East Carolina group and continued advances will allow us to decide whether this will find a routine place in the practice of mitral valve surgery.

I.L.K.

41

Mitral Valve Repair: Ischemic

David H. Adams, Farzan Filsoufi, Lishan Aklog, and Sacha P. Salzberg

Introduction

Severe coronary artery disease and myocardial infarction can be complicated by mitral regurgitation (MR). Commonly referred to as ischemic MR, in most instances it results from either left ventricular remodeling after myocardial infarction or, less frequently, acute ischemia. This entity should be distinguished from ischemic coronary artery disease and concomitant MR due to other underlying etiologies such as degenerative mitral valve disease, rheumatic disease, and endocarditis. For several years, because of a lack of understanding of the precise pathophysiology of ischemic MR, much of the medical and surgical literature failed to distinguish between these different clinical entities. Early clinical series included heterogeneous groups of patients and produced contradictory results that led to unclear conclusions and guidelines with respect to medical and surgical management of these patients. More recently, laboratory research and clinical outcome analysis have significantly improved the understanding of this complex disease and its medical and surgical management. This better understanding of the pathophysiology of ischemic MR and increased awareness of its negative effect on long-term survival are the principal factors that may explain the recent rise in the number of patients referred for surgical correction of ischemic MR at the time of coronary revascularization. In this chapter we review ischemic MR with regard to its pathophysiology, clinical presentations, diagnosis, indication for surgery, and management.

Definition

Carpentier's Functional Classification of Mitral Regurgitation

Careful attention to classification of mitral valve disease is critical when evaluating patients with ischemic MR. We prefer to use Carpentier's functional classification to describe the mechanism of MR (Fig. 41-1). This classification is based on the opening and closing motions of the mitral leaflets in relation to the annular plane. Patients with type I dysfunction have normal leaflet motion, and MR is due to annular dilation or leaflet perforation (Fig. 41-1, top). There is increased leaflet motion in patients with type II dysfunction, with the free edge of at least one of the leaflets overriding the plane of the annulus during systole (leaflet prolapse) (Fig. 41-1, middle). The most common lesions responsible for type II dysfunction are chordal elongation or rupture and papillary muscle elongation or rupture. Finally, type III dysfunction implies restricted leaflet motion, with the free margins of portions of one or both leaflets pulled restricted below the plane of the annulus into the left ventricle, reducing leaflet mobility and coaptation during systole, and leading to MR. Patients with type IIIa dysfunction have restricted leaflet motion during both diastole and systole. The most common lesions are leaflet thickening/retraction, chordal thickening/shortening or fusion, and commissural fusion. Type IIIb dysfunction is caused by restricted leaflet motion during systole. Left ventricular dysfunction and dilation

with apical and posterolateral papillary muscle displacement causes this type of valve dysfunction (Fig. 41-1, bottom).

Ischemic MR can result from type I, II, or IIIb dysfunction (Table 41-1). Isolated type I dysfunction with annular dilation is uncommon but may occur in basal myocardial infarction. Type II dysfunction after myocardial infarction results from papillary muscle rupture, which usually involves the posteromedial papillary muscle or occurs when a fibrotic papillary muscle elongates and causes leaflet prolapse, particularly in the commissural area. In rare instances, an isolated chordal rupture can cause type II dysfunction. Carpentier's type IIIb dysfunction is the *most common and significant* form of ischemic MR (Table 41-1).

Type IIIb Ischemic Mitral Regurgitation

Pathophysiology

Normal mitral valve function involves a complex three-dimensional interaction among the leaflets, annulus, subvalvular apparatus, and left ventricular wall. Several anatomic and pathophysiologic changes are associated with the pathogenesis of ischemic MR. They include ventricular changes (wall-motion abnormalities, dilation with increased sphericity), subvalvular changes (papillary muscle infarction, displacement, or tethering), and annular changes (distortion, dilation). The initiating insult in ischemic MR is ventricular,

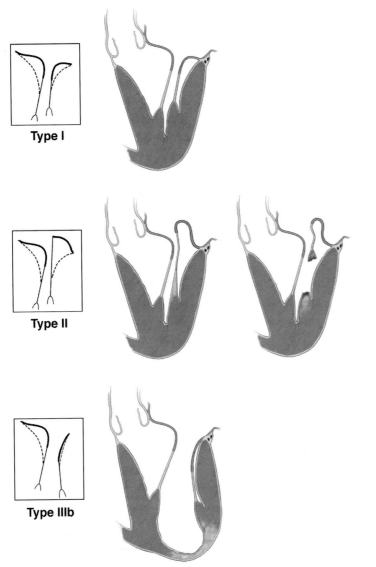

Figure 41-1. Carpentier's functional classification in ischemic mitral regurgitation (MR). **(Top)** Type I has normal leaflet motion, and MR is on the basis of annular dilation, which may occur in the setting of basal infarction. **(Middle)** Type II dysfunction implies excess leaflet motion with the free edge of the leaflet(s) traveling above the annular plane during systole, which may occur after myocardial infarction due to papillary muscle rupture (acute) or papillary elongation (chronic). **(Bottom)** Type IIIb is the most common form of ischemic MR, and results from restricted leaflet motion during systole secondary to apical and lateral papillary muscle displacement. (Adapted from DH Adams, F Filsoufi. Another chapter in an enlarging book: Repair degenerative mitral valves. J Thorac Cardiovasc Surg 2003;125:1197.)

specifically left ventricular remodeling after myocardial ischemia or infarction. This remodeling converts the shape of the left ventricle from ellipsoidal to spherical, which subsequently leads to regional annular and subvalvular distortion and ultimately to poor leaflet coaptation. It appears that left ventricular sphericity is more important than the actual ventricular volumes or ejection fraction in the progression of ischemic MR. The primary ventricular alteration leading to ischemic MR is papillary muscle dis-

placement. The pattern of displacement is complex and cannot simply be described as apical tethering. The papillary muscle tips are displaced away from the midseptal (anterior) annulus, that is, posterolaterally, apically, and away from each other. The tethering distance has been shown to correlate with the severity of ischemic MR. Papillary muscle tethering leads to *apical tenting* of the leaflets (restriction of the motion of the free margins of the leaflets), which prevents them from rising to the plane of the annulus

to coapt with one another (Fig. 41-2). This has been well documented using qualitative and quantitative echocardiographic methods in clinical practice. Tethering of the secondary chordae results in "sea-gull" deformation of the body of the leaflet, further impairing coaptation. Annular dilation is a common *associated finding* in chronic ischemic type IIIb MR. However, the degree of dilation can vary and does not necessarily correlate with the degree of MR. Laboratory data support the notion that annular dilation is not a fundamental component in the pathogenesis of ischemic MR. It has been demonstrated that mild degrees of annular dilation observed during acute occlusion of the left anterior descending or distal left circumflex in an animal model did not result in ischemic MR. The aforementioned changes in left ventricular geometry, papillary muscle position, and annular dimensions interact to result in poor leaflet coaptation during systole, which is the final common pathway for type IIIb ischemic MR.

Clinical Presentation

Type IIIb ischemic MR can occur in an acute or chronic setting. *Acute postinfarction ischemic MR*, without papillary muscle rupture, can be documented in many patients by physical examination, ventriculography, or echocardiography. Moderate to severe MR is present in up to 13% of these patients. Acute severe type IIIb ischemic MR often presents with a sudden onset of shortness of breath and/or angina. In most patients, this incident is preceded by an acute myocardial infarction (MI), which may be silent particularly in diabetic patients. A minority of patients will present with symptoms of severe heart failure and/or low cardiac output. Although MR resolves over time in some patients, it will persist in others and lead to *chronic postinfarction ischemic MR*. In some patients, chronic ischemic MR will first appear up to 6 weeks (median 7 days) after MI, as the infarcted left ventricle remodels. Risk factors for postinfarction ischemic MR include advanced age, female gender, prior acute MI, large infarct size, recurrent ischemia, multivessel coronary artery disease, and congestive heart failure.

In patients with chronic ischemic MR, two clinical scenarios are commonly encountered. Patients may present with moderate to severe MR, symptoms of congestive heart failure, or worsening left ventricular function and are referred primarily for mitral valve intervention. The preoperative coronary angiogram shows significant multivessel coronary artery disease that may

Table 41-1 Pathophysiological Triad in Ischemic Mitral Regurgitation		
Dysfunction	Lesions	Chronic/Acute
TYPE I	Annular dilation	Chronic
TYPE II	Chordal rupture	Acute
	Papillary muscle rupture	Chronic
	Papillary muscle elongation	Acute
TYPE IIIb	Papillary muscle displacement	Acute or chronic
	Leaflet tethering	

or may not have been symptomatic. These patients often have clear evidence of prior myocardial infarction and at least moderate left ventricular dysfunction. Other patients present with symptomatic multivessel coronary artery disease and are referred for coronary artery bypass grafting with a varying degree of MR on preoperative ventriculography or echocardiography. An acute coronary syndrome or chronic stable angina is often the dominant presenting symptom in these patients. In addition, they may present with symptoms of shortness of breath and/or congestive heart failure.

Diagnosis

Patients often present with changes on their electrocardiogram (ECG), and in most series a prior myocardial infarction may be noted in >80% of patients with chronic ischemic MR. When ECG changes are noted, inferior wall infarctions are more common than anterior or lateral infarcts. Most patients are in sinus rhythm; however, following atrial enlargement, p-wave abnormalities and atrial fibrillation may occur in the chronic setting. Conduction abnormalities are uncommon in these patients. In the acute setting, the chest x-ray may show evidence of pulmonary interstitial edema. With disease progression, enlargement of the cardiac silhouette (left atrial enlargement, ventricular dilation) is a common finding. Cardiac catheterization should be performed in all patients to determine the extent and severity of coronary artery disease. Left ventriculography is useful for assessing left ventricular function and segmental wall motion in selected patients, but has no role in assessing mitral valve dysfunction.

Two-dimensional echocardiography/Doppler is essential in determining the mechanism and the severity of MR and left ventricular wall motion abnormalities and function. Carpentier's functional classification should be used to classify the underlying mechanism of MR. During echocardiography the transgastric view best visualizes the different segments of the mitral valve. The severity of MR can be determined by semiquantitative measurements using jet geometry and area in multiple views. The severity of mitral regurgitation is graded on a scale from 0 to 4+ (1+, trace; 2+, mild; 3+, moderate; and 4+, severe MR). The direction of the jet is a good indicator of the mechanism of MR. With restricted leaflet motion (type IIIb) the direction of the jet is often toward the restricted leaflet, or central if associated annular dilation is present. In type II dysfunction (leaflet prolapse) the direction of the jet is opposite to the prolapsing leaflet. More recently, quantitative Doppler methods have been developed that allow quantitative grading of MR. This quantitative grading is based on the calculation of regurgitant volume (the difference between the mitral and aortic stroke volumes) and effective regurgitant orifice (ratio of regurgitant volume to regurgitant time velocity integral). Intraoperative transesophageal echocardiography (TEE) can be used to determine the mechanism of MR; however several studies have shown downgrading of the severity of MR in patients with type I or IIIb dysfunction. The mechanism underlying this phenomenon is almost certainly the unloading effect of general anesthesia, which results in arterial and venous dilation, decreasing afterload and preload, respectively.

Surgical Indications

Severe Ischemic Mitral Regurgitation

As mentioned, most patients presenting with severe ischemic MR have symptoms of congestive heart failure or worsening left ventricular function. In addition, they often have severe three-vessel coronary artery disease. Medical management of these patients is associated with poor clinical outcomes, and it is now well established that these patients should undergo a combined mitral valve procedure and myocardial revascularization, provided that the operative mortality is acceptable.

Mild to Moderate Ischemic Mitral Regurgitation

In this clinical scenario, often patients are referred for myocardial revascularization secondary to symptomatic coronary artery disease. The preoperative finding of mild to moderate type IIIb ischemic MR is often incidental, and the decision to intervene on the valve is controversial.

Recent studies have suggested that CABG alone does not completely correct ischemic MR. Our work concluded that CABG alone

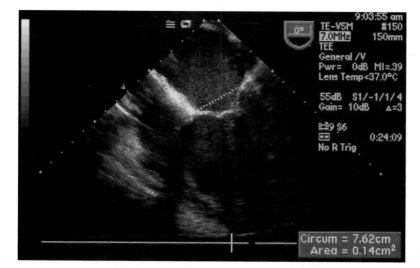

Figure 41-2. Transesophageal echocardiography image of type IIIb ischemic mitral regurgitation showing severe leaflet restriction below the annular plane (*white line*).

was not the optimal therapy for many patients with moderate ischemic MR.. One hundred thirty-six patients with moderate ischemic MR underwent CABG alone. Among the 68 patients who underwent early postoperative transthoracic echocardiography, 40% showed no improvement and were left with moderate or severe (3 to 4+) residual ischemic MR, and an additional 50% of patients had some improvement but were left with mild (2+) residual ischemic MR. Other reports suggests that CABG alone can decrease MR severity, especially in patients with mild ischemic MR and poor left ventricular function, but it has an inconsistent and relatively weak effect on moderate (3+) ischemic MR, leaving many patients with 2+ or greater residual MR.

Although no prospective, randomized studies have addressed the effect of a concomitant mitral valve procedure in patients with ischemic MR undergoing surgical coronary revascularization, many studies have documented a consistent reduction of MR grade early postoperatively, and some have suggested a potential survival benefit. We believe that patients with mild to moderate ischemic MR (2 to 3+) should undergo concomitant mitral valve repair at the same time as myocardial revascularization, unless preoperative risk factors suggest that the additional operative morbidity and mortality would be prohibitive (i.e., extensive mitral annular calcification, or strong indication for off-pump CABG in patients with heavily diseased aortas).

Surgical Management

Perioperative Considerations

Standard techniques of monitoring are used in patients undergoing a combined mitral valve repair and CABG. A Swan-Ganz catheter should be inserted in every patient, particularly in the presence of left ventricular (LV)/right ventricular dysfunction or pulmonary hypertension. Initially a TEE should be performed to determine the mechanism of MR, to assess LV function, and to determine the quality of repair and de-airing of the cardiac cavities at the completion of the procedure. As discussed, TEE should not be used to assess MR severity, except by provocative testing (volume loading, afterload enhancement). An epiaortic scan of the ascending aorta is recommended to rule out the presence of atherosclerotic lesions before aortic cannulation. An external defibrillator is placed in re-do operations for subsequent defibrillation. A double-lumen

endotracheal tube is inserted in right thoracotomy approaches.

Surgical Approaches and Cardiopulmonary Bypass

Median sternotomy is the surgical approach of choice in patients undergoing combined mitral valve repair and CABG, as well as in the reoperative setting. The population of patients referred for reoperative mitral surgery after a prior CABG increased in the last decade. The choice of cannulation sites and the indications for peripheral bypass before sternotomy are important determinants to avoiding any major complications during reoperative surgery. Femoral vessel exposure is recommended if severe mediastinal adhesions are suspected (recent reoperation, multiple previous sternotomies, mediastinitis, mediastinal radiation) and in patients with patent grafts. Femoral vessel cannulation with peripheral bypass at the time of sternotomy may be indicated in selected patients with patent left internal mary artery graft, severely dilated ascending aorta, and severe right ventricular dilation.

A right *anterolateral thoracotomy* may be used in selected patients referred for isolated ischemic MR with prior CABG and patent grafts, particularly internal thoracic arteries. The patient is rotated 30 degrees to the left side, and a 12-cm to 15-cm right anterolateral thoracotomy is performed through the fourth intercostal space. Because the right thoracotomy approach does not require extensive mediastinal dissection, it is also an interesting alternative if dense mediastinal adhesions are suspected (e.g., previous mediastinitis). Right thoracotomy is contraindicated in patients with previous right-sided chest surgery, severe chronic obstructive pulmonary disease (COPD), and moderate to severe aortic insufficiency. Direct cannulation of the ascending aorta or femoral or axillary arteries and percutaneous or direct femoral vein and superior vena cava cannulation are performed. Cardiopulmonary bypass is instituted using vacuum-assisted drainage.

Myocardial Protection

Mitral valve surgery is performed on cardiopulmonary bypass with intermittent antegrade or a combined antegrade and retrograde blood cardioplegic arrest. We favor a modified Buckberg approach with warm induction, cold maintenance, and warm reperfusion. Further myocardial protection can be obtained by moderate systemic hypothermia between 28°C to 30°C and local hypothermia with topical ice. In reoperative

mitral valve surgery, specifically through a right anterolateral thoracotomy, it is often difficult to cross-clamp the ascending aorta. Therefore, other types of myocardial management such as beating-heart or moderate to deep hypothermia and fibrillatory arrest should be considered as long as there is no more than trace to mild aortic regurgitation.

Exposure of the Mitral Valve

After completion of coronary bypass grafting, the careful exposition of the mitral valve is essential before undertaking valve analysis and any type of mitral valve surgery. Our preferred approach is the interatrial approach through *Sondergaard's groove*. The interatrial groove is incised and the two atria are dissected and divided up to the fossa ovalis. This dissection exposes the roof of the left atrium, which is incised close to the mitral valve (Fig. 41-3A, B). A trans-septal approach can be useful in selected patients with small left atrium or prior aortic valve replacement to achieve adequate exposure of the mitral valve.

Mitral Valve Repair

Mitral valve repair is the procedure of choice for correction of type IIIb ischemic mitral regurgitation. The main goal of valve repair is to restore a large surface of coaptation by aggressively reducing the septolateral dimension of the valve with a downsized remodeling (complete, rigid, or semirigid ring) annuloplasty.

Segmental Valve Analysis

The valvular apparatus is examined with a nerve hook to assess tissue pliability and identify leaflet restriction according to segmental valve analysis (Fig. 41-3C). The anterior paracommissural scallop of the posterior leaflet (P1) constitutes the reference point. Applying traction to the free edge of other valvular segments and comparing them to P1 determines the extent of leaflet restriction. Using two hooks, it is then possible to confirm leaflet restriction (type IIIb dysfunction) due to posterior papillary muscle displacement, most commonly affecting P2 and P3 segments. The mitral annulus is examined to assess the severity of *associated annular dilation*, which is common and may be asymmetric in type IIIb ischemic MR.

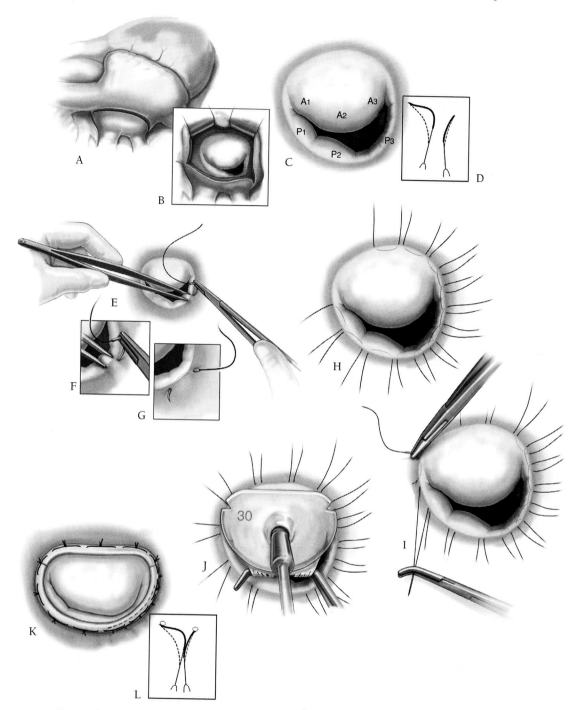

Figure 41-3. Surgical approach to ischemic mitral regurgitation. **(A)** Incision in Sondergaard's groove with inferior extension between the right inferior pulmonary vein and the inferior vena cava. **(B)** Exposure of the valve. **(C, D)** Typical findings with leaflet restriction predominantly in the P2–P3 region. **(E, F, G)** One places 2-0 braided annular sutures into the mitral annulus, taking advantage of the full curve of the needle, with the angle directed toward the ventricle to ensure passage through the annulus. **(H, I)** The sutures in the annulus at the position of the anterior commissure and trigone are placed last, taking advantage of previously placed sutures to expose this area. **(J)** Sizing the annulus with a Carpentier-Edwards sizer is based primarily on the surface area and height of the anterior leaflet. **(K)** After placement of a full remodeling Carpentier-McCarthy-Adams IMR Etlogix ring, surface of coaptation is restored (below the plane of the annulus). (Revised From A Carpentier, DH Adams, F Filsoufi (in press). Carpentier's Reconstructive Valve Surgery. Philadelphia: WB Saunders)

Undersized Remodeling Ring Annuloplasty for Type IIIb Ischemic Mitral Regurgitation

Remodeling annuloplasty using an undersized ring is the technique of choice in type IIIb dysfunction. Most commonly, 2-0 braided sutures are used to implant an annuloplasty ring. In general, sutures in the septal and lateral portions of the annulus should be placed using a backhand orientation, and sutures in the anterior and medial portions of the annulus are placed with a forehand orientation (Fig. 41-3E). The full curve of the needle should be used to encourage deep, wide placement of individual sutures along the annulus (Fig. 41-3F,G). Because of the potential increased tension in the setting of type IIIb dysfunction with associated annular dilation, it is preferable to place the sutures very close together along the annulus, and suture crossover may be warranted (Fig. 41-3H). The anterior commissure is usually the most difficult area to expose and is usually approached last after placement of sutures along the septal, medial, and lateral portions of the annulus to place tension on prior sutures to expose this area of the annulus (Fig. 41-3I). Once sutures are placed around the annulus, standard ring sizers are used to select an appropriate ring size (Fig. 41-3J). Placing gentle traction on marginal chords in the A-2 portion of the anterior leaflet with a hook allows the height and surface area of the anterior leaflet to be measured. An additional measurement to consider is the intercommissural distance. Because leaflet restriction in ischemic MR results in less leaflet tissue available for coaptation, it is necessary to downsize a *complete remodeling ring* such as the Carpentier Edwards Physioring by one or two sizes or to use a true-sized Carpentier-McCarthy-Adams IMR Etlogix ring (see later discussion) to ensure an adequate surface of coaptation following annuloplasty (Fig. 41-3K). Systolic anterior motion will not occur despite aggressive downsizing, because the restricted posterior leaflet cannot displace the anterior leaflet into the outflow tract. After a ring is selected (typical size 24 mm to 28 mm) the interrupted annular sutures are passed through it, respecting the associated geometry of the annulus. The individual sutures are then tied, securing the ring to the annulus (Fig. 41-3K). Once the downsized remodeling annuloplasty is completed, a saline test is used to confirm the line of coaptation along the margin of the leaflets (Fig. 41-3L). Nearly the entire orifice is occupied by the anterior leaflet, allowing the entire restricted posterior leaflet to contribute to coaptation.

De-airing Process

Careful de-airing at the end of the procedure is essential. Carbon dioxide insufflation is used in all patients to reduce intracardiac air. A small vent should be left across the mitral valve to facilitate de-airing after closure of the left atrium. When most of the air is expelled from the heart, the aortic cross-clamp is removed safely. Additional de-airing is performed during the rewarming period. The aortic vent is maintained on suction until the patient is totally weaned from CPB and complete air removal is confirmed by TEE.

Residual Mitral Regurgitation

As mentioned, we strongly recommend the use of remodeling annuloplasty (complete, rigid, or semirigid ring) in patients with ischemic MR. The observation of residual or recurrent MR in patients with ischemic MR after the use of flexible annuloplasty systems or suture annuloplasty techniques as well as new anatomic autopsy studies provide support for our position.

In one study, midterm results on 100 patients undergoing combined CABG/mitral annuloplasty using a Duran flexible ring in patients with ischemic MR included a 29% rate of >grade 2 recurrent ischemic MR at a mean follow-up of 36 months. More recently, the Cleveland Clinic experience with undersized Cosgrove-Edwards flexible posterior annuloplasty bands was reported to be a 30% incidence of recurrent ischemic MR 3 to 4+ at 18 months. In contrast, other authors recently reported on the efficacy of a *downsized remodeling annuloplasty*, in 51 patients with 3 to 4+ ischemic MR absent or trivial recurrent MR in all patients at 18-month follow-up. Finally, a human autopsy study showed a significant increase in the *intertrigonal distance* in mitral valves from patients with MR in ischemic cardiomyopathy versus controls, which reinforces the importance of using a complete remodeling annuloplasty ring in ischemic MR.

A recent clinical imaging study has provided precise anatomic and morphologic descriptions of type IIIb ischemic MR. In this study, three-dimensional echocardiography was viewed to further refine analysis of leaflet restriction (type IIIb) in ischemic versus dilated cardiomyopathy. The authors observed a significant difference in mitral valve deformation between the two patient groups. The pattern of mitral valve deformation from the posteromedial to the anterolateral commissure was asymmetric in the ischemic group, whereas it was symmetric in patients with dilated cardiomyopathy. These differences in mitral valve geometry emphasize the fact that in patients with ischemic cardiomyopathy, the P2 and P3 segments are the most restricted, causing an asymmetric mitral orifice and suggesting that downsizing with a symmetric ring may not be the optimal approach to mitral valve repair in ischemic MR.

New Developments: Carpentier-McCarthy-Adams IMR Etlogix Ring

In hope of achieving a better understanding of the pathophysiologic events in ischemic MR and to potentially reduce the incidence of residual MR, a new remodeling annuloplasty, the Carpentier-McCarthy-Adams IMR Etlogix ring, was recently developed by Edwards Lifesciences (Irvine, CA). This new prosthetic ring combines the principles of undersizing with the specific asymmetric deformation observed in type IIIb ischemic MR (Fig. 41-4C). Compared to a symmetric Carpentier Edwards Physioring (Fig. 41-4D), this new design leads to increased leaflet coaptation due to the reduced anteroposterior (AP) dimension (Fig. 41-4C, D2 and D3 dimensions) in patients with ischemic MR. The new ring downsizes the D3 dimension two sizes and the D2 dimension by one size when compared to the Physioring. This makes it possible to select a true-sized IMR Etlogix ring based on the anterior leaflet surface area measured with a standard Carpentier-Edwards sizer while achieving precise remodeling with optimal coaptation in the P2–P3 region (Fig. 41-4D, E). Furthermore, this remodeling ring contains a titanium core, which allows complete fixation of the septolateral dimension during the entire cardiac cycle.

We first implanted the IMR Etlogix ring in December 2003. Fifteen patients (14 male/1female, mean age of 66 years) presented with >3+ ischemic MR. The mean ejection fraction was 31%, and all patients were in New York Heart Association (NYHA) classes III and IV. They underwent a successful mitral valve repair with the IMR Etlogix ring (mean size 28 mm), and concomitant procedures included CABG, left-atrial maze, tricuspid valve repair, and patent foramen ovale closure. Expected operative mortality calculated by Euroscore for this cohort was 19% (range 4–47), and the plication, and septolateral "cinching" have been shown to have beneficial effects in animal models.

Results

Operative Mortality

Concomitant mitral valve surgery/CABG has historically carried a much higher mortality rate than isolated CABG or isolated mitral valve surgery. Several authors have demonstrated that early and late outcomes of combined mitral valve and coronary artery bypass surgery depend strongly on the underlying etiology, to the extent that it can be determined in retrospective analyses, with significantly worse outcome in ischemic disease. Although the reported operative mortality for mitral valve replacement at the time of CABG has remained relatively high, the outcomes for mitral valve repair appear to be improving over time; most recent series report operative mortalities well under 10%. For 2002, the Society of Thoracic Surgeons database reported an 8% operative mortality for mitral valve repair/CABG (down from 12% in 1993) and 11.5% mortality for mitral valve replacement/CABG (down from 17% in 1993). We reviewed early outcomes following CABG and mitral annuloplasty for moderate (3+) ischemic MR and found that observed operative mortality decreased from 14% to 3.7% during the 1990s. The latter was not significantly different from the 2.9% mortality reported previously in an unmatched but contemporaneous group of patients undergoing CABG alone for moderate ischemic MR.

Late Outcomes

Multiple reports over the last 20 years suggest that late survival in patients with ischemic MR undergoing mitral valve surgery is suboptimal and significantly worse than in those with degenerative or rheumatic mitral valve disease. Medium-term (3- to 5-year) survival in these studies ranged from 50% to 80% depending on the risk profile. Recent studies have sought to directly compare outcomes of CABG alone or CABG/mitral valve surgery in patients with ischemic MR.

In one study, 99 patients with 2 to 3+ ischemic MR and ejection fractions less than 30% split evenly between CABG alone and CABG/mitral valve surgery (nearly all repairs). Although the groups were comparable with regard to preoperative characteristics, concomitant mitral valve surgery led to improved ejection fraction, decreased

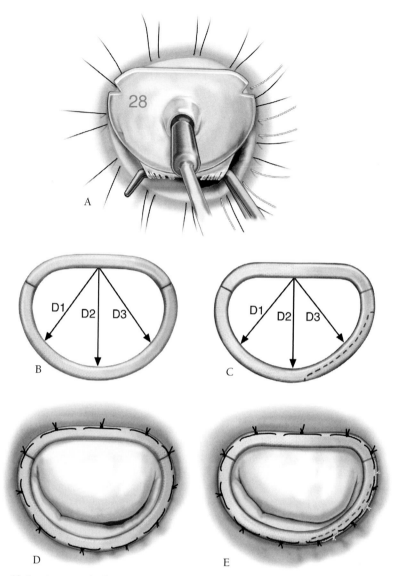

Figure 41-4. Asymmetric downsizing with the Carpentier-McCarthy-Adams IMR Etlogix annuloplasty ring. **(A)** True sizing of the annulus based on the surface area and height of the anterior leaflet. Difference in dimensions of **(B)** a true-sized symmetric remodeling ring (Carpentier-Edwards Physioring) and **(C)** the IMR Etlogix ring. Here D1 is similar, but D2 is equivalent to a one-size-smaller Physioring, and D3 is equivalent to a two-size-smaller Physioring. **(D, E)** Asymmetric downsized remodeling in IIIb dysfunction enhances coaptation in the area of P2–P3 leaflet restriction. (Revised From A Carpentier, DH Adams, F Filsoufi (in press). Carpentier's Reconstructive Valve Surgery. Philadelphia: WB Saunders)

observed operative mortality was 0%. Predischarge transthoracic echocardiography in all patients showed a significant reduction in mean MR grade (from 3.5 to 0.6; $p > .05$), although longer follow-up will be required to determine whether this new design prevents recurrent ischemic MR.

Although we suspect that routine use of a remodeling annuloplasty and more aggressive and strategic downsizing will likely decrease the incidence of residual MR after CABG/annuloplasty, it is possible that a small group of patients may exist in whom a remodeling annuloplasty alone is insuf-

ficient to correct ischemic MR. Adjunctive techniques may play a role here, but clinical experience is limited. Poor coaptation of individual scallops of the posterior leaflet can occur with leaflet restriction, and clefts (P1P2 or P2P3) should be closed if this is suspected or a corresponding jet is noted on saline testing. Posterior leaflet extension, especially over the P3 scallop, has been used in patients with severe posterior leaflet restriction. Ischemic MR has been treated with papillary muscle repositioning using a pledgeted suture attached to the annulus. Resection of secondary chordae, ventricular left ventricular dimensions, and improved 3-year survival. Another study reviewed 60 patients with moderate ischemic MR undergoing CABG alone ($n = 30$) and CABG/annuloplasty ($n = 30$) from 1998 to 2001. All patients underwent follow-up echocardiography at 12 and 36 months postoperatively. Before surgery, the groups were substantially homogenous. At follow-up the CABG/annuloplasty patients had a lower NYHA classification, fewer signs and symptoms of congestive heart failure, and better echocardiographic parameters (smaller LV volume, ejection fraction, and pulmonary artery pressures). In this series, the preoperative annular size was seen to be a risk factor for postoperative heart failure events. The authors concluded that the combined approach for patients with moderate MR leads to a better clinical status and better hemodynamic profile.

Overall, these data suggest that concomitant mitral valve surgery might improve late outcomes in patients with ischemic MR especially if it can be performed with little additional operative risk and a low incidence of residual MR.

Type II Ischemic Mitral Regurgitation

As mentioned, a minority of patients may present with type II ischemic MR. In this functional type of MR, the motion of one or two leaflets is excessive and the free edge of the leaflet over-rides the plane of the orifice during systole. Leaflet prolapse results from partial or complete rupture of one papillary muscle, papillary muscle elongation, or, more rarely, chordal rupture.

Pathophysiology

Papillary muscle rupture is an increasingly rare mechanical complication of myocardial infarction, which carries an excessive mortality without early diagnosis and appropriate expeditious medical and surgical management. Papillary muscle rupture can occur during the acute phase of myocardial infarction; however, most patients present within 2 to 7 days after myocardial infarction. The rupture involves most often the posteromedial papillary muscle (75% vs. 25% for anterolateral papillary muscle). The vulnerability of the posteromedial papillary muscle is explained by its singular vascular blood supply (either the right coronary artery or the circumflex artery in right- or left-dominant systems, respectively). In contrast, the anterolateral

papillary muscle is supplied by two major coronary arteries including the left anterior descending and the circumflex arteries. Complete papillary muscle rupture will result in bileaflet prolapse with severe mitral regurgitation. Partial rupture of one papillary muscle involving one or more heads remains the most common lesion in patients with type II ischemic MR. Myocardial infarction often involves a limited area of the myocardium, which may explain the relatively well preserved left ventricular function in most patients. Chronic *papillary muscle elongation* with leaflet prolapse due to remote myocardial infarction is also rare, and results from fibrotic transformation of a papillary muscle after myocardial infarction.

Clinical Presentation and Diagnosis

Patients with papillary muscle rupture often present with sudden development of congestive heart failure and cardiogenic shock. This rapid deterioration of clinical status suggests the diagnosis of a mechanical complication of myocardial infarction. It is important to note that the sudden appearance of a systolic murmur and hemodynamic compromise may result from acute severe ischemic MR secondary to papillary muscle rupture as well as from ventricular septal rupture.

Clinically, it is very difficult to distinguish between these two entities despite differences in the characteristics of murmurs (the systolic murmur associated with ventricular septal rupture is loud, prominent at the left sternal border, and associated with a thrill, whereas the systolic murmur of ischemic mitral regurgitation due to papillary muscle rupture is softer, intense at the apex, and without thrill). Extensive myocardial infarction with cardiogenic shock associated with varying degrees of ischemic mitral regurgitation without papillary muscle rupture (acute type IIIb) is also part of the differential diagnosis. Preoperative examinations including two-dimensional transthoracic echocardiography, TEE, and cardiac catheterization are crucial to making the accurate diagnosis of ischemic MR due to papillary muscle rupture and to evaluating left ventricular function and the severity of coronary artery disease.

Medical and Surgical Treatment

The principal goal of preoperative medical management is hemodynamic stabilization

(preservation of cardiac output and arterial pressure to maintain peripheral organ perfusion). This is best achieved with the use of inotropic agents and prompt insertion of an intra-aortic balloon pump. However, this stabilization phase should not delay surgical intervention on these critically ill patients. Based on the preoperative investigations, the surgical procedure should combine the correction of mitral regurgitation and myocardial revascularization.

Chordal-sparing mitral valve replacement is the procedure of choice in most patients. This technique preserves postoperative left ventricular function, contributing to improved long-term survival of these patients.

Mitral valve repair using classic Carpentier's techniques can be applied to patients with papillary muscle elongation. Papillary muscle shortening is best performed by resecting the appropriate length of papillary muscle and suturing the fibrous cuff supporting the chords to the papillary muscle. Four or five circumferential simple sutures without pledgets should be used for this fixation. If the elongation involves only one papillary muscle head resulting in the prolapse of one segment of the valve (e.g., P3-segment prolapse), more conventional techniques of repair such as leaflet resection combined with sliding plasty or annular plication can be performed safely. Papillary tip transposition, sewing the fibrous tip of the elongated muscle to a papillary tip at the normal height, can also be considered.

Results for Type II Ischemic Mitral Regurgitation

Operative mortality has traditionally been high. In a consecutive series of 21 patients who underwent mitral valve surgery (replacement, $n = 19$; repair, $n = 2$) and concomitant coronary artery bypass grafting (52% were urgent/emergent), operative mortality was 19%. The principal postoperative complications were stroke (6%) and renal failure requiring hemodialysis (18%). In this series actuarial survival at 1, 5, and 10 years was 81%, 68%, and 56%, respectively. The survival rates seen in this series compare well to that in a similar study, which demonstrated a survival rate at 55% after 7 years. Even though early mortality is high in the acute setting, aggressive surgical treatment does improve long-term outcome because this allows the correction of an acute hemodynamic compromise.

Summary

Ischemic MR is a progressive and dynamic disease with important clinical implications for patients with coronary artery disease in both the acute and chronic setting after myocardial infarction. Our knowledge of the pathophysiology of ischemic MR has grown substantially over the last few years, and today the mechanism(s) of mitral valve dysfunction secondary to ischemia as well as surgical treatment strategies are well defined. Mitral valve repair by a downsized remodeling annuloplasty should be performed in patients with moderate ischemic MR at the time of myocardial revascularization, with the expectation of low residual and recurrent rates of MR in the postoperative setting. Ongoing studies regarding adjunctive surgical procedures designed to optimize ventricular geometry will likely represent the next advance in the surgical management of ischemic MR.

SUGGESTED READING

Adams DH, Filsoufi F, Aklog L. Surgical treatment of the ischemic mitral valve. J Heart Valve Dis 2002;11(Suppl 1):S21.

Aklog L, Filsoufi F, Flores KQ, et al. Does coronary artery bypass grafting alone correct moderate ischemic mitral regurgitation? Circulation 2001;104(12 Suppl 1):I68.

Bax JJ, Braun J, Somer ST, et al. Restrictive annuloplasty and coronary revascularization in ischemic mitral regurgitation results in reverse left ventricular remodeling. Circulation, 2004;110(11 Suppl 1):II103.

Gillinov AM, Wierup PN, Blackstone EH, et al. Is repair preferable to replacement for ischemic mitral regurgitation? J Thorac Cardiovasc Surg 2001;122(6):1125.

Grigioni F, Enriquez-Sarano M, Zehr KJ, et al. Ischemic mitral regurgitation: Long-term outcome and prognostic implications with quantitative Doppler assessment. Circulation 2001;103(13):1759.

Hueb AC, Jatene FB, Moreira LF, et al. Ventricular remodeling and mitral valve modifications in dilated cardiomyopathy: New insights from anatomic study. J Thorac Cardiovasc Surg 2002;124(6):1216.

Kwan J, Shiota T, Agler DA, et al. Geometric differences of the mitral apparatus between ischemic and dilated cardiomyopathy with significant mitral regurgitation: Real-time three-dimensional echocardiography study. Circulation 2003;107(8):1135.

Reece TB, Tribble CG, Ellman PI, et al. Mitral repair is superior to replacement when associated with coronary artery disease. Ann Surg 2004;239(5):671;discussion, 675.

Tibayan FA, Rodriguez F, Zasio MK, et al. Geometric distortions of the mitral valvular-ventricular complex in chronic ischemic mitral regurgitation. Circulation 2003;108 (Suppl 1):II116.

EDITOR'S COMMENTS

The authors have done a truly excellent job in describing surgery for ischemic mitral valve disease. I agree completely with their concept of a complete ring. I also agree that coronary bypass alone is probably not enough for patients who have an anatomic as opposed to an ischemic lesion. Most ischemic mitral regurgitation is due to an anatomic lesion caused by chronic ischemic changes. There are a couple of minor differences in our views. The authors appropriately differentiate between ischemic mitral regurgitation and patients who have other mitral valve abnormalities and associated coronary disease. However, I am not certain that the differentiation is that clear. I have seen many individuals who clearly had a myxomatous valve as well as an anatomic lesion appropriate to ischemic disease as well. These are often very complex valves to repair, because the mechanisms are so different and surgical treatment is not as predictable.

A second difference is the concept of the type II mechanism, in which, as the authors clearly delineate, the individual's papillary muscle elongates. Certainly, the ruptured papillary muscle is a well-known entity, and the authors cover that well. However, I cannot say for certain that I have ever truly seen an elongated papillary muscle from ischemic disease. I wonder whether in those situations if, in fact, another pre-existing mechanism is in place. Overall this is an excellent chapter on this complex disease.

I.L.K.

42

Acquired Valvular Heart Disease: Mitral Valve Replacement

Kwok L. Yun and D. Craig Miller

Anatomic Considerations

The mitral valve and the subvalvular apparatus are composed of the annulus, valve leaflets, chordae tendineae, papillary muscles, and left ventricular wall. Abnormalities in any one of these structural components can lead to valvular dysfunction. The mitral valve has two main leaflets: the posterior and the anterior. The posterior leaflet consists usually of three discrete scallops (anterolateral, middle, and posteromedial, termed P_1, P_2, and P_3 by Carpentier), but the fetal subcommissures separating them can be variably complete. One or two commissural scallops exist near each commissure. The normal mitral orifice area is 4 cm^2 to 6 cm^2. The mitral annulus is a dynamic structure that varies in size and shape throughout the cardiac cycle, including substantial size reduction during late diastole (presystolic "sphincteric" action) due to "atriogenic" properties. Part of the anterior mitral annulus is in continuity with the aortic annulus, demarcated by the left and right fibrous trigones (the right trigone is also known as the central fibrous body of the heart). The anterior annulus is relatively fibrous and fixed; however, contrary to traditional thinking that the anterior annulus does not undergo pathologic annular dilation, it is now known (as discussed, e.g., by Heub et al., McCarthy, and Tibayan et al.) that it does dilate in patients with idiopathic dilated or ischemic cardiomyopathy, leading to functional mitral regurgitation (FMR) or ischemic mitral regurgitation (IMR). The atrioventricular node and bundle of His are

adjacent to the right fibrous trigone and can be injured during mitral valve operations. Each leaflet receives chordae tendineae from both the anterolateral and the posteromedial papillary muscles. The majority of the first-order (or primary or marginal) chordae tendineae insert near the free margin of the leaflets; these first-order chordae prevent leaflet prolapse and maintain competency of the valve. The second-order chordae (or "strut" chords) insert in the middle of the leaflets near the junction between the smooth and rough zones and are responsible for "valvular-ventricular interaction," which optimizes left ventricular (LV) systolic function. The third-order (or "basal") chordae insert in the base of the leaflets, predominately on the posterior leaflet.

After the first successful implantation of a caged-ball valve prosthesis by Starr in 1961, conventional mitral valve replacement (MVR) with complete excision of the native valve leaflets and subvalvular apparatus became the accepted orthodox surgical MVR technique. Lillehei and coworkers, however, introduced a technique of MVR in 1964 in which the mitral leaflets and chordae tendineae were preserved using Starr-Edwards ball valves. In a small series of 14 patients, the operative mortality rate was lower if the chordae were spared compared to the historical rate in those pioneering days of open-heart surgery. Because of the greater complexity and time associated with chordal-sparing methods and concerns that the retained subvalvular apparatus might interfere with the movement of the prosthetic components of mechanical valves, conventional MVR with complete excision of the mitral subvalvular apparatus re-

mained the standard MVR technique for another two decades. Thromboembolism and anticoagulant-related hemorrhagic complications in patients with mechanical prostheses and the limited long-term durability of bioprosthetic valves in the mitral position spawned the development of reliable mitral valve repair techniques, which was associated with improved clinical outcomes. This experience suggested that LV systolic function might be optimized if the mitral subvalvular apparatus was preserved during MVR. John W. Kirklin's 1972 dictum that elimination of systolic unloading into the low-impedance left atrium in patients with mitral regurgitation after MVR always increases LV afterload, thereby increasing LV systolic wall stress and decreasing LV ejection performance, was subsequently proven not to be true if the chordae tendineae were preserved. Conversely, chordal excision during MVR is associated with increased postoperative LV end-systolic volume and wall stress, along with a decline in ejection fraction. Not all pathologic conditions of the mitral valve are amenable to repair, however, including extensive leaflet involvement from rheumatic disease, severe leaflet destruction secondary to infective endocarditis, extreme anterior leaflet prolapse, and when the leaflet tissue is irreversibly damaged. As a result, numerous different chordal-sparing MVR techniques have been devised and investigated in clinical and experimental studies; today, total (anterior and posterior leaflet) chordal-sparing MVR is the technique of choice for patients with mitral regurgitation when the durability of valve repair is judged not to be satisfactory or when valve repair is not feasible.

Diagnostic Considerations

The electrocardiogram is not generally useful, but can detect atrial fibrillation or signs of ischemic heart disease. P-Wave abnormalities can be indicative of left atrial enlargement; right ventricular hypertrophy may also be evident in advanced mitral valve disease in patients with secondary pulmonary hypertension. In patients with left atrial enlargement, a chest x-ray can show a "double density" on the right side of the cardiac silhouette, along with pulmonary congestion, redistribution of the pulmonary vasculature, and basal interstitial edema with lymphatic engorgement (Kerley B lines) in advanced cases of chronic mitral regurgitation.

Transthoracic echocardiography (M-mode, two-dimensional [2D], and color Doppler flow mapping) is the most important diagnostic technique for evaluating mitral valve pathology and its consequences. M-Mode and 2D echocardiography measure left atrial and ventricular dimensions accurately; furthermore, left atrial thrombus can be detected and left ventricular systolic wall motion assessed. In cases of FMR due to dilated cardiomyopathy or ischemic heart disease (IMR), apical leaflet tenting or tethering during systole is evident (Carpentier type IIIb restricted systolic leaflet motion), which prevents adequate leaflet coaptation. Frequently, this apical tethering is associated with pronounced annular dilation, which results in incomplete mitral leaflet coaptation (IMLC) and Carpentier type I leaflet motion. The extent of involvement by the disease process and the degree of mitral regurgitation and/or stenosis can be readily determined. Mitral leaflet thickening and abnormal motion are assessed using M-mode and 2D echocardiography to confirm prolapse of the leaflets or ruptured chordae. Doppler velocity measurements are used to estimate transvalvular gradient, mitral valve area, and right ventricular systolic pressure. For those with mitral insufficiency, color Doppler determines the severity of regurgitation and the mechanism of mitral regurgitation, as assessed by the shape, timing, origin, magnitude, and direction of the color regurgitant jet(s). Color M-mode echocardiography is the preferred method for determining the timing of the leak during systole. The combination of echocardiographic methods can identify the structural abnormality responsible for the mitral regurgitation. In general, the regurgitant jet is directed away from the involved leaflet. Rarely, a transesophageal echocardiogram (TEE) is also necessary to delineate the complete pathologic anatomy of the mitral valve when the transthoracic images are not satisfactory.

Cardiac catheterization is very seldom necessary today to assess the reversibility of elevated pulmonary artery pressures using vasodilator drug or inhaled nitric oxide interventions and measuring cardiac output. In patients with mitral regurgitation, a prominent V-wave is seen in the pulmonary capillary wedge pressure tracing. In addition, regurgitant fraction can be calculated from the angiographic stroke volume and thermodilution cardiac output, but the best way to do this is cardiac magnetic resonance imaging. Finally, preoperative coronary angiography is performed in patients older than 50 years of age, those with symptoms of ischemic heart disease, and individuals with multiple arteriosclerosis risk factors. Cardiac catheterization in patients with mitral regurgitation due to mitral valve prolapse has essentially been replaced by echocardiography because they tend to be young patients, but in exceptional circumstances or in the elderly, visualization of the coronary artery anatomy is required.

Indications for Operation

Mitral Stenosis

Any patient with symptomatic mitral stenosis (with or without pulmonary hypertension, right heart failure, or hemoptysis) is considered an operative candidate unless he or she is a suitable candidate for percutaneous balloon valvotomy. It is generally agreed that operation is indicated for individuals in New York Heart Association (NYHA) functional class III or IV and those with critical mitral stenosis by echocardiographic criteria (mitral valve orifice <1.0 cm^2) and severe pulmonary hypertension (>60 mm Hg), regardless of symptoms. Although the onset of atrial fibrillation usually exacerbates symptoms, it is only a relative indication for operation; conversely, the development of systemic embolization should prompt early surgical consideration. Prophylactic operation may also be necessary for women with asymptomatic, severe mitral stenosis who plan to become pregnant, due to the increased hemodynamic burden during the third trimester.

Mitral Regurgitation

Acute mitral insufficiency accompanied by hemodynamic compromise that cannot be easily managed medically mandates urgent mitral valve repair or replacement. On the other hand, most patients stabilize with medical therapy. Patients with advanced class III or IV congestive heart failure symptoms as a result of chronic mitral regurgitation generally have depressed left ventricular systolic function; operation is indicated, and probably should have been offered much earlier. In contrast, the optimal timing for surgical treatment of patients with asymptomatic or minimally symptomatic chronic mitral regurgitation is debatable. Determination of left ventricular dimensions and measurement of right ventricular systolic pressure during exercise are the most useful objective approaches in terms of prognosis and determining therapy. For those with no or minimal symptoms, early operation is warranted if there is severe mitral regurgitation, the valve looks repairable, or there is evidence of progressive left ventricular dilation or any degree of systolic left ventricular dysfunction. Echocardiographic indicators include ejection fraction <60%, end-systolic diameter >40 mm. The evidence also favors operation for new onset of atrial fibrillation or pulmonary hypertension (>50 mm Hg at rest or >60 mm Hg with exercise). If the echocardiographic findings indicate that a high likelihood of valve repair does not exist and MVR is probably necessary, asymptomatic or minimally symptomatic patients should be treated medically and followed with serial echocardiograms.

Perioperative Management

Mitral Stenosis

Congestive heart failure symptoms due to mitral stenosis are controlled with sodium restriction, diuresis, and nitrates. Manifestations of pulmonary hypertension may require more aggressive diuresis. Patients with atrial fibrillation are treated by slowing the ventricular rate and prophylactic low-intensity anticoagulation with warfarin, unless contraindicated. Addition of beta-blockers or calcium-channel antagonists may be necessary for management of tachycardia during stress or physical activity. Because this is a flow-limiting lesion, either commissurotomy or MVR is the treatment of choice, unless the mitral stenosis is due to "soft" rheumatic changes without extensive subvalvular pathology and is amenable to percutaneous balloon valvuloplasty.

Mitral Regurgitation

Patients with severe, acute mitral regurgitation due to papillary muscle or chordal rupture as a result of myocardial ischemia/infarction or endocarditis frequently present in profound low–cardiac-output states and pulmonary edema. Attempts should be made to stabilize the patient's hemodynamics with inotropic agents and arteriolar vasodilators before operation. Intraaortic balloon counterpulsation can also be helpful. Congestive heart failure symptoms can usually be managed adequately with the use of diuretics and oral vasodilators in patients with chronic mitral regurgitation. Lowering peripheral vascular impedance decreases the regurgitant volume into the left atrium and increases forward cardiac output. As with patients with mitral stenosis, the ventricular rate in patients in atrial fibrillation is slowed medically.

Operative Technique

An essential step during mitral valve procedures is adequate exposure of the valve; surprisingly, limited surgical residency training and practice experience make this difficult for surgeons who do not perform a large number of mitral valve procedures each year. The final determination of whether mitral valve repair is technically feasible or whether valve replacement is necessary can only be made after comprehensive assessment of all of the components of the valve and the subvalvular apparatus. The heart is generally approached via a median sternotomy or lower ministernotomy. In selected patients with multiple previous cardiac procedures, with or without patent coronary artery bypass grafts or previous chest radiotherapy for neoplasms, a right anterolateral thoracotomy incision through the fourth intercostal space can provide adequate visualization of the mitral valve; however, potential disadvantages include (1) limited access to the ascending aorta for cannulation and cross-clamping, (2) left ventricular distention and a bloody field if aortic regurgitation is present, and (3) limitations in de-airing. In patients with patent single or bilateral mammary arterial or multiple vein grafts, a simple technique is to ignore the grafts and not cross-clamp the

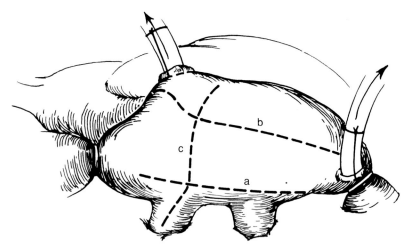

Figure 42-1.   Three options for exposing the mitral valve, which is of key importance. It can be exposed via **(a)** a standard vertical left atriotomy in Sondergaard's groove anterior to the right pulmonary veins; **(b)** the extended vertical trans-septal biatriotomy approach, which is popular when using a small incision; or **(c)** the Khonsari oblique biatriotomy technique. See Figs. 42-2 to 42-4 for further details.

aorta; instead, moderate (22°C to 24°C) systemic hypothermia keeping the perfusion pressure high ("hypothermic fibrillatory arrest") is used if the aortic valve is fairly competent.

After sternotomy, the right side of the pericardium is firmly suspended from the skin to rotate the right side of the heart anteriorly; no pericardial retraction sutures are used on the left side, allowing the left heart to rotate posteriorly. The heart is cannulated for cardiopulmonary bypass (CPB). Usually, bicaval cannulation and caval tourniquets are used (total CPB) to eliminate systemic venous return, which rewarms the heart during aortic cross-clamping. Systemic cooling to 28°C to 30°C is initiated on CPB. The aorta is then cross-clamped and the heart arrested with cold blood cardioplegia delivered retrograde via the coronary sinus. Myocardial protection is provided by intermittent retrograde cold blood cardioplegic solution and topical cooling employing a Daily myocardial cooling jacket (Daily Medical Products, San Diego, CA). For patients with severe pulmonary hypertension, antegrade-grade cold blood cardioplegia can enhance right ventricular myocardial protection. The initial dose of cold cardioplegic solution required to lower the myocardial temperature to 10°C is usually about 1,000 mL. Supplemental doses of retrograde cold blood cardioplegic solution are given intermittently every 20 to 30 minutes, even though the myocardial temperature usually remains <10°C by virtue of the Daily cooling jacket.

Surgical exposure of the mitral valve is achieved by one of three incisions (Fig.

42-1). The most commonly used is a vertical left atriotomy incision in Sondergaard's groove anterior to the right pulmonary veins (Fig. 42-2). The incision can easily be extended cephalad and caudad beneath the superior and inferior venae cavae, respectively, if needed, after the pericardial reflections are taken down. With cephalad extension, care is taken not to injure the sinus node artery, which courses across the top of the interatrial septum. Inferiorly, the incision is extended underneath the inferior vena cava aiming toward the left inferior pulmonary vein. In difficult re-do operations or patients with a small left atrium, adequate exposure of the mitral subvalvular apparatus can be problematic. In these cases, visualization of the mitral valve structures can be provided by either an extended vertical trans-septal biatriotomy (Fig. 42-3) or an oblique biatriotomy approach (Fig. 42-4). With the extended trans-septal technique, a vertical right atriotomy is directed superiorly toward the right atrial appendage to meet the interatrial septum. The fossa ovalis is then opened longitudinally and carried cephalad to connect to the right atriotomy incision. The incision is then extended for 2 cm to 3 cm onto the dome of the left atrium. The oblique biatriotomy method developed by Khonsari involves opening the right superior pulmonary vein approximately 1 cm from the interatrial groove. The incision is then extended obliquely and inferiorly across the interatrial groove and the right atrial free wall to expose the atrial septum and fossa ovalis. The septum is then opened down to the anterior limbus of the fossa ovalis in the same direction. One of these latter two

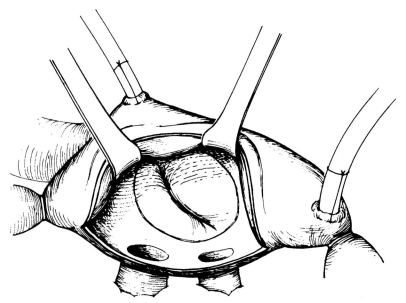

Figure 42-2. Conventional vertical left atriotomy incision is made anterior to the right pulmonary veins in Sondergaard's groove and extended cephalad and caudad beneath the venae cavae.

approaches is preferred if concomitant tricuspid annuloplasty is necessary. After the atriotomy is made, a sump vent is usually inserted into the left atrium and positioned dependently near the left superior pulmonary vein. Once it is determined that mitral valve reconstruction is not possible or is judged not to be the most prudent course of action, MVR is performed using one the following techniques.

Conventional Mitral Valve Replacement

Conventional MVR is preceded by complete removal of the mitral leaflets and the subvalvular apparatus (Fig. 42-5). This is reserved only for patients with advanced rheumatic disease with excessive scarring and calcification. The leaflets are excised, leaving 1 mm to 2 mm of leaflet tissue along the annular circumference. The chordae tendineae are divided near the tips of the papillary muscles. Irrespective of the type of procedure, the size of the mitral annulus is measured as the valve size that fits easily into the left ventricle; care not to oversize the valve is very important. The annulus is then ringed with a series of 2-0 SH or SH-1 braided polyester horizontal mattress sutures with a width of approximately 8 mm to10 mm. Pledget reinforcement of the sutures is not routine, but is used when friable or destroyed annular tissue is encountered in association with severe endocarditis, with re-do MVR, and in patients with the Marfan syndrome. It is important that the sutures not be placed too deeply into the annulus to avoid injury to the circumflex coronary artery, the aortic valve leaflets, or the conduction system. The sutures are placed in an everting fashion (atrium to ventricle) for mechanical valve prostheses, but usually from the ventricular to the atrial aspect for bioprosthetic valve substitutes. Next, the sutures are passed through the sewing ring of the prosthesis, which is then lowered into place. If a bioprosthesis is used, it is oriented such that the largest leaflet is situated facing the left ventricular outflow tract, thereby avoiding ejection flow obstruction from one of the struts. Bileaflet mechanical valve prostheses are inserted in the antianatomic position with the pivot guards located towards the 12:00 and 6:00 positions. After the bioprosthesis is seated on the mitral annulus, the leaflets near the valve struts are inspected with a small dental mirror to ensure that they have not been entrapped by looped valve sutures. This step is crucial for the newer pericardial bioprosthesis, which has low struts that are angled inward. The sutures are then tied and cut; unrestricted motion of the bioprosthetic or mechanical valve leaflets is then reconfirmed.

Chordal-Sparing Mitral Valve Replacement

When only the posterior leaflet is preserved (note that this technique is not as effective as preservation of both leaflets and chordae), the anterior leaflet is excised as described for conventional MVR. For bioprosthetic valves, the posterior valve sutures are passed from the ventricular to the atrial side in the annulus with attention not to trap any bundles of chordae tendineae inadvertently. Alternatively, the sutures can "reef in" excessive leaflet tissue and plicate this layer to the annulus. When a mechanical prosthesis is used, the sutures are placed from the

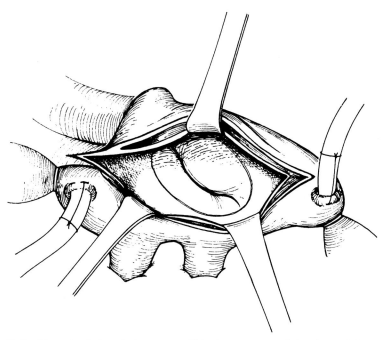

Figure 42-3. The extended vertical trans-septal biatriotomy approach involves a right atriotomy incision downward starting at the right atrial appendage. The interatrial septum is then incised down to the fossa ovalis and extended cephalad onto the dome of the left atrium.

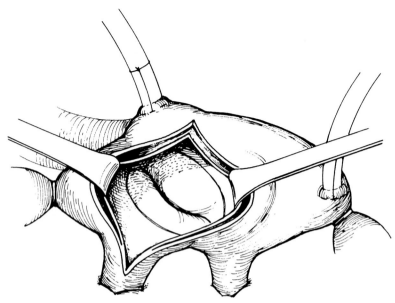

Figure 42-4. The Khonsari oblique biatriotomy incision extends from the right superior pulmonary vein onto the right atrial free wall to expose the septum, which is then opened down to the fossa ovalis (Reprinted with permission from S Khonsari, CF Sintek. Transatrial approach revisited. Ann Thorac Surg 1990;50:1002).

can be imbricated into the mitral annulus with the valve sutures to shorten overall chordal length (Fig. 42-6, inset). Alternatively, the central portion (closer to the annulus) of the redundant posterior leaflet can be partially excised in a crescent shape and then the leaflet reattached to the annulus during suture fixation of the mitral prosthesis (Fig. 42-6). When a bileaflet mechanical prosthesis is used, it is preferable to orient the valve such that the pivot guards are in the septal-lateral (or "anteroposterior") direction, or the "antianatomic" position, to ensure symmetric opening of both leaflets and to help prevent retained chordae from interfering with complete closing or opening of the prosthetic leaflets.

The best approach is to preserve the first- and second-order chordae to *both* the anterior and posterior leaflets, and various methods of preserving the anterior leaflet chordal attachments have been introduced over the years. Using the technique originally devised by David for a bioprosthesis, one makes an incision at the base of the central portion of the anterior leaflet, 2 mm to 3 mm from the annulus (Fig.42-7). The incision is extended obliquely toward the free margin of the anterior leaflet, thereby leaving intact most chordae attached to the

atrial to the ventricular side and back out the posterior leaflet 2 mm to 5 mm from the annulus. If the posterior leaflet is myxomatous or excessively redundant or the chordae tendineae are elongated, the posterior leaflet

Figure 42-5. Conventional mitral valve replacement with complete excision of the leaflets and the entire subvalvular apparatus, as used in the past and in cases of advanced rheumatic disease. The mitral prosthesis is implanted using a series of horizontal mattress sutures.

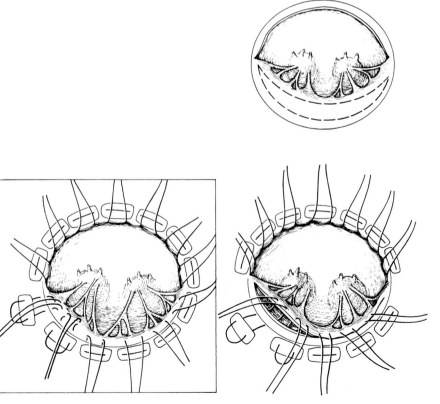

Figure 42-6. Preservation of the posterior leaflet by either imbricating the leaflet **(inset)** with the valve sutures or by excising a crescent-shaped portion of the leaflet and reattaching the free edge of the leaflet using the valve sutures.

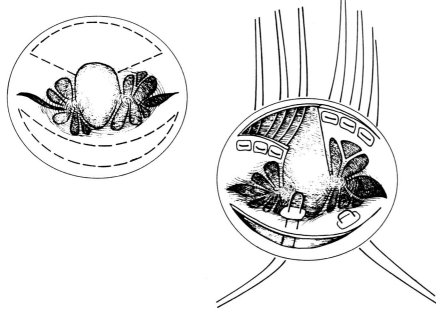

Figure 42-7.   Preservation of the anterior leaflet and its chordal attachments can be accomplished by excising a central trapezoidal segment of the anterior leaflet and resuspending the residual leaflet to the anterior annulus using the mitral valve suture (after David et al.). This method works well for bioprostheses.

mechanical valve, such as the Medtronic-Hall or Sorin valve. In this technique, the anterior leaflet is split into two halves radially from the free edge to the annulus. It is then completely detached from the anterior mitral annulus, and the two segments are transposed toward the posterior annulus, with the ventricular side facing the atrium. Uniform tension is exerted on the anterior leaflet chordal attachments, and any excessive myxomatous leaflet tissue extending above the plane of the posterior annulus is excised. Calcific material that may interfere with the valve mechanism is débrided. A series of 2-0 pledgeted braided polyester sutures is placed through the repositioned and trimmed anterior leaflet, the posterior leaflet (imbricating any redundant tissue), and finally the posterior annulus (Fig. 42-9). After the annular sutures are placed, the tilting disk valve is oriented such that the major orifice faces the middle of the anterior mitral annulus. In this manner, the downward excursion of the disk during diastole and closing motion during systole are anteriorly directed, away from the transposed anterior chordae and leaflet.

anterior leaflet. Thus, a trapezoidal central section (corresponding to the "bare area" devoid of major chordal insertions) of the anterior leaflet is excised. The portions of the residual anterior leaflet on each side are then resuspended to the annulus using the valve sutures. The posterior leaflet and its chordae are spared as previously described.

Using the method developed by Miki and associates from Nara, Japan, for a bileaflet mechanical valve, one makes a similar incision in the anterior leaflet, and the middle portion of the anterior leaflet, which is usually devoid of first-order and second-order chordal insertion, is resected. Thus the leaflet is divided into the lateral and medial segments attached to the anterolateral and posteromedial papillary muscles, respectively (Fig. 42-8). If part of the leaflet is excessively thickened, it is debulked with a blade. These two segments of anterior leaflet are then shifted and resuspended to the mitral annulus near the corresponding commissures with 2-0 braided polyester sutures placed from the ventricular to the atrial side (noneverting). The sutures are reinforced by Teflon pledgets. The midpoint of the central scallop of the posterior leaflet is divided radially toward the annulus and imbricated as necessary to allow insertion of a prosthesis of the appropriate size.

Feikes and colleagues designed a chordal-sparing procedure that is particularly well suited for MVR with a tilting disk

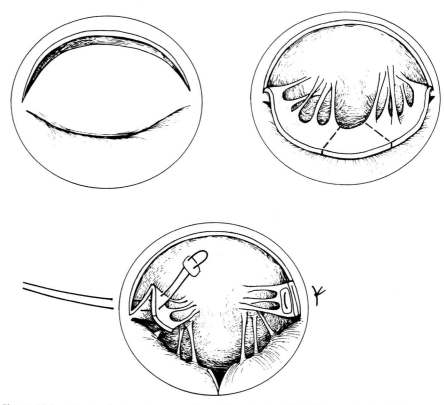

Figure 42-8.   Nara technique of preservation of the anterior leaflet. The anterior leaflet is detached from the annulus and then the central portion (*dashed lines*) is resected. The anterior and posterior remnants of the anterior leaflet are reattached to the annulus near the respective commissures (as described by Miki et al.). The middle scallop of the posterior leaflet is divided radially toward the annulus to allow implantation of an appropriately sized prosthesis.

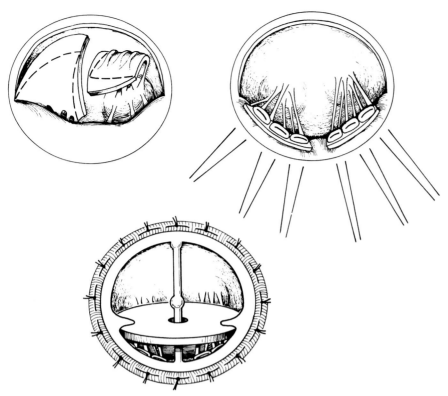

Figure 42-9. Chordal-sparing MVR technique (as described by Feikes et al.) for insertion of a tilting-disk mechanical prosthesis. The anterior leaflet is detached from the anterior annulus and divided into two halves. Excessive myxomatous leaflet tissue is excised (*dash lines*). The two segments are then transposed to the posterior annulus and then reattached along with the posterior leaflet using the valve sutures. The valve is oriented such that the major orifice is located anteriorly such that the downward excursion of the disk during diastole is away from the bulk of the retained subvalvular apparatus.

To preserve the subvalvular apparatus in an anatomic manner (e.g., circumferentially) without repositioning the anterior chordae or leaflets, Khonsari developed a technique that allows resection of sufficient valvular tissue to avoid left ventricular outflow tract obstruction and interference with prosthetic valve function. The original Khonsari I procedure was developed for patients with rheumatic mitral valve disease and retains the entire posterior leaflet in situ; any redundant tissue is plicated by passing the annular valve sutures through the free edge of the leaflet. The anterior leaflet is subdivided into two to five chordal segments or "buttons" (depending on the size of the leaflet) (Fig. 42-10); each button is connected to first-order or second-order chordae. If the leaflet is very thickened and calcified as in advanced rheumatic valve disease, wedges of tissue between chords can be resected to trim down the buttons. Each button is resuspended in its anatomic position with everting pledgeted valve sutures. Excessive tissue within these chordal buttons that cannot be safely excised is extracted and held on the atrial side (outside

the sewing ring) when the valve is seated and the sutures are tied, thus preventing this tissue from protruding beneath the prosthesis, which may cause outflow tract obstruction or interfere with the mechanical valve opening or closing mechanism.

Normal valvular-ventricular geometry, however, can be simulated more closely, especially if the anterior leaflet is relatively pliable without extensive fibrosis or scarring. Here the Khonsari II technique produces an elegant result. The leaflet is detached 2 mm to 3 mm from the annulus (from the left to the right trigone), and a central, elliptical-shaped portion of leaflet is excised, leaving a 5- to 10-mm rim of leaflet free edge attached to most of the first-order chordae tendineae and second-order "strut" chordae (Fig. 42-11). This strip of leaflet is then reattached to the annulus in its normal anatomic location with the everting valve sutures.

Instead of reattaching the rim of anterior leaflet to the annulus with the valve sutures, one can close the defect in the anterior leaflet primarily using a running 4-0 polypropylene suture (Fig. 42-12), as described by

Rose and Oz. This serves the same purpose in terms of debulking the anterior leaflet and displacing it away from the subvalvular region and toward the annulus while preserving the anterior leaflet first- and second-order chordae. This suture line is reinforced with the pledgeted everting valve sutures.

If the leaflets are malleable, a simpler method of preserving both the anterior and posterior chordae tendineae is to excise a circumferential crescent of valve tissue from the posterior leaflet as well as the anterior leaflet. Rather than resuspending the first- and second-order chordae with everting sutures, one can pass the valve sutures through the leaflet remnant and then through the annulus from the ventricular to the atrial side (Fig. 42-13). This option is useful when using a bioprosthetic valve.

Finally, preservation of the chordae tendineae may not be always be possible, for example, in patients undergoing repeat MVR where the chordae were previously excised or in those with severe mitral stenosis due to rheumatic disease, where the mitral subvalvular apparatus is markedly diseased with dense fibrosis and calcification of the leaflets, fusion of the chordae tendineae, and foreshortening of the chordal apparatus. When it is determined that the rheumatic changes are too advanced, both the anterior and posterior leaflets are excised entirely. The fused chordae are resected at the papillary muscle tips, except for the third-order or basal chords. Papillary-annular continuity can be reconstituted with 4-0 expanded polytetrafluoroethylene (e-PTFE) sutures to produce artificial chordae tendineae extending from the papillary muscle heads to the mitral annulus (Fig. 42-14), as performed by David. Two sutures are placed at the fibrous tip of the anterolateral and posteromedial papillary muscles in a mattress fashion. Appropriate artificial chordae length varies according to the size of the left ventricular cavity. The new chordae should be taut but not tight. In the normal heart, the distance from the papillary muscle tip to the mitral annulus generally ranges between 22 mm to 23 mm in systole. The two sutures originating from the posteromedial papillary muscle are passed through the annulus at the 2-o'clock and 5-o'clock positions and those from the anterolateral papillary muscle are placed at the 7-o'clock and 10-o'clock positions. Each suture is passed through the annulus in two or three places, and after length adjustment of the multiple ePTFE chordae using a fine nerve hook, the suture is tied. This is followed by implantation of the prosthesis as described for conventional MVR.

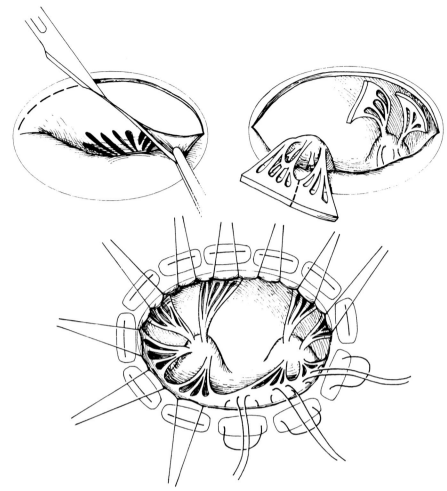

Figure 42-10. Khonsari I technique of chordal-sparing MVR. In cases of rheumatic disease where the leaflets are very thickened and/or calcified and the subvalvular apparatus is obliterated, the second-order chordae tendineae are preserved in individual bundles. The anterior leaflet is subdivided into two to five "buttons" containing larger chordae, which are then reattached to the annulus in their anatomic position with the pledgeted valve sutures.

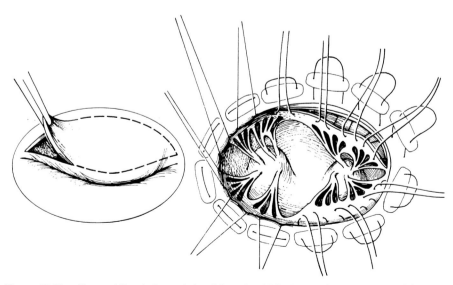

Figure 42-11. Khonsari II technique of chordal-sparing MVR. Anatomic preservation of the anterior chordal structures. A central ellipse of the anterior leaflet is excised, and the free edge is then reattached to the annulus in the normal anatomic location using the valve sutures.

Management of the Calcified Mitral Annulus

In the presence of extensive annular calcification in elderly patients, those with rheumatic disease, and some with severe Barlow's syndrome, insertion of a prosthesis in the anatomic position can be difficult. Characteristically, the calcification involves the entire posterior annulus from trigone to trigone in a "horseshoe" configuration, extends to a variable extent into the left ventricular myocardium, and can occasionally be completely circumferential, incorporating the entire anterior annulus. Extensive débridement can lead to atrioventricular disruption, injury to the circumflex coronary artery, and heart block. Partial debridement may cause fracture of the remaining calcified bar and injure the left ventricular free wall or lead to a paravalvular leak. Attempts to place the sutures on a heavy needle forcefully through the densely calcified annulus can create myocardial tears. Conversely, inadequate decalcification makes it difficult to seat the prosthesis in good apposition with the annulus, which may result in paravalvular leak and does not allow a prosthesis of adequate size to be used.

Despite meticulous débridement of the posterior annulus, up to and including complete unroofing of the atrioventricular groove to the epicardial fat, radical decalcification generally results in relatively poor quality tissue for holding valve sutures. In these situations, reconstruction of the mitral annulus can be performed with either fresh autologous pericardium or glutaraldehyde-fixed bovine pericardium. A pericardial patch is tailored in a semicircular fashion approximately 2 cm larger than the defect in the mitral annulus. The margin of the patch is sutured to the endocardium of the left ventricle with a continuous 4-0 or 3-0 polypropylene suture (Fig. 42-15). The corresponding valve sutures are secured to the patch and reinforced with Teflon pledgets. The reconstruction is then completed by suturing the remaining margin of the patch to the left atrial wall.

When extensive mitral annular calcification precludes orthotopic MVR and radical débridement is not performed, the mitral leaflets themselves can be used to secure the prosthesis while preserving the subvalvular apparatus (Fig. 42-16). Each needle of a series of 2-0 SH braided polyester pledgeted mattress sutures is passed through the leaflet tissue adjacent to the annular calcification from the left atrium to the left ventricle and

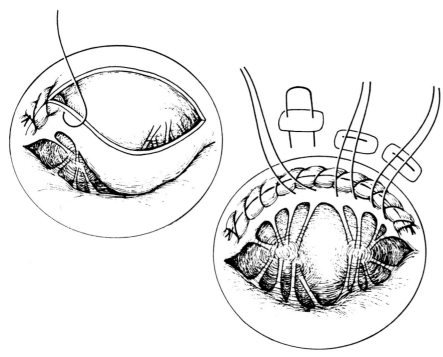

Figure 42-12. Another method of anatomic preservation of the anterior chordae. The anterior leaflet can be debulked and shifted toward the annulus by excising the central portion of the leaflet and closing the defect using a running polypropylene suture before the valve is implanted (Reprinted with permission from EA Rose, MC Oz. Preservation of anterior leaflet chordae tendineae during mitral valve replacement. Ann Thorac Surg 1994;57:768).

then continued through the leaflet to the left atrial side of the leading edge of the leaflet. The suture is then "double backed" through the central portion of the leaflet between the annulus and the free edge in a double-layered fashion, thereby producing radial plication with maximal incorporation of leaflet tissue into the valve sutures. Alternatively, the pledgeted horizontal mattress sutures can be taken in a noneverting fash-

ion from the calcified leaflet across the annulus to the left atrial surface. Conventional suture methods are used anteriorly, if possible. In this manner, the prosthetic valve is centrally seated and papillary-annular continuity is maintained. The major disadvantages of this technique are placement of sutures through very diseased valve tissue and being forced to implant a much smaller prosthesis than desired. An alternative operative approach to the heavily calcified mitral annulus is to implant the mitral prosthesis at the intra-atrial level (Fig. 42-17), which is a derivative of Yacoub's original "top hat" procedure for homograft MVR or tricuspid valve replacement (TVR). A similar method developed in Syria uses a pulmonary autograft valve mounted inside a tubular synthetic graft for MVR, termed the "Ross-II procedure." The circumference of the prosthetic sewing ring is enlarged with a polyethylene terephthalate (Dacron) collar (approximately 1.0 cm to 1.5 cm in width) with a running 4-0 polypropylene suture. Without débriding the mitral annular calcification, the prosthesis is secured with an inner row of 2-0 braided polyester mattress sutures placed in the left atrial wall 0.5 cm to 1.5 cm lateral to the mitral annulus; this suture line is then reinforced with a running 4-0 polypropylene suture between the free edge of the Dacron collar and the atrial wall. When only a portion of the mitral annulus is calcified, a partial collar is used to attach the prosthesis intra-atrially at the corresponding affected site; and the remainder of the prosthesis is sewn to the annulus in standard fashion. This intra-atrial "top hat" technique increases the effective annular perimeter and allows insertion of a larger prosthesis; however, transfer of systolic intraventricular pressure to the left atrial wall where it is sutured to the Dacron collar can potentially disrupt the suture line, and potentially thrombus can form in this cul de sac.

Reconstruction of the Mitral Annulus

In patients with endocarditis or after multiple previous mitral valve replacements, the mitral annulus can be extensively damaged such that a new prosthesis cannot be securely seated by passing the valve sutures normally through destroyed or very friable annular tissue. As described by David, the whole circumference can be reconstructed with a strip of bovine pericardium 2 cm wide and the length estimated by multiplying the annular diameter by π. It is sewn to the fibrous tissue below the aortic valve anteriorly and to the left ventricular endocardium

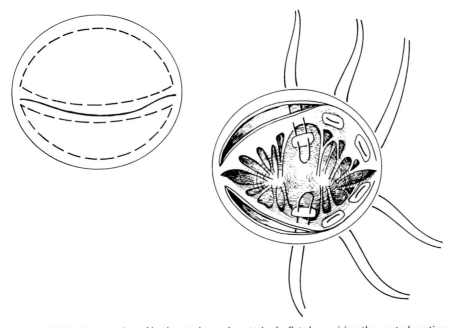

Figure 42-13. Preservation of both anterior and posterior leaflets by excising the central portion of both leaflets and then resuspending the chords using noneverting valve sutures. This method works well when using a bioprosthesis and is most applicable when extreme bileaflet prolapse is encountered that the surgeon does not want to repair.

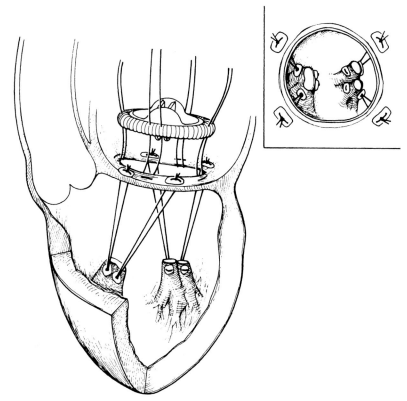

Figure 42-14. Papillary-annular continuity can be recreated using expanded polytetrafluoroethylene (ePTFE) sutures as artificial chordae tendineae. The sutures are placed into the papillary muscle tips and reattached to the annulus at the 2-, 5-, 7-, and 10-o'clock positions. Each suture is locked on itself after the length is adjusted with a fine nerve hook.

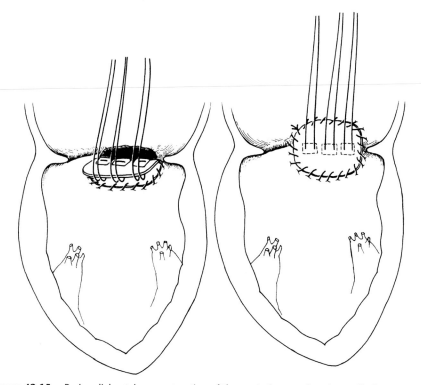

Figure 42-15. Pericardial patch reconstruction of the posterior annulus after radical débridement of annular calcification or destroyed annulus secondary to endocarditis. The corresponding valve sutures are secured to the patch before its suturing to the left atrial wall to complete the annular reconstruction.

posteriorly. The ascending aorta may need to be opened to facilitate suturing underneath the aortic valve and to prevent injury to the noncoronary or left aortic cusps. In the most advanced cases where infection has destroyed the intertrigonal fibrous mitral-aortic continuity, the entire base of the heart (left atrium, left ventricle, and ascending aorta) is opened widely into one common chamber. After reconstructing the posterior mitral annulus and area where mitral-aortic continuity had been with bovine pericardium, both aortic and mitral valves are replaced and the aorta patched closed. We term this the "meat cleaver" procedure, but reasonable success has been achieved in such very challenging circumstances.

Weaning from Cardiopulmonary Bypass

Rewarming of the patient is initiated when the valve sutures are being tied. The left atriotomy is closed with a running 3-0 or 4-0 polypropylene suture. A 1,500-mL "hot shot" of warm blood cardioplegia is given retrograde before releasing the cross-clamp. The caval snares are released, and venous return to the pump is restricted to fill the heart. The left ventricle is de-aired through the left atrial suture line by manually inflating the lungs to force air out of the pulmonary veins, massaging and/or invaginating the left atrial appendage, and needle aspirating the right superior pulmonary vein, left atrial dome, and left ventricular apex. A vent is inserted into the aortic root. With the patient in a steep Trendelenburg position, the aortic cross-clamp is released, and continuous cardiotomy suction is placed on the vent in the ascending aorta. The heart should not be elevated or manually massaged too vigorously after MVR to avoid iatrogenic atrioventricular groove disruption or left ventricular free wall rupture; when elevating the heart, the surgeon's entire hand should be placed behind the heart with the fingers extending into the transverse pericardial sinus to protect the left atrioventricular groove. After full rewarming and resuscitation of the heart, CPB is discontinued. De-airing is continued with the mitral valve opening vigorously and the heart ejecting using the aortic vent and by needle aspiration until all microcavitation targets seen on TEE are gone. Transesophageal echocardiography is used in all cases to determine the adequacy of de-airing and to ascertain that the prosthetic valve mechanism is functioning normally without interference by retained chordal structures, there

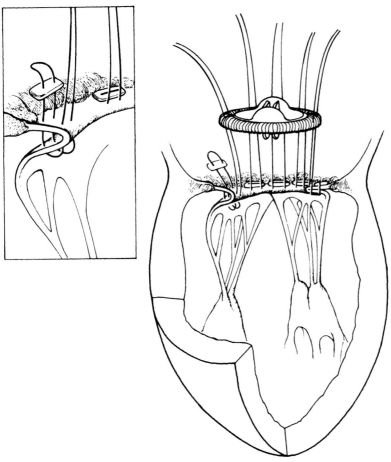

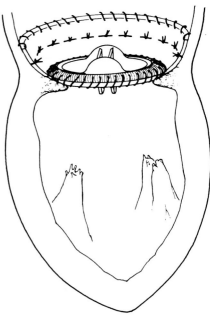

Figure 42-17. Intra-atrial insertion of the mitral prosthesis is an extra-anatomic technique that can be considered when dense annular calcification or annular destruction from multiple previous valve replacements (with or without prosthetic endocarditis) is present. The prosthetic sewing ring is enlarged circumferentially by sewing a polyethylene terephthalate (Dacron) circular flange or collar to the valve. This Dacron collar is sutured to the atrial wall with an inner row of interrupted mattress sutures with pledgets used on the atrial surface. The free margin of the Dacron flange is then secured to the atrial endocardium using a running 4-0 polypropylene suture.

Figure 42-16. When dense mitral annular calcification is encountered, normal suturing methods for valve implantation are not possible. Exclusion of the calcified mitral annulus by securing the prosthesis to the leaflet tissue adjacent to the annular calcification is one alternative. This technique also preserves the entire subvalvular apparatus.

are no periprosthetic leaks, and left ventricular outflow tract (LVOT) obstruction is not present. The patient is then decannulated, temporary bipolar ventricular pacing wires are placed, a mediastinal drainage tube is positioned, and the sternum is closed.

Surgical Complications

Left Ventricular Rupture

Myocardial rupture is quite rare, but is usually a lethal complication of MVR. It probably results from excision or stretching of the papillary muscle in a thin, fragile left ventricle. It may also occur in the setting of an acute or subacute myocardial infarction, particularly in the elderly. With contemporary low-profile mechanical valves and stented bioprostheses, all of the papillary muscles can be left intact without interference with the valve mechanism. Since the revival of chordal-sparing MVR

techniques, the incidence of this complication has fallen substantially. This further suggests that the integrity of the mitral subvalvular apparatus provides structural support to the left ventricular free wall in addition to optimizing postoperative left ventricular systolic pump function.

Left ventricular rupture can also be caused by a strut of a bioprosthetic valve eroding into or protruding through the posterior left ventricular wall. This serious complication occurs most commonly in elderly patients or as a result of excessive lifting of the heart after implantation of the prosthesis. Maintaining papillary-annular continuity provides a substantial degree of protection from this devastating complication.

Treatment of myocardial rupture involves immediate reinstitution of CPB. After the prosthesis is removed, the perforation is repaired with a bovine pericardial patch sewn to the LV endocardium, and the valve is re-replaced. If LV myocardial rupture is recognized after weaning from CPB in the op-

erating room, the prognosis is grave; if it occurs in the intensive unit, it is usually fatal.

Atrioventricular Disruption and Circumflex Artery Injury

Overly aggressive débridement or decalcification of the posterior mitral leaflet and annulus may lead to atrioventricular groove hematoma, disruption, and/or cardiac rupture. The circumflex coronary artery can also be injured if the valve sutures are placed too deeply into the posterior annulus. This complication requires a saphenous vein bypass to the circumflex artery distribution.

Entrapment of the Aortic Valve Cusp and Injury to the Atrioventricular Conduction Pathway

Placement of valve sutures too deep between the anterior commissure and the right fibrous trigone (across the anterior annulus) can inadvertently injure either the noncoronary or left aortic valve cusps. Similarly, the atrioventricular node and bundle of His can be injured by suture bites taken too deeply between the right trigone and the posterior commissure. The latter is usually related to radical annular débridement for endocarditis or a calcified annulus, thereby leaving minimal tissue for placement of sutures.

Aortic cusp trauma is recognized on removal of the aortic cross-clamp when the left ventricle distends due to aortic regurgitation and is confirmed by TEE. Treatment entails reapplying the cross-clamp, opening the left atrium and aorta, removing the mitral prosthesis or a single offending suture, repairing the injured aortic cusp, and reimplantating the prosthesis or adding a new valve suture. In contrast, permanent injuries to the conduction pathway may not be detected until many days postoperatively, when a permanent pacemaker is required.

Left Ventricular Outflow Tract Obstruction

A mitral prosthesis may interfere with ejection of blood from the left ventricle due to use of a very large stented bioprosthesis or a large high-profile mechanical valve. This complication is manifested by a bisferiens arterial pulse tracing (double opening of the aortic valve) and is readily identified using TEE. With contemporary low-profile bileaflet mechanical prostheses, this problem is relatively rare. Treatment requires the replacement of the mitral prosthesis with a low-profile valve in extreme cases. When using chordal-sparing techniques, LVOT obstruction can be caused by retained anterior mitral valve leaflet tissue and is identified as systolic anterior leaflet motion (SAM) of the anterior leaflet and chordae associated with LVOT turbulence and a gradient on TEE. Initial management includes discontinuing any inotropic agents, volume loading, adding beta-blockers, and increasing left ventricular afterload with vasopressors (e.g., phenylephrine). This medical therapy is monitored using TEE and usually is effective, as is also the case for SAM and LVOT obstruction after mitral repair. If left ventricular outflow tract obstruction persists, aortotomy and transaortic excision of the offending subaortic mitral tissue can be required.

Perivalvular Leak

Perivalvular leak with substantial mitral regurgitation may result from tearing of friable annular or retained leaflet tissue by the valve sutures. It can also be caused by poor seating of the mitral prosthesis into an extensively calcified annulus. The diagnosis is made using TEE, but judging the severity of the leak can be difficult. In questionable cases, TEE reinterrogation after protamine administration may be necessary. Perivalvular leaks must be differentiated from the usual symmetric pattern of "closing jets" seen with bileaflet mechanical valves. If an unacceptably large leak is suspected, it should be treated at that time by re-do MVR using pledgeted sutures (or intra-atrial insertion of a new prosthetic valve in the case of a heavily calcified annulus) and not ignored.

Postoperative Management

Anticoagulation

Warfarin anticoagulation is usually advised for 3 months in patients in normal sinus rhythm who received a bioprosthesis, and indefinitely for those with mechanical valve substitutes or individuals with a bioprosthesis who are in atrial fibrillation.

Mitral Stenosis

In the early postoperative period, prolonged ventilatory support can be necessary in patients with mitral stenosis due to long-standing pulmonary hypertension and lung disease. The degree of reversibility of the pulmonary hypertension is not predictable. Although the left ventricle is protected from both pressure and volume overload in patients with mitral stenosis, cardiac performance may be compromised secondary to right ventricular failure due to inadequate right ventricular protection. A combination of inotropic and pulmonary vasodilator drugs plus hyperventilation to lower the partial pressure of arterial carbon dioxide ($PaCO_2$) into the low 30-mm Hg range can optimize right ventricular afterload (lower pulmonary artery [PA] impedance) and improve cardiac output. Infusing the vasodilator drugs through a right-sided line and the inotropic drugs systemically via a left atrial line can help. Inhaled nitric oxide is the treatment of choice for refractory pulmonary hypertension (right ventricular afterload mismatch), which must be distinguished from right ventricular pump failure. In the former, the pulmonary pressures are high, the right-sided pressure step-up between mean right atrial (RA) and mean PA pressure is large, and right atrial pressure usually is only mildly elevated; in the latter circumstances, the pressure step-up is low because RA pressure is high and PA pressure has fallen (and eventually becomes nonphasic). In severe cases of right ventricular pump failure, the RA and PA pressure tracings appear similar.

Mitral Regurgitation

Postoperative management regarding ventilatory support and pulmonary hypertension is similar to that following MVR for mitral stenosis. Correction of mitral regurgitation (with elimination of systolic left ventricular unloading into the left atrium), however, may unmask significant left ventricular systolic dysfunction that was present preoperatively. Inotropic support along with arterial afterload-reducing agents (systemic vasodilators) is the treatment of choice. Infrequently, intra-aortic balloon counterpulsation may also be necessary to improve both myocardial and systemic perfusion and lower LV afterload even further. Low–cardiac-output states occur less frequently when MVR is performed using chordal-sparing techniques.

SUGGESTED READING

Bonow RO, Carabello BA, Chatterjee K, et al. ACC/AHA 2006 Guidelines for the management of patients with Valvular Heart Disease. J Am Coll Cardiol 2006;48:e1.

Coselli JS, Crawford ES. Calcified mitral valve annulus: Prosthesis insertion. Ann Thorac Surg 1988;46:584.

David TE. Mitral valve replacement with preservation of chordae tendineae: Rationale and technical consideration. Ann Thorac Surg 1986;41:680.

David TE, Feindel CM, Armstrong S, et al. Reconstruction of the mitral annulus: A ten year experience. J Thorac Cardiovasc Surg 1995;110:1323.

Feikes HL, Daugharthy JB, Perry JE, et al. Preservation of all chordae tendineae and papillary muscle during mitral valve replacement with a tilting disc valve. J Cardiac Surg 1990;2:81.

Heub AC, Jatene FB, Moreira LF, et al. Ventricular remodeling and mitral valve modifications in dilated cardiomyopathy: New insights from anatomic study. J Thorac Cardiovasc Surg 2002;124:1216.

Khonsari S, Sintek CF. Transatrial approach revisited. Ann Thorac Surg 1990;50:1002.

Kirklin JW. Replacement of the mitral valve for mitral incompetence. Surgery 1972;72:827.

Kumar N, Saad E, Prabhakar G, et al. Extended transseptal versus conventional left atriotomy: Early postoperative study. Ann Thorac Surg 1995;60:426.

McCarthy PM. Does the intertrigonal distance dilate? Never say never. J Thorac Cardiovasc Surg 2002;124:1078.

Miki S, Kusuhara K, Ueda Y, et al. Mitral valve replacement with preservation of chordae tendineae and papillary muscles. Ann Thorac Surg 1988;45:28.

Nataf P, Pavie A, Jault F, et al. Intraatrial insertion of a mitral prosthesis in a destroyed or calcified mitral annulus. Ann Thorac Surg 1994;58:163.

Okita Y, Miki S, Ueda Y, et al. Replacement of chordae tendineae using expanded polytetrafluoroethylene (ePTFE) sutures during mitral valve replacement in patients with severe mitral stenosis. J Cardiac Surg 1993;8:567.

Rose EA, Oz MC. Preservation of anterior leaflet chordae tendineae during mitral valve replacement. Ann Thorac Surg 1994;57:768.

Sintek CF, Pfeffer TA, Kochamba GS, et al. Mitral valve replacement: Technique to preserve the subvalvular apparatus. Ann Thorac Surg 1995;59:1027.

Tibayan FA, Rodriguez F, Langer F, et al. Does septal-lateral annular cinching work for chronic ischemic mitral regurgitation? J Thorac Cardiovasc Surg 2004;127:654.

Yun KL, Sintek CF, Miller DC, et al. Randomized trial comparing partial versus complete chordal-sparing mitral valve replacement: Effects on left ventricular volume and function. J Thorac Cardiovasc Surg 2002;123:707.

EDITOR'S COMMENTS

Yun and Miller have done an excellent job in describing mitral valve replacement. Basically, I agree with all the technical aspects they discussed. Obviously, the best situation occurs when the valve can be repaired. However, I asked these authors to review replacement, and this is what they focused on.

I would like to emphasize two issues that they discussed. The first one is the approach in a person who has hostile sternum using a right thoracotomy. This has been a lifesaving technique for us. A cross-clamp is not necessary. We prefer, obviously, that the patient be cooled and the heart to fibrillate so as to avoid any ejection of air. This is an excellent approach in a multiple re-do operation. It's also particularly helpful if the heart has to be approached in a hurry when a sternotomy is not easily possible. Unfortunately, wide-open aortic insufficiency is a contraindication.

A second and very difficult issue is the calcification of the annulus. The authors discussed anchoring the prosthesis within the mitral valve tissue as well as débridement of calcification. Another solution has been anchoring the prosthesis to a graft above the mitral annulus to avoid decalcification. We have found that the atrial tissue does not hold well, and we do our best to avoid this approach.

I.L.K.

43

Reoperative Mitral Replacement

G. Randall Green, Scott A. Buchanan, Reid W. Tribble, and Curtis G. Tribble

Choice of Approach

After the decision has been made to undertake a mitral valve operation in a patient who has previously undergone cardiac surgery, an approach to the operation must be selected. The choices of incision include re-do median sternotomy and right anterolateral thoracotomy. Each approach has advantages as well as disadvantages, which are derived from such factors as the nature and number of previous operations, the time interval since they were carried out, the presence of patent coronary grafts, and the degree of expected disease in the patient's aortic valve, great vessels, and lungs.

Factors that lead us to choose anterolateral thoracotomy include the presence of recently placed or undiseased patent coronary artery grafts, especially mammary arteries, which could be injured during re-do median sternotomy. Patients who have undergone multiple previous sternotomies, aortic valve replacement, or replacement of the ascending aorta may be more safely approached via an anterolateral thoracotomy, which avoids pitfalls related to adhesions, the presence of an aortic valve prosthesis, or a fragile sternum. Patients with a history of mediastinitis or mediastinal irradiation may also be more easily approached via the right chest.

By contrast, re-do median sternotomy is preferred in patients who require concomitant cardiac operations in addition to mitral valve procedures. Patients with significant aortic insufficiency are often better served by sternotomy, because aortic cross-clamping and venting can be difficult from the right chest. The presence of aortoiliac disease that prevents the use of femoral bypass makes re-do sternotomy more attractive. Pathologic conditions involving the right lung and

pleura such as severe chronic obstructive pulmonary disease, active pulmonary infection, or pleural adhesions push us to choose re-do median sternotomy rather than anterolateral thoracotomy to avoid expected adhesions and the possibility of contaminating the new valve through exposure to a nonsterile portion of lung or pleural space.

In our early experience with re-do mitral valve operations, we tended to favor the right anterolateral thoracotomy approach. Reoperative cardiac surgery has now become more routine, however, leading to extensive experience documenting the safety of re-do median sternotomy. Most surgeons are now convinced that median sternotomy provides optimal exposure of all parts of the heart, allows any technique of myocardial protection to be used, and permits optimal venting of both the left and right sides of the heart. With carefully selected exceptions, the majority of patients at our institution who require reoperation on the mitral valve undergo repeat median sternotomy.

Other preoperative considerations include finding the old operative note, reviewing the most recent cardiac catheterization to make decisions about grafting of coronaries, and obtaining a computed tomography scan to determine graft location, especially the internal mammary artery grafts.

Technique of Anterolateral Thoracotomy

The patient is positioned on a beanbag with 30 degrees of left down rotation and slight flexion to the left to splay the right rib

cage (Fig. 43-1). The entire chest and groins are prepared into the sterile field. The incision should be truly anterolateral, beginning near the sternum and carried laterally through the fifth interspace to the anterior axillary line. The skin incision need not be overly generous, because the intercostal musculature of the interspace may be divided much more posteriorly, allowing for increased rib retraction. The costal cartilages may be notched to enhance exposure. The right internal mammary artery is identified, divided, and carefully suture ligated. Rib retractors are inserted and the lung gently retracted posteriorly with laparotomy pads and malleable retractors. Double-lumen endotracheal ventilation is not mandatory in this setting, though some prefer it, because the lung may be easily retracted until cardiopulmonary bypass is instituted.

The heart is exposed by opening the pericardium laterally and anterior to the phrenic nerve (Fig. 43-1). This dissection can be tedious and time consuming because of dense adhesions, particularly in the region of the previously cannulated right atrial appendage. Strict avoidance of blunt dissection in favor of sharp dissection will minimize the chance of injury to the myocardium or its blood supply. The pericardial space is best approached posteriorly near the right pulmonary veins or inferiorly over the diaphragm, where there are often few adhesions. There is no need to take down the adhesions overlying the ventricles except for a small area on the diaphragmatic surface of the heart to permit the attachment of pacing wires at the end of the procedure. Similarly, the pericardium may be left on the right atrium, where it will serve as thick, pledget-like material for the purse strings placed directly through it before cannulation.

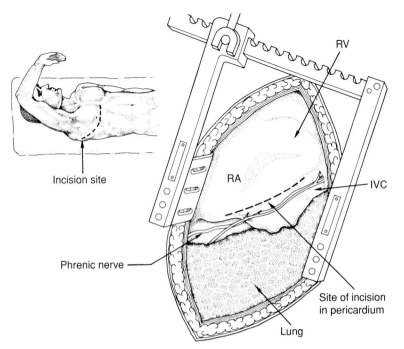

Figure 43-1. The incision site. (IVC = inferior vena cava; RA = right atrium; RV = right ventricle.)

Exposure of the superior and inferior venae cavae is necessary to apply caval cannula tapes. Protection of the phrenic nerve is of paramount importance. The phrenic nerve is particularly vulnerable in this dissection, because it descends along the side of the superior vena cava and at its position just anterior to the right hilum. The ascending aorta is dissected out if feasible, because it can often be used for cannulation, and de-airing through the aorta eventually will be necessary. The interatrial groove must be fully exposed all the way back to the true interatrial septum. This simple maneuver mobilizes the right atrium off the roof of the left atrium and markedly enhances exposure of the mitral valve (Fig. 43-2). At this point, the table is rolled to the patient's left to create a direct line of vision onto the mitral valve.

Technique of Re-Do Median Sternotomy

The patient is placed supine on the operating room table with the arms tucked. The external defibrillator pads are placed over the patient's right scapula and left chest. The cardiopulmonary bypass circuit is set up in the room and ready for expedient institution of bypass should it become necessary during the early part of the operation. We place a femoral arterial line before beginning the case to facilitate rapid insertion of

an arterial cannula if this becomes necessary. Cannulas should be available to perfuse any patent saphenous or mammary grafts that could be injured on entering the mediastinum. A sterile field is created from the patient's chin to the feet, allowing access not only to the patient's femoral vessels, but also to the right axillary artery and the saphenous veins, which may need to be harvested.

The re-do sternotomy is carried out in the standard manner by removing each of the old wires and using the oscillating saw to cut through the anterior and posterior tables of the sternum. Care is taken to elevate the sternum from the anterior surface of the heart during sternal division. Curved Mayo scissors are used to divide any remaining portions of the posterior sternal table. If the anterior mediastinum is extensively adherent to the undersurface of the sternum, the sternal wires may be divided anteriorly, leaving the wire intact beneath the posterior table of the sternum. The oscillating saw is then used to safely divide the posterior table of the sternum down onto each of the wires. The wires are then removed, and the remainder of the perforated posterior table is divided with curved Mayo scissors. A small 3- or 4-in. pediatric sternal retractor or articulating laminectomy retractor may be used to wedge open the lower portion of the sternum, facilitating division of the remaining connective tissue elements of the posterior table. If the CT shows the right ventricle (RV) is adherent to the posterior sternum, bilateral IMA retractors can be

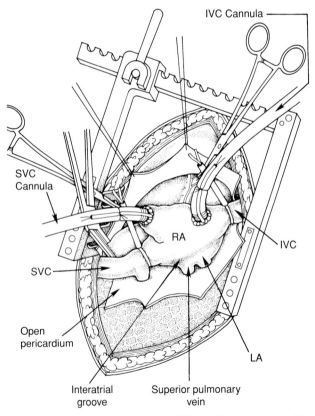

Figure 43-2. Anterolateral thoracotomy exposure. (IVC = inferior vena cava; LA = left atrium; RA = right atrium; SVC = superior vena cava.)

used to elevate the costal margins. Dissection can then proceed from the inferior portion of the incision under direct vision using sharp dissection and cautery. The sternum can be divided incrementally when using this approach.

After the sternotomy is completed, electrocautery is helpful in establishing the area under the sternum for placement of the sternal retractor and for subsequent sternal closure. The pleura of both the right and left chest are widely opened, allowing placement of the sternal retractor. An early priority is to clear the ascending aorta of adhesions so that cannulation can be achieved on short notice. Dissecting above and below the innominate vein can often facilitate finding the aorta. This part of the aorta has usually not been dissected out at the first operation. If emergent institution of cardiopulmonary bypass is necessary before dissection of the aorta, Seldinger cannulation of the aorta may be most expedient. Similarly, small areas on the right atrium should be selected and cleared of adhesions to facilitate expedient purse-string and venous cannula placement. Pericardium that is particularly adherent to the right atrium may be left in place to serve as pledget material along the atrial purse strings. The remaining dissection priorities include the superior and inferior venae cavae, the right pulmonary veins, and the interatrial groove as previously noted. The left side of the heart does not need to be cleared of adhesions nor does the left side of the pericardium need to be suspended. The heart should be allowed to drop back into the left chest as much as is feasible.

Institution of Cardiopulmonary Bypass

Bicaval cannulation is carried out using standard cannulas and purse-string techniques. However, correct placement of the superior vena cava cannula depends on the intended atrial incision. The superior vena cava cannula is placed in the region of the previously cannulated right atrial appendage when an interatrial groove approach is planned. Alternatively, the cannula is placed in the lateral wall of the right atrium when a transplant-type transatrial transseptal incision will be used. When placing the atrial purse strings, the surgeon must avoid placing them too close to the venae cavae or sinoatrial (SA) node. Direct cannulation of the superior vena cava is also acceptable.

The arterial perfusion setup includes an arterial cannula for either the aorta or for an alternative site, such as the axillary artery or femoral artery. We prefer to use the aortic position whenever possible. However, we do not hesitate to use alternative sites when access to the aorta is difficult or the aorta is diseased. When alternative sites of arterial perfusion are necessary, fibrillatory cardiac arrest rather than cardioplegic arrest may be needed. After bypass has been established, constant vigilance is maintained for pump-related problems along with a willingness to alter the approach to bypass as required. Dissection of the aorta for clamping is often easiest on the right lateral and posterior portions. After this is accomplished, the pulmonary artery can be dissected free from the aorta to allow safe clamping.

Myocardial Protection

We favor combined antegrade-retrograde induction of cold blood cardioplegia for all re-do mitral valve operations. This approach optimizes myocardial protection. In addition, retrograde coronary flow also helps to purge air from the coronary circulation before the aorta is unclamped. Antegrade infusion is administered through the aortic root using a dual-lumen cardioplegia/venting device. Patients with aortic valve insufficiency could undergo intracoronary delivery of cardioplegic perfusion by the surgeon's performing an aortotomy with insertion of the hand-held perfusion catheter into the coronary or bypass graft ostia. This is usually reserved for the situation in which exclusive use of retrograde cardioplegia is clinically insufficient. Retrograde cardioplegic perfusion is delivered using a standard retrograde cardioplegia catheter inserted through the right atrium with its tip in the coronary sinus. Cardioplegic perfusion can be administered in a continuous or intermittent manner. We prefer the intermittent administration of cardioplegic perfusate. When hypothermic fibrillation is used for myocardial protection (as in the setting of alternative sites of arterial perfusion), the temperature must be kept at <28°C to prevent intraoperative cardioversion while the heart is open. Topical cooling of the right ventricle can be used as an adjunctive measure of myocardial protection. Topically applied saline slush must not be left in contact with the phrenic nerve, because this has been shown to cause injury.

The degree of systemic hypothermia used during cardiopulmonary bypass is largely dependent on the preference of the individual surgeon. We generally use temperatures of 28°C to 32°C, except as noted during fibrillatory arrest. The ventricle is protected from distention as long as it is beating. At the onset of fibrillation, however, the aorta should be clamped or the left heart should be opened or vented to prevent distention and resulting stretch injury to the myocardium.

Choice of Atriotomy

The optimal approach to the mitral valve provides an unencumbered view of the complete mitral annulus and subvalvular apparatus without damage to the surrounding structures. A number of atrial incisions that afford this exposure have been described. The surgeon should be familiar with several approaches because the choice of incision will vary from case to case depending on the anatomy encountered at operation. Many patients with mitral valve disease will have an enlarged left atrium, which makes exposure of the mitral valve relatively straightforward. In the setting of a large left atrium, the horizontal left atriotomy provides excellent visualization of the valve structures. If the left atrium is small or if dense adhesions are present within a previously dissected interatrial groove, other techniques may be used. These include the superior septal exposure of the mitral valve, also known as the "transplant incision"; the transatrial oblique approach, which traverses the right superior pulmonary vein; and the Carpentier transatrial approach. As previously noted, the positioning of the atrial cannulas is determined after the choice of atrial incision has been made.

In most cases, exposure of the mitral valve using the horizontal left atriotomy is adequate. A number of tricks can be used to aid in this exposure. First, the right atrium is dissected away from the left atrium in Waterston's groove as far as possible (Fig. 43-3). In the primary operation, this is done by incising the fat pad in the interatrial groove and sweeping the overlying right atrium medially. If an extensive interatrial groove dissection was performed at the initial operation, dissecting the groove again can be difficult. Under these conditions, the surgeon may choose another approach. Often, however, surgeons doing mitral valve surgery do not perform extensive interatrial groove dissections, leaving this plane fresh for re-do operations. Additionally, the pericardial reflections should be incised inferiorly and superiorly to allow both vena cavae to move

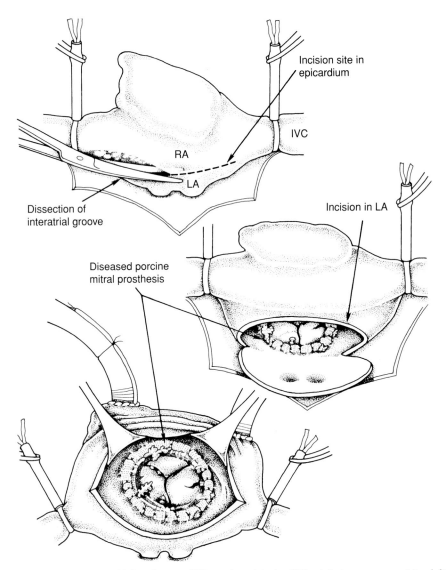

Figure 43-3. Horizontal left atriotomy. (AV = atrioventricular; IVC = inferior vena cava; LA = left atrium; RA = right atrium.)

anteriorly and to the patient's left, further exposing the mitral valve. The atriotomy itself may be extended superiorly and inferiorly (Fig. 43-3). The incision can also be extended across the dome of the left atrium toward the atrial appendage, especially with good mobilization of the superior vena cava. A more extensive incision at this time minimizes the chance of tearing or stretching the heart during the operation. The horizontal left atriotomy provides excellent exposure of the mitral apparatus in the majority of patients (Fig. 43-3).

The superior-septal approach to the mitral valve is based on the atrial incisions used for recipient cardiectomy during heart transplantation. After cardiopulmonary bypass is initiated, the caval tapes are tightened to allow the right atrium to be opened. The in-

cision is started in the mid-lateral wall of the right atrium between the two cannulation sites, carried anteriorly through the right atrial appendage, and continued posteriorly toward the superior end of the interatrial septum (Fig. 43-4). Retracting the anterior edge of the right atrium to the left exposes the fossa ovalis, which is incised (Fig. 43-4). This septal incision is extended cephalad to join the right atrial incision. The superior aspect of the left atrium is next incised, beginning at the confluence of the two previous incisions and extending across the dome of the left atrium toward the left atrial appendage (Fig. 43-4). The artery to the sinus node is usually cut when the atrial incisions are joined across the top of the septum. This devascularization of the SA node may lead to sinus node dysfunction post-

operatively, although a permanent problem with SA nodal function has not been frequently observed in our practice. Care is taken to leave 1 cm to 2 cm of right atrial tissue on the ventricular side of the incision to facilitate closure. Retraction of the right ventricle, the right atrium, and the roof of the left atrium to the left exposes the mitral valve apparatus. Stay sutures or retractors can be placed to maintain this exposure. A pledgetted polypropylene suture in the floor of the left atrium also helps to expose the valve by pulling the posterior mitral annulus anteriorly and superiorly toward the surgeon. Similarly, pledgetted sutures in the trigones can bring the annulus toward the surgeon.

The superior pulmonary vein exposure of the mitral valve can be useful in patients with a small left atrium. The atriotomy is made at the junction of the superior pulmonary vein and the left atrium and extended anteriorly along the right atrial free wall between the two cannulation sites (Fig. 43-5). The incision is then extended into the interatrial septum to the limbus of the fossa ovalis (Fig. 43-5). Retractors can then be inserted into the left atrium to expose the mitral valve (Fig. 43-5).

The transatrial approach proposed by Carpentier combines the advantages of the horizontal left atriotomy with the transseptal "transplant incision." The surgeon first incises the left atrium parallel to the interatrial groove as with the horizontal left atriotomy. The incision is next extended across the free wall of the right atrium toward the inferior vena caval cannula (Fig. 43-6). Additional exposure of the left atrium is then achieved by dividing the interatrial septum toward the coronary sinus. A stay suture placed at the opening of the coronary sinus serves to mark the limit of the septal incision (Fig. 43-6). Additional stay sutures retract the septum and expose the diseased mitral prosthesis (Fig. 43-6).

Strategies for Dealing with an Aortic Prosthesis Already in Place

If the patient has an aortic prosthesis already in place, a number of decisions must be made. If the valve is a porcine valve, it should be replaced at the time of this operation. If the valve is a durable mechanical valve, an approach to the mitral valve should be chosen that will not harm the aortic prosthesis. In this situation we favor median

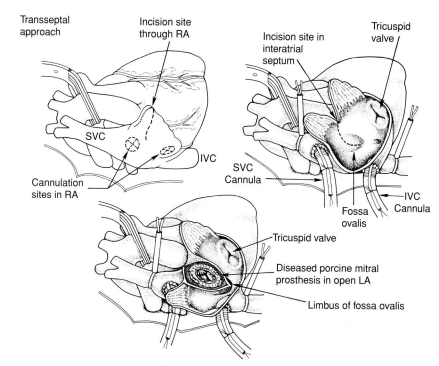

Figure 43-4. Trans-septal atriotomy. (IVC = inferior vena cava; LA = left atrium; RA = right atrium; SVC = superior vena cava.)

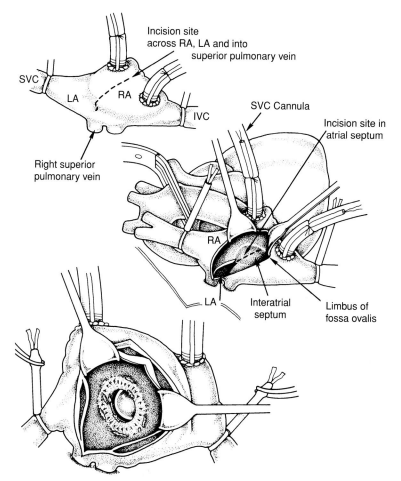

Figure 43-5. Transatrial oblique atriotomy. (IVC = inferior vena cava; LA = left atrium; RA = right atrium; SVC = superior vena cava.)

sternotomy with the transseptal approach or anterolateral thoracotomy.

Removal of the Old Prosthesis

In patients who have previously undergone mitral valve repair using a rigid annuloplasty ring, the metal skeleton of the ring must be removed to allow appropriate sealing of the annulus around the new prosthesis. This can be accomplished by incising the cloth covering on the ring and dividing the wire with a wire cutter. The wire is then pulled out, leaving the well-incorporated cloth covering in place (Fig. 43-7). Although it is ideal to remove all prosthetic material, flexible annuloplasty rings may be left in place as long as they appear to be well incorporated into the annulus. The ring should be completely removed, however, if there is any doubt about its incorporation into the annulus (Fig. 43-7).

The removal of prosthetic material in patients who have previously undergone valve replacement is facilitated by knowing whether the old prosthesis was implanted with everting sutures with pledgets on the atrial side or with an inverting technique with pledgets on the ventricular side. Each suture should be carefully removed, one at a time, accounting for each pledget. Pledgets left behind may seem to exhibit good ingrowth, but their stability should not be trusted. After the sutures and pledgets are removed, the old sewing ring is grasped with a Kocher clamp and dissected from the underlying annulus with a knife, a vascular spatula, or an elevator (Fig. 43-8).

Some surgeons have recently advocated leaving the sewing ring of an old porcine valve in place, with simple excision of the valve leaflets followed by mounting of a new mechanical prosthesis within the old ring. This approach has the advantage of avoiding dissection of the old sewing ring, but it has the disadvantage of potential leaking, which could occur between the old and new sewing rings. Interrupted sutures are then used to seat the prosthesis followed by a continuous suture to seal the two sewing rings.

Reconstruction of the Annulus

Once the old valve has been explanted and sent for culture, the annulus must be inspected. If injury to the annulus occurred during removal of the old valve or if infection was present, the annulus will need to be repaired or reconstructed. Small defects may be repaired with pledgeted sutures used to replace the valve if placed straddling the injured area of annulus. Larger defects in the

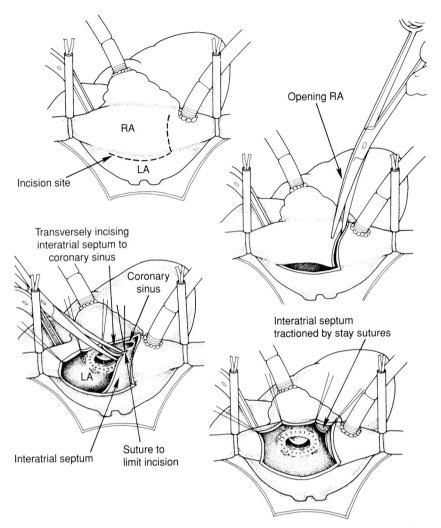

Figure 43-6. Carpentier transatrial approach. (LA = left atrium; RA = right atrium.)

annulus that are in essence points of atrioventricular discontinuity must be repaired using a patch to avoid tension. Autogenous or bovine pericardium may be used as patch material. These pericardial patches are secured with a running 4-0 or 5-0 polypropylene suture (Fig. 43-9).

Heavy calcification within the annulus may need to be addressed. Often, inadequate débridement of calcium during the primary operation is the reason a second mitral valve procedure is required. Sutures cannot be placed easily through calcium deposits, and seating a valve in the irregular and rocky terrain of a heavily calcified mitral annulus is difficult at best. For these reasons, we favor removal of the calcium in a manner quite similar to the techniques used in aortic annular débridement or in carotid endarterectomy (Fig. 43-10). Despite the observation that calcium deposits frequently extend deep into the posterior atrioventricu-

lar groove, we believe that virtually complete removal is warranted.

It is thought that maintaining the connection between the annulus and the papillary muscles is beneficial to future cardiac function. An intact posterior leaflet achieves this goal in the majority of patients. The anterior leaflet may, therefore, be completely excised without losing the connection of both papillary muscles to the annulus. Techniques for maintaining continuity of the major strut chordae to the anterior annulus, however, are not difficult to incorporate in valve replacement and may prove superior to preservation of the posterior leaflet alone. Occasionally, the posterior leaflet must be reattached to the annulus with a running suture, a repair that will be strengthened by the valve implantation technique. Occasionally, continuity between the annulus and papillary muscles cannot be maintained for a variety of anatomic or mechanical reasons.

Nevertheless, good cardiac function can still be maintained, because the contribution of this connection to overall cardiac function is probably small in most patients.

Valve Implantation

When choosing between a porcine bioprosthesis and a mechanical prosthesis, the usual guidelines should be followed, although many of our reoperative mitral valve patients receive mechanical valves. When selecting a mechanical valve, several issues are important. The bileaflet valves, such as the St. Jude prosthesis, have good hemodynamic performance and reliable long-term clinical outcomes. The annulus, however, must be carefully checked for scar tissue, which could interfere with leaflet action. Characteristics such as a low profile and thick sewing ring are preferred when a bioprosthetic valve is necessary for replacement. The lower-profile valves are well suited for both hypertrophic and dilated ventricles, whereas a thick sewing ring appears to seal the irregular re-do annulus. The optimal suturing technique for valve implantation depends on the degree of thickening around the mitral orifice. Similar to primary valve replacement, everting interrupted sutures placed from the atrial side into the ventricle is appropriate if the valve orifice is not particularly thickened (Fig. 43-11). In cases where the annular tissue is very thickened, friable, infected, or otherwise untrustworthy, the sutures should be placed in a mattress fashion from the ventricular side to the atrial side using what is known as the subannular stitch technique (Fig. 43-12). We have found that using a continuous strip of polytetrafluoroethylene (Teflon) pledget material can be superior to using individual pledgets. A 3-mm wide strip of Teflon felt is cut and placed within the ventricle just under the lip of the mitral valve orifice. Sutures of 2-0 braided polyester fiber with large needles are placed sequentially through this pledget, then brought out through the atrium, and finally through the valve ring. The continuous pledget strip eliminates the need to "seat" each pledget appropriately, effectively repairs annular defects, and helps to spread the tension of the sutures uniformly around the orifice (Fig. 43-13). Consideration may also be given to using a running suture for implantation of the valve. Running sutures have been favored by some surgeons for all mitral valve implantations. A very long (54-in.) 2-0 suture with a large needle is

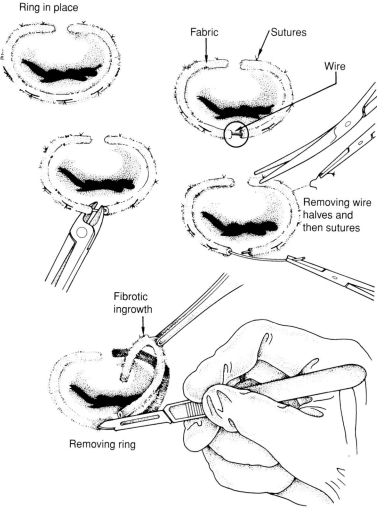

Figure 43-7. Annuloplasty ring removal.

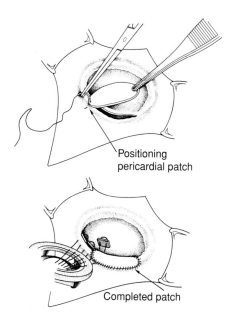

Figure 43-9. Patch repair of the annulus.

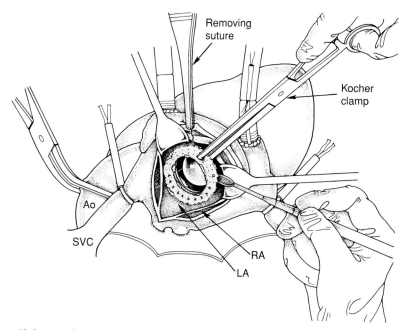

Figure 43-8. Prosthesis removal. (Ao = aorta; LA = left atrium; RA = right atrium; SVC = superior vena cava.)

used to suture the posterior portion of the valve first, using an "open" technique. The valve is then pulled down into place and the anterior portion of the valve is then sewn in (Fig. 43-14).

As sutures are being placed, the surgeon must be cognizant of surrounding structures that may be injured (Fig. 43-15). The circumflex coronary artery will be to the left on the posterior side of the mitral annulus, and the coronary sinus will be to the right on the posterior side on the annulus. The atrioventricular node will be to the right on the anterior portion of the annulus, and the aortic valve will be to the left on the anterior portion of the mitral annulus (Fig. 43-16). Secure placement of valve sutures is of critical importance. It would be preferable to have to insert a permanent pacemaker or to repair or ligate an injured coronary sinus than to undertake a second re-do valve replacement because of inadequate suture placement. Perhaps the most worrisome event is an injury to the circumflex artery. Fortunately, this artery is located fairly deep in the atrioventricular groove and well away from the mitral annulus. If an injury is suspected as the stitch is placed, however, the needle should be removed and replaced more superficially. Transesophageal echocardiography could then be used to monitor the function of the lateral wall. If injury has in fact occurred, a vein graft to a lateral wall vessel after implantation of the valve could be carried out. Protection of the lateral wall myocardium during such an event would

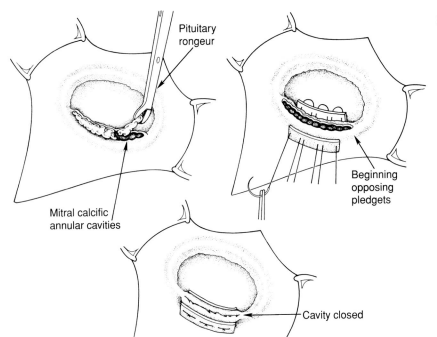

Figure 43-10   Primary repair of the annulus.

Pituitary rongeur

Mitral calcific annular cavities

Beginning opposing pledgets

Cavity closed

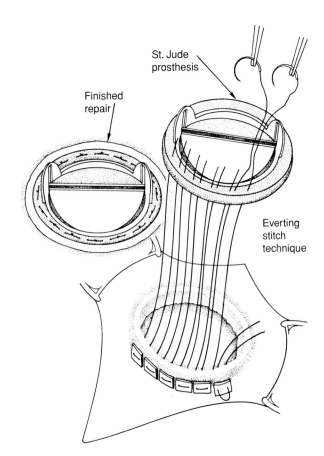

St. Jude prosthesis

Finished repair

Everting stitch technique

Figure 43-11.   Valve implantation with an everting stitch.

Figure 43-12 Valve implantation with a subannular stitch.

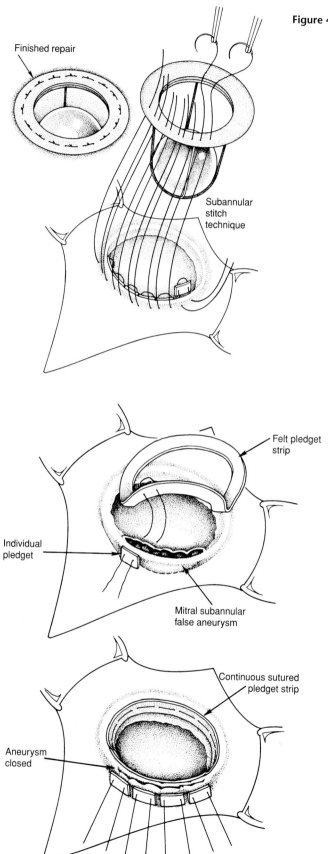

Finished repair

Subannular stitch technique

Felt pledget strip

Individual pledget

Mitral subannular false aneurysm

Continuous sutured pledget strip

Aneurysm closed

Figure 43-13. The continuous pledget strip technique.

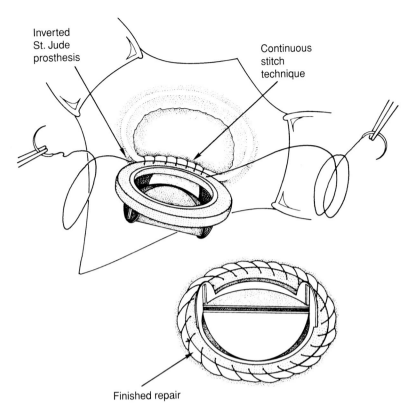

Figure 43-14. Valve implantation with a continuous suture.

be well maintained if retrograde cardioplegia were in use.

In checking the valve once it has been implanted, the surgeon must be sure that the valve has seated properly. Before the sutures are tied, an attempt should be made to inspect the ventricular side of the valve with a dental mirror when feasible. This will be possible in valves such as the Starr, Medtronic Hall, and pig valves, but not with the St. Jude valve. It is particularly important to be sure that the sutures have not become entangled around the struts of a porcine valve, if such a valve has been used, and that the string holding these struts together has been appropriately cut. This potential complication has recently been designed out of several valves by drawing in the valve struts on the applicator prior to release at which the struts take their normal position. Finally, the atriotomy is closed using a running 4-0 or 3-0 polypropylene suture in a single layer.

In finishing the operation, the surgeon must carry out a defined and specific strategy for de-airing the heart. Air is removed from the left ventricle by lifting it gently and placing a needle through the apex while "stealing" blood from the cardiopulmonary circuit (Fig. 43-17). Rendering the mitral prosthesis temporarily incompetent with a red rubber catheter causes the ejection of additional air out of the left ventricle into the atrium (Fig. 43-18). The two most effective methods for de-airing the aorta are (1) to make a small aortotomy with a No. 11 blade on the anterior surface of the aorta through which air can vent and (2) to place the cardioplegia catheter on high suction during the de-airing process. De-airing is aided if CO_2 insufflation is used throughout the case.

Before closure of the atria, the orifice of the left atrial appendage should be sewn shut with a 3-0 polypropylene purse-string suture (Fig. 43-19). (Alternatively, many oversew the appendage early in the operation in order not to forget this important step. Furthermore, the suture used for this may be left long to aid in exposing the annulus if it is difficult to visualize.) The maneuver minimizes the risk of clot formation or air entrapment within the appendage, which could result in later embolization. Air can be removed from the left atrium by allowing backbleeding through the atriotomy before the final suture line is tied. The heart is gently shaken to remove small air bubbles entrapped in various endocardial interstices, and a Valsalva's technique is used to remove air from the pulmonary veins. Perhaps most important in the de-airing sequence is examination of the heart with transesophageal echocardiography to confirm that de-airing has been successful.

The final stage of de-airing entails cycling on and off of cardiopulmonary bypass with the patient in the Trendelenburg position. Suction is maintained on the aortic root, or the aortotomy is kept open to allow air to escape. At the time of removing

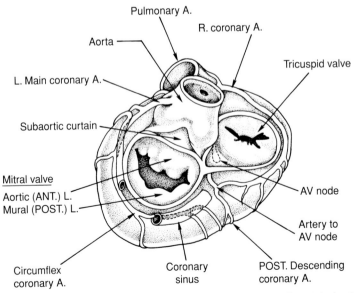

Figure 43-15. Cardiac anatomy. (A. = artery; ANT. = anterior; AV = atrioventricular; L. = left; POST. = posterior; R. = right.)

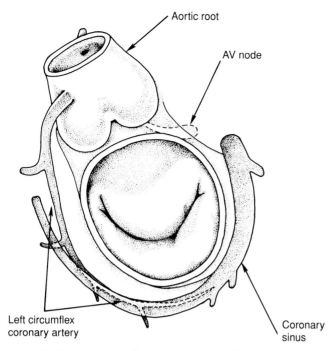

Figure 43-16. Perivalvular anatomic structures. (AV = atrioventricular.)

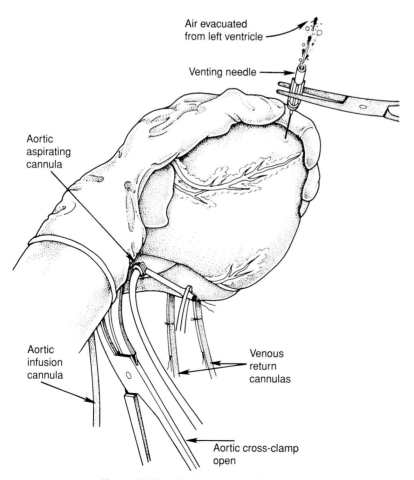

Figure 43-17. De-airing of the left ventricle.

the cross-clamp, the retrograde cardioplegia catheter infuses warm blood at a rate of approximately 150 mL/min for several minutes. We have found this maneuver to be an extremely effective method of preventing coronary air embolization at this critical juncture. Transesophageal echocardiography is used once again to check for the presence of residual air and for any evidence of perivalvular leak. If a significant perivalvular leak is present, the heart should be perfused for several minutes, reclamped, reprotected, and the leak repaired. An uncorrected perivalvular leak represents a serious problem for the patient, whereas a second period of myocardial ischemia will be reasonably well tolerated, particularly if the method of myocardial protection for the first period of ischemia was optimal.

Pacing wires are placed on both the atrium and the ventricle. Atrial wires should be placed in such a way as to be benign in their removal. Often, they can be placed on the tough atrial tissue where the purse strings for the cannulas have been. The ventricular wires should be placed as close to the apex as possible so that myocardial excitation-contraction begins at the apex in as physiologic a manner as possible. Wires placed inappropriately high on the ventricle can produce a sort of iatrogenic subaortic stenosis.

Closure

Closure of the median sternotomy is carried out in the standard manner. Particular attention needs to be paid to the sternum to be sure that it is intact and can hold wires. If the sternal bone is unhealthy or unable to hold sutures, it may be reinforced with vertical wires woven through the interspaces on either side of the sternum. Furthermore, it is essential that the fascia of the chest wall be closed securely. We consider this of equal importance to sternal closure in maintaining the stability of the chest wall. If a right anterolateral thoracotomy has been used, pericostal sutures are placed. We believe it is worthwhile to avoid trapping the intercostal nerve in the pericostal suture as it passes under the lower rib. Sutures may be placed directly through the rib using a rib punch, or the intercostal bundle can be dissected off the rib at the points where the pericostal sutures are to be placed. With the use of these techniques, postoperative pain can be lessened for some patients.

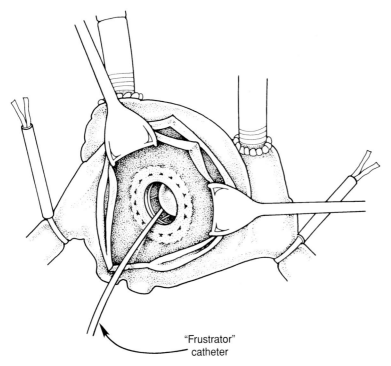

"Frustrator"
catheter

Figure 43-18. Rendering the prosthesis incompetent.

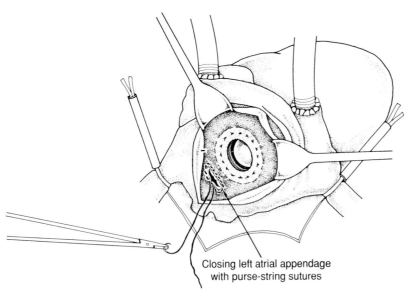

Closing left atrial appendage
with purse-string sutures

Figure 43-19. Exclusion of the left atrial appendage.

SUGGESTED READING

Berreklouw E, Ercan H, Schonberger JP. Combined superior-transseptal approach to the left atrium. Ann Thorac Surg 1991;51:293.

Cohn LH, Aranki SF, Rizzo RJ, et al. Decrease in operative risk of reoperative valve surgery. Ann Thorac Surg 1993;56:15.

Deloche A, Acar C, Jebara V, et al. Biatrial transseptal approach in case of difficult exposure of the mitral valve. Ann Thorac Surg 1990;50:318.

Najafi H, Guynn T, Najafi C, et al. Declining risk of reoperative valvular surgery. J Card Surg 1995;10:185.

Smith CR. Septal-superior exposure of the mitral valve. The transplant approach. J Thorac Cardiovasc Surg 1992;103:623.

Tribble CG, Killinger WA, Harman PK, et al. Anterolateral thoracotomy as an alternative to repeat median sternotomy for replacement of the mitral valve. Ann Thorac Surg 1987;43:380.

Tribble CG, Nolan SP, Kron IL. Anterolateral thoracotomy as an alternative to repeat median sternotomy for replacement of the mitral valve. Ann Thorac Surg 1995;59:255.

EDITOR'S COMMENTS

One of the more difficult cases for the less experienced surgeon is a re-do mitral valve replacement. This chapter is extensive in its detail in terms of the concept of right thoracotomy versus repeat sternotomy. Many tricks of the trade have been used and are well illustrated. The focus of my commentary is on whether right thoracotomy should be used. My belief has been that right thoracotomy should be used in those situations in which a very rapid entry is required or in which there are factors such as patent right internal mammary or left internal mammary artery to a coronary artery that may be injured by sternotomy. Right thoracotomy allows for excellent exposure of the mitral valve, but it does not allow one to visualize the heart extremely well nor to do any other procedures other than deal with the mitral valve. Therefore, the majority of repeat mitral operations that I have done have been done through the sternotomy as suggested by these authors. Their overall approach has been used at the University of Virginia and has been extremely successful in our hands.

I.L.K.

44

Tricuspid Valve

Benjamin B. Peeler

Introduction

Isolated surgery on the tricuspid valve in the adult population is required uncommonly because it is rare to encounter a patient with severe isolated tricuspid insufficiency. In adult practice, tricuspid valve insufficiency is most often secondary to left-sided valvular and/or myocardial disease with subsequent pulmonary hypertension, right ventricular hypertrophy, and dilation with subsequent annular enlargement. In these cases, the valve leaflets are structurally normal but fail to coapt appropriately, resulting in so-called functional tricuspid regurgitation. Operative indications in cases of functional regurgitation are often unclear for several reasons. First, the usually low pressure right-sided circulation is more tolerant to imperfect function of the tricuspid valve. Second, tricuspid valve regurgitation most often occurs in the setting of left-sided pathology, which serves as the primary surgical indication, resulting in an often long and complex procedure with higher risk. In addition, tricuspid valve function is dependent on the functional status of the right ventricle, with poor function and dilation resulting in failure of apposition of the structurally normal tricuspid valve leaflets. In most cases, some improvement in valve function can be expected after correction of left-sided pathology, thus in some cases obviating the need to extend the length of the operation. It is difficult to impossible, however, to accurately gauge which valves will improve and how much after correction of left-sided lesions, thus justifying a reasonably aggressive approach to concomitant repair of the tricuspid valve.

A more dangerous clinical scenario is encountered when the surgeon is asked to evaluate a patient with probably fixed pulmonary hypertension, right ventricular dysfunction, and severe tricuspid regurgitation with no real or active left-sided pathology but with right-sided failure symptoms. The prognosis in this especially high risk group of patients is related to the etiology of the right ventricular dysfunction (chronic pulmonary emboli, lung disease, etc.), and often their demise is only hastened by operation.

Primary leaflet abnormalities of the tricuspid valve are less common and are caused most commonly by infectious endocarditis and carcinoid heart disease. Ebstein's anomaly may also be first diagnosed in adulthood in its less severe forms. The more severe forms generally require surgical intervention in one form or another in the newborn period and/or childhood.

Evaluation and Operative Indications

Functional Tricuspid Regurgitation

In the adult, the tricuspid lesion most often requiring surgical therapy is functional tricuspid regurgitation secondary to left-sided cardiac pathology with subsequent pulmonary hypertension, right ventricular dilation, and subsequent annular dilation of the tricuspid valve. It is quite unusual to encounter a patient with isolated tricuspid valve regurgitation secondary to annular dilation with structurally normal tricuspid valve leaflets requiring surgery. Tricuspid annular dilation with resultant regurgitation in current practice is by far most often encountered secondary to left-sided cardiac pathology. Echocardiography is the most helpful modality in evaluating tricuspid valve regurgitation and reliably distinguishes between annular problems and primary leaflet problems. Transthoracic echocardiography usually provides excellent evaluation of the structure and hemodynamic function of the valve. Cardiac catheterization will often be done in these patients preoperatively, given considerations of age and often accompanying cardiac pathology. Although tricuspid valve regurgitation is poorly assessed by cardiac catheterization, assessment of right-sided hemodynamics during catheterization can be quite helpful.

Echocardiographic signs of severe tricuspid valve regurgitation include dilation of the right atrium, right ventricle, and inferior vena cava, along with a large color flow jet across the tricuspid valve.

The questions in cases of left-sided pathology with secondary tricuspid regurgitation are how much improvement in right ventricular and tricuspid valve geometry can be expected if left alone and when is tricuspid valve repair warranted. Given the relative technical simplicity of the procedure and the inherent difficulty in predicting postoperative improvement in tricuspid valve function after correction of left-sided lesions, we apply tricuspid valve annuloplasty aggressively to patients undergoing left-sided valvular surgery with tricuspid regurgitation (TR) graded 2+ or greater on preoperative echocardiography. Certainly patients undergoing second mitral valve operations with associated 2+ or greater tricuspid TR, patients with long-standing left atrial hypertension, typically rheumatics with 2+ or greater TR, and anyone likely to have persistent pulmonary hypertension and 2+ or greater TR should be strongly considered for concomitant tricuspid repair as part of their planned cardiac procedure.

In the rare patient with isolated tricuspid insufficiency, surgical correction is warranted when symptoms are refractory to maximal medical therapy. Often these patients will have difficult-to-treat congestive heart failure with significant peripheral edema and clinically significant passive congestion of the liver. Intensified diuretic administration often results in elevation in blood urea nitrogen (BUN) and creatinine rather than improvement in the patient's clinical status. Tricuspid valve repair in carefully selected patients may improve forward flow and improve the marked venous congestion that these patients suffer.

Carcinoid Heart Disease

Cardiac involvement occurs in the majority of patients with carcinoid syndrome, although clinically significant lesions are much less common. Right-sided cardiac structures including the tricuspid and pulmonic valves as well as the right ventricular endocardium are involved by far the most frequently. Right-sided structures are affected predominantly. Endocardial plaquing, the typical lesion seen in carcinoid heart disease, may involve either or both the pulmonic and tricuspid valves as well as the right ventricular endocardial surface. Tricuspid stenosis or regurgitation is equally likely in these patients. Evidence of tricuspid (and likely pulmonic) valve dysfunction and progressive right heart failure is the usual clinical presentation of patients considered for surgery. With current methods of treatment of malignant carcinoid tumors, significant survival rates (>50% at 5 years) can be expected. Thus, patients with valvular dysfunction and progressive heart failure should be considered for valve replacement if their tumor is not imminently life-threatening.

Endocarditis

Infectious endocarditis involving the tricuspid valve can occur as either an isolated valvular problem or as part of a multivalve process. The tricuspid valve is most frequently involved in cases of endocarditis secondary to intravenous drug abuse, occurring in nearly three fourths of these cases, whereas involvement of the mitral and aortic valve occurs in one fourth to one third of cases. Pulmonic valve involvement is much more rare, accounting for 1% or less of cases. Right-sided endocarditis is to be expected in intravenous drug abusers who present with fever and radiologic pulmonary infiltrates even in the absence of a significant murmur. Transthoracic echocardiography is quite accurate in evaluating tricuspid endocarditis.

Indications for surgery for right-sided endocarditis in intravenous drug abusers are limited compared to surgical indications for left-sided lesions. The tricuspid valve exists in a low-pressure circuit, and thus there is better tolerance for imperfect function. Second, the consequences of embolization from the tricuspid valve are less catastrophic than those from embolization from the left-sided valves. In addition, the risk of ongoing intravenous drug abuse with ongoing risks including reinfection and overdose as well as the risk of HIV infection also dictate a conservative approach to surgery in these patients. Two important indications for surgery for tricuspid valve endocarditis are (1) endocarditis caused by microorganisms that are difficult to eradicate such as fungal organisms or bacteria resistant to antibiotic therapy and (2) patients with tricuspid valve vegetations >2 cm, a dilated right ventricle, and recurrent pulmonary emboli or right-sided heart failure. When surgery is necessary, debridement of infected tissue and preservation of the native valve is preferred when at all possible. Patients usually have significant degrees of valve regurgitation, and restoration of complete competence is neither possible nor necessary. Complete excision of the valve has been favored by some surgeons because of the risk of reinfection of an implanted prosthetic valve by continued IV drug use. Some patients undergoing excision will eventually require prosthetic valve insertion secondary to poor cardiac output, whereas some fail immediately. Patients with any degree of pulmonary hypertension, sometimes related to extensive septic pulmonary emboli, will tolerate the absence of the tricuspid valve poorly. Valve excision without replacement should be avoided in these patients.

Ebstein's Anomaly

Ebstein's anomaly causes varying degrees of tricuspid regurgitation and may be clinically silent or present at any time in children or adults. The lesion is characterized by downward displacement of the septal and often posterior leaflets of the valve into the right ventricle (Fig. 44-1). This gives the characteristic "atrialized" appearance of the right ventricle. The annular circumference is often quite large, and the right atrium is quite enlarged. The anterior leaflet is generally large and sail-like. The quality of the anterior leaflet is at best relatively thin and pliable, but instead may be thickened and muscularized. The quality of the anterior leaflet is critical to the success of any attempted valve repair for Ebstein's anomaly. A thickened, muscularized anterior leaflet makes a poor substrate for Ebstein's repair.

Ebstein's anomaly of the tricuspid valve may present along a spectrum of severity and may become clinically significant at any time during life and require surgical intervention. In the neonatal period, transplantation or single-ventricle palliation (Starne's procedure) may be required. Adults with less severe forms of Ebstein's may nonetheless become symptomatic and require surgical intervention.

In adults presenting with Ebstein's anomaly, symptoms may include arrhythmias, fatigability, dyspnea, and cyanosis. In addition, patients with Ebstein's anomaly may have an associated atrial septal defect and may present with paradoxical embolus into the systemic circulation. Echocardiography is useful for characterizing the degree of valvular insufficiency and the quality of the leaflets, specifically the quality of the anterior leaflet when contemplating valve repair. Repair of the valve is obviously favored when possible. Replacement is necessary in some cases, however. Given the relatively young age of many adults requiring surgery for Ebstein's, mechanical valve replacement should be contemplated. Reports in the literature show similar rates of complication, including thromboembolism, in patients undergoing mechanical versus bioprosthetic tricuspid valve replacement.

Anatomy of the Tricuspid Valve

Fortunately, in most patients undergoing tricuspid valve surgery there is at least some degree of enlargement of the right atrium, which allows ample exposure of the valve. Bicaval cannulation is easily accomplished while still allowing for a generous right atriotomy. Certainly, superior vena caval cannulation should avoid injury to the sinus node, but this should be relatively straightforward. After right atriotomy is performed, the tricuspid valve is easily visualized with the septal leaflet lying closest to the surgeon, the anterior leaflet away from the surgeon, and the posterior leaflet closest to the inferior vena caval cannula (Fig. 44-2).

The anterior leaflet is quadrangular and is the largest of the three leaflets. Its chordae are derived from the anterior and posterior papillary muscles. The posterior leaflet generally is the smallest of the three leaflets and is triangular. Its chordae are also derived

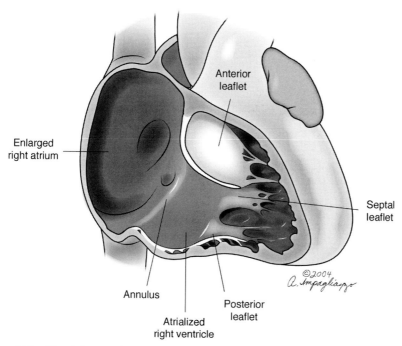

Figure 44-1. Ebstein's anomaly of the tricuspid valve, showing downward displacement of the septal and posterior tricuspid leaflets as well as "atrialization of the right ventricle."

from the anterior and posterior papillary muscles. The septal leaflet is semicircular, inserting into the top of the ventricular septum at its inlet and membranous portions. The membranous portion of the ventricular septum generally lies beneath the portion of the septal leaflet nearest to the anteroseptal commissure when looking in from the right atrium.

The position of the atrioventricular node in close proximity to the septal leaflet of the tricuspid valve is of major importance to the surgeon. The atrioventricular node lies in the apex of the triangle of Koch, which is bounded by the septal annulus of the tricuspid valve, the coronary sinus, and the tendon of Todaro (Fig. 44-2). The bundle of His continues on from the atrioventricular node to pierce the central fibrous body that runs along the posteroinferior margin of the membranous septum.

This close proximity of the atrioventricular node to the septal leaflet is of prime importance during tricuspid valve surgery. During tricuspid valve replacement it is safest to leave a small margin of septal leaflet tissue in order to place the valve sutures so as to avoid injuring the conduction system. Most rings used for tricuspid valve annuloplasty are designed to specifically avoid placement of sutures in this critical area by leaving a gap in the ring in this area.

Operative Setup

The setup for cardiopulmonary bypass for operations involving the tricuspid valve depends on whether the operation is performed for isolated tricuspid valve disease or combined mitral valve and tricuspid valve surgery. In both types of cases, double venous cannulation is performed; however, the exact placement of the upper venous cannula depends on which technique of exposure of the valves is to be used. For operations involving only the tricuspid valve, a standard right atriotomy is made parallel to the atrioventricular groove (Fig. 44-3A). Performing separate longitudinal left and right atriotomies in cases of combined mitral and tricuspid valve procedures is straightforward and provides excellent exposure. In the setup for this type of exposure, the superior vena cava cannula will be placed via the right atrial appendage preparing for a standard right atriotomy. Alternatively, the cannula may be placed directly into the superior vena cava. If, however, a superior trans-septal approach to the left atrium is to be used, the superior vena caval cannula can be placed more laterally on the right atrial wall as is done for orthotopic heart transplantation (Fig. 44-3B). Various combinations of antegrade and retrograde cardioplegia can be used according to the surgeon's preference. If left-sided valvular surgery is to be performed, it is performed first, the left atriotomy is closed, and the tricuspid valve procedure is performed as the patient is rewarmed. Some surgeons prefer to remove the aortic cross-clamp before the tricuspid portion of the operation. However, tricuspid valve procedures generally add little additional time, and I prefer the bloodless, motionless field afforded by leaving the aortic clamp on. Mild hypothermia is used for isolated tricuspid valve procedures and moderate hypothermia can be used for longer multiple valve procedures. After adequate cardioplegia has been delivered, in

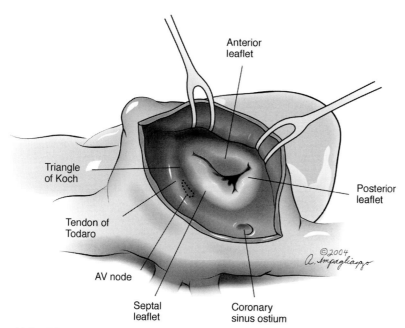

Figure 44-2. Tricuspid valve anatomy. Surgeon's view of the tricuspid valve as seen via right atriotomy. (AV = atrioventricular.)

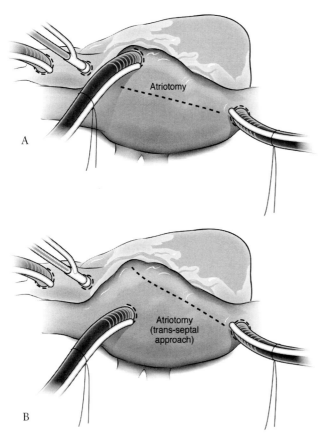

A

B

Figure 44-3. **(A)** Operative setup for standard right atriotomy parallel to the atrioventricular groove. **(B)** Operative setup for trans-septal approach to the mitral valve for operations involving both atrioventricular valves.

the case of an isolated tricuspid valve procedure, a standard right atriotomy is made parallel to the atrioventricular groove and far enough away from it to allow safe closure of the atriotomy without endangering the right coronary artery. After the atriotomy is made, exposure can be facilitated by suspending the edges of the atriotomy with silk stay sutures or by using a handheld or a self-retaining retractor system. The valve leaflets and subvalvular apparatus are inspected carefully, and the mechanism of tricuspid dysfunction is confirmed and dealt with accordingly.

Tricuspid Valve Annuloplasty

In considering repair of the tricuspid valve, we use the DeVega annuloplasty technique only rarely. This technique would be considered in cases that tricuspid regurgitation is secondary to a left-sided process and the amount of tricuspid regurgitation is 2+ or less by echocardiography with color flow Doppler.

For the DeVega annuloplasty (Fig. 44-4), 3-0 Prolene double-arm pledgeted sutures

are used. The inner suture line is begun approximately 3 mm off of the tricuspid annulus. The bites are approximately 3 mm in depth and 5 mm in length, skipping 5 mm between bites. This inner suture line proceeds in a clockwise fashion around the annulus to the posteroseptal commissure. The outer suture line is 3 mm outside the first and is placed in a similar fashion, in a clockwise direction to the posteroseptal commissure. A second Teflon pledget is passed onto the free ends of the suture. The suture is

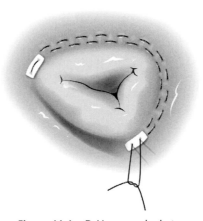

Figure 44-4. DeVega annuloplasty.

tightened down over a tricuspid ring sizer. A No. 29 sizer is generally adequate.

In isolated tricuspid regurgitation and for more severe forms of regurgitation with annular dilation in the presence of structurally normal leaflets, tricuspid ring annuloplasty is performed. We use the Carpentier-Edwards tricuspid annuloplasty ring, which is an incomplete ring leaving a gap in the area of the septal annulus adjacent to the conduction system. Sizing of the annuloplasty ring is done by referencing the intercommissural distance (anterior leaflet length). This can be done most accurately by distracting the chordae of the anterior leaflet adjacent to the commissures while using the ring sizers. Typically a No. 33 ring will be used for male patients and a No. 31 ring will be used for female patients.

Horizontal mattress sutures consisting of 2-0 Ticron with pledgets are used. No preset number of sutures is used for every case; rather a number suited to each particular patient is used. Typically there will be 3 mm to 4 mm between each suture in the annulus and 1 mm to 2 mm of space between each suture as it is placed through the annuloplasty ring. This will ensure even distribution of the annular plication around the circumference of the annuloplasty band. Each stitch enters the atrial tissue just outside the annulus and exits within the annulus (Figs. 44-5A, B). The suture is then placed through the inside of the ring to get the ring to seat in a directly annular position. The ring is lowered down to its annular position, and the sutures are tied and cut (Fig. 44-5C).

Tricuspid Valve Replacement

Tricuspid valve replacement may be indicated for infectious endocarditis, failed previous tricuspid repair, failing previously placed valve prosthesis, or the more rare instances of carcinoid heart disease or nonreconstructible rheumatic disease. In cases of endocarditis in drug-addicted patients, valvulectomy alone may be performed. In these cases, however, prosthetic replacement will be required if overt right heart failure is present or develops following the valvulectomy. Prosthetic replacement of the tricuspid valve with either a bioprosthetic or mechanical valve has been generally shown to be equally safe, although most would place a bioprosthetic valve in a drug-addicted patient with endocarditis. In patients who will require anticoagulation for

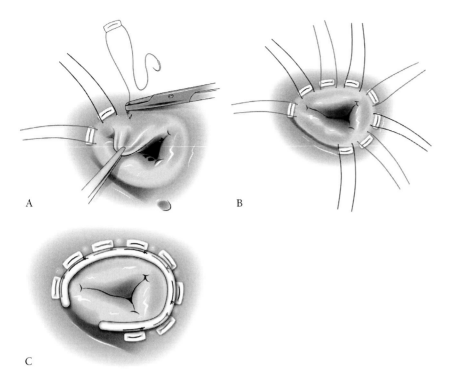

A

B

C

Figure 44-5. **(A)** Tricuspid valve annuloplasty. Placement of annuloplasty sutures in horizontal mattress fashion with needles passed through the annulus. **(B)** Tricuspid valve annuloplasty. Sutures in place. **(C)** Completed tricuspid valve annuloplasty using Carpentier-Edwards ring.

atrial fibrillation or the presence of a left-sided mechanical valve, a mechanical valve should be used in the tricuspid position.

The setup for tricuspid valve replacement is similar to that for a tricuspid valve repair. The valve is exposed, and the anterior and posterior leaflets are excised at their junction with the tricuspid annulus (Fig. 44-6A). The septal leaflet is excised leaving a 2-mm margin of septal leaflet adjacent to the annulus for suture placement to avoid injury to the conduction system. Excess chordal tissue is excised. Whether a bioprosthetic or mechanical valve is chosen, the suture placement is similar to the technique described for ring annuloplasty, that is, 2-0 Ticron pledgeted horizontal mattress sutures are placed with the needles entering just outside the tricuspid valve annulus and exiting from within the tricuspid annulus (Fig. 44-6B). In the area of the septal leaflet, the sutures are passed through the remnant of the leaflet to avoid injuring the conduction system. Alternatively, the sutures in this area can be placed below the annulus to protect the conduction system. The valve sutures are then passed through

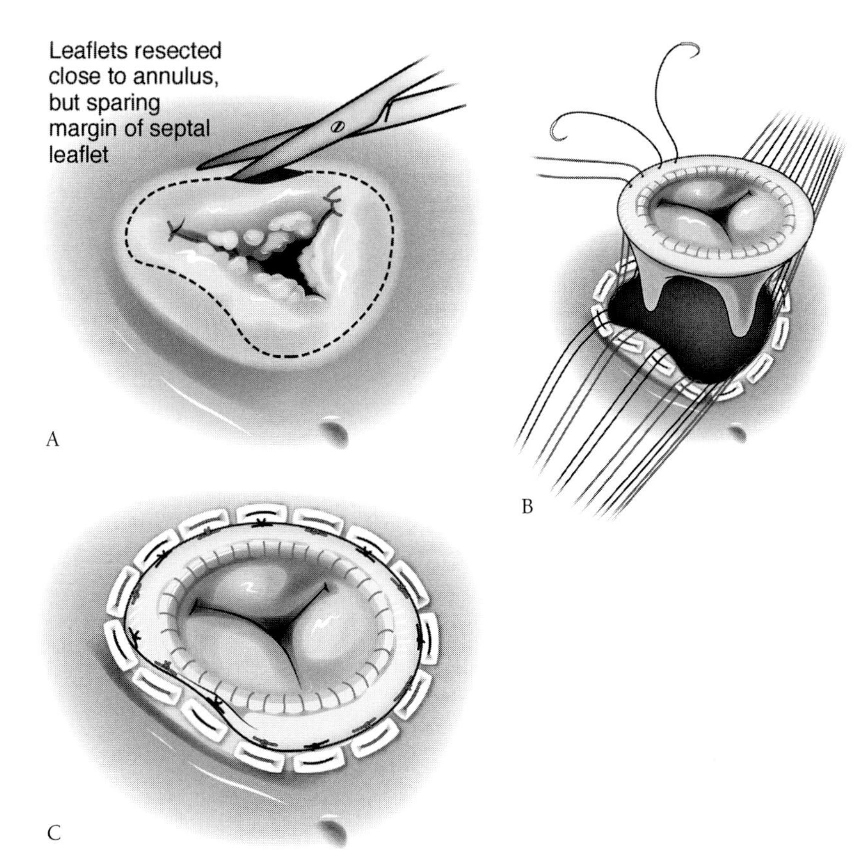

Leaflets resected
close to annulus,
but sparing
margin of septal
leaflet

A

B

C

Figure 44-6. **(A)** Tricuspid valve excision leaving a 2-mm margin of septal leaflet tissue adjacent to the annulus. **(B)** Suture placement for tricuspid valve replacement. **(C)** Completed tricuspid valve replacement.

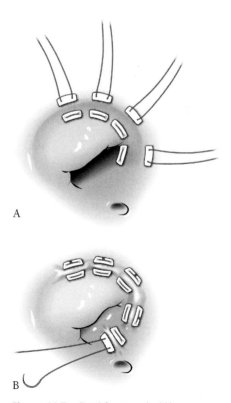

A

B

Figure 44-7. Danielson repair. **(A)** Pledgeted horizontal mattress sutures draw the tricuspid leaflets up to the tricuspid annulus. **(B)** Posterior annuloplasty suture lessens the annular circumference, creating a functional monocusp valve based on the anterior leaflet.

the sewing ring, the valve is lowered into position, and the sutures are tied and cut (Fig. 44-6C). In the case of placement of a bioprosthetic valve, the orientation of the valve is not critical because right ventricular outflow tract obstruction by one of the struts is unlikely.

Technique of Valve Repair for Ebstein's Anomaly

For repair of Ebstein's anomaly, the usual preparation is made for cardiopulmonary bypass. Double venous cannulation is used. Usually the right atrium is enlarged and cannulation of the superior vena cava via the right atrial appendage is used. Mild hypothermia is used. The aorta is cross-clamped and antegrade cardioplegia is delivered. Topical cold is applied to the heart. Once adequate myocardial preservation has been attained, a generous right atriotomy is made keeping in mind that in cases of a

markedly enlarged right atrium an ellipse of right atrial wall may be removed. The tricuspid valve and atrial septum are evaluated, and if an atrial defect is present, it is generally closed primarily after the tricuspid valve has been repaired. A cardiotomy sucker or vent catheter can be placed through the atrial septal defect during the tricuspid repair to facilitate visualization. The leaflets of the tricuspid valve are evaluated with particular attention to the morphology and quality of the anterior leaflet. Less satisfactory results can be predicted by the presence of a thickened muscularized anterior leaflet with fused or indistinct chordae. The Danielson and Carpentier methods of repair have both been used successfully; however, we have found the Carpentier repair to provide excellent results, given the appropriate candidate valve.

The Danielson repair (Fig. 44-7) in the adult involves the vertical plication of the atrialized portion of the right ventricle and creation of a functional monocusp valve based on the anterior leaflet. A portion of the right atrium is also removed to normalize its

size. Pledgeted horizontal mattress 3-0 Prolene sutures are placed from the downwardly displaced tricuspid valve to the tricuspid annulus. These sutures are tied down, drawing the tricuspid valve up to the tricuspid annulus and thus excluding the atrialized portion of the right ventricle. A 3-0 Prolene mattress posterior annuloplasty suture is also placed to reduce the annular circumference. Additional sutures may be placed to obliterate the remainder of the posterior tricuspid annulus. The atrial septal defect, if present, is closed.

The Carpentier repair (Figs. 44-8) uses longitudinal plication of the right ventricle and tricuspid annulus with resultant reduction in annular circumference. The anterior leaflet is detached along most of its annular circumference, and a sliding plasty is performed following annular plication using 4-0 Prolene running suture. This redistributes the anterior leaflet around much of the refashioned annulus. The result is effectively a monocusp valve that spans the tricuspid orifice. The repair is supported by placement of a Carpentier annuloplasty ring

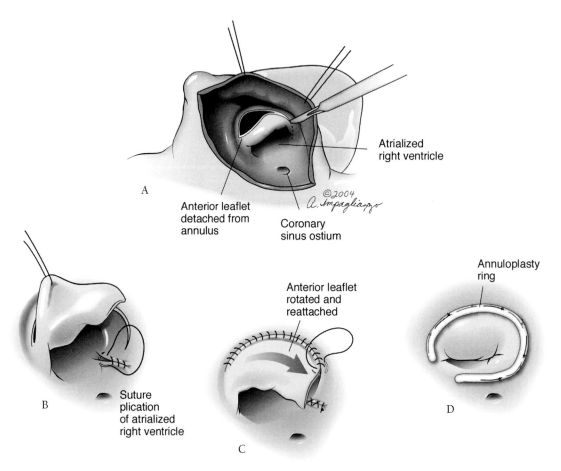

Figure 44-8.   Carpentier repair. **(A)** Anterior leaflet is detached from the tricuspid annulus. **(B)** Vertical plication of tricuspid annulus. **(C)** Redistribution and reattachment of the anterior leaflet to the remodeled tricuspid annulus. **(D)** Finished repair is supported by an annuloplasty ring.

using the method described previously in this chapter. Given an adequate annular reduction and an anterior leaflet of reasonable quality, a dramatic reduction in tricuspid regurgitation can be expected.

SUGGESTED READING

Cooley DA, Hallman GL, Leachman RD. Total anomalous pulmonary venous drainage: Correction with the use of cardiopulmonary bypass in 62 cases. J Thorac Cardiovasc Surg 1966;51:88.

Darling RC, Rothney VVB, Craig JM. Total pulmonary venous drainage into the right side of the heart. Lab Invest 1957;6:44.

Herlong JR, Jagger, JJ, Ungerleider RM. Congenital Heart Surgery Nomenclature and Database Project: Pulmonary venous anomalies. Ann Thorac Surg 2000;69:S56.

Katz MM, Kirklin IW, Pacifico AD. Concepts and practices in surgery for total anomalous pulmonary venous connection. Ann Thorac Surg 1978;25:479.

Kirklin JW, Ellis FH, Wood EH. Treatment of anomalous pulmonary venous connections in association with interatrial communications. Surgery 1956;39:389.

Neill CA. Development of the pulmonary veins: with reference to the embryology of anomalies of pulmonary venous return. Pediatrics 1956;18:880.

Van Praagh R, Corsirii L. Cor triatriatum: Pathologic anatomy and a consideration of morphogenesis based on 13 postmortem cases and a study of normal development of the pulmonary vein and atrial septum in 83 human embryos. Am Heart J 1969;78:379.

Warden HE, Gustafson RA, Tamay IJ, et al. An alternative method for repair of partial anomalous pulmonary venous connection to the superior vena cava. Ann Thorac Surg 1984;38:601.

EDITOR'S COMMENTS

Dr. Peeler has given a thorough and understandable approach to the tricuspid valve. I agree entirely with his approach, but would like to emphasize a couple of issues. First and foremost is that we all need to be aggressive in repairing tricuspid valves in patients with left-sided disease. I was taught as a resident that the tricuspid annulus would shrink in size after the repair of a left-sided lesion. Unfortunately, too many patients have prolonged and difficult postoperative courses with this approach. The addition of tricuspid valve repair has minimal morbidity and can be life saving in preventing right ventricular dysfunction and also organ dysfunction. Some surgeons have felt that a large tricuspid annulus should be repaired even in the absence of regurgitation.

The next question concerns the proper approach to the tricuspid valve. We favor doing a formal repair in most patients who have severe tricuspid regurgitation. However, other surgeons, particularly Cohn's group, (Brigham and Women's Hospital), Boston, feel that a suture annuloplasty is as effective as a ring. This is still not clear, but it certainly demonstrates that many approaches to the tricuspid valve are possible. In addition, I feel strongly that the tricuspid valve should essentially always be repaired. There are very few indications for tricuspid valve replacement. Tricuspid valve replacement in patients with endocarditis or tricuspid regurgitation leaves a very difficult situation with the possibility of multiple re-do operations. The repair is almost always possible and replacement should almost always be avoided.

I.L.K.

45

Aortic Valve Replacement

David A. Fullerton

Historical Perspective

Surgical attempts to correct aortic stenosis began in the early twentieth century. In 1912, Tuffier in Paris attempted transaortic digital dilation of a stenotic aortic valve. In 1947, Smithy (who died of aortic stenosis at 43 years of age) and Parker at the University of South Carolina described an experimental model of aortic valvotomy. Three years later in Philadelphia, Bailey reported successful aortic valvulotomy by insertion of a mechanical dilator across the stenotic valve of patients to open fused commissures. In 1952, Hufnagel and Harvey at Georgetown University placed the first prosthetic ball valve into the descending aorta of a patient with aortic insufficiency. Surgery on the aortic valve under direct vision required the development of cardiopulmonary bypass by Gibbon in 1954. In 1955, Swann performed the first successful aortic valvotomy using hypothermia and inflow occlusion. Initially, open aortic valve operations were limited to aortic valve commissurotomy and debridement of calcified aortic valve leaflets. Harken in Boston in 1960 and Starr in Portland in 1963, however, reported replacement of the aortic valve with a ball-valve prosthesis. In 1962, Ross in London successfully performed orthotopic homograft valve replacement. In 1967, Ross performed the first pulmonary autograft procedure (Ross procedure) for correction of aortic stenosis. In the mid-1960s, stent-mounted porcine aortic valves were implanted, but these formaldehyde-fixed valves rapidly degenerated. In 1974, Carpentier in Paris reported superior longevity of the glutaraldehyde-preserved porcine valve.

Surgical Anatomy of the Aortic Valve

The normal aortic valve is composed of three thin, pliable leaflets or cusps attached to the heart at the junction of the aorta and the left ventricle. The leaflets are attached within the three sinuses of Valsalva to the proximal aorta and joined together in three commissures that create the shape of a coronet. Because the coronary arteries arise from two of the three sinuses of Valsalva, the aortic leaflets are named after their respective sinuses as the left coronary leaflet, the right coronary leaflet, and the noncoronary leaflet. However, because of the oblique position of the aortic root, the sinuses themselves are rarely in a strict left or right position. The attachment of the leaflets to the left ventricular outflow tract is termed an annulus; however, in the strictest terminology this is not a true annulus because it is not truly circular: The points of attachment of the leaflets do not all lie in the same plane. There are two important surgical landmarks. First, the commissure between the left and noncoronary leaflets is positioned along the area of aortic-mitral valve continuity. Beneath this commissure is the fibrous subaortic curtain. The commissure between the noncoronary and the right coronary leaflets is positioned over the left bundle of His. Injury to this conduction bundle during aortic valve surgery may create heart block.

Aortic Stenosis

Etiology

Acquired aortic stenosis usually results from calcification of the aortic valve associated with advanced age. Although the process has traditionally been considered idiopathic, recent data suggest that an inflammatory process akin to atherosclerosis may play an important role in aortic valve calcification. In fact, several investigators report regression or slowed progression of aortic stenosis accomplished by administration of statin drugs. Mechanistic insight into the pathogenesis of calcific aortic stenosis has been provided by the demonstration that fibroblasts found within the aortic valve leaflets may change phenotype and become osteoblasts and thereby produce calcium. Although less common, rheumatic fever may also effect the aortic valve in a process similar to that by which it affects the mitral valve. In rheumatoid aortic stenosis, inflammation of the valve leaflets results in fusion of the commissures as well as the leaflets with thickening and calcium deposition. Retraction of the leaflets may make these valves both regurgitant and stenotic. With rheumatic fever, the inflammatory process rarely involves the aortic valve alone and usually involves the mitral valve as well. Regardless of etiology, the calcification, which develops on the aortic valve leaflets may extend beyond the leaflets onto the anterior leaflet of the mitral valve and upward along the intimal surface of the aorta. Occasionally, such extensive calcification may create coronary ostial stenosis.

Congenital valvular anomalies may be clinically significant at birth as with a unicusp or a dome-shaped valve. Patients born with a congenitally bicuspid aortic valve are uncommonly symptomatic in childhood but are prone to develop aortic stenosis early in adulthood. The bicuspid valve produces turbulent flow across the leaflets, which ultimately leads to fibrosis and calcification and stiffening of the leaflets. Patients with a bi-cuspid aortic valve are prone to develop aortic stenosis at an earlier age (fifth and sixth decades of life) than those with a tricuspid valve (seventh, eighth, and ninth decades).

Pathophysiology

In acquired aortic stenosis, there is a chronic, progressive narrowing of the aortic valve. As the valve narrows, the appropriate compensatory response of the left ventricle is hypertrophy. According to the law of Laplace, the wall stress of the left ventricle is normalized by increasing its thickness (hypertrophy). In fact, failure of this normal compensatory mechanism leads to ventricular failure. Nonetheless, as the ventricle hypertrophies, it becomes less compliant. The significance of this loss of compliance is that a higher left ventricular end-diastolic pressure is required to maintain the same volume of cardiac output. To achieve a sufficiently high left ventricular end-diastolic pressure (diastolic loading), the heart becomes increasingly dependent on the atrial kick; loss of the atrial kick, as occurs with atrial fibrillation, may result in a significant decline in cardiac output and acute hemodynamic decompensation.

Although left ventricular hypertrophy is an appropriate biological response to the increasing afterload, it does have detrimental effects. The combined effects of any of the following will culminate in increased myocardial oxygen demand: greater left ventricular muscle mass; decreased left ventricular compliance, which results in greater ventricular wall tension; higher systolic ventricular pressure; and longer systolic ejection time. At the same time, coronary artery blood flow is compromised by increased wall tension compressing the vessels by a higher left ventricular diastolic pressure, which lowers the coronary artery perfusion pressure. These factors contribute to an inadequate coronary artery perfusion of the subendocardium, which leads to chronic ischemia. In turn, chronic ischemia may lead to cell death and fibrosis.

Left ventricular hypertrophy may allow the heart to achieve a normal cardiac output under resting conditions. To do so, however, a pressure gradient across the valve is required, and as the valve area becomes smaller, the gradient across the valve from the left ventricle into the aorta increases. This relationship to flow across the valve, valve area, and transvalvular pressure gradient is expressed in the Gorlin formula as follows:

$$AVA \ (cm^2) = \frac{Flow \ across \ the \ valve}{44.5 \times \sqrt{Mean \ transvalvular \ gradient}}$$

AVA is the aortic valve area in square centimeters; aortic flow equals cardiac output in milliliters per minute divided by systolic ejection period in seconds per minute; and 44.5 is an empirical orifice constant. Although the Gorlin formula is very widely used on a clinical basis, the constant, 44.5, has never been scientifically verified.

The relationship of flow across the aortic valve and the transvalvular pressure gradient is shown in Fig. 45-1. As the valve area decreases to 1 cm² there is little change in the transvalvular gradient needed to generate a given flow and patients uncommonly experience symptoms. As the valve area decreases below 1 cm² the transvalvular gradient required to maintain the same aortic flow increases and patients typically become symptomatic.

Symptoms

The classic symptoms of aortic stenosis are angina, syncope, and heart failure. Heart failure is usually manifest by dyspnea on exertion. Patients typically do not develop symptoms until the valve area is approximately 1 cm². This is, however, quite variable because some patients become symptomatic before the valve area is 1 cm² and others remain aymptomatic with a valve area consistent with severe aortic stenosis.

Diagnosis

The diagnosis of aortic stenosis may be suggested by symptoms of angina, syncope, or heart failure. Heart failure may be overt, but far more commonly, it is manifest as a subtle loss of exercise tolerance or progressive dyspnea on exertion. On physical examination, the diagnosis may be suspected by the classic systolic murmur heard best at the base of the heart with radiation into the carotid arteries. With significant aortic stenosis, the murmur is associated with a slow, prolonged rise in the arterial pulse called pulsus parvus ettardus. The murmur of severe aortic stenosis is soft and high pitched and is often described as a "seagull" murmur.

Echocardiography is the mainstay of diagnosis. With color flow Doppler, the peak transvalvular gradient may be calculated from the velocity of blood traversing the valve by the following formula:

$$Gradient = 4V^2$$

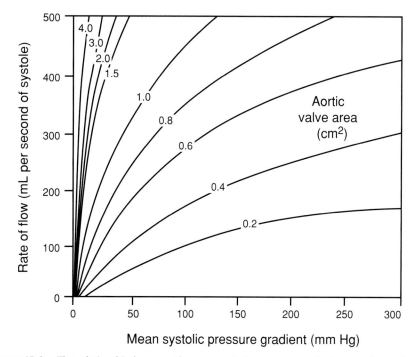

Figure 45-1. The relationship between the mean systolic pressure gradient across the aortic valve and the rate of flow across the aortic valve per second of systole, as predicted by the Gorlin formula. Once the valve area is reduced to about 0.7 cm², little increase in flow is achieved despite marked increases in mean gradient, and thus flow is "fixed," thereby defining "critical" aortic stenosis. (Reprinted with permission from JW Hurst, RB Logue, RC Schlant, et al. [eds], Hurst's The Heart: Arteries and Veins [3rd ed]. New York, McGraw-Hill, 1974;811.)

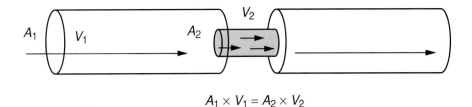

$$A_1 \times V_1 = A_2 \times V_2$$

Figure 45-2. Determination of aortic valve area using the continuity equation. For blood flow ($A_1 \times V_1$) to remain constant when it reaches a stenosis (A_2), velocity must increase to V_2. Determination of the increased velocity V_2 by Doppler ultrasound permits calculation of both the aortic valve gradient and solution of the equation for A_2. (Reprinted with permission from BA Carabello. Aortic stenosis. In MH Crawford [ed], Current Diagnosis and Treatment in Cardiology. Norwalk, CT: Appleton & Lange, 1995;87.)

where V is the maximal measured peak velocity in meters per second across the valve. The velocity across the normal aortic valve is approximately 1.0 m/sec. With mild aortic stenosis the velocity is increased to 2.5 to 2.9 m/sec. Velocity increases in moderate aortic stenosis to 3.0 to 4.0 m/sec, and to more than 4.0 m/sec in severe aortic stenosis.

The echocardiographic determination of the aortic flow velocity across the valve may also be used to calculate the aortic valve area using the continuity equation (Fig. 45-2). The normal aortic valve area is approximately 3 cm² to 4 cm². Very little gradient is created as the valve narrows until the area is reduced by approximately one half. Using the aortic valve area, one can characterize aortic stenosis as mild (area >1.5 cm²), moderate (area 1.0 cm² to 1.5 cm²), or severe (area <1.0 cm²). Normalized for patient body surface area, severe aortic stenosis is an aortic valve area ≤0.60 cm²/m².

Although the diagnosis can usually be made by echocardiography, cardiac catheterization may be used to verify the calculated gradient. The most accurate technique at cardiac catheterization is the simultaneous measurement of aortic and ventricular pressure rather than a "pullback" technique by which the catheter is withdrawn from the left ventricle into the aorta. Typically cardiac output is measured at the same setting, which allows a simplification of the Gorlin formula for estimating aortic valve area (AVA):

$$AVA = (\text{Cardiac output})^2$$
$$\div \text{Mean transvalvular gradient}$$

Natural History

Ross and Braunwald delineated the natural history of aortic stenosis. Over a period of years, the valve progressively narrows. As noted previously, little gradient is generated across the valve until the valve area has been reduced by approximately one half. During this "latent" period, patients are typ-

ically asymptomatic. It is noteworthy that the progressive narrowing of the valve is not linear; it occurs in an unpredictable, stepwise fashion. Patient survival is not significantly diminished until patients develop symptoms. Thereafter, survival is quite limited. The three principal symptoms of aortic stenosis are angina, syncope, and heart failure. With the onset of angina, the mean survival of a patient with aortic stenosis is 4.7 years. After a patient develops syncope, the mean survival is typically <3 years. Patients with dyspnea and heart failure have a mean survival between 1 and 2 years. Heart failure is the presenting symptom in at least one third of patients with aortic stenosis. Approximately 3% to 5% of patients who cross the threshold from asymptomatic to symptomatic die within weeks to months. Hence, it is extremely important to accurately identify the presence of symptoms. The presence of symptoms in a patient with aortic stenosis is an indication for an aortic valve replacement (AVR) (Fig. 45-3).

Aortic Regurgitation

Etiology

Aortic regurgitation may result from disease of the aortic valve leaflets or of the aortic root itself. Rheumatic fever may affect the leaflets by shortening the distance from the leaflet free edge to the annulus rather than by leading to commissural fusion. This prevents sufficient coaptation of the leaflets during diastole and results in a central leak. Congenital bicuspid aortic valves typically lead to aortic stenosis but may become more regurgitant if leaflet prolapse occurs. In addition, endocarditis may, of course, destroy leaflets.

Dilation of the aortic root produces aortic regurgitation despite normal leaflet morphology by precluding leaflet coaptation. With dilation of the sinotubular junction, the leaflet edges are distracted, which creates a central leak of the valve. The most common cause of this condition is annuloaortic ectasia, an idiopathic dilation of the aortic root and annulus; as the sinus of Valsalva and the proximal aorta dilate, diastolic coaptation of the leaflets is precluded, which results in valvular insufficiency. Similarly, myxoid degeneration of the aortic root may lead to dilation of the root as seen in Marfan syndrome, Ehlers-Danlos syndrome, and cystic medial necrosis. These conditions may lead to leaflet redundancy, progressive prolapse, and regurgitation. Finally, trauma or dissection of the aortic wall may produce

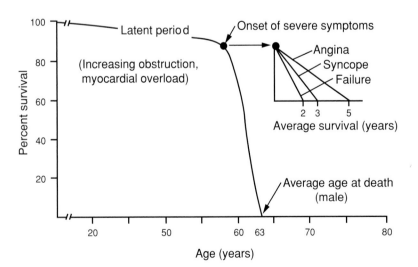

Figure 45-3. The natural history of medically treated aortic stenosis. (Reprinted with permission from J Ross, E Braunwald. Aortic stenosis. Circulation 1968;38:61.)

aortic regurgitation if it leads to loss of commissural suspension and leaflet prolapse.

Pathophysiology

The aortic valve leaks during diastole, which lowers diastolic pressure and widens the pulse pressure. Because coronary blood flow occurs primarily in diastole, the lower diastolic blood pressure lowers coronary perfusion pressure. Unlike aortic stenosis, in which the pathologic process is left ventricular pressure overload, the pathophysiology of aortic insufficiency derives from left ventricular volume overload. The increased left ventricular end-diastolic volume (preload) results from filling through the mitral valve as well as the incompetent aortic valve. In patients with chronic aortic insufficiency, the left ventricular end-diastolic volume may be greater than in any other form of heart disease. Because left ventricular compliance is often diminished, however, left ventricular end-diastolic pressure may or may not be elevated. With left ventricular dilatation, normal forward stroke volume and ejection fraction may be maintained by increased left ventricular end-diastolic and end-systolic volumes. According to the law of Laplace, this left ventricular dilation increases the left ventricular wall tension required to develop systolic pressure. Such increased wall stress not only increases myocardial oxygen demand, but also initiates left ventricular hypertrophy and increases left ventricular wall mass. Ultimately, myocardial fibrosis occurs.

With well-compensated aortic insufficiency, exercise may be tolerated because peripheral vascular resistance declines, thus lowering left ventricular afterload and increasing effective forward flow. At the same time, heart rate increases, which shortens diastolic time and thereby decreases regurgitant flow. Because the left ventricle ultimately decompensates, however, the left ventricular end-diastolic volume increases, even without an increase in aortic regurgitant volume. The end-systolic volume increases as the forward stroke volume declines because ventricular emptying is impaired; the ventricle fails. In severe aortic regurgitation, increased myocardial oxygen demand exceeds myocardial oxygen supply, which causes ischemia despite normal coronary arteries. Increased left ventricular mass and wall tension occur concurrently with low diastolic pressures (low coronary perfusion pressure). Consequently, and particularly with exercise when the diastolic period shortens, coronary blood flow may not meet demand.

Diagnosis

Compensatory mechanisms of aortic regurgitation permit patients to remain symptom-free for long periods of time. When these compensatory mechanisms begin to fail, however, left ventricular dysfunction becomes manifest and patients experience symptoms of heart failure. Symptoms, generally the result of an elevation in left atrial pressure, include dyspnea on exertion, orthopnea, and paroxysmal nocturnal dyspnea. Nocturnal angina occurs occasionally as a result of a slow heart rate and exceedingly low diastolic pressure with resultant poor coronary blood flow.

On physical examination, patients with aortic regurgitation may have distinctive findings resultant to wide pulse pressure. The peripheral pulses rise and fall abruptly (Corrigan's or "water hammer" pulse), the head may bob with each systole (DeMusset's sign), and the capillaries may visibly pulsate (Quincke's sign). Auscultation reveals a high-frequency decrescendo diastolic regurgitant murmur. A middle or late diastolic rumble may be heard (Austin-Flint murmur) and represents rapid antegrade flow across the mitral valve, which closes prematurely as a result of rapid ventricular filling secondary to aortic regurgitation. Finally, the diastolic blood pressure is typically low.

Doppler echocardiography is the most accurate technique for confirming the diagnosis of aortic regurgitation as well as for quantifying its severity. As with mitral regurgitation, the severity is graded as mild, moderate, or severe.

Natural History

Because of the compensatory mechanisms discussed previously, patients with chronic aortic regurgitation may be symptom-free for long periods of time. In fact, patients with mild to moderate aortic regurgitation have an excellent long-term prognosis; the 10-year survival after diagnosis is approximately 90%. Studies in which patients with severe aortic regurgitation were managed conservatively reveal a 10-year survival of 50% or less. Once symptoms of congestive heart failure occur, survival is markedly diminished; almost 50% of patients with left ventricular failure die within 2 years.

Operative Technique

The standard surgical approach for AVR is via a median sternotomy (Fig. 45-4). Cardiopulmonary bypass is established by aortic and right atrial cannulation. After initiation of cardiopulmonary bypass, the aortic root is vented and a left ventricular vent is inserted via the right superior pulmonary vein. If the aortic valve is competent, cardiac arrest may be achieved by antegrade cardioplegia with subsequent administration of cardioplegia in retrograde fashion. Otherwise, all cardioplegia may be administered retrograde. The myocardial temperature is monitored in the interventricular septum and kept below 10° by administration of cold blood cardioplegia every 20 minutes throughout the period of aortic occlusion. I routinely cool the patient to a bladder temperature of 28°C.

There are several important technical caveats. First, it is important to prevent the introduction of air into the left atrium with the insertion of a left ventricular vent via the right superior pulmonary vein. This can be done by temporarily pinching the venous line, thereby filling the left atrium with blood. I typically vent the aortic root before placing the left ventricular vent to evacuate any air that might be introduced. Second, the ascending aorta in patients undergoing aortic valve replacement may be very thin because of poststenotic dilation, advanced age, annuloaortic ectasia, and so on. Hence, aortic cannulation stitches must be placed very carefully to avoid tearing the aorta. I often use felt pledgets to reinforce each bite of the aortic cannulation stitches to minimize this problem. Third, in operations for aortic regurgitation, the heart is prone to ventricular fibrillation once cardiopulmonary bypass has been initiated. If the heart fibrillates, the left ventricle will immediately distend, which may sometimes be lethal. To avoid this, I avoid systemic cooling until the left ventricular vent has been placed. The heart typically fibrillates soon after the initiation of systemic cooling, at which point I immediately cross-clamp the aorta and administer retrograde cardioplegia.

After cardiopulmonary bypass has been initiated, the plane between the aorta and pulmonary artery is dissected. This is important to optimize visualization of the aortic valve and to facilitate aortic closure. One of the most important technical nuances of this operation is to identify the surface anatomy of the right coronary artery as it originates from the right sinus of Valsalva. This may be done by gentle dissection of the fat pad overlying the right sinus of Valsalva. If the aortotomy is too close to the right coronary ostium, the os may be damaged or distorted with aortic closure or by the valve itself. As the patient is systemically cooled, the

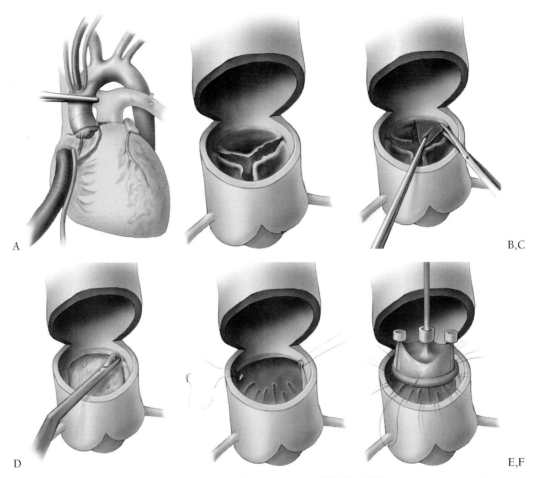

A   B,C

D   E,F

Figure 45-4. Operative technique: aortic valve replacement. **(A)** The initial transverse aortotomy is made 3 cm to 4 cm distal to the right coronary artery. The valve is visualized, and the aortotomy is extended at least 1 cm distal to the zenith of the commissure between the right and noncoronary leaflets. **(B)** The aortotomy is extended to the halfway point over the noncoronary leaflet. It is then opened down toward the annulus, stopping at least 1 cm from the annulus itself. **(C)** The leaflets are removed. **(D)** The calcified annulus is debrided with a Rongeur. It is helpful to place a small gauze sponge in the left ventricle to help catch any flecks of calcium during the debridement. **(E)** Interrupted horizontal pledgeted sutures are placed with pledgets in the subannular position. **(F)** After the sutures are brought through the valve sewing ring, the valve is seated and the sutures tied.

heart will fibrillate. The aortic cross-clamp is then applied, and cardioplegia is administered.

A small, transverse aortotomy is made approximately 3 cm to 4 cm distal to the origin of the right coronary artery. Through this initial aortotomy, one can visualize the aortic valve. The aortotomy is then extended transversely across the anterior surface of the aorta. It is important to stay approximately 1 cm distal to the zenith of the commisures of the aortic valve leaflets. Having extended the aortotomy to the patient's right, once the incision is exactly over the halfway point of the noncoronary leaflet, one directs the aortotomy incision in the axis of the aorta down toward the aortic annulus. This portion of the aortotomy incision should stop at least 1 cm distal to the aortic annulus.

The aortic valve is best visualized with the operating table in a bit of reverse Trendelenburg position and rotated a bit to the patient's left. Traction sutures are then placed through the top of each commissure and snapped to the surgical drapes. This brings the aortic valve up toward the surgeon. The aortic valve leaflets are then excised with scissors. After the leaflets have been removed, a moist gauze sponge is placed in the lumen of the left ventricle to help catch any small pieces of calcium. A Rongeur instrument is then used to gently debride the annulus of calcium. During this process, it is helpful for the assistant to follow along with an open-tipped suction catheter to help sweep up any small pieces of calcium. After the annulus has been sufficiently debrided of calcium, the sponge is removed from within

the ventricle, and the lumen of the left ventricle is liberally irrigated with cold saline to flush out any calcium debris. The annulus is then sized.

The appropriate valve size is chosen by measuring the annulus with valve sizers. It is very important not to attempt to place an oversized valve. Regardless of the choice of prosthesis, I routinely implant a valve one size smaller than what the patient's annulus might accept as judged by valve sizers. Horizontal pledgetted mattress sutures are placed in the aortic annulus with the pledgets in the subannular position. After all the sutures have been placed, the aortic valve prosthesis is brought to the field and the sutures passed through valve sewing ring. To facilitate symmetric suture placement, it is helpful to mark the sewing ring in thirds.

Table 45-1 Independent Risk Factors for Operative Mortality (Odds Ratios) for Aortic Valve Replacement (AOR)

Risk Factor	AVR	AVR+CABG
Salvage status	7.12	7.00
Dialysis-dependent renal failure	4.32	4.60
Emergency status	3.46	1.89
Nondialysis renal failure	2.20	2.11
First reoperation	1.70	2.40

CABG = coronary artery bypass grafting.

After the sutures are passed through the sewing ring, the valve is seated into the aortic annulus, and the sutures are tied. To minimize difficulty in seating the valve, the sutures at each of the three commissures should be tied first. Next, a suture midway between each commissure should be tied. In this manner, the surgeon may be assured that the valve will seat appropriately.

After the valve is sewn in place, the aortotomy is closed with 5-0 polypropylene sutures in two layers. The first layer is a running horizontal mattress stitch, and the second is an over-and-over running stitch.

In anticipation of removing the aortic cross-clamp, I typically infuse warm blood in retrograde fashion. The purpose of this is to flush air out of the coronary arteries and to begin increasing the myocardial metabolic rate before reanimating the heart. During this infusion, it is helpful to begin de-airing the left ventricle by partial occlusion of the venous line and the resumption of ventilation while the left ventricular and aortic vents are on suction. After the retrograde administration of 500 cc of warm blood, the aortic cross-clamp is removed. With the heart reanimated, one should assess the adequacy of the de-airing maneuvers by transesophageal echo. The usual maneuvers include filling the heart while on cardiopulmonary bypass, rotating the operating table from right-to-left, and using Valsalva maneuvers to express air out of the pulmonary veins. When the surgeon is satisfied that the left heart is completely de-aired, the left ventricular vent is removed and the patient is weaned from cardiopulmonary bypass.

Surgical Outcomes

According to the Society of Thoracic Surgeons (STS) National Cardiac Surgery Database, approximately 70,000 valve operations are performed in the United States annually. The operative mortality rate in the STS database for isolated AVR is approximately 4%. The operative mortality rate for combined AVR/coronary artery bypass grafting (CABG) is approximately 6.8%. Other large databases, including the New York State Department of Health Cardiac Surgery Reporting System and the Department of Veteran Affairs Cardiac Surgery Database, have found very similar mortality rates for cardiac valve operations.

The inherent risks, as in all surgical procedures, are influenced by patient-specific risk factors, and large databases such as those mentioned provide the statistical power to identify patient-specific factors contributing to the risks of valve surgery. Table 45-1 lists some the major patient-specific risk factors for the most common valve operations from the STS database.

Choice of Prosthetic Aortic Valve

The operative risks of cardiac valve replacement are unassociated with the choice of prosthesis. Furthermore, the hemodynamic performances of contemporary valves are similar. Traditionally, the choice of aortic valve prosthesis has focused on whether a patient would be committed to the risks of lifelong anticoagulation (mechanical valve) or the presumed need for reoperation for structural valve deterioration (bioprosthetic valve). However, this approach is an oversimplification, and the choice of prosthetic valve must be patient specific. In addition to appropriate consideration of a given patient's comorbidities, one of the most important considerations is the age of the patient at valve implantation. In this light, it is important to recognize that approximately 80% of all valve replacements in the United States are performed in patients older than the age of 60 years.

The 10-year survival for patients following aortic valve replacement ranges from 40% to 70%, with an average in the literature of 50%. The type of prosthesis does not affect survival, but other patient-specific factors such as age at operation and presence or absence of coronary artery disease do affect survival after valve replacement. Regardless of the type of prosthetic valve implanted, approximately one third of patients die of valve-related causes. Given that valve-related complications occur at a frequency of about 3% to 6% per year, it is important to ask whether the risks in a given patient may be minimized by the choice of a mechanical versus a bioprosthetic valve.

As shown in Fig. 45-5, the principal causes of valve-related death after valve implantation include thromboembolism, reoperation, bleeding, and prosthetic valve endocarditis (PVE). The risk of PVE is not different between mechanical and tissue valves. It is approximately 4% spread over the patient's lifetime. However, if PVE does occur, it is associated with a 50% mortality rate.

The leading cause of valve-related death is thromboembolism. Largely because mechanical valves are thrombogenic, the risk of thromboembolism is greater with mechanical valves. At 10 years after AVR, the risk of thromboembolism is 20% for mechanical valves and 9% for bioprosthetic valves.

Because a mechanical valve obligates the patient to chronic anticoagulation therapy (warfarin sodium), the choice of a prosthetic valve must consider the risks of chronic anticoagulation. The risk of bleeding complications from chronic anticoagulation is between 1% and 2% per year. In fact, 4% of valve-related deaths result from bleeding (Fig. 45-5). Mechanical valves should be avoided in patients with contraindications to anticoagulation because of occupation or because of coexistent medical conditions. Likewise, patients who are medically noncompliant or whose level of anticoagulation may not be closely monitored should not receive mechanical valves.

Ten percent of valve-related deaths result from reoperation. It was traditionally assumed that after implantation of a tissue valve, patients would require reoperation for structural valve deterioration within approximately 10 years. Mechanical valves were therefore recommended for patients with a life expectancy longer than 10 years. This reasoning requires refinement. First, placement of a mechanical valve does not eliminate the potential for subsequent valve reoperation. Although mechanical valves will not structurally fail, approximately 10% of mechanical aortic valves require reoperation within 5 to 10 years, primarily for

Cause of Valve-Related Death

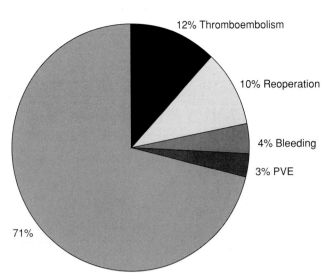

12% Thromboembolism

10% Reoperation

4% Bleeding

3% PVE

71%

Figure 45-5. Causes of valve-related deaths. Mortality following valve replacement is valve-related in approximately 30% of patients. (Reprinted with permission from DA Fullerton, AH Harken, Acquired Heart Disease: Valvular. In CM Townsend Jr, RD Beauchamp, BM Evers, et al. [eds]. Sabiston Textbook of Surgery. The Biological Basis of Modern Surgical Practice (17th ed]. Philadelphia: Elsevier Saunders, 2004;1898.)

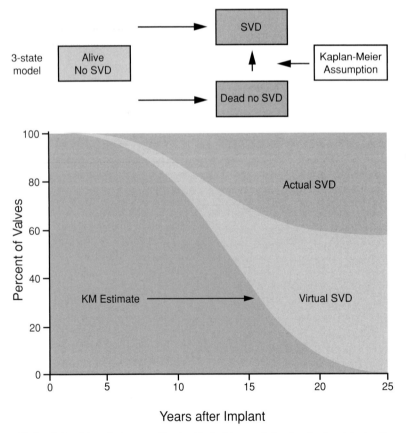

Figure 45-6. Actuarial analysis overestimates the incidence of structural valve deterioration (SVD). Kaplan-Meier methodology uses the assumption that patients who died before SVD would eventually have had SVD. The group of patients in this group is labeled "virtual SVD." (Reprinted with permission from GL Grunkemeier, YX Wu. Interpretation of nonfatal events after cardiac surgery: Actual versus actuarial reporting. J Thorac Cardiovasc Surg 2001;122:2160.)

perivalvular leak, endocarditis, or nonstructural valve dysfunction such as scar tissue or pannus in-growth. Second, the structural durability of newer bioprosthetic valves is superior to that of prior generations of valves. Third, it is now appreciated that the appropriate statistical methodology for analysis of structural valve deterioration of bioprosthetic valves utilizes *actual* rather that *actuarial* statistics (Fig. 45-6). Use of these statistical methods does confirm that the durability of a bioprosthetic valve placed in the aortic position is inversely related to the patient's age at the time the valve is implanted. They also demonstrate that the incidence of reoperation for structural valve deterioration of a bioprosthetic valve is less than 15% for patients older than 60 years (Fig. 45-7).

The Asymptomatic Patient

Asymptomatic Aortic Stenosis

The management of asymptomatic aortic stenosis is controversial. Although the survival of patients with asymptomatic aortic stenosis is generally considered to be excellent, some do carry a low but real risk of sudden death. In the asymptomatic patient, this risk must be weighed against the perioperative risks of aortic valve replacement as well and the longitudinal risks of the valve prosthesis itself. The challenge for the surgeon is to identify those asymptomatic patients who should have aortic valve replacement.

The Risks without Operation

The risk of sudden death in asymptomatic patients has traditionally been considered quite low, usually less than 1%, but has been reported as high as 9%. Most of these data were generated prior to an era when the degree of aortic stenosis could be accurately quantified. Contemporary studies have employed thorough echocardiographic evaluation of the aortic stenosis and used clinical endpoints of death or AVR to examine outcomes in asymptomatic patients. In a rigorous study of nonoperated patients with asymptomatic aortic stenosis, the incidence of sudden death was approximately 6%. Furthermore, one must also consider that the mortality is 3% to 4% soon after the onset of symptoms. Perhaps because of this, the mortality among patients awaiting aortic valve replacement for aortic stenosis may be as high as 7% over 6 months.

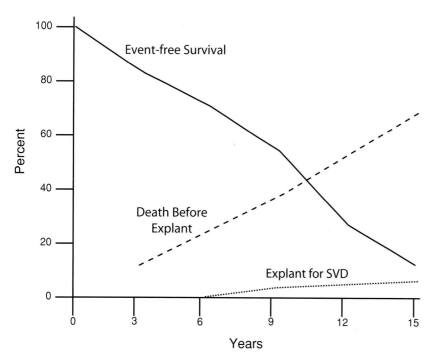

Figure 45-7. After aortic valve replacement with a bovine pericardial bioprosthesis, the risk of undergoing reoperation for structural valve deterioration (SVD) is less than 15% at 15 years. (Reprinted with permission from MK Banbury, DM Cosgrove 3rd, JA White, et al. Age and valve size effect on the long-term durability of the Carpentier-Edwards aortic pericardial bioprosthesis. Ann Thorac Surg 2001;72:753.)

Unmasking the Symptoms

Given a patient with significant aortic stenosis by echocardiogram, it is therefore important to determine that the patient is truly asymptomatic. This may be objectively confirmed by exercise stress testing (treadmill). Although it is unnecessary and risky in the symptomatic patient with aortic stenosis, exercise testing has been found to be safe in asymptomatic patients. A modified Bruce protocol should be employed under careful observation. An exercise test is considered positive if symptoms occur, systolic blood pressure falls by >10 mm Hg, dysrhythmias occur, or ST-segment changes are noted. Given a positive exercise test, the patient should be considered symptomatic and offered surgery. As many as 66% of asymptomatic patients may have a positive stress test.

Outcomes of Patients with a Negative Stress Test

After a negative stress test, patients must be closely followed for hemodynamic progression of aortic stenosis. On average, the aortic flow velocity increases by 0.3 m/sec per year and the aortic valve area decreases by 0.1 cm² per year. However, the flow velocity is largely dependent on ventricular contractility, and should ventricular function decline, velocity may not change. Furthermore, ex-

tremely wide individual variability is noted in the hemodynamic progression of aortic stenosis, which makes it difficult to predict the clinical course of a given patient.

Several characteristics have been identified that help to stratify asymptomatic patients. Otto and colleagues identified aortic flow velocity as the most important patient-specific variable. The highest-risk group were those asymptomatic patients with an

aortic flow velocity of >4 m/sec because only 21% were alive without valve replacement at 2 years (Fig. 45-8).

In addition to an absolute aortic flow velocity >4 m/sec, longitudinal follow-up may reveal patients with a rapidly increasing flow velocity on serial echocardiograms; these patients are at risk for cardiac events. It was noted in one study that among patients who remained asymptomatic, the average rate of progression of aortic flow velocity was 0.14 m/sec per year. Among patients who experienced cardiac events, however, it was 0.45 m/sec per year.

Patient age and aortic valve calcification may also be important. Among asymptomatic patients, all of whom had aortic flow velocity >4 m/sec, those older than age 50 years were much more likely to experience cardiac events in follow-up. Interestingly, in this same group, moderate or severe aortic valve calcification was strongly associated with subsequent cardiac events (Fig. 45-9).

From a practical standpoint, I have found the following helpful. For the patient who appears to be asymptomatic following a carefully obtained history, an exercise stress is obtained. Patients with a positive stress test are offered surgery. If the stress test is negative, I have found the recommendations of the European Society of Cardiology helpful, and recommend AVR if the aortic flow velocity is >4 m/sec, the aortic valve has moderate or severe calcification, and the rate of progression of aortic flow velocity is >0.3 m/sec per year. I also recommend aortic valve replacement if the left ventricular ejection fraction (LVEF) is <50% because this implies ventricular dysfunction secondary to aortic stenosis.

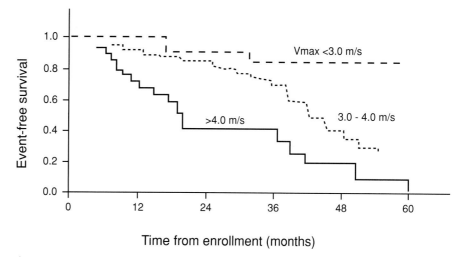

Figure 45-8. An aortic flow velocity of >4 m/sec predicts a rapid decline in event-free survival among patients with asymptomatic aortic stenosis. (Reprinted with permission from CM Otto, IG Burwash, ME Legget, et al. Prospective study of asymptomatic valvular aortic stenosis. Circulation 1997;95:2262.)

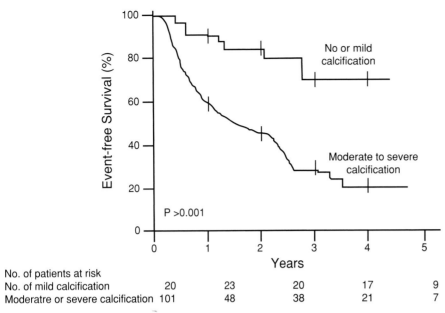

Figure 45-9. Significant aortic valve calcification predicts a rapid decline in event-free survival among patients with asymptomatic aortic stenosis. (Reprinted with permission from R Rosenhek, T Binder, G Porenta. Predictors of outcome in severe, asymptomatic aortic stenosis. N Engl J Med 2000;343:611.)

Asymptomatic Aortic Regurgitation

Aortic valve replacement is clearly indicated in the patient with symptomatic aortic regurgitation. Conversely, the natural history of asymptomatic severe aortic regurgitation is not well defined. Ten years after the diagnosis of severe aortic regurgitation, as many as 75% of patients will have died or undergone AVR. It is now clear that on diagnosis, certain subsets of asymptomatic patients with severe aortic regurgitation should be offered AVR. The recommendation for AVR should be based on left ventricular size and function.

There is consensus that the asymptomatic patient with severe aortic regurgitation with subnormal LVEF at rest should undergo AVR. This consensus is based on a 25% progression per year to heart failure or death in these patients. Evidence of left ventricular dilation is strongly associated with progression to heart failure or death; a left ventricular end-systolic dimension of >55 mm (or >25 mm/m^2) or a left ventricular end-diastolic dimension of >80 mm is an indication for AVR. Likewise, if longitudinal echocardiographic follow-up reveals either "rapid" diminution in LVEF or a "rapid" increase in left ventricular dimensions, AVR is indicated. Although it is normal at rest, myocardial performance may be found to be abnormal with exercise. Hence, exercise stress testing may be used to unmask myocardial contractile dysfunction; a fall in

LVEF with exercise of >5% is a strong relative indication for surgery.

Low-Gradient Aortic Stenosis

Among the most challenging patients with aortic stenosis are those with a low transvalvular gradient and severe left ventricular dysfunction. Low-gradient aortic stenosis is defined as <30 mm Hg. Treated medically, the survival of these patients is usually <2 years; the 1- and 4-year survivals are 41% and 15%, respectively. Because this subset represents <5% of patients with aortic stenosis, the clinical outcomes of aortic valve replacement in these patients have not been well characterized. Historically, the operative mortality rate for aortic valve replacement in this group of patients was quite high, leading some authors to recommend against surgery.

When the patient with severe left ventricular dysfunction associated with low-gradient aortic stenosis is first seen it may be difficult to know whether the left ventricular dysfunction is primary or secondary. The pathogenesis of left ventricular dysfunction secondary to aortic stenosis is derived from afterload mismatch. With significant aortic stenosis, the left ventricle compensates for pressure overload by hypertrophy, thereby normalizing wall stress. In this manner, LVEF and cardiac output are initially maintained. When the ventricle is no longer

able to compensate for the increased wall stress, left ventricular systolic function declines secondary to afterload mismatch. The transvalvular pressure gradient may be low despite the presence of severe aortic stenosis. Provided the left ventricle still has the ability to contract (contractile reserve), clinical outcomes with aortic valve replacement are quite good; operative mortality is low and left ventricular function improves after AVR.

On the other hand, the left ventricular dysfunction may be primary rather than secondary to the aortic stenosis. The dysfunctional left ventricle may be unable to open a mildly calcified aortic valve fully if the stroke volume is significantly decreased. This condition is termed "relative aortic stenosis." These patients have a cardiomyopathy (ischemic or otherwise) with only mild aortic stenosis.

For the surgeon and the patient, the principal questions relate to the risks of an operation and whether the patient will be improved afterward. The answers must rely on a paucity of data regarding the clinical outcomes of patients with low-gradient aortic stenosis and severe left ventricular dysfunction. Carabello and colleagues were the first to provide insight into this situation. In 1980, they reported their experience with 14 patients undergoing aortic valve replacement with aortic stenosis, low LVEF, and heart failure. Four of the 14 patients had transvalvular gradients <30 mm Hg and either died or did poorly after AVR. Conversely, those patients with a higher transvalvular gradient despite severe left ventricular dysfunction did well on relief of severe aortic stenosis. The authors therefore highlighted the fact that despite severe preoperative left ventricular dysfunction, some patients recovered ventricular contractile function postoperatively and did well, whereas others did not. They concluded that a preoperative transvalvular gradient helped identify those who would not benefit from surgery.

Over the ensuing 25 years, surgeons have been very cautious about offering AVR to these patients because of the associated poor outcomes. In 1990, Lund reported that among patients undergoing AVR, prognosis was inversely related to the preoperative gradient; those with gradients <35 mm Hg faired very poorly. In 1993, Brogan and colleagues reported a 33% operative mortality among patients who underwent AVR with a low-gradient and left ventricular dysfunction (6 of 18 patients). However, among the 12 operative survivors, 10 showed significant clinical improvement. The authors

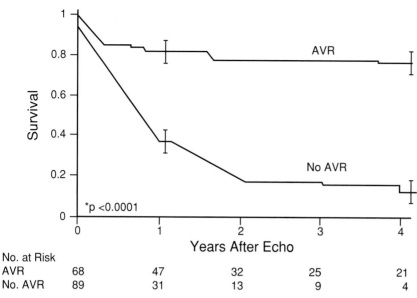

Figure 45-10. Aortic valve replacement (AVR) may significantly improve survival in patients with severe left ventricular dysfunction and low transvalvular gradient. (Reprinted with permission from JJ Pereira, MS Lauer, M Bashir, et al. Survival after aortic valve replacement for severe aortic stenosis with low transvalvular gradients and severe left ventricular dysfunction. J Am Coll Cardiol 2002;39:1356.)

concluded that some patients in this subset do benefit from AVR. Connolly and colleagues confirmed this observation in 2000. Among 52 patients, the operative mortality was 21% and 5-year survival was less that 50%. Nonetheless, some patients showed significant improvements in functional status and LVEF. Pereira and colleagues reported an observational study of 68 patients undergoing AVR compared with a cohort of 89 managed medially in 2002. In these highly selected patients, the operative mortality rate was 8% with 1- and 3-year survivals following AVR of 82% and 78%, respectively. Among the medically treated group, the survival at 3 years was only 15% (Fig. 45-10).

Taken together, the data suggest that patients with low-gradient aortic stenosis and severe left ventricular dysfunction may be stratified according to the severity of aortic stenosis and the contractile reserve of the left ventricle. This can be accomplished with a pharmacologic challenge with dobutamine. During an infusion of dobutamine up to 40 µg/kg/min the hemodynamic response may be monitored by echocardiography or cardiac catheterization. In response to dobutamine infusion, stroke volume and thereby cardiac output should increase, raising the transvalvular gradient. An increase in stroke volume of at least 20% is considered evidence of contractile reserve.

Among 21 patients with low-gradient aortic stenosis, Nishimura and colleagues identified 15 with contractile reserve in response to dobutamine. The operative mortality was 7% (1 patient) among those with contractile reserve. On the other hand, 2 of 6 patients (33%) without preoperative contractile reserve died perioperatively with

AVR, and 2 more died beyond 30 days postoperatively from heart failure. In a large multicenter study, Monin and colleagues evaluated 136 patients with low-gradient aortic stenosis with dobutamine challenge using echocardiography. Contractile reserve was found in 92 patients and absent in 44 patients. Sixty-four of the 92 patients with contractile reserve underwent aortic valve replacement with an operative mortality of 5%. Conversely, 31 of the 44 patients without contractile reserve underwent AVR with an operative mortality of 32%. Monin and colleagues further characterized the extremely poor prognosis of patients with low-gradient aortic stenosis treated medically with and without contractile reserve (Fig. 45-11).

I have come to rely heavily on the echocardiographic appearance of the aortic valve. If the valve is densely calcified with severely restricted leaflet motion, I feel confident that the patient has severe aortic stenosis. Conversely, if the leaflets are not badly calcified or the leaflet motion subjectively seems better than the patient's clinical condition suggests, I examine the hemodynamics during dobutamine infusion.

A doubutamine stress echocardiogram is useful in two ways. First, if the stroke volume (and thereby cardiac output) increases

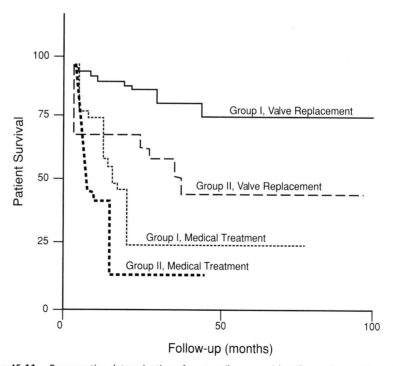

Figure 45-11. Preoperative determination of contractile reserve identifies patients with aortic stenosis with severe left ventricular dysfunction and low transvalvular gradient who will benefit from aortic valve replacement with a low perioperative mortality. (Reprinted with permission from JL Monin, JP Quere, M Monchi, et al. Low-gradient aortic stenosis. Operative risk stratification and predictors for long-term outcome: A multicenter study using dobutamine stress hemodynamics. Circulation 2003;108:319.)

by at least 20%, the patient has contractile reserve. If the increase in stroke volume is associated with an increase in transvalvular gradient, I feel confident that the patient will survive aortic valve replacement with a postoperative improvement in LVEF and functional status. However, if no increase in stroke volume and transvalvular gradient is noted with dobutamine, the patient has no contractile reserve or may not have severe aortic stenosis. Aortic valve replacement is not recommended.

"Prophylactic" Aortic Valve Replacement

Whether to replace the aortic valve of patients with mild to moderate aortic stenosis undergoing coronary artery bypass surgery may be a difficult and controversial decision. In 1994, Collins and colleagues reported a high operative mortality rate (18.2%) in patients undergoing AVR who had had prior coronary artery bypass surgery. Shortly thereafter, several other groups reported similar results. Following these reports, an international trend toward "prophylactic" AVR began for patients with mild to moderate aortic stenosis undergoing coronary artery bypass surgery. The decision to perform a "prophylactic" AVR has always been controversial, and significant variation in the management of these patients continues.

Proponents of "prophylactic" aortic valve replacement at the time of CABG argue the aortic stenosis will inevitably progress, committing the patient to a second operation associated with a high morbidity and mortality. Those favoring an expectant approach argue that "prophylactic" AVR unnecessarily commits an unacceptable number of patients to the risks of valve-related morbidity and mortality. Although progression from asymptomatic to symptomatic aortic stenosis in a relatively short time is clinically recognized, it is very difficult to identify those patients likely to do so. At the core of the argument is the need for an understanding of the natural history of mild to moderate aortic stenosis and the contemporary risks of AVR after previous CABG.

The natural history of mild to moderate aortic stenosis is not well defined. Horstkotte and Loogen reported that by 10 years, only 8% of patients with mild aortic stenosis (AVA >1.5 cm^2) progressed to severe aortic stenosis. Likewise, Turina and

colleagues reported that at 10 years, only 15% experienced death or AVR. These data suggest that the natural history of mild aortic stenosis is fairly benign. The natural history of moderate aortic stenosis (AVA 1.0 cm^2 to 1.5 cm^2) is more difficult to define but is clearly worse than that of mild aortic stenosis. Turina and colleagues reported an event-free survival of 100% at 3 years but only 35% at 10 years in patients with moderate aortic stenosis. More recently, Rosenhek and colleagues reported a more ominous natural history for patients with mild to moderate aortic stenosis (aortic flow velocity 2.5 to 3.9 m/sec). Of 176 patients followed for an average of 48 months, 33 underwent aortic valve replacement; 34 patients died. The 5-year event-free survival was 60%. The strongest predictors of patient events were aortic valve calcification, a peak aortic flow velocity at study entry of >3 m/sec, age >50 years, and coronary artery disease. The data from Rosenhek are consistent with those of Otto and clearly indicate that patients with moderate aortic stenosis may experience hemodynamic progression during relatively short follow-up.

The operative mortality rate reported for AVR subsequent to CABG has significantly diminished in recent years. Advances in

myocardial protection and surgical and anesthetic techniques as well as greater collective experience with cardiac reoperations have contributed to improved outcomes. In recent series, the mean interval between CABG and subsequent AVR is typically 7 to 9 years. In these reports, the operative mortality rate of the AVR at reoperation has been approximately 7% and not significantly different from the operative mortality associated with AVR/CABG done in the same institutions, which suggests that an expectant approach is warranted.

These data suggest that patients with mild aortic stenosis at the time of CABG (AVA >1.5 cm^2; aortic flow velocity <2.5 m/sec) have an excellent prognosis from their aortic valve and should not have AVR. It has been mathematically estimated that "prophylactic" AVR in these patients leads to a significantly higher mortality over 10 years (Fig. 45-12). On the other hand, patients older than age 65 years who undergo CABG with moderate aortic stenosis and an AVA of <1.2 cm^2 and/or an aortic flow velocity of >3 m/sec associated with significant aortic valve calcification are likely to have symptomatic aortic stenosis within the next several years. In this subset of patients it is reasonable to perform AVR with CABG at the initial operation.

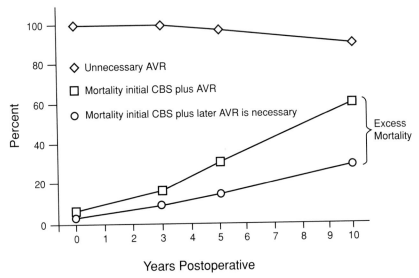

Figure 45-12. Projected patient outcomes in those with severe coronary artery disease that undergo coronary bypass surgery and also have mild aortic stenosis. Because the likelihood of needing an aortic valve replacement (AVR) is low over the subsequent 10 years, most AVRs would be unnecessary. The mortality associated with valve-related complications in patients undergoing an unnecessary AVR leads to a net mortality greater than a strategy of AVR subsequent to coronary bypass surgery (CBS) should it become necessary. (Reprinted with permission from SH Rahimtoola. Should patients with asymptomatic mild or moderate aortic stenosis undergoing coronary artery bypass surgery also have valve replacement for the aortic stenosis? Heart 2001;85:337.)

Aortic Valve Replacement with a Patent Internal Mammary Artery

Aortic valve replacement in patients who have had previous coronary artery grafting, particularly if the internal mammary artery (IMA) graft is patent, can be technically challenging. It is associated with mortality rates of 6% to 17%, considerably higher than first-time aortic valve replacement procedures. Contributing to this mortality rate is the fact that the IMA may be damaged during the procedure, or its presence may compromise myocardial protection during the procedure.

To minimize the risk of injury to the IMA, some advocate moderate to deep systemic hypothermia (20°C) while on cardiopulmonary bypass, aortic occlusion, administration of cardioplegia, but avoidance of dissection of the IMA pedicle. Others also leave the IMA open during the period of aortic occlusion but administer continuous retrograde cardioplegia. With either technique, flow through the IMA may wash out cardioplegia and warm the heart during the procedure. A third option is to utilize deep hypothermia and circulatory arrest.

Although these techniques may be helpful in situations in which the IMA is densely adherent to the posterior sternum and cannot be safely dissected, it is preferable to dissect out the IMA and occlude it during aortic cross-clamping. The IMA may be isolated even before re-sternotomy using a supraclavicular incision. With interruption of IMA flow, the surgeon may be confident that cardioplegia will not be washed out and the heart will be made uniformly cold.

It may also be difficult to expose the aortic valve through the standard aortotomy because of the presence of saphenous vein grafts anastomosed to the proximal aorta. In my practice, I have found it helpful to cannulate the axillary artery in these cases. In so doing, the aorta may be cross-clamped just proximal to the innominate artery, which provides several more centimeters of ascending aorta unencumbered by the aortic cannula. This extra length of ascending aorta then permits an aortotomy incision (which avoids proximal anastomoses) to be made in the axis of the aorta, directed posteriorly along the patient's right. Excellent exposure of the aortic valve is achieved without injury to previously placed proximal anastomoses.

The Small Aortic Annulus

In choosing the appropriate size of aortic valve prosthesis, the surgeon strives to leave the patient with minimal gradient across the valve. When this is done, the increased left ventricular mass index (developed in compensation for aortic stenosis) typically resolves following AVR. Traditional concern has surrounded the potential for a high residual transvalvular gradient should too small a prosthesis be implanted, creating the phenomenon of "patient–prosthesis mismatch." This concern has led to a persistent controversy over the management of the small aortic annulus.

Whereas some authors have demonstrated that implantation of small aortic valves has no effect on long-term survival, others have suggested otherwise. One factor confounding the interpretation of these data is the fact that the sizing of prosthetic valves is inconsistent from one manufacturer to the next. A 19-mm valve may vary in effective orifice area (EOA) from 1.0 cm² to 1.3 cm². Another confounding factor is the fact that the population of patients (in particular with regard to patient age, gender, and size) varies from one report to the next.

The patient's size (body surface area, BSA) and age must be considered when choosing the appropriate aortic valve prosthesis. Acknowledging some of the uncertainties provided by the literature in this area, one should avoid implantation of an aortic prosthesis when the calculated EOA/BSA is <0.8 cm²/m². This recommendation is derived from the fact that an aortic valve area of 0.6 cm²/m² is considered severe aortic stenosis. Use of this guideline is helpful because it places the consideration of valve size in the context of the patient's hemodynamic needs rather than in absolute terms.

The implication of this strategy is the anticipation that a patient with a larger BSA will require a higher flow rate across the valve (cardiac output) than will a patient with a smaller BSA. Knowledge of the patient's BSA and the EOA of given sizes of a particular type of prosthesis permits an estimation of the valve size needed to leave the patient with an appropriate EOA/BSA ratio (Fig. 45-13). Because "patient–prosthesis mismatch" may not affect a difference in survival for 5 to 7 years, other patient-specific factors must be considered such as age and activity level; a 60-year-old distance runner will require a larger EOA than an 80-year-old sedentary person. Nonetheless, this strategy

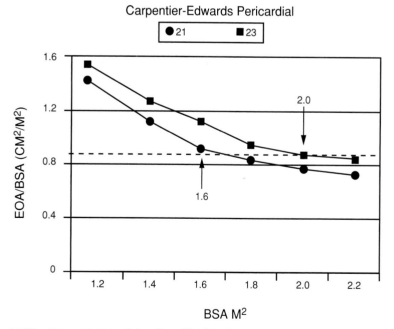

Carpentier-Edwards Pericardial

Figure 45-13. Demonstration of the effect of body surface area (BSA) on patient–prosthesis mismatch for Edwards Life Sciences pericardial valves of 21 mm and 23 mm. An indexed effective orifice area (EOA/BSA) of 0.9 cm²/m² is achieved when a 21-mm valve is placed in a patient with a BSA of 1.6 m². Similarly, patient–prosthesis mismatch occurs when a 23-mm valve is inserted into a patient with BSA of >2.0 m². (Reprinted with permission from V Rao, WRE Jamieson, J Ivanov, et al. Prosthesis–patient mismatch affects survival after aortic valve replacement. Circulation 2000;102:III-5.)

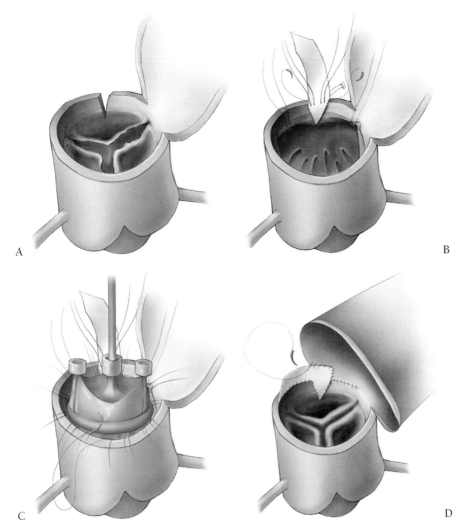

Figure 45-14.   Operative technique: aortic annulus enlargement. **(A)** The aortotomy incision is extended across the aortic annulus at the midpoint of the noncoronary leaflet. **(B)** Vascular patch material is partially sewn in place. **(C)** The valve is implanted. Across the patch material, the pledgetted valve sutures are placed from "outside-in." **(D)** The patch material is brought anteriorly to close the aorta.

serves as a useful guide in choosing valve size.

To successfully implant an appropriate size of valve, it may be necessary to enlarge the aortic annulus. Most reported series of aortic valve replacement indicate that annular enlargement is uncommonly performed, and may be associated with a higher operative mortality rate. Several techniques have been described for aortic annular enlargement. My preferred method is as follows (Fig. 45-14):

1. Enlarge the annulus at the midway point of the noncoronary leaflet. This is accomplished by extension of the aortotomy incision.
2. Extend this incision into the fibrous apron between the mitral and aortic annuli, but it is unnecessary to incise the mitral annulus or the anterior leaflet of the mitral valve.
3. Beginning at the apex of the incision, sew a fashioned piece of woven Dacron in place. The patch material is typically 2 cm wide. A pledgetted 5-0 polypropylene suture is brought through the patch material, then the roof of the left atrium, then the apex of the aortic incision, and then tied. The patch material is sewn to the aorta for a distance of about 2 in.
4. The valve stitches are placed. In the area over the patch material, four pledgeted sutures are brought from outside-in through the patch material. *Technical caveat:* At each edge of the patch, a horizontal mattress stitch is brought outside-in with one needle through the aorta and the other through the patch material. Between these two stitches, two additional valve sutures are typically placed. I prefer to use 4-0 polypropylene for these four valve sutures because the needle holes through the patch material are small and bleeding is less.
5. The patch material is then brought anteriorly to complete aortic closure. *Technical caveat:* If the patch material is too wide over the anterior aorta, the proximal aorta may be displaced anteriorly. When this is done, the orifice of the right coronary may be displaced and kinked. This may be avoided by cutting the patch material no wider than about 1.5 cm to 2 cm in this area. After the aorta is closed, one should test for hemostasis by administration of antegrade cardioplegia. A small amount of oozing through the patch material is to be expected until heparin reversal. However, any bleeding sites, particularly near the apex of the patch closure, should be repaired before release of the aortic cross-clamp.

SUGGESTED READING

Banbury MK, Cosgrove DM III, White JA, et al. Age and valve size effect on the long-term durability of the Carpentier-Edwards aortic pericardial bioprosthesis. Ann Thorac Surg 2001;72:753.

Borer JS, Bonow RO. Contemporary approach to aortic and mitral regurgitation. Circulation 2003;108:2432.

Byrne JG, Karavas AN, Filsoufi F, et al. Aortic valve surgery after previous coronary artery bypass grafting with functioning internal mammary artery grafts. Ann Thorac Surg 2002;73:779.

Grover FL, Edwards FH. Similarity between the STS and New York State databases for valvular heart disease. Ann Thorac Surg 2000;70:1143.

Grunkemeier GL, Wu Y. Actual versus actuarial event-free percentages. Ann Thorac Surg 2001;72:677.

Kuralay E, Cingoz F, Gunay C, et al. Supraclavicular control of patent internal thoracic artery graft flow during aortic valve replacement. Ann Thorac Surg 2003;75:1422.

Lung B, Gohlke-Barwolf C, Tornos P, et al. Working Group Report. Recommendations on the management of the asymptomatic patient with valvular heart disease. Eur Heart J 2002;23:1253.

Monin JL, Quere JP, Monchi M, et al. Low-gradient aortic stenosis. Operative risk stratification and predictors for long-term outcome: A multicenter study using dobutamine stress hemodynamics. Circulation 2003;108:319.

Nishimura RA, Grantham JA, Connolly HM, et al. Low-output, low-gradient aortic stenosis in patients with depressed left ventricular systolic function. The clinical utility of the dobutamine challenge in the catheterization laboratory. Circulation 2002;106:809.

Otto CM, Burwash IG, Legget ME, et al. Prospective study of asymptomatic valvular aortic stenosis. Circulation 1997;95:2262.

Rahimtoola SH. Should patients with asymptomatic mild or moderate aortic stenosis undergoing coronary artery bypass surgery also have valve replacement for the aortic stenosis? Heart 2001;85:337.

Rao V, Jamieson WRE, Ivanov J, et al. Prosthesis–patient mismatch affects survival after aortic valve replacement. Circulation 2000;102: III-5.

Rosenhek R, Binder T, Porenta, G. Predictors of outcome in severe, asymptomatic aortic stenosis. N Engl J Med 2000;343:611.

Sommers KE, David TE. Aortic valve replacement with patch enlargement of the aortic annulus. Ann Thorac Surg 1997;63:1608.

Task Force on Practice Guidelines (Committee on Management of Patients with Valvular Heart Disease). ACC/AHA guidelines for the management of patients with valvular heart diseases: A report of the American College of Cardiology/American Heart Association. J Am Coll Cardiol 1998;32:1486.

EDITOR'S COMMENTS

Dr. Fullerton has provided a complete discussion of aortic valve replacement. I am particularly pleased and impressed with his indications regarding aortic valve replacement. The surgeon must truly be the expert on the medical and surgical management of valvular heart disease particularly as it relates to when to operate and when not to. This is part of our curriculum and heritage and I cannot overemphasize this point. Dr. Fullerton has given a complete discussion of the timing of operation and the risks. I agree basically with his approach to aortic valve replacement. In general, I favor tissue valves except in those patients who truly fear for reoperation. I agree fully that in elderly patients at the coronary artery bypass moderate aortic stenosis should be treated with aortic valve replacement. Aortic valve reoperations are reasonably safe these days even with patent bypass grafts. However, it is easier to avoid a second operation.

Finally, I have begun to favor the ministernotomy approach for aortic valve replacement in patients who do not need associated coronary artery bypass. The operation is essentially the same as that done through a standard sternotomy with the exception of use of femoral percutaneous venous cannulation. This surgical exposure is excellent, and I believe the same operation can be done with a smaller incision.

I.L.K.

46

Aortic Valve Replacement: Ross Procedure

Ronald C. Elkins

Pulmonary autograft replacement of the aortic valve, first performed by Ross in 1967, is being utilized by an increasing number of surgeons worldwide as their operation of choice in young children and adults with active lifestyles. It is viable, can grow, has the potential to be a permanent valve replacement, does not require anticoagulation, and has the hemodynamic characteristics of a normal aortic valve. With increased experience during the last 15 years, indications for its use have widened to include neonates, patients with endocarditis, and patients with associated ascending aortic disease. Routine echocardiographic surveillance of patients after a Ross operation has allowed the identification of failure modes, which has led to modifications of the operation that include avoidance of mismatch between the aortic and pulmonary annulus, management of ascending aortic dilation or aneurysm formation, suggested indications for choice of implant procedure, and patient selection. Concern for the relatively early failure mode of allograft reconstruction of the right ventricular outflow tract in some patients as well as the limited availability of allografts has led to alternate choices of valves or procedures. Several investigators are evaluating the use of decellularized allografts and xenograft valves and conduits to reduce the immunologic response to the allograft in hopes of improving durability. The Ross operation will continue to change as additional long-term data about indications, operative technique, and late results become known.

Indications

Patients with a life expectancy of more than 20 years and isolated aortic valve disease requiring surgical intervention are candidates for the Ross procedure. Patients who cannot be safely anticoagulated or who do not desire lifetime anticoagulation, and patients who because of their relatively young age are not candidates for aortic valve replacement using an aortic homograft, are considered for the Ross procedure. Recently there has been increasing enthusiasm for the use of pulmonary autograft replacement of the aortic valve in those patients with aortic valve endocarditis because the pulmonary autograft is the only valve replacement that is viable and the surgeon can avoid the use of prosthetic material or nonviable biologic tissue. Recently developed techniques allow use of the pulmonary autograft in patients requiring aortic valve replacement when there is a significant discrepancy in size between the aortic valve annulus and the pulmonary valve annulus. Patients with a small aortic annulus and significant subvalvular obstruction can have an extended Ross procedure (Ross procedure with a Konno myotomy and myomectomy). Patients with aortic insufficiency and significant aortic annulus dilation are candidates for an aortic annuloplasty with a reduction in the size of the aortic annulus, fixation of the size of the aortic annulus appropriate for the patient's body surface area, and replacement of the aortic valve with a Ross procedure as a root replacement.

Contraindications

Patients with Marfan syndrome or other genetic disorders known to affect fibrillin or elastin of the aortic valve are not candidates for a Ross procedure because the pulmonary valve is likely to be affected by the disease process. Patients with significant immune-complex disease (juvenile rheumatoid arthritis, lupus erythematosus, and active rheumatic heart disease) as the etiology of their aortic valve disease have had early failure or degeneration of the pulmonary autograft valve, and these patients are not considered candidates for a Ross procedure. Patients with annuloaortic ectasia who require replacement of the aortic valve and the ascending aorta may be candidates for a Ross procedure, especially if the aortic valve is bicuspid. Patients with a normal trileaflet aortic valve are more likely candidates for a valvuloplasty and replacement of the ascending aorta as described by David.

Operative Technique

After median sternotomy and suspension of the heart with a pericardial cradle, aortic cannulation should be accomplished near the origin of the innominate artery or more distally if resection of the ascending aorta is required. Bicaval cannulation with the superior vena caval cannula inserted directly in the superior vena cava provides improved exposure and, if necessary, cannulation of the coronary sinus under direct vision for retrograde cardioplegia. Before institution of bypass, the aortic fat pad is dissected to identify the origin of the right coronary artery, and the adventitial plane between the aorta and the pulmonary artery is dissected until the origin of the right pulmonary artery can be identified. Myocardial protection is provided with moderate systemic hypothermia (30°C to 32°C), surface cooling of the myocardium with ice slush, and a combination of antegrade and retrograde blood cardioplegia, maintaining a myocardial temperature below 12°C. With the aorta cross-clamped and the heart arrested, a transverse

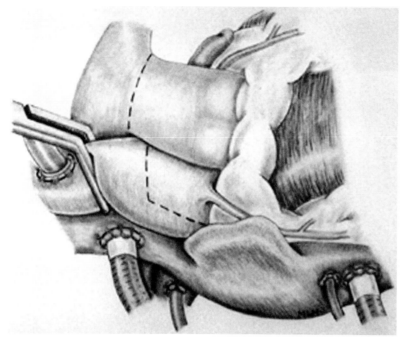

Figure 46-1. Cannulation: Distal aorta, bicaval cannulation with the superior vena caval cannula placed through a purse string in the vena cava, the left ventricular vent through the right superior pulmonary vein, and the retrograde cardioplegia cannula through the right atrium. All illustrations are oriented as seen by a surgeon standing on the right side of the patient.

valves will have minor (1 mm or 2 mm) fenestrations, as does the normal aortic valve. In patients with a bicuspid aortic valve, the pulmonary valve is also bicuspid in 2% to 3%, and we do not recommend using these valves as an autograft. (Some surgeons have used a bicuspid pulmonary valve for an autograft, but the mid-term late results of this have shown early degeneration in our patients.) If the pulmonary valve is abnormal, the pulmonary artery can be closed, and the surgeon can proceed to replace the aortic valve with a homograft, a prosthetic valve, or a bioprosthesis based on the patient's and surgeon's choice. With a normal pulmonary valve, the surgeon divides the pulmonary artery and begins to enucleate the pulmonary artery and its contained valve by dissecting posteriorly, staying adjacent to the pulmonary artery (Fig. 46-4). It is frequently advantageous to divide the posterior pericardial reflection of the pericardium on the pulmonary artery and enter the transverse sinus. The left main coronary artery should be protected, and a small probe in this artery will help an inexperienced surgeon in its identification. The dissection is continued posteriorly, staying adjacent to the pulmonary artery until left ventricular myocardium is encountered. The surgeon then looks into the pulmonary artery, beneath the pulmonary valve, and identifies a point 3 mm to 4 mm below the pulmonary annulus. A right-angled clamp is used to identify this point on the anterior free wall of the right ventricle (Fig. 46-5). A right

aortotomy is made 1.5 cm to 2.0 cm distal to the origin of the right coronary artery (Fig. 46-1). The aortotomy is extended to the patient's right until the midpoint of the noncoronary sinus is seen and then extended into this sinus, stopping 2 mm to 3 mm from the aortic annulus. Stay sutures are placed on the edges of the aortotomy to provide wide exposure of the aortic valve. The aortic valve is inspected, and any dysplasia involving the aortic annulus or the coronary sinuses or abnormality involving the position and relationship of the coronary orifices is noted. The aortic valve is excised at the level of the annulus, and the annulus is measured. In patients without significant aortic annulus dysplasia, with three coronary sinuses of near equal size and coronary ostium that are in a normal position (about 120 degrees from each other), and with an aortic annulus that is 20 mm to 25 mm in diameter, we implant the pulmonary autograft as an intra-aortic implant using the inclusion cylinder technique. In patients who do not meet these criteria, we implant the pulmonary autograft as a root replacement. These two operative techniques are described separately.

imal to the origin of the right pulmonary artery (Fig. 46-2). The pulmonary artery is divided anteriorly, and the pulmonary valve is inspected. It should be a three-leaflet valve without fusion of any commissures and should not have any major fenestrations (Fig. 46-3). Many of the pulmonary

Inclusion Cylinder

After inspection and excision of the aortic valve, the pulmonary artery is opened prox-

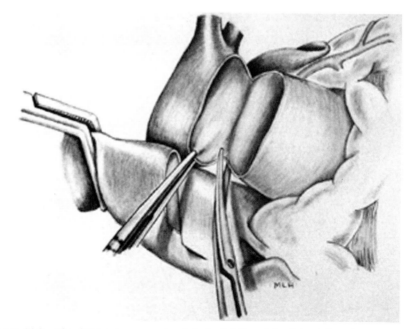

Figure 46-2. The distal pulmonary artery is incised at the origin of the right pulmonary artery. A transverse arteriotomy is made that is adequate for careful inspection of the pulmonary artery.

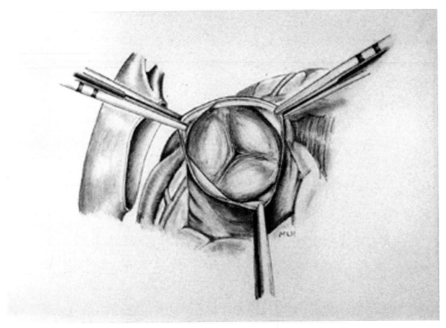

Figure 46-3. The normal trileaflet pulmonary valve with three equal sinuses and no significant fenestrations or other abnormalities of the leaflets.

ventriculotomy is made with a knife, ensuring that it is caudal to the pulmonary valve. The right ventriculotomy is then extended toward the patient's left, with the pulmonary annulus in view, and the ventriculotomy is continued 3 mm to 4 mm below the annulus. As the left anterior descending coronary artery is approached, the surgeon stops and begins the dissection on the patient's right. The pulmonary artery and its contained valve are enucleated from the outflow tract of the right ventri-

cle as the surgeon divides right ventricular myocardium and joins the previous posterior dissection. Frequently, the pulmonary artery and aorta are very adherent near the anterior fibrous trigone, an area of common conal tissue. Posteriorly the right ventricular muscle is dissected from the remaining septal musculature in a horizontal plane (Fig. 46-6). This dissection should be done carefully, with traction being maintained on the pulmonary artery to avoid injury to the first septal coronary artery. The anatomy of the first septal coronary artery has recently been redescribed for the normal heart and hearts with aortic stenosis. The artery branches from the left anterior descending coronary artery at the level of the first diagonal and courses toward the middle papillary muscle of the tricuspid valve and moderator band. It runs in the lower margin of the septomarginal trabecula. In patients with a small anterior extension of the septomarginal trabecula, the first septal perforator may be very close to the nadir of the posterior cusp of the pulmonary valve, and extreme caution should be used to avoid injury to this vessel.

When the pulmonary artery and valve have been enucleated from the right ventricular outflow tract, the proximal muscle rim is trimmed so that 2 mm to 3 mm of muscle is left proximal to the valve annulus. If the autograft is to be implanted as an intra-aortic inclusion cylinder, all adventitia is carefully dissected from the pulmonary artery. (This adventitia is left intact if the autograft is to be implanted as a root replacement.) The pulmonary autograft is not mechanically sized because it will dilate to almost any size because the annulus of the pulmonary valve is primarily muscle and will dilate readily. Implantation of the autograft is begun by orienting the pulmonary valve so that the posterior sinus will become the left coronary sinus of the autograft. A 4-0 polypropylene suture is placed through the pulmonary annulus at the nadir of the hinge mechanism of the pulmonary leaflet, and this stitch is then brought through the nadir of the aortic annulus in the left coronary sinus, adjacent to the left coronary ostium (Fig. 46-7A). A second suture is then placed through the nadir of the pulmonary sinus that will become the right coronary sinus and in the nadir of the aortic annulus of the right coronary sinuses, adjacent to the right coronary orifice. A third suture is then positioned from the base of the remaining sinus of the pulmonary valve, and this suture is positioned in the aortic annulus in the noncoronary sinus so that the aortic annulus is trifurcated by the three sutures. The sinuses of the pulmonary valve

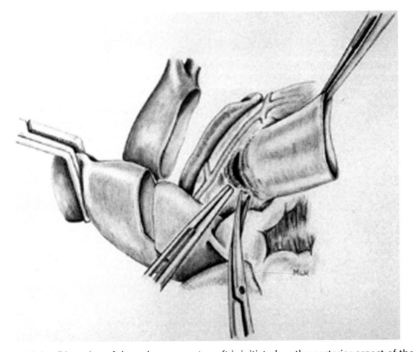

Figure 46-4. Dissection of the pulmonary autograft is initiated on the posterior aspect of the proximal pulmonary artery. Dissection is continued in this plane, adjacent to the pulmonary artery, until septal myocardium is encountered. The left main coronary artery and left anterior descending coronary artery are protected.

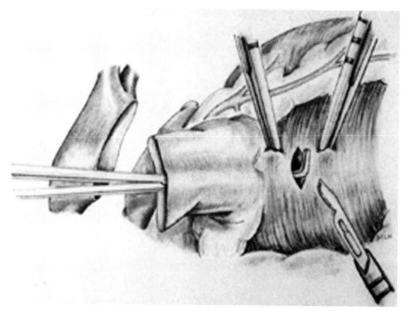

Figure 46-5. Identification of the anterior right ventriculotomy is facilitated by placing a right-angled clamp through the pulmonary valve and indenting the myocardium 3 mm to 4 mm below the pulmonary valve annulus.

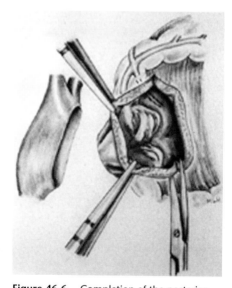

Figure 46-6. Completion of the posterior enucleation of the pulmonary autograft from the outflow tract of the right ventricle. Note the usual location of the first large septal perforating coronary artery. It arises adjacent to the first diagonal coronary artery of the left anterior descending coronary artery and traverses the septal musculature toward the conal papillary muscle of the tricuspid valve.

are almost equal in size, and the sinuses of the aortic valve are rarely equal, so some adjustment must be made in the positioning of the sutures in the aortic annulus. After these sutures are placed to orient the valve, additional interrupted sutures are inserted between the pulmonary artery and the aortic outflow tract in a plane that connects the three orienting sutures. This plane does not parallel the scalloped annulus of either the aortic valve or the pulmonary valve, but is in a horizontal plane below the annulus in the interleaflet triangles, below the commissural attachments. With these sutures gathered into three equal groups, the pulmonary valve is seated, and the artery and valve are allowed to invert into the left ventricle to facilitate tying and dividing the sutures (Fig. 46-7B). The pulmonary artery and valve are reinverted and inspected to ensure that inadvertent injury to the valve leaflets has not occurred. Commissural attachment is secured with horizontal mattress sutures of 4-0 polypropylene placed 1 mm above the pulmonary valve commissures and placed through the aorta at a height above the aortic commissures determined by exerting equal tension on the pulmonary artery and the aorta. This height is usually 3 mm to 5 mm above the aortic valve commissure. With the pulmonary artery and valve as a cylinder, it is relatively easy to ensure that the valve is suspended with an equal amount of tension on each commissure and symmetrically oriented in the aorta. These three sutures are tagged and not tied until the coronary artery anastomoses have been completed. The left coronary artery is implanted by removing a 4.5- to 5.0-mm button of pulmonary artery from the sinus overlying the left coronary ostium (Fig. 46-7C). The ostium of the left coronary artery is anastomosed to the open-

ing in the pulmonary artery with a continuous suture of 5-0 polypropylene. A similar technique is used for attachment of the right coronary orifice to the pulmonary artery.

With the coronary ostia attached, the commissural sutures are tied to secure firm attachment of the pulmonary valve commissures to the aortic wall. The pulmonary artery is trimmed 2 mm distal to the commissural sutures in preparation for the distal anastomosis. The distal suture line is accomplished with a continuous suture of 4-0 polypropylene. Beginning at the commissure between the left and right coronary sinuses, the suture is placed full thickness through the pulmonary artery and aorta and tied on the adventitial side of the aorta (Fig. 46-7D). The ends of the suture are then brought into the lumen of the aorta, and a continuous suture technique is used, ensuring a smooth anastomosis between the pulmonary artery and the aorta. To complete this suture line, the aortotomy closure in the noncoronary sinus must be completed. A 4-0 suture is used to close the aortotomy and it is initiated in the noncoronary sinus (see Fig. 46-7D). The suture line includes a full-thickness bite of the pulmonary artery so that a potential space in the noncoronary sinus between the pulmonary artery and the aorta is obliterated, and the aortic closure is reinforced by the pulmonary artery in this sinus. When the aortotomy closure reaches the distal anastomosis of the pulmonary autograft, the distal suture line of the pulmonary autograft is completed by bringing the ends through the aortic wall and tying the suture. The transverse aortotomy closure is completed, air is evacuated from the ascending aorta, and the cross-clamp is removed. Competency of the autograft valve can be tested at this time by evaluating the amount of regurgitant flow coming through the left ventricular vent and by noting whether there has been a significant decrease in the mean aortic pressure with removal of the aortic cross-clamp.

With a successful implantation of the pulmonary autograft, attention is now directed to reconstruction of the right ventricular outflow tract. We prefer to use a pulmonary homograft, and always try to use a homograft that is larger than the patient's aortic annulus. We select a homograft that is from a donor of similar age and usually try to use a homograft that is between 22 mm and 27 mm. The pulmonary homograft is selected and thawed during the implantation of the autograft and can be kept cold and moist or simply placed in the pericardial well until used. The pulmonary homograft is trimmed by

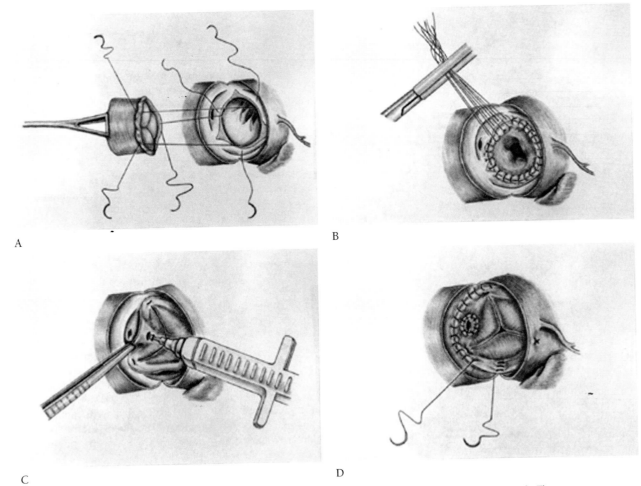

A

B

C

D

Figure 46-7. **(A)** Placement of three polypropylene sutures to orient the pulmonary autograft. The posterior sinus of the pulmonary autograft becomes the new left coronary sinus. **(B)** The autograft is inverted into the left ventricle, and the proximal sutures are tied and divided. **(C)** The pulmonary autograft is reinverted. Horizontal mattress sutures are placed to secure the height and position of the autograft (but not tied until the right and left coronary arteries are implanted). An aortic punch (4 mm or 5 mm) is used to create an opening in the autograft to allow attachment of the coronary artery ostia. **(D)** Completion of coronary artery anastomosis. Commissural stay sutures are tied and divided, and the distal suture line is initiated at the commissure between the left and right coronary arteries. This is continued to the aortotomy extension into the noncoronary sinus. This portion of the aortotomy is closed with a running suture line with the suture including a full-thickness "bite" of the noncoronary sinus of the pulmonary autograft.

removing any excess myocardium proximal to the valve and by trimming the branch pulmonary arteries as necessary. The pulmonary homograft is always implanted in its normal anatomic orientation. The proximal suture line is completed first with continuous 4-0 polypropylene. This suture line must be completed with some care because deep bites into the ventricular septum could lead to injury to the first septal perforator (Fig. 46-8). After the posterior portion of the proximal suture line is completed, rewarming can be instituted and the anterior portion of this suture line completed. Before the distal suture line is completed, hemostasis must be accomplished in the area

of dissection where the pulmonary autograft was harvested. This dissection plane frequently has several small coronary arteries and small coronary venules that must be controlled with the cautery or fine sutures. After hemostasis is secured, the distal suture line is completed. It is possible to narrow the distal pulmonary arteries, especially the right, with this anastomosis. Care to avoid "purse stringing" the anastomosis and avoiding tension on the right pulmonary artery will minimize the likelihood of this occurrence.

After bypass has been discontinued, intraoperative echocardiographic assessment of autograft function is obtained before de-

cannulation. In general, minimal to trace autograft insufficiency can be identified by color-flow Doppler echocardiography. This represents an excellent result, and experience suggests that this degree of insufficiency will not significantly increase with time. Autograft insufficiency of 2+ or 3+ suggests that a technical error has been made. Careful echocardiographic assessment or direct assessment will usually demonstrate leaflet prolapse, and in our experience this has been secondary to failure to properly suspend or orient the three commissures. This can usually be corrected by taking down the distal autograft suture line and resuspending the commissures. In our

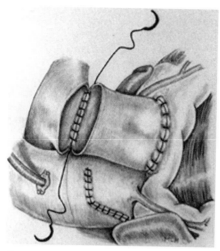

Figure 46-8. Completion of the closure of the aortotomy. The aortic cross-clamp is removed. The pulmonary homograft reconstruction of the outflow tract is accomplished with two continuous sutures of polypropylene. The proximal suture line is completed first.

experience, the most common error is associated with the commissure between the right and the noncoronary sinuses. Using the described inclusion cylinder technique, we have not found it necessary to adjust or redo any valves nor have we had to abandon the use of a pulmonary autograft.

Root Replacement

The root replacement has become the most popular technique for insertion of the pulmonary autograft, and if continued follow-up demonstrates that the pulmonary root adapts to the increased pressure load of the systemic circulation without dilation and autograft valve insufficiency, it will become the technique of choice. We use the root replacement in patients with a small aortic annulus (<20 mm) or a dysplastic aortic annulus or in patients with valve and subvalvular obstruction. Patients with a true bicuspid aortic valve and coronary arteries that are 180 degrees apart, marked distortion of one or more coronary sinuses, or significant dilation of the annulus or sinotubular junction of the aorta are also candidates for a root replacement.

The root replacement has become our primary technique for the Ross procedure, and 409 patients are operative survivors. Actuarial freedom from autograft degeneration (reoperation on the autograft valve, severe autograft valve insufficiency not due to infection, autograft valve stenosis and valve-related death) is 88% ± 4% at 13 years. In

the 86 patients having an intra-aortic technique for their Ross procedure, the actuarial freedom from autograft degeneration is 78% ± 6% at 13 years (Wilcoxon p= .0024).

The techniques of cannulation and bypass are identical to those used for an intra-aortic implant. After the pulmonary autograft has been enucleated from the right ventricular outflow tract, it is prepared by trimming the proximal myocardium so that it extends only 2 mm to 3 mm proximal to the pulmonary annulus. All adventitia is left on the pulmonary artery to provide additional substance to the autograft. The aorta is transected transversely 1 cm to 2 cm distal to the origin of the right coronary artery. The two coronary arteries are mobilized with generous cuffs of aorta for later implantation to the autograft (Fig. 46-9A). The remaining aorta is then excised, leaving a 2- to 3-mm cuff of aorta above the level of the aortic valve annulus. The aortic annulus is left intact to provide some support, especially in the left coronary and noncoronary sinuses in the portion of the aortic annulus between the two fibrous trigones. Any subvalvular obstruction is excised, and, if indicated, a left ventricular myomectomy can be accomplished. The pulmonary autograft is oriented so that its posterior sinus can become the left coronary sinus (Fig. 46-9B). A 4-0 polypropylene suture is placed from the nadir of this sinus to the aortic annulus at the ostium of the left coronary artery. A similar suture is placed in the sinus that will become the right coronary sinus, and a third suture is placed in the remaining sinus and is used to trifurcate the aortic annulus. Interrupted 4-0 sutures are then placed from the autograft to the aortic annulus in a plane connecting these orienting sutures. The plane is at the level of the annulus in the nadir of the coronary sinuses but is below the annulus in the interleaflet triangles. The suture line must seat the autograft into the left ventricular outflow tract so that the autograft annulus has the support of the left ventricular myocardium. The autograft should be sutured to the fibrous trigone at the edge of the anterior leaflet of the mitral valve and to the valve leaflet between the trigones. In the region of the membranous septum, the suture line remains on the aortic annulus to avoid the conduction system. When all sutures have been placed, the autograft is seated and the sutures are tied. To enhance hemostasis, this suture line is usually tied over a strip of pericardium, or, if we wish to fix the size of the annulus, we use a strip of woven polyethylene terephthalate (Dacron). After completion of this suture line, the left coronary artery is implanted to a

5-mm opening made in the pulmonary autograft with an aortic punch (Fig. 46-9C). The aorta is trimmed around the coronary ostium to match this opening, and the suture line is continuous 5-0 polypropylene. The distal suture line is then completed with a continuous 4-0 suture. It may be necessary to trim either the aorta or the pulmonary artery. If there is a significant discrepancy between the size of the aorta and that of the pulmonary artery, an aortoplasty can be performed. If there is aneurysmal dilation of the ascending aorta, the aneurysm can be resected and replaced with an appropriate vascular graft. After the distal anastomosis is completed, the autograft is distended with cardioplegic perfusate, the left coronary anastomosis is inspected for any leaks, and the site for the right coronary implant is selected. To assist in selecting the site for the right coronary implantation, a marking suture to identify the commissure between the left and right coronary sinuses is helpful. It may also assist in avoiding accidental injury to the pulmonary valve when making the opening in the pulmonary artery. The right coronary should be implanted under some tension because distention of the right heart after bypass is discontinued can cause kinking of this vessel if the right coronary is inset close to the proximal anastomosis (Fig. 46-9D). The right coronary implantation is similar to that of the left coronary, and after it is completed, air is evacuated from the autograft and the cross-clamp is removed. Assessment of autograft function is similar to the evaluation used with the intra-aortic implant.

Use of the pulmonary autograft as a root replacement has been associated with immediate good results with the absence of significant valvular insufficiency in all patients. Early failure has been seen when the pulmonary autograft has been used in patients with significant aortic annular dilation and there is a significant size discrepancy between the aortic annulus and the pulmonary annulus. The learning curve of this operation has been associated with a greater risk of operative death, primarily from hemorrhage. The integrity of each of the four anastomoses must be assessed before reconstruction of the right ventricular outflow tract and while the patient is cannulated so that perfusion pressure can be manipulated when the autograft is being sutured.

The pulmonary homograft insertion to complete the operation is similar to the technique used for the previously described intra-aortic implant. Echocardiography is used to assess autograft function as well as homograft function.

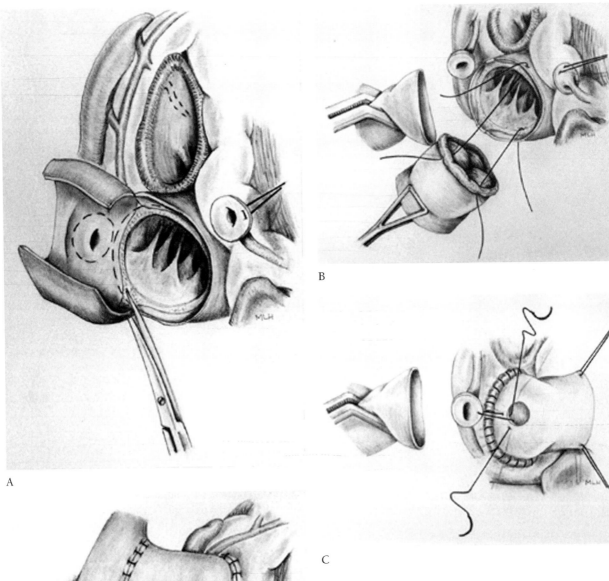

A

B

C

D

Figure 46-9. **(A)** Generous cuffs of aorta are left attached to the right and left coronary ostia. Minimal mobilization of these coronary arteries is performed. The remaining proximal aorta is excised, transecting the aorta below the aortic annulus in the interleaflet triangle. **(B)** The pulmonary autograft is in an anatomic position with the posterior sinus of the autograft becoming the new left coronary sinus. (The stay suture in this sinus is not shown for clarity.) The remaining sutures for orientation are placed to position the new right coronary sinus and to trifurcate the aortic annulus. **(C)** The left coronary artery is implanted with a continuous suture of polypropylene. **(D)** Completion of the pulmonary autograft root implantation with selection of the site of implantation of the right coronary artery with the autograft distended. The pulmonary homograft reconstruction of the outflow tract of the right ventricle is done with two continuous suture lines.

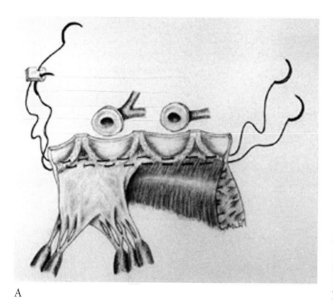
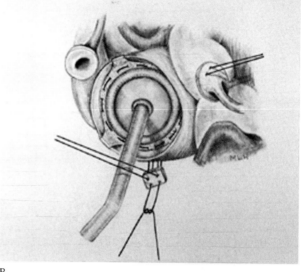

A   B

Figure 46-10. **(A)** Purse strings of 2-0 or 3-0 polypropylene are placed at the annulus in the nadir of the coronary sinus and subannular in the interleaflet triangle. The sutures are brought external to the aorta in the noncoronary sinus, and a felt pledget is used for reinforcement. **(B)** The annulus is sized with a Hegar dilator or a valve sizer, and the sutures are tied. This adjusts the aortic annulus size to one appropriate for the patient's body surface area.

Pulmonary Autografts in Aortic Annular Dilation

Pulmonary autograft insertion in patients with significant aortic annular dilation (aortic annulus ≥27 mm or an annulus with a Z-value of >+2 when compared with body surface area) has been associated with early failure as a result of progressive autograft insufficiency and dilation of the autograft root. However, these are frequently patients in whom a Ross operation would otherwise be appropriate. They are frequently young, have a bicuspid aortic valve with severe aortic insufficiency, have significant dilation of their aortic annulus, and may have an ascending aortic aneurysm. Recently, we used a reduction aortic annuloplasty with an external cuff of Dacron to fix the size of the aortic annulus appropriate for the size of the pulmonary autograft. When indicated, the ascending aorta is replaced with a collagen-impregnated Dacron graft.

After excision of the aortic valve and confirmation of the size of the aortic annulus, two purse-string sutures of 3-0 polypropylene are placed at the aortic annulus at the level of the nadir of the coronary sinuses and below the aortic annulus in the interleaflet triangle in the noncoronary-left triangle and the left-right triangle. In the triangle between the right and noncoronary sinus, adjacent to the membranous septum, the

suture line remains adjacent to the aortic annulus to avoid the conduction system. These sutures are brought outside the lumen of the aorta in the noncoronary sinus (Fig. 46-10). These sutures are tied over a polytetrafluoroethylene (Teflon) felt pledget, and the size of the aortic annulus is adjusted to the anticipated normal annulus size based on the patient's body surface area. The autograft root replacement is accomplished as previously described except that the proximal sutures must be passed around the annuloplasty sutures and are then tied over an external 3-mm ring of woven Dacron (Fig. 46-11). In those patients with active endocarditis and a dilated aortic annulus, aortic annulus reduction is accomplished with a suture annuloplasty but the fixation ring is glutaraldehyde-fixed bovine pericardium.

This technique of annulus reduction and fixation has been used in 170 patients since the initial use in 1995. Actuarial freedom from autograft degeneration in this group of patients is 96% ± 3% at 7 years. This is similar to the autograft performance for this time frame in those patients having a Ross operation as a root replacement who did not require annulus reduction or annulus fixation. In all adult patients and children of adult size, annulus fixation with a Dacron cuff has been used routinely since 1997 except in patients with endocarditis. In those patients, autologous pericardium or glutaraldehyde-fixed bovine pericardium has been used

for annulus fixation. Glutaraldehyde-fixed bovine pericardium has been used in patients with endocarditis that involved the native aortic annulus. When the proximal suture line has been tied over strips of autologous pericardium to enhance hemostasis it has not been found to provide fixation of the aortic annulus in our patients.

Surgical Results and Current Thoughts

The operative mortality of aortic valve replacement depends on the patient population, and in healthy young adults approaches 1%. A Ross operation can be performed by surgeons who have considerable experience with it with a similar operative risk; however, in general, the operative risk for a Ross operation is slightly higher. The operative risk as reported in the International Ross Registry is 3.3% in 4,205 patients. In our experience of 518 patients, the operative mortality is 4.2% for all patients. The 22 operative deaths in this series were reviewed to assess the operative events most likely associated with their outcome in the hope of providing information that would be helpful to surgeons early in their Ross experience. There were 9 operative deaths in neonates and very young

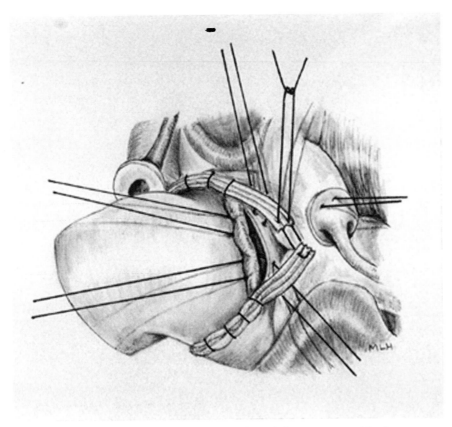

Figure 46-11. The proximal sutures of the autograft are tied over a narrow strip of woven Dacron to "fix" the aortic annulus size. The proximal sutures are placed such that the suture includes the previously placed annuloplasty sutures.

children. The 3 neonate deaths were in critically ill children following a failed aortic balloon valvuloplasty with severe aortic insufficiency and progressive ventricular dysfunction. Two patients were on extracorporeal membrane oxygenation support at the time of their Ross operation. These patients probably should have had an aortic valvuloplasty as a salvage procedure, and, if this had been successful, they might have become candidates for a Ross operation at a later date. One patient died of malalignment of the left coronary anastomosis to the autograft root. This calls attention to the need for very careful alignment of the coronary buttons with the recognition that the autograft root will distend and dilate when it is placed in the systemic circulation, and the coronary buttons should be placed relatively high on their respective sinuses to avoid any possibility of kinking when the root is distended. Four patients with aortic and left ventricular outflow tract obstruction died following a Ross-Konno operation; 2 of these were related to severe pulmonary hypertension. One patient died related to a prolonged period of circulatory arrest used to reconstruct the transverse arch and resection of a pre-

viously placed left ventricular aortic graft, and the other died of ventricular dysfunction associated with recurrent ventricular arrhythmia. In review of the adult deaths, only two details of operative management warrant comment: intraoperative bleeding from the autograft anastomosis and coronary implantation. The avoidance of intraoperative bleeding is a key to a successful Ross operation. Anastomotic suture lines must be performed carefully, and prior to discontinuing cardiopulmonary bypass they must be carefully inspected, and they must be secure. Any repair to a suture line must be accomplished while on bypass so that systemic pressure can be controlled and repairs accomplished with the autograft root relatively flaccid. The use of pledgeted sutures is discouraged because they tend to pull through the thin-walled pulmonary root. Some surgeons recommend the use of sealants or glue on the autograft suture line, but I have not utilized these because I prefer accurate small sutures placed and tied with the distending pressure in the pulmonary root below 50 mm Hg. The second detail relates again to attention to the implantation of the coronary buttons. Either the right or left coronary

may be malaligned, particularly in patients who have had prior aortic surgery, and surgical adhesions and scarring may involve the aorta or the proximal coronary arteries. The most common error of which I am aware is to implant the coronary button low in the coronary sinus, and with distention of the pulmonary root, kinking can develop with resultant inadequate coronary perfusion.

In our 518 patients (age 1 day to 62 years, median 25 years), followed up to 16.9 years (median 5.3 years) the actuarial survival is 77% ± 8% at 16 years. There have been 17 late deaths. Five were sudden and presumed to be possibly valve-related deaths, 10 were non–valve-related, 1 was due to late fungal mediastinitis, and 1 was related to reoperation for replacement of an allograft aortic valve in a patient with early failure of the autograft valve from systemic lupus erythematosus.

Actuarial freedom from autograft valve degeneration (severe autograft valve insufficiency not due to infection, autograft valve reoperation, and valve-related death) in the 495 operative survivors was 81% ± 5% at 16 years. Actuarial freedom from autograft valve reoperation was 80% ± 5% at 16 years. Autograft valve reoperation occurred in 36 patients. Reoperation was required for management of autograft valve insufficiency in 30, and for sinus dilation without significant insufficiency in 6. Autograft insufficiency was due to annulus dilation in 17 patients before the use of annulus reduction and fixation or annulus fixation in those patients with a normal-sized annulus. In the remaining patients autograft insufficiency was secondary to the use of an abnormal pulmonary valve in 3 patients (bicuspid in 2 and quadricusp in 1), technical errors in 3 early in our learning curve, endocarditis in 4, and leaflet prolapse in 2. Two additional reoperations have been required on the left ventricular outflow tract for subvalvar obstruction. In 1 patient the subvalvar obstruction was a recurrent membrane, and the other patient developed a new subvalvar membranous obstruction 3 years after his Ross operation. Autograft valve replacement was required in 24 patients, and the actuarial freedom from replacement of the autograft valve was 83% ± 5% at 16 years (Fig. 46-12).

Because the Ross operation requires reconstruction of the right ventricular outflow tract (for which we used a pulmonary allograft valve in all but three patients in whom an aortic allograft was used), this reconstruction may later require reoperation for pulmonary stenosis or insufficiency. Actuarial freedom from replacement of the

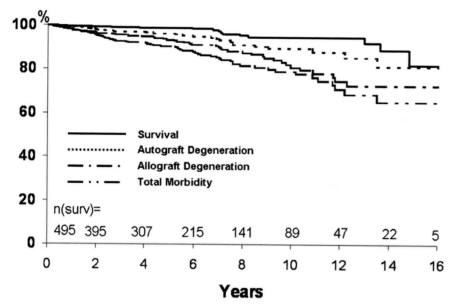

Figure 46-12.   Actuarial freedom from late death (82% ± 8%), autograft valve degeneration (81% ± 5%), allograft valve degeneration (73% ± 5%), and all valve-related morbidity (65% ± 6%) at 16 years.

pulmonary allograft is 86% ± 4% at 16 years. The actuarial freedom from allograft degeneration—allograft reoperation, severe allograft insufficiency, intervention by balloon valvuloplasty with or without stent placement, or echocardiographic gradient of ≥50 mm—is 73% ± 5% at 16 years. In the patients with an echocardiographic gradient, the obstruction has been in the conduit and not at the valve level in most patients.

Survival and valve morbidity and mortality are different in this series of Ross operations from those in several recently reported similar-sized series of aortic valve replacement with a prosthetic or bioprosthetic valve. Actuarial survival in our series of operative survivors was 82% ± 8% at 16 years. In two published series of aortic valve replacements using the most popular mechanical valve prosthesis, survival was 61% ± 5% in one group of 666 patients (age <65 years) at 15 years and 37% ± 5% in another group of 418 patients, age 20 to 84 years (mean 55 ± 15 years) at 15 years. Survival with a bioprosthetic stented aortic tissue valve was 55% ± 6% in a series of patients <65 years of age at 15 years; in a series of aortic pericardial valves in 310 patients, age 21 to 95 years (mean 64 ± 11 years), survival was 42% ± 4% for isolated aortic valve replacement at 12 years.

The rate of valve-related morbidity is quite different for this series of Ross operations because there have been no late thromboembolic events, and because the patients are not anticoagulated, there are no

bleeding events related to anticoagulation. The incidence of late endocarditis has been very low, occurring in 11 patients during follow-up. The actuarial freedom from postoperative endocarditis was 95% ± 2% at 16 years. Endocarditis involved the autograft valve in 8 patients, the pulmonary allograft in 2, and a Dacron graft replacing an ascending aortic aneurysm in 1. Actuarial freedom from valve-related morbidity (autograft valve degeneration, autograft valve reoperation, allograft valve reoperation, endocarditis, and valve-related death) was 65% ± 6% at 16 years. In the prosthetic valve series, valve-related morbidity and mortality was reported in one group as 61% ± 6% at 15 years and in the older age group as 42% ± 4% at 15 years. In the stented tissue valve series it was 39% ± 5% in patients younger than 65 years, and in the pericardial valve (isolated aortic valve replacement) series it was 65% ± 5% at 12 years. These series clearly do not have similar-aged patients with similar risk factors, and their late valve-related complications are different. In the Ross operation, the risk of reoperation is high because two valves are at risk and one of these nonviable. The patient electing for a Ross operation (or the patient's parents in the case of a child) must understand this risk and be willing to accept it to avoid the risk of thromboembolism and anticoagulation-related bleeding associated with a prosthetic aortic valve, or the risk of thromboembolism and a lower risk of structural valve degeneration if the patient

were to have a bioprosthetic valve. Because the Ross operation has very good results in terms of survival and nondebilitating complications at 16 years when compared to other choices, it remains an excellent choice for the adult and the parents of a young child who wish to avoid anticoagulation and are willing to accept the risk of reoperation.

SUGGESTED READING

Banbury MK, Cosgrove III DM, Lytle BW, et al. Long-term results of the Carpentier-Edwards pericardial aortic valve: A 12-year follow-up. Ann Thorac Surg 1998;66:S73.

David TE, Feindelm CM. An aortic valve-sparing operation for patients with aortic incompetence and aneurysm of the ascending aorta. J Thorac Cardiovasc Surg 1992;103:617.

Elkins RC, Knott-Craig CJ, Ward KE, et al. Pulmonary autograft in children: Realized growth potential. Ann Thorac Surg 1994;57:1387.

Elkins RC, Santangelo K, Stelzer P, et al. Pulmonary autograft replacement of the aortic valve: An evolution of technique. J Card Surg 1992;7:108.

Gerosa G, McKay R, Ross DN. Replacement of the aortic valve or root with a pulmonary autograft in children. Ann Thorac Surg 1991;51:424.

Khan SS, Trento A, DeRobertis M, et al. Twenty-year comparison of tissue and mechanical valve replacement. J Thorac Cardiovasc Surg 2001;122:257.

Kouchoukos NT, Davila-Roman VG, Spray TL, et al. Replacement of the aortic root with a pulmonary autograft for aortic valve disease in children and young adults. N Engl J Med 1994;330:1.

Melo JQ, Abecasis ME, Neves JS, et al. The large septal arteries in normal hearts, in aortic valve disease, and in tetralogy of Fallot. Ann Thorac Surg 1995;60:S626.

Oswalt JD, Dewan SJ. Aortic infective endocarditis managed by the Ross procedure. J Heart Valve Dis 1993;2:380.

Ross D, Jackson M, Davies J. Pulmonary autograft aortic valve replacement: Long-term results. J Card Surg 1991;6:529.

Ross DN. Replacement of aortic and mitral valves with a pulmonary autograft. Lancet 1967;2:9568.

Stelzer P, Jones DJ, Elkins RC. Aortic root replacement with pulmonary autograft. Circulation 1989;80:III-209.

Zellner JL, Kratz JM, Crumbley III AJ, et al. Long-term experience with the St. Jude Medical valve prosthesis. Ann Thorac Surg 1999;68:1210.

EDITOR'S COMMENTS

Dr. Elkins has given a detailed description of the Ross procedure. He clearly has vast experience and emphasizes the critical importance of the technical details. I agree entirely with his description and his enthusiasm for this procedure. I would like to emphasize a couple of points.

The most important is that the Ross procedure is not for everybody. It usually is done in younger patients without significant comorbidities. There are other good tissue valve substitutes for older patients. I also agree that this is an extremely safe procedure.

The major technical point that I would like to emphasize is the issue of implantation of the right coronary artery. Although our group has not had difficulty with this, we have heard multiple horror stories regarding this particular issue. As Dr. Elkins has clearly stated, the major issue here is implanting it in too low a position. This can cause it to kink. To avoid this complication, we use a slightly different technique than Dr. Elkins described. We implant the left coronary and then the distal aortic suture line. We then take the cross-clamp off temporarily so we can see exactly where the right coronary artery has to be implanted. This is almost always higher than what one would predict in the arrested heart. Using this technique, we have avoided too low an implantation site.

One last technical detail relates to the distal pulmonary artery anastomosis. We have tended to do this before doing the distal aortic suture line. This makes the pulmonary anastomosis incredibly easy and adds a very short amount to the cross-clamp time.

We are very happy with the Ross procedure for children and young adults. The risk of operation is low, and it provides an excellent functional valve without risk of anticoagulation.

I.L.K.

C

Coronary Artery Disease

47

Coronary Artery Bypass Grafting Using Cardiopulmonary Bypass

Robert S.D. Higgins and R. Anthony Perez-Tamayo

Introduction

Atherosclerotic heart disease is the leading cause of death in the United States. Among the most spectacular advances in modern medicine has been the development of the ability to treat this disease. Since its inception in the early 1960s, cardiopulmonary bypass has facilitated the development of procedures for performing coronary artery bypass and for allowing surgeons around the world to treat this devastating disease by enhancing myocardial blood flow, preventing complications related to heart disease, and enhancing overall survival and quality of life in ways seldom matched by other medical advances.

Advances in anesthetic techniques and the surgical management of patients with left ventricular dysfunction have created an environment in which the majority of the approximately 600,000 coronary artery bypass patients undergo these procedures yearly with a risk-adjusted operative mortality of <3% (Fig. 47-1). Additional adjuncts utilized in these procedures such as transesophageal echocardiography, newer inotropic agents, and hemostatic agents have created a platform for continued growth and development of innovative techniques. In conjunction with safe and effective myocardial revascularization, aortic and mitral valve repairs, ablative therapies for supraventricular arrhythmias, and ventricular restorative procedures can be safely performed with improved outcomes. Most of these advances would not have been possible without the development of the cardiopulmonary bypass apparatus.

It is evident, however, that with the evolution of alternative means of revascularizing the myocardium, including angioplasty, drug-eluting stents, and off-pump technologies, the profile of patients referred for coronary artery revascularization will challenge the next generation of cardiothoracic surgeons in many ways. Older patients with advanced disease, left ventricular dysfunction, and multiple comorbidities, including previous revascularization, as well as incomplete and inadequate attempts to revascularize the myocardium using interventional techniques will lead to even greater challenges with greater potential morbidity and mortality in referral centers. In this chapter, we highlight key aspects of the evolution of cardiopulmonary bypass, emphasizing the secondary effects of this procedure from a physiologic standpoint, review the indications for coronary revascularization, and discuss the conduct of the coronary artery bypass operation with specific emphasis on postoperative physiology, management, complications, and outcomes.

Evolution of Coronary Artery Bypass Grafting

In 1912, James Herrick of the Rush Medical College in Chicago, in collaboration with the pathologist Ludvig Hektoen, published a paper in the *Journal of the American Medical Association* entitled "Clinical Features of Sudden Obstruction of the Coronary Arteries." His report encompassed observations that others, including Osler, Dock, Hammer, and Fothergill, had made in the centuries since William Heberden's complete description of angina pectoris and its natural history in 1768. It was the first real unifying description of the full syndrome of myocardial ischemia and its pathologic correlation with coronary occlusion.

The history of the treatment of coronary artery disease has many branches that intertwine with coronary artery bypass grafting (CABG), approaches that, seen from the modern perspective, are at their worst false starts and at their best early explorations of as-yet-controversial treatment options such as transmyocardial revascularization and coronary endarterectomy. A by no means exhaustive list of these approaches includes palliative measures such as sympathectomy that claim the honor of being the first surgical attacks on the disease. The list also includes methods of indirect revascularization including pericardial and cardiac poudrage, grafting of pectoral muscle, omentum, jejunum, skin, or spleen to myocardium, direct implantation of vessels such as the left internal mammary artery (LIMA) into myocardium, and redirection of collateral flow by interventions including ligation of such structures as the mammary arteries, the coronary sinus, and the bronchial arteries.

This summary concentrates on those developments most crucial to the evolution of CABG using cardiopulmonary bypass (CPB), although the development of CABG is independent in most regards of that of CPB.

Modern treatment of coronary artery disease begins with Alexis Carrel's Nobel Prize–winning research in vascular anastomosis and his suggestion of coronary surgery for

Risk-Adjusted Isolated CAB Operative Mortality

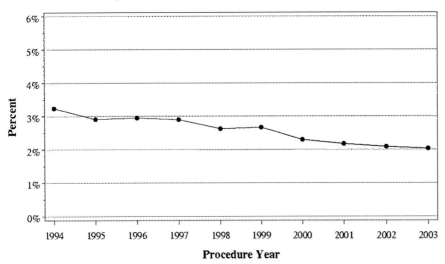

Figure 47-1. Risk-adjusted isolated coronary artery bypass (CAB) operative mortality. (Data Analyses of the Society of Thoracic Surgeons National Adult Cardiac Surgery Database Fall 2003 Site Report Images.)

the treatment of angina. He performed experimental bypass of coronary arteries in canines using arterial conduit, although his procedure resulted in arrest and required support using manual cardiac massage during the anastomosis. He felt that the anastomosis needed to be performed in <3 minutes, and suggested that tube connector devices were necessary. During the 1930s and 1940s, Beck and others attempted to improve myocardial perfusion with a number of indirect revascularization techniques. The culmination and the longest-lived of these procedures was the direct implantation of the internal mammary artery into the myocardium, experimental work reported by Vineberg in 1946, which was followed by his clinical work in 1950.

Much of the animal research into direct coronary revascularization during this time had a minimal impact because it was unpublished or was presented in relatively isolated forums. During the 1940s, Murray performed a number of unpublished animal experiments with coronary division, primary repair, and reversed saphenous vein graft interposition. The Russian transplant pioneer Vladimir Demikhov performed the first experimental anastomosis of the LIMA to the left anterior descending (LAD) in dogs using a three-way tube in 1953, although this work was not known outside the then Soviet Union. That year saw the first clinical use of Gibbon's screen oxygenator cardiopulmonary bypass machine. The toxicities inherent to early CPB in the era before the bubble and hollow fiber oxygenators

and the association of CPB with hypothermia made its use unusual in the early history of coronary revascularization. When May performed the first experimental closed retrograde coronary endarterectomy and Bailey the first clinical example of this procedure in 1955 and 1956, respectively, these were done without CPB. In the latter year, Thal performed the first sutured LIMA-LAD anastomosis in a beating heart animal model. Julian, in 1957, experimented with CPB to perform CABG using IMA and other arterial conduits.

Senning performed experiments in 1958 using an open endarterectomy technique and long-patch angioplasty with split free mammary patch. In 1959, Dubost used CPB to reconstruct the coronary ostia in a patient with syphilitic aortitis. Goetz used a nonsuture tantalum ring technique to anastomose the right internal mammary artery (RIMA) to the right coronary artery (RCA) in 1960. The next year, Senning built on his laboratory experience to perform coronary endarterectomy and patch angioplasty with saphenous vein graft (SVG) strips using hypothermia. This patient was the first to have a coronary operation guided by a coronary angiogram, performed at that time with a nonelective technique. Before that time, occlusion had been inferred on clinical grounds and confirmed with palpation.

There is some irony in the observation that the first SVG CABG, performed by Sabiston in 1962, was on a reoperative patient. Sabiston had endarterectomized

the patient's RCA the year before. This interposition graft procedure was complicated by the death of the patient from a stroke on the third postoperative day. The first sutured anastomosis mammary bypass (LIMA-LAD) was performed in the Soviet Union by Kolesov the following year, with long-term relief from angina. In 1964, Garrett performed a left coronary circulation SVG bypass to allow a patient to be weaned from CPB. Unfortunately, all three landmarks were virtually unknown to the medical community. The first forays into SVG CABG were not reported until 1973, and Kolesov's work was presented only at a conference in Leningrad, a plenum whose conclusion was that coronary revascularization had no future. Kolesov's work was not published in English until 1967.

The work of Sones with direct coronary catheterization and angiography in 1962 began a new era in revascularization, and did much to establish Cleveland Clinic's pre-eminence in the field. Effler had been performing endarterectomy and pericardial patch angioplasty with the assistance of hypothermia and CPB at the Cleveland Clinic in 1964, so all elements were in place for the exciting developments of 1967, when Favaloro took his experimental work with SVG interposition coronary grafts out of the laboratory. The interposition technique, like endarterectomy before it, did not lend itself well to ostial or branch point disease. Favaloro developed the technique into the end-to-side bypass graft, which required fewer coronary anastomoses. It is interesting to note the relative contemporary acceptance of the indirect revascularization techniques: Favaloro's first combinations of the SVG CABG and the IMA were to use one or both IMAs as Vineberg vessels. Later he and his group performed combined SVG and IMA CABG, alone and then in the setting of other procedures such as valve replacement and aneurysmectomy. The Cleveland Clinic's wealth of experience with CABG provided a platform for Lytle to document the clinical observation of superior patency of mammary grafts in 1984.

In many ways the final milestone to mention is the introduction of percutaneous transluminal coronary angioplasty (PTCA) by Gruntzig in 1979. The CABG, whose technical difficulty required some of its first incarnations to employ metal tubes for revascularization, is increasingly being supplanted by the technically easier insertion of metal tubes after PTCA (Table 47-1).

Table 47-1	Timeline
1768	Heberden: Complete description of angina pectoris and its natural history
1899	Francois-Franck: Suggestion of surgical sympathetic denervation for treatment of angina
1910	Carrel: Pioneered vascular anastomosis techniques, suggested coronary surgery for relief of angina, performed experimental CABG
1912	Herrick (in collaboration with Ludvig Hektoen): Unifying description of the full syndrome of myocardial ischemia and its pathologic correlation with coronary occlusion
1916	Jonnesco: First cardiac sympathectomy
1935	Beck: Cardiopericardiopexy
1940s	Murray: Unpublished experimental work with coronary division, primary repair, and reversed SVG interposition
1945	Bigelow: Hypothermia in cardiac surgery
1946	Vineberg: Experimental work with direct implantation of LIMA into myocardium
1948	Beck: Arterialization of coronary sinus and staged partial ligation
1950	Vineberg: First human Vineberg procedure
1952	Dodrill: Combined right and left heart bypass to perform experimental and clinical cardiac surgery
1953	Demikhov: Anastomosis of LIMA to LAD in canines using three-way tube
1953	Gibbon: First clinical use of CPB (screen oxygenator)
1955	May: Experimental retrograde closed coronary endarterectomy
1956	Bailey: Closed coronary retrograde coronary endarterectomy
1956	Thal: Experimental sutured anastomosis LIMA-LAD beating heart
1957	Julian: Experimental CABG using IMA and other arterial conduits utilizing CPB
1958	Senning: Experimental open coronary endarterectomy with long-patch angioplasty using split free mammary patch
1959	Dubost: Coronary ostium reconstruction in patient with syphilitic aortitis using CPB
1960	Goetz: First mammary CABG (RIMA to RCA) using nonsuture tantalum ring technique
1961	Senning: Coronary endarterectomy, patch angioplasty using SVG strips under hypothermia, first patient with coronary operation guided by coronary angiogram
1962	Sones: Direct coronary catheterization and angiography
1962	Conolly: Transaortic endarterectomy of RCA ostium under CPB
1962	Sabiston: First SVG CABG (*note*: re-do), not reported until 1974
1963	Kolesov: First sutured mammary CABG (LIMA-LAD) (work presented at a Leningrad plenum whose conclusion was that surgery for CAD had no future)
1964	Garrett: SVG CABG on CPB (to wean from CPB), not reported until 1973
1964	Effler: Endarterectomy, pericardial patch angioplasty using hypothermia and CPB
1967	Favaloro: Extensive experimental and clinical work with SVG interposition coronary grafts, progressing to CABG, CABG with SVG, and Vineberg (simultaneous with Johnson)
1968	Green: Sutured LIMA to LAD CABG
1969	Reed: Sutured LIMA to LAD, CPB and fibrillation utilized
1970	Favaloro: CABG with SVG and IMA, alone and later in combination with valve replacement, aneurysmectomy
1979	Gruntzig: Percutaneous transluminal coronary angioplasty

CABG = coronary artery bypass grafting; CAD = coronary artery disease; CPB = cardiopulmonary bypass; IMA = internal mammary artery; LAD = left anterior descending; LIMA = left internal mammary artery; RCA = right coronary artery; RIMA = right internal mammary artery; SVG = saphenous vein graft.

Indications for Cardiopulmonary Bypass

Coronary artery disease develops from the progression of atherosclerosis, which produces an obstruction in the coronary arteries. When the myocardium is rendered ischemic, angina, myocardial infarction, left ventricular dysfunction, valvular dysfunction secondary to papillary muscle ischemia, and congestive heart failure can occur. The goal, then, of myocardial revascularization is to restore myocardial blood flow and prevent complications of atherosclerotic heart disease.

The indications for myocardial revascularization include the following:

- The relief of angina that is unresponsive to medical therapy.
- Unstable angina (angina at rest) that is unresponsive to medical therapy.
- Postinfarction angina, unstable angina, or acute ischemia by electrocardiographic criteria after percutaneous angioplasty.
- Mechanical complications of myocardial infarction including postinfarction ventricular septal defect, mitral valve insufficiency secondary to papillary muscle dysfunction, and ventricular free rupture.
- Congestive heart failure complicating acute myocardial ischemia or severe coronary artery disease.
- Cardiogenic shock after myocardial infarction.

Additional anatomic or physiologic indications for myocardial revascularization include the following:

- Left main coronary artery stenosis greater than 50%.
- Left main equivalent disease: significant stenosis (>70%) of proximal LAD and proximal circumflex artery.
- Acute occlusion of the coronary artery after percutaneous angioplasty or stent placement.
- Three-vessel coronary artery disease with left ventricular dysfunction (left ventricular ejection fraction [LVEF] <50%).
- Coronary anomalies that may predispose to sudden death from acute coronary occlusion, for example, anomalous origin of the circumflex artery from the right coronary artery or right coronary sinus.

Effects of Cardiopulmonary Bypass Machine

The effect of the cardiopulmonary bypass machine on a patient undergoing CABG is a function of the inflammation generated by blood contact with a foreign surface, the anticoagulation and reversal this requires, the aortic cannulation used to deliver oxygenated blood, the temperature ranges used during bypass, and the myocardial ischemia during cross-clamping. This section focuses on the inflammatory effects of foreign surface blood contact, which occurs to its greatest extent in the oxygenator portion of the CPB circuit.

The primary protein systems involved in the inflammatory response are the contact system, the intrinsic and extrinsic coagulation systems, the fibrinolytic system, the complement system, and the cytokines. The cellular elements primarily involved are the platelets, endothelial cells, neutrophils, monocytes, and lymphocytes. Each protein system is an amplifying cascade, with key agents crossing over between systems and feeding back to promote or inhibit the cascade. Each cellular element interacts with each of the others and with each protein system in a fashion that defies easy summary. Although heparin is necessary to prevent the most immediately lethal endpoint of these cascades, thrombin production, it inhibits coagulation at the final points of the cascade and does not effectively diminish the inflammatory mediators that have been amplified before that point.

The exposure of blood to foreign surfaces activates the contact system, whose key agent, kallikrein, interacts with high-molecular-weight kininogen and factors XII and XI to produce bradykinin and to activate the intrinsic coagulation system, ultimately producing thrombin. Kallikrein and bradykinin activate the fibrinolytic system through activation of prourokinase and release of tissue plasminogen activator from endothelial cells. Kallikrein activates neutrophils, releasing toxic agents that strongly potentiate all of the inflammatory cascades. Kallikrein crosses over to the complement system by forming complexes with C1.

Blood/foreign surface contact also directly activates the classic and alternative pathways of the complement system. These pathways terminate in the cytocidal membrane attack complex and in the anaphylatoxins C3a, C4a, and C5a, potent vasoactive substances that are chemotactic for neutrophils as well as being neutrophil activators. The heparin/protamine complex is known to produce a large spike in C4 and C2 that is thought to be behind the vasodilation and hypotension seen with protamine administration in 50% of patients.

The activated neutrophil is characterized by a dramatic morphologic change with the development of pseudopodia and degranulation. The granules release a variety of substances cytotoxic in and of themselves and toxic by production of oxygen free radicals such as neutrophil elastase, cathepsin G, lysozyme, and myeloperoxidase.

Monocytes are markedly activated on contact with wound and pericardial tissues, and to a lesser extent in their passage through the CPB circuit. The activated monocyte expresses the strongly procoagulant tissue factor, setting off the extrinsic coagulation pathway. Activated monocytes release inflammatory cytokines including interleukins (ILs) 1, 2, 4, 6, 8, 10, and the

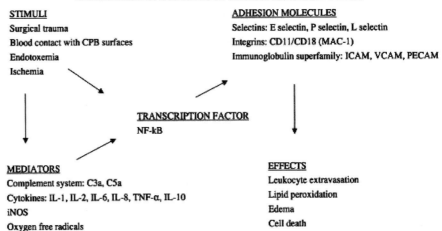

Figure 47-2. Schematic of the inflammatory process induced by cardiopulmonary bypass (CPB). The key role of NF-κB leading to endothelial cell and leukocyte activation is highlighted. (ICAM = intercellular adhesion molecule; IL = interleukin; iNOS = inducible nitric oxide synthase; PECAM = platelet-endothelial cell adhesion molecule; TNF-α = tumor necrosis factor-α; VCAM = vascular cell adhesion molecule.) (Reprinted with permission from D Paparella, TM Yau, E Young. Cardiopulmonary bypass induced inflammation: Pathophysiology and treatment. An update. Eur J Cardiothorac Surg 2002;2:232.)

inhibitory 12, which act to increase nitric oxide release by endothelial and smooth muscle cells by upregulation of inducible nitric oxide synthetase, leading to greater endothelial permeability and vasodilation. Monocytes are also a rich source of tumor necrosis factor-α (TNF-α), which, through renal vasoconstriction in the setting of glomerular fibrin deposition, leads to decreased glomerular filtration rate. TNF-α separately increases vascular permeability. When exposed to TNF-α, the cardiomyocyte releases sphingosine, which interferes with calcium egress from the sarcoplasmic reticulum, acting as a negative inotrope.

A key amplification mechanism that has been the focus of much recent attention is the nuclear transcription factor designated NF-κB (Fig. 47-2). A variety of stimuli such as cytokines, TNF-α, oxidative stress, C3a, C5a, oxygen radicals, and oxidative stress cause a phosphorylation of NF-κB and its dissociation from an inhibitory protein. After it migrates to the nucleus, it binds to DNA and induces the expression of numerous inflammatory agents, including cytokines, inducible nitric oxide synthase (iNOS), and adhesion molecules. Adhesion molecules binding to activated integrins on leukocytes, in concert with selectins found on leukocytes, platelets, and endothelial cells, act to make the rolling leukocyte adherent to the endothelial cell, aiding in its activation, transendothelial migration, and degranulation. At the same time, platelet-leukocyte aggregates, brought together by

platelet and leukocyte selectins, cause microvascular obstruction and end-organ damage (Fig. 47-3).

The integration of this maelstrom of inflammatory cascades is the clinical picture of the postoperative patient after CABG using CPB: bleeding secondary to the consumption of coagulation factors and activation of fibrinolysis; microvascular obstruction secondary to fibrin, fat, platelets, gaseous microemboli, leukocyte-platelet aggregates, vasoconstriction, and local edema; and organ dysfunction secondary to microvascular obstruction, tissue edema, and in the case of the heart, direct myocardial suppression. The vector sum of opposing tendencies toward vasoconstriction and vasodilation in different tissue beds will tend to produce a picture of evanescing microvascular vasoconstriction followed by sharp systemic vasodilation secondary to complement effects and patient rewarming.

The morass of noxious agents generated by CPB during CABG cannot help but prompt comparison to off-pump CABG and certain on-pump beating heart preparations that do not employ an oxygenator, the major culprit in blood–foreign surface interaction. These comparisons should be made in the light of two observations. The first is that there appears to be great variability between patients in the acuity and specific nature of their inflammatory responses that has confounded investigations in this area. The second consideration is that the particular differences between inflammation in

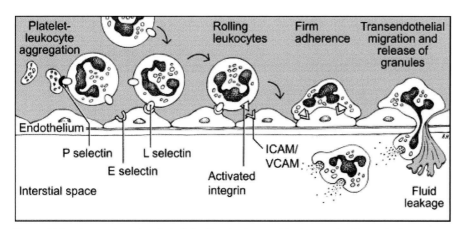

Figure 47-3. Interaction of endothelial cells, platelets, and leukocytes leading to leukocyte extravasation, granule release, and fluid leakage into the interstitial space. (ICAM = intercellular adhesion molecule; VCAM = vascular cell adhesion molecule.) (Reprinted with permission from D Paparella, TM Yau, E Young. Cardiopulmonary bypass induced inflammation: Pathophysiology and treatment. An update. Eur J Cardiothorac Surg 2002;2:232.)

off-pump and on-pump CABG in the most common forms of these procedures may not be due to the absence of the oxygenator in the OPCAB, but to the presence of the native lung as a scavenger and filter in that setting. Some inflammatory markers such as TNF-α, IL-8, IL-10, and elastase are clearly elevated in CABG-CPB versus OPCAB; however, this elevation is confined to the surgery itself and the very early postoperative period. By 24 hours after procedure there is no difference in these markers (Fig. 47-4). Likewise, reduced platelet consumption and decreased fibrinolytic activation are seen during and immediately after OPCAB, but are no different from levels seen after CABG-CPB at 24 hours. No differences between OPCAB and CABG-CPB in platelet or endothelial activation markers are seen at any time. It has been difficult to tease out real clinical differences in outcomes between OPCAB and CABG beyond advantages in blood transfusion requirement and intensive care unit length of stay. Most of the inflammation generated after either procedure seems to be primarily determined by the tissue injury involved with the surgical approach itself, the elements of which do not differ substantially in these techniques.

Conduct of Coronary Artery Bypass Surgery on Bypass

Preoperative Assessment

Historically, patients referred for coronary artery bypass surgery have had critical anatomic lesions such as left main steno-sis or multivessel coronary artery disease. As the indications for coronary artery bypass surgery have evolved to encompass a much different patient population than was previously referred, the medical condition of patients undergoing cardiac surgery is of particular importance to the operating surgeon. Preoperative conditions that require consideration include any medical condition that would predispose the patient to bleeding, either on cardiopulmonary bypass or in the perioperative and postoperative period; potential causes for deterioration of renal function; a history of preoperative cerebral vascular disease or ongoing cerebral vascular symptoms such as transient ischemic attacks or the presence of carotid bruits; electrolyte disturbances that may cause postoperative arrhythmias; preoperative infectious disease complications such as pneumonia, urinary tract infection, or dental abscesses; significant pulmonary dysfunction such as a forced expiratory volume in 1 second of <1.0 liter in patients with chronic obstructive pulmonary disease; and overall malnutrition secondary to cardiac cachexia and/or chronic disease states. Each of these factors may have a deleterious effect on patient outcome, and they should be considered and/or treated before any decision to take the patient to the operating room.

There are a number of specific risk factors that have been noted to have a significant effect on postoperative outcome. It is generally accepted that every surgeon considering myocardial revascularization using cardiopulmonary bypass should take into consideration the presence of these factors and incorporate this information into the discussion of risk and benefit with patients and their advocates before surgery. Risk factors for morbidity and mortality after coronary artery revascularization include the following:

- Elevated serum creatinine, chronic renal dysfunction.
- Emergency surgery.
- Severe left ventricular dysfunction.
- Reoperation.
- Coexistent ischemic mitral valve insufficiency.
- Advanced age, >75 years.
- Chronic obstructive pulmonary disease.
- Diabetes mellitus.
- Cerebral vascular disease.
- Body surface area <1.6.

Any patient with one or a combination of these risk factors or disease states determined before surgery may have an increased risk of postoperative complications such as prolonged intubation, cerebral vascular accident, renal dysfunction, and congestive heart failure leading to poor outcome. Furthermore, infectious complications such as mediastinitis, pneumonia, and endocarditis may also be increased in patients with poorly controlled diabetes mellitus, malnutrition, and severe pulmonary disease.

Intraoperative Management

After preoperative assessment of the patient's overall condition and a carefully planned anesthetic assessment, it is imperative that members of the operative team including anesthesiologists, perfusionists, nurses, and operating surgeons communicate effectively about the operative plan, projected use of conduits such as saphenous vein, radial artery, and the internal mammary artery, and any other intervention that might affect patient outcome. Of increasing importance are the appropriate selection of prophylactic antibiotics in surgical interventions and the timing of the administration of these drugs prior to incision. Antibiotics most appropriately used to cover gram-positive organisms administered within 1 hour of skin incision have provided the greatest benefit from a prophylactic standpoint. It has been our practice to also document the presence of femoral pulses and mark these pulses in case of postoperative left ventricular dysfunction requiring intra-aortic balloon pump counterpulsation. After appropriate monitoring devices have been inserted and anesthesia has been induced with endotracheal intubation, transesophageal echocardiography may be performed to assess left

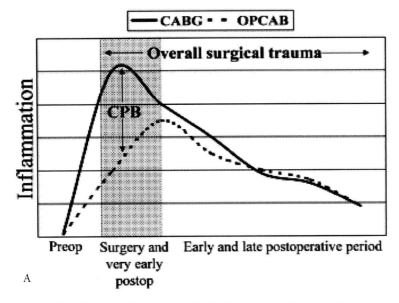

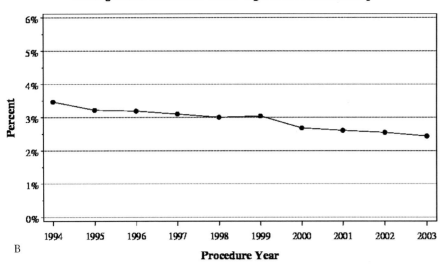

A

B

Figure 47-4. **(A)** During surgery and the very early hours of the postoperative period, some proinflammatory mediators peak to significantly higher levels in on-pump coronary artery bypass grafting (CABG) than off-pump coronary artery grafting (OPCAB) patients. However, during the following postoperative period, the differences in terms of the inflammatory state progressively fade and finally cancel out. (CPB, cardiopulmonary bypass.) (Reprinted with permission from P Biglioli, A Cannata, F Alamanni, et al. Biological effects of off-pump vs. on-pump coronary artery surgery: Focus on inflammation, hemostasis and oxidative stress. Eur J Cardiothorac Surg 2003;24:269.) **(B)** Unadjusted isolated coronary artery bypass mortality (Data Analyses of the Society of Thoracic Surgeons National Adult Cardiac Surgery Database Fall 2003 Site Report Images.)

ventricular function and the presence of mitral valvular insufficiency. Intraoperative transesophageal echo may also provide important information at the time of weaning from cardiopulmonary bypass. Recent evidence suggests that attention to surgical technique and the use of antifibrinolytic agents such as aminocaproic acid, serine protease inhibitors (aprotinin), and heparin-coated devices (Carmeda) may assist in the provision of a hemostatic

operation. There is also evidence that aprotinin may have important perioperative anti-inflammatory effects.

With respect to platelet antiaggregating drugs such as aspirin as well as the more aggressive medications now commonly used in all patients with coronary artery disease (Clopidogrel and Plavix) that bind to the glycoprotein IIB/IIIA platelet receptors, there is a growing body of evidence that suggests that perioperative antiplatelet ther-

apy may enhance outcome. These enhancements must be balanced against the potential risk of postoperative mediastinal hemorrhage. We recommend that patients on glycoprotein IIB/IIIA platelet receptor antagonists discontinue this medication several days before elective surgery, unless they have an urgent or emergency indication for surgery. The effects of these medications can be counteracted with the infusion of platelets in the postoperative period, if necessary. Aspirin therapy is initiated immediately after open-heart surgery within hours of the return to the intensive care unit.

Surgical Techniques

Of critical importance in planning the myocardial revascularization procedure is the intent of complete revascularization by bypassing all severe stenoses with >50%-diameter occlusion. Successful procurement of the saphenous vein to be used for revascularization is of paramount importance. Similarly, a successfully harvested left internal thoracic artery is the cornerstone of most myocardial revascularization procedures requiring bypass of the left anterior descending artery. Careful review of the preoperative angiograms gives the informed surgeon a clear understanding of what conduit may be necessary to fulfill the objective of complete revascularization, and this should be discussed with surgical assistants as they prepare for the procedure. Alternative conduits such as the right internal mammary artery and the radial artery are also commonly used when considering complete arterial revascularization. Theoretical advantages of complete arterial revascularization are, of course, that these arteries are well suited to the purpose of improving myocardial perfusion, and they are less prone to postoperative occlusion or anastomotic hypertrophic response.

The left internal mammary or thoracic artery is usually mobilized after performing the median sternotomy. The externally positioned retractor, developed by Favaloro, has been used as an effective tool to provide visualization of this artery located several centimeters lateral to the edge of the sternum. The internal thoracic artery either can be mobilized as a pedical or be skeletonized, using the electrocautery and scissors. The internal thoracic artery is mobilized from the xiphoid up to the level of the second intercostal space, where the left phrenic nerve can be identified. Similar techniques can be used to harvest the right internal thoracic artery when bilateral mammary operations are planned. For fear of sternal wound complications, bilateral mammary artery revascularization may be contraindicated in patients who have severe pulmonary function limitations and those who are diabetic. The left and right internal thoracic arteries can be used as pedical grafts or as free mammary grafts if inadvertent injury occurs during the harvesting procedure or if they are too short to reach the distal left anterior or right coronary arteries.

The greater saphenous vein has historically been an excellent conduit for myocardial revascularization. It does, however, require diligent and careful dissection to prevent injuries to the vein and creation of wound complications. Historically, a large, continuous incision over the entire length of the saphenous vein has been employed, although many surgical teams now employ multiple small incisions and/or endoscopic techniques to procure the vein. The vein is often prone to spasm during dissection, and so a careful assessment of its adequacy should occur at the initiation of the dissection and at its completion after the vein has been removed. After side branches have been ligated with either sutures or hemoclips, it is reversed with the placement of a small infusion cannula to flush the vein with heparinized saline solution. The vein is then gently distended at low pressure with this solution to preserve endothelial integrity, and hemostasis is ensured where evulsed or leaking side branches can be suture ligated. It has been our practice to mark the vein at this time to prevent twisting, and it is stored in a heparinized solution until the distal anastomoses are completed.

The radial artery has been used by many as an effective conduit in patients with inadequate vein or mammary arteries, with the ultimate goal of complete arterial revascularization. Preoperative assessment of arterial perfusion of the hand is necessary before dissection. An Allan's test to determine the completeness of the radial and ulnar arterial trees is performed in the nondominant hand. The arm is then positioned on an arm board at the side of the field, and the incision is carried over the radial pulse at the wrist and extended proximally over the brachioradialus muscle. The deep fascia is then opened at the wrist, exposing the radial vascular pedicle, and the incision is then extended proximally, exposing the muscles of the arm. Important landmarks include the lateral antebrachial cutaneous nerve and the superficial radial nerve. Dissection of the artery is then completed from the wrist proximally, and branches are doubly ligated and con-

trolled in the usual fashion. A small catheter is then placed into the distal artery, and the artery is flushed with heparinized solution of Ringer's lactate. Because of the propensity for vasoconstriction in this artery, many experienced surgeons utilize the infusion of a calcium-channel blocker (Diltiazem) in the perioperative period to prevent acute radial artery vasospasm. The incision in the leg (and radial artery, when used) is then closed with absorbable sutures in continuous layers, and compression dressings are applied usually before completion of the procedure.

Institution of Cardiopulmonary Bypass

After harvesting of the appropriate conduit, the operating surgeon checks the adequacy of the conduit and then proceeds to the institution of cardiopulmonary bypass. Heparin is administered as the dissection of the internal thoracic artery is completed. The internal thoracic artery can then be divided, and the adequacy of flow in the artery can be determined at that time. The pericardium is opened, and pericardial stay sutures are placed. Two circumferential purse-string sutures are placed in the sites for cannulation in the ascending aorta. A single circumferential suture is placed in the right atrial appendage and a pledgeted purse-string suture is placed in the ascending aorta for the cardioplegia cannula and vent. If retrograde cardioplegia is to be utilized, then a purse string is placed in the right atrial wall. Care must be taken to select a cannulation site in the ascending aorta to allow adequate room for the placement of the cardioplegia delivery system and the aorta cross-clamp as well as for proximal anastomoses of the saphenous vein grafts. Direct palpation may be adequate to assess the cannulation site to avoid atherosclerotic aortic disease. However, epiaortic ultrasounds may also be an important adjunct if the adequacy of the aorta cannot be assessed by direct palpation. A single two-stage venous cannula placed in the right atrium with the tip in the inferior vena cava is adequate for venous drainage in a standard coronary artery bypass procedure. Bicaval cannulation may be necessary if additional procedures such as mitral valve repair are considered. After it is confirmed that the patient is adequately anticoagulated based on the activated clotting time, cardiopulmonary bypass can be initiated. The adequacy of venous drainage can be assessed by the perfusion staff as well as by direct examination of the right side of the heart, and the adequacy of arterial flow is also de-

termined before discontinuing mechanical ventilation.

It has been our practice to allow the patient's temperature to drift rather than use active systemic cooling through the cardiopulmonary bypass circuit because we anticipate that the procedure will be fairly straightforward. More profound systemic cooling may be appropriate in patients with left ventricular dysfunction or those requiring combined complex procedures. Blood-based cold cardioplegia is then administered through the aortic root cannula or through the retrograde cannula placed in the coronary sinus as the cardiopulmonary bypass flow is decreased and the aorta cross-clamp is placed. Topical hypothermia has been used to sustain and/or augment myocardial protection while the aortic cross-clamp is in place. After successfully establishing electrical and mechanical arrest (10 cc/km infusion of cardioplegia), attention is turned to identification of appropriate distal coronary artery bypass targets. These targets can be identified before the institution of cardiopulmonary bypass as well. The sequence of anastomoses often depends on the indications for myocardial revascularization.

The internal thoracic artery is used whenever possible because of its demonstrated long-term patency and affect on outcome. If the patient has an urgent or emergency indication for revascularization such as an acute anterior myocardial infarction, then an expedient saphenous vein graft to the left anterior descending artery may be the most appropriate anastomosis completed. This allows for the infusion of cardioplegia through the saphenous vein graft immediately after completing the anastomosis.

In the standard operating sequence, the branches of the right coronary artery or the marginal branches of the circumflex artery are initially bypassed, followed by the anastomosis of the left internal mammary artery to the left anterior descending artery. In these circumstances, an assistant is often used to retract the heart laterally for the circumflex circulation or cephalad for the right posterior descending or posterolateral circulation. With stabilization of the distal coronary artery, the artery is opened, and the anastomosis is completed with a suture passed through the artery or vein and continued to the heel of the anastomosis. This sequence is then followed around the full circumference of the anastomosis. At the completion of the anastomosis, additional cardioplegia is delivered via the saphenous vein graft before tying the polypropylene suture. Additional saphenous vein grafts or sequential anastomoses can then be completed to proximal branches of the circumflex, diagonal branch, or left anterior descending artery. After completing the distal anastomoses, rewarming is initiated, and the proper length and alignment of the graft are determined as the aortic cross-clamp is removed. If the ascending aorta is free of significant atherosclerosis, a partial occluding clamp is then placed on the ascending aorta and proximal anastomotic openings are made using an appropriately sized punch in the aorta. The proximal anastomoses are then sutured to the aorta using a similar suture technique on the lateral surface of the ascending aorta. Alternatively, if the aorta is diseased, the proximal anastomoses can be performed with the aortic cross-clamp in place to prevent a second clamping of the ascending aorta. After air is evacuated from the ascending aorta and the saphenous vein grafts, the aortic clamp or side-biting clamp is removed, and reperfusion of the myocardium is completed.

Weaning from Cardiopulmonary Bypass

As the patient is fully rewarmed, mechanical ventilation is initiated with the resumption of a normal sinus rhythm. If bradycardia or temporary heart block develops, then pacing wires are placed in the right atrium and right ventricular outflow tract for temporary pacing. In addition, electrolyte abnormalities such as hypomagnesemia and hypokalemia are treated. The transesophageal echo can be of great help in identifying regional or global myocardial dysfunction as the perfusionist leaves blood in heart to allow ejection. By using the transesophageal echo, the patient is then weaned from cardiopulmonary bypass as a greater percentage of the overall hemodynamic support is provided by the native ventricular function. Gradual reduction of venous return and incremental volume loading of the heart assist in this process until cardiopulmonary bypass is discontinued. Additional inotropic agents may be necessary if the patient has pre-existing myocardial dysfunction or congestive heart failure. After successful cessation of cardiopulmonary bypass, anticoagulation is reversed by administration of protamine. The activated clotting time normalizes as the infusion of protamine is completed. As a general rule of thumb, weaning from cardiopulmonary bypass should incorporate a stepwise method addressing heart rate, rhythm, preload, afterload, and, finally, the inotropic state of the ventricle in sequence.

Postoperative Physiology and Management

The postoperative physiology of the patient who has undergone CABG using CPB is generally quite predictable. This has allowed the development of management algorithms for each organ system that permit the frontline health care practitioner a great deal of autonomy in directing the patient through the "fast-track" care map.

The use of short-duration, fast-acting anesthetic and paralytic agents during the procedure frees the patient from any cardiosuppressant action of these drugs and allows for a prompt extubation. It should be possible to extubate >90% of patients by the sixth postoperative hour. Sedation in the postoperative period is used sparingly, therefore, and, when necessary, agents with very short half-lives are used, such as dexmedetomidine (Precedex) or propofol (Diprivan).

Synchronized intermittent mandatory ventilation (SIMV) mode weaning with physiologic positive end-expiratory pressure and pressure support settings are used, and the patient is extubated with appropriate spontaneous tidal volumes and mental status. Pulmonary toilet and endotracheal suction to clear secretions are crucial before and after extubation. The weaning protocol should proceed without regard to preoperative ejection fraction, preoperative myocardial ischemia, the presence of IABP, postoperative vasoactive drips, inotropes, or anything but obvious extremes in chest tube output. In controlled circumstances, in patients who were not difficult intubations, the benefits of early extubation outweigh the inconveniences of reintubation should a return to the operating room for bleeding be required.

As previously mentioned, the vasoconstriction present during the CPB run gives way to vasodilation. After CPB has been discontinued, and particularly after the administration of protamine, as much of the volume contained within the circuit should be reinfused as is possible. After this pump blood has been returned, some form of colloid should always stand ready for infusion, cell-saver blood, hetastarch, or albumin. This relative hypovolemia most frequently manifests as hypertension and blood pressure lability. The uninitiated intensive care unit staff will treat the hypertension with additional doses of sedative and vasodilators that will prolong the extubation process and create hypotension. These overcontrol swings will continue until volume is administered. The vasodilation is extended mildly by the afterload-reducing properties of dobutamine, and much more markedly with milrinone, which often requires the administration of phenylephrine (Neo-Synephrine) in concert.

When the rate of vasodilation exceeds that of volume administration, vasoconstrictive agents such as phenylephrine should be used. By 6 to 12 hours after CPB, the need for vasoconstriction should pass. An extremely profound vasodilation, usually resistant to phenylephrine, sometimes known as "vasoplegia," has been described in roughly 10% of the CABG patient population. This has been associated with low-ejection-fraction patients and/or those with angiotensin-converting-enzyme inhibition or intravenous heparin administration for prolonged periods preoperatively. Low levels of vasopressin and excessive inducible nitric oxide synthetase activity have been found in these patients. An early warning may take the form of a phenylephrine requirement during CPB. Intravenous vasopressin infusion in doses of 1.5 to 6 units/hr have been effective in treating the vasoplegic state, and there is also growing support in the literature for administration of methylene blue as a nitric oxide inhibitor at 1.5 to 3.0 mg/kg over 1 hour. It should be kept in mind that coronary perfusion through bypass grafts, particularly those using arterial conduit, is driven by mean arterial pressure to a far greater extent than it is limited by vasoconstrictors.

Inotropic requirements are dealt with first by ensuring appropriate volume loading, correcting ionized calcium levels, and securing a regular atrial rhythm when possible. The appropriate inotropic agent is then selected by considering the degree of systemic arterial tone, pulmonary arterial tone, right ventricular contractility, and degree of left ventricular hypertrophy. If systemic vascular resistance (SVR) is low, epinephrine's combination of alpha- and beta-adrenergic stimulation may make it the drug of choice. If SVR is high, then agents such as dobutamine and milrinone have the advantage of inotropy with afterload reduction. In patients with right ventricular dysfunction and/or pulmonary hypertension, milrinone is felt to have unique properties of right ventricular inotropy and pulmonary vasodilation. Epinephrine is a potent pulmonary vasodilator and a good alternative in this setting. Severe left ventricular hypertrophy (LVH) is typified by the short-axis transesophageal echocardiographic view wherein the bases of the papillary muscles almost come together despite normal or supranormal filling pressures. Dobutamine, milrinone, or dopamine should be used only by extreme necessity in these patients because their resultant increased adrenergy will accentuate the diastolic dysfunction seen in these patients. Milrinone, and at the first available opportunity, beta-blockade, will have a welcome beneficial effect.

Fluid management during the first 6 to 12 hours after CPB will usually involve volume administration as intravascular volume is drawn into the third space through a temporarily leaky endothelial barrier and as diuretics given on pump take effect. To minimize edema and third-space losses, colloid volume is preferred. Blood products as necessary are the best colloid, then hetastarch or albumin solutions. Increased blood loss has been attributed to hetastarch, imputed to binding of the starch molecule to the platelet surface. Thromboelastography of patients randomized to CPB circuit priming with different-weight hydroxyethyl starch solutions and albumin have shown slower and less stable clot formation with hetastarch, although differences in these values and in postoperative blood loss have not been dramatic. Other clinical work has demonstrated a moderate advantage to albumin over hetastarch in terms of postoperative blood loss, but this advantage must be balanced with the infectious and financial drawbacks of albumin. To many clinicians, the addition of a mild antiplatelet effect during the immediate postoperative period might be seen as advantageous.

As endothelial tone returns with the resolution of inflammation, the third-space fluid will re-enter the intravascular volume, around 12 to 24 hours after bypass. This increased hydrostatic pressure often manifests as mild pulmonary dysfunction from edema, turgor, and effusion. At 12 to 24 hours, diuresis with scheduled-dose furosemide should begin, with potassium supplementation to maintain serum potassium at ≥ 4.5 mEq/dl. Although it will lag by approximately 12 hours, the progress of diuresis can be followed by the ratio of serum blood urea nitrogen to creatinine.

Prophylaxis for atrial fibrillation begins with diuresis to euvolemia and potassium supplementation to serum values of 4.5 mEq/dl. In addition, beta-blockade should be initiated at the earliest time possible, usually postoperative day 1. The dose of beta-blocker should be incremented to the highest level the heart rate and blood pressure permit. Systematic attention to these details should at least halve the incidence

of postoperative atrial fibrillation from 25%. If atrial fibrillation occurs, the treatment focuses on rate control, then on conversion to sinus rhythm. A detailed discussion of the treatment options is beyond the scope of this chapter. Amiodarone provides good rate control and is very effective for the restoration of sinus rhythm. Unless contraindicated, anticoagulation is begun simultaneously with subcutaneous fractionated heparin and Coumadin, though some may choose to allow 24 hours for sinus rhythm to return before beginning these medications. Elective synchronized electrocardioversion is another option.

All patients recovering from CABG should initiate a lifetime course of the following key medications, almost without exception: aspirin, a beta-blocker, an angiotensin-converting-enzyme inhibitor, and a cholesterol-lowering agent. Patients with nonmammary arterial grafts should receive nitrates or calcium-channel blockers for at least 6 weeks. Finally, aggressive perioperative diabetic management using intravenous insulin therapy has been reported to have significant positive effect on early and late outcome.

Complications

Neurologic

Neurologic complications after coronary artery bypass grafting fall into two categories. Type I events tend to be more dramatic: focal deficits, stupor, and coma. Type II represents a vague set of cognitive dysfunctions, usually identified only with sophisticated neuropsychologic testing. The study of these complications and the measures that can be taken to avoid them are necessarily confounded by the rarity of type I events and the subtlety of type II pathology. Incidence of type I events is typically around 1%, whereas type II neurologic complications have ranged widely in series from 5% to 30% and as high as 90% of CABG patients. A few consistent observations can be abstracted from the controversies in the literature on type II neurologic damage. Serum markers of brain injury like neuron-specific enolase and S100 β do increase with CPB. These markers do not reliably correlate with performance on neuropsychologic testing. There does not seem to be any real difference in performance on such testing at any time interval after CABG with CPB in patients compared to nonsurgical controls or surgical controls, even when the surgical group is pa-

tients who have undergone OPCAB. Whatever type II neurologic damage has occurred seems to be transient and has clears up by 3- and 12-month follow-up. The etiology of the neurologic damage in the spectrum between type I and type II complications is either hypoperfusion or, much more commonly, embolic phenomena. Strategies for combating hypoperfusion essentially concentrate on delivery of higher mean arterial pressures or the provision of truly physiologically pulsatile waveforms during CPB. The subject of macroembolic and microembolic phenomena is much more complicated.

At least one third of type I events are caused by hemodynamically significant carotid artery disease. The risk of perioperative stroke after CABG has been quoted as increasing with the degree of asymptomatic stenosis, with a risk of <2% with <50% stenosis; 10% with stenoses from 50% to 80%; and 11% to 19% in patients with stenosis >80%. Endarterectomy should precede CABG in these and in symptomatic carotid disease patients. When performed with CABG under the same anesthetic period, a mortality of 3.5% and a reduced perioperative stroke rate of 4% can be achieved with the combined procedure with a 5-year freedom from stroke of 88% to 96%.

Beyond the concept of endarterectomy preceding CABG in patients with symptomatic carotid disease, few measures intended to prevent emboli result in any clinically verifiable advantage. Counts of microemboli have been used as a surrogate for brain damage, but have not consistently been correlated with findings on neuropsychologic testing. We can adopt measures that have been shown to cause fewer microemboli with the understanding that any microembolus is a bad thing, but we cannot expect to make a clinical difference. Measures include the use of epiaortic ultrasound to plan cannulation and proximal sites, dispersal aortic cannulae, and a single aortic cross-clamp technique as opposed to separate side-biting clamp application for proximal anastomosis. Excessive manipulation of the CPB circuit by the perfusionist has been associated with more numerous gaseous microemboli. Gaseous microemboli are also brought out of solution by too rapid a rewarming on CPB. A variety of microemboli including lipid droplets are generated by return of pericardial shed blood to the circuit by cardiotomy suction. Cell-saver suction and additional filtration of the washed blood can markedly reduce this source of microemboli.

Bleeding

The incidence of return to the operating room for bleeding should be around 1% to 2%. Apart from routine preoperative measurement of coagulation parameters, steps taken to reduce intraoperative blood loss include cessation of anticoagulation, fibrinolytics, and antiplatelet agents stronger than aspirin for the longest period possible prior to surgery. Fractionated heparin is stopped the night before surgery. Clopidogrel is stopped at least 5 days prior to surgery. Though the incidence of significant bleeding is increased with aspirin, the benefits in early graft patency seem to outweigh the risks, so this medication is continued even to the day of surgery. Aprotinin in its full dose has been repeatedly shown to reduce intra- and postoperative blood loss. Its anti-inflammatory properties should be examined in the light of the fact that the doses required for kallikrein inhibition are 100-fold greater than those for plasmin inhibition.

Chest tube output thresholds for re-exploration are often left up to surgical judgment. The key determination is whether bleeding is from coagulopathy or from technical failure. In the time lag during which conventional assessments of coagulation parameters of PT, PTT, fibrinogen, and platelet counts are obtained, much blood can be lost, and many unnecessary units of blood products are empirically transfused. The ideal test would be a point-of-care thromboelastography, synthesizing the various branches of the coagulation cascade and establishing whether the patient can form a clot. A bleeding patient with a normal thromboelastogram would have to be returned to the operating room. Correction of abnormal coagulation could be attempted in those with abnormal values prior to re-exploration.

Infection

Deep sternal wound infection is a devastating complication that occurs in 1% to 2% of patients. Although ultimately attributable to a break in sterile technique, there are several factors that have been repeatedly demonstrated to increase the risk of this complication. These are diabetes, obesity, reoperation, severe chronic obstructive pulmonary disease, and the use of bilateral mammaries in the setting of diabetes. The presence of these factors is a clinical circumstance usually outside the surgeon's control. There are a few interventions within the surgeon's control that have been shown to make a difference.

To begin with, clipping is preferable to shaving surgical sites from body hair. If shaving must be employed, it should not occur before the patient's entry into the operating suites. The only antibiotic dose that has any effect is one whose serum level peaks at the time of incision. No quantity, frequency, or duration after surgery has otherwise been shown to affect the incidence of infection. Tight glucose control, preferably using an insulin drip, is a key element of prevention of sternal wound infection.

It is sometimes difficult to know whether infection leads to sternal instability or instability leads to infection. Sternal precautions with ambulation are therefore a crucial part of pre- and postoperative patient education. Patients should protect their sternum as they cough. Coughing should be a voluntary maneuver as part of a program of pulmonary toilet with incentive spirometry and not an involuntary reflex. A persistent cough should be aggressively managed with antitussives, even to the point of suppression with codeine.

Renal Dysfunction

Of the 4% of CABG patients who experience postoperative renal dysfunction, one fifth will require dialysis. Postoperative renal dysfunction is associated with a high mortality: 20% overall, and more than half of those who require dialysis. Risk of postoperative renal failure is higher in those with prior nephropathy, diabetes, and congestive heart failure. Once renal dysfunction has occurred, two schools of thought exist as to its management. The more traditional approach relies on diuretics such as furosemide to "convert" oliguric to nonoliguric renal failure, which carries a far lower mortality. The mechanism most commonly quoted for this "conversion" is the clearance of debris from tubules affected by acute necrosis with flow of urine. The opposing viewpoint suggests that the diuretic dose exacerbates the renal damage by demanding increased metabolic activity at a time when the nephron is already injured. This approach advises maximizing renal blood flow by maintaining preoperative-level mean arterial pressures and providing renal and splanchnic vasodilators, like renal-dose dopamine or fenoldapam. If fluid overload requires it, low-impact continuous dialysis is used, venovenous if necessary.

Outcomes

The results of coronary artery bypass surgery using cardiopulmonary bypass have improved significantly since the early 1970s when the first randomized trials demonstrated significant survival advantages with myocardial revascularization. Three major studies conducted during that period demonstrated that surgery provided superior relief of angina and improvement of functional capacity with a reduction in the incidence of fatal myocardial infarctions. They also showed that patients with left main disease or three-vessel coronary artery disease and moderate left ventricular dysfunction had survival advantages after surgery. Although the Coronary Artery Surgery Study, the Veterans Administration Cooperative Study, and the European Coronary Surgery Study were landmark publications, in retrospect, they suffered from a number of critical limitations that bear mentioning. Specific limitations include male-selective patient populations <65 years of age, shortcomings in the "intention-to-treat" study design, which allowed for patient results to be collated with initial randomizations, a limited utilization of the internal mammary artery as the conduit of choice, and a variety of other changes in surgical and anesthetic management techniques.

The Society of Thoracic Surgeons (STS) created a national voluntary cardiac surgery database as a means of supporting national quality improvement efforts in 1989. Since that time, this database has grown to include more than 600 hospitals and clinical information from two million surgical procedures and become the most accurate, state-of-the-art database regarding the results of coronary artery bypass surgery. As the most recent STS database report highlights, based on a risk-adjustment model that has been validated over the last several years, operative mortality for coronary artery bypass procedures was 2.59% (95% confidence intervals). Furthermore, the risk of permanent stroke was 1.5%, the risk of renal failure was 3.49%, the risk of deep sternal wound infection was 0.5%, and the risk of prolonged ventilation was 7.1% (Table 47-2).

The results and outcomes of this database report not only underscore the improvements in outcomes after coronary artery bypass surgery, but they also highlight the overall value of risk-adjusted databases as predictors of outcome and essential tools for quality assessment and improvement. In spite of these remarkable trends in reported outcomes using this voluntary database, the actual results of CABG procedures may, in fact, be worse if one were to take into account the remainder of coronary bypass

Table 47-2   Society of Thoracic Surgeons Cardiac Surgery Database: Risk-Adjustment Model with 95% Confidence Intervals

Operative mortality for coronary artery bypass grafting	2.59%
Risk of permanent stroke	1.5%
Risk of renal failure	3.49%
Risk of deep sternal wound infection	0.5%
Risk of prolonged ventilation	7.1%

procedures not reported to the voluntary database.

It is evident that as the management of atherosclerotic heart disease evolves with the growing influence of percutaneous angioplasty procedures and stent utilization, a greater percentage of patients may be managed initially with these procedures before surgery. Subsequent referrals to surgical practices will involve much more complicated patients who have been subjected to many procedures in the context of multiple cardiovascular comorbidities. It is in this light that we turn to specific patient populations who may not be candidates for percutaneous procedures, but rather are referred to surgeons for definitive surgical therapy with increasing potential morbidity and mortality.

Patients with cardiogenic shock and heart failure secondary to acute myocardial infarction are among the most challenging patient populations to manage. Cardiogenic shock is among the leading causes of death in patients hospitalized with myocardial infarction. It complicates approximately 10% of cases of acute myocardial infarction and is associated with a 70% to 80% mortality. Given these observations, a number of investigators have attempted to prospectively assess the benefit of early emergency revascularization versus an initial medical stabilization in patients with cardiogenic shock. Revascularization was accomplished either by coronary artery bypass or angioplasty. Intra-aortic balloon counterpulsation was also used to support patients in a number of cases. Interestingly, overall mortality at 30 days did not differ significantly between the revascularization and medical therapy groups (46.7% and 56.0%, respectively). However, the 6-month mortality was lower in the revascularization group compared to the medical therapy group (50.3% vs. 63.1%, $p < .027$). Long-term outcomes after coronary artery bypass grafting in car-

diogenic shock using multivariate analysis of survival confirmed a very high hospital mortality at 35% in this shock group. These outcomes challenge every surgical practice to balance their resources carefully against early high mortality and modest survival improvements at 6 months, 1 year, and 10 years.

Patients with stable or chronic heart failure or ischemic cardiomyopathies represent another challenging group of patients for coronary artery bypass surgery. A clearer understanding of the pathophysiology of heart failure provides a greater appreciation for the nuances of coronary revascularization in these patients. As we learn more about adaptive mechanisms in heart failure and the affect on sympathetic activation and parasympathetic withdrawal, we can use many strategies before routine surgical intervention to enhance outcome. These factors also mandate additional management techniques such as mitral reconstruction and left ventricular remodeling in addition to myocardial revascularization. A number of centers have demonstrated improved survival in patients with severe left ventricular dysfunction. Success in this group of patients requires an accurate assessment of myocardial viability and dysfunctional areas. Preoperative quantification of viable myocardium is of critical importance to identify patients who may benefit from revascularization or other surgical procedures instead of heart transplantation. Nuclear techniques that show preserved tracer uptake and metabolism in viable myocardium, echocardiographic methods that detect the residual contractual reserve, and inotrope (dobutamine) stress echocardiography may have a higher specificity and therefore gain in clinical utility in these patients.

Given the appropriate assessment and documentation of potential improvements in myocardial function with preoperative testing, myocardial revascularization in patients with ischemic cardiomyopathy can be performed with acceptable morbidity and mortality. However, long-term improvements in outcome may be determined by the patient's preoperative congestive heart failure in spite of adequate revascularization as well as pharmacologic therapies employed after surgery.

Patients with diabetes mellitus have been demonstrated to have diffuse and progressive coronary artery disease compared to patients without diabetes. Given the progressive and diffuse nature of this disease, percutaneous strategies often leave the myocardium at risk for recurrent is-

chemia in spite of adequately treating focal, high-grade stenosis. In 1996, the Bypass Angioplasty Revascularization Investigation (BARI Trial), a randomized trial, found that an initial strategy of coronary artery bypass grafting as compared to percutaneous transluminal coronary angioplasty significantly improved 5-year survival among patients with medically treated diabetes. These benefits were sustained over many years with a 50% reduction in risk out to 5 years of follow-up. Furthermore, in subsequent analysis of the BARI patient cohort, these survival advantages were demonstrated in patients who had previous coronary artery bypass surgery as compared to coronary angioplasty, particularly in the context of an acute myocardial infarction.

Among the most important aspects of patient outcome has been the observation that patients undergoing cardiopulmonary bypass are at risk for central nervous system complications including embolic complications and stroke. The significance of these neurologic complications has been emphasized in a number of recent landmark publications and they are among the most often-cited reasons for avoiding cardiopulmonary bypass. The etiology of embolic neurologic events arising from severely atherosclerotic ascending aorta has been well documented, and a number of investigators and surgeons have used techniques such as intraoperative ultrasound scanning of the ascending aorta before cross-clamping and/or cannulation, transesophageal echocardiography of the aorta, and a number of physiologic manipulations to enhance cerebral circulation through the management of pH on bypass. Aprotinin, a nonspecific protease inhibitor, is an effective hemostatic agent that prevents blood loss and preserves platelet function during cardiopulmonary bypass procedures requiring cardiopulmonary bypass. It also has a number of anti-inflammatory effects and has been demonstrated to inhibit enzymatic intermediaries involved in the generalized inflammatory response to cardiopulmonary bypass. Recent data analyzing the aprotinin patient database demonstrated that the incidence of stroke and neurologic complications was reduced in high- and low-dose-aprotinin groups relative to placebo. This is the subject of further prospective clinical trials underway in cardiac surgery. Ultimately, the reduction of central nervous system complications by the use of anti-inflammatory medications or other techniques will be an important consideration in limiting the intermediate and long-term effects of cardiopulmonary bypass.

Future Considerations

Since 1953 when Dr. John Gibbon pioneered the use of the heart-lung machine, coronary artery bypass grafting has evolved as the definitive therapy for atherosclerotic heart disease and has demonstrated remarkable benefits to patients in terms of long-term outcome and improvements in quality of life with low morbidity and mortality. Subsequent efforts to enhance the performance of these procedures center around ways to avoid neurologic complications as well as to facilitate surgical techniques to decrease the amount of time on cardiopulmonary bypass. Although innovative techniques for constructing proximal and distal anastomoses continue to evolve, the introduction and development of minimally invasive direct coronary bypass surgery has initiated a technical revolution in the field. It has been suggested that off-pump coronary artery bypass procedures will be performed to a greater or lesser extent based on the operating surgeon's facility and comfort with the technical aspects of this procedure. At the farthest end of the spectrum is the emergence of robotically assisted coronary procedures, which some day may be the next breakthrough.

SUGGESTED READING

American College of Cardiology/American Heart Association. Guidelines for coronary artery bypass graft surgery: Executive summary and recommendations: A report of the American College of Cardiology/American Heart Association Task Force on Practice Guidelines. Circulation 1999;100:1464.

Biglioli P, Cannata A.,Alamanni F, et al. Biological effects of off pump vs. on pump coronary artery surgery: Focus on inflammation, hemostasis and oxidative stress. Eur J Cardiothorac Surg 2003;24:260.

Bolling S, Dicstein M, Levy J, et al. Management strategies for high risk cardiac surgery: improving outcomes in patients with heart failure. Heart Surg Forum 2000;3:337.

Cameron A, Davis KB, Green G, et al. Coronary artery bypass surgery with internal thoracic artery grafts—Effects on survival over a 15 year period. N Engl J Med 1996;334:216.

Edmunds LE. Inflammatory response to cardiopulmonary bypass. Ann Thorac Surg 1998;66:S12–6.

Furnary A, Gao G, Grunkemeier G, et al. Continuous insulin infusion reduces mortality in patients with diabetes undergoing coronary artery bypass grafting. J Thorac Cardiovasc Surg 2003;125:1007.

Grigore A. Neurological Outcome Research Group and CARE Investigators of the Duke Heart Center: Prospective randomized trial of normotheric versus hypothermic cardiopul-

monary bypass on cognitive function after coronary artery bypass graft surgery. Anesthesiology 2001;95:1110.

Hachman J, Sleeper L, Webb J, et al. Early revascularization in acute myocardial infarction complicated by cardiogenic shock. N Eng J Med 1999;341:625.

Hangler HB, Nagele G, Danzmayr M, et al. Modification of surgical technique for ascending aortic atherosclerosis: Impact on stroke reduction in coronary artery bypass grafting. J Thorac Cardiovasc Surg 2003;126:391.

Jones E, Weintraub W. The importance of completeness of revascularization during long term follow-up after coronary artery operations. J Thorac Cardiovasc Surg 1996;112:227.

Koster A, Fischer T, Praus M, et al. Hemostatic activation and inflammatory response during cardiopulmonary bypass. Impact of heparin management. Anesthesiology 2002;97:837.

Levin RL, Degrange MA, Bruno GF, et al. Methylene blue reduces mortality and morbidity in vasoplegic patients after cardiac surgery. Ann Thorac Surg 2004;77:496.

Mangano D. Aspirin and mortality from coronary bypass surgery. N Engl J Med 2002;347:1309.

Mekontso-Dessap A, Houel R, Soustelle C, et al. Risk factors for post-cardiopulmonary bypass vasoplegia in patients with preserved left ventricular function. Ann Thorac Surg 2001;71:1428.

Morris J, Smith L, Jones R, et al. Influence of diabetes and mammary artery grafting on survival after coronary bypass. Circulation 1991; 84:111:275.

Murashita T, Makino Y, Kamiturbo Y, et al. Quantitative gated myocardial perfusion single photon emission computed tomography improves the prediction of regional functional recovery in kinetic areas after coronary bypass surgery: useful tool for evaluation of myocardial viability. J Thorac Cardiovasc Surg 2003;126:1328.

Olsen MA, Lock-Buckley P, Hopkins D, et al. The risk factors for deep and superficial chest surgical site infections after coronary artery bypass surgery are different. J Thorac Cardiovasc Surg 2002;124:136.

Paparella D, Yau T, Young E. Cardiopulmonary bypass induced inflammation: Pathophysiology and treatment. An update. Eur J Cardiothoracic Surg 2002;21:232.

Puskas J, Thourani V, Marshall J, et al. Clinical outcomes, angiographic patency, and resource utilization in 200 consecutive off-pump coronary bypass patients. Ann Thorac Surg 2001;71:1477.

Puskas J, Williams W, Mahoney E, et al. Off pump vs. conventional coronary artery bypass grafting: Early and 1-year graft patency, cost, and quality-of-life outcomes. JAMA 2004;241:1841.

Rosenfeldt FL, He GW, Buxton BF, et al. Pharmacology of coronary artery bypass grafts. Ann Thorac Surg 1999;67:878.

Shah P, Hare D, Raman J, et al. Survival after myocardial revascularization for ischemic cardiomyopathy. A prospective ten

year follow-up study. J Thorac Cardiovasc Surg 2003;126:1320.

SOLVD Investigators. Effect of enalapril on survival in patients with reduced left ventricular ejection fraction and congestive heart failure. N Engl J Med 1991;325:293.

Van Dijk D, Jansen E, Hifman R, et al. Cognitive outcome after off-pump and on-pump coronary artery bypass graft surgery. A randomized trial. JAMA 2002;287:1405.

Van Dijk D, Keizer AMA, Diephuis JC, et al. Neurocognitive dysfunction after coronary artery bypass surgery: A systematic review. J Thorac Cardiovasc Surg 2000;120:632.

Villareal R, Hariharan R, Liu B, et al. Postoperative atrial fibrillation and mortality after coronary artery bypass surgery. J Am Coll Cardiol 2004;43:742.

EDITOR'S COMMENTS

Coronary artery bypass surgery is the most commonly performed cardiac surgical procedure, although there has been a decrease in its use due to the improvement of stenting and a more aggressive percutaneous approach to multivessel coronary disease. Therefore, it is incumbent on the surgeon to get the best graft patency possible. It really does not matter which technique is used, as long as a safe and successful operation is performed. This chapter reviews prevention and treatment of surgical complications.

I would like to emphasize a few points. We have basically gone away from the use of partial occlusion clamps in the majority of operations involving bypass. It reduces embolization from the aorta and perhaps reduces the small but finite risk of aortic dissection during this operation. The second question is that of what conduits to use. We try to use bilateral internal mammaries except in the elderly, obese patient, and, in some cases, when the patient is an insulin-dependent diabetic. There is no question that there is an increased wound complication rate with the use of bilateral mammaries in diabetics. However, in a young person, this may be a worthwhile risk due to the long-term patency of bilateral internal mammary arteries. Another alternative is the radial artery. Although we use these frequently, it is still not clear whether they are better long term than vein grafts. Some studies are looking at this, but the long-term (10 year) results are not in yet. Finally, what about vein grafts? Although they are not as ideal as internal mammary arteries, they are still very important conduits. Our preference is to use endoscopic techniques to avoid wound complications. This has meant a great deal to our patients and clearly is cost effective.

I.L.K.

48

Coronary Artery Bypass: Hypothermic Ventricular Fibrillation

Cary W. Akins

Hypothermic ventricular fibrillation without aortic occlusion is one of the methods of myocardial preservation continuously in use since the earliest days of surgical myocardial revascularization for ischemic heart disease. The basic principles of the method were developed and substantiated by laboratory research in the late 1960s and early 1970s, with several minor modifications added in more recent years. Although most cardiac surgeons have converted to one of the various forms of hyperkalemic cardioplegic arrest for myocardial protection, hypothermic ventricular fibrillation without aortic occlusion remains a very useful, reliable technique with reproducible results.

Indications and Contraindications

Hypothermic ventricular fibrillation without aortic occlusion has been successfully used with all types of primary and reoperative myocardial revascularization, as well as resection of left ventricular aneurysms. There are virtually no contraindications to using this technique of myocardial preservation whenever coronary artery bypass grafting is chosen as the best treatment option for a patient.

The only pathologic condition that can compromise this approach is the presence of significant aortic regurgitation. However, when aortic regurgitation is severe enough to interfere with coronary grafting done by this method, the regurgitation is usually severe enough to warrant either aortic

valve repair or replacement. In addition, this method can be used in the presence of ascending aortic calcification as long as a site can be found in the arterial tree to insert an aortic perfusion cannula. One also needs a source of arterial inflow for the bypass conduits, that is, usually one proximal vein graft anastomosis or a patent internal mammary artery.

Preoperative Preparation of the Patient

Very little should or needs to be changed in the usual medical management of patients before performing coronary bypass grafting during hypothermic ventricular fibrillatory arrest. Medications that are needed to maintain the patient in a nonischemic state, including beta-blockers, calcium-channel blockers, and anticoagulants, can be continued as needed to the time of operation. I feel strongly that getting the patient to the operating room in a nonischemic state, even if that requires intra-aortic balloon pumping, is an important determinant of the results of coronary artery bypass grafting. If the operation is going to be an elective procedure, aspirin may be stopped before hospitalization. However, the continuation of aspirin to the time of operation in recent years has not been associated with increased re-exploration for bleeding, but has been associated with a greater use of platelet transfusions.

Basic Operative Principles of Hypothermic Ventricular Fibrillation

The philosophic reasoning behind hypothermic ventricular fibrillation without aortic occlusion is a simple hydraulic argument: If a mean aortic root perfusion pressure of 80 to 100 mm Hg can be provided while the intracavitary pressure in the left ventricle is kept low, an adequate perfusion gradient across the coronary vascular bed will be maintained. Modest levels of hypothermia are used to lower global myocardial oxygen requirements to provide an increment of protection during the local vessel occlusion required for distal anastomoses and also to lower total body oxygen demand to provide a margin of safety for rare problems with the cardiopulmonary bypass circuit. Because proximal anastomoses can be constructed before the institution of cardiopulmonary bypass, as each distal anastomosis is completed and blood flow in the conduit is established, the area of the myocardium served by that graft is reperfused.

The basic tenets of the use of hypothermic ventricular fibrillation without aortic occlusion for myocardial preservation are the following:

1. Institution of intravenous nitroglycerin after the induction of anesthesia up to a dose of 1 μg/kg per minute, as tolerated by the patient.
2. Administration of beta-blocking agents after the induction of anesthesia to

lower the pulse rate to less than 60 beats per minute, as tolerated by the patient, if the patient is not adequately beta-blocked preoperatively.

3. Early administration of heparin during the harvesting of the internal mammary artery and before aortic cannulation.

4. Performance of one or more proximal anastomoses of saphenous vein to the aorta before atrial cannulation and the institution of cardiopulmonary bypass.

5. Addition of mannitol to the crystalloid bypass priming solution for its osmotic and free-radical scavenging effects.

6. Systemic hypothermia on cardiopulmonary bypass, usually to about 30°C.

7. Maintenance of the mean systemic perfusion pressure on cardiopulmonary bypass of 80 to 100 mm Hg, either with the adjustment of cardiopulmonary bypass flow rates or the administration of pharmacologic agents: phenylephrine (Neo-Synephrine) to increase peripheral vascular resistance or nitroprusside (Nipride) to lower peripheral resistance.

8. Elective electrical initiation, but not electrically sustained, ventricular fibrillation if the heart does not spontaneously fibrillate with cooling.

9. Routine venting of the left ventricle via the right superior pulmonary vein, preferably with a catheter that allows continuous monitoring of the left ventricular pressure.

10. Avoidance of cross-clamping the aorta.

11. Local coronary artery isolation with vinyl loops to perform distal vein or internal mammary artery anastomoses to the coronary artery.

12. Initial grafting of the most ischemic zone first, if possible.

13. Grafting of the diseased left lateral circumflex coronary arteries before internal mammary grafting to the left anterior descending system to avoid excessive traction on the mammary pedicle.

14. Complete revascularization whenever possible.

15. Initiation of rewarming on cardiopulmonary bypass while the last distal anastomosis is being completed.

Operative Technique

Primary Revascularization

Although many of the aspects of the technique of coronary artery bypass grafting, in particular the actual performance of the proximal and distal anastomoses, do not need to be different than those used with other methods, there are certain technical steps that can be used to achieve good, reproducible results. After median sternotomy is completed, one or both internal mammary arteries are isolated. At the same time, any venous conduit or other arterial conduits can also be harvested. In recent years, we have converted almost exclusively to endoscopic harvesting of saphenous vein, which has been associated with fewer leg complications and greater patient satisfaction. Just before the distal end of the mammary artery is divided, the appropriate dose of heparin for systemic heparinization for cardiopulmonary bypass is given. The mammary is then divided to assess the adequacy of flow. The distal end of the mammary pedicle is occluded with a noncrushing, soft-jawed clamp, and the pedicle is wrapped in a papaverine-soaked sponge.

After the pericardium is opened and a cradle is created to support the heart, cannulation of the ascending aorta is achieved just proximal to the innominate artery. If atherosclerotic plaques are identified by palpation or intraoperative echocardiography, the site of cannulation may need to be altered. Just before the aortic perfusion cannula is connected to the appropriate line from the heart-lung machine, I remove a small quantity of the patient's own heparinized blood to use when checking the saphenous vein for any leaks before performing the proximal vein-to-aorta anastomoses. I use an aortic perfusion cannula that has a second pressure-monitoring lumen to allow the display of accurate aortic pressures during bypass and while weaning from bypass.

The branches of the saphenous vein are carefully ligated with 4-0 silk. Other areas of bleeding on the vein may be secured with 7-0 polypropylene sutures. The necessary length of the venous conduits is then assessed, the vein segments are divided, and the ends are secured with noncrushing, soft-jawed clamps. All proximal vein anastomoses can be performed prior to bypass. Frequently, however, if there is some uncertainty about the exact length of the vein segments to be used, only one proximal anastomosis is performed prior to bypass, and subsequent proximal anastomoses are alternated with distal anastomoses on bypass.

My usual preference is to attempt to revascularize each of the major coronary distributions—namely, anterior descending, left circumflex, and right—with one piece of conduit, if possible. Since I average about 4.5 grafts per patient, this means that multiple sequential grafts are preferred over individual conduits to each artery. I use sequential grafts preferentially to avoid using too much conduit with each operation and to limit the number of proximal anastomoses and, thus, the amount of aorta used.

For the anterior surface of the left ventricle, sequential internal mammary grafts are used for the diagonal and left anterior descending arteries if possible. Occasionally a more lateral course of the diagonal artery or the limited length and caliber of the internal mammary artery may necessitate grafting diseased diagonal arteries either with individual vein grafts or as part of sequential vein grafts to the left lateral wall vessels.

I prefer to place grafts going to arteries on the left side of the heart on the left side of the ascending aorta. If the patient needs only one venous or free arterial graft to the left lateral arteries and there is sufficient room on the aorta, I prefer to place the proximal anastomoses quite high so that future operations for either recurrent coronary artery disease or new valvular heart disease will not be compromised by low-lying saphenous vein grafts. Venous or free arterial grafts that are intended to revascularize the right side of the coronary circulation are placed on the right side of the ascending aorta.

If the aorta is judged to be relatively free of atherosclerotic disease, a side-biting clamp is applied to the ascending aorta for the performance of the proximal anastomoses. The patient's systolic pressure, electrocardiogram, and filling pressures from the Swan-Ganz pulmonary artery catheter are then assessed for a few moments to watch for any signs of instability before a hole is created in the aorta. Not infrequently, the patient's systolic pressure may rise with the application of the side-biting clamp. If the pressure rises significantly, the anesthesiologist may have to administer a pharmacologic agent to lower the pressure while the proximal anastomosis is performed.

Although any standard technique for the proximal anastomoses is acceptable, I prefer to create a hole in the ascending aorta with a punch and then sew the vein to the aorta with one running 5-0 polypropylene suture. If a free arterial graft is used, 6-0 polypropylene suture may be used if the artery is small. Adequate flow is assessed in each conduit attached to the aorta before the patient is placed on cardiopulmonary bypass.

Venous cannulation is usually delayed until the proximal anastomoses have been completed. This sequence keeps the venous line out of the way during the performance of the proximal anastomoses. In addition, the irritation of the heart caused by placing the sutures for the venous cannulation or the insertion of the cannula itself can cause the patient to develop atrial fibrillation, an arrhythmia I wish to avoid until I am ready to begin cardiopulmonary bypass. In the past I usually used two separate venous cannulas if the heart needed to be retracted to reach the lateral or posterior ventricular walls. However, to standardize the perfusion equipment in our operating rooms in more recent years, I now routinely use a two-stage venous cannula without problems.

The level of systemic cooling can be varied somewhat depending on the intended length of the operation or the severity of the coronary artery disease. However, for most patients a temperature of 30°C is used because higher temperatures are occasionally associated with the resumption of sinus rhythm. As the heart cools on bypass, ventricular fibrillation will usually occur spontaneously. If necessary, a brief application of direct current from an electrical fibrillator is used to initiate, but never to maintain, ventricular fibrillation.

After the heart fibrillates, a left ventricular vent catheter is inserted. For virtually all patients, I insert the vent catheter directly into the left ventricle through the right superior pulmonary vein. The catheter has a second pressure-monitoring lumen that is attached to a transducer, and the pressure is displayed continuously on the monitoring screen for the perfusionist. This allows the perfusionist to vary the level of suction on the vent to keep the intracavitary left ventricular pressure at a level usually between 0 and 5 mm Hg while the heart is fibrillating on bypass. This pressure channel also provides a direct measurement of left ventricular end-diastolic pressure or, when it is pulled back into the left atrium, left atrial pressure to aid with weaning the patient from cardiopulmonary bypass after the revascularization is completed.

The choice of which arterial system to revascularize first depends on several factors. If the surgeon knows which area of the myocardium is most ischemic, as judged from electrocardiographic changes during ischemia or from preoperative nuclear imaging studies during stress testing, that area usually is addressed first. However, if the most ischemic area is the anterior wall and the surgeon intends to revascularize that area with the internal mammary artery, diseased left circumflex arteries are revascularized first so that there will not be excessive traction on the internal mammary artery pedicle while the heart is retracted to revascularize circumflex branches.

If there is not clear evidence of which myocardial zone is most ischemic, several other features enter into the judgment of the sequence of revascularization. Generally speaking, occluded arteries are revascularized first because the local isolation required to perform the distal anastomosis will not, in the case of occluded arteries, cause the myocardium distally to become ischemic. This is particularly true if the occluded artery receives collateral flow from another patent artery. For example, if an occluded right coronary artery is fed by collaterals from a diseased left anterior descending coronary artery, the right coronary artery is bypassed first. The reason for this sequence is that during the time the right coronary artery is locally isolated for the distal anastomosis, its distal bed will still be perfused through the collateral supply from the anterior descending because the aorta is not occluded. Then, when the left anterior descending is isolated for grafting, blood supplied via the patent graft to the right coronary artery can flow through the collateral channels in a retrograde fashion to supply the myocardium in the left anterior descending distribution. This limits even the short-term local ischemia that can occur with isolation of the distal artery for grafting and emphasizes the advantage that accrues from re-establishing coronary blood flow with the completion of each distal anastomosis.

Local isolation of the distal coronary artery is achieved by gently passing a fine-pointed right-angled clamp around the coronary artery and pulling through a hollow vinyl loop, which can be put on just enough tension to stop or adequately diminish coronary flow. I try to include some of the periarterial fat and epicardium in the vinyl loop to minimize direct trauma to the coronary artery. I also try to avoid encircling the coronary artery with the vinyl loop to prevent a crush injury.

The isolated coronary artery is then opened with a scalpel. The arteriotomy is lengthened to the appropriate size with the use of fine ophthalmic scissors. I usually probe the distal lumen gently with calibrated metallic probes. Release of the vinyl loops briefly also gives a good estimation of antegrade and retrograde collateral flow.

One feature of the performance of the conduit-to-distal-coronary anastomosis about which I feel strongly is the principle of having a few interrupted sutures at the ends of the anastomosis. This avoids the purse-string effect that can occur if too much tension is placed on a single monofilament suture. My standard vein-to-distal-coronary

anastomosis is constructed with five 7-0 polypropylene sutures. With the vein held about 1 to 2 in. away from the coronary artery, the back row of sutures is begun at one end and run continuously down one side in an open fashion. I always place the sutures so that the passage of the needle through the coronary artery is done from the lumen to the adventitia.

When the first side of the anastomosis is completed, the vein is gently lowered down to the coronary artery. Two simple interrupted sutures are then placed at the ends of that side of the anastomosis, and the running suture is tied to each of these. The ends of those sutures are then divided. Then two additional interrupted sutures are placed at each end of the other side of the anastomosis, and these sutures are then run to meet in the middle of that side. Just before the anastomosis is tied down, the vinyl loops are released and the arterial anastomosis is probed for patency. The clamp is removed from the vein graft to flush any air or debris from it, and the sutures are tied as the assistant briefly occludes the flow from the vein with a forceps.

For internal mammary and other arterial distal anastomoses, I use a somewhat different suture technique. I prefer to avoid manipulation of the arterial conduit with forceps as much as possible. Three interrupted sutures are placed at the heel of the anastomosis, with the internal mammary artery held back from the coronary artery by its pedicle fascia. The internal mammary artery is then lowered down to the coronary artery and all three sutures tied. The two side sutures are left with a long end. Starting on either side, one of the side sutures is run toward the toe of the anastomosis. Then the other side suture is run down its side of the anastomosis toward the toe. Finally, three interrupted simple sutures are placed at the distal end of the anastomosis. The side sutures are tied to the corresponding sutures on each side of the distal end. Again, the vinyl loops are released and the distal anastomosis is probed for patency. I then release the clamp on the mammary artery and gently probe the area that was clamped. Unlike the venous anastomosis, the final sutures are tied without compressing the mammary artery to avoid the development of spasm at the compression site.

Rewarming of the systemic blood is begun during the performance of the last distal anastomosis. If necessary, the heart is defibrillated when the systemic blood return temperature is about 34°C and after a bolus of lidocaine has been administered. If two venous lines have been used, during rewarming the venous cannulas are pulled back into the right atrium to ensure that flow through the vena cavae is not obstructed. Atrial and ventricular pacing wires are routinely placed. The vent catheter is pulled back into the left atrium to monitor left atrial pressure as the patient is weaned from cardiopulmonary bypass.

Reoperative Revascularization

Reoperative coronary bypass grafting poses several problems not encountered with primary revascularization. This is particularly true if there are some patent but atherosclerotically diseased vein bypass grafts. Patent arterial bypass grafts do not pose a problem for myocardial protection with hypothermic ventricular fibrillation because the aorta is not occluded, and the heart is not electrically arrested.

Embolization of atheromatous debris from stenotic vein grafts into the coronary arteries is a well-defined complication of reoperative coronary grafting and is to be avoided if at all possible. Because division of all diseased but patent grafts at the start of the operation is not appropriate with this technique, the sequence of revascularization must be individualized for each patient's pathologic condition.

If possible, proximal vein or free arterial segments are anastomosed to the aorta before cardiopulmonary bypass. This can be accomplished either by placing the anastomoses in unused areas of the aorta or by placing them at the site of old occluded vein bypass grafts, which are excised. Care is taken not to manipulate old diseased grafts or to occlude old patent vein grafts with the partial aortic occlusion clamp.

The sequence of revascularization depends on how many proximal anastomoses can be performed before cardiopulmonary bypass is established. Very often, if only one, or possibly no, proximal anastomoses can be safely accomplished before cardiopulmonary bypass, the sequence of grafting becomes the alternation of proximal and distal anastomoses until all the areas are revascularized.

Complete dissection of the heart from the pericardium is not initially performed if it might lead to embolization of atheromatous debris. After a diseased vein bypass graft has been divided and a new proximal anastomosis is constructed, the area of the myocardium served by that graft is mobilized and the standard distal anastomosis is created, as described. On some occasions, I will perform the new distal vein-to-coronary artery anastomosis first, followed by the vein-to-aorta proximal anastomosis. The actual sequence of the two anastomoses is not important if the proximal anastomosis cannot be constructed before the institution of cardiopulmonary bypass.

If the distal end of the vein-to-coronary artery anastomosis and the native coronary distal to the old anastomosis are free of disease, I may retain 2 mm to 3 mm of the old vein graft and construct my distal anastomosis to that instead of creating a new arteriotomy in the coronary artery.

As with primary grafting, left lateral wall vein graft bypasses are usually redone before a new internal mammary graft is inserted into anterior wall vessels to avoid excessive traction on the mammary pedicle.

Patient Management after Cardiopulmonary Bypass

The management of the patient after either primary or reoperative coronary revascularization has been completed is generally directed at several issues. Maintenance of adequate coronary perfusion pressure in the early hours after bypass is important and may require the use of norepinephrine in the setting of adequate cardiac output and diminished peripheral vascular resistance. Pure inotropic agents are rarely needed. Filling pressures are continuously monitored either with a preoperatively placed Swan-Ganz catheter or with a catheter placed into the left atrium through the ventricular venting site in the right superior pulmonary vein.

The removal of excess fluid acquired during the operation, particularly during cardiopulmonary bypass, is achieved by encouraging a brisk diuresis, occasionally with the use of intravenous diuretics. The patient's pulmonary function as well as other organ systems benefit significantly from the removal of the excess fluid. Low-dose dopamine may be used to improve renal perfusion in patients with compromised renal function. For patients with severe renal dysfunction, a continuous low-dose infusion of a mixture of furosemide and mannitol can be very helpful in improving diuresis and avoiding the need for early dialysis.

Intravenous nitroglycerin is usually continued until the patient is fully rewarmed and extubated, when it can be discontinued if the electrocardiogram shows no ischemic changes. Anticoagulation with a single dose of aspirin daily is begun as soon as the postoperative bleeding has ceased.

Potential Advantages and Disadvantages of Hypothermic Ventricular Fibrillation

Whenever the cardiac surgeon is faced with several choices for an operative procedure, such as which type of myocardial protection to use during coronary artery bypass grafting, it is useful to consider the potential advantages and disadvantages of each method. In comparison with other methods of myocardial protection, the relative potential advantages of hypothermic ventricular fibrillation include the following:

1. The avoidance of aortic cross-clamping and cannulation for the delivery of cardioplegic solutions may minimize trauma to the ascending aorta.
2. The avoidance of cannulation of the coronary sinus for the retrograde administration of cardioplegic solutions is avoided, minimizing trauma to that area of the heart.
3. Global myocardial ischemia created by aortic occlusion is avoided, which is a feature that can be of particular importance in the setting of acute myocardial ischemia.
4. Coronary bypass grafts can be performed in any sequence; for example, internal mammary grafting does not have to be delayed until the end of the revascularization.
5. The fluid and potassium loads attendant with the use of cardioplegic methods are avoided.
6. During reoperative myocardial revascularization, myocardial protection in the presence of patent bypass grafts, especially arterial conduits, is simplified.
7. During revascularization operations in which an intra-aortic balloon pump is in place, the myocardium is continuously benefited by the salutary effects of pulsatile perfusion while on cardiopulmonary bypass because the aorta is not occluded.
8. The technique is simpler, quicker, less cumbersome, and cheaper than cardioplegic methods.

The relative disadvantages of hypothermic ventricular fibrillation compared to other methods include the following:

1. Partial occlusion of the ascending aorta is necessary to perform proximal anastomoses of saphenous vein or free arterial grafts to the aorta.

2. Although global myocardial ischemia is avoided, distal anastomoses of the various conduits to the coronary arteries require local occlusion of the coronary artery to limit blood flow into the operative field, which creates the potential for local short-term myocardial ischemia in the absence of adequate collateral blood supply.

3. Local isolation of the coronary arteries for the distal anastomosis creates the potential for damage to the coronary vessels.

4. Retraction of the heart to expose lateral and posterior wall coronary arteries may be more difficult because of the continuous coronary perfusion, although this may not be much different than methods employing continuous coronary perfusion of cardioplegic solutions.

5. The site for the distal anastomosis may be more bloody, but probably not much more so than with cardioplegic methods that employ continuous perfusion of blood cardioplegic solutions.

Brief Review of Clinical Results

Since joining the staff of the Massachusetts General Hospital in 1977, I have used hypothermic ventricular fibrillation without aortic occlusion as essentially my sole method of myocardial preservation during myocardial revascularization or left ventricular aneurysm resection. In more than 5,000 cases of isolated coronary artery bypass grafting done with this technique during that period, I have averaged about 4.5 grafts per patient, and the total hospital mortality rate has been 1.9%. For primary coronary grafting, including emergency cases, the hospital mortality rate has been 1.5%. For reoperative revascularization, including emergency cases, the hospital mortality rate has been 5.2%.

Acknowledgment

This work was supported in part by a grant from the John F. Welch/GE Fund for Cardiac Surgical Research.

SUGGESTED READING

Akins CW. Noncardioplegic myocardial preservation for coronary revascularization. J Thorac Cardiovasc Surg 1984;88:174.

Akins CW. Resection of left ventricular aneurysm during hypothermic fibrillatory arrest without aortic occlusion. J Thorac Cardiovasc Surg 1986;91:610.

Akins CW. Early and late results following emergency isolated myocardial revascularization during hypothermic fibrillatory arrest. Ann Thorac Surg 1987;43:131.

Akins CW. Myocardial preservation with hypothermic fibrillatory arrest for coronary grafting. J Mol Cell Cardiol 1990;22:S44.

Akins CW. Hypothermic fibrillatory arrest for coronary artery bypass grafting. J Card Surg 1992;7:342.

Akins CW, Carroll DL. Event-free survival following nonemergency myocardial revascularization during hypothermic fibrillatory arrest. Ann Thorac Surg 1987;43:628

Grotte GJ, Levine FH, Kay HR, et al. Effect of ventricular fibrillation and potassium-induced arrest on myocardial recovery in hypothermic hearts. Surg Forum 1980;31:296.

Krukenkamp I, Badellino M, Levitsky S. Effects of ischemic ventricular fibrillation on myocardial mechanics and energetics in the porcine heart. Surg Forum 1990;41:239.

Yaku H, Goto Y, Futaki S, et al. Ventricular fibrillation does not depress postfibrillatory contractility in blood-perfused dog hearts. J Thorac Cardiovasc Surg 1992;103:514.

EDITOR'S COMMENTS

I had asked Dr. Akins to update this chapter from the previous edition. I recognize full well that the vast majority of surgeons do not use this technique for coronary bypass operations. However, Dr. Akins clearly has expertise in this technique and has excellent results. The reason to include the use of this technique is that it is important in the armamentarium of any cardiac surgeon. The technique can be used in individuals with atherosclerotic aortas where the bypass technology might be required. Avoiding cross-clamping and a beating heart might be preferable in these situations.

I.L.K.

49

Off-Pump Coronary Artery Bypass Surgery

Howard K. Song and John D. Puskas

Introduction

Over the last 10 years, there has been increasing interest in performing coronary artery bypass grafting (CABG) without the use of cardiopulmonary bypass. This growth in off-pump coronary artery bypass surgery (OPCAB) has been largely driven by increasing recognition of the deleterious effects of cardiopulmonary bypass and the desire to avoid the diffuse inflammatory response, multiorgan dysfunction, and neurocognitive complications that may follow. Increasing clinical experience with OPCAB has allowed analysis of outcomes following the procedure and demonstrated improved clinical outcomes in both prospective and large, risk-adjusted, retrospective comparisons among various patient populations.

Approximately 25% of CABGs performed in the United States in 2002 were performed off-pump, and some centers report a significantly higher percentage of OPCAB cases. This growth has been facilitated in large part by improvements in exposure and retraction techniques and the development of specialized stabilizers and positioners that allow experienced surgeons to conduct complex off-pump coronary revascularizations that were not previously feasible without the use of cardiopulmonary bypass. With current techniques and instruments, OPCAB can now be performed in the vast majority of patients needing coronary revascularization.

Even among cardiovascular surgeons not routinely performing coronary revascularization off-pump, there are newly recognized clinical scenarios, such as a patient with severe atherosclerosis of the ascending aorta, for whom use of OPCAB techniques is strongly favored. OPCAB is itself a fa-cilitating technology for surgeons developing minimally invasive approaches to coronary revascularization. Over a brief period of time, OPCAB has therefore evolved into a requisite component of the armamentarium of the modern cardiovascular surgeon interested in continuously improving outcomes and preserving the confidence of the clinical community in CABG surgery.

Clinical Outcomes after Off-Pump Coronary Artery Bypass Surgery

Clinical outcomes after OPCAB have been studied for a number of years by surgeons interested in developing the technique. These studies in general can be divided into two categories. Smaller, prospective, randomized studies directly comparing outcomes following off-pump and on-pump CABG have the advantage of avoiding selection bias; however their typically small enrollment limits the statistical power that may be necessary to detect incremental improvements in complication rates that are already low with conventional on-pump CABG. Larger, risk-adjusted, retrospective studies, though prone to selection bias, have the advantage of greater statistical power that may detect small advantages in outcomes and identify areas that would benefit from further study. Familiarity with the results of both types of studies is therefore useful.

Prospective, Randomized Studies

Patient outcomes following OPCAB have been studied by several prospective, ran-domized studies. A consistent finding among all of these studies is that OPCAB in experienced hands is a safe and efficacious method for performing coronary revascularization. No study has demonstrated a disadvantage for OPCAB with respect to mortality or adverse cardiac events when compared to conventional CABG. On the contrary, use of OPCAB has been found in these studies to provide a number of advantages in the early postoperative period leading to decreased resource utilization (Table 49-1). The magnitude of the overall clinical benefit to the patient from avoiding cardiopulmonary bypass is a point of contention.

Exposure of circulating blood to the large foreign surface of a cardiopulmonary bypass circuit leads to the broad activation of plasma protein systems and cellular blood components, which triggers a whole-body inflammatory response, coagulation cascade activation, and fibrinolytic activity. As expected, avoidance of cardiopulmonary bypass by OPCAB is associated with a decreased inflammatory response after surgery as measured by neutrophil activity, cytokine levels, and complement activation. The overall incidence of postoperative infections, including sternal wound infections, has been found to be lower in patients following OPCAB, suggesting a clinically relevant consequence of reducing the inflammatory response after bypass surgery.

Neutrophil activation has been implicated in the pathogenesis of pulmonary dysfunction after cardiopulmonary bypass, which is common and usually manifests as reduced lung compliance and impaired gas exchange. Patients undergoing OPCAB have reduced ventilatory requirements, leading to streamlined critical care management and reduced overall length of hospital

Table 49-1   Benefits of Off-Pump Coronary Artery Bypass Grafting Demonstrated in Prospective, Randomized Studies

Myocardial protection
   Reduced release of cardiac enzymes
   Decreased need for inotropic support
   Fewer postoperative arrhythmias
Pulmonary function
   Decreased requirement for mechanical ventilation
Renal protection
   Improved preservation of glomerular filtration and renal tubular function
Coagulation
   Decreased coagulopathy
   Decreased transfusion requirement
Inflammation
   Reduced release of cytokines
   Reduced complement activation
   Decreased incidence of postoperative infections
Neurocognitive function
Improved early postoperative neurocognitive function
Resource utilization
   Decreased total resource utilization

stays postoperatively. The use of OPCAB also mitigates the measurable coagulopathy associated with cardiopulmonary bypass. A repeated finding in several studies has been a reduced transfusion requirement for red blood cells and other blood components as well as a higher hematocrit at discharge. This advantage has led to reduced transfusion-related costs and has contributed to reduced resource utilization overall.

The technique of OPCAB by necessity leads to periods of regional myocardial ischemia, which raises the possibility that myocardial damage during OPCAB may be more severe than that associated with conventional on-pump CABG. This has been studied prospectively in a number of trials by measuring myocardial enzyme release postoperatively. Enzyme release has consistently been found to be lower in patients undergoing OPCAB than in those undergoing on-pump CABG. This finding indicates superior myocardial protection for patients undergoing OPCAB, most likely because periods of global ischemia are avoided. Myocardial stunning also appears to be attenuated. Evidence corroborating this interpretation comes from the observation that patients undergoing OPCAB have a decreased need for inotropic support and fewer arrhythmias in the postoperative period.

End-organ protection also is a potential area of benefit for patients undergoing

OPCAB. The whole-body inflammatory response initiated by cardiopulmonary bypass leads to a degree of end-organ dysfunction in virtually every organ system studied. Avoidance of this inflammatory response, superior myocardial protection, and decreased inotrope requirement are mechanisms by which superior end-organ protection may be achieved by OPCAB. With regard to renal function, glomerular filtration and renal tubular function were found to be better preserved in patients undergoing OPCAB in the one randomized trial in which these endpoints were studied.

Neurocognitive outcomes following OPCAB have been intensively studied. Demonstration of a definitive advantage for OPCAB or conventional CABG is complicated by the complex interaction among embolic, inflammatory, and hemodynamic phenomena that all may contribute to impaired neurocognitive function in the postoperative period. For example, in the randomized trial described by Puskas, Williams, Duke, et al., all patients undergoing OPCAB or conventional CABG were screened for atherosclerosis of the ascending aorta by epiaortic ultrasound. Those patients assigned to the conventional CABG group who were subsequently found to have severe atherosclerosis of the ascending aorta and were therefore at high risk for an atheroembolic event were allowed to cross over to the OPCAB group to avoid any manipulation of the diseased aorta. Patient care was therefore not compromised in the study, but an opportunity to compare embolic phenomena in the two patient groups was lost. An advantage for patients undergoing OPCAB has been demonstrated by two studies in the early postoperative period; however one study found this effect to be limited in duration and negligible 12 months after surgery.

OPCAB presents unique technical challenges to the surgeon, who must master the exposure and stabilization techniques that make beating-heart surgery possible. Because of this, graft patency in patients undergoing OPCAB has been an area of concern throughout the development of the field. In the largest randomized study in which graft patency was systematically studied, there were no differences in patency rates in any coronary distribution for patients undergoing OPCAB or conventional CABG. A smaller study subsequently demonstrated reduced patency rates for patients undergoing OPCAB 3 months after surgery. Individual operator variability may explain the differences between these studies because surgeons in the latter study performed

OPCAB on only 13% of their patients in the period before their randomized trial. The surgeon in the prior study has routinely performed OPCAB in his practice, and OPCAB accounts for >90% of his CABG practice. Approximately 25% of CABGs performed in the United States in 2002 were performed off-pump, and this proportion has been steadily growing. The issues of operator dependence and safe adoption of OPCAB into clinical practice have been studied. Although there is a significant learning curve for OPCAB, through careful patient selection, this period can be managed and safely traversed while maintaining excellent clinical outcomes.

Risk-Adjusted, Retrospective Studies

Whereas randomized, prospective trials are the most rigorous method by which an emerging therapy such as OPCAB can be evaluated, larger, retrospective, risk-adjusted studies with greater statistical power serve to identify potential areas of benefit that merit further investigation. This is particularly true for OPCAB, where large, prospectively collected databases can be used to analyze outcomes of clinical scenarios that are less common. Operative mortality is an example of a (thankfully) rare clinical event that has been studied by several large retrospective studies in which the expected risk of death was risk-adjusted for patient comorbidities. Although the conclusion of the majority of these studies was that OPCAB is safe and not associated with increased risk-adjusted mortality, two such studies did demonstrate significant improvement in mortality. Three of these studies showed significant reduction in risk-adjusted rates of morbid complications in patients undergoing OPCAB.

Outcomes following OPCAB have also been studied in subpopulations of patients at higher risk for adverse outcomes. Data from a growing number of these large observational studies is accumulating that suggest that patients designated as high risk by the presence of various comorbidities have better outcomes when their CABG surgery is performed off-pump. For example, OPCAB patients with poor left ventricular function have been observed in several large observational studies to have lower morbidity and mortality. Patients with advanced age are another high-risk subgroup that has increasingly been found to benefit from off-pump coronary revascularization. Other high-risk subgroups potentially benefiting from OPCAB include female patients and patients with obesity, diabetes mellitus, and renal insufficiency.

Preoperative Considerations

The patient selection process for OPCAB benefits from careful consideration of a number of preoperative variables. Although OPCAB is now performed routinely in some clinical practices, the tendency to automatically or blindly assign patients to OPCAB should be resisted. Preoperative factors favoring OPCAB must be weighed carefully against relative or absolute contraindications for the procedure. Rational and systematic consideration of these factors maximizes the likelihood of a technically successful procedure while limiting the chance for adverse events.

Surgeon

Any preoperative decision-making should begin with the individual surgeon's training, experience, and attitudes toward OPCAB. OPCAB surgery presents a unique set of technical challenges to the cardiovascular surgeon, who otherwise would be operating in a motionless and bloodless field. It has been estimated that OPCAB is feasible in up to 90% of patients presenting for first-time CABG surgery. Clearly, the proportion of patients having surgery off-pump is significantly lower than this, so individual surgeon preference and attitude toward the procedure is having a large effect on patient selection for the OPCAB.

Surgeon interest in and commitment to OPCAB is usually tied to a conviction that the technical challenges inherent in the procedure are worth overcoming so that the patient may benefit from avoidance of cardiopulmonary bypass. An individual surgeon's decision-making therefore is determined by the degree of technical challenge presented by an individual patient and the extent to which that patient may benefit from OPCAB. This balance varies widely from surgeon to surgeon and patient to patient. Surgeons who have incorporated OPCAB into up to 90% of their coronary revascularization practice may feel that, for them, the technical challenge of OPCAB is worth overcoming to derive an incremental benefit, for example, in transfusion and ventilator requirements, for low-risk patients. Other surgeons may feel that the technical challenge may be worth overcoming only for patients at high risk for an adverse event, such as those with poor left ventricular function

or advanced age. Despite this spectrum of attitudes and commitment to OPCAB, there is increasing recognition that there are certain subgroups of patients, such as those with severe atherosclerosis of the ascending aorta, for whom OPCAB is strongly advised.

Individual surgeon experience in OPCAB is an important determinant in patient selection for OPCAB. The unique technical challenges of OPCAB grafting and its relative unfamiliarity have raised concern that adoption of OPCAB may lead to poorer outcomes during each surgeon's learning curve. This issue has been studied. With careful patient selection, OPCAB surgery can be gradually assimilated into clinical practice while preserving and ultimately improving clinical outcomes. Very early in a surgeon's experience, it is recommended that patients with depressed left ventricular function, left main disease, and three-vessel disease be excluded from selection for off-pump surgery. As surgeon experience with specialized techniques and retractors grows, more-complex and higher-risk cases can be performed safely off-pump. Over time, OPCAB can be applied to a broad spectrum of clinical settings, including patients with advanced age, multivessel disease, depressed left ventricular function, left main disease, and complete arterial revascularization. Gradual assimilation of OPCAB thereby develops surgeon familiarity and comfort with the technique, allowing its broader application to an increasing pool of patients who derive benefit from avoiding cardiopulmonary bypass.

Patient

Once surgeon experience and comfort with OPCAB is established, the preoperative decision-making can focus on patient factors. With patience and persistence, OPCAB can be performed in the vast majority of patients needing coronary revascularization. Patients for whom OPCAB may be inappropriate are those in cardiogenic shock, those suffering from ischemic arrhythmias, and those with thoracic anatomy that severely limits the ability to rotate the heart, for example, those with pectus excavatum or previous left pneumonectomy (Table 49-2). Relative contraindications include intramyocardial coronary arteries and unusually small or calcified coronary arteries. These targets may be safely bypassed off-pump only with the benefit of considerable experience. On the other hand, patients with left main coronary lesions and recent myocardial infarction can safely have coronary revascularization performed off-pump

and should be considered candidates for the procedure.

The preoperative evaluation of the patient proceeds with a complete history and physical exam. If radial artery harvest is contemplated, patients with inconclusive Allen's tests undergo radial and ulnar artery duplex examinations. Criteria for preoperative carotid duplex examination include left main disease, peripheral vascular disease, carotid bruits, history of cerebrovascular accident, history of heavy tobacco use, and age >65 years. If significant carotid disease is detected, further workup is pursued, and typically staged carotid endarterectomy followed by coronary revascularization are performed.

Beyond the routine history and physical exam, the remainder of the preoperative evaluation may focus on identifying characteristics that may make the patient a particularly good candidate for OPCAB surgery. As discussed, a number of studies have demonstrated reduced morbidity and mortality in patients undergoing OPCAB who are at high risk for adverse events following CABG surgery. These studies define high-risk patients as those carrying one or more comorbidities known to increase risk after coronary revascularization. Individual risk factors have also been identified that may increase the benefit patients derive from avoidance of cardiopulmonary bypass.

Left ventricular dysfunction appears to be one such risk factor, perhaps due to improved myocardial protection afforded by avoiding global ischemia. OPCAB is not only safe for patients with advanced age, but it also has been associated with improved outcomes in this group. Patients with chronic renal insufficiency may have superior renal protection with off-pump coronary revascularization compared to conventional CABG, reducing the incidence of acute renal failure and postoperative hemodialysis.

The role of atherosclerotic lesions of the ascending aorta in perioperative stroke

Table 49-2   Contraindications to Coronary Artery Bypass
Off-Pump
Absolute contraindications
Cardiogenic shock
Ischemic arrhythmias
Anatomic factors preventing rotation of the heart
Previous left pneumonectomy
Severe pectus excavatum
Relative contraindications
Intramyocardial coronary arteries
Small or calcified coronary arteries

has become increasingly evident over the last decade. OPCAB surgery combined with clampless proximal anastomosis techniques are becoming a new standard by which patients with severe atherosclerosis of the ascending aorta at high risk for postoperative stroke should be managed. Routine intraoperative use of epiaortic ultrasound is an invaluable tool for identifying patients with severe atherosclerosis of the ascending aorta so that their stroke risk can be effectively managed.

Two subgroups of patients conspicuous by their absence from the literature summarized previously are those with severe chronic obstructive pulmonary disease and those with end-stage liver disease. Cardiopulmonary bypass is well documented to produce pulmonary dysfunction related primarily to neutrophil activation. Avoidance of cardiopulmonary bypass with the use of OPCAB techniques is therefore an appealing approach to avoid pulmonary complications postoperatively in this challenging group. Similarly, avoidance of coagulation cascade activation and fibrinolysis during coronary revascularization in patients with significant hepatic dysfunction would seem to be a rational approach. Data for these subgroups, however, are lacking, and this area would benefit from further investigation.

Patients with the specific comorbidities of depressed left ventricular function, advanced age, chronic renal insufficiency, and severe atherosclerosis of the ascending aorta are therefore viewed in our institution as potentially benefiting the most from OPCAB surgery. Surgeons not routinely performing OPCAB should consider patients carrying these comorbidities carefully when planning a coronary revascularization procedure. Tipping the decision-making more toward OPCAB for high-risk patients has the potential to improve outcomes in this challenging group and for the overall population of patients undergoing coronary revascularization.

Intraoperative Management

The planned conduct of an OPCAB surgery introduces a number of new patient care issues to the staff of an operating room. An important underlying concept to ensuring patient safety and the smooth conduct of the procedure is communication among the surgeon, operating room staff, and anesthesiologists. During an OPCAB case, there may be anticipated or unanticipated changes in patient hemodynamics, changes in the operative plan, and departure from the expected order of distal or proximal anastomoses. Effective communication helps team members to anticipate or react to changes promptly to ensure a safe outcome.

Anesthesia

Much of the anesthetic management of patients during OPCAB surgery is common to the management of patients having conventional CABG surgery. All patients undergoing OPCAB require invasive monitoring. At a minimum, an arterial line and a central venous line are required. Significantly depressed left ventricular function mandates a Swan-Ganz catheter. Monitoring of pulmonary artery pressures can be particularly useful during retraction of the heart for construction of distal anastomoses because pulmonary artery pressure elevations are frequently the first sign of hemodynamic compromise prior to ischemic arrhythmias and cardiovascular collapse.

In addition to the routine monitoring and safe anesthetic induction desired in all CABG procedures, there are a number of anesthesia management issues that are specific to OPCAB. In contrast to conventional CABG procedures, maintenance of normothermia is critically important throughout the case because the ability to actively rewarm the patient by cardiopulmonary bypass is forfeited. Significant hypothermia adversely affects coagulation, is arrhythmogenic, and delays postoperative extubation. Efforts to maintain normothermia should therefore begin before induction. The preoperative holding area and operating room should be kept warm. Warm blankets should be kept on the patient during induction until the patient is ready to be prepped. All intravenous fluids and blood products administered to the patient should be warmed. At our institution, an adhesive pad system is routinely applied that continuously circulates warm water to the patient's back and flank (Arctic Sun; Medivance, Inc., Louisville, CO). This system is more effective than conventional warming methods alone in preventing hypothermia during OPCAB surgery. A sterile convective forced-air warming system is placed over the patient's legs after saphenous vein conduit is harvested (Bair Hugger; Arizant Healthcare, Eden Prairie, MN).

Another challenge in the intraoperative anesthetic management of patients undergoing OPCAB is maintenance of hemodynamic stability during the lifting and retracting of the heart necessary to obtain exposure to coronary targets. Significant alterations in blood pressure and cardiac output occur, particularly with rightward retraction of the heart for lateral wall exposure. Acutely, this is typically related to decreases in preload and left ventricular filling that are diminished because the vena cavae, right ventricular outflow tract, and pulmonary veins may be kinked with this maneuver. An effective first-line treatment for this response is the administration of intravenous fluids. An assessment of the patient's intravascular volume status is made before manipulation of the heart and preload is optimized in this way. To compensate for the acute changes in preload that occur during heart manipulation, placement of the patient in steep Trendelenburg and reverse Trendelenburg positions can rapidly alter preload conditions to favor different hemodynamic states. Patient positioning is particularly useful when moment-to-moment changes in blood pressure are desired, for example, when rightward displacement of the heart is anticipated (Trendelenburg position) or when moderate hypotension is desired before placement of a partial occluding vascular clamp on the ascending aorta (reverse Trendelenburg position).

As experience with OPCAB has evolved, the use of inotropes and vasopressors to maintain hemodynamic stability has been liberalized. Early in our experience, adjustment of preload conditions with intravenous fluid was the primary means by which stable blood pressures were maintained. To limit the intravenous fluid load given to patients intraoperatively, low to moderate doses of alpha agents such as norepinephrine are now routinely given as an adjunct. This practice has led to more favorable volume status in the postoperative period and has not had untoward effects on myocardial protection. It is unusual for patients to have a significant inotrope or vasopressor requirement beyond the immediate perioperative period.

Familiarity with the OPCAB procedure on the part of the anesthesia team is obviously critical to the safe conduct of the operation. Patient care issues specific to OPCAB are thereby anticipated and addressed before they adversely affect the outcome of the procedure. Communication between the anesthesia team and the surgeon before and during the operation is important, particularly when changes in the surgeon's operative plan occur. Effective communication between the anesthesia team and the surgeon allows the surgeon to devote more attention to the technical aspects of the procedure.

Surgery

The surgeon should come to the operating room with an operative plan that optimizes the likelihood for a successful outcome but also should remain flexible enough to change the operation substantively as intraoperative findings dictate. This is one area where OPCAB and conventional CABG procedures differ significantly. OPCAB procedures frequently require significant intraoperative decision-making that results in departure from the routine. The following describes how a typical OPCAB case is performed in a patient requiring multivessel bypass.

Preparation

All patients for whom OPCAB is planned receive an aspirin suppository (1,000 mg) after induction of anesthesia and before being prepped for surgery. Unlike the case when patients undergo on-pump CABG surgery, aspirin use up to the day of surgery has not been associated with increased bleeding-related complications in patients undergoing OPCAB. The early graft patency of patients undergoing OPCAB may be jeopardized by the absence of cardiopulmonary bypass-related coagulopathy. In fact, patients undergoing OPCAB may be in a relatively hypercoagulable state in the immediate postoperative period, as is the case for patients undergoing general surgical procedures. For this reason, we administer aspirin perioperatively and clopidogrel in the immediate postoperative period for platelet inhibition and to improve early graft patency.

After the patient is draped, pacing cables and internal defibrillator paddles are handed off the field so they will be immediately available in the event that pacing or defibrillation is needed at any time during the procedure. On occlusion of the right coronary artery, particularly when there is not a well-developed network of collaterals, it is not infrequent that symptomatic bradyarrhythmias are encountered. Immediate availability of pacing cables and defibrillator paddles usually limits the duration of hemodynamic compromise and salvages the OPCAB procedure.

The chest is opened in the usual fashion through a midline sternotomy incision. Left and/or right internal mammary artery pedicles (LIMA/RIMA) are harvested with the use of an upward-lifting Favaloro retractor. Other radial artery or saphenous vein conduits are harvested simultaneously by endoscopic techniques. Heparin is given (1.5 mg/kg) to achieve a target activated

clotting time of >350 seconds. Heparin is re-dosed every 30 minutes to maintain this level of anticoagulation. Re-dosing of heparin in OPCAB cases may be necessary more frequently than in conventional CABG cases because heparin metabolism is more rapid in normothermic OPCAB patients.

After heparinization, the mammary pedicle is divided and a mixture of papaverine and lidocaine is injected intraluminally and allowed to dwell there for 15 to 30 minutes. A sternal retractor (OctoBase; Medtronic, Inc., Minneapolis, MN) designed to act as a platform for OPCAB stabilizers and positioners (Octopus 4.3 and Starfish 2; Medtronic, Inc.) is placed in the chest. A wide, inverted T-shaped pericardiotomy is performed, dividing the pericardium along the diaphragm toward the right and left phrenic nerves. It is important to divide the pericardium extensively from the diaphragm to facilitate cardiac displacement. The left and right pericardiophrenic artery and vein branches are carefully clipped and divided to avoid postoperative hemorrhage. The left pleural space is opened widely; opening the right pleural space will facilitate cardiac displacement, but has been less necessary since the introduction of the Starfish cardiac positioning device. Care is taken during the dissection to clip any large vessels encountered and to avoid the phrenic nerves. It is also important to divide the diaphragmatic muscle slips that insert on the right side of the xiphoid to allow elevation of the right sternal border, creating space for rightward cardiac displacement. Excision of a large right-sided pericardial fat pad, if present, also provides additional room. Placement of two rolled towels under the right limb of the retractor elevates the right sternal edge, which allows the heart to be positioned toward the right without compression against the sternum or retractor.

Several heavy pericardial sutures are then placed to provide traction and exposure. One or two sutures are placed on the left pericardium above the phrenic nerve. It is important to divide the left side of the pericardium off the diaphragm widely so that traction on these stitches will lead to rightward rotation of the heart along the axis of the vena cavae and allow visualization of the lateral wall of the left ventricle.

The most important traction suture is a deep posterior pericardial suture placed approximately two thirds of the way between the inferior vena cava and left pulmonary vein at the point where the pericardium reflects over the left atrium. Care should be taken with placement of this suture to avoid the underlying descending thoracic aorta,

esophagus, left lung, and pulmonary veins. The suture is covered with a soft rubber catheter to prevent laceration of the epicardial surface of the heart. The purpose of this deep traction suture is to elevate the heart up and out of the pericardial well to facilitate exposure of the coronary targets. When this suture is retracted toward the patient's feet, it elevates the base of the heart toward the ceiling and points the apex vertically with remarkably little change in hemodynamics. When the deep pericardial traction suture is retracted toward the left shoulder, the heart rotates from left to right. A variety of cotton slings can be applied at the base of this suture to aid in displacing the heart into the right pleural cavity. The slings may be particularly helpful during OPCAB in the setting of cardiomegaly.

Epiaortic ultrasound is performed on all patients before manipulation of the aorta. This procedure adds only 1 to 2 minutes to the operative time and is the most sensitive means of detecting atherosclerotic lesions of the ascending aorta intraoperatively. More important, it allows the surgeon to individualize placement of aortic clamps and proximal anastomosis devices to minimize the risk of atheroembolism. Its use has led to the reduction of postoperative stroke in patients at high risk for atheroembolism. A finding of grade IV or grade V atherosclerosis precludes application of a clamp to the ascending aorta. Use of a clampless surgery system that allows construction of a hand-sewn anastomosis (Heartstring; Guidant Corporation, Indianapolis, IN) is possible when relatively uninvolved areas of the ascending aorta are detected by epiaortic ultrasound. When atherosclerotic involvement is diffuse, the innominate artery, LIMA, or RIMA is used for proximal bypass graft in-flow.

The heart is allowed to roll with gravity into the left or right chest, facilitated by table rotation, tension on traction sutures, and occasionally a cotton sling. The heart should never be compressed against the sternum or pericardium. Right pericardial traction sutures are released when exposing the left side of the heart, and similarly left pericardial traction sutures are released when exposing the right coronary artery. Pericardial sutures on both the right and left sides are never under tension simultaneously when displacing the heart to expose coronary targets. Gentle application of these techniques maintains stable hemodynamics while providing excellent exposure.

When grafting of the lateral wall or inferior wall is planned, a cardiac positioning device (Starfish 2; Medtronic, Inc., Minneapolis, MN) is also used. This device uses suction to attach to the epicardial surface of the heart and elevates and displaces the heart to provide exposure of coronary targets with little hemodynamic compromise. Its hemodynamic advantage comes from the fact that it rotates the heart along the axis of the vena cavae while elevating it out of the pericardial well, thereby avoiding compression or kinking of the atria, vena cavae, and pulmonary veins. This device aids in exposure and presentation and is not designed for coronary stabilization. It is used in conjunction with a coronary stabilizer and facilitates exposure, especially in cases of cardiomegaly and depressed left ventricular function. It may be applied anywhere on the epicardial surface of the heart, and is frequently moved away from the apex to facilitate exposure of various coronary artery targets.

On rare occasions when bradycardia and cardiomegaly coexist, ventricular distension hinders effective cardiac displacement. In this situation, temporary epicardial atrial pacing may significantly reduce cardiac size by decreasing diastolic filling time and improve target vessel exposure.

Sequence of Grafting

In OPCAB surgery, the chosen sequence of grafting is important to maintain hemodynamic stability and avoid critical ischemia. It is therefore an important factor in the success of the operation. As a general rule, the collateralized vessel or vessels are grafted first and then reperfused by performing the proximal anastomoses or releasing flow through the IMA. The last coronary target grafted is the collateralizing vessel. This strategy avoids interrupting vital flow from the collateralizing vessel to the collateralized territory until after the collateralized vessel has been grafted.

At times the proximal anastomoses may be performed early in the operative sequence to aid in early reperfusion of a collateralized vessel. Performing the proximal anastomoses first may make estimation of graft length more difficult. The anticipated length is measured with a silk tie so that conduit can be appropriately cut in this circumstance. If the LIMA-to-left anterior descending (LAD) artery graft must be performed first, it may be necessary to leave a long mammary pedicle to avoid tension on the LIMA anastomosis during subsequent displacement of the heart to expose other target vessels.

A preferred sequence of grafting is as follows:

1. Perform the anastomosis to the completely occluded or most collateralized vessel first. The collateralizing vessel can then be safely grafted. This strategy minimizes myocardial ischemia.

2. The LIMA-to-LAD artery anastomosis should be performed first if the LAD is collateralized or in cases of tight left main stenosis. This anastomosis is performed last when the LAD is the collateralizing vessel.

3. The proximal anastomosis can be performed first or early after the distal anastomosis if the target is a critical, collateralized vessel. This allows simultaneous perfusion during subsequent occlusion of the collateralizing vessel and minimizes overall myocardial ischemia.

4. Beware of a large right coronary artery. The right coronary artery, particularly if large and dominant, can cause significant problems when occluded during OPCAB. Acute occlusion of a moderately stenotic right coronary artery may lead to severe hemodynamic compromise secondary to bradycardia. The surgeon must be prepared to use an intracoronary shunt or epicardial pacing promptly to correct bradycardia and interrupt a downward spiral leading to cardiovascular collapse.

5. Beware of mitral regurgitation in OPCAB. Prolonged displacement of the heart in the setting of mitral regurgitation can lead to severe hemodynamic compromise. Attempts should be made to address acute ischemic mitral regurgitation early in the operative sequence. This is accomplished by grafting and perfusing the culprit vessel responsible for presumed papillary muscle dysfunction.

6. Finally, graft sequence should be individualized, depending on anatomic patterns of coronary occlusion and collateralization, myocardial contractility, atherosclerosis of the ascending aorta, conduit availability, and graft geometry.

Cardiac Displacement and Presentation of Coronary Targets

It is important to understand that the cardiac displacement techniques for exposure of the inferior and lateral coronary arteries are different. The lateral wall vessels are approached by rolling the apex of the heart under the right sternal border (Fig. 49-1). As previously described, the right pleural cavity may be opened, and the traction sutures on the right pericardium are released. The left-sided traction sutures are pulled up taut on the sternal retractor (OctoBase; Medtronic, Inc.), and the table is rotated sharply to the right to assist in rolling the heart under the right sternal border. The deep stitch is pulled toward the patient's left shoulder and secured to the drapes. The coronary stabilizer (Octopus 4.3; Medtronic, Inc.) is mounted on the right side of the sternal retractor and its arm reaches across the heart, aiding in both the presentation and stabilization of the obtuse marginal coronary arteries. The Starfish cardiac positioner may be applied to the left lateral wall of the heart rather than the apex.

For the inferior wall vessels, such as the posterior descending artery, left ventricular branch of the right coronary artery, or posterolateral obtuse marginal branch, the deep traction stitch is pulled toward the patient's feet and clamped to the drapes (Fig. 49-2). The coronary stabilizer is attached to the left limb of the sternal retractor. The patient is placed in Trendelenburg position with the bed tilted to the patient's right. The base of the heart is elevated and the apex is oriented vertically toward the ceiling. The Starfish cardiac positioner may be applied to the apex of the heart and helps to elevate the heart.

In contrast to targets on the lateral and inferior walls, the anterior wall vessels (LAD and diagonals) are exposed with very little manipulation of the heart (Fig. 49-3). The deep traction stitch is secured to the drapes on the patient's left side, and the coronary stabilizer is brought over the anterior wall from the caudal or left side of the sternal retractor. An apical positioner is not routinely used for grafting of the anterior wall. Care is taken to divide the pericardium to allow the LIMA pedicle to fall posteriorly into the left chest, medial and posterior to the apex of the left lung.

Coronary Stabilization and Grafting

The current generation of coronary stabilization devices rely on suction rather than compression to maintain epicardial tissue capture. This characteristic allows the device to achieve coronary stabilization at the mechanical median of the cardiac cycle, rather than compressing the cardiac chambers excessively. Thus, stabilization is maintained while mechanical interference with ventricular function is minimized. Once the device is applied, a few seconds may be needed for the heart to recover. If hemodynamics is compromised, the degree of compression should be reduced and the mechanical median of the cardiac cycle should be more clearly identified by allowing the stabilizer arm to become flexible while still maintaining suction. The suction is maintained to avoid losing tissue capture. After

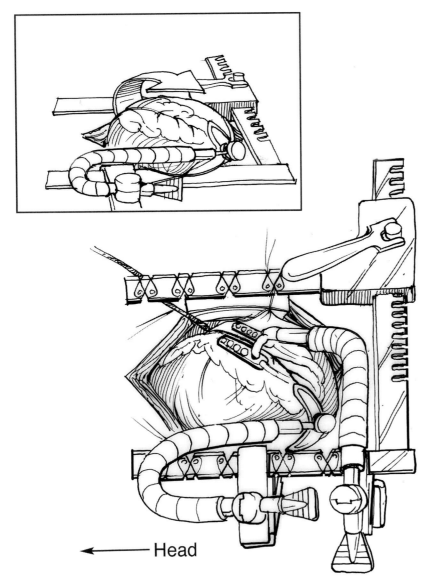

← Head

Figure 49-1. Cardiac displacement and presentation of lateral wall coronary targets. The cardiac positioner is applied to the apex or left lateral wall of the heart and lifts the heart out of the pericardial well and rolls it to the right **(insert)**. Left-sided pericardial traction sutures and the deep stitch are placed under tension to assist in rolling the heart under the right sternal border. The coronary stabilizer reaches across the heart from the right side of the sternal retractor, aiding in both the presentation and the stabilization of the lateral wall coronary targets.

assurance before committing to the anastomosis by creating an arteriotomy. Once the distal anastomosis is underway, it is critical for the anesthesia team to continuously communicate with the surgeon. Changes in hemodynamics should be quickly addressed. Bradyarrhythmias are promptly treated with epicardial pacing.

The target vessel is occluded by applying the minimum necessary tension on the vessel loop. This tension is directed in such a manner that the vessel is lifted out of surrounding epicardial fat, further improving exposure of the target. The target vessel is opened with a coronary knife and the arteriotomy is extended with coronary scissors. The field is kept free of blood by dispersing retrograde bleeding from the distal end of the arteriotomy with a humidified CO_2 blower (Clearview Blower/Mister; Medtronic, Inc.). It is important that the surgeon's assistant blow on the target only when the surgeon is placing the needle through the tissue of the conduit or target vessel. This minimizes the potential trauma to the target vessel that can occur with excessive use of the blower. Excellent visualization is critical for a precise anastomosis. Magnification of 3.5×, a headlight, and Castro Viejo needle drivers are used for all anastomoses. An 8-0 monofilament suture is used to optimize precision, unless severe calcification mandates use of a heavier needle.

Myocardial Protection

Concern for myocardial protection during OPCAB stems from the understanding that the brief periods of coronary occlusion necessary to visualize the target vessels during construction of distal anastomoses cause regional ischemia and some degree of myocardial injury that not only may affect the ischemic region, but also may cause accumulated global dysfunction after sequential occlusions imposed during multivessel bypass grafting. In animal models of simulated OPCAB, even brief periods of ischemia lead to contractile dysfunction, endothelial injury in the target vessel, and apoptosis that contributes to postrevascularization pathology. Strategies for protecting the myocardium from ischemic and reperfusion injury have therefore been developed to improve acute and potentially longer-term outcomes following OPCAB procedures.

Myocardial protection during OPCAB has evolved as techniques for performing the procedure have been refined. Before the development of suction-based stabilizers, intermittent pharmacologic arrest and profound bradycardia were induced during

the appropriate position for the stabilizer arm is determined, it is tightened once more. The malleable pods of the Octopus 4.3 allow the surgeon to spread the epicardium adjacent to the coronary targets, significantly improving visualization of the coronary artery. Epicardial fat retractors are rarely necessary. The malleable pods can be bent or rotated independently to accommodate irregular epicardial surfaces.

After optimal exposure is obtained, a soft silastic vessel loop (Quest Medical, Allen, TX) is placed around the target vessel for occlusion. The loop is placed proximal to the planned site of anastomosis—never distally,

to avoid trauma to the runoff of the bypass graft. Care should be taken when the vessel loop is placed to avoid entering the ventricle or damaging epicardial veins. When this occurs, a superficial epicardial suture generally stops bleeding. The vessel loop may be directed out of the surgeon's field of view with the aid of a loose pericardial suture acting as a pulley.

When the target vessel is poorly collateralized, an interval of test occlusion lasting 2 to 5 minutes can be used to determine how regional myocardial ischemia will be tolerated once the anastomosis is underway. This gives the surgeon some measure of

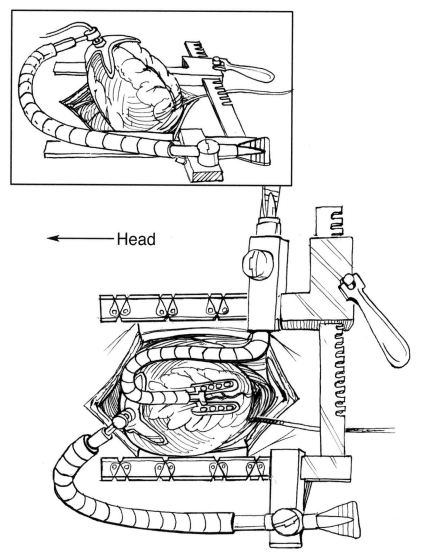

◄── Head

Figure 49-2. Cardiac displacement and presentation of inferior wall coronary targets. The cardiac positioner is applied to the apex of the heart and elevates the heart out of the pericardial well, exposing the inferior wall of the heart **(insert)**. The deep traction stitch is pulled toward the patient's feet to assist in lifting the base of the heart out of the pericardial well. The coronary stabilizer is attached to the left limb of the sternal retractor.

of vasopressors is part of careful anesthetic management. During target vessel occlusion, however, this practice is an important component of myocardial protection because perfusion to ischemic myocardium via collaterals is dependent on this perfusion pressure. Another myocardial protection strategy that may be taken for granted is the careful use of traction sutures, apical heart positioners, and coronary stabilizers that provide adequate exposure of the target vessel without excessively compressing the cardiac chambers and causing undue hemodynamic compromise. When ideally placed, these devices do not interfere with the cardiac cycle, vasopressor requirements are minimized, and overall myocardial oxygen demand is minimized. This careful positioning of the heart should be considered a routine strategy for myocardial protection. Finally, selection of the order in which distal anastomoses are constructed during a multivessel OPCAB procedure is another strategy by which the surgeon can limit the degree of regional ischemia to which the heart is subjected. Occlusion of a collateralized target vessel first in the operative sequence allows this territory to be perfused via collaterals during construction of the anastomosis. Subsequently occluded territories can then be perfused via reversed flow in the collaterals through completed grafts.

Construction of one or more proximal anastomoses early in the operative sequence is an adjunct to the thoughtful selection of the order in which distal anastomoses are constructed. Construction of a proximal anastomosis prior to the first distal anastomosis allows immediate reperfusion of the ischemic territory after target vessel occlusion and construction of the distal anastomosis. If this target vessel is collateralized, then a subsequently constructed distal anastomosis to the collateralizing target vessel can be performed with the benefit of reversed collateral flow originating from the first bypass graft. An advantage of grafting the LAD with an in situ LIMA pedicle first in the operative sequence is that this anastomosis requires minimal lifting of the heart, and subsequent target vessels can be exposed and grafted with the benefit of collateral flow from the LIMA-to-LAD anastomosis without interrupting the operative sequence to perform a proximal anastomosis.

An intracoronary shunt may be placed if significant hemodynamic compromise occurs after target vessel occlusion despite use of the routine measures described. The shunts (ClearView Intracoronary Shunts; Medtronic, Inc.) range in size from 1.0 mm to 3.0 mm. When appropriately sized for

the procedure with adenosine and short-acting beta-blockers. In addition to reducing motion of the target vessel, this strategy achieved some degree of myocardial protection by reducing myocardial oxygen demand. These maneuvers have largely passed from common clinical practice with the widespread application of second- and third-generation suction-based coronary stabilizers.

Ischemic preconditioning has also enjoyed brief popularity as a cardioprotective strategy during OPCAB. The theoretical benefit of brief occlusion and reperfusion before the long occlusion period necessary to construct a coronary anastomosis was supported by abundant laboratory evidence

showing improved myocardial protection in the region served by the occluded coronary artery. Ischemic preconditioning has not been universally shown to attenuate myocardial contractile dysfunction or stunning, and its clinical use in OPCAB has been questioned. As the number of bypass grafts routinely performed during off-pump cases has increased, the enthusiasm of surgeons for performing repeated episodes of ischemic preconditioning for each coronary artery has diminished.

A number of other myocardial protection strategies developed early in the experience of OPCAB remain in routine use. Maintenance of good systemic blood pressure by optimizing preload conditions and the use

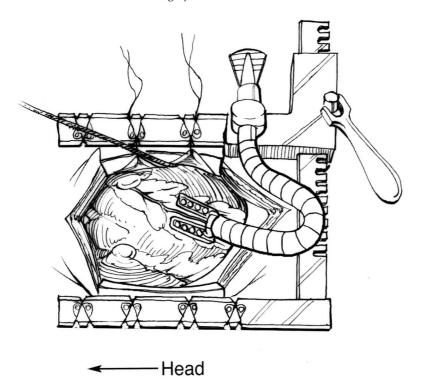

◄——Head

Figure 49-3. Cardiac displacement and presentation of anterior wall coronary targets. Left-sided pericardial traction sutures and the deep stitch are placed under tension and the coronary stabilizer is brought over the anterior wall from the caudal or left side of the sternal retractor. An apical positioner is not routinely used for grafting of the anterior wall.

the target vessel, they are easily placed and removed and provide significant flow and a reasonably bloodless field. Though used infrequently, they are kept available in the operating room for all cases in the event of their urgent need. Intracoronary shunts may be particularly useful with large right coronary arteries and bradyarrhythmias, intramyocardial vessels where placement of an occlusive vessel loop may be hazardous, and critical anatomy where occlusion of an important collateralizing vessel may lead to global myocardial ischemia and hemodynamic collapse. The shunt is removed and the coronary artery is de-aired prior to tying the suture on the distal anastomosis and flow is re-established.

With experience and gentle application of the principles described, the vast majority of patients tolerate OPCAB grafting of all coronary targets. However, the cumulative effect of sequential coronary occlusions can occasionally lead to a downward spiral of hemodynamics. At times, it may be helpful to provide accessory perfusion to the myocardium while other vessels are occluded. Perfusion-assisted direct coronary artery bypass (PADCAB) directly perfuses myocardium subtended by a bypassed coronary artery by providing controlled flow down the conduit. Inflow to the circuit and

pump is provided by a catheter placed in the ascending aorta or femoral artery. Use of a computer-controlled blood delivery system (Quest Medical MPS; Quest Medical, Allen, TX) allows for exact control of coronary perfusion pressure. Pharmacologic additives and temperature control may accentuate its protective effects. Unlike other protective strategies, including proximals-first grafting and shunts, the coronary perfusion pressure with PADCAB is independent of systemic pressure. This technique is especially helpful with collaterized targets because coronary flow can be driven through collaterals with suprasystemic pressure to supply adjacent myocardium. One can also measure and document graft patency and flows through the circuit. Multiple grafts can be perfused simultaneously with the use of a multilimbed perfusion set. It is important to not discontinue flow through all grafts simultaneously when proximal anastomoses are performed. Each conduit should be disconnected from the multilimbed perfusion set separately to perform its proximal anastomosis. We use PADCAB selectively to minimize regional ischemia and improve myocardial protection in cases of critical coronary anastomosis and profound cardiac dysfunction. PADCAB may also be used more liberally early in a surgeon's OPCAB

experience to optimize hemodynamics and broaden the application of OPCAB.

Although it is not strictly a form of myocardial protection, intra-aortic balloon pump (IABP) counterpulsation is a form of circulatory support that effectively preserves hemodynamics during OPCAB surgery for patients who are marginal candidates for the procedure. Patients at high risk for OPCAB failure due to severe proximal multivessel coronary artery disease, recent myocardial infarction, and severe ventricular dysfunction who also have comorbid disease making the avoidance of cardiopulmonary bypass desirable are candidates for this support. The IABP improves hemodynamic stability and virtually eliminates the need for inotropic support during exposure and occlusion of target vessels in this challenging subpopulation of patients (84). This strategy thereby allows surgeons to safely extend the benefits of OPCAB surgery to high-risk patients who would otherwise be marginal candidates for the procedure.

Even as OPCAB has been extended to a larger population of high-risk patients needing coronary revascularization, the intraoperative conversion rate of patients for whom OPCAB is planned to conventional on-pump CABG is low. This frequency has been estimated to be <4% by other authors. In general, OPCAB cases unexpectedly requiring conversion to cardiopulmonary bypass fall into one of two categories, elective and emergent. Causes for elective conversion are generally technical and include the inability to identify intramyocardial coronary targets and the unexpected finding of small or calcified targets. Occasionally, elective conversion is prompted by ventricular arrhythmias that are repeatedly induced with lifting of the heart for target vessel exposure. Although it is frustrating to the surgeon, elective conversion to on-pump CABG does not necessarily portend a poorer prognosis for the patient. On the other hand, emergent conversion is associated with a significantly higher risk for patient morbidity and mortality. Patient risk factors for emergent conversion to bypass include previous CABG and congestive heart failure. A thoughtful operative plan, careful exposure, and appropriate application of myocardial protection strategies keep the frequency of emergent conversion to bypass low and limit patient exposure to its accompanying risks.

Proximal Anastomoses

Proximal anastomoses to the aorta are routinely performed with an aortic partial occlusion clamp. The systolic blood pressure is lowered to <95 mm Hg before application of the clamp. This maneuver has rarely been complicated by aortic dissection with hypertension being a predisposing factor. Once the clamp is applied, aortotomies are made with a 4.0-mm aortic punch. Vein graft anastomoses are created with 6-0 monofilament suture and arterial grafts with 7-0 monofilament suture. Any graft taken as a "T" off an IMA is anastomosed with 8-0 monofilament. The aortic root is de-aired through the most anterior anastomosis after the clamp is removed, before tying this suture. The vein grafts are kept occluded until they are de-aired with a 25-gauge needle. Arterial grafts are not punctured but are allowed to backbleed prior to clamp removal.

As described previously, placement of the partial occluding aortic clamp is guided by the results of routine epiaortic ultrasound scanning. Clamping is not performed in the presence of diffuse grade III or any grade IV or grade V atherosclerotic involvement of the ascending aorta. When an uninvolved segment of the ascending aorta can be identified that would yield acceptable graft geometry, we typically use a clampless proximal aortotomy system (Heartstring; Guidant Corp.) that allows creation of a beveled, hand-sewn anastomosis. If atherosclerotic involvement of the ascending aorta is diffuse, precluding use of the Heartstring device, the proximal anastomosis is taken off of an IMA pedicle.

After completion and reperfusion of all grafts, protamine is administered (0.75 to 1.0 mg/kg) to partially correct the activated clotting time to approximately 150 seconds. As hemostasis is being achieved, three chest drains (Blake Drains; Johnson and Johnson, L.L.C., Piscataway, NJ) are placed, one in each pleural space and one in the mediastinum. Temporary epicardial pacing wires are placed only if the patient requires epicardial pacing immediately before chest closure. The chest is closed in the standard fashion with sternal wires and running absorbable sutures in the fascia, subcutaneous, and subcuticular layers.

Postoperative Care

The postoperative care of patients who have undergone OPCAB surgery does not differ in many respects from that of patients undergoing conventional CABG surgery. The requirement for close monitoring of patient cardiopulmonary status, renal function, and chest tube drainage is similar. However, there are a number of important differences that caregivers must be aware

of to take advantage of the opportunity for expedited care that OPCAB surgery can offer.

Patients who have undergone OPCAB surgery have a decreased need for inotropic support in the postoperative period, most likely because of avoidance of global ischemia and reduced myocardial stunning. The intravenous fluid requirement for patients who have undergone OPCAB surgery is also reduced because the systemic inflammatory response and capillary leak related to cardiopulmonary bypass is avoided. Massive volume resuscitation in the early postoperative period should be avoided in favor of low-dose vasopressors that may be necessary secondary to intravenous sedation. OPCAB patients typically are volume loaded intraoperatively and are more likely to be euvolemic in the immediate postoperative period than conventional CABG patients. Judicious use of intravenous fluids during this period avoids problems with volume overload.

Postoperative hemorrhage and transfusion requirements are reduced in OPCAB patients because of reduced fibrinolytic pathway activation and coagulation factor and platelet consumption. We do not routinely check platelet counts or clotting times in the immediate postoperative period for this reason. In the absence of preexisting coagulopathy, chest tube drainage is typically low. Persistent or massive hemorrhage in the postoperative period should prompt early evaluation for surgical bleeding because this is unlikely to be related to factor or platelet deficiency in an OPCAB patient.

Patients who have undergone OPCAB surgery are in a relatively hypercoagulable state as opposed to manifesting the coagulopathy that is typical after cardiopulmonary bypass. This state has the potential to adversely affect graft patency in the postoperative period. As described earlier, we address this preoperatively with the rectal administration of aspirin after induction of anesthesia. After surgery we continue aspirin administration daily as with patients undergoing conventional CABG surgery. In addition, we start clopidrogrel 75 mg/day in the immediate postoperative period once chest tube drainage has been low for three consecutive hours.

The incidence of deep venous thrombosis (DVT) may be higher in patients undergoing OPCAB due to the absence of coagulopathy postoperatively. We do not routinely use additional DVT prophylaxis other than that described unless the patient has additional risk factors, such as obesity. For patients who cannot be immediately extubated

and mobilized, subcutaneous heparin and sequential compression stockings are prescribed if not contraindicated.

One of the major benefits of OPCAB surgery to the health care system is the potential for OPCAB patients to have reduced resource utilization. An area where this advantage can be exploited is in reducing length of mechanical ventilation and intensive care unit stay. OPCAB patients have been reliably demonstrated to have a decreased need for mechanical ventilation postoperatively. To realize this benefit for the patient and the health system, caregivers should be cognizant of this and be immediately prepared to wean and extubate patients as their need for mechanical assistance is diminished. With appropriate anesthesia planning and staffing, patients can generally be extubated in the operating room after an OPCAB procedure or within 30 minutes of arrival in the intensive care unit. When this is not feasible, clinical pathways that set objective criteria and goals facilitate the timely progression of ventilator weaning and extubation that minimizes patient exposure to ventilator-related complications and maximizes efficiency and cost-effectiveness.

Further benefits can be realized by omitting the intensive care unit stay altogether from the postoperative course. In our institution, selected OPCAB patients not requiring invasive hemodynamic monitoring are transferred directly to the cardiac step-down unit after their surgery. These are typically patients with normal left ventricular and respiratory function who are extubated in the operating room or in a post-anesthesia care unit. Of course, proper nurse training and staffing in a dedicated cardiac step-down unit are necessary for patients to safely recover in this environment. When an intensive care unit stay is required, use of clinical pathways that set objective criteria and goals for subsequent transfer to the stepdown unit and discharge from the hospital also increase the efficiency and timeliness with which patient care is delivered. Periodic and systemic evaluation of patient care pathways will assure that the important potential gains in cost-effectiveness provided by OPCAB surgery are realized.

Future Directions for Off-Pump Coronary Artery Bypass Surgery

Until recently, OPCAB surgery was performed rarely and only by a few surgeons. Only patients with certain coronary anatomy were even considered candidates for the procedure. In a brief period, OPCAB has evolved into a routinely performed operation that can be applied to virtually the entire spectrum of patients requiring coronary revascularization. OPCAB surgery is now well recognized as having specific advantages to the patient compared to conventional CABG and is becoming the gold standard of care for certain clinical situations, such as management of the atherosclerotic aorta. For many surgeons, OPCAB surgery has become an important component of the armamentarium with which to attack a wide array of clinical challenges.

OPCAB surgery has matured and been accepted by the clinical community to the extent that it has become a facilitating technology for further advances in cardiovascular surgery. Minimally invasive approaches to surgical coronary revascularization are now by definition OPCAB procedures. These evolving procedures will continue to be dependent on OPCAB techniques to construct anastomoses. At our institution, endoscopic techniques for LIMA harvesting are being combined with atraumatic minithoracotomies through which minimally invasive coronary revascularization is performed to the anterior wall. This procedure is extending the benefits of LIMA-to-LAD grafting to patients who would otherwise not be referred for sternotomy due to comorbid conditions.

Application of this procedure to patients with multivessel disease is also done in combination with percutaneous revascularization of other territories to yield so-called "hybrid" procedures. Hybrid procedures are being evaluated rigorously to determine what subpopulation of patients with multivessel disease may benefit from this approach. Patients with multivessel disease being treated with percutaneous techniques alone because of high operative risk represent a group for whom hybrid procedures may increasingly be used.

Further advances in miniaturization and the development of robotics and anastomotic devices will expand our ability to revascularize patients with more complex coronary anatomy by less invasive means. These techniques will continuously be evaluated against emerging stent technologies and other percutaneous techniques. The continued confidence of the clinical community in surgical revascularization rests in our ability to continue to decrease the morbidity of our procedures without compromising long-term outcomes. Although it is difficult to predict technological advances and it is limiting to place arbitrary boundaries on what it may achieve, it is reasonable to predict that OPCAB surgery will continue to drive innovation in cardiovascular surgery in the coming years and provide a means by which these goals can be achieved.

SUGGESTED READING

Al-Ruzzeh S, Ambler G, Asimakopoulos G, et al. Off-pump coronary artery bypass (OP-CAB) surgery reduces risk-stratified morbidity and mortality: A United Kingdom multi-center comparative analysis of early clinical outcome. Circulation 2003;108:II1.

Angelini GD, Taylor FC, Reeves BC, et al. Early and midterm outcome after off-pump and on-pump surgery in Beating Heart Against Cardioplegic Arrest Studies (BHACAS 1 and 2): A pooled analysis of two randomised controlled trials. Lancet 2002;359:1194.

Ascione R, Lloyd CT, Underwood MJ, et al. Economic outcome of off-pump coronary artery bypass surgery: A prospective randomized study. Ann Thorac Surg 1999;68:2237.

Ascione R, Williams S, Lloyd CT, et al. Reduced postoperative blood loss and transfusion requirement after beating-heart coronary operations: A prospective randomized study. J Thorac Cardiovasc Surg 2001;121:689.

Calafiore AM, Teodori G, Di Giammarco G, et al. Multiple arterial conduits without cardiopulmonary bypass: Early angiographic results. Ann Thorac Surg 1999;67:450.

Cleveland JC Jr, Shroyer AL, Chen AY, et al. Off-pump coronary artery bypass grafting decreases risk-adjusted mortality and morbidity. Ann Thorac Surg 2001;72:1282; discussion 1288.

Craver JM, Murrah CP. Elective intraaortic balloon counterpulsation for high-risk off-pump coronary artery bypass operations. Ann Thorac Surg 2001;71:1220.

Diegeler A, Hirsch R, Schneider F, et al. Neuromonitoring and neurocognitive outcome in off-pump versus conventional coronary bypass operation. Ann Thorac Surg 2000; 69:1162.

Edgerton JR, Dewey TM, Magee MJ, et al. Conversion in off-pump coronary artery bypass grafting: An analysis of predictors and outcomes. Ann Thorac Surg 2003;76:1138; discussion 1142.

Hoff SJ, Ball SK, Coltharp WH, et al. Coronary artery bypass in patients 80 years and over: Is off-pump the operation of choice? Ann Thorac Surg 2002;74:S1340.

Khan NE, De Souza A, Mister R, et al. A randomized comparison of off-pump and on-pump multivessel coronary-artery bypass surgery. N Engl J Med 2004;350:21.

Lev-Ran O, Loberman D, Matsa M, et al. Reduced strokes in the elderly: The benefits of untouched aorta off-pump coronary surgery. Ann Thorac Surg 2004;77:102.

Mack M, Bachand D, Acuff T, et al. Improved outcomes in coronary artery bypass grafting with beating-heart techniques. J Thorac Cardiovasc Surg 2002;124:598.

Magee MJ, Coombs LP, Peterson ED, et al. Patient selection and current practice strategy for off-pump coronary artery bypass surgery. Circulation 2003;108:II9.

Magee MJ, Jablonski KA, Stamou SC, et al. Elimination of cardiopulmonary bypass improves early survival for multivessel coronary artery bypass patients. Ann Thorac Surg 2002;73:1196; discussion, 1202.

Plomondon ME, Cleveland JC Jr, Ludwig ST, et al. Off-pump coronary artery bypass is associated with improved risk-adjusted outcomes. Ann Thorac Surg 2001;72:114.

Puskas JD, Vinten-Johansen J, Muraki S, et al. Myocardial protection for off-pump coronary artery bypass surgery. Semin Thorac Cardiovasc Surg 2001;13:82.

Puskas JD, Williams WH, Duke PG, et al. Off-pump coronary artery bypass grafting provides complete revascularization with reduced myocardial injury, transfusion requirements, and length of stay: A prospective randomized comparison of two hundred unselected patients undergoing off-pump versus conventional coronary artery bypass grafting. J Thorac Cardiovasc Surg 2003;125:797.

Puskas JD, Williams WH, Mahoney EM, et al. Off-pump vs conventional coronary artery bypass grafting: early and 1-year graft patency, cost, and quality-of-life outcomes: A randomized trial. JAMA 2004;291:1841.

Roach GW, Kanchuger M, Mangano CM, et al. Adverse cerebral outcomes after coronary bypass surgery. Multicenter Study of Perioperative Ischemia Research Group and the Ischemia Research and Education Foundation Investigators. N Engl J Med 1996;335:1857.

Sabik JF, Gillinov AM, Blackstone EH, et al. Does off-pump coronary surgery reduce morbidity and mortality? J Thorac Cardiovasc Surg 2002;124:698.

Song HK, Petersen RJ, Sharoni E, et al. Safe evolution towards routine off-pump coronary artery bypass: Negotiating the learning curve. Eur J Cardiothorac Surg 2003;24:947.

Van Dijk D, Jansen EW, Hijman R, et al. Cognitive outcome after off-pump and on-pump coronary artery bypass graft surgery: A randomized trial. JAMA 2002;287:1405.

Van Dijk D, Nierich AP, Jansen EW, et al. Early outcome after off-pump versus on-pump coronary bypass surgery: results from a randomized study. Circulation 2001;104:1761.

Zamvar V, Williams D, Hall J, et al. Assessment of neurocognitive impairment after off-pump and on-pump techniques for coronary artery bypass graft surgery: Prospective randomised controlled trial. BMJ 2002;325:1268.

EDITOR'S COMMENTS

Song and Puskas have done an excellent job analyzing off-pump coronary bypass surgery. This is one of the major innovations in thoracic surgery over the last 5 years.

Dr. Puskas has studied this area as scientifically as possible and has performed one of the major randomized studies in this field. What do we know about off-pump coronary bypass surgery? We know that patients who receive this modality have their length of stay reduced by about 1 day and a reduced blood transfusion is required. It is difficult to sort out whether there are differences in neurologic outcomes. There is at least one study that would suggest reduced graft patency, although Puskas's group has not demonstrated this. Finally, there appear to be fewer bypass grafts per patient in several of the studies.

The issue with off-pump surgery is not that it has to be better than standard coronary artery bypass surgery, but rather that it should be as good. Clearly, graft patency is what the coronary bypass operation is all about. Anyone who can attain excellent graft patency can do the procedure by any modality that they prefer. The technical issues with off-pump relate to some anatomic factors, the occasional need for a partial occlusion clamp in the ascending aorta, and perhaps a little bit more intraoperative instability. No matter what the individual practitioner feels about off-pump versus on-pump, this technology is critical to everyone's practice. Patients with calcified ascending aortas may do better if one uses off-pump technology. I think these authors have done an excellent job in discussing the issues and the technical aspects. There will be more refinements as time goes on.

I.L.K.

50

Robotic Coronary Artery Bypass Surgery

Saqib Masroor, L. Wiley Nifong, and W. Randolph Chitwood, Jr.

Minimally Invasive Coronary Artery Bypass Surgery

The Concept

Coronary artery bypass grafting (CABG) has been performed traditionally through a median sternotomy using cardioplegic arrest. The concept of minimally invasive surgery as applied to CABG suggests either the elimination of cardiopulmonary bypass or the minimization of trauma incurred from surgical access. Clearly, the ideal goal is to be able to perform an excellent anastomosis through a tiny incision using an endoscope on a beating heart. The deleterious effects of cardiopulmonary bypass and large incisions, especially in elderly patients, are reasons alone for changing. Moreover, the successes in general surgery, orthopedics, urology, and gynecology have inspired cardiac surgeons to consider endoscopic access in their operations. The evolution of coronary surgery using robotic methods parallels that of off-pump coronary surgery. In the last few years coronary artery stabilizers and robotic devices have improved greatly. Through multiple parallel advances in technology and iterations in technique, robotic coronary surgery has become practical. With the recent Food and Drug Administration (FDA) approval of robotic devices for this indication, robotic coronary surgery has just begun to be accepted as a safe, enabling method for CABG. Robotic devices have been quite efficient in minimally invasive harvesting of the internal thoracic artery (ITA); however, technique and technology still need to be improved regarding the coronary anastomosis.

Evolution of Technology and Techniques

The first off-pump coronary bypass operation (OPCAB) was reported by Kolessov, after he anastomosed the left ITA to the left anterior descending coronary artery without using cardiopulmonary bypass. The development of safe extracorporeal circulation and cardioplegia techniques impeded the progress of OPCAB. Except for a few isolated reports in the 1970s, it was not until 1985 that a systematic series of OPCAB operations was reported by Buffolo and Benetti. Motivated mainly by the desire to lower operative costs, these surgeons became facile in performing multivessel coronary surgery without using the heart-lung machine. At that time, target vessel stabilization was achieved solely through stay suture deployment and by pharmacologically (β-blocker) induced bradycardia. These early operations required a great deal of improvisation, patience, and talent to perform with acceptable results. Calafiore's LAST operation (left anterior small thoracotomy) was an important evolutionary step in the movement toward both off-pump and robotic coronary surgery. The LAST procedure was almost identical to that done by Kolessov, reported more than 25 years earlier. Using a fifth intercostal space left anterior minithoracotomy, Calafiore harvested the ITA directly and anastomosed it to the left anterior descending artery (LAD) on a beating heart. For several years the spotlight remained on the MIDCAB or single-vessel minimally invasive direct-vision coronary artery bypass operation. Obviously, a single-vessel operation was of limited application, and the advent of improved coronary stents, and especially drug-eluting stents, called for even less ap-

plication. At that time few surgeons adopted off-pump methods, and early reports by Gundry additionally eclipsed acceptance of off-pump coronary surgery. He reported that of 112 patients undergoing beating-heart coronary surgery, 20% of them required either an interval angioplasty or a second operation. Industrial engineers and surgeons then began to design devices that would immobilize coronary artery segments better on a beating heart. Acceptance of off-pump methods by cardiac surgeons as a mainstream procedure came only after the development of effective stabilizers. Through the work of the Utrecht group, suction stabilization became an effective method for both accessing and stabilizing all three coronary vessels. From their work, off-pump coronary artery bypass surgery was used more widely. With better stabilization, the OPCAB became effective for grafting lateral and inferior coronary arteries, albeit still through a median sternotomy.

The left anterior thoracotomy in the classic MIDCAB was very painful for patients because of the extreme rib cartilage retraction used to harvest the ITA under direct vision. Closed-chest thoracoscopic ITA harvesting decreased the morbidity of this operation. However, regardless of the stabilization method, it still was impossible to perform a distal anastomosis thoracoscopically on a beating heart using long hand instruments. A hand-sewn distal anastomosis directly through a minithoracotomy again became the least invasive choice and became used successfully with excellent results. Initially, this operation was limited to anterior wall revascularization, as lateral and inferior surfaces remained inaccessible. To treat multivessel disease, Angelini suggested a hybrid approach in which the ITA was harvested endoscopically and anastomosed to the ITA through the incision. This was followed by percutaneous revascularization of the remaining stenotic vessels. Although hybrid approaches have been used by some groups to treat multivessel coronary disease, in general most surgeons still prefer to revascularize the heart completely using minimally invasive surgical methods.

Minimally Invasive Coronary Operations

The following terms are used to describe various less invasive coronary operations:

Minimally invasive direct coronary artery bypass (MIDCAB). This operation is really the same as a single-vessel LAST procedure. The ITA is harvested through a small anterior thoracotomy under direct-vision, and the LAD anastomosis is performed through the same incision.

Endoscope-assisted coronary artery bypass (Endo-ACAB). Here, the ITA is harvested with an endoscope, using the voice-controlled camera of the Automated Endoscopic System for Optimal Positioning Robotic System (AESOP; Computer Motion, Inc., Goleta, CA) placed through a port, and the distal anastomosis is constructed through a minithoracotomy.

Multivessel small thoracotomy CABG (MVST). Single or bilateral ITA harvesting is performed using a robotic surgical system. Through a minithoracotomy and using hand-sewn methods, multiple distal anastomoses are constructed with ITAs and radial artery composite Y-grafts.

Totally endoscopic coronary artery bypass (TECAB). Both ITA harvesting and the distal anastomosis are performed using a robotic system. Usually this is on an arrested heart; however, several groups have perfected this method for beating-heart coronary surgery (BH-TECAB).

Robotic (Computer-Assisted) Coronary Artery Bypass Operations

With the advent of computer-enhanced tele-manipulation systems, a completely closed chest coronary artery bypass operation became possible. In 1999 Carpentier and Loulmet first demonstrated the possibility of using robotic technology to perform minimally invasive cardiac surgery. Using both the Zeus (Computer Motion, Inc., Goleta, CA) and da Vinci (Intuitive Surgical, Inc., Sunnyvale, CA) robotic systems, groups in Europe and North America demonstrated the feasibility of totally endoscopic (robotic/computer-assisted) coronary artery bypass grafting (TECAB). These operations were difficult to perform, but proved to be safe and effective when performing an ITA to single-vessel coronary artery anastomosis. With the da Vinci system, both the left and right ITAs could be harvested from the right chest, which made two-vessel ITA-coronary grafting possible. Tried initially on the arrested heart, the robot-assisted coronary bypass became compatible with off-pump surgery after the development of better stabilizers and robotic instruments. These procedures continue to be limited to patients with single vessel disease, generally involving the LAD or its diagonal branches. For patients with multivessel disease necessarily involving the lateral and posterior wall, hybrid revascularization procedures are one option and the multivessel small thoracotomy (MVST) operation is another.

The next leap to providing less traumatic multivessel surgery came about with the development of the endoscopic heart positioner (Medtronic Corp., Minneapolis, MN) This suction device allows safe closed-chest exposure of both lateral and inferior wall coronary artery sites with limited hemodynamic compromise. Through a 6-cm left minithoracotomy, bilateral ITA grafts with composite radial artery branches can be anastomosed to the LAD/diagonal, the obtuse circumflex marginal (OMB), and/or the posterior descending branches (PDA) coronary arteries. In the MVST operation the ITA is harvested using robotic assistance, and the distal coronary and the proximal T-graft anastomoses are performed under direct vision using conventional suturing techniques. Mechanical anastomotic devices may facilitate robotic coronary surgery; however, they remain a few years away. This chapter will relate mostly to robot-assisted coronary surgery on the beating heart. Arrested-heart techniques are similar, except for the added thoracic work space afforded by cardiopulmonary perfusion.

Robotic Technology

Robotic technology similar to that being used in coronary surgery is discussed in detail in Chapter 40. The da Vinci system is the only FDA-approved robotic device to perform these operations. Although surgeons have become dexterous, adaptive, and fast, they are also prone to geometric inaccuracy and fatigue. Robots are precise, untiring, and translate no tremor to distant operative target sites. A typical surgeon can perform an anastomosis with an accuracy of ± 0.1mm to 0.2 mm. When operating on a 1-mm target vessel in an arrested heart, this translates into an error margin of 10% to20% with every stitch in the anastomosis. In a beating heart these inaccuracies are amplified and become formidable. Here, target vessel motion can reach amplitudes of 1 mm, or the size of the vessel itself, even after stabilization. In addition, the eye loses the ability to track objects moving at frequencies of >90 Hz. Moreover, long endoscopic instruments transduce and amplify tremor and also plague surgeons with instrument collisions. To operate freely in a three-dimensional space, six degrees of hand-movement freedom are required. Typical long endoscopic instruments provide only four degrees of freedom. Therefore, a beating-heart closed-chest sewn coronary artery anastomosis becomes impossible when using standard endoscopic instruments. Comparatively, the da Vinci robotic system can provide an anastomotic accuracy of up to 0.005 mm because of the operative freedom combined with tremor filtration, motion scaling, and better ergonomic instrument control. Moreover, through a clutching mechanism, the surgeon can adjust his or/her hands to a more effective position with regard to the operative field and without moving the instrument tips.

Multivessel Small Thoracotomy Coronary Artery Bypass Grafting

ITA Anatomic Considerations

The ITA branches from the subclavian artery (Fig. 50-1) and descends along the anterior thorax (ventral), just lateral to the sternum, and deep (dorsal) to the costal cartilages, where it often is covered by the endothoracic fascia. Caudally slips of the transversus thoracic muscle may cover ITA arterial branches. At the level of the sixth intercostal space, the ITA divides into the superior epigastric and musculophrenic arteries. The former artery continues medially in the rectus abdominus muscle. The latter navigates the costal margin, branching into the lower anterior intercostal arteries, which supply part of the diaphragm. From the cardiac surgeon's standpoint, important branches include the pericardiophrenic artery and the anterior intercostal branches. The

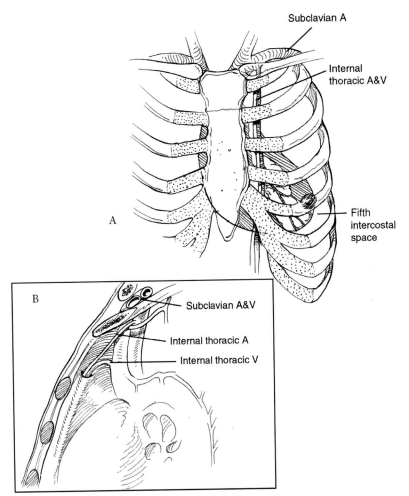

Figure 50-1. **(A)** The relationship of the internal thoracic artery and the internal thoracic vein to the sternum. **(B)** The anatomic relationship of the internal thoracic artery to the subclavian artery and vein and the internal thoracic vein. (A = artery; V = vein.)

pericardiophrenic artery accompanies the phrenic nerve and supplies the pleura, pericardium, and diaphragm. The anterior intercostal arteries run laterally to join the posterior intercostal arteries. Internal thoracic veins (ITVs) drain corresponding arterial tributaries. The anterior intercostal veins that run along the third to seventh intercostal spaces, flow into the ITVs and then drain into the brachiocephalic vein. The first two anterior intercostal veins drain directly into the brachiocephalic vein. The right ITV is larger than the left and deviates and is in close proximity to the phrenic nerve in the superior mediastinum.

Patient Selection

All patients with a target vessel diameter of 1.75 mm or greater may be considered for a computer-assisted MVST. Relative contraindications to using these methods include a prior left thoracotomy, severe left main coronary disease, ventricular arrhythmias, an intramyocardial LAD, small target vessels, diffuse coronary disease, cardio-

megaly, poor pulmonary function, significant obesity (body mass index >35 kg/m^2), an emergency operation, and reoperations. TECAB candidates should be selected along similar criteria.

To predict inability to tolerate single-lung ventilation, preoperative pulmonary testing should be done in patients with a history of severe pulmonary disease. Patients with carotid bruits and/or a history of stroke or transient ischemic attacks should have carotid ultrasound/Doppler examinations to rule out significant extracranial arterio-occlusive disease. Preoperative angiographic assessment of the ITA is helpful to document vessel size, especially if a T- or Y-graft side branch is being planned.

Conduit Options for Multivessel Revascularization

Single-vessel LAD or diagonal branch disease has been treated by the MIDCAB approach for several years in some institutions. Whether the ITA is harvested under direct

vision, using an endoscope, or with robotic assistance, an excellent conduit can be delivered. Depending on the surgeon's experience and patient's coronary anatomy, the following conduit options can be used either for MVST or TECAB operations:

1. Bilateral internal thoracic arteries:
   - Right ITA (RITA) to LAD
   - Left ITA (LITA) to circumflex marginal vessels (OM)
2. Bilateral internal thoracic arteries with a radial artery extension:
   - LITA to LAD
   - Radial artery composite extension on the in situ RITA to graft an OM or PDA
3. Bilateral internal thoracic arteries with a radial artery T- or Y-graft:
   - LITA to LAD and/or diagonal
   - Radial artery T/Y side graft from RITA to the OM or PDA branches
4. Bilateral internal thoracic arteries with a free RITA as a T- or Y-graft:
   - LITA to LAD and/or diagonal
   - Free RITA as a T- or Y-graft from LITA to OM and/or PDA

Operating Room Preparation

The left side should be elevated 30 degrees using a molded bean bag. Transcutaneous defibrillator patches are placed across the maximal ventricular mass, and an active body-warming system pad is placed on the back. The latter has avoided significant hypothermia in our OPCAB and MVST patients. If a radial artery is to be harvested, the nondominant arm is extended on an arm board. For both LITA and RITA harvesting, the da Vinci instrument cart is positioned on the right side of the patient. RITA grafts are harvested by crossing the anterior mediastinum and placing the robotic instruments in the right thorax. The typical setup for a right-hand-dominant person undergoing LITA-to-LAD bypass is shown in Fig. 50-2. The surgeon operates comfortably from the console on the left side while the table-side surgeon changes instruments tips that include an electrocautery, clip appliers, scissors, tissue graspers, and needle holders.

Anesthesia and Monitoring

A dual-lumen endotracheal tube is positioned to provide single-lung ventilation. Transesophageal echocardiography (TEE) is used to assess cardiac wall motion and ventricular filling continuously during cardiac manipulation. Hypotension usually can be managed by the combination of volume loading through the Trendelenburg position and with fluid boluses. Pharmacologic support is the second choice for blood pressure

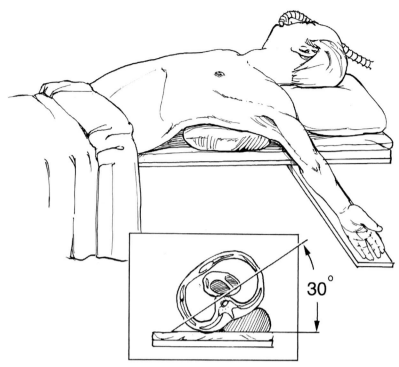

Figure 50-2. The patient is positioned for robotic coronary bypass surgery. The left arm is extended on an arm board with the left shoulder pushed posteriorly toward the table.

control, and low-dose norepinephrine and dopamine can be helpful. Short-acting narcotic anesthesia is used to enable early extubation. As is any off-pump operation, the anesthesiologist must be vigilant and react quickly to smooth out hemodynamic fluctuations. This eliminates distractions for the surgeon and provides an optimal operative field.

Internal Thoracic Arterial Harvest

The right lung should be deflated with the left ventilated independently. Robotic arm ports should be positioned in the third, fifth, and seventh intercostal spaces along the mid-axillary line (Fig. 50-3). Through these respective ports, the right instrument

arm, camera, and left instrument arm will be inserted. First, the 30-degree da Vinci camera is inserted through a 12-mm port placed in the fifth intercostal space and just lateral to the nipple. Thereafter, the left chest cavity is examined to identify anatomic landmarks for safe instrument-arm port insertion. To compress both the nonventilated and ventilated lung during bilateral ITA harvesting, carbon dioxide is insufflated into the left hemithorax continuously (10 to 12 torr).

First, the ITA should be visualized in the superior mediastinum. Next, the subclavian artery, phrenic nerve, and internal thoracic vein should be defined. The phrenic nerve is in closest proximity to the LITA at the subclavian artery, just as the latter exits the thoracic inlet. Multiple areas of encircling fat or muscle fibers may obscure the LITA pathway along the journey toward the diaphragm. Under endoscopic vision, the right robotic arm trocar then is placed in the third intercostal space. Similarly, the left instrument-arm trocar is placed through the seventh intercostal space. After completion of the ITA harvest, the camera port will become the lateral margin of the minithoracotomy. Instrument arms are introduced into the chest through the ports and always under endoscopic vision. The thoracic geometry greatly influences ITA robotic instrument access. A small anteroposterior chest dimension increases ITA harvest difficulty.

With tissue forceps in the left arm and the cautery in the right, costodiaphragmatic attachments are divided to increase work space between the sternum and cardiac apex (Fig. 50-4). When harvesting bilateral ITAs, retrosternal mediastinal tissues are dissected first and the pleura is opened along the RITA course. ITA dissection is begun opposite either the second or third rib, where it is seen most clearly. With the tip of the robotic cautery as a blunt dissector, the ITA is freed from the chest wall as a pedicle. Low-energy cautery settings have three benefits: (1) less smoke production, (2) less chance of ITA thermal injury, and (3) better coagulation of side branches before division. Dissection of the ITA begins laterally with pedicle dissection and continuing in a caudal (inferior) direction. The pedicle is deflected laterally as each interspace is freed of the artery, and all arterial branches either are cauterized or clipped. Minor venous bleeding can be controlled by manual compression. It is important not to exert excessive downward (dorsal) force on the ITA with robotic instruments. Intimal tears and avulsions can originate from a stressed arterial branch and result in an ITA dissection. The ITA pedicle

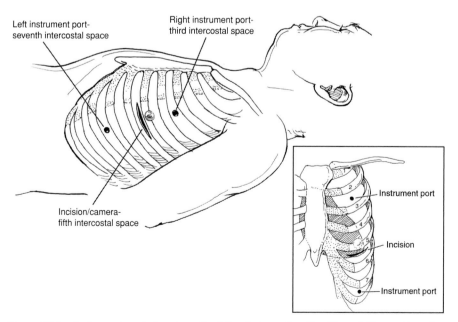

Figure 50-3. Instrument-port sites along the left anterior axillary line. The minithoracotomy is an extension of the camera-port site.

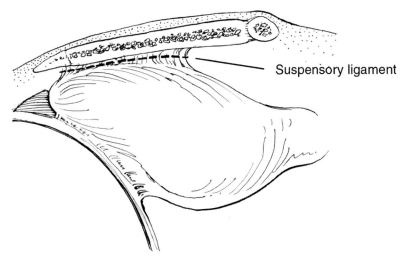

Figure 50-4. Pericardial suspensory ligaments attached to the retrosternal border. Lysis of these attachments "drops" the heart in a dorsal direction.

should be mobilized from the second to the seventh interspace.

During ITA dissection it is important to be gentle and employ what we call "visual tactility." One can gauge tissue tension using visual cues and determine when tearing is about to occur. The current robotic system provides no tactile feedback. When retracting straight structures, as in the early part of ITA dissection, there should be no sudden right-angle tension on the artery (Fig. 50-5). Subtle traction should change the course of the artery sufficiently. It is important to not "dig a hole" into an interspace, but to operate along a long linear segment of the pedicle. Often it is better to expose several branches over a long distance rather to control each branch as it appears. Only large branches, including the first intercostal or pericardiophrenic branches, usually require clipping. Only after entire LITA exposure is the medial endothoracic fascia divided, allowing the vascular pedicle to "drape" from the chest wall.

Target Vessel Exposure

With the chest remaining closed, the pericardium should be opened widely 4 cm to 5 cm anterior to the phrenic nerve. When opening with the cautery, the pericardium should be "tented" away from the left ventricle to avoid risk of injury and/or arrhythmias. For maximal LAD exposure, the distal pericardial incision is continued as a "T incision" inferiorly. After LAD and diagonal branches are identified, the target site can be marked with a clip. At this point robotic instruments are removed, chest wall bleeding is contained, and the 5-cm minithoracotomy is made. A soft-tissue retractor is

placed for initial exposure but followed by a low-profile chest wall retractor. After heparinization, the ITA is divided distally and flow adequacy determined.

Graft-Coronary Anastomosis

Radial artery segment T- or Y-grafts are constructed from each ITA using 7-0 polypropylene suture. A small incision in the fifth intercostal space provides the best LAD access. From here traction on the pericardial edge displaces the heart to expose the mid-LAD and diagonal branches. By retracting the posterolateral edge inferiorly, diagonal branches can be exposed. Right and OM coronary target exposure is gained using the heart positioner. The cardiac apex lies in the fifth intercostal space just medial to the left nipple. The endoscopic positioner consists of a suction cup on a long shaft. The suction cup provides vacuum grip on the cardiac apex. After this device is deployed, the shaft can be manipulated to rotate the cardiac apex in different directions (Fig. 50-6). It is inserted through a small subxiphoid incision made just to right of the lower sternum in the retrosternal space of the upper abdomen. By lifting the cardiac apex upward and displacing it toward the left shoulder, the right coronary artery and posterior descending branch can be exposed (Fig. 50-7). Positioning for right-sided coronary grafting still remains the most difficult. By rotating the apex downward and toward the right hip, the lateral wall with the OMB branches is exposed (Fig. 50-8).

When grafting circumflex and right coronary branches, a transthoracic stabilizer

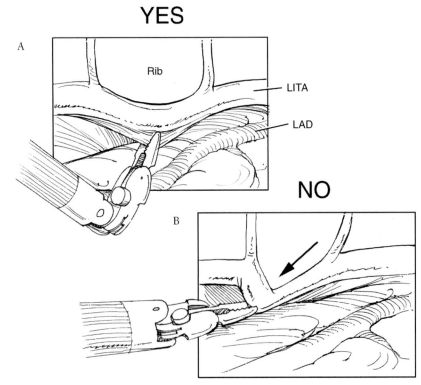

Figure 50-5. Internal thoracic arterial harvest is done by gentle deflection of the mid-artery away from the chest wall. If during the dissection the artery is pulled at acute angles, there is a greater risk of a branch tearing or an intimal dissection. (LAD = left anterior descending; LITA = left internal thoracic artery.)

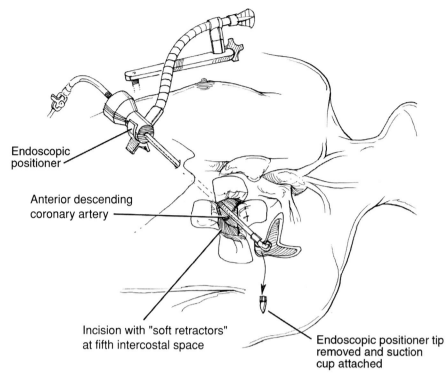

Endoscopic positioner

Anterior descending coronary artery

Incision with "soft retractors" at fifth intercostal space

Endoscopic positioner tip removed and suction cup attached

Figure 50-6. The endoscopic heart positioner is placed just under the xiphoid and passed through the minithoracotomy, where the suction tip is attached.

is passed through the chest wall via the left instrument port (Fig. 50-9). For LAD and diagonal vessel grafting a suction stabilizer may be placed directly through the incision. Just before making the arteriotomy, Silastic slings are used to occlude the proximal coronary artery. Generally, we do not oc-clude the distal artery but handle collateral blood flow using a CO_2 blower. The primary LITA-LAD anastomosis is done first. Continuous polypropylene sutures first are placed along the right side of the ITA. Generally, five stitches are completed before parachuting the right side of the ITA. Generally, five

stitches are completed before parachuting the ITA onto the LAD arteriotomy. Suturing is continued in a counterclockwise direction. Diagonal branches can be grafted using either a sequential side-to-side LITA or radial artery Y-graft technique. At this time we measure graft flow using the transit-time flow measurement.

On completion of all anastomoses, flow is measured in each graft and half-dose pro-tamine sulfate is administered. A large Blake drain is placed in the left pleural space through the left instrument port, and an-other is passed into the pericardial cavity via the subxiphoid port site. The minithoraco-tomy incision is closed in multiple layers, using braided polymer paracostal, fascial, subcutaneous, and subcuticular stitches. Closure of the right instrument port site should be done with a simple absorbable subcuticular suture.

The following operative tips should be helpful:

- The ITA dissection should be started on a rib where there are no branches and minimal risk of bleeding.
- The ITA pericardiophrenic branch lies very close to the phrenic nerve. In the event of bleeding, the artery should be clipped and not cauterized.
- The ITA may be covered the transver-sus thoracic muscle below the third inter-costal space. If confused with fibers from the diaphragm, premature ITA ligation or division can occur.
- Prior to making the minithoracotomy, port sites and the chest wall should be evalu-ated endoscopically for bleeding.
- The anterior ventricular wall should be revascularized first.
- When dissecting the distal ITA, the right instrument arm may conflict with the pa-tient's left shoulder. The assistant surgeon can push down on the left shoulder or lift up on the port to resolve this conflict.
- If the cautery does not reach the most distal ITA, instruments can be switched as the left arm reaches a few centimeters more distally.
- It is critical to confirm target vessel iden-tity before making the arteriotomy. Diag-onal branches can be mistaken easily for the LAD.

Postoperative Care

Patients can be extubated in the operating room, but most are extubated within 6 hours of surgery. The pulmonary artery catheter is removed soon after extubation, the time at which we transfer them to the step-down

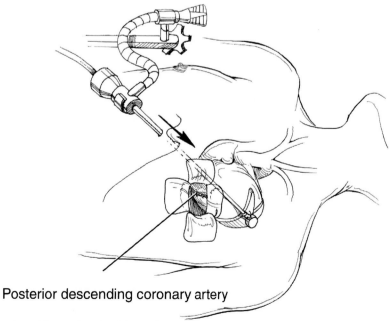

Posterior descending coronary artery

Figure 50-7. The suction tip of the endoscopic positioner has been deployed on the cardiac apex, and the heart is being positioned for grafting the posterior descending coronary artery.

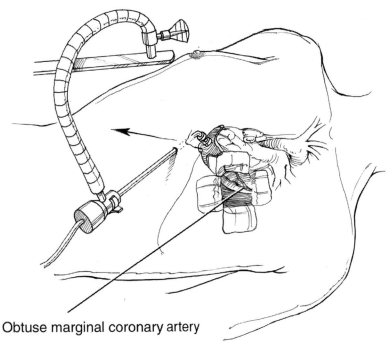

Obtuse marginal coronary artery

Figure 50-8. The endoscopic heart positioner is deflected toward the right and caudad to expose the obtuse circumflex coronary arteries.

unit. Blake drains are removed on the first postoperative day, and most patients are discharged after 2 to 3 postoperative days.

Beating Heart Totally Endoscopic Coronary Artery Bypass Grafting

The BH-TECAB operation (Fig. 50-10) is very similar to the MVST, except for the absence of a thoracotomy. The entire operation is done closed chest on a beating heart. Once LAD is exposed, an arteriotomy is made on the posterior surface of the ITA. The endoscopic stabilizer is introduced through a subxiphoid port and the LAD target site is immobilized. Self-locking Silastic occluders are applied to the proximal and distal LAD, and a 6-mm to 7-mm arteriotomy is made. The first two stitches are taken at the heel of the anastomosis, and then sutures

are placed along the LAD medial (back) wall. The ITA remains draped from the chest wall while these initial sutures are placed (Fig. 50-11). Subsequently, the ITA is divided, and the spatulated end is parachuted onto the LAD. The medial wall (away from the camera) is sutured first from inside out on the ITA and outside in on the LAD (Fig. 50-12A–D). On reaching the anastomotic "toe," the suture is tightened and locked before the lateral side is sewed (closer to camera), tying it at the heel (Fig. 12 E–G). Toe and heel sutures must be snugged tightly because "loose-stitch" bleeding on the anastomotic medial side is very difficult to control. Once hemostasis is confirmed, the stabilizer is released and withdrawn from the thorax. After stabilizing the diagonal artery and without disturbing the LAD anastomosis, a sequential ITA anastomosis can be constructed. A small chest tube or Blake drain is introduced through the left instrument-port site under endoscopic vision. Patency of the graft is verified by angiography 24 hours postoperatively. Intraoperative angiography via the radial artery has been described as a reliable technique for verifying postoperative ITA graft flow.

Robot-Assisted Coronary Surgery: Clinical Outcomes

Whereas the robot-assisted MIDCAB has been performed by many surgeons, the MVST is a recent development, made possible by the development of the endoscopic heart positioner. Whether it is done endoscopically or with the da Vinci system, outcomes uniformly have been successful with robot-assisted IMA harvesting. Vassiliades reported 66 consecutive Endo-ACAB patients with no mortality or reoperations and a 2.2-day mean stay. Three patients were converted to a sternotomy because of intramyocardial LADs and 1 because of inadequate ITA size. Of 46 patients who had angiograms 5.8 months (mean) after surgery, 97.8% (N = 45) had patent grafts. Fifteen other patients with positive preoperative nuclear or transthoracic Doppler scans converted to negative ones after surgery, rendering an effective ITA patency of 98.3%.

Hybrid operations that combine a robot-assisted ITA graft with a percutaneous coronary intervention have been encouraging. Stahl reported 54 patients with a robot-assisted LAD/diagonal MIDCAB combined with percutaneous interventions of additional vessels. Of 63 ITA grafts and 58

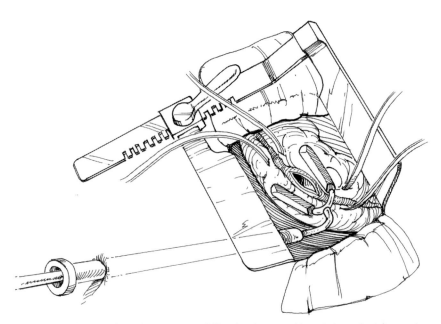

Figure 50-9. The transthoracic coronary stabilizer has been positioned along the left anterior descending margins and Silastic occluders have been deployed for a multivessel small thoracotomy procedure.

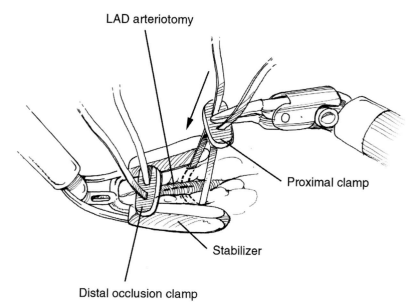

Figure 50-10. In a totally endoscopic coronary bypass operation (TECAB) Silastic occluders are locked using small plastic clips. This maneuver provides a bloodless field in the closed-chest operation. LAD = left anterior descending.

percutaneous transluminal coronary angioplasty (PTCA)/stent procedures, the event-free survival was 87.1% with 100% of ITA grafts patent. Recurrent symptoms in 10 patients led to follow-up angiography that identified 2 patients with in-stent restenoses and 1 with a stent occlusion.

Recently, Subramanian reported 30 MVST patients who were operated on using either an anterior thoracotomy ($n = 23$) or the transabdominal approach ($n = 7$). An average of 2.6 grafts were done, and the ITA was used in all patients. A RIMA was used in 21 patients and either a radial or gastroepiploic artery was used in 10 patients. The target vessels included the LAD/diagonal ($n = 37$), circumflex ($n = 32$), and RCA/PDA ($n = 12$) branches. There was no mortality, and 15 patients were discharged home within 24 hours. A composite OM radial

graft occluded in 1 patient, who required urgent reoperative vein grafting. In another patient an ITA-radial artery composite graft failed 6 months after the surgery, and the patient then had a successful native LAD PTCA.

An FDA-sponsored multicenter arrested heart TECAB trial was completed recently. Of the 75 patients enrolled, 8 were excluded intraoperatively. Two patients were converted to a sternotomy intraoperatively because of an ITA injury. Hybrid procedures were done in 11 patients. For the successful 65 TECAB patients mean cardiopulmonary bypass and cross-clamp times were 118 and 71 minutes, respectively. The mean hospital length of stay was 5.2 days. Of the 58 patients catheterized 3 months later, 52 (90%) patients had patent grafts, and 6 (10%) had an anastomotic stenosis of >50%. Four of the latter patients underwent a percutaneous reintervention. There were no operative mortality or strokes, but there was one perioperative myocardial infarction. Freedom from adverse events was 90% at 3 months after surgery. Anastomotic times fell markedly with experience and approximated 20 minutes near the end of the study. This study showed that single-vessel LAD grafting could be done robotically on an arrested heart in a completely closed chest.

In comparison, BH-TECAB has only been done in a few academic centers worldwide. Recently Wimmer-Greinecker reported 28 patients undergoing a BH-TECAB. In all patients a single-vessel ITA-to-LAD bypass was performed with mean operative and ischemic times of 208 and 24 minutes, respectively. Of these, 6 patients required conversion either to a MIDCAB or sternotomy either because of bleeding, poor-quality target vessel, or ITA injury. Significant postoperative complications included one re-exploration for bleeding, two reoperations for graft stenosis, and one for grafting a diagonal branch mistakenly. These data suggest clearly that this procedure is in the early stages of development, and considerable improvements in technique and adjunctive technologies are required for widespread expansion of the BH-TECAB.

Future Directions

Despite the introduction into cardiac surgery of safe robotic telemanipulation technology, early clinical experience has defined and continues to elucidate the limitations. Understanding current limitations as well as patient demands will drive future

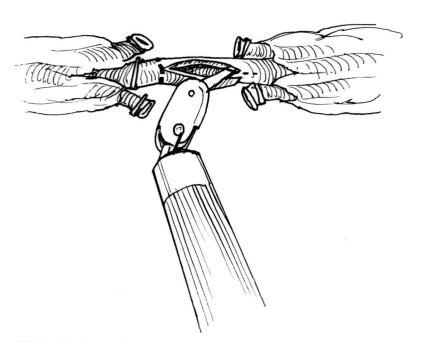

Figure 50-11. The internal thoracic artery graft is left in situ, after freeing it from the chest wall, and is being prepared for grafting the left anterior descending.

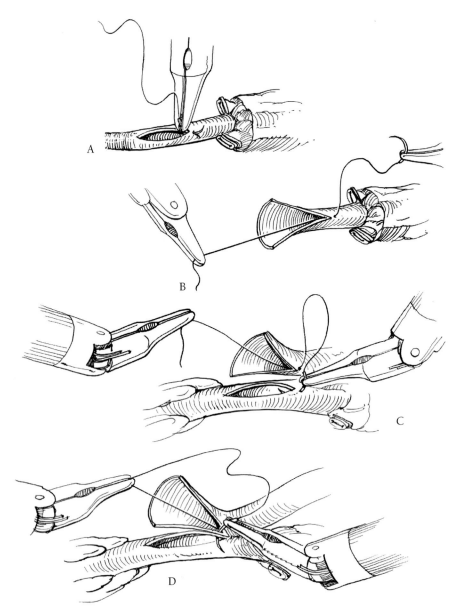

Figure 50-12. **(A–D)** Sutures are placed robotically first through the heel of both the internal thoracic artery (ITA) graft and left anterior descending coronary. Subsequently, the ITA is divided and lowered to the anastomotic plane, and the suture line is carried along the distal (back) wall, away from the camera, toward the toe of the anastomosis. The left robotic instrument is used to maintain suture tension and a tight approximation. **(E–G)** The suture is carried around to toe of the anastomosis and continued along the medial (camera) side to be tied at the heel. *(continued)*

technological developments. Assessment of tissue integrity and composition by robotic means remains a problem, and this alone blunts many surgeons' interest in robotic surgery. However, tactile feedback is being addressed in some robotic surgical systems, and instrument-tip strain sensors eventually may allow a more controlled application of operative force. Smaller (5-mm) arms now are in production and should provide more operative work space by avoiding collisions. Similar reductions in the size of three-

dimensional cameras present a much greater engineering challenge. To achieve this goal, optical (endoscopic) transmission of analog light to a large extracorporeal sensor will have to be replaced by intrathoracic three-dimensional microchips.

For both the MVST and BH-TECAB, design improvements in endoscopic stabilizers and positioners would facilitate robotic coronary surgery. Current positioners are very bulky and cannot be conformed for optimal cardiac presentation. Endoscopic sta-

bilizers are still positioned and controlled manually by the patient side surgeon. A robot-controlled endostabilizer could improve stabilization of target sites in difficult geometric regions. Smaller stabilizers would help surgeons to minimize the size of the incision and avoid collisions with ribs above and below the thorax entrance site. Additional robotic arms will facilitate robot-assisted coronary surgery. One instrument can hold the ITA while the other two perform the anastomosis. Distal anastomotic connectors have the potential also of facilitating a robotic coronary anastomosis. Nevertheless, the development of coronary connectors has lagged far behind advances in surgical robotics, and connector technology appears to be at least 5 years from significant clinical application. Arterial–arterial graft connectors will present the greatest challenge. In Europe magnetic vascular couplers for the distal anastomosis have been used successfully in BH-TECABs.

As an alternative to using clip appliers during IMA preparation, micro-bipolar cautery tips are being developed. An ultrasonic robotic cautery is needed to facilitate safe, bloodless ITA harvest; however, any instrument articulation prevents focused sound delivery to the tip. Endoscopic ultrasonic probes would be helpful for identifying target vessels, especially when they are covered by epicardial fat or are intramyocardial. Moreover, intrathoracic graft flow analysis would be possible. Because tangential vision of target vessels can be misleading, mapping systems would be ideal for confirming the appropriate vessel to be grafted. For preoperative planning, multidetector computed tomographic scanning may be used to confirm the position of the coronary target. Steerable or alternative-viewing-angle scopes also might optimize target vessel visualization during closed-chest beating-heart surgery.

As with any new procedure, there is a significant learning curve with robot-assisted coronary bypass. However, once ITA harvesting is mastered, the different approaches to performing the distal anastomosis are relatively safe and easy to learn. Constructing the distal anastomosis with the robot on a beating heart is still difficult and limited to a few academic institutions. However, with the ongoing research in robot science as well as development of adjunctive technologies, the future of robot-assisted coronary bypass surgery holds promise for cardiac surgeons and their patients.

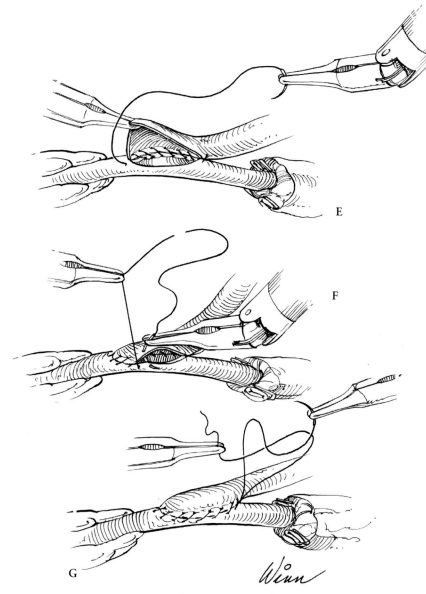

Figure 50-12. *(Continued)*

SUGGESTED READING

Acuff TE, Landreneau RJ, Griffith BP, et al. Minimally invasive coronary artery bypass grafting; a new method using an anterior mediastinotomy. Ann Thorac Surg 1996;61:135.

Angelini GD, Wilde P, Salerno TA, et al. Integrated left small thoracotomy and angioplasty for multivessel coronary artery revascularization. Lancet 1996;347:747.

Benetti FJ, Ballester C. Use of thoracoscopy and a minimal thoracotomy, in mammary-coronary bypass to left anterior descending artery, without extracorporeal circulation: Experience in 2 cases. J Cardiovasc Surg 1995;36:529.

Boyd WE, Rayman R, Desai ND, et al. Closed-chest coronary artery bypass grafting with the use of a computer-enhanced surgical robotic system. J Thorac Cardiovasc Surg 2000;120:807.

Calafiore AM, DiGiammarco G, Teodori G, et al. Left anterior descending coronary artery grafting via left anterior small thoracotomy without cardiopulmonary bypass. Ann Thorac Surg 1996;61:648.

Carpentier A, Loulmet D, Aupecle B, et al. Computer-assisted cardiac surgery. Lancet 1999;353:379.

Damiano RJ, Ehrman WJ, Ducko CT, et al. Initial United States clinical trial of robotically assisted endoscopic coronary artery bypass grafting. J Thorac Cardiovasc Surg 2000;119:77.

Detter C, Boehm DH, Reichenspurner H, et al. Robotically assisted coronary artery surgery with and without cardiopulmonary bypass—From first clinical use to endoscopic operation. Med Sci Monit 2002;8:MT118.

Dogan S, Aybek T, Andressen E, et al. Totally endoscopic coronary artery bypass grafting on cardiopulmonary bypass with robotically enhanced tele-manipulation: A report of forty-five cases. J Thorac Cardiovasc Surg 2002;123:1125.

Elbeery JR, Brown PM, Chitwood WR Jr. Intraoperative MIDCABG arteriography via the left radial artery: A comparison with Doppler ultrasound for assessment of graft patency. Ann Thorac Surg 1998;66:51.

Falk V. Manual control and tracking—A human factor analysis relevant for beating heart surgery. Ann Thorac Surg 2002;74:624.

Gundry SR, Romano MA, Shattuck OH, et al. Seven year followup of coronary artery bypasses performed with and without cardiopulmonary bypass. J Thorac Cardiovasc Surg 1998;115:1273.

Herzog C, Dogan S, Diebold T, et al. Multidetector row CT versus coronary angiography: Preoperative evaluation before totally endoscopic coronary artery bypass grafting. Radiology 2003;229:200.

Jansen EW, Borst C, Lahpor JR, et al. Coronary artery bypass grafting without cardiopulmonary bypass using the octopus method: Results in the first one hundred patients. J Thorac Cardiovasc Surg 1998;116:60.

Kappert U, Cichon R, Schneider J, et al. Closed chest bilateral mammary artery grafting in double-vessel coronary artery disease. Ann Thorac Surg 2000;70:1699.

Kappert U, Schneider J, Cichon R, et al. Development of robotic enhanced endoscopic surgery for treatment of coronary artery disease. Circulation 2001;104(Suppl I):I102.

Klima U, Falk V, Maringka M, et al. Magnetic vascular coupling for distal anastomosis in coronary artery bypass grafting: A multicenter trial. J Thorac Cardiovasc Surg 2003;126:1568.

Koransky ML, Tavana ML, Yamaguchi A, et al. Quantification of mechanical stabilization for the performance of off-pump coronary artery surgery. Heart Surg Forum 2003;6:224.

Loulmet D, Carpentier A, d'Attellis N, et al. Endoscopic coronary artery bypass grafting with the aid of robotic assisted instruments. J Thorac Cardiovasc Surg 1999;118:4.

Mohr FW, Falk V, Diegeler A, et al. Computer-enhanced robotic cardiac surgery-experience in 148 patients. J Thorac Cardiovasc Surg 2001;121:842.

Newman R. A systematic approach to minimally invasive coronary artery bypass surgery. Presented at the STS/AATS Tech-Con 2004, January 24–25, 2004, San Antonio, TX.

Stahl KD, Boyd WD, Vassiliades TA, et al. Hybrid robotic coronary artery surgery and angioplasty in multivessel coronary artery disease. Ann Thorac Surg 2002;74:S1358.

Subramanian VA, Patel NU, Patel NC, et al. Robotic assisted multivessel MidCAB with port-access stabilization and cardiac positioning: Paving the way for outpatient CABG? Presented at the 40th Annual Meeting of the Society of Thoracic Surgeons, January 26–28, 2004, San Antonio, TX.

Taylor RH, Jenson M, Whitcomb L, et al. A steady-hand robotic system for microsurgical augmentation. Int J Robotics Res 1999;12: 1201.

Vassiliades TA, Rogers EW, Nielsen JL, et al. Minimally invasive direct coronary artery bypass grafting: Intermediate-term results. Ann Thorac Surg 2000;70:1063.

Wimmer-Greinecker G, Aybek T, Mierdl S, et al. Totally endoscopic robotic-assisted coronary artery surgery. Presented at the STS/AATS Tech-Con 2004, January 24–25, 2004, San Antonio, TX.

EDITOR'S COMMENTS

I included this chapter because I believe robotic coronary surgery is in its infancy but needs to be discussed. I really don't know how frequently this modality will be used in the future, but I felt there was no one better to discuss this than Dr. Chitwood and his group. This type of surgery is possible. The robot has most frequently been used to take down internal mammaries in order to limit the incision. Anastomoses with the robot have been difficult but the technology is evolving. There is also the potential of using these with hybrid procedures in that some vessels may end up being stented and then an internal mammary artery to the LAD bypass done. It is too soon to tell how important this will be in the individual surgeon's armamentarium.

I.L.K.

D

Surgery for Heart Failure

51

Left Ventricular Reconstruction

Constantine L. Athanasuleas and Gerald D. Buckberg

Introduction

Ventricular remodeling is a natural process after infarction as the remote, noninfarcted muscle undergoes changes in shape and volume. Excessive ventricular dilation may impair systolic and diastolic function and cause congestive heart failure. The prognosis of patients with ischemic cardiomyopathy is closely related to ventricular volume.

Early reperfusion of the occluded coronary artery limits dilation in the majority of patients, yet still occurs in about 20%. The epicardial layer often remains viable because the wave of necrosis, which progresses from endocardium to epicardium, is halted. This results in akinesia of the infarcted ventricular segment rather than dyskinesia, which is encountered with transmural necrosis. Excision or plication of a dyskinetic ventricular segment is a well-established operation, but few surgeons approach an akinetic segment, probably because of the retained viable epicardial surface.

Surgical ventricular restoration (SVR) returns ventricular shape and volume toward normalcy. The operation excludes the infarcted segments usually by placement of an endocardial patch (Fig. 51-1).

Preoperative Evaluation

Candidates for operation typically have a history of remote infarction months to years before operation and symptoms of advanced congestive heart failure (New York Heart Association class III or IV). Electrocardiography confirms prior infarction in all cases. Such patients may or may not have angina, but because coronary artery disease is the major causative factor, coronary angiogra-phy is essential. Evaluation of left ventricular size and function is crucial in assessing operability and determining adjunctive procedures. This is done with echocardiography, ventriculography, or magnetic resonance imaging (MRI). Each method has advantages and limitations.

Echocardiography is readily available. It can be used to confirm ventricular enlargement by measurement of the short axis and to calculate ejection fraction. Volume determination, however, is less reliable by this method. The extent of regional asynergy of the infarcted segment can be visualized, as can the wall motion and thickness of the remote noninfarcted segments. An asynergic (noncontracting region with either akinesia or dyskinesia) area of $\geq 35\%$ warrants intervention. Normal motion of the lateral and inferior walls in the case of anterior ventricular restoration is an encouraging finding.

Ventriculography in the right anterior oblique (RAO) view confirms asynergy of the anterior and apical segments but does not reveal septal or lateral wall motion that must compensate for the noncontractile region. These are best viewed in the left anterior oblique (LAO) view. Ejection fraction can be easily calculated and ventricular volumes measured in systole and diastole. If only an RAO view is available, volume will generally be underestimated, but will at least confirm significant enlargement. Left ventricular end-systolic volume index (LVESVI) of ≥ 60 mL/m^{2}is our threshold for surgical restoration.

If there is akinesia or severe hypokinesia of the remote no-infarcted segments, then myocardial viability tests are needed to determine the degree of reversible ischemia. Although thallium may be useful, MRI with delayed gadolinium enhancement is very predictive of viability and return of function in hypokinetic areas after coronary revascularization (Fig. 51-2). MRI images allow determination of regional wall thickening and calculation of ejection fraction. MRI is also the best method of measuring ventricular volume.

The preoperative workup is not complete without assessment of mitral valve function. Late failure of ventricular restoration is linked to untreated mitral regurgitation at the initial operation. Global left ventricular enlargement can cause mitral regurgitation that occurs at rest or with exertion. The associated anatomic changes include annular dilation, decreased leaflet coaptation, and widening of the papillary muscle insertion sites due to scar. The mitral valve function should be determined preoperatively by history, physical examination, and echocardiography. We recommend mitral repair if there is 2 to 4+ mitral regurgitation or if the mitral annulus exceeds 35 mm in diameter even in the absence of mitral regurgitation. In such cases there is usually limited leaflet coaptation, which may be functionally significant. The vast majority of mitral interventions in the RESTORE registry were repairs. Replacement was required in <1% of patients. Scarring of the lateral and/or inferior segments from prior infarctions was the usual reason for replacement. In such cases, because of limited long-term survival, a bioprosthetic valve is recommended.

Operative Technique

Transesophageal echocardiography is employed in all cases to assess regional wall movement and mitral valve function. After sternotomy, the aorta is cannulated, as are both vena cavae if mitral valve intervention is anticipated. A left ventricular vent is

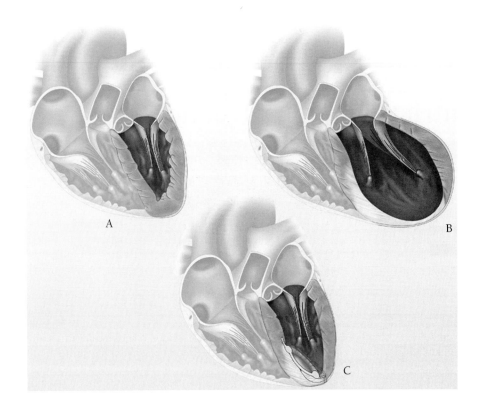

Figure 51-1. **(A)** The normal heart. **(B)** Ventricular dilation secondary to anteroseptal infarction. **(C)** Ventricular restoration with intracardiac patch.

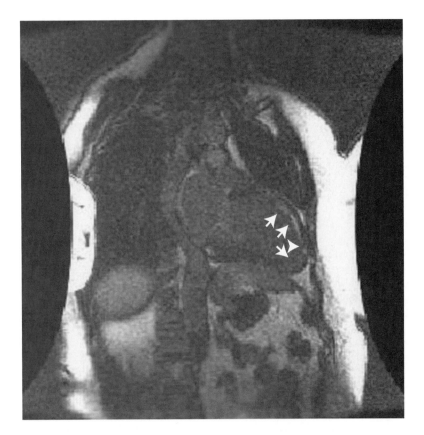

Figure 51-2. Magnetic resonance imagining with delayed gadolinium enhancement, demonstrating area of thinning and necrosis.

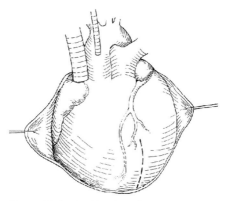

Figure 51-3. Incision into the anterior ventricular scar.

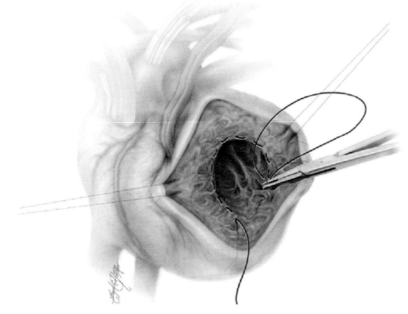

Figure 51-5. Placement of an encircling Fontan suture, which isolates the noncontracting segment.

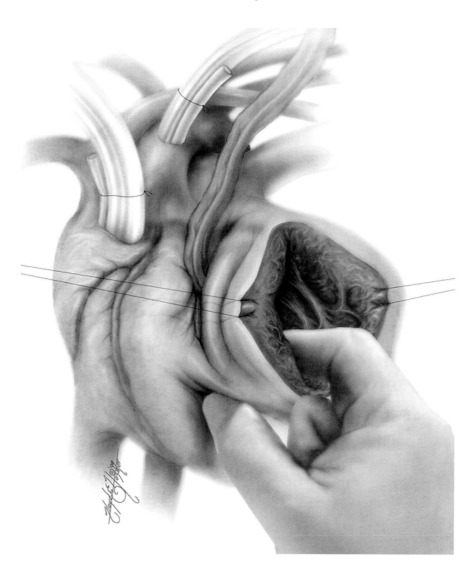

Figure 51-4. Palpation defines the boundary between contracting and noncontracting segments.

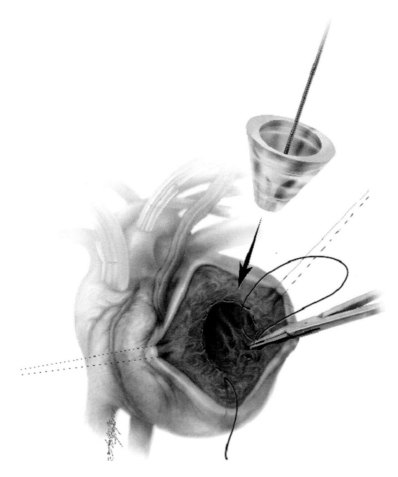

Figure 51-6. Placement of a device to determine patch size.

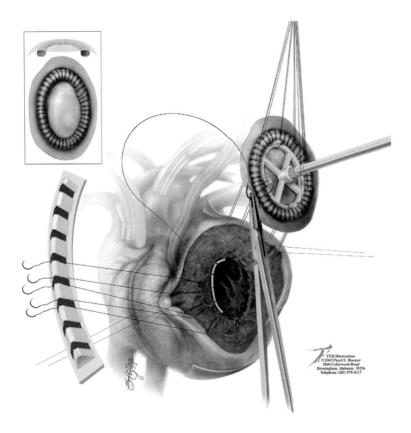

Figure 51-7. Placement of sutures around the oval opening and through the patch.

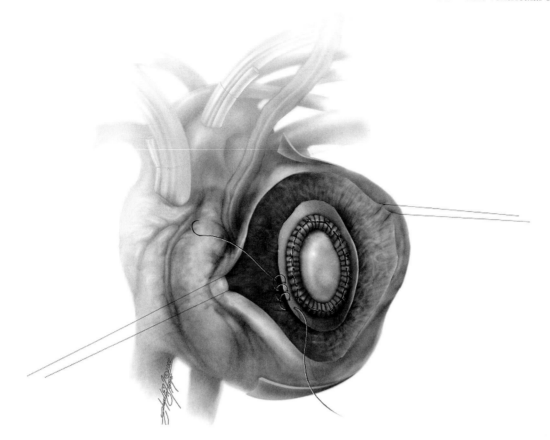

Figure 51-8.   A rim suture secures hemostasis.

inserted via the right superior pulmonary vein while the heart is still beating. Cardiopulmonary commences with core cooling to 34°C. Coronary bypass is performed in the arrested heart after aortic cross-clamping and administration of antegrade and retrograde cold blood cardioplegia. Induction warm cardioplegia is utilized if there is ongoing ischemia or unstable preoperative hemodynamics. The details of cardioplegia content and administration by the "integrated myocardial management" method have been widely tested and described elsewhere.

The mitral valve is approached after coronary revascularization in the cardioplegia-arrested heart. We prefer to the repair the mitral valve through an atrial septal incision.

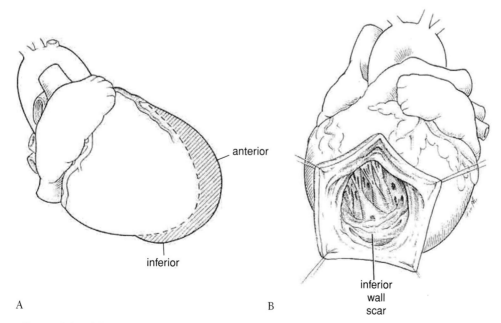

anterior

inferior

A   B

inferior
wall
scar

Figure 51-9.   **(A)** Distal inferior wall scar from "wraparound" left anterior descending infarction. **(B)** Interior view of inferior wall scar.

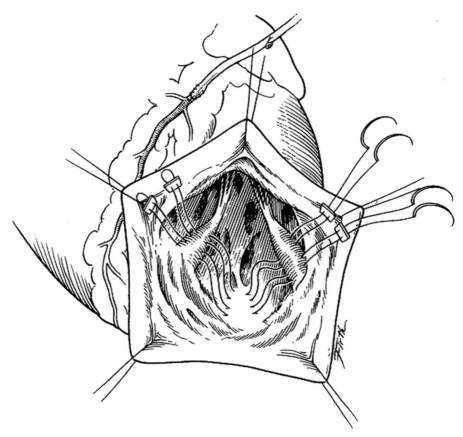

Figure 51-10.   Narrowing the widened inferior wall scar by bringing the papillary heads together.

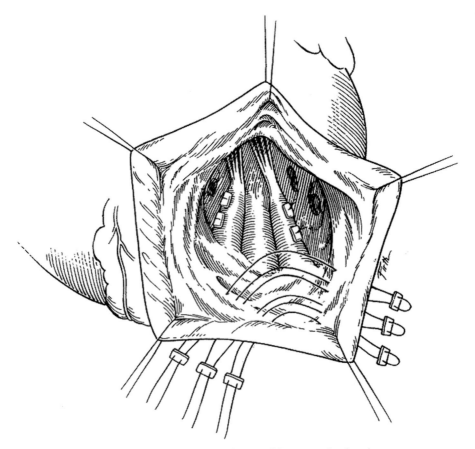

Figure 51-11.   Imbrication of the inferior wall by externally placed sutures.

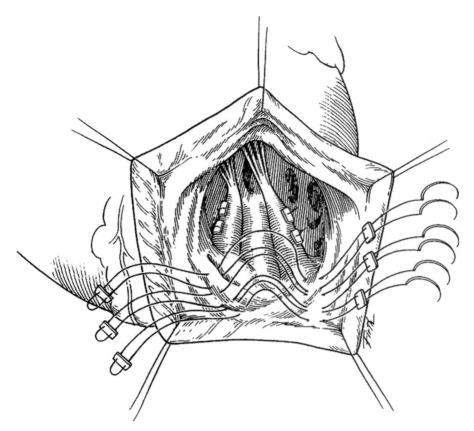

Figure 51-12. Imbrication of the inferior wall by internally placed sutures.

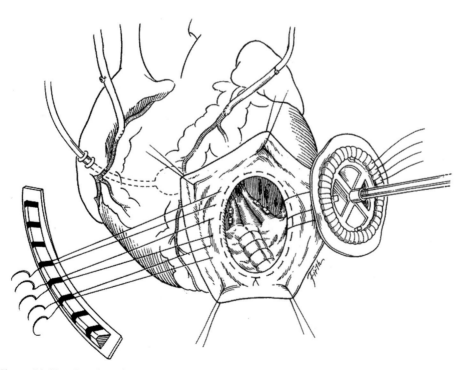

Figure 51-13. Creation of a conical ventricular chamber by placing an oblique Fontan suture at the newly created apex, and placement of an oval patch that is anchored high on the septum.

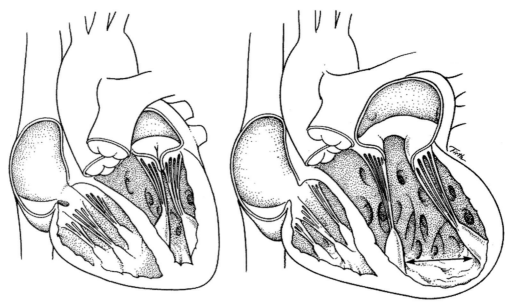

Figure 51-14. **(Left)** Normal chamber. **(Right)** Dilated chamber with displacement of the papillary insertions.

Global left ventricular enlargement secondary to anterior infarction usually causes central regurgitation. The mitral leaflet morphology is normal. In such cases a ring annuloplasty is performed with downsizing of the annulus to 28 mm to 30 mm. A complete ring is recommended because the anterior intratrigonal distance is usually increased by the annular dilatation.

After coronary bypass and mitral valve intervention, the aortic cross-clamp is removed and the heart resumes contraction. This form of myocardial protection is termed the "open-beating" method of myocardial protection and has been found to be advantageous in patients with ischemic cardiomyopathy. Mean arterial pressure is maintained at ≥80 mm Hg because of the empirical

observation that contractility is optimum at these pressures. Suction is applied to the ventricular vent, and we observe for dimpling of the anterior ventricle. This occurs when there is thinning of the dyskinetic or akinetic ventricle. Its absence, however, does not change the decision to open the ventricle. In spite of a normal epicardial surface, the *preoperative* functional assessment

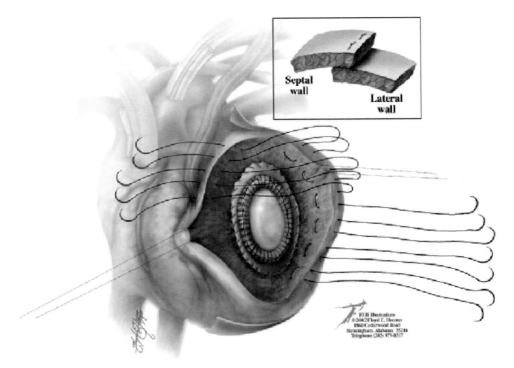

Figure 51-15.   Sliding of the lateral segment beneath the medial segment.

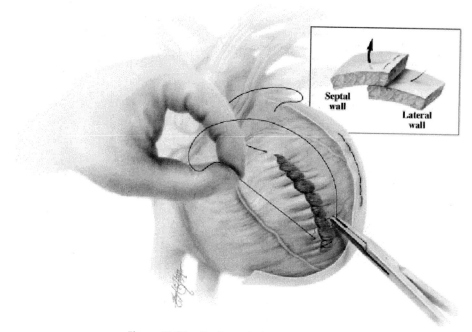

Figure 51-16. Final ventricular running suture.

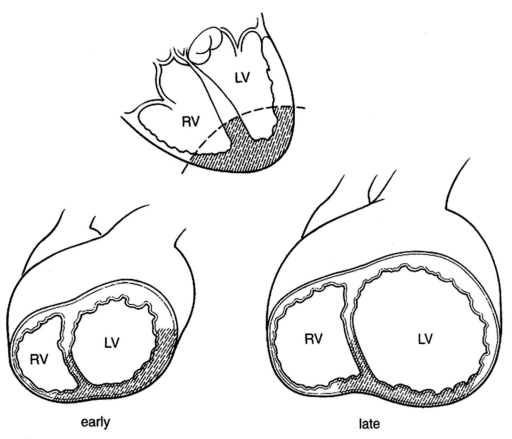

Figure 51-17. Area of damage with inferior infarction (*hatched*) in longitudinal and saggital views. Note **(bottom right)** the enlargement of remote muscle. (LV = left ventricle; RV = right ventricle.)

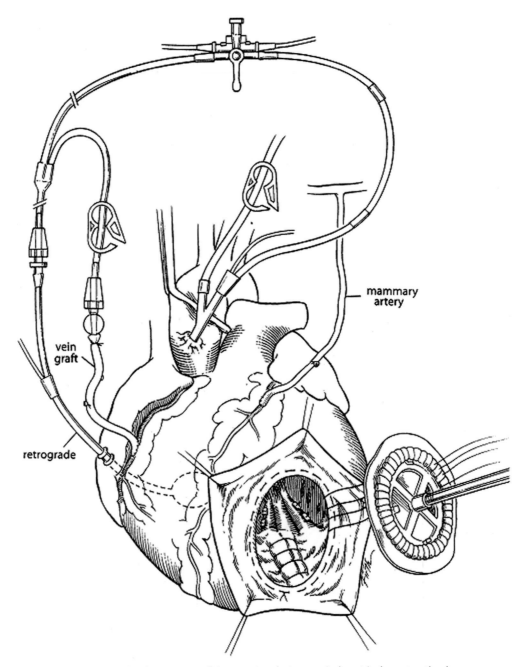

mammary
artery

vein
graft

retrograde

Figure 51-18. Beating-heart myocardial protection during surgical ventricular restoration in a patient with aortic insufficiency. Note the clamped aorta, with perfusion via the internal mammary artery, vein grafts, and retrograde via the coronary sinus. This method is used with either anterior or inferior repairs.

of the ventricle determines the need for restoration.

The beating method is preferred over the cardioplegic technique, and this is especially important in patients whose regional segment is akinetic and there is thick-walled heart. On ventriculotomy, the scar may be trabecular or absent in the early postinfarction phase. Consequently, it is impossible to make visual identification of the damaged area and its point of connection to non-

scarred muscle. Conversely, this distinction is made easily by palpation.

Anterior Ventricular Restoration

An incision is made anteriorly approximately 2.5 cm to 3.0 cm lateral to the left anterior descending artery (Fig. 51-3). Stay sutures hold the muscle apart. Palpation is a

very effective and easy method of determining the extent of myocardial necrosis. The muscle is grasped between the thumb and forefinger. Contraction is defined as thickening and can readily be appreciated (Fig. 51-4). A monofilament suture of 2-0 polypropylene is passed through the endocardium of the left ventricle at the junction of contracting and noncontracting segments. This so called "Fontan suture" is then tightened to form an oval opening or ledge

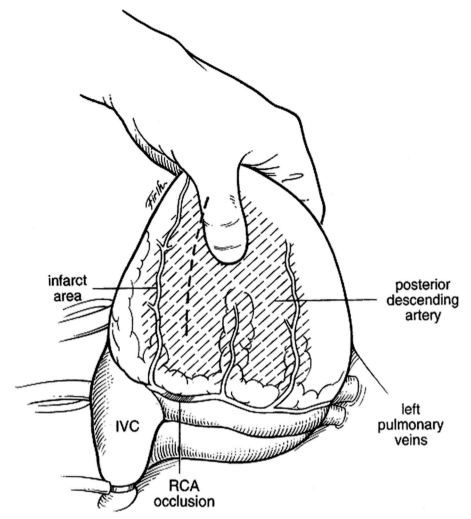

Figure 51-19. Elevated apex, with marking of damaged region (*hatching*) and region of incision, 2 cm to 3 cm from the posterior descending artery. (IVC = inferior vena cava; RCA = right coronary artery.)

onto which a patch can be secured (Figs. 51-5 and 51-6).

The septal endocardium, if sufficiently scarred, can be dissected and thus peeled away and used as a septal patch. Alternatively, a Dacron or bovine pericardial patch can be used to cover this opening. We prefer the latter and have employed a patch with modifications of the sewing ring to secure homeostasis when placed against a trabeculated surface. Interrupted pledgeted braided 2-0 sutures are first placed on the septal side (Fig. 51-7). Then a strip of bovine pericardium is placed on the lateral ventricular surface, and mattressed sutures are placed through the lateral ventricle from epicardium to endocardium. Sutures are placed in holders as they are during valve procedures. The patch is brought onto the field and the

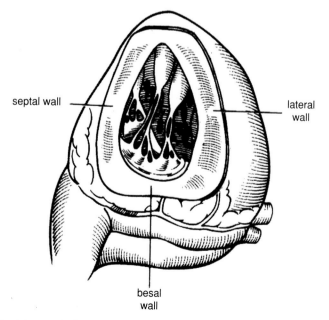

Figure 51-20. Intraventricular exposure, with identification of the areas to be excluded, which include the septum, base, adjacent to the mitral ring, and the lateral, wall.

sutures evenly spaced through the sewing ring. The patch is lowered into place, and the sutures are tied and cut. Before securing the last sewing ring suture, the lungs are insufflated and the ventricular vent discontinued to permit filling of the ventricle. The patient is placed in Trendelenburg position to prevent any expulsion of air into the systemic circulation. The rim of patch outside the sewing ring is then sewn to the endocardium with a running 3-0 polypropylene suture to prevent leakage (Fig. 51-8). At this point the ventricle is full and beating and hemostasis can be checked and corrected.

An important aspect of initial suture placement is recognition of the future alignment of the patch. To achieve a final elliptical shape, the Fontan suture should be placed high onto the septum. This creates an oblique orientation of the patch with respect to the mitral valve annulus. Failure to achieve this places the patch parallel to the mitral annulus and creates a more spherical than elliptical ventricle.

A modification of the standard technique is needed when the anterior scar extends beyond the apex to involve the distal inferior wall. This segment may be scarred because the infarction involved a long left anterior descending artery that wraps around the apex (Fig. 51-9). With wraparound anterior infarctions, displacement of the bases of the papillary muscles are usually posteriorly and cephalad. Figure 51-10 shows that coaptation from within the ventricle will narrow the widening between papillary muscle bases. An elliptical ventricle is created by imbricating the inferior wall by placing sutures either from within the ventricle, or from outside the ventricle to its interior (Figs. 51-11 to 51-13). This imbrication suture also narrows the widened papillary muscle insertion sites and is an integral part of mitral valve repair because it increases leaflet coaptation (Fig. 51-14).

Closure of the residual excluded scar is done in layers. The first layer is a series of mattressed sutures placed from the edge of the lateral ventricle from inside to outside.

These sutures are then brought through the septal side from inside to outside, thereby sliding the lateral wall under the septal segment (Fig. 51-15). This "vest over pants"-type closure eliminates any dead space distal to the patch. Finally, a running polypropylene suture is used to complete hemostasis (Fig. 51-16).

In the absence of left-bundle-branch block, the akinetic septum above the scared region resumes normal contraction after restoration. Use of the "integrated method" of myocardial protection normally assures recovery of septal function, a critical factor in right ventricular recovery. We have found temporary biventricular synchronous pacing useful in patients with preoperative left-bundle-branch block because the septum is usually dyskinetic from this excitation contraction dyssyncrony, which causes mitral insufficiency from early systolic bulging. Biventricular pacing places the distended septum in mid line position, and thus limits functional mitral insufficiency.

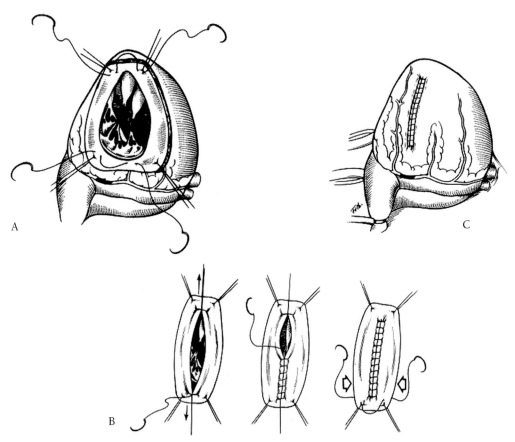

Figure 51-21. **(A)** Placement of the initial basal and apical sutures with direct closure. Note the site of basal suture placement, approximately 1.5 cm from the annulus of the mitral valve, and into an adjacent septal muscle, intended to make a V shape at the apex. **(B)** Closure of the apical and basal sutures **(left)** to create a V shape at both ends. Traction helps in the closure line as the closure is started, **(center)** and is completed **(right)**. **(C)** Closed ventricle.

The surgical method involves using a temporary epicardial lead placed high on the lateral wall close to the atrioventricular groove in the region of the obtuse marginal artery. Transesophageal echocardiography confirms improved contractility with the use of this method. In many patients, a permanent lead can be also placed and routed into a subcutaneous pocket under the left clavicle for subsequent placement of a biventricular pacemaker.

Inferior Ventricular Restoration

Restoration of the inferior ventricle follows the same general principles. Here the infarction process has usually involved the circumflex and posterior descending arteries. The basal, free wall, and septal anatomy components of inferior lesions are shown in Fig. 51-17. Mitral regurgitation is present in the majority of these cases because the base of the heart is dilated to widen the mitral annulus, and the papillary muscles may become scarred. Because repair is less proven in this situation, we would prefer replacement of the mitral valve with a bioprosthesis.

Exposure of the inferior scarred segment is generally more difficult in the beating heart, but the use of apical suction devices, as used in off-pump coronary bypass, has made this easier. Normally, we use bicaval cannulation when inferior lesions are corrected because elevation of the ventricle can impede venous return, and this distortion may also produce aortic insufficiency. We normally use the beating technique but make some changes. If aortic regurgitation is anticipated, the aortic clamp is left in place; proximal grafts are perfused, rather than connected to the aorta, the internal mammary artery graft is opened, and retrograde normal blood perfusion is delivered to the beating heart during repair, in the same manner as used for anterior scar, as shown in Fig. 51-18.

For inferior lesions, the incision (Fig. 51-19) is made lateral to the posterior descending artery directly into scarred tissue.

It is carried to within 1 cm of the mitral annulus and distally to the apex (Fig. 51-20). The incision is kept on the septal side of the papillary muscle to avoid cutting the base of the papillary muscle attachment to the mitral valve. The mitral valve may be is replaced through this incision.

The operation excludes noncontracting segments including a portion of the septum. Restoration can be done either by direct closure in large scarred defects that collapse during ventricular venting, as shown in Fig. 51-21, or with use of the patch. With inferior lesions, the patch shape should be triangular, as Dor has described. We use Teflon backed by bovine pericardium. Because the defect requiring closure is triangular, the patch is fashioned into a triangle as well. We narrow the triangular cardiac defect by "re-triangulation," which is accomplished by placement of a series of imbricating sutures along the edge of the scar, as shown in Fig. 51-22. When they are tightened, the ventricular chamber size is reduced. The new patch conforms to the size of this opening, as defined in Fig. 51-23. The residual ventricle is

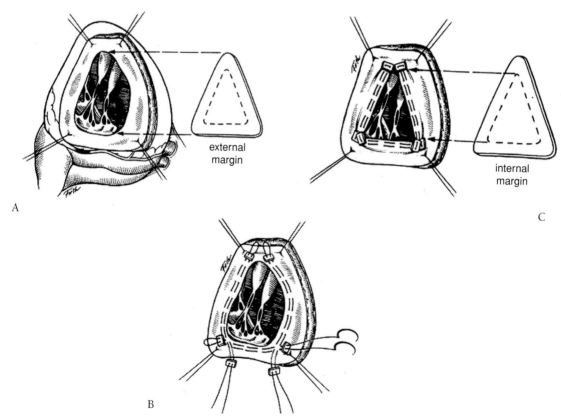

Figure 51-22. **(A)** The open ventricle defines the areas of basal, septal, and lateral wall exposure, showing a triangular defect. The patch is placed adjacent to the ventriculotomy site, with an external surface that closely matches the open ventricular area. **(B)** The Prolene imbrication sutures are placed into the triangular borders. **(C)** The sutures are secured to reduce the size and match the internal triangle of the patch.

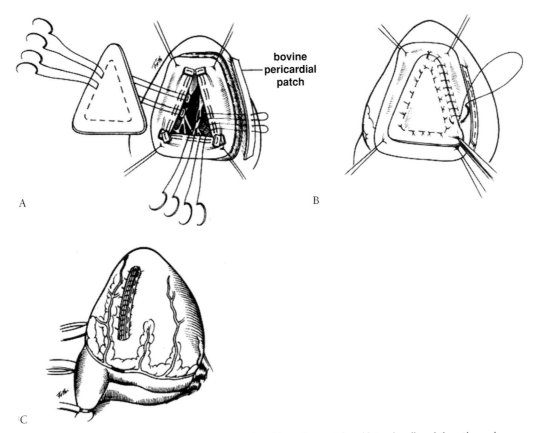

Figure 51-23.   **(A)** The mattress sutures are placed into the septal and lateral wall and then through the patch, as described in the text. **(B)** The patch is secured in place, and a running suture is started on the ledge of the patch to ensure hemostasis. **(C)** The closure.

closed with a simple running polypropylene suture.

Postoperative Care

Monitoring of volume is crucial in the early postoperative period by Swan-Ganz catheter or left atrial line or both. Volume should be expanded to assure an adequate preload because the ventricle is stiffer after patch placement. In patients who present with decompensated heart failure with pleural effusions and reduced cardiac indices, intra-aortic balloon counterpulsation may be initiated early.

The use of antiarrhythmic medication is controversial, but we prefer the use of perioperative amiodarone in all patients with subsequent electrophysiologic testing a few weeks postoperatively to assess the need for implantable defibrillators. Generally these have not been needed, presumably because reduced left ventricular volume decreases arrhythmias by reducing wall stress.

The remainder of postoperative care is routine. Beta-blockers and angiotensin-converting-enzyme inhibitors are added as tolerated. Cholesterol is monitored and aggressively treated if elevated. Warfarin is administered for 3 months to maintain an International Normalized Ratio of 2.0. Aspirin is also prescribed if concomitant coronary bypass is performed.

SUGGESTED READING

Athanasuleas CL, Stanley AW, Buckberg GD, et al. Surgical anterior ventricular endocardial restoration (SAVER) for dilated ischemic cardiomyopathy. Semin Thorac Cardiovasc Surg 2001;13:448.

Beyersdorf F, Doenst T, Athanasuleas C, et al. The beating open heart for rebuilding ventricular geometry during surgical anterior restoration. Semin Thorac Cardiovasc Surg 2001;13:42.

Buckberg GD. Defining the relationship between akinesia and dyskinesia and the cause of left ventricular failure after anterior infarction and reversal of remodeling to restoration. J Thorac Cardiovasc Surg 1998;116:47.

Di Donato M, Sabatier M, Dor V, et al. Effects of the Dor procedure on left ventricular dimension and shape and geometric correlates of mitral regurgitation one year after surgery. J Thorac Cardiovasc Surg 2001;121:91.

Dor V. Left ventricular aneurysms: the endoventricular circular patch plasty. Semin Thorac Cardiovasc Surg 1997;9:123.

Dor V. Reconstructive left ventricular surgery for post-ischemic akinetic dilatation. Semin Thorac Cardiovasc Surg 1997;9(2):139-145.

Menicanti L, Dor V, Buckberg GD, et al. Inferior wall restoration: anatomic and surgical considerations. Semin Thorac Cardiovasc Surg 2001;13:504.

Migrino RQ, Young JB, Ellis SG, et al. End-systolic volume index at 90 to 180 minutes into reperfusion therapy for acute myocardial infarction is a strong predictor of early and late mortality. The Global Utilization of Streptokinase and t-PA for Occluded Coronary Arteries (GUSTO)-I Angiographic Investigators. Circulation 1997;96:116.

White HD, Norris RM, Brown MA, et al. Left ventricular end-systolic volume as the major determinant of survival after recovery from myocardial infarction. Circulation 1987;76(1):44.

EDITOR'S COMMENT

I asked these authors to write this chapter because Dr. Buckberg was the individual who popularized this procedure first developed by Dr. Buckberg came to the University of Virginia to help us with our first such operation. This type of reconstruction for patients with heart failure is an incredibly important aspect of surgical therapy. The techniques have been well worked out, and the results continue to improve. Dr. Buckberg's approach has been found to be excellent, as attested by the results that he and many other authors have published. We differ just a little bit with our approach. These authors have kept the heart beating and palpate where the beating heart ends to determine where the Fontan stitch goes.

We think that at least theoretically there are disadvantages with this approach. We believe that this clot in the apex of the heart potentially could be embolized with manipulation. We also feel that it is more difficult to suture in a beating heart. Our preference is to use running sutures, which reduces the amount of time for the restoration, and we think that it is easier to do this with aortic cross-clamp. We have demonstrated in the literature equivalent results to the technique described by these authors.

There are some secondary issues as well. The most important thing that we can do is optimize the size of the heart for the individual patient. These authors use the beating-heart technique, but others have used balloon catheters based on the patient's weight. I think most of these techniques are not exact enough. In the future we should be able to tell exactly to what size and shape an individual's heart can be restored based on preoperative imaging. We should be able to deal with most of the mitral regurgitation if we can place the papillary muscles in the proper position. I believe this technology is one of the most exciting developments in the last 5 years and I believe will be part of every surgeon's armamentarium.

I.L.K.

52

Mitral Valve Repair for Cardiomyopathy

Martinus T. Spoor and Steven F. Bolling

Introduction

The management of patients with congestive heart failure (CHF) has become an international heath care problem and it is one of the world's leading causes of hospitalization and mortality. In our aging population, advances in basic cardiac care that have extended average life expectancy have also left more people living with chronic cardiac disease than ever before. Despite improvements in medical management, approximately 50% of patients with CHF die within 3 years of presentation. Secondary mitral regurgitation (MR) is a complication of end-stage cardiomyopathy and may affect up to 60% of all heart failure patients as a preterminal or terminal event. In the United States alone, 5 million people (2.2% of the total population) are suffering with heart failure, with 550,000 new cases diagnosed each year. Less than 3,000 of the 53,000 patients who die annually are offered transplantation, which many consider to be the standard treatment for select patients with severe CHF and end-stage heart disease. Transplantation is limited by donor availability and its inapplicability in the older patient or those with comorbid medical conditions and will likely never have a major epidemiologic impact. In an effort to solve this problem, alternative medical and surgical strategies are evolving.

Anatomy and Pathology

To address the issue of heart failure and MR, one needs to understand the complex anatomy of the mitral valve. Mitral valve competence depends on the coordinated function of the components of the mitral apparatus: the leaflets, annulus, papillary muscles, chordae tendinae, and entire left ventricle (LV).

The mitral valve is the "inlet" to the LV. The mitral valve consists of two leaflets, the anterior (aortic) and posterior (mural) leaflets. The two leaflets are separated at the annulus by the posteromedial and anterolateral commissures. The anterior leaflet is semicircular and spans the distance between the two commissures. It is attached to the anterolateral wall of the LV in direct continuity with the fibrous skeleton of the heart and with the left and part of the noncoronary aortic valve leaflets. The posterior leaflet is rectangular and is divided into three portions by clefts in the leaflet.

The mitral annulus represents the junction of the fibrous and muscular tissue that joins the left atrium and ventricle. The average human mitral annular cross-sectional area is 5 cm² to 11 cm². The annulus has two major collagenous structures: the right fibrous trigone (located at the intersection of the membranous septum, mitral and tricuspid valves, and aortic root) and the left fibrous trigone (located at the posterior junction of the mitral valve and left coronary leaflet of the aortic valve). During systole the annulus assumes an elliptical shape and is able to contract and decrease in diameter, whereas in diastole it assumes a more circular shape. Annular flexibility allows for increased leaflet coaptation during systole and increased annular orifice area during diastole. The anterior aspect of the annulus, which is in continuity with the fibrous skeleton of the heart, has limited flexibility, whereas the posterior aspect of the annulus, which is not attached to any rigid surrounding structures, has more flexibility. In MR, dilation typically occurs along the more flexible posterior aspect of the annulus.

The anterolateral and posteromedial papillary muscles arise directly from the apical and mid portions of the ventricular wall and give rise to chordae tendinae that attach to both leaflets. The anterolateral papillary muscle receives a dual blood supply from the left anterior descending and from either a diagonal or marginal branch of the circumflex artery. In contrast, the posterolateral papillary muscle has a singular blood supply, either from the right coronary or the circumflex artery, and is therefore more susceptible to ischemia and infarction. The posterior aspect of the LV wall and the papillary muscles together play a very important role in valvular competence and leaflet coaptation. The dynamics of both papillary muscles closely mimics the dynamics of the LV. During LV contraction, the leaflets are pulled downward and together. The LV wall geometry and mechanics play a more significant role in valve competence than the papillary muscles alone. Dilation of the LV may alter the alignment and tension on the papillary muscles and therefore may contribute to valvular incompetence (Fig. 52-1).

The chordae tendinae are comprised of fibrous connective tissue and attach the leaflets to either the papillary muscles or the LV wall directly. The chordae are divided into three groups. The primary chordae attach directly to the free edge of the leaflet and ensure that the leaflets coapt without prolapse or flail. The secondary chordae are more prominent on the anterior leaflet, attach to the leaflet along the line of coaptation, and are important in maintenance of ventricular function. Tertiary chordae are only present on the posterior leaflet and attach directly to the ventricular wall or to the trabeculae carnae. In addition, there are commissural chordae, which arise directly

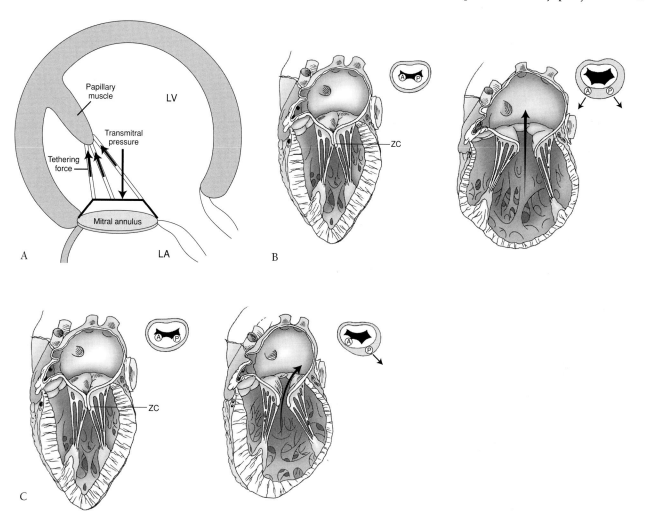

Figure 52-1. Valvular pathology in secondary mitral regurgitation. **(A)** Left ventricular dilation alters the alignment of the papillary muscles and contributes to the development of valve incompetence. In secondary mitral regurgitation, the transmitral pressure exceeds the tethering forces of the papillary muscles. **(B)** Geometric changes of the left ventricle producing central MR. **(C)** Asymmetric geometric ventricular changes secondary to myocardial infarction. (LA = left atrium; LV = left ventricle; ZC = zone of coaptation.)

from either of the papillary muscles and attach to both leaflets.

Maintenance of the chordal, annular, and subvalvar continuity and mitral geometric relationships is important in the preservation of overall ventricular function and may be even more important in patients with compromised function. Secondary MR is observed in patients with either idiopathic or ischemic cardiomyopathy and can be caused by many factors. In patients with nonischemic dilated cardiomyopathy, in the absence of intrinsic mitral valve disease, MR is due to a progressive dilation of the annular-ventricular apparatus with altered ventricular geometry and subsequent loss of leaflet coaptation. In patients with ischemic cardiomyopathy, the mechanisms that contribute to MR are more complex. They may include a combination of dilation of the

annular-ventricular apparatus and LV wall/ papillary muscle dysfunction, again with the net result being failure of leaflet coaptation. A large leaflet area is required for coaptation because mitral leaflet area is 2 times greater than the area of the mitral orifice. As more leaflet tissue is used for coverage of the enlarging orifice, a critical reduction in tissue available for coaptation is reached, such that leaflet coaptation becomes ineffective, and a central regurgitant jet of functional or secondary insufficiency develops. Therefore, the most significant determinants of mitral valve coaptation, leaflet orifice area, and MR are the dimensions of the mitral valve annulus. The LV dimension is less important in functional MR because chordal and papillary muscle length are not significantly altered in people with idiopathic cardiomyopathy with or without MR.

Pathophysiology

MR leads to a cycle of continuing volume overload of the already dilated ventricle, progression of annular dilation, increased LV wall tension, increasing degrees of MR, and worsening CHF. Patients with MR refractory to medical therapy have a poor long-term survival. In a study of 28 patients with cardiomyopathy and an ejection fraction of <25%, the 1-year survival without transplantation was 46%.

The pathophysiology of acute MR (from chordal rupture, endocarditis, blunt chest trauma, or myocardial infarction) is different from that of secondary MR. In acute MR, the left atrium is relatively normal with low compliance, and the acute increase in left atrial pressure can lead to pulmonary edema. This is not the case in secondary MR, where the compensatory changes occur slowly and lead to a gradual increase in left atrial and pulmonary venous compliance, and therefore the signs of pulmonary congestion may not become apparent until much later in the process.

In MR, the regurgitant volume ejected into the left atrium is dependent on mitral orifice size, ventricular-to-atrial pressure gradient, and heart rate. The regurgitant flow into the left atrium increases left atrial pressure, which leads to atrial enlargement and an increase in compliance and decreases forward systemic flow. Left atrial pressures rise during systole and decline in diastole. At end diastole, left atrial pressure will remain mildly elevated, representing a flow gradient. In this setting, with only mild elevations in left atrial pressures, increases in pulmonary vascular resistance usually do not occur, and therefore acute pulmonary edema is not frequently seen.

Various interventions can alter the size of the regurgitant orifice area. An increase in preload or afterload or a decrease in contractility will result in dilation of the LV and an increase in regurgitant orifice area. In a study of patients with severe CHF who were managed medically (with diuretics, nitrates, and afterload-reduction agents), the observed decrease in filling pressure and systemic vascular resistance led to a reduction in the MR associated with their failure. This was attributed to reduction in the regurgitant orifice area related to the decrease in LV volume and annular distension. This complex relationship between mitral annular area and leaflet coaptation may explain why performing a "valvular" repair with an undersized annuloplasty ring can help with a "muscular" problem. This represents a ventricular solution for a ventricular problem (Fig. 52-2).

In MR, the impedance to LV emptying (afterload) is reduced and allows the ventricle to adapt to the regurgitant volume by increasing total cardiac output to maintain an adequate forward output. The increases in LV preload, wall tension, diastolic volume, and stroke volume represent ventricular adaptations to severe MR. The increase in preload eventually leads to LV dilation and a change in the shape of the ventricle from an ellipse to a sphere. There is a significant decrease in the efficiency of work expended by the LV to produce flow that ultimately does not contribute to effective forward cardiac output. In these patients, maintenance of forward flow becomes difficult because up to 50% of the stroke volume is ejected into the left atrium before the aortic valve even opens. With elimination of the regurgitant volume, the ventricle no longer has to expend an excessive amount of work on flow that is going in the reverse direction. In cases of severe myocardial dysfunction, the positive effects of the elimination of the regurgitant flow may be even more pronounced. In secondary MR, ventricular mass also increases, and the degree of LV hypertrophy correlates with the amount of chamber dilation. The ratio of LV mass to LV end-diastolic volume remains normal. In the setting of decreased afterload, the ejection fraction (a clinical measure of pump performance) may remain in the normal range even in the presence of significantly impaired intrinsic LV contractility. Many of the commonly used indices of cardiac pump performance are dependent on both preload and afterload, and therefore are not as reliable in the setting of MR. LV end-systolic volume is a better parameter because it does reflect changes in systolic ventricular function and is independent of preload and varies directly with afterload.

Secondary MR also affects coronary flow characteristics. A recent study assessed coronary flow in patients before and after mitral valve reconstruction. Coronary flow reserve was limited in patients with MR due to an increase in baseline coronary flow and flow velocity, which was related to LV volume overload, hypertrophy, and preload (LV wall stress). The restriction in coronary flow reserve improved following valve reconstruction because of a reduction in the baseline coronary flow and flow velocity once the LV preload, work, and mass were reduced. Based on this study, in patients with secondary MR, a restriction in the coronary flow reserve would seem probable and an improvement in flow reserve and velocity would be expected following mitral valve repair. Ultimately mitral valve repair in this setting would lead to an improvement in LV geometry.

In the setting of chronic CHF, cardiac reserve is depressed, and a number of compensatory mechanisms are activated and may account for many symptoms of failure and contribute to its further progression. Some of these mechanisms are responsible for the vasoconstriction seen in heart failure and include stimulation and activation of the neuroendocrine and sympathetic nervous systems. Increases in circulating norepinephrine levels are documented in CHF. Norepinephrine is released and binds to the β-adrenoceptors and results in a positive inotropic response. In CHF, there is an excessive release of norepinephrine from the myocardium, a corresponding increase in plasma levels, and a reduction in its myocardial stores. Following long-term exposure to elevated levels of norepinephrine, the numbers of β-adrenoceptors become downregulated, which results in a reduced positive inotropic effect of β-adrenoceptor agonists. In addition, studies have shown that proinflammatory cytokines (tumor necrosis factor-α [TNF-α], interleukin-1 [IL-1], IL-2, and IL-6) may be responsible for the myocardial depression in heart failure. TNF-α has been shown to be produced by the heart under stress, has negative inotropic effects, and may play a role in the development of LV dysfunction, dilated cardiomyopathy, hypotension, and pulmonary edema, all of which can be seen in advanced CHF.

Clinical Presentations

Patients with mild to moderate MR may remain asymptomatic for years as the LV adapts to its increased workload. In contrast, patients with secondary MR usually

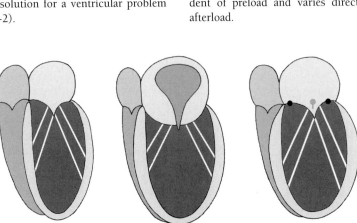

Figure 52-2.   Rationale for annuloplasty in secondary mitral regurgitation. As the left ventricle dilates, there is an increase in the regurgitant orifice area and the mitral annulus dilates. An undersized annuloplasty ring facilitates the return of the zone of coaptation to a more normal dimension to correct for the regurgitation.

present with symptoms related to the underlying cardiomyopathy and CHF. Symptoms of decreased cardiac output and pulmonary congestion develop (weakness, fatigue, and dyspnea). These symptoms worsen with the further progression of MR. On physical examination, the cardiac impulse may be hyperdynamic and there is a characteristic blowing apical holosystolic murmur that may radiate to the axilla, back and into the neck.

Diagnostic Techniques

Chest X Ray

An enlarged cardiac silhouette is a common radiographic finding in patients with secondary MR and is indicative of LV and left atrial enlargement. Congestive findings in the pulmonary parenchyma are less prominent.

Electrocardiogram

Atrial fibrillation is common. Findings consistent with left atrial enlargement and ventricular hypertrophy are typical.

Echocardiogram

Echocardiography provides a noninvasive means of assessing ventricular function and the severity of MR. Color Doppler analysis yields a semiquantitative analysis of MR. This assessment of the degree of MR is based on the relative comparisons of size and area of the regurgitant jet to the size and area of the left atrium. The Doppler jet is sensitive to load conditions, driving pressure, jet eccentricity, and left atrial size, and therefore can lead to an incorrect estimation of the extent of MR. Proximal flow convergence analysis, which allows for calculation of the regurgitant volume by measuring the flow proximal to the mitral valve orifice, is a useful tool in the assessment of the extent of MR. Transesophageal echocardiography (TEE) is superior to transthoracic echocardiography in that it better defines the details of mitral valve pathology and anatomy and the severity of the regurgitation (Fig. 52-3).

Cardiac Catheterization

Cardiac catheterization is not necessary to establish the diagnosis of secondary MR; however, it provides data regarding secondary processes and associated cardiac pathology. Although left ventriculography does not permit a truly accurate assessment of the mitral valve or subvalvar apparatus, it does allow a calculation of ejection fraction.

Management

The mainstay of medical management of patients with cardiomyopathy and secondary MR is the treatment of the underlying CHF with the use of diuretics and afterload-reduction agents. Reducing the aortic ejection impedance reduces the regurgitant volume into the left atrium and relieves pulmonary congestion. This strategy reduces LV volume and increases forward stroke volume, which results in a smaller regurgitant orifice area. An area of current investigation for newer modalities of medical treatment include the use of recombinant agents directed at TNF-α and the specific TNF-α receptors.

Historically, the surgical approach to patients with MR was mitral valve replacement, and little was understood of the adverse consequences that interruption of the annulus-papillary muscle continuity had on LV systolic function. This procedure was associated with high mortality rates. It is in this population of patients that the concept of the "pop-off" effect of MR originated; that is, reversal of blood flow was somehow beneficial to the patient in failure. It has been demonstrated in a number of studies that preservation of the annulus-papillary muscle continuity is of paramount importance to preservation of LV function. It was the excision of and disruption of the subvalvar apparatus that accounted for the significant loss of systolic function due to the destruction of the LV that led to the poor outcome in the earlier patients who underwent valve replacement. Preservation of the mitral apparatus and LV in mitral valve repair has been demonstrated to enhance and maintain LV function and geometry with an associated decrease in wall stress. This procedure has been shown to be safe with good long-term outcomes. In fact, it has been shown that there is no "pop-off" effect, but the mortality ascribed to these patients from mitral replacement was in fact due to disruption of the subvalvar apparatus and loss of LV function.

Because the availability of transplantation for end-stage cardiomyopathy is limited, there has been recent interest in the altered geometry of the LV in patients with severe dysfunction. This innovative work was initially described by Batista, who stated that all mammalian hearts share the same ratio of mass, M, to the cube of the radius, R, regardless of the size of the heart ($M/R^3 = 4$). Batista proposed that for those hearts that do not comply with this relationship, an operative procedure should be performed to restore the ratio back to normal. Surgeons have attempted to renormalize this relationship by LV myoreduction surgery (the Batista procedure). Batista initially reported an operative mortality of 5%,

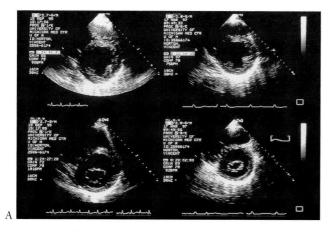
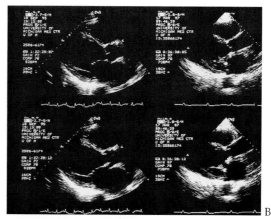

Figure 52-3. Transesophageal echocardiogram. Transesophageal echocardiography and color Doppler analysis demonstrating annular dilation and the presence of secondary mitral regurgitation.

a 30-day mortality of 22%, and a 2-year survival of 55%. Unfortunately, complete and long-term follow-up was not available. This procedure has met with varying degrees of success in the United States and worldwide. The Cleveland Clinic series of 62 patients reported a 3.5% in-hospital mortality, with 7 late deaths, and a 1-year actuarial survival of 82%. It is significant that in all of these cases, a mitral valve repair or replacement occurred routinely as part of the myoreduction procedure. It is therefore difficult to discern the exact role that correction of MR plays in the overall success of the procedure.

At the University of Michigan, from 1993 to 2003, 215 patients with end-stage cardiomyopathy and refractory MR underwent mitral valve repair with an undersized annuloplasty ring. The range in age was 30 to 87 years (64 ± 12 years). Ejection fraction was 6% to 30% (20.8% ± 6%). Preoperative New York Heart Association (NYHA) class was 3.1 ± 0.9. A large number of patients (64 of 215, 30%) had a previous open-heart procedure. Thirty-day mortality was 4.7% (10 of 215) for all mitral repairs. Postoperative low-cardiac-output syndrome was 2.3% (5 of 215). Complication rates were low, with a cerebrovascular accident (CVA)/transient ischemic attack (TIA) rate of 2% (4 of 215), a prolonged ventilation rate of 6% (14 of 215), a total infection rate of 5% (11 of 215), a rate of renal failure requiring dialysis of 1% (2 of 215), and a rate of reoperation for bleeding of 0.5% (1/215). Average intensive care unit stay was 2.67 days and average hospital stay was 7.8 days. The 1- and 2-year actuarial survival rates were 80% and 70%, respectively. These encouraging results have been confirmed in other studies. Bitran noted a decrease in heart failure symptoms and a decrease in NYHA functional class in 115 patients. Chen published a report of 81 patients undergoing mitral valve surgery for mitral valve regurgitation in dilated cardiomyopathy. In this series LV ejection fraction (LVEF) increased from 24% to 32% and there was an improvement in NYHA class from 3.3 to 1.6. Survival in this study was 73%, 58%, and 38% at 1, 3, and 5, years, respectively. More recently Calafiore and associates published a series of 49 patients. In this study LVEF improved from 27% to 30% and NYHA functional class improved from 3.5 to 2.2. Survival was 90%, 87%, 78%, and 73% at 1, 3, 5, and 10 years, respectively. Interestingly, in this report actuarial survival was 83% for mitral valve repair versus 70% for mitral valve replacement and improvement of NYHA class at 5 years was 76% in MV repair and 65% in MV replacement. Bishay and

colleagues looked at 44 patients who underwent isolated mitral valve surgery. In this series LVEF improved from 28% to 36% and NYHA functional class decreased from 2.9 to 1.2. Survival was 89%, 86%, and 67% at 1, 2, and 5 years, respectively. Furthermore, they noted a decrease in the left ventricular chamber sphericity. Although all of these series have had failures associated with return of MR, new techniques such as new three-dimensional shaped rings, plication of the papillary muscles, attachment of the posterior papillary muscle to the annulus, and jacketing the heart all are aimed at reducing failure rates by changing LV geometry.

In patients undergoing mitral valve reconstruction for myopathy there is reestablishment of a more normal LV mass-to-volume ratio without the loss of myocardial mass. The average LV volume at 24-month follow-up in this study was >200 ml, still quite large, whereas with the LV myoreduction procedure Batista demonstrated acute reduction of volumes to 90 ml to 100 ml at the time of operation. In a recent study that assessed acute cardiovascular changes that occur with the Batista procedure, significant elevations in LV end-diastolic pressure and end-diastolic elastance were noted, indicative of persistent postoperative depressed diastolic function. There is no loss of ventricular mass with mitral valve reconstruction alone; however, an appropriate mass/volume ratio is restored. In addition, a decrease in sphericity index and LV volume measurements was demonstrated postoperatively, and it is in these patients that the negative cycle of CHF is interrupted and the surgical unloading of the LV is achieved. These patients may be undergoing a slow self-remodeling from the alteration of the angulation of the base of the heart, stabilization of the mitral annulus, or LV unloading, each of which contributes to a more favorable ventricular geometry. There is an acceptable surgical mortality, both at 30 days and 1 year, for mitral valve reconstruction, which is equivalent to or lower than what has been reported for LV myoreduction procedures. Furthermore, in one of the largest and best-documented series, Franco-Cereceda and coworkers from the Cleveland Clinic described 62 patients with idiopathic cardiomyopathy who underwent mitral valve repair and concomitant partial left ventriculectomy. Survival was 80% at 1 year and 60% at 3 years. However, 18% of patients required left ventricular assist device (LVAD) support, and 72% of this subpopulation underwent eventual transplantation. The authors pointed out that LVAD and transplantation accounted for the high

1-year survival because freedom from composite events was only 49%.

Prognosis

For patients with idiopathic or ischemic dilated cardiomyopathy, mortality is directly related to severity of ventricular systolic dysfunction and volume. In addition, increased chamber sphericity, the presence of MR, and an increase in LV end-diastolic volume are markers of a poor prognosis. In review of these types of patients, 1-year mortality has been reported to be between 54% and 70%. Mitral valve surgery for secondary MR relieves symptoms, increases long-term survival, helps prevent further progression of LV dysfunction, and improves overall ventricular function.

Summary

Secondary MR is a significant complication of end-stage cardiomyopathy. The MR is thought to occur due to progressive dilation of the annular-ventricular apparatus, altered ventricular geometry, loss of leaflet coaptation, and LV wall/papillary muscle dysfunction. In secondary MR, there is an increase in preload and a decrease in afterload, which eventually leads to LV dilation and remodeling. Medical management consists primarily of diuretics, beta blockers, and afterload reduction, which results in poor long-term quality of life and survival. Mitral reconstruction via an annuloplasty ring effectively corrects MR in cardiomyopathy patients, is a safe procedure in a high-risk population, and has an acceptable operative mortality rate. Both survival and functional status have improved for these patients. The effects of this procedure with severe myocardial dysfunction may be attributed to a decrease in the regurgitant orifice area, better effective forward flow, and an increase in coronary flow reserve. These changes all contribute to restoration of the normal LV geometric relationship. Although longer-term follow-up is necessary, mitral reconstruction offers a new strategy for end-stage cardiomyopathy.

SUGGESTED READING

Akasaka T, Yoshida K, Hozumi T, et al. Restricted coronary flow reserve in patients with mitral regurgitation improves after mitral reconstructive surgery. J Am Coll Cardiol 1998;32:1923.

Akins CW, Hilgenberg AD, Buckley MJ, et al. Mitral valve reconstruction versus replacement for degenerative or ischemic mitral regurgitation. Ann Thorac Surg 1994;58:668.

Anguita M, Arizon JM, Bueno G, et al. Clinical and hemodynamic predictors of survival in patients aged <65 years with severe congestive heart failure secondary to ischemic or non-ischemic dilated cardiomyopathy. Am J Cardiol 1993;72(5):413.

Batista R. Partial left ventriculectomy—The Batista procedure. Thorac Surg 1999;15(Suppl. 1):S12.

Batista RJV, Verde J, Nery P, et al. Partial left ventriculectomy to treat end-stage heart disease. Ann Thorac Surg 1997;64:634.

Bolling SF, Deeb GM, Brunsting LA, et al. Early outcome of mitral valve reconstruction in patients with end-stage cardiomyopathy. J Thorac Cardiovasc Surg 1995;109:676.

Bolling SF, Pagani FD, Deeb GM, et al. Intermediate-term outcome of mitral reconstruction in cardiomyopathy. J Thorac Cardiovasc Surg 1998;115:381.

Boltwood CM, Tei C, Wong M, et al. Quantitative echocardiography of the mitral complex in dilated cardiomyopathy: the mechanism of functional mitral regurgitation. Circulation 1983;68:498.

Bristow MR, Ginsburg R, Minobe W, et al. Decreased catecholamine sensitivity and beta-adrenergic receptor density in failing human hearts. N Engl J Med 1982;307:205.

Carabello BA, Williams H, Gash AK, et al. Hemodynamic predictors of outcome in patients undergoing valve replacement. Circulation 1986;74:1309.

David TE, Uden DE, Strauss HD. The importance of the mitral apparatus in left ventriuclar function after correction of mitral regurgitation. Circulation 1983;68(3 Pt 2):II76.

Dowling RD, Koenig SC, Ewert DL, et al. Acute cardiovascular changes of partial left ventriculectomy without mitral valve repair. Ann Thor Surg 1996;67:1470.

Fann JI, Ingels NB, Miller DC. Pathophysiology of mitral valve disease and operative indications. In Edmunds LH (ed), Cardiac Surgery in the Adult. New York: McGraw-Hill, 1997;959.

Harding SE, Brown LA, Wynne DG, et al. Mechanisms of β adrenoceptor desensitization in the failing human heart. Cardiovasc Res 1994;28:1451.

Herrera-Garza EH, Stetson SJ, Cubillos-Garzon A, et al. Tumor necrosis factor-α: A mediator of disease progression in the failing human heart. Chest 1999;115:1170.

Huikuri HV. Effect of mitral valve replacement on left ventricular function in mitral regurgitation. Br Heart J 1983;49:328.

Kawaguchi HK, Kitabatake A. Alterations of signal transduction system in heart failure. Japan Heart J 1997;38:317.

McCarthy JF, McCarthy PM, Starling RC, et al. Partial left ventriculectomy and mitral valve repair for end-stage congestive heart failure. Eur J Cardiothorac Surg 1998;13:337.

Rosario LB, Stevenson LW, Solomon SD, et al. The mechanism of decrease in dynamic mitral regurgitation during heart failure treatment: Importance of reduction in the regurgitant orifice size. J Am Coll Cardiol 1998;32:1819.

Sarris GE, Cahill PD, Hansen DE, et al. Restoration of left ventricular systolic performance after reattachment of the mitral chordae tendineae. The importance of valvular-ventricular interaction. J Thorac Cadiovasc Surg 1988;95:969.

Starling MR, Kirsh MM, Montgomery DG, et al. Impaired left ventricular contractile function in patients with long-term mitral regurgitation and normal ejection fraction. J Am Coll Cardiol 1993;22:239.

Stevenson LW, Fowler MB, Schroeder JS, et al. Poor survival of patients with idiopathic cardiomyopathy considered too well for transplantation. Am J Med 1987;83:871.

Thomas, JD. How leaky is that mitral valve? Simplified Doppler methods to measure regurgitant orifice area. Circulation 1997;93:548.

Tischler MD, Cooper KA, Rowen M, et al. Myocardial function/valvular heart disease/hypertensive heart disease: Mitral valve replacement versus mitral valve repair: A Doppler and quantitative stress echocardiographic study. Circulation 1994;89:132.

Torre-Amione G, Kapadia S, Benedict C, et al. Proinflammatory cytokine levels in patients with depressed left ventricular ejection fraction: A report from the Studies of Left Ventricular Dysfunction (SOLVD). J Am Coll Cardiol 1996;27:1201.

EDITOR'S COMMENTS

Bolling and his group were the first to demonstrate that one could safely repair the mitral valve in patients with dilated cardiomyopathy. It had previously been thought that this would be too dangerous a procedure with patients with limited ventricular reserve. Interestingly, mitral regurgitation is what makes patients with cardiomyopathy symptomatic. As the mitral valve begins to leak, the patient truly decompensates. We had been taught, as noted in this chapter, that mitral regurgitation was considered a good thing as a "pop-off" valve. It turned out that this concept was absolutely incorrect. Conversely, mitral valve replacement in patients with cardiomyopathy probably is a bad thing. The mortality is quite high and mitral valve repair, as the authors noted, is the way to go.

Where exactly does mitral valve repair fit in patients with cardiomyopathy? Clearly it can be done safely. It makes patients less symptomatic and may improve ventricular function in some patients. However, it probably does not markedly increase the lifespan of these patients because the late cause of death is arrhythmias. We use this modality in our heart failure population, and patients certainly do well and feel better. However, long-term survival is limited by the underlying cardiac function.

I.L.K.

53

Ventricular Assist

Nicholas C. Dang, Mehmet C. Oz, and Yoshifumi Naka

Background

Ventricular assist devices (VADs) have evolved in parallel with advances in cardiac transplantation. The introduction of cyclosporine in the 1980s and continued refinements of surgical technique established heart transplantation as the most effective therapy for patients with end-stage heart disease, including those with congestive heart failure. However, heart transplantation is the solution for a select few, about 10% of patients die annually while waiting for a heart, and organ supply continues to be limited, with only about 2,000 hearts available each year. Therefore, alternatives to cardiac transplantation have emerged almost necessarily. The alternative that has proven to be the most successful and holds the most promise is the ventricular assist device.

The development of VADs began in earnest in the early 1960s when Hall and colleagues designed an intrathoracic left ventricular bypass pump. This device featured an outer air chamber that, when compressed by pulsed air externally, collapsed the inner blood chamber and propelled blood forward. Since then, VADs have undergone dramatic refinement and modification to evolve into the present generation of devices (Table 53-1). The majority of VADs are dedicated to supporting the left ventricle (left ventricular assist devices [LVADs]) because of the predominant number of heart failure cases that are left-sided, but the use of right-sided VADs (RVADs) and biventricular assist devices (BIVADs) is also well established. The predominant VAD design incorporates a pulsatile mechanism, and these are classified as either extracorporeal or fully implantable, depending on the intended duration of support. The most commonly utilized among these include the Thoratec ventricular assist system (VAS; Thoratec Laboratories Corp., Berkeley, CA), the ABIOMED BVS 5000 (ABIOMED Cardiovascular Inc., Danvers, MA), the HeartMate IP-1000 (pneumatically actuated; Thoratec Corp., Pleasanton, CA), the HeartMate VE (vented electric) LVAS, and the Novacor LVAS (Baxter Healthcare Corp., Oakland, CA).

Gaining in momentum and invested effort are the continuous-flow devices, which include the smaller, more streamlined axial-flow pumps. Numerous studies of animal models using support with axial flow pumps for upward of 6 months failed to show any detrimental effects clinically, biochemically, or microscopically. The theoretical advantages of continuous-flow pumps include, in addition to the aforementioned smaller size, fewer moving parts, absence of valves, smaller blood-contacting surfaces, reduced energy requirements, and the elimination of a compliance chamber. The most prominent among this group of VADs are the HeartMate II (Thoratec Corp., Pleasanton, CA), the De-Bakey/NASA LVAD (MicroMed Inc., Houston, TX), and the Jarvik 2000 (Jarvik Heart Inc., New York, NY). Despite the differences in design, all LVADs strive to achieve the same purpose: mechanically unload the failing left ventricle and supply oxygen to adequately meet the demands of the body.

Mechanical unloading of the left ventricle by way of VADs results in a number of important physiologic and molecular changes. Because the LVAD is able to increase cardiac output (outflow) above what was previously achieved by the native failing left ventricle, more blood is returned to the systemic circulation, and there is increased venous return to and increased cardiac output from the right ventricle. This enhanced right ventricular cardiac output is also augmented by the LVAD's reduction of pulmonary pressure afterload. Myocardial work is diminished and subendocardial perfusion is optimized, which allows the heart to rest and recover. During LVAD support, left ventricular distension is decreased, which leads to increases in sarcoplasmic reticulum calcium content, a decrease in G-protein receptor kinase expression, and subsequent reverse remodeling. Furthermore, the neurohormonal activation and catabolic state normally associated with heart failure is suppressed as plasma levels of epinephrine, norepinephrine, angiotensin II, arginine vasopressin, interleukin-6 and interleukin-8, and tumor necrosis factor (TNF)-α levels are all noted to decrease. This suspension and reversal of the heart failure milieu prevents further deterioration and sets the stage for myocyte recovery.

LVADs are beneficial in three distinct groups of patients. The first group comprises patients who require ventricular assistance to allow the heart to rest and recover its function. The degree of myocardial injury is felt to be reversible and myocardial function is expected to recover following a short period of support (<2 weeks). Most often, this group consists of patients who suffer from acute viral myocarditis, acute myocardial infarction, and postcardiotomy shock with failure to wean from cardiopulmonary bypass. Generally, these patients receive an extracorporeal LVAD unless it is felt they will require longer period of support, in which case the extracorporeal device is replaced by a fully implantable one. In theory, although LVAD support within this group should facilitate myocardial recovery and subsequent device explantation, this has not been our experience. The rate of explantation in our

Table 53-1 Types of Ventricular Assist Devices

Paracorporeal pulsatile
ABIOMED BVS 5000
Thoratec VAD
Intracorporeal pulsatile
HeartMate LVAS
Implantable Pneumatic LVAD (IP-1000 LVAD)
Vented Electric LVAD (VE-LVAD)
Novacor LVAS
CardioWest Total Artificial Heart (TAH)
AbioCor Total Artificial Heart (TAH)
Arrow LionHeart LVAS
Centrifugal and axial flow blood pumps (nonpulsatile)
Extracorporeal membrane oxygenation
MicroMed DeBakey VAD
Jarvik 2000
HeartMate II LVAS
Terumo Duraheart LVAS
Arrow CorAide LVAS
Berlin Heart INCOR
CardiacAssist TandemHeart
Impella VAD

LVAD = left ventricular assist device; LVAS = ventricular assist system; VAD ventricular assist device; VE = vented electric.

patient population is exceedingly low, with fewer than 5% of this group undergoing successful device removal. The reasons for this are not entirely clear and warrant further evaluation. However, novel therapies such as pharmaceutical adjuncts and stem cell implantation hold promising potential for myocardial recovery in the future.

The second group of patients who benefit from LVAD implantation consists of those who suffer from long-standing end-stage heart failure or severe acute myocardial infarction and are not expected to recover adequate myocardial function. These patients require mechanical circulatory support solely as a bridge to transplantation. Implantable LVADs are used in these instances to permit greater patient mobility, rehabilitation, and discharge to home. We generally advocate LVAD support times of at least 3 months before transplantation, if feasible, to optimize end-organ perfusion.

Previously, patients with irreversible heart failure who were ineligible for cardiac transplantation had only optimal medical management as a therapeutic option. Prognosis for this group was dismal, with a 1-year survival rate approximating 25%. The recent Randomized Evaluation of Mechanical Assistance for the Treatment of Congestive Heart Failure (REMATCH) trial sought to compare outcomes in these patients receiving either HeartMate LVAD therapy or optimal medical management (angiotensin-converting-enzyme inhibitors [ACEIs], digoxin, diuretics, and beta-blockers) and found that LVAD therapy doubled the 1-year survival rate of medical therapy alone, in addition to achieving a significant improvement in quality of life and functional status. The HeartMate LVAD was subsequently approved by the Food and Drug Administration (FDA) for use as a form of permanent, destination therapy. This surgical alternative defines the third group of patients for whom LVADs bear application, one that will likely expand in parallel with the growing number of patients living with congestive heart failure.

Patient Selection and Preoperative Evaluation

Patient selection is of critical importance in determining the clinical outcomes of those who receive LVADs. In general, there are no absolute hemodynamic criteria that dictate when to initiate support. However, several important clinical factors should be considered (Table 53-2). Cardiogenic shock that may warrant LVAD insertion is diagnosed on the basis of hemodynamic parameters coupled with clinical signs: cardiac index <2.0 L/min/m^2, systolic blood pressure <85 mm Hg, central venous pressure >16 mm Hg, pulmonary capillary wedge pressure >20 mm Hg, oliguria <30 mL/hr, altered mental status, capillary refill >2 seconds, and cool extremities, all despite maximal pharmacotherapy, intra-aortic balloon pump, or both. Moreover, specific preop-

Table 53-2 Indications for Left Ventricular Assist Device Insertion

Cardiogenic shock
CI <2.0 L/min/m^2
SBP ≤85 mm Hg
CVP >16 mm Hg
PCWP >20 mm Hg
SVO$_2$ $<50\%$
UOP <30 mL/hr
Maximal inotropic/pressor support (IABP assistance)

CI = cardiac index; CVP = central venous pressure; PCWP = pulmonary capillary wedge pressure; SBP = systolic blood pressure; SVO$_2$ = mixed venous oxygen saturation; UOP = urinary output.

Table 53-3 Preoperative Left Ventricular Assist Device Risk Factor Score

Preoperative Variable	Weight Value
Ventilatory status	4
Postcardiotomy shock	2
Previous LVAD	2
CVP >16 mm Hg	1
PT >16 secs	1

CVP = central venous pressure; LVAD = left ventricular assist device; PT = prothrombin time.

erative factors have been shown to adversely affect survival following LVAD insertion (Table 53-3). These include ventilatory dependence, postcardiotomy shock, previous LVAD (e.g., ABIOMED BVS 5000), prothrombin time (PT) >16 seconds, and central venous pressure >16 mm Hg. LVAD implantation scores can be derived from these five clinical variables and classified as low (0 to 4), medium (5 to 7), or high (8 to 10), with an inverse relationship between score and clinical stability. By assigning preoperative scores to all patients being evaluated for LVAD implantation, particularly in the acute setting, we are able to predict those who will likely suffer poor outcomes and we can effectively allocate comprehensive care resources to those who are more likely to benefit from this mode of therapy. Proper patient selection weighs heavily on overall patient survival, total hospital and intensive care unit (ICU) length of stay, resource utilization, and cost of treatment.

It is evident from the previous discussion that accurate assessment of end-organ dysfunction plays a critical role. Hepatic dysfunction is often the result of congestion from right-sided heart failure, in turn evoked by left ventricular failure and increased pulmonary resistance. Hepatic synthesis is impaired, primarily in the way of coagulation factors, but also with respect to albumin, wound-healing proteins, and immunologic factors. This degree of organ compromise can have profound effects both in the immediate and long-term postoperative periods because the propensity for bleeding is increased substantially and the likelihood of infection is also elevated. Preoperative renal dysfunction is common in patients being evaluated for LVADs, most often as a result of the low-flow state associated with advanced heart failure. Although LVAD support can sometimes alleviate acute renal failure by restoring adequate blood flow to the kidneys, patients who require renal replacement therapy (e.g., hemofiltration or hemodialysis) at any time during hospitalization are known to have adverse clinical outcomes, including decreased rate of bridge to transplantation. Despite this observation, the presence of acute renal failure requiring dialysis is not an absolute contraindication to LVAD implantation, and clinical evaluation needs to take into consideration the degree and duration of cardiogenic shock as well as the patient's baseline renal function.

Certain concomitant cardiac factors also require attention in terms of patient selection. The valvular defects that warrant correction prior to device implantation are mitral stenosis and aortic regurgitation. Mitral stenosis, if severe, can limit filling of the device. Aortic insufficiency decreases net forward flow because the blood that is pumped into the aortic root by the device flows backward through the incompetent valve. In fact, mild to moderate aortic insufficiency can become severe on LVAD support because mechanical unloading of the left ventricle increases the aortic-ventricular pressure gradient during diastole, promoting backward flow. Patients with mechanical aortic valve prostheses should have the mechanical valve closed during device placement to prevent thrombus from being showered to the systemic circulation with occasional valve openings.

The presence of coronary artery disease does not contribute significantly to hemodynamic performance while patients are on LVAD support, although it is often the very reason why certain patients receive LVADs (e.g., acute myocardial infarction, postcardiotomy shock following failed coronary bypass operation). Angina sometimes persists despite adequate device function. Right ventricular ischemia following implantation can cause right ventricular failure and decreased flow to the LVAD. Moreover, ongoing ischemia limits the potential for myocardial recovery and device weaning.

Arrhythmias are common in patients with cardiomyopathies, and these continue to occur even after device implantation. Atrial fibrillation and flutter can limit right ventricular filling but are reasonably well tolerated in LVAD patients because device outflows are not markedly altered. For atrial arrhythmias, early cardioversion is indicated to prevent thrombus formation. Ventricular fibrillation is also reasonably tolerated, and adequate but slightly decreased LVAD flows are maintained during the chronic stage, presumably owing to the fact that the device is able to fill regardless of native ventricular activity. Anticoagulation should be in-

---

Table 53-4
Contraindications to Left Ventricular Assist Device Placement

Sepsis
Severe neurologic deficit, including major cerebrovascular accident
Metastatic cancer
Irreversible hepatic failure
Irreversible renal failure
Severe chronic obstructive pulmonary disease or respiratory failure
Compliance problems
Comorbidities that would prove to be life limiting
Contraindication to cardiac transplantation (bridge to transplant patients only)

---

stituted in all patients with persistent atrial and ventricular arrhythmias to minimize the risk of thrombus formation with subsequent systemic embolization.

Several clinical conditions exist that should preclude LVAD placement (Table 53-4). In general, patients who should not be considered for LVAD therapy include those who suffer from irreversible hepatic, renal, or respiratory failure. The presence of a previous neurologic event with significant residual deficit also precludes implantation, as does the coexistence of severe obstructive or restrictive pulmonary disease. The latter comorbidity, in particular, is often associated with elevated pulmonary vascular resistance unresponsive to pulmonary vasodilator therapy, which can impair proper device performance, result in right-sided heart failure, and prohibit heart transplantation in those who are candidates. Other relative contraindications to HeartMate LVAD placement include sepsis, body mass index (BMI) <18 or >35 kg/m², body surface area (BSA) <1.5 m², high surgical risk (e.g., ascending aorta calcification), heparin-induced thrombocytopenia (HIT), and the presence of another acute medical condition (e.g., gastrointestinal hemorrhage). Each patient should be considered on an individual basis to determine the acuteness of cardiac decompensation and the need for LVAD as well as the risks associated with accepting various comorbidities.

Economic Considerations

As a technological advance that has enormous potential effects on many patients liv-

ing with congestive heart failure, LVADs require a comprehensive analysis of cost data and a discussion of proper resource allocation. The cost and utilization of health care resources depend on the device and the indication for implant. In general, LVAD therapy should be regarded in terms of the same medical and societal values assigned to other life-saving procedures in both the acute and chronic settings.

Although LVADs have clearly been shown to improve survival for certain patients, few reports have analyzed the costs related to this survival benefit. A recent study looked specifically at the cost of hospital resource use and its predictors among the destination therapy LVAD patients involved in the REMATCH trial. Cost data were available for 52 of 68 study patients randomized to receive an LVAD and included Medicare data, standard billing forms (UB-92), and line-item bills obtained from each participating clinical center. The mean cost for the primary LVAD hospitalization was $210,187 ± 193,295. When costs were compared between hospital survivors and nonsurvivors, mean costs jumped from $159,271 ± 106,423 to $315,015 ± 278,713. The principal drivers of implantation cost (incurred from time of randomization to time of discharge from acute care facility) were sepsis, pump housing infection, and perioperative bleeding. Sepsis alone drove the predicted cost of hospitalization in a patient suffering no major complications from $119,874 to $263,822. The combination of all three adverse events escalated these costs even further to $869,199.

The average cost of the LVAD was $62,308 ± 11,651, accounting for 29.64% of the total cost, and the average cost of the intensive care unit (ICU) stay was $50,262 ± 82,076, accounting for 23.91% of the total cost. The average annual readmission cost per patient for the entire LVAD cohort was $105,326, and was $99,118 for the 27 patients who survived >1 year.

These cost data suggest that LVAD therapy in a chronic, end-stage heart failure patient population is comparable to other life-saving organ replacement procedures, such as liver transplantation and even heart transplantation. Thus, a transition is due to occur that will take LVAD therapy from a payer perspective of experimental surgery to a legitimate, life-saving procedure. Such momentum hinges on further progress, however. As an evolving technology, LVADs have considerable margin for improvement in areas such as device design, patient selection, nutritional optimization, surgical technique, antimicrobial therapy, and management of perioperative coagulopathy.

Surgical Procedure

The specific procedures for the implantation of each device vary, but the basic principles are similar. The following discussion describes our operative strategies for the placement of the Thoratec HeartMate LVAS. Device assembly and setup takes place on a back table in the operating room under sterile conditions. The inflow and outflow valve conduits, as well as the outflow graft, require preclotting to maintain hemostasis and minimize the likelihood of inadvertent air entry during device startup. The Thoratec Heart-Mate uses a Dacron (Dupont, Wilmington, DE) outflow graft, whose external surface is coated evenly with combination cryoprecipitate and thrombin or other standard preclotting agent. Patient nonheparinized autologous blood is also a viable alternative. After the valve conduits have undergone sequential rinsing, their external surfaces are also preclotted with combination cryoprecipitate and thrombin (Fig. 53-1). Care is taken not to preclot the internal surfaces, especially in the area of the porcine valves.

The preclotted inflow and outflow conduits are attached to the main LVAD housing unit and hand-tightened securely. The pump is primed with sterile normal saline through the inflow valve conduit until the device is full. The inflow conduit is covered with a cut fingertip of a sterile rubber glove, and the outflow conduit is covered with the hexagonal-shaped, solid, white thread protector to prevent contamination

of the device interior. The driveline is covered with vancomycin-soaked (cefazolin-gentamicin in vancomycin-allergic patients) laparotomy pads.

Transesophageal echocardiography is always performed intraoperatively to properly assess cardiac function, determine chamber proportions, and identify any anatomic abnormalities (e.g., patent foramen ovale, aortic insufficiency, mitral stenosis) that may warrant surgical correction during LVAD placement. Echocardiography can also confirm adequate left ventricular decompression once the LVAD is activated. Pulmonary artery catheterization is useful for monitoring patient hemodynamics and fluid status intraoperatively. Thermodilution-based cardiac output can be measured and compared with LVAD flows. Generally, a difference of >20% between the right heart output and the LVAD flow suggests significant aortic insufficiency, which will need to be corrected surgically. The echocardiogram is repeated following implantation and actuation of the LVAD to confirm proper coordination between the native heart and the device. Sometimes certain flow abnormalities, such as aortic insufficiency or right-to-left shunt from a patent foramen ovale, only become evident after the LVAD is initiated, owing to dramatic left ventricular decompression and resultant altered pressure differences between chambers.

To begin the operative procedure, a midline incision is made, extending from the sternal notch to a point just above the umbilicus with division of the linea alba. Median sternotomy is completed, and the heart is exposed before LVAD pocket creation to permit quick access in the instance of acute hemodynamic instability. Pump placement

can be carried out either intra-abdominally or preperitoneally, and there are advantages and disadvantages to each approach. Intra-abdominal pump placement is sometimes preferable in thin patients in whom driveline tunneling may not result in adequate tissue ingrowth or erosion of the device through the skin is a potential concern. Some of the associated disadvantages of intra-abdominal pump placement include abdominal adhesions, gastric or bowel compression, bowel obstruction and perforation, herniation of the device through the diaphragm into the pericardial space, and erosion of abdominal viscera. Preperitoneal pump placement is preferred in patients who have undergone previous abdominal surgery or who have short torsos. The major advantages of this technique include the avoidance of abdominal adhesions, posterior dislocation of the stomach, and complications related to direct contact between the device and the abdominal viscera. Potential disadvantages include wound dehiscence, pocket fluid collection or hematoma leading to pocket infection, and driveline exit site infection. With these factors taken into consideration, we have adopted the practice of performing preperitoneal placement in the majority of patients. This particular approach will be described.

With the midline incision extending to a level just above the umbilicus, the preperitoneal fat is cleared from the rectus sheath, and this space is extended to the right of the linea alba by approximately 2 cm to 3 cm (Fig. 53-2). The area under the right costal margin (space of Larrei) is also dissected using electrocautery to further extend the plane. If necessary, any terminal branches of the right internal mammary artery should be ligated to avoid postoperative bleeding. The additional margin on the right facilitates subsequent abdominal closure and allows adequate room for the outflow valve conduit and graft to sit without impingement. The muscular attachment of the right hemidiaphragm to the medial edge of the sternum is also divided to provide room for the crossing outflow graft. Superiorly, dissection is taken to the undersurface of the diaphragm where the apex of the heart can be palpated just lateral to the inferior phrenic vessels. These vessels are generally ligated because they can be injured during transdiaphragmatic placement of the inflow cannula, and visualization of the bleeding is often difficult after device insertion. Further dissection is carried out laterally and inferiorly to create additional space for the device and can be extended as far posterior as the spleen. A plastic HeartMate sizer device is

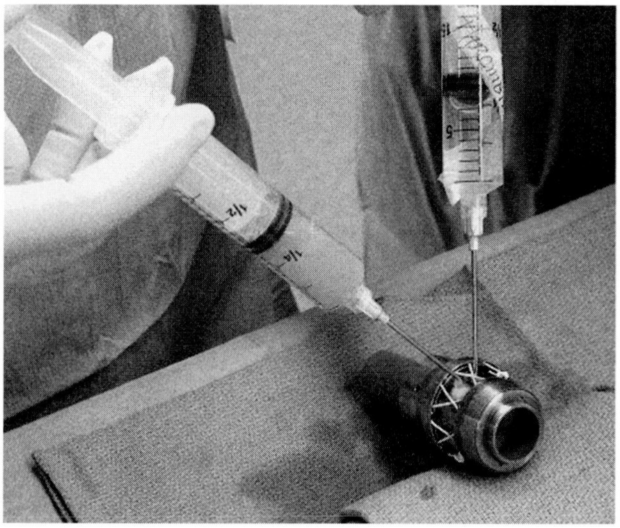

Figure 53-1. Preclotting the inflow valve conduit.

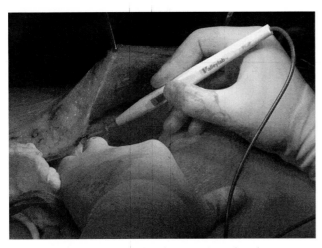

Figure 53-2.   Creating the preperitoneal pocket.

often placed into the pocket to determine whether enough room is available for the actual LVAD. The pocket is bounded anteriorly by the posterior rectus sheath and transversalis fascia and posteriorly by the preperitoneal fat and peritoneum. If the peritoneum is entered during the dissection process, the defect is repaired with 3-0 Vicryl sutures to prevent any herniation of abdominal contents. If the proper plane is difficult to develop, the rectus sheath can be entered and the posterior sheath left as a patch over that area of peritoneum. In some patients, a synthetic patch can be placed above the peritoneum to promote anterior displacement of the device. This prevents posterior compression of the underlying stomach, which can result in abdominal discomfort, early satiety, and partial outlet obstruction in some patients. In other patients where abdominal closure is anticipated to be tight due to narrow body girth, for example, a polypropylene or Marlex mesh (C.R. Bard, Inc., Murray Hill, NJ) can be placed above the device at the end of the procedure. This bridges together the edges of the abdominal fascia and permits the abdomen to be closed without excessive tension.

The driveline is attached to the inferolateral aspect of the device and will course from within the preperitoneal pocket below the umbilicus to its exit site just superior to McBurney's point (approximately three fingerbreadths below the right costal margin in the midclavicular line). An approximately 1.3-cm circular exit site incision (similar to that used for an ostomy) is made first, and dissection is carried down to the level of the anterior rectus sheath. The incision should be large enough to accommodate the driveline tunneler, but not so large as to permit laxity of the percutaneous tube at the exit site. The tunneling device is passed subcutaneously and directed inferiorly to a point

just below the umbilicus. Once the tunneler enters the most inferior aspect of the LVAD pocket, the entry point should be examined to assure there is no bleeding from any vessels associated with the rectus muscles. The swiveling bullet on the end of the percutaneous tube is screwed onto the tunneler, and the entire driveline is brought back through the subcutaneous tunnel (Fig. 53-3). Before actually tunneling the driveline, one needs to ensure that the tunneling shroud has been firmly applied to the vent holes of the percutaneous tube. This prevents material from entering the vent holes during the tunneling process. At least 2.5 cm of the smaller-diameter polyester velour covering the percutaneous tube should remain within the subcutaneous tunnel prior to exiting the skin to facilitate tissue adherence and minimize the risk of exit site infection. The exteriorized driveline is covered with antibiotic-moistened lap pads until connection with the system controller is required during electrical actuation of the LVAD. The percutaneous tube can be anchored at the exit site medially and laterally with a heavy monofilament suture, but these

should be removed at 4 to 6 weeks postoperatively.

A full cardiopulmonary bypass dose of heparin is administered, and standard aortic and dual stage venous cannulae are placed. Bicaval venous cannulation can be used if access to the right atrium is necessary (e.g., to close a patent foramen ovale). Cardiopulmonary bypass is initiated without cardioplegic arrest (unless concomitant procedures are to be performed). The left ventricular apex is elevated with laparotomy pads and its characteristic dimple is identified before coring. With the left ventricle distended, a small, 0.5-cm incision is made into the center of the anticipated coring site using a No. 11 blade. The HeartMate coring knife is slid over a 14-F Foley catheter (C.R. Bard, Inc., Covington, GA), which serves as a ventricular vent, and the catheter is inserted into the left ventricular apex. The Foley catheter balloon is filled with 5 ml of normal saline, and gentle traction is maintained on the catheter towards the apex. The cutting edge of the coring knife is applied to the epicardium and rotated back and forth until the ventricular cavity is entered. During this process, the Foley catheter is used as a centering guide and the coring knife is aimed toward the mitral valve inflow and lateral wall of the left ventricle. This avoids angling the inflow cannula toward the interventricular septum. Metzenbaum scissors are used to completely excise any residual muscle or scar tissue. The left ventricular cavity is inspected for the presence of retained core tissue or thrombus; loose thrombi are removed and adherent mural thrombi are generally left in place.

The apical sewing ring is positioned such that the felt portion is directed toward the heart and the silicone, tubular portion is facing outward. The plastic centering device is kept in place until the inflow valve conduit is

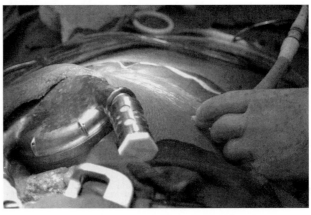

Figure 53-3.   Tunneling the driveline.

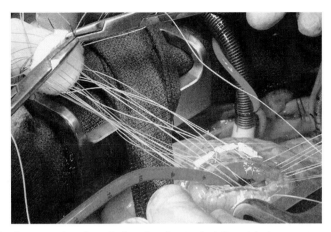

Figure 53-4. Anastomosing the apical sewing ring to the left ventricular apex.

ready to be inserted. A minimum of 12 pledgeted 2-0 TI-CRON sutures (Tyco Healthcare Group LP, Norwalk, CT) are placed partial thickness into the myocardium in circumferential fashion around the core. Full-thickness bites should be taken if the myocardium is scarred, attenuated, or friable, as in the post–myocardial infarction setting, for example. The sutures should be distanced approximately 1.5 cm from the perimeter of the core, and then placed into their corresponding positions on the felt sewing cuff (Figs. 53-4 and 53-5). Polar coordinates are marked on the felt of the sewing ring to assure proper alignment. Each suture should be tied with six or seven knots snug enough to cause slight dimpling of the myocardial cuff.

An incision must be made in the diaphragm to permit connection of the left ventricular apex and the LVAD inflow valve conduit. We prefer to use a 28-mm end-to-end anastomosis (EEA) stapling device for this purpose. A cruciate incision is made in the diaphragm opposite the left ventricular apex and just lateral to the inferior phrenic vessels. The stapler is introduced from the side of the preperitoneal pocket and deployed, and the core of diaphragmatic tissue is removed. This EEA stapler size is sufficiently large to accommodate the inflow valve conduit. The pericardium is entered and reflected to the left. A direct window is now evident between the left ventricular apex and the preperitoneal pocket. Before inserting the titanium inflow valve conduit into the apical sewing ring, the plastic centering device needs to be removed. The inflow cannula is passed through the hole in the left hemidiaphragm and into the silicone portion of the ring until the entire sintered titanium surface is fully seated against the

edge of the cuff (Fig. 53-6). Proper positioning of the LVAD should orient the inlet cannula toward the mitral valve while avoiding kinking of the inflow conduit and malrotation of the native heart. The green TI-CRON suture on the sewing ring is tied down tightly over the inflow cannula until the silicone sleeve visibly puckers. This ensures that the connection will be snug and leak-resistant. We reinforce this connection even further by tying down two umbilical tapes. Finally, BioGlue (CryoLife, Inc., Kennesaw, GA) is applied over the plastic ring at the green TI-CRON suture penetration sites. As attention is next turned to creating the aortic anastomosis, the pump itself is covered with antibiotic-soaked laparotomy pads.

The anastomosis should be positioned with consideration for the subsequent operation, which is most often cardiac transplantation. The graft should be positioned high enough to permit aortic-aortic anastomosis for transplant but low enough to facilitate placement of an aortic cross-clamp. A partial occlusion clamp is placed on the right lateral aspect of the proximal ascending aorta and a longitudinal aortotomy is made (Fig. 53-7). The incision can be widened by trimming extra tissue from either edge. An aortic punch is also used to round out the apices of the aortotomy and open the incision further. The outflow graft is cut to a length that accommodates the size of the patient. Care must be taken not to leave the graft too long because this could lead to kinking and the development of high pressures and low LVAD outflow. Nor should the graft be trimmed too short, especially if anticipated device removal or replacement is to be attempted through an extrathoracic approach. In general at least two thirds of the length of the outflow valve conduit should sit below the right costal margin once the pump is in place. The optimal graft length in most adults ranges between 12 cm and 14 cm. Before beginning the aortic anastomosis, one needs to make sure that the securing nut overlies the outflow graft; this is necessary to assure firm connection of the outflow graft to the housing unit later.

The anastomosis is created in a graft-to-aorta end-to-side fashion using 4-0 Prolene sutures (Fig. 53-8). Four horizontal mattress anchor sutures are placed in the 12-o'clock, 3-o'clock, 6-o'clock, and 9-o'clock positions, respectively, and each is run in continuous fashion clockwise to the next stitch. The anastomosis is sometimes buttressed with a strip of bovine or autologous pericardium, although it has been our preference to apply BioGlue over the suture line

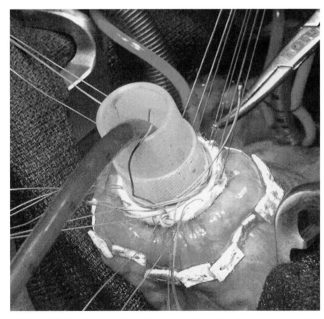

Figure 53-5. Completion of the apical sewing ring anastomosis.

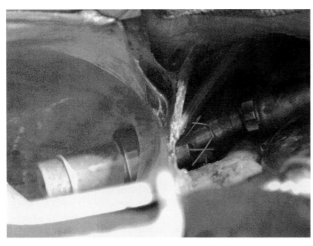

Figure 53-6. Passing the inflow valve conduit through the left hemidiaphragm.

in most instances (Fig. 53-9). A cross-clamp is placed on the outflow graft, although not on the overlying bend relief. The aortic clamp is removed, and de-airing precautions are taken with the patient in Trendelenburg position. The outflow graft connector is inspected and confirmed to be clean and free of thrombus. The presence of thrombus can preclude a water-tight seal, leading to potential serious hemorrhage. Bleeding from this connection can be reinforced and tamponaded with circumferential heavy silk ties onto the bend relief.

Throughout the implant procedure, large pockets of air are often retained within the pump, and therefore it is imperative to de-air the heart and the device in proper sequence. One removes the white thread protector on the outflow graft bend relief and the hexagonal white cap from the outflow conduit. One backfills the graft with blood from the aorta,

then reapplies the cross-clamp to the graft. The left heart is filled by increasing return from cardiopulmonary bypass; this allows blood to flow passively from the left ventricle into the device and through the outflow conduit. The outflow graft is now connected to the outflow valve conduit and the securing nut is screwed in a clockwise direction until it can no longer turn any. The cross-clamp is removed from the outflow graft, and an 18-gauge needle is inserted into the graft at its highest point to serve as an air vent. A partial occlusion clamp is applied distal to the de-airing hole. The hand pump is connected to the vent adapter, which, in turn, is connected to the percutaneous tube. Before the hand pumping process is initiated, cardiopulmonary bypass flow is reduced by at least 2 liters/min of blood flow to the ventricle. The patient is kept in steep Trendelenburg position while hand pumping is

begun. The handles are squeezed to collapse the black bulb and the bulb is slowly allowed to fully inflate after each pumping cycle. The lungs are inflated and the device is hand-pumped to remove the remaining air. De-airing is continued until no air is seen by transesophageal echocardiogram, at which time the outflow graft partial cross-clamp is removed. After this is completed, the 18-gauge needle can be removed from the graft and its insertion site repaired with a 4-0 Prolene suture.

The hand pump is removed from the vent adapter, and the percutaneous tube is connected to the system controller. The white power connector of the system controller cable is connected to the white connector of the power base unit (PBU) cable. Inotropic and pressor support is started before completely weaning from bypass and activating the LVAD. In the setting of elevated pulmonary pressures, we prefer to use dobutamine and milrinone to augment filling of the LVAD. The use of inhaled nitric oxide has also been beneficial in reducing pulmonary pressures in select patients. Norepinephrine and arginine vasopressin are added to maintain mean arterial blood pressure >65 mm Hg. The LVAD is begun at 50 beats per minute (bpm) in "fixed rate" mode. The target stroke volume is between 70 mL and 80 mL. When the LVAD is electrically activated, rapid reduction of cardiopulmonary bypass flow ensues, ensuring ample blood flow to the device without overdistending the right side of the heart. The black connectors of the PBU and system controller are connected in the same manner as the white connectors. One continues to wean the patient off of cardiopulmonary bypass while slowly increasing the LVAD fixed rate to maintain adequate filling. Once cardiopulmonary bypass is weaned off and the patient is deemed hemodynamically stable, the LVAD is switched from "fixed rate" mode to automatic ("auto") mode. Depending on the clinical condition of the patient, this transition may not be feasible until 24 to 48 hours in the postoperative period. The automatic mode more closely resembles the physiologic response of the heart; the device ejects blood when the pump is at least 97% full or when it senses a decreased rate of filling. Thus, the pump reacts to an increase in the patient's activity level by increasing its output.

Before chest and abdominal closure, the pump housing needs to be anchored within the LVAD pocket (Fig. 53-10). Heavy, nonabsorbable sutures are used to attach the device to the abdominal wall or fascia via the eyelets on the titanium housing. Failure to

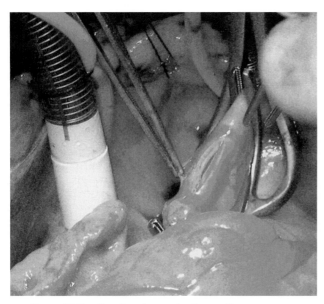

Figure 53-7. Creating the proximal ascending aortotomy.

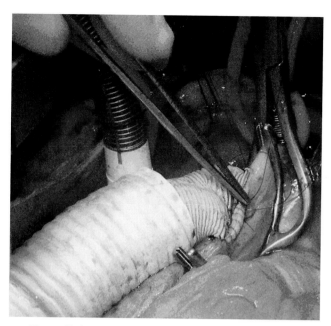

Figure 53-8. Sewing the outflow graft-aorta anastomosis.

thrombin (Gen Trac, Inc., Middleton, WI). This paste is mixed in the operating room and applied to the LVAD pocket and around the sternum before chest and abdominal closure. The vancomycin has antimicrobial action directed primarily against staphylococcal species, and the MCH and thrombin provide a solid, hemostatic lattice.

In some patients with thin torsos, abdominal closure is difficult because of excessive tension imposed by the device within the preperitoneal pocket. To ameliorate this problem, we sometimes place a midline, Marlex mesh to bridge the defect created in the linea alba and abdominal fascia. This strategy is also useful in any patient in whom abdominal herniation is a concern. Moreover, the additional space created by the mesh affords further anterior displacement of the device, thereby minimizing the potential for posterior compression of the stomach. This may allow for placement of devices into smaller recipients, in general.

anchor the LVAD in place can lead to movement or migration within the body and potential adverse consequences. Pocket drains are also placed to minimize the likelihood of pocket hematomas or fluid collections. We prefer to use two Blake drains placed superior and inferior to the pump. These drains are kept in place until they put out <100 mL per 24-hour period. This generally occurs between the postoperative days 3 and 7. In the chest, both anterior and posterior peri-

cardial chest tubes are placed, along with pleural chest tubes, if necessary.

Additional measures are taken to reduce the likelihood of postoperative sternal wound and LVAD pocket infection. We favor the use of a paste created from a combination of 1 g of vancomycin, 2 g of microfibrillar collagen hemostat (MCH) (Avitene, Davol, Inc., Cranston, RI) or INSTAT MCH (Ethicon, Inc.; Johnson & Johnson, Piscataway, NJ), and 20,000 units of bovine-origin

Potential Complications and Postoperative Care

The most common complications associated with LVAD therapy include perioperative bleeding, right-sided heart failure, acute renal failure, infection, and thromboembolism. All of these confer significant morbidity and mortality in both the early and late postoperative periods. Table 53-5 reflects our cumulative experience of these complications using the HeartMate LVAD. Indeed, many of these factors are also the major drivers of hospitalization costs, either through the direct utilization of resources to correct them or through the additional time spent in the ICU and operating room. The following discussion elaborates on the development of postoperative complications and highlights our perioperative strategies for countering them (Table 53-6).

The incidence of perioperative bleeding ranges between 25% and 60% at most centers, with a reoperative rate upward of 50%. The frequency of bleeding occurs independent of whether the specific device used requires systemic anticoagulation. Device-induced alterations of the balance between coagulation and fibrinolysis have been implicated. For the HeartMate LVAD, this process may evolve from the direct contact made between the LVAD prosthetic membrane and blood elements. In the early postoperative period, hemostasis is influenced primarily by activation of the intrinsic contact-dependent fibrinolysis system with consumption of contact

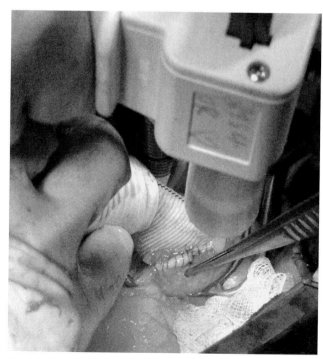

Figure 53-9. Applying BioGlue to the outflow graft-aortic anastomosis suture line.

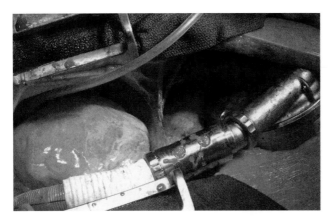

Figure 53-10.   HeartMate left ventricular assist device in situ.

factors and increased levels of plasmin–α2-antiplasmin (PAP) complexes. Other factors that contribute to high bleeding rates include preoperative hepatic insufficiency, preoperative malnutrition, reoperative surgery, prolonged cardiopulmonary bypass times, extensive surgical dissection, and renal failure–induced platelet dysfunction. The risk for major hemorrhage has decreased significantly with the routine intraoperative use of the serine protease inhibitor aprotinin and preoperative administration of vitamin K in certain patients. This practice has led to a decreased rate of blood product transfusion and consequent incidence of right-sided heart failure and immune sensitization. Research efforts are investigating the synthesis of anticoagulants that operate at higher levels in the coagulation cascade (factors IX and Xa), thereby minimizing the extent of postoperative bleeding.

Right heart failure occurs in approximately 20% to 30% of patients following LVAD implantation, necessitating subsequent placement of a right VAD (RVAD) in certain instances. The causes for right-sided circulatory failure are multifactorial and are felt to be related to anatomic, intraoperative, and perioperative factors. From an anatomic perspective, mechanical unloading of the left ventricle by the LVAD causes bowing of the interventricular septum away from the right ventricle. Although this mechanism theoretically improves diastolic compliance, if peak left ventricular pressure is reduced, the interventricular septum tends to bulge into the left ventricle, reducing the efficiency of right ventricular contractility. Moreover, as the LVAD enhances forward flow to the systemic circulation, it can increase venous return beyond the capacity of the right ventricle. The incidence of right heart failure is usually associated with intra- and perioperative bleeding and subsequent blood product transfusion. Such resuscitation increases the production of cytokines such as interleukin-1β, interleukin-6, interleukin-10, and tumor necrosis factor-α, the collective effects of which can induce pulmonary

hypertension. This scenario is often compounded by an additional degree of pulmonary vasoconstriction mediated by cardiopulmonary bypass-related generation of thromboxane A2. We maintain a low threshold to initiate therapy with inhaled nitric oxide, which substantially reduces pulmonary artery pressures and averts the need for RVAD placement in many patients.

Acute renal failure is a common complication following LVAD placement, although the incidence is more pronounced in those with some degree of renal insufficiency preoperatively. At our institution, acute renal failure occurs in upward of 40% of LVAD recipients. The etiology is almost always acute tubular necrosis (ATN), a consequence of low-flow states that can occur within the intra- and postoperative periods. These conditions are often reversible if adequate LVAD flows can be maintained, but some patients will require temporary support with continuous venovenous hemodialysis (CVVHD) within the ICU setting.

As many as 28% to 66% of patients develop some form of infection while on LVAD support, although the use of smaller axial flow pumps has reportedly decreased those rates significantly. The most common types of infections involve the LVAD driveline, the preperitoneal pocket, the device itself, and the sternal and abdominal wounds. Bacteremia and sepsis also occur not infrequently and contribute to even further morbidity and mortality. Numerous factors account for the high propensity toward infection in this patient population. First, the operation involves placement of a large, cumbersome foreign-bodied device into patients who are generally elderly and

Table 53-5 Postoperative Complications Associated with the HeartMate Left Ventricular Assist Device	
Complication	**Number (%)**
Bleeding	47 (23.60%)
Right heart failure	24 (12.18%)
Acute renal failure	83 (42.13%)
Infection	87 (44.16%)
Driveline	10 (5.08%)
Pocket	30 (15.23%)
Device	11 (5.58%)
Wound	33 (16.75%)
Bacteremia	25 (12.69%)
Sepsis	28 (14.21%)
Thromboembolism	24 (12.18%)

Total number of patients = 197.

Table 53-6 Optimal Clinical Management Strategies within the Perioperative Period		
Preoperative	**Intraoperative**	**Postoperative**
IABP	Aprotinin	Nitric oxide
Early LVAD implantation	BioGlue	Phosphodiesterase inhibitors (milrinone)
Optimization of fluid status	Nitric oxide	Aggressive use of RVADs for RV failure
Broad-spectrum antibiotics	Phosphodiesterase inhibitors (milrinone)	Avoidance of excessive blood products
Nutritional supplementation	Screening for PFO	CVVH
	INSTAT antibiotic paste	Use of abdominal binder
		Early mobilization
		Physical rehabilitation
		Early enteral feeding and nutritional supplementation

IABP = intra-aortic balloon pump; PFO = patent foramen ovale; RVAD = right ventricular assist device; RV = right ventricle; CVVH = continuous venovenous hemofiltration.

therefore relatively immunocompromised. With the HeartMate unit, the device traverses two body cavities and incorporates a sizeable incision, and therefore the potential for wound and LVAD pocket infections is substantial. Second, many LVAD recipients are severely malnourished on entering surgery. Much of this derives from the overall catabolic state associated with chronic heart failure, and crucial proteins and amino acids are shunted away from the pathways required for maintenance of immune integrity. Postoperatively, these malnourished patients are placed at a significant disadvantage in terms of wound healing, immune response, or both. Third, there is evidence to suggest that the biosynthetic membrane used in certain pulsatile LVADs, by making direct contact with elements of the blood circulation, induces circulating CD4 T-cell apoptosis. This process generates progressive defects in cellular immunity and places patients at an increased risk of serious infection. The mainstay of treatment for all infections remains judicious use of antibiotics in conjunction with operative debridement and device replacement, when necessary. We also advocate use of an abdominal binder to reduce the risk of driveline infection as a result of exit site trauma. Further technological advances will steer toward the development of smaller, totally implantable devices that minimize the degree of host–environment interface. Aggressive perioperative nutritional supplementation with immune-enhancing compounds (arginine, glutamine, oligonucleotides, omega-3 fatty acids) is necessary to promote proper wound healing and maintain adequate immune defenses.

The incidence of thromboembolic events ranges from 5% to 11% and hinges on a tight balance between the coagulation and fibrinolysis pathways. The general observation has been that the early postoperative period is complicated by bleeding and the later course is complicated by thromboembolic phenomena. This phenomenon poses a difficult dilemma when managing recipients with VAD types that require postoperative anticoagulation. The HeartMate LVAD is unique in that it features a textured, blood-contacting surface (sintered titanium microspheres on the metallic surface and integrally textured polyurethane on the pusher-plate diaphragm) that is promptly covered by a densely adherent neointima after implantation. This biosynthetic membrane reduces the risk of thromboembolization and minimizes the necessity for systemic anti-coagulation. For the majority of LVADs that do in fact require anticoagulation (including the newer axial flow devices), most centers use a combination of heparin and low-molecular-weight dextran and transition to oral warfarin when the chest tubes have been removed. A regimen of aspirin or dipyridamole, both antiplatelet agents, is also administered in many of these patients, yet is the only mode of antithrombotic therapy in HeartMate LVAD recipients.

Conclusion

With the prevalence of congestive heart failure ever increasing worldwide and the total number of donor hearts for cardiac transplantation remaining constant, the current place for VADs is firmly established. Ventricular assist devices have effectively expanded their role to include serving as a means of bridge to transplantation, bridge to recovery, and destination therapy. Although the efficacy of VADs continues to be hampered in part by the development of numerous postoperative complications, further device modification and improvements in perioperative care promise to enhance clinical outcomes. These devices will remain an attractive alternative for patients with end-stage heart failure refractory to optimal medical therapy, but they may also bear application to a broader class of less severe heart failure patients in the future. Thus, as technology responds to the demands imposed by medical illness, it, in turn, has the potential to dramatically shape the face of heart failure.

SUGGESTED READING

Gelijns AC, Richards AF, Williams DL, et al. Evolving costs of long-term left ventricular assist device implantation. Ann Thorac Surg 1997;64:1312.

Goldstein DJ, Moazami N, Seldomridge JA, et al. Circulatory resuscitation with left ventricular assist device support reduces interleukins 6 and 8 levels. Ann Thorac Surg 1997;63:971.

Goldstein DJ, Oz MC (eds). Cardiac Assist Devices. Armonk, NY: Futura, 2000.

Goldstein DJ, Oz MC, Rose EA. Implantable left ventricular assist devices. N Engl J Med 1998;339:1522.

James KJ, McCarthy PM, Thomas JD, et al. Effect of the implantable left ventricular assist device on neuroendocrine activation in heart failure. Circulation 1995;92(Suppl 9):II-191.

John R, Lietz K, Schuster M, et al. Immunologic sensitization in recipients of left ventricular assist devices. J Thorac Cardiovasc Surg 2003;125:578.

Kaltenmaier B, Pommer W, Kaufmann F, et al. Outcome of patients with ventricular assist devices and acute renal failure requiring renal replacement therapy. ASAIO J 2000;46:330.

Oz MC, Gelijns AC, Miller L, et al. Left ventricular assist devices as permanent heart failure therapy: The price of progress. Ann Surg 2003;238:577; discussion 583.

Oz MC, Goldstein DJ, Pepino P, et al. Screening scale predicts patients successfully receiving long-term implantable left ventricular assist devices. Circulation 1995;92(9 Suppl): II-169.

Rao V, Oz MC, Flannery MA, et al. Revised screening scale to predict survival after insertion of a left ventricular assist device. J Thorac Cardiovasc Surg 2003;125:855.

Rose EA, Gelijns AC, Moskowitz AJ, et al. Randomized Evaluation of Mechanical Assistance for the Treatment of Congestive Heart Failure (REMATCH) Study Group. Long-term mechanical left ventricular assistance for end-stage heart failure. N Engl J Med 2001;345:1435.

Slater JP, Williams M, Oz MC. Implantation techniques for the TCI HeartMate left ventricular assist systems. In Cox JL (ed). Operative Techniques in Thoracic and Cardiovascular Surgery, Vol 4, No 4. Orlando, FL: Saunders, 1999;330.

EDITOR'S COMMENTS

The Columbia group has had some of the most extensive experience with the use of ventricular assist devices. This chapter describes is a very practical approach to placement and care of the ventricular assist device. In our institution we have used ventricular assist mostly as a bridge to transplantation. We have not used it very much as rescue therapy or as destination therapy. Although we are approved for destination therapy, finding the proper patients for that indication is not easy. The use of ventricular assist device as a bridge for transplantation is a very straightforward approach and clearly has saved lives by maintaining the health of the future transplant recipient. It has provided excellent results in terms of long-term survival. The more difficult issue is salvage of the patient who does not do well after cardiopulmonary bypass. As the authors noted, the worst results are in patients who have other organ failure. Unfortunately, this is what we deal with in such salvage cases. Clearly the technology of the devices has to improve to resolve that particular problem.

The best present use of ventricular assistance is as a bridge to transplantation.

I.L.K.

54

Surgery for Complications of Myocardial Infarction

Mark F. Berry and Timothy J. Gardner

Introduction

Surgical intervention is often required to manage acute mechanical complications of myocardial infarctions. These mechanical complications, which are responsible for 15% to 20% of deaths after acute myocardial infarction, have historically been considered to include free ventricular wall rupture, acute ventricular septal defects, and acute ischemic mitral regurgitation. An acute myocardial infarction complication increasingly considered to be mechanical and amenable to surgical intervention is "pump failure," or cardiogenic shock refractory to maximal medical treatment and revascularization. Surgical techniques used for this complication include ventricular assist device implantation and transplantation.

Free Ventricular Wall Rupture

Incidence and Pathogenesis

Free ventricular wall rupture is found in approximately one fourth of patients who die within 3 weeks of an acute myocardial infarction. Overall, free wall rupture occurs in up to 11% of patients after acute infarction. Rupture location depends on the site of the infarct, with the rupture tract most commonly occurring between viable and necrotic myocardium. Rupture usually occurs after acute expansion of a transmural infarction. Infarct hemorrhage may play a role because revascularization with thrombolytic therapy but not angioplasty has been found to be independently associated with rupture of both the free wall and the septum.

Clinical Presentation and Diagnosis

Free wall rupture has acute, subacute, and chronic presentations. Acute rupture usually results in death within minutes. Subacute rupture represents 20% to 40% of the cases of free wall rupture, and presents as cardiac tamponade progressing to shock. Echocardiography evaluating for a pericardial effusion in the presence of ventricular wall defects in a patient with tamponade physiology after acute infarction is used for diagnosis. Chronic rupture is rare and involves a contained ventricular leak that results in a pseudoaneurysm. Most patients have symptoms of congestive heart failure, chest pain, or dyspnea, although 12% to 23% are asymptomatic. More than two thirds of patients have a murmur, and virtually all patients have nonspecific electrocardiogram abnormalities. Most patients have cardiomegaly on chest x-ray. Angiography, echocardiography, computed tomography scans, radionuclide scans, and magnetic resonance imaging can be used to identify the pseudoaneurysm.

Natural History

Acute rupture rarely allows time for intervention and is invariably fatal. Patients with subacute rupture have a median survival of 8 hours after symptom onset, with a range from 45 minutes to 6.5 weeks. Only 17 cases of survival without surgery for subacute rupture have been reported. The natural history of chronic rupture is not well defined. One study identified 290 patients reported in the literature as having a left ventricular pseudoaneurysm, 139 of which had resulted from a myocardial infarction. Of 31 patients treated conservatively, 15 died at <1 week

from infarction and the other 16 survived long term, which suggests that chronic pseudoaneurysms are relatively stable.

Preoperative Treatment and Operative Timing

Acute rupture is generally not amenable to any attempts at repair. Emergent operative repair is needed for any patient with a subacute rupture, and the patient must be brought immediately to the operating room. Pericardiocentesis at the time of echocardiography can provide short-term hemodynamic improvement in some patients, allowing some degree of stability while preparing for surgery. Inotropic agents, fluid infusion, vasoconstrictors, and an intra-aortic balloon pump can also be used to maintain hemodynamics during transfer to the operating room.

Timing of surgical repair for chronic rupture depends on the interval between infarction and diagnosis. Patients who are within a few months of infarction are thought to have a high risk for rupture and should undergo urgent cardiac catheterization to evaluate the extent of coronary artery disease followed by operative repair of the pseudoaneurysm. The need for surgery in patients who present after an extended period after infarction depends on whether the pseudoaneurysm is >3 cm, expanding, or symptomatic, or if the patient has mitral regurgitation and/or severe coronary artery disease that requires intervention.

Operative Technique

Patients with subacute rupture are rapidly prepared for a standard median sternotomy, with close monitoring of hemodynamics during anesthesia induction because significant hypotension can occur. Close hemodynamic monitoring is also required when the pericardium is decompressed because hypertension can occur and possibly worsen the rupture size and the amount of bleeding. The tear location and status and the patient status determine the need for cardiopulmonary bypass. Cardiopulmonary bypass is instituted in all hemodynamically unstable patients. Bypass is also used if the rupture cannot be exposed adequately without excessive compromise of circulation or if the

bleeding from the rupture cannot be controlled or prevents adequate repair.

Subacute rupture can be repaired by various techniques, which should be kept as simple as possible. Sutures should not be placed into friable myocardium. Epicardial repair can be performed by placement of a patch of pericardium, Dacron, or polytetrafluoroethylene felt over the ventricular defect; the patch is sutured to healthy myocardium along the periphery of the infarct (Fig. 54-1A). The rupture can also be closed directly with horizontal mattress

sutures buttressed with Teflon felt strips and a patch secured over the repair (Fig. 54-1B). Biocompatible glue can also be used to further reinforce the patch over the defect (Fig. 54-1C). Simple epicardial repair is not appropriate when a intraventricular defect such as septal rupture or papillary muscle rupture also exists. Operative options in these cases require cardiopulmonary bypass and aortic cross-clamping with infarct excision and defect closure using a patch or infarct exclusion, which are described in detail in the following sections.

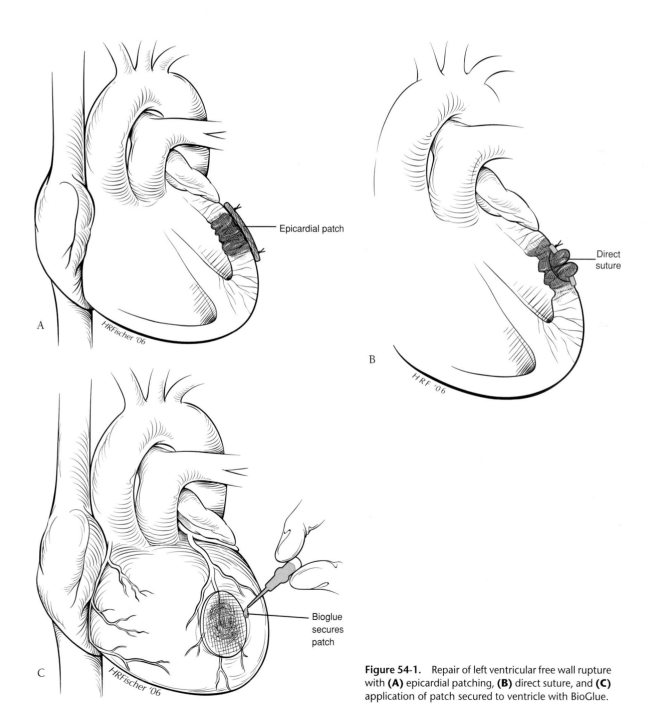

Figure 54-1. Repair of left ventricular free wall rupture with **(A)** epicardial patching, **(B)** direct suture, and **(C)** application of patch secured to ventricle with BioGlue.

The decision to repair a chronic ventricular rupture is partially based on the presence of either mitral dysfunction or coronary disease. Cardiopulmonary bypass is instituted, and the chronic rupture site is repaired similarly to an acute rupture. Anterior pseudoaneurysms can usually be closed directly because of the presence of fibrotic edges. Posterior pseudoaneurysms are closed with a patch so ventricular geometry is not distorted. Even for cases in which the primary purpose of the operation is to repair a large or expanding pseudoaneurysm, cardiopulmonary bypass is indicated to allow adequate exposure for repair and to also prevent the systemic embolization of thrombotic material from within the pseudoaneurysm cavity.

Survival

Most reports of surgical intervention for subacute rupture involve a limited number of patients. These reports, however, indicate that a significant number of patients can be saved from this lethal condition with prompt diagnosis and intervention. In one series, 2 of 5 patients who were extremely unstable and underwent emergent repair of a subacute rupture survived long term. In another series of 5 patients treated similarly, there were 4 survivors. In a series of 6 patients treated with a sutureless patch over an 8-year period, 5 patients survived to leave the hospital. The experience with surgical management of chronic rupture is also limited and largely anecdotal. In one series, 8 of 12 patients treated for a chronic rupture were long-term survivors. All deaths occurred in patients with poor ventricular function or mitral valve disease.

Ventricular Septal Defect

Incidence and Pathogenesis

An acute ventricular septal defect (VSD) is an uncommon but lethal complication of infarction. A VSD that occurs within 4 to 6 weeks of infarction is considered acute. Even though the septum is involved in up to 70% of all infarcts, acute VSD historically has complicated only 1% to 2% of all infarctions, with recent evidence suggesting that the incidence is now <1%. This decreased incidence may reflect the success of interventions that limit muscle necrosis and prevent transmural infarctions. However, the time between infarction and the VSD occurrence appears to be becoming shorter.

Because infarct hemorrhage may play a role in septal rupture, thrombolysis may accelerate the time course of VSDs in those patients in which they occur.

Patients with acute postinfarction VSD have an average age of 62.5 years; the male-to-female ratio is 3:2, although the incidence may be rising in women. Acute VSD usually occurs after occlusion of a coronary artery that results in a full-thickness infarction that is on average larger (25% of the total left ventricular wall mass) than an infarction that is not complicated by a VSD (15%). The infarcts in patients who develop a postinfarction VSD more commonly involve both ventricles than the infarcts in those patients who do not develop a VSD. The typical patient has single-vessel disease with poor collateral flow and presents with an anterior infarct. Although this complication may occur as early as a few hours and as late as a few weeks after infarction, the diagnosis is most commonly made within 4 days of the onset of infarction symptoms. The time of septal rupture correlates with the period when necrotic muscle from the infarction has not been adequately replaced by fibrous connective tissue. Defect size ranges from 0.3 cm to 4.0 cm, with an average of 1.7 cm.

Historically, acute septal defects were described primarily in the anteroapical septum as a result of left anterior descending artery occlusion. Recent data, however, suggest that the proportion of posterior VSDs is rising, and these now represent one third to one half of VSDs. Posterior VSDs result from occlusion of a dominant right coronary artery or a dominant circumflex artery. Defects are classified as either simple or complex. Simple defects are usually located anteriorly. Complex defects are usually located inferiorly and have a worse prognosis. Multiple VSDs occur in 5% to 11% of cases. One third of cases involve mitral valve regurgitation, which results from either papillary muscle infarction (15% of cases) or left ventricular dysfunction and mitral annular dilation. The mitral regurgitation seen due to left ventricular dysfunction generally resolves with repair of the VSD, whereas papillary muscle rupture requires valve replacement.

Clinical Presentation and Diagnosis

An acute VSD typically presents with recurrent chest pain, a new holosystolic murmur and palpable left sternal thrill, and hemodynamic deterioration a few days after acute infarction. Septal rupture causes left-to–right shunting that can result in heart failure. Clinical presentation varies from

an asymptomatic murmur to cardiogenic shock. Symptoms occur due to both ventricular dysfunction and the shunting caused by the VSD. Failure occurring with an anterior VSD is usually the result of both the VSD and extensive left ventricular infarction, whereas failure occurring with a posterior VSD is usually due to extensive right ventricular infarction. Infarct location on the electrocardiogram (ECG) correlates highly with VSD location. The ECG often shows a rightward QRS axis shift and a right-bundle-branch block, and approximately one third of patients get a transient atrioventricular conduction block before septal rupture.

The clinical appearance of an acute VSD is very similar to that of acute mitral regurgitation. Physical exam and the electrocardiogram are used to distinguish between the two entities. The murmur associated with a VSD is most prominent at the left sternal border and is often accompanied by a thrill, whereas the murmur from acute mitral regurgitation is best heard at the apex and has no thrill. In addition, acute mitral regurgitation is more commonly associated with inferior infarctions and no conduction abnormalities. Echocardiography has a very high sensitivity and specificity in identifying the presence, size, and location of a VSD and shows a diagnostic trans-septal flow jet, as well as an echo-free area of the septum.

Demonstrating a 9% step-up in oxygen saturation from the right atrium to the pulmonary artery during right heart catheterization with pulmonary artery placement also confirms shunt presence due to VSD.

Natural History

Patients with a postinfarction VSD treated medically have a 1-year mortality as high as 97%. One fourth of patients die within 24 hours, and 80% die within 4 weeks. Death usually occurs as a result of end-organ failure due to shock.

Preoperative Therapy and Operative Timing

Because early surgical repair of acute VSDs had a very high mortality, surgical repair was previously delayed for 4 to 6 weeks to allow hemodynamic stabilization and fibrosis of the infarct to facilitate suturing around the VSD. Although some patients survived this delayed management, it became clear that only low-risk patients survived to surgical repair. Surgical intervention is now recognized as required before cardiogenic shock results in irreversible end-organ damage, and operative timing for repair is dictated by the patient's hemodynamic status.

Completely stable patients, comprising only a small proportion of patients, should have elective repair sometime during their hospitalization for the acute infarction.

Patients requiring pharmacologic support for heart failure require intervention within 12 to 24 hours of diagnosis. A patient in cardiogenic shock is a true surgical emergency and needs immediate repair. Patients who have already developed multisystem failure or sepsis are extremely high risk for emergency surgery and likely require further attempts at stabilization, with antibiotics as needed, before attempted repair.

The preoperative treatment goal is to divert blood systemically and maintain cardiac output, blood pressure, and coronary flow. Diuretics, inotropes, and vasodilators can minimize the left-to-right shunt; however, vasodilators are often not tolerated due to systemic hypotension. Vasoconstrictors increase afterload and can worsen left-to-right shunting and should be avoided if possible. An intra-aortic balloon pump (IABP) may improve cardiac output by reducing afterload and decreasing shunting and is mandatory in management of VSD patients who present in shock. However, IABP use has peak improvement within 24 hours and then no further benefit, so surgery should not be delayed beyond this time.

The role of preoperative coronary angiography is not completely clear; delaying surgical repair to perform cardiac catheterization during a period of patient instability is risky. In addition, the use of coronary angiography and coronary artery bypass grafting did not show improved short-term or long-term survival in a study of 179 patients with postinfarction VSD. However, routine coronary angiography detected significant coronary artery disease beyond the vessel that resulted in the acute infarction in 28 patients in another study of 54 patients with acute postinfarction VSDs. These patients underwent concomitant revascularization and experienced similar early and late survival compared to patients without associated coronary disease, suggesting that revascularization controlled the added risk of associated coronary disease. In another recent multi-institutional review, 42 of 65 patients who had coronary bypass grafting at the same time as VSD repair had significantly better survival both in the short-term and at 4 years. Given that coronary angiography can be performed very rapidly, a reasonable policy is to perform angiography with a limited amount of contrast in all patients who can be temporarily stabilized. Patients who are in severe shock should proceed directly to surgery for VSD repair.

Operative Technique

Several techniques can be used to repair acute postinfarction VSDs. Regardless of the specific technique utilized, a number of technical guidelines have been developed. A median sternotomy is performed with expeditious establishment of cardiopulmonary bypass using bicaval venous drainage. Cardioplegia should be first administered antegrade followed by retrograde via the coronary sinus to achieve optimal myocardial protection. In addition, patients with critical coronary stenoses identified preoperatively should undergo revascularization prior to VSD repair in order to maximize myocardial protection. A transinfarct approach to the VSD should be used. Because surgical success is completely dependent on adequate VSD closure, thorough evaluation for multiple defects must be performed both pre-operatively and intraoperatively. In patients with associated significant mitral regurgitation, mitral valve replacement is needed only if frank papillary muscle rupture has occurred. The septal defect and the infarctectomy must be closed without tension, which generally necessitates the use of prosthetic material. Finally, all suture lines must be buttressed with pledgets or Teflon felt.

Apical septal ruptures can be repaired using the technique of apical amputation described by Daggett (Fig. 54-2). An incision through the infarct is made, and all necrotic muscle of both ventricles and the septum is debrided. The remaining apical parts of the ventricles and septum are reapproximated by a row of interrupted mattress sutures using buttressing strips of felt.

Operative procedures to repair acute anterior VSDs include both infarctectomy and infarct exclusion. For the infarctectomy technique, a transinfarct incision is made, and infarct debridement with thorough trimming of left ventricular margins to viable muscle with more conservative trimming of the right ventricle is performed to simply allow adequate visualization of the septal defect margins (Fig. 54-3A). Small defects can be closed using a plication technique (Fig. 54-3B). The VSD is closed by approximating the anterior edge of the septum to the right ventricular wall with mattress sutures buttressed with felt strips. The ventricular incision is also closed with mattress sutures over felt. Larger defects require reconstruction of the septum and ventricular walls with prosthetic material to reduce postrepair tension (Fig. 54-3C). Sutures are first passed from right to left through the septum, and then additional sutures are

passed from the epicardial surface to the endocardial surface of the right ventricle. The anchored sutures are then passed through the patch and tied to close the VSD with the patch secured on the left side of the septum. The debrided infarct of the free ventricular wall is similarly closed with a patch as needed.

Infarct excision can distort ventricular geometry and has high potential for right heart dysfunction. David developed a procedure involving infarct exclusion rather than excision. A patch sutured to healthy myocardium excludes both the infarct and the VSD, preserving left ventricular geometry and function (Fig. 54-4). A transinfarct incision is made parallel to the left anterior descending coronary artery in the apex of the left ventricle. A patch tailored to the shape of the left ventricular infarction is sutured first to the endocardium of a noninfarcted portion of the septum and then to the noninfarcted endocardium of the anterolateral ventricular wall. The ventriculotomy is then closed over strips of felt.

Closure of posterior septal defects is technically challenging. The left side of the heart should be vented via the right superior pulmonary vein and the heart retracted as if preparing for a posterior bypass. As with anterior defects, repair can be performed with infarctectomy or infarct exclusion techniques. For the infarctectomy technique, a transinfarct incision is made, and the left ventricular portion of the infarct is thoroughly debrided to expose the septal defect. The papillary muscles should be inspected, and mitral valve replacement should be performed if papillary muscle rupture has occurred. As with anterior VSD repair, the portion of the right ventricle involved in the infarct is more conservatively trimmed to simply allow adequate visualization of the septal defect margins (Fig. 54-5A). Septal defects close to the adjacent ventricular free wall and not associated with significant loss of septal tissue can be repaired by approximating the septal rim of the posterior defect to the right ventricular free wall using buttressed mattress sutures (Fig. 54-5B). Larger defects require patch closure of both the septal defect and the infarct (Fig. 54-5C). Sutures are first passed from right to left through the septum, and then additional sutures are passed from the epicardial surface to the endocardial surface of the right ventricle. All placed sutures are then passed through the patch and tied to close the VSD.

David's infarct exclusion method can also be used to repair posterior defects (Fig. 54-6). An incision through the midportion of the inferior wall a few millimeters from

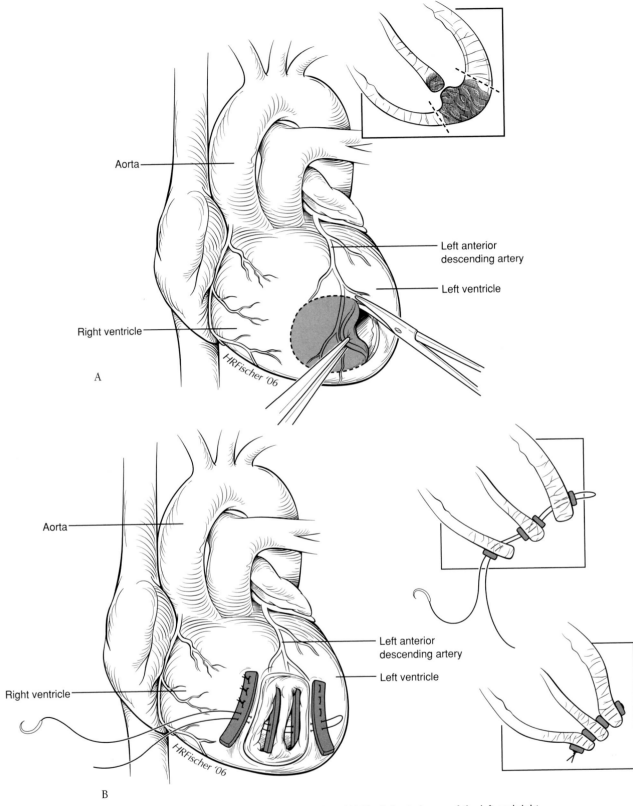

Figure 54-2.   Repair of apical ventricular septal defect. **(A)** The infarcted apex of the left and right ventricles is amputated to expose the septal defect. **(B)** The left ventricle, septal apex, and right ventricle are reapproximated with interrupted, buttressed mattress sutures.

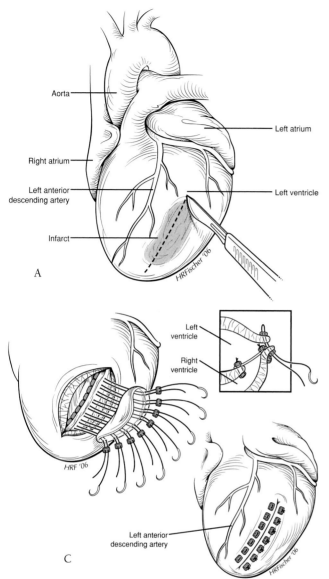

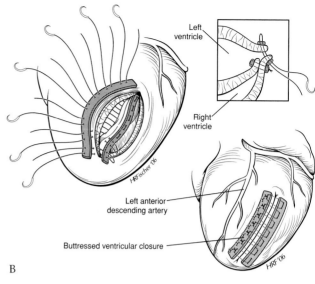

A

B

C

Figure 54-3. **(A)** A transinfarct incision is made in the left ventricle parallel to the left anterior descending coronary artery to repair an anterior postinfarction ventricular septal defect. **(B)** A small defect is repaired using the plication technique. The septal defect is closed by first approximating the anterior edge of the septum to the right ventricular wall with mattress sutures buttressed with felt strips, followed by buttressed closure of the ventricular incision. **(C)** Prosthetic material is used for reconstruction of the septum to reduce postrepair tension in repair of a large defect. The patch is first secured to the left side of the ventricular septum using pledgeted sutures passed from right to left through the septum and then the patch. Sutures are then passed from the epicardial surface to the endocardial surface of the right ventricle and then through the patch and tied. The debrided infarct of the free ventricular wall is closed with buttressed sutures.

the posterior descending artery is extended proximally toward the mitral annulus and distally toward the apex of the ventricle. The base of a patch tailored in a triangular shape is sutured to the fibrous annulus of the mitral valve with a continuous suture starting at a point corresponding to the level of the posteromedial papillary muscle and moving medially toward the septum until reaching noninfarcted endocardium. The suture is then interrupted with trimming of any excess patch material. The medial margin of the triangular patch is sewn to healthy septal endocardium with a continuous suture. The lateral side of the patch is sutured to the posterior wall of the left ventricle along a line corresponding to the medial margin of the base of the posteromedial papillary muscle. Sutures placed into infarcted myocardium require full-thickness

bites buttressed with felt on the epicardial surface. The infarct incision is closed in two layers of buttressed sutures, leaving the infarcted right ventricular wall undisturbed.

Survival

Although survival for treatment of an acute postinfarction VSD has improved significantly over time, operative mortality in most large series is between 30% and 50%. In the largest published series, involving 179 patients, survival at 1, 5, and 10 years was found to be 60%, 49%, and 31%, respectively. The observation that mortality is not significant between 1 and 5 years indicates that those patients who survive the perioperative period have reasonable long-term survival. The technique of infarct exclusion has been associated with both a low operative

mortality of 14% and an actuarial survival of 66% at 6 years, which is significantly better than all previous series.

Acute Ischemic Mitral Regurgitation

Incidence and Pathogenesis

Ischemic mitral regurgitation (MR) is mitral insufficiency caused by myocardial infarction. From 17% to 55% of patients have either echocardiographic evidence of MR or a new mitral systolic murmur early after acute infarction. The MR is mild or disappears in many patients, but is moderate-severe or severe in as many as 4% of patients. Overall, acute severe MR complicates 0.4% to 0.9% of acute myocardial infarctions.

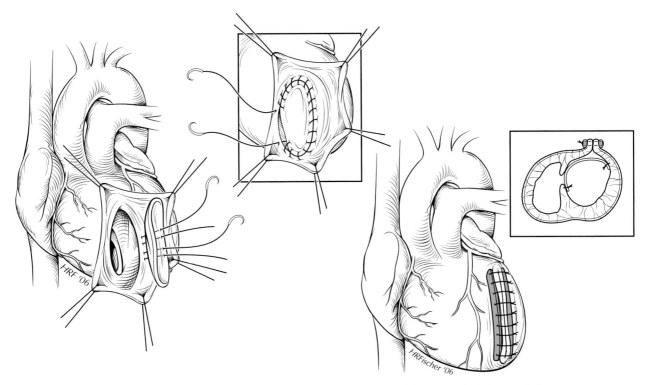

Figure 54-4.   Repair of an anterior postinfarction ventricular septal defect using the infarct exclusion technique. After a transinfarct incision is made to expose the defect, a patch that is tailored to the shape of the left ventricular infarction is sutured to the endocardium of the noninfarcted portion of the septum and then sutured to the noninfarcted endocardium of the anterolateral ventricular wall. The ventriculotomy is then closed with buttressed sutures.

Acute ischemic MR is actually a myocardial problem, not an intrinsic valve problem. Of the six components of the mitral valve (the leaflets, chordae tendinae, annulus, papillary muscles, left ventricle, and left atrium), the leaflets, chordae, and annulus are not acutely affected by a myocardial infarction. Myocardial injury involving papillary muscle rupture or displacement causes acute severe MR. The posterior papillary muscle, which has a single blood supply from the circumflex coronary artery, is involved 6 to 12 times more frequently in acute severe MR than the anterior papillary muscle, which is supplied by both the left anterior descending and circumflex coronary arteries. The MR is also usually more severe when the posterior papillary muscle is affected by the infarction.

Papillary muscle rupture results in a flail valve leaflet and generally occurs 2 to 7 days after infarction, with a mean of 4 days. Trunk rupture leads to complete dehiscence of the papillary muscle and the rapid onset of severe MR, pulmonary edema, and shock. Tip rupture of smaller papillary muscle heads also causes severe MR but results in less severe clinical deterioration initially, although the subsequent course is

unpredictable. Complete trunk rupture usually occurs within the first week after the acute infarction, whereas partial rupture can be delayed for as long as a few months. Both types of rupture are highly lethal conditions without surgical intervention.

Acute ischemic MR due to papillary muscle displacement results from a number of small geometric changes in left ventricular shape, size, and wall motion that lead to incomplete coaptation of intrinsically normal leaflets. Papillary muscle ischemia alone usually causes a murmur but not severe MR with significant hemodynamic compromise. In the absence of papillary muscle rupture, left ventricular wall ischemia in conjunction with papillary muscle ischemia is required to cause severe MR. Severe MR resulting from papillary muscle displacement, although generally more compatible with short-term survival than severe MR resulting from rupture, can cause a impairment of cardiac function similar to papillary muscle rupture and also almost always requires surgical intervention to ensure long-term survival.

Both papillary muscle rupture and displacement result in regurgitant flow into the left atrium during systole, with volume over-

load of the left atrium during systole and the left ventricle during diastole. The regurgitant flow causes an increase in stroke volume and a decrease in cardiac output. In acute MR, there is usually a marked increase in pressure in the noncompliant left atrium. This pressure increase actually helps to decrease the left ventricular–left atrial pressure gradient and may decrease the regurgitant volume.

Clinical Presentation and Diagnosis

Patients who develop acute MR after acute infarction typically have acute chest pain or shortness of breath with the appearance of a systolic murmur 2 to 7 days after the initial infarction. Acute severe MR due to either papillary muscle rupture or displacement leads to pulmonary edema and cardiogenic shock that is usually more abrupt and severe than that resulting from an acute VSD. Patients have a mean age of 60 years, usually have a history of hypertension, and are more commonly male. Chest x-rays usually show a normal-sized heart and pulmonary edema. Right heart catheterization generally shows elevated pulmonary artery pressures and tall

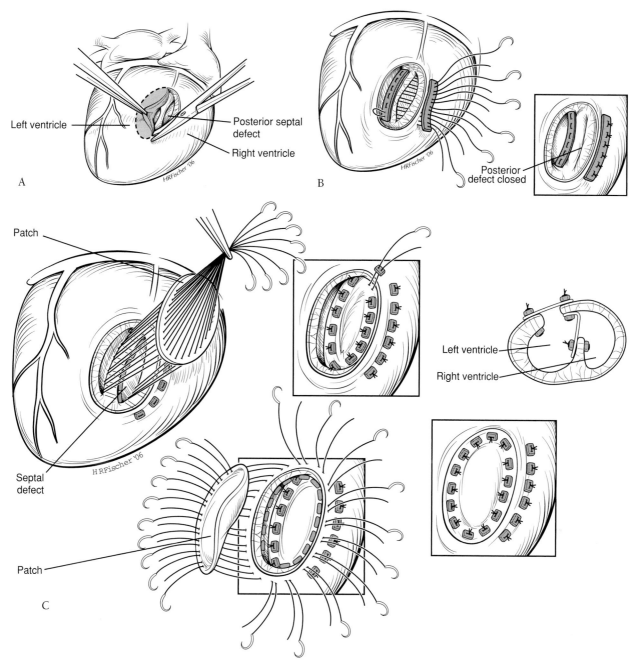

Figure 54-5. **(A)** A transinfarct incision is made, and the left ventricular portion of the infarct is debrided to expose the septal defect. **(B)** The infarctectomy technique is used to repair small posterior septal defects. The septal rim of the posterior defect is approximated to the right ventricular free wall using buttressed mattress sutures. **(C)** Large posterior defects are repaired using patch closure with the infarctectomy technique. Sutures are first passed from right to left through the septum, and then additional sutures are passed from the epicardial surface to the endocardial surface of the right ventricle. All placed sutures are then passed through the patch and tied to close the ventricular septal defect. The debrided infarct of the free ventricular wall is then closed with a patch and buttressed sutures.

V waves, but there is no oxygen step-up in the pulmonary artery.

As described, the clinical appearance of acute MR is very similar to that of an acute VSD. Again, physical exam and the electrocardiogram can distinguish acute MR from an acute VSD. The holosystolic murmur associated with acute MR is best heard at the apex, has no thrill, and is associated with an atrial gallop (S_4), whereas the murmur associated with a VSD is most prominent at the left sternal border and is commonly accompanied by a thrill. Acute MR is more commonly associated with an inferior infarction and the absence of conduction abnormalities than an acute VSD.

Echocardiography with Doppler color flow mapping is the preferred diagnostic

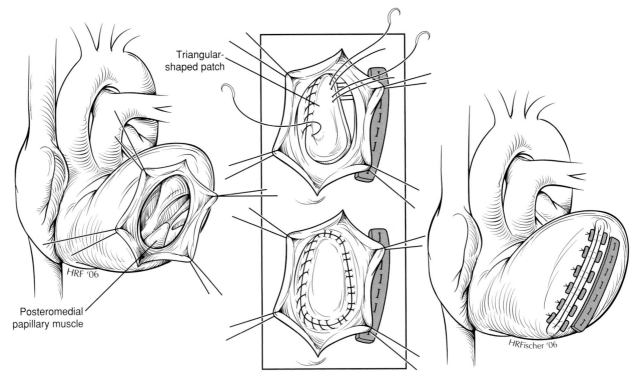

Figure 54-6.   Repair of a posterior postinfarction ventricular septal defect using the infarct exclusion technique. An incision is made in the inferior wall of the left ventricle a few millimeters from the posterior descending artery. The base of a triangular patch is sutured to the fibrous annulus of the mitral valve with a continuous suture from the level of the posteromedial papillary muscle toward the septum until one reaches noninfarcted endocardium. The suture is then interrupted with trimming of any excess patch material. The medial margin of the triangular patch is sewn to healthy septal endocardium with a continuous suture. The lateral side of the patch is sutured to the posterior wall of the left ventricle along a line corresponding to the medial margin of the base of the posteromedial papillary muscle. The infarct incision is then closed in two layers of buttressed sutures.

tool for acute severe MR. Transthoracic echocardiography is useful for assessing the degree of MR and can confirm wall motion abnormalities. In the case of papillary muscle rupture, echo can demonstrate flail mitral leaflets and also possibly a mass attached to the chordae, which is the ruptured portion of the papillary muscle. Even if a flail leaflet is not seen, the diagnosis of acute papillary muscle should be suspected if intact systolic function is seen in the clinical setting of acute pulmonary edema and shock. Transthoracic echocardiography can be a reliable diagnostic test for direct transfer to surgery when there is no question in the diagnosis. Transesophageal echocardiography is the tool of choice when the diagnosis is in question because it more definitively assesses the degree of MR and wall motion abnormalities while also assessing the posterior papillary muscle. Transthoracic echocardiography also does not always reliably distinguish papillary muscle rupture versus displacement.

Natural History

Acute severe ischemic mitral regurgitation is associated with a mortality of 24% at 30 days, 42% at 6 months, and 52% at 1 year. For an acute papillary muscle rupture, approximately 50% of patients die within 24 to 48 hours without surgical intervention.

Preoperative Therapy and Operative Timing

Acute ischemic MR that is not severe requires no specific treatment other than that used to treat the infarction. Immediate surgery is indicated for patients with severe MR and cardiogenic shock or congestive heart failure (CHF). Attempts are made to stabilize hemodynamics while surgery is arranged. As the size of the regurgitant orifice is increased by increased afterload and volume overload, inotropes, vasodilators, and an IABP can decrease the regurgitant flow and increase cardiac output.

As with acute VSDs, the role of preoperative coronary angiography for acute severe MR is not entirely clear. Delaying surgical repair to perform cardiac catheterization in a potentially unstable patient can be risky. Revascularization also prolongs both surgery and the duration of cardiopulmonary bypass and likely has no impact on immediate survival, particularly in the case of a ruptured papillary muscle, although it may be beneficial in those patients who cannot be weaned off bypass. However, given the etiology of myocardial infarction as the cause of MR and the fact that approximately half of the patients with acute ischemic MR have three-vessel coronary disease, identifying and bypassing associated coronary lesions can improve long-term prognosis. Given that coronary angiography can now be performed rapidly so that surgical intervention is not delayed, a reasonable policy, as with acute VSDs, is to perform angiography with a limited amount of contrast in all patients who can be temporarily stabilized medically or with the use of a balloon pump.

Patients who cannot be stabilized must go directly to surgery.

Operative Technique

Transesophageal echocardiography must be used in the operating room to guide and assess surgical results. A standard median sternotomy is performed with expeditious establishment of cardiopulmonary bypass. Bicaval cannulation with caval tourniquets is used to minimize systemic venous return, which could warm the heart and decrease myocardial protection during aortic cross-clamping. An alternative approach such as via a right thoracotomy with bypass established by peripheral cannulation is not appropriate in these emergency situations, except possibly in cases in which a patient has had a previous sternotomy and is known to have patent midline bypass grafts. The patient is cooled systemically to 28°C. The heart is arrested with cold cardioplegia solution delivered retrograde via the coronary sinus after the aorta is cross-clamped, and cold blood cardioplegia is delivered both antegrade and retrograde intermittently to maximize myocardial protection. The left atrium is opened to decompress the heart, and patients with associated critical coronary stenoses should then have the distal anastomoses completed.

Mitral valve exposure must allow full evaluation of all components of the valve and the subvalvular apparatus so that a decision to either repair or replace the valve can be made. The sternotomy must be well centered, with the right side of the pericardium suspended to sternal fascia. An incision is made in the left atrium near the right superior pulmonary vein, parallel to the interatrial groove, extended behind the superior vena cava and below the inferior vena cava, which must be fully dissected (Fig. 54-7). The superior vena cava is dissected to the level of the innominate vein to maximize mitral exposure. The azygos vein is divided as needed during dissection of the superior vena cava to prevent tearing due to traction during valve exposure.

Although the feasibility of valve repair should be assessed, repair in the setting of acute severe MR is very difficult. Given that these patients are usually in extremis, the possible benefits of repair instead of replacement are generally not worth the risk that surgery and bypass time could be significantly prolonged if revising or even replacing the initial repair is ultimately required. In the case of a ruptured papillary muscle, repair by reimplantation of the ruptured muscle with the placement of sutures into freshly

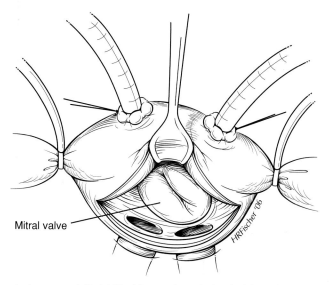

Figure 54-7. An transverse left atrial incision made at the level of the right superior pulmonary vein and extended behind the superior vena cava and below the inferior vena cava fully exposes the mitral valve.

ischemic, friable tissue is quite precarious and generally not advisable, although sometimes for distal partial papillary muscles the disrupted fibrous tip of the papillary segment can be reimplanted into an adjacent noninfarcted papillary muscle or adjacent noninfarcted ventricular myocardium (Fig. 54-8).

Because of the difficulties in performing mitral valve repair, mitral valve replacement is almost always required for patients in the setting of acute severe ischemic MR. As many chordal attachments to the annulus as possible should be preserved when replacing the valve to maintain the mitral subvalvular apparatus and optimize postoperative left ventricular geometry and function (Fig. 54-9A). Although the need for chronic anticoagulation and questions of valve durability may not be particularly great concerns in the setting of emergency surgery, the surgeon must choose between a mechanical valve and a bioprosthetic valve. Some recommend that a mechanical valve be used in patients already chronically anticoagulated. Otherwise the surgeon must consider the patient's age and comorbid conditions to evaluate whether the patient is likely to outlive a bioprosthetic valve if he or she survives his or her current state. The valve chosen is sutured to the annulus with interrupted sutures (Fig. 54-9B,C). For a bioprosthetic valve, the sutures can be passed from the ventricular to the atrial side within the annulus. For a mechanical valve, the sutures are placed from the atrial to the ventricular side. The atrium is closed with a running suture, and proximal coronary anastomoses are completed.

Survival

The 30-day mortality for surgical repair for acute severe MR is 18% to 27%. The 1-, 5-, and 10-year survival rates are 75% to 81%, 65% to 68%, and 32% to 56%, respectively. The relatively stable long-term mortality observed in these series indicates that although this condition is highly lethal, left ventricular function is usually maintained, particularly in the case of a ruptured papillary muscle, and surgical correction can indeed be life-saving. Operative risk factors for mortality include advanced age, preoperative shock, other comorbidities, infarction size, and operative delay.

Pump Failure

Incidence and Pathogenesis

Cardiogenic shock occurs in 6.7% of patients after acute myocardial infarction, and predominant left ventricular failure is the cause of shock in >75% of these cases. Cardiogenic shock results from a cycle of progressive myocardial damage and necrosis beyond the initial infarct. The overall incidence is decreasing due to better medical and interventional treatments for an acute myocardial infarction. Failure occurs when left ventricular function is <30% of normal or when the abnormally contracting segment is >25% of the left ventricular circumference. Complete regional myocardial ischemia usually results in only 60% to 70% necrosis of the cardiomyocytes in the ischemic area, which probably explains why the decrease in function seen in these

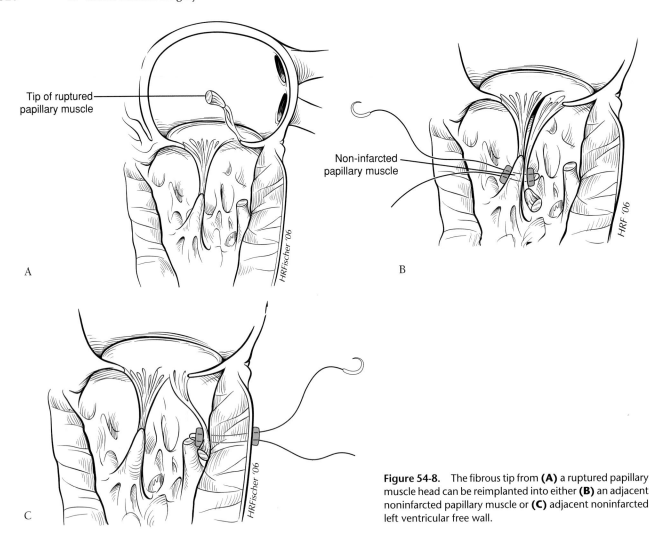

Tip of ruptured papillary muscle

A

Non-infarcted papillary muscle

B

C

Figure 54-8.   The fibrous tip from **(A)** a ruptured papillary muscle head can be reimplanted into either **(B)** an adjacent noninfarcted papillary muscle or **(C)** adjacent noninfarcted left ventricular free wall.

instances is only transient for 24 to 72 hours in two thirds of cases. When the damage involves <35% to 40% of the left ventricle, the usual clinical scenario is left ventricular dysfunction and pulmonary congestion but no evidence of end-organ hypoperfusion. Cardiogenic shock occurs when >35% to 40% of the left ventricle is involved in the infarct.

Clinical Presentation, Diagnosis, and Natural History

Patients in cardiogenic shock have left ventricular dysfunction and end-organ hypoperfusion manifested by oliguria, decreased mental status, and cold, clammy skin. Pulmonary congestion may or may not be present. Cardiac index is <1.8 liters/min/m^2, systolic blood pressure is generally <80 to 90 mm Hg, and pulmonary capillary wedge pressure is >18 mm Hg. Echocardiography shows severe left ventricular dysfunction without evidence for any of the mechanical complications described. Patients

with persistent cardiogenic shock after acute myocardial infarction despite maximal therapy have mortalities of 35% to 80%.

Preoperative Treatment and Operative Timing

The treatment goal of a patient in cardiogenic shock is to increase both coronary and end-organ perfusion and maintain oxygenation. Volume is used to keep the pulmonary capillary wedge pressure >15 mm Hg. Inotropes and vasopressors are used as needed to maintain blood pressure. If tolerated, vasodilators are useful in reducing afterload. An IABP reduces afterload to decrease left ventricular work and myocardial oxygen demand while diastolic aortic pressure is increased to improve coronary blood flow to the myocardium. Any patient who does not respond to these measures must be taken for cardiac catheterization and restoration of coronary blood flow with either angioplasty and/or stenting or surgically with

coronary artery bypass grafting. Revascularization does not significantly reduce mortality at 30 days but does have a significant survival benefit at 6 months. Patients who remain in cardiogenic shock refractory to these maximal measures require additional circulatory assistance to prevent otherwise certain death. A new treatment paradigm in suitable patients with "pump failure" is implantation of a ventricular assist device, which unloads the left ventricular to greatly reduce myocardial oxygen consumption and may salvage critical myocardial mass and act as a bridge to recovery (Fig. 54-10A). For those patients who do not recover adequate myocardial function, this technique can act as a bridge to transplantation. The ventricular assist device is implanted as quickly as possible when it becomes clear that the patient's status is not improving with maximal conventional therapy; otherwise, univentricular failure can progress to biventricular failure, and end-organ dysfunction may become permanent.

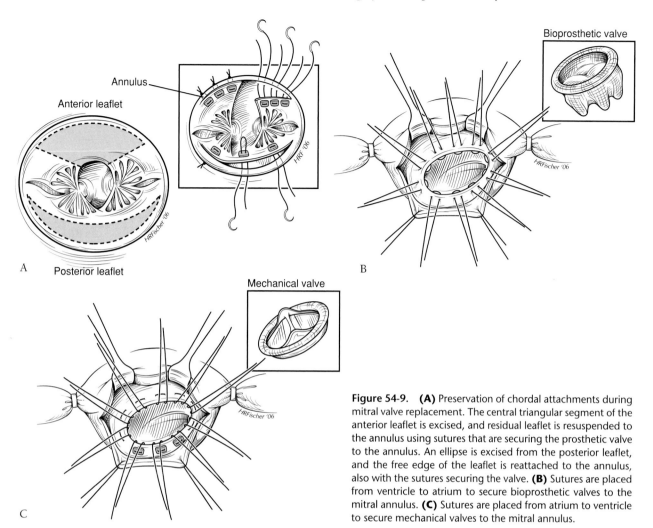

Figure 54-9. **(A)** Preservation of chordal attachments during mitral valve replacement. The central triangular segment of the anterior leaflet is excised, and residual leaflet is resuspended to the annulus using sutures that are securing the prosthetic valve to the annulus. An ellipse is excised from the posterior leaflet, and the free edge of the leaflet is reattached to the annulus, also with the sutures securing the valve. **(B)** Sutures are placed from ventricle to atrium to secure bioprosthetic valves to the mitral annulus. **(C)** Sutures are placed from atrium to ventricle to secure mechanical valves to the mitral annulus.

Operative Technique and Survival

A median sternotomy is performed, and the patient is prepared for bypass and heparinized. Device preparation is performed according to the manufacturer's protocols. The outflow tract for the assist device is sewn into the aorta; this can either be done before institution of bypass using a side-biting aortic clamp to reduce bypass time or after instituting bypass if partial clamping off bypass is not tolerated by the patient. The assist device inflow tract is sewn into the heart while on bypass. The inflow tract can be sewn into either the left atrium or the left ventricle. Left ventricular cannulation may prevent left ventricular stasis and therefore reduce the risk of subsequent thrombus formation. If device flows are not adequate, a right ventricular assist device should also be implanted. Anticoagulation is reversed at the end of the case, and heparin is started 24 hours later if signifi-

cant post–device insertion bleeding has not occurred.

Short-term (days to weeks), intermediate-term (weeks to months), and long-term (months to years) ventricular assist devices are available. Patients suffering from refractory postinfarction cardiogenic shock generally should have a short-term device such as the Abiomed BVS 5000 initially implanted. These devices can be implanted at virtually any cardiac center, although a tertiary care institute that performs heart transplantations should be available for patient transfer if indicated. Assist-device weaning is begun after the patient begins to demonstrate end-organ recovery. Device flows are reduced with minimal to moderate pharmacologic support while hemodynamics is closely monitored. Consideration can be given for explanting the device if the patient's hemodynamic status is stable on moderate amounts of pharmacologic support; otherwise, the device is maintained. If the patient is not weaned from assistance within

1 week and is a transplant candidate, then the short-term device should be exchanged in the operating room for a longer-term implantable device to act as a bridge to transplantation. If additional myocardial recovery does not occur, transfer to a transplant center is indicated. If the patient is not a transplant candidate, then the original device should be maintained until a decision is made that further support is futile or patient death or recovery occurs.

Multiple series show success in treating patients with acute infarction and refractory cardiogenic shock with a left ventricular assist device. In one series, 22 of 25 patients were successfully bridged to transplant, with 6 early post-transplant mortalities and 1-, 2-, and 5-year survival rates of 71%, 71%, and 51%, respectively. In another series, 10 of 15 patients were successfully bridged to transplant with this strategy, with 1 patient having the device explanted without requiring transplant. Six of 7 patients in another series were successfully bridged to transplant,

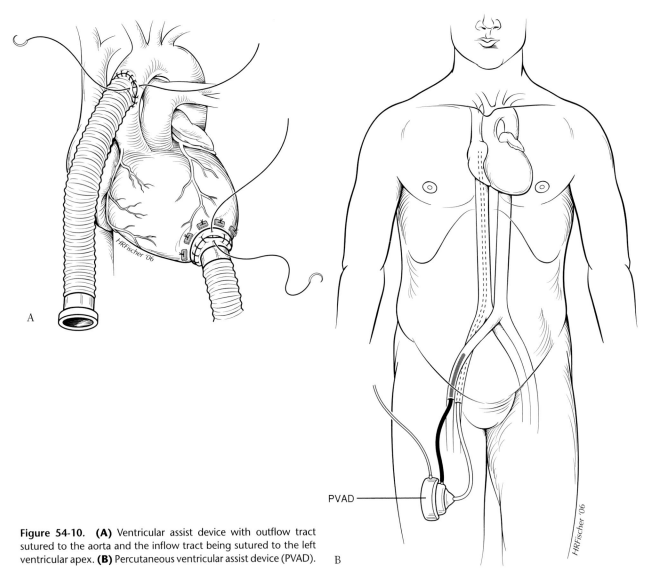

Figure 54-10. **(A)** Ventricular assist device with outflow tract sutured to the aorta and the inflow tract being sutured to the left ventricle apex. **(B)** Percutaneous ventricular assist device (PVAD).

PVAD

A

B

with 5 well at a median follow-up of nearly 900 days.

A percutaneous ventricular assist device as described by Thiele has also been used for patients with acute myocardial infarction and delayed recovery of myocardial function and continued shock after revascularization. This method uses percutaneous left atrial-to-femoral artery bypass, with the venous cannula introduced via the femoral vein and a trans-septal puncture and the arterial cannula introduced via the femoral artery and advanced into the iliac artery (Fig. 54-10B). This device, which is deployed in the cardiac catheterization laboratory, provides up to 4.0 liters/min of assisted cardiac output to allow unloading of the left ventricle. In one study of 18 patients, support was maintained an average of 4 days, with a 30-day mortality of 44%.

Double-bridge mechanical resuscitation has also been used to treat acute cardiogenic shock. With this technique, extracorporeal membrane oxygenation (ECMO) is used acutely for the treatment of profound cardiogenic shock with an early bridge to a ventricular assist device before transplantation. In one study, 9 of 23 patients were transferred to ventricular assist device, with 7 transplanted, 3 of 23 weaned off ECMO, and 11 of 23 withdrawn from support due to severe neurologic injury or multi-organ failure. In a similar study, 7 of 14 patients were transferred to ventricular assist device, with 1 directly transplanted.

SUGGESTED READING

Agnihotri AK, Madsen JC, Daggett WM. Surgical treatment of complications of acute myocardial infarction. In Cohn LH, Edmunds LH (eds), Cardiac Surgery in the Adult. New York: McGraw-Hill, 2003.

Chitwood WR. Mitral valve repair: Ischemic. In Kaiser LR, Kron IL, Spray TL (eds), Mastery of Cardiothoracic Surgery. Philadelphia: Lippincott-Raven, 1998.

David TE, Dale L, Sun Z. Postinfarction ventricular septal rupture: repair by endocardial patch with infarct exclusion. *J Thorac Cardiovasc Surg* 1995;110:1315.

Gorman RC, Gorman JH, Edmunds LH. Ischemic mitral regurgitation. In Cohn LH, Edmunds LH (eds), Cardiac Surgery in the Adult. New York: McGraw-Hill, 2003.

Gudbjartsson T, Aranki S, Cohn LH. Mechanical/bioprosthetic mitral valve replacement. In Cohn LH, Edmunds LH (eds), Cardiac Surgery in the Adult. New York, McGraw-Hill, 2003.

Pennington DG, Smedira NG, Samuels LE, et al. Mechanical circulatory support for acute heart failure. *Ann Thorac Surg* 2001;71:S5.

Thiele H, Lauer B, Hambrecht R, et al. Reversal of

cardiogenic shock by percutaneous left atrial-to-femoral arterial bypass assistance. *Circulation* 2001;104:2917.

Yun KL, Miller DC. Mitral valve replacement. In Kaiser LR, Kron IL, Spray TL (eds), Mastery of Cardiothoracic Surgery. Philadelphia: Lippincott-Raven, 1998.

EDITOR'S COMMENTS

One of the most difficult patients to treat is the patient in shock due to a complication of myocardial infarction. Berry and Gardner have outlined a practical approach to surgery for this condition. Regardless of surgical skills, so much of the survival is dependent on the time the patient has been in shock prior to therapy. In addition, in patients with ventricular septal defect, the tissue is often so poor that it is difficult to properly close the defect. Our group is generally in agreement with the approach described by the authors. We treat VSDs just as these authors have noted. The only slight difference is in the rare inferior septal defect that one can approach through the atrium and avoid ventriculotomy. However, it has to be a small defect that can be easily visualized through the tricuspid valve.

We fully agree with the approach on the mitral valve as well. There have been reports of repairing these valves. We have found this to be a difficult situation and prefer mitral valve replacement. This is really the only situation in which we do not attempt to directly repair a leaking valve. The reason of course is that if the infarcted muscle comes loose after a repair, then it is a much longer pump run for a patient who has previously been in shock. We believe that these complications are becoming less frequent. Perhaps earlier recognition angioplasty, and thrombolytic therapy have played a role. Despite this, every practicing surgeon has to have the ability to look after these lesions

I.L.K.

E

Thoracic Aortic Disease

55

Annuloaortic Ectasia

Tirone E. David

Annuloaortic Ectasia

Denton Cooley introduced the term "annuloaortic ectasia" in 1961 to describe an aortic root aneurysm due to Erdheim's cystic medial necrosis in a patient without the stigmata of Marfan syndrome. Although annuloaortic ectasia is often associated with aortic root aneurysm, it may also occur in patients without aneurysm but aortic insufficiency with bicuspid or tricuspid aortic valve and in those with subaortic ventricular septal defect. Conversely, not all patients with aortic root aneurysm have annuloaortic ectasia. The term annuloaortic ectasia is now used to define a dilated aortic annulus, which is often encountered in patients with connective disorders of the aortic root. The aortic valve may be bicuspid or tricuspid. This chapter is dedicated to surgery for aortic root aneurysm with or without annuloaortic ectasia.

Aortic root aneurysm is caused by dilation of the aortic sinuses, which often progresses to involve the sinotubular junction and ascending aorta. The aortic annulus may also dilate. Aortic root aneurysm is usually caused by connective tissue disorders such as in Marfan syndrome and its forme frusta. Patients with congenital bicuspid aortic valve may also develop aortic root and ascending aortic aneurysm due to an abnormality of the connective tissue. Dilation of the aortic sinuses does not cause aortic valve dysfunction as long as the aortic annulus and the sinotubular junction remain unchanged. However, if the aortic annulus and/or the sinotubular junction dilate, the aortic cusps are pulled apart with resulting central aortic insufficiency. The stress on the aortic cusps increase as the aortic root dilates and the cusps become thinner,

overstretched, and may develop stress fenestration in the commissural areas. This structural alteration in the aortic cusps usually parallels the increase in diameter of the aortic root. Thus, patients with large aortic root aneurysm (e.g., >60 mm) are more likely to have cusp damage, which may preclude a satisfactory aortic valve repair. For this reason, if reconstruction of the aortic root with preservation of the aortic valve is contemplated, surgery should be performed before the aortic root reaches 60 mm. We recommend aortic root reconstruction when the diameter of the aortic sinuses reaches 50 mm in patients with Marfan syndrome and 55 mm in others. In addition to aortic insufficiency and its sequelae, patients with aortic root aneurysm are at risk of aortic dissection and/or rupture of the ascending aorta. Patients with aortic root aneurysm and family history of aortic dissection should be operated on even before the root reaches 50 mm in diameter.

There are two types of operations to treat patients with aortic root aneurysm: aortic valve–sparing operations and composite replacement of the aortic valve and ascending aorta with a conduit containing a heart valve.

Aortic Valve–Sparing Operations

The two most common aortic valve–sparing operations are remodeling of the aortic root and reimplantation of the aortic valve. To perform these operations, the surgeon has to have a good knowledge of the functional anatomy of the aortic valve and how the various pathologic processes alter its structure and function.

Given the anatomic and functional relationship of the aortic cusps with the surrounding structures, the aortic valve is best described as aortic root. The aortic root has four anatomic components: the aortic annulus, the aortic cusps, the aortic sinuses or sinuses of Valsalva, and the sinotubular junction. The aortic annulus attaches the aortic root to the left ventricle. The aortic root is attached to the ventricular myocardium in approximately 45% of its circumference and to fibrous structures (the anterior leaflet of the mitral valve and the membranous septum) in the remaining 55%. The aortic annulus has a scalloped shape. The three triangular spaces beneath the scallop-shaped aortic annulus are part of the left ventricular outflow tract but are important for the function of the aortic valve. The triangle beneath the right and left cusps is made of ventricular muscle and it is seldom affected by connective tissue disorders of the aortic root. The other two triangles are fibrous structures, and, as such, flatten and acquire a broader base in patients with dilated aortic annulus.

The aortic cusps have a semilunar shape with a base and a free margin, and extend from commissure to commissure. The length of the base of the aortic cusps is approximately 1.5 times longer than its free margin. In normal adults, the average length of the base of the aortic cusp is 48 mm, the free margin is 32 mm, the cusp height is 14 mm, and the commissural height is 19 mm.

The ridge immediately above the commissures is called sinotubular junction, and it is functionally important for the aortic root because it suspends the aortic cusps. Dilation of the sinotubular junction causes the free margins of the cusps to move away from each other, and eventually they cannot coapt centrally with consequent aortic insufficiency.

The arterial walls contained within the aortic annulus and sinotubular junction are the aortic sinuses. Isolated dilation of the aortic sinuses has no effect on aortic valve competence. The aortic sinuses are important to maintain coronary artery blood flow during the entire cardiac cycle and to create eddies and currents to facilitate closure of the aortic cusps during diastole.

The aortic root is very elastic in young patients and expands considerably during systole and shortens during diastole. The transverse diameter of the aortic annulus at its nadir is approximately 15% to 20% larger than the diameter of the sinotubular junction in young patients. However, as the amount of elastic fibers in the arterial wall decreases with age, the aortic root becomes less compliant. The diameter of the sinotubular junction increases in older patients and tends to become equal to or slightly larger than the transverse diameter of the aortic annulus.

Remodeling of the Aortic Root

The three aortic sinuses are excised leaving approximately 5 mm of arterial wall attached to that aortic annulus and around the coronary artery orifices as illustrated in Fig. 55-1. A reduction aortic annuloplasty should be performed if there is annuloaortic ectasia. This can be accomplished by suturing a strip of Dacron fabric on the outside of the left ventricular outflow tract along its fibrous components as shown in Fig. 55-2. Most of the reduction in the transverse diameter of the aortic annulus should be in the triangles beneath the commissures of the noncoronary aortic cusp. A tubular Dacron graft of diameter equal to an imaginary circle that contains all three commissures of the aortic valve when it is closed is selected. This graft is tailored in such way as to recreate the aortic sinuses as illustrated in Fig. 55-3. The width of these neoaortic sinuses should be proportional to the size of the aortic cusps and their height should be equal to or taller than the diameter of the graft. The three commissure of the aortic valve are resuspended into this tailored graft, and the neoaortic sinuses are sutured to the aortic annulus with a continuous 4-0 polypropylene suture as shown in Fig. 55-3. At this stage, the aortic cusps are carefully inspected for the level of coaptation of the cusps. The three cusps should coapt at the same level and several millimeters above the level of

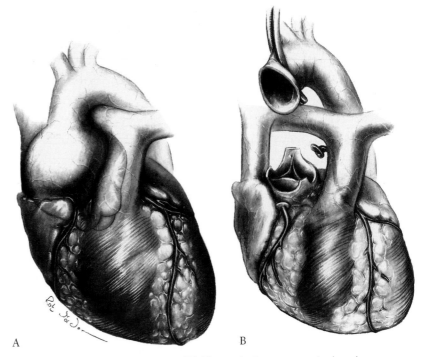

Figure 55-1.   (A) Aortic root aneurysm. **(B)** The aortic sinuses are excised, and coronary arteries are detached from the aortic root leaving 5 mm or 6 mm of arterial wall attached to the aortic annulus and around the coronary arteries. (Reprinted with permission from TE David. Remodeling of the aortic root and preservation of the native aortic valve. Oper Tech Cardiac Thorac Surg 1996;1:44.)

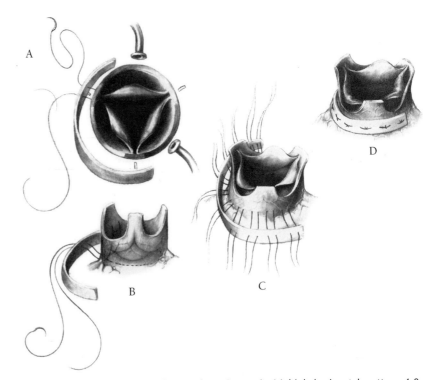

Figure 55-2.   Aortic annuloplasty for annuloaortic ectasia. Multiple horizontal mattress 4-0 polyester sutures are passed from the inside to the outside of the fibrous components of the left ventricular outflow tract **(A)** through a single horizontal plane **(B)**. The sutures are passed through a strip of Dacron fabric so as to reduce the bases of the triangles beneath the commissures of the noncoronary aortic cusp **(C)**. The sutures are tied on the strip of Dacron fabric **(D)**. (Reprinted with permission from TE David. Remodeling of the aortic root and preservation of the native aortic valve. Oper Tech Cardiac Thorac Surg 1996;1:44.)

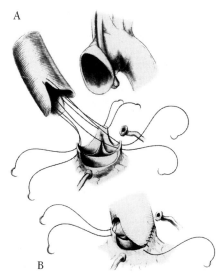

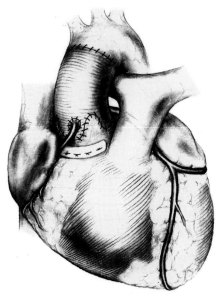

Figure 55-3. Remodeling of the aortic root. **(A)** The three commissures of the aortic valve are resuspended into a tailored tubular Dacron graft with neoaortic sinuses. **(B)** The neoaortic sinuses of Dacron are sutured to the junction between the remnants of the aortic sinuses and aortic annulus.

Figure 55-4. Remodeling of the aortic root. The graft used to reconstruct the aortic root is anastomosed to the distal ascending aorta.

the aortic annulus. If one or more cusps appear to be coapting at a lower level than the other two, its free margin should be shortened by plication of its central portion along the nodule of Aranti as described later. Next, the coronary arteries are reimplanted into their respective neoaortic sinuses. Injecting cardioplegia under pressure into the reconstructed aortic root by clamping the graft distally can now assess valve competence. If the left ventricle does not distend, the aortic valve must not have more minimal aortic insufficiency. The graft is sutured to the distal ascending aorta and the operation is completed (Fig. 55-4).

Remodeling of the aortic root is a physiologically sound operative procedure because it re-creates the aortic sinuses and allow for relatively normal aortic annulus and cusp motion. However, the commissural areas and the sinotubular junction are fixed and do not change during the cardiac cycle as they do in the normal aortic root. The problem with this operation is that the aortic annulus may dilate in certain patients, particularly if they have Marfan syndrome or a more severe form of degenerative disorder of the connective tissue. The aortic annuloplasty described in Fig. 55-2 does not seem to prevent the fibrous tissue between the suture lines from dilating. For this reason we favor reimplantation of the aortic valve to treat patients with aortic root aneurysm with or without annuloaortic ectasia.

Reimplantation of the Aortic Valve

The three aortic sinuses are excised leaving 5 mm of arterial wall attached to the aortic annulus and all around the coronary artery orifices as illustrated in Fig. 55-1. Sizing the diameter of the graft to be used for reim-

plantation of the aortic valve may be a bit more complicated than for the remodeling of the aortic root because the graft lies on the outside of the aortic root. Although we have tried several different formulas, the simplest and most reliable is to use the height of the aortic cusps because it is a variable that cannot be altered during the procedure. Thus, we use a graft of diameter equal to twice the average height of the cusps. Because most aortic cusps have a height of 14 mm to 16 mm, grafts of diameter 28 mm to 32 mm are usually used. If the three aortic cusps have similar size, three equidistant marks are made in one of the ends of the graft to correspond to each commissure. If the cusps have different sizes, the spaces between those three marks should reflect those differences. A small triangular segment is excised along the mark in the graft that corresponds to the commissure between the right and left cusps because that part of the aortic annulus is subtended by the muscular interventricular septum as shown in Fig. 55-5. Next, multiple horizontal mattress of 4-0 polyester sutures are passed from the inside to the outside of the left ventricular outflow tract, immediately below the aortic annulus. These sutures are placed in a single horizontal plane along the fibrous component of the left ventricular outflow tract and following the scalloped shape of the aortic annulus along the muscular component (Fig. 55-5). If the fibrous portion

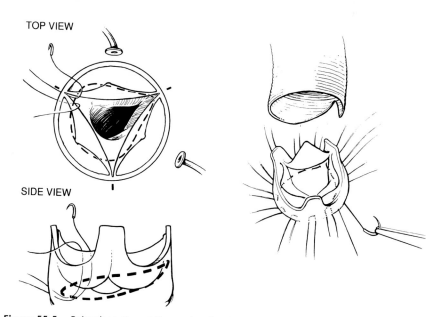

TOP VIEW

SIDE VIEW

Figure 55-5. Reimplantation of the aortic valve. **(Right)** A small triangular segment is cut from one of the ends of the Dacron graft to correspond to the commissure between the left and right cusps. **(Left)** Multiple horizontal mattress sutures are passed from the inside to the outside of the left ventricular outflow tract along a single horizontal plane immediately below the aortic annulus along its fibrous components and following the scalloped shape of the annulus along the muscular interventricular septum.

is very thin, small Teflon felt pledgets are used in these sutures. The sutures are then passed from the inside to the outside of the tailored end of the Dacron graft. If the aortic annulus is larger than the graft, reduction is carried out by distributing the sutures closer together in the graft than in the left ventricular outflow in the spaces beneath the commissures of the noncoronary aortic cusp. The aortic valve is placed inside the graft, and the left ventricular outflow tract sutures are tied on the outside. The graft is cut in the length of 5 cm or 6 cm. The three commissures and the graft are pulled gently upward, and each commissure is secured to the graft with a transfixing 4-0 polypropylene suture from the inside to the outside of the graft but these sutures are left untied. These three sutures are pulled apart gently, and the level of coaptation of the cusps and the level and alignment of the commissure are inspected. It is important to remember that the three commissures must be correctly aligned within the graft, and the level where they are sutured in the graft will determine the shape of the reconstructed aortic annulus. Next, the three sutures are tied on the outside of the graft, and one of the arms of the polypropylene suture is brought inside the graft and used to secure the remnants of the aortic sinuses and aortic annulus against the graft by passing the needle through the junction between aortic annulus and aortic sinus from the inside to the outside of the graft and back from the outside of the graft to inside at the level where the rim of the remaining aortic sinus lies. This suture line should be hemostatic and should remodel the aortic annulus into a smooth scallop shape. The aortic cusps are inspected, and if the free margin of one cusp appears to coapt at a lower level than the other two, it should be shortened as will be described. The left and right coronary arteries are reimplanted into their respective neoaortic sinuses. Valve competence can be assessed at this time by applying a clamp to the upper end of the graft and injecting cardioplegia under pressure. If there is no ventricular distension during this maneuver, it is unlikely that there is more than trace aortic valve insufficiency. The distal end of the graft is sutured to the ascending aorta (Fig. 55-6).

The main criticism of this operative technique has been that it places the aortic valve inside a straight tube without sinuses of Valsalva. The absence of aortic sinuses may increase mechanical stress on the aortic valve and shorten the durability of the repair. It has been shown that the velocity of opening and closing of the aortic cusps is increased

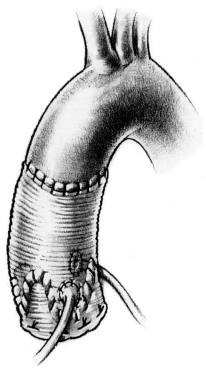

Figure 55-6. Reimplantation of the aortic valve. The Dacron graft is secured to the left ventricular outflow tract with the first row of interrupted sutures. The aortic annulus and remnants of the aortic sinuses are secured to the graft with a continuous suture. The coronary arteries are reimplanted into their respective neoaortic sinuses.

compared to that of the aortic valve. Although we have numerous patients who had this operation and >10 years of follow-up with no signs of deteriorating aortic valve function, the issue of absent aortic sinuses can be addressed by tailoring the graft during the performance of this operation. Actually, there is a commercially available Dacron graft with sinuses of Valsalva, but we believe that it remodels the aortic annulus to a spherical shape, which is incorrect and may accelerate cusp wear. We do not use this commercially available graft and prefer to reimplant the aortic valve into a straight tube, which correctly remodels the aortic annulus, and then create neoaortic sinuses.

If neoaortic sinuses are to be created, the tubular Dacron graft chosen to reconstruct the aortic root should be 2 mm to 4 mm larger than needed. Thus, grafts of 30 mm to 36 mm are usually used. Three marks are placed in one of its ends to correspond to each commissure of the aortic valve. A small triangular piece is removed to correspond to the commissure between the left and right cusps. This end of the graft is then plicated in three areas to correspond to the nadir of

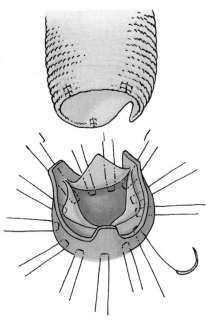

Figure 55-7. Reimplantation of the aortic valve with creation of neoaortic sinuses. A graft 4 mm larger than needed is used, and three plications of 4 mm each are made in one of its ends to reduce its diameter by 4 mm and create a curvilinear shape at the level of the nadir of the aortic annulus.

the cusps. These plications reduce the diameter of the graft to the original size that is needed for the reconstruction as illustrated in Fig. 55-7. For every linear plication of 3 mm, the diameter of the graft is reduced by 1 mm (the perimeter of a graft is equal to its diameter times π). Next, the graft is secured to the left ventricular outflow tract as described when a straight tube is used. The three commissures are resuspended within the graft and the aortic annulus, and remnants of the aortic sinuses are sutured to the graft. Darts are placed between the commissures to create neoaortic sinuses as shown in Fig. 55-8. Folding the graft in a vertical fashion and stitching with a continuous polypropylene suture makes these darts. The three cusps are carefully inspected, and if there is prolapse, the free margin of the prolapsing cusp is shortened accordingly. The coronary arteries are reimplanted into their respective sinuses and the graft is anastomosed to the distal ascending aorta (Fig. 55-9). This procedure produces three neoaortic sinuses with a correctly scalloped aortic annulus into a cylinder, which is the shape of the normal aortic annulus. The opening and closing of the aortic cusps resembles that of the normal aortic valve although the velocity is still higher than normal, but similar to that obtained when remodeling of the aortic root is performed.

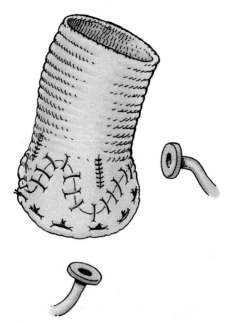

Figure 55-8. Reimplantation of the aortic valve with creation of neoaortic sinuses. After the aortic valve is sutured to the graft and the coronary arteries are reimplanted, longitudinal darts are created between the commissures to create neoaortic sinuses.

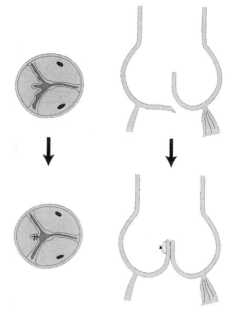

Figure 55-10. Repair of aortic cusp prolapse. The central portion of the free margin is plicated with interrupted sutures to shorten its length.

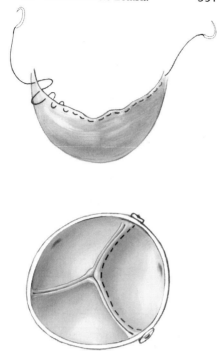

Figure 55-11. Reinforcement of the free margin of the aortic cusp. A 6-0 expanded polytetrafluoroethylene suture is woven on a single or double layer along the free margins and anchored on the outside wall of the aortic root.

Repair of Aortic Cusp Prolapse

Elongation of the free margin of an aortic cusp causes prolapse, which can be corrected by plicating its central portion. The nodule of Aranti is folded toward the aortic side and plicated with a 5-0 polypropylene suture. If additional shortening is needed, another suture is applied 1 mm or so from the first toward the commissures of the prolapsing cusp and the free margin is further shortened. Plication of the free margin raises the level of coaptation of the cusp and corrects its excessive motion as illustrated in Fig. 55-10.

If a fenestration is present in a commissural area or the free margin is flimsy and elongated, in addition to shortening its length as described, the free margin can be reinforced by weaving a 6-0 expanded polytetrafluoroethylene suture from commissure to commissure and anchoring the suture on the outside the aorta or graft as shown in Fig. 55-11.

Replacement of the Aortic Root

Patients with aortic root aneurysm and damaged aortic cusps should have replacement with a conduit containing a valve. This conduit can be a commercially available tubular Dacron graft containing a mechanical

valve or a biologic or bioprosthetic aortic root. Aortic root replacement with pulmonary autograft or with aortic valve homograft is described in detail elsewhere in this textbook. There are commercially available glutaraldehyde-fixed porcine aortic roots that can also be used for aortic root replacement using the same techniques as for aortic valve homograft. I will describe the technique we have used for replacement with mechanical valves and with stented bioprosthetic valve.

The aortic valve is excised and the aortic annulus debrided from all calcium, scar, or other abnormality. The aortic sinuses are excised leaving a few millimeters of arterial wall attached to the aortic annulus and 5 mm around the coronary arteries. The coronary arteries should be mobilized only enough to allow for reimplantation without tension. As the left main coronary artery is mobilized, a small vein is always found near the outside of the aortic annulus. If this vein is damaged during dissection, it should be ligated because bleeding from this area can be troublesome after reimplantation of the left coronary artery. The transverse diameter of the aortic annulus is measured and a commercially available conduit containing a mechanical valve is selected. Most patients with aortic root aneurysm have dilated aortic annulus, and patient–prosthesis mismatch

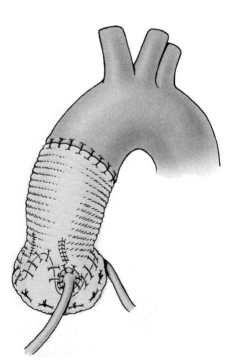

Figure 55-9. Reimplantation of the aortic valve with creation of neoaortic sinuses. The distal end of the graft is sutured to the ascending aorta.

is not a problem. We prefer to secure the sewing ring of the mechanical valve to the aortic annulus with inverting horizontal mattress of 2-0 polyester sutures with pledgets. If the aortic annulus is relatively small for the patient's body surface area, we use simple interrupted sutures because this technique allows for implantation of a larger valve than the technique of inverting sutures. Next, the coronary arteries are reimplanted. A round opening is created in the graft in an area that allows for the coronary artery button to be sutured without tension or kinking. This is particularly important for the right coronary artery because the position of the right ventricle changes when the heart begins to work and the coronary artery may kink or be distorted. The diameter of the round openings in the Dacron graft for the reimplantation of the coronary arteries should not be more than twice that of the diameter of the coronary artery, particularly in patients with Marfan syndrome, to reduce the risk of late coronary artery button aneurysm. We use continuous 5-0 polypropylene suture for the reimplantation of the coronary arteries. We do not believe that Teflon felt is needed in this anastomosis. The graft is sutured to the distal ascending aorta with a continuous 4-0 polypropylene suture as illustrated in Fig. 55-12. The graft should not be longer than 6 cm to 7 cm to replace the entire ascending aorta. It should be proportionally shorter if it is anastomosed to the mid-portion of the ascending aorta.

If a stented bioprosthetic valve is used, a graft of appropriate diameter is selected, and the bioprosthesis and graft are secured simultaneously to the aortic annulus with multiple interrupted 2-0 polyester sutures with pledgets in the ventricular side of the annulus because there is no risk of the pledgets interfering with the function of the bioprosthetic valve. If bioprosthetic valve failure is a consideration because of the patient's age, the valve should be sutured to the graft before it is secured to the aortic annulus. The bioprosthetic valve is sutured 10 mm from the end of the graft, and the graft alone is sutured to the aortic annulus. This modification allows for future re-replacement of the bioprosthetic valve without taking down the coronary arteries from the graft. The coronary arteries are reimplanted as described.

Postoperative Complications and Late Outcomes

Bleeding is probably the most common early complication of aortic root surgery, particularly when aortic valve–sparing operations combined with transverse arch and/or mitral valve repair are performed. These operations are associated with long cardiopulmonary bypass times, and the patients often develop coagulopathy, particularly if they have Marfan syndrome or present as an emergency such as acute type A aortic dissection. Antifibrinolytic agents such as tranexamic acid and particularly aprotinin are helpful, but transfusion of platelets, cryoprecipitate, and fresh-frozen plasma is often necessary.

Low-cardiac-output syndrome has been practically abolished with current methods of myocardial protection except when there is concomitant myocardial infarction. Ventricular dysrhythmias, heart block, stroke, and wound infection are uncommon.

In the first 200 consecutive aortic valve–sparing operations for aortic root aneurysm in our hospital the operative mortality was 1.5%, and the series included patients with acute type A aortic dissection, reoperations, and combined procedures. The operative mortality for aortic root replacement among 452 consecutive patients was 4%, and it also included aortic dissections, reoperations, and patients with aortic root abscess. Advanced age, New York Heart Association functional class 4, urgent/emergent surgery, and the need for circulatory arrest were independent predictors of operative mortality for aortic root replacement.

The late outcomes of aortic valve–sparing operations have been extremely encouraging. Valve-related complications are rare. The 10-year survival was 82% for all patients and 96% for those with Marfan syndrome. The 10-year freedom from reoperation in the aortic valve was 96%, and there was no difference in patients with Marfan syndrome. Late development of aortic insufficiency is the Achilles heel of aortic valve–sparing operations, and approximately one third of our patients developed moderate aortic insufficiency. However, we have found that the dilation of the aortic annulus in patients who had remodeling of the aortic root was the main cause of late valve dysfunction. For this reason, we favor the reimplantation of the aortic valve in all patients with aortic root aneurysm because it results in a more stable aortic valve repair.

The late outcomes of aortic root replacement are also very satisfactory. In our series of 452 patients the 10-year survival was 74%, and older age, left ventricular ejection fraction <40%, coronary artery disease, endocarditis, and re-do surgery were independent predictors of late death. These patients were also at similar risk of thromboembolism, endocarditis, and hemorrhagic complications as other patients with prosthetic aortic valves.

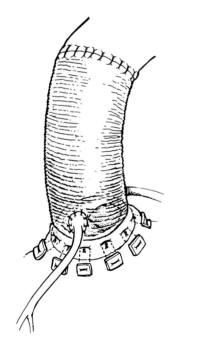
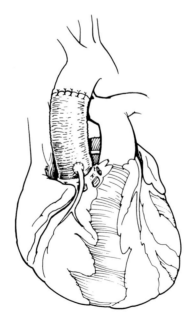

Figure 55-12. Aortic root replacement with a commercially available conduit containing a mechanical valve.

SUGGESTED READING

David TE. Remodeling of the aortic root and preservation of the native aortic valve. Oper Tech Cardiac Thorac Surg 1996;1:44.

David TE. Surgery of the aortic valve. Curr Probl Surg 1999;36:421.

David TE, Armstrong S, Ivanov J, et al. Results of aortic valve-sparing operations. J Thorac Cardiovasc Surg 2001;122:39.

David TE, Feindel CM, Webb GD, et al. Long-term results of aortic valve-sparing operations for aortic root aneurysm. J Thorac Cardiovasc Surg 2006;132:347:54.

de Oliveira NC, David TE, Ivanov J, et al. Results of surgery for aortic root aneurysm in patients with Marfan syndrome. J Thorac Cardiovasc Surg 2003;125:789.

Sioris T, David TE, Ivanov J, et al. A Comparative study on separate and composite replacement of the aortic valve and ascending aorta. J Thorac Cardiovasc Surg 2004;126:260.

EDITOR'S COMMENTARY

Dr. David has developed most of the techniques for sparing the aortic valve in treatment of annuloaortic ectasia. We have used his work, and this has become a major part of our treatment of ascending aortic disease. As Dr. David describes, we too favor aortic valve reimplantation in most situations. We still use the remodeling technique in patients with annuloaortic ectasia and competent bicuspid aortic valves. The only situation where we differ is in the patient with acute aortic dissection and annuloaortic ectasia. In these situations we have preferred the Bentall procedure because of all the hematoma around the root and the difficulty in sparing the valve. In those patients with aortic dissection and a normal root the valve is resuspended followed by a graft at the sinotubular junction.

Dr. David's technique is durable. We have had two situations where aortic insufficiency occurred years after aortic valve reimplantation. We believe this occurred because the small amount of aortic tissue left behind continued to grow and pushed the valves into the ventricle. Both patients underwent aortic valve replacement through their reconstructed root.

There is no question that this technique is the treatment of choice in patients undergoing surgical treatment of annuloaortic ectasia.

I.L.K.

56

Aortic Dissection

Alberto Pochettino and Joseph E. Bavaria

Introduction

Aortic dissection is a catastrophic disease with a reported incidence of >2,000 cases per year in the United States. Over the last decade, improved understanding of the dynamics of aortic dissection has led to a lower morbidity and mortality in selected centers, despite an unchanged overall mortality of 25% as reported by the International Registry of Aortic Dissection or of 20% as noted by the prospectively randomized evaluation of CryoLife BioGlue in acute type A dissection.

Appropriate treatment is best managed by a team approach because the aortic dissection process can affect any part of the circulation and potentially cause malperfusion of the heart, the brain, the spinal cord, the gastrointestinal tract, the kidneys, and the extremities. A more focused understanding of the causes of death and morbidity of aortic dissection has allowed us to devise a better operation to prevent them and has led to improved outcomes. Further refinements in management, such as the use of the operating room as the diagnostic suite, can lead to even better survival.

Classification

Aortic dissection develops from a tear within the intima of the aortic wall. Blood flows across this "entry point" into a weakened media, splitting the medial layer along the direction of flow and creating a new, "false" channel within the aortic media. This new channel progresses downstream, and significant pressure/mechanical stress is exerted by the advancing column of blood on the aortic branches encountered in its path. An

individual branch will either tear, leading to a communication from the false lumen into the original, "true" lumen of the aorta, or close off, causing a so-called malperfusion of the organ supplied by the given arterial branch. The multiple torn branches down the path of the false lumen become known as re-entry points or "fenestrations." The false lumen thus does not become a blind pouch with the potential for thrombosis, but is kept patent by the many re-entry points of variable size. If the re-entry points are, in aggregate, small or restrictive, a pressure gradient will develop between the false and the true lumen. This pressure differential will cause the false lumen to expand in an amount commensurate to the gradient, causing the true lumen to contract. A new equilibrium is eventually reached with equalization of pressure within the two lumens, typically leaving a small true lumen and a larger false channel. This final equilibrium point is reached within minutes to hours from the time of the original tear, such that the dissection is established and relatively stable by the time the patient reaches medical attention, with a false lumen extending from the entry site most often all the way down to the aortic bifurcation.

Although the final initiating event in an aortic dissection is an intimal disruption, the disease is not an intimal disease. Endothelial cells and their basement membrane do not possess significant intrinsic tensile strength, and their disruption is due to a lack of appropriate mechanical support from the medial layer. The media can be abnormal secondary to a genetic structural abnormality as in Marfan syndrome, in which abnormal fibrillin causes loss of elasticity in the medial layer. More often, other, less clearly identified genetic conditions can predispose to abnormalities in the media that lead to dis-

section. These less well defined heterogeneous abnormalities are often grouped in the category of annuloaortic ectasia, in which different abnormalities in the media lead to the common end pathway of dilation of the aortic diameter with thinning of the aortic wall. Atherosclerotic disease will also damage the media in a variable pattern. Wall weakness in atherosclerotic disease is more often combined with sustained high blood pressure, leading to increased stress on the abnormal aortic wall. Within this hypertensive background, a paroxysm of increased arterial blood pressure will incite the initial tear.

Anatomic classifications of aortic dissection are based on the location of the initial tear (Fig. 56-1). The first classification scheme was designed by DeBakey, who separated dissections into the following types:

Type I. The process involves the ascending aorta, the aortic arch, the descending thoracic and often the abdominal aorta.

Type II. The dissection involves the ascending aorta, but stops at the level of the aortic arch and does not involve the aorta beyond the subclavian artery take-off.

Type III. The dissection starts distal to the subclavian artery and extends to the entire thoracic aorta (IIIa) or the thoracic and abdominal aorta (IIIb).

The following Stanford classification has became more commonly used primarily because of its therapeutic implications:

Type A dissection involves the ascending aorta and will most often extend into the descending thoracic as well as abdominal aorta. The subset of DeBakey II is included in this Stanford type.

Type B dissection starts beyond the aortic arch usually at the subclavian artery and

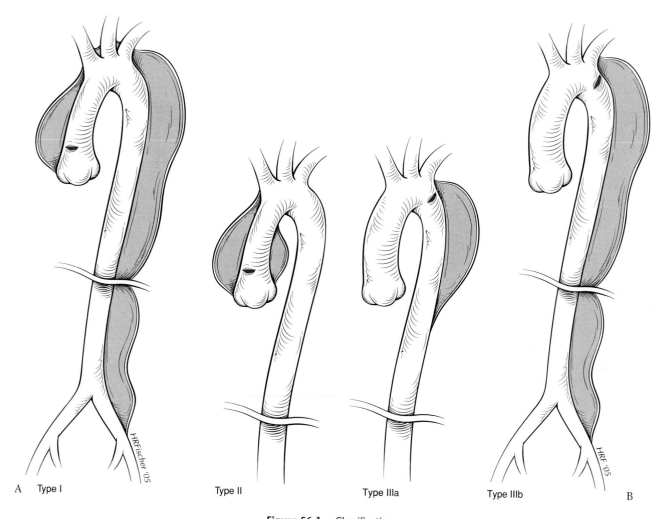

A   Type I   Type II   Type IIIa   Type IIIb   B

Figure 56-1.   Classification.

progresses distal, thus not involving the ascending aorta or the aortic arch.

The power and popularity of the Stanford classification are due primarily to the very different natural histories of the two types of dissection and the requirement of very different surgical approaches to successfully treat them. A type A dissection carries a high risk of early mortality and morbidity if not treated surgically. A type B dissection has a much lower early mortality, with early surgical treatment providing no clear advantage or even a higher mortality over observation alone. Because a type A dissection is so ominous early in the process, this represents a surgical emergency. Type B dissection is a much lower risk aortic process with a relatively low risk of rupture. The primary acute problems caused by type B dissections are malperfusion syndromes of those organs in the path of the descending thoracic, the abdominal aorta, or even the iliac arteries.

Clinical Presentation and Diagnostic Evaluation

The aortic media has a high density of nerve endings, so when medial disruption takes place, the acute onset of sharp pain is a nearly uniform presenting symptom. The heavier the atherosclerotic degeneration of the media, the less acute and sharp might be the pain described by the patient during the dissection progression. In a type A dissection, the pain is classically described by acute onset of chest pain, which then migrates to the upper back and indeed is often described as extending/progressing down to the lower back and even the groins depending on the dynamics of growth of the false lumen. Once the false lumen is fully established and has stabilized, the acute pain may change into a more persistent and dull pain, which is often not as easy to localize and may involve the chest and back in variable

patterns with additional elements of nausea, abdominal pain, diaphoresis, and shortness of breath. The presence of a new focal neurologic deficit suggests aortic arch malperfusion. Flank pain can also be described, especially in patients who are suffering an acute malperfusion of one of the kidneys. Signs and symptoms of venous hypertension suggest pericardial tamponade and are usually accompanied by poorly perfused extremities, sweaty and clammy appearance, and presyncopal symptoms all consistent with a low cardiac output state. Additional presenting symptoms can be the sudden onset of a cold and pulseless extremity, most commonly the right lower extremity. A right upper extremity vascular impairment is often associated with a neurologic event, especially in a patient with an incomplete circle of Willis. These patients can have a catastrophic hemispheric infarct with a dense contralateral paralysis. Rarely, paraplegia can be a presenting symptom. This is usually associated with signs of spinal shock, which, compounded with other cardiovascular effects of the acute dissection, can further complicate the early assessment of the patient. Abdominal pain can occur in either type A or type B dissection, and it is often associated with stenosis or occlusion of either the celiac or the superior mesenteric arteries.

In a relatively young patient without significant risk factors for atherosclerotic disease, the index of suspicion for aortic dissection should be very high when any of these symptoms are described. Screening tests should include a chest x ray and an electrocardiogram (ECG). ECG is often nondiagnostic, and occasionally it may show inferior wall changes suggestive of right coronary artery compromise by the dissection. Chest x ray is a very nonspecific exam and it may show a dilated mediastinum or a large cardiac silhouette possibly due to an acute pericardial effusion.

The next screening test, when readily available, should be a transthoracic echocardiogram focusing on the ascending aorta and the aortic valve. A transthoracic echo may be difficult to carry out and poor windows may limit its usefulness, but if the aortic root is clearly visualized, a variable degree of aortic valve insufficiency with a dilated root or the suggestion of an intimal flap will suggest the diagnosis of type A dissection.

In most emergency departments, a computed tomography (CT) scan with contrast can be obtained within a few minutes of admission into the emergency system and it is often the next test obtained before an echocardiogram. An echo will often require cardiology staff evaluation, which will take often longer than a trip to the CT scanner. Most modern CT scans with contrast will make the diagnosis of aortic dissection with exceptional accuracy and will often be the only test required prior to proceeding to definitive treatment. Rarely, in a CT scan, particularly when the intravenous contrast is not well timed, the ascending aorta can show artifactual lines that might be interpreted as a type A dissection; these scans represent the few false-positive studies.

After a screening transthoracic echo suggestive but not diagnostic of an aortic dissection, a transesophageal echocardiogram (TEE) can nearly always make an accurate diagnosis of the type of dissection present. Although there is no need to delay definitive treatment by adding TEE to a diagnostic contrast CT scan, TEE in our recent experience is as accurate as any other diagnostic study and allows rapid evaluation of an unstable patient.

Although contrast magnetic resonance imaging (MRI)/magnetic resonance angiography (MRA) provides excellent images of any dissection, it is not often readily available and it usually requires long acquisition times with the patient not as closely monitored because of the technical requirement of the high magnetic field. We do not advocate it as a primary modality except when a TEE is not readily available and the patient has evidence of renal dysfunction. MRI can be extremely valuable in following a type B dissection after the initial diagnosis or in evaluating any chronic dissection.

Whereas aortography was once considered the standard diagnostic modality for aortic dissection, over the last decade we have dropped the aortogram from our diagnostic evaluation. When obtained, aortography will only show the presence of a dissection flap and will not provide the anatomic detail a standard CT scan with contrast, a transesophageal echocardiogram, or an MRI/MRA can provide. Aortography is only obtained when an aortic dissection is not suspected on presentation and the patient is taken to the cardiac catheterization lab to be evaluated for suspected coronary disease. Taking a patient with acute aortic dissection to the cardiac catheterization lab carries a very high mortality. Suspicion of coronary disease leads to the use of platelet-inhibiting agents, anticoagulants, and occasionally fibrinolytics, all of which can transform a contained rupture into a free disruption or can increase the diffuse blood extravasation occasionally noted in a dissected, extremely thin aorta. Furthermore, a trip to the catheterization lab will typically cause significant and dangerous delay in definitive treatment, and the catheter manipulations performed can cause dangerous direct damage to the freshly dissected aorta.

A question occasionally arises over the value of elective coronary evaluation after making the diagnosis of type A dissection. Retrospective reviews suggest that the incidence of coronary disease in this population is sufficiently low that more patients are placed at risk by the delay and technical risks of a cardiac catheterization than are saved by the discovery of occult coronary disease. The only exception may be in patients who have undergone previous coronary bypass surgery, in which case knowledge of coronary disease and graft position and patency can contribute to a safer operation. When the technology of intraoperative coronary angiogram becomes practical, that may become an option for all patients.

Once the diagnosis of a type A dissection is suggested by any screening test, the patient should not be delayed in the emergency department by further testing, but should be transferred to an appropriate institution that can proceed with expeditious surgical repair. Over the last several years, our policy has been that any patient with a documented or highly suspected type A dissection should be transferred immediately to the operating room to minimize any delay. As soon as the patient arrives at the operation room, if sufficient suspicion or good studies are available, the patient is placed under general anesthesia and a transesophageal echocardiogram is obtained. If dissection is demonstrated by TEE in the ascending aorta, the patient undergoes emergency surgery. With this policy, 5% to 10% of patients admitted directly to the operating room are found to have a negative TEE and are then transferred to MRI to further document the anatomic details of their type B dissection or any other aortic pathology.

Acute Type A Dissection

Patients with an acute type A dissection have a risk of death traditionally estimated at 80% in the first 48 hours from their presentation. Some more recent data suggest that the early mortality may be as low as 60% in patients without a concomitant root aneurysm and with aggressive use of antihypertensive medications, especially beta-blockers. Either way, medical therapy has no role in acute type A dissection except to allow a safer transfer to a center with experience in complex aortic repair. In the past, the goal of surgery seemed to focus on placing a short segment of Dacron graft in the ascending aorta in the hope of obliterating the false lumen both proximally into the aortic root and distally into the arch and beyond. That principle often led to recurrent malperfusion proximally (myocardial infarctions and recurrent aortic insufficiency [AI]) and distally (cerebrovascular accidents) as well as a moderate distal early rupture rate. Furthermore, a high incidence of long-term failure was seen with dissecting aneurysms of both the root and the distal ascending aorta and aortic arch.

As better understanding of the risk factors for early complications and death was gained, a better operation could be designed. The idea of focusing on eliminating downstream dissection in the acute setting may be intrinsically flawed. False lumen obliteration at the arch rarely closes the dissection downstream, because of multiple distal

≥ = Size of annulus in older pts.

fenestrations, and focusing on this often shifts attention from what really matters in acute type A dissection. Our review of the data on the cause of death in acute type A dissection allowed us to identify four primary causes of early death and to design an operation that would address them appropriately and directly:

1. Aortic rupture. The ascending aorta is subjected to more stress than any other portion of the aorta. It is the site of the majority of medial degeneration and thus intimal tears. Once dissection has occurred, the ascending aorta is at very high risk of early rupture. This risk is magnified when the aortic root and ascending aorta are dilated because the tension exerted on the remaining media and adventitia increases, according to Laplace's law, by the square of the diameter. To prevent this lethal complication, the ascending aorta needs to be completely replaced.

2. Congestive heart failure due to acute onset of aortic valve insufficiency. Aortic valve support is lost due to prolapse of the intimal layer at the level of one or more commissures. The most commonly affected is the noncoronary to right coronary sinus commissure, followed by the noncoronary to left coronary sinus, and least common is the right to left coronary commissure. To eliminate aortic valve regurgitation, the operation should include either a repair or a replacement strategy as necessary. The most common repair technique consists in aortic valve resuspension to re-establish normal commissural support (Fig. 56-2). Furthermore, the sinotubular junction may be dilated and may need to be brought back to a geometrically normal size. The ascend-

ing aortic graft is sized to best return the sinotubular dimension to its normal state.

3. Acute myocardial infarction due to malperfusion of the coronary arteries. Very few patients with left main coronary compromise survive to reach medical attention. Right coronary malperfusion is much more common. At surgery, the root needs to be repaired definitively to treat ongoing coronary stenosis/occlusion or to prevent future coronary compromise or late root dilation. The incidence of aortic root dissection is quite high, especially in the noncoronary sinus, where the great majority of the aortic root will often be dissected down to the annulus. The second-most-commonly dissected sinus is the right coronary sinus with often some element of coronary malperfusion. Occasionally, the left coronary sinus of Valsalva will be also dissected, and although in the past that was considered to be an indication for root replacement, as long as the intima within the root is intact and the valve leaflets are otherwise normal, dissection of the left coronary sinus can be also managed by repair techniques. Our preferred technique consists in reinforcing any dissected component of the root with an appropriately fashioned Teflon felt sheet placed between the intima and the adventitia, becoming essentially a neo-media. (Fig. 56-3) The Teflon neo-media is fashioned to allow an appropriate opening for the coronary ostia and is secured in place either with a running monofilament fine suture of 4-0 or 5-0 at the level of the sinotubular junction or by utilizing a small amount of biologic glue, CryoLife BioGlue being the most commonly used in our recent expe-

rience (Figs. 56-4 and 56-5). It is important to use a minimal amount of glue because they all have the potential of causing long-term wall damage, especially of the adventitial layer. Long-term results with CryoLife BioGlue have been satisfactory, but further data are needed. Over the last 10 years, repair of a nondilated dissected root with Teflon neo-media has been safe and effective, with excellent and highly reproducible physiologic results leading to sparing of the aortic root in >80% of acute type A dissections, with no incidence of redissection or dilation of the repaired root and no postrepair coronary malperfusions. Alternative procedures include complete valve-sparing root replacement, in which the valve is placed within an appropriately fashioned Dacron graft, and aortic root replacement with a biologic or mechanical option.

4. Stroke due to malperfusion of the aortic arch vessels. The innominate artery is the most commonly dissected of the arch vessels, followed by the left common carotid and at a much lower rate by the left subclavian artery. Replacement of most or all of the aortic arch with reinforcement of the arch vessels ensures true lumen patency and prevents most perioperative strokes, occasionally even reversing preoperative focal neurologic deficits. We usually resect all of the lesser curvature of the aortic arch leaving a strip of arch tissue comprising the three-arch vessels connected to the descending thoracic aorta. Teflon felt strips can be placed between the intima and the adventitia as a neo-media to achieve two goals: first, to restore true lumen perfusion within the arch vessels to prevent postoperative malperfusion syndromes, and second, to reinforce the arch anastomosis suture line, preventing distal disruption. Between 80% and 90% of false lumen beyond the arch will be widely patent after the complete hemiarch repair has been achieved. That does not represent failure of the arch reconstruction. The re-entry fenestrations at the time of surgery are in aggregate so large that it is unrealistic to hope that closing the proximal entry site will ubiquitously result in thrombosis of the false lumen. Our observation is that closure of the false lumen only occurs in limited dissections such as DeBakey type II or when dissections occur in the setting of atherosclerotic disease, in which variably fibrosed and calcified media may prevent the usual extension of the dissection and limit re-entry sites; in these patients obliterating the entry point in

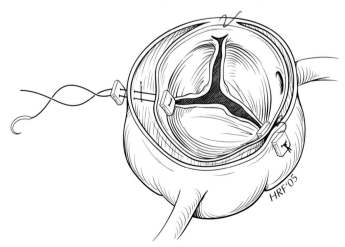

Figure 56-2. Aortic valve resuspension.

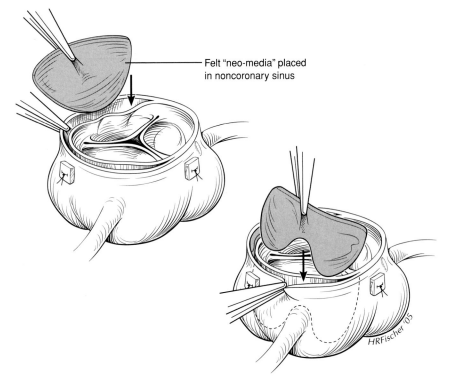

Felt "neo-media" placed in noncoronary sinus

Figure 56-3. Aortic root repair.

the presence of low flow from the few exit sites may cause false lumen thrombosis.

A successful operation for acute type A dissection will leave the patient with a reconstructed or replaced root, a well-functioning aortic valve, a completely replaced ascending aorta, a partially or completely replaced aortic arch with true lumen patency in the arch vessels, and a distal "type B–like" residual aorta (Fig. 56-6). The patient in most instances will have been shifted from a dissection with a high likelihood of death (type A) to a dissection with a very low risk of early rupture and only a moderate risk of long-term aneurysm formation in the residual dissected aorta (type B).

Detailed Surgical Technique

Once the diagnosis of an acute type A dissection is established, the patient is anesthetized under endotracheal general anesthesia. Minimal arterial monitoring consists in using a right radial artery catheter and if feasible also a left radial artery line. The most common arch vessel to suffer malperfusion is the innominate artery; thus the right radial artery would provide early warning of the most likely malperfusion syndrome affecting the brain. If time allows, a left radial artery catheter can give further information about the presence of downstream, less common arch malperfusions. A pulmonary artery catheter is routinely placed to optimize preoperative hemodynamics, but, more important, for postoperative management. High filling pressures correlate with bloody pericardial effusion and tamponade. High central venous pressure (CVP) with low left-sided filling pressures and low pulmonary artery (PA) pressures are highly suggestive of right ventricular (RV) ischemia secondary to right coronary artery (RCA) malperfusion. If a patient is unstable, large-bore intravenous and arterial lines are placed, deferring the PA catheter to a more controlled time. Whenever possible, electroencephalogram (EEG) monitoring should be placed to both monitor for any asymmetry of perfusion at the level of the cerebral cortex and serve as a criterion for achieving adequate cooling to maximize safety for the brain and improve surgical efficiency. It is clear, however, that many acute dissections will occur when EEG monitoring may not be available. In our institution we have been fortunate to achieve emergent neurologic monitoring in approximately 60% of patients presenting with an acute dissection. The patient's chest, abdomen, and both lower extremities are then prepped and draped. In a patient without significant atherosclerotic disease, the most expeditious method for obtaining arterial access for bypass is through a cut-down over the common femoral artery. Malperfusion syndromes of the lower extremities will affect as many as 20% of patients, most commonly the right leg. If both femoral arteries have good pulses, either side can be cannulated. If the patient has signs of poor perfusion to both lower extremities and/or has significant evidence of atherosclerotic disease by significant past history, CT scan, or TEE, our approach has been to cut down

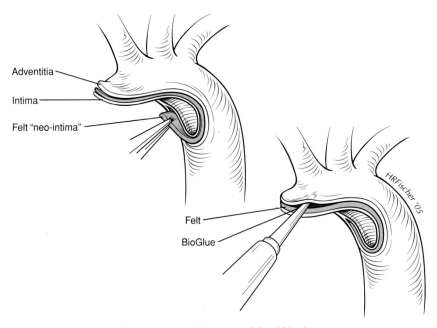

Adventitia

Intima

Felt "neo-intima"

Felt

BioGlue

Figure 56-4. Obliteration of distal false lumen.

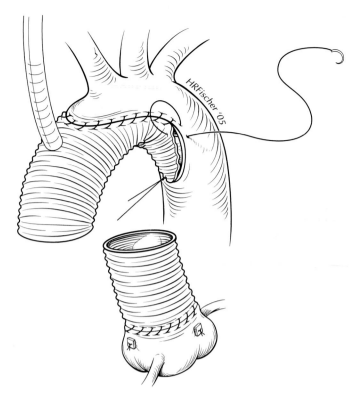

Figure 56-5. Distal graft anastomosis.

on the right axillary artery. A 8-mm Dacron graft is anastomosed first in an end-to-side fashion to the vessel. The arterial cannula is then secured to the Dacron graft. At the end of the procedure the Dacron is oversewn close to the anastomosis.

It is usually preferable to obtain peripheral arterial access before performing the sternotomy. In a setting where two surgeons can work simultaneously, the chosen artery can be exposed at the same time as the sternotomy. In an unstable patient the

femoral artery has the clear advantage over the axillary artery of allowing two surgical teams to work simultaneously without having to share the same limited thoracic space. Once the sternotomy is performed, the pericardium is opened. It is common to find a variable amount of blood-tinged pericardial fluid or even a moderate amount of blood under tension. Often the ascending aorta will be moderately dilated because aneurysm is a major risk factor leading to an ascending aortic dissection. We find the most common area of ascending aortic leak to be the mid-ascending aorta. Most often blood enters the areolar tissue between the main pulmonary artery and the ascending aorta, sometimes dissecting down onto the right ventricular outflow tract, which may look quite discolored by blood and thrombus extending often all the way down to the right atrial ventricular groove. It is important early in the process not to disturb this discoloration or dissected tissue because it is easy to convert this process into a free rupture. With arterial access obtained peripherally, the right atrium is cannulated in the usual fashion. We routinely place a retrograde cardioplegia cannula at this time into the coronary sinus, as well as a superior vena caval (SVC) cannula, which we will use during the circulatory arrest period for retrograde cerebral perfusion either alone or as an adjunct to antegrade cerebral perfusion. The patient is then placed on full cardiopulmonary bypass. During the institution of bypass very close monitoring of arterial waves from the right radial and, if available, the left radial artery is used to detect an arch malperfusion syndrome potentially caused by placement on cardiopulmonary bypass. When available, EEG is also closely monitored for hemispheric asymmetry. When EEG monitoring is not available, carotid artery interrogation can be performed by a handheld probe connected to the same echo machine used for TEE. All our anesthesiologists have become extremely proficient with this simple common carotid artery evaluation. The detection of poor or no perfusion in one of the carotid arteries will prompt appropriate action by the surgical team. If a malperfusion syndrome is documented by ultrasound, EEG, or a persistent radial artery pressure differential, the patient is weaned off bypass and a different arterial cannulation site is often necessary to resolve the problem.

Occasionally two cannulation sites may be necessary, presumably one supplying the true lumen and the other the false lumen. As soon as adequate cardiopulmonary bypass is noted and no malperfusion syndrome

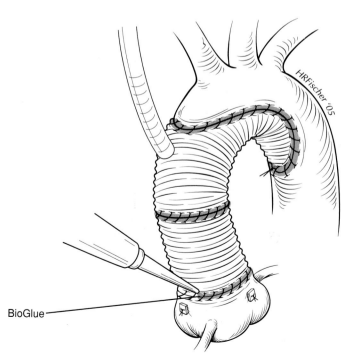

BioGlue

Figure 56-6. Completed repair.

is documented by EEG, arterial pressures, carotid ultrasound, and monitoring of the backpressure of the arterial cannulas, the left ventricle is vented via the right superior pulmonary vein. In many of these patients significant aortic valve insufficiency will be present. Core cooling is then begun with the goal of achieving flat-line EEG if available or, based on our experience with several hundred monitored circulatory arrest cases, cooling is continued to either achieve a nasopharyngeal temperature of 12°C or for a total period of 50 minutes, whichever is reached first. Our data suggest that at this level 100% of patients will have a flat-line EEG. Patients with more severe atherosclerotic disease will likely require longer periods of cooling to achieve uniform end-organ cooling, and furthermore, because adjunctive techniques of retrograde cerebral perfusion or selective antegrade perfusion may be less effective, a deeper level of cooling in this population will make the circulatory arrest period safer.

Very soon after the cooling phase is begun, the patient's heart will fibrillate. Aortic cross-clamp is then applied to the mid-ascending aorta. Although in the past there may have been reluctance to cross-clamp a dissected ascending aorta, over the last 10 years no aortic disruption has resulted from cross-clamping, even in patients with severe collagen vascular disease such as Marfan or Ethan-Danlos syndrome. Clearly the aortic cross-clamp should be placed well below the innominate artery take-off to allow for a greater margin of safety because sometimes more than one cross-clamp may be necessary to fully control this friable, diseased, and often-dilated ascending aorta. At the time of ascending aortic clamping it is again very important to assess for malperfusion syndromes. It is possible, especially when perfusing from the femoral artery, that the application of the cross-clamp may close the largest communication between true and false lumen in the ascending aorta, precipitating an aortic arch malperfusion. Monitoring lines in the right and left radial arteries, EEG monitoring of both hemispheres, and common carotid artery Doppler interrogation may show significant asymmetry. If a malperfusion syndrome is documented, expeditious surgical correction is necessary. Cardiopulmonary bypass is turned off with the patient in deep Trendelenburg position. The aortic cross-clamp is removed, and the ascending aorta is opened proximal to the clamp site to visualize the dissection flap extending into the aortic arch. The dissection flap is then cut deeply into the aortic arch, creating a wide communication between true and false lumen at the arch. The cross-clamp is then reapplied to the distal ascending aorta as cardiopulmonary bypass is restarted slowly, making sure to avoid cerebral air emboli. Although such episodes are rare, occurring in 3% to 4% of our dissection experience, the maneuvers described have been successful in avoiding neurologic injuries that might have led to mortality if they had been unrecognized and left untreated.

After the ascending aorta is cross-clamped without distal malperfusions, it is divided at the level of the right pulmonary artery and cold blood cardioplegia is given both by retrograde coronary sinus infusion and antegrade via direct coronary ostia cannulation. The right coronary is commonly involved in the dissection process, and cannulation for cardioplegia gives the first opportunity to assess for the presence of false lumen–induced stenosis or occlusion or even for the presence of complete disruption. If cardioplegia extravasation is demonstrated in the very proximal portion of the right coronary, a segment of saphenous vein should be obtained by a second surgical team to bypass the right coronary arterial system in case a right button ostial repair proves impossible. Left main coronary problems are rare (if they occur, they are usually fatal out of hospital), and if they are noted at this point in the operation, additional vein grafts can be obtained to deal with them.

Next, the aortic root is exposed to assess whether it is reparable. If the intima within the aortic root is intact and the aortic valve leaflets are normal, the root is usually reparable. Mild dilation of the sinotubular junction up to about 30 mm in maximum diameter can be tolerated with an adequate repair. If the aortic root is severely aneurysmal, consideration of either a valve-sparing root replacement or a mechanical or biologic root replacement should be planned at this time. With normal leaflets and intact root intima, the aortic root is mobilized circumferentially, ensuring adventitial root integrity. The aorta is then transected approximately 3 mm above the sinotubular junction, and three Teflon pledgeted monofilament sutures are placed approximately 2 mm above each of the three commissures. These resuspension sutures allow re-establishment of appropriate commissural geometry. Attention is directed next to the sinuses of Valsalva. The noncoronary sinus is nearly always dissected down to the annulus. Any debris or thrombus within the noncoronary-sinus false lumen is cleared. Teflon felt is then fashioned to completely fit within the dissected space of the noncoronary sinus and is then inserted between the intima and the adventitia as a "neo-media." It is secured in place either by using 5-0 or 4-0 monofilament sutures at the level of the sinotubular junction or by placing a few precise drops of CryoLife BioGlue. Attention is next directed to the right coronary sinus of Valsalva. This is involved in >50% of acute type A dissections and often requires a very similar repair technique to that used in the noncoronary sinus. Teflon felt is placed between the intima and the adventitia, fashioned in such a way to avoid any narrowing of the right coronary lumen as it courses through the dissected sinus. The left coronary sinus of Valsalva is then inspected. It is rarely involved in the dissection, but when it is, it is treated in a similar fashion as the right coronary sinus with a similar Teflon felt inserted between the intima and the adventitia and secured in the same fashion.

If the aortic root is not reconstructible either because of pre-existing root disease or because of significant intimal root destruction and/or leaflets disease or tears, the coronary ostia are mobilized for root replacement. Although valve-sparing root replacement might be an option, we have rarely used this in acute type A dissection, and it should be reserved for patients <50 years old, often with collagen vascular disease and normal leaflets. A mechanical valved conduit remains an excellent option in most patients <60 years old. A biologic root replacement, primarily with a porcine root, should be considered in anyone >60 years of age because the avoidance of Coumadin greatly simplifies postoperative management, and furthermore, patients in this age group who have suffered an acute type A dissection are not likely to outlive their biologic prosthesis.

Usually, adequate cooling will be reached before the completion of root replacement. To maximize overall operative efficiency, all proximal work is stopped once flat-line EEG, 12°C nasopharyngeal temperature, or 50 minutes of cooling is reached, and attention is directed to the aortic arch. Antegrade cardiopulmonary bypass is interrupted, and retrograde cerebral perfusion is begun via the snared SVC cannula. Flows of 150 to 250 cc/min are typically used to a target jugular venous pressure of 20 to 25 mm Hg. Jugular venous pressure is measured via the right internal jugular sheath used to introduce the PA catheter. The ascending aortic cross-clamp is removed and the aorta is assessed. The goal now is to excise the remainder of the ascending aorta and to prevent arch malperfusion once antegrade cardiopulmonary bypass is reestablished. The remainder of the ascending aorta is therefore debrided. The majority of the undersurface of the arch is excised. The details of the true and false lumen relationships are assessed carefully because there can be significant individual variation. The amount of aortic arch removed depends in large part on the relationship of the arch vessels to the arch false lumen. In general, the entire lesser curvature of the arch and the majority of the anterior and posterior aortic arch are excised leaving a lip of aortic tissue encompassing the left subclavian, left common carotid, and innominate artery. A thin Teflon felt strip is placed within the false lumen areas around the arch vessels and as necessary into the dissected portions of the residual proximal descending thoracic aorta. Again, the primary goal here is to prevent arch malperfusion with the secondary goal to create a layer that would hold sutures well for aortic arch reconstruction. The strip of Teflon felt is secured between the intima and the adventitia around the arch vessels and the dissected portion of the proximal descending thoracic aorta with a few drops of CryoLife BioGlue or with a few interrupted or short running of 4-0 or 5-0 monofilament nonabsorbable sutures. A Dacron graft is then appropriately beveled and sewn to the reinforced arch tissue using running 4-0 monofilament sutures. Multiple interrupted pledgeted monofilament reinforcement sutures are placed wherever necessary to further buttress the suture line. De-airing maneuvers are performed, greatly aided by retrograde cerebral perfusion.

Occasionally the aortic arch disruption is so severe that a total aortic arch replacement is necessary. Selective antegrade cerebral perfusion can be carried out via manually inflated balloon-tip cannulas inserted in the innominate and the left common carotid arteries. A Dacron graft is sewn to the neomedia reinforced proximal descending thoracic aorta usually using the elephant-trunk technique. The arch graft is then sewn either to a reinforced island containing the arch vessels or to the individual branches as necessary. Before resuming antegrade cardiopulmonary bypass, de-airing maneuvers are then performed with the aid of retrograde cerebral perfusion. In our experience only 10% of acute type A dissections required total aortic arch replacement, with another 5% requiring a separate graft to the innominate artery only.

After either a "hemiarch" or a "total arch repair" the Dacron graft is directly cannulated, and antegrade cardiopulmonary bypass is re-established. We feel it is very important at the end of the arch reconstruction

to cannulate the aorta in antegrade fashion at the arch Dacron graft, even if the patient was initially cannulated via the right axillary artery. Antegrade reperfusion after arch repair minimizes potential malperfusion or arch suture-line disruptions. Between 50% and 60% of distal arch vessels have a patent false lumen in acute type A dissections. If flow were re-established via the right axillary artery in the setting of a distal innominate artery dissection, a right common carotid artery malperfusion could develop. Furthermore, the innominate artery false lumen may still have a sufficient distal entry point to sufficiently pressurize the arch suture line to cause disruption of the reconstructed aortic arch. Direct cannulation of the aortic arch graft should prevent such local perfusion anomalies, minimizing the risk of arch suture-line disruption and maximizing true lumen flow. A few minutes are taken early after full flow is established to assess the arch suture line and ensure adequate hemostasis. This may be the only opportunity to treat significant bleeding points from the reconstructed aortic arch because there is nothing worse than a leaking arch anastomosis. Full rewarming is then allowed to begin.

The appropriate size of Dacron graft to restore normal sinotubular junction geometry is selected and it is then sewn to the reinforced sinotubular junction with 4-0 nonabsorbable monofilament suture. If a root replacement was underway prior to the arch reconstruction, it is now completed. The proximal reconstruction is then tested by infusing cardioplegia solution into the repaired or replaced aortic root to assess for the presence of significant aortic valve insufficiency as well as suture-line hemostasis. The proximal reconstruction is then sewn to the arch graft with running monofilament suture. Cardiac de-airing maneuvers are performed, and the heart is the allowed to reperfuse. During reperfusion, the peripheral arterial cannulation site is appropriately repaired. After full rewarming, the patient is weaned off cardiopulmonary bypass. Early post pump, it is important to assess for significant aortic valve insufficiency. Any more than trace or 1 + AI will result in poor long-term valve durability. If the patient can tolerate going back on cardiopulmonary bypass, 2+ and higher AI should be fixed now, either by valvular replacement within the repaired root or by complete root replacement if necessary.

After the cardiac repair is noted to be satisfactory, the systemic vascular system is assessed to exclude new malperfusion syndromes or to reassess preoperative ischemic

regions. Greater than 50% of preoperative limb ischemias will resolve after adequate proximal aortic repair. If one limb remains pulseless with good perfusion in the contralateral limb, a femoral–femoral bypass can be performed. If both lower extremities continue to have poor pulses at this stage, an axillary–femoral or axillary–bifemoral reconstruction is favored over opening the abdomen and subjecting the patient to very morbid additional surgery. This latter outcome is very rare, and in the near future stent grafting may provide an effective and durable treatment for abdominal and bilateral lower extremity malperfusions.

Acute Type B Dissection

Most patients with an acute type B dissection have a much lower risk of dying from the process than do those with a type A dissection. The early risk of rupture in the descending thoracic or abdominal aorta is much less than 10%, and in the chronic phase the risk remains low unless associated with aneurysmal dilation. The major early morbidity and mortality are due to malperfusion syndromes. These may require surgical intervention. The ultimate malperfusion syndrome is the development of a pseudo-coarctation, in which the true lumen is severely narrowed by a pressurized thrombosed or sluggishly flowing false lumen (Figs. 56-7 and 56-8). All downstream vessels will suffer from impaired perfusion.

Surgical interventions in type B dissection need to be tailored to the specific problems encountered by the individual patient. Unlike patients with type A dissection, most patients with type B dissection are more likely to have significant atherosclerotic disease, with the tear often within a ruptured plaque. In severely atherosclerotic aortas, dissection extension may occasionally be quite limited due to the fibrotic media resisting establishment of a false lumen.

The mainstay of early therapy for uncomplicated acute type B dissection remains medical management primarily consisting of strict blood pressure control. Beta-blocking agents provide excellent control of absolute systolic pressure and also minimize aortic wall stress by minimizing the blood pressure rate of rise (dP/dT). In the early phase intravenous control is usually achieved with esmolol and labetalol. Additional intravenous vasodilators can be used including calcium-channel blockers such as nicardipine. We try to avoid nitroprusside, except for very short periods very early in the stabilization process. After

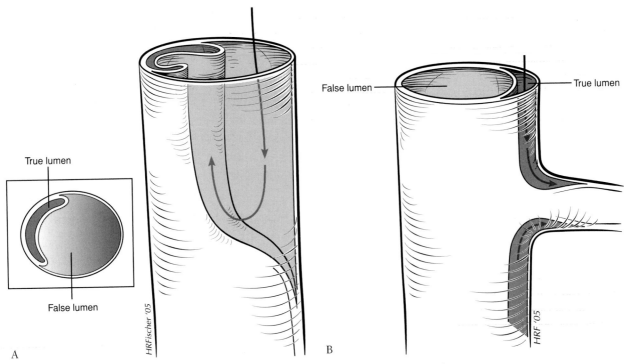

Figure 56-7. **(A)** Pseudo-coarctation. **(B)** Malperfusion syndrome.

the patient is past the acute phase, oral agents are titrated to maintain ideal blood pressure and heart rate levels. That often includes long-acting beta-blockers like metoprolol or Metoprolol SR as well as a calcium-channel blocker such as Amlodipine or nifedipine. If renal function remains normal, angiotensin-converting-enzyme (ACE) inhibitors can be used as well as occasionally ganglionic blockers such as Captopril. Many of these patients may have presented with a very malignant pattern of hypertension and often require chronically three or four drugs including beta-blockers, calcium-channel blockers, ganglionic blockers, plus or minus ACE inhibitors and diuretics.

It is very important to minimize aortic stress early in the process primarily to avoid rupture, control pain, stabilize treated or mild malperfusions, and allow stabilization of the weakened aorta. Once the patient is in the chronic state, tight blood pressure control is maintained to limit aneurysmal degeneration. Many of these patients, as noted already, have severe atherosclerotic distal vascular beds, including cerebrovascular intracranial disease, as well as renovascular and occlusive disease in their abdominal visceral and lower extremity beds. These patients may not respond favorably to "normalization" of their blood pressure. Often a balance has to be reached between minimizing aortic disruption and allowing

adequate perfusion of very extensively diseased vascular beds.

The goals of surgical intervention in type B dissection need to be individualized and well defined prior to proceeding to surgery. If a patient has a contained or free rupture, the goal of surgery should be the excision of the ruptured segment. Although rare, one should look for evidence of aortic disruptions early in the course. More commonly, treatment needs to focus on regional malperfusions. The most time-tested and expeditious method of surgically dealing with malperfusion is through extra-anatomic bypass because direct surgery to the acutely dissected thoracic or abdominal aorta can be treacherous and often leads to significant morbidity and mortality.

The new technology of stent grafting is likely to revolutionize the management and treatment of acute type B aortic dissection. Endovascular stent grafting of the true lumen may already represent the most appropriate treatment of pseudo-coarctation and mesenteric malperfusion. Endovascular fenestration, often with bare stents, has also been utilized to increase flow to poorly perfused vascular beds. The historical experience of placing short interposition grafts within the descending thoracic aorta in uncomplicated type B dissections to obliterate the false lumen downstream has not worked well with the majority of false lumens remaining patent at the price of a moderate

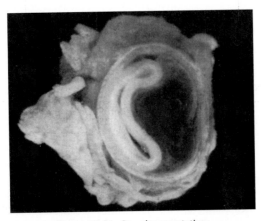

Figure 56-8. Pseudo-coarctation.

operative morbidity and mortality risk. Downstream fenestrations are multiple and well established by the time the patient is taken to surgery. However, the availability of very early intervention by stent graft technology can be much more effective in chronically obliterating the distal false lumen at minimal morbidity and mortality. The present preliminary experience consists in landing a stent graft across the intimal entry point at the level of the subclavian artery and then covering at a minimum the proximal one third or up to the entire descending thoracic aortic true lumen. Distal re-entry points may still be few and poorly established in the very early phase, allowing such interventions to be successful. Even a partial success in obliterating type B dissections may lead to a significant decrease in the long-term sequelae of dissecting aneurysms. A number of stent graft protocols are in the design stage in the United States to establish just how safe and effective a strategy of very early stent graft placement might be in acute type B dissections. A number of European institutions are already managing complicated type B dissections with short stent graft placement at the entry tear routinely obliterating the take-off of the left subclavian artery. Early results appear satisfactory, yet most patients with type B dissections do very well early in their course with blood pressure control alone. Therefore, only long-term follow-up will allow us to assess the true benefit of such therapy. One additional extension of such a strategy may be applied to the treatment of acute type A dissection. In the future, a stent graft may be deployed routinely in the proximal descending thoracic aorta via the open aortic arch at the original surgery. This may significantly increase the likelihood of obliterating the distal false lumen, with minimal added operative risk, and, it is hoped, sparing many patients from late dissecting aneurysms.

Special Cases: Intramural Hematomas and Retrograde Extensions of Type B Dissections

Occasionally both type A and type B dissections may present with either a partially or a completely thrombosed false lumen. A partially thrombosed type A dissection may have a lower risk of rupture or malperfusion especially when the ascending aorta is not dilated. The data supporting such an assertion, however, are very limited, and furthermore the risk of urgent surgery for a type A dissection in our hands is lower than that reported from observing a partially thrombosed dilated ascending aortic dissection. Our approach has been to treat such patients with a thrombosed false lumen in the ascending aorta in the same fashion as those with a standard type A dissection, thus proceeding to surgery without delay. Often these patients have a higher degree of atherosclerotic disease, which may account for the lack of further progression of their dissection or for the early thrombosis due to sluggish false lumen flow secondary to minimal re-entry sites. A type B dissection with thrombosed false lumen should be treated in the same fashion as a standard type B dissection, with primary medical treatment. However, a partially thrombosed false lumen when pressurized is more likely to compromise true lumen flow and lead to pseudo-coarctation. Appropriate assessment and potential stenting or extra-anatomic bypass of the pseudo-coarctation should be considered.

Aortic dissection may rarely arise in the aortic arch and then progress both retrograde and antegrade. This process may on occasion be difficult to classify within the Stanford system, and it may be difficult to decide whether the initial management should be surgical or medical. Most of these patients will have significantly atherosclerotic aortas with the false lumen becoming pressurized early in the descending thoracic aorta exerting significant retrograde forces to extend the dissection retrograde as the path of least resistance. If the retrograde extension ends at the level of the aortic arch and does not involve significant portions of the ascending aorta, the primary additional risk to a standard type B dissection is a cerebrovascular accident. The risk of rupture should be relatively low. Although our management remains individualized, we would initially observe patients with this type of retrograde extension and treat them as patients with type B dissections. If, however, the ascending aorta becomes involved, either acutely or during follow-up, these patients should be treated as patients with a standard type A dissection because they do suffer from the same risks of rupture, aortic valve insufficiency, and aortic root compromise leading to coronary malperfusion. We find, furthermore, that these patients have a higher surgical risk because the aortic arch is often completely destroyed and very difficult to piece back together. These are the class of patients in whom an often very technically challenging total arch replacement may need to be performed, with an attendant higher mortality and a higher incidence of neurologic complications.

Long-Term Follow-up and Chronic Dissections

Any patient with a valve-sparing repair or replacement of aortic root needs lifelong surveillance to monitor the long-term durability of aortic valve function. Patients with less than 1+ AI at the time of primary surgery have had an extremely durable repair using the technique described. If the valve fails, regurgitation is typically the problem, and an aortic valve replacement alone is often sufficient because the aortic root has been reinforced sufficiently to make the incidence of root dilation very low.

All patients who have undergone proximal repair for an acute type A dissection will need lifelong surveillance of the residual aorta. Approximately 90% will have a residual type B–like dissection beyond the completion of the arch repair. This residual dissection is at risk for aneurysm formation. If a dissecting aneurysm develops, these patients are candidates for repair based on standard aneurysm management criteria. We find that 30% to 40% of patients will require downstream aneurysm surgery after proximal type A repair over a 5-year follow-up, and the risk will be higher the younger is the patient, with a risk as high as 70% to 90% in patients with collagen-vascular disease. Any patient who requires a distal aortic arch and descending thoracic aortic replacement must have a very careful evaluation for the presence of significant aortic valve insufficiency. Full cardiopulmonary bypass through the left chest with hypothermia leading to fibrillation can be very problematic in the presence of more than 1+ aortic valve insufficiency. It is difficult to control the ascending aorta from the left chest, and significant left ventricular distension can occur, even with a well-positioned left ventricular vent. This can lead to cardiac and pulmonary dysfunction at the completion of the distal arch and descending thoracic replacement. To prevent such problems, the aortic valve may need to be replaced before the distal aortic repair.

Occasionally a patient will survive an undiagnosed acute type A dissection and will present months to years later with a large ascending dissecting aortic aneurysm with variable amount of AI. Such a patient is treated surgically in an urgent fashion because the risk of rupture is higher than with a nondissected ascending aneurysm of equal size. These aneurysms may have grown quite rapidly and present occasionally with compression symptoms to surrounding structures. At surgery no attempt should be made to obliterate the distal false lumens because many distal vascular beds will have become dependent on false lumen flow. The dissection flap should be resected as far as reachable to maintain free flow in all distal lumens. Depending on the sinus involvement and the chronicity, valve resuspension techniques may not be effective. If the aortic leaflets appear to be relatively preserved, a valve-sparing root replacement may be a good option. In the chronic setting, total arch replacement with branched arch grafts is more often required and carries a significantly lower morbidity and mortality compared to the acute setting.

Conclusion

In the last decade we have gained a much better understanding of the aortic dissection process, which has allowed us to define specific goals for our surgical treatment and led to significantly improved results. An early mortality of approximately 10% for treatment of acute type A dissections has been achieved because of multiple factors such as improvements in diagnostic techniques, expeditious transfer to the operating room before cardiovascular collapse, better physiologic understanding of intraoperative malperfusion syndromes especially affecting the arch vessels, intraoperative neurologic monitoring leading to real-time surgical maneuvers to reverse abnormalities, precise repair or replacement of the aortic root, and precise and durable anastomoses at the level of the arch. Type B dissections have remained a relatively low-risk early process

where medical management remains the mainstay. The availability of stent graft technology may allow further improvement in the early management of complicated type B dissections and may significantly minimize late-dissecting aneurysms. Combining the described type A dissection repairs with intraoperative deployment of a stent graft to the residual downstream dissection may allow further improvement in the long-term outcome for these patients. Much has been accomplished, yet there is still room for further improvement and refinement in our techniques and understanding.

SUGGESTED READING

Bavaria JE, Pochettino A, Brinster DR, et al. New paradigms and improved results for the surgical treatment of acute type a dissection. Ann Surg 2001;234:336.

Bavaria JE, Woo YJ, Hall RA, et al. Circulatory management with retrograde cerebral perfusion for acute type A aortic dissection. Circulation 1996;94(Suppl9):II1730.

David TE, Armstrong S, Ivanov J, et al. Surgery for acute type A aortic dissection. Ann Thorac Surg 1999;67:199.

Fann JI, Smith JA, Miller DC, et al. Surgical management of aortic dissection during a 30-year period. Circulation 1995;92(Suppl 9): II113.

Hagan PG, Nienaber CA, Isselbacher EM, et al. The international registry of acute aortic dissection (IRAD). New insights into an old disease. JAMA 2000;283:897.

Januzzi JL, Marayati F, Mehta RH, et al. Comparison of aortic dissection in patients with and without Marfan's syndrome (results from the International registry of aortic dissection). Am J Cardiol 2004;94:400.

Kallenbach K, Leyh RG, Salcher R, et al. Acute aortic dissection versus aortic root aneurysm: comparison of indications for valve sparing aortic root reconstruction. Eur J Cardiothorac Surg 2004;25:663.

Kitamura M, Hashimoto A, Akimoto T, et al. Operation for type A aortic dissection: Intro-

duction of retrograde cerebral perfusion. Ann Thorac Surg 1995;59:1195.

Mehta RH, Bossone E, Evangelista A, et al. International Registry of Acute Aortic Dissection Investigators. Acute type B aortic dissection in elderly patients: Clinical features, outcomes, and simple risk stratification rule. Ann Thorac Surg 2004;77:1622; discussion 1629.

Motallebzadeh R, Batas D, Valencia O, et al. The role of coronary angiography in acute type A aortic dissection. Eur J Cardiothorac Surg 2004;25:231.

EDITOR'S COMMENTS

The University of Pennsylvania group has developed the most-organized approach to the transfer and care of acute aortic dissection. This is the main reason I asked them to present this chapter. They give an excellent overview of the etiology, diagnosis, and surgical treatment. In general, we do all the things they suggest. However, we have moved away from the various biologic glues recently due to published reports demonstrating poor long-term results and arterial wall injury. Like the authors, we tend to be conservative about root replacement except when the root is truly enlarged. We avoid valve-sparing roots in most of those situations with the exception of the case in which the aorta is not totally torn apart in a very young patient. We perhaps differ in not using nearly as much felt as the authors suggest, and believe that we can get a better closure without the use of Teflon felt sheets. However, this is a very individual choice. In spite of improvements in our understanding and diagnosis, the mortality remains quite high. In patients with shock the mortality can approach 30% to 50% at reputable centers. This does not relate to surgical issues, but rather to multiorgan failure, which continues to markedly worsen the results.

I.L.K.

57

Descending Thoracic and
Thoracoabdominal Aneurysms

John A. Kern and Irving L. Kron

Since the initial description in 1955 by Etheridge and in 1956 by DeBakey of successful repair of thoracic and thoracoabdominal aneurysms, great changes have occurred in the techniques used to surgically reconstruct the thoracic and thoracoabdominal aorta. Patient outcomes have improved considerably, from Crawford's reported 26% 30-day mortality in 1965 to recent report of 2% 30-day mortality over 162 cases at the same institution. In addition to improvements in perioperative patient management techniques that have occurred over that time, there is a greater understanding of the comorbid factors that are likely to affect patient outcomes and of the importance of the rapid restoration of distal organ perfusion after application of the aortic cross-clamp. Hospitals with considerable experience in dealing with these challenging aortic problems are able to achieve low mortality and morbidity figures, reflecting the surgical team's expertise in assessing the individual patient's unique needs and appropriately applying surgical techniques gathered by individual experience over previous cases.

In this chapter we address the current problems confronting a surgeon who operates on a patient with a chronic thoracic or thoracic or thoracoabdominal aneurysm and outline the surgical techniques available in the endeavor to achieve a safe and lasting aortic repair.

Anatomic Considerations

This chapter concerns aspects of aneurysm surgery for aneurysms arising between the aortic isthmus and the infrarenal aorta. The Crawford classification (Fig. 57-1) defines thoracoabdominal aortic aneurysms as follows: type I, proximal descending thoracic aorta to the upper abdominal aorta; type II, proximal descending thoracic aorta to below the renal arteries; type III, distal half of the descending thoracic aorta into the abdomen; and type IV, most or all of the abdominal aorta. Many surgeons use the term "extent" rather than "type." The branches of the aorta in this region may be classified as either visceral or somatic. The aorta gives off paired somatic branches beginning as the third intercostal arteries and continuing to the fourth lumbar arteries. From these intercostal or lumbar arteries, most commonly in the region T9 to L2, arises the artery or arteries that feed the descending anterior spinal artery and supply the lower spinal cord and cauda equina. Visceral branches are given off ventrally as celiac axis, superior mesenteric, and inferior mesenteric arteries and laterally as the paired and sometimes multiple renal arteries.

A surgeon undertaking operative repair of thoracic or thoracoabdominal aneurysms must understand the proximity of the visceral arteries to the aneurysm and, if they are involved, how these arteries are to be reconstructed with a graft or reimplantation. The major difficulty in dealing with the somatic aortic branches is not their number but deciding which is important and should be revascularized. Fortunately, with modern perfusion techniques, most major aortic branches can be reconstructed with little additional time and morbidity. Preoperative identification of the spinal artery and its vessel of origin has not proved to be rou-tinely feasible and practical by current angiographic or other radiological techniques. The anterior spinal artery originates most commonly between T9 and L2 but may arise higher or lower. Thus, indirect methods of identifying important intercostal or lumbar arteries must be used as a guide to finding and preserving the blood supply to the spinal cord.

The aorta passes between the crura of the diaphragm at T12 level. A thoracoabdominal aneurysm by definition will straddle the diaphragm, which must therefore be taken down at least partially and then reconstructed without damaging its function. The anatomic distribution of the phrenic nerves as they ramify on the abdominal surface of the diaphragm as they supply its fibers must be understood by the surgeon.

Diagnostic Considerations

There are a number of different causes of thoracic or thoracoabdominal aneurysms. Although syphilis was once a common cause of aneurysm disease, it is now exceedingly rare. The most common cause of aneurysm in the United States now is atherosclerosis. All common risk factors for atherosclerosis and heart disease can predispose patients to an increased risk of aneurysm formation. Hypertension can also predispose patients to aortic dissections, which over time will almost invariably become aneurysmal. Patients with Marfan syndrome, cystic medial necrosis, and other connective tissue disorders are at risk for aneurysm formation.

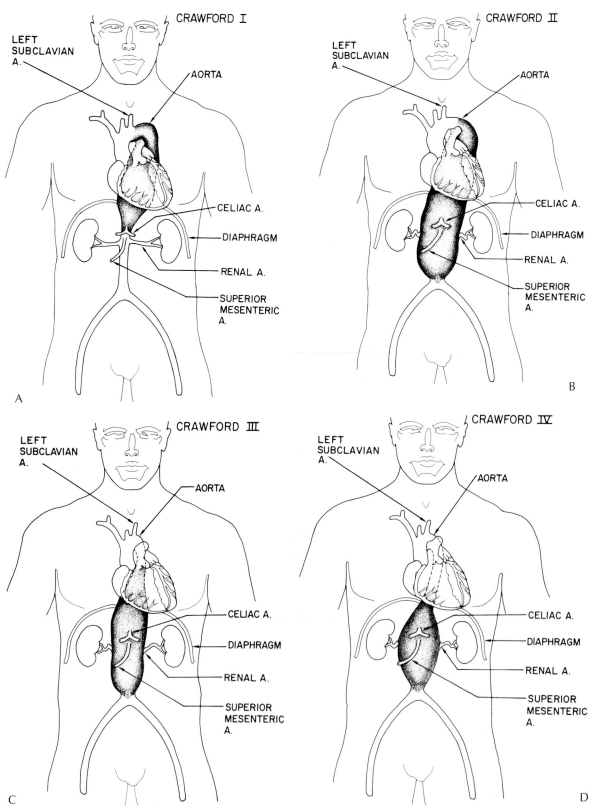

Figure 57-1.   Crawford classification of thoracoabdominal aneurysms. **(A)** Type I. **(B)** Type II. **(C)** Type III. **(D)** Type IV. (A. = artery.)

Patients with undiagnosed thoracic aortic trauma may present years later with late aneurysm formation. There are of course a variety of ways in which a patient with a thoracic or thoracoabdominal aneurysm may present to medical care. The patient may have a chest x-ray film or more commonly a computed tomographic (CT) scan for an unrelated reason, and an abnormality of the mediastinum or the aorta is detected. The patient previously may have undergone surgery for abdominal aortic or ascending aortic aneurysm disease and thus be known to be at risk for further aortic disease. The patient may have suffered from symptoms of an aortic dissection in the past with back pain and hypertension. Occasionally the patient will present with indirect signs of an aortic aneurysm, such as hoarseness caused by recurrent laryngeal nerve dysfunction or distal ischemic events caused by embolism of atherosclerotic material or laminated thrombus. Infrequently the patient may have a symptom or sign of an impending rupture, such as severe back pain, pleural effusion, or retroperitoneal hematoma.

Complete diagnosis is usually made from a contrast-enhanced CT scan of the chest and or abdomen. The scan will accurately supply information about the size of the aneurysm, the presence of hematoma or bleeding, and the degree of laminated thrombus or atheroma. Thin-slice CT angiography (CTA) with associated image reconstruction has nearly supplanted standard catheter-based angiography in fully diagnosing aortic pathology and aneurysm disease. Properly timed contrast bolus is critical, and care must be taken when measuring the diameter of the aorta on the source axial images because the tortuosity of the aorta must be taken into account. Although aortography remains the gold standard in determining the relationship of the aneurysm to aortic branches and whether these branches are stenosed or occluded, CTA is rapidly evolving as a fast and less invasive way of diagnosing all aortic pathology. Most aspects of intervention, whether surgical or endovascular, can be planned off of a well-done CTA, thereby obviating the need for distal subtraction angiography.

Magnetic resonance angiography (MRA) has also evolved over the last decade and is another modality available to diagnose aortic aneurysm disease and allow planning of an appropriate intervention. MRA is attractive because it uses no nephrotoxic contrast and is therefore often the diagnostic modality of choice for patients with renal insufficiency. The few contraindications to MRA

and the need for a radiologist skilled in post imaging processing may limit the utility of this technique in the acute diagnosis of aortic aneurysm disease.

Because of the significant operative risks associated with repair of thoracic and thoracoabdominal aortic aneurysms, the size generally accepted in an asymptomatic patient before recommending surgery is 6 cm. A diameter greater than this carries an appreciable risk of rupture, and if the patient is fit enough to tolerate the procedure, then elective repair should be planned. Consideration also needs to be given to the disease process causing the aneurysm, the diameter of the aneurysmal aorta with respect to normal aorta, and any evidence of growth by >5 mm over a 6-month period. These factors may alter the 6-cm rule and promote earlier operation or continued careful observation. In the preoperative evaluation careful attention should be paid to the presence of ischemic heart disease, obstructive lung disease, and renal impairment. If any of these conditions is present, efforts should be made to maximize available therapy before surgery in order to minimize collateral morbidity.

Operative Procedure

Anesthesia and Monitoring

The patient will undergo general anesthesia with double-lumen endotracheal intubation. A single-lumen tube can be used for lower thoracic thoracoabdominal aneurysms. Large-bore peripheral intravenous access with 14-gauge cannulas, a radial arterial pressure line, and central venous pressure monitoring are mandatory. Use of a pulmonary artery catheter may be advisable in some patients as well as transesophageal echocardiography. A Foley bladder catheter should be placed for continuous urine measurement, and continuous electrocardiographic (ECG) monitoring and pulse oximetry should also be used. For those patients receiving left heart bypass, a femoral arterial line is useful to help maintain balanced pressures while on bypass. When adequate monitoring and control of ventilation have been established, the patient is rolled to expose the left lateral chest wall and flank. Although a posterolateral thoracotomy is used for exposure of thoracic aneurysms, a full lateral position is not used. The pelvis should be half-rolled anteriorly to allow access to the left femoral vessels. The patient should be positioned over the break of the operating table on a

beanbag with all pressure points padded. An axillary roll is used, and the table is flexed to open the intercostal spaces and allow access to the aorta.

Incision and Operative Exposure

Thoracic Aneurysms

The thoracic aorta can be exposed over its entire length through use of a single thoracotomy incision. We use a long posterolateral thoracotomy, dividing the latissimus dorsi and some of serratus anterior. Ventilation of the left lung should be discontinued before entry into the pleural cavity. The level of intercostal entry into the pleural cavity is tailored according to the case in hand. Aneurysms confined to the upper or middle thoracic aorta may be adequately exposed through one intercostal space, especially if one of the ribs is divided posteriorly. For more extensive aneurysms, we prefer a fourth interspace entry to expose the aorta up to the distal arch and the left subclavian artery, and a second interspace entry, utilizing the same skin incision, in the seventh or eighth intercostal space. Care is taken to avoid injuring the lung when the pleura is opened. The lung is retracted anteriorly under sponges and a slung whisk to expose the aorta. The pleura over the aorta is divided to expose the aneurysm and the aorta. Care should be taken to identify both the vagus nerve throughout its transit of the pleural cavity and the phrenic nerve proximally, where dissection of the aortic arch may endanger it. Identifying its proximal extent and dissecting out the aorta at the aneurysm neck effects control of the aneurysm. The aorta should be taped either just proximal or just to the origin of the left subclavian artery and enough room made around the aorta with careful sharp dissection to allow for application of the crossclamp. If any lymph vessels, especially the thoracic duct, are seen during this dissection, they should be avoided. If a lymph leak is identified, it should be controlled at this time.

The aorta distal to the aneurysm also is dissected out and taped. If a second intercostal entry is to be made because of the extent of the aneurysm, the intercostal retractor is removed from the upper entry, the lower pleural entry is performed, and the retractor is inserted here. The lower dissection is performed, and the retractor is moved back to the upper incision for application of the cross-clamp. No attempt is made to dissect out the length of the aneurysm. Such dissection is unnecessary for the repair and may cause hazardous bleeding.

Thoracoabdominal Aneurysms

The incision we use starts posterolaterally over the ribs at the level of the eighth or ninth interspace. The incision goes obliquely, crossing the costal margin over the ninth interspace, and curves inferiorly to run parallel to the midline to a level below the umbilicus. The abdominal portion of the incision stays lateral to the midline. The pleural cavity is entered with the left lung deflated. The muscles of the abdominal wall are divided in the line of the incision, but the peritoneal cavity is not entered. Peritoneum and transversalis fascia are often closely applied at the lateral edge of the rectus muscle, and special care should be exercised here to avoid entering the peritoneal cavity.

A curving incision is made to take down the diaphragm and yet preserve its function. The diaphragm is divided to the chest wall under the incision at the costal margin, and a 3-cm lip is then left attached to the inner aspect of the ribs as the incision curves posteriorly. This circumferential incision is continued to the crura; the left crus can be divided to expose the aorta beneath. Many surgeons use this circumferential incision to avoid injury to the phrenic nerve; however, we have also recently begun to use a radial incision with no appreciable increase in postoperative pulmonary complications. Others have reported this same observation. We have also found it possible to not completely divide the diaphragm, but keep it partially intact and work above and below the diaphragm and pass the graft through the natural hiatus. This may also improve postoperative pulmonary performance.

With use of progressive retraction and blunt dissection, the peritoneum and its contents can be moved forward and the retroperitoneum exposed. Use of a self-retraining retractor will facilitate obtaining and maintaining this exposure. The aorta and its branches lie medial to the iliopsoas muscle bundle. We prefer to mobilize the left kidney from its bed on the psoas muscle, but if desired, it can be left in place. Sharp dissection over the anterior aspect of the aorta is then required to identify the anterior visceral branches and allow enough mobility for their reimplantation if required (see later discussion). The aorta should then be dissected out and taped above and below the aneurysm to prepare for aortic clamping.

Control of Hemodynamic Instability during Aortic Cross-Clamping

Proximal aortic clamping, especially between the left common carotid and left subclavian arteries, is associated with a severe, sudden increase in afterload. Cross-clamp release precipitates sudden afterload reduction, with relative hypovolemia and acute systemic hypotension. Several strategies are available to modulate these hemodynamic changes.

Pharmacologic Manipulation

Before application of the cross-clamp, adequate warning should be given to the anesthesiologist. Aggressive lowering of the systemic blood pressure and afterload acutely is achieved through rapid infusion of nitroglycerine or sodium nitroprusside. The cross-clamp is applied when systolic blood pressure has been lowered to 70 to 80 mm Hg. The blood pressure will rise acutely with aortic clamping and should be kept within normal limits during clamping. Again, adequate notice should be given to the anesthesiologist before cross-clamp release. To prepare for unclamping, all dilators should be turned off, sodium bicarbonate and calcium administered, and rapid infusion of volume given. Pressor agents such as phenylephrine may also be administered shortly before cross-clamp release. These measures may help to minimize post–clamp release hypotension.

Slow Clamp Application and Release

Progressive clamp application and release over 2 to 4 minutes may help to blunt the acute afterload changes that aortic clamping causes. To accurately assess distal ischemia, cross-clamp time should be measured from the first squeeze on the clamp to its complete release. Unfortunately, in some cases, despite the most aggressive use of dilators, volume, and clamp techniques, severe hemodynamic instability and hypotension may occur.

Extracorporeal Circulation

Redistribution of blood flow through the use of extracorporeal circuits may be used to reduce afterload and to continue perfusion of organs distal to the cross-clamp. The simplest method is to use a passive aorto-aortic shunt. More sophisticated and effective methods include left atriofemoral bypass and femorofemoral cardiopulmonary bypass.

1. Left atriofemoral bypass (Fig. 57-2). Blood is drawn from the left atrium by

way of a cannula introduced through the atrial appendage or more commonly the left inferior pulmonary vein. With use of a heparin-bonded circuit to reduce the amount of heparin necessary, the blood is pumped through a centrifugal or roller pump and returned to the femoral artery or to the aorta below the level of the distal clamp if the aorta is not diseased at this level. The amount of flow through the system can be adjusted to achieve a small increase in blood pressure with aortic cross-clamping and a small drop with clamp release. We favor this method for distal perfusion; our recommendation is that it be used in most cases of type I and II extent aneurysms and even some type III aneurysms. Patients who will benefit most from this technique are those with some degree of heart disease and who have brittle hemodynamics and those with extensive aneurysm who are likely to require longer cross-clamp times for difficult anastomoses or multiple-vessel reimplantation. The arterial limb of the bypass circuit can be Y'd off to allow a multihead cannula to be used for perfusion of visceral arteries to minimize ischemic time to critical organs. Studies have been unable to show, in the entire group of patients undergoing thoracic or thoracoabdominal aneurysm repair, a reduction in the risk of ischemic paraplegia through use of distal perfusion. However, outcomes are probably improved if distal perfusion is used in patients with clamp times >30 minutes.

The left femoral artery is exposed and taped before heparinization. Opening the pericardium exposes the left atrial appendage, and a purse string is place around it. Alternatively, the base of the inferior pulmonary vein may be used for cannulation. We prefer this technique and avoid opening the pericardium and the more fragile atrial appendage. When the aorta is ready for cross-clamping, heparin (100 units/kg) is administered to achieve an activated clotting time of around 200 seconds. Small-diameter pediatric arterial and venous cannulas are inserted and secured. Generally, pump flows of 2 to 2.5 liters/min are all that are required. As the aorta is about to be clamped, the pump is activated and blood is drawn from the left atrium and returned to the femoral artery. Initially, high pump flows should be used to drop preload as the clamp is being applied to the aorta and afterload increases above the clamp. Pump flows can

LEFT ATRIOFEMORAL BYPASS

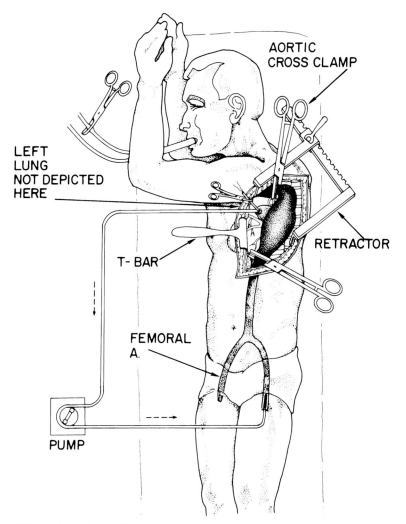

AORTIC
CROSS CLAMP

LEFT
LUNG
NOT DEPICTED
HERE

RETRACTOR

T- BAR

FEMORAL
A.

PUMP

Figure 57-2.   Left atriofemoral bypass for distal aortic perfusion.

then be adjusted to achieve a satisfactory blood pressure above and below the clamps.

When the clamp is to be released the pump can be stopped and preload increased to alleviate hypotension. We prefer to minimize the components in the atriofemoral pump circuit and do not routinely include a heat exchanger.

2. Femorofemoral cardiopulmonary bypass (Fig. 57-3). This may be used as an alternative approach to distal body perfusion. A long venous cannula such as a Bio-Medicus-Medtronic (Medtronic Inc., Atlanta, GA) is introduced via the femoral vein toward the right atrium to achieve satisfactory venous drainage. Bypass is begun shortly before the aorta is cross-clamped. Mild systemic hypothermia may be used to facilitate spinal cord protection, and the circuit may be used to fully rewarm the patients at the comple-

tion of the procedure. Longer activated clotting times than with atriofemoral bypass are required because the circuit is more complex and contains an oxygenator/heat exchanger. Additional volume may be added to the reservoir to allow for rapid transfusion after cross-clamp release, and the circulation can be supported with high pump flows to prevent any hypotension after cross-clamp release.

Femorofemoral cardiopulmonary bypass is a particularly useful technique if it is not technically possible to place a proximal clamp due to a heavily calcified aorta. In these situations the patient is cooled to 15°C to 18°C and circulatory arrest is used to make the proximal anastomosis possible. Care must be taken to properly vent the left ventricle once fibrillation occurs if aortic insufficiency is present.

Spinal Cord Preservation

Protection of the spinal cord remains the most controversial and troublesome aspect of thoracic and thoracoabdominal aortic surgery. In the largest series reported to date, Svensson and associates noted a 16% incidence of paraplegia or paraparesis in 1,509 patients who had undergone repairs for the treatment of thoracoabdominal aortic disease. The complexity of the repair was found to be a significant predictor of spinal cord injury. Repairs of type I, II, III, and IV aneurysms were associated with paraplegia or paraparesis rates of 15%, 31%, 7%, and 4%, respectively. Other authors have also reported an increased frequency of spinal cord injury in patients undergoing complex repairs.

Repairs limited to the descending thoracic aorta are generally associated with a lower incidence of spinal cord injury. However, any alteration to distal aortic perfusion, whether with aortic cross-clamping alone or in combination with some form of distal aortic perfusion, is associated with complex changes in spinal cord flow, many of which are mediated through the renin–angiotensin system. Most authors agree that the presence of dissection or the need for emergent operation increases the risk of spinal cord injury. The data regarding the influence of aortic cross-clamp times on the likelihood of spinal cord injury are mixed. Svensson and coauthors showed a dramatically increased risk with clamp times of >60 minutes when compared with clamp times of <30 minutes. In the series of Hollier and associates, however, all 5 cases of postoperative paraplegia underwent repairs with cross-clamp times of <20 minutes. Najafi observed no postoperative spinal cord injury in 31 patients who underwent repairs with mean cross-clamp times of 58 minutes. However, distal aortic perfusion with partial femorofemoral cardiopulmonary bypass was used in all patients. Svensson concluded that cross-clamp times of 40 minutes were not associated with spinal cord injury if distal aortic perfusion was used. Hence, the use of distal aortic perfusion may have offset any influence cross-clamp times had on spinal cord injury.

Spinal cord ischemia in the perioperative period can result from perioperative hypotension, distal aortic hypotension after aortic occlusion, the interruption of critical intercostal and lumbar arteries, thromboembolism and embolism of intercostal arteries, and postoperative hypotension and hypoxia. At normothermia, the supply of adenosine triphosphate, the fuel for membrane-bound calcium homeostasis

PARTIAL FEMORAL–FEMORAL CARDIOPULMONARY BYPASS

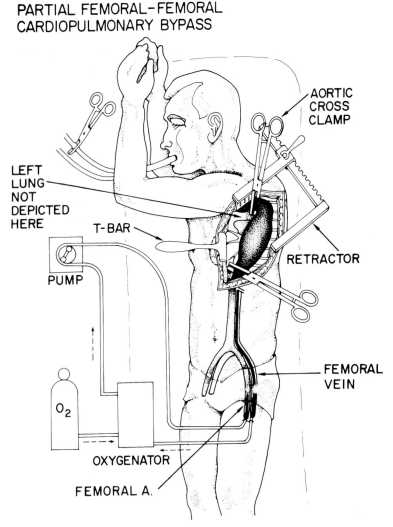

Figure 57-3. Femorofemoral partial cardiopulmonary bypass for distal aortic perfusion.

pumps, is exhausted after 3 to 4 minutes of ischemia. In addition, reperfusion of ischemic spinal cord may result in further injury as a result of the action of oxygen free radicals.

The methods available for improving spinal cord protection are the following:

1. Distal aortic perfusion. The techniques for atriofemoral bypass and partial or total femorofemoral cardiopulmonary bypass have been described (see the prior section Extracorporeal Circulation). As noted, there are mixed data regarding the protection afforded to the spinal cord using these techniques. Although additional measures such as monitoring spinal cord evoked potentials may give additional information, the degree of protection afforded by this information may not be improved. This may be because important arteries of supply to the spinal cord are occluded either temporary

or permanently during the cross-clamp period.

2. Intrathecal vasodilators. Several investigators, including Svensson and colleagues, have used vasodilators such as papaverine delivered intrathecally to improve spinal cord blood flow and improve spinal cord protection in experimental animals. One nonrandomized trial using intrathecal papaverine in humans reported a decreased incidence of spinal cord injury.

3. Reattachment of intercostal and lumbar arteries. Despite the theoretical appeal, reimplantation of multiple intercostal vessels was reported by Crawford in a series of 605 patients to increase the risk of spinal cord injury, possibly because of prolonged clamp times. Hollier reported on 24 consecutive patients who underwent thoracoabdominal aortic aneurysm repair using spinal fluid drainage and intercostal reimplantation

without a single incident of postoperative paraplegia. This number of patients is not sufficient to allow us to conclude that this technique is completely protective.

4. Decreasing cerebrospinal fluid (CSF) pressure. CSF drainage to reduce intrathecal pressure that increased after aortic cross-clamping was originally championed by Cooley and Blaisdell. Several experimental studies reported a low incidence of postoperative paraplegia using this technique. A prospective, randomized trial by Crawford and associates found no benefit in using CSF drainage; however a more recent prospective, randomized trial by Coselli and associates found a statistically significant decrease in the rate of spinal cord injury in patients undergoing CSF drainage. In Coselli's report, all patients had either type I or II thoracoabdominal aneurysms and all received left heart bypass, permissive mild hypothermia, and reattachment of what were felt to be any patent critical intercostals. One hundred forty-five patients were randomized between CSF drainage and no CSF drainage. In this trial, the group undergoing CSF drainage had a spinal cord injury rate of 2.6% compared to 13.0% in the group not undergoing CSF drainage ($p = .03$). Because of the results of this randomized trial and the low risk of CSF drainage, most surgeons operating on thoracic and thoracoabdominal aneurysms have begun to use the technique of CSF drainage.

5. Hypothermia. General and topical hypothermia have both been reported to be effective mechanisms for improving spinal cord tolerance to ischemia. Profound systemic hypothermia may be associated with hemorrhagic and pulmonary complications; however, several surgeons still routinely use full cardiopulmonary bypass and hypothermia as a matter of routine. Topical cooling of the spinal cord has been championed by Cambria with excellent results. This technique uses the instillation of cold saline solution into the epidural space and requires extra equipment and some additional expertise. As a result it has not been widely used.

6. Pharmacologic agents. Calcium-channel antagonists, steroids, barbiturates, cocaine-derived local anesthetic agents, N-methyl-D-aspartate (NMDA) receptor agonists, and other agents have all been reported as adjuncts to improving spinal cord tolerance to ischemia; none has been proved to be clearly beneficial

clinically. Most recently we have been investigating the protective effects of adenosine and adenosine-derived A2A agonists. These agents appear to show great promise in animal studies of spinal cord ischemia and are soon approaching clinical trials.

7. Minimizing aortic cross-clamp times. Short periods of aortic occlusion have been reported to be generally associated with a lower risk of postoperative paraplegia than have prolonged cross-clamp times. Adequate use of preoperative imaging studies will allow planning of an efficient operation. For these reasons emergent operations for thoracic and thoracoabdominal aortic aneurysms have always been associated with higher spinal cord injury rates.

Our favored approach to spinal cord protection is to minimize the clamp time in conjunction with left heart bypass and CSF drainage for all extent I and II aneurysms and for selected extent III's and any thoracoabdominal aneurysms requiring complex reconstructions. It is hoped that minimizing clamp time and carefully planning clamp placement to avoid clamping a segment of aorta with significant atheroma or mural thrombus will decrease the chance of embolization to the spinal cord and viscera. Minimizing hemodynamic instability and maintaining perfusion through all possible collateral channels by using left heart bypass for distal perfusion may also limit the rate of spinal cord injury. Beveling the anastomosis to maintain perfusion to or revascularizing large critical paired intercostal and lumbar arteries at the T11-L1 level may also be beneficial and is something we try to do whenever feasible without unduly extending total clamp time.

In the rare situation where aortic clamping is hazardous or impossible, such as in aneurysms extending proximally into the arch or in those with totally calcified aortas, others and we have had favorable experience using femorofemoral cardiopulmonary bypass and hypothermic circulatory arrest to complete the proximal anastomosis. The graft can then be cannulated and perfusion and warming commenced to the great vessels and to the legs, and potentially even the viscera, while the distal anastomosis is completed. Cannulation strategy may need to be altered to minimize the risk of embolic stroke in those patients with extensive atheroma, and the axillary artery may be the preferable arterial cannulation site in these patients.

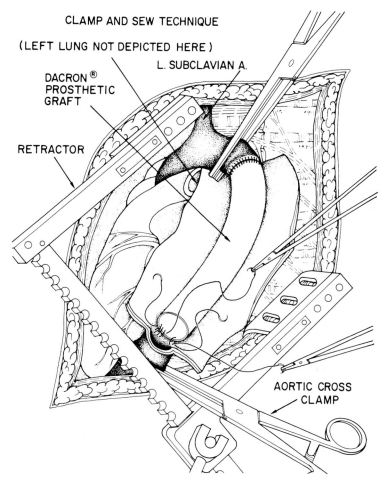

Figure 57-4. Clamp-and-sew technique, with rapid construction of aortic anastomoses, to minimize aortic cross-clamp time. (A. = artery; L. = left.)

Selecting the Aortic Graft

Either with the aid of a sizing device or by measuring the aortic diameter proximally and distally, the graft should be selected and opened onto the sterile field before the aorta is clamped. Since the advent of zero-porosity polyethylene terephthalate (Dacron) grafts, preclotting of the graft and bleeding though the graft have ceased to be issues of concern. The advent of side-arm grafts has also facilitated complex reconstructions and revascularization of visceral and even intercostal vessels.

The suture material to be used in fashioning the anastomoses should be selected and loaded ready to use before aortic clamping. In most situations we favor a long, double-armed 3-0 polypropylene suture for each aortic anastomosis.

Fashioning the Aortic Anastomoses

When the dissection has been completed and the aorta has been cross-clamped, the aneurysm is incised longitudinally with a large-bladed knife close to the intended site of anastomosis. The aortotomy is then extended proximally and distally with scissors to expose the lumen of the aneurysm and to allow evacuation of any laminated thrombus. In long aneurysms, we advise keeping the aortic clamps as close to one another as possible to minimize the possibility of an important artery of spinal cord supply being excluded from the circulation. In these cases the distal clamp can be moved to the site of the distal anastomosis at the completion of the proximal suture line. Alternatively, in cases where the decreasingly popular technique of clamp-and-sew (Fig. 57-4) is being used, the distal aorta may not be clamped at all. The field is kept clear using a cell-saving sucker. Care must be taken when using the sequential clamping technique to try to always clamp relatively nondiseased segments of aorta to minimize the potential for embolization.

Tube Graft Placement

Proximally the aortotomy is cut to fashion a transverse anastomosis site. In chronic

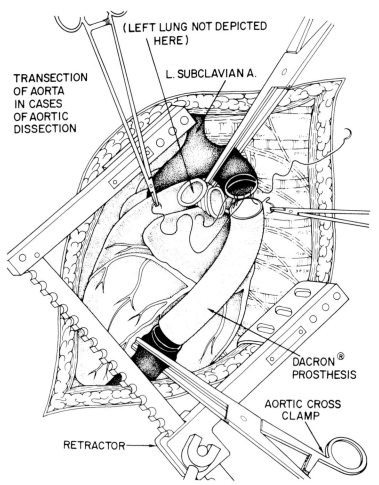

TRANSECTION
OF AORTA
IN CASES
OF AORTIC
DISSECTION

(LEFT LUNG NOT DEPICTED
HERE)

L. SUBCLAVIAN A.

DACRON®
PROSTHESIS

AORTIC CROSS
CLAMP

RETRACTOR

Figure 57-5. Transection of the aorta in cases of aortic dissection to ensure that all aortic layers are incorporated into the anastomosis. (A. = artery; L. = left.)

dissections especially, we prefer to transect the aorta completely to identify each of the layers of the aorta so that they can be incorporated accurately into the anastomosis (Fig. 57-5). It may also facilitate the anastomosis in chronic atherosclerotic aneurysm disease to transect the aorta, but this should be avoided if extensive additional dissection is required to accomplish this.

Side towels are used to cover all retractors and clamps, and the graft is brought onto the field and the proximal anastomosis is begun with the graft; then the aorta picked up for the first four sutures as a parachute stitch. The graft is then brought down to the aorta and the anastomosis rapidly completed, taking large bites of aorta in an attempt to effect hemostasis. We prefer to run the suture toward ourselves beginning with the back wall until we reach the anterior part of the suture line. The other arm of the suture is then brought up from below also coming toward us. In general, it does not matter whether one goes outside-in or inside-out on the aorta, as long as large bites and rapid though accurate suture placement is achieved.

When the anastomosis has been completed, the graft is clamped 4 cm to 5 cm below the suture line and the proximal aortic cross-clamp is released. The suture line is quickly inspected, and only gross bleeding points should be of concern at this stage. If a large bleeding point is found, it should be repaired with a standard-length 3-0 polypropylene suture as a mattress, pledgeted with polytetrafluoroethylene (Teflon).

Attention is then turned to the distal suture line. In thoracic aneurysms where the chest has been entered through two different intercostal spaces, the retractor should be moved rapidly from the upper to the lower space. The aortotomy is extended down the aorta to the distal neck of the aneurysm and again squared off horizontally at the site selected for the anastomosis. For the distal anastomosis, we favor transecting the aorta only for aortas with chronic dissection flaps. In subacute dissections, we prefer to cut a long tongue away from the flap and sew the graft to the outer layer of the aorta alone, thus ensuring the perfusion of both true and false lumens distally. The distal anas-

tomosis is performed using the same methods described for the proximal. Adequate warning should be given to the anesthesiologist about impending cross-clamp release as the anastomosis nears. With the use of left heart bypass, as the distal clamp is removed, flows are decreased and stopped and minimal hemodynamic comprise should be seen.

Reimplantation of Intercostal Arteries

Intercostal arteries of particularly large size that are identified during the dissection before aortic clamping should be marked for potential reimplantation or revascularization through an on-lay patch sewn to the main graft; however, this technique may predispose to late aneurysm formation. If during the opening of the aneurysm the intercostals are found to be occluded, reimplantation is not necessary. Large intercostals found in the region of the anastomoses should be preserved and incorporated into the anastomosis if possible. Large patent intercostals with weak, dark backbleeding represent the strongest case for separate intercostal reimplantation. In these cases, the aortic anastomoses proximal and distal should be completed and the cross-clamps released. The intercostal or intercostals must then be mobilized as a button or as tongue of aortic wall if there are multiple vessels to be reimplanted. A partial occlusion clamp can then be applied to the aortic graft and the anastomosis performed with 4-0 or 5-0 polypropylene. Alternatively, the intercostals can be reimplanted after performing the proximal anastomosis while maintaining perfusion distally through left heart bypass. The clamp is then moved below the reimplanted intercostals, and the distal anastomosis is completed.

Reimplantation of Celiac, Mesenteric, and Renal Arteries

In extensive thoracoabdominal aortic aneurysm disease, all of the visceral arteries may need to be reimplanted. In these situations we prefer to mobilize the celiac axis, the superior mesenteric artery, and the right renal artery together as one large Carrel patch (Fig. 57-6). For extensive disease requiring complex reconstructions, we favor distal aortic perfusion (see prior discussion). The aortic cross-clamps can be moved sequentially distally as each anastomosis is completed in an attempt to minimize the segment of aorta and associated viscera that is excluded from the circulation. In these cases the proximal aortic anastomosis should be completed first,

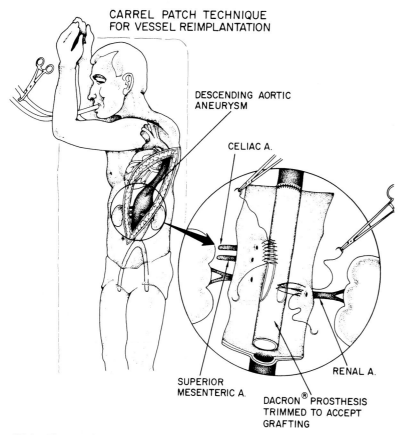

CARREL PATCH TECHNIQUE
FOR VESSEL REIMPLANTATION

DESCENDING AORTIC
ANEURYSM

CELIAC A.

SUPERIOR
MESENTERIC A.

DACRON® PROSTHESIS
TRIMMED TO ACCEPT
GRAFTING

RENAL A.

Figure 57-6. The Carrel patch technique for reimplantation of visceral vessels. (A. = artery.)

with clamps applied to the aorta just above and below the anastomotic site. When the proximal anastomosis is completed, the graft is clamped just below the anastomosis, the proximal aortic clamp is removed, and the distal aortic clamp is moved to a site below the arteries to be reimplanted. The Carrel patches for these vessels are then fashioned and corresponding patches cut from the aortic graft, and each of the reimplantation anastomoses is performed with 3-0 or 4-0 polypropylene. The proximal clamp on the graft is then moved to a point below these anastomoses. The distal aortic clamp may be moved farther down, and the final aortic anastomosis performed. With this technique the segment of aorta excluded from perfusion, either from above or below, is minimized, thus reducing the risks of spinal cord or organ ischemia.

In many cases, the aneurysm may extend close to the visceral vessels but not actually completely involve their origins. In these situations we favor a distal aortic anastomosis that is cut obliquely in such a way as to preserve a tongue of aorta anteriorly from which the visceral vessels arise (Fig. 57-7). This tongue of tissue can be incorporated into the aortic anastomosis so that in effect visceral vessel reimplantation has

been performed without requiring a separate anastomosis.

New multi–side-branched grafts may be useful when there is significant splaying of the origins of the visceral vessels due to the aneurysm or if the visceral vessels have associated origin occlusive or aneurysmal disease that would preclude direct reimplantation. A multihead perfusion catheter off the arterial line of the left heart bypass circuit can be used to perfuse all visceral arteries individually through coronary sinus balloon catheters while they are sequentially revascularized using the individual side-arm grafts.

Completing the Operation

When the graft has been inserted, all the anastomoses completed, and the clamps removed, care should be taken to ensure that there is hemostasis at each of the suture lines. Adequacy of distal perfusion should be ensured. If left atriofemoral bypass or femorofemoral partial cardiopulmonary bypass has been used for distal perfusion, this should be discontinued and withdrawn with the patient adequately warmed, in a satisfactory rhythm, and with adequate blood pressure. Protamine sulfate then can be admin-

istered and the cannulation sites repaired. Wherever possible the Dacron graft should be wrapped within the sac of the aneurysm to prevent later fistulization to lung or intestine. It is especially important that tissue of some type is interposed between the graft and the intestine when repairing thoracoabdominal aneurysms; retroperitoneal tissue is usually available, but if it is deficient, then greater omentum can be used. When the graft has been covered and hemostasis secured, drains are placed in the pleural cavity at the apex and base. We prefer large-caliber (32 F to 36 F), soft, round tubes for the pleural space but have recently begun using smaller-diameter (19 F to 24 F) channel drains. We do not routinely drain the retroperitoneum. In cases where there is persistent generalized oozing from raw surfaces, topical hemostatic agents can be used, and for these reasons antifibrinolytic agents are being used more frequently as a matter of routine. The collapsed lung is reinflated and the operative field copiously irrigated to remove residual clot or debris from within the aneurysm. We prefer to oppose the ribs with multiple interrupted, heavy, absorbable sutures, taking care to avoid the intercostal neurovascular bundles. Drilling holes through the lower rib may be the most affective way to prevent disabling intercostal neuralgia. The soft tissues are then approximated in layers.

Postoperative ventilation is required in all these patients until normothermia is achieved, acidosis has been reversed, and hemodynamic variables including postoperative bleeding are controlled and stable.

Results

A steady reduction in operative mortality and morbidity from the earliest reports in the late 1950s has occurred. In the large series of 1,509 thoracoabdominal aortic aneurysm repairs reported by Svensson and colleagues in 1993, the 30-day survival rate was 92%. The 30-day survival rate in the 210 consecutive patients most recently operated on was 97%. They reported that the factors influencing mortality were increasing age, preoperative creatinine level, presence of chronic lung disease or coronary artery disease, concurrent proximal aortic aneurysms, and total aortic cross-clamp time. Factors reported as significant in influencing the likelihood of spinal cord injury included total aortic clamp time and extent of aorta replaced. Similar figures for mortality and morbidity have been reported for patients

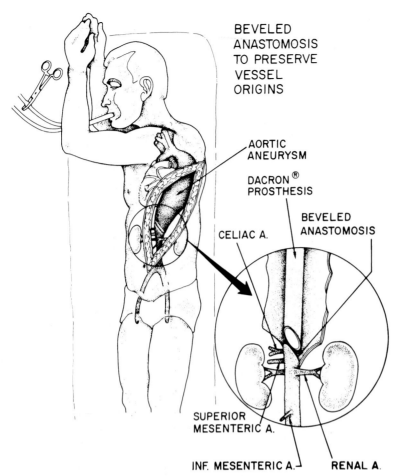

BEVELED
ANASTOMOSIS
TO PRESERVE
VESSEL
ORIGINS

AORTIC
ANEURYSM

DACRON®
PROSTHESIS

BEVELED
ANASTOMOSIS

CELIAC A.

SUPERIOR
MESENTERIC A.

INF. MESENTERIC A.   RENAL A.

Figure 57-7.   Oblique fashioning of the anastomosis may allow reimplantation of visceral vessels without a separate anastomosis. (A. = artery.)

undergoing repairs of the descending thoracic aorta.

We consider the factors most important in effecting a safe operation for thoracic and thoracoabdominal aortic disease to be a careful assessment of the patient's overall condition, especially noting chronic lung disease or coronary artery disease; planning of an operation that replaces in one sitting the shortest segment of aorta possible; assessment before aortic cross-clamping of the likely complexity of the repair and planning for distal aortic perfusion if appropriate as well as CSF drainage; and rapid and precise anastomotic techniques that minimize cross-clamp times and allow smoother management of hemodynamic instability.

Endovascular Thoracic Aortic Aneurysm Repair

The last decade has brought forth significant change in therapy for aortic aneurysm disease. Although devices for the endovascular repair of abdominal aortic aneurysms have been Food and Drug Administration approved, thoracic aortic stent grafts are still being evaluated in clinical trials. Although a few institutions have some experience with side-branch endografts for the repair of thoracoabdominal aneurysms, this technology is still years away from mainstream clinical application.

Many thoracic aneurysms are of appropriate anatomy for endograft therapy; however, other factors must be evaluated before attempting an endovascular repair. There must be an appropriate neck or landing zone both proximal and distal to the aneurysm. Although many surgeons have experience in placing endografts in the aortic arch and covering the left subclavian and performing a carotid-to-subclavian bypass if needed, this strategy clearly increases the complexity of the procedure and lends itself to increased complication rates, especially the rate of stroke.

Patients being considered for endograft therapy of a thoracic aortic aneurysm must also undergo evaluation of their entire aorta, iliac, and femoral vessels as routes for delivery of the device. In general, the iliac and femoral vessels must be 7 mm or larger and relatively free of significant calcium and tortuosity. The abdominal and thoracic aorta through which one must navigate the device should also be relatively free of significant tortuosity; however, there are techniques and stiff guidewires that can permit safer negotiation of tortuous vessels. We have found an emerging relative contraindication to endovascular therapy to be a severely tortuous aorta with significant atheromatous debris or laminated thrombus. This situation clearly predisposes the patient to significant risk of distal embolization. The reported incidence of spinal cord injury during endovascular repair of thoracic aortic aneurysms is 3% to 5% and clearly is a result of spinal cord ischemia caused by covering critical intercostals with the device or from embolization to the intercostals.

Because the outcomes after endovascular therapy of thoracic aortic aneurysms are not fully understood, and because the surgery itself to place these devices is not without risk, one should not change the criteria for repairing thoracic aortic aneurysms just because a "less invasive" mode of therapy exists.

SUGGESTED READING

Cambria RP, Davison JK, Carter C, et al. Epidural cooling for spinal cord protection during thoracoabdominal aneurysm repair: A five-year experience. J Vasc Surg 2000;31:1093.

Cassada DC, Gangemi JJ, Rieger JM, et al. Systemic adenosine A2A agonist ameliorates ischemic reperfusion injury in the rabbit spinal cord. Ann Thorac Surg 2001;72:1245.

Cassada DC, Tribble CG, Kaza AK, et al. Adenosine analogue reduces spinal cord reperfusion injury in a time-dependent fashion. Surgery 2001;130:230.

Cassada DC, Tribble CG, Long SM, et al. Adenosine A2A analogue ATL-146e reduces systemic tumor necrosis factor-alpha and spinal cord capillary platelet-endothelial cell adhesion molecule-1 expression after spinal cord ischemia. J Vasc Surg 2002;35:994.

Coselli JS, LeMaire SA, Koksoy C, et al. Cerebrospinal fluid drainage reduces paraplegia after thoracoabdominal aortic aneurysm repair: Results of a randomized clinical trial. J Vasc Surg 2002;35:631.

Cox GS, O'Hara PJ, Hertzer NR, et al. Thoracoabdominal aneurysm repair: A representative experience. J Vasc Surg 1992;15:780.

Francel PC, Long BA, Malik JM, et al. Limiting ischemic spinal cord injury using a free radical scavenger 21-aminosteroid and/or cerebrospinal fluid drainage. J Neurosurg 1998;79:742.

Gangemi JJ, Kern JA, Ross SD, et al. Retrograde perfusion with a sodium channel antagonist provides ischemic spinal cord protection. Ann Thorac Surg 2000;69:1744.

Hansen CJ, Bui H, Donayre CE, et al. Complications of endovascular repair of high-risk and emergent descending thoracic aortic aneurysms and dissections. J Vasc Surg 2004;40:228.

Herold JA, Kron IL, Langenburg SE, et al. Complete prevention of postischemic spinal cord injury by means of regional infusion of hypothermic saline and adenosine. J Thorac Cardiovasc Surg 1994;107:536.

Mauney MC, Blackbourne LH, Langenburg SE, et al. Prevention of spinal cord injury after repair of the thoracic or thoracoabdominal aorta. Ann Thorac Surg 1995;59:245.

Nafaji H. Descending aortic aneurysmectomy without adjuncts to avoid ischemia. Ann Thorac Surg 1993;55:1042.

Safi HJ, Miller CC, Huynh TTT, et al. Distal aortic perfusion and cerebrospinal fluid drainage for thoracoabdominal and descending thoracic aortic repair: Ten years of organ protection. Ann Surg 2003;238:372.

Svensson LG, Crawford ES, Hess KR, et al. Experience with 1509 patients undergoing thoracoabdominal aortic operations. J Vasc Surg 1993;17:357.

Svensson LG, Crawford ES, Hess KR, et al. Variables predictive of outcome in 832 patients undergoing repairs of the descending thoracic aorta. Chest 1993;104:1248.

EDITOR'S COMMENTS

The surgical treatment of thoracic and thoracoabdominal aortic aneurysm has undergone significant refinement since the initial description in the 1950's. However, repair of a thoracoabdominal aortic aneurysm today remains challenging and is associated with significant morbidity and mortality. Successful outcome requires that three fundamental concepts be addressed during operative repair: (1) control of hemodynamics during aortic cross clamping, (2) spinal cord protection, and (3) distal organ (visceral) perfusion. The refinement of cardiopulmonary bypass technology has had a significant impact in optimizing each of these. Using either partial or full cardiopulmonary support, we are able to achieve total circulatory control, and, in effect, complete control of the operation. The majority of reports in the literature today emphasize the use of a some variant of circulation management technique to optimize outcome of the reconstruction of the thoracoabdominal aorta.

We routinely utilize partial left heart bypass to manage the circulation during repair of types I, II, and III thoracoabdom-

inal aneurysms. Similar to the Kern, our group prefers to cannulate the left inferior pulmonary vein for left atrial access, and the left femoral or iliac artery for arterial access. This technique allows for reconstruction of the aorta in a staged, segmental fashion (i.e. proximal anastomosis, intercostal reimplantation, mesenteric anastomosis, separate left renal anastomosis, and distal aortic anastomosis), as the clamp site is moved from proximal to distal. Just as important, this technique allows us to maintain control and "protection" of the proximal anastomosis, limits the afterload placed on the heart (if a high cross clamp site), and avoids extreme swings in the hemodynamics by controlling distal flow in his circuit. Concurrently, we recognize that distal visceral and spinal cord ischemia is kept to a minimum. If the situation requires that an open proximal anastomosis be performed, full cardiopulmonary bypass with hypothermia must be employed. The most important consideration with this technique is that only minimal aortic insufficiency may be tolerated. Even with mild to moderate aortic insufficiency, the left ventricular vent may not be able to keep up with the regurgitant flow. Pre-operative planning with echocardiography is absolutely essential if the surgeon intends to use full cardiopulmonary bypass with hypothermia. Similar to the authors, in general we do not recommend simple aortic cross clamping, as it likely increases the rate of paraplegia (especially if cross-clamp times are >30 minutes). Adjunctive methods for spinal cord protection were discussed in the chapter and deserve mention here. Refinement in spinal cord protection have contributed greatly to the improvement of outcomes for thoracic aortic reconstruction. The influence of CSF drainage on paraplegia rates has made a significant impact on most surgeons' practice and we routinely employ this technique. In the hands of an experienced anesthesia team, CSF drain placement has very low morbidity and the potential benefit on paraplegia incidence certainly justifies the small risk. In addition, we routinely utilize neuromonitoring specifically electroencephalography (EEG)/somatosensory evoked potentials (SSEP) to guide our management of the distal circulation. Finally, in aortic pathology not associated with development of collaterals (i.e., transection, dissection), we routinely reimplant the intercoastal arteries.

Endovascular approaches for thoracic and thoracoabdominal aneurysms is a rapidly emerging field and deserves men-

tion. There is currently no FDA approved product for repair of thoracoabdominal aortic aneurysm. Only a handful of centers currently are involved in clinical trials. Due to the involvement of the mesenteric vessels and the requirement of fenestrated and/or branched grafts, treatment of a thoracoabdominal aneurysm with stent graft technology remains a very challenging task and far from clinical mainstream practice. Much more investigation and refinement in devices will be needed before we know the full potential and impact. For an isolated descending thoracic aortic aneurysm, endovascular aortic stent graft repair has become a viable option to open repair. There is currently one FDA approved device with several others likely to be approved soon. As with open repair, endovascular repair also is associated with a risk of paraplegia. The amount of coverage of aorta appears to be the major determinant of paraplegia risk, as most of these devices require at least two centimeters of aortic landing zone proximal and distal to the aneurysmal aorta. Thoracic aneurysms that require coverage from the left subclavian artery to the celiac artery (i.e. total pavement) are obviously at highest risk. Furthermore, we are now seeing patients with previous abdominal aortic aneurysm repair (either open, or stent graft repair) who present for thoracic aortic stent graft repair. This represents another ever growing population of patients with significant risk of paraplegia. In these selected groups of patients, we routinely use adjunctive methods of spinal cord protection (i.e., CSF drain, EEG/SSEP). In our experience, intraoperative events detected with neuromonitoring have altered our management of the distal circulation and CSF drainage similar to our experience during open repair. Endovascular stent graft therapy is a technology in evolution and is being applied to other aortic pathology as well. (i.e. transection, dissection, arch aneurysm, hybrid operations). The short and intermediate-term results are promising, but long term data will be needed to assess the durability of this technology.

There is no question thoracic and thoracoabdominal aortic aneurysms represent a complex group of patients, and operative repair of these aneurysms presents significant challenges. These procedures probably are best performed by surgeons with extensive experience in complex aortic reconstruction who can offer each patient the best surgical option, be it open repair or an endovascular approach.

Wilson Szeto and L.R.K

58

Arch Aneurysms

Joseph S. Coselli, John Bozinovski, and Scott A. LeMaire

Etiology and Pathology

Aneurysms can occur anywhere along the aorta, but isolated arch aneurysms are uncommon and are usually associated with ascending and/or descending aneurysms. Aortic aneurysms most commonly are due to medial degeneration with resulting loss of elastic fibers as in idiopathic cystic medial degeneration and in Marfan and Ehlers-Danlos syndromes. Other causes of arch aneurysms include atherosclerosis, infection, inflammation, trauma, chronic dissection, and poststenotic dilation.

Loss of elastic integrity causes weakening of the aortic wall. The weakened aortic wall dilates circumferentially, resulting in the more common fusiform aneurysm, or in a localized area that manifests as a saccular aneurysm. As the aorta dilates, wall tension increases according to LaPlace's formula (tension = pressure × radius/twice the wall thickness). The increase in wall tension further dilates the vessel, leading to even greater wall tension and dilation in a progressive manner. The significance of progressive dilation is illustrated by the finding that the incidence of rupture is <10% for aneurysms 35 mm to 49 mm, 18% for those 50 mm to 59 mm, and >25% for aneurysms >60 mm.

Diagnosis

Symptoms of aortic arch aneurysms include locally compressive effects or those arising from the vessel itself. Locally compressive effects manifest according to the structures involved. Chest wall compression can present as a dull, aching, retrosternal, or mid-scapular pain. Compression of the trachea may have accompanying stridor, whereas stretch on the recurrent laryngeal nerve will cause hoarseness. The patient may have dysphagia from esophageal compression, or plethora and edema of the upper body in the case of superior vena cava syndrome from compression of this structure. Dyspnea, either due to compression on the lung or as a result of congestive failure from the mass compressing cardiac structures, may also be seen. Less commonly, compression of the sympathetic chain could result in a Horner syndrome.

Symptoms arising from the vessel per se include thromboembolic events, such as stroke and visceral and limb ischemia, aortic insufficiency from associated root enlargement, or congestive heart failure and myocardial infarction from compression of the coronary arteries. Rupture of the vessel usually is accompanied by severe pain. If the rupture is contained by the adventitia, this may be the only symptom. A rupture into the pleural cavity is more common on the left and can cause dyspnea, pleuritic chest pain, and hypotension. Aneurysms, however, can rupture into any of the surrounding structures such as the mediastinum, esophagus, trachea, or bronchial tree. Aneurysms of the aorta can also give rise to dissection of the aorta. This topic is addressed in detail in another chapter. It should be noted that most diagnosed aneurysms are asymptomatic, having been identified during chest x-ray or computed axial tomography scan obtained for other reasons.

Diagnostic modalities used to investigate aortic aneurysms include chest roentgenography, electrocardiography, echocardiography, computed tomography, angiography, and magnetic resonance imaging. Radiographic findings in patients with aortic aneurysm include widened mediastinum, tracheal or endotracheal tube displacement, depression of the left main stem bronchus, esophageal or nasogastric tube displacement, irregular aortic contour, opacification of the aortopulmonary window, and left pleural fluid collection in the case of rupture.

An electrocardiogram may show evidence of cardiac ischemia as a sequela of the aneurysm or due to associated atherosclerotic coronary artery disease. Coronary angiography should be done in all patients going for elective surgery of the aorta if they have symptoms of, or risk factors for, coronary artery disease or if they are advanced in age.

Echocardiography is used to assess the aorta and cardiac function preoperatively and intraoperatively. Transthoracic imaging of the aorta is limited by the constraints of available imaging planes, and its intraoperative use is less suitable than transesophageal imaging, which also has its limitations in evaluation of the aortic arch due to acoustic shadowing from the trachea. Computed tomography allows one to image the entire aorta, head and neck vessels, and surrounding structures. This gives valuable information regarding relationships to bony structures, presence of pericardial effusion, characteristics of the aneurysm, and its relationship to the great vessels. Computed tomography can reconstruct images to produce a three-dimensional representation of the aorta, giving the surgeon a better understanding of what to expect in the operating room; however, it is generally not necessary. Computed tomography has the added advantage that it is less expensive and more readily available than magnetic resonance imaging. The disadvantages of computed tomography are the renal toxicity induced by the contrast and the inability to assess valvular competency or branch artery stenosis.

Angiography is generally not used on a routine basis, having been supplanted by the less invasive computed tomography and magnetic resonance angiography. It can be of use in trying to further delineate a suspected aneurysmal leak, and it should be obtained in those patients who are already undergoing left heart catheterization for evaluation of coronary artery disease. Its use is probably better suited to evaluation of aortic dissection and traumatic ruptures and patients suspected of major branch vessel stenosis or obstruction. Disadvantages include contrast use, risk of cerebral vascular and peripheral vascular embolic events, and risk of injury to the aorta and vessel of access.

Indications

Because aortic arch aneurysms usually occur with ascending and/or descending aortic aneurysms, the need for surgery is frequently determined by the size of the aorta at these other sites, as discussed in their respective chapters. The decision to include the arch in the repair is sometimes difficult. One must consider the patient's age, comorbidities, and cardiac function in addition to the characteristics of the aneurysm itself to make a decision on whether the benefits of arch replacement outweigh the risks. Arch repair involves a prolonged cardiac ischemic time and a period of circulatory arrest or low-flow cerebral perfusion, potentially jeopardizing the patient's recovery.

An arch that is >6 cm in diameter, or twice the normal size, is generally accepted as an indication for arch replacement. In patients with connective tissue disorders or chronic dissection of the aorta or in younger patients, replacement of the arch should be done sooner. Other indications are rapid expansion of the vessel, presence of symptoms, pseudoaneurysms, or mycotic aneurysms.

Preoperative

Pertinent preoperative investigations in patients undergoing planned surgery of the aorta are determined by a thorough history and physical examination. Not to the exclusion of other systems, there should be a focus on associated coronary artery, renal,

carotid, and pulmonary diseases. Patients with a history of angina, otherwise unexplained dyspnea, or previously diagnosed coronary artery disease need to be further evaluated. These patients, along with those with risk factors for coronary artery disease or ECG evidence of coronary lesions, should have a cardiac workup that may include a stress test, nuclear imaging, and coronary angiography.

Patients placed on cardiopulmonary bypass are at increased risk for renal dysfunction including the risk of dialysis requirement. This is especially true of those with pre-existing renal dysfunction and patients undergoing a period of circulatory arrest. Baseline creatinine and blood urea nitrogen are obtained preoperatively. Patients with depressed renal function should have their exposure to intravenous contrast used in imaging the aorta and coronary arteries kept to an absolute minimum with coordination of investigations if more than one study is required. If both angiography and computed tomography are to be obtained, it is better to perform the angiogram first. The computed tomography scan can be done afterward without additional contrast while still providing good images of the aortic and great vessel lumens.

With the association of aortic disease and carotid lesions, it is necessary to identify those patients with occlusions and significant stenosis in the carotid arteries especially if antegrade cerebral perfusion via an axillary, innominate, or single carotid artery is planned. Patients with an atherosclerotic aorta, symptoms of cerebral vascular events, or syncopal and presyncopal episodes need to have noninvasive screening via duplex ultrasonic scanning. Significant lesions as suggested by Doppler studies need to be further evaluated using angiography to optimize surgical management.

The association in patients of diseases of the aorta and obstructive pulmonary disease is strong partly due to smoking, which contributes to the presence of each. Evaluation of pulmonary function includes arterial blood gas analysis and spirometry; however, it is important to point out that no single value from these tests should be used to determine that risk of surgery is prohibitive. There is a linear relationship between partial arterial carbon dioxide pressure ($PaCO_2$) and postoperative risk of respiratory failure and an inverse linear relationship between forced expiratory volume in 1 second (FEV_1), forced expiratory volume at 25% vital capacity ($FEV_{25\%}$), forced expiratory volume at 25% to 75% vital capacity ($FEV_{25-75\%}$), partial arterial oxygen pressure

(PaO_2), and postoperative risk of respiratory failure.

Perioperative

Intravenous lines, including internal jugular venous access, are obtained. The radial artery is monitored for blood pressure and blood gas analysis. In patients planned for circulatory arrest, an additional femoral arterial line is established because pressure measurements in the peripheral radial artery are usually dampened in the immediate period after circulatory arrest. Patients undergoing operation via median sternotomy are intubated with a single-lumen endotracheal tube, whereas those having thoracotomy or thoracoabdominal incisions are intubated with a double-lumen endobronchial tube. Transesophageal echocardiography probes are placed before heparinization and manipulated as little as possible during systemic anticoagulation. Nasoesophageal temperature probes are placed to monitor cooling and rewarming.

Techniques

There are numerous approaches that can be used to address an arch aneurysm. We do not catalogue them all here; rather, we describe those that we commonly use. It is important that the surgeon develops a consistent approach that allows the anesthesiologist, perfusionist, and nurses to function as a team and that limits circulatory arrest and cardiac ischemic times. The guiding principle should be the economy of steps, avoiding unnecessary activities, especially during circulatory arrest.

Hemi-arch

There are times when operating on the ascending aorta that an aneurysm extends to the proximal portion of the arch without involving the great vessels. In these situations it may be preferable to perform the aortic replacement as a so-called "hemi-arch" procedure or "open distal anastomosis." This requires a period of circulatory arrest when performing the distal anastomosis. Commonly, arterial inflow for the bypass circuit is established using the ascending aorta, the femoral artery, or the axillary artery. The choice depends on factors such as the extent of the diseased aorta to be repaired, age of the patient, presence of atherosclerotic disease, anticipated difficulty of repair, and duration of circulatory arrest.

Ascending aortic cannulation is a safe and easy technique with which all cardiac surgeons are familiar. It has a drawback in arch surgery compared to the axillary inflow technique, in that it does not lend itself as well to antegrade cerebral perfusion during circulatory arrest. Antegrade cerebral perfusion can still be used by employing separate perfusion cannulae deployed into the head vessels, but these can be cumbersome in a somewhat limited surgical field.

After sternotomy, pericardiotomy, and heparinization, the ascending aorta is cannulated in a region that will be excised. Venous cannulation is obtained either with a single two-stage venous cannula or by bicaval cannulation if retrograde cerebral perfusion is to be used or access to the mitral valve. In the case in which no antegrade cerebral perfusion is to be used it is preferable to give either a short period of retrograde cerebral perfusion to flush out gaseous and particulate embolic debris prior to reestablishing cardiopulmonary bypass or to flow retrograde into the superior vena cava during circulatory arrest. This will be described here. However, in straightforward cases it is not unreasonable to keep the circuit and operation as simple as possible by using a single venous cannulation technique without cerebral perfusion. In anticipation of retrograde cerebral perfusion the bypass circuit is established with a connection between the arterial arm of the circuit and the superior vena cava cannula (Fig. 58-1A). This connection from the arterial to the venous cannula is clamped during cardiopulmonary bypass (Fig. 58-1A) and opened during circulatory arrest by placing clamps as shown in Fig. 58-1B, thereby providing retrograde flow to the head.

Cardiopulmonary bypass is initiated and ventilation is discontinued once an adequate activated clotting time (ACT >480 seconds) is achieved. We routinely place a retrograde cardioplegia cannula in the coronary sinus and a sump drain into the left ventricle via the right superior pulmonary vein, into the left atrium and across the mitral valve. Once the sump is in place, cooling can safely begin. In the absence of aortic valve insufficiency, cooling can begin with little risk of ventricular distension occurring before the sump is placed. As soon as ventricular fibrillation ensues, the ventricle is observed for distension. If the sump is positioned and working properly, this should not be an issue, but one must be ready to clamp and arrest the heart should this not be the case.

We generally cool all the way to electroencephalogram (EEG) silence and begin work on the distal aorta. With an incompetent aortic valve, it is not unusual to clamp the aorta if it is not too large or atherosclerotic, deliver a dose of cardioplegia, and begin proximal aortic repair while cooling. Rather than cooling to a predetermined temperature, cooling is performed until the EEG shows absence of brain wave activity, and then cooling continues for an additional 5 minutes. Usually this corresponds to a core temperature of 18°C or less. The head is packed in ice at this time to assist in cerebral cooling. Once adequate cooling has been achieved, pentobarbital (2 g/70 kg) is given intravenously. Three minutes are allowed to elapse for pentobarbital to be taken up by the tissue, after which whole-body cardiopulmonary bypass is discontinued and the clamps are adjusted to permit retrograde cerebral perfusion as

described. The superior vena cava cannula is snared using a tourniquet, and flows of 200 to 400 mL/min are used to maintain a proximal venous pressure of 25 mm Hg or less.

The patient is placed in Trendelenburg position, the aorta is opened, and cardioplegia is given into the ostia. Cardioplegia is administered every 10 minutes into the ostia, coronary sinus, or both. The aneurysmal segment of aorta is excised, beveling the incision along the lesser curvature of the arch, leaving the uninvolved great vessels still attached to the aorta. The aorta is sized, and a graft with an 8-mm side arm is cut near the take-off of the side arm, beveling it to fit the distal aorta. Running 3-0 polypropylene suture is used to create the distal anastomosis (Fig. 58-2A). The entire circumference is then reinforced with pledgeted 4-0 polypropylene sutures. This step should add minimal time to the duration of circulatory arrest and has decreased the incidence of bleeding on the posterior aspect of the anastomosis along the lesser curvature, which is very difficult to access after the graft is in place.

Flow into the superior vena cava is stopped, and the snare is removed. The arterial circuit is then attached to the side arm of the graft, which is preattached by the manufacturer. The clamps are adjusted, allowing resumption of whole-body cardiopulmonary bypass. Flow is slowly restarted by allowing the graft to fill while the patient is still in Trendelenburg position. Placing the pump suckers into the proximal part of the unclamped graft greatly assists in de-airing by allowing air to escape for a prolonged time while keeping the field dry. When one is satisfied that air has been removed, the

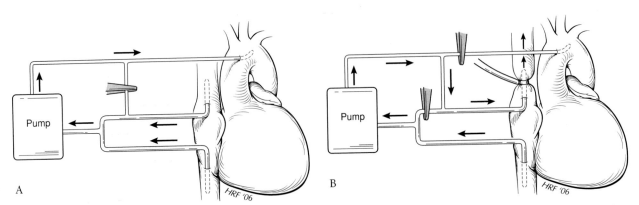

Figure 58-1. **(A)** Circuit setup during cardiopulmonary bypass in anticipation of retrograde cerebral perfusion. Arrows indicate the direction of blood flow. **(B)** During retrograde cerebral perfusion, the clamps are applied as shown to allow perfusion to the head via the superior vena cava. The superior vena cava is snared using a tourniquet.

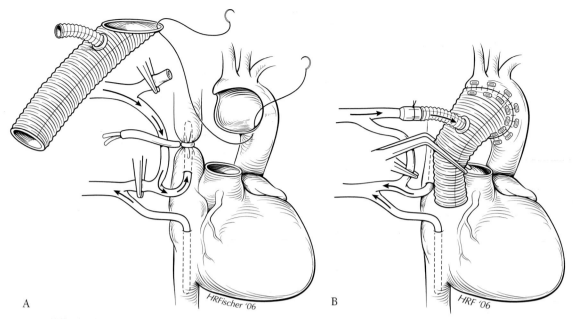

Figure 58-2. **(A)** The arterial cannula is removed, and the aneurysmal aorta is excised. A beveled offset sidearm graft is anastomosed to the beveled undersurface of the aortic arch. Retrograde cerebral perfusion is shown. **(B)** The anastomosis is reinforced with interrupted 4-0 pledgeted suture. The side arm of the graft is connected to the arterial arm of the bypass circuit. The clamps are repositioned to resume antegrade flow, and after the aorta and graft are de-aired, the graft is clamped, allowing restoration of full-flow cardiopulmonary bypass.

graft is clamped proximal to its side arm and full flow is restored (Fig. 58-2B). The graft is cut to size, and the proximal anastomosis is performed using running 4-0 or 3-0 polypropylene suture. A de-airing 18-gauge needle is placed in the graft, and suction on the sump drain is stopped, leaving volume in the patient. The lungs are given manual ventilation to dislodge air, and once blood is seen to eject from the de-airing needle the patient is placed in deep Trendelenburg position. Flows from the bypass circuit are reduced, and the cross-clamp is removed. Suction on the sump is resumed to decompress the heart, and full flows in the bypass circuit are resumed. The de-airing needle is left in place until no air is seen on echocardiographic examination of the left heart. The retrograde cardioplegia cannula and the sump drain are removed, and the patient is then weaned from cardiopulmonary bypass.

Rewarming can be initiated immediately after cardiopulmonary bypass is restarted, but it is occasionally prudent to delay rewarming if extensive reconstruction is required proximally. The difference in perfusate and core body temperature is kept to <10°C until a core body temperature of 27°C is achieved, and then the perfusate is kept at 37°C for the remainder of rewarming. Separation from cardiopulmonary bypass occurs after an esophageal temperature of 36°C has been achieved. When one is ready to remove the arterial cannula, the side arm of the graft is clamped between two hemostats and cut. A heavy silk suture is used to tie off the side arm graft flush with the aortic graft, and then a suture ligature is used to provide definitive obliteration of the side arm lumen. If the side arm is not tied flush with the graft, future computed tomography scans might be interpreted as an anastomotic leak or rupture because contrast may enter the residual side arm.

The foregoing procedure can be accomplished in the same manner using femoral artery cannulation in place of ascending aortic cannulation. Just as with aortic cannulation, separate head vessel cannulae and/or retrograde cerebral perfusion techniques can be used. The advantages of femoral arterial cannulation include its ease of use, the ability to establish cardiopulmonary bypass before sternotomy in the case of high-risk reoperation, and the ability to place a cross-clamp snug up to the innominate artery and arch in those cases where that extra length on the ascending aorta would allow the procedure to be done without circulatory arrest. The disadvantages include risk of vascular injury or dissection, risk of cerebral and visceral ischemia due to retrograde

flow in an atherosclerotic aorta, cerebral or visceral embolization, absence of antegrade cerebral perfusion without separate head vessel cannulation, and risk of limb ischemia.

Alternatively and with increasing frequency, we use axillary inflow to perform these cases. This technique is described in the following section on total arch replacement and has the same advantages described for femoral artery cannulation with the addition of allowing easy establishment of selective antegrade cerebral perfusion. Unlike femoral artery cannulation, there is no retrograde aortic flow, and the procedure provides the best cerebral protection of all perfusion techniques. Although small, there is a risk of brachial plexus and vascular injury inherent to this procedure.

Total Arch

Aneurysms that involve the aortic arch always need a period of circulatory arrest or low-flow selective perfusion, usually in combination with varying degrees of hypothermia, to perform the repair. Right radial and femoral arterial pressures are transduced. It has become our preferred approach to cannulate the right axillary artery. An incision made in the deltopectoral groove usually provides better access to the artery than an infraclavicular incision, and this is performed before sternotomy. In the groove, the thoracoacromial artery will be out of the way and the pectoralis major muscle can be preserved. The 4-cm to 6-cm incision is taken down to the pectoralis major with electrocautery, and then the muscle is spread along its fibers to expose the pectoralis minor muscle. This is divided to expose the artery that lies immediately behind the muscle. Here, the lateral and medial cords of the brachial plexus lie superior and inferior to the vessel, respectively, and care is taken to avoid injury to the plexus. The vessel is taken pliable, and a 3-cm to 4-cm segment of the vessel is freed, after which a vessel loop is passed around it. The sternum and pericardium are then opened. Heparin (4 mg/kg) is given intravenously. The axillary artery is lifted using the vessel loop, and a partial occlusion clamp is placed on the artery, to which an 8-mm graft is anastomosed using running 6-0 polypropylene suture. The graft is clamped, and the partial occlusion clamp is removed. The graft is attached to the arterial arm of the bypass circuit and secured in place with a plastic band and a heavy silk tie (Fig. 58-3).

For venous cannulation we usually use a single two-stage venous cannula because we have been using selective antegrade cerebral perfusion, but bicaval cannulas and retrograde cerebral perfusion can also be used. After an adequate ACT is established, cardiopulmonary bypass is instituted and ventilation is discontinued. The patient is cooled, and a retrograde cardioplegia catheter and a left ventricular sump drain are inserted. To assist in cerebral protection, the head

is packed in ice. The innominate artery is encircled with a tourniquet in preparation for snaring when cardiopulmonary bypass is discontinued. The patient is cooled to EEG silence, and then cooling continues for an additional 5 minutes.

Once EEG silence has been achieved, pentobarbital (2 g/70 kg) is given intravenously and allowed to circulate for a few minutes. The patient is placed in Trendelenburg position, whole-body cardiopulmonary bypass is discontinued, and the innominate artery is snared with the previously placed tourniquet. Flows of 500 to 1,000 mL/min into the axillary artery are used to perfuse the brain antegrade. Flow is adjusted to maintain the right radial arterial line pressure of at least 60 to 70 mm Hg. The aorta is opened through a longitudinal incision, and cardioplegia is given directly into the coronary ostia. Subsequent doses of cardioplegia are given every 10 minutes into the ostia, coronary sinus, or both. The aorta and arch are inspected, and the aneurysmal segment of aorta is excised, leaving an island of aorta attached to the great vessels. An appropriately sized graft is obtained.

The distal anastomosis is performed using running 3-0 polypropylene suture. Blood returning from the left subclavian and left common carotid arteries may obscure the field; however, intermittent suctioning with the pump suckers is usually all that is necessary to enable adequate visualization. Occasionally, flow into the axillary artery can be temporarily discontinued if visualization becomes a problem. Another option is to place occlusion balloon catheters into the

origins of these vessels. We use a retrograde cardioplegia catheter for this. Although they add some complexity to the circuit, these catheters can be used to deliver antegrade flow as well. This may be the ideal approach because flow into the axillary artery alone relies on intact collateral flow from the circle of Willis to perfuse the entire brain. The distal anastomosis is secured circumferentially with interrupted pledgeted 4-0 polypropylene sutures (Fig. 58-4A).

The great vessels that were left attached to the aorta are then anastomosed to the opening created in the side of the graft using running 3-0 polypropylene suture. Again, blood may obscure visualization, and one of the aforementioned approaches may be needed to counter this. With the patient still in Trendelenburg position, the snare on the innominate artery is released, and blood is allowed to fill the graft to remove air from the head and neck vessels while still flowing at 500 to 1,000 mL/min. Theoretically, there should be minimal air in these vessels if antegrade flow into the axillary artery was nearly continuous. The graft is then clamped proximal to the arch, and full flow is resumed (Fig. 58-4B). If no other procedures besides the proximal anastomosis are required, rewarming can begin. The proximal anastomosis is performed with running 3-0 polypropylene suture. De-airing manoeuvres are performed as described. After rewarming, the patient is separated from cardiopulmonary bypass.

Elephant Trunk Procedure

Aneurysms of the ascending aorta and arch sometimes extend a variable distance into the descending thoracic aorta and may even involve the abdominal aorta. It is possible to replace the entire aorta during a single procedure, but this carries significant risk. Alternatively, it may be preferable to perform the repair as a staged procedure. Referred to as the elephant trunk procedure, the ascending aorta and arch are first replaced, followed by a second operation to replace the distal part of the aneurysm. The setup and conduct of the initial operation are identical to those described for total arch repair except for the following. After circulatory arrest is established and the aneurysm is excised the distal anastomosis is performed, with the graft invaginated within itself mimicking an intussusception. The entire graft is placed within the descending aorta with the free ends sitting distally in the aorta. The folded edge is anastomosed to the aorta using running 3-0 polypropylene suture creating the distal anastomosis. The graft is then pulled from inside itself leaving one

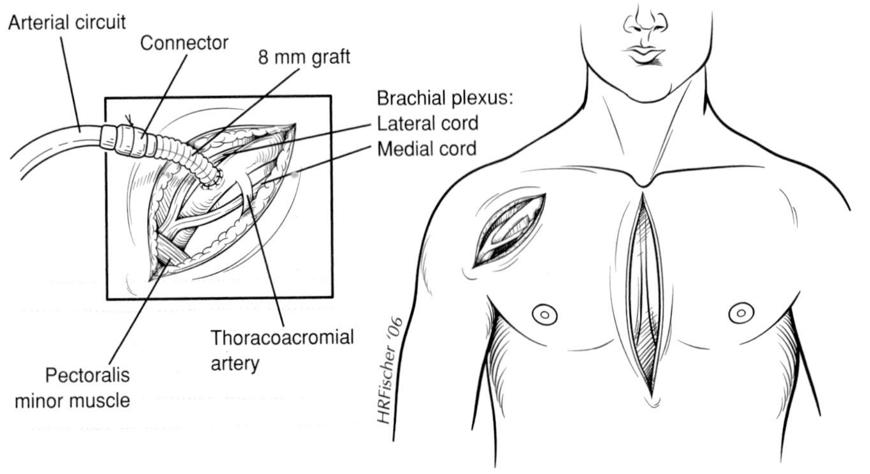

Figure 58-3.   Cannulation of axillary artery via 8-mm graft. The thoracoacromial artery defines the medial extent of the dissection.

Labels in figure: Arterial circuit; Connector; 8 mm graft; Brachial plexus: Lateral cord, Medial cord; Thoracoacromial artery; Pectoralis minor muscle; HRFischer '06

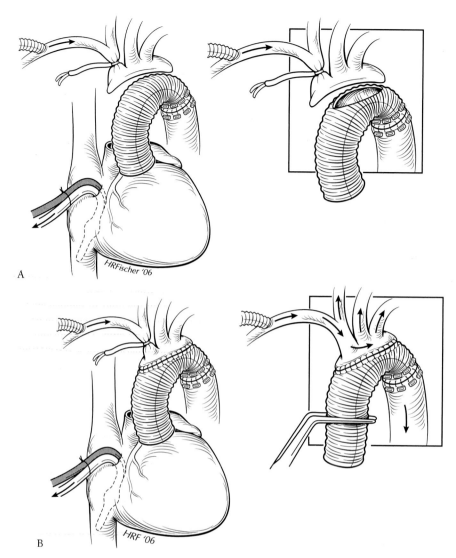

A

B

Figure 58-4. **(A)** The distal anastomosis is performed with 3-0 running polypropylene suture and reinforced with 4-0 interrupted pledgeted suture. A hole is then cut in the graft to correspond to the island of vessels left attached to the aorta. **(B)** The island of aorta with the great vessels attached is anastomosed to the graft. The aorta and graft are de-aired by removing the snare on the innominate artery and filling the vessel while the patient is in Trendelenburg position. The graft is then clamped, restoring full-flow cardiopulmonary bypass.

latissimus dorsi and serratus anterior muscles, and the lung is deflated.

If the aneurysm extends below the diaphragm, the incision is extended toward the umbilicus in a curvilinear fashion. We do not remove a rib, and only occasionally need to notch the rib for completion of elephant trunk procedures. The costal margin and rectus abdominus muscle are divided, connecting the thoracotomy to the abdominal incisions. The retroperitoneal reflection is dissected with electrocautery, mobilizing the spleen, descending colon, and left kidney, thereby exposing the abdominal aorta. An arcuate incision in the diaphragm is made staying approximately 1 cm to 2 cm from the tendonous portion, where the neurovascular bundle runs, and leaving a 3-cm to 4-cm margin attached to the chest wall to facilitate repair using No. 1 polypropylene suture on closure. A Richardson retractor on the upper rib and Omni retractors on the lower rib, with gentle reflection of the abdominal contents to the right by the surgical assistant, provides exposure for these thoracoabdominal incisions.

We use left heart bypass for Crawford extents I and II thoracoabdominal aneurysms. For this, we use a circuit with a centrifugal pump but no heat exchanger or oxygenator. The dose of heparin is reduced to 1 mg/kg. The pericardium overlying the left inferior pulmonary vein is opened, and a pledgeted 4-0 polypropylene purse-string suture is placed in the vessel, which is then cannulated. The aorta is cannulated distally in the descending thoracic portion, or in the abdominal portion in the case of thoraco-abdominal aneurysms. Flow is initially run at 500 mL/min until the cross-clamp is applied, after which flows are adjusted (usually 2 to 2.5 L/min) to maintain a right radial mean arterial pressure of 60 to 70 mm Hg, and a femoral arterial pressure of at least 50 to 60 mm Hg. The aorta is clamped in a place that includes the free-floating arm of the elephant trunk graft. A metallic clip placed during the initial procedure on the distal, free-floating end of the graft will show up on imaging and allows the surgeon to see where the distal end of the graft extends. This can be confirmed intraoperatively using trans-esophageal echocardiography. Because the graft should extend some distance into the descending aorta, the clamp does not have to be applied flush against the arch (Fig. 58-6A). A second clamp is placed on the aorta proximal to the arterial cannula. The aorta is opened in its aneurysmal segment, and the free-floating portion of the graft is seized and clamped (Fig. 58-6B). The first clamp is removed, which allows the graft to

end sitting freely in the descending aorta; the other end will become the arch and ascending aorta (Fig. 58-5). A hole is cut in the side of the graft to which the great vessels are attached, and the remainder of the operation is performed as described in the previous section. If the patient has indications for replacement of the descending thoracic aorta, it is performed approximately 3 to 6 weeks later as the second stage of the operation. If symptoms suggest more urgent indications, then the procedure can be done sooner.

For the second-stage procedure, the patient is intubated with a double-lumen endobronchial tube. Pressures are transduced

from right radial and femoral arterial lines. We use a cerebrospinal fluid (CSF) drain for all Crawford extents I and II thoracoabdominal aneurysms. An intrathecal catheter is placed in the intervertebral space between L3 and L4, or L4 and L5. While the aorta is cross-clamped, the CSF is allowed to drain to keep pressure between 5 and 10 mm Hg, and not more than 50 mL of fluid is removed. The patient is then positioned on the right side with the thorax 75 degrees to the bed and hips 45 degrees, providing exposure to the vessels in the groin in the event that they are needed to establish cardiopulmonary bypass. A posterolateral thoracotomy incision is made in the sixth interspace, dividing the

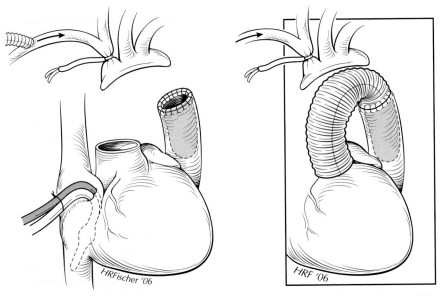

Figure 58-5. The aorta and invaginated graft are anastomosed together. The interior arm of the invaginated graft is then delivered from the aorta. The remainder of the procedure is performed as for a total arch.

be pulled a little inferiorly because it has a tendency to condense due to its corrugated structure. Communication with the anesthesiologists is essential so that they may make adjustments to preload, afterload, and contractility before and upon clamping the aorta.

An appropriately sized graft is anastomosed to the free-floating arm of the elephant trunk graft using 3-0 polypropylene suture. It is not necessary to routinely reinforce this anastomosis because the graft-on-graft connection is quite hemostatic. Left heart bypass is discontinued, and the arterial cannula is removed. The distal clamp is also removed, and backbleeding from the aorta is dealt with using suction to a cell-saver system (Fig. 58-6C). The remainder of the aneurysmal segment of aorta is splayed open, and large intercostal vessels below T6 that have poor backbleeding are identified. An island of aortic tissue surrounding these vessels is anastomosed using running

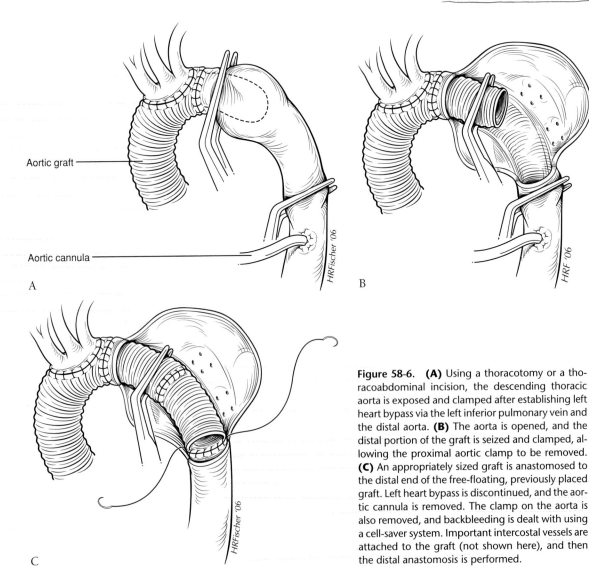

Figure 58-6. **(A)** Using a thoracotomy or a thoracoabdominal incision, the descending thoracic aorta is exposed and clamped after establishing left heart bypass via the left inferior pulmonary vein and the distal aorta. **(B)** The aorta is opened, and the distal portion of the graft is seized and clamped, allowing the proximal aortic clamp to be removed. **(C)** An appropriately sized graft is anastomosed to the distal end of the free-floating, previously placed graft. Left heart bypass is discontinued, and the aortic cannula is removed. The clamp on the aorta is also removed, and backbleeding is dealt with using a cell-saver system. Important intercostal vessels are attached to the graft (not shown here), and then the distal anastomosis is performed.

Aortic graft

Aortic cannula

A

B

C

3-0 or 4-0 polypropylene suture to a hole created in the side of the graft. Intercostal vessels with vigorous backbleeding are oversewn. The proximal clamp is then moved below this anastomosis providing perfusion to the spinal cord. If the aneurysm ends before these important intercostals branch off, this end-to-side anastomosis is not done and the distal anastomosis is performed. In fact, if the aneurysm extends only a small distance, ending before T7, then left heart bypass may not be necessary and a "clamp and sew" technique can be employed provided a very short cross-clamp time is assured.

If the aneurysm extends inferior to the celiac, superior mesenteric, and renal vessels, they are reattached. This is addressed in the chapter on thoracoabdominal aortic aneurysms. The graft is then cut to size, and the distal anastomosis is performed using running 3-0 or 4-0 polypropylene suture, during which time the anesthesiologist is alerted to the impending removal of the clamp within minutes so that appropriate adjustments to preload, afterload, contractility, and acid-base status can be made. The patient is placed head down, and the remaining clamp is slowly removed. The cannula in the left inferior pulmonary vein is removed, protamine is given, and meticulous care is directed to achieve a hemostasic field, after which the wound is closed.

Reverse Elephant Trunk Procedure

In cases of extensive aneurysmal disease of the aorta, such as that described previously, there are instances where either the aortic segment distal to the subclavian artery is disproportionately larger than the proximal segment or the distal segment is producing symptoms. It then becomes necessary to address the distal portion of the aorta first. Replacing the descending thoracic aorta, or the thoracoabdominal aorta, as may be the case, and then performing a second procedure at a later time can accomplish this. Furthermore, to reduce the risk of injury to the esophagus, pulmonary artery, and vagus and recurrent laryngeal nerves that can be obscured by adhesions, the procedure can be done using the reverse elephant trunk technique.

In this technique the initial procedure is identical to the second procedure of the elephant trunk technique just described, except that the graft is invaginated into itself and the anastomosis is between the aorta and the folded edge of the graft (Fig.

58-7A). The remainder of the initial procedure is carried out as described above (Fig. 58-7B). After an appropriate period of convalescence the patient is brought back for the second stage of the procedure. This is identical to the first stage of the elephant trunk procedure with the following alteration: after cardiopulmonary bypass is discontinued and the aortic clamp is removed, the invaginated portion of the previously placed graft is pulled up from the descending aorta into the operative field (Fig. 58-7C). This portion is then used to replace the arch by suturing the island of aorta left attached to the great vessels to the side of the graft (Fig. 58-7D). The graft is clamped proximal to the great vessels, and cardiopulmonary bypass is restored (Fig. 58-7E). The proximal portion of the graft is then used to replace the aneurysmal ascending aorta, and the remainder of the operation follows that described for the first stage of the elephant trunk procedure.

Cerebral Protection

Various techniques are available to the surgeon to protect the brain during operations on the aortic arch. Whenever possible, we use deep hypothermic circulatory arrest, cerebral perfusion, ice packs around the head, aggressive blood sugar control, steroids, mannitol, and barbiturates. Regardless of adjunctive measures, the most important factor in limiting cerebral injury is an expeditious surgery with a short period of cerebral ischemia; this should be the center of every surgeon's strategy of cerebral protection.

The utility of hypothermia is derived from its reduction in cellular metabolic activity and oxygen demand. For every $10°C$ drop in temperature, the metabolic activity of the brain drops by twofold to threefold. This is translated into periods of "safe" arrest times. Traditionally, a core temperature of $18°C$ was thought to provide approximately 30 minutes of safe arrest time. Although this does not hold true for everyone, it is used as a guide when planning a repair using hypothermic circulatory arrest. We use EEG activity to assess the effectiveness of cerebral cooling in reducing brain wave activity. It is assumed that by decreasing brain wave activity to levels that can not be detected, we are optimizing the decrease in metabolic demand, thereby avoiding, or at least limiting, ischemic injury to the brain. It is interesting to note that at $15°C$, a temperature at which nearly all people have no detectable brain wave activity, metabolic activity is still

15% to 20% of baseline. To assess how effectively cerebral cooling reduces metabolic demand, jugular venous bulb saturations can be monitored. An oxygen saturation of >95% suggests that extraction of oxygen at the capillaries is reduced owing to a decrease in the need for oxygen, which is due to cerebral cooling.

Providing cerebral perfusion also influences the oxygen demand-and-supply relationship, extending the period of safe "circulatory arrest." Of the two options, retrograde and antegrade cerebral perfusion, it appears that the latter may be better. Nonetheless, retrograde cerebral perfusion still provides benefits. These most likely are due to cooling the brain by flowing cold blood through the sagittal sinuses, effectively mimicking an in situ cooling jacket, and flushing out embolic air and debris. It is unlikely that retrograde cerebral perfusion provides any nutritive flow to cerebral tissues. Antegrade cerebral perfusion does provide nutrient flow to the brain extending the time the surgeon has to repair the arch. Some have used antegrade cerebral perfusion to decrease the extent of cooling, performing repairs at higher core temperatures. Caution should be exercised when doing this, for two reasons. First, the benefits of profound hypothermia. and selective antegrade cerebral perfusion are probably additive; by cooling to higher temperature, the overall benefit of adding antegrade cerebral perfusion may be lost. Second, the lower body and spinal cord are not being perfused and are more prone to injury when not using profound hypothermia.

Another aspect of hypothermia-assisted surgery that has recently generated interest is delayed rewarming. Improved cerebral arterial blood flow has been observed in patients subjected to a period of cold reperfusion before rewarming. Reasons for this observation are unknown. Theoretically, this benefit would transfer to patients subjected to selective antegrade cerebral perfusion because they are being perfused continuously prior to rewarming.

Strategies to manage pH are discussed elsewhere in this book. Basic principles are that as the patient is cooled, CO_2 becomes more soluble in gas, thereby pulling to the right the equilibrium in the equation

$$H^+ + HCO_3 \leftrightarrow H_2CO_3 \leftrightarrow H_2O + CO_2$$

Hydrogen ion concentration falls, increasing the pH, which makes the blood more alkalemic. Adding CO_2 to the system as the patient cools, known as pH-stat management, keeps the pH at 7.4 for any given temperature. Warming the sample to $37°C$

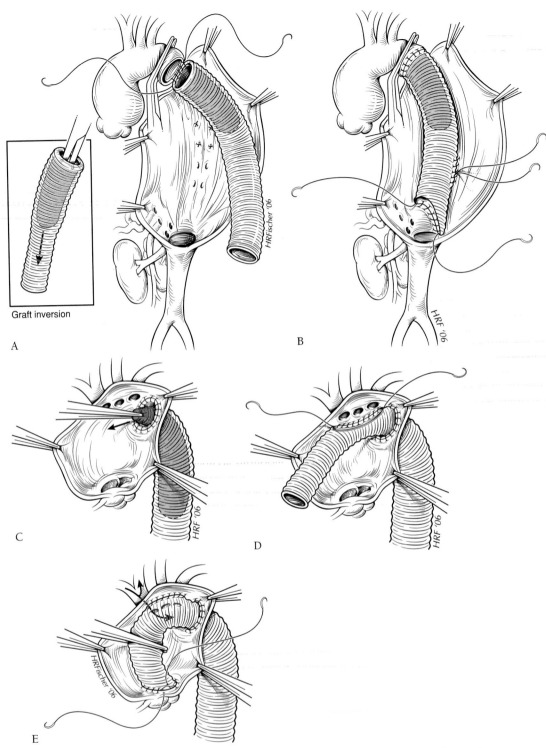

Figure 58-7. **(A,B)** The initial steps of the reversed elephant trunk technique: **(A)** After aortic clamping, the aneurysm is opened, the graft is inverted on itself (*arrow in inset*), and the folded edge is sutured end to end to the proximal descending aorta. **(B)** After completion of the proximal anastomosis, the intercostal arteries have been reattached to an opening in the side of the graft. In this circumstance, the distal anastomosis is being constructed as a bevel at the level of the visceral and renal vessels. **(C–E)** Second stage of the reversed elephant trunk procedure: **(C)** The invaginated graft is delivered into the field after circulatory arrest is established. **(D)** A hole is created in the graft, which is then anastomosed to the aorta surrounding the great vessels. **(E)** The graft is clamped proximal to the great vessels and cardiopulmonary bypass is restored either through the axillary or, femoral artery or by cannulating the or directly.

would make it acidemic. On the other hand, alpha-stat management adds nothing to the system, allowing the blood to be alkalemic at cooler temperatures. Warming the sample to 37°C would return the pH to 7.4.

pH-stat management uncouples cerebral autoregulation of blood flow, thereby enhancing cerebral blood flow. This "luxurious" flow likely assists in cerebral cooling but has the potential of delivering a larger volume of embolic debris to the brain. CO_2 crosses membranes freely, and as it enters the cell it shifts to the left the equilibrium in the foregoing equation, resulting in an intracellular acidosis and loss of enzymatic function. Alpha-stat management maintains cerebral autoregulation, avoiding the benefits and detriments of luxurious blood flow. Although there are arguments for the use of each, the optimal approach may be to use a combination of both, cooling under pH-stat management and then switching over to alpha-stat management. We use an alpha-stat management strategy.

Steroids are thought to be of benefit by attenuating the systemic inflammatory response associated with cardiopulmonary bypass, decreasing permeability of the blood–brain barrier, decreasing cerebral edema, stabilizing cell membranes, decreasing capillary permeability, and improving colloid oncotic pressure. Most commonly, methylprednisolone is administered intravenously at a dose of 15 to 30 mg/kg. In addition to the dose, the timing of administration may have an effect on the beneficial effects seen with steroids. Giving the dose hours before surgery may be of greater benefit than dosing while on cardiopulmonary bypass. It has been difficult for our institution to obtain a steady supply of methylprednisolone, and we have substituted dexamethasone. Our practice is to give 100 mg of intravenous dexamethasone for every 70 kg of weight before initiating cardiopulmonary bypass.

Mannitol is also of benefit in reducing cerebral edema associated with cardiopulmonary bypass and circulatory arrest. It is given into the pump prime at a dose of 25 g. Pentothal is given intravenously at a dose of 2 g/70 kg after EEG silence has been achieved. It is given 3 minutes to circulate and perfuse brain tissue, after which cardiopulmonary bypass is discontinued. Lidocaine is also of use in these cases. Intravenous lidocaine (200 mg/70 kg) is given as the patient is cooled. We believe that it lowers the fibrillation threshold as the patient cools, and it has allowed us to achieve lower core temperatures before fibrillation

ensues. Another dose is given as the clamp is released to prevent or delay fibrillation on rewarming. Lidocaine may also provide a degree of cerebral protection.

Tight control of blood sugar is believed to improve cerebral protection. In the absence of oxygen delivery to the brain during hypothermic circulatory arrest, the cells, which still have a measurable level of metabolic activity, use the anaerobic pathway to generate energy. This anaerobic glycolysis generates lactate, which causes intracellular acidosis, enzymatic dysfunction, cellular injury, and neurotransmitter release. By preventing hyperglycemia, some of the deleterious effects of anaerobic glycolysis may be avoided or attenuated, potentially improving cerebral function.

Postoperative Care

The postoperative care of these patients is, for the most part, not unlike that for other cardiac surgical patients. A few points are worthy of mention. We usually remove the femoral arterial catheter on the first postoperative day because by this time the radial artery should be measuring accurately. As stated earlier, it is usually spasmodic after a period of circulatory arrest, especially when axillary inflow has been used. Another point is that it is occasionally seen that patients exposed to profound hypothermia, especially those exposed to complete circulatory arrest, take longer to fully awake than their counterparts. Therefore, close attention to neurologic status is that much more important with these patients. In addition, the delay in awakening afterward lengthens the period of mechanical ventilation and warrants more vigilance on the patient's respiratory status. As always, attention should be directed as appropriate to limb perfusion in cases of femoral artery cannulation.

Results

The early mortality following elective repair for diseases of the transverse aortic arch is significantly affected by the higher incidence of neurologic injury and has been reported to range from 6% to 20%. In treating 1,142 patients for aortic arch pathology, we encountered 616 (53.9%) with nondissection disease, 221 (19.4%) with acute dissection, and 305 (26.7%) with chronic dissection. The average age of our patients was 65.3 ± 11.2 years; 60% (686) were male patients. Chronic arterial hypertension and aortic valvular insufficiency were common, representing 65.6% and 55.9%, respectively, of cases. Mean cardiopulmonary bypass and circulatory arrest times were 127 ± 48 minutes and 34 ± 11 minutes, respectively. The overall operative mortality was 7.9% (90 patients) represented by a 6.6% 30-day mortality and a 7.7% in-hospital mortality. Major morbidity following arch replacement included neurologic injury or stroke occurring in 43 patients (3.8%). Postoperative renal failure requiring hemodialysis occurred in 13 patients (1.1%); in 7 patients the need for dialysis was temporary. Three hundred and forty-eight (30.5%) patients had pulmonary complications, 162 (14.2%) had cardiac complications, and 38 (3.3%) required reoperation for bleeding. Adverse outcome, which includes death, stroke, and hemodialysis, occurred in 126 patients (11.0%). Results based upon perfusion technique are listed in Table 58-1.

Elephant Trunk Technique

Over a $15\frac{1}{2}$-year period, 205 consecutive patients presented with extensive aneurysms that involved the entire thoracic aorta. Only 8 (4%) of these patients underwent single-stage repair of the ascending aorta, transverse aortic arch, and descending thoracic aorta. Forty-nine (24%) of the patients underwent staged repair using

Table 58-1 Results of 1,142 Aortic Arch Aneurysm Repairs			
Perfusion	Number of Patients (%)	Stroke (%)	Operative Mortality (%)
RCP	695 (60.9)	17 (2.4)	32 (4.6)
ACP	43 (3.8)	0	2 (4.7)
ACP + RCP	138 (12.1)	2 (1.4)	2 (1.4)
HCA alone	266 (23.3)	24 (9.0)	54 (20.3)
Total	1,142 (100)	43 (3.8)	90 (7.9)

ACP = antegrade cerebral perfusion; HCA = hypothermic circulatory arrest; RCP = retrograde cerebral perfusion.

the reversed elephant trunk procedure, in which the descending thoracic component is repaired first; these patients are described in the next section. One hundred forty-eight consecutive patients (72%) underwent total aortic arch replacement using the elephant trunk technique and are the focus in this section. These 148 patients comprised 13% of the 1,135 aortic arch repairs performed by our team during this period.

After the first stage of repair, operative mortality was 12% (18/148). Two of the 15 early deaths were caused by rupture of the descending thoracic aorta. The first patient ruptured 15 days after surgery; an attempt at emergency repair was unsuccessful. The other patient ruptured on postoperative day 27 after suffering from respiratory failure and could not be resuscitated. Seven (5%) patients suffered strokes, 5 (3%) underwent reoperation for bleeding, and 14 (9%) developed acute renal failure requiring dialysis. Pulmonary complications were the most common and were often exacerbated by vocal cord paralysis, which occurred in 37 (25%) patients. One patient suffered bilateral vocal cord paralysis requiring permanent tracheostomy.

Of the 130 patients who survived stage one, 32 (25%) subsequently died without undergoing distal aortic repair. In most cases, the cause of death was unknown. There were 3 deaths due to distal aortic rupture. Nineteen (15%) surviving patients have not undergone the second stage of repair. In most cases, the remaining aneurysm has not yet reached sufficient size to warrant repair. Thus far, 79 (61%) patients have undergone the second-stage distal aortic repair; 76 of these were performed at our institution.

Operative mortality following the second stage of repair was 4% (3/76). Two (3%) patients suffered paraplegia, 2 patients had a stroke, 2 required reoperation for bleeding, and 3 needed dialysis for acute renal failure. There were 6 new cases of vocal cord paralysis. Long-term survival after completing the second stage of repair was 70% at 5 years and 59% at 8 years.

Reversed Elephant Trunk Technique

Thirty-eight patients underwent planned two-stage replacement of the entire thoracic aorta using a reversed elephant trunk technique. There were 21 male patients and 17 female patients; the mean age was 64.6 years. Fifteen patients (39%) had chronic aortic dissection and 22 patients (58%) had fusiform medial degenerative disease; 1 patient (3%) presented with acute dissec-

tion superimposed on pre-existing aneurysmal disease and was operated on emergently. Forty-five percent of patients were symptomatic at presentation, with back pain the primary symptom. Emergent or urgent operations were required in 13 patients (34%) with acute presentation, including 3 (8%) with contained rupture. Patients with symptomatic or extensive critical coronary artery disease, along with patients with severe valvular pathology, were excluded from this approach and required an initial approach via median sternotomy addressing aortic and cardiac issues. The extent of the initial operation included 3 (8%) descending thoracic, 14 (37%) Crawford extent I, and 21 (55%) Crawford extent II. Fifty percent of patients had previously undergone aortic operations, including 12 proximal aortic repairs, 1 descending thoracic repair, 1 extent IV thoracoabdominal, and 5 abdominal aortic repairs.

In 12 of 28 patients (43%) the second stage was performed with a mean interval of 3.9 months (range: 1.6 to 14 months) after the initial procedure. All 12 second-stage procedures included total replacement of the transverse aortic arch. Concomitant procedures included coronary artery bypass grafting in 2 patients, aortic valve annuloplasty in 3 patients, and aortic root homograft replacement in 1 patient. In addition, 1 patient underwent concomitant innominate artery bypass and 1 patient underwent innominate artery, left common carotid, and left subclavian artery bypass. Sixteen patients have not yet received a second-stage intervention. The reasons for this delay are multiple and include the following: The proximal aneurysm has not yet reached a size for which operative intervention is recommended ($n = 12$); postoperative complications from the initial procedure are prohibitive (stroke, paraparesis) ($n = 3$); and the patient is not interested in undergoing another major operation ($n = 1$).

During the initial procedure on the descending thoracic or thoracoabdominal aorta, there were no intraoperative deaths. The median clamp time was 45 minutes, left heart bypass was used in 27 patients (71%), and cerebrospinal fluid drainage was used in 23 patients (61%). Intercostal artery reattachment was performed in 30 patients (79%). Postoperative complications included paraparesis in 1 patient (3%) who underwent emergent extent II thoracoabdominal aortic aneurysm repair. This patient was ambulating with the assistance of a walker at discharge and is reportedly walking on his own at follow-up. One patient

developed a stroke, 4 patients (11%) had cardiac complications, and 2 patients (5%) required hemodialysis. The 4 patients with cardiac complications experienced atrial fibrillation ($n = 2$) and myocardial infarction ($n = 2$). There were 6 (16%) early deaths. Four patients died during follow-up before repair of the ascending/transverse aortic arch for the completion of the reversed elephant trunk. Causes of 3 of these late deaths are unknown; they occurred at 21.3, 32.8, and 45.4 months respectively, after initial repair. The fourth late death was due to respiratory failure at 14.3 months after initial repair.

Twelve of the remaining 28 patients (43%) underwent completion procedures at an average of 3.9 months after initial repair. There were no intraoperative deaths after the completion procedure. There was no incidence of stroke or paraplegia/paraparesis after the second-stage procedures. Pulmonary complications occured in 3 patients (25%), and 1 patient (8%) developed severe encephalopathy. There was 1 (8%) in-hospital death due to multiple organ failure (MOF) 3.5 months after completion repair. Four late deaths occurred; 1 due to MOF at 5.3 months postoperatively and 3 due to unknown causes at 1.3, 34, and 96.5 months postoperatively, respectively. Cumulative 5-year survival for the entire group of 38 patients was $51.3 \pm 10.8\%$.

Acknowledgement

The authors gratefully acknowledge Stephen N. Palmer, PhD, ELS, for providing editorial support.

SUGGESTED READING

Coady MA, Rizzo JA, Elefteriades JA. Developing surgical intervention criteria for thoracic aortic aneurysms. Cardiol Clin 1999;17:827.

Coselli JS. Aneurysms of the transverse aortic arch. In Baue AE (ed), Glenn's Thoracic and Cardiovascular Surgery, 6th ed. Norwalk, CT: Appleton & Lange, 1996:2239.

Coselli JS. Retrograde cerebral perfusion via superior vena caval cannula for aortic arch aneurysm surgery. Ann Thorac Surg 1994;57:1668.

Coselli JS, Buket S, Djukanovic B. Aortic arch surgery: current treatment and results. Ann Thor Surg 1995;59:19.

Coselli JS, Crawford ES, Williams TW Jr, et al. Treatment of postoperative infection of ascending aorta and transverse aortic arch. Ann Thorac Surg 1990;50:868.

Coselli JS, LeMaire SA, Carter SA, et al. The reversed elephant trunk technique used for treatment of complex aneurysms of the entire thoracic aorta. Ann Thorac Surg 2005; 80:2165.

Coselli JS, Poli de Figueiredo LF. Surgical techniques for symptomatic aortic arch disease. In Calligaro KD, DeLaurentis DA, Baker WH (eds), Management of Extracranial Cerebrovascular Disease. Philadelphia: Lippincott-Raven, 1996:93.

Crawford ES, Coselli JS. Replacement of the aortic arch. Semin Thorac Cardiovasc Surg 1991;3: 194.

Crawford ES, Coselli JS, Svensson LG, et al. Diffuse aneurismal disease (chronic aortic dissection, Marfan, and mega aorta syndromes) and multiple aneurysm: Treatment by subtotal and total aortic replacement emphasizing the elephant trunk operation. Ann Surg 1990;211: 521.

Crawford ES, Kirklin JW, Naftel DC, et al. Surgery for acute ascending aortic dissection: Should the arch be included? J Thorac Cardiovasc Surg 1992;104:46.

Ehrlich MP, Fang WC, Grabenwoger M, et al. Impact of retrograde cerebral perfusion on aortic arch aneurysm repair. J Thorac Cardiovasc Surg 1999;118:1026.

Ergin MA, Galla JD, Lansman L, et al. Hypothermic circulatory arrest in operations on the thoracic aorta. Determinants of operative mortality and neurologic outcome. J Thorac Cardiovasc Surg 1994;107:788.

Kouchoukos NT, Mauney MC, Masetti P, et al. Single-stage repair of extensive thoracic aortic aneurysms: Experience with the arch-first technique and bilateral anterior thoracotomy. J Thorac Cardiovasc Surg 2004;128:669.

Lass J, Jurmann MJ, Heinemann M, et al. Advances in aortic arch surgery. Ann Thorac Surg 1992;53:227.

LeMaire SA, Coselli JS, Carter SA. The elephant trunk technique for staged repair of complex aneurysms of the entire thoracic aorta. Ann Thorac Surg 2006;81:1561.

McCullough JH, Zhang N, Reich DL, et al. Cerebral metabolic suppression during hypothermic circulatory arrest in humans. Ann Thorac Surg 1999,67:1895.

Michenfelder JD, Milde JH. The relationship among canine brain temperature, metabolism and function during hypothermia. Anaesthesiology 1991;75:130.

Rodriguez RA, Austin EH, Audenaert SM. Postbypass effects of delayed rewarming on cerebral blood flow velocities in infants after total circulatory arrest. J Thorac Cardiovasc Surg 1995;110:1686.

Shum-Tim D, Tchervenkov CI, Jamal AM, et al. Systemic steroid pretreatment improves cerebral protection after circulatory arrest. Ann Thorac Surg 2001;72;1465.

Svensson LG, Crawford ES, Hess KR, et al. Deep hypothermia with circulatory arrest: Determinants of stroke and early mortality in 656 patients. J Thorac Cardiovasc Surg 1993;106: 19.

Ueda Y, Miki S, Kusuhara K, et al. Surgical treatment of aneurysm or dissection involving the ascending aorta and aortic arch, using circulatory arrest and retrograde cerebral perfusion. J Cardiovasc Surg 1990;31: 553.

EDITOR'S COMMENTS

Coselli and colleagues have described a definitive approach to aortic arch aneurysms. This is an extremely detailed approach and will be helpful to anyone performing this kind of surgery. We have essentially used all of the techniques described by the authors. Their results really are excellent for these extraordinarily complex patients.

We have some minor differences. We agree essentially with the cannulization techniques described by the authors. We have frequently cannulated temporarily the ascending aorta in the aneurysmal segment as long as it is free of atherosclerosis. Once the arch aneurysm is resected, the sidearm graft can be used and the procedure completed. However, use of selective antegrade perfusion noted with the axillary artery approach is an attractive one, and we are just beginning to use this on a routine basis. We tend to use 4-0 polypropylene sutures for our arch anastomosis. We worry about 3-0 in fragile tissue. Coselli and his group make up for this with the use of a separate layer of 4-0 pledgeted polypropylene sutures, and I believe this provides similar hemostasis.

Finally, the issue of ascending aortic atherosclerosis is a difficult one, particularly in patients with aneurysmal disease. These patients are at the highest risk for stroke, and we have not yet figured out a way to completely avoid that complication in such patients. Clearly, in those patients axillary cannulation has a large role, and a no-touch technique is required to avoid stroke.

I.L.K.

59

Acute Traumatic Aortic Transection

Daniel Martinez, Scott Johnson, O. L. Miller, and John Calhoon

The treatment of acute traumatic aortic transection continues to be a challenge for thoracic surgeons. Initially, 80% of patients with this injury will die in the field. The survival of the remaining 20% depends on the skill and surgical judgment of the thoracic surgeon and the multidisciplinary team. Rarely is acute traumatic aortic transection an isolated injury; associated injuries to other organs are common and may take initial priority. Prudent surgical judgment has to be exercised from initial evaluation through the process of resuscitation, diagnosis, and ultimate treatment. Once the patient enters the emergency room with acute traumatic aortic transection, untreated, overall mortality increases with every hour. Treatment may include nonoperative therapy, at least initially, depending on the severity and priority of other injuries. Therefore, each patient needs to be treated individually because there is no one specific method for treating and managing this type of injury.

After the diagnosis of acute traumatic aortic transection is made, a thoracic surgeon should become involved with the case. It is imperative that he or she take charge of the management and direct appropriate care for the patient. The thoracic surgeon should approach the treatment of acute traumatic aortic transection with respect for the lethality of this condition as well as the possible complications/sequelae of paraplegia, renal failure, and respiratory insufficiency.

Many have championed a particular technique for repairing this injury. However, each technique has its advantages and also its inherent risks. The techniques vary in how they attempt to minimize the alarming complications of paraplegia and renal failure. However, no one has demonstrated conclusively that one technique has any advantage over the simple clamp-and-sew

technique. It may be necessary to apply methods of different techniques according to the injury itself, associated injuries, and the hemodynamic condition of the individual patient.

Incidence and Natural History

Eighty percent of acute traumatic aortic transections occur as a result of motor vehicle collisions. Other causes include kicks, falls from heights, and crush injuries. Most series report that 20% of motor vehicular accident fatalities are a result of thoracic aortic transection. The incidence is higher in the young adult population and has an increased male-to-female ratio.

More than one half of the transections occur at the aortic isthmus. Injury to the ascending aorta is seen in about 20% of the cases, and there are very few survivors from this injury. Another 20% of patients have multiple sites of injury, and very few of these patients survive. The mechanism of injury in aortic transection is thought to be the combination of deceleration and sheer forces concentrated at the fixed portions of the aorta, these being the descending aorta at the isthmus and the arch of the aorta.

The natural history of acute traumatic aortic transection is such that immediate death is seen in 80% to 90% of cases. Patients who survive the initial injury have an intact adventitia and mediastinal pleura, which allows containment of the injury and the continued flow of blood to the distal aorta. It is not uncommon to find a completely separated aorta within this adventitial hematoma. Of the 10% to 20% of patients who survive initially, one half,

if left untreated, die within 24 hours. Of those who live 24 hours, it is estimated that about 5% per day die in the next 2 weeks. Only a few patients survive to develop untreated chronic traumatic thoracic aortic aneurysms.

Diagnosis

With a history of any deceleration injury, there should be a suspicion for possible acute aortic transection. Symptoms on arrival at the emergency room in a conscious patient range from nonspecific complaints to those of chest pain, intrascapular pain, hoarseness, dyspnea, dysphasia, and frank paralysis. Physical examination findings include rib fractures, sternal fractures, and even imprints of the steering wheel on the chest. The cervical and thoracic spines are also vulnerable, and these should be carefully examined. Hypertension in the arms, so-called coarctation syndrome, has been reported. It is important to carefully examine the pulses in the upper and lower extremities and check for any differences. A baseline neurologic examination is extremely important in these patients because paraplegia may be present preoperatively and may be due to other causes such as spinal fractures and dislocations. On arrival at the emergency room, an initial chest radiograph should be obtained as soon as the patient's cervical spine is cleared. An upright posteroanterior (PA) film is desirable. If this is not possible, then the most-upright anteroposterior (AP) film possible is the best alternative. Supine chest radiographs usually reveal a widened mediastinum. Any abnormality seen in the mediastinum on an upright PA chest film should raise the suspicion for aortic transection and prompt further investigation. Various specific radiographic findings associated with aortic transection include mediastinal widening, obscurity of the aortic knob, obliteration of the AP window, tracheal deviation, depression of the left mainstem bronchus, widening of the paravertebral stripe, deviation of the esophagus (seen most commonly as deviation of the nasogastric tube), and a left hemothorax. Fractures of the first rib and/or scapula should raise the suspicion of an aortic injury due to the extreme force required to fracture these bones.

A history of a deceleration injury in conjunction with an abnormal mediastinum seen on the chest radiograph should prompt further investigation.

The gold standard for diagnosing a transected thoracic aorta is arteriography. In some institutions contrast-enhanced computed tomographic (CT) scanning is used as a screening tool. Such scans may be more advantageous in patients who have a suggestive history and a mediastinum that appears normal. In patients with a widened mediastinum, a CT scan may help to rule out possible aortic injury. Magnetic resonance imaging (MRI) has also been advocated, but there is less experience in this area, and it may be cumbersome to obtain in the acute trauma situation. Recently, transesophageal echocardiography (TEE) has been shown to be a useful diagnostic tool, but this test may not be readily available in all institutions, and its accuracy is operator dependent. With TEE, there is also a risk of free aortic rupture due to patient gagging causing increase in intrathoracic pressure. In our experience, TEE has been most useful when the patient was sent to the operating room emergently for other life-threatening injuries and there remains a question regarding the diagnosis of acute thoracic aortic transection. Intraoperatively, TEE is useful in helping to rule in or out aortic injury. Operative exploration may be justified without the use of arteriography in the acute setting based on the clinical picture along with other radiologic findings such as that seen on plain radiographs, CT scans, and intraoperative TEE findings.

Associated injuries are common, and acute traumatic aortic transection is rarely seen as an isolated entity. Injuries to other organ systems (intracranial, intra-abdominal), including major fractures (spine, pelvis), must be considered and treated if a successful outcome is to be obtained. When associated injuries are present, the thoracic surgeon should be involved with the treatment and prioritization of these injuries.

In a patient with stable vital signs and a suspected aortic tear (and no signs of an impending intracranial or intra-abdominal catastrophe) an arteriogram should be performed. If this confirms the diagnosis, an immediate thoracotomy and repair of this injury should be undertaken. Signs of intracranial hemorrhage in association with signs of increased intracranial pressure obviously need to be addressed before repair of the transected aorta is attempted. When hemodynamically unstable patients present with causes believed not secondary to an aortic transection, the other sites of hemorrhage need to be identified and managed first. Usually hemodynamic instability results from intra-abdominal hemorrhage, which can usually be confirmed by diagnostic peritoneal lavage. Obviously, in this case, a laparotomy should precede repair of the transected aorta. Patients should be taken immediately to the operating room for laparotomy and control of major intra-abdominal hemorrhage. If they stabilize, they then can be taken to the angiography suite later and returned to the operating room for a thoracotomy if a transected aorta is confirmed, especially if the intraoperative TEE findings are ambiguous. It is imperative that the thoracic surgeon be directly involved with decision-making regarding these patients and aware of all injuries. Obviously, each patient needs to be individualized so that care can be expedited in an orderly manner appropriate to the injuries.

Medical Therapy

The use of antihypertensive therapy was first applied in the management of descending thoracic aneurysms and has expanded to use in the management of acute traumatic aortic injuries. This therapy decreases the wall stress tension in the aorta by means of beta-blockade and, if necessary, vasodilating agents. Prospective studies have demonstrated a decrease in the incidence of spontaneous rupture with the institution of appropriate antihypertensive therapy. This is an important aspect in the management of multiply injured patients where other life-threatening injuries need to be addressed first, prior to aortic repair.

It is our policy to initiate a short-acting beta-blocker and afterload-reducing agent as needed when the patient has been adequately resuscitated and there is a high index of suspicion for an aortic tear. This allows the trauma team to address any other life-threatening injuries or hemorrhage that is occurring, correct any coagulopathy that

may be present, address the associated pulmonary contusions and/or closed head injuries that are frequently present, and treat any metabolic derangements that may develop. The overall goal is to convert what has traditionally been treated emergently into more of a semi-elective procedure after many of the foregoing abnormalities have been treated and corrected, at which time the patient has a better chance for survival. Several studies have supported the concept of delaying repair in these multiply injured patients and treating other life-threatening conditions first, which reduces overall mortality. Even patients initially deemed nonoperative candidates due to severe injuries such as brain or pulmonary injuries may eventually become operative candidates. In any event, most patients benefit from the institution of aggressive medical management and antihypertensive therapy.

Surgical Management

The surgical preparation of a patient with an acute traumatic aortic transection should be done in an orderly fashion. Every attempt to approach this problem as elective surgery should be made if the patient is stable. Although time is of the essence, an assessment for all major injuries and a baseline neurologic examination should be performed. Routine laboratory studies should be obtained and blood sent for typing and cross-match. In addition, the operating room should be mobilized and prepared to care for the multiply injured patient.

As a part of the preoperative preparation for operation, it is of paramount importance that the patient and the family be thoroughly counseled about the procedure and specifically about the perioperative risks of paraplegia. This is a lethal injury, and the possibility of death from other injuries or from the transected aorta should be thoroughly discussed with the family. The other major risks of the operation should be discussed. These include the possibility of infection, renal failure, respiratory distress syndrome, vocal cord paralysis, and complications from other associated injuries.

If the diagnosis of acute aortic transection is made, it is best that these patients not be over-resuscitated. Adequate pain control and antihypertensive therapy are critical because any hypertensive event can precipitate tearing of the tenuous adventitia and mediastinal tissues holding the hematoma intact. It may be necessary to sedate a patient to control anxiety or combativeness. Antihypertensive therapy should be continued up to the induction of anesthesia. However, hypotension should be avoided because of its association with the development of paraplegia.

In preparation for surgery, it is important that the thoracic surgeon and anesthesiologist be in constant communication before and during the operation and that a two-way dialogue be established from the very start of the procedure. If at all possible, a double-lumen endotracheal tube should be placed for the procedure because this will greatly facilitate exposure of the injury. If there is a question of a cervical spine injury, it should be ruled out before the patient is taken to the operating room. A cervical collar makes anesthetic intubation difficult and limits access to the neck should the placement of additional intravenous lines be necessary. Large-bore intravenous lines and some type of central access such as a subclavian or internal jugular venous catheter should be placed. A cardiopulmonary perfusionist should be available, especially if partial left heart bypass or some other type of bypass becomes necessary. In addition, in preparation for potential rapid blood loss, a rapid-infusion transfusion system and a qualified person to run this system should be available. A Foley catheter should be inserted to monitor urinary output. The blood pressure in the upper extremities should be monitored through a right radial artery catheter, because during the repair the left subclavian artery will need to be occluded and inaccurate readings will be obtained from a left radial artery catheter. Usually, an arteriogram will have been obtained in the majority of cases. We prefer arteriography to be performed through the right groin, and at the conclusion of the arteriogram, a monitoring catheter should be left in the right femoral artery. In the operating room, this catheter is attached to a transducer to allow continuous lower body/extremity blood pressure monitoring throughout the operative repair. The left groin is left free in case access is needed for bypass procedures or for other lines. A pulmonary artery catheter for measuring pulmonary artery pressures, wedge pressures, or cardiac output may be desirable in some instances but is not mandatory for the procedure. If the situation warrants, such a catheter could be placed through a previously placed Swan introducer sheath at a later time during the operation or even postoperatively. Our preference is to place a Swan sheath for its size and to use a true Swan-Ganz catheter only when hemodynamic questions arise. We do not routinely monitor cerebral spinal fluid (CSF) pressure, because this adds time and complexity

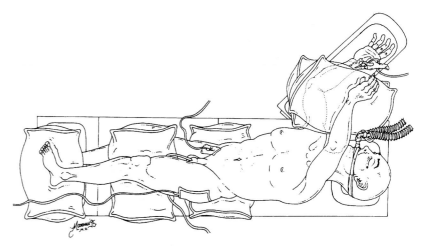

Figure 59-1.   The patient properly positioned for left posterolateral thoracotomy. The right radial arterial line and right femoral arterial line are in place. The left groin should be somewhat exposed in case access for cardiopulmonary bypass is necessary. A double-lumen endotracheal tube is in position and secured.

to the procedure with little known benefit in the acute trauma setting. All patients receive prophylactic antibiotic therapy mainly aimed at prevention of *Staphylococcus aureus* infection in anticipation of potentially placing a prosthetic graft in the aortic position. Discussions with the operating room personnel including the scrub nurse and the circulating nurse are mandatory for orderly progression of the operation. Several sizes of aortic grafts should be in the room and made available. Our routine is to size the aorta intraoperatively, either visibly or with sizers, which generally gives us an accurate idea of what size of graft to use. Our graft preference is a pretreated woven graft, which does not require preclotting.

After all the preoperative plans have been made, the patient is taken to the operating room, placed in the supine position, and anesthetized. The induction of anesthesia and intubation is a very critical point in the procedure. Every attempt should be made to avoid severe blood pressure fluctuations, because any hypertension can precipitate a rupture and turn an "elective" procedure into an emergent one. After a double-lumen tube is placed, one should ensure that all intravenous lines are adequately taped and that adequate monitoring of hemodynamic status for both the upper and lower body (i.e., above and below the injury) and urine output is present. The patient is then placed in the right lateral decubitus position. Positioning and padding of the extremities are to be performed at this juncture. In addition, we like to position the patient so the left groin is available in case the femoral artery or femoral vein needs to be exposed during the procedure.

The patient is prepared and draped. Our preference is to use an antiseptic-impregnated plastic drape to keep as much skin covered as possible considering the probability of a prosthetic graft being used during the procedure (Fig. 59-1).

A full posterolateral thoracotomy incision is made from just below the left nipple all the way up between the scapula and the spine. Both the latissimus dorsi and serratus anterior are divided, and the fourth intercostal space should be chosen for entering the pleural cavity. It is our preference to go high, using the fourth interspace. A fifth interspace incision is usually too low and makes the exposure difficult. This is a very important part of the operation, because an inappropriate choice of intercostal space will make the exposure and the repair unnecessarily difficult. It is usually not necessary to excise a rib. However, if exposure is inadequate on opening of the chest cavity, our procedure has been to cut 1 cm or so of rib out (posteriorly, behind the paraspinous ligament) below our initial incision to allow us additional exposure as needed.

Once the pleura is entered, the anesthesiologist should work toward deflating the left lung. The down lung (i.e., right lung) should be checked for adequate ventilation. The anesthesiologist should be allowed time to get the tube positioned if necessary to obtain good oxygenation and ventilation; it is worth the time and effort. After the lung is deflated, often a formidable, large pulsating hematoma will be seen in the mediastinum (Fig. 59-2). As with any vascular procedure, proximal and distal control is necessary to properly perform the operation.

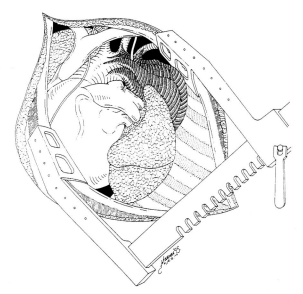

Figure 59-2. Surgeon's view through a wide posterolateral left thoracotomy incision. The left lung has been deflated. The hematoma is in broad view, and the vagus nerve and phrenic nerves are identified.

The surgeon should proceed very deliberately and with the utmost care to obtain proximal and distal control. Distal control is usually obtained first, because this is easiest to perform and is associated with the least chance for a misadventure, which might precipitate free rupture. It is important when dissecting around the distal aorta to avoid the intercostal artery branches, which are paired and come off each side. It is preferable to not sacrifice any intercostals but to go between the intercostals and encircle the aorta with an umbilical tape (Fig. 59-3). The umbilical tapes are placed to provide a

handle in case of sudden rupture and to facilitate the placement of vascular clamps. It is much easier to pull up on these tapes and place a clamp on the aorta than to try to get both a hand and a vascular clamp in the wound. The other advantage of a tape is to ensure that when the clamp is placed, it is completely around the aorta. Attention is then turned superiorly. The subclavian artery can be palpated easily. Usually, there is some hematoma over this, but not to any great degree. Control of the subclavian artery is very important and should be obtained even when the angiogram suggests

that the injury is distal to its takeoff. This is again accomplished carefully, making sure to stay away out of the hematoma. We prefer a Rommel tourniquet on the subclavian artery, because it takes up very little space in the surgical field and is more than adequate to provide hemostasis during the repair. Placement of the proximal aortic clamp is one of the most important technical parts of this operation. It is preferable to place this clamp distal to the left carotid, but well proximal to the takeoff of the left subclavian artery. Although aortic transections are usually distal to the takeoff of the left subclavian artery, this extra portion of aorta is often necessary to obtain a good repair. In addition, intimal tears may extend further proximally than can be appreciated by the angiogram. Attempts to obtain control distal to the take-off of the left subclavian artery are often met with rupture of the pseudo-aneurysm, because, invariably, the hematoma is entered or friable aortic tissue is encountered in this region. When a clamp is placed distal to the left subclavian, the tear will often extend into the clamp, and it may be necessary to obtain more proximal control. The vagus nerve runs in this area, with the recurrent branch as well. The recurrent branch is almost never seen because of the hematoma, but the vagus can usually be seen stretched by the hematoma. By staying anterior to this nerve, one should easily be able to obtain proximal control of the aorta. A finger can usually be placed gingerly between the left carotid and the left subclavian around the aorta in this area to create a proximal clamp site (Fig. 59-4). At this point, an umbilical tape is passed to provide a handle to place the clamp at a later time (Fig. 59-5). One should be aware that multiple aortic tears are possible. The tear at the isthmus is sometimes associated with a tear in the arch, the ascending aorta, or the great vessels, and this should be anticipated and watched for as well. On rare occasions, the clamp will have to be placed between the innominate and left carotid to gain adequate proximal control.

When proceeding with partial left heart bypass, it is necessary to establish a drainage line and a return line to the patient. Many sites are available for this. Our preference is to use the juncture of the left atrium with the superior pulmonary vein (or, alternatively, via the left atrial appendage) for drainage and the descending aorta distal to our distal clamp for return. The lung should be retracted laterally and the pericardium opened with care to avoid injury to the phrenic nerve. We usually open the pericardium posterior to the phrenic nerve immediately anterior to the pulmonary veins, but

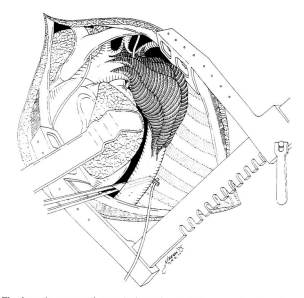

Figure 59-3. The lung is retracted superiorly and anteriorly, exposing the descending thoracic aorta, which is encircled away from the hematoma. The intercostal vessels should be avoided.

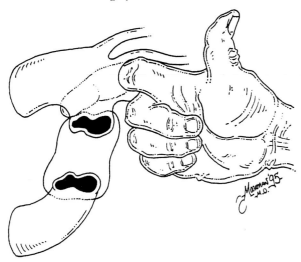

Figure 59-4. The transverse arch between the carotid and the subclavian is carefully encircled with a finger, with care being taken to avoid the hematoma itself.

occasionally have opened it anterior to the phrenic nerve. The surgeon should inspect the pericardium before deciding on which side of the phrenic nerve to incise the pericardium. Usually the left atrial appendage can be identified easily because it beats within the pericardium. In the decubitus position, there is almost an up-and-down motion of the appendage. When the pericardium is opened, the left atrial appendage almost "pops" up into the wound (Fig. 59-6). On occasion, the pericardium can be ruptured from the blunt trauma, and access can be obtained through the rupture. The tip of the appendage is often very friable, and, if handled with pick-ups, it may easily tear; it is for this reason that we have made it

our preference in recent years to obtain venous drainage at the confluence of the left superior pulmonary vein and the left atrium. This area takes sutures well and is less likely to tear. To avoid tears in the left atrial appendage, we immobilize the appendage with a Glover clamp and place a purse string of 2-0 braided polyester suture. The tip of the appendage is amputated, and a venous drainage catheter is placed into the left atrium. Depending on the size of the patient, a 26-, 28-, or 30-F wire-reinforced venous cannula is selected. With a 28-F drainage catheter, flows can be obtained in the 3- to 4-liter range without difficulty. During the placement of this catheter in the atrium, communication between the anesthesiolo-

gist and the surgeon is important as the clamp is removed from the appendage. A Valsalva maneuver is performed to prevent entry of air into the left side of the heart. The clamp is removed, the cannula is placed, and a Rommel tourniquet is secured and tied to the cannula (Fig. 59-7). The connection to the inlet tubing of the pump is freed of air.

Distal perfusion can be obtained in several areas. If at all possible, the descending aorta well away from the injury is usually easily accessible through the thoracotomy wound. A purse-string suture is placed with 2-0 Ethibond similar to a cannulation stitch for placing a patient on cardiopulmonary bypass (Fig. 59-8). The cannula we use is a 24-F flexible aortic cannula. Alternatively, if descending aortic cannulation is not feasible, an incision is made in the left groin, which should have been prepared at the start of the operation. The femoral artery is dissected and a femoral artery cannula inserted. In patients with multiple injuries or fractures with possible delayed or remote bleeding, this circuit can be used without heparin or a very minimal amount of heparin, such as 5,000 units.

At this point, a graft is chosen. We prefer to use sizers for adequate estimation of the aortic dimensions. We have used both knitted and preclotted woven grafts. Because the knitted grafts are easier to sew, we either preclot them before heparinization or select a presealed graft of appropriate size. Appropriate vascular clamps are chosen to be used for the proximal and distal control. Before the clamps are placed for repair of the transection, mannitol (12.5 g to 25 g [0.25 to 0.5 mg/kg]) is administered to maximize renal perfusion.

Once all the above steps are accomplished, the proximal aortic clamp is applied (Fig. 59-9). Proximal hypertension is alleviated by increasing left heart assist to unload the left heart. The distal clamp is applied, and then the snare on the subclavian artery is secured. The operation should proceed expeditiously but in an orderly manner. The hematoma is opened, usually met with a disconcerting amount of blood, which is not unusual and should be anticipated. With the clamps properly placed, active bleeding should not be seen from any of the clamp sites. Bleeding from intercostal collaterals is expected and anticipated; however, this should not be a cumbersome amount. If the clamps are not placed all the way across the aorta, time will be wasted in obtaining proximal or distal control, and a large amount of blood will be lost. Once the hematoma is entered, the site of the tear will be obvious.

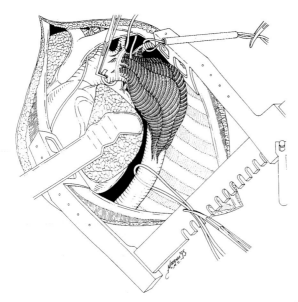

Figure 59-5. With blunt dissection of the plane complete, the transverse aorta is encircled proximal to the ligamentum arteriosum between the subclavian and the carotid. A tourniquet has been placed on the left subclavian and secured.

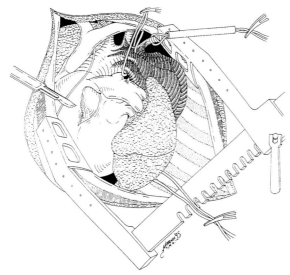

Figure 59-6. An incision is made over the left atrial appendage, which is generally visible through the pericardium. Care should be taken to avoid the phrenic nerve, and usually the incision is posterior to it.

In the case of complete transection, the stumps may be retracted and separated by several centimeters. Once the free ends are identified, the edges of both sides should be freshened, excising to good tissue (Fig. 59-10). Sometimes a primary repair may be possible. However, in the majority of cases a graft will be needed to bridge the gap without undue tension. Sometimes bleeding from intercostals can be problematic, and these can be controlled with bulldog clamps, hemoclips, or silk ligatures as needed. We try not to sacrifice any intercostals unless they are involved directly in the tear and cannot be salvaged. We prefer to address the proximal aorta first because this will probably be the harder anastomosis as a result of relatively limited exposure around the ligamentum and the friable and unpredictable nature of the tissue in this area. Our preference is to use a double-arm 4-0 polypropylene suture without pledgets and to perform the anastomosis in a simple running manner. Care should be taken not to place the sutures blindly and deep in this area because the esophagus and recurrent laryngeal nerve are immediately adjacent and posteromedial to this area. After the proximal anastomosis is completed, the graft is stretched and cut to length. An important point is to cut the graft appropriately. Too long a graft will lead to kinking; too short a graft will create tension and tearing of the aorta as sutures are placed. The distal suture line is then done with a running 4-0 Prolene suture. Just before the anastomosis is completed, the distal clamp is removed to check for hemostasis and to de-air the aorta (Fig. 59-11). The anastomosis is completed and the proximal clamp removed after de-airing. Weaning from left heart assist, if it has been used, is done simultaneously with removal of the proximal clamp. Sometimes, hypotension will develop, which requires reapplication of a clamp either partially or totally to restore the proximal blood pressure; then, as volume is added, an adequate pressure proximally and distally can be maintained. This is an important part of the procedure, during which the surgeon, the perfusionist, and the anesthesiologist need to communicate effectively. At this point, the proximal and distal suture lines can be further examined. Sometimes bleeding is seen and can be controlled with simple sutures. However, bleeding from needle holes or just oozing from distal suture lines should be watched; if heparin has been administered, it should be reversed with protamine to allow these sites to clot. Usually, packing the area and waiting 5 to 10 minutes will reveal complete hemostasis. At this point, the bypass circuit, if used, can be removed and the previously placed purse strings tied to ensure hemostasis. Before the thoracotomy is closed, we cover the graft, especially the suture lines, with mediastinal pleura using absorbable sutures to exclude the graft site from the lung.

Over the years, our technique for repair has evolved from one in which all cases were done in a clamp-and-sew manner to one in which we nearly routinely use left heart bypass from the left atrium to the descending aorta or to the left femoral artery using a centrifugal pump with very little heparinization. However, when this is not technically feasible, we do not hesitate to perform the clamp-and-sew technique. We do not use passive shunts because flow cannot be regulated, which makes it difficult to know how much flow is being directed to the distal aorta. The other advantage of using a centrifugal type of left heart assist is the ability to warm or cool the blood, because a heat exchanger can be easily added to the circuit. We do not believe that any one technique in particular has conclusively been proven to prevent paraplegia. It is our opinion that expeditious and timely repair of this lesion is the most important aspect in preventing this complication. Much has been made of the 30-minute ischemia period as a contributing factor to paraplegia. However, there have been many cases reported of clamp times much longer than this with

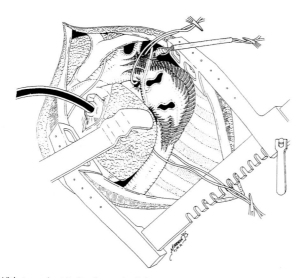

Figure 59-7. With tourniquets in place, the left atrial appendage is cannulated through purse-string sutures and connected to the venous end of the pump after it is de-aired.

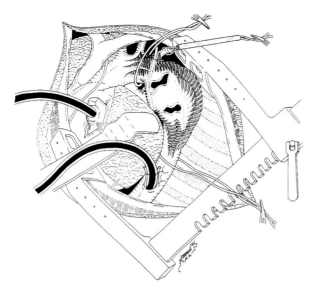

Figure 59-8. Arterial access is achieved in the descending aorta well away from the hematoma below the tape placed for distal control through purse-string sutures. Alternatively, the femoral artery may be cannulated.

no evidence of paraplegia. The complication of paraplegia is probably multifactorial, and time represents only one factor. However, partial left heart assist may benefit in other ways, because it does maintain distal perfusion pressure and allow us to unload the left heart and avoid hypertension proximal to the clamp. It, therefore, may help to avoid the use of vasodilating agents such as nitroprusside, which have been known to cause decreased blood flow to the spinal cord. Most importantly, it maintains perfusion to the lower body and kidneys during the period of cross-clamping. It also allows the opportunity to either cool or warm the patient in an expeditious manner. Although it does add complexity to the operation, we believe that its benefits are well worth the effort. However, in the case of free aortic rupture, we do not hesitate to revert to the clamp-and-sew technique, which is a time-honored and proven technique. In summary, there is no one technique that has been shown to be superior in all cases; each has its advantages, disadvantages, and indications for application.

Surgical Outcome

Acute traumatic aortic transection is a lethal injury. Approximately 80% of patients die at the time of the initial injury. Perioperative mortality can be high, ranging up to 30% in some series depending on initial injury severity scores. Patients can succumb intraoperatively from uncontrollable hemorrhage either because of rupture of the aneurysm or an inability to control the aorta proximally or distally. Patients can also die intraoperatively from associated injuries at distal sites. With the use of adjuncts to surgery, such as femorofemoral bypass, atriofemoral bypass, and descending aorta bypass, the attendant use of anticoagulation may increase hemorrhagic complications elsewhere in the body. Our preference is simplicity of repair aided by a simple bypass circuit. Most clinical series are relatively small, and it is difficult to compare across institutions. Even in our institution, numerous techniques have been used, which dilutes the numbers from which statistical comparisons and conclusions can be drawn.

Paraplegia or parapareses are probably the most serious complications seen postoperatively. The incidence is variable in reported series, ranging from only a few percent to 20% to 25%. Paraplegia should be noted preoperatively, and its presence or absence should be documented postoperatively as soon as the patient is able to cooperate with a neurologic examination. For unknown reasons, paraplegia can occur remote from the operation, even days later. Although adjuncts to prevent the complication of paraplegia have been advocated, there is still controversy surrounding these, and no technique has been proven to prevent paraplegia or decrease mortality, probably because the development of paraplegia is multifactorial. One cause may be related to clamp time. Although a clamp time of >30 minutes may be associated with an increased incidence of postoperative paraplegia, this is certainly not absolute. In addition, a clamp time of <30 minutes does not necessarily guarantee that postoperative paraplegia will not occur. Preoperative, intraoperative, or postoperative hypotension may also be a contributing factor. In addition, intercostal arteries that may be injured at the time of the injury or ligated to facilitate repair may play a role in its development. The possibility of a pharmacologic role, as blood is shunted away from the spinal cord in the presence of vasoactive substances used to control proximal blood pressure, could also contribute. The arterial blood supply of the spinal cord comes segmentally from the intercostal arteries via the radicular arteries to the posterior and anterior spinal arteries. The

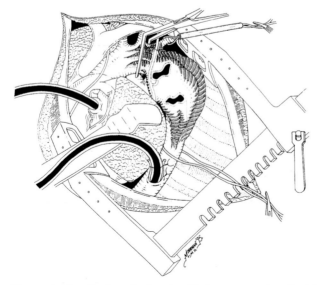

Figure 59-9. The proximal aortic clamp is placed on the transverse arch as the left heart bypass circuit is initiated. Pump flows are adjusted as the clamp is placed to ensure adequate proximal and distal aortic perfusion pressures.

jured trauma patient, we find less appeal with this approach. If a patient develops late (1 to 3 days out) paralysis or parapareses, we advocate immediate spinal fluid drainage based on the foregoing aneurysm data in hopes of avoiding a permanent injury.

We believe that in experienced hands an expeditious (but not hurried) repair will lead to the best results. We also believe that death, paraplegia, vocal cord paralysis, and other "complications" may actually be sequelae of the injury itself in most cases.

Renal failure can also be seen after successful surgery for repair of a transected aorta and may be related to clamp time, hypotension, or both. Severe sepsis and adult respiratory distress syndrome (ARDS) are occasionally seen in these patients as well. Not unlike other major trauma, isolated aortic injury is rare, and multiple other injuries contribute to the development of these complications.

Specific complications from the surgery include vocal cord paralysis as a result of injury to the recurrent laryngeal nerve. Upper-extremity hypertension can sometimes be present postoperatively, and the presence of decreased blood pressure in the lower extremities with high pressure in the upper extremities might indicate a suture line stricture; aortography or MRI should be performed in these cases to clarify the problem. Other complications rarely seen are pseudo-aneurysm in the suture lines, phrenic nerve palsy, pericarditis, chylothorax, and wound infection. Aortoesophageal or aortobronchial fistulas have been reported as late complications, but such reports are rare.

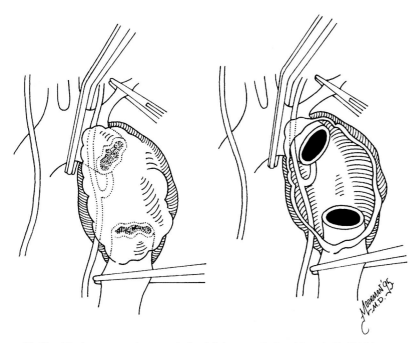

Figure 59-10. The hematoma is opened after left heart assist is achieved. The friable aortic edges are carefully débrided to good tissue, any intercostal bleeders are controlled, and the recurrent nerve is avoided.

spinal artery is frequently incomplete, particularly in the lower thoracic areas, which makes perfusion dependent on the lower intercostal or lumbar arteries. This unpredictable blood supply to the spinal cord may play a major role in the development of paraplegia and may explain its appearance in some cases with short clamp times and its absence in other patients with long clamp times.

Cooling the patient 3°C to 4°C to 34°C to 35°C has been suggested to be protective of the spinal cord, but it is impractical in a trauma patient, because many of these patients are already hypothermic as a result of shock and/or transfusion of room-temperature blood products and fluids. However, one should not try to actively warm these patients above 34°C to 35°C until the repair is complete. The role of cerebrospinal fluid drainage in the surgical management of thoracoabdominal aneurysms as an adjunct for spinal cord protection has been extensively studied, with recent studies demonstrating a beneficial effect. However, in a multiply in-

Endovascular Aortic Stents

The use of endovascular aortic stents in the management of acute traumatic aortic injury is an attractive alternative surgical option in high-risk patients. One attractive aspect of endovascular stenting is that it is a less invasive procedure that does not require a posterior lateral thoracotomy. There are recent published case reports and small studies demonstrating the technical feasibility and short-term success with the use of stents. Aside from the complications associated with endovascular stents, which include endo leaks, subclavian arterial occlusion, and paraplegia, these studies generally lack long-term follow-up to clearly justify their use routinely, especially in those

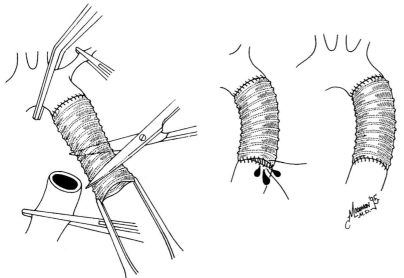

Figure 59-11. With the proximal anastomosis completed, the graft is trimmed to appropriate length, and torsion is avoided. Before the clamps are removed, de-airing should be performed by releasing the inferior clamp and backbleeding the graft.

patients whose life-threatening injuries have been corrected, are hemodynamically stable, and are otherwise considered to be reasonably good surgical candidates. As technology for aortic stenting improves and long-term results become comparable over time, endovascular stenting may replace the open surgical technique in selected patients. However, at this time, we believe that it should only be considered in certain high-risk patients with favorable anatomy, and should generally still be considered experimental in most situations. Nonetheless, it is certainly worth studying in high-volume centers facile with its use in elective situations.

Conclusion

Acute aortic transection continues to be one of the most challenging injuries for a thoracic surgeon to treat and requires good surgical skill and prudent clinical judgment for a successful outcome. The injury is particularly lethal in the setting of other associated injuries. A multidisciplinary approach to treating the multiply injured patient is necessary. It is hoped that in time, improved methods of surgical technique and of spinal cord protection can be developed that will help to minimize paraplegia and other postoperative complications seen in patients who have undergone surgical repair. Endovascular stenting may eventually play a role in treating this injury in selected patients, but should be considered experimental in most patients.

SUGGESTED READING

Cohen A, Crass J. Traumatic aortic injuries: Current concepts. Semin Ultrasound CT MRI 1993;14:71.

Coselli JS, LeMaire SA, Koksoy C, et al. Cerebral spinal fluid drainage reduces paraplegia after thoracoabdominal aortic aneurysm repair: Results of a randomized clinical trial. J Vasc Surg 2002;35:631.

Cowley R, Turney S, Hankins J. Rupture of thoracic aorta caused by blunt trauma. J Thorac Cardiovasc Surg 1990;100:652.

Duhaylongsod FG, Glower DD, Wolfe WG. Acute traumatic aortic aneurysm: The Duke experience from 1970–1990. J Vasc Surg 1992;15:331.

Eddy C, Rusch V, Marchioro T. Treatment of traumatic rupture of the thoracic aorta. Arch Surg 1990;125:1351.

Fabian TC, Davis KA, Gavant ML, et al. Prospective study of blunt aortic injury: Helical CT is diagnostic and antihypertensive therapy reduces rupture. Ann Surg 1998;227:666.

Iannelli G, Piscione F, DI Tommaso, et al. Thoracic aortic emergencies: Impact of endovascular surgery. Ann Thorac Surg 2004;77:591.

Katz N, Blackstone E, Kirkland J. Incremental risk factors for spinal cord injury following operation for acute traumatic aortic transection. J Thorac Cardiovasc Surg 1981;81:669.

Kodali S, Jamieson W, Lei-Stephens M. Traumatic rupture of the thoracic aorta: A twenty year review 1969–1989. Circulation 1991;84(Suppl):40.

Lebl DR, Dicker RA, Spain DA, et al. Dramatic shift in the primary management of traumatic thoracic aortic rupture. Arch Surg 2006;141:177.

Lee R, Stalman G, Sharp K. Treatment priorities in patients with traumatic rupture of the thoracic aorta. Am Surg 1992;58:37.

Marty-Ane CH, Berthet JP, Branchereau P. Endovascular repair for acute traumatic rupture of the thoracic aorta. Ann Thorac Surg 2003;75:1803.

Mattox KL, Holzman M, Laurens R. Clamp repair: A safe technique for treatment of blunt injury to the descending thoracic aorta. Ann Thorac Surg 1985;40:456.

Parmley L, Mattingly T, Manion W. Non-penetration traumatic injury of the aorta. Circulation 1958;17:1086.

Pate JW, Gavant ML, Weiman DS, et al. Traumatic rupture of the aortic isthmus: Program of selective management. World J Surg 1999;23:59.

Peterson BG, Matsumura JS, Morasch MD, et al. Thoracic aortic emergencies: impact of endovascular surgery. Ann Thorac Surg 2004;77:591.

Thompson CS, Rodriguez JA, Ramaiah VG, et al. Acute traumatic rupture of the thoracic aorta treated with endoluminal stent grafts. J Trauma 2002;52:1173.

Turney S. Blunt trauma of the thoracic aorta and its branches. Semin Thorac Cardiovasc Surg 1992;4:209.

EDITOR'S COMMENTS

The authors have described a careful approach for the treatment of acute aortic transection. This disease can be a complicated one, even in experienced hands. It certainly is much more difficult for the individual who rarely handles this problem. Certainly, in a patient with multiple injuries, delaying repair will allow for a better chance for recovery.

I would like to focus on just a few details. The authors have, just as we have, changed to routine left atrial-to-aortic artery bypass. We had excellent results with the clamp-and-sew technique, but the problem was that even one spinal cord injury was too many. Our approach for left atrial aortic cannulation is slightly different. We use a small pediatric extracorporeal membrane oxygenation (ECMO) cannula in the inferior pulmonary vein and also cannulate the aorta directly with another small ECMO cannula. This allows for adequate flow with small purse strings and easy decannulization. We had some injuries to the left atrial appendage and now prefer to avoid the left atrial appendage.

The authors also bring up the issue of stent graft. We have a very large stent graft program and are not sure where this technique would fit with acute aortic transections. We have tended to manage urgent operations with an open surgical approach. However, in the patient who has other injuries and needs a delayed approach, stent graft repair is a great idea.

I.L.K.

F

Transplantation

60

Heart Transplantation

Christopher T. Salerno and Edward Verrier

Introduction

The techniques developed by Norman Shumway and Richard Lower at Stanford University set the stage for heart transplantation to become the therapy of choice for patients with end-stage heart failure. The introduction of transvenous endomyocardial biopsy and the advent cyclosporine immunosuppression dramatically increased patient survival and marked the beginning of the modern era of successful cardiac transplantation. Heart transplantation is now a widely accepted therapeutic option for end-stage cardiac failure, with >2,700 procedures performed annually.

Recipient Selection

Patients with end-stage heart disease who are being considered as potential candidates for cardiac transplantation should be evaluated by a multidisciplinary committee to ensure an equitable, objective, and medically justified allocation of the limited donor organs. This process should select patients with the greatest chance of postoperative survival and rehabilitation. The primary objective of the recipient selection process is to identify patients with irreversible cardiac disease not amenable to other therapy (optimization of medical therapy, revascularization, ventricular remodeling, valve repair/replacement, biventricular pacing). It is desirable to identify patients who will most likely resume a normal active life and be compliant with the rigorous postoperative medical regimen. Recent successes and the introduction of improved immunosuppression have significantly expanded the eligibility criteria. Patients with New York Heart

Association class III or IV symptoms despite optimal medical therapy should be considered for cardiac transplantation. Most patients present with end-stage heart failure due to ischemic heart disease or idiopathic dilated cardiomyopathy. However, the spectrum of known causes of end-stage cardiomyopathy include infectious (viral), inflammatory, toxic, metabolic, and familial etiologies. Patients selected for cardiac transplantation should have a predicted 2-year survival of <60%. Other, less common indications for cardiac transplant include refractory angina, life-threatening arrhythmias, and chronic cardiac allograft rejection. Contraindications to cardiac transplant are primarily based on comorbid illnesses. Examples of widely accepted contraindications include active infection, irreversible renal or hepatic dysfunction and fixed pulmonary hypertension (pulmonary artery systolic pressure >60 mm Hg, transpulmonary gradient >15 mm Hg, pulmonary vascular resistance >6 Wood units).

Preoperative Recipient Evaluation

Evaluation for cardiac transplantation begins with a comprehensive history and physical examination, chest roentgenogram, and lab work including complete blood count, coagulation screen, erythrocyte sedimentation rate, uric acid level, liver function tests, fasting lipid panel, and infectious disease serologies (hepatitis A, B, and C, herpes simplex virus, Epstein-Barr virus, varicella-zoster virus, human immunodeficiency virus, rapid plasma reagin, rubella, measles, *Toxoplasma*). All patients should undergo an exercise test with maximal oxygen consumption (Vo_2) measurement. A

right heart cardiac catheterization study should be performed to rule out irreversible pulmonary hypertension. For patients with ischemic cardiomyopathy, coronary angiography should be reviewed or repeated to confirm the inoperability of coronary artery disease. For patients with nonischemic cardiomyopathies and prolonged or atypical symptoms, endomyocardial biopsy should be performed to rule out the possibility of a medically treatable illness.

Most centers also include nutritional labs, thyroid function studies, fasting and postprandial blood sugar, creatinine clearance, 12-lead electrocardiogram, echocardiogram, pulmonary function tests, panel reactive antibody screen, HLA typing, vascular screening exams (abdominal ultrasound, carotid and lower extremity Doppler flow studies), esophagogastroduodenoscopy, psychosocial evaluation, dental evaluation, financial analysis, and screening studies for malignancy (stool guaiac, prostate-specific antigen, mammogram, Papanicolaou smear).

Patients listed for transplantation should be examined routinely for re-evaluation of recipient status. Repeat right heart catheterization is indicated when follow-up echo studies suggest worsening or persistent pulmonary hypertension.

Donor Availability and Allocation

Donor organ availability is the primary factor limiting the application of heart transplantation. As a result, 20% to 40% of patients on the waiting list die before transplantation. Organ allocation is based on recipient priority status, time on the waiting list, and proximity. Highest priority is given to local status 1 patients with the longest accrued waiting time. The allocation system is designed to provide the most critically ill patient with a heart while minimizing allograft ischemic time. Although only 25% of patients are classified as status 1 at time of listing, 48% progress to status 1 by the time of transplantation. The mean waiting period for a status 2 candidate is currently >1 year, whereas status 1 patients wait a mean of 60 days.

Donor Selection

Potential cardiac donors undergo a rigorous screening evaluation. The local organ procurement agency should provide the implanting program with patient's age, height, weight, gender, blood type, hospital course, cause of death, routine laboratory data, and viral serologies. Additional required data include electrocardiogram, chest roentgenogram, arterial blood gas, and echocardiogram. Coronary angiogram is indicated in a selective fashion. The presence of advanced donor age (male donors >45 years of age, female donors >50 years of age), risk factors for atherosclerotic coronary artery disease (tobacco abuse, diabetes, significant family history), and occasionally the mechanism of death should be evaluated to determine the need for coronary angiogram. When a member of the transplant team arrives for organ procurement, a secondary screening is performed. This secondary screening allows the recovering surgeon to confirm and review the data presented by the procurement agency. The most important donor screening occurs in the operating room at the time of organ procurement. The heart is examined to identify ventricular or valvular dysfunction, previous infarction, coronary atherosclerosis, or myocardial contusion. If direct examination of the heart is unremarkable, the procurement surgeons proceed with donor cardiectomy.

Matching potential recipients with the appropriate donor is based primarily on blood group compatibility and patient size. As a rule, ABO barriers should not be crossed in heart transplantation because incompatibility frequently results in fatal hyperacute rejection. Donor weight should be within 20% of recipient weight except in pediatric patients, where closer size matching is required. If the recipient has elevated pulmonary vascular resistance (>4 Wood units), a larger donor is preferred to reduce the risk of right ventricular failure in the

early postoperative period. When the percentage (or panel) reactive antibody (PRA) is ≥10% to 15%, a prospective negative T-cell cross-match between recipient and donor sera is recommended before transplantation. Some centers also insist on a negative B-cell cross-match before transplantation. A positive cross-match is an absolute contraindication to transplantation. A cross-match is always performed retrospectively, even if the PRA is absent or low. Retrospective studies have also demonstrated that better matching at the HLA-DR locus results in fewer episodes of rejection and infection and an overall improved survival. Because of current allocation criteria and limits on ischemic time of the cardiac allograft, prospective HLA matching is not always logistically possible.

Donor Heart Procurement

During the secondary donor screening, the location of central and arterial lines should be noted. The location of these lines may affect the conduct of the organ harvest. It is important to continually monitor the donor's volume status and urine output during the harvest to maintain organ function. The donor is positioned in the supine position and widely prepped from chin to knees. To facilitate both thoracic and abdominal organ recovery, the harvest is begun with a midline incision from sternal notch to pubis, including a median sternotomy. The pericardium is incised and a pericardial well is created. The heart is examined as described. After this inspection the harvesting surgeon should notify the implanting surgeon regarding the suitability of the heart for transplantation.

The heart is then mobilized for cardiectomy. It is important for the harvesting surgeon to know whether any extended lengths of vessels will be necessary to facilitate implantation. For our preferred method of implantation, the bicaval technique, an extended length of superior vena cava (SVC) is required. The SVC is mobilized from the right atrium to the innominate vein. SVC mobilization usually includes dissection of the right pulmonary artery and ligation of the azygous vein. If additional caval length is required, the innominate vein can be harvested en bloc. The inferior vena cava (IVC) is dissected and mobilized circumferentially. Encircling the SVC and IVC with umbilical tapes or heavy suture may assist with retraction during cardiectomy. The aorta is

dissected from the pulmonary artery and isolated with umbilical tape. If hemodynamic instability is encountered during the harvest, clamping of the abdominal aorta at the iliac bifurcation may be helpful. Once the mobilization of the abdominal organs is complete the donor is given 30,000 U of heparin intravenously. A purse-string suture is placed in the ascending aorta, through which an antegrade cardioplegia catheter is placed. The central venous pressure line is pulled back to beyond the caval-innominate junction. After assurance is given that the abdominal team is ready to proceed, the superior vena cava is clamped or ligated distal to the azygous vein (which avoids sinoatrial nodal injury) (Fig. 60-1).

If the abdominal IVC is vented, the inferior vena cava is clamped at the level of the diaphragm. The heart is vented by transecting the left inferior pulmonary vein (or left atrial appendage if the lungs are being concomitantly harvested) and incising the anterior IVC proximal to the clamp. The aortic cross-clamp is applied, and the heart is arrested with cold cardioplegic solution. Adequate perfusion pressure is assessed by palpating the aortic root. The left ventricle should also be monitored to assure that it does not become dilated. Rapid cooling of the heart is achieved with 10 liters of topical cold saline (4°C). After a successful arrest, cardiectomy is initiated by completing the transection of the IVC (Fig. 60-2). The heart is wrapped in an ice-soaked lap pad, and the apex of the heart is elevated. Proceeding from inferior to superior, first on one side and then the other, one divides the remaining intact pulmonary veins and branch pulmonary arteries. The procedure is modified to retain adequate left atrial cuffs and pulmonary arteries for both lungs and the heart, if the lungs also are being procured. The ascending aorta and superior vena cava are transected last. The underlying disease of the recipient should be taken into account when determining the required length of aorta and superior vena cava.

After explanation, the allograft is carefully taken to the back table and placed in a basin of cold saline for inspection and final preparation. The heart is examined for evidence of a patent foramen ovale, vascular injuries (or inadequate length), and valvular abnormalities. Any positive findings should be disclosed to the implanting surgeon. The donor heart is then sequentially placed in two sterile bowel bags, each filled with cold saline, a sterile saline-filled air-tight container, and finally a standard cooler of ice for transport.

by mimicking the intracellular milieu. Examples of commonly used solutions include University of Wisconsin and Euro-Collins extracellular solutions, which are characterized by low to moderate potassium and high sodium concentrations and avoid the theoretical potential for cellular damage and increased vascular resistance associated with hyperkalemic solutions. Stanford, Hopkins, and St. Thomas Hospital solutions are representative extracellular cardioplegic solutions. Some centers choose to augment their solution with highly oncotic additives (mannitol, lactobionate, raffinose, and histidine), which theoretically counteract intracellular osmotic pressure to reduce hypothermia-induced cellular edema in the allograft. Several other groups report using other additives, including Krebs-cycle substrates and free radical scavengers. During graft implantation, myocardial preservation can be augmented with continued use of topical cold saline and retrograde blood cardioplegia.

Orthotopic Heart Transplantation

Nearly all heart transplants are performed in an orthotopic fashion. The technique has changed little from what was originally described by Shumway and Lower in the 1960s. The transplant surgeon must be well organized to avoid any technical or nontechnical mishaps. Special attention should be paid to assuring that an ABO mismatch does not occur. At our center, the operative surgeon must confirm the donor and recipient blood type prior to incision. Patients who have been fully anticoagulated preoperatively should be corrected with a combination of vitamin K and fresh-frozen plasma. After the organ procurement team has confirmed that the donor allograft is acceptable, the recipient is taken to the operating room and placed under general anesthesia. Preferentially, central line placement should avoid the right internal jugular to minimize difficulties with future myocardial biopsies. High-dose narcotics are usually the primary agents for induction and maintenance anesthesia. Inotropic and vasoactive agents should be readily accessible for the rapid management of induction-induced hypotension. Inhaled agents may be added, but their potential myocardial depressant effects limit widespread use in this patient population. Antibiotics should be given at least 30 minutes before skin incision. At our center, we selectively use aprotinin or

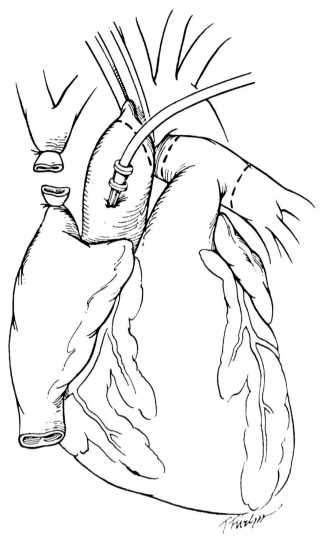

Figure 60-1. Standard donor cardiectomy. Dotted lines identify aortic and pulmonary artery sites of division.

Several common pitfalls have been identified. Avoiding the following mistakes is vital to successful organ harvest:

1. Failure to monitor the heart closely during multiorgan dissection.
2. Failure to heparinize.
3. Right or left ventricular distension.
4. Failure to adequately cool the heart during harvest and transport.

Organ Preservation

Most preservation techniques of the cardiac allografts permit a "safe" ischemic period of 4 to 6 hours, because ischemia times >4 hours have traditionally been associated with poorer outcomes. Multiple factors contribute to postoperative myocardial dysfunction including insults associated with sub-optimal donor management, hypothermia, ischemia-reperfusion, and depletion of energy stores. The preservation method used by >90% of transplant centers is a single flush of a cold crystalloid cardioplegic solution followed by hypothermic storage. No single preservation regimen has demonstrated consistent, clinically significant superior myocardial protection. Hypothermia is the cornerstone of organ preservation, and some experimental evidence suggests that 4°C provides the best protection. Perfusion of the donor heart with a cardioplegic solution to achieve electromechanical arrest is an invaluable adjunct to topical hypothermia. Crystalloid solutions are classified as "intracellular" or "extracellular." Intracellular solutions, characterized by moderate to high concentrations of potassium and low concentrations of sodium, purportedly reduce hypothermia-induced cellular edema

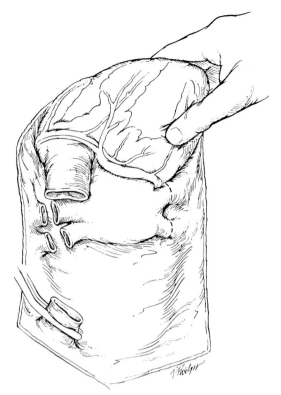

Figure 60-2. Standard donor cardiectomy. After transaction of the inferior vena cava the heart is retracted cephalad and the pulmonary veins are transected.

aminocaproic acid therapy to minimize perioperative blood loss.

Operative Preparation of the Recipient

The heart is exposed via a median sternotomy and vertical pericardiotomy. If the patient has had prior cardiac surgery, a femoral arterial line may be placed in case cardiac decompensation requires the emergent placement of an intra-aortic balloon pump or the initiation of peripheral CAPB. In a patient with a left ventricular assist device, peripheral arterial cannulation may be preferential, because this often makes the arterial graft anastomosis more straightforward. The patient is heparinized and prepared for cardiopulmonary bypass. In most cases, the aortic cannula is inserted just proximal to the origin of the innominate artery. Bicaval cannulation is performed with venous cannulae placed at the inferior vena cava–atrial junction and directly into the superior vena cava. Umbilical tape snares are passed around the superior and inferior vena cava. Bypass is initiated, the caval snares are tightened, and any additional cardiac mobilization is performed. Af-

ter the donor heart has arrived, the ascending aorta is cross-clamped and the cardiectomy is performed. The aorta and main pulmonary artery are transected above the semilunar valves. Most centers now perform a bicaval atrial anastomosis, and hence the superior and inferior vena cava are transected at the caval–atrial junction. A generous amount of right atrium should be retained inferiorly to facilitate the right atrial–IVC anastomosis. The left atrium is entered anterior to the right pulmonary veins and then incised along the atrioventricular groove to leave an adequate cuff for allograft implantation. Great care should be taken to avoid injury to the left superior pulmonary vein when excising the left atrial appendage. If a biatrial anastomosis is required, a right atrial cuff can be preserved.

To facilitate implantation, the proximal 1 cm to 2 cm of aorta and pulmonary artery are separated from one another with electrocautery. A weighted sucker placed in the left atrial remnant will keep the field free of blood and augments donor heart myocardial protection. Some centers routinely flood the operative field with CO_2 to assist with graft de-airing.

Timing of donor and recipient cardiectomies is critical to minimize allograft

ischemic time and recipient bypass time. Frequent communication between the procurement and transplant teams permits optimal coordination of the procedures. Ideally, the recipient cardiectomy is completed at the time, of cardiac allograft arrival. At our institution we have a protocol that mandates five telephone calls: first when the recovery team arrives at the harvest site and assesses the donor, next after visualization of the organ in the operating room, then before cross-clamp at the harvest site, next on leaving the remote site. and finally when arriving locally. At any time, the implantation team should be allowed to slow down the harvest process as needed to minimize organ ischemia time.

Implantation

The donor heart is removed from the transport cooler and placed in a basin of cold saline. The aorta and pulmonary artery are separated using either electrocautery or sharp dissection. The left atrial cuff is prepared by connecting the pulmonary vein orifices and excising excess atrial tissue (Fig. 60-3). The cuff is tailored to the size of the recipient's left atrium. The tricuspid apparatus and intraatrial septum are inspected. There have been several recent reports suggesting that there should be a low threshold for performing a donor tricuspid annuloplasty at the time of transplantation. Recipients are predisposed to increased right-sided heart pressures in the early postoperative period owing to pre-existing pulmonary hypertension and volume overload. Both conditions are poorly tolerated by the recovering right ventricle. To avoid refractory arterial desaturation associated with right-to-left shunting, patent foramen ovale is oversewn.

Implantation begins with an end-to-end left atrial anastomosis (Fig. 60-4). A 54-in., double-armed 4-0 polypropylene suture is passed through the recipient left atrial cuff at the level of the left superior pulmonary vein and then through the donor left atrial cuff near the base of the atrial appendage. The allograft is lowered into the recipient mediastinum, and the suture is continued in a running fashion caudally and medially to the inferior aspect of the intraatrial septum. The second arm of the suture is run along the roof of the left atrium and down the intraatrial septum. Any size discrepancy between donor and recipient atria should be continually assessed and corrected. At our center, we often leave a weighted sucker in the left atrium (as a vent) at the completion of the suture line. The suture line is temporarily controlled with a Rummel tourniquet. After completion of all the anastomosis, the heart is de-aired, the vent is removed, and the suture line is secured. Some centers introduce a bubble-free cold line into the left atrial appendage for continuous hypothermic saline lavage (50 to 75 mL/min) and evacuation of intracardiac air.

After completing the left atrial anastomosis, attention is turned to the inferior vena cava anastomosis. As described, retention of recipient right atrium helps to facilitate this anastomosis. An end-to-end donor-to-recipient anastomosis should be performed using a 4-0 polypropylene suture. Again, great care should be taken to correctly manage any size discrepancy. This is often the most difficult of the five anastomoses and often is more easily performed from the right side of the table. Next, an end-to-end SVC-to-SVC anastomosis is constructed using a 5-0 polypropylene suture. We prefer to lock the posterior row of this anastomosis to minimize the risk of purse-stringing. When prolonged ischemia is expected after the completion of the two caval anastomoses, a dose of cardioplegia can be administered in either an antegrade or retrograde fashion.

Next, an end-to-end pulmonary artery anastomosis is performed. It is crucial that the pulmonary artery ends be trimmed to eliminate any redundancy that might cause kinking and lead to right heart dysfunction. Using a 4-0 polypropylene, one starts the anastomosis at approximately 3 o'clock on the recipient pulmonary artery from outside to inside. The posterior wall of the anastomosis is then performed from the inside of the vessel while the anterior wall is completed from the outside. If adjunctive hypothermia was used, the patient is rewarmed at this time. Finally, an end-to-end aortic anastomosis is performed in a similar fashion. If a significant donor–recipient size mismatch is encountered when performing the aortic anastomosis, this may be handled by either beveling the aorta or creating a vertical aortotomy. In cases where prolonged ischemia times are encountered, the aortic anastomosis can be performed first and the pulmonary artery anastomosis can be performed with the cross-clamp off. The caval tapes are then released and the heart is filled with blood. Before the aortic anastomosis is secured, the lungs are ventilated and the heart is manipulated to facilitate de-airing through the anastomosis. An aortic root vent/cardioplegia needle is then placed. If desired, a dose of warm cardioplegia can be administered before removal of the cross-clamp. Lidocaine is given, and

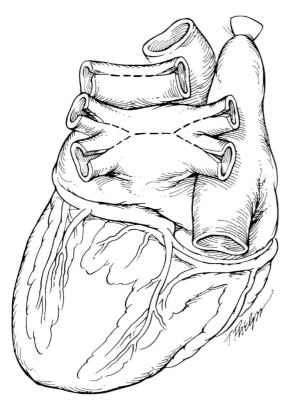

Figure 60-3. Allograft preparation for orthotopic transplant. The pulmonary vein orifices are joined to form a left atrial cuff.

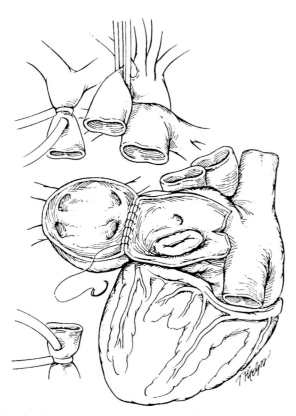

Figure 60-4. Bicaval orthotopic heart transplant starts with the left atrial anastomosis.

the patient is placed in a steep Trendelenburg position. The aortic cross-clamp is removed, and de-airing is continued via the root vent until no air is visible on transesophageal echocardiography.

Several maneuvers are performed during the resuscitation phase. Atrial and ventricular pacing wires are placed, pleural and mediastinal chest tubes are placed, the pulmonary artery catheter is advanced into proper position, and a thorough exploration for bleeding is undertaken. The patient is than weaned from cardiopulmonary bypass with the assistance of inotropes and nitric oxide as indicated. After removal of the cannulae and assurance of hemostasis, the wound is closed in the standard fashion.

To assure excellent results, it is crucial to be hypervigilant during the early resuscitation period. This is especially important in cases with recipient pulmonary hypertension, prolonged organ ischemia, or when using a slightly undersized donor heart. In these cases, right ventricular failure may be potentiated by subtle changes in cardiac volume, acid–base status, or pulmonary artery pressure. The cardiac surgeon should work closely with the anesthesiologist to assure that all metabolic derangements are promptly corrected (e.g., hyperglycemia, hyper- or hypokalemia, respiratory or metabolic acidosis, hypocalcemia). Volume resuscitation should be closely monitored, especially when blood products are required to correct a coagulopathy. Pulmonary hypertension can be mitigated with the rational use of inotropes, nitric oxide, and ventilator management. Finally, per the local protocol, immunosuppressive therapy should be started in the operating room.

Alternative Techniques for Orthotopic Heart Transplantation

Although most centers now perform the bicaval anastomosis, the original biatrial technique described by Shumway and Lower and revised by Barnard can often prove useful. We prefer the bicaval technique due to the associated increase in 5-year survival (81% vs. 62%), decreased risk of tricuspid regurgitation, reduced postoperative dependence on diuretics and inotropes, and lower incidences of atrial dysrhythmias, conduction disturbances, mitral and tricuspid valve incompetence, and right ventricular failure. To perform a right atrial cuff anastomosis, a

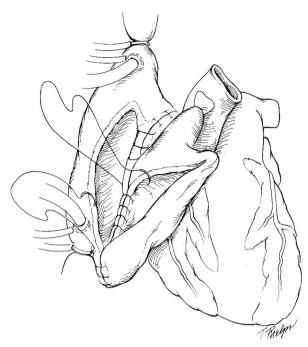

Figure 60-5. Biatrial orthotopic heart transplant. After completion of the left atrial anastomosis, full-thickness bites are taken through the interatrial septum. Note the curvilinear incision made in the right atrium.

curvilinear incision is made from the inferior vena caval orifice toward the right atrial appendage of the allograft (Fig. 60-5). The right atrial anastomosis is performed in a running fashion similar to the left with the initial suture placed at the most superior aspect of the intra-atrial septum.

Some centers have advocated total-heart transplantation, which involves complete excision of the recipient heart with bicaval end-to-end anastomosis and bilateral pulmonary venous anastomosis.

Recipients with Congenital Anomalies

Transplantation in adults with previous palliative procedures for congenital anomalies is uncommon; however, it is critical that a generous donor cardiectomy be performed so that sufficient tissue is available for optimal reconstruction. Several authors have described techniques detailing heart transplantation in recipients with "L" transposition, hypoplastic left heart, previous Fontan procedures, and situs inversus. In most situations, an allograft cardiectomy that includes the branch pulmonary arteries, aortic arch, and innominate vein is required. The details of these specific reconstructions are well described in the

literature and beyond the scope of this text.

Re-Do Sternotomy

At least 30% of heart transplant recipients will have had a previous median sternotomy. Use of preoperative chest x-rays or computed tomographic imaging may help to determine whether a potential space exists posterior to the sternum. External defibrillation pads should be placed before making an incision. In patients with previous coronary artery bypass surgery, an angiogram should be reviewed to determine which, if any, grafts are still open. If the proximal aorta must be retained, the stumps of any existing bypass grafts must be oversewn to minimize the risk of pseudo-aneurysm formation. In patients who have had multiple previous median sternotomies or are re-do transplants, it may help to expose the femoral vessels. If emergent bypass is required, it may help to start with a single venous cannula and transition to bicaval cannulation after control of the situation has been achieved.

The sternum is divided with an oscillating saw (anterior table) and Mayo scissors (posterior table). The right atrium, superior and inferior vena cava, and aorta are then mobilized to facilitate cannulation.

The remainder of the heart is than mobilized, and a low threshold for early use of cardiopulmonary bypass is observed. The implantation is performed in the standard fashion.

Transplant after Ventricular Assist Device

A growing number of patients will be status post a ventricular assist device (VAD) at the time of transplantation. These patients can provide many additional challenges. Femoral arterial cannulation is often preferred in these patients due to the risk of re-entry injury and to facilitate the aorta–aorta anastomosis. If one chooses to primarily cannulate centrally, the outflow graft from the VAD often provides a flexible site for temporary arterial cannulation. After the initiation of cardiopulmonary bypass, the VAD is turned off, the aorta is cross-clamped, and the native cardiectomy is performed. It is often advantageous to amputate the left ventricular apex to facilitate cardiectomy and remove the VAD after reperfusion of the allograft.

Heterotopic Heart Transplantation

Heterotopic cardiac transplantation, the intrathoracic placement of an allograft in series with patient's heart, is rarely performed today. The procedure was first used clinically by Barnard in 1974. Today, the procedure may be indicated in cases with marked elevated pulmonary vascular resistance (pulmonary artery systolic pressure >60 mm Hg and no pulmonary vasoreactivity) or when a donor heart is too small to sustain the recipient. Even in these selected cases, results have not been equivalent to orthotopic heart transplantation, with reported 1- and 5-year survival rates of 83% and 66%, respectively.

Similar to the cardiectomy performed for patients with congenital disease, the maximal lengths of aorta, superior vena cava, and pulmonary arteries are procured. The inferior vena cava and the right pulmonary veins are oversewn, and a common left pulmonary vein orifice is created (Fig. 60-6). A linear incision is made along the long axis of the posterior right atrium extending 3 cm to 4 cm into the superior vena cava. The recipient is cannulated in a bicaval fashion as described, and the pericardium and right pleura are incised to permit placement of the allograft in

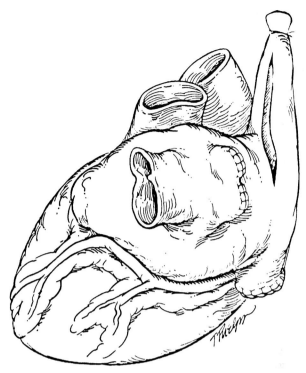

Figure 60-6. Preparation of heart for heterotopic heart transplant.

the right chest. The sequence of anastomosis is as follows: donor to recipient left atrium, donor superior vena cava to recipient right atrium, end-to-side aortic–aortic anastomosis, and finally, an end-to-side anastomosis joining the pulmonary arteries of donor and recipient (Fig. 60-7). The pulmonary artery anastomosis often requires the use of an aortic homograft or synthetic graft conduit permitting the donor heart to reside within the right pleural space.

Postoperative Management

Postoperatively, the transplant recipient is usually admitted to a private room in the intensive care unit (ICU). Traditional "protective isolation" with elaborate positive-pressure air filtration systems has been abandoned by most centers because recent studies demonstrate no benefit over mask and hand-washing regimens. Contact with individuals with communicable diseases should be avoided.

Intensive care monitoring is analogous to that of any patient who has undergone cardiac surgery. A radial artery catheter, left internal jugular venous catheter, continuous telemetry, pulse dosimeter, oceanography, and Foley catheter are essential components

for optimal postoperative care. Occasionally, a Swan-Ganz catheter is indicated in patients with increased pulmonary vascular resistance or if donor allograft dysfunction is anticipated. If the patient remains hemodynamically stable, all invasive monitoring lines and Foley catheter should be removed by 48 to 72 hours to minimize the risk of nosocomial infection. Chest tubes are removed on the first postoperative day if drainage is <25 mL/hr.

Donor myocardial performance is transiently depressed in the immediate postoperative period. Allograft injury associated with donor hemodynamic instability and the hypothermic, ischemic insult of preservation contributes to the reduced ventricular compliance and contractility characteristic of the newly transplanted heart. With a biatrial anastomosis, abnormal atrial dynamics owing to the mid-atrial anastomosis exacerbates the reduction in ventricular diastolic loading. An infusion of isoproterenol or dobutamine is initiated routinely in the operating room to provide temporary inotropic support. The positive chronotropic effect of isoproterenol is also therapeutic for the bradyarrhythmias that frequently complicate the early post-transplant period.

In patients with high pulmonary artery pressures or right heart failure, inhaled nitric oxide is a therapeutic alternative. Intra-aortic or pulmonary artery balloon

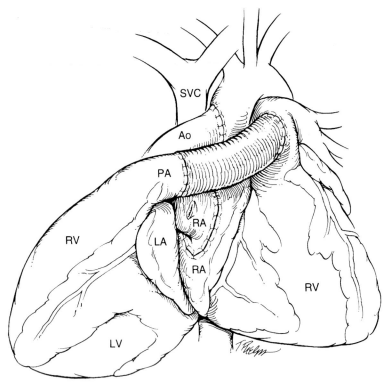

Figure 60-7. Heterotopic heart transplant. An interposition graft has been used for the pulmonary artery anastomosis. (Ao = aorta; LA = left atrium; LV = left ventricle; PA = pulmonary artery; RA = right atrium; RV = right ventricle; SVC = superior vena cava.)

counterpulsation and right ventricular assist devices have been utilized in patients unresponsive to medical therapy. Restoration of normal myocardial function usually permits the cautious weaning of inotropic support within 2 to 4 days.

Sinus or junctional bradycardia occurs in more than half of transplant recipients. The primary risk factor for sinus node dysfunction is prolonged organ ischemia. Adequate heart rate is achieved with isoproterenol infusion and/or temporary epicardial pacing. Most bradyarrhythmias resolve over 1 to 2 weeks, although placement of a permanent pacemaker is necessary in 2% to25% of patients; few are still pacer dependent at 6 months.

Most patients undergo an endomyocardial biopsy on approximately day 7 and are discharged shortly thereafter. All patients have close outpatient follow-up with intensive monitoring of their immunosuppression, antibiotic prophylaxis, and endomyocardial biopsies.

Results

Cardiac transplantation continues to have an operative mortality of approximately 5%, due to primary graft nonfunction, acute rejection, sepsis, and pre-existing recipient comorbidities. Most patients will have an acute rejection episode during the first posttransplant, which is most often treated with corticosteroids. Patients with recurrent or refractory rejection are often treated with polyclonal antibodies, alternate immunosuppression, or antimetabolites. Chronic rejection is manifest by allograft coronary artery disease, for which the only available therapy is re-transplant. The use of calcineurin inhibitors (cyclosporine, FK506) is associated with a 3% to 10% incidence of chronic renal failure. The overall 1-year patient survival is now between 80% and 90%, with a 3-year survival of >75%. There is every reason to believe that, with continued improvements in immunosuppression and treatment of transplant-related illnesses, these data will improve.

SUGGESTED READING

Bolman RM. Cardiac transplantation: The operative technique. Cardiovasc Clin 1990;20: 133.

Edwards NM, Garrido M. Advances in Cardiac Transplantation. In Franco KL, Verrier ED (eds), Advanced Therapy in Cardiac Surgery. Hamilton, Canada: BC Decker, 2003.

Fleisher KJ, Baumgartner WA. Heart. In Kaiser LR, Kron IL, Spray TL (eds), Mastery of Cardiothoracic. Philadelphia: Lippincott-Raven, 1998;501.

Gamel AE, Yonan NA, Grant S, et al. Orthotopic heart transplantation: A comparison of standard and bicaval Wythenshawe techniques. J Thorac Cardiovasc Surg 1995;109:721.

Kirklin JK, McGiffen DC, Pinderski LJ, et al. Selection of patients and techniques of heart transplantation. Surg Clin North Am 2004;84: 257.

Kirklin JK, Young JB, McGiffen DC. The Heart Transplant Operation. In Kirklin JK, Young JB, McGiffen DC (eds), Heart Transplantation. Philadelphia: Churchill Livingston, 2002.

Lower RR, Shumway NE. Studies on the orthotopic homotransplantations of the canine heart. Surg Forum 1960;11:18.

Miniati DN, Robbins RC. Techniques in orthotopic cardiac transplantation: A review. Cardiol Rev 2001;9:131.

Shumway SJ, Operative Techniques in Heart Transplants. In Shumway SJ, Shumway NE (eds), Thoracic Transplantation. Cambridge, MA: Blackwell Science, 1995.

Smith CR. Techniques in cardiac transplantation. Prog Cardiovasc Dis 1990;32:383.

Yacoub M, Mankad P, Ledingham S. Donor procurement and surgical techniques for cardiac transplantation. Semin Thorac Cardiovasc Surg 1990;2:153.

EDITOR'S COMMENTARY

The authors have given an excellent overview of cardiac transplantation. This is one of the most satisfactory operations that a surgeon can do. One can take a critically ill patient and in a short time leave him or her with normal cardiac function. The minor amounts of controversy relate to whether bicaval anastomosis should be performed versus biatrial. Certainly this is dependent on the style of the center as well as the ischemic time that is required. A more controversial issue is whether routine tricuspid valve annuloplasty should be performed. There have been recent studies that demonstrate the efficacy of this approach in reducing right ventricular failure. Regardless of which surgical technique is used, the major issue is attaining adequate donor supply. There has been an extreme shortage of donors in our institution. Therefore a major issue is who should be listed for transplantation. In general, we reserve transplantation for patients with nonischemic cardiomyopathy because there are really no other alternatives. Patients with ischemic cardiomyopathy are likely, at least at the first operation, to get some attempt at nontransplant surgical therapy such as coronary bypass or left ventricular restoration.

I.L.K.

61

Heart-Lung Transplantation

Bruce A. Reitz and Abdulaziz Alkhaldi

Introduction

Heart-lung transplantation represents the last hope for a small group of patients with severe combined end-stage disease. It was performed successfully at Stanford University in 1981, and these patients were the first to be completely supported by transplanted lung grafts. The Registry of the International Society for Heart and Lung Transplantation reports that >3,000 heart-lung transplants have been performed worldwide. In the earlier years, this included patients with primarily lung disease, such as emphysema or cystic fibrosis; more recently, it has been restricted to end-stage disease of both organs, such as patients with congenital heart disease and pulmonary vascular disease (Eisenmenger syndrome), or severe primary pulmonary vascular disease with end-stage right heart failure. About 50 heart-lung transplant procedures are performed yearly in the United States and another 50 worldwide.

Recipient Selection

The primary objective in recipient selection is to identify individuals with progressively disabling cardiopulmonary or pulmonary disease who still possess the capacity for full rehabilitation after transplantation. Heart-lung transplantation has a greater potential for technical complications than either heart transplant or lung transplant alone, so that it is particularly important to have stricter recipient selection criteria to assure a reasonable chance of a successful outcome. To this end, older recipients (>60 years of age) have not usually been selected for heart-lung transplantation, whereas they are frequently

candidates for heart transplant. Significant multisystem disease is a contraindication, although combined heart-lung and liver transplantation has been successfully performed. Contraindications include renal dysfunction, active malignancy, infection with HIV, hepatitis B, or hepatitis C, severe liver disease, cachexia or obesity, drug or alcohol abuse, and inability to cooperate with treatment programs. Patients who have had previous thoracic surgery are evaluated on a case-by-case basis. Multiple previous thoracotomies or pleurodesis are not absolute contraindications, although they might represent higher risk for surgical teams without significant experience in performing the operation. A patient who is acutely ill in the intensive care unit and specifically on mechanical ventilation is generally considered to be too ill to undergo heart-lung transplantation.

Patients accepted for transplantation are listed on the National Transplant Registry on the basis of diagnosis, time on the waiting list, and ABO blood group. Because heart-lung transplant recipients are in competition with critically ill heart recipients who may have a more urgent status, the number of potential donors offered is low. The additional requirement for lung volumes of approximately equal or slightly smaller size further limits the potential donor pool. Like lung transplantation alone, patient height is a reasonable predictor for lung volume, and donors of significantly greater height should be avoided. The presence of preformed reactive antibodies (PRA) at a level of >25% requires a prospective specific cross-match between the donor and recipient. The presence of a significantly elevated PRA will require specific measures, either pretransplant or post-transplant, to reduce the likelihood of hyperacute rejection of the donor organs, such as plasmapheresis and alternative immunosuppression.

Organ Procurement and Preservation

Like all thoracic organ donors, heart-lung block donors have sustained irreversible brain death but retain near-normal heart and lung function. Standard donor evaluation is performed, including physical examination, chest x-ray, 12-lead electrocardiogram (ECG), arterial blood gases, and serologic screening. A donor age of <50 years is preferred. Coronary angiography may be indicated in donors >40 years of age or with cardiac risk factors. Meticulous fluid management prevents excessive pulmonary edema and improves pulmonary and myocardial function. The last decade has seen significant progress toward better donor management, such that initially poor lung and heart function can be improved with aggressive treatment. Because of the already greater technical complexity of the heart-lung transplant operation, good donor organ function is extremely important. The criteria for donor selection are listed in Table 61-1.

The donor operation is performed via a median sternotomy, as shown in Fig. 61-1. Some harvests may also be done with a bilateral transverse thoracotomy as shown, depending on the requirements of the abdominal organ teams. Both pleural spaces are immediately opened with inspection of both lungs for atelectasis or major hemorrhage. The heart is inspected with palpation of the coronary arteries. The lungs are briefly deflated, and the pulmonary ligaments are

Table 61-1   Heart-Lung Donor Selection Criteria
Age <50 years
Smoking history <20 pack-years
Arterial oxygen pressure of 140 mm Hg on a fraction of inspired oxygen of 40% or 300 mm Hg on a fraction of inspired oxygen of 100%
Normal chest x-ray
Sputum free of bacteria, fungus, or significant numbers of white blood cells on Gram and fungal staining
Bronchoscopy showing absence of purulent secretions or signs of aspiration
Absence of significant thoracic trauma
HIV-negative

divided using electrocautery. After completely dissecting and removing the thymic remnant, the pericardium is removed to within about 2 cm of the phrenic nerves bilaterally. Umbilical tapes are placed around the ascending aorta and both venae cava. The pericardium overlying the trachea is incised vertically, and the trachea is encircled in the superior part of the mediastinum at least five or six complete tracheal rings above the carina. This maneuver can be facilitated by ligating and dividing the innominate vein.

An infusion of prostaglandin E_1 is started approximately 15 minutes before applying the aortic cross-clamp, beginning at a rate of 20 ng/kg/min, followed by incremental increases, to a target rate of 100 ng/kg/min.

Careful monitoring of the mean arterial blood pressure should assure that it remains above 50 mm Hg. Ventilation continues with a fraction of inspired oxygen (FiO_2) of 40% and a small amount of positive end-expiratory pressure (PEEP) (3 cm to 5 cm of water). Infusion lines are placed in the ascending aorta and the main pulmonary artery, as shown in Fig. 61-2. The donor is then heparinized, the superior vena cava is ligated, and a straight Potts clamp is placed across the inferior vena cava. After the heart empties, the aortic cross-clamp is applied, and 10 mL/kg of cold crystalloid cardioplegia is rapidly infused into the aortic root. We prefer the Stanford formulation, but several other cardioplegia solutions are available. The inferior vena cava is then in-

cised, and the tip of the left atrial appendage is amputated (Fig. 61-2), to avoid cardiac and lung distention from the return of the pulmonary perfusion. While antegrade cardioplegia is being delivered, a separate pulmonoplegia is flushed through the main pulmonary artery at a rate of 15 mL/kg/min for a period of 4 to 5 minutes. Ice-cold saline or Physiosol solution (Abbott Laboratories, North Chicago, IL) is immediately poured over the heart and lungs. During the cardioplegia and pulmonoplegia infusions, ventilation is maintained with half-normal tidal volumes of room air. On completion of these infusions and topical cold application, all solutions are aspirated from the thoracic cavity, and the lungs are fully deflated.

The heart-lung block is dissected free from the esophagus, commencing at the level of the diaphragm and continuing cephalad to the level of the carina. Dissection is kept close to the esophagus, and care is taken to avoid injury to the trachea, lung, and great vessels. The posterior hilar attachments are divided and the lungs inflated to a half-normal tidal volume, and the trachea is stapled at the highest point possible with a TA-55 stapler (United States Surgical, Norwalk, CT) at least four rings above the carina. The trachea is then divided above the staple line, and the entire heart-lung block is removed from the chest. After the heart-lung block is removed from the donor, it is wrapped in sterile gauze pads and immersed in ice-cold saline at between 2°C and 4°C, placed in several sterile plastic bags, and then placed in a sterile plastic container. This is placed in an ice-filled insulated box and transported to the transplant center. Because nonpressurized aircraft might be employed, we believe it is important to avoid overdistention of the lung before stapling of the trachea, to prevent overexpansion during transport.

With current preservation techniques and careful and atraumatic excision of the heart-lung block, procurements from as far as 1,000 miles from the transplant center and ischemic times up to 6 hours are reasonably well tolerated. The additional use of corticosteroids in the donor and white cell filtration before lung reperfusion in the recipient are also measures that contribute to improved preservation.

Recipient Operation

The heart-lung transplant operation is composed of two phases of equal importance.

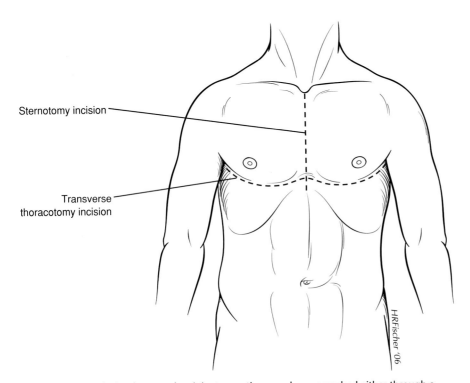

Figure 61-1. Both the donor and recipient operations can be approached either through a median sternotomy or a bilateral transverse thoracotomy in the fourth intercostal space. Sternotomy is preferred, but bilateral transverse thoracotomy does provide better exposure of the posterior mediastinum and the apical spaces of both lungs.

Sternotomy incision

Transverse thoracotomy incision

HRFischer '06

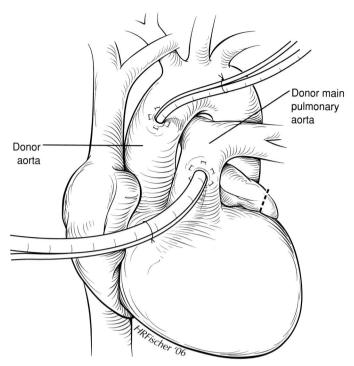

Donor main
pulmonary
aorta

Donor
aorta

HRFischer '06

Figure 61-2.   After dissection and inspection of the donor organs, an infusion catheter is placed in the mid-ascending aorta and the mid-portion of the main pulmonary artery for the administration of cardioplegia solution and pulmonoplegia solution. The dashed line on the tip of the left atrial appendage shows the place that the heart is opened to allow decompression of the solution perfusing the lungs.

excision. This helps to prevent injury to the esophagus while dissecting in the posterior mediastinum. A median sternotomy is employed for the majority of recipients, with transverse bilateral thoracotomy helpful for patients who have had extensive previous thoracotomies or pleurodesis (Fig. 61-1). In that situation, the bilateral thoracotomies offer better access to the posterior mediastinum and the apical areas of the thoracic cavity for a more meticulous dissection and better hemostasis. Otherwise, the median sternotomy is preferable for better chest wall mechanics postoperatively.

Two useful adjuncts that are helpful in maintaining good hemostasis are the infusion of aprotinin (Bayer HealthCare, West Haven, CT) to decrease the systemic inflammatory response of bypass and the Argon Beam Coagulator (ConMed, Corp, Utica, NY) for control of diffuse bleeding from chest wall adhesions. Both have been helpful in controlling blood loss and reducing the amount of blood factor components given postoperatively.

After sternotomy, both pleural spaces are opened widely just below the sternal edges. Anterior mediastinal thymic remnants and the anterior pericardium are carefully dissected and removed. The ascending aorta is dissected free and encircled with umbilical tape, followed by the superior vena cava and the inferior vena cava, as shown in Fig. 61-3. Cannulation for cardiopulmonary bypass consists of a cannula in the high ascending aorta and separate vena caval cannulas, as seen in Fig. 61-4. Once cardiopulmonary bypass has been initiated, the aorta is cross-clamped and tapes are placed down around the vena cava. The heart is then excised by dividing the great vessels just above the aortic and pulmonary valves in a manner quite similar to cardiectomy for heart transplantation (Fig. 61-5). When bilateral caval anastomosis will be used, we do like to leave a portion of posterior right atrium that connects the superior and inferior vena cava to prevent them from retracting once the cardiectomy has been performed. The left atrium is divided across its mid-portion, leaving the pulmonary veins intact. Mobilization of the lungs is begun with separation of the pulmonary ligaments bilaterally. The pleural reflections over the anterior mediastinum are carefully opened, and dissection of the pulmonary veins is begun. As much as possible of the dissection of the hila can be performed before cardiopulmonary bypass, but cardiopulmonary bypass should be started if hemodynamic instability develops. Any pleural adhesions are divided using electrocautery with meticulous hemostasis.

The first is safe excision of the native organs with excellent hemostasis, followed by implantation of the donor organs and continued attention to excellent hemostasis.

Anesthetic monitoring includes arterial pressure, pulse oximetry, continuous electrocardiography, temperature, and urine output. A standard endotracheal tube is used, and transesophageal echocardiography may be helpful during the early stages of the operation, but should be removed during the time of recipient organ

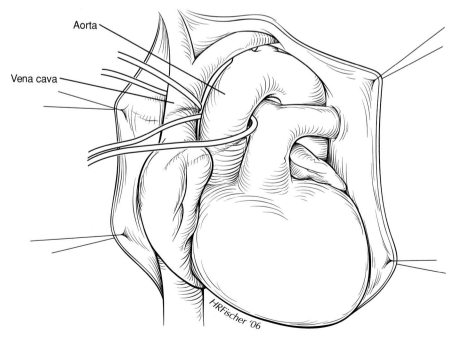

Aorta

Vena cava

HRFischer '06

Figure 61-3.   After sternotomy, both pleural spaces are opened widely, just below the sternal edges. The aorta and vena cava are dissected and encircled with umbilical tapes.

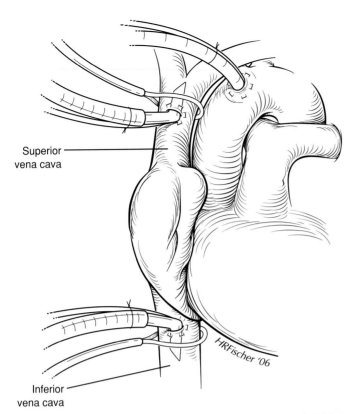

Superior
vena cava

Inferior
vena cava

HRFischer '06

Figure 61-4. After the median sternotomy, both pleural spaces are opened widely just below the sternal table. The ascending aorta and both vena cava are dissected free and encircled with umbilical tapes. Cannulation for cardiopulmonary bypass includes a typical arterial return line in the high ascending aorta and a right-angled venous cannula in the superior vena cava and the inferior vena cava.

After cardiectomy, bilateral pneumonectomies are performed. The pulmonary veins and pulmonary artery are divided by stapling, as shown in Fig. 61-6. In some particularly scarred hila, the electrocautery can also be used to divide the pulmonary veins and arteries.

In some patients, there may be significant bronchial artery collaterals, as well as other mediastinal vessels in the lymphatic and peribronchial tissue. All of these have to be carefully controlled with either the electrocautery or ligaclips. The right and left mainstem bronchi are stapled using the TA-30 (United States Surgical, Norwalk, CT), dividing distally and then removing the lungs. At this point, very careful control of any bleeding in the posterior mediastinum is essential.

The next steps in preparing the recipient for implantation consist in creating openings for both the right and left hila in the lateral pericardial walls and dissecting the main bronchi back to the distal trachea, to divide the trachea and prepare it for the implantation.

Anterior to the pulmonary veins bilaterally, the left and right pericardium are opened and enlarged superiorly and inferiorly to provide enough room for the donor lungs. Careful identification of the right and left phrenic nerve should provide adequate protection against injury. By grasping the stapled ends of the right and left bronchus and using the electrocautery, careful dissection right against the bronchus can separate it from the posterior mediastinum and dissect it back into the central posterior mediastinum, where they meet at the carina (Fig. 61-7). Dividing the right pulmonary artery remnant just anterior to the trachea will help facilitate this exposure. We believe it is important to leave a portion of the left pulmonary artery intact adjacent to the underside of the aorta near the ligamentum arteriosum to preserve the left recurrent laryngeal nerve. It is also important to stay right on the bronchus and not to injure the tissue immediately posterior to the carina, where the phrenic nerves will be passing anterior to the esophagus. A common error is to divide or traumatize the vagii at this location, causing a high vagotomy with gastric paresis post-transplant. Again, multiple bronchial vessels must be identified and carefully ligated using ligaclips or controlled

with the electrocautery. Patients with Eisenmenger syndrome have fairly large bronchial collaterals, which are identified and ligated. Once perfect hemostasis has been obtained, the trachea is divided at the carina with a #15 blade. The surgeon should keep in mind that the membranous trachea should not be pulled down excessively and then divided, because this may remove a fair amount of the recipient posterior wall unnecessarily. Additional tracheal collaterals should be controlled at this point. The chest is now prepared to receive the heart-lung graft.

The donor heart-lung block is removed from its transport container and prepared by opening the trachea just below the staple line and carefully obtaining a swab culture, irrigating, and then aspirating the retained mucus. The suction used for this purpose should be kept separate from the suctions used for the recipient operation. The cultures obtained are sent for fungal and bacterial examinations. The donor trachea is then trimmed down to leave just one cartilaginous ring intact above the carina. All of the peritracheal tissue should be retained as much as possible to facilitate post-transplant vascularization of the anastomosis. Excessive dissection of this tissue will lead to possible necrosis or stricture, especially if a long left bronchial remnant remains with extensive skeletonization. Care should be taken to leave adequate tracheal tissue in the membranous portion posteriorly when transecting the donor trachea.

The heart-lung graft is then lowered into the chest, passing the right lung beneath the right phrenic nerve pedicle. The left lung is gently manipulated under the left phrenic nerve pedicle. An alternative technique that leaves one or both lungs anterior to the phrenic nerves has been described by Copeland's group. This maneuver facilitates rotation of the heart-lung block for better exposure during the post-bypass phase of the operation to inspect the posterior mediastinum for bleeding points. We have used this method, and find that it can be quite helpful when inspecting for bleeding post–cardiopulmonary bypass.

Positioning of the donor organs before beginning the anastomosis is shown in Fig. 61-8. The implantation begins with anastomosis of the trachea. In the adult patient, this is performed using continuous 3-0 polypropylene suture, as shown in Fig. 61-9A. For children or neonates, appropriately smaller polypropylene suture is used. The posterior membranous portion is sutured first from the inside and from the left to the right, followed by completion of the anastomosis anteriorly, as shown in Fig. 61-9B.

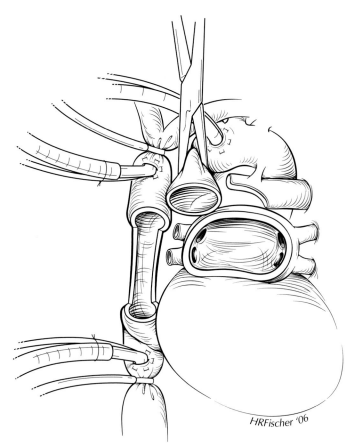

HRFischer '06

Figure 61-5. Cardiectomy is performed in a manner quite similar to that for isolated heart transplantation. We prefer to leave an intact portion of posterior and medial right atrial wall that will connect the superior and inferior vena cava– and prevent their retraction, facilitating the anastomosis.

The heart is wrapped with a sterile gauze pad, and topical myocardial hypothermia is initiated for the heart, with secondary topical cooling of both lungs.

Next, the bicaval venous anastomosis is performed beginning with the inferior vena cava, as seen in Fig. 61-10. The donor interatrial septum should be looked at through the opening of the inferior vena cava to see whether a patent foramen ovale is present and needs closure. The inferior vena cava–right atrial junction is joined with a continuous 4-0 polypropylene suture. This is performed along the back wall of the right atrium, where the posterior atrial wall is intact, between the superior vena cava and inferior vena cava of the recipient. It is then continued along the free edge of the recipient inferior vena cava anteriorly. When this is completed, we usually proceed with anastomosis of the ascending aorta in a standard fashion using 4-0 polypropylene suture. Finally, the superior vena cava is appropriately trimmed and sutured to the recipient vena cava using 5-0 polypropylene, with care to prevent purse-stringing of this anastomosis by leaving it intentionally looser. Excessive

tension in this suture line will cause some stricture and possible later thrombosis.

Before release of the aortic cross-clamp, the amputated left atrial appendage is over-sewn, and the pulmonoplegia site in the pulmonary artery is also repaired. A bubble vent in the anterior aorta is put to coronary suction as the tapes are removed from the vena cava, and blood is allowed to return into the heart and lung block. Just before this maneuver, we initiate white cell filtration of the cardiopulmonary bypass circuit to reduce the exposure of recipient white blood cells to the donor lungs. The aortic cross-clamp is then removed so the heart will be reperfused.

The reperfusion and resuscitation of the heart-lung may require 30 to 45 minutes. De-airing and complete dilution of the pulmonoplegia solution are essential. Gentle ventilation with room air is performed prior to coming off of cardiopulmonary bypass. Weaning is initiated with an FIO_2 of 50% and adjusted based on the oxygen saturation measured peripherally. Some low-dose dopamine or isoproterenol may be helpful to maintain heart rate and improve renal per-

fusion. Methylprednisolone (500 mg intravenously) is given after protamine is administered. The appearance of the completed transplant is shown in Fig. 61-11. Drains are left in both chest cavities and the mediastinum, and closure is routine.

Clinical Management in the Early Postoperative Period

The early postoperative management for heart-lung transplant recipients includes careful fluid and ventilatory management. The primary objective is to maintain adequate perfusion and gas exchange while minimizing intravenous fluid, cardiac work, and barotrauma. Careful and gentle pulmonary and endotracheal suctioning should be used to remove mucus and prevent atelectasis. Standard ventilatory weaning is initiated after the patient is deemed to be stable, awake, and alert. Typically, extubation is feasible within the first 24 hours after transplantation. As with all heart transplant recipients, some degree of transient sinus node dysfunction may be present in about 10% to 20% of patients. The use of isoproterenol or temporary cardiac pacing will usually lead to resolution within 1 week.

If pulmonary dysfunction develops, as manifested by an increasing requirement for FIO_2 with development of a diffuse interstitial infiltrate on chest roentgenogram, then the presence of a reperfusion injury should be considered. In addition, some element of obstruction of a pulmonary vein should be considered, because it has been reported after heart-lung transplantation. This can be detected by transesophageal echocardiography. If primary graft dysfunction continues, the use of inhaled nitric oxide or temporary extracorporeal membrane oxygenation (ECMO) may be considered. Postoperative hemorrhage and the need for excessive blood product replacement will magnify any pulmonary dysfunction, again pointing out the importance of careful intraoperative hemostasis.

Immunosuppressive Management

The immunosuppression for heart-lung transplant recipients begins intraoperatively and continues for the patient's lifetime. The drug protocols used are similar to those for other lung transplant recipients. We have

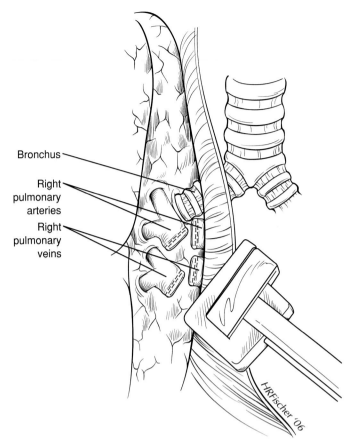

Figure 61-6. Dissection of the lung hilum includes identification of the pulmonary veins and pulmonary artery, and stapling them on the recipient side, as a way to help control some of the mediastinal collateral adventitial vessels. Finally, the bronchus is also stapled to help maintain sterility of the thoracic cavity. The trachea will be divided and opened just before the tracheal anastomosis is performed.

seen significant benefits from the use of induction therapy using rabbit anti-thymocyte globulin, with delay in the use of maintenance steroids for 2 weeks post-transplant. During this time, cyclosporine is initiated early postoperatively and switched to oral administration when extubation has occurred. Methylprednisolone is administered intraoperatively at graft reperfusion and continued for the first 24 hours at 125 mg intravenously every 8 hours. After 2 weeks, prednisone is started at a daily oral dose of

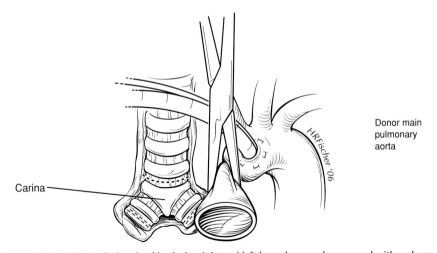

Figure 61-7. The stapled ends of both the right and left bronchus can be grasped with a clamp and gently retracted to facilitate the retrograde dissection back to the carina and to the point of the incision in the trachea.

0.6 mg/kg and gradually tapered over the next month to 0.2 mg/kg/day.

Infection Prophylaxis

In heart-lung transplantation, as in lung transplantation, very meticulous antiviral and antifungal prophylaxis are important components of postoperative management. Cytomegalovirus prophylaxis (CMV) with ganciclovir is used by most centers in any CMV-negative recipient receiving an allograft from a CMV-positive donor. Fungal prophylaxis against mucosal *Candida* infection includes use of daily Nystatin mouthwash. *Pneumocystis carinii* prophylaxis consists of trimethoprim-sulfamethoxazole or aerosolized pentamidine. *Aspergillus* colonization is inhibited by the use of aerosolized amphotericin B early postoperatively. Recipients who are toxoplasma-negative and receive grafts from toxoplasma-positive donors receive pyrimethamine prophylaxis for at least the first 6 months after transplantation.

Graft Surveillance

Routine clinical follow-up to monitor and modify the need for immunosuppressive drugs requires regular surveillance. This consists of serial pulmonary function tests, arterial blood gases, and bronchoscopic evaluation beginning at 2 weeks post-transplant. Further surveillance bronchoscopies and biopsies are obtained on a regular schedule.

Postoperative Complications

The importance of a meticulous and atraumatic operative procedure is highlighted by the fact that most of the early morbidity and mortality can be directly related to the quality of the donor organs and the need for excessive blood product administration due to postoperative hemorrhage. The most common cause of early death is due to primary graft failure or infection, together with multisystem organ failure due to poor primary graft function or excessive bleeding. This leads to a relatively high early postoperative mortality of 16% in our series of more than 200 heart-lung transplants.

If present, pulmonary dysfunction and multisystem organ failure are managed in a conventional manner, as for all critically about 67% of heart-lung patients having pulmonary rejection within the first year and only approximately 15% experiencing heart graft rejection.

Chronic Rejection or Late Complications

The major long-term limitation of heart-lung transplantation, similar to isolated lung transplants, is the presence of chronic lung rejection presenting as obliterative bronchiolitis (OB). The diagnosis is confirmed with lung histology obtained by bronchoscopy, characterized by a dense eosinophilic submucosal scar, which partially or totally obliterates the lumen of small airways, accompanied by a decrease of arterial oxygen pressure, a decrease of the forced expiratory volume in 1 second, and a decrease of the forced expiratory rate between 25% and 75% of forced vital capacity. The only therapy is an augmentation of immunosuppression, which may be helpful in reducing the ongoing progression, but usually does not reverse the disease.

Retransplantation

When terminal respiratory failure develops secondary to OB or when chronic coronary artery disease develops (rarely) in long-term recipients, retransplantation of

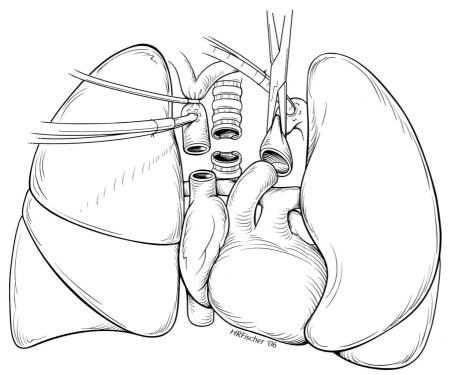

Figure 61-8. The donor heart-lung block has been lowered into the thoracic cavity, positioning the right and left lung either anterior or posterior to the phrenic pedicle. The initial anastomosis performed will be the trachea.

ill postoperative patients. Careful attention to preservation of the graft, judicious fluid administration, and minimizing the need for excessive blood products postoperatively will reduce the incidence of this syndrome.

Fortunately, as in heart or lung transplant–only recipients, acute rejection episodes and graft failure due to rejection are extremely unusual. The lung is more likely to experience rejection than is the heart, with

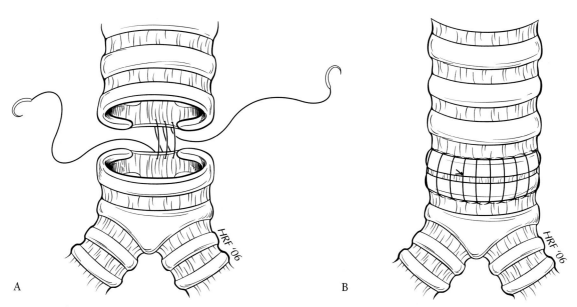

A   B

Figure 61-9.   **(A)** The tracheal anastomosis is started along the posterior wall at the junction between the cartilaginous portion and the membranous portion. A 3-0 polypropylene suture is used in a continuous running anastomosis from left to right and inside the trachea, being converted to an external suture line anteriorly. **(B)** The completed tracheal anastomosis is shown, with just one complete ring above the carina.

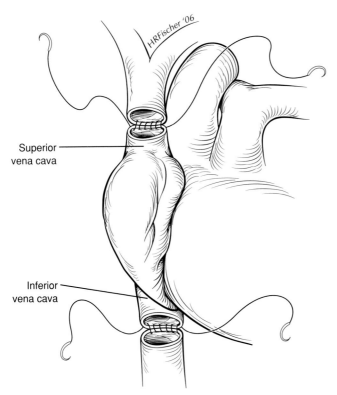

Figure 61-10.   The inferior vena cava anastomosis is started along the posterior wall and sutured from left to right. It is continued anteriorly, with care to avoid severe purse-stringing. Usually this opening is large enough that this is not as much of a concern as with the superior vena cava.

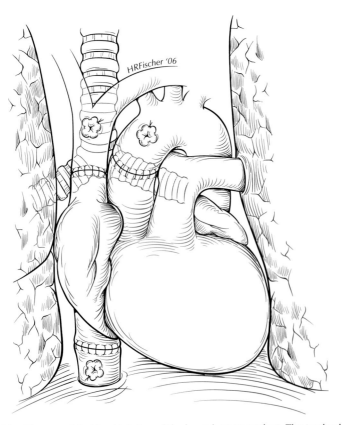

Figure 61-11.   The completed implantation of the heart-lung transplant. The tracheal anastomosis lies in the space between the superior vena cava and posterior to the ascending aorta. Angled chest drains are placed bilaterally and a straight drain in the anterior mediastinum. The chest closure is routine.

the heart-lung block, the lung alone, or of the heart alone has been performed. These operations represent technical challenges, but have been reported to be successful in recipients who are otherwise in reasonably good physiologic condition. The same principles of meticulous donor procurement and preservation, attention to hemostasis, and careful perioperative management are essential. The major cause of death after retransplantation procedures remains multisystem organ failure.

Airway Complications

Fortunately, the heart-lung graft facilitates revascularization of the tracheal anastomosis through the early development of coronary-to-bronchial collaterals. This has resulted in a very low rate of primary tracheal dehiscence, as well as a low rate of tracheal stenosis, which is usually due to ischemia. In fact, tracheal complications have tended to develop only in patients who required extended postoperative ventilation and increased PEEP. When complications develop, the diagnosis is made by bronchoscopy and can be treated by reoperation or bronchoscopy with dilation or airway stenting.

Domino-Donor Procedures

In patients who require a double-lung transplant, the strategy of performing a heart-lung transplant with donation of the recipient heart has been described as the "domino-donor transplant," with good results for both the heart-lung recipient and the heart recipient. These operations must be done with complete bicaval anastomosis so that an adequate donor heart is procured. Otherwise, the procedures are as already described.

Heart–Single-Lung Transplant

A small number of patients with congenital heart disease have been reported who have unilateral pulmonary vascular disease or severe developmental changes in one lung, which have been successfully transplanted with a heart–single-lung block. This strategy has also been used when severe scarring of one thoracic cavity has made it impossible to safely remove one of the recipient's lungs.

A single bronchial anastomosis with appropriate pulmonary vein and pulmonary artery anastomosis are then performed. Good long-term results can be obtained.

Long-Term Results

The long-term survival for heart-lung patients has gradually improved with better operative and postoperative management. Newer immunosuppressive drugs and better antimicrobial prophylaxis, particularly for cytomegalovirus, have been major factors. In the last 10 years at Stanford, the 1-, 5-, and 10-year survival rates were 77%, 56%, and 40%, respectively, in 100 patients. The currently longest-living heart-lung transplant recipient is 21.5 years post-transplant, with normal heart and lung function.

Conclusion

The evolution of heart-lung transplantation for end-stage cardiopulmonary disease has depended on careful operative technique. It can be a very straightforward operation in some patients and a very demanding and difficult procedure in others. The importance of appropriate donor organ procurement and preservation cannot be overemphasized. Meticulous hemostasis and the use of all possible measures to reduce postoperative hemorrhage are essential to good outcomes. Patients who experience successful procedures can look forward to long-term survival equivalent to any recipient of a bilateral lung graft, with very satisfactory and rewarding return to normal activities. Future improvements in immunosuppression and the ability to induce immunologic tolerance will continue the evolutionary improvement of heart-lung transplantation therapy.

SUGGESTED READING

Balsam LB, Yuh DD, Robbins RC, et al. Heart-lung and lung transplantation. In Cohn LH, Edmunds LH (eds), *Cardiac Surgery in the Adult.* New York: McGraw-Hill, 2003:1461.

Hardesty RL, Griffith BP. Procurement for combined heart-lung transplantation. Bilateral thoracotomy with sternal transection, cardiopulmonary bypass, and profound hypothermia. J Thorac Cardiovasc Surg 1985;89:795.

Jamieson SW, Stinson EB, Oyer PE, et al. Operative technique for heart-lung transplantation. J Thorac Cardiovasc Surg 1984;87:930.

Lick SD, Copeland JG, Rosado LJ, et al. Simplified technique of heart-lung transplantation. Ann Thorac Surg 1995;59:1592.

Hertz MI, Boucek MM, Deng MC, et al. The Registry of the International Society for Heart and Lung Transplantation: Introduction to the 2004 Annual Reports. J Heart Lung Transplant 2004;23:789.

Novick RJ, Stitt LW, Al Kattan K, et al. Pulmonary retransplantation: Predictors of graft function and survival in 230 patients. Ann Thorac Surg 1998;65:227.

Reichenspurner H, Girgis RE, Robbins RC, et al. Obliterative bronchiolitis after lung and heart-lung transplantation. Ann Thorac Surg 1995;60:1845.

Reitz BA, Wallwork JL, Hunt SA, et al. Heart-lung transplantation: Successful therapy for patients with pulmonary vascular disease. N Engl J Med 1982;306:557.

Stoica SC, McNeil KD, Perreas K, et al. Heart-lung transplantation for Eisenmenger syndrome: Early and long-term results. Ann Thorac Surg 2001;72:1887.

Straznicka M, Follette DM, Eisner MD, et al. Aggressive management of lung donors classified as unacceptable: Excellent recipient survival one year after transplantation. J Thorac Cardiovasc Surg 2002;124:250.

Vricella LA, Karamichalis JM, Ahmad S, et al. Lung and heart-lung transplantation in patients with end-stage cystic fibrosis: The Stanford experience. Ann Thorac Surg 2002;74:13.

EDITOR'S COMMENTS

Dr. Reitz is truly the world expert on heart-lung transplantation. He developed the operation at Stanford in 1981, and he set the standard for this procedure. This chapter thoroughly examines the donor and recipient operations. The difficulty for us has been obtaining appropriate heart-lung blocks. Typically, either the lungs or the heart are offered, and on the East Coast it has been very difficult to get the entire block. Our focus therefore has been on single- or double-lung transplantation and repair of the cardiac defect for Eisenmenger syndrome. Having said that, there are obviously patients who would benefit from heart-lung transplantation. These include patients with end-stage pulmonary disease and unrepairable cardiac problems. Therefore, these techniques must be available for those patients.

I.L.K.

G

Arrythmias

62

The Maze Procedure for the Surgical Treatment of Atrial Fibrillation

John M. Stulak and Hartzell V. Schaff

Background

Early Approaches

The earliest approach to the elimination of medically refractory atrial fibrillation/flutter (AF) was atrioventricular (AV) nodal ablation with permanent pacemaker (PPM) implantation. Catheter-based techniques simplified this approach, but AV node ablation corrected the rhythm disturbance while leaving the patient at risk for embolic complications from left atrial thrombi. Another early surgical approach to AF was left atrial isolation, which provided a regular ventricular rhythm without the need of a pacemaker, but again the procedure did not prevent thromboembolic sequelae because the left atrium continued to fibrillate. The corridor procedure isolated a pathway from the sinoatrial (SA) node to the AV node, but it did not restore atrioventricular synchrony. Subsequently, Cox and colleagues developed the maze procedure, which addressed all the adverse consequences of AF including rhythm, hemodynamics, and thromboembolic risk. The Cox maze procedure quickly proved to be the most effective means of eliminating AF and its morbid complications.

Maze I and Maze II Procedures

Two modifications to the original maze procedure were made to minimize chronotropic insufficiency and mechanical dysfunction of the left atrium. The original maze I procedure included several incisions around the SA node including one that crossed the area immediately anterior to the junction of the superior vena cava (SVC) and right

atrium. This lesion led to chronotropic insufficiency during stress and exercise. To prevent re-entry of conduction around the base of the right atrium, the maze I operation had an incision extending from the base of the resected right atrial appendage, across the septum, and across the dome of the left atrium to the base of the resected left atrial appendage. This incision was modified and relocated more posteriorly such that the medial aspect of the SVC was the endpoint. The result of repositioning this incision more posteriorly resulted in the relocation of the atrial septal incision more posteriorly.

Postoperative left atrial dysfunction appeared to be the result of interatrial conduction delay. Conduction travels from the SA node to the left atrium through Bachmann's bundle, and this thick area of conduction tissue was disrupted by the incision across the dome of the atria in the maze I and II incisions. Thus, conduction to the left atrium was delayed and arrived almost simultaneously with the retrograde impulse of the left ventricle, subsequently abolishing effective atrial mechanical function. To address this problem, Cox and his colleagues modified the maze II procedure by moving the atrial dome incision so that it was located posterior to the SVC. With this incision in a more posterior location, only one incision ended at the junction of the distal SVC and right atrium, thus the risk of SVC narrowing was lessened, and a patch was no longer necessary in this location. In addition, this modification enhanced exposure of the left side of the heart. Therefore, the maze III procedure was simplified technically and addressed the two major prob-

lems, chronotropic insufficiency and left atrial dysfunction, that plagued the first two procedures.

Indications

Although medical treatment is the first-line therapy for most patients with AF, surgical management may be appropriate for several patient groups. Operation to ablate AF should be considered for younger patients with limiting symptoms, particularly those who have failed medical treatment or who are intolerant of medications. A significant number of young patients prefer a curative procedure rather than lifetime treatment with drugs that have bothersome side effects. In addition, there are patients who have a medical contraindication to systemic anticoagulation, or a strong personal preference to avoid chronic warfarin therapy.

Furthermore, there is a small subset of patients who have suffered a thromboembolic stroke while on anticoagulation with Coumadin, and these patients should be considered for a Cox maze procedure because operation includes removal of the left atrial appendage and thus greatly reduces risk of left atrial thrombus formation. As will be discussed later, there are select patients with left ventricular (LV) dysfunction who may benefit from surgical treatment of AF in the setting of tachycardia-induced cardiomyopathy. Another group of patients who may benefit from surgical ablation of atrial arrhythmias are those patients with congenital heart disease that results in right atrial dilation. In these patients, we selectively include a right-sided maze procedure

599

at the time of intracardiac repair with incisions limited to the right atrium and interatrial septum.

Perhaps the largest group of patients who may benefit from surgical treatment is those patients with valvular heart disease and associated AF who require valve repair or replacement. In these patients, elimination of the arrhythmia allows discontinuation of chronic anticoagulation if the valve is repaired or a bioprosthesis is used.

Technique

For most patients, we continue to prefer the standard "cut-and-sew" maze operation with two technical modifications made to the procedure described by Cox et al. (Fig. 62-1). Numerous other modifications of the Cox maze procedure have been proposed, and most of these involve use of alternate energy sources and creation of alternate atrial lesion sets; these new approaches are aimed at simplifying the operation and shortening the time needed to create atrial ablation lines.

Cox Maze III Modifications

On the medial aspect of the right atrium, we avoid incision and apply a linear cryolesion from the cut edge of the appendage to the tricuspid valve (Fig. 62-2a). This avoids division of the frequently seen branch of the right coronary artery that supplies the SA node. We have found that the risk of postoperative sinus node dysfunction can be reduced by using a cryolesion instead of an incision in this location. In the left atrium,

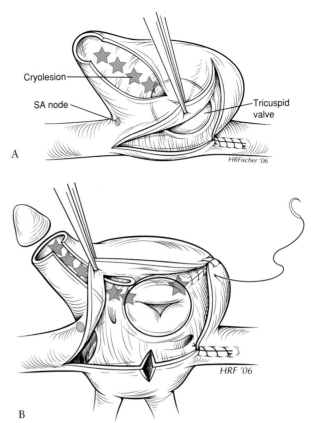

Figure 62-2. **(A)** Right atrial modification. On the medial aspect of the right atrium, instead of making an incision from the cut edge of the atrial appendage to the tricuspid valve annulus, we prefer a line of cryolesions. Often a branch of the right coronary artery supplies the sinoatrial node, and the cryolesion reduces the risk of vascular injury and sinus node dysfunction.
(B) Right-sided maze incisions. The incisions applied with a right-sided maze procedure are those that were originally described by Cox with the addition of an incision in the atrial septum and cryolesions placed at the tricuspid valve annulus both anteriorly and inferiorly.

we prefer to extend the incision that encircles the pulmonary veins to the orifice of the left atrial appendage and then close the orifice transversely as part of the encircling incision. Alternatively, cryolesions can be used as part of the lesion encircling the pulmonary veins to avoid the conjunction of the encircling suture line and left atrial appendage suture line (Fig. 62-3). The principal advantage of the "cut and sew" technique over other methods is that full-thickness lesions are assured, particularly around the pulmonary veins. This is particularly important because of the recent recognition that pulmonary venous tissue is the origin of AF in many patients.

Alternate Energy Sources

Many surgeons use alternate energy sources to create atrial lesions, and several methods have been described for maze-like procedures in the beating heart on cardiopulmonary bypass. Indeed, some surgeons are attempting to ablate AF by application of

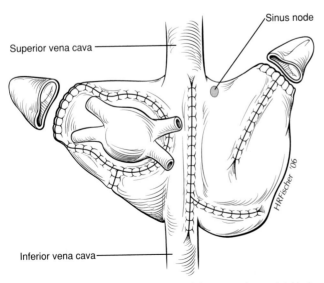

Figure 62-1. Posterior view of the heart. Depiction of the cut-and-sew atrial lesions created in the Cox maze procedure.

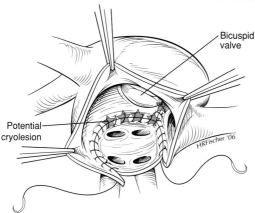

Figure 62-3. Left atrial modification. We often include the orifice of the left atrial appendage in closing the pulmonary vein–encircling incision, and do not use two separate incisions with their junction at this point because of bleeding that is commonly encountered at this location (not shown). Alternatively, a line of cryolesions can be used as part of the pulmonary vein–encircling lesion in an attempt to avoid the conjunction of two suture lines at this location (shown).

various energy sources to the epicardial atrial surface in the beating heart.

The largest clinical experience using alternate energy sources is with radiofrequency (RF) ablation, which employs alternating current to transfer energy to atrial tissue. Studies have documented success of this technology in the catheterization laboratory, leading surgeons to apply RF directly to the heart during cardiac surgery. Several different instruments have been developed to create atrial lesions including rigid unipolar probes with cooled tips, flexible unipolar probes, and bipolar clamps with and without irrigation. Radiofrequency probes can be applied to the endocardial or epicardial surfaces of the atrium in a unipolar configuration. Potential disadvantages of this method are inconsistent depth of injury, leading to nontransmural lesions, and injury to surrounding mediastinal structures.

Bipolar RF probes configured as clamps minimize the potential for injury to surrounding structures and produce transmural lesions more consistently than unipolar probes. Animal studies suggest a higher success rate in producing transmural lesions with irrigated delivery of RF compared to performing ablation without irrigation. This can be attributed to the prevention of char accumulation on the tissue surface due to the cooling effect of the irrigant. The energy is driven deeper into the tissues under these conditions. Both nonirrigated and irrigated RF devices have sensing systems that indicate when transmurality is achieved.

Lesion Sets

Availability of the new technologies has led to numerous alternate lesion sets aimed at

elimination of re-entrant atrial fibrillation and flutter. These lesion sets include bilateral isolation of the pulmonary veins, with either exclusion or excision of the left atrial appendage, and some variation of a connecting incision between the pulmonary vein lesion sets and the mitral valve annulus. Some authors believe that omission of the connecting incision between the pulmonary vein isolation lesion and the mitral valve annulus leads to increased atrial arrhythmias in the early postoperative period.

Another modification has been termed the minimaze procedure, and essential elements include a pulmonary vein–encircling incision, an atrial isthmus lesion to the orifice of the left atrial appendage, and lateral left atrial incisions without cryolesions. This method is advocated as a simpler approach, which does not seem to compromise effectiveness in controlling AF.

More recently, a "triangle-like" lesion set using saline-irrigated, cooled-tip RF ablation (SICTRA) has been described to facilitate the creation of atrial lesions. The left and right pulmonary veins are isolated within the confines of the triangle, as well as the suture closure of the left atrial appendage. One vertex of the triangle meets at the midportion of the posterior mitral valve annulus. This simplified lesion set is reported to result in a shorter duration of operative time, and, at last follow-up, 80% of patients were in stable sinus rhythm. This method conserves atrial tissue, thus addressing the concern that loss of atrial tissue correlates directly with the loss of atrial contraction postoperatively. Right atrial lesions are not included in this procedure.

Outcomes

Success with the standard Cox maze procedure has varied in published reports. In general, approximately 90% of patients who undergo the Cox maze operation are free from AF at last follow-up, with new pacemakers required in 10% to 15% of patients. At the Mayo Clinic, we have performed approximately 600 operations for AF, and through June 2006, over 400 patients have undergone the standard biatrial maze procedure with modifications as described previously. In over 125 additional patients, we have used an isolated right atrial maze procedure to eliminate AF associated with congenital heart disease affecting the right-sided cardiac chambers (e.g., Ebstein anomaly or isolated acquired tricuspid valve disease).

Our experience is similar to others in that operative risk is low, 1.5% overall, which includes patients having concomitant intracardiac repair; risk of operation for isolated AF is less than 1%, which is comparable to the risk of closure of an atrial septal defect (ASD). New permanent pacemakers were required in <10% of patients, and the indication in almost all was sick sinus syndrome. This incidence of pacing postoperatively is lower than expected based on the original reports of the Cox maze operation. In the earlier experience, clinicians were hesitant to allow patients to remain in junctional rhythm early postoperatively, but in many such patients, a stable sinus mechanism will return. Thus, some patients may have had pacemakers implanted prematurely. In addition, technical modifications to the original Cox maze operation may reduce injury to the SA node.

Preoperatively, patients are counseled that this operation reliably eliminates AF in most individuals, but it does not necessarily restore sinus rhythm. In older patients especially, there is an underlying incidence of sick sinus syndrome, and when AF is eliminated, permanent pacemakers may be necessary to manage sinus node dysfunction. It is also important that conduction disturbances may also develop in those patients who require concomitant intracardiac procedures at the time of surgery for AF; 80% of patients undergoing the standard biatrial maze procedure at Mayo Clinic have combined procedures.

In our experience, approximately 90% of patients are free from AF on dismissal from the hospital. This includes patients with sinus rhythm, paced rhythm, or junctional rhythm with an adequate rate. It is important to recognize that the Cox maze procedure, like other cardiac operations, predisposes patients to transient atrial fibrillation in the early postoperative period.

Surgical cure of AF appears to be durable, and at last follow-up (median, 42 months), overall freedom from AF is approximately 90%. When outcome is analyzed in a product limit estimate (Kaplan-Meier), freedom from AF was 76% at 5 years and 51% at 10 years. In our experience, late outcome and cure of AF depend on preoperative characteristics. At last follow-up (median, 41 months), 93% of patients with preoperative lone paroxysmal AF were free from their arrhythmia, with an actuarial freedom from AF of 90% at 5 years and 64% at 10 years. Patients with preoperative lone chronic AF had 83% freedom from AF at a last follow-up (median, 28 months), with an actuarial freedom from AF of 80% at 5 years and 62% at 10 years. The Cox maze operation is less durable for patients undergoing combined Cox maze and mitral valve surgery, with 70% of patients free from AF at last follow-up (median, 33 months) and an actuarial freedom from AF of 68% at 5 years and 41% at 10 years.

These results highlight some of the difficulties in assessing follow-up in patients who have undergone the Cox maze procedure. The first lies in the method of evaluation. The electrocardiogram is a "snapshot" in time and has limited ability to detect those patients that may have transient atrial arrhythmias in the follow-up period. The ideal method for assessment of recurrent arrhythmias is Holter monitoring; however, widespread use for routine follow-up is not feasible. After clinical evaluation and follow-up are obtained, the second difficulty is in how the results of the procedure are reported. "Rhythm at last follow-up" may underestimate the recurrence atrial arrhythmias in the follow-up period and thus overestimate the success of the procedure. Conversely, actuarial methods used to delineate time-related events, "freedom from AF," define *any* recurrent arrhythmia as a failure of the procedure, and thus they may underestimate the true success. As new instruments and lesion sets are being used and scrutinized, outcomes should be reported in a standardized fashion. Other factors that contribute to confusion in assessing results of surgical methods for treating AF are viable terminology (intermittent vs. paroxysmal, etc.) and differing patient populations.

Postoperative Management

Protocols for the postoperative management of patients who have undergone a Cox maze operation vary. For arrhythmia control, some centers use antiarrhythmic drugs, such as amiodarone, prophylactically in all patients and maintain this for 3 months. We prefer to use these medications selectively in patients who experience atrial or ventricular arrhythmias during hospitalization. We monitor potassium and magnesium levels and maintain them in the high-normal range. Postoperative atrial fibrillation is treated promptly with amiodarone, and electrical cardioversion is used as needed. If atrial fibrillation occurs early after operation and is treated with amiodarone, we continue the drug for 3 months.

It is important to use diuretics liberally early after operation. Removal of the atrial appendages during the Cox maze procedure eliminates an important source of atrial natriuretic peptide, and this, along with elevations of aldosterone and antidiuretic hormone early postoperatively, predisposes the patient to fluid retention.

We recommend systemic anticoagulation with Coumadin for 3 months postoperatively, but there is no consensus on the need for anticoagulation beyond this interval. Some clinicians prefer to continue Coumadin, believing that risk of thromboembolism is not reduced sufficiently to avoid systemic anticoagulation. Others argue that if AF is eliminated and ventricular function is normal , the risk of an intracardiac source of thromboemboli in a postoperative patient without a left atrial appendage is very low. Thus, the additional risk and inconvenience of using Coumadin is not justified.

Although a number of patients in our series had evidence of a junctional rhythm postoperatively, with some subsequently dismissed in this rhythm, we do not routinely use antiarrhythmic medications or stimulants, such as theophylline, as have been suggested. A significant number of such patients will regain a stable sinus rhythm, and it has been reported that a period of up to 50 weeks is required until this occurs. Persistent junctional rhythm may reflect sinus node dysfunction, and this will predispose the patient to recurrent arrhythmias and stroke. In these patients, a PPM should be considered.

The Cox Maze Procedure and Mitral Valve Surgery

A large group of patients to be considered for Cox maze operation are those with valvular disease and associated AF in whom repair or replacement of the valve with a bioprosthesis could result in avoidance of both antiarrhythmic medication and chronic anticoagulation with warfarin. Up to 40% of patients who undergo mitral valve repair or replacement have associated chronic AF, and addressing the mitral valve disease alone fails to restore sinus rhythm in the majority of patients. Chronic enlargement of the left atrium in these patients creates a substrate for the development of AF, and consequently, these patients have high rates of failure when AF is treated with drugs or catheter-based ablative techniques. The routine addition of the Cox maze procedure to mitral valve surgery was not embraced initially because of concern regarding the potential increased morbidity and mortality added to a procedure that already resulted in a low risk of postoperative thromboembolism. However, if sinus rhythm did not return after successful mitral valve surgery, patients continued to require antiarrhythmic medications and chronic anticoagulation with warfarin. Although warfarin therapy decreases risk of stroke in AF, its chronic use carries a risk of bleeding as high as 3%/year. In addition, careful clinical follow-up and dose adjustment are necessary for optimal therapeutic efficacy.

Because the pulmonary veins provide a trigger for AF in approximately 90% of patients with paroxysmal arrhythmia, pulmonary vein isolation alone would be expected to cure a majority of patients with this type of AF. However, it will fail as an ablative procedure in those 10% of patients in whom the pulmonary veins do not contribute the substrate for AF. In patients with chronic AF, the goal of treatment shifts from isolating the trigger of the arrhythmia (pulmonary veins in paroxysmal AF) to ablating the macroreentrant pathways responsible for its maintenance. Chronic AF leads to atrial remodeling and the development of macroreentrant pathways that sustain electrical re-entry. Allesie et al. pointed out that "atrial fibrillation begets atrial fibrillation." In this setting, the arrhythmia is not dependent on stimuli from the pulmonary veins, and, as such, pulmonary vein isolation may be inadequate treatment. This remodeling is present in a significant portion of patients with mitral valve regurgitation, especially those who have evidence of left atrial enlargement. Again, in such patients with mitral valve regurgitation and chronic AF, pulmonary vein isolation would not be expected to be as effective as a standard Cox maze procedure.

Handa et al. reported that the Cox maze operation is a safe adjunct to mitral valve repair for patients with preoperative AF. In this study from our clinic, the addition of the Cox maze procedure was particularly useful in patients with chronic AF of more than 3 months duration preoperatively. Freedom from AF was achieved in 82% of patients who underwent combined maze and mitral valve repair compared to 53% in patients who underwent mitral valve repair alone. Morbidity and mortality were not increased by the addition of the maze procedure, and 75% of patients regained sinus rhythm by last follow-up. In this series, only the omission of the maze procedure and the presence of chronic AF were predictors of arrhythmia recurrence.

Some groups advocate only left-sided maze lesions to ablate AF in patients having mitral valve surgery in an attempt to keep morbidity and mortality at a minimum. Handa et al. found no significant difference in perioperative morbidity and mortality in patients who underwent mitral valve surgery alone and those who had an additional maze procedure. It is very unlikely that the omission of the right-sided atrial lesions would have lessened the already low complication and death rate that was observed when the biatrial procedure was performed.

Tachycardia-Induced Cardiomyopathy

Surgical treatment of AF should also be considered in patients with tachycardia-induced cardiomyopathy. Rapid heart rate caused by AF can lead to cardiomyopathy, and multiple reports have documented that LV dysfunction caused by supraventricular tachycardia can be cured or improved by conversion to sinus rhythm. Furthermore, ventricular dysfunction may resolve with control of tachycardia by the simple ablation of the AV node and insertion of a pacemaker. In our review, 99 patients who underwent the maze procedure had no evidence of associated valvular or congenital heart disease, and LV dysfunction (EF <60%) was present in 37 of them. Patients were stratified into severe (EF ≤35%), moderate (EF 36%–45%), and mild LV dysfunction (EF 46%–55%) categories to study the specific effects of the Cox-maze procedure given each degree of LV impairment.

The majority of these patients had poor control of heart rate preoperatively despite aggressive medical management. Notably, two thirds had symptoms of heart failure, and 45% of patients exhibited severe or moderate LV dysfunction. Late after operation, all but one patient was free of AF, and

Table 62-1 Summary of Studies Documenting Improvement in Left Ventricular Function after Performing Ablation of Atrial Fibrillation in the Setting of Tachycardia-Induced Cardiomyopathy

Study	Pts	Procedure	Preop	Postop	P value
Kieny et al., 1992	12	Cardioversion	32 ± 5	53 ± 10	<0.001
Van Gelder et al., 1993	8	Cardioversion	36 ± 13	53 ± 8	<0.05
Twidale et al., 1993	14	AV ablation/pacer	42 ± 3	47 ± 4	<0.05
Mayo (all pt), 2006	34	Cox-maze	46 ± 10	53 ± 3	<0.001
36%–45%	8	Cox-maze	44 ± 2	53 ± 10	<0.05
≤35%	11	Cox-maze	31 ± 4	53 ± 7	<0.05

AVN = atrioventricular nodal; EF = ejection fraction; Postop = postoperative; PPM = pacemaker implantation; Preop = preoperative; Pts = number of patients.

73% of patients were free of antiarrhythmic medications. It is significant that LV function improved early postoperatively, as was evident on dismissal echocardiogram, and this improvement in ventricular function persisted at late follow-up. Furthermore, the greatest improvement was seen in those patients with the most severe impairment preoperatively (Table 62-1). Thus, as has been described with correction of other forms of tachycardia-induced cardiomyopathy, surgical treatment of AF can reverse this process, and the procedure does not impair ventricular function further or prevent improvement of ventricular function in the setting of tachycardia-induced cardiomyopathy. Greater than 35% of patients in our experience had paroxysmal AF preoperatively, so this form of the arrhythmia should be considered as a possible cause of LV dysfunction.

Atrial fibrillation impairs hemodynamic function by several mechanisms. First, the arrhythmia results in loss of atrioventricular synchrony and atrial contraction. This may reduce ventricular filling and thereby reduce cardiac output. The consequence of loss of atrial contraction may be especially pronounced in patients with impaired diastolic filling as is seen in the presence of hypertrophied ventricles, restrictive cardiomyopathy, and mitral valve stenosis. Fluctuation in the RR interval changes the diastolic filling interval, producing a variable stroke volume. In animals, cardiac output is reduced 15% when ventricular rhythm is irregular compared to a regular rhythm at the same rate.

Second, in addition to these mechanical consequences, AF can lead to tachycardia-induced cardiomyopathy. Cardiomyopathy caused by tachycardia is commonly thought to be associated with chronic arrhythmias having rates >120 beats per minute. Our experience suggests that ventricular dysfunction may be associated with resting heart

rates considerably lower than this, and, furthermore, paroxysmal AF can lead to ventricular dysfunction.

It is important to identify patients with tachycardia-induced cardiomyopathy because ventricular dysfunction can be reversed by control of the arrhythmia. Improvement in LV function has been documented in patients having cardioversion (medical or electrical) to sinus rhythm and in patients having rate control with ablation of the atrioventricular node coupled with implantation of a transvenous pacemaker (Table 62-1).

It was previously stated that LV dysfunction was the only contraindication to the Cox maze procedure. However, tachycardia-related cardiomyopathy is not uncommon in patients with AF, and our experience suggests that surgical treatment of AF should be considered in select patients with cardiomyopathy, particularly those in whom onset of tachycardia precedes or is known to coincide with development of LV dysfunction. In addition, our results demonstrate that even patients with moderate LV impairment benefit in terms of ventricular function after the procedure.

Atrial Arrhythmias in Congenital Heart Disease

Congenital heart disease (CHD) resulting in right atrial dilation is commonly associated with atrial tachyarrhythmias, particularly AF. To reduce the incidence of persistent late atrial arrhythmias in this patient population, which already exhibits a limited physiologic reserve, we use a concomitant right-sided modification of the Cox maze procedure at the time of intracardiac repair (Fig. 62-2). Because many repairs for CHD are reoperations in patients with AF, the right-sided maze procedure has the advantage of minimizing dissection of adhesions, thus resulting in shorter cardiopulmonary bypass time compared to the standard bi-atrial maze procedure. In addition, avoiding suture lines in the left atrium minimizes the risk of bleeding behind the heart, where hemostasis can be difficult.

In our experience from 1993 to June 2006, over 100 patients, median age of 43 years, underwent a right-sided Cox maze procedure at the time of repair for congenital heart disease. AF was paroxysmal in >80% of patients, and median preoperative duration of arrhythmia was approximately 3 years. The most common diagnoses were Ebstein anomaly, isolated ASD, and tetralogy of Fallot. At dismissal, approximately 90% were free from AF, with approximately 70% of patients leaving the hospital in sinus rhythm. New pacemakers were necessary in 15 patients, all but 1 for sick sinus syndrome. At a mean follow-up of 33 months, 77% of patients with preoperative chronic arrhythmias were free from AF and 96% of patients with preoperative paroxysmal arrhythmias were free from AF. The addition of a right-sided maze procedure at the time of repair for congenital heart anomalies causing right atrial enlargement appears to reduce late arrhythmia recurrence without increasing morbidity or mortality.

The Cox maze operation is the gold standard for the surgical treatment of AF (primarily arising from the left atrium) that is refractory to maximal medical therapy. The original concept was that incisions should be made in both the left and right atria to control the arrhythmia. A potential disadvantage of a right-sided maze procedure is that in some patients, the left atrium may contribute an additional substrate for AF. Our patients were selected on the basis of right atrial dilation and a normal left atrial size.

Although previous studies showed that the incidence of late recurrence of AF is *modestly* reduced by CHD repair alone, which includes restoring a competent tricuspid valve combined with right reduction atrioplasty, this study demonstrated that late results are *substantially* improved by the addition of a concomitant right-sided maze.

Atrial Fibrillation and Hypertrophic Cardiomyopathy

Atrial fibrillation occurs in up to 30% of patients with hypertrophic obstructive car-diomyopathy (HOCM), and the development of this arrhythmia in the setting of significant diastolic dysfunction can result in profound clinical deterioration due to loss of the atrial component of left ventricular filling. Patients who undergo septal myectomy can have dramatic relief of symptoms and improved exercise capacity; a number of these patients will be left with underlying diastolic dysfunction, however, and there is controversy regarding the usefulness of the Cox maze procedure in patients with paroxysmal AF and HOCM who undergo septal myectomy. In this patient population, there is concern that although sinus rhythm is restored, atrial incisions may impair contractility, thus decreasing LV filling and cardiac output. Chen et al. suggested that the Cox maze procedure can be safely included at the time of septal myectomy for HOCM, given that 80% of patients were in sinus rhythm at last follow-up. Although 2 patients in their study developed recurrent atrial arrhythmias, they were successfully treated with a combination of antiarrhythmic medications and cardioversion. Twenty percent of patients in this series required new PPM. We have used a concomitant Cox maze procedure in 11 patients with AF undergoing septal myectomy for HOCM. This combined approach was successful in ablating AF without increasing morbidity or mortality compared to a maze procedure alone. So, as reported for the combination of various other procedures with the Cox maze procedure, ablation of AF at the time of septal myectomy for HOCM does not appear to increase operative morbidity beyond what is expected for an isolated maze procedure.

Recurrent Atrial Fibrillation after the Cox Maze Procedure

Atrial fibrillation is most frequently encountered in patients with mitral valve disease. Despite documented success of the Cox maze procedure in this patient population, it fails to free all patients from their arrhythmia. Furthermore, of all subgroups of patients who undergo the Cox maze procedure, it is in this group that the maze procedure is least durable. There has been a wide variability in reported outcomes in patients undergoing combined mitral valve and Cox maze surgery. Cox and colleagues reported 98% cure of AF, whereas the experience at our clinic demonstrates 70% freedom from AF at almost 3 years. Numerous other centers have reported long-term AF prevalence after the Cox maze operation that lies scattered throughout this range. Some of these disparities in outcome clearly may be due not only to the conduct of the Cox maze operation and preoperative patient selection, but also the method of reporting success because there is no standard means of assessing or reporting success.

As demonstrated by several studies, patient characteristics heavily influence the long-term postoperative return of AF after the Cox maze procedure. The most commonly implicated risk factors include duration of preoperative AF, advanced age, and left atrial enlargement. Examining the relationship of increased left atrial size and postoperative return of AF, some studies demonstrate a clear cutoff for left atrial size above which success of ablation of AF is significantly compromised. Others have observed a more continuous relationship with no clear extent of left atrial size above which the maze procedure would be rendered totally ineffective. There are different approaches reported for patients with a dilated left atrium undergoing the maze procedure. Some combine left reduction atrioplasty and report >90% success. This also may contribute to disparate results in reported outcome for this patient population.

Left atrial enlargement is also extremely important in patients undergoing cardiac surgery without evidence of AF. Postoperative AF is frequent after cardiac surgery in general and is associated with increased morbidity and mortality and increased hospital stay and costs. Furthermore, it has been demonstrated that in patients undergoing mitral valve surgery, postoperative AF is independently associated with subsequent stroke, congestive heart failure, and late occurrence of AF. Because increased left atrial volume has been shown to predict the development of AF in nonsurgical populations, it stands to reason that increased preoperative size and volume would be an accurate marker for the development of postoperative AF. This would allow for valuable preoperative risk stratification and heightened anticipation of postoperative AF.

Left atrial volume is regarded as a marker of duration and severity of cardiovascular disease. An enlarged left atrium reflects the result of a significant remodeling process and represents an arrhythmogenic substrate. Currently for the prevention of postoperative AF, beta-blocking agents and, more aggressively, amiodarone are recommended. However, the current therapy is largely pharmacologic and although these interventions have decreased the prevalence of postoperative AF, this has not translated into a change in time-related onset of AF, AF duration, or duration of hospital stay, whereas it has introduced the possibility of adverse drug-related events.

Because preoperative risk stratification has been more clearly defined to target patients who would potentially benefit from preventive therapy against development of postoperative AF, the concept of a prophylactic Cox maze procedure has been introduced. Clearly, patients with a dilated left atrium undergoing mitral valve surgery or any other cardiac surgical procedure are at increased risk for postoperative AF, and so in this setting, preemptive ablation of the arrhythmogenic substrate may prove as effective prevention. It has been shown in patients undergoing mitral valve surgery that the addition of a full, cut-and-sew Cox maze procedure does not significantly add to the morbidity and mortality compared with mitral valve surgery alone. This is a new, potential application of the maze procedure and is being investigated.

Future Perspectives

Our results reflect the outcome in patients who underwent the standard biatrial maze procedure, which, as mentioned, employs surgical incisions and cryothermy to create the atrial lesions. As discussed previously, the new instruments developed to facilitate surgical ablation of AF and the new lesion sets may achieve similar rates of AF control as the traditional cut-and-sew methods. However, equivalency has not yet been proven, and future comparative studies are necessary. In addition, studies of other patient groups are necessary such as patients without preoperative AF who have enlarged left atria and undergo valvular surgery. Late postoperative AF is not uncommon in such patients, and performing a "prophylactic" maze procedure during the initial operation may reduce this risk. Furthermore, studies are needed to understand the role of the maze procedure in patients with AF who undergo coronary artery bypass surgery.

SUGGESTED READING

Albage A, van der Linden J, Bengtsson L, et al. Elevations in antidiuretic hormone and aldosterone as possible causes of fluid retention in the Maze procedure. Ann Thorac Surg 2001; 72(1):58.

Chen MS, McCarthy PM, Lever HM, et al. The effectiveness of atrial fibrillation surgery in patients with hypertrophic cardiomyopathy. Am J Cardiol 2004;93(3):373.

Cox JL. Atrial fibrillation I: A new classification system. Thorac Cardiovasc Surg 2003;126: 1686.

Cox JL, Ad N, Palazzo T. Impact of the maze procedure on the stroke rate in patients with atrial fibrillation. J Thorac Cardiovasc Surg 1999; 118:833.

Cox JL, Ad N, Palazzo, et al. Current status of the maze procedure for the treatment of atrial fibrillation. Semin Thorac Cardiovasc Surg 2000;12:15.

Cox JL, Boineau JP, Scheussler RB, et al. Five-year experience with the maze procedure for atrial fibrillation. Ann Thorac Surg 1993;56:814.

Cox JL, Boineau JP, Scheussler RB, et al. Modification of the maze procedure for atrial flutter and atrial fibrillation. I. Rationale and surgical results. J Thorac Cardiovasc Surg 1995;110:473.

Cox JL, Canavan TE, Schuessler RB, et al. The surgical treatment of atrial fibrillation. J Thorac Cardiovasc Surg 1991;101:406.

Cox JL, Jaquiss RDB, Scheussler RB, Boineau JP. Modification of the maze procedure for atrial flutter and atrial fibrillation. II. Surgical technique of the maze III procedure. J Thorac Cardiovasc Surg 1995;110:485.

Cox JL, Sundt TM III. The surgical management of atrial fibrillation. Annu Rev Med 1997;48:511.

Fasol R, Meinhart J, Binder T. A modified and simplified radiofrequency ablation in patients with mitral valve disease. J Thorac Cardiovasc Surg 2005;129:215.

Gillinov AM, McCarthy PM. Advances in the surgical treatment of atrial fibrillation. Cardiol Clin 2004;22(1):147.

Haissaguerre M, Jais P, Shah DC, et al. Spontaneous initiation of atrial fibrillation by ectopic beats originating in the pulmonary veins. N Engl J Med 1998;339:659.

Handa N, Schaff HV, Morris JJ, et al. Outcome of valve repair and the Cox maze procedure for mitral regurgitation and associated atrial fibrillation. J Thorac Cardiovasc Surg 1999;118: 628.

Kieny JR, Sacrez A, Facello A, et al. Increase in radionuclide left ventricular ejection fraction after cardioversion of chronic atrial fibrillation in idiopathic dilated cardiomyopathy. Eur Heart J 1992;13:1290.

Luschsinger JA, Steinberg JS. Resolution of cardiomyopathy after ablation of atrial flutter. J Am Coll Cardiol 1998;32(1):205.

Melo JQ, Santiago T, Gouveia RH, Martins AP. Atrial ablation for the surgical treatment of atrial fibrillation: Principles and limitations. J Card Surg 2004;19:207.

Oh JK, Holmes DR, Hayes DL, et al. Cardiac arrhythmias in pts with surgical repair of Ebstein's anomaly. J Am Coll Cardiol 1985;6: 1351.

Packer DL, Brady GH, Worley SJ, et al. Tachycardia-induced cardiomyopathy: a reversible form of left ventricular dysfunction. Am J Cardiol 1986;57:563.

Theodoro DA, Danielson GK, Porter CJ, Warnes CA. Right-sided maze procedure for right atrial arrhythmias in congenital heart disease. Ann Thorac Surg 1998;65:149.

Twidale N, Sutton K, Bartlett L, et al. Effects on cardiac performance of atrioventricular node catheter ablation using radiofrequency current for drug-refractory atrial arrhythmias. Pacing Clin Electrophysiol 1993;16:1275.

Van Gelder IC, Crijins HJ, Blanksma PK, et al. Time course of hemodynamic changes and improvement of exercise tolerance after cardioversion of chronic atrial fibrillation unassociated with cardiac valve disease. Am J Cardiol 1993;72:560.

Editor's Comments

I believe that Schaff and colleagues have the largest contemporary series of patients undergoing a cut-and-sew maze procedure for atrial fibrillation. They have superb results as witnessed by this chapter. They discuss the physiology in detail and how these lesions should be applied. Clearly, the results are better than those achieved with more limited procedures using alternate energy sources. The difficulty is to decide the least that needs to be done during a maze procedure and what should be done for different patient subsets. This is an evolving field, and the answer is not available.

The area that I find most difficult to decide on concerns those patients who have cardiomyopathy and atrial fibrillation. As the authors noted, in many cases atrial fibrillation can lead to cardiomyopathy. However, it is well known that cardiomyopathy itself can lead to some mitral regurgitation due to any annular dilation. As the atrium enlarges, atrial fibrillation can occur. The authors note that one must be certain that atrial fibrillation precedes the cardiomyopathy. This is the subset that I'm certain has the highest risk for poor postoperative outcomes.

I.L.K.

63

Surgical Treatment of Atrial Fibrillation

A. Marc Gillinov

The Epidemic of Atrial Fibrillation

Atrial fibrillation (AF) is the most common sustained cardiac arrhythmia. More than 2 million Americans suffer from AF, and this number is expected to double in the next three decades. Responsible for billions of dollars in health care expenditures each year, AF is associated with adverse clinical consequences that include reduced survival, stroke and other thromboembolism, tachycardia-induced cardiomyopathy, and symptoms related to rapid and irregular heart rates. For these clinical and economic reasons, there is great interest in developing effective treatments for AF.

Although medical therapy is the most common treatment for patients with AF, recent data reveal that it is frequently ineffective at restoring sinus rhythm and leaves patients at relatively high risk for cardiovascular morbidity and mortality. Disappointing results with medical strategies of rate and rhythm control have helped to foster the development of new interventional catheter and surgical therapies. Although often successful, catheter-based ablation of AF is limited to a relatively small number of patients treated by highly skilled electrophysiologists. In contrast, virtually all cardiac surgeons are capable of performing surgical procedures to ablate AF.

Developed by Cox and colleagues, the Cox-Maze III procedure is the surgical standard for management of AF. This procedure, which has excellent long-term results extending over more than a decade, has recently given way to a variety of simpler operations that employ alternate energy sources

and lesion sets to treat AF. A brief description of current thinking concerning the pathophysiology of AF helps to clarify the rationale for these new procedures.

Pathophysiology of Atrial Fibrillation

In recent years, there has been considerable progress in enhancing our understanding of the pathogenesis of AF, and this increased knowledge has directly affected approaches to ablation. Initial studies by Cox and others demonstrated that AF is characterized by macro-reentrant circuits in both atria. Designed to interrupt these macro-reentrant circuits, the Cox-Maze III procedure consists in precisely placing incisions and cryolesions in both atria. These lines of conduction block segment the atria, reducing the available contiguous atrial area and volume. The lesions of the Cox-Maze procedure thereby prevent formation and propagation of the macro-reentrant circuits of AF, consequently terminating the arrhythmia. Of note, the Cox-Maze procedure also includes excision of the left atrial appendage, a procedure that may reduce the risk of thromboembolism.

Both electrophysiologic research and clinical experience have augmented our understanding of AF. It is now generally accepted that the pathogenesis of AF involves both initiation and maintenance of the arrhythmia; a variety of different mechanisms may be responsible for initiation and maintenance of AF. It is certain that, like clinical presentation, the pathogenesis of AF varies among patients. The extent to which mechanisms of focal activity, re-entry and auto-

nomic nerve activation contribute to the initiation and maintenance of AF is disputed. Thus, it is difficult to tailor an AF ablation procedure to a patient's particular electrophysiologic profile. Although the electrophysiologic mechanisms of AF require further investigation, the anatomic basis of AF is increasingly clear, and it is this anatomic knowledge that has influenced surgical approaches to ablation.

Endocardial electrophysiologic mapping data demonstrate that the pulmonary veins and posterior left atrium are the critical anatomic targets for ablation in humans with isolated AF. In addition, mapping studies support the importance of the left atrium and pulmonary veins in the pathogenesis of AF in patients with valvular heart disease. For many patients with permanent AF, regular and repetitive activation can be identified in the posterior left atrium in the regions of the pulmonary vein orifices and left atrial appendage. Although routine intraoperative mapping is currently not feasible for guiding intraoperative AF ablation, an anatomic approach based on our understanding of pathophysiology and on empiric results is reasonable. In fact, such an anatomic (rather than map-guided) approach is rapidly becoming the standard for catheter-based ablation of AF.

It is generally agreed that surgical ablation must include left atrial lesions and treatment of the left atrial appendage. However, the choice of left atrial lesion set and the importance of right atrial lesions are matters of controversy and study. The Cox-Maze III procedure, which includes extensive lesions in both atria, offers important insights for guiding the development of new procedures.

The Cox-Maze Procedure

Surgical Technique

Aside from a slight modification in the right atrium that utilizes bipolar radiofrequency and the addition of a right atrial isthmus lesion, we employ the lesions and techniques described by Dr. Cox. The Cox-Maze III procedure can be performed either through a median sternotomy or partial lower sternotomy. Cardiopulmonary bypass is established using bicaval and ascending aortic cannulation. The heart is arrested with antegrade cardioplegia, and a retrograde cardioplegia catheter is placed directly after construction of a right atriotomy. If coronary artery bypass grafting is required, distal anastomoses are completed before the Cox-Maze III procedure. Valvular lesions are addressed after the Cox-Maze III procedure.

The Cox-Maze III procedure is started by opening the left atrium anterior to the right pulmonary veins, as for a mitral valve opera-tion. The right atrium is opened with an incision that extends from the tricuspid annulus (2 o'clock position as the surgeon views the valve) toward the fossa ovalis. The interatrial septum is then incised with scissors, placing one jaw of the scissors inside the left atrium and the other jaw inside the right atrium. A self-retaining retractor is then placed to facilitate completion of the left atrial lesion set.

The pulmonary vein–encircling incision is continued with scissors, bringing the incision to the level of the left inferior

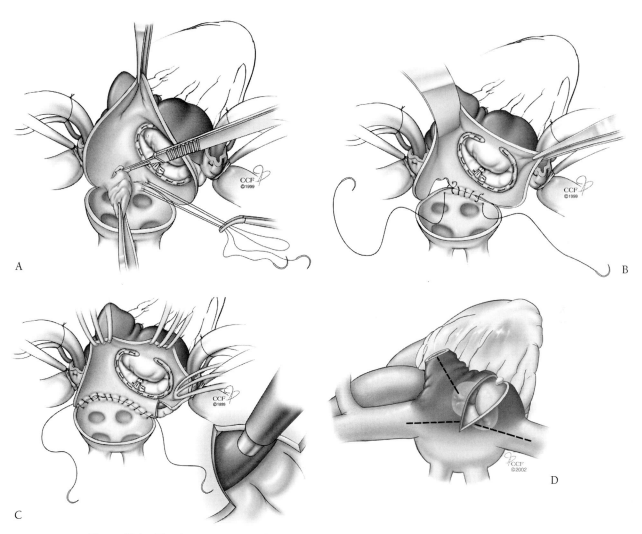

Figure 63-1. The Cox-Maze III procedure with bipolar radiofrequency application in right atrium. **(A)** The left atrium is opened anterior to the left pulmonary veins, and the pulmonary vein–encircling incision is carried to the level of the left inferior pulmonary vein. A stay suture is placed at this point. The left atrial appendage is excised sharply. **(B)** The pulmonary vein–encircling incision is completed and then partially closed. **(C)** An incision is created to the mitral annulus, exposing the anterior surface of the coronary sinus. Cryolesions are created at the mitral annulus and coronary sinus. **(D)** There is a single long incision in the right atrium heading from the tricuspid annulus to the fossa ovalis; a cryolesion is created at the tricuspid annulus at the 2 o'clock position. Through this incision, bipolar radiofrequency lesions are created to the superior vena cava and to the inferior vena cava (*dashed lines*). A stab incision is created in the right atrial appendage, and a bipolar radiofrequency lesion is created in the appendage (*dashed line*).

pulmonary vein (Fig. 63-1A). A stay suture is placed here to facilitate later closure. The pulmonary vein–encircling incision is then completed, disconnecting the
pulmonary veins from the left atrium. In addition, the left atrial appendage is excised.
The incision around the pulmonary veins
is then partially closed, incorporating the
region of the left atrial appendage in this suture line (Fig. 63-1B). At the level of the P2
segment of the mitral valve, an incision is
carried from the pulmonary vein–encircling
incision up to the mitral annulus. This incision begins full thickness but includes only
endocardium and underlying muscle as the
annulus and coronary sinus are approached.
The anterior surface of the coronary sinus
is exposed. A large cryolesion is created at
the mitral annulus and coronary sinus; this
lesion is performed using nitrous oxide–
based cryothermy at −60°C for 2 minutes
(Fig. 63-1C). Then all left atrial incisions and the interatrial septum are
closed.

We prefer to create the right atrial lesions with the heart arrested (Fig. 63-1D).
The previously placed right atrial incision
is carried all the way to the tricuspid annulus, and a 2-minute cryolesion is created at
the 2 o'clock position of the tricuspid annulus. Then a stab incision is created in the
right atrial appendage. One jaw of a bipolar radiofrequency clamp is introduced into
this stab incision and directed toward the
patient's back, creating a lesion in the right
atrial appendage that ends 1 cm from the
previously placed right atriotomy. The direction of the bipolar radiofrequency clamp
is then reversed, and a lesion is created
toward the tricuspid annulus. The bipolar
radiofrequency clamp is then used to create a lesion from the right atriotomy to the
superior vena cava. A second lesion is created from the right atriotomy to the inferior
vena cava. Finally, a cryolesion is created on
the right atrial isthmus, extending from the
tricuspid annulus to the orifice of the inferior vena cava. The right atrial incisions
are closed after removing the aortic cross-
clamp. The final left atrial lesion set of the
Cox-Maze III includes a pulmonary vein–
encircling incision, a connecting incision
to the stump of the excised left atrial appendage, and a connecting lesion to the mitral annulus that incorporates cryolesions at
the mitral annulus and at the coronary sinus
(Fig. 63-2).

Before weaning the patient from cardiopulmonary bypass, it is prudent to examine the region of the left atrial appendage for
bleeding because this is most easily repaired
while on bypass. Nodal rhythms are com-

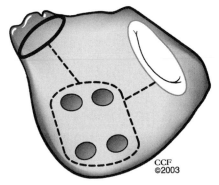

Figure 63-2.   Left atrial lesion set of the
Cox-Maze III procedure. Dashed lines indicate
surgical incisions. The pulmonary veins are
encircled by a surgical incision, and there is a
connecting incision to the mitral valve
annulus. The left atrial appendage is excised,
and this incision is connected to the
pulmonary vein–encircling incision.

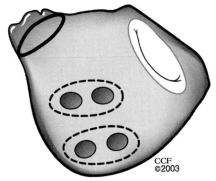

Figure 63-3.   Bilateral pulmonary vein
isolation with excision of the left atrial
appendage. The pulmonary veins are isolated
as two separate ovals that include wide areas
of left atrial tissue. The left atrial appendage is
excised sharply.

mon after separation from bypass, and most
patients leave the operating room paced
atrially.

Results

The Cox-Maze procedure is the only ablation technique for which long-term results
are available. Reported late freedoms from
AF range from 75% to 98% at 5 to 10 years
after surgery. Disparities in results from different groups may be related to different
follow-up methodologies and different definitions of success. Risk factors for recurrent AF after a Cox-Maze procedure include
longer duration of preoperative AF and left
atrial enlargement, pattern of AF (paroxysmal vs. permanent), and need for concomitant procedures that do not affect results. In
addition to restoring sinus rhythm, the Cox-
Maze procedure virtually eliminates the risk
of late stroke. This beneficial effect may
relate in part to excision of the left atrial
appendage.

Alternate Approaches to Surgical Ablation

Pulmonary Vein Isolation

Because of the important role of the
pulmonary veins and the left atrial in the
pathogenesis of paroxysmal AF, pulmonary
vein isolation may be used to treat paroxysmal AF. A variety of energy sources have
been employed to perform pulmonary vein
isolation. The pulmonary veins can be isolated with two separate oval-shaped lesions
(Fig. 63-3) or, alternatively, as a single,

large, boxlike lesion. Either approach is acceptable.

With the use of bipolar radiofrequency,
pulmonary vein isolation is simple. When
performed through a sternotomy as a concomitant procedure, pulmonary vein isolation is generally accomplished after cardiac
arrest. Blunt dissection is used to dissect the
posterior surface of the pulmonary veins. Fat
along the anterior surface of the pulmonary
veins is dissected with cautery to enable the
surgeon to perform a wide pulmonary vein
isolation that includes adjacent left atrial
tissue; on the left side, this includes dissection of the ligament of Marshall. A bipolar radiofrequency clamp is then introduced
about the pulmonary veins (Fig. 63-4). The
clamp is advanced toward the left atrium,
isolating as much atrial tissue as possible
and ensuring that energy is not delivered directly to pulmonary vein tissue because this
may cause pulmonary vein stenosis. Each
set of pulmonary veins is isolated with two
parallel applications of the bipolar radiofrequency clamp to ensure that there are no
gaps. The left atrial appendage is excised
with scissors, and its stump is oversewn with
two layers of running polypropylene suture.
In addition to pulmonary vein isolation, we
recommend creation of a cryolesion on the
right atrial isthmus to prevent development
of right atrial flutter.

When applied to patients with mitral
valve disease and paroxysmal AF, wide pulmonary vein isolation is extremely effective.
One year after pulmonary vein isolation,
90% of patients with paroxysmal AF are free
of AF. In contrast, this approach is far less
effective in patients with mitral valve disease and permanent AF, leaving nearly 50%
of patients in AF 1 year after ablation.

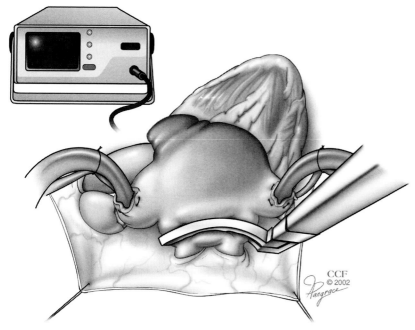

Figure 63-4. Isolation of the right pulmonary veins with a bipolar radiofrequency clamp (Atricure Inc., West Chester, Ohio). Under direct vision, the clamp is placed on the left atrial cuff adjacent to the pulmonary veins. With two parallel 5- to 15-second applications, the pulmonary veins and a wide left atrial cuff are isolated.

Pulmonary Vein Isolation with Connecting Lesions

In patients with permanent (continuous) AF, a more extensive lesion set is employed in the left atrium, reproducing the pattern of the Cox-Maze III (Fig. 63-5). The pulmonary veins are isolated as described earlier. A lateral left atriotomy is constructed anterior to the right pulmonary veins. Bipolar radiofrequency is used to create connecting lesions between the superior pulmonary veins and between the inferior pulmonary veins. Bipolar radiofrequency is also used to

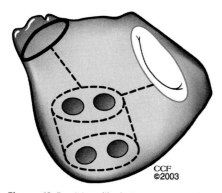

Figure 63-5. Maze-like lesion set created with bipolar radiofrequency and cryothermy (for lesion to the mitral annulus). The lesion to the mitral annulus is created with cryothermy. The left atrial appendage is excised.

create a connecting lesion from the stump of the excised left atrial appendage to the left inferior pulmonary vein. A connecting lesion from the left pulmonary veins to the P3 region of the mitral annulus is created with cryothermy or unipolar radiofrequency; for this lesion, we favor cryothermy because of possible proximity of the circumflex coronary artery. Finally, cryothermy is used to create a lesion on the right atrial isthmus.

When applied to patients with permanent AF and mitral valve disease, this approach is associated with approximately 80% freedom from AF at 1 year. Adjunctive measures, such as left atrial reduction in those with left atrial enlargement, may improve results.

Isolated Atrial Fibrillation and Minimally Invasive Epicardial Ablation

The aforementioned techniques have been applied primarily in patients with AF who require cardiac surgery for other reasons, most commonly for mitral valve disease. However, there is increasing interest in the surgical treatment of isolated AF. Patients with isolated AF have a variety of

treatment options, including medical management (rate or rhythm control), catheter ablation, and surgical ablation. Potential advantages of surgical treatment include reliable creation of transmural lesions, freedom from collateral damage to adjacent structures like the esophagus, direct or endoscopic visualization eliminating the possibility of pulmonary vein stenosis, negligible periprocedural risk of stroke, and ability to excise the left atrial appendage. There are several minimally invasive approaches to surgical AF ablation. All have in common the use of endoscopy and/or small incisions and no need for cardiopulmonary bypass.

Our favored approach to the patient with isolated AF is bilateral video-assisted thoracoscopic pulmonary vein isolation with excision of the left atrial appendage. Bilateral, keyhole access is obtained in the third intercostal space, and the pulmonary vein is dissected with video assistance and specially designed instrumentation; the segments are then isolated using bipolar radiofrequency (Fig. 63-6A). Isolation is confirmed by recording pulmonary vein electrograms that demonstrate conduction block. In addition, autonomic fibers contained in fat pads adjacent to the pulmonary veins may be ablated with cautery. On the left side, the left atrial appendage is excised with an endoscopic stapler (Fig. 63-6B). Procedural times are generally 2 to 4 hours, and hospital length of stay is currently 2 to 3 days for most patients. Early results are excellent, with >90% of patients free of AF at 6 months after ablation.

Postablation Care

Periprocedural AF occurs in 30% to 60% of patients after surgical ablation. Like AF after routine cardiac surgery, this arrhythmia is usually transient; by 3 months after surgery, AF has abated in 85% to 95% of patients. When postablation AF occurs, patients are treated with standard antiarrhythmic drugs for 4 to 6 weeks. We perform a single cardioversion in hospital if medical therapy fails to restore sinus rhythm. All patients are discharged with Coumadin (target INR 2) for 6 months and a transtelephonic monitor. Rhythm strips are obtained monthly and at the time of any symptoms. If the patient remains in AF, electrical cardioversion is performed at 3 months and, if necessary, again at 6 months. A full evaluation including Holter monitoring is recommended at 6 months after surgery. If patients have no evidence of AF at 6 months, Coumadin is discontinued. Conversely, if patients have

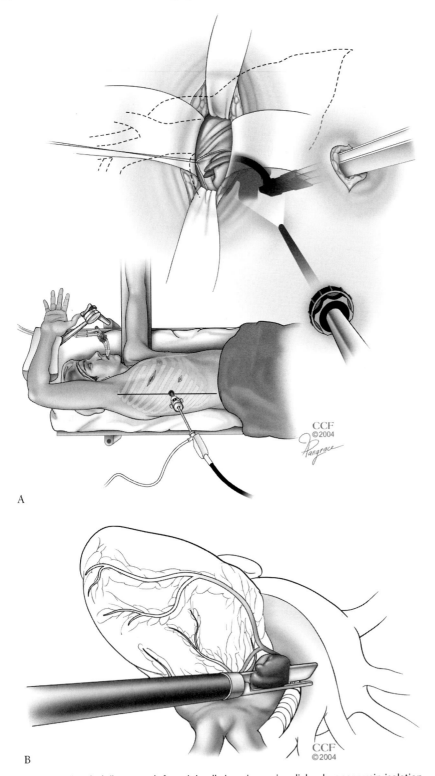

A

B

Figure 63-6. "Keyhole" approach for minimally invasive, epicardial pulmonary vein isolation with excision of the left atrial appendage. **(A)** Access to right pulmonary veins through a keyhole incision with endoscopic guidance. A bipolar radiofrequency clamp is used to isolate the left atrial cuff adjacent to the right pulmonary veins. **(B)** Stapled excision of the left atrial appendage after isolation of the left pulmonary veins using a similar technique to that displayed for the right pulmonary veins.

recurrent AF at 6 months, we recommend catheter-based electrophysiologic study and ablation if possible.

Current Clinical Algorithm

Tables 63-1 and 63-2 present our current approach to the patient with AF. In patients having concomitant surgery, the lesion set is tailored to the clinical pattern of AF. If the AF is paroxysmal, we perform wide pulmonary vein isolation, making sure to incorporate a large area of left atrium adjacent to the pulmonary veins; in addition, we excise the left atrial appendage and perform a cryolesion on the right atrial isthmus. If the AF is permanent, we favor a left atrial lesion set that resembles that of the Cox-Maze III procedure. In such patients, if maximum left atrial diameter exceeds 5 cm, we favor a cut-and-sew Cox-Maze III to reduce atrial size. Patients with permanent AF also receive a right atrial isthmus lesion.

In the patient with isolated AF that is paroxysmal, we perform minimally invasive pulmonary vein isolation with excision of the left atrial appendage. In the patient with permanent AF, we offer a classic Cox-Maze III procedure, generally accomplished via a limited skin incision and a partial or full sternotomy.

Future Directions

In the near future, advances in our understanding of AF and ablation instrumentation will affect surgical procedures and results. Real-time, intraoperative electrophysiologic mapping will enable precise identification of anatomic regions that require ablation and postprocedure electrophysiologic assessment of lesions created. Such targeted (rather than empiric) ablation strategies will improve results by enabling procedures that treat the patient's particular electrophysiologic pathophysiology. In addition, intraoperative assessment of results will guide the surgeon, enabling more confident creation of lesions that effectively block conduction.

In order to facilitate minimally invasive, epicardial ablation, new devices for dissection and ablation are under development. These devices will ensure safe and directed epicardial delivery of ablation energy through ports or very small incisions. Surgical management of the left atrial appendage will be achieved with devices specifically designed for this purpose, increasing the ease

Table 63-1   Atrial Fibrillation Ablation with Concomitant Cardiac Surgical Procedure

Procedure	Paroxysmal AF	Persistent or Permanent AF
Low-risk, simple cardiac procedure	Wide PVI/ LAA excision	PVI/left atrial connecting lesions/LAA excision or Cox-Maze III
High-risk or complex cardiac procedure	Wide PVI/ LAA excision	PVI/left atrial connecting lesions/LAA excision

AF = atrial fibrillation; LAA = left atrial appendage; PVI = pulmonary vein isolation.

Table 63-2   Atrial Fibrillation Ablation in Patients with Lone Atrial Fibrillation

Paroxysmal AF	Persistent or Permanent AF
Minimally invasive PVI/LAA excision	Cox-Maze III or minimally invasive PVI/left atrial connecting lesions/ LAA excision

AF = atrial fibrillation; LAA = left atrial appendage; PVI = pulmonary vein isolation.

and safety of this component of the procedure. With these near-term advances, minimally invasive epicardial AF ablation will become widely available, extending the possibility of surgical AF ablation to large numbers of patients.

SUGGESTED READING

Cox JL, Ad N. New surgical and catheter-based modifications of the Maze procedure. Semin Thorac Cardiovasc Surg 2000;12:68.

Cox JL, Ad N, Palazzo T. Impact of the Maze procedure on the stroke rate in patients with atrial fibrillation. J Thorac Cardiovasc Surg 1999;108:833.

Cox JL, Ad N, Palazzo T, et al. Current status of the Maze procedure for the treatment of atrial fibrillation. Semin Thorac Cardiovasc Surg 2000;12:15.

Damiano RJ Jr. Alternative energy sources for atrial ablation: Judging the new technology. Ann Thorac Surg 2003;75:329.

Gillinov AM, Blackstone EH, McCarthy PM. Atrial fibrillation: Current surgical options and their assessment. Ann Thorac Surg 2002;74:2210.

Gillinov AM, McCarthy PM: Advances in the surgical treatment of atrial fibrillation. Cardiol Clin 2004;22:147.

Gillinov AM, McCarthy PM, Blackstone EH, et al. Surgical ablation of atrial fibrillation with bipolar radiofrequency as the primary modality. J Thorac Cardiovasc Surg 2005;129:1322.

Wolf RK, Schneeberger EW, Osterday R, et al. Video-assisted bilateral pulmonary vein isolation and left atrial appendage exclusion for atrial fibrillation. J Thorac Cardiovasc Surg 2005.

EDITOR'S COMMENTS

I made a decision to include two chapters on atrial fibrillation ablation. I believe this is a very important and growing part of our specialty. Dr. Gillinov's approach is a little bit different from the Mayo approach. He uses appropriately other energy sources. I believe that the majority of surgeons in this country are using alternative energy sources for the Maze procedure. I think Dr. Gillinov's approach is a thoughtful and reproducible one. I am not sure as of yet exactly what lesions are truly necessary, but further study will tell us the best approaches. I use Dr. Gillinov's approach. At this point, I believe it is the most easily reproducible one.

I.L.K.

H

Other Cardiac

64

Cardiac Tumors

Himanshu J. Patel, Francis D. Pagani, and Richard L. Prager

Historical Background

Realdo Columbus first described a cardiac tumor as an anatomic finding in Padua, Italy, in 1559. Centuries later, in 1931, the first classification system similar to what is in current use was reported by Yater. In his monograph, he reported nine cases of primary cardiac tumors from pathologic examination. However, it was not until 1934 that the first antemortem diagnosis of a cardiac tumor (sarcoma) was made by Barnes, who used electrocardiography and a biopsy of a lymph node. Twelve years later, Mahaim's classic paper described over 400 cardiac tumors.

The era of operative treatment of cardiac neoplasms was ushered in by Beck in 1936, when he successfully removed a teratoma located on the right ventricular surface. Bahnson is credited with removal of the first right atrial myxoma with inflow occlusion, but the patient died postoperatively on day 24. Following the advent of cardiopulmonary bypass in the 1953, left-sided intra-cardiac neoplasms were successfully removed first by Crafoord in Sweden in 1954. By 1964, removal of 60 intracardiac neoplasms had been reported. The addition of cardiac echocardiography allowed easier antemortem diagnosis, and thus resulted in an increase in number of tumor resections.

Epidemiology and Classification

Cardiac neoplasms can be divided into primary and secondary types. Primary tumors are typically more common, but the overall incidence is still quite low, at 0.15% to 0.2% in autopsy series. Most primary cardiac tu-

mors are benign (70%; Table 64-1). More than half of the primary cardiac neoplasms in adults are myxomas.

Malignant primary cardiac tumors (Table 64-2) are more frequently seen in adults than in children. Of malignant cardiac tumors, metastatic malignancies (Table 64-3) comprise the majority of those noted. Virtually every neoplasm has been shown to metastasize to the heart. The most frequent primary malignancies are leukemic neoplasms (54%), melanoma (34%), and bronchogenic carcinoma (10%), with others including sarcoma, breast, and esophageal carcinoma. Primary cardiac malignancies are uncommon, and most frequently are sarcomas.

Myxomas

Myxomas are the most frequently seen adult cardiac neoplasm. They usually occur sporadically, but have been reported in autosomal-dominant inherited forms in 5% of cases. The typical sporadic tumor is seen in women aged 30 to 60 years, and is solitary in nature. The familial form is more likely seen in younger patients, often male, and multicentric in nature. The two types can be differentiated on the basis of DNA ploidy, with the familial type having an abnormal ploidy.

Myxomas are typically located in the atria (most commonly on the limbus of the fossa ovalis) (Fig. 64-1A), but can arise in the ventricles. The tumors are variable in their gross pathologic appearance (Fig. 64-1B), and can be papillary or smooth, pedunculated or sessile, but are often quite friable. They are usually white or yellow, and may be covered with thrombus. On cut sections, they frequently contain areas of

hemorrhage. They are typically 5 cm to 6 cm in size, but have been reported to reach up to 15 cm. Histopathologically, they have an acid mucopolysaccharide matrix and contain smooth muscle cells, capillaries, and reticulocytes. Calcification is reported more frequently in right atrial myxomas. These tumors typically grow outward into the cardiac chambers, and rarely invade into the walls of the heart. However, those tumors that are biatrial in location are thought to be a result of bidirectional growth of the myxoma because they are usually attached to the same point on the atrial wall. Usually they are limited to the subendocardial region at their base. The subendocardial multipotential mesenchymal cell is considered the precursor cell for myxoma, thus accounting for the variable cell types seen in the tumor.

The natural history of myxomas is of rapid growth. Although these tumors are considered to be benign, there have been reports of extensive local extension, as well as metastatic spread. The familial type is more likely to be recurring and more aggressive.

The clinical presentation patterns of myxomas relate to their potential to cause obstruction (congestive heart failure, atrial fibrillation, fatigue, and syncope), embolization, and constitutional symptoms (myalgias, fevers, arthralgias, and weakness). Occasionally, they can present with evidence of infection, with a syndrome not unlike infective endocarditis. Physical findings can include signs of right- or left-sided congestive failure, the early diagnostic "tumor plop," or diastolic rumbles.

The workup of a suspected myxoma includes echocardiography as the most useful test for diagnosis. Although surface echocardiograms can identify the pathology in most cases, the transesophageal echocardiogram (Fig. 64-1C) gives the best images

Table 64-1 Benign Cardiac Neoplasms

Myxoma
Papillary fibroelastoma
Lipoma
Teratoma
Rhabdomyoma
Pheochromocytoma
Fibromas
Atrioventricular node mesothelioma
Neurofibroma
Lymphangioma
Granular cell tumor

Table 64-3 Metastatic Cardiac Neoplasms

Leukemia
Bronchogenic carcinoma
Melanoma
Sarcoma
Breast cancer
Esophageal cancer
Ovarian cancer
Prostate cancer
Renal cell carcinoma (hypernephroma)
Lymphoma

and provides details regarding the location and attachment areas for tumors even as small as 2 mm. This aids in planning the operative approach. We also request left heart catheterizations to aid in diagnosis of coronary disease in patients older than the age of 45 years or even younger if they have significant risk factors or symptoms. Computed tomography (CT) and magnetic resonance imaging (MRI) are rarely utilized at our center for suspected myxomas because in the setting of a myxoma, they typically do not add additional information. However, if there is suspicion that the tumor may not be a myxoma, cardiac-gated CT scans or cardiac-gated MRI may better delineate the extent of involvement of adjacent structures by the tumor. It is important to exclude endocarditis as a cause of cardiac mass.

The indication for operation in patients with a myxoma is the presence of one. Given the risk of embolization (8% to 10%) or obstruction, we typically perform the operation in an urgent fashion following establishment of diagnosis. These patients are usually operated on during the same hospitalization. Initial attempts are made to diurese the patients while obtaining necessary workup, but the surgery is typically not delayed. Anticoagulation with heparin is important to institute during the time of evaluation because it is felt to decrease the risk of embolization.

Table 64-2 Malignant Primary Cardiac Neoplasms

Angiosarcoma
Rhabdomyosarcoma
Liposarcoma
Malignant mesothelioma
Malignant fibrous histiocytoma
Lymphoma
Malignant teratoma
Malignant pheochromocytoma
Thymoma
Osteosarcoma

Operative Approach

Median sternotomy is the incision of choice. However, in this era of minimally invasive surgery, other options include anterolateral thoracotomy (fourth intercostal space), partial sternotomy (with a "J" or "T" extension), or in female patients, a submammary incision. We utilize a "no-touch" technique to minimize the risk of embolization until the aortic cross-clamp is in place. Cannulation for cardiopulmonary bypass is performed with bicaval inflow, and if the tumor is in the typical location in the left atrium, left ventricular venting through the left superior pulmonary vein is not performed, to avoid dislodging tumor material. The patient's temperature is allowed to drift down to 32°C to 34°C degrees, and the heart is arrested with cold blood antegrade cardioplegia. We often use a biatrial approach, having exposed the left atrium through the interatrial groove. The right atrial incision is a standard one, approximately 1 cm parallel to the atrioventricular groove. This exposure usually results in adequate immediate visualization of the tumor (Fig. 64-1A). If the tumor is small, it may be delivered through the left atriotomy with minimal manipulation. When it is larger, gentle application of pressure to the right ventricular (RV) outflow tract area may aid in exposing the stalk of the tumor. The tumor is then removed with a 0.5-cm to 1-cm margin of tissue, taking care not to injure the mitral annulus, the area of conduction tissue, and the tricuspid annulus. The defect is closed primarily if the stalk is ≤1 cm and with a patch (pericardium or Gore-Tex) if the stalk is larger. It should be emphasized that adequate resection with negative margins is the key in resection of this tumor to avoid the risk of recurrence. A copious amount of saline is then used to irrigate the ventricular cavity, and the atria are closed in a routine fashion. After de-airing the heart, the patient is weaned from cardiopulmonary bypass.

If the tumor is in the right atrium, cannulation may be done in a bicaval fashion or with a superior vena cava cannula and a femoral vein cannula. A standard right atriotomy is made, and the tumor is then resected. If the tumor extends to the entrance of the inferior vena cava into the pericardium, deep hypothermic circulatory arrest may be needed to aid in complete resection.

Operative mortality is typically <5%, with the majority of deaths occurring in the older patient population (>70 years of age). Morbidity can be related to embolic phenomena (e.g., stroke). Atrial fibrillation is commonly seen both preoperatively and postoperatively in these patients, and may require anticoagulation (given the raw surface of the atria in this scenario). Recurrence is estimated to be <5% in patients with sporadic myxomas, but up to 25% in patients with the familial form. Therefore, all patients should continue to get routine echocardiographic follow-up after myxoma resection.

Papillary Fibroelastomas

These benign tumors typically occur on valves or adjacent endocardium and comprise 7% to 10% of cardiac neoplasms. They are usually asymptomatic, but can present with embolic phenomena (stroke) or with obstruction (coronary artery). Their gross pathologic appearance consists of a frondlike mass with multiple projections, and they are typically small. These tumors should be resected, especially if they are found on the left side of the heart. When they are located on valvular elements, after resection, every effort should be made to repair rather than replace the valve.

Lipomas

Lipomas can occur at any age in any location within the pericardium. These tumors are typically slow growing and present with obstructive or compressive symptoms. Grossly, these tumors are like lipomas seen elsewhere in the body, being well-encapsulated and containing mature adipocytes. Resection is indicated in the presence of symptoms. Tumors found incidentally are resected at the time of other cardiac operations, assuming that the addition of this procedure confers minimal added risk. These tumors are not thought to recur, so a large negative margin is likely not necessary.

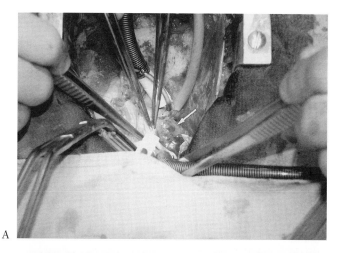

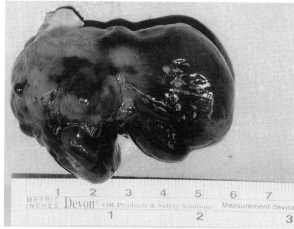

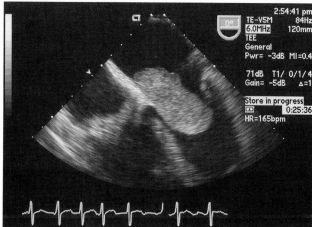

Figure 64-1. **(A)** Typical operative approach, using median sternotomy and cardiopulmonary bypass using a bicaval inflow technique. The exposure of the tumor is via a biatrial approach, and the tumor (*white arrow*) is readily delivered via the left atriotomy. **(B)** Gross pathologic appearance of this myxoma, which consists of large, mottled-tan hemorrhagic tissue, somewhat gelatinous and myxoid, measuring 6 cm in maximal dimension. **(C)** Transesophageal echocardiogram of this tumor in vivo. Note the "ballvalve" obstruction of the mitral valve caused by the tumor. The attachment is to the left atrial wall, along the fossa ovalis.

When these tumors exist in a nonencapsulated form in the interatrial septum, the condition is called lipomatous hypertrophy of the interatrial septum. This entity is often difficult to separate from neoplasm, but the addition of MR imaging allows identification of masses with fat, intense signals. Very little is known about the natural history of this entity, and typical indications for resection have not been identified but may include arrhythmias occurring with this pathology. If this lesion is found intraoperatively or preoperatively on transesophageal echocardiography, resection is not felt to be necessary.

Rhabdomyoma

The most frequently seen tumor in children is rhabdomyoma (45% to 60% of cardiac tumors in children vs. <1% of cardiac tumors in adults). The natural history of this entity is not well characterized. It will often present in the first few days of life with symptoms of obstruction. The diagnosis is established on echocardiography. This neoplasm is usually multicentric, occurring with equal frequency in either ventricular chamber. Tuberous sclerosis is sought for because greater than one half of patients with rhabdomyoma have this hereditary disorder. Once the diagnosis is established, surgery is indicated unless the patient has tuberous sclerosis. The prognosis is poor in most patients, and especially if they have associated tuberous sclerosis.

Fibromas

Fibromas are cardiac tumors that present often in children. They are usually located in the ventricular chambers and are solitary. Presenting symptoms are secondary to obstruction or arrhythmias. Because these tumors can calcify, they are occasionally identified on chest x-rays. Complete surgical resection is the goal for cure, but debulking can be associated with long-term survival.

Cardiac Pheochromocytomas

Less than 2% of pheochromocytomas occur in the thoracic cavity. Those occurring in the intrapericardial location are often located in the dome of the left atrium. The diagnosis is suspected on clinical manifestations and laboratory confirmation of catecholamine oversecretion. Localization is obtained with the ^{131}I-metaiodobenzylguanidine (MIBG) scan. A CT scan is the next most appropriate test for identifying the extent of involvement of adjacent structures. We also obtain transesophageal echocardiograms in all patients to evaluate the cardiac chambers and valves, as well as obtain information about the extent of tumor. Finally, cardiac catheterization is performed in selected patients to identify significant coronary disease. Management first consists in controlling the hyperadrenergic syndrome (beta-blockade, followed by alpha-blockade and if necessary intravenous hydration). The tumors are then removed using cardiopulmonary bypass. Complete resection is the goal.

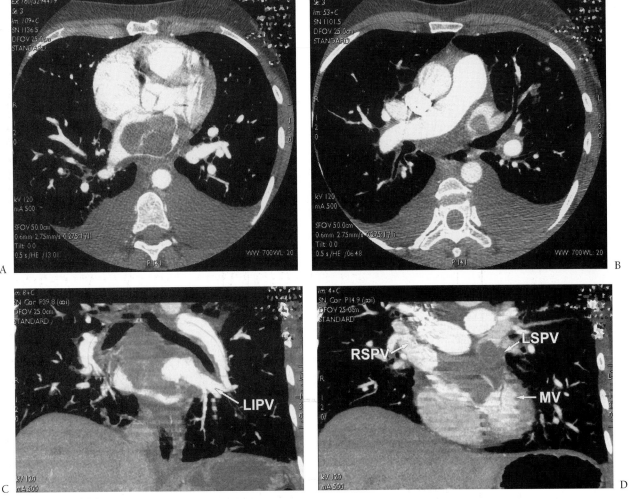

Figure 64-2. Selected cuts of a cardiac gated thoracic computed tomography scan demonstrating this large angiosarcoma arising from the left atrial wall. **(A)** Neoplasm filling approximately 80% of the left atrial volume. **(B)** Tumor extension into the left superior pulmonary veins. **(C, D)** Saggital and coronal views, respectively, each showing extension into the pulmonary veins. (LIPV = left inferior pulmonary vein; LSPV = left right superior pulmonary vein; MV = mitral valve; RSPV = right superior pulmonary vein.)

Primary Malignant Cardiac Neoplasms

Primary cardiac malignancies are rare and almost always a type of sarcoma. In order of decreasing frequency, the types include angiosarcoma (Fig. 64-2), rhabdomyosarcoma, malignant mesothelioma, and fibrosarcoma. They can arise in any location, and are often disseminated widely at the time of diagnosis. Presenting symptoms include congestive heart failure and arrhythmias. The preoperative workup includes a search for extracardiac spread. Operative therapy is reserved for those in whom metastases are absent, and some centers advocate adjuvant chemotherapy. If tumors are not resectable, chemotherapy and radiation therapy may be considered.

Angiosarcomas are more often located on the right. At the time of presentation, these tumors are often quite advanced in stage, with metastasis most frequently to lung, liver, and brain. Prognosis is poor, with median survival rates of <1 year without resection. Surgical intervention is typically done to establish diagnosis and provide palliation. The therapy often consists in tumor debulking, and patients typically do not obtain long-term benefit.

Rhabdomyosarcomas are often multiple and involve valvular structures. Like angiosarcomas, surgery is considered if the tumor is small and has no evidence of metastasis, but survival is usually limited.

There have been recent reports of orthotopic heart transplantation as a therapeutic option in patients with cardiac neoplasms (sarcoma, pheochromocytoma, lymphoma,

myxoma). In malignant tumors, reported median survival has been 12 months. However, this remains a controversial option, given the scarcity of donor organs, the need for rapid treatment in patients after presentation, and, finally, the unknown effect of immunosuppression on future malignant and metastatic potential.

Metastatic Cardiac Neoplasms

Metastatic tumors typically involve the pericardium, followed by epicardial, myocardial, and endocardial involvement in decreasing frequency. The mode of metastasis is dependent on primary tumor. Melanoma, sarcoma, and pulmonary

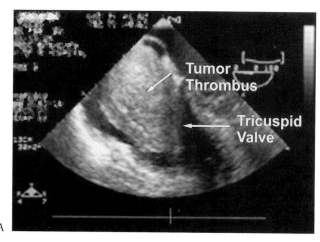
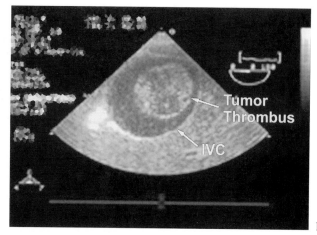

Figure 64-3. Two cuts of a transesophageal echocardiogram of a renal cell carcinoma with tumor thrombus extension into the right atrium. **(A)** Tumor thrombus extending up the inferior vena cava (IVC). **(B)** Tumor thrombus encroaching onto the tricuspid valve.

malignancies spread by hematogenous routes. Direct extension is frequently seen in association with pulmonary, breast, thymic, and esophageal cancers.

Symptoms occur infrequently in metastasis, but when they do occur, they usually result from pericardial effusions. The therapy in this setting is a palliative subxiphoid pericardial drainage procedure. This procedure often results in durable symptomatic relief. Some authors advocate a formal "pericardial window" procedure to allow drainage into the left chest. We believe that this approach is not significantly different from simple subxiphoid drainage because the left lung often adheres to the "window," thus eliminating the possibility of continuous drainage of pericardial fluid into the left chest. Moreover, this procedure may require general anesthesia (with double-lumen intubation), whereas a subxiphoid approach can be performed under local anesthesia.

Renal Cell Carcinomas

Renal cell carcinomas (hypernephromas) are an important group of metastatic tumors to the heart. About 5% of all hypernephromas present with direct vena caval extension to the right atrium (Fig. 64-3A). In such cases, symptoms of caval obstruction, including lower body anasarca, gastrointestinal intolerance, and ascites predominate. If complete resection is performed and there is an absence of distant metastasis, 5-year survival can be 75%. Other tumors that extend from the abdomen into the right atrium

include hepatic, adrenal, and gynecologic tumors.

Our approach to these tumors is a multidisciplinary one with urologists or surgical oncologists. Preoperative workup includes chest, abdomen, and pelvic CT scanning, transesophageal echocardiography, and left and right heart catheterization in selected patients. Tumors that are confined to Gerota's fascia with extension into the vena cava or right atrium without regional lymph node or distant metastasis have the best prognosis, but only distant metastasis is an absolute contraindication to surgery.

The patients are prepared and draped from the neck to the upper thighs. The abdominal team starts with an exploratory laparotomy and mobilization of the kidney. After the kidney is mobilized and the retroperitoneum is hemostatic, a median sternotomy is performed and the patient is placed on cardiopulmonary bypass. The patient is cooled to 18°C, and neuroprotective agents (Solu-Medrol, pentobarbital, and mannitol) are administered. The ascending aorta is cross-clamped, and cardioplegia is delivered in an antegrade manner. Bypass is discontinued, and the right atrium is incised with an extension down to the inferior vena cava. We typically do not use adjunctive retrograde cerebral perfusion because resection of the tumor is accomplished usually in <20 minutes. In a combined fashion, the abdominal and thoracic teams resect all tumor and thrombus. Bypass is then initiated, the cross-clamp is removed, and the patient is then rewarmed. The incisions in the vena cava and right atrium are closed. After ade-

quate rewarming, the patient is weaned from bypass.

Summary

Operative therapy of cardiac neoplasms generally comprises a small portion of all cardiothoracic surgical practice. These pathologic entities often require considerable clinical judgment for both diagnosis and treatment. However, because a significant percentage of these tumors can be treated with good results, they often provide surgeons a chance to dramatically alleviate symptoms in patients debilitated by these neoplasms.

SUGGESTED READING

Bissada NK, Yakout HH, Babanouri A, et al. Long term experience with management of renal cell carcinoma involving the inferior vena cava. Urology 2003;61:89.

Chitwood WR Jr. Cardiac neoplasms: Current diagnosis, pathology and therapy. J Card Surg 1988;3:119.

Gowdamarajan A, Micheler RE. Therapy for primary cardiac tumors: Is there a role for heart transplantation. Curr Opin Cardiol 2000;15: 121.

McAllister HA Jr, Fenoglio JJ Jr. Tumors of the Cardiovascular System. In Hartman WH, Cowan WR (eds), Atlas of Tumor Pathology (2nd series, fascicle 15). Washington DC: Armed Forces Institute of Pathology, 1978.

Miralles A, Bracamonte MD, Soncul H, et al. Cardiac tumors: Clinical experience and surgical results in 74 patients. Ann Thorac Surg 1991;52:886.

Orringer MB, Sisson JC, Glazer G, et al. Surgical treatment of cardiac pheochromocytomas. J. Thorac Cardiovasc Surg 1985;89:753.

Prager RL, Dean RH, Turner B. Surgical approach to intracardiac renal cell carcinoma. Ann Thorac Surg 1982;33:74.

Reardon MJ, Smythe WR. Cardiac Neoplasms. In Cohn LH, Edmunds LH (eds), Cardiac Surgery of the Adult. New York.McGraw-Hill, 2003;1373.

Reynen K. Cardiac myxomas. N Engl J Med 1995; 333:1610.

Shahian DM. Papillary fibroelastomas. Semin Thorac Cardiovasc Surg 2000;12:101.

Spotnitz WD, Blow O. Cardiac tumors. In Kaiser LR, Kron IL, Spray TL (eds), Mastery of Cardiothoracic Surgery. New York: Lippincott-Raven, 1998;565.

Vander Salm TJ. Unusual primary tumors of the heart. Semin Thorac Cardiovasc Surg 2000, 12:89.

EDITOR'S COMMENTS

Cardiac tumors are a relatively unusual condition in cardiac surgery, and therefore this chapter, by definition, is an overview. It is quite complete, and the approach is a rational one. We have a great deal of experience basically with two of these areas: the myxoma and the renal cell carcinoma with caval involvement. Our approach to the myxoma is very similar to that of the Michigan group. We rarely use a right atrial approach, however, and believe that the majority of the left-sided tumors can be taken down through the left atrium including the stalk. The authors are quite right to focus on the no-touch technique. These tumors can embolize and can be a disaster if they do.

We agree entirely with their approach to hypernephromas. We have seen many tumors confined to the cava below the diaphragm where the tumor can be removed without circulatory arrest. However, short-term arrest is extremely helpful in tumors involving the right atrium. This is a very effective therapy for these patients, with often long-term survival.

I.L.K.

65

Acute Pulmonary Embolus

Thoralf M. Sundt

It is ironic that the heart-lung machine is rarely used today in treatment of the very condition that stimulated its creation: acute pulmonary embolism. Dr. Gibbon was inspired to his life's work as a research resident at the Massachusetts General Hospital in 1931 as he sat at the bedside of a young woman dying of a massive pulmonary embolism. Have we wrongfully relinquished this part of our surgical heritage?

Acute pulmonary embolism is a remarkably common phenomenon, particularly among hospitalized individuals. The majority of acute pulmonary emboli results in little morbidity, and most are likely entirely unrecognized. Massive pulmonary embolism, however, may lead to hemodynamic collapse and death via a combination of mechanical obstruction of central right ventricular outflow and a peripheral vasospastic response in the remaining unobstructed vasculature. Although such massive emboli represent a relatively small proportion of acute events, they account for significant mortality and morbidity each year by virtue of the frequency with which pulmonary embolism occurs.

Unfortunately, surgical embolectomy is seldom even entertained as an option in the management of these patients. The only mention of surgical embolectomy in the American College of Chest Physicians (ACCP) Consensus Committee on Pulmonary Embolism in their 1996 Special Report on the Management of Venous Thromboembolic Disease reads as follows: "The selection of intravenous thrombolytic therapy, reduced-dose thrombolytic therapy . . ., open embolectomy, catheter tip embolectomy, or catheter-tip fragmentation depends upon the experience of the physician and the availability of the procedure." The 1998 update of this report mentions surgery not at all! The guidelines of the British Thoracic Society published in 2003 discuss thrombolysis and "invasive approaches (thrombus fragmentation and IVC filter insertion)" as options for the management of massive pulmonary embolism, but dismiss surgical embolectomy out of hand as an option few centers can offer. Indeed in 1989, the *British Journal of Hospital Medicine* published a vigorous debate as to whether there is *any* place for surgical embolectomy in the management of acute pulmonary embolism.

Why is this so? Apart from logistical issues regarding the availability of surgical centers with on-site cardiac surgical support, published mortality rates for acute pulmonary embolectomy have ranged from 20% to 60%, making it difficult to argue that the surgical results were any better than the natural history. A more charitable view recognizes that the condition of the patient prior to the surgical procedure has a profound effect on operative results. It will surprise no surgeon that preoperative cardiac arrest doubles the mortality rate. Similarly, the time interval between diagnosis and operation has a profound effect on surgical risk. This becomes, of course, a self-perpetuating problem, with many physicians, on the basis of the reported high risk of the procedure, reluctant to refer patients for surgery unless profound hemodynamic instability is present. It is only fair to add, however, that inadequate surgical embolectomy is likely a contributor to excessive mortality as well.

A critical assessment of the data reveals that there is in fact a small but definite place for surgical therapy in the management of massive pulmonary embolism. As surgeons we must take responsibility for true "around-the-clock" availability and for performing the lowest-risk procedure with the best-possible results. I believe that a small number of technical points are important for achieving the latter by both minimizing the intraoperative insult to the struggling right ventricle and optimizing the relief of outflow obstruction. This argument is supported by the results recently reported from Brigham and Women's Hospital by Aklog and colleagues in which 29 patients underwent embolectomy during a 2-year period with only 11% mortality in the first 30 days. It is my objective here to elucidate these principles.

Diagnosis

The diagnosis of acute pulmonary embolism has generally already been made by the time the surgeon has been called. Still, it is important to be familiar with the diagnostic modalities. Of course, a history consistent with massive pulmonary embolism, such as the postoperative orthopedic patient in a long-leg cast or pelvic surgical patient after prostatectomy or hysterectomy, can be quite helpful. The serum D-dimer enzyme-linked immunosorbent assay is almost universally elevated in the presence of acute pulmonary embolus and is frequently used in emergency rooms as a screening test. Nuclear scintigraphy has almost been entirely replaced by high-resolution computerized tomographic (CT) scanning. An adequate scan requires an appropriately timed bolus of contrast material, and a scan performed for other reasons may not image the pulmonary arteries adequately to rule out the diagnosis. CT scanning has the added advantage providing some information about other intrathoracic pathology such as aortic dissection, although again the timing of the bolus, if appropriate for imaging the pulmonary arteries, will not be ideal for the other structures. The place of nuclear scintigraphy lies principally with the evaluation of pregnant women and patients allergic to contrast agents or with a marginal renal function.

Perhaps the most important recent diagnostic development from a surgical standpoint is transesophageal echocardiography. This modality can identify embolic material in the pulmonary vasculature, but far more important is its ability to identify thrombus in transit, including paradoxical embolus in transit, and to permit evaluation of right ventricular dysfunction. Certainly any patient who has not had a transesophageal echo preoperatively should have one in the operating room if such is available.

Indications for Surgery

When called to evaluate the patient at the bedside for possible embolectomy it is important to remember that the pathophysiology of pulmonary hypertension in acute pulmonary embolism entails the release of serotonin from platelets, histamine from tissues, and circulating thrombin. Hypoxia due to ventilation/perfusion mismatch and increased dead space will also worsen pulmonary vasoconstriction. Therefore, one must ensure that oxygenation has been optimized before determining that a patient must go to the operating room.

It is widely accepted that systemic hypotension despite inotropic support is an indication for aggressive intervention—surgical, radiological, or lytic—as is persistent, refractory hypoxemia. As noted, however, operative risk is markedly elevated once the patient is in cardiogenic shock. Accordingly, the challenge is to stratify patients early with regard to risk of poor outcome with anticoagulant therapy alone. At the time of the 1996 ACCP Consensus Committee Special Report there remained significant disagreement regarding right ventricular dysfunction as an indication for intervention. It is increasingly recognized today, however, that right ventricular dysfunction is a harbinger of hemodynamic decompensation, an event that may unfold quite precipitously, abruptly closing the window of opportunity on a patient that has been otherwise "holding on" for several hours.

For patients not requiring surgical intervention, heparin is of course the cornerstone of therapy. Individuals with heparin-induced thrombocytopenia may require the use of a hirudin analogue. In either case oral warfarin will be indicated for 3 to 6 months.

Thrombolytics have taken center stage in the aggressive treatment of the unstable patient. This is in part due to their wide availability and the familiarity many physicians have with their use in the context of treating acute coronary syndromes. Thrombolytics are not without risk, however. In the International Cooperative PE Registry the risk of cerebral events with thrombolytics was 3%. Thabut's meta-analysis of thrombolytic studies reported in 2002 found no improvement in mortality rate when thrombolytics were used in unselected patients as compared with heparin but an almost twofold increased risk of hemorrhage (risk ratio 1.76, confidence interval 1.04 to 2.98).

Catheter embolectomy is another option. Endovascular techniques include clot fragmentation, clot aspiration, and rheolytic therapy. The mortality rate associated with these interventions, however, has been 25% to 30%. Not surprisingly, they have not caught on.

It is our view that surgical intervention performed before hemodynamic collapse has an operative risk no higher than that of thrombolytic therapy in most cases. Surgery is clearly the option of choice when there is clot in transit present in the right atrium or, even more compelling, trapped in a patent foramen ovale. Operative intervention may be contraindicated, however, in the patient in full arrest who cannot be pharmacologically resuscitated. There has been some experience with the institution of percutaneous extracorporeal membrane oxygenation in this subset of patients, with anecdotal survivors; however, this is far from the standard of care. In addition, the group from Brigham and Women's hospital suggested that the very elderly (>80 years of age) are also poor candidates for operation.

Anatomic Considerations

The anatomy of the pulmonary vasculature should be familiar to all cardiothoracic surgeons. What may be less well appreciated, however, is the remarkable access available to the lobar vessels via median sternotomy. All lobar and segmental vessels can be accessed via incisions in the pulmonary arteries from within the pericardial space as one would during pulmonary thromboendarterectomy. This is an important point because it has been my experience that a true saddle embolus lodged at the pulmonary bifurcation without distal fragments is relatively uncommon. More often, the embolic material has passed out the main pulmonary vessels and is impacted in the orifices of the lobar vessels.

Operative Procedure

Pulmonary embolectomy is accomplished on normothermic cardiopulmonary bypass without cardioplegic arrest to minimize further insult to the right ventricle and to permit complete removal of thrombus bilaterally under direct vision. There are some older reports of pulmonary embolectomy under simple inflow occlusion, and this remains an option if cardiopulmonary bypass is unavailable: however a much more complete job can be performed with the aid of the pump without risking hypoperfusion of end organs during the procedure. The pump run is invariably quite brief.

Once the decision has been made to proceed with surgical intervention, the patient should be expeditiously transported to the operating room. Anesthetic monitoring includes an arterial blood pressure line. An internal jugular introducer should be placed, but insertion of a pulmonary artery catheter at the beginning of the case should be avoided. Intraoperative transesophageal echocardiography is a routine in our institution and greatly facilitates intraoperative decision-making particularly with regard to exploration of the right atrium and evaluation for clot in transit.

The groin vessels should be prepped into the field in case postoperative extracorporeal membrane oxygenation is necessary. We prefer a full sternotomy to permit complete inspection of the right atrium. Bicaval cannulation will permit exploration of the right atrium if necessary. Of note, on more than one occasion, I have observed poor venous return from the inferior vena cava line only to find clot in transit impacted in the cannula orifice. For this reason the superior vena cava cannula is placed first so that partial bypass may be initiated if clot is dislodged from the inferior vena cava. Jakob has even advocated routine massage of the lower extremities and abdomen and open aspiration of the inferior vena cava return with cardiotomy suckers to extract additional material in transit.

Normothermic cardiopulmonary bypass is instituted, and tapes are passed around the superior vena cava and inferior vena cava. If a patent foramen ovale or paradoxic embolus in transit has been identified by transesophageal echo, a brief episode of

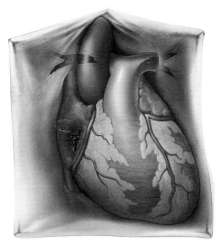

Figure 65-1. Paradoxical embolus in transit can be identified by transesophageal echo. When such is identified, the left atrium must be opened before making any attempt to remove the thrombus. This may be accomplished via simultaneous standard right and left atriotomies or, as shown here, a Dubost incision extending vertically across the right atrial free wall and Waterston's groove into the left atrium. This permits the surgeon to open the septum into the patent foramen while controlling the thrombus. This should be performed with a brief episode of cardioplegic arrest at the beginning of the procedure, providing the remainder of the bypass run for the struggling right heart to reperfuse and recover.

cardioplegic arrest should be instituted. In such instances I have opened the right and left atria via a Dubost incision through both atrial free walls and the septum to assure control of the distal clot (Fig. 65-1). After

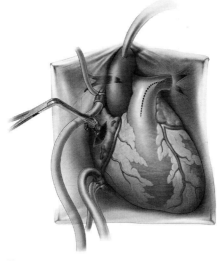

Figure 65-3. Common duct stone forceps are ideally suited for extraction of the thrombus.

the patent foramen ovale and left atrium have been closed, the cross-clamp may be removed, permitting maximum time on bypass for reperfusion.

If no patent foramen ovale is identified, it is preferable to perform the entire procedure without cardioplegic arrest. Clot in transit in the right atrium can easily be removed with the heart beating (Figs. 65-2 to 65-4). If right atrial exploration is not required, a bullet-tip sucker can be dropped into the right atrium via a stab wound with a purse-string suture. This will reduce the amount of blood passing through the right ventricle and into the pulmonary artery.

Clot in the pulmonary arteries should be removed under direct vision. This can be

accomplished via the same incisions used for the relief of chronic pulmonary thromboembolic disease during pulmonary thromboendarterectomy. It cannot, however, be accomplished solely via an incision in the main pulmonary artery.

Embolic material lodged in the left lung should be removed under direct vision via a pulmonary arteriotomy beginning in the main pulmonary artery and extending out onto the left pulmonary artery to the level of the pericardial reflection (Fig. 65-5). Via this arteriotomy, the clot can be removed with stone forceps. It is also my preference to pass soft endotracheal suction catheters down the artery orifices while massaging the lungs in an effort to remove any small clot that has migrated distally (Fig. 65-6). Balloon-tipped embolectomy catheters should not be used. The pulmonary vessels are extraordinarily fragile and rapidly taper in diameter, making rupture of the vessels a very real possibility.

The incision in the right pulmonary artery is made between the aorta and superior vena cava again as one would when doing a pulmonary thromboendarterectomy for chronic disease. With a blunt-tipped,

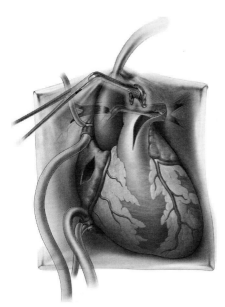

Figure 65-5. Thrombus in the left pulmonary artery is accessed via an incision beginning in the main pulmonary artery. Adequate access permitting direct visualization of the segmental vessels requires extension of the incision onto the left pulmonary artery itself. This may require division of the pericardial reflection over the ventral surface of the pulmonary artery. Some caution in the application of electrocautery is appropriate superiorly to prevent injury to the recurrent nerve. Again, common duct stone forceps are ideal for extraction of thrombus under direct vision.

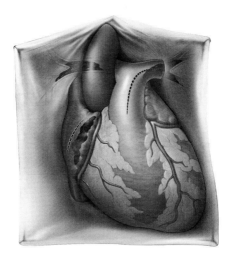

Figure 65-2. If embolus in transit is identified in the right atrium, this can be extracted via a standard right atrial incision without cardioplegic arrest. This approach provides optimal protection of the right ventricle during the procedure.

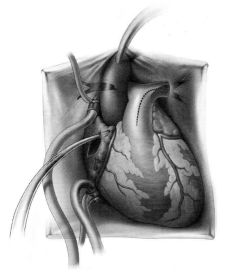

Figure 65-4. Any fragments of clot are easily extracted using a wide-mouthed sucker.

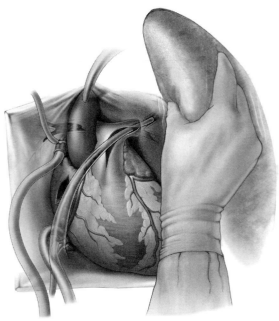

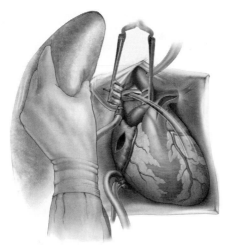

Figure 65-9.   Use of stone forceps is followed by use of suction devices.

Figure 65-6.   More-distal fragments of thrombus can be cleared with a wide-mouthed suction catheter or flexible endotracheal suction catheter. Massage of the lungs can be performed to milk thrombus proximally for removal. Balloon-tipped embolectomy catheters should not be introduced. The pulmonary vasculature is fragile, and the risk of rupture with such devices is real.

cerebellar-type retractor separating the aorta and superior vena cava, the transverse portion of the right pulmonary artery can be readily accessed (Fig. 65-7). A linear incision first in the posterior pericardium overlying the vessel and then in the vessel itself provides ready access to all of the lobar and segmental vessels. If one has not previously performed an arteriotomy such as this, one will be surprised how central the takeoff to the right upper lobe is. An incision such as this permits direct inspection of the right upper lobe branch, right middle lobe branch, and the segmental vessels to the right lower lobe. Again, clot is removed under direct vision using stone forceps (Fig. 65-8). This is followed with a flexible suction catheter and

massage of the lungs (Fig. 65-9). These arteriotomies are easily closed with running 4-0 Prolene (Fig. 65-10). Pericardial patch augmentation is seldom necessary. The patient is then weaned from cardiopulmonary bypass, with inotropic support for the right ventricle routine. A pulmonary artery thermodilution catheter can now be passed.

The final step in the procedure is insertion of an inferior vena cava filter via a purse-string suture on the right atrial appendage (Fig. 65-11). There is general agreement that an inferior vena cava filter is indicated in patients with contraindications to anticoagulation, if pulmonary embolism has recurred while on anticoagulant therapy, or if pulmonary embolism is sufficiently severe that recurrent pulmonary embolism would be life threatening. Although such filters do not prevent thrombosis and some argue are themselves a nidus of thrombosis, it is my practice to insert a filter in all patients with

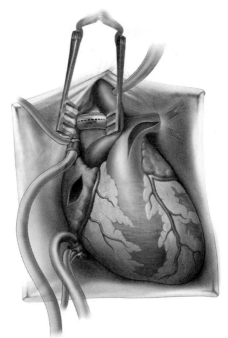

Figure 65-7.   The right pulmonary artery can be accessed directly between the aorta and superior vena cava.

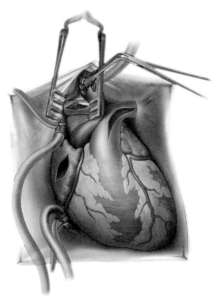

Figure 65-8.   This permits removal of thrombus again under direct vision.

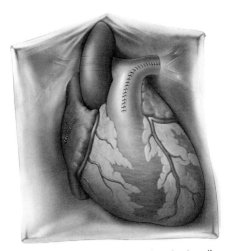

Figure 65-10.   Incisions are closed primarily.

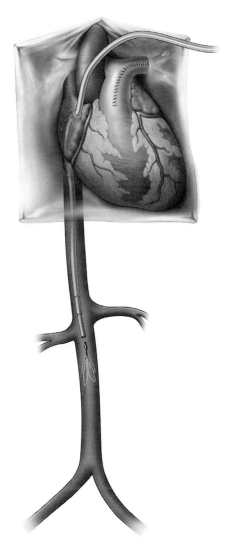

Figure 65-11. An inferior vena cava filter may be placed via a purse-string suture in the right atrial appendage.

chronic disease as well as anyone having an embolus severe enough to require emergent surgery.

Postoperative Considerations

Postoperatively, these patients frequently require significant inotropic support while the right ventricle recovers from surgery. On occasion, a temporary extracorporeal membrane oxygenation is necessary as well.

These patients should be aggressively anticoagulated postoperatively with heparin followed by warfarin for 6 months if a discrete precipitating event such as surgery or prior trauma is identifiable.

A search should certainly be made for factors predisposing these patients to pulmonary embolism, and efforts should be made toward secondary prevention. Surgeons should take part in encouraging patients in secondary prevention of modifiable factors such as obesity, tobacco abuse, use of oral contraceptives, or postmenopausal hormone replacement. If no causes are identified, consideration should be given to a search for occult malignancy. A consultation with a hematologist and systematic search for a prothrombotic state is routine. If no treatable cause is identifiable or patients have evidence of a hypercoagulable state, warfarin therapy is indicated for life.

SELECTED READING

ACCP Consensus Committee on Pulmonary Embolism. Opinions regarding the diagnosis and management of venous thromboembolic disease. Chest 1996;109:233.

ACCP Consensus Committee on Pulmonary Embolism. American College of Chest Physicians. Opinions regarding the diagnosis and management of venous thromboembolic disease. Chest 1998;113:499.

Aklog L, Williams CS, Byrne JG, et al. Acute pulmonary embolectomy: A contemporary approach. Circulation 2002;105:1416.

British Thoracic Society Standards of Care Committee Pulmonary Embolism Guideline Development Group. British Thoracic Society guidelines for the management of suspected acute pulmonary embolism. Thorax 2003;58:470.

Goldhaber SZ. Integration of catheter thrombectomy into our armamentarium to treat acute pulmonary embolism. Chest 1998;114:1237.

Goldhaber SZ, Elliott CG. Acute pulmonary embolism: Part I: Epidemiology, pathophysiology, and diagnosis. Circulation. 2003;108(22):2726.

Goldhaber SZ, Elliott CG. Acute pulmonary embolism: Part II: Risk stratification, treatment, and prevention. Circulation 2003;108:2834.

Goldhaber SZ, Visani L, De Rosa M. Acute pulmonary embolism: Clinical outcomes in the International Cooperative Pulmonary Embolism Registry [ICOPER]. Lancet 1999;353; 1386.

Jakob H, Vahl C, Lange R, et al. Modified surgical concept for fulminant pulmonary embolism. Eur J Cardiothorac Surg 1995;9:557.

Kucher N, Luder CM, Dornhofer T, et al. Novel management strategy for patients with suspected pulmonary embolism. Eur Heart J 2003;24:366.

Thabut G, Thabut D, Myers RP, et al. Thrombolytic therapy of pulmonary embolism: A meta-analysis. J Am Coll Cardiol 2002;40:1660.

Wood KE. Major pulmonary embolism: Review of a pathophysiologic approach to the golden hour of hemodynamically significant pulmonary embolism. Chest 2002;121:877.

EDITOR'S COMMENTS

I could not agree more with Sundt's approach to acute pulmonary embolus. I believe he covers all the high points. Pulmonary embolectomy has been thought of as a procedure of last resort, and as such the surgical results have been terrible. Once a patient arrests and develops cerebral anoxia the game is over. We agree entirely with Sundt that right ventricular dysfunction is a precursor to sudden death. A patient who is found by echo to have right ventricular dysfunction, a large pulmonary embolus, and hypotension likely does not have time or cardiac reserve for thrombolytic therapy or other nonsurgical approaches. This is a specific indication for a patient requiring cardiopulmonary bypass so the clot can be removed. A patient who can get to the operating room alive likely will survive pulmonary embolectomy. If the patient arrests prior to surgery, then the results are dismal.

From a surgical standpoint we agree entirely with Sundt. We agree embolectomy catheter should not be used because of the risk of perforation. We agree with the type of forceps he uses and have also opened both pleura to be able to milk the clot back from the lungs. A critical point is the use of an inferior vena cava filter right after surgery. This is important to avoid recurrent pulmonary emboli and starting the process over.

I.L.K.

66

Chronic Pulmonary Thromboembolism and Pulmonary Thromboendarterectomy

Michael M. Madani and Stuart W. Jamieson

Pulmonary thromboendarterectomy (PTE) for the treatment of chronic thromboembolic pulmonary hypertension (CTEPH) is an uncommon surgical procedure; however, it is the only curative option that provides immediate and permanent cure for this devastating disease. The condition is remarkably underdiagnosed, and as a result the procedure is uncommonly applied. Patients with chronic pulmonary hypertension secondary to thromboembolic disease may present with a variety of debilitating cardiopulmonary symptoms. However, once it is diagnosed, there is no curative role for medical management, and surgical removal of the thromboembolic material is the only therapeutic option.

The exact incidence of pulmonary embolism is unknown, but there are some valid estimates. Acute pulmonary embolism is the third-most-common cause of death (after heart disease and cancer). Approximately 75% of autopsy-proven pulmonary embolisms (PEs) are not detected clinically. It is estimated that pulmonary embolism results in approximately 650,000 symptomatic episodes in the United States yearly. The disease is particularly common in hospitalized elderly patients. Of hospitalized patients who develop PE, 12% to 21% will die in the hospital, and another 24% to 39% die within 12 months. Thus, approximately 36% to 60% of the patients who survive the initial episode live beyond 12 months, and they may present later in life with a wide variety of symptoms.

The mainstay of treatment of patients with deep vein thrombosis (DVT) and acute PE is medical management. In general, cardiac surgeons may rarely intervene in hospitalized patients who suffer a massive embolus that causes life-threatening acute right heart failure and severe hemodynamic compromise. In contrast, the only treatment for patients with chronic pulmonary thromboembolic disease is the surgical removal of the disease by means of pulmonary thromboendarterectomy. Medical management in these patients is only palliative, and surgery by means of transplantation is an inappropriate use of resources with less-than-satisfactory results.

The prognosis for patients with pulmonary hypertension is poor, and it is worse for those who do not have intracardiac shunts. Thus, patients with primary pulmonary hypertension and those with pulmonary hypertension secondary to pulmonary emboli fall into a higher-risk category than those with Eisenmenger syndrome and have a higher mortality rate. In fact, once the mean pulmonary pressure in patients with thromboembolic disease reaches ≥ 50 mm Hg, the 3-year mortality approaches 90%.

Surgical preferences are dependent on both the principal disease process and the reversibility of the pulmonary hypertension. With the exception of thromboembolic pulmonary hypertension, lung transplantation is the only effective therapy for patients with pulmonary hypertension, that is, when the disease reaches the end stage. Although it has been performed less frequently in the last few years, pulmonary transplantation is still used in some centers as the treatment of choice for patients with thromboembolic disease. However, a true assessment of the effectiveness of any therapy should take into account the total mortality after the patient has been accepted and put on the waiting list. Thus, the mortality for transplantation (and especially double-lung or heart-lung transplantation) as a therapeutic strategy is much higher than is generally appreciated because of the significant loss of patients awaiting donors. Bearing in mind, in addition, the long-term use of immunosuppressants with their associated side effects, the higher operative morbidity and mortality, the inferior prognosis even after successful transplantation, and the long waiting period, one can see that transplantation is clearly an inferior alternative to pulmonary thromboendarterectomy and should be considered an inappropriate and outdated form of therapy.

Incidence

Determining an accurate incidence of CTEPH is almost impracticable. Most patients with this condition do not have a clear history of DVT or pulmonary embolism. Furthermore, the majority (about 75%) of autopsy-proven pulmonary embolisms are not clinically diagnosed. This makes the exact incidence of this disease even more difficult to determine than that of acute pulmonary embolism. A conservative estimate only considers patients who do have an acute pulmonary embolism and survive the episode. There are approximately 500,000 such patients every year in the United States. The incidence of chronic thrombotic occlusion in the population depends on what proportion of patients fail to resolve acute embolic material. Recent studies have shown that of these patients, up to 3.1% will have symptomatic CTEPH at 1 year and 3.8% will have it at 2 years. If these figures are correct, and if one counts only patients with symptomatic acute pulmonary emboli, approximately 15,000 to 19,000 individuals would progress to chronic thromboembolic pulmonary hypertension in the United States each year. However, because many (if not most) patients diagnosed with chronic thromboembolic disease have no antecedent history of acute embolism, the true incidence of this disorder is much higher.

Regardless of the exact incidence or the circumstances, it is clear that acute embolism and its chronic relation, fixed chronic thromboembolic occlusive disease, are both much more common than generally appreciated and are seriously underdiagnosed. Calculations extrapolated from mortality rates and the random incidence of major thrombotic occlusion found at autopsy support a postulate that more than 100,000 people in the United States currently have pulmonary hypertension that could be relieved by operation.

Pathology and Pathophysiology

Most cases of chronic pulmonary emboli arise from previous acute embolic episodes, even though the majority of individuals with chronic pulmonary thromboembolic disease are unaware of a past thromboembolic event and give no history of deep venous thrombosis. Why some patients have unresolved emboli is not certain, but a variety of factors must play a role, alone or in combination.

For instance, the volume of acute embolic material may simply overwhelm the lytic mechanisms, and the total occlusion of a major arterial branch may prevent lytic material from reaching, and therefore dissolving, the embolus completely. Furthermore, repetitive emboli may not be able to be resolved. Other causes may relate to the fact that the emboli may be made of substances that cannot be resolved by normal mechanisms (already well-organized fibrous thrombus, fat, or tumor), and the lytic mechanisms themselves may be abnormal. In some groups, patients may actually have a propensity for thrombus or a hypercoaguable state.

In general, after the clot becomes wedged in the pulmonary artery, one of two processes occurs: (1) the clot may proceed to canalization, producing multiple small endothelialized channels separated by fibrous septa (i.e., bands and webs) or (2) it may continue to form to a solid mass of dense, fibrous connective tissue, without canalization, totally obstructing the arterial lumen.

In addition, chronic indwelling central venous catheters and pacemaker leads are sometimes associated with pulmonary emboli. Less frequent causes include tumor emboli; tumor fragments from stomach, breast, and kidney malignancies have also been demonstrated to cause chronic pulmonary arterial occlusion. Right atrial myxomas may also fragment and embolize.

Whatever the predisposing factors to residual thrombus within the vessels, the genesis of the resultant pulmonary vascular hypertension is more complex than appreciated. With the passage of time, the increased pressure and flow as a result of redirected pulmonary blood flow in the previously normal pulmonary vascular bed can create a vasculopathy in the small precapillary blood vessels similar to the Eisenmenger syndrome.

Factors other than the simple hemodynamic consequences of redirected blood flow are probably also involved in this process. For example, after a pneumonectomy, 100% of the right ventricular output flows to one lung, yet little increase in pulmonary pressure occurs, even with follow-up to more than a decade. In patients with thromboembolic disease, however, we frequently detect pulmonary hypertension even when <50% of the vascular bed is occluded by thrombus, and not uncommonly as early as a few months to 1 year after the initial episode. It thus appears that an array of sympathetic neural connections and hormonal changes may be responsible for setting off pulmonary hypertension in the initially unaffected pulmonary vascular bed. This process can occur with the initial occlusion in either the same or the contralateral lung.

Regardless of the cause, the evolution of pulmonary hypertension as a result of changes in the previously unobstructed bed is serious because this process may lead to an inoperable situation. Accordingly, with our accumulating experience in patients with thrombotic pulmonary hypertension and superior surgical outcomes, we have increasingly been inclined toward early operation so as to avoid these changes.

Clinical Presentation

There are no specific signs or symptoms associated with pulmonary hypertension as a result of chronic pulmonary thromboembolism, which explains the degree of underdiagnosis with this condition. The most common symptom associated with thromboembolic pulmonary hypertension, as with all other causes of pulmonary hypertension, is exertional dyspnea. Generally this dyspnea is out of proportion to any abnormalities found on clinical examination. Like complaints of easy fatigability, dyspnea that initially occurs only with exertion is often attributed to anxiety or being "out of shape." In patients with more advanced disease and higher pulmonary artery pressures, syncope or presyncope (light-headedness during exertion) is another common symptom.

Nonspecific chest pains occur in approximately 50% of patients with more severe pulmonary hypertension. Hemoptysis can occur in all forms of pulmonary hypertension, and probably results from abnormally dilated vessels distended by increased intravascular pressures. Peripheral edema, early satiety, and epigastric or right upper quadrant fullness or discomfort may develop as the right heart fails (cor pulmonale). Some patients with chronic pulmonary thromboembolic disease present after a small acute pulmonary embolus that may produce acute symptoms of right heart failure. A careful history brings out symptoms of dyspnea on minimal exertion, easy fatigability, diminishing activities, and episodes of angina-like pain or light-headedness. Further examination reveals the signs of pulmonary hypertension.

The physical signs of pulmonary hypertension are the same no matter what the underlying pathophysiology. Initially the jugular venous pulse is characterized by a large A wave. As the right heart fails, the V wave becomes predominant. The right ventricle is usually palpable near the lower left sternal border, and pulmonary valve closure may be audible in the second intercostal space. Occasional patients with advanced disease are hypoxic and slightly cyanotic. Clubbing is an uncommon finding.

As the right heart fails, a right atrial gallop usually is present, and tricuspid insufficiency develops. Because of the large pressure gradient across the tricuspid valve in pulmonary hypertension, the murmur is high pitched and may not exhibit respiratory variation. These findings are quite different from those usually observed in tricuspid valvular disease. A murmur of pulmonic regurgitation may also be detected.

Diagnostic Modalities

To ensure diagnosis in patients with chronic pulmonary thromboembolism, a standardized evaluation is recommended for all

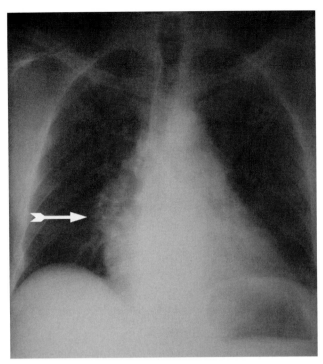

Figure 66-1.   Chest radiograph in a patient with chronic thromboembolic pulmonary hypertension. Note the bilaterally enlarged hilar shadows, prominent right atrium and superior vena cava, and small left atrium.

patients who present with unexplained pulmonary hypertension. This workup includes a chest radiograph. One should bear in mind that a large number of patients might present with a relatively normal chest radiograph, even in the setting of high degrees of pulmonary hypertension. The radiographic findings differ in patients with various degrees of pulmonary hypertension; however, an abnormal chest x-ray may show either apparent vessel cutoffs of the lobar or segmental pulmonary arteries, or regions of oligemia suggesting vascular occlusion. Central pulmonary arteries are also typically enlarged, and the right ventricle may be enlarged without enlargement of the left atrium or ventricle (Fig. 66-1).

The ventilation-perfusion lung scan is the essential test for establishing the diagnosis of unresolved pulmonary thromboembolism. An entirely normal lung scan excludes the diagnosis of both acute and chronic, unresolved thromboembolism. The usual lung scan pattern in most patients with pulmonary hypertension either is relatively normal or shows a diffuse nonuniform perfusion. When subsegmental or larger perfusion defects are noted on the scan, even when matched with ventilatory defects, pulmonary angiography is appropriate to confirm or rule out thromboembolic disease.

Pulmonary angiography is the gold standard for the diagnosis of chronic pulmonary

thromboembolism. In addition to identifying the level of obstruction and providing a surgical roadmap, right heart catheterization can be performed in the same setting, measuring right heart parameters and evaluating the degree of pulmonary hyper-

tension and pulmonary vascular resistance (PVR). Organized thromboembolic lesions do not have the appearance of the intravascular filling defects seen with acute pulmonary emboli, and experience is essential for the proper interpretation of pulmonary angiograms in patients with unresolved, chronic embolic disease. Typically, organized thrombi appear as unusual filling defects, webs, or bands or as completely thrombosed vessels that may resemble congenital absence of the vessel (Fig. 66-2). Organized material along a vascular wall of a recanalized vessel produces a scalloped or serrated luminal edge. Because of both vessel-wall thickening and dilation of proximal vessels, the contrast-filled lumen may appear relatively normal in diameter. Distal vessels demonstrate the rapid tapering and pruning characteristic of pulmonary hypertension.

In recent years, higher-resolution computed tomography (CT) scans of the chest have been used more frequently in the diagnosis of pulmonary embolism. The presence of large clots in lobar or segmental vessels generally confirms the diagnosis. In addition, in rare situations where occlusion of main pulmonary arteries is present or there are concerns of external compression, CT scans can helpful to differentiate thromboembolic disease from other causes of pulmonary vascular obstruction such as mediastinal fibrosis, lymph nodes, and tumors.

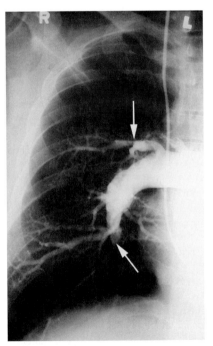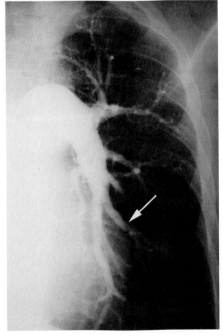

Figure 66-2.   Right and left pulmonary angiograms demonstrate intraluminal filling defects, abrupt cutoffs of branches, and bands (*white arrows*). Note lack of filling to the periphery.

Pulmonary angiography is the gold standard for the diagnosis and for planning the operative approach. In addition to pulmonary angiography, patients older than 45 years of age undergo coronary arteriography and other cardiac investigation as necessary. If significant disease is found, additional cardiac surgery is performed at the time of pulmonary thromboendarterectomy.

Pulmonary angioscopy may be performed in patients where the differentiation between primary pulmonary hypertension and distal small-vessel pulmonary thromboembolic disease is difficult. The pulmonary angioscope is a fiberoptic telescope that is placed through a central line into the pulmonary artery. The tip contains a balloon that is then filled with saline and pushed against the vessel wall. A bloodless field can thus be obtained to view the pulmonary artery wall. The classic appearance of chronic pulmonary thromboembolic disease by angioscopy consists of intimal thickening, with intimal irregularity and scarring, and webs across small vessels. The presence of embolic disease, occlusion of vessels, or thrombotic material is diagnostic.

Alternative Treatments

Medical therapy for CTEPH is of limited value and is palliative at best. There are a wide variety of pharmacologic agents in recent use for the treatment of primary pulmonary hypertension. These include calcium-channel blockers such as diltiazem or nifedipine, prostacyclins such as epoprostenol (Flolan, Remodulin), prostacyclin analogues, endothelin-receptor antagonists (Tracleer), and nitric oxide. However, thromboembolic disease represents a mechanical obstruction that is not amenable to drug therapy.

Right ventricular failure is generally treated with diuretics and vasodilators, and although some improvement may result, the effect is generally transient because the failure will not resolve until the obstruction is removed. Similarly, the prognosis is unaffected by medical therapy, which should be regarded as only supportive. However, because of the bronchial circulation, pulmonary embolization seldom results in tissue necrosis. Surgical endarterectomy therefore will allow distal pulmonary tissue to be used once more in gas exchange.

Chronic anticoagulation represents the mainstay of the medical regimen. Anticoagulation is primarily used to prevent future embolic episodes, but it also serves to limit the development of thrombus in regions of low flow within the pulmonary vasculature. Inferior vena caval filters are used routinely to prevent recurrent embolization. If caval filtration and anticoagulation fail to prevent recurrent emboli, immediate thrombolysis may be beneficial, but lytic agents are incapable of altering the chronic component of the disease.

The only other surgical alternative for these patients is transplantation. However, we consider transplantation to be inappropriate for treatment of this disease and believe it is an outdated form of surgical management for CTEPH. Considering the mortality and morbidity rates of patients on the waiting list, the higher risk of the operation, and the lower survival rate (approximately 80% at 1 year at experienced centers for transplantation vs. 95% for pulmonary endarterectomy), we believe that pulmonary thromboendarterectomy is the superior choice. Furthermore, pulmonary endarterectomy appears to be permanently curative, and the issues of a continuing risk of rejection and immunosuppression are not present.

Pulmonary Thromboendarterectomy

The first successful pulmonary "thromboendarterectomy" was performed by Allison in 1960, and took place in a patient who 12 days before had a thigh injury that had led to a pulmonary embolus. Allison used a sternotomy and surface hypothermia, but only fresh clots were removed. Since then, there have been many occasional reports of the surgical treatment of chronic pulmonary thromboembolism, but most of the surgical experience in pulmonary endarterectomy has been reported from the University of California, San Diego (UCSD), Medical Center. Braunwald commenced the UCSD experience with this operation in 1970, which now totals >2,000 cases. The operation to be described, using deep hypothermia and circulatory arrest, is now our standard procedure.

Indications

When the diagnosis of thromboembolic pulmonary hypertension has been firmly established, the decision for operation is made based on the severity of symptoms and the general condition of the patient. Early in the pulmonary endarterectomy experience, Moser and colleagues pointed out that there were three major reasons for considering thromboendarterectomy: hemodynamic, alveolo-respiratory, and prophylactic. The hemodynamic goal is to prevent or ameliorate right ventricular compromise caused by pulmonary hypertension. The respiratory objective is to improve respiratory function by removing a large ventilated but unperfused physiologic dead space. The prophylactic goal is to prevent progressive right ventricular dysfunction or retrograde extension of the obstruction, which might result in further cardiorespiratory deterioration or death. Our subsequent experience has added another prophylactic goal: the prevention of secondary arteriopathic changes in the remaining patent vessels.

The ages of the patients in our series have ranged from 7 to 86 years. A typical patient will have a severely elevated PVR level at rest, the absence of significant comorbid disease that is unrelated to right heart failure, and the appearances of chronic thrombi on angiogram that appear to be in balance with the measured PVR level. Exceptions to this general rule, of course, occur.

Although most patients have a PVR level in the range of 800 dynes/sec/cm^{-5} and pulmonary artery pressures less than systemic, the hypertrophy of the right ventricle that occurs over time makes pulmonary hypertension to suprasystemic levels possible. Therefore many patients (perhaps 20% in our practice) have a level of PVR in excess of 1,000 dynes/sec/cm^{-5} and suprasystemic pulmonary artery pressures. There is no upper limit of PVR level, pulmonary artery pressure, or degree of right ventricular dysfunction that excludes patients from operation.

We have become increasingly aware of the changes that can occur in the remaining patent (unaffected by clot) pulmonary vascular bed subjected to the higher pressures and flow that result from obstruction in other areas. Therefore, with the increasing experience and safety of the operation, we are tending to offer surgery to symptomatic patients whenever the angiogram demonstrates thromboembolic disease. A rare patient might have a PVR level that is normal at rest and elevated with minimal exercise. This is usually a young patient with total unilateral pulmonary artery occlusion and unacceptable exertional dyspnea because of an elevation in dead-space ventilation. Operation in this circumstance is performed to reperfuse lung tissue, re-establish a more normal ventilation/perfusion relationship (thereby reducing minute ventilatory requirements during rest and exercise), and preserve the integrity of the contralateral circulation. If one has not been previously implanted, an inferior vena caval filter is routinely placed several days before the operation.

Operative Techniques

Principles

Although the essential techniques of pulmonary thromboendarterectomy are quite similar to those of other open-heart operations, there are several guiding principles for this procedure. The disease is almost always bilateral, although the volume of chronic thromboembolic material may vary significantly between the two lungs. Furthermore, for pulmonary hypertension to be a major factor, both pulmonary arteries must be substantially involved. The surgery is therefore always bilateral. The only reasonable approach to both pulmonary arteries is through a median sternotomy incision. Historically, there were many reports of unilateral operation, and occasionally this is still performed, in inexperienced centers, through a thoracotomy. However, the unilateral approach ignores the disease on the contralateral side, subjects the patient to hemodynamic jeopardy during the clamping of the pulmonary artery, and does not allow good visibility because of the continued presence of bronchial blood flow. In addition, collateral channels develop in chronic thrombotic hypertension not only through the bronchial arteries, but also from diaphragmatic, intercostal, and pleural vessels. The dissection of the lung in the pleural space via a thoracotomy incision can therefore be extremely bloody. The median sternotomy incision, apart from providing bilateral access, avoids entry into the pleural cavities and allows the ready institution of cardiopulmonary bypass.

Cardiopulmonary bypass is essential not only to ensure cardiovascular stability when the operation is performed, but also to allow cooling of the patient for periods of circulatory arrest. Exceptional visibility of the pulmonary vasculature is required. A bloodless field is an absolute requirement to define an adequate endarterectomy plane and to then follow the pulmonary endarterectomy specimen deep into the subsegmental vessels. Because of the copious bronchial blood flow usually present in these cases, periods of circulatory arrest are necessary to ensure perfect visibility. Again, there have been sporadic reports of the performance of this operation without circulatory arrest. However, it should be emphasized that although

endarterectomy is possible without circulatory arrest, a complete and full endarterectomy is not. We always initiate the procedure without circulatory arrest, and depending on the collateral flow, a variable amount of dissection is possible before the circulation is stopped, but never complete dissection. The circulatory arrest periods are limited to 20 minutes, with restoration of flow between each arrest. With experience, the endarterectomy usually can be performed with a single period of circulatory arrest on each side.

A true endarterectomy in the plane of the media must be accomplished. It is essential to appreciate that the removal of visible thrombus is largely incidental to this operation. Indeed, in most patients, no free thrombus is present; on initial direct examination, the pulmonary vascular bed may appear normal to an inexperienced eye. The early literature on this procedure indicates that thrombectomy was often performed without a complete endarterectomy, and in these cases the pulmonary artery pressures did not improve, often with the resultant death of the patient.

Preparation and Anesthetic Considerations

The operative preparation and anesthetic concerns are for the most part quite similar to those for any open-heart procedure. Routine monitoring for anesthetic induction includes a surface electrocardiogram, cutaneous oximetry, and radial artery pressure lines. After induction a pulmonary artery catheter and a transesophageal echocardiographic probe are also inserted. We generally include a femoral arterial line for more accurate assessment during rewarming and on discontinuation of cardiopulmonary bypass. It is quite common for these patients to develop some degree of peripheral vasoconstriction that occurs after hypothermic circulatory arrest, thereby making radial pressure readings inaccurate. The femoral line is generally removed in the intensive care unit when the two readings are correlated.

Electroencephalographic recording is routinely performed to ensure the lack of cerebral activity before circulatory arrest is induced. The patient's head is enclosed in a cooling jacket, and cerebral cooling is begun after the initiation of bypass. Temperature measurements are made of the esophagus, tympanic membrane, urinary catheter, rectum, and blood (through the Swan-Ganz catheter). If the patient's condition is stable after the induction of anesthesia, up to

500 mL of autologous whole blood is withdrawn for later use, and the volume deficit is replaced with crystalloid solution.

Operative Techniques

After a median sternotomy incision is made, the pericardium is incised longitudinally and attached to the wound edges. Typically the right heart is enlarged, with a tense right atrium and a variable degree of tricuspid regurgitation. There is usually severe right ventricular hypertrophy. These patients are generally quite sensitive to any manipulation of the heart, and with critical degrees of obstruction, the patient's condition may become quite unstable.

Anticoagulation is achieved with the use of beef-lung heparin sodium (400 units/kg, intravenously) administered to prolong the activated clotting time beyond 400 seconds. Full cardiopulmonary bypass is instituted with high ascending aortic cannulation and two caval cannulae. These cannulae must be inserted into the superior and inferior vena cavae sufficiently to enable subsequent opening of the right atrium. The heart is emptied on bypass, and a temporary pulmonary artery vent is placed in the midline of the main pulmonary artery 1 cm distal to the pulmonary valve. This will mark the beginning of the left pulmonary arteriotomy.

When cardiopulmonary bypass is initiated, surface cooling with both the head jacket and the cooling blanket is begun. The blood is cooled with the pump-oxygenator. Cooling generally takes 45 minutes to 1 hour. When ventricular fibrillation occurs, an additional vent is placed in the left atrium through the right superior pulmonary vein. This prevents atrial and ventricular distension from the large amount of bronchial arterial blood flow that is common with these patients.

Generally the primary surgeon starts the operation on the patient's left side. During the cooling period, some preliminary dissection can be performed, with full mobilization of the right pulmonary artery from the ascending aorta. The superior vena cava is also fully mobilized. The approach to the right pulmonary artery is made medial, not lateral, to the superior vena cava (Fig. 66-3). All dissection of the pulmonary arteries takes place intrapericardially, and neither pleural cavity should be entered. An incision is then made in the right pulmonary artery from beneath the ascending aorta out under the superior vena cava and entering the lower lobe branch of the pulmonary artery just after the takeoff of the middle lobe artery (Fig. 66-4). It is important that

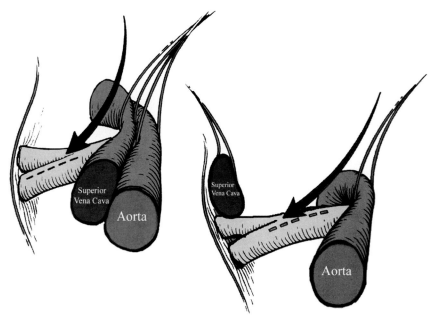

Figure 66-3. Surgical approach to the right pulmonary artery. The approach is medial to the superior vena cava, between the superior vena cava and the aorta. An approach lateral to the superior vena cava provides a restricted view.

the incision stays in the center of the vessel and continues into the lower rather than the middle lobe artery.

A modified cerebellar retractor is placed between the aorta and superior vena cava. Upon opening the pulmonary artery, a varying degree of loose thrombus may be pre-sent. The material is then removed to ensure good visualization of the vascular bed. It is most important to recognize, however, that first, an embolectomy without subsequent endarterectomy is quite ineffective regardless of the size of thromboembolic material, and second, in most patients with chronic thromboembolic hypertension, direct examination of the pulmonary vascular bed at operation generally shows no obvious embolic material. Therefore, to the inexperienced or cursory glance, the pulmonary vascular bed may well appear normal even in patients with severe chronic embolic pulmonary hypertension.

When the patient's temperature reaches 20°C, the aorta is cross-clamped and a single dose of cold cardioplegic solution (1 liter) is administered. Additional myocardial protection is obtained by the use of a cooling jacket. The entire procedure is now performed with a single aortic cross-clamp period with no further administration of cardioplegic solution.

If the bronchial circulation is not excessive, the endarterectomy plane can be found during this early dissection. However, although a small amount of dissection can be performed before the initiation of circulatory arrest, it is unwise to proceed unless perfect visibility is obtained because the development of a correct plane is essential. Recognizing the plane is perhaps the most crucial and technically challenging part of the operation.

When blood obscures direct vision of the pulmonary vascular bed, thiopental is administered (500 mg to 1 g) until the electroencephalogram becomes isoelectric. In most cases, the electroencephalogram is already isoelectric when the core temperature reaches 20°C. Circulatory arrest is then initiated, and the patient undergoes exsanguination. All monitoring lines to the patient are turned off to prevent the aspiration of air. Snares are tightened around the cannulae in the superior and inferior vena cavae. It is rare that one 20-minute period for each side is exceeded. Although retrograde cerebral perfusion has been advocated for total circulatory arrest in other procedures, it is not helpful in this operation because it does not allow a completely bloodless field, and with the short arrest times that can be achieved with experience, it is not necessary.

A microtome knife is used to develop the endarterectomy plane posteriorly because any inadvertent egress in this site could be repaired readily or simply left alone. Dissection in the correct plane is critical because if the plane is too deep, the pulmonary artery may perforate, with fatal results, and if the dissection plane is not deep enough, inadequate amounts of the chronically thromboembolic material will be removed, leaving the patient with residual pulmonary hypertension.

After the plane is correctly developed, a full-thickness layer is left in the region

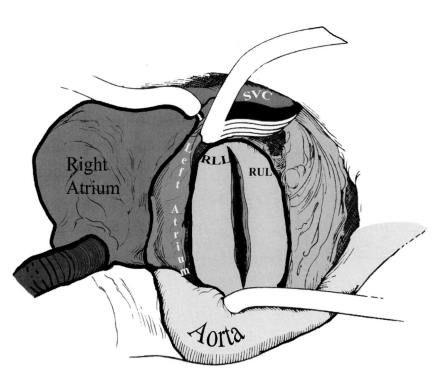

Figure 66-4. Exposure to the right pulmonary artery. Note how the incision is made between the superior vena cava (SVC) and the aorta. In addition, the right upper lobe (RUL) and the right lower lobe (RLL) takeoffs are shown.

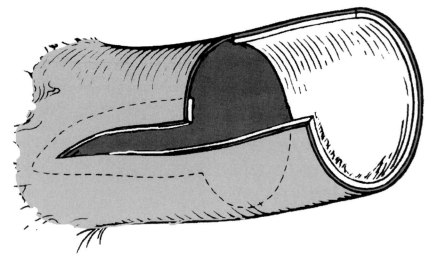

Figure 66-5. The plane of dissection is first raised posteriorly and continued toward the edge of the arteriotomy but trimmed short in the region of the incision. This results in a full-thickness artery for subsequent closure.

of the incision to ease subsequent repair (Fig. 66-5). The endarterectomy is then performed with an eversion technique. Because the vessel is everted and subsegmental branches are being worked on, a perforation here will become completely inaccessible and invisible later. This is why the absolute visualization in a completely bloodless field provided by circulatory arrest is essential. It is important that each subsegmental branch is followed and freed individually until it ends in a "tail" beyond which there is no further obstruction. Residual material should never be cut free; the entire specimen should "tail off" and come free spontaneously.

After the right-sided endarterectomy is completed, circulation is restarted, and the arteriotomy is repaired with a continuous 6-0 polypropylene suture. The hemostatic nature of this closure is aided by the nature of the initial dissection, with the full thickness of the pulmonary artery being preserved immediately adjacent to the incision.

After the completion of the repair of the right arteriotomy, the surgeon moves to the patient's right side. The pulmonary vent catheter is withdrawn, and an arteriotomy is made from the site of the pulmonary vent hole laterally to the pericardial reflection, avoiding entry into the left pleural space. Additional lateral dissection does not enhance intraluminal visibility, may endanger the left phrenic nerve, and makes subsequent repair of the left pulmonary artery more difficult (Fig. 66-6).

The left-sided dissection is virtually analogous in all respects to that accomplished on the right. The duration of circulatory arrest intervals during the performance of the

left-sided dissection is subject to the same restriction as the right.

After the completion of the endarterectomy, cardiopulmonary bypass is reinstituted and warming is commenced. If the systemic vascular resistance level is high, nitroprusside is administered to promote vasodilation and warming. The rewarming period generally takes approximately

90 minutes, but it varies according to the body mass of the patient.

The pulmonary artery is then closed, and the pulmonary vent is replaced. The heart is retracted upward and to the left, and a posterior pericardial window is generally made. The right atrium is then opened and examined. Any intra-atrial communication is closed. Although tricuspid valve regurgitation is invariable in these patients and is often severe, tricuspid valve repair is not performed. Right ventricular remodeling occurs within a few days, with the return of tricuspid competence. If other cardiac procedures are required, such as coronary artery or mitral or aortic valve surgery, these are conveniently performed during the systemic rewarming period. Myocardial cooling is discontinued after all cardiac procedures have been concluded. The left atrial vent is removed, and the vent site is repaired. All air is removed from the heart, and the aortic cross-clamp is removed.

When the patient has rewarmed, cardiopulmonary bypass is discontinued. Dopamine hydrochloride is routinely administered at renal doses, and other inotropic agents and vasodilators are titrated as necessary to sustain acceptable hemodynamics. The cardiac output is generally high, with a low systemic vascular resistance.

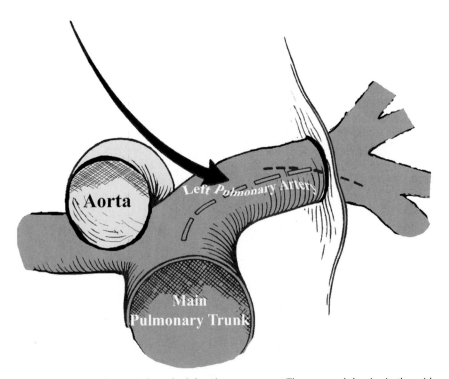

Figure 66-6. Surgical approach to the left pulmonary artery. The approach begins in the mid portion of the main artery and carried past the takeoff of the left upper lobe. The incision stays in the midline of the vessel as far as the pericardial reflection. A more distal incision provides limited view.

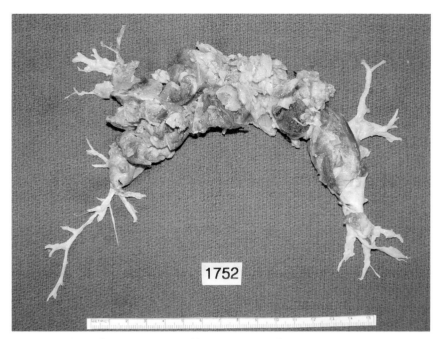

Figure 66-7. Surgical specimen removed from a patient with type I surgical classification. Note that the removal of fresh thromboembolic material leaves behind a large amount of obstructive disease.

Temporary atrial and ventricular epicardial pacing wires are placed.

Despite the duration of extracorporeal circulation, hemostasis is readily achieved, and the administration of platelets or coagulation factors is generally unnecessary. Wound closure is routine. A vigorous diuresis is usual for the next few hours, also a result of the previous systemic hypothermia.

There are four broad types of pulmonary occlusive disease related to thrombus that can be appreciated, and we use the following classification: Type I disease (approximately 20% of cases of thromboembolic pulmonary hypertension; Fig. 66-7) refers to the situation in which major vessel clot is present and readily visible on the opening of the pulmonary arteries. As mentioned earlier, all central thrombotic material has to be completely removed before the endarterectomy. In type II disease (approximately 70% of cases; Fig. 66-8), no major vessel thrombus can be appreciated. In these cases only thickened intima can be seen, occasionally with webs, and the endarterectomy plane is raised in the main, lobar, or segmental vessels. Type III disease (approximately 10% of cases; Fig. 66-9) presents the most challenging surgical situation. The disease is very distal and confined to the segmental and subsegmental branches. No occlusion of vessels can be seen initially. The endarterectomy plane must be carefully and painstakingly raised in each segmental and subsegmental branch. Type III

disease is most often associated with presumed repetitive thrombi from indwelling catheters (such as pacemaker wires) or ventriculoatrial shunts. Type IV disease (Fig. 66-10) does not represent primary thromboembolic pulmonary hypertension and is inoperable. In this entity there is intrinsic small-vessel disease, although secondary thrombus may occur as a result of stasis. Small-vessel disease may be unrelated to thromboembolic events ("primary" pulmonary hypertension) or occur in relation to thromboembolic hypertension as a result of a high-flow or high-pressure state in previously unaffected vessels similar to the generation of Eisenmenger syndrome. We believe that there may also be sympathetic "crosstalk" from an affected contralateral side or stenotic areas in the same lung.

Postoperative Care

Although much of the postoperative care is common to that of the more ordinary open-heart surgery patients, there are some important differences. Meticulous postoperative management is essential to the success of this operation. All patients are mechanically ventilated for at least 24 hours, and all patients are subjected to a maintained diuresis with the goal of reaching the patient's preoperative dry weight within 24 hours.

The electrocardiogram, systemic and pulmonary arterial and central venous pressures, temperature, urine output, arterial oxygen saturation, chest tube drainage, and fluid balance are monitored. A pulse oximeter is used to continuously monitor peripheral oxygen saturation. Management of cardiac arrhythmias and output and treatment of wound bleeding are identical to those for other open-heart operations. In addition,

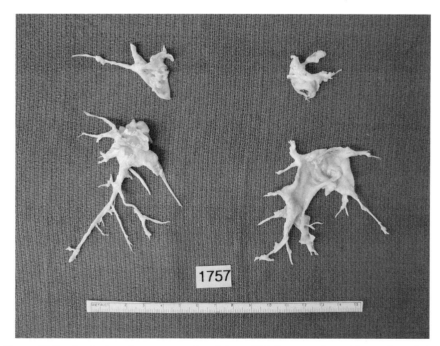

Figure 66-8. Surgical specimen removed on right and left from a patient with type II surgical classification. Note how the specimen ends in "feathered tails" in each of the branches.

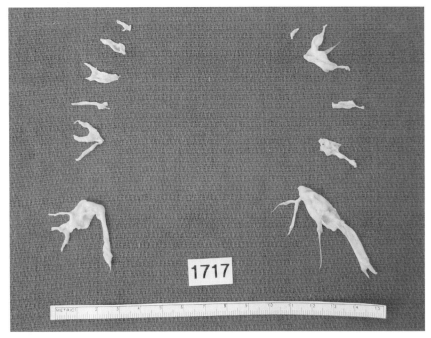

Figure 66-9. For this specimen, the plane of dissection was raised at each segmental level. The surgical classification is type III.

higher minute ventilation is often required early after the operation to compensate for the temporary metabolic acidosis that develops after the long period of circulatory arrest, hypothermia, and cardiopulmonary bypass. Although we used to believe that prolonged sedation and ventilation was beneficial and led to less pulmonary edema, subsequent experience has shown this not to be so. Extubation should be performed on the first postoperative day, if possible.

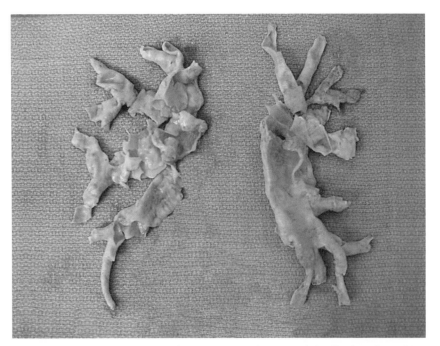

Figure 66-10. The surgical specimen from a patient with a surgical classification of type IV. Note that each branch ends abruptly in "trousers" rather than "feathered tails." This patient's postoperative hemodynamic numbers were unchanged despite the impressive appearance of the endarterectomy specimen.

Complications

Patients are subject to all complications associated with open-heart and major lung surgery (arrhythmias, atelectasis, wound infection, pneumonia, mediastinal bleeding, etc.), but also may develop complications specific to this operation. One such complication is the development of a "reperfusion response." This is a specific complication that occurs in most patients to some degree and is related to localized pulmonary edema. Reperfusion injury is defined as a radiologic opacity seen in the lungs within 72 hours of pulmonary endarterectomy. This unfortunately loose definition may therefore encompass many causes, such as fluid overload and infection.

True reperfusion injury that directly adversely impacts the clinical course of the patient now occurs in approximately 8% to 10% of patients. In its most dramatic form, it occurs soon after operation (within a few hours) and is associated with profound desaturation. Edema-like fluid, sometimes with a bloody tinge, is suctioned from the endotracheal tube. Frank blood from the endotracheal tube, however, signifies a mechanical violation of the blood–airway barrier that has occurred at operation and stems from a technical error. This complication should be managed, if possible, by identification of the affected area by bronchoscopy and balloon occlusion of the affected lobe until coagulation can be normalized.

One common cause of the reperfusion pulmonary edema is persistent high pulmonary artery pressures after operation when a thorough endarterectomy has been performed in certain areas, but there remains a large part of the pulmonary vascular bed affected by type IV change. However, the reperfusion phenomenon can also be encountered in patients after a seemingly technically perfect operation with complete resolution of high pulmonary artery pressures. In these cases the response may be one of reactive hyperemia, after the revascularization of segments of the pulmonary arterial bed that have long experienced no flow. Other contributing factors may include perioperative pulmonary ischemia and conditions associated with high-permeability lung injury in the area of the now denuded endothelium. Fortunately, the incidence of this complication is very much less common now in our series, probably as a result of the more complete and expeditious removal of the endarterectomy specimen that has come with the large experience over the last decade and the recognition that an aggressive diuresis is required postoperatively.

Management of the "Reperfusion Response"

Early measures should be taken to minimize the development of pulmonary edema with diuresis, maintenance of the hematocrit levels, and the early use of ventilatory peak end-expiratory pressure. Once the capillary leak has been established, treatment is supportive because reperfusion pulmonary edema will eventually resolve if satisfactory hemodynamics and oxygenation can be maintained. Careful management of ventilation and fluid balance is required. The hematocrit is kept high (32% to 36%), and the patient undergoes aggressive diuresis, even if this requires ultrafiltration. The patient's ventilatory status may be dramatically position sensitive. The inspired oxygen fraction (FiO_2) level is kept as low as is compatible with an oxygen saturation of 90%. A careful titration of positive end-expiratory pressure is carried out, with a progressive transition from volume-limited to pressure-limited inverse ratio ventilation and the acceptance of moderate hypercapnia. The use of steroids is discouraged because they are generally ineffective and may lead to infection. Infrequently, inhaled nitric oxide at 20 to 40 parts per million can improve the gas exchange. On occasion we have used extracorporeal perfusion support (extracorporeal membrane oxygenator or extracorporeal carbon dioxide removal) until ventilation can be resumed satisfactorily, usually after 7 to 10 days.

Conclusion

It is increasingly apparent that pulmonary hypertension caused by chronic pulmonary embolism is a relative common condition that is under-recognized and carries a poor prognosis. Medical therapy is ineffective in prolonging life and only transiently improves the symptoms. The only therapeutic alternative to pulmonary thromboendarterectomy is lung transplantation. The advantages of thromboendarterectomy include a lower operative morbidity and mortality and excellent long-term results without the risks associated with chronic immunosuppression and chronic allograft rejection. The mortality for thromboendarterectomy at our institution is now in the range of 4.5%, with sustained benefit. These results are clearly superior to those for transplantation in both the short and long term.

Although PTE is technically demanding for the surgeon, requiring careful dissection of the pulmonary artery planes and the use of circulatory arrest, excellent short- and long-term results can be achieved. Successive improvements in operative technique developed over the last two decades now allow pulmonary endarterectomy to be offered to patients with an acceptable mortality rate and excellent anticipation of clinical improvement. With this growing experience, it has also become clear that unilateral operation is obsolete and that circulatory arrest is essential.

We have performed >2,000 pulmonary endarterectomies at the University of California, San Diego, Medical Center, with almost all of these carried out since 1990. With our growing experience we are now able to offer this procedure to some very high-risk patients with a total overall mortality rate of about 4.5%. The vast majority of patients enjoy a dramatic hemodynamic improvement postoperatively. A reduction in pulmonary pressures and pulmonary vascular resistance to normal levels and a corresponding improvement in pulmonary blood flow and cardiac output are generally immediate and sustained. In general, these changes can be assumed to be permanent. Whereas before the operation, >95% of the patients are in New York Heart Association (NYHA) functional class III or IV, at 1 year after the operation, 95% of patients are in NYHA functional class I or II. In addition, echocardiographic studies have demonstrated that with the elimination of chronic pressure overload, right ventricular geometry rapidly reverts toward normal. Right atrial and right ventricular enlargement regresses. Tricuspid valve function returns to normal within a few days as a result of restoration of tricuspid annular geometry after the remodeling of the right ventricle, and therefore tricuspid repair is not part of the operation.

Even with increased awareness of this disease, coupled with our continuous effort in spreading our understanding and knowledge, the principal difficulty remains that this is an under-recognized condition. Increased understanding of both the prevalence of this condition and the possibility of a surgical cure should avail more patients of the opportunity for relief from this debilitating and ultimately fatal disease.

SUGGESTED READING

Dalen JE, Alpert JS. Natural history of pulmonary embolism. Prog Cardiovasc Dis 1975;17:259.

Fedullo PF, Auger WR, Channick RN, et al. Surgical Management of Pulmonary Embolism. In Morpurgo M (ed), Pulmonary Embolism. New York: Marcel Dekker,1994;223.

Jamieson SW. Pulmonary Thromboendarterectomy. In Franco KL, Putnam JB (eds), Advanced Therapy in Thoracic Surgery. Hamilton, Canada: BC Decker, 1998;310.

Jamieson SW, Kapelanski DP. Pulmonary endarterectomy. Curr Probl Surg 2000;37:165.

Jamieson SW, Kapelanski DP, Sakakibara N, et al. Pulmonary endarterectomy: experience and lessons learned in 1,500 cases. Ann Thorac Surg 2003;76:1456.

Madani MM, Jamieson SW. Pulmonary Thromboendarterectomy. In Edmunds LH, Cohn LH (eds). Cardiac Surgery in the Adult. New York: McGraw-Hill, 2003;1205.

Moser KM. Pulmonary vascular obstruction due to embolism and thrombosis. In Moser KM (ed), Pulmonary Vascular Disease. New York: Marcel Dekker, 1979;341.

Moser KM, Auger WF, Fedullo PF. Chronic major-vessel thromboembolic pulmonary hypertension. Circulation 1990;81:1735.

EDITOR'S COMMENTS

Not many centers in the world have the experience with this specific disease process that Dr. Jamieson and colleagues have, more than 2,000 cases. This is truly not part of the armamentarium of the typical cardiothoracic surgeon. However, this chapter is included because it represents the work of some institutions and knowledge of this disease process is very important. The authors have done an excellent job in terms of diagnosis and treatment of this process. Clearly, the huge differential is primary pulmonary failure versus chronic pulmonary thromboembolism. The authors have explained the logic for their approach, particularly the use of circulatory arrest. I applaud them for their excellent results.

I.L.K.

III

Congenital Cardiac Surgery

67

Anatomy and Classification of Congenital Heart Disease

Paul M. Weinberg

The hallmark of congenital heart disease is the variability in spatial relationships as well as interconnections among the various cardiac and vascular structures. To appreciate these types of abnormalities, it is first necessary to define certain terms that may have different meanings from those used to describe normal anatomy. When cardiac chambers are described, the terms *right* and *left* refer only to morphologic characteristics, which are further elaborated on later. They do not refer to the right–left frame of reference in the body. For example, right ventricle refers to a particular cardiac structure with specific morphologic features regardless of its location in the body. When the right–left frame of reference is intended, the terms *right sided* and *left sided* are used.

It is also important to recognize which structures are, by definition, part of a chamber and which are frequently associated with that chamber. For example, the normal right ventricle includes the infundibulum or outflow tract portion of the heart, whereas there are some hearts in which the infundibulum is partially or entirely related to the left ventricle (anatomically corrected malposition or double-outlet left ventricle). Therefore, the presence of infundibulum does not define the right ventricle, but rather is usually associated with it.

Another aspect that is central to a morphologic approach to congenital heart disease is the recognition of the differences among anatomic, physiologic, and surgical diagnoses. This chapter concerns itself entirely with anatomic descriptions and diagnoses. Some of the terms can also be used in a physiologic sense; it is vital that one not make the mistake of using them in-terchangeably. For example, anatomically, *transposition of the great arteries* means that the aorta arises above the morphologic right ventricle and the pulmonary artery above the left ventricle. This is true regardless of whether the right ventricle receives desaturated blood from the body or fully saturated blood from the lungs. *Transposition physiology*, however, refers to any anatomic situation in which the pulmonary artery receives blood of a higher saturation than the aorta. If a term is used without further clarification, it should always refer to anatomic diagnoses, whereas physiologic terms should always be stated as such—that is, *transposition physiology* or *physiologic mitral stenosis*.

Aims and Basic Principles of Classifying Congenital Heart Disease

The purpose of a classification system is to permit identification of all examples of anatomy, physiology, and surgery of congenital heart disease in a way that permits storage and retrieval from computerized databases. The aim of a classification system is really to classify entities, not names. As Shakespeare said, "What's in a name? That which we call a rose by any other name would smell as sweet." There seems to be a broad consensus on what the entities are. Rather than trying to win over everyone to the best nomenclature, classification systems should focus on the following five principles: (1) organization, (2) economy, (3) accuracy, (4) precision, and (5) quantification.

Organization

Organization is essential with any comprehensive classification system. Simple alphabetical listing of diagnoses is unhelpful because of the absence of a standardized nomenclature. Instead, diagnoses should be grouped by the organization of the heart according to a systematic method. In this way all possible diagnoses related to a given portion of the heart can be viewed at one time and the appropriate one selected.

Economy

Economy refers to saving the time of the physician who has to determine which diagnoses to use and saving computer space by avoiding redundant information. This is accomplished through mutual exclusivity. Diagnoses are grouped within organizational categories into subgroups in which diagnoses are mutually exclusive—only one diagnosis within that subgroup is possible. For example, only one atrial situs, one ventricular situs, one great artery situs, one atrial-to-atrioventricular valve (AVV) connection, one AVV-to-ventricle connection, and one ventriculoarterial alignment abnormality are possible. Additional diagnoses that are thought to relate a group of similar abnormalities are superfluous, and if ultimately shown to be incorrect (i.e., abnormalities not similar), can actually be counterproductive. Provision of redundant information during data entry wastes time and computer storage space.

Accuracy

Accuracy means that a given diagnosis has the same meaning every time it is used. The meaning does not change with context. In other words, a particular anatomic ventricular septal defect (VSD) has the same designation regardless of ventriculoarterial alignment and great artery position. The atrial situs designation is the same whether there is dextrocardia or levocardia. Dependence on context complicates data retrieval because a given diagnosis could have different meanings depending on what other diagnoses are present in each case.

Precision

Precision is the ability to classify fine anatomic detail if the information is available. Nonspecific diagnoses should be used only if more precise information is lacking. For example, a plain chest roentgenogram may indicate a right aortic arch (not further specified), but magnetic resonance imaging or angiography may show a right aortic arch with retroesophageal diverticulum. A dilution of information would occur if only "right aortic arch" were used as the diagnosis, whereas if one were searching for all right aortic arches, general as well as specific entities could be included.

Quantification

Quantification refers to the option of assigning an indication of severity to certain diagnoses. Sometimes the severity of a lesion is as important as the anatomic detail. Although an epidemiologist may consider all VSDs of a particular type equally significant, the clinician may want to distinguish small VSDs from large VSDs. In many cases the designation is arbitrary but may still be useful.

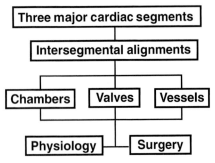

Figure 67-1. The hierarchy of cardiac diagnoses based on the segmental approach to diagnosis of Van Praagh.

Classification of Congenital Heart Disease: The Segmental Approach

The segmental approach to diagnosis of congenital heart disease was developed by Van Praagh to provide a systematic method for describing congenital heart defects. It fits the basic principles outlined here. Important features that distinguish Van Praagh's segmental approach from many other systems include the following:

1. Diagnoses are based on morphologic analysis. Although physiologic correction of defects is the primary goal of cardiac surgery, it is also clear that attention to the underlying morphology is important because it influences the surgical approach as well as long-term function.
2. The system is not situs dependent; each segment is diagnosed independently. Situs-dependent systems suffer from two shortcomings. If the situs is found to be different than initially thought, all of the dependent diagnoses change as well. If the situs is ambiguous or if the downstream connections are not one-to-one, as in double-inlet ventricles, the concept of a situs-dependent system breaks down.
3. There is a hierarchy of diagnoses (Fig. 67-1). Those entities at the top do not change the diagnoses or nomenclature of those below, but they have greater significance: Internal organization is more important than a stenotic valve in terms of classification.
4. There is a logical sequence to the analysis and description of the heart.

The cardiovascular system is thought of as having three major segments: visceroatrial situs, ventricular loop, and great artery situs. The situs or spatial organization of each of the segments can be described independently using morphologic features of the chambers and vessels. Adjacent segments are related to each other by intersegmental alignments. The three major segments can be thought of as the blueprints of each of the floors of a three-story house. They are not, in and of themselves, diagnoses, but rather define the outline of cardiac organization. The intersegmental alignments are analogous to stairways that connect adjacent floors.

After segments and intersegmental alignments have been determined, individual chamber, valve, and vessel diagnoses are made. Continuing the architectural analogy, one might consider the chamber, valve, and vessel abnormalities to be like the furnishings of individual rooms.

Cardiac Segments

Visceroatrial Situs

Visceroatrial situs describes the arrangement of the asymmetric abdominal viscera and vessels and of the atria. There are three forms of visceroatrial situs: solitus, inversus, and ambiguus. Situs solitus is characterized by a right-sided liver, left-sided stomach, and right-sided inferior vena cava (IVC). The atria display characteristic right atrial morphology of the right-sided appendage, left atrial morphology of the left-sided appendage, IVC entering the right-sided atrium, and the septum primum attached to the left side of the septum secundum. Situs inversus means the mirror image of solitus, namely left-sided liver and IVC, right-sided stomach, right atrial appendage on the left, left atrial appendage on the right, IVC entering a left-sided atrium, and the septum primum attached to the right side of the septum secundum. Situs ambiguus has some characteristics of situs solitus and some of situs inversus in the same person. For example, a liver that spans the abdomen from right to left (sometimes referred to as a "midline" liver), being both right sided and left sided, has characteristics of both solitus and inversus. Similarly, bilateral morphologic right or bilateral morphologic left atrial appendages means one solitus and one inversus. In the same way, a left-sided abdominal IVC that crosses to the right in the liver and enters a right-sided atrium with right atrial appendage morphology has features of both situs inversus (abdominal) and situs solitus (atrial). All these examples of combinations of situs solitus and situs inversus are termed situs ambiguus. This is the visceroatrial situs seen in the abdominal heterotaxy syndrome. Most but not all of these patients have splenic abnormalities: asplenia or polysplenia. The terms *bilateral right sidedness* and *bilateral left sidedness* are conveniences for remembering the constellation of abnormalities frequently seen with asplenia (bilateral right sidedness) or polysplenia (bilateral left sidedness) but do not carry the force of visceroatrial situs because there are numerous exceptions to the symmetry implied by those terms.

Ventricular Loop

Ventricular loop is the designation for the situs of the ventricles. There are two types: D loop and L loop. Unlike the atria, which are virtually always side by side, the ventricles,

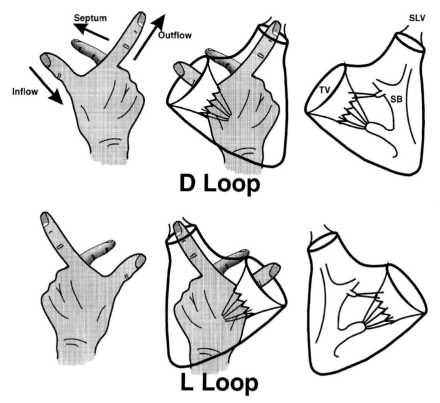

Figure 67-2. Ventricular loop and handedness. Ventricular loop or situs is determined by the internal organization of the ventricles. Right ventricular organization (right) is compared with the right hand: the thumb, index finger, and middle finger are held mutually orthogonal and represent ventricular inflow, outflow, and septum, respectively. Right-hand organization of the right ventricle is termed D loop; left-hand organization is termed L loop. (SB = septal band; SLV = semilunar valve; TV = tricuspid valve.)

while frequently so, may be oriented antero-posteriorly or superoinferiorly, still displaying one of two internal spatial organizations. Therefore a designation independent of a simple right–left frame of reference is necessary. Just as it is possible to distinguish a right hand from a left hand without seeing the rest of the body—that is, without a right–left frame of reference, so too it is possible to distinguish the two stereoisomers of ventricular organization. By focusing on ventricular inflow, outflow, and septum, it is possible to attribute chirality or handedness to the ventricular organization (Fig. 67-2). If one holds the hand with the thumb, index finger, and middle finger mutually orthogonal, with the thumb representing ventricular inflow, the index finger representing outflow, and the middle finger pointing to the septum, a right hand in the right ventricle indicates a D-loop arrangement of ventricles. If the left hand fits the right ventricle, there is an L loop. Just as a right hand can always be distinguished from a left, so too D-loop ventricles should not be mistaken for L-loop ventricles regardless of position of the heart or ventricles in three-dimensional space.

What if the right ventricle does not have all three components, inflow, outflow, and septum? For example, tricuspid atresia has no right ventricular inflow. The ventricles are always concordant with each other having adjacent inflows, adjacent outflows, and a septum common to both. Because of this, a right-handed right ventricle is matched with a left-handed left ventricle. Similarly, a left-handed right ventricle would go with a right-handed left ventricle. So, in the case of tricuspid atresia, one would simply determine the handedness of the left ventricle and interpret the ventricular loop as just described.

Great Artery Situs

Great artery situs refers to the spatial arrangement of the semilunar valves and great arteries. A special spatial arrangement exists when the great arteries are normally aligned with the ventricles (see the later section on intersegmental connections). Thus, a special segmental description is given in those cases in which the pulmonary artery arises above the right ventricle and the aorta normally above the left ventricle. If the two

great arteries spiral about each other in a clockwise fashion (viewed from the ventricles) so that the ascending aorta crosses the right pulmonary artery, this is designated solitus normal great arteries. If they spiral counterclockwise with the ascending aorta crossing the left pulmonary artery, they are termed inversus normal great arteries. For all other cases—transpositions and malpositions described under intersegmental connections—the great artery segment is called D if the aortic valve is to the right of the pulmonary valve, L if the aortic valve is to the left of the pulmonary, and A if the aortic valve is directly anterior (i.e., same sagittal plane) to the pulmonary.

Segmental Notation

The purpose of the segmental approach to diagnosis is not only to have designations for the various spatial arrangements of the cardiac structures, but also to have a concise way of communicating the basic organization of the heart when also listing the various intersegmental connections and chamber, valve, and vessel abnormalities mentioned later. This shorthand description of the cardiac organization is the segmental notation. Van Praagh conceived of each heart as representing a subset of all the possible spatial arrangements that could occur in nature. He borrowed mathematical set notation—braces {}—to accomplish this. Each heart can be described as a three-member subset of the whole with the first member of the set representing visceroatrial situs, the second, ventricular loop, and the third, great artery situs. Furthermore, the possibilities for each member of the set are designated by their first letter in capital form with the individual members separated by commas (Fig. 67-3).

Therefore, the visceroatrial segment can be described by S, I, or A for situs solitus, inversus, or ambiguus, respectively. Similarly, the second member, ventricular loop, is represented by D or L for D-loop or L-loop organization of the ventricles, respectively. The great artery notation is S or I, respectively, for solitus normal or inversus normal if the pulmonary artery arises above the right ventricle and aorta normally above the left ventricle, or D, L, or A, respectively, for aortic valve to the right, left, or directly anterior relative to the pulmonary valve. In cases where the information is insufficient to determine the particular segment, that member of the subset may be represented by the letter X.

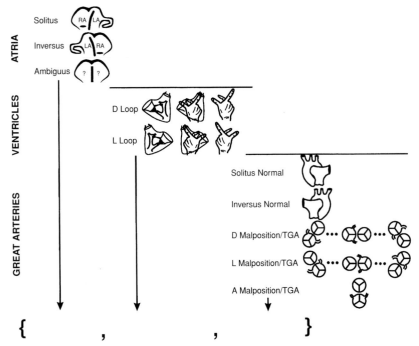

Figure 67-3. Segmental notation. Segmental notation consists of a three-member set in braces {}. The first member is the visceroatrial situs—solitus, inversus, or ambiguus; the second is the ventricular loop—D or L; and the third is the great artery situs—solitus normal, inversus normal, D, L, or A transposition or malposition. The meaning of those terms is discussed in the text and represented diagrammatically in the figure. Great artery situs diagrams with malposition or transposition of the great arteries (TGA) in the lower right represent the two semilunar valves viewed from above; the aorta is shown with coronary arteries. (LA = left atrium, RA = right atrium, ? = ambiguous morphology, a combination of solitus and inversus.)

aorta to the left of the pulmonary artery. Transposition of the great arteries {S,D,L} has situs solitus of viscera and atria, ventricular D loop, but transposed aorta to the left of the pulmonary artery rather than to the right as in the {S,D,D} form. This difference in segments does not imply different connections, but rather an altered spatial arrangement, which has implications for associated abnormalities (e.g., hypoplasia of the right ventricle, straddling tricuspid valve) as well as for surgical approaches. Figure 67-4 shows examples of spatial arrangements of atria, ventricles, and great arteries with their corresponding segmental notation. The segmental designation is a fundamental part of the overall cardiac diagnosis and is not meant to be a parenthetical—that is, extraneous or explanatory—supplement.

Intersegmental Alignments

Each pair of adjacent segments has a discrete set of intersegmental alignments. Under the principle of economy described earlier, intersegmental alignment diagnoses are mutually exclusive entities.

Atrioventricular Alignments

AV alignments are really a combination of atrial-to-AVV connection and AVV-to-ventricle connection. There are four basic

In the cases of normal arrangement of cardiac chambers and vessels, the segmental notation is {S,D,S} for visceroatrial situs solitus, ventricular D loop, and solitus normal great arteries. These would also be the segments in classic tetralogy of Fallot, and the same segmental notation would apply to classic tricuspid atresia with normally aligned great arteries. Thus it can be seen that the segmental description does not describe abnormalities of chambers, valves, or vessels nor does it describe intersegmental connections (except for normally aligned great arteries). Classic complete transposition of the great arteries has segments {S,D,D} because the atria and ventricles are normally arranged, but in the absence of normally aligned great arteries the segmental notation indicates that the aorta is to the right of the pulmonary artery at the level of the semilunar valves. The same segmental description could apply to a case of double-outlet right ventricle with the aorta to the right of the pulmonary artery. Classic physiologically corrected transposition of the great arteries has segments {S,L,L} indicating normal (solitus) arrangement of the atria but a ventricular L loop plus the

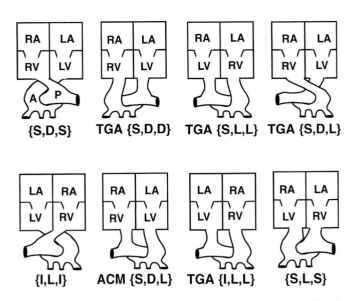

Figure 67-4. Examples of selected anomalies and their segmental notations. Box diagrams of the heart showing the position of the atria—right atrium (RA) and left atrium (LA); the ventricles—right ventricle (RV) and left ventricle (LV); and the great arteries—aorta (A) and pulmonary artery (P). The upper left diagram represents normal spatial relations and the lower left diagram represents normal relations in situs inversus of viscera and atria. The three examples of transposition of the great arteries (TGA) in the upper row are discussed in the text. The case of anatomically corrected malposition (ACM) in the lower row has the aorta arising abnormally from a left-sided infundibulum above the left ventricle. (TGA {I,L,L} = physiologically complete transposition in situs inversus; {S,L,S} = isolated ventricular inversion: physiologic transposition but with normal ventriculoarterial alignment.)

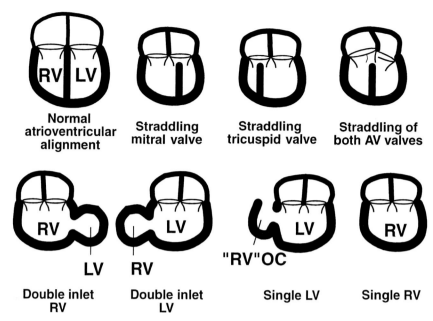

Figure 67-5. Atrioventricular (AV) alignments with two AV valves. All possible ways for two AV valves, one from each atrium, to connect with the ventricles. (Shown here only for D-loop ventricles; comparable connections for L loops exist, keeping in mind that the tricuspid valve is left sided and the mitral right sided. Similarly, the right ventricular outlet chamber ["RV" OC], not a ventricular sinus, is left sided in an L loop.) (LV = left ventricle.)

types of atrial-to-AVV connection: two AVVs, one from each atrium; one common AVV from both atria; right AVV atresia (i.e., no AVV from the right-sided atrium but one AVV from the left-sided atrium); and left AVV atresia. Each atrial-to-AVV connection has several possible AVV-to-ventricle connections: With two AVVs, each may enter one ventricle (normal), one or both may enter two ventricles (straddling AVV or AVVs), or both may enter one ventricle (double-inlet ventricle) (Fig. 67-5); with a common AVV, it may connect to both ventricles equally (balanced), unequally (unbalanced), or only one ventricle (common inlet) (Fig. 67-6); with AVV atresia, the other valve may enter the ipsilateral ventricle, the contralateral ventricle, or both ventricles (straddling AVV) (Fig. 67-7).

Ventriculoarterial Alignments

Ventriculoarterial alignments do not reflect anatomic reality. The ventricles are connected to the great arteries via the infundibulum or AV canal. (The normal right ventricle is connected to the pulmonary artery via the infundibulum, whereas the left ventricle is connected to the aorta via the AV canal, hence mitral-aortic fibrous continuity.) However, unlike the AV alignments, most classification systems have not used this relationship in developing their nomenclatures. Instead ventriculoarterial align-

ments tend to be based on a system in which each great artery is "assigned" to one, and only one, ventricle. When the ventricular septum is intact, the assignment is straightforward. In the presence of a relatively large VSD near the great arteries, the assignment can be problematic. All

such classification schemes have therefore adopted certain rules governing assignment of great arteries to ventricles. The rules are depicted in Fig. 67-8 and can be stated as follows:

1. The pulmonary artery is assigned to a ventricle if the pulmonary valve lies >50% above it.
2. Because the aorta *normally* may lie predominantly above the ventricular septum rather than above the left ventricular cavity, mitral valve-to-aortic valve fibrous continuity, if present, determines assignment of the aorta to the left ventricle, regardless of how far the aorta extends above the right ventricle. Mitral valve is defined as that valve on the side of the left ventricle or its remnant (compared to the right ventricle or its remnant).
3. If mitral-aortic fibrous continuity is not present, the 50% rule, as described previously for the pulmonary artery, applies.
4. With conotruncal anomalies and pulmonary atresia, it may not be feasible to assign the pulmonary artery to either ventricle; in those cases only the aorta is assigned: right ventricular aorta with pulmonary atresia or left ventricular aorta with pulmonary atresia. Based on these rules, the ventriculoarterial alignments are named according to Fig. 67-8.

As with any system of more or less arbitrary rules, there are potential problems or "exceptions." Here are a few. If there is

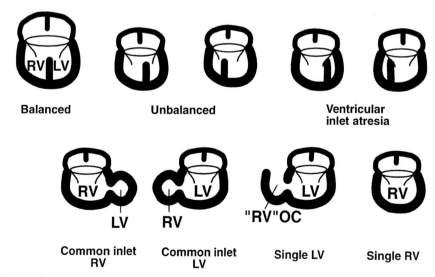

Figure 67-6. Atrioventricular (AV) alignments with a single, common AV valve. All possible ways for a common AV valve, one valve from both atria, to connect with the ventricles. (Shown here only for D-loop ventricles; comparable connections for L loops exist. The right ventricular outlet chamber ["RV" OC], not a ventricular sinus, is left sided in an L loop.) In ventricular inlet atresias, a leaflet of the common AV valve seals off the "septal defect," the only entrance into the ventricle. (LV = left ventricle.)

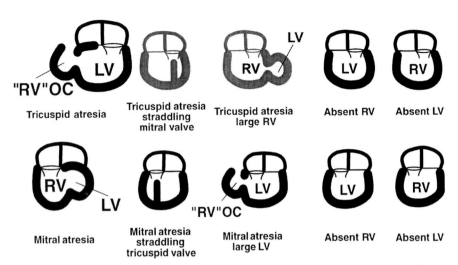

Figure 67-7. Atrioventricular (AV) alignments with right or left AV valve atresia. All possible ways for the valve contralateral to the atretic one to connect with the ventricles. (Shown here only for D-loop ventricles; comparable connections for L loops exist, keeping in mind that the tricuspid valve is left sided and the mitral right sided. Similarly, the right ventricular outlet chamber ["RV" OC], not a ventricular sinus, is left sided in an L loop.) Hypothetical but unreported cases are shown in gray. (LV = left ventricle.)

tenuous mitral-aortic fibrous continuity through a tiny VSD so that the aorta arises virtually exclusively above the right ventricle, it is assigned to the right ventricle. If there is no mitral valve but a common AVV instead, the previous rules apply to the portion of the common AVV attached to the left ventricle, as if it were a mitral valve. Finally, if there is no mitral valve because of AVV atresia, the 50% rule applies, but the aorta, if assigned to the left ventricle, is considered normally aligned unless there is clearly subaortic infundibular muscle. Thus, typical hypoplastic left heart with mitral atresia is considered to have normally aligned great arteries.

Anatomy of Congenital Heart Disease

Chamber, Valve, and Vessel Abnormalities

An exhaustive description of all chamber, valve, and vessel abnormalities is not within the scope of this chapter. The following sections indicate the characteristics that define the various structures and list some of the surgically important anatomic abnormalities.

Venae Cavae and Coronary Sinus

The superior vena cava (SVC) connects veins from the upper portion of the body to the heart. Normally there is a single, right-sided SVC that enters the right atrium,

but single SVCs can connect to a coronary sinus (CoS) or to the left atrium. Bilateral SVCs may be present, most commonly with a right SVC connecting to the right atrium and a left SVC connecting to a CoS and ultimately draining to the right atrium. However, each may connect to its ipsilateral atrium as in heterotaxy with asplenia, or rarely, both may connect to the same atrium. A venous structure that is in a similar position to the SVC but connects a pulmonary vein confluence to the innominate vein is not considered to be an SVC because it does not connect to the heart. Rather, the term *vertical vein* or *connecting vein* is appropriate.

The IVC enters the right atrium guarded medially by the left venous valve, which blends with the septum primum portion of the atrial septum, and laterally by the right venous (Eustachian) valve. The anterior commissure of these two venous valves forms the tendon of Todaro, which points to the AV node. The IVC is always single at the level of the heart. (Double IVC refers only to duplication of the infrarenal portion.) Although two IVC-like vessels may enter the heart either in the same atrium or one in each atrium, one vessel is invariably only a confluence of hepatic veins. Because the IVC is always single at the atrial level, it is used as a strong indicator of the right atrium (see later discussion). There are, however, two potentially ambiguous situations that render this unacceptable for all cases: so-called absent IVC and an IVC that enters both atria via a so-called sinus venosus type

atrial septal defect of the inferior caval variety. In absent IVC, the renal-to-hepatic portion of the IVC is absent so that the veins of the lower portion of the body (except the hepatic veins) are drained by the azygos vein to a SVC. Only the hepatic veins connect directly to the right atrium. In the IVC type of sinus venosus atrial septal defect, the right atrium cannot be defined by IVC entrance because it straddles the atrial septum.

The CoS usually enters the right atrium near the entrance of the IVC (Fig. 67-9). Its entrance is partially covered by the Thebesian valve, which may be an extension of the Eustachian valve or a separate structure. The AV node may extend into the mouth of the CoS. If there is a SVC connection to the CoS, its orifice will be quite large and could be mistaken for an atrial septal defect or occasionally for a common atrium. A large CoS ostium may also occur with anomalous connection of pulmonary veins or, rarely, hepatic veins to the CoS. Uncommonly, the CoS ostium may enter the left atrium, and rarely there may be no patent CoS ostium, in which case the CoS drains into an SVC remnant (vein of Marshall), which drains blood superiorly to the innominate vein. Surgical or catheter device occlusion of the vein of Marshall in this situation results in coronary venous obstruction.

Morphologic Right Atrium

The morphologic right atrium is characterized by a broad-based appendage that, on the exterior, blends almost imperceptibly with the venous portion of the atrium. Anderson pointed out that this is more definitively seen from the interior aspect as pectinate muscles extending all the way to the crux of the heart. The fact that pectinate muscles constitute a large portion of the effective right atrial cavity makes that chamber more compliant than the left atrium, whose appendage is more isolated from the main cavity. The septum secundum or the superior limbic band of the atrial septum is seen in front of the septum primum or the flap valve of the foramen ovale from the right atrial aspect. Typically, the IVC enters the right atrium with the exception of those situations noted previously under venae cavae. The SVC and CoS, being much more variable, cannot be used to define the right atrium. When the SVC does enter the right atrium, the crista terminalis forms the lateral aspect of the entrance internally. The external aspect of this structure is the sulcus terminalis, in which lies the sinus node.

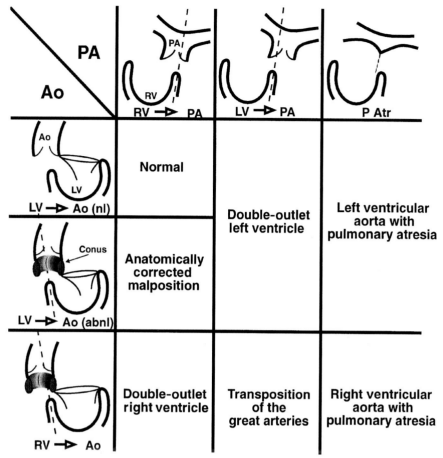

Figure 67-8. Ventriculoarterial alignments. The rules for assigning great arteries to ventricles discussed in the text are shown diagrammatically. For the pulmonary artery (PA) across the top row, the PA is said to arise from the right ventricle (RV) if its valve is >50% above the RV. It is assigned to the left ventricle (LV) if >50% above that. If there is pulmonary atresia (P Atr) without clear evidence of association with either ventricle, no assignment is made (far right column). For the aorta (Ao) the rules are depicted in the far left column. The Ao is assigned to the LV in a normal (nl) fashion if there is mitral valve-to-aortic valve fibrous continuity, regardless of the degree to which the aorta may be situated above the RV. If there is no mitral-aortic fibrous continuity such as occurs with subaortic conus, the aorta is assigned to the LV but as an abnormal (abnl) alignment if it arises >50% above the LV, or it is assigned to the RV if >50% above that. The ventriculoarterial alignments for each of the combinations of aortic and pulmonary assignment are given in the corresponding boxes.

Atrial Septum

The atrial septum has three portions (Fig. 67-9), most easily appreciated in the newborn but still identifiable in the adult heart: the septum primum, the septum secundum, and the canal septum. The septum primum or flap valve of the foramen ovale is the thin central portion of the septum. In the fetus and preterm infant it is so thin as to be transparent. At term, it is typically translucent and becomes somewhat thicker with advancing age but is always thinner than the other two components of the septum. It is this structure that is torn by balloon septostomy. Defects in or a deficiency of the septum primum are called ostium secundum atrial septal defects. The septum secundum, or the superior limbic band, is a thick, muscular ridge at the superior aspect of the atrial septum immediately medial to the SVC (if one enters the atrium directly). The septum primum usually has two points of attachment onto the left atrial side of the septum secundum with the space between the two being the foramen ovale. The superior aspect of the septum primum (between the two points of attachment) forms a half-moon shape. The third portion of the atrial septum is the AV canal septum, a thick, muscular tissue anterior to the septum primum extending to the level of the AVVs and actually continuing on to become the canal or so-called inlet portion of the ventricular septum. It is the canal septum that is deficient or absent in cases of common AV canal including the ostium primum atrial septal defect. Other apparent atrial septal defects are actually vessel ostia. Sinus venosus atrial septal defects are examples of either the right pulmonary vein straddling the atrial septum (SVC type) or the IVC straddling the septum (IVC type). CoS ostium-type ASD occurs when the CoS is unroofed into the left atrium. Atrial septal defect types are shown in Fig. 67-10.

Tricuspid Valve

By definition, the tricuspid valve is the right-sided AVV in a D loop or the left-sided AVV in an L loop. Because of the marked variability in morphology of the AVVs and the propensity for AVV morphology to be influenced by the ventricle into which they enter, the foregoing definition is used to avoid ambiguity in such circumstances as double-inlet ventricles in which both AVVs may appear morphologically similar. Having thus defined the tricuspid valve, it is nonetheless worth describing the commonly seen morphology. The classic three leaflets are anterior, posterior, and septal. Although the name implies three leaflets, this is not always the case. Frequently, the newborn has only two distinct leaflets with no commissure between the anterior and posterior leaflets. The most characteristic feature of the tricuspid valve is the similarity of depth (annulus to free edge) of all leaflets.

Morphologic Right Ventricle

The morphologic right ventricle has broad or coarse and relatively parallel trabeculations. If an AVV is present, there are chordal attachments onto the face (not simply the crest) of the ventricular septum as well as onto the free wall. There is typically a single large papillary muscle attached to the septal band by the moderator band.

Ventricular Septum

The right ventricular septal surface, like the rest of the right ventricle, shows coarse, parallel trabeculations. A large trabeculation called the septal band appears like an appliqué on top of the septum. At its inferior aspect, the septal band becomes the moderator band and that, in turn, becomes the main papillary muscle of the right ventricle. The "Y" is usually marked by the presence of the papillary muscle of the conus or muscle of Lancisi slightly posterior to the fork of the "Y." The infundibular septum normally fills the "Y" of the septal band. In cases of infundibular (conal) septal malalignment or hypoplasia, however, the "Y" is

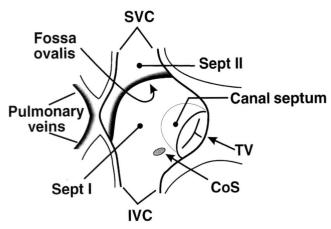

Figure 67-9. Right atrial septal surface. The opened right atrium viewed in anatomic position from the right lateral aspect shows the various components of the atrial septum. (CoS = coronary sinus; IVC = inferior vena cava; Sept I = septum primum, the flap valve of the foramen ovale; Sept II = septum secundum, the superior limbic band; SVC = superior vena cava; TV = tricuspid valve.) (Reprinted with permission from PM Weinberg. Morphology of Congenital Heart Disease. In RM Freedom [volume ed], E Braunwald [series ed], Atlas of Heart Diseases, Vol 12: Congenital Heart Disease. Philadelphia: Current Medicine, 1997.)

empty—that is, there is a VSD in its place, and the infundibular septum is not part of the ventricular septum. The right bundle branch runs along the septal band between the upper two thirds and the lower one third and extends onto the moderator band to the base of the main papillary muscle. The septal-moderator band complex marks the boundary between the sinus portion of the right ventricle below and the outflow tract above. Pathologic extension of the septal-moderator band complex can divide the two, resulting in subpulmonary stenosis—anomalous muscle bundle or so-called double-chambered right ventricle.

The left ventricular septal surface is smooth over the one-half to two-thirds basilar portion and has fine interdigitating trabeculations over the apical one-third to one-half portion. The left bundle branch penetrates the septum from the right ventricular side and divides into an anterior and a posterior fascicle, which run along the smooth portion of the left ventricular septal surface before traveling around the ventricular free wall or across the left ventricular cavity to the bases of the two left ventricular papillary muscles.

One interesting aspect of the ventricular septum is that, despite what the name implies, it is not necessarily located entirely between the ventricular cavities. In cases in which one ventricular sinus is hypoplastic (e.g., aortic atresia or pulmonary atresia with intact ventricular septum) or absent (e.g., tricuspid atresia, single left ventricle), a structure with the morphology of the ventricular septum lies between one ventricle and either an outlet chamber or the exterior of the heart. Hence, ventricular septum does not always imply two well-developed ventricular sinuses. Thus, a defect in that structure is a VSD even if the two chambers joined are not full-fledged ventricles, as in single left ventricle with right ventricular outlet chamber.

VSDs occur in five morphologic types based on location relative to landmarks in the ventricular septum, most easily recognized from the right ventricular septal surface (Fig. 67-11). The key landmarks are the septal band, the muscular or trabecular septum, the infundibular septum, and the annulus of the tricuspid valve. Conoventricular VSDs, also called perimembranous or paramembranous, are located between the conal (infundibular) septum and the muscular or trabecular septum but with conal septum still located in the fork of the "Y" of the septal band (Fig. 67-12). This is in the general location of the membranous ventricular septum but is often larger than the 1- to 3-mm diameter of the normal membranous septum. Conal septal malalignment VSDs, or malalignments for short, are located *in* the "Y" of the septal band because the infundibular septum is displaced *out* of the "Y." The AV canal-type VSD, also called *inlet-type VSD*, is located beneath the entire length of the AVV (either tricuspid or common AVV) that contacts or intersects the ventricular septum. The defect comes up to the valve—that is, there is no muscle between the defect and the valve. (VSDs with interposed muscle between the defect and the AVV are considered muscular; see later discussion.) Muscular VSDs are located in

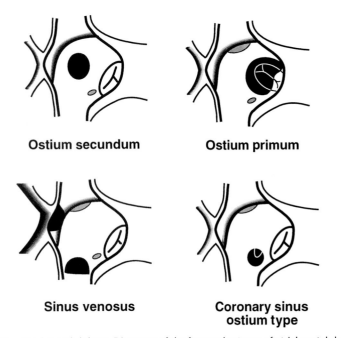

Figure 67-10. Atrial septal defects. Diagrams of the four major types of atrial septal defect in the same format as Fig. 67-9. The defects are shown in black. The sinus venosus type has two varieties: (1) the superior vena cava type adjacent to the pulmonary vein entrance and (2) the inferior vena cava type adjacent to the inferior vena cava entrance. (Reprinted with permission from PM Weinberg. Morphology of Congenital Heart Disease. In RM Freedom [volume ed], E Braunwald [series ed], Atlas of Heart Diseases, Vol 12: Congenital Heart Disease. Philadelphia: Current Medicine, 1997.)

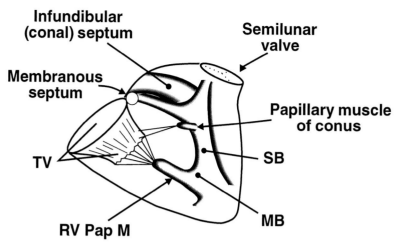

Figure 67-11. Right ventricular septal surface. The opened right ventricle viewed in anatomic position from a right anterior oblique aspect shows the landmarks used to describe the location of ventricular septal defects. (MB = moderator band; RV Pap M = main papillary muscle of the right ventricle; SB = septal band; TV = tricuspid valve.) (Reprinted with permission from PM Weinberg. Morphology of Congenital Heart Disease. In RM Freedom [volume ed], E Braunwald [series ed], Atlas of Heart Diseases, Vol 12: Congenital Heart Disease. Philadelphia: Current Medicine, 1997.)

the muscular or trabecular septum in any of the following general areas: posteroinferior to the main portion of the septal band, midmuscular; the inferior aspect of the muscular septum, inferomuscular; beneath the septal leaflet of the tricuspid valve but with a muscle bar separating the defect from the valve annulus, posterior muscular; apical muscular; and anterior to the main portion of the septal band, anterior

muscular. Muscular VSDs often have the appearance of multiple defects when viewed from the right ventricle or on angiograms or color Doppler ultrasound scans because of the lattice-like trabeculations of the right ventricle. However, such defects are usually single on the left ventricular side. Thus the term *multiple VSDs* should be reserved for multiple separate defects and not used for multiple streams from a single muscular

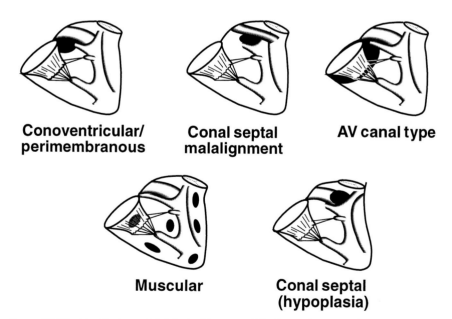

Conoventricular/ perimembranous   **Conal septal malalignment**   **AV canal type**

Muscular   **Conal septal (hypoplasia)**

Figure 67-12. Ventricular septal defects. Diagrams of the five major types of ventricular septal defect in the same format as in Fig. 67-11. The names of the specific varieties of muscular defects are given in the text. (AV = atrioventricular.) (Reprinted with permission from PM Weinberg. Morphology of Congenital Heart Disease. In RM Freedom [volume ed], E Braunwald [series ed], Atlas of Heart Diseases, Vol 12: Congenital Heart Disease. Philadelphia: Current Medicine, 1997.)

VSD. Conal septal hypoplasia VSDs are, like malalignment defects, located in the "Y" of the septal band but without malalignment. Any remnant of the infundibular septum is normally aligned with the septal band, but there is actual deficiency of the infundibular septum. In addition to these five main types, there are combinations of some of them: malalignment–conal septal hypoplasia, malalignment–canal type, malalignment–canal type–conal septal hypoplasia, and conoventricular–muscular.

In keeping with the principle of accuracy—independence from context—the definitions of the various VSDs are uninfluenced by associated conotruncal or other malformations. This is why the terms *subpulmonary, subaortic, beneath both* (doubly committed), or *beneath neither* (uncommitted) are not acceptable by themselves because a subaortic defect with normally aligned great arteries is in the same anatomic location as a subpulmonary defect with transposition of the great arteries. (These terms may be used in a supplementary fashion with an anatomic term to specify *great artery location* with double-outlet right or left ventricles.)

Pulmonary Valve

The pulmonary valve is normally a trileaflet valve with the infundibular septal commissure facing the aortic valve and all three commissures equally spaced around the valve's circumference. Pulmonary valvular stenosis, not part of a conotruncal anomaly, is typically a domed valve with all three commissures rudimentary and a central orifice, whereas pulmonary stenosis with a conotruncal anomaly is usually bicuspid or unicuspid with at least a rudimentary septal commissure.

Pulmonary Arteries

The pulmonary arteries refer to the main and proximal right and left branch pulmonary arteries. These in turn supply the peripheral pulmonary arteries. The morphologic right pulmonary artery courses anterior to the right mainstem, eparterial, bronchus. The morphologic left pulmonary artery crosses over the left mainstem, hyparterial, bronchus. Absent right or left pulmonary artery means the absence of the proximal pulmonary artery, not the entire pulmonary arterial tree. In such cases, the peripheral pulmonary artery may be supplied by a ductus arteriosus, a bronchial artery, some other systemic collateral vessel, or, rarely, a coronary artery. True pulmonary arteries always arise anterior to the tracheobronchial tree.

Therefore, a confluence behind the trachea is always some form of systemic collateral vessel.

Pulmonary Veins

Pulmonary veins, numbering from three to five, drain blood from the lungs and normally connect to the morphologic left atrium. Any other connection is considered an "anomalous pulmonary venous connection" regardless of the ultimate destination of the pulmonary venous blood. Hence, partial anomalous pulmonary venous connection or total anomalous pulmonary venous connection are anatomic terms, whereas partial anomalous pulmonary venous return or total anomalous pulmonary venous return are physiologic diagnoses, describing the destination of the blood, which may or may not be concordant with their anatomic counterparts.

Morphologic Left Atrium

The morphologic left atrium is best characterized by a discrete, narrow-based appendage, distinct from the venous portion. Pectinate muscles, being confined to the appendage portion, do not come near the crux of the heart as do the pectinate muscles in the right atrium. As mentioned previously, the absence of the accordion-like pectinate muscles from the main cavity of the left atrium renders it less compliant than the morphologic right atrium. This has implications for pressure changes engendered by AVV regurgitation, especially that which occurs acutely.

Mitral Valve

The mitral valve is defined as the left AVV in a D-loop heart and the right AVV in an L-loop heart. The rationale for this approach was described earlier under tricuspid valve. The usual mitral valve morphology is a bileaflet valve with the anterior leaflet deeper (from the annulus to the leaflet edge) than the posterior or mural leaflet. The anterior leaflet is shorter in circumferential length than the posterior leaflet.

Morphologic Left Ventricle

The morphologic left ventricle is characterized by fine, interdigitating trabeculations and absence of AVV chordal attachments to the ventricular septal surface. The left ventricle usually has two papillary muscles—anterolateral and posteromedial—arising from the ventricular free wall. The left ventricle does not usually have an infundibulum; however, this is not by way of definition. That is, the left ventricle, as defined, can give rise to the infundibulum. It must be emphasized that a left ventricular infundibulum, if present, is on the same side of the ventricular septum as the left ventricular sinus. When the infundibulum is on the opposite side of the ventricular septum as described earlier under "ventricular septum," it must be presumed to be a right ventricular infundibulum.

Aortic Valve

The aortic valve, like the pulmonary valve described earlier, is a trileaflet valve with evenly spaced commissures. Valvular stenosis is almost always caused by a bicuspid or unicuspid valve with one or two rudimentary commissures, respectively. Unicuspid valves have a funnel shape with an eccentric orifice. The commissure between the left coronary and noncoronary cusps is nearly always well developed.

Aorta

The aorta arises above the aortic valve and supplies at least one of the brachiocephalic vessels. Unlike the pulmonary artery, which may be atretic or even absent, the ascending aorta is virtually always patent down to the level of the valve even if the valve is atretic, because it carries at least coronary blood flow. The aortic arch is said to be left or right according to which bronchus it crosses over, regardless of the side of its origin from the heart. However, arch sidedness can be inferred very reliably from the fact that the first arch vessel almost always contains the carotid artery opposite the side of the arch.

Coronary Arteries

There are three main coronary arteries—the right (ventricular), the anterior descending, and the (left ventricular) circumflex—and one minor coronary artery, the infundibular or conal branch. The coronaries follow the ventricles. Thus, the right ventricular coronary can be right sided or left sided just as the right ventricle can be. Normally the anterior descending and circumflex coronaries arise from a single vessel named the left (ventricular) main coronary artery. Similarly, the right and conal branches arise from a single vessel, the right coronary. A common variant is for the right and conal branches to arise from separate orifices from the same sinus of Valsalva. However, other combinations are possible, particularly with conotruncal anomalies in which the spatial relationship between the aorta and the ventricles differs from normal. Hence, the anterior descending can arise from the conal branch of the right coronary as in some cases of tetralogy of Fallot, or the right and anterior descending can arise from one vessel and the (left ventricular) circumflex from the other, as frequently occurs in D transposition of the great arteries.

Conotruncal Anomalies

Conotruncal anomalies are defects involving the outflow tract (infundibular) portion of the heart, including the infundibular septum, the proximal great arteries, and the semilunar valves (Fig. 67-13). These anomalies are determined by the relative amounts of infundibular (conal) muscle beneath each semilunar valve plus the degree of expansion of each outflow tract. The normal conotruncus has subpulmonary but not subaortic conus with full expansion of both outflow tracts. A poorly expanded subpulmonary conus with no subaortic conus is the tetralogy conotruncus. A normally expanded subpulmonary conus with a poorly expanded subaortic area without subaortic conus is the interrupted aortic arch conotruncus. Subaortic conus without subpulmonary conus is typically seen with transposition of the great arteries. When the subaortic conus is poorly expanded, the conotruncus is that seen in transposition-VSD-coarctation. With a poorly expanded subpulmonary area, the conotruncus is characteristic of transposition-VSD-subpulmonary stenosis. Other conotruncal anomalies include bilateral conus with or without outflow obstruction and bilaterally deficient conus.

It is important to recognize the difference between conotruncal anomalies and ventriculoarterial alignments. There are three factors that determine ventriculoarterial alignment: (1) the relative amounts of subsemilunar infundibulum (conus)—the conotruncal anomaly, (2) the association of infundibulum with one or both ventricles, (3) and ventricular size. A subarterial conus carries the corresponding great artery anterior and superior, which tends to place it above the right ventricle. Absence of subarterial conus tends to result in origin above the left ventricle. However, association of the infundibulum with the left ventricle or hypoplasia of the right ventricle can vitiate the aforementioned tendency and result in association of the great artery in question with the left ventricle. Thus, nearly any conotruncus can be seen with nearly any ventriculoarterial alignment. Remember that the conotruncal anomaly is anatomic fact, whereas the ventriculoarterial alignment is a conceptual construct to describe

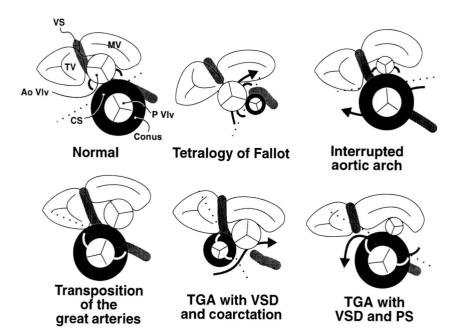

Normal   **Tetralogy of Fallot**   **Interrupted aortic arch**

Transposition of the great arteries   **TGA with VSD and coarctation**   **TGA with VSD and PS**

Figure 67-13. Conotruncal anomalies. Diagrammatic representation of normal conotruncus and representative conotruncal anomalies as if viewed from above. The aortic valve (Ao Vlv) is indicated by accompanying coronary arteries. A dotted line shows the plane of the infundibular or conal septum (CS) for comparison with the ventricular septum (VS). Note the leftward anterior deviation in tetralogy of Fallot relative to normal, the rightward anterior deviation in transposition (TGA) with ventricular septal defect (VSD) and coarctation, the posterior leftward deviation in interrupted aortic arch, and the posterior and rightward deviation in transposition with VSD and subpulmonary stenosis (PS). The large arrows represent the malalignment VSDs associated with displacement of the infundibular or conal septum. (MV = mitral valve; P Vlv = pulmonary valve; TV = tricuspid valve.) (Reprinted with permission from PM Weinberg. Morphology of Congenital Heart Disease. In RM Freedom [volume ed], E Braunwald [series ed], Atlas of Heart Diseases, Vol 12: Congenital Heart Disease. Philadelphia: Current Medicine, 1997.)

pulmonary venous connection to the ductus venosus, persistent left SVC to left-sided atrium, ectopic atrial rhythm, status post-modified (Gore-Tex tube graft) left Blalock-Taussig shunt, status post-Fontan operation with residual left pulmonary artery stenosis." In cases in which some of these headings are normal, those are simply omitted. For example, one could have "VSD and persistent left SVC to CoS" or "tricuspid atresia with VSD and pulmonary stenosis." One must always include the segmental notation if there is a ventriculoarterial alignment abnormality. It is also useful to include the segmental notation when there is a cardiac malposition even if the segments are normal because the segmental description clarifies the type of malposition instead of using additional, and frequently ambiguous, descriptions such as dextroposition and dextroversion.

SUGGESTED READING

Van Praagh R. The Segmental Approach to Diagnosis in Congenital Heart Disease. In Bergsma D (ed), Birth Defects: Original Article Series (Vol 8, No. 5). Baltimore: Williams & Wilkins, 1972;4.

Van Praagh R, Weinberg PM, Calder AL, et al. The Transposition Complexes: How Many Are There? In Davila JC (ed), Second Henry Ford Hospital International Symposium on Cardiac Surgery. New York: Appleton-Century-Crofts, 1977;207.

Van Praagh R, Weinberg PM, Smith SD, et al. Malpositions of the Heart. In Adams FH, Emmanouilides GC, Riemenschneider TA (ed), Moss' Heart Disease in Infants, Children, and Adolescents (4th ed). Baltimore: Williams & Wilkins, 1989;530.

Weinberg PM. Systematic approach to cardiac diagnoses. Pediatr Cardiol 1986;7:35.

Weinberg PM. Morphology of Congenital Heart Disease. In Freedom RM (volume ed), Braunwald E (series ed), Atlas of Heart Diseases, Vol 12: Congenital Heart Disease. Philadelphia: Current Medicine, 1997;4.1.

the proximity of each great artery to a ventricle.

Cardiac Malpositions

The heart is normally located within the thorax, in the mediastinum, extending predominantly into the left chest, although it crosses the midline slightly into the right chest. Locations outside this usual one are called cardiac malpositions. They fall into two broad categories: intrathoracic and extrathoracic. Intrathoracic malpositions include dextrocardia (i.e., the heart is predominantly in the right chest); mesocardia (i.e., the heart is predominantly in the midline); extreme levocardia (i.e., the heart is entirely in the left chest, more leftward than normal); absent pericardium, in which part or all of the heart lies in an abnormal position within one of the chest cavities; and pericardiodiaphragmatic defect, in which the heart is raised up above herniated liver, as if the heart were perched on a pitcher's mound. Extracardiac malpositions include ectopia cordis and thoracopagus conjoined twins.

Syntax for Cardiac Diagnoses

The convention for listing diagnoses is to use the following order:

Cardiac syndromes (e.g., hypoplastic left heart syndrome, heterotaxy syndrome with asplenia)

Cardiac malpositions (dextrocardia)

AV alignment abnormalities

Ventriculoarterial alignment abnormalities

Segmental notation

Chamber, valve, and vessel abnormalities beginning at the arterial end of the heart and proceeding to the venous end

Arrhythmias and physiologic diagnoses

Surgical diagnoses and residua in chronologic order

For example, one case showing all of these headings could be "heterotaxy syndrome with asplenia, dextrocardia, common AV canal, double-outlet right ventricle {A,D,D} with mirror-image right aortic arch, pulmonary stenosis, total anomalous

EDITOR'S COMMENTS

Complex forms of congenital heart disease are being seen with increasing frequency in most centers for congenital cardiac surgery in part because the relative success with surgical palliative interventions for congenital heart disease has improved and surgical therapy is being more widely applied to malformations that in the past were associated with very high mortality. Thus, it becomes increasingly important for cardiac surgeons and cardiologists to be able to communicate effectively the anatomic features of these complex defects. The anatomic classification scheme devised by Van Praagh and described in this chapter has advantages for creating a consistent description of certain features of the heart. Thus, the use of the Van Praagh classification system can accurately convey information about the situs of the heart, the situs or isomerism of the ventricles, and the position of the aortic origin. It must be emphasized, however, that these classification systems are primarily *anatomic*. Physiologic and surgical definitions and definitions of common complex malformations that have come into the terminology of congenital heart disease but are anatomically ambiguous must also be taken into account in any classification scheme or description of cardiac malformations. Thus, cardiac syndromes such as hypoplastic left heart syndrome, heterotaxy syndromes, and cardiac malpositions should be also used in descriptive terminology of cardiac malformations. These syndromes have surgical implications and can make communication simpler. The segmental notation scheme of Van Praagh then is complementary information. A hierarchical scheme of description is important because certain features are ambiguous. For example, double-outlet right ventricle with transposition of the great arteries is a relative misnomer because either

double-outlet right ventricle or transposition should be the primary diagnosis and the location of the great arteries can be described separately. Transposition of the great arteries has certain anatomic and certain physiologic abnormalities separate from double-outlet right ventricle.

Certain phrases have become commonly used that may be anatomically somewhat inaccurate but remain part of the nomenclature. For example, corrected transposition of the great arteries, isolated ventricular inversion, the Taussig-Bing heart, complete transposition of the great arteries, and AV canal are diagnoses that may be embryologically inaccurate, not anatomically descriptive, or may have physiologic connotations. Additional descriptors such as the concordancy or discordancy of AV or ventricular-arterial connections may be important. Although AV alignment and ventricular arterial alignment abnormalities and segments are defined in the Van Praagh system, the common conventional usage of concordant and discordant relationships may also aid in communication.

It is also important to recognize that the embryologic development of the heart is not completely understood, and specific gene defects identified with congenital heart malformations are rare. Thus, the anatomic classification system, surgical syndromes, and embryologic development are not necessar-

ily consistent. For a review of what is known about cardiac development, see Bharati S, Lev M. Embryology of the Heart and Great Vessels. In C Mavroudis and CL Backer (eds), Pediatric Cardiac Surgery. St. Louis: Mosby, 1994;1.

It is obviously fundamentally important that cardiologists and surgeons dealing with congenital heart disease be able to communicate accurately about cardiac diagnoses and anatomy. The multiple classification systems and descriptions cloud the ability to create databases that can accurately collect data on large numbers of patients internationally with congenital heart disease. Because of this problem, there has been a very active international effort among cardiologists, surgeons, and pathologists to create standard nomenclature for congenital heart disease diagnoses and surgery and to cross-map these diagnoses to other databases, such as the European Congenital Heart Database. The Herculean efforts involved in creating these common nomenclatures will ultimately provide a standardized list of anatomic diagnoses and operative procedures and enable data acquisition internationally and benchmarking of outcomes for congenital heart disease from one congenital heart center to another.

T.L.S.

68

Echocardiographic Evaluation of Congenital Heart Disease

Jack Rychik

Methodologies using ultrasonic imaging have been developed over the last two decades that allow for the assessment of both the form and the function of the heart. Because of its noninvasive nature and portability to the patient's bedside, cardiac ultrasound, or echocardiography, has become the imaging modality of choice in the initial diagnostic evaluation of infants and children suspected of having congenital heart disease. Structural abnormalities as well as alterations in flow and hemodynamics may be quickly and easily identified with a minimum of disturbance to the patient. Unlike angiography, in which images of opacified blood are radiographically exhibited and in which structural form is assumed from the visualization of nonopacified regions, echocardiography allows for direct, real-time imaging of cardiac structures based on their ultrasonic reflective properties. Multiple advantages are inherent in this diagnostic tool. Ultrasonic imaging is safe and radiation free. Views and sweeps of the heart from different angles and positions may be performed freely to conceptually reconstruct a three-dimensional image. Echocardiography may be used serially at different points in time or used continuously as a monitoring tool during procedures or interventions. Familiarity with the principles used to generate the echocardiographic image and its limitations will aid in the appropriate interpretation and clinical application of ultrasound in the surgical management of infants and children with congenital heart disease.

Principles of Ultrasound Physics and Applications

Ultrasonic Frequencies

Ultrasonic energy is generated by the delivery of electrical impulses to piezo-electric crystals, which resonate at a set frequency. The range of ultrasound frequencies used for conventional cardiac imaging is 2.0 MHz to 7.5 MHz. The choice of a particular frequency for imaging is based on its tissue penetration and resolution characteristics. High-frequency ultrasound is dissipated quickly in tissue and can be propagated only for short distances, whereas low-frequency ultrasound penetrates greater distances before attenuation. Alternatively, high-frequency ultrasound allows for greater resolution of structure. This concept is illustrated by the formula: wavelength = velocity/frequency, where the velocity of ultrasound in biologic tissue is constant at 1,540 m/sec. To ultrasonically resolve two points in space, they must be the distance of at least one wavelength from each other; hence, the higher the frequency, the smaller is the wavelength and the greater is the ability to resolve points that are in close proximity. For example, using 2.0-MHz ultrasound, one can resolve two points that are a minimum of 0.78 mm apart. If the objects are any closer, they will not be resolved and will appear as one. At 7.5 MHz, two points can be resolved at a minimum of 0.21 mm apart, hence resolution

is greater. In practice, high-frequency transducers are chosen for use in newborns and small children to maximize resolution, whereas in older children and adolescents lower frequencies are used to maximize penetration.

The Doppler Principle

In 1842, Christian Johann Doppler described the change in frequency of energy emission of an object in motion in relation to its velocity of motion toward or away from a stationary observer as follows:

$$F_d = 2VF_o(\cos Y)/c$$

where F_d is the frequency shift, F_o is the emitting frequency, Y is the angle of incidence between the direction of motion of the object and the emitted frequency, V is the velocity of motion of the object, and c is the velocity of the energy in the medium (a constant). In the setting of reflected ultrasound, this principle can be used to assay for the velocity of blood flow moving through the chambers of the heart. Rearranging the equation, we obtain

$$V = F_d F_o(\cos Y)c/2$$

Hence, the velocity of blood flow can be derived from the Doppler frequency shift of reflected ultrasound from moving blood if the emitting frequency and the angle of incidence between the direction of motion of blood and the interrogating ultrasound beam are known. In the clinical setting, it is cumbersome to measure the angle of incidence between flow direction and the ultrasound beam. Every effort is therefore made to align the ultrasound beam parallel to the direction of blood flow; angle Y is thereby assumed to be 0 (cosine of $Y = 1$). Doppler velocity assessments based on this assumption continue to be valid for angles of incidence of ≤ 20 degrees because the cosine of 20 remains close to unity; however, at angles > 20 degrees this assumption is not valid, and Doppler-derived velocities may be underestimated.

Information relating to velocity and direction of blood flow can be obtained via pulsed-wave, continuous-wave, or color Doppler techniques. In the pulsed-wave Doppler technique, ultrasound crystals fire pulses of energy and then stop to "listen" for reflected sound. This technique permits the spatial determination of velocity by allowing for interrogation of flow within a selected region of interest. Distance is calculated from the time it takes for reflected ultrasound to return to the transducer during the listening phase. Pulsed-wave Doppler is limited by its inability to assess peak velocities when there are significant disturbances of flow and velocities are high. Once a region of disturbed flow is identified, continuous-wave Doppler may be applied to determine the peak velocity in the region. However, continuous-wave Doppler will assess all velocities within a line of interrogation—velocities within as well as proximal to and distal to the site of interest. Hence, spatial localization of disturbed flow is diagnosed via pulsed-wave Doppler, whereas the peak velocity of the disturbed flow is measured by continuous-wave Doppler.

Color Doppler is a pulsed-wave method in which flow within a region is assigned a color based on velocity and direction and is displayed as an overlay onto the two-dimensional image. By convention, flow toward the transducer is designated as varying shades of red, whereas flow away from the transducer is blue.

Modified Bernoulli Theorem

Based on the concept of exchange of potential energy into kinetic energy, the velocity of flow between cardiac structures can be used to calculate the pressure difference, thereby providing hemodynamic information. Bernoulli showed that the difference in potential energy, or pressure, between two sites is equal to the kinetic energy loss in addition to the energy losses caused by inertial and frictional forces. If the loss of energy because of inertia or friction is assumed to be minimal, as can be done when assessing flow across a discrete, short segmental narrowing, then these

contributing variables may be ignored and the modified Bernoulli formula applied to calculate the pressure difference between upstream point 1 (proximal point) and downstream point 2 (distal point):

$$P_1 - P_2 = 4\left(V_2^2 - V_2^2\right)$$

If the proximal blood flow velocity is ≤ 1.0 m/sec, as is the case within most of the structures of the normal heart, the formula can be further simplified to

$$\text{Pressure difference} = 4V_2^2$$

Hence, the pressure difference across an area of discrete stenosis can be calculated based on the peak velocity across the region of narrowing obtained by Doppler echocardiography. Systolic pressure gradients derived from peak velocity data reflect the peak instantaneous pressure gradient, which usually occurs during the upstroke of systole and not at peak systole. This is why Doppler-derived gradients may be higher than cardiac catheterization gradients in which peak-to-peak pressure gradients are measured. Lesions in which the time for reaching peak pressure is delayed in one chamber relative to the other will add to a further exaggeration of differences between the catheter-derived and Doppler-derived gradients. For example, in aortic stenosis, peak ascending aorta pressure is reached much later than peak left ventricular pressure. Hence, whereas the peak-to-peak (catheter) gradient may be 40 to 50 mm Hg when comparing the two time-delayed peaks, the peak instantaneous (Doppler echocardiography) gradient, which will likely occur during early systole when aortic pressure is low and left ventricular pressure is rapidly on the rise, may be up to 30 to 40 mm Hg higher. The mean gradient, which can be calculated from the echocardiogram by integrating the sum of the peak instantaneous gradients within the systolic cycle, is most likely the best reflection of the afterload work imposed on the ventricle; however, clinical correlates were developed in the era before echocardiography, and the standard for grading and treatment of valvular stenosis of a congenital cause today is still based on the peak-to-peak gradient assessment.

Approach to Imaging Children with Congenital Heart Disease

Echocardiographic evaluation of a child with possible heart disease should be per-

formed in a standardized, systematic fashion with identification of all segments of the anatomy from multiple planes. Once the anatomic structure is fully understood, physiologic information via the Doppler methodologies may be obtained. To facilitate the study, patients younger than 3 years of age should be sedated. A complete study consists of two-dimensional views and sweeps (incremental views obtained while rotating the transducer through a plane or on an axis), starting with subcostal imaging in which the liver is used as an acoustic window to the heart and ending with the suprasternal windows (Table 68-1).

Abdomen and Situs

The echocardiographic study commences with a determination of situs. A transverse view of the abdomen just below the sternum at the level of the diaphragms should display the position of the liver, stomach, inferior vena cava, and descending aorta (Fig. 68-1). In situs solitus, the following should be noted: (1) The liver and the inferior vena cava traversing throughout the body of the liver are to the right of the spine; (2) the stomach is to the left of the spine; and (3) the aorta is retroperitoneal and lies just anterior and slightly to the left of the spine. In situs inversus, the mirror image is found, whereas in heterotaxia (asplenia or polysplenia), the liver is usually in the midline, and the inferior vena cava and aorta may be on the same side of the spine either to the right or the left. In polysplenia, the inferior vena cava may be interrupted at the infrarenal level, with no inferior vena cava seen at the level of the diaphragms. In this case, a dilated azygos vein should be sought in the retroperitoneal space adjacent to the spine, which will be carrying inferior venous return to the superior vena cava. A dilated superior vena cava confirms this finding. At all times, the hepatic venous drainage into the atria should be identified. The size of the hepatic veins should be noted because inordinate dilation may be a sign of (1) right atrioventricular (AV) valve insufficiency, stenosis, or atresia or (2) infradiaphragmatic total anomalous pulmonary venous connection.

Atria, Ventricles, and the Atrioventricular Connection

Identification of atrial and ventricular morphology is an important part of the echocardiographic examination. The atria are identified by their appendage morphology. The right atrial appendage has a wide inlet and a broad-based triangular appearance; the left atrial appendage has a narrow inlet

Table 68-1   Views and Sweeps for Echocardiographic Imaging of the Child with Suspected Congenital Heart Disease

Imaging Window	Transducer Position	Angling	Structures Best Visualized
Transverse abdominal view	Below the xiphoid process	Posterior, at a straight line perpendicular to the spine	Diaphragms, liver, stomach, aorta, IVC
Frontal subcostal sweep	Below the xiphoid process	Posterior to anterior in a coronal plane, parallel to long axis of patient	Atrial appendages, atrial, vent and great arterial relationships
Left axial oblique sweep	Below the xiphoid process	30 degrees left oblique from frontal starting from right shoulder sweeping toward apex of the heart	Pulmonary veins, atrial sept and large portion of vent sept on-end, LV outflow tract and aorta
Sagittal subcostal sweep	Below the xiphoid process	At 90 degrees from the frontal, sweeping from right to left	SVC, IVC, atrial sept, conal sept, muscular and apical vent sept
Right anterior oblique view	Below the xiphoid process	30 degrees right oblique from frontal	RV inflow and outflow, conal septum, pulmonary artery
Apical "four-chamber" view	Apex of the heart, sixth intercostal space, medial to the left anterior-axillary line	Superiorly, aimed toward the right shoulder	Atrioventricular relationship, mitral and tricuspid valves, muscular and apical sept
Apical "two-chamber" view	Rotate 90 degrees clockwise from apical "four-chamber"	Superiorly, aimed toward the right shoulder and anteriorly	Left atrium, mitral valve, LV inflow, vent sept, LV outflow, aorta
Parasternal long-axis sweep	Third-fourth intercostal space, just to the left of the sternum	Plane cuts through long axis of the heart from right shoulder to the left hip. Sweep is from direction of right hip to left shoulder.	Tricuspid valve, RV inflow, LV inflow and outflow, vent sept, RV outflow and pulmonary valve
Parasternal short-axis sweep	Rotate 90 degrees clockwise from long-axis sweep	Plane cuts through short axis of the heart starting at level of great vessels. Sweep is from cephalad to caudad, toward the apex	Aortic and pulmonary valves, RV inlet and outlet, mitral valve apparatus, anterior portion of muscular sept, apical sept
Suprasternal frontal view	Suprasternal notch	Parallel to long axis of the patient, aimed caudad	SVC and innominate vein, arch sidedness, branch pulmonary arteries, pulmonary veins
Suprasternal sagittal view	Suprasternal notch	Perpendicular to long axis of the patient, aimed caudad	Aortic arch, descending aorta, left pulmonary artery

IVC = inferior vena cava; LV = left ventricle , RV = right ventricle ; sept = septum; vent = ventricular; SVC = superior vena cava.

and a long, fingerlike appearance. The left ventricle is identified by the presence of (1) smooth trabeculations along the septal surface, (2) two papillary muscles, (3) an AV valve with two leaflets opening with a "fish-mouth" appearance, and (4) no valve chordal attachments to the ventricular septum. The right ventricle is identified by the presence of (1) coarse septal trabeculations, (2) a single papillary muscle, (3) a trileaflet AV valve, and (4) chordal attachments to the ventricular septum. In a "D-looped" ventricle, the right and left atria connect normally to their respective right and left morphologic ventricles. In an "L-looped" ventricle, the right atrium connects to a morphologic left ventricle that functions as the pulmonary ventricle, whereas the left atrium connects to a morphologic right ventricle that func-

tions as the systemic ventricle. Because the AV valves follow the ventricles, the systemic AV valve in this case is a tricuspid valve, which may at times appear abnormal and regurgitant.

Atrial and Ventricular Septal Defects

Three types of atrial septal defects (ASDs) are possible:

1. Secundum ASD is a deficiency in the septum primum. These are usually located centrally, may be of varying size, and, if small, may be difficult to distinguish from a patent foramen ovale (Fig. 68-2). A defect measuring >6 mm in diameter on a subcostal long axial

oblique or sagittal sweep should be considered one of significance. Defects <5 mm may be considered a large patent foramen ovale and may spontaneously become smaller with time. Occasionally even an anatomically small defect may be physiologically significant (large left-to-right shunt), and surgical closure may be indicated.

2. Primum ASD is part of the spectrum of common AV canal defects. In addition to the atrial deficiency, there is a cleft in the mitral valve and possibly a ventricular septal defect (VSD) of varying size. The atrial septal deficiency is large, located inferiorly and anteriorly, and best seen in the subcostal long axial oblique sweep and in the apical view (Figs. 68-3 and 68-4).

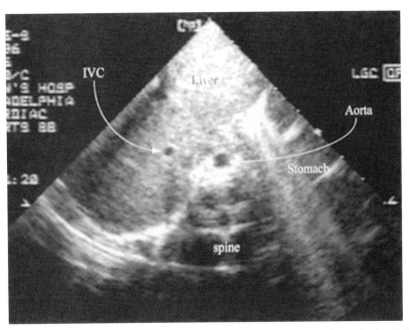

Figure 68-1. Cross-sectional image of the abdomen from anterior to posterior at the level of the diaphragms. This is the starting position for the pediatric echocardiographic examination. This patient has situs solitus with the liver and inferior vena cava (IVC) on the right; the stomach and aorta are on the left.

3. Sinus venosus ASD is a deficiency in the atrial septum at the level of the venous connections to the atria and is large. A superior defect is located at the orifice of the superior vena cava into the right atrium, hence echocardiographically, the defect creates the appearance of the superior vena cava overriding the atrial septum. Normally the right pulmonary veins drain posteriorly, and they should

be clearly delineated relative to the defect because anomalous connection to the superior vena cava may occur. In an inferior defect, the inferior vena cava overrides the septum and the flow may be directed toward the left atrium. In a subcostal sagittal sweep, the position of the inferior vena cava and the presence of a Eustachian valve and its relationship to the atrial deficiency should be noted in order not to confuse the vena caval orifice with ASD.

Because it is a thin structure and false image drop-out is possible, the atrial septum should always be imaged in multiple planes perpendicular to the ultrasound beam. Secondarily the right atrium, right ventricle, and pulmonary arteries may appear dilated, and pulmonary artery flow velocities may be elevated in relation to the right-sided volume load. Echocardiography provides all of the information that is sufficient to refer patients for surgery without the need for cardiac catheterization in this lesion.

The ventricular septum is a complex three-dimensional structure made up of tissue of varying morphology as well as embryologic origin; hence, there are a variety of types of VSDs. The conoventricular VSD is the most common and is located on the right ventricular side in the region adjacent to the septal leaflet of the tricuspid valve; on the left ventricular side it is located close to and beneath the aortic valve. It may be of varying size and in fact may be partially filled in with tricuspid valve tissue, forming an "aneurysm." The presence of aneurysm tissue on echocardiographic examination may indicate a high likelihood for spontaneous diminution or closure. Displacement of the conal or infundibular septum results in a malalignment-type VSD. These defects are located anteriorly, are usually large, do not close spontaneously, and, in the face of posterior or anterior infundibular displacement, result in left ventricular or right ventricular outflow tract obstruction (muscular subaortic stenosis or tetralogy of Fallot), respectively. Deficiency of the infundibular septum may occur with or without displacement, resulting in a conoseptal hypoplasia VSD. Because of the proximity of this defect to the aortic valve annulus, prolapse of the right aortic cusp with deformity of the aortic valve architecture and subsequent insufficiency may occur. An AV canal VSD may be part of the common AV canal anomaly in which a primum ASD and a common AV valve are present, or it may exist alone. It is usually large and located posteriorly at the

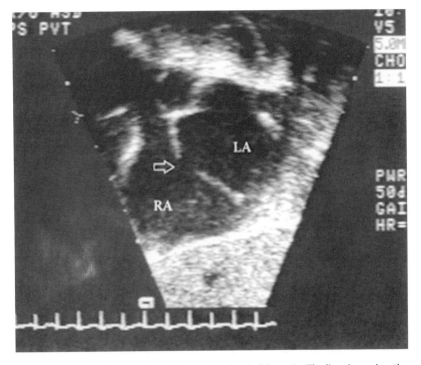

Figure 68-2. Subcostal image, frontal view at the level of the atria. The liver is used as the acoustic window. The arrow points to a secundum-type atrial septal defect. (LA = left atrium; RA = right atrium.)

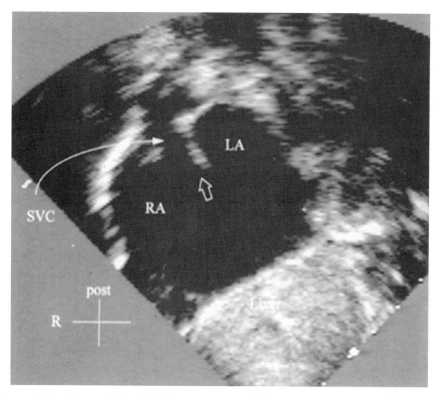

Figure 68-3. Subcostal, left axial oblique sweep view of the atria in a child with a large primum atrial septal defect. The arrow points to the inferior rim of the remnant of atrial septum (the septum secundum). (LA = left atrium; post = posterior; R = right; RA = right atrium: SVC = superior vena cava.)

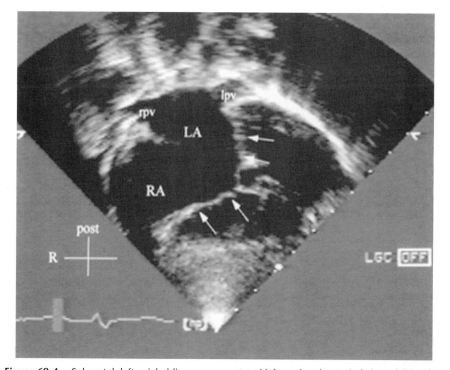

Figure 68-4. Subcostal, left axial oblique sweep rotated leftward and anteriorly in a child with a primum atrial septal defect demonstrating a large interatrial communication and connection of the pulmonary veins. The arrows point to the common atrioventricular valve. (LA = left atrium; lpv = left pulmonary vein; post = posterior; R = right; RA = right atrium; rpv = right pulmonary vein.)

"inlet" portion of the right ventricle. In the common AV canal spectrum, the VSD may be filled in with valve tissue, which may partially or completely occlude the defect. A muscular VSD may exist in the anterior trabecular zone or in the middle portion, apex, or posterior aspect of the septum. These are defects that are rimmed circumferentially by muscular tissue and may be of varying size (Figs. 68-5 and 68-6). In the presence of a large VSD such as in tetralogy of Fallot, an additional small or moderate-sized muscular defect has been reported in up to 5% to 10% of cases and may be difficult to detect because flow is preferentially across the larger defect. Once the larger defect is closed, the smaller defects may then play a greater physiologic role and cause morbidity related to increased left-to-right shunt in the postoperative period. Hence, a careful search for additional muscular defects, particularly in the anterior trabecular zone of the right ventricle, should be undertaken in all patients with a large VSD.

Part of the assessment of the physiologic effect of a VSD is an estimate of the right ventricular pressure. Assessing the velocity of tricuspid regurgitation will allow for the calculation of the peak gradient between the right ventricle and the right atrium (Fig. 68-7A,B). By adding the value of right atrial pressure, which in the absence of direct monitoring may be assumed to be 5 to 10 mm Hg, one can obtain an estimate of right ventricular pressure. In addition, a less accurate but somewhat useful method of assessing right ventricular pressure is to measure peak velocity across a native VSD or a residual defect after repair. Problems with this method commonly arise when the flow jet across the defect is irregularly shaped because of an irregular orifice shape, and hence, the modified Bernoulli equation may not be valid. Because the Doppler technique measures the peak instantaneous pressures within the cardiac cycle, a right-bundle-branch block, which may be common after closure of a VSD, may create a period in early systole in which a large pressure gradient is present, and a high peak velocity will be obtained. This may create the spurious finding that right ventricular pressures are low when in fact peak right ventricular pressure, which is delayed relative to the left ventricle, may be extremely high. Cardiac catheterization is at times indicated before referral for surgery of patients with VSDs. If a defect appears anatomically large on echocardiography in conjunction with signs and symptoms of congestive

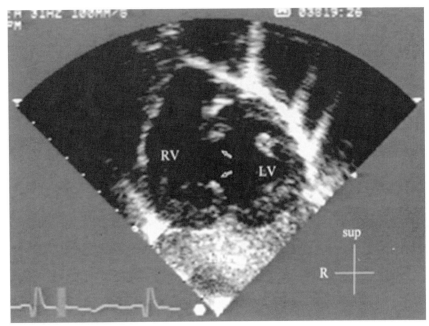

Figure 68-5. Subcostal, frontal sweep demonstrating a large muscular ventricular septal defect. The arrows point to the muscular edges of the defect. (LV = left ventricle; R = right; RV = right ventricle; sup = superior.)

heart failure and if there is no suspicion of pulmonary vascular disease (i.e., the patient is <6 months of age), cardiac catheterization is unnecessary and repair should be undertaken. Invasive catheter assessments are indicated when the defect appears restrictive, when calculation of the degree of shunt helps in decision making, and in circumstances in which a calculation of the vascular resistances would help.

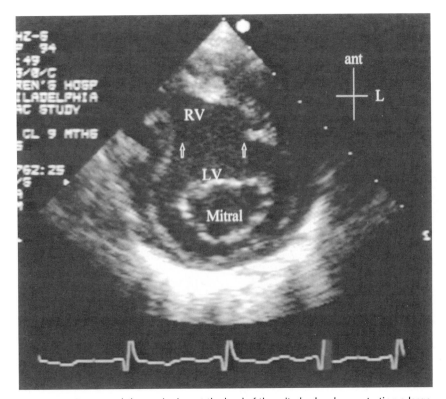

Figure 68-6. Parasternal short axis view at the level of the mitral valve demonstrating a large midmuscular ventricular septal defect. (ant = anterior; L = left; LV = left ventricle; RV = right ventricle.)

Conotruncal Anomalies

Conotruncal anomalies involve defects of the infundibulum (conus) and the great arteries. The conus is a smooth-walled region of muscle normally situated beneath the pulmonary valve, raising it above the level of the aortic valve and positioning it anterior and to the left of the aorta. The aortic valve annulus is hence, normally in fibrous continuity with the mitral valve and is the characteristic that defines the aorta as arising from the left ventricle. This relationship is easily visible in many different echocardiographic planes. Conotruncal defects arise when displacement of the infundibular septum is present and when the normal relationship of the great arteries is disturbed.

Tetralogy of Fallot is a common form of conotruncal anomaly in which a large malalignment VSD is present with anterior displacement of the infundibular septum into the right ventricular outflow tract (Fig. 68-8). In addition, distal pulmonary artery stenosis and hypoplasia are present. Key parts of the echocardiographic evaluation include an examination of (1) the nature and degree of the infundibular and pulmonary arterial narrowing, (2) the branch pulmonary artery architecture, (3) the presence of additional muscular defects, and (4) the location and course of the coronary arteries. The coronary artery anatomy is important because in approximately 5% to 10% of cases the anterior descending artery will arise from the right coronary artery and course across the infundibulum in the region where a surgical incision may be anticipated. If all four aforementioned points of anatomy are well delineated by echocardiography, cardiac catheterization is not necessary in this lesion.

Transposition of the great arteries is a defect in which the aorta arises from the right ventricle and the pulmonary artery from the left ventricle (Fig. 68-9). Echocardiographic evaluation should include determination of (1) the nature and size of the interatrial communication as a source of mixing, (2) the presence or absence of left ventricular outflow tract obstruction, (3) the relative position of the great arteries one to the other, and (4) the coronary artery anatomy, in order to anticipate the technique of coronary reimplantation at the time of arterial switch repair. In most circumstances, echocardiographic evaluation is sufficient to refer infants with this lesion for surgery without cardiac catheterization. In the past, balloon atrial septostomy, which may be needed to increase the degree of intercirculatory mixing and raise

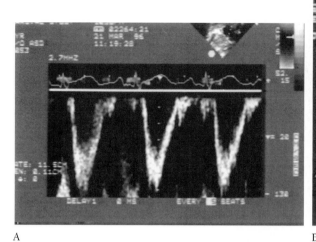
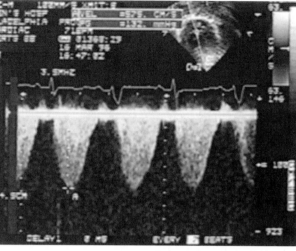

A

B

Figure 68-7. **(A)** An example of pulsed-wave Doppler spectral tracing obtained from sampling in the normal pulmonary artery. Note the presence of laminar flow—blood cells within the sample all moving at the same velocity at any one point in the cardiac cycle; hence, a smooth curve is generated with central clearing underneath. The peak velocity is 1.3 m/sec. **(B)** An example of an estimate of right ventricular pressure via assessment of tricuspid regurgitation velocity in a child with pulmonary hypertension. Continuous-wave Doppler is used. Note the lack of central clearing underneath the spectral curve, indicating turbulent flow. The tricuspid regurgitation peak velocity is markedly elevated, with calculated right ventricular pressure of 132 mm Hg above the right atrial V-wave pressure.

the arterial oxygen level, has been done under fluoroscopic guidance. At present, this can be safely performed with echocardiographic guidance (transthoracic or transesophageal), obviating the need to move a critically ill infant to the cardiac catheterization laboratory.

Double-outlet right ventricle is a class of anomalies of the conotruncal type in which both great vessels arise from the right ventricle. Associated lesions dictate a wide spectrum of variability in physiology for this lesion. A VSD is almost always present, and in addition there may be (1) left ventricular hypoplasia with mitral stenosis or atresia (physiologically similar to hypoplastic left heart syndrome), (2) infundibular narrowing of the pulmonary outflow tract with VSD flow directed toward the aorta (physiologically similar to tetralogy of Fallot), or (3) infundibular narrowing of the aortic outflow tract with VSD flow directed toward the pulmonary artery (physiologically similar to transposition of the great arteries). Key points that must be delineated echocardiographically are (1) the relative position of the great arteries one to the other, (2) the presence or absence of conus beneath either of the great vessels and the associated degree of outflow obstruction, (3) direction of flow from the VSD to the great vessels, (4) the size of the VSD, which may be restrictive, and (5) chordal attachments of the AV valves, which may be to the infundibular septum or across the VSD.

Venous Connections and Extracardiac Vessels

The suprasternal window allows for visualization of abnormalities of the pulmonary veins, superior vena cava, and aortic arch. All four pulmonary veins should be

Figure 68-8. Subcostal sagittal sweep in an infant with tetralogy of Fallot. The arrow points to the hypertrophied infundibular septum, which is malaligned anteriorly, encroaching on the right ventricular outflow tract. Just beneath the infundibular septum is the ventricular septal defect. (Ant = anterior; Ao = aorta; LA = left atrium; RA = right atrium; RV = right ventricle; Sup = superior.)

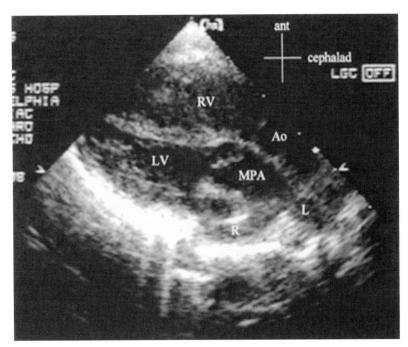

Figure 68-9.   Parasternal long-axis view in an infant with D transposition of the great arteries. Note that the vessel arising from the left ventricle bifurcates proximally into two branches, indicating it is the pulmonary artery. (ant = anterior; Ao = aorta; MPA = main pulmonary artery; L = left; LV = left ventricle; R = right; RV = right ventricle.)

identified entering the left atrium from the suprasternal frontal plane. Venous structures originating from the left atrium in which flow appears to be directed superiorly toward the innominate vein or caudad toward the diaphragm should suggest an anomalous pulmonary venous connection. A left superior vena cava should be sought in patients who are candidates for cavopulmonary connection surgery. Typically, this vessel crosses anterior to the left pulmonary artery and enters the coronary sinus posteriorly. Aortic arch sidedness is determined by identifying each of the branches arising off the arch from proximal to distal. In a left aortic arch, the first vessel arising off the arch is the right innominate artery bifurcating into the right carotid and subclavian arteries, followed by the left carotid, then left subclavian arteries. In a suprasternal frontal sweep, if the first vessel off the arch is the left innominate artery, the arch is right sided. The branching pattern of the first vessel should be noted to be sure that it bifurcates into a carotid and a subclavian. If it does not bifurcate, the possibility of an aberrant subclavian artery should be entertained. Patency of the ductus arteriosus may present by itself or in association with other lesions, whereby its function is to augment the systemic or pulmonic circulations. Doppler sampling of the flow patterns in the ductus arteriosus will aid in

understanding the physiology. In a ductus arteriosus by itself or in association with lesions in which there is impediment to pulmonic flow (tetralogy of Fallot, critical pulmonic stenosis), the direction of flow will be from the aorta to the pulmonary artery (left to right) continuously throughout the cardiac cycle. In lesions in which severe left-sided obstruction is present (critical aortic stenosis, coarctation of the aorta, hypoplastic left heart syndrome), the role of the ductus is to support the systemic circulation, hence, flow in systole will be from the pulmonary artery to the aorta (right to left) with reversed flow left to right into the pulmonary circulation during diastole because of lower pulmonary vascular resistance relative to systemic. Right-to-left flow across the ductus without an associated lesion is an ominous sign reflecting the presence of abnormally elevated pulmonary vascular resistance.

Intraoperative Transesophageal Echocardiography and Postoperative Imaging

As a result of the miniaturization of ultrasound probes, transesophageal echocardiographic (TEE) imaging may be performed

in infants as small as 3 kg in weight. Information concerning surgical repair is immediately available in the operating room before closure of the chest wall. TEE is useful in assessing the outcome after closure of a VSD, repair of an outflow tract obstruction, and repair of AV valve insufficiency and in observing for abnormalities of myocardial function. Quantitative hemodynamics such as pressure gradients and degrees of valvular insufficiency, however, must be interpreted cautiously in the operating room because body temperature, cardiopulmonary bypass, inotropes, and an open chest wall may be variables that transiently influence the vascular resistances or myocardial mechanics. Information obtained in this setting may not always predict the patient's steady-state outcome under different conditions in the intensive care unit or beyond.

Conventional transthoracic echocardiography has been shown to be effective in detecting residual lesions and in providing sufficient information in approximately 85% of cases for surgeons to reoperate on the same admission. Color Doppler echocardiography is an exquisitely sensitive tool that has demonstrated the presence of residual left-to-right shunting in up to 38% of cases after closure of a large VSD. Quantitative assessment of the size of these defects in children younger than 2 years of age shows the vast majority of them to be small, peripatch leaks that are <4 mm in diameter and are of no hemodynamic consequence. Residual lesions with color jet diameters of >4 mm should suggest a significant residual defect that may need further intervention. At approximately 1 year follow-up, two thirds of these small residual defects will have disappeared on further echocardiographic study.

SUGGESTED READING

Chang AC, Vetter JM, Gill SE, et al. Accuracy of prospective two-dimensional Doppler echocardiography in the assessment of reparative surgery. J Am Coll Cardiol 1990;16:903.

Chin AJ. Non-Invasive Imaging of Congenital Heart Disease Before and After Surgical Reconstruction. Armonk, NY: Futura, 1994.

Chin AJ, Vetter JM, Seliem M, et al. Role of early postoperative surface echocardiography in the pediatric cardiac intensive care unit. Chest 1994;105:10.

Rychik J. Aortic stenosis or atresia with associated hypoplasia of the left ventricle: imaging before and after reconstructive surgery. Echocardiography 1996;13:318.

Rychik J, Norwood WI, Chin AJ. Doppler color flow mapping assessment of residual shunt after closure of large ventricular septal defects. Circulation 1991;84:III-153.

EDITOR'S COMMENTS

As is well described in this chapter, noninvasive imaging modalities for congenital heart disease have become increasingly sophisticated, such that much hemodynamic information can now be obtained in addition to anatomic information. Thus, in most congenital heart surgery centers, including our own, cardiac catheterization is reserved for patients in whom complete anatomic information has not been obtained by noninvasive modalities or for specific hemodynamic determinations (such as shunt calculations and measurement of vascular resistances) in which it has not been possible to calculate gradients or estimate ventricular pressures from echocardiographic images. Occasionally, catheterization may be necessary to confirm or refute calculations of gradients across cardiac valves when imaging is suboptimal or when decisions for surgery are equivocal. However, the use of "diagnostic cardiac catheterization" is decreasing in frequency, and most cardiac catheterizations now include at least some component of intervention, including electrophysiologic determinations, drug evaluation studies, or an assessment of the reversibility of pulmonary vascular resistance.

An understanding of the standard views and methods of evaluation by echocardiography and a good understanding of echocardiographic imaging are important for congenital cardiac surgeons not only for preoperative diagnosis, but also for postoperative evaluation of surgical repairs. Intraoperative echocardiography, usually by the transesophageal technique, has now become a common source of information on the suitability of cardiac repairs. Although in some centers echocardiography is used selectively to evaluate VSD patches for the presence of residual leaks or for evaluation of residual valvular insufficiency after AV canal repairs or tricuspid valvuloplasties, in other centers echocardiography is used routinely in all cardiac cases to assess the quality of the operative intervention and to rule out any additional hemodynamic lesions. (RM Ungerleider, JA Kislo, WJ Greeley, et al. Echocardiography during congenital heart operations, experience from 1000 cases. Ann Thorac Surg 1995;60:S539.) The hypothesis associated with the use of intraoperative echocardiography in the immediate evaluation of postoperative anatomy is that if residual lesions are identified, then addressing these at the initial operation would improve the morbidity or mortality in the postoperative period. Our experience with intraoperative echocardiography for assessing AV canal defects has shown that its routine use is associated with a significant reduction in the rate of reoperation for AV canal defects over time because significant residual valvular regurgitation can be addressed promptly. This approach has also decreased the risk of pulmonary hypertensive problems after repair (CE Canter, TL Spray, CB Huddleston, E Mendeloff. Intraoperative evaluation of atrioventricular septal defect repair by color flow Doppler echocardiography. Ann Thorac Surg 1997;63:592). The argument certainly can be made that intraoperative TEE is an integral part of any congenital cardiac operation as more complex repairs are being performed frequently in newborns and infants.

Recent echocardiographic techniques, including three-dimensional imaging, have improved the ability to provide anatomic information on mechanisms of valvar regurgitation and more three-dimensional geometric information that can aid in guiding cardiac surgical repair.

T.L.S.

69

Cardiac Magnetic Resonance Imaging

Mark A. Fogel

Introduction and General Comments

Magnetic resonance imaging (MRI) has been playing an increasingly important role in the pre- and postoperative management of patients with congenital heart disease. It is complementary to echocardiography and cardiac catheterization and can add significant information that can change the care of the child. In most instances, all anatomic data necessary for diagnosis and much physiologic information may be obtained via MRI. It is evident, then, that choosing the correct imaging modality or combination of imaging modalities is important.

Table 69-1 displays the distinct advantages MRI has over both echocardiography and cardiac catheterization as well as its limitations. Because patient size plays an important role in the ability of echocardiography to visualize structures, MRI has a distinct advantage in the older child, adolescent, and adult. In complex congenital heart disease, the overlapping of structures in angiography or the "sweeps" used in echocardiography may not be enough to conceptualize the total anatomic picture. With MRI, because images can be obtained in contiguous, parallel slices, computers can off-line stack these images one atop the other and slice the volumetric data set in any plane desired (called multiplanar reconstruction or oblique sectioning), yielding the salient points of the anatomy. Even curved planes are used clinically. This same ability allows a three-dimensional shaded surface display or volume-rendered three-dimensional image to be created that can itself be sectioned in any plane, viewed from any angle, and have individual structures removed to reveal the necessary information. An MRI image is typically averaged over multiple heartbeats (unlike echocardiography and angiography, a single MRI image can be averaged over two to many hundreds of heartbeats), and, therefore, functional analysis by MRI can give a better handle on long-term performance (the image itself is an average, and the physician does not have to do this averaging in his or her head as in echocardiography). However, "real-time" as well as "interactive" cardiac MRI is now coming into routine clinical use, and this allows for imaging typical of echocardiography and cardiac catheterization. Furthermore, there are abilities such as magnetic blood and tissue tagging that allow calculation of regional wall strain, motion, and visualization of velocity profiles that are unique to MRI. Delayed enhancement, another example of a unique cardiac MRI capability, allows for identification of myocardial scar tissue. On the other hand, pacemakers in general cannot be placed in the scanner without scrambling the electronics inside (although new research in this area has suggested that some selected patients can be scanned even with a pacemaker), and coils can give major artifacts. There is a lot to sort out in the choice of imaging modalities.

The detailed physics of magnetic resonance image generation is beyond the scope of this text. However, the general concept is not. A powerful magnet is used the align the spins of the hydrogen atoms in the body, and a radiofrequency pulse (electromagnetic energy) combined with a special magnetic field that creates a magnetic "gradient" is used to perturb a small percentage of these molecules in a specific part of the body into a higher-energy state. When the radiofrequency pulse is turned off, the hydrogen atoms from that part of the body return to their normal state, releasing energy in the process. This energy is then collected and analyzed by a complex series of mathematical computations to yield one line of imaging data (the image is divided into a checkerboard [matrix]; each box is called a pixel, and a line of imaging data is a row of pixels). Generally, anywhere between 64 and 512 lines of data make up an image. To allow for "noise" in the system (false data) and to mitigate artifacts from breathing, each line can be obtained two or three times and averaged (with breath-holding techniques, this is typically not necessary). To image the heart, the scanner uses the electrocardiogram (ECG) (or pulse recording) to determine what part of the heartbeat in which to obtain the image.

By timing the radiofrequency pulses differently and changing their magnitude, one can generate different types of images. There are many types of cardiac MRI in clinical use as shown in Fig. 69-1. To define anatomy (Fig. 69-1A), double-inversion (DI) dark-blood MRI yields high-resolution images of myocardial tissue and blood vessel walls, and the blood remains signal poor. Steady-state free-precession (SSFP) imaging also yields high-resolution images of myocardial tissue and blood vessels; however, the blood is bright. Cine MRI (see later discussion) can be used to delineate morphology as well, including valve morphology.

Although static images were the mainstay of cardiac MRI, many other techniques have come into clinical use for morphology, including contrast-enhanced imaging. A contrast, typically a gadolinium-based agent, is injected, and a T_1-weighted, three-dimensional sequence is used to obtain a three-dimensional image of the cardiovascular system. These images can then be formatted as multiple two-dimensional images, as a shaded surface display

Table 69-1   Magnetic Resonance Imaging Advantages and Limitations

Advantages over catheterization	Noninvasive
	No ionizing radiation
	No contrast agent needed to delineate cavities and lumina
	Measures flow in parallel circuits
	No overlapping structures
Advantages over echocardiography	No limit to patient size
	Not limited by patient "windows"
	No artifacts from calcification, surgical patches, or prosthetic valves
	Compared with transesophageal echocardiography, is noninvasive
	Identifies areas of perfusion defects
Advantages over echocardiography and catheterization	Averages functional data over hundreds of heartbeats
	Three-dimensional imaging after ROUTINE acquisition
	Ability to magnetically "tag" myocardial tissue and blood (calculation of myocardial strain and wall motion, and visualizing velocity profiles)
	Ability to assess velocity at different points across the ventricular cavity or blood vessel
	Does not rely on geometric assumptions to calculate mass, volume, etc.
	Identifies areas of scarred or fibrosed myocardium
	Tissue characterization including cardiac tumors
	Myocardial iron and oxygen levels (beginning to become clinically utilized)
Limitations	Unable to image patients with pacemakers
	Artifacts from wires, clips, coils
	Respiration can cause blurring of images at times
	Lying still, sedation still necessary
	Limited imaging of valves and chordae, although this has been improving for many years
	Many studies must be "gated" to the electrocardiogram; certain circumstances may make recognizing the "R" wave a problem
	Cannot be done at the bedside; equipment is large
	Measuring pressures still clinically experimental; turbulent flow can make gradient calculations unreliable

(SSD), a maximum intensity projection (MIP), or a volume-rendered object (VRT) (Fig. 69-1A).

Cardiac MR goes beyond anatomy, however (Fig. 69-1B–D). Cine (also called gradient echo) MRI (Fig. 69-1B) produces a high signal from blood and a lower-amplitude signal from tissue, and usually is used for determination of cardiac motion, cardiac index, and blood flow and for functional analysis. If turbulent blood flow is present, cine MRI will show a signal void in the region of turbulence, and is used to detect valvular regurgitation, stenosis, or blood vessel stenosis. Alternatively, cine MRI can obtain static images at various levels of the body, "labeling" blood as signal-intense regions. This may be used, for example, to find collateral vessels off the aorta in a patient with tetralogy of Fallot and pulmonary atresia. Cine MRI can be of the spoiled gradient-echo type (SGE) or of the steady-state free-precession type.

The MRI signal that is generated usually contains both amplitude information and phase information. Phase-encoded velocity uses this phase information to encode velocity data that can be used to determine the velocity of blood (or tissue) as well as flow to any organ (such as cardiac output or relative flow to each lung) (Fig. 69-1C). The velocity maps come in two forms: (1) through plane velocity mapping, in which velocity is encoded into and out of the plane of the image, and (2) through in-plane velocity mapping, in which velocity is encoded in the plane of the image (similar to Doppler echocardiography). The advantage of through-plane velocity mapping is that if a blood vessel is imaged in cross section, all the pixels that encode velocity in the blood vessel can be summed over the entire cross section of the vessel and integrated over the entire cardiac cycle to obtain flow (as in liters/minute, not just velocity).

Myocardial tissue tagging (Figs. 69-1B and 69-2) is another MRI technique, which "magnetically labels" the walls of the myocardium and divides it into "cubes of magnetization." This allows for the calculation of regional wall strain, radial motion, and torsion. This can be of the two-dimensional tagging type, in which a "grid" is laid down on the myocardium (spatial modulation of magnetization [SPAMM]), or of the one-dimensional type, in which just a series of parallel lines is laid down. Finally, blood tagging is similar to tissue tagging, except that the blood is labeled, allowing for visualization of velocity profiles as well as calculation of cardiac index. Either only a thin stripe is laid down on the blood vessel to label it (bolus tagging) or a large stripe is laid down on the blood, to detect shunt flow (Fig. 69-1B).

Recently, examination of regional myocardial perfusion and viability has come into routine clinical use in cardiac MRI (Fig. 69-1D). With gadolinium enhancement, cardiac MRI assesses regional wall perfusion by using a "first-pass" injection technique. Typically, short-axis views of the ventricle are obtained, and the sequence setup is such that the heart is imaged relatively motionless. Gadolinium is injected intravenously while the scanner continuously images the ventricle (up to four or five short-axis slices may be imaged at once), and the gadolinium bolus is followed from right ventricular cavity to left ventricular cavity to ventricular myocardium. Defects in perfusion show up as dark portions of the myocardium, whereas the rest of the ventricle is signal intense. It is usually used in conjunction with a coronary vasodilator, such as adenosine. Lung perfusion can also be assessed qualitatively using time-resolved gadolinium techniques (Fig. 69-1C).

Infarcted myocardium is less of an issue in congenital heart disease than it is in adults, although native lesions such an anomalous left coronary artery from the pulmonary artery or operations that scar the myocardium (e.g., most repaired tetralogy of Fallot) may manifest myocardial infarction and scarring. Gadolinium is avidly taken up by scarred myocardium and can remain in the scarred tissue for an extended period of time; it is subsequently "washed" out by coronary blood flow in perfused myocardium. Put another way, the signal intensity–time curves separate, with the infarcted myocardium gadolinium curve remaining highly signal intense after 5 minutes, whereas normal myocardium becomes much less so. Cardiac MR sequences

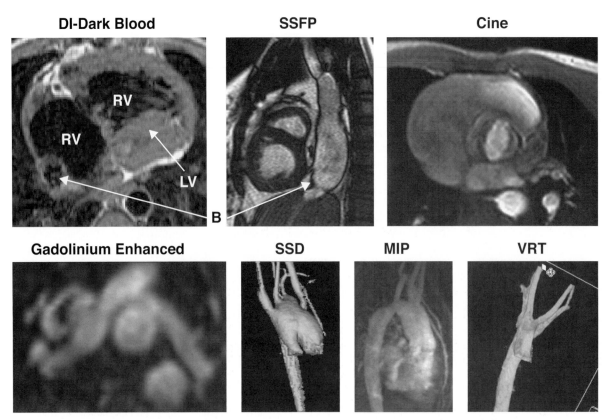

Figure 69-1. Types of cardiac MRI in common use. **(A)** Anatomy: The upper leftmost panel is a double inversion (DI) dark-blood image of a patient with hypoplastic left heart syndrome who is after Fontan procedure. Note that the blood is "black" and myocardial and vascular tissue give off signal. In this image, the left ventricle (LV) is just a "hunk of muscle." The Fontan baffle (B) is imaged in short axis. The upper middle image is a steady-state free-precession (SSFP) image of a patient with superoinferior ventricles after Fontan procedure; note how bright the blood is. The upper rightmost image is from a patient with bicuspid aortic valve, taken using a spoiled gradient-echo (SGE) sequence with a high flip angle, making the blood very bright flowing into the plane of the image. This is equivalent to a parasternal short-axis view by echocardiography. The bottom images are all gadolinium-enhanced (contrast) studies, shown in different ways: The lower leftmost image is a two-dimensional reformatted view of the pulmonary arteries in a Lecompte maneuver after arterial switch repair for transposition of the great arteries. The second and third images from the left are respectively a shaded surface display (SSD) and a maximum intensity projection (MIP) of a reconstructed aorta for hypoplastic left heart syndrome. The rightmost image is a volume-rendered technique (VRT) image of a patient with a right aortic arch and a diverticulum of Kommerel. (*Continued*)

take advantage of this ability to image infarcted myocardium, which is unique in noninvasive imaging. Signal intensity differences between normal and infarcted myocardium of up to 500% have been achieved. The technique has been shown to accurately delineate the presence, extent, and location of acute and chronic myocardial infarction as well as fibrous tissue (Fig. 69-1D). In addition, various cardiac tumors can take up gadolinium, whereas others will not, and cardiac MRI uses this property, along with T_1-weighted images, T_2-weighted images, and fat saturation to predict what type of tumor is present (Fig. 69-1D).

Coronary imaging, as with perfusion and viability, is less of an issue in congenital heart disease; however, there remains a substantial portion of patients who have lesions that need to be addressed. Cardiac MRI generally uses three-dimensional, fat-saturated sequences along with navigator techniques (an MRI technique that monitors diaphragmatic motion) to allow for cardiac imaging in even small infants (Fig. 69-1D).

Imaging Approach

The imaging approach to the patient with congenital heart disease is the same in MRI as it is in echocardiography, which was

outlined previously in this chapter. However, there are various views that are used in the MRI evaluation of congenital heart disease that any physician in the care of children with heart disease should be aware of. The following text describes the various techniques and when they are performed in the study. Not all techniques are run on every patient, and the study is tailored to the individual patient.

The initial images obtained are contiguous, tomographic slices in the transverse (also called "axial") plane (images are oriented anteroposterior and right–left). This allows for one complete volumetric data set to be obtained so that if the study is

SGE **SSFP** **SPAMM**

Bolus Tagging **Blood Tagging** **1-D Tissue**

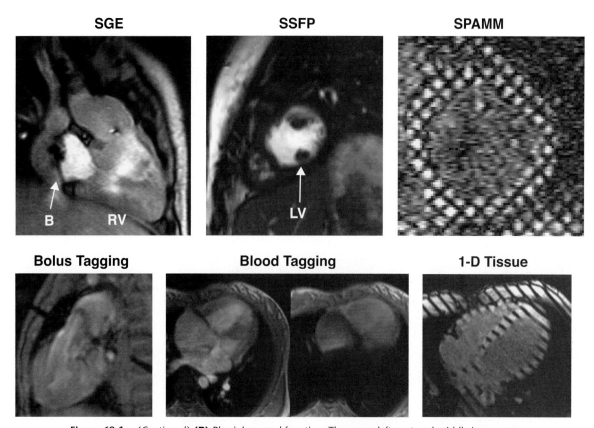

Figure 69-1. (*Continued*) **(B)** Physiology and function: The upper leftmost and middle images are cine images using SGE and SSFP, respectively, of single-ventricle patients. The leftmost image demonstrates the Fontan B and the right ventricle (RV) in long axis of a patient with hypoplastic left heart syndrome. The upper middle image demonstrates the left ventricular short axis in a patient with tricuspid atresia. The upper rightmost image is a tissue-tagging image (spatial modulation of magnetization [SPAMM]) of the normal human LV in short axis. Note how the checkerboard created by the pulse sequence divides the tissue into "cubes of magnetization." The lower panels all demonstrate a form of magnetic tagging: The leftmost panel is blood (bolus) tagging of the ascending aorta in the candy-cane view. This is a modification of tissue tagging with only one stripe laid down. Black arrowheads show the velocity profile, and black arrows show the site of initial tagging. The lower middle panel demonstrates another form of blood tagging, used for shunt detection, in which the tagged blood is "black" and the signal void can be followed (left image without the tag, right image with the tag). This is a patient with an ostium primum atrial septal defect. The lower rightmost image is a form of myocardial tagging in which only a single set of parallel stripes is laid down on the myocardium (normal patient in this case). (*Continued*)

terminated prematurely (e.g., due to patient instability), multiplanar reconstruction and three-dimensional shaded surface displays can still be generated off-line and used in the analysis of the anatomy. This view depicts the following structures (preoperatively): short axes of the ascending and descending aorta, pulmonary and aortic annulus, vena cavae, azygous vein, trachea, and esophagus, the long axes of the transverse aortic arch, main and branch pulmonary arteries, pulmonary veins, and a slightly off-axis apical four-chamber view.

The next set of images obtained is determined by the region of interest. For example, if a coarctation of the aorta or the systemic venous pathway of a Fontan patient is being imaged, an off-axis sagittal image is used to obtain the "candy-cane" view of the aorta or the long axis of the systemic venous pathway (parallel to the path of flowing blood). If a double aortic arch is being imaged or the left ventricular outflow tract is assessed, a set of straight or slightly off-axis coronal images is obtained to yield the short axes of the right and left aortic arches, the long axes of the amalgamation of these structures into ascending and descending aorta, and the long axis of the left ventricular outflow tract. This can be performed using either dark- or bright-blood technique.

Once the anatomy is sorted out, cine MRI is the next performed to determine ventricular performance, valve function, or shunts that may be present and to aid in determining stenosis of the great vessels. This series of scans is also used to confirm the anatomic information obtained by static imaging (e.g., hypoplasia of the branch pulmonary arteries should show the signal void of turbulence on cine MRI). The static images are used as a localizer for cine MRI imaging (e.g., using the four-chamber view on the static images to obtain the left ventricular short axis for shortening), another reason that the static images are obtained first.

The next set of images typically run comprises phase-encoded velocity maps, which are used for flow and velocity information.

Phase Encoded Velocity Mapping

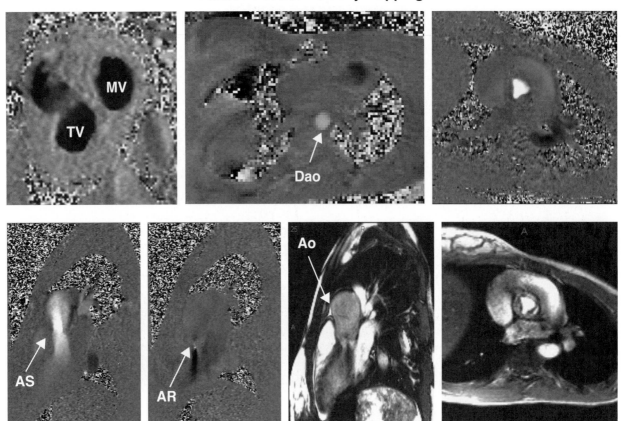

Figure 69-1. (*Continued*) **(C)** Velocity mapping: Each pixel has a velocity measurement associated with it and encodes velocity into and out of the plane of the image for the through-plane version and in the plane for the in-plane version. Direction is encoded as either increased signal (*white*) in one direction or decreased signal (*black*) in the other direction. Summation of the multiplication of pixel areas by their respective velocities yields flow in the through-plane version. Through-plane velocity mapping: The upper leftmost image is a velocity map across the atrioventricular valves in a patient with transposition of the great arteries, whereas the upper middle panel is an axial phase-encoded velocity map of the descending aorta (DAo). The upper rightmost and lower rightmost panels demonstrate the velocity map and anatomic image, respectively, across a normal trileaflet aortic valve. In-plane velocity mapping: The bottom lower leftmost and middle two images are in-plane velocity maps (lower left and second from left) and the anatomic image (third from left) of the left ventricular outflow tract of a patient with aortic stenosis and insufficiency. The lower leftmost image is for systole, the second and third from left for diastole. (*Continued*)

Which vessel to interrogate depends on the lesion, but typically, a minimum is to place velocity maps across the aorta and pulmonary artery. This serves two purposes: (1) with no shunts present, the cardiac output of the aorta should equal the cardiac output of the main pulmonary artery, and (2) with a shunt present, the pulmonary-to-systemic blood flow ratio (Qp/Qs) may be obtained. Our laboratory recommends obtaining right and left pulmonary artery flow when calculating a Qp/Qs as well because both flows should add up to flow in the main pulmonary artery. These quantitative internal checks are usually performed in cardiac MRI and are among the unique features of the technique. In addition, ventricular pressure estimates and gradients can be calculated using through-plane and in-plane velocity mapping as one would in Doppler echocardiography.

Gadolinium injection is then performed to obtain a three-dimensional volumetric set of the cardiovascular system. The injection can be done in two ways: (1) Bolus tracking: A special sequence is used to track the bolus of contrast through the cardiovascular system in real time, and when it reaches the region of interest (e.g., branch pulmonary arteries in a patient with tetralogy of Fallot), the three-dimensional sequence is then run automatically. (2) Test dose technique: A sequence is used to determine how long it takes a small test dose of contrast to reach the region of interest from the time of injection. The three-dimensional sequence is then run after the full dose of contrast is injected, delayed by the amount of time determined by the test dose (this has the advantage of making it possible to have the patient hold his or her breath).

A number of other techniques can be run in between these sets of sequences or in place of them. Myocardial tagging or blood tagging can be done after the cine sequences. If perfusion is the goal of the study, this is usually done close to the beginning of

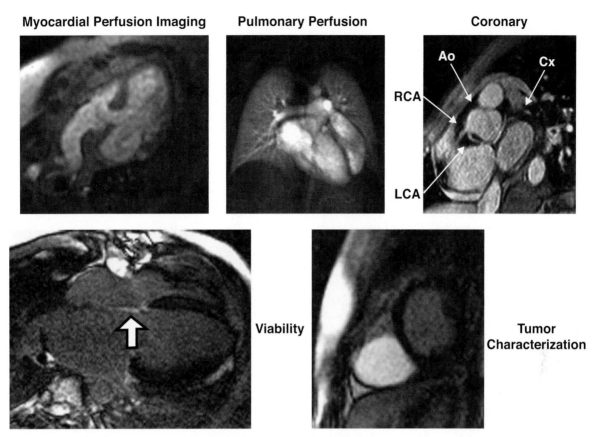

Figure 69-1. (*Continued*) **(D)** Perfusion, viability and coronary imaging: Perfusion imaging uses gadolinium injection, and visualization of the myocardial "blush" indicates the degree of myocardial perfusion. The upper leftmost image is a perfusion image of a patient with tricuspid stenosis and a functional single left ventricle. Pulmonary perfusion can also be visualized with time-resolved gadolinium injections as in the upper middle image of a patient with inverted ventricles after a "double switch." Coronary imaging of a patient with a single coronary artery and the left coronary artery coursing behind the aorta is shown in the upper rightmost image. Delayed enhancement imaging, in the lower images, can help to detect scar tissue (left, image of a patient after endocardial cushion defect repair and fibrous tissue on the patch [*arrow*]) or to characterize tumors (right, image of a patient with an RV fibroma). (Ao = aorta, AR = aortic regurgitation, AS = aortic stenosis, Cx = circumflex coronary artery, MV = mitral valve, LCA = left coronary artery, RA = right atrium, RCA = right coronary artery, RV = right ventricle, TV = tricuspid valve.)

the exam but after all dark-blood sequences. Coronary imaging can take a long time, and this would also be performed after the initial static images and some cine imaging. Viability (delayed enhancement imaging) is performed from 5 to 10 minutes after gadolinium injection, so this needs to be kept in mind during the planning of the scans.

One of the distinct advantages of MRI is that it does not rely on geometric assumptions to calculate volume, mass, and so on as other imaging modalities do. This is extremely important in congenital heart disease, in which bizarre, misshapen cardiovascular structures cannot be modeled by geometry. Furthermore, MRI is exquisitely sensitive to turbulence and can detect even small amounts of regurgitation or stenosis.

Cardiac Magnetic Resonance Imaging: Major Uses for Anatomy

In certain situations, cardiac MRI imaging is so vastly superior to other imaging modalities that it is steadily becoming the standard of care. There are five broad categories in which MRI has found an increasing important role (both pre- and postoperatively) in the anatomic diagnosis of congenital heart disease: (1) great artery anatomy, (2) imaging extracardiac conduits and intracardiac baffles, (3) complex spatial relationships, (4) venous connections both pre- and postoperatively, and (5) general morphologic evaluation and miscellaneous *but important* individual diseases not included

in the other categories; this includes (a) valve morphology, (b) tissue characterization (such as characterizing right ventricular dysplasia and identifying myocardial scar tissue or cardiac tumors), and (c) coronary imaging.

Great Artery Anatomy: Preoperative and Postoperative

Aorta

Lesions of the aorta commonly evaluated by MRI are classified as either ring or nonring abnormalities (Fig. 69-3). A vascular ring is an aortic malformation in which vascular structures (or former vascular structures) completely surround the trachea and

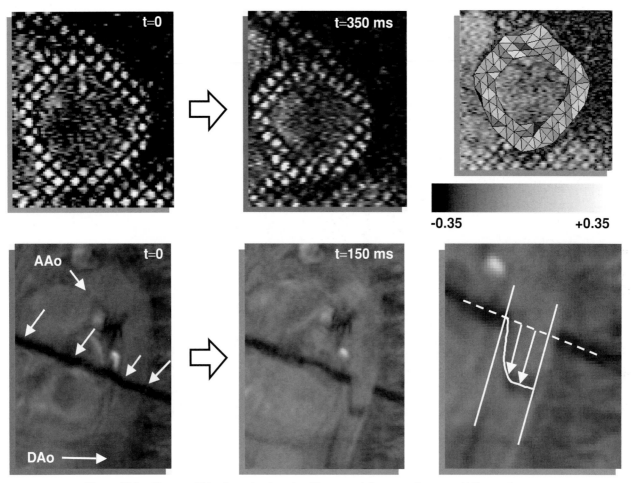

Figure 69-2.   Tissue and blood-tagging imaging. The upper leftmost and upper middle panels display short-axis tissue tagging of the normal left ventricle at end-diastole (t = 0) and 350 msec into systole (t = 350 ms). Note the deformation of the "cubes of magnetization" at 350 msec. Strain is calculated, coded in grayscale (underneath the upper rightmost panel), and superimposed onto the anatomic image (upper rightmost panel). Wall motion can also be displayed graphically (not shown). Lower leftmost and lower middle panels display blood (bolus) tagging in the descending aorta (DAo) in the candy-cane view at end-diastole (t = 0) and 150 msec into systole (t = 150 ms), respectively. White arrows represent the site of initial tagging, and the white arrowhead is the tag in the DAo. Note the velocity profile of the DAo in the lower middle panel. The lower rightmost panel is a magnification of the site of tagging in the DAo, showing how velocities at each point across the vessel diameter are measured. With the appropriate mathematical calculation, planimeterizing of the area underneath the velocity profile yields the regional cardiac index. (AAo = ascending aorta.)

esophagus, possibly compromising these structures (diverticulum of Kommerell). An advantage of cardiac MRI, in imaging the trachea and bronchi as it relates to the vascular ring, is that it allows the physician to examine the bronchoarterial relations and find the reason for and assess the amount of airway compression.

In the MRI evaluation of a vascular ring, the initial axial images can almost always make the diagnosis, and a set of contiguous coronal images complements the axial ones as an orthogonal view (useful in assessing the diameter of the vascular structures, which may ultimately affect the surgical management). Sometimes, a three-dimensional reconstruction is also useful in assessing the size of the various components of the vascular ring and in the evaluation of tracheal or bronchial compression.

In a double aortic arch (Fig. 69-3, lower panels), the ascending aorta splits into two arch vessels that cross over both bronchi and branch pulmonary arteries, coalescing behind the trachea and esophagus to form the descending aorta. The aorta totally surrounds the trachea and esophagus, and surgical management entails ligation and division of the smaller of the two arches, which is more commonly the left one.

Because this is performed by thoracotomy, cardiac MRI is crucial in determining the surgical management by assessing which arch is smaller to know which hemithorax to enter (Fig. 69-3, lower panels).

Right aortic arch complexes may form rings, depending on where regression in the embryonic aortic arches occurs. For example, in a right aortic arch with a retro-esophageal diverticulum of Kommerell and an aberrant left subclavian artery, the components of the ring are as follows: anterior and right lateral portions formed by the aorta, posterior portion from the diverticulum, and left lateral portion formed

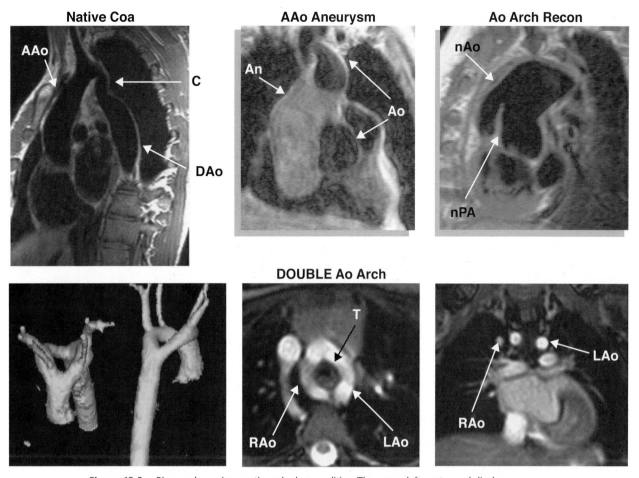

Figure 69-3. Ring and nonring aortic arch abnormalities. The upper leftmost panel displays an off-axis sagittal image of a native coarctation (C) (Coa). The upper middle panel is a coronal image of a patient with Marfan syndrome who had aortic root and ascending aortic (AAo) dilation and required a "wrap" of homograft around the AAo. The native AAo ruptured into the potential space between the native AAo and the homograft, resulting in the aneurysm (An). The signal-intense region is because of stagnant blood. The upper rightmost panel is also an off-axis sagittal image, but of a patient who underwent an aortic-to-pulmonary anastamosis. Note how well it can be visualized. The lower panels are demonstrations of a dominant double aortic (Ao) arch. The leftmost panel demonstrates two views of a shaded surface display of the double aortic arch, and the middle panel is an off-axis two-dimensional axial view of the right aortic arch (RAo) and left aortic arch (LAo). Note how the trachea (T) is surrounded. The lower rightmost image is a coronal view of the both arches in short axis (cross section). (DAo, descending aorta; nAo = native ascending aorta, nPA = native pulmonary artery, Recon = reconstruction.)

by the left ligamentum arteriosum and left pulmonary artery. The lower right panel of Fig. 69-1A is a volume-rendered image of such a lesion.

With nonring aortic arch abnormalities, as with ring abnormalities, the initial axial images can generally yield the diagnosis or at least lead one in the correct direction. Instead of a set of coronal images, a set of oblique sagittal images is obtained parallel to the path of flowing blood, allowing the whole arch to be visualized in one picture.

Of the nonring aortic arch abnormalities, assessment of the aortic arch for coarctation (Fig. 69-3, upper panel) is one of the

most frequent referrals seen. Four extremity blood pressures and an image of the coarctation by MRI are all that is necessary for the diagnosis and referral for surgery. Postoperatively, MRI is used to assess the presence of coarctation in patients with aortic arch reconstruction or may be used as a follow-up in patients who have had coarctation repair, monitoring for recurrence of coarctation or aneurysm formation. Other nonring aortic abnormalities include interruption of the aortic arch, supravalvar aortic stenosis (e.g., as in Williams syndrome), or dilation of the ascending aorta because of valvar aortic stenosis (Fig. 69-1A,C), postoper-

assessment of the adequacy of an aortic-to-pulmonary anastomosis in patients who require left ventricular outflow reconstruction (lower middle panels, Fig. 69-1, and upper right panel, Fig. 69-3), or ascending aortic aneurysm formation such as after a "wrap" procedure (in which the ascending aorta is wrapped by homograft for support) (Fig. 69-3).

Pulmonary Artery

Initial assessment of the pulmonary arteries is performed from the axial images, followed by long-axis views of the individual branch pulmonary arteries (Fig. 69-4). Pulmonary

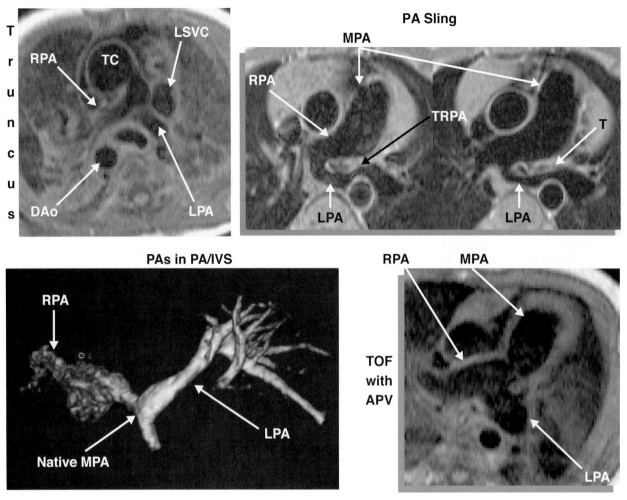

Figure 69-4. Pulmonary artery abnormalities. The upper left panel displays an axial image of a patient with truncus arteriosus (TC) type A1, which visualizes the origin of the main pulmonary artery (MPA) from the TC, branching into right (RPA) and left (LPA) pulmonary arteries. This patient also had a left superior vena cava (LSVC). The upper right panels displays two axial images (progress inferiorly from left to right) of a patient with anomalous origin of the left pulmonary artery (LPA) from the right pulmonary artery (RPA): a PA sling. Note how the LPA courses behind the trachea (T), compressing it. The lower left panel is a volume-rendered image of the pulmonary arteries in a patient with tetralogy of Fallot with pulmonary atresia. Note the diminutive main pulmonary artery (MPA) segment. The lower right panel is an axial image of an infant with tetralogy of Fallot (TOF) with absent pulmonary valves (APV). Note the dilation of both the RPA and LPA. (DAo = descending aorta.)

artery lesions imaged by MRI fall into three basic categories. Stenosis or hypoplasia of one or both branch pulmonary arteries (Fig. 69-4) or main pulmonary artery (e.g., pre- and postoperative tetralogy of Fallot or tricuspid atresia) is one category in which the data are important preoperatively to help predict outcome and may affect the conduct of the surgery because pulmonary artery augmentation may be necessary. Pulmonary artery size is thought to be one of multiple prognosticators of surgical outcome in patients with single-ventricle lesions leading to Fontan reconstruction. MRI can characterize the geometry and size of the arteries and determine branch pulmonary artery dis-

continuity (ideally imaging in three orthogonal planes) and, the amount of collaterals present from the aorta, and, if pulmonary atresia is present, it can determine how far the main pulmonary artery extends to the base of the heart.

Aneurysmal dilation of the pulmonary arteries is the second category (Fig. 69-4). This occurs classically in patients with tetralogy of Fallot with absent pulmonary valve leaflets, but may also occur in patients with pulmonary artery hypertension or the poststenotic dilation of pulmonic stenosis. MRI can yield the size and geometry of the pulmonary arteries and the amount of respiratory compromise. The last category

is anomalous origin or course of the pulmonary arteries (Figs. 69-1A and 69-4). This category includes, for example, anomalous origin of the left pulmonary artery from the right pulmonary artery (a pulmonary artery "sling"), in which tracheal embarrassment may occur, anomalous origin of the right pulmonary artery from the ascending aorta (hemitruncus), and the situation in which one great artery arises from the base of the heart and gives rise directly in its ascending portion to the systemic, pulmonary, and coronary circulations (truncus arteriosus). In addition, postoperative assessment of patients after arterial switch procedure and the Lecompte maneuver (Fig. 69-1A, lower left

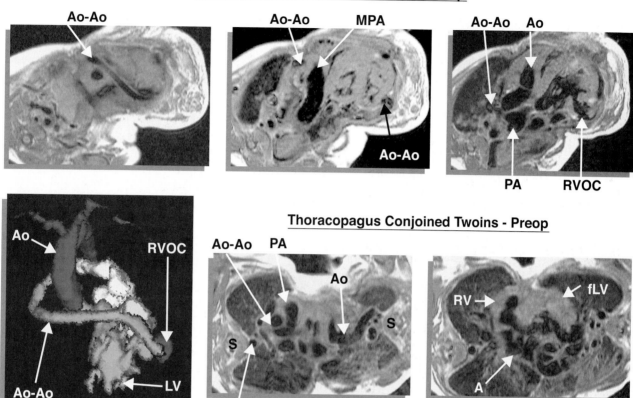

Figure 69-5. Complex spatial relationships and extracardiac conduits. These are axial images of thoracopagus conjoined twins both preoperatively (preop) and postoperatively (postop). A physiologic repair of this defect required an aortic-to-aortic (Ao-Ao) conduit placement, visualized on the top three panels (progresses inferiorly from right to left). One image could not obtain the entire extent of the conduit; however, a major portion of it is shown in the upper leftmost panel. The aorta from the right infant originated from the right ventricular outflow chamber (RVOC), which can be seen in the upper rightmost panel. The lower leftmost panel is a three-dimensional shaded surface display of the conduit. Note how the full extent of the conduit may be visualized in three dimensions, along with its origination in the RVOC and connection to the aorta. The preoperative axial images are shown for comparison in the lower middle and rightmost panels. The infants shared a left ventricle (fLV), and the atria (A) were fused. The infant on the right had a rudimentary RVOC. Note how in the bottom middle image, the ascending aorta (AAo) and the descending aorta (DAo) are seen in cross section and the main pulmonary artery (MPA) and the left pulmonary artery (PA) are seen in long axis on the left infant and the aortic arch is visualized in the right infant. (RV = right ventricle, S = spine.) (Three-dimensional reconstruction courtesy of Dr. Paul Weinberg.)

panel) falls into this category. In all cases, MRI can and should be used to delineate size, geometry, and site of origin.

Extracardiac Conduits and Baffles

Echocardiography may be hampered in imaging these structures because extracardiac conduits frequently pass immediately underneath the sternum or near the lungs and parts of the intracardiac baffle are posterior in the atria or ventricle. Cardiac MRI can usually succeed in situations in which echocardiography fails.

Extracardiac conduits (Fig. 69-1B, Fontan extracardiac baffle; and Figs. 69-5, 69-6A, and 69-7) fall into a few categories. A right ventricular-to-pulmonary artery conduit (e.g., a Rastelli procedure), an apical left ventricular-to-pulmonary artery conduit (e.g., {I,L,L}, severe pulmonic stenosis, and two good-size ventricles) or an apical left ventricular-to-descending aorta conduit (e.g., severe aortic stenosis) are examples of *ventriculoarterial* conduits (Fig. 69-6A). An example of a *venoatrial* conduit is a Baffes procedure (Fig. 69-6A), and an example of an *arterioarterial* conduit is an aortic-to-aortic conduit used in

reconstructing the heart of thoracopagus conjoined twins (Fig. 69-5). Another example, shown using a shaded surface display in Fig. 69-6C, is an ascending-to-descending aortic conduit to bypass a coarctation of the aorta.

Intracardiac baffles (Fig. 69-6B) can also be categorized. *Atrial* baffles, which function to channel venous blood to arteries or the ventricles, include the Fontan reconstruction for single-ventricle complexes (Figs. 69-1B and 69-6B), an atrial baffle to direct pulmonary venous blood to the left atrium in anomalous venous connection (see later discussion and Fig. 69-8),

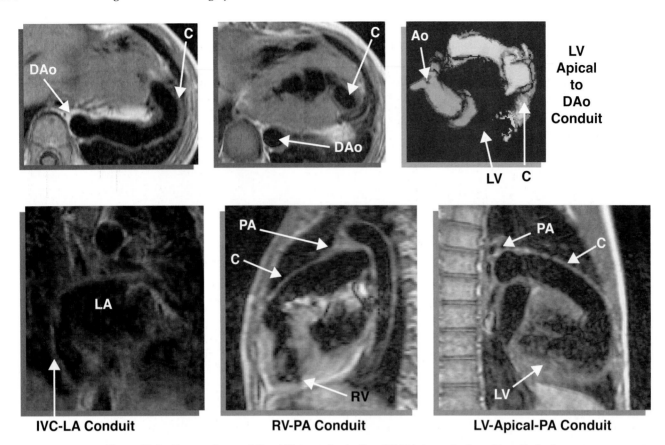

Figure 69-6.   Extracardiac conduits and intracardiac baffles. **(A)** This is a collection of four kinds of extracardiac conduits. The top images are a three-dimensional shaded surface display in grayscale (right image, looking from a transverse view) and axial images (leftmost and middle panels) of a patient with severe subaortic and aortic stenosis who underwent placement of a left ventricular (LV) apical-to-descending aortic (DAo) conduit (C). The bottom leftmost panel is a coronal image of the inferior vena cava-to-left atrial (IVC-LA) conduit of a Baffes procedure for transposition of the great arteries. The bottom middle image is a right ventricle-to-pulmonary artery (RV-PA) conduit of a patient who underwent repair of tetralogy of Fallot with pulmonary atresia and now has residual stenosis (note how narrow the proximal portion of the conduit is). The bottom rightmost image is of a patient with situs inversus totalis, a right ventricular aorta with pulmonary atresia {I,L,L}, who underwent placement of an LV apical-to-pulmonary artery (PA) conduit. Note how well magnetic resonance imaging visualizes the entire extent of the conduits. (*Continued*)

and the Mustard and Senning procedures (which have been performed in the past) for the transposition of the great arteries. The Rastelli procedure, performed for transposition of the great arteries with ventricular septal defect and pulmonic stenosis, is an example in which a *ventricular* baffle is placed.

After contiguous axial images are performed, which can be used to follow the conduit and baffle in short axis, double oblique-angled images are usually necessary to obtain the long axis of the conduit or baffle in one image. Sometimes, this may be impossible and the physician must be satisfied with two or three images of the conduit in long axis to obtain its full extent. Stenosis, regurgitation, or leaks across the baffle can be detected by cine MRI.

Complex Spatial Relationships

The orientation of various cardiovascular structures relative to each other and the rest of the body can be sorted out by MRI more easily than with other imaging modalities (Figs. 69-1 and 69-5 through 69-8). The ability of MRI to obtain parallel, contiguous, tomographic slices, creating three-dimensional shaded surface displays and the use of multiplanar reconstruction gives the physician a powerful tool with which to analyze the complex geometry.

As with conduits and baffles, contiguous axial images are performed that can be used to follow the various cardiovascular structures and in general to yield a first approximation of the anatomy. Afterward, double

oblique-angled images (coronal angled to sagittal angled to axial) are usually necessary to further delineate the morphology and regions of interest identified on the axial images. Confirmation of certain diagnoses can be made using cine MRI.

The case of superoinferior ventricles with criss-cross atrioventricular relations is an example of complex spatial relationships (Figs. 69-1A and 69-7). In this lesion, the two ventricles are oriented superoinferiorly instead of anteroposteriorly and right–left, with the ventricular septum lying parallel to the axial plane. Furthermore, in connecting atria to ventricles, the atrioventricular valves appear to cross each other, hence the name criss-cross. To depict the ventricular relationship, coronal or sagittal

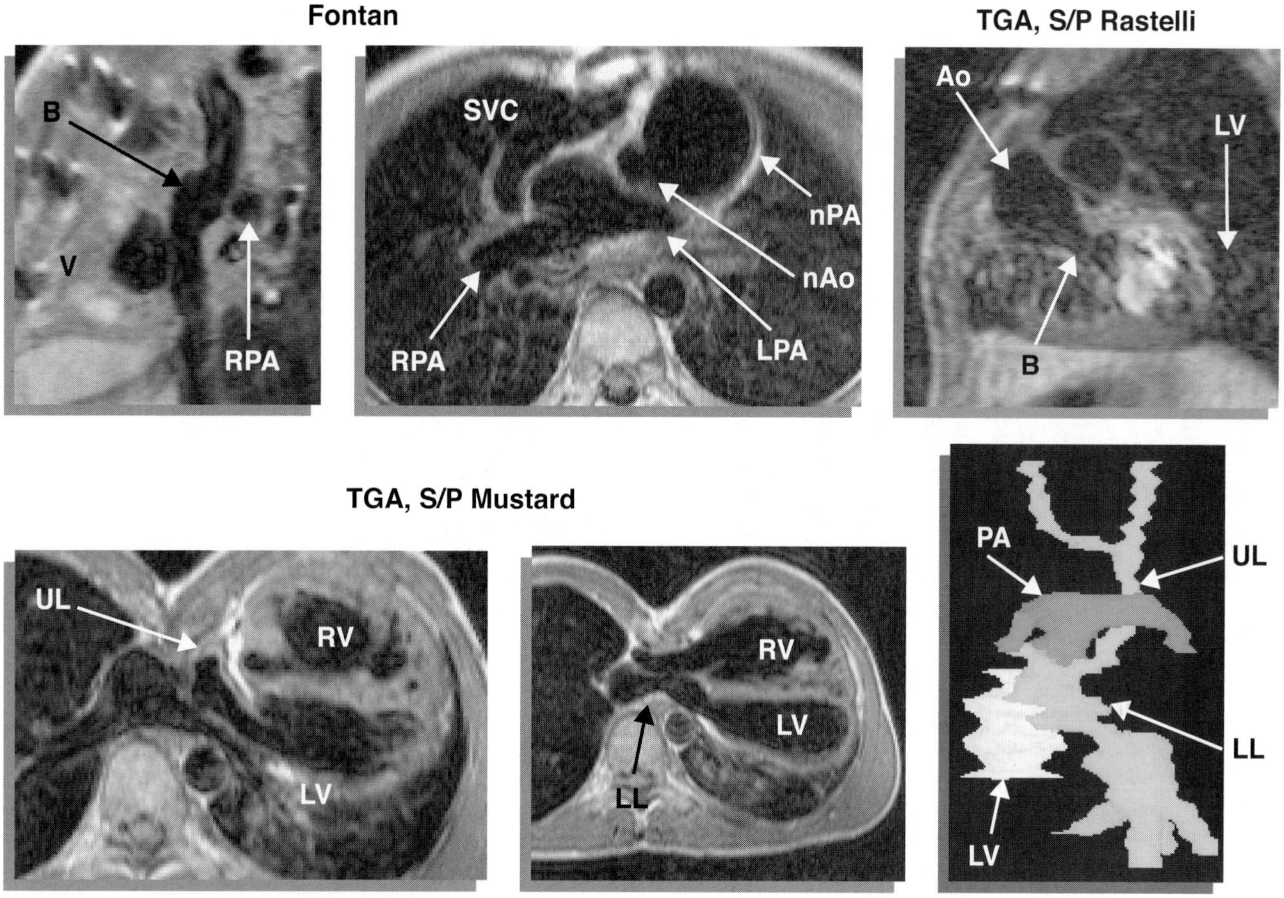

Fontan

TGA, S/P Rastelli

TGA, S/P Mustard

Figure 69-6. (*Continued*) **(B)** Baffles: Fontan, Rastelli, and Mustard. The upper leftmost and center images are off-axis sagittal and axial images, respectively, of components of the Fontan reconstruction for single-ventricle complexes. The upper leftmost image shows the long axis of the baffle (B), which creates a systemic venous and pulmonary venous pathway. An axial image (upper middle panel) at the level of the baffle and right pulmonary artery (RPA) shows the anastamosis of the superior vena cava (SVC) to the RPA. The proximal left pulmonary artery (LPA), native aorta (nAo), and native pulmonary artery (nPA) are also seen. The upper rightmost image is an off-axis sagittal spin-echo image of the LV outflow tract created by the ventricular baffle (B) in a patient with transposition of the great arteries (TGA), ventricular septal defect, and pulmonic stenosis who is status post (S/P) a Rastelli procedure. The left ventricular outflow tract is small and stenotic. A cine MRI through this left ventricular outflow tract is shown in Fig. 69-1. The lower leftmost and lower middle panels are axial images, and the lower rightmost panel is a three-dimensional shaded surface display of a patient with transposition of the great arteries shown after a Mustard procedure. The shaded surface display shows the systemic venous pathway, left ventricle (LV), and pulmonary artery (PA). Note how both the upper limb (UL) and lower limb (LL) of the systemic venous pathway are easily visible from the axial view and the three-dimensional course seen from the shaded surface display. These limbs baffle superior and inferior vena cava blood to the LV while pulmonary venous blood goes around the baffle into the right ventricle (RV). (*Continued*)

images are used, whereas the criss-cross of the atrioventricular valves can be shown by the standard axial images. Off-axis coronal and sagittal images can be used the delineate the criss-cross in the superoinferior plane.

The case of thoracopagus conjoined twins is another example of a complex spatial relationship (Fig. 69-5). The twins are joined at the thorax, and cardiac fusion may occur at one or multiple levels. Echocar-diography is difficult postnatally because of acoustic windows; actually, prenatal imaging is usually better than postnatal imaging. MRI is used to sort out the various cardiac structures, including the complex venous anatomy (e.g., status of the inferior vena cavae), ventricular morphology [e.g., fused central (usually left ventricular morphology) ventricle] and abdominal viscera (status of the liver). For all lesions in this category, three-dimensional shaded surface displays as well as multiplanar reconstruction are useful in conceptualizing the anatomy.

Venous Connections: Preoperative and Postoperative

At times, these may be difficult to visualize by echocardiography because of their position in the chest or poor

Coarctation, After Ascending to Descending Aortic Conduit

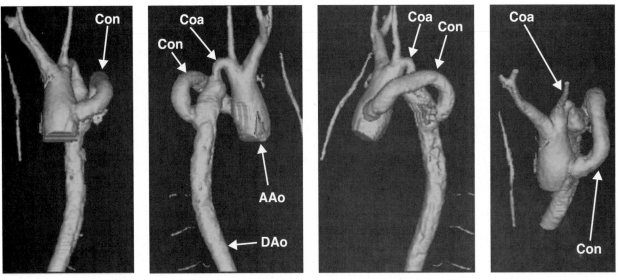

Figure 69-6. (*Continued*) **(C)** Ascending (AAo) to descending aortic (DAo) conduit (Con) to bypass a coarctation (Coa). The shaded surface displays demonstrate this type of extracardiac conduit. The three leftmost images are the shaded surface display turned around the superoinferior axis, and the rightmost image shows the aorta and the conduit tipped up.

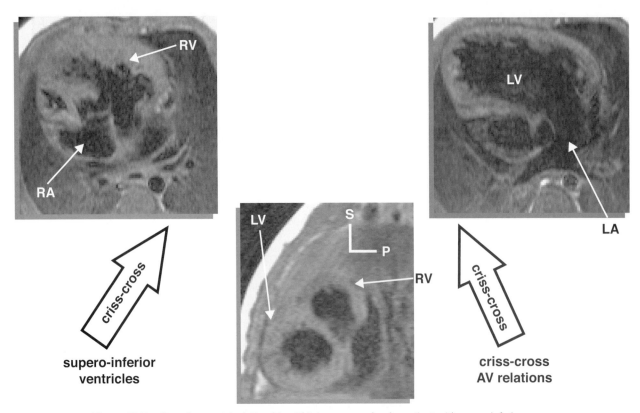

Figure 69-7.   Complex spatial relationships. This is an example of a patient with superoinferior ventricles with criss-cross atrioventricular (AV) relations. The bottom panel is an off-axis sagittal view of the short axis of the right ventricle (RV) superiorly (S) and the left ventricle (LV) inferiorly. The upper left panel displays an axial image of the right atrium (RA), which is superior, and to the right, emptying into the leftward and superior RV. A moderate ventricular septal defect is present. In the upper right panel (inferior to the image in the upper left panel), the left atrium (LA), which is inferior and to the left, crosses the path of blood from RA to RV and empties into the rightward and inferior LV, which depicts the criss-cross nature of the atrioventricular valves. (P = posterior.)

RSVC to LA, LSVC to CS   **LPV → VV → P, RPV → VV → RSVC**

Scimitar Syndrome

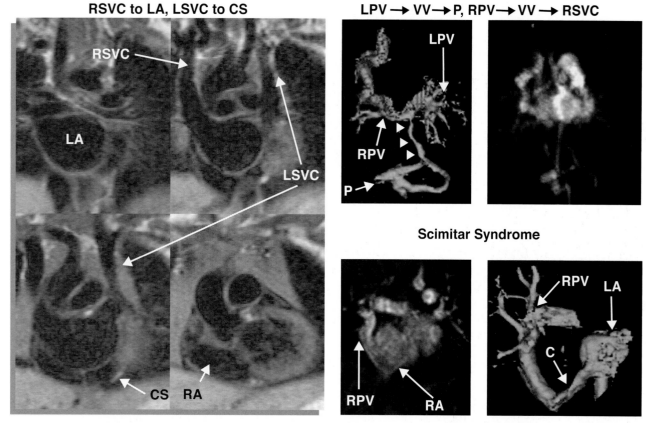

Figure 69-8. Venous anomalies. The left panel displays four coronal images (successively anterior from left to right and from top to bottom) of a patient with anomalous connection of the right superior vena cava (RSVC) to the left atrium (LA) and the presence of a left superior vena cava (LSVC) connected to the coronary sinus (CS). Note how well the RSVC to LA is visualized (top right image). The right upper panels demonstrate total anomalous pulmonary venous connection of an unusual type: a vertical vein (VV) drains above and below the diaphragm with the connection above the diaphragm to the RSVC and the connection below the diaphragm draining to the portal system (P). Because of the anatomy and the narrowing of the VV as it crosses the diaphragm, the left pulmonary drains (LPV) empty mostly into the P and the right pulmonary veins (RPV) drain to the RSVC. The image on the left is a three-dimensional shaded surface display, and the image on the right is a still frame of a time-resolved gadolinium injection. The right lower images are of a patient with Scimitar syndrome, in which there is partial anomalous pulmonary venous connection of the right lower pulmonary vein to the right atrium in this instance. The left image of this set is a gadolinium injection demonstrating the large RPV in a coronal view, and the right image is a shaded surface display of an atrial baffle repair of this lesion. Note how well this vein is visualized. (V = ventricle.)

echocardiographic windows (Fig. 69-8). Cardiac MRI is a useful tool in delineating these connections.

Systemic Veins

Sometimes, isolated lesions of the systemic veins may have marked physiologic consequences, such as when the right or a persistent left superior vena cava connects to the left atrium, causing cyanosis (Fig. 69-8, left panel). Other anomalies of the systemic veins may be associated with intracardiac lesions and will affect the conduct of surgery, necessitating the need to be aware of these lesions preoperatively (e.g., if a patient with

hypoplastic left heart syndrome has a persistent left superior vena cava not identified before Fontan reconstruction, deoxygenated blood will enter the pulmonary venous pathway, mix with the oxygenated blood, and cause cyanosis). The necessity for identifying this lesion is obvious, and therefore it is important to diagnose it at MRI. Because most systemic veins run in a superoinferior plane, coronal images are obtained after the contiguous axial images, delineating the vein along its long axis. This allows confirmation of the connections, assessment of the size of the vessel, and identification of any areas of stenosis.

Pulmonary Veins

Axial images can delineate the pulmonary venous anatomy and can also follow the vertical vein along its course through the thorax or abdomen. Off-axis coronal images can be obtained to confirm the diagnosis by visualizing the pulmonary veins in long axis.

There are a number of anomalies of pulmonary veins, and their importance is obvious. They are dealt with elsewhere in this book. Examples shown in Fig. 69-8 (on the right) are of a patient with total anomalous pulmonary venous connection (upper right panels) with a vertical vein that connects to the portal system as well as the right superior vena cava. There is a narrowing of the vein as it crosses the diaphragm, which creates the physiology of the left pulmonary veins draining mostly to the portal system and the right pulmonary veins draining to the right superior vena cava. A patient with Scimitar syndrome, who has an anomalous large, single right pulmonary venous connection to the right atrium, is also shown along with the conduit placed to repair this lesion (Fig. 69-8, lower right panels).

General Morphology and Miscellaneous Diseases

MRI can also be used for general morphologic evaluation as well. It can be of great utility in the older child, adolescent, and adult for this, and because of the wide field of view, a single MRI study may serve the purpose of multiple other studies. For example, in heterotaxy syndrome, in which defining the morphology and sidedness of the trachea, liver, gastrointestinal tract, and finding

a spleen is important, an MRI may suffice. A chest x-ray, abdominal ultrasound, echocardiogram, abdominal computed tomography scan, and possibly a liver-spleen scan might have to be performed otherwise.

MRI may also add another dimension to the lesion under study because of its reliance on the magnetic properties of the tissue. For example, in an intracardiac myxoma or tumor (Fig. 69-9, top left panel), the acoustic contrast (by echocardiography) may not be the same as the contrast

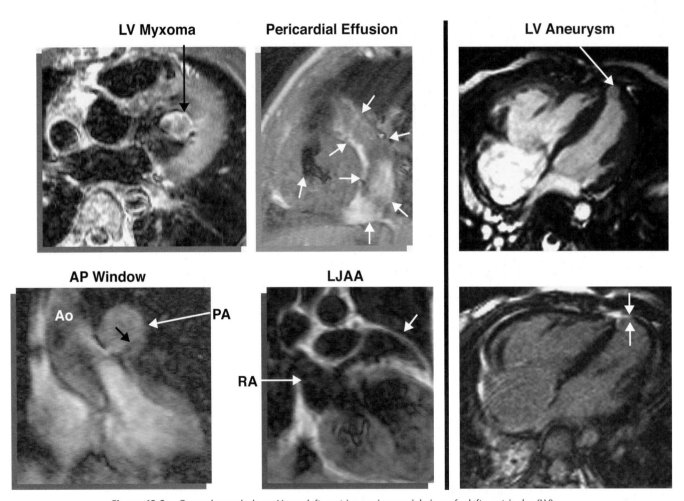

Figure 69-9. General morphology. Upper leftmost image is an axial view of a left ventricular (LV) myxoma in the LV outflow tract that enhanced with gadolinium (*arrow*). The upper middle panel is a short-axis image of a patient with hypoplastic left heart syndrome after a Fontan procedure who has a very large, circumferential pericardial effusion (*arrowheads*). The lower leftmost panel is a coronal image of a patient with an aorticopulmonary (AP) window. This was missed on the dark-blood images; however, cine magnetic resonance imaging (MRI) depicts the turbulent jet of shunting blood in systole from aorta (Ao) to pulmonary artery (PA) (*black arrowhead*). The lower middle image is also a coronal image but of a patient with left juxtaposition of the atrial appendages (LJAA), diagnosed here by the right atrial (RA) appendage on the left side (*arrowhead*). This patient also had tricuspid atresia, transposition of the great arteries, and pulmonic stenosis with a hypoplastic right ventricle. The rightmost images are cine **(upper)** and delayed enhancement **(lower)** images of a patient after repair of double outlet right ventricle with an apical left ventricular aneurysm (*arrows*). This aneurysm ballooned in systole on cine MRI and demonstrated increased signal on delayed enhancement imaging, indicating that it was myocardial scar tissue.

on MRI [using different pulse sequences and injecting gadolinium (which magnetically enhances vascular structures) to demarcate the extent of the tumor and its water content]. Another example is a left ventricular aneurysm, which is demonstrated on steady-state free-precession imaging in the upper right panel of Fig. 69-9. This apical left ventricular aneurysm demonstrates delayed enhancement after gadolinium injection (Fig. 69-9, lower right panel), implying that it is made up of scar tissue.

Other examples of common lesions for which MRI is used or have been diagnosed incidentally are shown in Fig. 69-1 and Fig. 69-9. A pericardial effusion (Fig. 69-9, upper middle panel) and single ventricle lesions (Fig. 69-1) are fairly straightforward to recognize on MRI. An aortopulmonary window is visualized by the turbulent jet of blood shunting from aorta to pulmonary artery in the coronal and axial views by cine MRI (Fig. 69-9, lower left panel). Occasionally, a dark-blood scan can identify this lesion as well and the shunt can be quantified using phase-encoded velocity mapping. Finally, left juxtaposition of the atrial appendages can be visualized in the coronal and (less well) axial planes, findings of which generally include a ventricular and/or atrial septal defect, tricuspid atresia or stenosis, a hypoplastic right ventricle, pulmonic stenosis, and bilateral infundibulum.

With the advent of faster imaging sequences and improvements in hardware as well as software, capabilities of cardiac MRI for examining generalized anatomy have expanded greatly. For example, valve morphology (category 5a referred to earlier) can be performed by cardiac MRI, which is approaching echocardiography. An example is shown in the upper panel of Fig. 69-1A, with a bicuspid aortic valve. MRI can use en face imaging to view this type of morphology using either steady-state free-precession imaging or spoiled gradient-echo sequences with a high flip angle. Even phase-encoded velocity mapping can be used to determine valve morphology, as for the trileaflet aortic valve shown in Fig. 69-1C.

In addition to valve morphology, tissue characterization has begun to play an increasingly important role in cardiac MRI (category 5b referred to earlier). It has been suggested that this tool be used to identify patients with right ventricular dysplasia by characteristics such as (1) fatty substitution of the myocardium, (2) ectasia of the right ventricular (RV) outflow tract, (3) dyskinetic bulges or dyskinesia of RV wall motion, (4) a dilated right ventricle, (5) a dilated right atrium, and (6) fixed RV wall thinning

with decreased RV wall thickening. Tumor characterization is also an important use of cardiac MRI and is based on viewing tissue characteristics by T_1 and T_2 weighting (with and without fat saturation), signal intensity during and after gadolinium injection (Fig. 69-1D and 69-9), and the contraction pattern on myocardial tissue tagging. Finally, identification of myocardial scar tissue by use of delayed enhancement 5 to 10 minutes after gadolinium injection (Fig. 69-1D and 69-9) is useful for determining ventricular performance, myocardial perfusion (see later discussion), or an etiology for arrhythmia, to mention a few examples.

Coronary imaging by MRI is a major emphasis in adults with heart disease; in addition, it has much applicability in pediatrics as well (category 5c referred to earlier). This is typically performed in pediatrics by obtaining a three-dimensional volume data set using steady-state free-precession imaging or spoiled gradient-echo sequences using a navigator technique, which monitors diaphragmatic motion and allows acceptance of data from only one part of the respiratory cycle (i.e., no need for breath-holding). There are the better-known coronary anomalies found in pediatrics, such as anomalous left coronary artery from the pulmonary artery, but others, such as single coronary arteries (Fig. 69-1D), origin of the left coronary artery from the right sinus of Valsalva, or its mirror image, also need to be delineated. The status of the coronary arteries in coronary transplantation, which occurs in such surgeries as the Ross procedure or the arterial switch procedure for transposition of the great arteries, can also be assessed with this technique. Other cardiac MRI techniques can be used in conjunction with structural imaging of the coronaries such as delayed enhancement to evaluate for myocardial infarction (see earlier discussion) or perfusion imaging (see later discussion).

Cardiac Magnetic Resonance Imaging: Major Uses for Physiology and Function

Some of the applications of MRI for physiology and function are extremely clinically useful (e.g., accurate measurement of ventricular volume in a patient with borderline left ventricular size to determine whether it can support the systemic circulation) and play an important role in the management of

patients. Others arise in physiology or ventricular function/fluid mechanics research or are still in the experimental or development stage clinically. Still others are on the verge of acceptance (e.g., assessment of myocardial iron stores using the T_2^* technique). Nevertheless, the physician caring for patients with congenital heart disease should be aware of all of these capabilities because the research ones will no doubt enter clinical practice in the near future. Here I present just the most common uses in practice and in research.

The various techniques may be used in conjunction with each other. For example, to obtain the mitral regurgitant fraction in a patient with mitral insufficiency, cine MRI is used to obtain left ventricular end-diastolic volume, stroke volume. and total cardiac output. Phase-encoded velocity mapping in the aorta measures forward stroke volume, and the subtraction of this forward stroke volume from the total stroke volume measured by cine MRI is the mitral regurgitant volume (which, if divided by the total stroke volume, is the mitral regurgitant fraction).

A feature unique to MRI is the capability of making internal checks in obtaining quantitative data. To use the example just given, phase-encoded velocity mapping across the mitral valve in diastole should yield the same flow volume as the mitral regurgitant volume calculated in the example. Similarly, in patients without intracardiac shunting, velocity mapping across the main pulmonary artery should equal velocity mapping across the aorta. All this strengthens the accuracy of MRI for the assessment of physiology and function.

Another unique feature of MRI is that the image can be built up over multiple heartbeats and averages (unlike echocardiography and angiography, a single MRI image can be averaged over two to many hundreds of heartbeats). Some might call this a disadvantage; however, it should be noted that using this approach, functional analysis by MRI can give a better handle on long-term performance. The image itself is an average, and this average over many heartbeats is built into the image—the physician does not have to do this averaging in his or her head as in echocardiography.

Cine Magnetic Resonance Imaging Uses

As noted in the introduction, cine MRI (steady-state free-precession imaging and spoiled gradient-echo sequences) is used to image cardiac motion and blood flow (Fig. 69-1). Blood is signal intense in this pulse sequence, myocardial tissue is less so, and turbulence yields a signal void in the blood.

To assess ventricular shortening, a single-level short-axis view or multiple levels of the short axis of the ventricle can be obtained. This may be complemented by cine in the apical four-chamber view or the ventricular long-axis view. Regional wall motion abnormalities can be grossly visualized in this manner. Furthermore, some investigators have been using dobutamine infusions to assess the myocardium in a stressed state. Most software on present-day scanners can give a temporal resolution of about 20 msec. Newer techniques allow for "real-time" visualization of ventricular performance or "interactive scanning,," in which the real-time technique can be used but the user can change planes instantaneously, similar to echocardiography. ECG gating is not a requirement in these instances, and this makes cine MRI very useful in patients with arrhythmias. Modifications of existing techniques use "arrhythmia-rejection" algorithms to successfully image the heart in patients with arrhythmias. Clearly, a physician versed in all the nuances of cardiac MRI is needed to choose the best imaging for the particular task at hand.

Ventricular volume, mass, stroke volume, ejection fraction, and cardiac index may be accurately assessed by cine MRI. As mentioned earlier, this technique does not rely on any geometric assumptions, which is an advantage with the bizarre ventricular shapes found in congenital heart disease. Multiple contiguous cine MRI runs are performed throughout the entire ventricle at the same temporal resolution (scans usually take approximately 5 to 10 minutes), and the data are then sorted by time. The results are multiple full-volume data sets at down to 20-msec intervals. Ventricular volume at a given time (usually end-diastole and end-systole are the times of interest) is obtained by tracing the endocardial borders on all images at that time (done on a computer with a video cursor and a mouse), planimeterizing the areas, multiplying by the slice thickness, and adding them up. Ventricular mass is obtained by tracing the epicardial borders on all images, planimeterizing the areas, multiplying by the slice thickness, adding them up, and then subtracting the ventricular volume. Stroke volume is simply the ventricular volume at end-diastole minus the ventricular volume at end-systole (usually defined by closure of the semilunar valve). Once this is known, ejection fraction is calculated in the usual fashion. Cardiac index is simply the stroke volume multiplied by heart rate

during the study divided by body surface area.

Cine MRI, as noted, can also be used to visualize turbulence of blood flow. This is especially useful when valvar regurgitation or stenosis is present. Grading the regurgitation is similar to color Doppler echocardiographic imaging, although the "volume amount" of regurgitation may be calculated using phase-encoded velocity techniques alone or in combination with cine MRI techniques as noted later. Similarly, valvar stenosis may be detected using cine MRI, and peak velocities may be measured using phase-encoded velocity techniques. One must be cautious when using the signal void because this can be made greater or smaller by manipulation of MRI parameters (such as the echo time).

Cine MRI is useful in many disease states in congenital heart disease. Postoperative ventricular performance is a common application. Assessment of ventricular performance in patients with single ventricle, tetralogy of Fallot, and transposition of the great arteries is a common use cine cardiac MRI. Accurate assessment of regurgitant fraction in patients with left atrioventricular valve insufficiency in a postoperative endocardial cushion defect repair is another example. Another useful application is visualization of dynamic obstruction to the left ventricular outflow tract in the older patient with transposition of the great arteries after an atrial inversion operation.

Phase-Encoded Velocity Mapping

This technique uses phase information obtained at MRI to encode velocity. This may be done in images perpendicular to flow or parallel to flow (Fig. 69-1C). In the images perpendicular to flow (e.g., obtaining a cross-sectional area of the vessel), adding up all the velocities in each pixel in a given cross section of blood vessel and multiplying by the area of each pixel, yields the flow at that given period of time. Adding up all phases of the cardiac cycle yields the flow during one heartbeat. Multiplying by the heart rate yields the cardiac output. As with cine MRI, most software on present-day scanners can give a temporal resolution of up to 20 msec. "Real-time" velocity mapping that can yield real-time flow measurements (i.e., flow vs. time, not just velocity vs. time as in echocardiography) is being tested. Cardiac output can be measured to assess ventricular function in such lesions as single ventricles or transposition of the great arteries after atrial inversion. Regur-

gitant fractions can be measured by simply placing a velocity map across a great vessel and measuring both forward and reverse flow. This is important, for example, in a patient after tetralogy of Fallot repair with a transannular patch.

As with echocardiography, velocities obtained at MRI are useful for obtaining a non-invasive estimate of the pressure using the Bernoulli equation (see Chapter 68). Similarly, to obtain, for example, the amount of atrioventricular valve regurgitation, one only needs to take an image perpendicular to the atrioventricular valve in systole to obtain volumetric data (as described earlier). An alternative method for assessing atrioventricular valve regurgitation is imaging perpendicular to the atrioventricular valve during diastole (volumetric amount of inflow) (see Fig. 69-1C) and perpendicular to the semilunar valve during systole (volumetric amount of outflow) and subtracting outflow from inflow to obtain the amount of regurgitation. Similarly, one can use a combination of cine MRI techniques (measure ventricular volume at end-diastole and end-systole to obtain the total amount of blood ejected by the ventricle) and phase-encoded velocity mapping (the amount of forward flow from the ventricle) to measure the volumetric amount of regurgitation. Furthermore, because MRI can obtain velocities perpendicular to flow, velocities in different regions of the blood vessel at a given level may be obtained, and this is used in fluid mechanics research of the cardiovascular system.

Flow can be measured to different organs or parts of organs. A Qp/Qs ratio can be obtained in patients with an atrial or ventricular septal defect simply by placing velocity maps across the aorta and pulmonary arteries. Cerebral blood flow can be measured by velocity mapping across the jugular veins. Right and left pulmonary blood flow can be measured by placing velocity maps across the right and left pulmonary arteries, respectively, and the same information can be obtained as from a nuclear scan. This is useful in patients with single ventricles, for example, or with tetralogy of Fallot.

Myocardial Tissue and Blood Tagging

A unique ability of MRI is the ability to magnetically tag tissue or blood. This makes use of cine MRI (on most machines, although some use spin-echo) in combination with a special technique that destroys all the spins in a given plane (resulting in a line of signal void). The result is a "slicing up" of the myocardium into "cubes

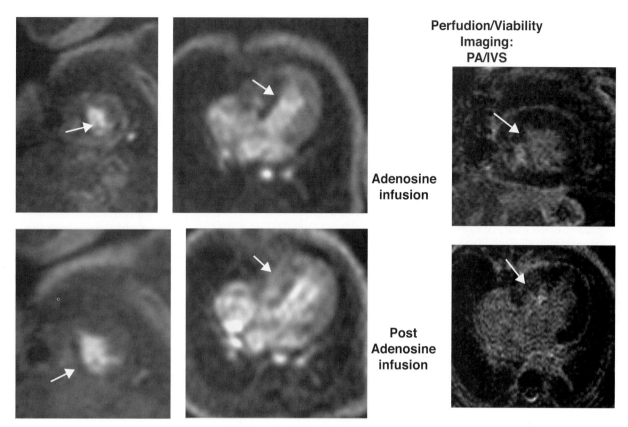

Perfudion/Viability Imaging: PA/IVS

Adenosine infusion

Post Adenosine infusion

Figure 69-10. Perfusion and viability. The patient has pulmonary atresia with intact ventricular septum (PA/IVS). Images with **(upper leftmost and middle)** and without **(lower leftmost and middle)** adenosine infusion show a perfusion defect in the ventricular septum (*arrows*). The leftmost images are short-axis views, and the middle images are "four-chamber" views. The rightmost panels are delayed enhancement images, which show the area of the perfusion defect to be myocardial infarction (*bright area, arrows*). The top image is a short-axis view, and the bottom image is a "four-chamber" view.

of magnetization" or labeling (with a signal void from it and hence a black line on the cine image) the blood. Once the slicing into "cubes of magnetization" is performed at end-diastole, images can be obtained as often as every 20 msec, and the distortion of these cubes (in systole or diastole) allows for calculation of regional strain, ejection fraction, and wall motion (Fig. 69-2). Qualitatively, regional wall motion can also be assessed, and this can be used in instances in which there are questionable areas of contraction on cine imaging.

In blood tagging, however, the more useful technique is to tag before each image (similar to myocardial tagging, images can be obtained as often as every 20 msec), and cardiac index can be calculated and velocity profiles can be visualized (Figs. 69-1 and 69-2). This can also be used for shunt detection (e.g., isolation of atrial septal defects; see Fig. 69-1B). As with phase-encoded velocity mapping, individual regions of the blood vessel may be isolated to evaluate for flow dynamics. It may also be useful for measuring forward flow (cardiac index) for

valvular regurgitation calculations (see earlier discussion).

Myocardial Perfusion

Regional myocardial perfusion is an important parameter in the assessment of the myocardium in adults; there is a place for this in pediatrics as well. Manipulation of the coronaries in procedures mentioned earlier such as repair of transposition of the great arteries or the Ross procedure can lead to perfusion abnormalities. Anomalies of the coronaries such as in anomalous origin of the left coronary artery from the pulmonary artery or in hypoplastic left heart syndrome can also lead to perfusion defects. Regional wall-motion abnormalities, for example, may be caused by a lack of blood supply to a certain region of the myocardium. Cardiac MRI, using gadolinium enhancement has the ability to assess regional wall perfusion by using a "first-pass" injection technique. Typically, short-axis views of the ventricle as described in the cine MRI section are obtained, and the sequence setup

is such that the heart is imaged relatively motionless in diastole. Gadolinium is injected intravenously while the cardiac MRI scanner continuously images the ventricle (up to four or five short-axis slices may be imaged at once) and the gadolinium bolus is followed from right ventricular cavity to left ventricular cavity to ventricular myocardium. Defects in perfusion show up as dark portions of the myocardium, whereas the rest of the ventricle is signal intense. This is typically performed with and without an adenosine infusion and then followed 5 to 10 minutes later with delayed enhancement imaging. The patient in Fig. 69-10 has pulmonary atresia with intact ventricular septum. Images with and without adenosine show a perfusion defect in the ventricular septum (Fig. 69-10, arrows), and delayed enhancement shows this area to be myocardial infarction.

Conclusion

Cardiac MRI has advanced considerably in the last 20 years, and the next 20 years holds even more promise for additional capabilities. It is gaining widespread use, but there is a long way to go. It is an extremely useful and complementary technique to other imaging modalities and has supplanted some to become the gold standard in certain areas. Recognition of this fact should play a role in the practice of twenty-first-century medicine.

SUGGESTED READING

Bank ER. Magnetic resonance of congenital cardiovascular disease. An update. Radiol Clin North Am 1993;31:553.

Beerbaum P, Korperich H, Barth P, et al. Noninvasive quantification of left-to-right shunt in pediatric patients. Phase-contrast cine magnetic resonance imaging compared with invasive oximetry. Circulation 2001;103:2476.

Fleenor JT, Weinberg PM, Kramer SS, Fogel M. Vascular rings and their effect on tracheal geometry. Pediatr Cardiol 2003;24:430.

Fogel MA. Assessment of cardiac function by MRI. Pediatr Cardiol 2000;21:59.

Fogel MA, Baxter B, Weinberg PM, et al. Midterm follow-up of patients with transposition of the great arteries after atrial inversion operation using two- and three-dimensional magnetic resonance imaging. Pediatr Radiol 2002;32:440.

Fogel MA, Durning S, Wernovsky G, et al. Brain versus lung: Hierarchy of feedback loops in single ventricle patients with superior cavopulmonary connection. Circulation 2004;110(Suppl II):II-147.

Fogel MA, Hubbard A, Weinberg PM. A simplified approach for assessment of intracardiac baffles and extracardiac conduits in congenital heart surgery with two- and three-dimensional magnetic resonance imaging. Am Heart J 2001;142(6):1028.

Fogel MA, Ramaciotti C, Hubbard AM, Weinberg PW. Magnetic resonance and echocardiographic imaging of pulmonary artery size throughout stages of Fontan reconstruction. Circulation 1994;90:2927.

Fogel MA, Weinberg PM, Fellows KE, Hoffman EA. A study in ventricular–ventricular interaction: Single right ventricles compared with systemic right ventricles in a dual chambered circulation. Circulation 1995;92:219.

Fogel MA, Weinberg PM, Haselgrove J. Non-flow dynamics in the aorta of normal children: A simplified approach to measurement using magnetic resonance velocity mapping study. J Mag Reson Imaging 2002;15:672.

Fogel MA, Weinberg PM, Hoydu A, et al. Effect of surgical reconstruction on flow profiles in the aorta using magnetic resonance blood tagging. Ann Thorac Surg 1997;63:1691.

Fogel MA, Weinberg PM, Rychik J, et al. Caval contribution to flow in the branch pulmonary arteries of Fontan patients using a novel application of magnetic resonance presaturation pulse. Circulation 1999;99:1215.

Powell AJ, Maier SE, Chung T. Phase-velocity cine magnetic resonance imaging measurement of pulsatile blood flow in children and young adults: In vitro and in vivo validation. Pediatr Cardiol 2000;21:104.

Taylor AM, Dymarkowski S, Hamaekers P, et al. MR coronary angiography and late-enhancement myocardial MR in children who underwent arterial switch surgery for transposition of the great arteries. Radiology 2005;234:542.

Videlefsky N, Parks WJ, Oshinski J, et al. Magnetic resonance phase-shift velocity mapping in pediatric patients with pulmonary venous obstruction. J Am Coll Cardiol 2001;38:262.

EDITOR'S COMMENTS

Cardiac MRI imaging has become extremely sophisticated, and with new techniques, much additional *hemodynamic* information can be added to the *morphologic* information from MRI scanning. In addition, the ability to three-dimensionally reconstruct MRI images has provided a very useful anatomic description of cardiac anomalies, including abnormalities of the aortic arches and vascular rings. The MRI scan is now the most useful imaging modality for evaluation of these lesions, and barium swallow determinations are now most commonly used as screening modalities. The ability to assess not only great vessel anatomy, but also airway and esophageal anatomy by MRI has distinct advantages in assessment in these patients. In addition, assessing abnormalities of chest wall anatomy may be useful in determining whether simple division of vascular rings or more complex vascular reconstruction or aortopexies may be necessary to completely relieve obstruction.

One of the greatest limitations to cardiac MRI is the fact that it is somewhat cumbersome in the management of very small infants, who require anesthesia to prevent motion during the scans. The limits of resolution of the scans also are important for imaging in very small children. Nevertheless, the unique ability of MRI to create three-dimensional images of cardiac anatomy with associated images of blood flow and ventricular function, make hemodynamic evaluations of ejection fraction and blood flow velocity, and assess regurgitant volumes is making this modality an increasingly important tool in the assessment of congenital heart disease.

Recently, fast multislice computed tomography angiography has been added to MRI as a good modality for three-dimensional reconstruction of vascular images in children with congenital heart disease. This technique has the advantage of very rapid acquisition times, making anesthesia less important. An additional advantage is excellent resolution even in relatively small children and the ability to evaluate the airways, including the possibility of virtual bronchoscopy. A disadvantage of this technique is the relatively large radiation dose necessary to acquire the images.

T.L.S.

70

Hemodynamic Assessment and Transcatheter Therapy for Congenital Heart Disease

Nancy D. Bridges and Jonathan J. Rome

Advances in noninvasive imaging have done away with the need for preoperative cardiac catheterization in the management of many heart lesions. Whether a patient facing surgical repair of a complete common atrioventricular canal defect, a simple paramembranous ventricular septal defect, or tetralogy of Fallot, for example, requires cardiac catheterization is a judgment that depends on the individual circumstances and the preferences of the patient's surgeon and cardiologist. This discussion of heart catheterization in children therefore focuses not on which lesions require a heart catheterization for a complete evaluation, but rather on what information is desired when it has been decided that a heart catheterization should be undertaken. The emphasis is on hemodynamic evaluation.

As with noninvasive evaluation, the conclusion drawn from a heart catheterization will be no better than the quality of the data collected and the interpretation applied to those data. Often, the timing of or manner in which a particular measurement is made is as important as the measurement itself. Thus, it behooves the surgeon to be able to read beyond the first page of a heart catheterization report to evaluate the quality of the conclusions that are presented.

Basic Principles of Hemodynamic Evaluation

Invasive hemodynamic assessment involves calculation of flows and resistances, shunt calculations, and measurement of pressure and flow gradients.

Calculation of Flows

Operationally, the simplest method of measuring flow is to use a thermodilution catheter. This method uses temperature decrement to calculate the column of flow out of the chamber in which the proximal port is positioned and is most reliable when there is a mixing chamber between the proximal and distal ports. Thus, when a thermodilution catheter is positioned so that the proximal port is in the right atrium and the distal port is in the pulmonary artery, the flow measured is the flow out of the right atrium and the intervening mixing chamber is the right ventricle. Obviously, in the normal case in which there are no shunts, the flow out of the right atrium is equal to both the systemic and pulmonary flows. However, because most children with congenital heart disease do have right-to-left, left-to-right, or bidirectional shunting, thermodilution is often not an appropriate method of determining cardiac output in these patients.

More often, the Fick principle is used for calculation of flow. The essence of the Fick principle is that, in instances in which it is not possible to measure flow directly, flow can be calculated by use of a measurable indicator, which is added or subtracted at a known rate.

The unknown flow rate F (mL/min) is given by

$$F(mL/min) = R(mg/min)/[I_2 - I_1(mg/mL)]$$

where I_1 and I_2 are the indicator concentrations (mg/mL) at the two ends of the flow pathway and R is the rate (mg/min) at which indicator is added or subtracted.

In a hemodynamic study, the unknown flow rate is systemic or pulmonary blood flow; the indicator is oxygen; and the rate of change of the indicator is the oxygen consumption. Oxygen content is measured indirectly by multiplying the hemoglobin concentration times the spectrophotometrically measured percentage of oxygen saturation of hemoglobin. Oxygen consumption is either measured in a flowthrough hood or assumed on the basis of age and heart rate, using standardized tables. Thus, the equation for calculation of pulmonary blood flow is

$$Q_P = (O_2 \text{ consumption})/ \\ (\text{pulmonary vein } O_2 \text{ content} \\ -\text{pulmonary artery } O_2 \text{ content})$$

and the equation for calculation of systemic blood flow is

$$Q_S = (O_2 \text{ consumption})/ \\ (\text{aortic } O_2 \text{ content} \\ -\text{venous } O_2 \text{ content})$$

Effective flow is the term used for the deoxygenated blood that flows through the pulmonary circuit or the oxygenated blood that flows through the systemic circuit. Q_P effective equals Q_S effective and is calculated by taking the difference between the mixed venous and pulmonary venous oxygen contents and dividing that into the oxygen consumption:

$$Q_{\text{eff}} = (O_2 \text{ consumption})/ \\ (\text{pulmonary venous } O_2 \text{ content} \\ -\text{mixed venous } O_2 \text{ content})$$

Calculation of Shunts

The volume of blood that is shunted from left to right is equal to the total pulmonary flow minus the effective pulmonary flow ($Q_P - Q_{eff}$). The volume of blood that is shunted from right to left is equal to the total systemic flow minus the effective systemic flow ($Q_S - Q_{eff}$).

Because of the great variation in size among pediatric patients, flows are always indexed to body surface area.

Calculation of Resistance

For the purposes of hemodynamic assessment, resistance is the change in mean pressure divided by the flow. Thus, pulmonary vascular resistance (R_P) is the difference between the pulmonary venous and pulmonary arterial pressures divided by the total pulmonary flow:

R_P = (mean pulmonary vein pressure
    −mean pulmonary arterial pressure)/Q_P

and the systemic vascular resistance is the difference between the systemic arterial and right arterial pressures divided by systemic flow:

R_S = (mean arterial pressure
    −mean right atrial pressure)/Q_S

The resulting units, liters per minute per millimeters of mercury, are termed *Wood's units*, after the cardiologist Paul Wood. As with flows, vascular resistance is generally indexed to body surface area in pediatric patients.

Flow Gradients

In the cardiac catheterization laboratory, gradients across stenotic valves or vessels are generally measured as "peak-to-peak" gradients. This measurement is often inaccurately referred to as the PSEG, or peak systolic ejection gradient. The peak-to-peak gradient is a different entity than the maximal instantaneous gradient that is estimated noninvasively by Doppler studies. Whether a gradient is expressed as peak-to-peak, maximal instantaneous gradient, or mean gradient, it is not a meaningful number unless one has some idea of the amount of flow that is producing the gradient. For example, a patient with critical aortic stenosis who is in low cardiac output may have a relatively low measured gradient across a severely narrowed valve orifice.

Hemodynamic Evaluation of Patients with a Left-to-Right Shunt Lesion

Patients with left-to-right shunt lesions (ventricular septal defect, complete or partial common atrioventricular canal defect, patent ductus arteriosus) undergo cardiac catheterization to address the following related questions:

1. What is the magnitude of the left-to-right shunt? Does it justify surgical repair?
2. What is the status of the pulmonary vascular bed? Is the pulmonary vascular resistance sufficiently low that a complete repair is possible?

In general, a pulmonary-to-systemic shunt ratio of 2:1 in association with a pulmonary vascular resistance less than about 8 Wood's units (indexed) is an indication for repair. This is a very general guideline from which one may deviate in some circumstances. For example, a lesion producing a shunt ratio of less than 2:1 may well warrant repair in the presence of symptoms, dysrhythmias, or ventricular dysfunction; a patient with an elevated R_p who is responsive to vasodilators such as oxygen, calcium-channel blockers, or nitric oxide may yet be a candidate for cardiac repair.

Hemodynamic Evaluation of Patients with a Right-to-Left Shunt Lesion

In patients with right-to-left shunt lesions (critical pulmonary stenosis status post–surgical or transcatheter correction, pulmonary atresia with intact ventricular septum status post–aortopulmonary shunt, Ebstein anomaly, tetralogy of Fallot with pulmonary atresia status post–right ventricular outflow reconstruction with an open ventricular septal defect, single-ventricle status post–fenestrated Fontan palliation), there is often some uncertainty as to the adequacy of the right heart or pulmonary vascular bed. Specifically, the question is whether one normal cardiac output can pass through the right heart with acceptable systemic venous and right ventricular pressures. If not, the presence of an atrial- or ventricular-level combination will often permit adequate cardiac output with

acceptable hemodynamic values at the expense of oxygenation. Often, an attempt will be made to temporarily occlude the site of right-to-left shunting during the heart catheterization to assess the hemodynamic sequelae. Increased heart rate, increased systemic venous pressure, and decreased cardiac output with occlusion of an atrial-level communication are all signs of right heart insufficiency.

Hemodynamic Evaluation of Patients with Complete Mixing Lesions and Functional Single Ventricle

The "ideal" surgical palliation for children with functional single-ventricle lesions is the modified Fontan operation with or without an atrial-level right-to-left shunt. This type of surgical palliation requires that the pulmonary vascular resistance be low (<4 Wood's units) because the separation of the circulations is accomplished by using the functional single ventricle to pump systemic blood flow, whereas pulmonary blood flow occurs passively across a pressure gradient. Early in life (i.e., in the first year), the goal of management is to provide adequate but limited pulmonary blood flow. In cases of functional single ventricle with pulmonic stenosis, no intervention may be needed in the first few months of life. More often, the desired hemodynamics will be achieved via placement of a pulmonary artery band or an aortopulmonary shunt. Frequently, these forms of arterial pulmonary blood flow are traded for a venous shunt (classic Glenn shunt, bidirectional cavopulmonary anastomosis, or "hemi-Fontan") some time in the first year of life. Cardiac catheterization before the Fontan operation is performed to assess whether "Fontan physiology" is possible in a given patient. Thus, important questions to be addressed at cardiac catheterization are as follows:

1. What is the pulmonary vascular resistance? A patient with a pulmonary vascular resistance greater than about 4 Wood's units is likely to be hemodynamically unstable after a modified Fontan or venous shunt type of operation with high central venous pressures and low cardiac output.
2. What is the pulmonary artery pressure? Elevated pulmonary artery pressure is not

necessarily a contraindication to a modified Fontan operation provided that it is measured in the setting of elevated pulmonary blood flow. However, a mean pulmonary artery pressure greater than about 15 mm Hg in the setting of normal or diminished pulmonary blood flow bodes poorly for the outcome after conversion to Fontan physiology.

3. What is the ventricular filling pressure? After a modified Fontan operation, blood flows passively across the pulmonary vascular bed. The central venous pressure will therefore be determined by the ventricular filling pressure and the pulmonary vascular resistance. Elevated ventricular filling pressure may be present as a result of chronic volume overload or ventricular hypertrophy; the latter case in particular is associated with poor outcome after Fontan palliation.

Hemodynamic Assessment of Semilunar Valve Stenosis or Insufficiency (Without Shunt)

Pulmonary Valve

The severity of pulmonary valve stenosis is graded according to the peak-to-peak gradient across the valve (trivial, <25 mm Hg; mild, 25 to 49 mm Hg; moderate, 50 to 79 mm Hg; severe, >80 mm Hg). In general, the presence of a peak-to-peak gradient of =40 mm Hg is an indication for treatment. As mentioned previously, however, gradient is meaningless if not evaluated in the context of flow; thus, a gradient of 35 mm Hg may represent severe pulmonary stenosis if there is ventricular dysfunction, tricuspid insufficiency, an atrial-level right-to-left shunt, low pulmonary blood flow, or some combination thereof. The same gradient may represent very mild obstruction in the face of moderate or severe pulmonic insufficiency. All of these things are considered in the hemodynamic evaluation of right ventricular outflow tract obstruction, whether subvalvar, valvar, or supravalvar.

Pulmonary insufficiency is difficult to assess quantitatively in the cardiac catheterization laboratory. A ventricularized pulmonary artery tracing—that is, one in which the diastolic pressure approximates that of the right ventricle—indicates severe pulmonic insufficiency.

Aortic Valve

Although cardiologists will generally grade adult aortic stenosis according to the calculated valve orifice, pediatric cardiologists more often refer to the peak-to-peak transvalvar gradient. The preceding comments regarding assessment of pulmonic stenosis apply equally to the assessment of aortic stenosis: cardiac output, left ventricular function, and mitral and aortic valve insufficiency must all be evaluated to arrive at an accurate assessment of left ventricular outflow tract obstruction. Left ventricular outflow tract obstruction may be subvalvar, valvar, or supravalvar.

Aortic valve insufficiency is assessed in a semiquantitative fashion in the cardiac catheterization laboratory by angiography. A wide arterial pulse pressure may represent important aortic valve insufficiency but may also be seen with aggressive afterload reduction.

Hemodynamic Assessment of Atrioventricular Valve Stenosis or Insufficiency

Tricuspid Valve

Isolated tricuspid stenosis is extremely rare; more often, tricuspid stenosis is seen in the context of right heart hypoplasia and pulmonic stenosis or atresia. Tricuspid stenosis cannot be assessed in the presence of pulmonic atresia because there will be little or no flow across the tricuspid valve in these cases. The presence of a patent foramen ovale that allows right-to-left shunting or right ventricular diastolic dysfunction (both of which are common in right heart hypoplasia) makes assessment of the degree of tricuspid stenosis problematic. Complete evaluation requires balloon occlusion of the atrial communication and simultaneous measurement of right atrial and right ventricular pressures; this may not be technically feasible (e.g., the atrial communication is too large to be occluded) or may not be tolerated by the patient. A more general assessment of right heart competency may be obtained by occluding the atrial communication with a balloon and noting any resultant changes in right atrial pressure, cardiac index, and heart rate.

Angiographic assessment of tricuspid insufficiency requires attention to the technical details. The catheter in the right ventricle of necessity crosses the tricuspid valve; if

the catheter stents the valve open or if some of the holes of the catheter are in the right atrium at the time the injection is made, the valve will appear to be more insufficient than it really is. In addition, non-sinus beats (e.g., ventricular premature contractions stimulated by the injection of contrast) will often be associated with induced atrioventricular valve insufficiency.

Mitral Valve

Mitral stenosis is generally graded in terms of calculated valve area by cardiologists treating adults and in terms of anatomy and valve gradient by cardiologists treating children. Both the mean valve gradient (arrived at by digitizing the area between the left atrial or pulmonary artery wedge pressure tracing and the left ventricular pressure tracing during the period when the mitral valve is open) and the gradient between the a-wave and the left ventricular end-diastolic pressure as well as the absolute left atrial pressure are generally considered in assessing mitral stenosis. Because gradients are meaningful only when considered in association with flow, the presence of an atrial communication with left-to-right shunting interferes with the evaluation of mitral stenosis; the atrial communication must be balloon occluded while the measurements are made. A mean left atrial pressure that is >25 mm Hg is generally associated with moderate to severe reactive pulmonary hypertension.

Mitral insufficiency is assessed in a semiquantitative fashion by angiography. This is more reliably accomplished than in the case of the tricuspid valve because the catheter with which the picture is taken usually does not cross the mitral valve and the shape of the left ventricle is such that it accommodates a catheter more easily than does the right. However, entanglement of the catheter in the mitral valve apparatus or stimulation of ventricular premature contractions can result in induced mitral insufficiency.

Transcatheter Therapy for Congenital Heart Disease

Introduction

Catheter-directed treatments have assumed a major role in the care of patients with congenital cardiovascular defects. These techniques have replaced surgery as the primary mode of therapy in some instances.

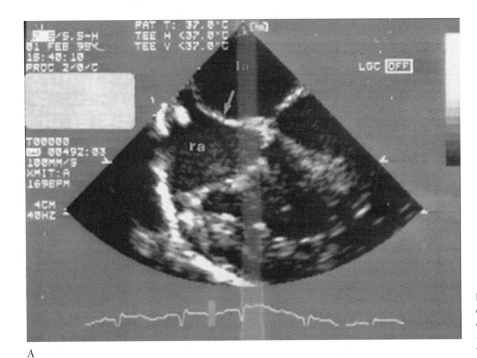

A

Figure 70-1. Transesophageal echocardiogram in cross-sectional plane demonstrating balloon atrial septostomy. **(A)** Intact atrial septum (*arrow*) bowing from left to right.

In many others, optimal treatment combines staged transcatheter and surgical intervention. It is therefore essential that the congenital heart surgeon have a working knowledge of interventional cardiology. This section introduces catheter interventions for patients with congenital cardiovascular defects, highlighting therapies particularly useful in combination with surgery.

Catheter interventions can be classified into septostomy procedures, dilations, closures, and retrievals. Another commonly performed intervention, radiofrequency ablation, is more appropriately dealt with as part of a discussion of cardiac dysrhythmias.

Septostomy Procedures

Balloon atrial septostomy was described in 1966 by Rashkind and Miller for palliation of cyanosis in D-transposition of the great arteries. Even with use of prostaglandin E1, many infants with transposition require septostomy procedures to ameliorate compromising cyanosis. The procedure is also performed to relieve left atrial hypertension in infants with left atrioventricular valve stenosis or atresia. The basic technique has changed little since it was first described. A septostomy catheter is advanced through either umbilical or femoral vein into the right atrium and across the foramen ovale. The balloon is filled with fluid and the catheter

pulled quickly across the foramen, tearing septum primum. Balloon septostomy may often be done at the bedside under echocardiographic guidance (Fig. 70-1).

In many situations balloon septostomy is not the best way to create an atrial communication. Balloon septostomy is ineffective if septum primum is too thick (patients >6 weeks of age and many newborn patients with hypoplastic left heart syndrome) and in cases where the left atrium is too small or posterior deviation of septum primum is present. In these populations, a atrial septal defect (ASD) is best created by other means. The intact atrial septum may be traversed either by the standard transseptal puncture technique (Brockenbrough procedure) or with the aid of a specially designed radiofrequency perforation system (Nykanen Catheter, Baylis Medical Corp., Mississauga, ON). Once the atrial septum has been crossed, a hole may be created by static balloon angioplasty or, in the case of the very thick atrial septum, endovascular stent deployment. These procedures may be indicated for relief of cyanosis in patients with mixing lesions and left atrial outlet obstruction, for augmentation of systemic blood flow in patients with right heart failure, or for left atrial decompression in patients on extracorporeal support for left heart dysfunction. When the technique is used to palliate right heart failure (transient right ventricular dysfunction after repair of tetralogy of Fallot or primary

pulmonary hypertension) the procedure results in systemic arterial desaturation. The goal is therefore to create a restrictive ASD to augment systemic output without excessive cyanosis. This is best accomplished by graded balloon angioplasty of the atrial septum. Similar techniques may be used to create a fenestration after Fontan surgery if necessary.

Balloon Valvuloplasty

Inflation balloon angioplasty was developed in 1974 by Gruntzig for treatment of atherosclerotic peripheral arterial stenoses. Advances in equipment and technique have allowed the application of balloon dilation to a variety of valvar and vascular stenoses in patients of all ages.

Pulmonic Valve Stenosis and Atresia

The first congenital lesion treated with balloon dilation was pulmonic stenosis. Balloon valvuloplasty for pulmonic stenosis is usually curative and generally regarded as the treatment of choice in patients of all ages. In older children and adolescents, the procedure is straightforward. After hemodynamic evaluation, a right ventricular angiogram is performed to assess anatomy and measure the pulmonary annulus dimension. Dilation is accomplished by advancing the balloon catheter over a guide wire that has been positioned in the distal pulmonary artery tree through the stenotic valve. The balloon size

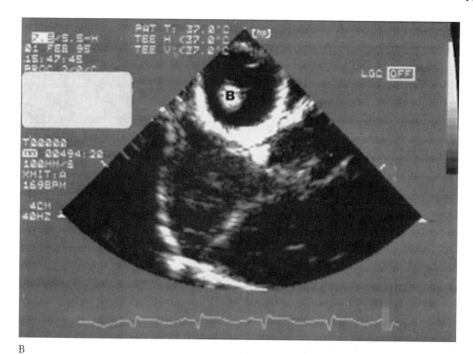

B

C

Figure 70-1. (*Continued*) **(B)** Balloon inflated in left atrium just before septostomy. **(C)** After septostomy an atrial septal defect is present in septum primum. (B = septostomy balloon; d = atrial septal defect; la = left atrium; ra = right atrium.)

is chosen to be 120% to 140% of the annulus diameter. As the balloon is inflated, the stenotic valve creates a waist, which then disappears. Failures may occur when (1) the pulmonary valve is thickened, non-doming, and often muscularized (so-called dysplastic valve common in Noonan syndrome) and (2) where valvar stenosis is part of complex obstruction involving infundibulum, valve annulus, or supravalvar region.

Dilation for critical pulmonary stenosis in the newborn is successful in the majority of cases. Moderate cyanosis is common after dilation due to atrial right-to-left shunting. Cyanosis diminishes as right ventricular compliance improves. Severe cyanosis after valvuloplasty should prompt further evaluation. When inadequate relief of right ventricular outflow obstruction is present after technically adequate balloon valve di-

lation, right ventricular outflow patch augmentation is required, usually in combination with a systemic-to-pulmonary artery shunt.

Balloon valvuloplasty is also applicable to some newborns with pulmonary atresia and intact ventricular septum. Before intervention these children require diagnostic evaluation to determine that the right ventricle and particularly the infundibulum are of adequate size as well as to rule out the presence of a right ventricular dependent coronary circulation (see Chapter 87). If an infant is deemed a suitable candidate, the pulmonary valve is perforated with a radiofrequency catheter (see prior discussion) and then dilated in the standard manner (Fig. 70-2). Patients undergoing this intervention very frequently develop cyanosis with constriction and closure of the ductus arteriosus. When this occurs they may be managed in one of several ways: In cases in which the right ventricle is deemed well developed, the patients may be maintained on prostaglandins for a time to allow improvement in right ventricular compliance. When the right heart is more significantly hypoplastic a stable source of additional pulmonary blood flow is added either via surgical shunt or stenting of the ductus arteriosus.

Aortic Stenosis

Treatments for aortic stenosis, which include surgical valvuloplasty, valve replacement, pulmonary autograft, and balloon valvuloplasty, should all be considered palliative. Balloon dilation of aortic stenosis generally results in adequate gradient relief with only minimal increase in aortic regurgitation. Reported failure rates vary from 0% to 10%, and significant increases in aortic regurgitation occur in approximately 10% of patients. The duration of successful palliation varies from months to decades, although most (if not all) patients will subsequently develop restenosis, progressive regurgitation, or both. Intermediate-term results after balloon and surgical valvuloplasty are comparable, and thus balloon valvuloplasty is generally recommended as the first treatment for patients with aortic stenosis and little regurgitation. Aortic valvuloplasty is usually performed via a retrograde approach from the femoral artery. After measurement of the transvalvar gradient, aortic root injection and ventriculography are performed for valve anatomy, degree of insufficiency, and annulus measurement. The valve is dilated by advancing the angioplasty balloon over a guide wire positioned in the left

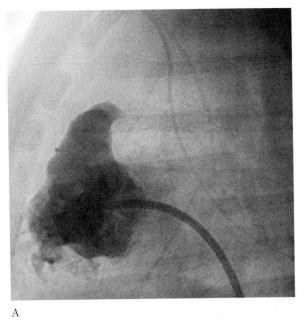

A

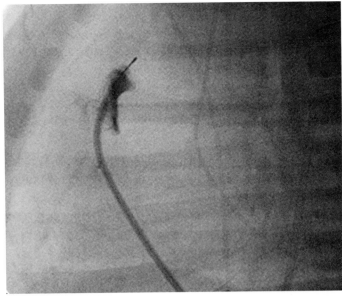

B

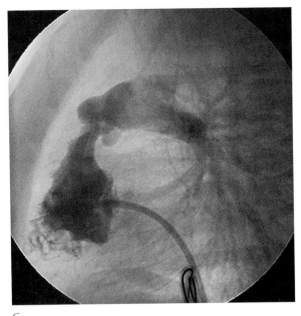

C

Figure 70-2. **(A)** Lateral projection of a right ventricular injection in a newborn demonstrates a tripartite right ventricle with a well-developed infundibulum and valvar pulmonary atresia. A Nykanen catheter (*arrow*) (Baylis Medical, Ontario) has been advanced through a guide catheter to the atretic valve, which has been perforated by the application of radiofrequency energy. **(B)** After subsequent balloon valvuloplasty, repeat ventriculography shows dense opacification of the main pulmonary artery.

ventricle (Fig. 70-3). Balloon size is chosen to be equal to or slightly less than annulus diameter. The risk of significant aortic insufficiency increases when the balloon-to-annulus ratio exceeds 110%.

Special considerations apply to critical aortic stenosis in the newborn. This lesion has traditionally been very difficult to treat, with high mortality. However, improvements in stratifying patients to appropriate treatment as well as in the treatments themselves have resulted in markedly decreased mortality. The approach to such patients is primarily dependent on left ven-

tricular function and anatomy: when the left ventricle is inadequate to support systemic circulation, patients require treatment as hypoplastic left heart syndrome. Several reports have established criteria for stratification of patients to biventricular repair versus Norwood procedure. Balloon aortic valvuloplasty is the treatment of choice when left ventricular size (including mitral valve, ventricular volume, and aortic valve sizes) and function are deemed adequate to support systemic circulation. When the left ventricular volume and mitral valve are adequate but the aortic valve is hypoplas-

tic, the primary Ross procedure may be the optimal strategy. After successful valvuloplasty, ventricular function generally recovers enough to allow discontinuation of ventilatory and intravenous inotropic support within a few days. When this cannot be accomplished, either left heart size and/or function are inadequate or left ventricular outflow obstruction persists. In the former circumstance, early surgery with the Norwood procedure is the only approach likely to lead to long-term survival. When persistent obstruction persists despite a technically adequate balloon procedure it is

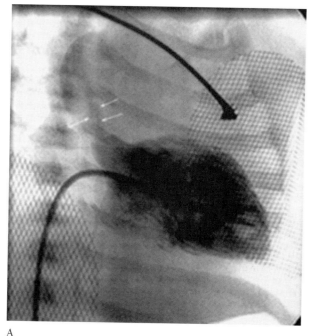

A

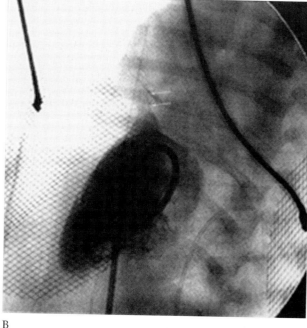

B

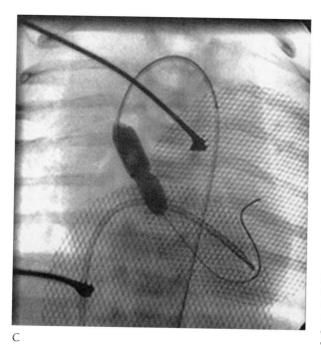

C

Figure 70-3. A left ventriculogram in a newborn with critical aortic stenosis demonstrates a narrow jet (*arrows*) in both right anterior oblique **(A)** and long axial oblique **(B)** projections, typical of a unicommisural aortic valve. **(C)** A valvuloplasty balloon advanced over a guide wire through the aortic annulus is inflated revealing a waist from the stenotic valve.

usually the result of annular hypoplasia and may be successfully treated by autograft root replacement.

Other Valvular Lesions

Balloon dilation has been applied to mitral, tricuspid, and bioprosthetic stenoses. In contrast to the excellent outcome after balloon dilation for rheumatic mitral stenosis, results after dilation in infants and children with congenital mitral stenosis are mixed and restenosis is common. Nonetheless, bal-

loon valvuloplasty is an appropriate first-line treatment in certain anatomic subtypes of congenital mitral stenosis because these lesions respond poorly to surgical valvuloplasty. Dilation may be reasonably attempted in patients with either "typical" congenital mitral stenosis or multiple orifice mitral valve. Neither parachute mitral valve nor supravalvar mitral ring should be dilated—in the former because success has never been demonstrated, and in the latter because surgical therapy is clearly superior. Results after dilation of bioprosthetic valves and subaor-

tic stenosis have by and large been disappointing.

Balloon Angioplasty and Endovascular Stenting

Balloon dilation has been used for more than a decade to treat native and postoperative aortic, pulmonary artery, and venous obstructions. Balloon-expandable endovascular stents are used to treat pulmonary artery stenoses, venous obstructions, and aortic coarctation. In balloon angioplasty, the vessel is dilated to a diameter significantly greater than the expected final size. Relief of obstruction is generally due to intimal and medial disruption at the site of stenosis. Vascular integrity after successful angioplasty depends on an intact adventitia. As a general rule, dilation should not be performed within 6 weeks to 2 months after surgical dissection of the region.

Aortic Arch Obstructions

Balloon angioplasty for native coarctation and postsurgical recoarctation has similar results, with residual gradients of <20 mmHg in 80% to 90% of cases. Restenosis is more common after dilation of native coarctation, largely due to a particularly high rate of restenosis when dilation is performed in young infants. Balloon angioplasty is the treatment of choice for recoarctation of the aorta after previous surgical repair. Given the high restenosis rate after dilation, data suggest that surgery is the optimal treatment for native coarctation in the very young infant. For native coarctation in older infants and children, dilation is an acceptable alternative to surgery. Endovascular stenting for coarctation is now a widely used form of therapy for native and recurrent coarctation in older children and adults. The early

results of this form of therapy have been documented in several small series with very good success rates. In most reported series complication rates are low but not insignificant. In particular, dissection and aneurysm formation have been reported. These complications are associated with technical issues such as stent migration. In addition, it appears that older adults are at higher risk for these complications. Large outcome studies are underway and have not yet been reported, and long-term follow-up is not yet available for this treatment. Patients undergoing stent for coarctation should have ongoing medical follow-up.

Results of dilation for restenosis after interrupted aortic arch and hypoplastic left heart surgery are comparable to simple recoarctation, although risks tend to be higher, particularly in patients with palliated heart defects. Risks of balloon aortoplasty include femoral artery injury, vascular disruption, and aneurysm formation.

Branch Pulmonary Artery Stenosis

The success of pulmonary angioplasty is quoted at approximately 80% when defined as an increase in vessel diameter of >50% (Fig. 70-4). In patients with complex or multiple pulmonary artery narrowings, angioplasty procedures may be relatively lengthy. Lesions are dilated from distal

to proximal in the pulmonary artery tree, approaching the most severe stenoses first to minimize hemodynamic instability during balloon inflation. Wires are positioned in the largest distal branches, and dilations are performed with short balloons to minimize risk of aneurysm formation. Potential vascular complications include perforation, aneurysm formation, dissection, and thrombosis. Mortality rates for the procedure may be as high as 0.5% to 1%. Patients require careful follow-up because restenosis may occur, although the mechanism is unknown. Endovascular stenting has proven to be a very effective treatment for branch pulmonary artery obstruction. Stents are deployed on angioplasty balloons advanced through long sheaths to the site of the stenosis (Fig. 70-5). Disadvantages of endovascular stenting include the need for redilation to accommodate growth, restenosis from neointima formation (most significant in small-diameter stents), and prothrombotic potential of the foreign body (particularly in low-flow vessels). In general, stents are most effective in the treatment of proximal branch pulmonary artery obstructions, where it is rare for angioplasty alone to completely relieve vascular obstruction.

Branch pulmonary artery narrowings may occur in isolation. More commonly these lesions occur in association with other

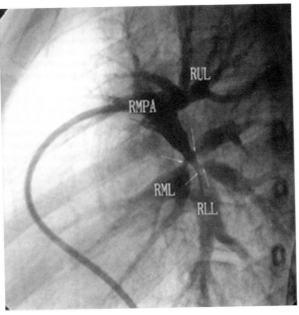
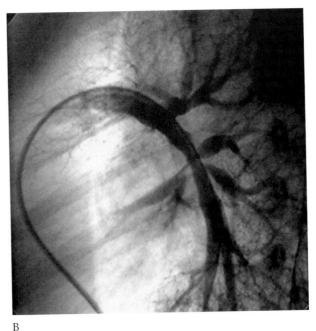

A   B

Figure 70-4. **(A)** Lateral projection of right pulmonary artery angiogram demonstrating multiple stenoses (*arrows*) at origins of lobar and segmental branches. **(B)** Repeat angiogram in the same vessel after balloon angioplasty of right main and lower lobe pulmonary arteries demonstrates significant increased diameter of stenotic segments. (RLL = right lower lobe pulmonary artery; RML = right middle lobe; RMPA = right main pulmonary artery; RUL = right upper lobe.)

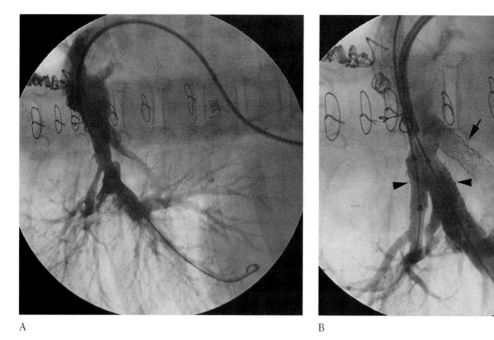

Figure 70-5. **(A)** Right pulmonary arteriogram in a patient with multiple complex branch pulmonary artery stenoses with tetralogy of Fallot, pulmonary atresia, and multiple aortopulmonary collaterals after unifocalization. **(B)** Lateral projection of cineangiogram demonstrating a severe stenosis of the proximal left pulmonary artery (*arrow*).

defects, either congenitally (tetralogy of Fallot, particularly with pulmonary atresia, truncus arteriosus) or as a result of prior surgery (pulmonary artery banding, shunt procedures, and arterial switch operations). Treatment often requires a combination of catheter and surgical intervention. Dilation in the early postoperative period and surgery that involves dissection of freshly dilated vessels may be equally risky. Thus it is essential that balloon angioplasty and surgery be staged to minimize such risks. Catheter intervention should nonetheless be considered for the occasional patient who develops signs of right heart failure immediately postoperatively from previously unrecognized or inadequately treated pulmonary artery distortion. Such situations must be approached case by case, comparing risks of surgical versus catheter approaches. Endovascular stenting is the preferred transcatheter treatment in these patients because the risk of vascular disruption is lower than with angioplasty.

Complex branch pulmonary artery obstruction due to multiple stenoses in series and parallel remains among the most difficult problems in the care of children with complex congenital heart defects (Fig. 70-5). Therapy includes standard balloon angioplasty, cutting balloon angioplasty, and the use of stents. Although stents usually result in the most complete resolution of stenoses, their use in more distal vessels is limited because of the risk of "jailing" multiple branching segmental arteries, effectively reducing the arborization of an already compromised pulmonary artery tree.

Systemic and Pulmonary Veins

Balloon angioplasty or stent placement for systemic venous obstructions may be very effective and has been particularly useful in patients with systemic venous pathway obstruction after Mustard or Senning operations. Treatment of pulmonary vein stenoses by angioplasty has generally been disappointing. Although dilation often results in initial angiographic and hemodynamic improvement, restenosis is rapid and inevitable. Endovascular stenting of pulmonary vein stenosis has been somewhat more successful. The duration of success depends on the underlying disorder. Thus, some patients with discrete obstruction of large normal pulmonary veins after previous procedures (usually older individuals after lung transplantation or repair of partially anomalous pulmonary venous return with anastomotic narrowing, or stenosis after radiofrequency ablation for atrial flutter) will have lasting improvement with stenting. However, infants with pulmonary vein stenosis invariably develop restenosis either from neointimal proliferation within the stent or progressive vascular disease in the more peripheral pulmonary veins. There has been interest in the use of antimetabolites and sirolimus-eluting stents in this disease, but the efficacy of these methods is unknown.

Conduits and Shunts

Endovascular stents can be very useful for relief of obstruction in surgical conduits and shunts. Progressive obstruction in conduit reconstruction of the right ventricular outflow tract is to be expected as infants grow. However, in many cases the process is accelerated due to external compression or shrinkage of homograft conduit from host inflammatory response. In these instances the conduit can often be stented back to near its original diameter, prolonging the life of the prosthesis (Fig. 70-6). The wide availability of coronary stents mounted on very low profile balloons allows treatment of surgical shunt obstruction or occlusion even in very small children (Fig 70-7).

Closure Procedures

A variety of techniques have been developed for closure of vascular connections and intracardiac defects. The versatility of these techniques has allowed their use in a wide range of congenital lesions.

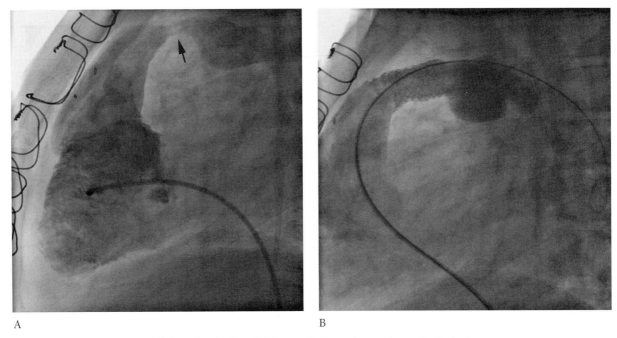

A   B

Figure 70-6. **(A)** Lateral projection of right ventricular angiogram in a patient who has severe obstruction of a homograft conduit (*arrow*). **(B)** Repeat angiogram in this patient after stenting of the homograft shows relief of obstruction.

Embolizations

Steel or platinum coils are most commonly used for embolization in patients with congenital cardiovascular defects. The devices are relatively inexpensive and versatile. After careful angiographic definition of vessel size and anatomy, the delivery catheter is advanced into the structure to be embolized. One or more coils are then deployed through the catheter. Efficacy of the procedure generally exceeds 90%. The most common complication of the procedure is embolization of the coil to the distal vasculature, and errant coils are usually removable by transcatheter retrieval. Other, less common complications include vascular injury at catheter entry site, hemolysis from partially occlusive coils, and endovascular infection.

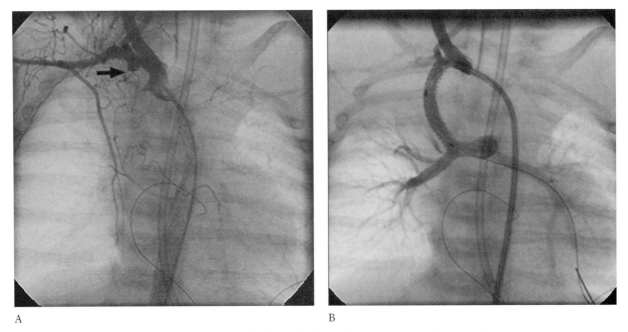

A   B

Figure 70-7. **(A)** Retrograde pigtail catheter injection in innominate artery demonstrating completely occluded right modified Blalock-Taussig shunt (*arrow*). **(B)** Restored patency of shunt after stenting.

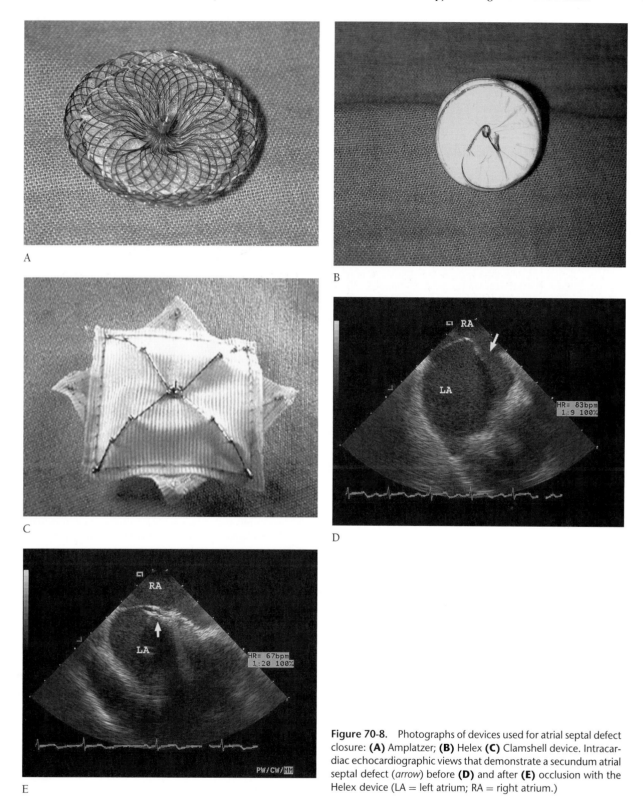

Figure 70-8. Photographs of devices used for atrial septal defect closure: **(A)** Amplatzer; **(B)** Helex **(C)** Clamshell device. Intracardiac echocardiographic views that demonstrate a secundum atrial septal defect (*arrow*) before **(D)** and after **(E)** occlusion with the Helex device (LA = left atrium; RA = right atrium.)

Transcatheter coil embolization is often an adjunct to surgery. Instances in which this method has proven useful include aortopulmonary collateral arteries in tetralogy of Fallot with pulmonary atresia, chest wall pulmonary collateral vessels in cyanotic patients undergoing modifications of the Fontan operation, persistent left superior vena cavae or other decompressing veins in patients undergoing bidirectional Glenn or Fontan procedures, and previously placed surgical shunts in patients with multiple sources of pulmonary blood flow. In addition, coil embolization may be used as definitive therapy for some lesions. The technique has been widely used for treatment of persistent patent ductus arteriosus and has been proven to be

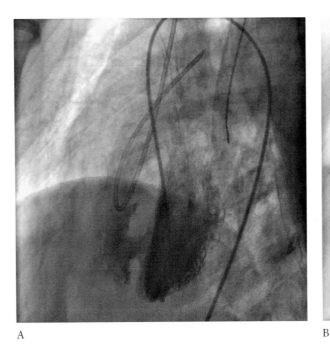

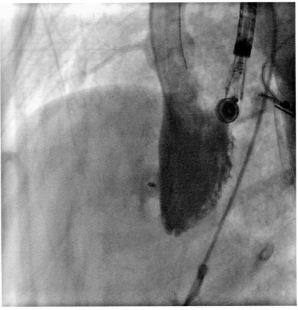

A

B

Figure 70-9. **(A)** Retrograde pigtail injection into left ventricle demonstrates a large muscular VSD. **(B)** After deployment of an Amplatzer Muscular VSD device the defect is effectively closed with trivial residual shunt through the Dacron of the device.

efficacious in treatment of coronary cameral fistulae.

Device Closures

Devices designed for closure of defects including patent ductus arteriosus, atrial septal defects, and ventricular septal defects have been developed and tested for almost 30 years. Many such devices are in routine clinical use, and several others are in clinical trials. The majority of transcatheter device procedures are performed for closure of atrial communications—either typical secundum atrial septal defects or patent foramen ovale in patients with prior stroke. The most widely used device for closure of atrial defects is the Amplatzer Septal Occluder. This, the only device approved in the United States for closure of secundum ASD, has been used in tens of thousands of cases worldwide. It is composed of a woven frame of superelastic nitinol in which have been sewn three disks of woven Dacron (Fig. 70-8). The device is attached via a microscrew to a delivery cable. The assembly is advanced through a delivery sheath that has been positioned through the defect to be closed. It is then deployed such that it straddles the defect. The Helex Septal Occluder is approved in Europe and under clinical trial in the United States (Fig. 70-8). This device is composed of Gore-Tex that has been sewn to a single helical strand of nitinol. When

advanced out of its delivery catheter, the device forms two disks, one on each side of the atrial septum. This device is easily repositioned and retrieved but is not suitable for large defects. The Amplatzer PFO Occluder and the CardioSeal Septal Occluder have Humanitarian Device Exemptions for closure of patent foramen ovale in patients who have had strokes and failed anticoagulant therapy. The CardioSeal Occluder has full approval in the United States for muscular ventricular septal defect (VSD) closure. It was the first of these devices to be developed, is a double-umbrella design, and is quite versatile (Fig. 70-8). The majority of secundum atrial septal defects can be successfully closed by catheter-delivered devices. Typically, the procedure is performed with combined echocardiographic (transesophageal or intracardiac) and fluoroscopic guidance. Though fewer data have been accumulated for transcatheter closure of ventricular septal defects, results are encouraging for certain lesions. Because of impingement on atrioventricular or semilunar valves, the devices are not suited for closure of atrioventricular canal or malalignment defects. Both the CardioSeal Occluder (approved) and the Amplatzer muscular VSD Occluder (investigational) have been used successfully for closure of muscular and postoperative peripatch septal defects (Fig. 70-9). The large, stiff delivery sheath requires patients larger than approximately 5 kg in weight

for standard endovascular device delivery. In smaller children, intraoperative closure via a sheath placed perventricularly has been successfully used to close difficult defects. The Amplatzer Membranous VSD Occluder is in clinical trial for closure of membranous VSD. Initial results in patients >8 kg in weight demonstrate effective closure of suitable defects.

Retrievals

Several specialized catheter systems have been designed for intravascular retrievals. These devices include snares, baskets, and grabber catheters. Most can be advanced through small introducers and are therefore applicable even in small infants. With the exception of large, noncollapsible endovascular devices (expanded stents), most errant catheters and intravascular foreign materials can be successfully removed without the need for surgery. In children undergoing heart surgery, this approach is particularly useful for removal of fractured, retained lines.

Summary and Conclusions

Transcatheter therapies are available for many cardiovascular lesions. The patient with complex lesions may require several operations and interventional catheterizations. In these cases, outcome is optimal when surgeon and cardiologist, both educated in the range of therapeutic options, construct treatment strategies in a collaborative and prospective manner.

SUGGESTED READING

Bridges ND, Freed MD, Mandell V. Cardiac catheterization and angiography. In: Emmanouilides GC, Riemenschneider TA, Allen HD, Gutgesell HP (eds), *Moss and Adams Heart Disease in Infants, Children, and Adolescents, Including the Fetus and Young Adult* (5th ed). Philadelphia: Williams & Wilkins, 1995.

Lock JE, Keane JF, Perry SB (eds). *Diagnostic and Interventional Catheterization in Congenital Heart Disease.* Boston: Kluwer Academic, 2000:199.

Rome JJ. Percutaneous catheter interventions. In Yang SC, Cameron DE (eds). *Current Therapy in Thoracic and Cardiovascular Surgery.* Philadelphia: Mosby, 2004.

Rome JJ, Kreutzer J. Pediatric interventional catheterization: Reasonable expectations and outcomes. Pediatr Clin North Am 2004;51:1589.

EDITOR'S COMMENTS

The advent of transcatheter approaches for the treatment of many cardiovascular lesions in children has resulted in the need for close cooperation between surgeons and interventional cardiologists in planning operative therapies. Because the results with balloon dilation of the aortic valve in critical aortic stenosis in newborns are similar to those of open surgical valvotomy, there is little added benefit to a surgical approach in these patients. It should be emphasized that the results are no better with transcatheter approaches, and there remains significant mortality in these newborns. A certain proportion of patients will have significant residual aortic valve stenosis or insufficiency and ultimately require additional intervention. Because of the success of balloon dilation of aortic stenosis in young patients, however, it is rare to require pulmonary autograft valve replacement or other surgical approaches to the aortic valve in infancy. Most patients can be at least satisfactorily palliated with balloon dilation, and then if significant insufficiency or recurrent stenosis not amenable to additional balloon dilation occurs, pulmonary autograft aortic valve replacement can be undertaken in early childhood. As noted by Drs. Bridges and Rome, the long-term results of even pulmonary autograft

valve replacement are unknown, and therefore all of these procedures should be considered palliative at the present time.

Hemodynamic evaluation at cardiac catheterization is important for determining operability in many patients with complex congenital heart disease with significant shunts. A shunt calculation in many of these patients of 2:1 or greater is an indication for surgical repair. However, there is evidence that the presence of even modest shunts should prompt operative or transcatheter correction because the long-term effects on pulmonary vascular resistance of even a modest shunt are still variable. Therefore, in most situations a left-to-right shunt ratio of 1.5:1 or greater should be considered an indication for operative or transcatheter intervention, and even minor ductus arteriosus patency should be considered an indication for surgical or coil closure because subacute bacterial endocarditis is still a risk factor in these patients. Even ASD with a modest left-to-right shunt should not be considered a completely benign lesion because some of these patients will develop pulmonary vascular changes even with a relatively small defect. It appears that there are some patients who have a particular predisposition to vascular disease, and even a modest left-to-right shunt may exacerbate the development of progressive pulmonary vascular obstructive disease in these patients. In addition, as patients increase in size and age, shunts are not fixed; therefore, a significant shunt may be present in a patient with an ASD who at one isolated determination may have a relatively modest left-to-right shunt. As growth occurs, the shunt can increase significantly. With the relatively low risk of intervention in the current era, in my opinion, even modest shunts should be addressed.

Interventional devices useful for some forms of congenital heart disease are being investigated, and the long-term value of these catheter interventions is undetermined. It seems apparent, however, that coils or occlusion devices for ductus arteriosus will gain increasing use and have particular value in older patients who have a small ductus arteriosus that has the risk of development of subacute bacterial endocarditis and in whom the operative risk for intervention is relatively great compared with the potential benefit.

The usefulness of occluder devices for ASD is unknown, although it is probably inevitable that these devices will be improved such that they can be applied to most patients with moderate-sized secundum ASDs with an adequate atrial rim. The relative ben-

efit of these devices for closure of the defects and the risk of recurrent defects or late device failure are unknown. However, it is of interest that, at least at the present time, use of atrial septal occluder devices has not been associated with a significant incidence of pericardial effusion, which is the cause of the greatest morbidity after surgical closure of ASD. The reasons for this difference are not apparent. With surgical closure of ASD, no prosthetic material or mechanical struts are implanted, and the operative risk is extremely low. However, an incidence of pericardial effusion that requires treatment in approximately 5% to 20% of patients is noted in ASD closure, and the reason for this high occurrence of pericardial effusion is unknown. Transcatheter devices have resulted in high closure rates with a low incidence of recurrence or infection and have become the procedure of choice for small to moderate-sized secundum ASDs.

The larger Amplatzer devices that have been used for larger-sized secundum atrial septal defects are quite large in the atrium. Some of the transcatheter devices have resulted in significant complications. There have been several reports of infection, thromboembolism, and erosion of the devices into the base of the sinus of the aortic valve or the atrial wall, resulting in rupture of sinus of Valsalva into the atrium. It appears that the incidence of these complications is low; however, the larger devices seem to occupy much more space in the heart, and therefore longer follow-up will definitely need to be obtained before these devices are proved to have similar safety and efficacy as the smaller devices for small to moderate-sized atrial septal defects.

Another interesting area of investigation is balloon dilation and transcatheter stenting of coarctation of the aorta. Although results with dilation of the native infant coarctation are suboptimal and certainly no better than for surgical therapy, the long-term results remain to be determined. Balloon dilation of recurrent coarctation has become accepted standard therapy in most patients. The incidence of aneurysm formation and other long-term complications requires longer follow-up. It is certainly possible to argue that in an older patient with a normal-sized aorta, primary stenting of coarctation may result in relief of gradient and improvement in hypertension with no greater morbidity or mortality than surgical intervention. Stenting in younger patients, however, may be suboptimal because growth may require additional dilation of the stent to prevent relative stenosis.

Catheter intervention for residual defects after surgical intervention is an exciting new area for continued application. Patients with multiple ventricular septal defects are particularly amenable to this type of approach. Although most apical defects and perimembranous defects can be directly addressed with standard surgical techniques, muscular ventricular septal defects are often obscured from right ventricular or transatrial approaches and require left ventricular incisions. Although it is advantageous to avoid left ventricular apical incisions, the overall results of apical ventriculotomies have been good. In patients with multiple defects, however, a primary surgical approach to the defects in the apical and perimembranous regions and then subsequent catheter closure if necessary of residual muscular defects is reasonable. Because most multiple ventricular septal defects are generally amenable to surgical and transcatheter closure, we have taken the approach that patients with multiple defects in general should not undergo pulmonary artery banding. Avoidance of banding may prevent hypertrophy of ventricular muscle, which can obscure margins of muscular defects and make later repair more difficult. Cooperation and communication between the catheterizing interventional cardiologists and surgeons can result in optimal outcomes in these patients.

An area of increasing interest is that of "hybrid" treatment options for various forms of congenital heart disease. In the hybrid approaches, transcatheter and surgical procedures are done simultaneously. There has been an increasing experience with the perventricular approach to muscular VSD closure in the operating room, with excellent short-term results. The ability to access the VSD directly through the ventricular wall results in a very straight catheter course and ease of implantation of these devices. In addition, there has been increasing interest in use of hybrid therapies for first-stage palliation in hypoplastic left heart syndrome.

In these approaches the ductus arteriosus is stented over its entire length and bands are surgically placed on the pulmonary arteries. Currently investigational are the use of internal banding devices that can be inserted to limit pulmonary blood flow and avoid surgery and the need for cardiopulmonary bypass. These innovative interventions are in the experimental stages but may take an increasing role in the future in certain complex patients with single-ventricle physiology.

The availability of stents for maintaining ductal patency has also led to greater interventional use as an alternative to aortopulmonary shunts in the newborn. Patients with pulmonary atresia and intact ventricular septum may undergo a radiofrequency perforation of the valve plate with balloon dilation and placement of a ductal stent to avoid the need for surgery. Nevertheless, the long-term outcomes for patients with these strategies have not been determined, and in most cases the ductal stenting needs to be performed in a somewhat restrictive ductus to allow the stent to anchor adequately. There have been cases of stent migration and stenosis, and the hemodynamic characteristics of a central stent may be suboptimal in terms of protection from pulmonary vascular resistance over the short term. Nevertheless, increased experienced is being gained with the use of these interventional devices.

Although they are not yet readily available in the United States, the Amplatzer perimembranous VSD occluder devices are being used more extensively in Europe. Relatively large series of VSD closures with these devices are being reported. Although the closure rates appear to be quite good, there is an incidence of late development of complete heart block that needs to be addressed with additional long-term follow up. Nevertheless, many of these defects could have device closure with appropriate patient selection.

As transcatheter interventions become more sophisticated, the communication between interventional cardiologists and surgeons becomes even more critical. In many cases, transcatheter interventions can be undertaken in conjunction with surgical therapy to occlude shunts that may be difficult to access intraoperatively, to occlude additional sources of pulmonary blood flow in patients who are undergoing the Fontan procedure, or to occlude decompressing veins after staged palliation for single ventricle. In some cases, intraoperative transcatheter interventions may be useful for stenting pulmonary arteries (e.g., in patients with compression of the left pulmonary artery after staged reconstruction for hypoplastic left heart syndrome), which can significantly improve flow to the lungs after the bidirectional Glenn or hemi-Fontan procedure or completion Fontan procedures. In many cases, such as patients with discontinuous pulmonary arteries and a ductal source of pulmonary blood flow to one lung, early, complete operative repair can be undertaken but with a very high risk of stenosis of the pulmonary arteries because of involution of ductal tissue after neonatal life. These patients should be referred for transcatheter dilation early and scheduling of these procedures should be considered part of the operative intervention.

It should be noted that diagnostic catheterization has particular value in patients with residual lesions after surgical intervention because many of these lesions cannot be directly identified by echocardiography. Postoperatively, echocardiographic windows may be inadequate, and therefore catheterization may be necessary to identify the exact anatomy of the residual lesion. As emphasized by the authors, surgical outcomes in complex congenital heart disease with often multiple operative interventions are optimal when both surgeons and cardiologists construct treatment strategies in a collaborative and prospective manner.

T.L.S.

71

Palliative Operations for Congenital Heart Disease

Carl L. Backer and Constantine Mavroudis

With continuing advances over the years in neonatal cardiopulmonary bypass and surgical techniques, the chapter on palliative procedures in all textbooks on congenital heart surgery has grown shorter and shorter. There seem to be progressively fewer indications for palliative operations, although there is a select, small group of patients for whom (at least with our current understanding of cardiovascular physiology) palliation apparently always will be required. In addition, there has been a recent resurgence in the use of certain palliative techniques performed in conjunction with transcatheter procedures: the "hybrid" approach. The history of cardiac surgery has been one of an evolution from operations that were solely palliative to ones in which there is complete correction in the neonatal period with one procedure. Recognition of the complications associated with palliative operations and the realization that neonates and infants do not necessarily fare worse than older children during open-heart surgery have provided the impetus for primary corrective surgery at an earlier age. In this process, many previously commonly performed palliative procedures are now considered completely obsolete and are no longer indicated. It is important, though, for the practicing congenital heart surgeon to understand these palliative procedures because there are many patients who have had these operations in the distant past who require later surgical intervention. The two primary palliative procedures still frequently used are the aortopulmonary shunts (Table 71-1) for patients with diminished pulmonary blood flow and cyanosis and pulmonary artery banding for certain patients with excessive pulmonary blood flow and congestive heart failure. The pulmonary artery band has recently undergone a rebirth in its use as

part of the hybrid approach to the treatment of infants with hypoplastic left heart syndrome. The importance of the initial palliative procedure cannot be overemphasized. A poorly performed aortopulmonary shunt that destroys a pulmonary artery may prohibit the child from having a completion Fontan correction. Hence, although these are older and seemingly less important procedures, they must be performed well to ensure a smooth eventual corrective procedure.

Aortopulmonary Shunts

Classic Blalock-Taussig Shunt

The Blalock-Taussig shunt (Table 71-2) was the first aortopulmonary shunt; it was performed in 1944 by Alfred Blalock of the Johns Hopkins University Medical Center. The classic Blalock-Taussig shunt is a direct end-to-side anastomosis of the transected subclavian artery to the pulmonary artery. Legend has it that Helen Taussig, the pediatric cardiologist at Johns Hopkins University, observed that the condition of infants and children with severe forms of tetralogy of Fallot worsened after their patent ductus arteriosus closed. She traveled to Boston and asked Robert Gross if he could create an artificial ductus in these children. He supposedly told her that he was in the business of closing the ductus, not creating new ones. She then met with Blalock, the chairman of the department of surgery at her institution. Blalock had successfully created a left subclavian artery-to-pulmonary artery anastomosis 6 years earlier while developing a canine model of pulmonary hypertension at Vanderbilt University. Taussig suggested to Blalock that he apply his experimental

procedure to the many patients that she saw in her clinic who had cyanosis from insufficient pulmonary blood flow. The first operation was performed on November 29, 1944, on a 15-month-old girl with the diagnosis of tetralogy of Fallot and severe pulmonary stenosis. After that first successful case, hundreds of cyanotic children went to Baltimore for "the operation." Within the next 2 years, more than 500 patients had undergone the Blalock-Taussig shunt. During this time, there was an early mortality of 16%, and 6% of the patients were considered inoperable. This procedure was very commonly used until the introduction of the modified Blalock-Taussig shunt, which uses an interposition graft of Gore-Tex, avoiding sacrifice of the subclavian artery.

The anastomosis for the classic Blalock-Taussig shunt is classically constructed on the side opposite the aortic arch. When there is a left aortic arch, there is typically a right innominate artery, and using the subclavian artery on this side provides a gentle curve down to the pulmonary artery. With a right aortic arch and mirror-image branching, the left innominate artery provides a similar gentle curve to the pulmonary artery. In contrast, the other subclavian artery for each arch would require an angulation of the artery of nearly 180 degrees to effect the anastomosis. Figure 71-1 illustrates the anatomy for exposure of the subclavian and pulmonary arteries through a right thoracotomy (see inset). The branches of the right subclavian artery are ligated and divided along with the distal subclavian artery, and the subclavian artery is pulled through the loop formed by the right recurrent laryngeal nerve. The carotid artery is freed to provide more mobility. The end of the subclavian artery is spatulated, so the anastomosis

693

Table 71-1   Aortopulmonary Shunts

Blalock-Taussig shunt
Modified Blalock-Taussig shunt
Waterston/Cooley shunt
Potts shunt

is 1.5 to 2.0 times larger than the subclavian artery per se. The anastomosis is constructed to the main pulmonary artery, with care taken to avoid the complication of performing the anastomosis to the right upper lobe branch. The subclavian artery will then be in a groove just posterior to the superior vena cava and the phrenic nerve (Fig. 71-2).

The classic Blalock-Taussig shunt does not require prosthetic material and provides a precise amount of pulmonary blood flow limited by the orifice of the subclavian artery. In addition, the shunt grows with the patient, providing more pulmonary blood flow as the child grows. However, the Blalock-Taussig shunt sacrifices the subclavian artery, which in a small number of cases can result in hand or arm ischemia. In addition, the affected arm is usually shorter than the contralateral arm, is always somewhat cool to the touch, and will not have a palpable pulse. Finally, even with mobilization of the carotid artery and division of the inferior pulmonary ligament, the subclavian artery may still be so short as to cause the pulmonary artery to be "pulled" up and kink. Takedown of the classic Blalock-Taussig shunt at the time of complete correction through a median sternotomy involves dissection posterior to the superior vena cava. The artery then can be encircled and double ligation performed (Fig. 71-3).

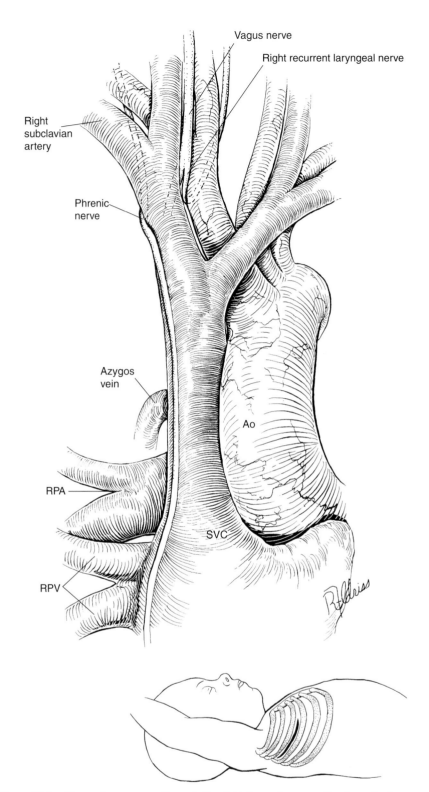

Figure 71-1.   The anatomy as seen through the right thorax in preparation for a classic or modified Blalock-Taussig shunt. **(Inset)** Right thoracotomy. (Ao = aorta; RPA = right pulmonary artery; RPV = right pulmonary vein; SVC = superior vena cava.)

**Table 71-2
Blalock-Taussig Shunt**

Date/surgeon	1944/Alfred Blalock
Technique	Direct anastomosis, subclavian artery to pulmonary artery
Most common indications	Tetralogy of Fallot Pulmonary atresia Tricuspid atresia (right-sided obstructive lesions)
Advantages	Precise amount of pulmonary blood flow Grows with the patient
Disadvantage	Sacrifices subclavian artery

Modified Blalock-Taussig Shunt

The use of a polytetrafluoroethylene (PTFE) tube for an aortopulmonary shunt was first reported by Gazzaniga and associates in 1976. Three infants with pulmonary atresia underwent aorta-to-pulmonary artery shunt using an interposed 4-mm PTFE tube. DeLeval coined the term *modified*

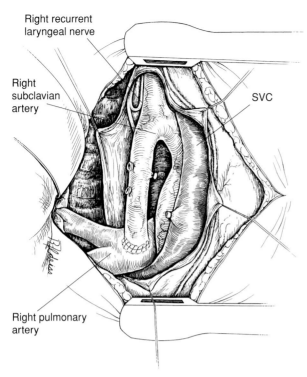

Figure 71-2. The classic Blalock-Taussig shunt. (SVC = superior vena cava.)

Table 71-3 Modified Blalock-Taussig Shunt	
Date/surgeon	1975/Marc DeLeval
Technique	Interposition of polytetrafluoroethylene graft between subclavian artery and pulmonary artery
Most common indications	Right-sided obstructive lesions (tetralogy of Fallot, pulmonary atresia, tricuspid atresia)
Advantages	Flow limited by subclavian orifice
	Does not sacrifice subclavian artery
Disadvantage	Seroma formation

Blalock-Taussig shunt when he reported on 99 patients operated on between 1975 and 1979 having a prosthesis of Dacron (13) or PTFE (86) interposed between the subclavian and pulmonary arteries (Table 71-3).

Shunt failure rate was 6%, and mortality was 8%. The advantages of the modified Blalock-Taussig shunt, which has now become the shunt of choice at most congenital heart surgery centers, include (1) preservation of the circulation to the affected arm, (2) regulation of the shunt flow by the size of the systemic (subclavian or innominate) artery, (3) high early patency rate with minimal tissue ingrowth of even a small-diameter expanded PTFE arterial prosthesis (Gore-Tex; W.L. Gore & Associates, Inc., Flagstaff, AZ), and (4) guarantee of adequate shunt length. One disadvantage of the modified Blalock-Taussig shunt is the occasional excessive leaking of serous fluid through the interstices of the fabric of the PTFE. This may result in excessive and prolonged chest tube drainage, localized seroma formation around the graft, or both. This complication occurs in 10% to 15% of patients.

The modified Blalock-Taussig shunt can be performed through a right or left thoracotomy or a median sternotomy. In the last 5 years we have almost exclusively used a median sternotomy approach. This facilitates the use of cardiopulmonary bypass support if the child has significant oxygen desaturation during the procedure. This of course is much easier with a median sternotomy approach. Cardiopulmonary bypass should always be readily available for such an instance when a shunt is performed. There are several other advantages to the median sternotomy approach. A patent ductus arteriosus can be ligated as soon as the shunt is opened or when the patient is placed on cardiopulmonary bypass. The lungs are not compressed by the exposure through a thoracotomy (which can affect the O_2 saturations). If a thoracotomy approach is used, the side selected depends on the subclavian and pulmonary artery anatomy, the presence and location of a ductus arteriosus, and the great-vessel relationship. The disadvantages (relatively minor) of the

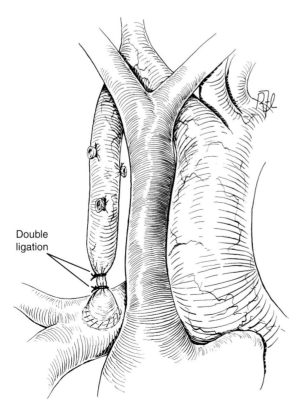

Figure 71-3. Takedown of a classic Blalock-Taussig shunt with double ligation.

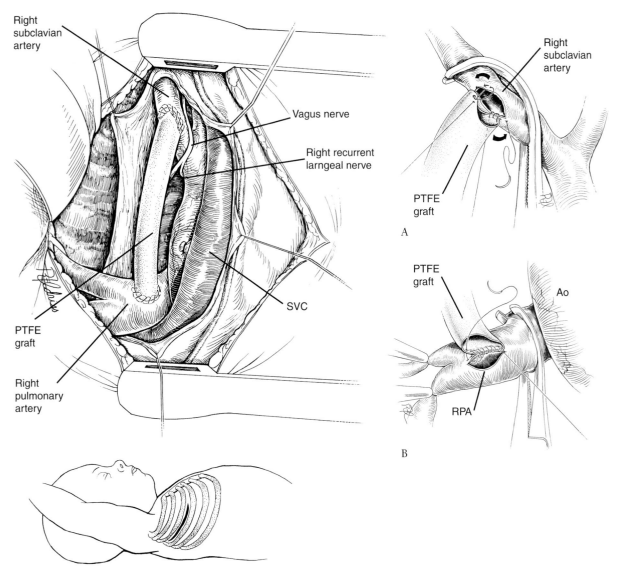

Figure 71-4.   The modified Blalock-Taussig shunt using a polytetrafluoroethylene (PTFE) graft. **(Inset)** Right thoracotomy. **(A)** Right subclavian artery anastomosis. **(B)** Right pulmonary artery anastomosis. (Ao = aorta; RPA = right pulmonary artery; SVC = superior vena cava.)

median sternotomy are the adhesions with reoperation.

With a thoracotomy approach the latissimus dorsi muscle is divided; the serratus anterior is mobilized and spared. The thorax is entered through the fourth interspace. The lung is retracted anteriorly and inferiorly (Fig. 71-4). The mediastinal pleura is opened posterior to the superior vena cava and phrenic nerve. The azygos vein is doubly ligated and divided. The subclavian artery is encircled with a vessel loop, with care being taken to avoid the right recurrent laryngeal nerve, which passes around the distal innominate artery at the takeoff of the subclavian and common carotid arteries. The right pulmonary artery is dissected free, with care being taken to identify the right upper lobe branch and main pulmonary artery continuation to the right lower and middle lobes. The right upper lobe and the distal right pulmonary artery branches are encircled with vessel loops, which can then be occluded with small Rommel tourniquets. The patient is administered 1 mg/kg of heparin intravenously.

The size of the PTFE graft selected is based on the size of the patient. We use only the "stretch" PTFE. We use a 5-mm graft for neonates weighing >4.0 kg and a 4-mm graft for neonates weighing between 2.5 and 4.0 kg. A 3.0 mm shunt is used for infants weighing <2.5 kg. The PTFE is cut to size before the clamps are placed; the clamps distort the relative distance between the subclavian and pulmonary arteries. The graft is usually cut to give it a gentle curve, which allows for some patient somatic growth. It should not kink or distort the pulmonary artery, which can easily happen if the length is not accurate. The vessel loop is used to pull the subclavian artery, and a segment of the vessel is then occluded with a small Castaneda clamp. The PTFE graft is beveled as illustrated in Fig. 71-4A, and an arteriotomy is created in the inferior aspect of the subclavian artery. The PTFE graft is anastomosed to the opening in the subclavian artery with 7-0 polypropylene suture and a parachute technique. The clamp on the subclavian artery is left in place until the pulmonary artery anastomosis is completed. Repositioning the clamp to the PTFE graft may increase the risk of blood stasis and shunt thrombosis. The proximal pulmonary artery is controlled with another small Castaneda clamp. The Rommel tourniquets are snugged on the right upper and right distal pulmonary arteries. A longitudinal arteriotomy is created in the superior aspect of the right pulmonary artery. With a single 7-0 polypropylene suture, the PTFE graft is anastomosed to the pulmonary artery (Fig. 71-4B). The distal Rommel tourniquets are released first, then the clamps on the pulmonary and the subclavian arteries.

There should be a nearly instantaneous rise of approximately 10% to 15% in the patient's oxygen saturation as monitored by pulse oximetry. A thrill should be palpable in the shunt and in the distal pulmonary artery. It is important to maintain adequate systemic arterial pressure before, during, and after the operation to prevent early shunt thrombosis. This may require the use of inotropic support (dopamine, dobutamine). Bleeding is controlled with absorbable gelatin sponge (Gelfoam) soaked with topical thrombin. The heparin is not routinely reversed with protamine unless there is excessive bleeding from the suture lines. The graft should lie in a groove posterior to the superior vena cava, where it is accessible at the time of takedown for intracardiac repair through a median sternotomy approach. The chest is closed in layers with a single chest tube directed posteriorly and superiorly. We routinely sedate and ventilate the child for the first 24 hours postoperatively. In our experience, the incidence of early shunt occlusion from thrombosis and the hospital mortality are 3% each for the modified Blalock-Taussig shunt.

The takedown at the time of intracardiac repair through a median sternotomy is quite easily performed, particularly if the shunt was placed on the right side (Fig. 71-5). The shunt can be identified by dissecting the medial aspect of the superior vena cava posteriorly. Locating a shunt on the left side is more difficult, but it can be identified either by dissecting along the left pulmonary artery, along the aorta to the shunt, or by entering the pleural space and approaching the shunt laterally. The dissection will first encounter a thick fibrous "peel," which typically forms around the PTFE graft. After the plane between the "peel" and the PTFE graft is entered, the dissection proceeds relatively quickly and easily and enough graft length can be achieved for double hemoclip

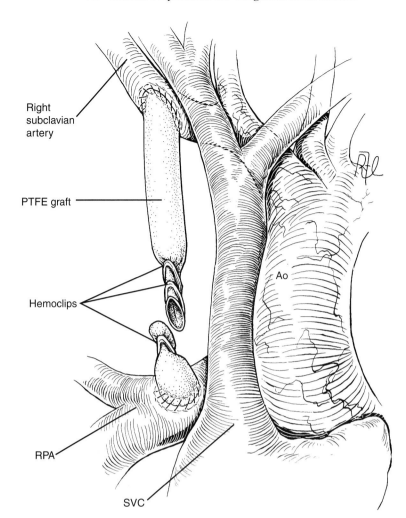

Figure 71-5. Takedown of a modified Blalock-Taussig shunt with the hemoclip and division technique. (Ao = aorta; PTFE = polytetrafluoroethylene; RPA = right pulmonary artery; SVC = superior vena cava.)

application proximally and single hemoclip distally. The graft should be divided between the hemoclips to prevent distortion of either the subclavian artery or the pulmonary artery as the patient grows and the distance between these two vessels naturally increases. No attempt is made to remove the proximal portion of the graft. In some patients the distal graft will require removal to facilitate performing a bidirectional Glenn anastomosis. However, if the operation involves repair at the site of the main pulmonary artery, the distal graft can be left in place and typically does not cause a residual peripheral pulmonary artery stenosis.

As mentioned earlier, our preference is to perform the modified Blalock-Taussig shunt through a median sternotomy approach. This is particularly useful for the child who is having uncontrollable episodes of oxygen desaturation despite sedation, paralysis and full ventilation, and administration of phenylephrine (Neo-Synephrine). Cardiopulmonary bypass with a single atrial cannula and cooling to 32°C will allow the Blalock-Taussig shunt to be performed in a safe and unhurried fashion, with the heart beating in normal sinus rhythm throughout the procedure. We and others have adopted the median sternotomy as the standard approach for a modified Blalock-Taussig shunt, believing that the safety factors outweigh the adhesions at reoperation.

Waterston/Cooley Shunt

In 1962, Waterston (Table 71-4) first reported an aortopulmonary shunt that was an anastomosis between the posterior ascending aorta and the anterior right pulmonary artery. This procedure was performed through a right thoracotomy with the anastomosis posterior to the superior

Table 71-4 Waterston/Cooley Shunt	
Date/surgeon	1962/David Waterston 1966/Denton Cooley
Technique	Waterston: right thoracotomy, anastomosis of ascending aorta to right pulmonary artery posterior to superior vena cava Cooley: right thoracotomy, anastomosis anterior to superior vena cava
Most common indications	Right-sided obstructive lesions
Advantages	Technically "easier" than modified Blalock-Taussig shunt No prosthetic material Preserves subclavian artery
Disadvantages	Right pulmonary artery distortion Possibility of excessive or inadequate shunt flow

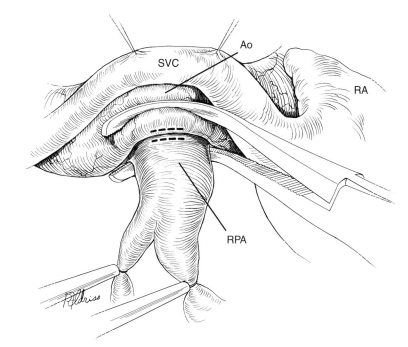

Figure 71-6.   Preparation for a Waterston anastomosis. (Ao = aorta; RA = right atrium; RPA = right pulmonary artery; SVC = superior vena cava.)

vena cava. Denton Cooley reported the same technical shunt but performed it anterior to the superior vena cava. After mobilizing the proximal and distal right pulmonary artery, the distal pulmonary artery branches can be controlled with small Rommel tourniquets. Proximally, a Castaneda clamp is used to occlude both a portion of the ascending aorta and the right pulmonary artery. The aorta is rotated slightly anteriorly with a forceps so that a posterior rather than a lateral portion of its wall is exteriorized by the clamp for the anastomosis. As illustrated in Fig. 71-6, matching incisions are made in the posterior aorta and anterior pulmonary artery. These incisions are between 3 mm and 4 mm in length, depending on the size of the patient. An anastomosis is then created with running polypropylene suture as illustrated in Fig. 71-7. The tourniquets are released and the clamp is removed, and the oxygen saturation should increase appropriately.

A major problem with the Waterston shunt is that it is not as controlled a shunt as either the classic or the modified Blalock-Taussig shunts. If the incisions in the aorta and pulmonary artery are too long and the anastomosis is too large, there will be excessive pulmonary blood flow with a risk of pulmonary vascular disease. If the incisions are too short and the opening is too small, there will be inadequate pulmonary blood flow. A second problem with the Waterston

anastomosis is that as the patient grows and the aorta rotates, the anastomosis tends to put traction on the right pulmonary artery and actually to kink and distort the right pulmonary artery. This may cause preferential flow to one lung. For this reason, almost all patients who have takedown of a Waterston shunt will require a major reconstruction of the right pulmonary artery.

The Waterston shunt (Fig. 71-8) is taken down at the time of intracardiac repair of the primary cardiac lesion through a median sternotomy. It is important to dissect out the shunt area and pulmonary arteries before cardiopulmonary bypass to occlude the shunt on initiation of cardiopulmonary bypass to prevent pulmonary runoff with inadequate systemic perfusion. Alternatively, the right and left pulmonary arteries can be snared or clamped. The repair is done with the patient on cardiopulmonary bypass with the aorta cross-clamped distal to the shunt. After cardioplegic solution has been administered (occluding the shunt or pulmonary arteries to prevent cardioplegic solution runoff), the aorta is separated from the right pulmonary artery with an incision made along the original anastomotic line. Typically, the aorta in these patients is large, and the opening in the aorta can be closed primarily with running suture. The cross-clamp can then be temporarily removed and a PTFE or pericardial patch used to patch open the area of the right pulmonary artery

where focal stenosis is usually created by the shunt. Another approach to the Waterston shunt at the time of takedown (originally described by Cooley) is to open the aorta anteriorly after the cross-clamp has been applied and inspect the opening from within the aorta itself. The aorta can also be completely divided to provide better exposure of the right pulmonary artery. The Waterston shunt has fallen out of favor because of the previously mentioned disadvantages and has been replaced in most centers by the modified Blalock-Taussig shunt. However, there are still a number of patients (now constantly declining) who have had this shunt who will require eventual takedown as described.

Potts Shunt

The Potts shunt is described here for almost solely historical purposes. The Potts shunt (Table 71-5) is an anastomosis between the descending thoracic aorta and the left pulmonary artery performed through a left lateral thoracotomy incision; it was first reported by Willis J. Potts from Children's Memorial Hospital in Chicago. The first operation was performed on September 13, 1946. The child was 21 months of age and weighed 8.3 kg. She had been cyanotic since 3 months after birth and had multiple hypercyanotic spells. She was intensely cyanotic and clubbed. The Potts shunt was performed

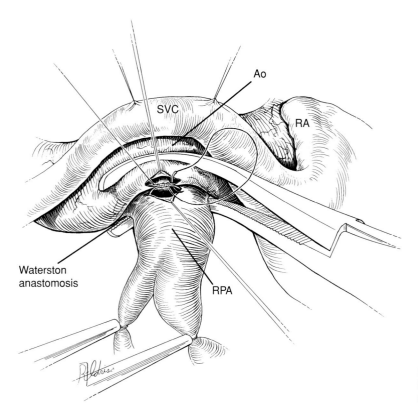

Figure 71-7. Construction of a Waterston anastomosis. (Ao = aorta; RA = right atrium; RPA = right pulmonary artery; SVC = superior vena cava.)

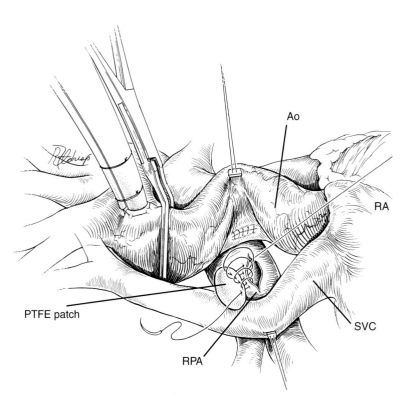

Figure 71-8. Takedown of a Waterston anastomosis with cardiopulmonary bypass and a polytetrafluoroethylene (PTFE) patch. (Ao = aorta; RA = right atrium; RPA = right pulmonary artery; SVC = superior vena cava.)

Table 71-5   Potts Shunt

Date/surgeon	1946/Willis Potts
Technique	Anastomosis of left pulmonary artery to descending thoracic aorta
Most common indications	Right-sided obstructive lesions
Advantages	"Easier" anastomosis than classic Blalock-Taussig shunt
	No prosthetic material
	Preserves subclavian artery
Disadvantages	Left pulmonary artery aneurysm formation
	Risk of stroke with shunt takedown
	Excessive pulmonary blood flow, pulmonary hypertension
	Cannot be performed with right aortic arch

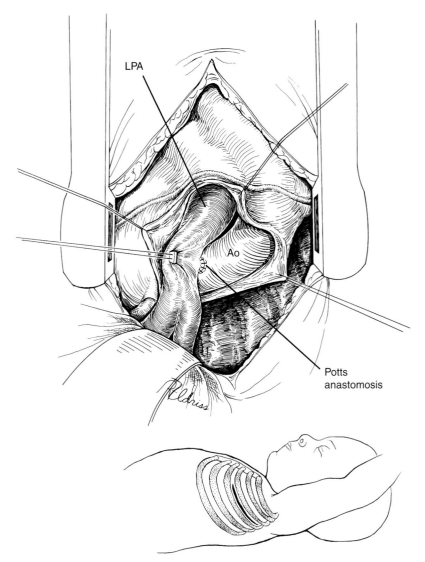

Figure 71-9. Potts anastomosis. **(Inset)** Left thoracotomy. (Ao = aorta; LPA = left pulmonary artery.)

using a special clamp developed by Potts that only partially occluded the descending thoracic aorta. The proximal and distal left pulmonary arteries were occluded. The anastomosis was performed between parallel 4-mm incisions made in the descending thoracic aorta and the posterior left main pulmonary artery. The completed shunt is shown in Fig. 71-9.

The Potts anastomosis was widely used at Children's Memorial Hospital in the late 1940s and 1950s. Between 1946 and 1967, 659 such shunts were performed. However, there were several serious complications that developed from the Potts shunt. Many children developed large aneurysms of the left pulmonary artery. Another complication was that the Potts shunt was frequently either too small and the patient remained cyanotic, or it was too big and caused congestive heart failure. The final and most significant problem with the Potts shunt was the difficulty in taking down the shunt at the time of complete correction of the intracardiac lesion. Initial attempts at simply ligating the shunt resulted in uncontrollable hemorrhage in the operating room or in the immediate postoperative period. The preferred technique now is to use deep hypothermia and circulatory arrest, with adequate precautions taken to avoid air embolism to the cerebral circulation with the descending aorta opened. After cardiopulmonary bypass is initiated through a median sternotomy with aortic or femoral arterial cannulation, the aortic-pulmonary

anastomosis is digitally occluded with a finger from outside the pulmonary artery to limit the left-to-right shunt and improve the efficiency of cooling (Fig. 71-10). The head vessels are encircled with vessel loops. The aorta is cross-clamped, and the heart is arrested with cardioplegic perfusion. The head vessels are snared, and the patient is placed on circulatory arrest. Only then can the left pulmonary artery be safely opened anteriorly (Fig. 71-11). Under circulatory arrest, the communication between the pulmonary artery and the aorta can be visualized and closed with a PTFE patch. The circulation can then be resumed, taking standard precautions to prevent air embolus to the cerebral circulation, venting air out the patch occluding the Potts shunt before the knot is tied.

Other complications during Potts shunt takedown can occur because of the poten-

tial for aneurysm formation of the left pulmonary artery and the difficulty with gaining access to a very posterior anastomosis from the anterior mediastinum. Because of the complications of left pulmonary artery aneurysm, excessive pulmonary blood flow and resultant pulmonary hypotension, and the difficulties in taking down the Potts shunt, this procedure is essentially no longer performed at congenital heart surgery centers. This has been true for many years, and there are very few patients alive with a Potts shunt intact.

Pulmonary Artery Banding

Pulmonary artery banding (Table 71-6) was first suggested by Muller and Dammann in 1952 for children with a large left-to-right shunt or single ventricle. For many years, pulmonary artery banding was the preferred

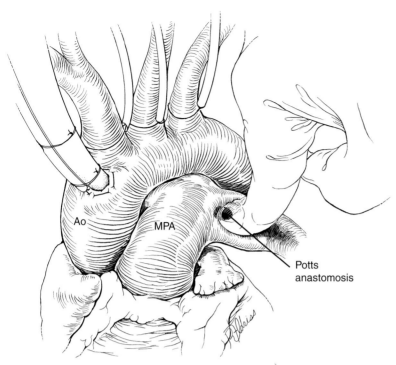

Figure 71-10. Takedown of a Potts anastomosis with digital occlusion of the Potts anastomosis during cooling and ascending aortic cannulation. (Ao = aorta; MPA = main pulmonary artery.)

Table 71-6 Pulmonary Artery Band	
Date/surgeon	1952/William Muller
Technique	Band sequentially tightened around pulmonary artery
Most common indications	Excessive pulmonary blood flow not amenable to primary repair (Swiss-cheese ventricular septal defect, tricuspid atresia type IIc) Prepares left ventricle for arterial switch
Advantage	Performed without cardiopulmonary bypass
Disadvantages	Causes pulmonary artery distortion; may cause ventricular hypertrophy Band can migrate and occlude right pulmonary artery

initial palliation for any small child with a large left-to-right shunt and increased pulmonary blood flow, that is, ventricular septal defect, atrioventricular canal, or truncus arteriosus. However, as improvements in neonatal cardiopulmonary bypass and surgical techniques have taken place, pulmonary artery banding has fallen out of favor for almost all lesions with the exception of a very few precise defects, which include (1) Swiss-cheese muscular ventricular septal defects, (2) multiple ventricular septal defects with coarctation, and (3) single ventricle (i.e., tricuspid atresia type IIc) with increased pulmonary blood flow in anticipation of an eventual Fontan procedure; and (4) to prepare the left ventricle of a patient with transposition of the great arteries for the arterial switch procedure either (a) after presentation after 4 to 6 weeks of age or (b) after prior atrial repair.

There has recently been a resurgence of interest in the use of pulmonary artery banding for infants with hypoplastic left heart syndrome. There are two strategies that have incorporated the use of pulmonary artery banding. One new approach is the "hybrid Norwood" using bilateral pulmonary artery banding and a catheter-delivered stent in the ductus as the first stage of the classic three-stage approach. The other use for pulmonary artery bands is as part of a strategy for patients slated for orthotopic cardiac transplantation. Bilateral pulmonary artery bands are placed with a stent in the ductus to avoid prostaglandin E1 administration while awaiting a donor heart. Another "twist" for pulmonary artery banding that I will review is the modification using an "intraluminal" pulmonary artery band.

Pulmonary artery banding in a child with normally related great vessels can be performed either through a left lateral thoracotomy or a median sternotomy incision. We prefer the median sternotomy approach. Many of the same advantages noted for a

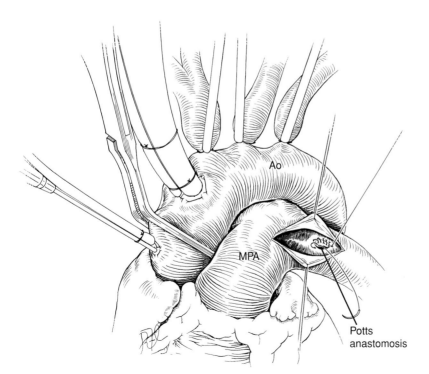

Figure 71-11. Takedown of a Potts anastomosis with placement of a polytetrafluoroethylene (PTFE) patch in the left pulmonary artery under circulatory arrest. (Ao = aorta; MPA = main pulmonary artery.)

modified Blalock-Taussig shunt apply to use of a median sternotomy for pulmonary artery banding. The left thoracotomy is used with simultaneous coarctation repair. The bands we use are either Teflon-impregnated Dacron (infants) or a strip of PTFE (older children). The pericardium is opened anterior to the phrenic nerve through a lateral left thoracotomy incision (Fig. 71-12). Stay sutures are placed to hold the pericardium

open. The left atrial appendage generally sits just at the site where the band is to be applied and can be retracted with a stay suture. Encircling a dilated, thin-walled pulmonary artery can possibly lead to inadvertent entering of the pulmonary artery and thus needs to be done with great care. The safest way to encircle the pulmonary artery is by the subtraction technique. This is illustrated in Fig. 71-12A. The band is first placed around

both the aorta and the main pulmonary artery proximally (Fig. 71-12B). This initial maneuver also avoids the complication of encircling only the left pulmonary artery. A plane is then developed between the aorta and the pulmonary artery with a combination of sharp dissection and electrocautery. A right-angled clamp is then passed around the aorta (not the pulmonary artery) and the free end of the

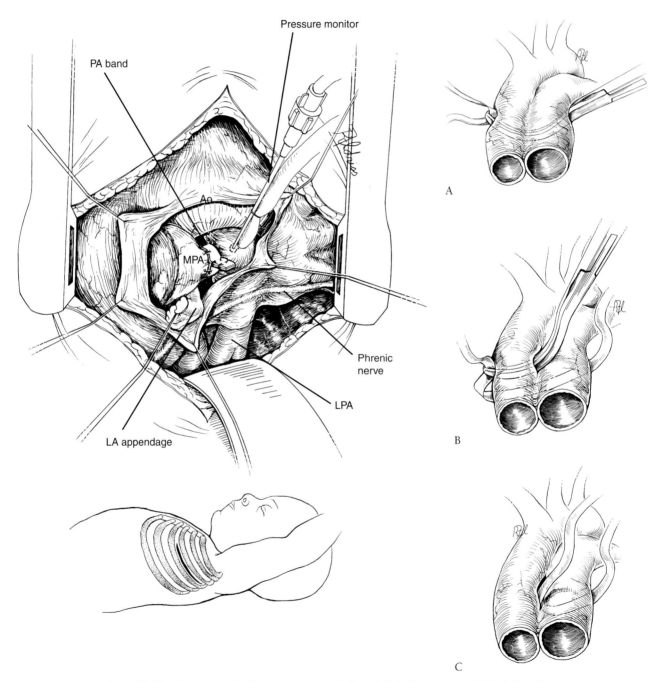

Figure 71-12.   Placement of pulmonary artery band. **(Inset)** Left thoracotomy. **(A)** Encircling the aortopulmonary trunk. **(B)** Encircling the aorta. **(C)** Final location of the pulmonary artery band. (Ao = aorta; LA = left atria; LPA = left pulmonary artery; MPA = main pulmonary artery; PA = pulmonary artery.)

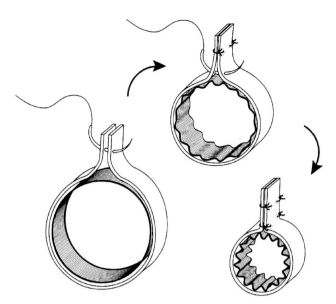

Figure 71-13. Details of sequential tightening of the pulmonary artery band.

band is grasped (Fig. 71-12C). This is then pulled around the aorta and (by subtraction technique) encircles the pulmonary artery. The band is then sequentially tightened by placing interrupted sutures in the band, as illustrated in Fig. 71-13. A catheter is placed in the distal pulmonary artery to monitor the distal pulmonary artery pressure in comparison with the aortic pressure.

Placement and tightening of the band in general results in an elevation of the aortic systolic blood pressure by 10 to 20 mm Hg. The distal main pulmonary artery systolic pressure should be reduced to <50% of the measured aortic systolic blood pressure. For a patient who is going to eventually undergo a Fontan procedure, the lowest possible distal main pulmonary artery pressure that can be achieved with acceptable oxygen saturations is desired. Oxygen saturations for a patient who is going to undergo biventricular repair can be left at about 90% to 95%. For the patient who eventually is going to undergo a Fontan operation, the oxygen saturation should preferably drop to between 80% and 85%. It should be kept in mind that as the child grows, the band will automatically become "tighter" and further reduce the distal pulmonary artery pressure. After the band has been tightened to the desired degree, it is fixed to the proximal pulmonary artery with several interrupted sutures to prevent distal migration of the band and encroachment on the right pulmonary artery. A possible complication of band placement is the aforementioned encroachment, which tends to pinch off the right pulmonary artery while allowing excessive blood flow to the left pulmonary artery. This results in se-

vere proximal right pulmonary artery stenosis and left pulmonary artery hypertension. After the band has been secured in place, the pericardium is irrigated with saline, so there is less chance of intrapericardial adhesions at the time of intracardiac repair. The pericardium is approximated with several interrupted polypropylene sutures, with care being taken to avoid injury to the phrenic nerve. The chest is closed in the

usual fashion with a single pleural drainage tube.

Pulmonary artery band takedown is performed at the time of intracardiac repair through a median sternotomy. The patient is placed on cardiopulmonary bypass. Generally, the intracardiac repair is performed first, and the pulmonary artery reconstruction can be done while the patient is being warmed. All portions of the band should be removed because even a small portion of Dacron band left posteriorly can create scarring, which can cause late pulmonary artery stenosis. Removing the band completely, however, is not always adequate for providing pulmonary blood flow without pulmonary stenosis because the pulmonary artery wall does not necessarily rebound open. The area of banding usually must be either patched anteriorly or excised. The patch technique is illustrated in Fig. 71-14. A patch of either pericardium or PTFE is used to provide an opening for the pulmonary blood to flow over the posterior scarred area and into the right and left pulmonary arteries without hemodynamic obstruction to flow. This sometimes requires use of a "pantaloon" patch with extension into the right and left anterior sinuses of Valsalva. The other technique of pulmonary artery band takedown is illustrated in Fig. 71-15. This involves resecting

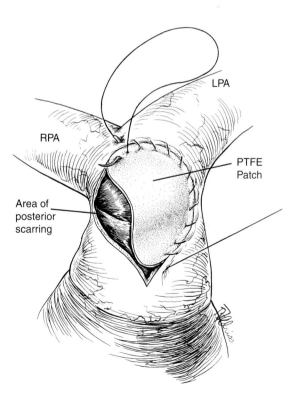

Figure 71-14. Takedown of a pulmonary artery band with anterior polytetrafluoroethylene (PTFE) patch placement. (LPA = left pulmonary artery; RPA = right pulmonary artery.)

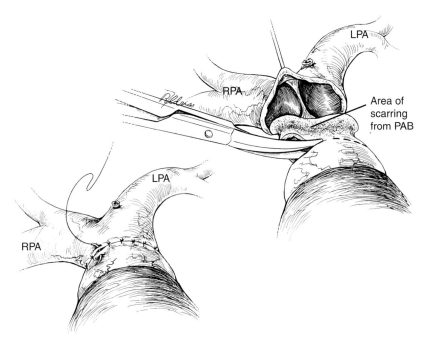

Figure 71-15.   Takedown of a pulmonary artery band with pulmonary artery transection, removal of the band site, and end-to-end reconstruction with interrupted absorbable suture. (LPA = left pulmonary artery; PAB = pulmonary artery band; RPA = right pulmonary artery.)

the area where the band was positioned and then doing an end-to-end anastomosis between the two remaining pulmonary arterial segments with interrupted, absorbable, fine monofilament suture. The distal right and left pulmonary arteries must be completely mobilized and the ligamentum arteriosum ligated and divided to provide a tension-free anastomosis. Although most surgeons have used a patch anteriorly, this usually still results in a mild main pulmonary artery stenosis and residual murmur. The use of transection of the site of the band and direct end-to-end anastomosis in most cases results in no gradient and no residual murmur. If the band is only in place for a few weeks, pulmonary artery reconstruction may not be necessary.

Another method of pulmonary artery band placement is the "intraluminal" technique (Fig. 71-16). This technique is used only in patients who require cardiopulmonary bypass for other, simultaneous procedures. The technique utilizes a Gore-Tex patch with a calibrated precut hole in the center that is sutured as a patch in the main pulmonary artery. It results in a consistent and significant reduction in pulmonary artery pressure and flow. It essentially eliminates the problem of band "slipping" with resultant pinching of the right pulmonary artery. One of the advantages of this "band" is that it can be dilated with transcatheter techniques if the patient should become pro-

gressively cyanotic with growth. Pulmonary artery band takedown is performed by incising the pulmonary artery and resecting the Gore-Tex patch and then performing an end-to-end anastomosis. Many of the patients, however who have the intraluminal band go on to a bidirectional Glenn (Fontan strategy), in which case the pulmonary artery is transected at the site of the patch.

Miscellaneous Palliative Procedures

Miscellaneous palliative procedures include atrial septectomy (Table 71-7), either the surgical Blalock-Hanlon atrial septectomy or the transcatheter Rashkind balloon septostomy, and palliative Glenn and Mustard operations. The Blalock-Hanlon atrial septectomy was first performed in 1950 and was done through a right thoracotomy. A portion of the right and left atria is occluded with a single clamp. The atria are then opened within the confines dictated by the clamp with two parallel incisions, one on either side of the septum, and a portion of intra-atrial septum is grasped, pulled up, and excised from within the clamp. The clamp is then repositioned so that the atrial septum falls back into the atrial cavity and the clamp is only holding the cut edges of the atrium, and the atrial suture

line is closed. This procedure is generally no longer performed, and most patients now who require an atrial septal defect undergo Rashkind balloon septostomy. The Rashkind septostomy is typically performed in an infant with transposition of the great arteries and intact ventricular septum. A balloon-tipped catheter is passed up the femoral vein across the patent foramen ovale and into the left atrium. The balloon is initially inflated in the left atrium and then rapidly pulled across the septum into the right atrium, tearing the atrial septum. For patients with a thick atrial septum that is recalcitrant to Rashkind balloon septostomy, open atrial septectomy with cardiopulmonary bypass is the safest procedure. The atrial septectomy can be performed either during a short period of aortic cross-clamping or with induced electrical fibrillation of the heart. The entire atrial septum within the fossa ovalis can be excised, with the surgeon taking care to avoid injury to the atrioventricular node or cutting outside the heart. Rashkind balloon septostomy in the cardiac catheterization laboratory now is the preferred approach for most cases.

Some patients with complex cyanotic congenital heart disease and suboptimal anatomy for complete correction undergo a Glenn operation or a Mustard procedure for palliation of their cyanotic heart disease. These patients will have an elevation in their oxygen saturations after these palliative procedures, but are not completely corrected.

Conclusion

In summary, the primary palliative operations for congenital heart disease are aortopulmonary shunts and the pulmonary artery band. We prefer a median sternotomy approach for both techniques. The aortopulmonary shunt of choice is the modified Blalock-Taussig shunt. Pulmonary artery banding is selected for very few patients now, but is still indicated for patients with Swiss-cheese muscular ventricular septal defects and infants with single ventricle and increased pulmonary blood flow, who are candidates for the Fontan procedure. There has been a resurgence in the use of pulmonary artery banding for infants with hypoplastic left heart syndrome either as a replacement for the Norwood procedure or as part of a heart transplant strategy. Surgeons need to be aware of the techniques used to create a Waterston or Potts anastomosis and the possible complications of these shunts to care

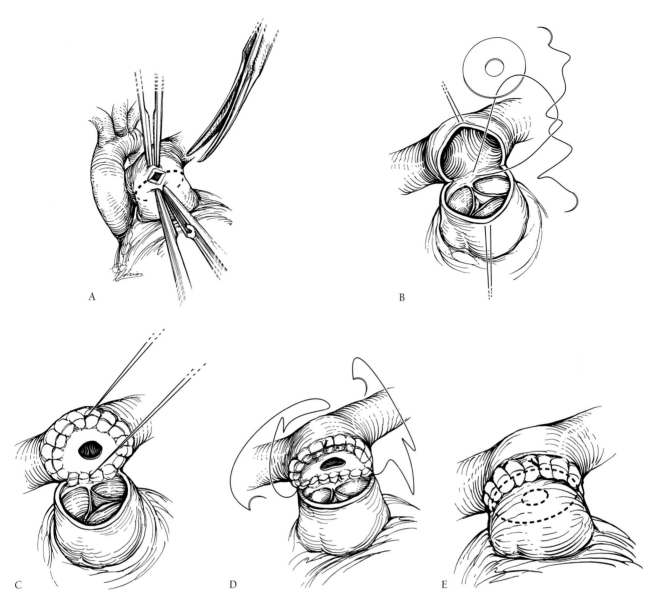

Figure 71-16. Technique of "intraluminal" pulmonary artery banding. **(A)** The main pulmonary artery is opened circumferentially approximately 5 mm above the pulmonary valve commissure. **(B)** The incision is extended 180 to 270 degrees circumferentially around the pulmonary artery. **(C)** A Gore-Tex patch with a calibrated hole punched in the middle (2.7 mm, 3.6 mm, or 4.0 mm) is sutured in place with running continuous suture. **(D)** The pulmonary artery is re-anastomosed. **(E)** The completed intraluminal pulmonary artery band.

Table 71-7	Atrial Septectomy
Technique	Right thoracotomy; Blalock-Hanlon atrial septectomy:1950 Rashkind balloon: 1966 Open septectomy on cardiopulmonary bypass
Most common indications	Restrictive atrial septal defect in transposition of the great arteries; restrictive atrial septal defect with single ventricle

for those patients who have had these procedures in the past.

SUGGESTED READING

Blalock A, Hanlon CR. Surgical treatment of complete transposition of the aorta and pulmonary artery. Surg Gynecol Obstet 1950;90:1.

Blalock A, Taussig HB. The surgical treatment of malformations of the heart in which there is pulmonary stenosis or pulmonary atresia. JAMA 1945;128:189.

Cooley DA, Hallman GL. Intrapericardial aortic-right pulmonary arterial anastomosis. Surg Gynecol Obstet 1966;122:1084.

DeLeval MR, McKay R, Jones M, et al. Modified Blalock-Taussig shunt. J Thorac Cardiovasc Surg 1981;81:112.

Gazzaniga AB, Elliott MP, Sperling DR, et al. Microporous expanded polytetrafluoroethylene arterial prosthesis for construction of aortopulmonary shunts: experimental and clinical results. Ann Thorac Surg 1976;21:322.

Mitchell MB, Campbell DN, Boucek MM, et al. Mechanical limitation of pulmonary blood flow facilitates heart transplantation in older infants with hypoplastic left heart syndrome. Eur J Cardiothorac Surg 2003;23:735.

Muller WH Jr, Dammann JF Jr. The treatment of certain congenital malformations of the heart by creation of pulmonic stenosis to reduce pulmonary hypertension and excessive pulmonary blood flow: A preliminary report. Surg Gynecol Obstet 1952;95:213.

Odim J, Portzky M, Zurakowski D, et al. Sternotomy approach for the modified Blalock-Taussig shunt. Circulation 1995;92(9 Suppl): II-256.

Piluiko VV, Poynter JA, Nemeh H, et al. Efficacy of intraluminal pulmonary artery banding. J Thorac Cardiovasc Surg 2005;129:544.

Potts WJ, Smith S, Gibson S. Anastomosis of aorta to pulmonary artery: Certain types in congenital heart disease. JAMA 1946;132:627.

Rashkind WJ, Miller WW. Creation of an atrial septal defect without thoracotomy: A palliative approach to complete transposition of the great vessels. JAMA 1966;196:991.

Vogt PR, Akinturk HI, Michel-Behnke I, et al. Replacement of stage I Norwood by ductal stenting and bilateral pulmonary artery banding. J Thorac Cardiovasc Surg (in press).

Waterston DJ. Treatment of Fallot's tetralogy in infants under the age of 1 year. Rozhl Chir 1962;41:181.

EDITOR'S COMMENTS

As the authors noted, palliative procedures have become less important for patients with congenital heart disease because early primary repair has become the standard approach to treatment. A small number of patients, however, still require palliative shunts or pulmonary artery banding. Most typically, shunting is required as a component of more complex reconstructions, such as the Norwood operation for hypoplastic left heart syndrome. Isolated shunting is still required for certain patients with single-ventricle physiology with limited pulmonary artery blood flow, who require immediate intervention in infancy as staged palliation to later Fontan procedures. Similarly, pulmonary artery banding may be required in certain patients with excessive pulmonary artery flow in infancy, who also are candidates for later single-ventricle repairs. Early limitation of pulmonary blood flow to prevent elevation of pulmonary vascular resistance is very important.

The standard Blalock-Taussig shunt takes advantage of growth of the subclavian artery, which may improve the pulmonary artery blood flow into early infancy and childhood. However, the sacrifice of a subclavian artery, with limitation of use of that artery for monitoring purposes and reduction in limb growth, has limited the usefulness of the standard Blalock anastomosis. In most centers, PTFE-modified Blalock-Taussig shunts, which do not require the sacrifice of a subclavian vessel, are preferentially used. We have generally used smaller

PTFE grafts of 3.5 mm to 4.0 mm in most neonates and infants because in most cases additional surgical intervention, either for complete repair or additional palliation, will occur before the child is 6 months of age, and therefore long-term patency is not necessary.

We have chosen sternotomy as the primary approach for almost all palliative operations, including the systemic-to-pulmonary shunt and pulmonary artery banding. For shunting procedures, the side of the aortic arch is not of concern if a median sternotomy approach is used, and, in addition, the shunt can be placed to the main pulmonary artery if necessary in very small infants with this technique. Access to the patent ductus for ligation to remove competitive flow is always possible through the sternotomy approach. An additional advantage of a sternotomy for aortopulmonary shunting is the possibility of creating a more central shunt from the main aorta to the pulmonary artery if the innominate vessel is small or there is an aberrant right subclavian artery making the first branch from the ascending aorta the right carotid artery. Use of the carotid artery for the proximal anastomosis of the modified Blalock-Taussig shunt is possible; however, often there is limitation to flow by the size of the vessel, and therefore placement more centrally on the ascending aorta may be an advantage. An additional advantage of the sternotomy approach is the fact that thoracotomies in children may be associated with late development of scoliosis, and in cyanotic patients significant aortopulmonary collateral vessels may develop from the chest wall into the lung, which can be problematic at reoperations or if potential cardiopulmonary replacement is necessary as at final palliation.

Left modified Blalock-Taussig shunts are discouraged because of difficulty in isolating the shunt at reoperation; often the left phrenic nerve is intimately adherent to the shunt, making left phrenic nerve injury more common with dissection to ligate the shunt at reoperation. We therefore prefer right modified Blalock-Taussig shunts through a sternotomy approach if at all possible. Adhesions are generally not a major issue at reoperation. Division of right modified Blalock-Taussig shunts can be accomplished easily at the time of a modified Fontan or Glenn procedure, whereas division of left-sided modified Blalock-Taussig shunts can still be associated with pulmonary artery distortion at the shunt insertion site, which can be complex and difficult to repair, requiring pulmonary arterioplasty, often out into the hilum of the left lung. Waterston shunts are not a preferred ap-

proach for palliation. There may still be isolated circumstances where a Waterston-type approach may be used in patients with tetralogy of Fallot and pulmonary atresia with very diminutive central pulmonary arteries, as advocated by Roger Mee. In these cases, the central pulmonary confluence can be directly anastomosed to the back of the aorta in a Waterston-type fashion to encourage pulmonary arterial growth. In most cases, these procedures are performed with cardiopulmonary bypass and even a brief period of circulatory arrest to allow for the best possible alignment of the pulmonary bifurcation to the back of the ascending aorta and to prevent kinking during growth.

For pulmonary artery banding, the variations in location of the great vessels allow approach to the pulmonary arteries safely through a sternotomy incision in all cases, and we therefore reserve the left thoracotomy approach for pulmonary artery banding to selected patients where additional surgery on the ductus arteriosus or coarctation is necessary.

The authors described the use of the Blalock-Hanlon atrial septectomy, which is a closed technique for removing the atrial septum. As they stated, the Rashkind balloon septostomy has virtually replaced the Blalock-Hanlon operation. In patients in whom the atrial septum is particularly thick or in cases in which the capacity is lacking to perform a Rashkind balloon septostomy or atrial septal defect stenting in the catheterization laboratory or when restrictive atrial septal flow remains and operative intervention is necessary, it is preferable to use open techniques to widely excise the atrial septum. In patients with bilateral superior vena cavae and restrictive atrial septal defect, it may be necessary to cut back the roof of the coronary sinus into the left atrium to achieve a wide opening of the atrial septal wall and avoid recurrent obstruction even after open septectomy.

Although palliative operations for congenital heart disease are relatively uncommonly performed, there may be a resurgence of interest in these techniques, as noted by the authors, for certain kinds of neonatal conditions, including hypoplastic left heart syndrome. The recognition that neonates are particularly sensitive to neurologic injury has led to interest in avoiding neonatal operations requiring cardiopulmonary bypass if possible. Delaying intervention into early infancy (6 to 8 weeks) may potentially decrease the risk of neurologic injury, although data have not yet been accumulated to define whether the additional risks of abnormal physiology may outweigh the potential benefits in neurologic outcome. Early primary repair has become the standard approach for lesions where it can be accomplished in the newborn or infant period, and therefore this "hybrid" approach represents a relatively radical change in the approach to newborns with congenital heart disease. However, if data continue to accumulate suggesting that there is a specific neurodevelopmental advantage in avoiding early operation, then palliative procedures, either operative or in the catheterization laboratory, may take on a greater role.

There has been much interest in ductal stenting as an alternative to surgical aortopulmonary shunt creation. Ductal stenting provides a stable source of pulmonary blood flow; however, there continue to be issues with the ability to create a stable shunt size with the use of ductal stenting techniques and the potential for stent migration and for stent ingrowth and obstruction if the stent does not completely extend across the entire length of ductal tissue. Hybrid approaches using intraoperative pulmonary banding and ductal stenting for hypoplastic left heart syndrome are gaining increasing interest, although the results are not superior to standard surgical approaches. In the past, banding of the pulmonary arteries had been used for patients with truncus arteriosus; however, the difficulties in placing bands on small pulmonary arteries accurately and the potential for occlusion of the artery or significant distortion, making repair more difficult have led to abandonment of this technique. It is therefore interesting that it is being resurrected for patients with hypoplastic left heart syndrome as a potential way to avoid early surgical morbidities. There have even been attempts to create endovascular pulmonary artery bands with calibrated openings in a endovascular plug that can be delivered in the catheterization laboratory. As these techniques evolve, the relative risks and benefits of these more modern palliative approaches and hybrid approaches remain to be evaluated.

Although the authors describe pulmonary artery banding as being useful for patients with Swiss-cheese muscular ventricular septal defects and complex ventricular septal defect (VSD) with coarctation, in most cases primary repair of multiple VSDs has been accomplished with good results. Therefore, pulmonary artery banding is reserved for patients with multiple ventricular septal defects in whom direct operative intervention is not considered possible, such as true "Swiss-cheese" defects or isolated ventricular "noncompaction" in which little true septum is present. The problem with pulmonary artery banding in these patients is the development of significant right ventricular hypertrophy, which may obscure the margins of the VSDs at the time of operative intervention. In addition, after banding, angiography may suggest that most muscular ventricular septal defects have become small or closed, whereas when ventricular hypertrophy regresses after pulmonary artery debanding, residual VSD lesions may be significant. We believe that generally it is best to address these VSDs early and that in most cases, direct closure can be accomplished. With the advent of transcatheter interventions, small residual or moderate residual defects can be addressed in the catheterization laboratory, and, on occasion, device delivery in the operating room via a transventricular puncture may aid in complete closure of VSDs that are difficult to access via the right atrium.

Complex VSDs with coarctation can often be addressed by primary coarctation repair and VSD closure at a single operation. Although results with coarctation repair and pulmonary artery banding for significant ventricular septal defects are excellent with later repair of the defect and debanding, the progression of techniques of infant repair allows one-stage repair of both defects in most circumstances.

Pulmonary artery banding is now used most commonly in patients with single ven-

tricle with increased pulmonary blood flow to prepare the patient for an eventual Fontan procedure and as a secondary procedure to prepare the left ventricle in patients with late presentation of transposition of the great arteries or for right ventricular failure after the Mustard operation in anticipation of a takedown and an arterial switch procedure. Remotely adjustable banding devices are being developed for this purpose. The authors stated that simple removal of pulmonary artery banding is rarely sufficient to allow relief of pulmonary outflow obstruction. We and others have noted that if second operations are undertaken early, then pulmonary artery debanding can often be accomplished with complete relief of residual obstruction. As the trend toward early intervention for complete repair continues, it may be possible to use very short terms of pulmonary artery banding in most patients with single-ventricle physiology with takedown of the band and performance of a hemi-Fontan or bidirectional Glenn procedure by 3 to 6 months of age. A similar scenario can be used for most patients with multiple VSDs, as noted by the authors. We have not elected to use pulmonary artery banding for atrioventricular canal defects because the use of a band results in significant right ventricular hypertrophy, which may complicate the actual repair of the intracardiac defect. Even in very small patients, primary repair of atrioventricular canal defects has been associated with excellent results; therefore, banding is very rarely indicated.

Knowledge of palliative approaches to congenital heart disease is still essential for congenital heart surgeons to permit the appropriate staging of patients to complete repair. In addition, as noted by the authors, knowledge of the range of palliative operations is particularly important so that successful takedown can be accomplished at time of complete repair.

T.L.S.

72

Anomalies of Systemic Venous Drainage

Sanjiv K. Gandhi and Ralph D. Siewers

Introduction

This chapter discusses abnormalities of position and connection of the major systemic venous channels that drain into the heart. Although an understanding of the morphogenesis of the venous system is important, a classification of venous anomalies that is helpful to the surgeon is most appropriately based on anatomic considerations. Thus, this chapter is organized on an anatomic basis, and the anomalies of the venous system within each anatomic segment are addressed. Few of these venous anomalies are intrinsically pathologic to the circulation. However, many, if not most, present important surgical considerations during the palliation or correction of the fundamental cardiac condition. Diagnosis of these abnormal systemic venous connections can usually be made echocardiographically, although angiography, computed tomography, and magnetic resonance imaging serve as adjunctive and very useful modalities.

Where appropriate, the relative frequency of presentation and incidence of the major venous anomalies is provided. This incidence is based on the Cardiology Patient Database at Children's Hospital of Pittsburgh (CHP), which numbers >34,200 patients entered from 1955 to 1979. The information is based on a diligent coding of all cardiovascular anomalies in this patient database. Further information from the Children's Hospital of Pittsburgh Heart Museum database is also used when appropriate to illustrate certain relationships between classes of congenital heart defects and anomalies of the systemic venous circulation.

Anomalies of the Superior Caval Veins

Bilateral Superior Caval Veins Draining to the Systemic Venous Atrium

The superior caval drainage embryologically begins by means of paired cardinal veins (Fig. 72-1). After development of the left brachiocephalic (innominate) vein at week 7 of gestation, the left superior vena cava (SVC) usually involutes and becomes the ligament of Marshall. The most common anomaly of the superior caval circulation is the persistence of the left SVC. This is readily recognized during cardiac catheterization or echocardiography and is frequently seen with absence of the left innominate vein. Small bridging veins between the right and left SVCs may be present, thus joining the superior cavae. The presence of a left SVC may cause the right SVC to be somewhat smaller than usual, but the relative size of either the right or left vein is variable. In the usual circumstance, with rare exception, if there are no lateralization abnormalities, the left SVC drains into the coronary sinus and thus into the systemic or morphologic right atrium. It produces no physiologic abnormalities in its isolated condition and only becomes important when it is associated with other cardiac anomalies that require surgical correction or during cardiac transplantation.

The presence of bilateral SVCs, with the left caval vein entering the coronary sinus, is by far the most common major venous anomaly in the CHP database. It was found in 0.8% of all the patients and in >4% of the specimens in the heart museum. Seventeen percent of these patients had ventricular septal defects, and 10% to 15% had coarctation, tetralogy of Fallot, or atrioventricular septal defects. A slightly smaller percentage had atrial septal defects, double-outlet right ventricle, transposition of the great vessels, and various forms of single-ventricle anatomy.

The left SVC originates at the junction of the left jugular and left subclavian veins. It is located anterior to the aortic arch and left pulmonary artery. Before entering the pericardial space, it accepts the hemiazygos vein, then runs inferiorly and medially into the posterior atrioventricular groove and joins the coronary sinus passing between the left pulmonary veins and the left atrial appendage (Fig. 72-2).

When the right atrium must be opened during open cardiac surgical procedures, provision must be made for management of the right and left SVC drainage. Short periods of occlusion of one, either the right or the left SVC, are tolerated nicely, but long procedures usually require cannulation of not only the right superior vein, but also the left. It is believed that venous pressures proximally in the left SVC system that are <30 mm Hg when the left SVC is occluded are well tolerated during most surgical procedures.

There are several options for managing drainage of the left SVC. This may be managed by cannulation through the coronary sinus from within the right atrium or directly with surgical cannulation of the left SVC using techniques similar to those on the right side. Bilateral SVCs, when joined by a bridging vein reminiscent of the left innominate vein, allow for the usual right SVC cannulation and simple (temporary) occlusion of the left SVC. The presence or absence of a

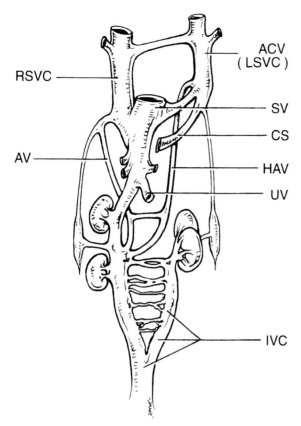

Figure 72-1. Composite schematic of the venous embryology. (ACV = anterior cardinal vein; AV = azygos vein; CS = coronary sinus; HAV = hemiazygos vein; IVC = inferior vena cava; LSVC = left superior vena cava; RSVC = right superior vena cava; SV = sinus venosus; UV = umbilical vein.)

Although persistence of the left SVC, which drains through an intact coronary sinus into the right atrium, is not intrinsically a pathologic state, a defect in the common wall between the coronary sinus and the left atrium will produce a variable degree of interatrial communication and often must be surgically repaired. These defects in the partition may be small and relatively minor and become of greater significance only in association with complex disease. However, almost complete absence of this partition causes mixing and bidirectional shunting at the atrial level with the resultant systemic desaturation. It is difficult to diagnose various forms of unroofing of the coronary sinus when in association with a persistent left SVC. However, during the surgical repair of interatrial septal defects and other lesions in association with the persistence of the left SVC, the integrity of the coronary sinus with its drainage into the right atrium should be ascertained. Surgical options may include ligation of the SVC if a left innominate vein is present and then a repair of the coronary sinus interatrial communication in the usual way, or simply a patching of the coronary sinus/left atrial defect to maintain left superior caval drainage into the right atrium through the coronary sinus. This condition is discussed in detail in Chapter 75.

Isolated Left Superior Caval Vein

The presence of a left SVC may rarely be associated with the absence of the right SVC. When this occurs, there is a right brachiocephalic (innominate) vein that joins the

left innominate vein is readily determined early during the operation when a midsternal approach is taken.

The augmented blood flow through the coronary sinus enlarges the coronary sinus, and this becomes an important echocardiographic manifestation of the presence of a left SVC that drains via the coronary sinus. Knowledge that a left SVC is present in the face of a coronary sinus orifice that appears normal is a tip that the left SVC may drain directly into the left atrium or that the coronary sinus may be "unroofed." An enlarged or dilated coronary sinus is an important consideration during the surgical repair of specific heart defects, the most important one perhaps being the repair of an atrioventricular septal defect. In this abnormality, which was present in 15% of our patients with a left SVC draining into the coronary sinus, the large and dilated coronary sinus changes somewhat the anatomic relationships during the surgical repair. In some centers, the placement of the septal patch, because of concern over conduction system injury, will leave the coronary sinus orifice on the pulmonary venous side of the reconstructed atrial septum. This, of course,

would not be acceptable with a left SVC draining via the coronary sinus, resulting in a significant right-to-left shunt, unless the SVC could be moved or perhaps closed if bridging veins to the right SVC were present.

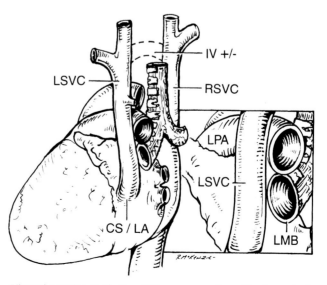

Figure 72-2. Bilateral superior caval veins. (CS = coronary sinus; IV = innominate vein; LA = left atrium; LMB = left main bronchus; LPA = left pulmonary artery; LSVC = left superior vena cava; RSVC = right superior vena cava.)

left SVC. We found 15 cases (0.05%) in the CHP database and 5 additional cases in the Heart Museum. The most commonly associated anomalies were ventricular septal defects, atrial septal defects, and atrioventricular septal defects. Rarely, the coronary sinus may also be unroofed in association with this entity. It is said that arrhythmias, including sinus node dysfunction, atrioventricular block, supraventricular tachycardia, and bundle-branch block, are more common under the circumstance of an absent right SVC. During cardiopulmonary bypass, the isolated left SVC must be cannulated directly for the management of venous return if the atrium must be opened.

Left Superior Caval Vein Draining Directly into the Left Atrium

A left SVC may drain directly into the left atrium. Drainage of the vena cava to the left atrium (either the left or the right SVC) was found in <0.2% of the patients in the CHP Cardiology Patient Database. Forty percent of these were patients with atrial isomerism, and 15% also were associated with an atrioventricular septal defect. When the left SVC connects directly to the left atrium, it is usually in association with abnormalities of lateralization with either right or left atrial isomerism. It is slightly more common for the SVC to drain directly into the left atrium in cases of right isomerism. In addition, the left SVC may drain directly into the left atrium without other serious cardiac malformations, causing right-to-left shunting. When this becomes hemodynamically significant, correction of the shunt may require interatrial baffling of the orifice of the left SVC to the systemic atrium or translocation of the left SVC to the right atrium or right SVC. It should be recalled that in left isomerism, a solitary left SVC may drain directly to the systemic or right-sided atrium or through the coronary sinus.

Left superior caval drainage into the left-sided atrium must be surgically addressed when the systemic and pulmonary venous circulations are to be separated. This most commonly is encountered during the palliation or repair of various forms of the functionally univentricular heart. Under those circumstances, the left SVC may be directly connected to the left pulmonary artery (left bidirectional Glenn anastomosis) as part of a staged or total cavopulmonary connection. Interatrial tunneling of the venous return from the atrial orifice of the left SVC to the right (systemic) atrium may compro-

mise or complicate the intracardiac repair of many defects, especially atrioventricular septal defects. Removal of the left SVC from the left atrium and direct attachment to the right-sided atrium or right SVC may be more efficacious. Cryopreserved homograft tissue may also be used as a patch or conduit to help achieve this extracardiac correction. Another option, in the presence of normal pulmonary hemodynamics, is to attach the left SVC directly to the left pulmonary artery, even when a biventricular repair is contemplated. This will correct the right-to-left shunt and still provide decompression of the left superior caval system.

Presence of a Levoatrial Cardinal Vein

The levoatrial cardinal vein is occasionally confused with the persistence of the left SVC. However, it differs from a left SVC in several ways. The levoatrial cardinal vein is thought to result from the persistence of anatomic channels that connect the capillary plexus of the embryonic foregut to the cardinal veins. It is usually found with a normally present left innominate vein. It ascends from the left atrium or a confluence of pulmonary veins dorsal to the left pulmonary artery, passing between the left pulmonary artery and the left bronchus (Fig. 72-3). When this vein receives pulmonary venous return, the passage of the

levoatrial cardinal vein between these two large and potentially fixed structures causes obstruction to the anomalously draining pulmonary venous return.

The levoatrial cardinal vein is most usually recognized in association with left atrioventricular valve stenosis or atresia and with a restrictive or absent interatrial opening. It may provide the only exit for pulmonary venous blood that arrives through normally connected pulmonary veins into the left-sided atrium in patients with left ventricular inflow obstruction. It provides an exit into the systemic venous circulation. An analysis of the CHP Cardiology Patient Database found that 0.04% of the patients had a levoatrial cardinal vein. Fifty percent of the patients had either right or left isomerism, and a small proportion of the patients had other associated anomalies, including double-outlet right ventricle, tetralogy of Fallot, ventricular septal defect, and atrioventricular septal defect.

The levoatrial cardinal vein has little surgical significance. It does not provide a useful venous pathway beyond the early neonatal period, and even then it is too small or obstructive. However, it must be recognized and closed during corrective surgery that demands a separation of the systemic and pulmonary venous circulations. For example, persistence of this vein following a bidirectional Glenn anastomosis would provide an unacceptable collateral route of decompression for the superior venous circulation.

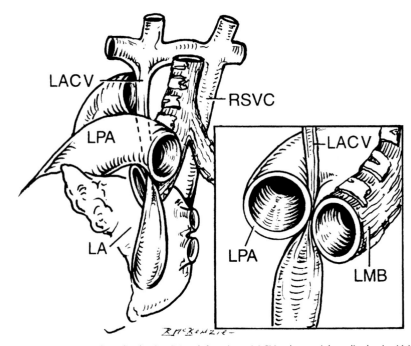

Figure 72-3. Levoatrial cardinal vein. (LA = left atrium; LACV = levoatrial cardinal vein; LMB = left main bronchus; LPA = left pulmonary artery; RSVC = right superior vena cava.)

Right Superior Caval Vein to the Left (Pulmonary) Atrium

A right SVC that connects directly to the left atrium has been reported as an isolated anomaly and may cause a right-to-left shunt of approximately 30%. In this situation, the right SVC passes medially and dorsally to the aortic root, connecting to the cephalic portion of the left atrium. It may receive one or more pulmonary veins (Fig. 72-4). These patients often escape a diagnosis in infancy, but cyanosis usually worsens and a diagnosis will likely be established. There are open and closed techniques for the connection of the right superior cava to the right atrial appendage, removing it from its posteriorly located position with its attachment to the left atrium. The association of partial anomalous pulmonary venous return into the abnormally located right SVC must be recognized. If this is an isolated situation draining a small portion of the right lung, the anomalous pulmonary veins may be left alone. If a large portion of the right pulmonary venous return is connected to the anomalously draining right SVC, the portion of the right SVC containing the anomalous pulmonary veins should be left attached to the left atrium and only the more proximal part of the right SVC attached to the right atrium.

There have been several cases in which the right SVC has been noted to drain into both atria. This is conceptually identical to the superior type of sinus venosus interatrial defect, in which the right SVC "overrides" the atrial septum and offers drainage into both the right and left atria. Correction of this anomaly is usually achieved with enlargement, if necessary, of the interatrial opening (the sinus venosus defect) and baffling of the anomalously connected right-side pulmonary vein or veins to the left of the atrial septum. This sinus venosus defect repair functionally corrects the SVC drainage solely into the right atrium.

Aneurysmal Dilation of the Superior Caval System

Aneurysmal dilation of portions of the superior caval system may occur. These malformations are usually localized and may involve the SVC on either the right or left side. They also have been found in the left innominate vein and in the right and left internal jugular veins. There is usually no need for surgical involvement or correction unless they produce symptoms because of mass or displacement. Thrombus formation and emboli are theoretical concerns but have not been recognized. We have resected one such aneurysm, believed to be a congenital malformation, of the internal jugular vein in a child who had symptoms of fullness and respiratory effort on assuming the supine position. The symptoms were thought to be caused by displacement of the trachea because of the mass effect of the large internal jugular vein and were relieved by simple resection of the hugely dilated vein.

Retroaortic Innominate Vein

Occasionally, the surgeon will encounter what appears to be an absence of the left innominate vein. However, on opening the pericardium, a large vein may be found passing across the upper pericardial space, connecting the left internal jugular and subclavian veins to the right SVC. This vein passes dorsal to the ascending aorta, and its course parallels the right pulmonary artery. It is not thought to be associated with any specific cardiac abnormality; however, most patients with a retroaortic innominate vein have a congenital cardiac malformation. It has been noted with a left SVC, but this association is uncommon. There are no specific surgical connotations associated with this interesting finding other than an awareness of its occurrence so that it may be protected during dissection and not be confused with other structures.

Anomalies of the Inferior Caval Vein

Anomalies of the inferior vena cava (IVC) are less common than anomalies of the SVC. The Cardiology Patient Database at CHP indicates an incidence of 0.3%. Slightly >1% of the hearts in the museum collection were associated with IVC anomalies. Other than lateralization abnormalities, atrioventricular septal defect was the only cardiac malformation with an apparent association with abnormalities of the IVC. Fully 15% of the patients with interruption of the IVC in our database have this anomaly.

Absence of the Hepatic Segment of the Inferior Caval Vein

Clearly the most noteworthy form of IVC anomaly is absence of the hepatic segment of the IVC with azygos or hemiazygos continuation of the lower portion of the IVC to the superior caval system. This malformation, referred to as an interrupted IVC, may occur in situs solitus or in the context of a lateralization abnormality.

Azygos Continuation to the Right Superior Caval Vein

In the absence of lateralization abnormalities, IVC blood return to the heart is through

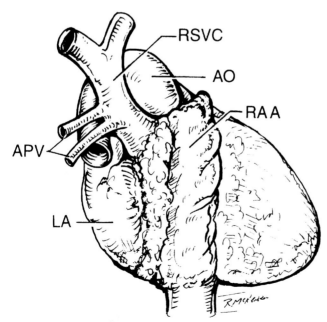

Figure 72-4. Right superior caval vein connected to the left atrium, with partial anomalously draining pulmonary veins. (AO = ascending aorta; APV = anomalous pulmonary veins; RAA = right atrial appendage; LA = left atrium; RSVC = right superior vena cava.)

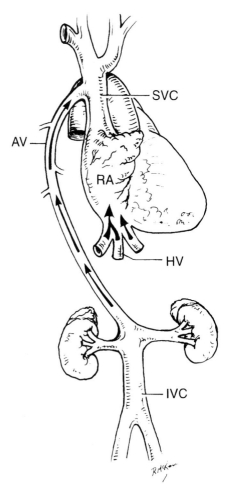

Figure 72-5. Absence of the hepatic segment of the inferior vena cava (IVC) (IVC interruption with azygos continuation). (AV = azygos vein; HV = hepatic veins; RA = right atrium; SVC = superior vena cava.)

an azygos vein continuation to the right SVC from the infrahepatically interrupted IVC (Fig. 72-5). Rarely, the continuation is via the left (hemi) azygos system to the right SVC, even without lateralization abnormalities. It is the most common inferior caval anomaly, and, aside from surgical consideration during the repair of other cardiac anomalies, it is of no major consequence. The hepatic veins usually connect singly through a short suprahepatic confluence resembling a normal IVC to the right atrium. On rare occasions there may be several separate hepatic vein connections to the atrium, and in the absence of heterotaxy they connect to the right atrium.

Closure of the azygos vein, for instance, during a right subclavian-to-pulmonary artery shunt should not be performed when the IVC is congenitally interrupted. The tip-off to the surgeon, unless it is known preoperatively, would be an unusually large azygos

vein. During the creation of a bidirectional Glenn shunt, the azygos vein is ordinarily ligated. With IVC continuation via the azygos vein, however, the shunt will direct all of the systemic venous blood, save the hepatic venous return, into the pulmonary artery circuit. This has been called the "Kawashima operation," and it is intrinsically attractive as a form of palliation for some patients with a functionally univentricular heart. However, it is occasionally associated with the development or enlargement of intrahepatic venous communications between the hepatic venous and systemic venous circuits, and it may provide a progressive decompression of the systemic venous flow away from the pulmonary circuit. Additionally, the development of arteriovenous pulmonary connections (fistulae) is much more common when the pulmonary circuit is deprived of hepatic venous blood flow. Most patients with a bidirectional SVC-to-pulmonary artery connection in the presence of azygos continuation of an interrupted IVC will eventually require baffling of some or all of the hepatic veins to the pulmonary artery—a completion of the modified Fontan operation.

Interruption of the Inferior Caval Vein in Visceral Heterotaxy

Fifty percent (37 patients) of the CHP database patients with IVC interruption had lateralization abnormalities. All but one are left isomerism with the IVC continued into a left SVC by means of the hemiazygos vein. The surgical considerations are the same as those that apply to the right-side continuation with the azygos vein. Exceptions depend on how the left SVC connects with the atrial mass, either directly or by means of the coronary sinus.

In patients with right isomerism, interruption of the IVC is extremely rare, and the azygos vein anatomy is of much less concern. However, there is a tendency for the hepatic veins to connect directly to the atrial mass, either on the right or the left side. This direct connection of the hepatic veins is very common, of course, in left isomerism because of the higher frequency of IVC interruption in this cardiac defect. The hepatic vein anatomy is much more variable in right isomerism and must be delineated carefully in anticipation of procedures designed to separate the pulmonary and systemic venous drainage and during cardiac transplantation.

Left Atrial and Biatrial Connection of the Inferior Caval Vein

The IVC may connect directly to the left atrium, with or without the presence of an interatrial communication. The inferior form of the sinus venosus interatrial defect provides the situation in which the IVC "over-rides" the atrial septum and streaming from the IVC delivers a large amount of inferior caval blood into the left atrium. This anomaly is invariably associated with some degree of partial anomalous pulmonary venous return from the right lung. Depending on the relative degree of "over-ride," the patient may be hypoxic, but shunt studies will miss the diagnosis unless done from the IVC.

Surgical correction of this anomaly involves correction of the interatrial communication with baffling of the IVC to the right side of the atrial septum. In circumstances in which there is a direct connection without interatrial communication, the inferior caval blood flow may be directed to the systemic venous atrium either by reconnection of the IVC or by means of an interatrial baffle construction. This anomaly with an intact atrial septum is extraordinarily unusual.

Other Abnormalities of the Inferior Caval Vein

Duplication of the IVC below the renal veins is not infrequent, but it has no relation to congenital abnormalities of the heart. Its presence or the presence of a left infrarenal IVC that crosses sharply to the right at a subhepatic level may cause the cardiologist some problems during catheterization. The surgeon may experience difficulty during the unusual circumstance of passing large cardiopulmonary bypass venous cannulae from the femoral approach in circumstances when bypass is necessary before the chest is opened or when transthoracic IVC cannulation is not feasible.

Congenital membranous obstruction of the IVC as it enters the right atrium has also been described, and, similar to Budd-Chiari syndrome, may present with liver dysfunction. Resection of such membranes can be performed using cardiopulmonary bypass.

Rarely, the IVC may be completely absent, and the venous return from the lower body is through small paravertebral venous channels that communicate through the azygos systems.

Pulmonary Vein Connection to the Systemic Veins

Anomalous connection of a portion or all of the pulmonary veins to either the superior or inferior caval systems may occur. Other than enlargement from increased flow, the systemic vein anatomy and connections are usually normal in this circumstance. The subject is addressed in Chapter 93.

Total Anomalous Systemic Venous Connection

There are reports of patients with absence of both the right superior and infrahepatic caval veins with azygos continuation to a left SVC and then to the left atrium. Surgical considerations pertain to separation of the pulmonary venous and systemic venous drainage. It is postulated that most of these patients have some form of lateralization abnormality.

Anomalies of the Coronary Sinus

The coronary sinus receives venous blood from the cardiac veins and is usually the major venous pathway of the coronary circulation. A minor group of cardiac veins (venae cordis minimae) provides a variable degree of additional drainage directly into the cardiac chambers, predominantly the right atrium. The anterior cardiac vein drains directly into the right atrium, and the recognizable thebesian foramina provide outlets for either the minor cardiac veins or the sinusoidal systems of the heart with their drainage into the right atrium and, to some extent, into the right ventricle. Because of these alternative pathways, long-standing (slow onset) obstruction of the coronary sinus or absence of the coronary sinus, most frequently seen in right isomerism, is well tolerated without impairment of the coronary circulation.

Whereas the phenomenon of "unroofing" (partial or complete absence of the common wall between the left atrium and the coronary sinus) of the coronary sinus is found more commonly in patients with a left SVC draining via the coronary sinus, it may also occur in situations of a solitary (normal) right SVC and, in either circumstance,

provides an interatrial communication by means of the coronary sinus (coronary sinus atrial septal defect).

The coronary sinus may be entirely absent in an otherwise normal heart, although this is quite unusual. More commonly, the coronary sinus is absent in the lateralization abnormalities, most frequently with right isomerism. In addition, the coronary sinus may be small and underdeveloped with the predominance of the venous drainage of the coronary system through the minor venous channels directly into the right atrium and right ventricle.

Although stenosis or hypoplasia and agenesis of the coronary sinus are well tolerated as a developmental anomaly, acute closure or narrowing of the structure with a sudden rise in cardiac venous pressure is associated with myocardial edema and may be implicated in myocardial dysfunction. It has, however, been difficult to document whether the lateral tunnel approach to the Fontan procedure, which leaves the coronary sinus draining into the lower-pressure atrium, carries any functional benefit. Narrowing or obstruction of the coronary sinus should be guarded against, and preferably one should avoid leaving the coronary sinus in an acutely increased venous pressure situation such as the classic right atrium-to-pulmonary artery connection with the Fontan procedure.

Coronary sinus diverticula and aneurysms have also been described. They are often associated with accessory atrio-

ventricular pathways and consequently with arrhythmias.

The most important anomaly of the coronary sinus is related to its enlargement because of flow increases caused by a left SVC connection or by an anomalous pulmonary venous connection. The latter is addressed in Chapter 93 as one form of anomalous pulmonary venous return. The dilated coronary sinus should alert the surgeon to these possibilities.

Anomalies of the Valves of the Venous Sinus

A consideration of the morphogenesis of the valves of the sinus venosus is fundamental to the understanding of atrial anatomy and the systemic and pulmonary venous connections to the atrial mass. Involution of the right venous valve leaves remnants we recognize as the thebesian and eustachian valves, guarding the coronary sinus and the IVC, respectively. Failure of various degrees of the involution process may leave harmless remnants we recognize as a Chiari network in the right atrium or may produce a fully developed membrane that partitions the systemic atrium and may severely restrict the fetal development of the right heart structures because of its consequences for venous flow patterns in the right atrium.

Persistence of the right venous valve of the sinus venosus to form a variously

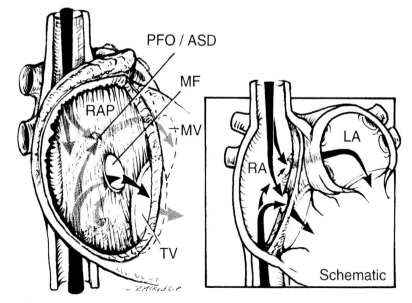

Figure 72-6. Persistence of the right atrial venous valve (cor triatriatum dexter). (ASD = atrial septal defect; LA = left atrium; MF = membrane fenestration; MV = mitral valve; PFO = patent foramen ovale; RA = right atrium; RAP = right atrial partition [persistent venous valve]; TV = tricuspid valve.)

fenestrated right atrial partition (cor triatriatum dexter) divides the atrium into a venous portion, which receives the systemic veins and coronary sinus and communicates with the left atrium through a patent foramen ovale or atrial septal defect, and a trabeculated portion, which communicates with the right atrioventricular valve (Fig. 72-6). Seriously restrictive partitions are usually associated with and are considered one cause of tricuspid stenosis or hypoplasia, right ventricular hypoplasia, or pulmonary stenosis or atresia.

An interesting and more benign and treatable form of persistence of the right valve of the sinus venosus is the occasional windsock-shaped fibrous structure that attaches in a parachute-like fashion to the former attachment points of the right venous valve along the terminal crest and the eustachian and thebesian valves. This windsock structure may, during ventricular diastole, be filled with blood and travel through the tricuspid valve into the right ventricle and even out the right ventricular outflow tract and through the pulmonary valve. It may be confused with an abnormality of the tricuspid valve, a possible vegetation of a structure of the right side of the heart, or a pedunculated right atrial tumor. We have resected three of these interesting lesions, each of which occurred without associated cardiac abnormalities other than patent foramen ovale. They provide interesting echocardiographic findings for the cardiologist, and may produce long-term problems with trauma to the tricuspid or pulmonary valves. It has been speculated that they may cause arrhythmias because of their movement throughout the right heart system in addition to progressive interference with systemic venous return and may be associated with thrombus formation. These structures should be removed when identified.

SUGGESTED READINGS

Fischer DR, Zuberbuhler JR. Anomalous Systemic Venous Return. In Anderson RH, McCartney FJ, Shinebourne EA, Tynan M (eds), Paediatric Cardiology (Vol 1). Edinburgh: Churchill Livingstone, 1987;497.

Freedom RM, Benson LN. Anomalies of Systemic Venous Connections, Persistence of the Right Venous Valve and Silent Cardiovascular Causes of Cyanosis. In Freedom RM, Benson LN, Smallhorn JF (eds), Neonatal Heart Disease. London: Springer, 1992;485.

Gatzoulis MA, Shinebourne EA, Redington AN, et al. Increasing cyanosis early after cavopulmonary connection caused by abnormal systemic venous channels. Br Heart J 1995;73:182.

Geva T, Van Praagh S. Abnormal Systemic Venous Connections. In Allen HD, Gutgesell HP, Clark EB, et al. (eds), Moss and Adams' Heart Disease in Infants, Children, and Adolescents (6th ed). Philadelphia: Lippincott, Williams, & Wilkins, 2001;773.

Ho SY, Cook A, Anderson RH, et al. Isomerism of the atrial appendages in the fetus. Pediatr Pathol 1991;11:589.

Nsah EN, Moore GW, Hutchins GM. Pathogenesis of persistent left superior vena cava with a coronary sinus connection. Pediatr Pathol 1991;11:261.

Rubino M, Van Praagh S, Kadoba K, et al. Systemic and pulmonary venous connections in visceral heterotaxy with asplenia. J Thorac Cardiovasc Surg 1995;110:641.

Slavik Z, Lamb RK, Webber SA, et al. A rare cause of profound cyanosis after Kawashima modification of bidirectional cavopulmonary anastomosis. Ann Thorac Surg 1995;60:435.

EDITOR'S COMMENTS

Anomalies of systemic venous return to the heart are often ignored in texts on congenital heart abnormalities. Although the majority of systemic venous return abnormalities are of no particular physiologic consequence, an understanding of venous anatomy and development and the variations of venous connections to the heart is critically important for congenital cardiovascular surgery in which cavopulmonary anastomoses and separation of pulmonary and systemic venous return are required, as in the Fontan operation.

As noted in the chapter, the most common venous anomaly is a left SVC that drains through the coronary sinus into the systemic venous atrium. This venous anomaly, although physiologically unimportant, can have significant consequences if unrecognized at the time of cardiac operation. Although it is possible to snare the left SVC temporarily, we have preferred not to snare an undrained left SVC in most patients, and would utilize circulatory arrest at the time of cardiac repair in most lesions short of simple ASD closure if the presence of a left-sided vena cava draining to the coronary sinus is known. Although presence of a left SVC entering the coronary sinus was thought to complicate cardiac transplantation, in fact, the vein can be left in situ and cardiac transplantation performed in the usual fashion with only minor modification, as described in Chapter 95 on pediatric cardiac transplantation. One problem we have seen on occasion

with a left SVC entering the coronary sinus in patients who have elevations of right atrial pressure and pulmonary hypertension is the presence of a dilated coronary sinus, which can impinge on the wall of the left atrium and create what appears echocardiographically and functionally to be a cor triatriatum with limitation of free flow from the pulmonary venous confluence across the mitral valve. This abnormality has on occasion resulted in exploration of the left atrium at the time of cardiac repair without finding any abnormality of the left atrium. The coronary sinus, when decompressed on bypass with the heart under cardioplegic arrest, eliminates the ridge seen on echocardiography, and the defect can be quite obscure.

As is apparent from the summary presented in this chapter, knowledge of the possible venous connections to the heart and recognition that the venous drainage must be identified at the time of atrial repairs and cavopulmonary connections are important for the management of children with congenital heart disease. Minor unrecognized systemic venous connections after cavopulmonary anastomoses can create decompression of the SVC and result in significant arterial desaturation. Thus, in patients with cavopulmonary anastomoses in whom significant desaturation is noted postoperatively, a search in the catheterization laboratory for other systemic venous pathways to the atrium should be undertaken and coil embolization performed to eliminate these decompressing channels. In spite of the theoretical need to ligate the azygos vein in patients who undergo SVC anastomosis for a hemi-Fontan procedure for single ventricle, we have found in many patients that the azygos vein can be left open without producing significant desaturation despite relative elevation of superior vena caval pressures. Thus, it would appear that development of significant systemic venous collaterals to the left or right atrium in patients with cavopulmonary anastomoses is likely related to elevated resistance to pulmonary blood flow.

The authors noted that there are often abnormalities of the coronary sinus drainage in patients with lateralization abnormalities. On occasion the absence of the coronary sinus can be associated with direct drainage of the major cardiac veins into the right atrium from the epicardial surface. In these situations, care must be taken not to divide these veins when performing a right atriotomy for access to the intracardiac lesions. Often these patients have associated left juxtaposition of the atrial appendages, which makes the right atrial wall smaller than normal and limits access to the right side of the heart.

Perhaps the major surgical issue with anomalies of systemic venous return is the situation of a left superior vena cava that enters the left atrium directly. In these cases it may be difficult to reconnect the left superior vena cava to the right atrial chamber. Various techniques have been described including detachment of the left superior vena cava and anastomosis to the right superior vena cava, recreating an innominate vein. Often, however, the size of the great arteries and space limitations in the superior mediastinum prevent there being enough length for this reconstruction to be accomplished without tension. Other approaches have involved detaching the left superior vena cava and reattaching it to the dome of the right atrium if there is not compression by the pulmonary artery or aorta. In some cases it may be possible to create an intra-atrial baffle that redirects the flow from the superior vena cava as it enters the roof of the left atrium over to the right side of the heart. In situations where there is left juxtaposition of the atrial appendages, we have found it useful to divide the left superior vena cava and then anastomose it to the appendage of the right atrium, which is now on the left side, adjacent to the left superior vena cava. In situations where the left superior vena cava cannot reach the right-sided structures adequately, there have been reports of ligation of the left superior vena cava without serious sequelae, although at least transient left facial and arm edema is often present and chylothorax may be a problem. In situations of single ventricle or if the pulmonary artery pressure is expected to be low, another alternative is to perform a left bidirectional Glenn shunt, which allows the left superior vena caval flow to go directly to the pulmonary arteries.

T.L.S.

73

Patent Ductus Arteriosus

Redmond P. Burke

Anatomic Considerations

Persistence of the fetal ductus arteriosus, a common, straightforward, completely repairable cardiac lesion, presents a rather difficult therapeutic dilemma. Options include open division or ligation via left thoracotomy or sternotomy, transcatheter device occlusion, and ligation via video-assisted thoracoscopic surgery (VATS). Open division represents the gold standard, with almost 50 years of experience to support this technique. Direct anatomic control and visualization minimize the risk of hemorrhage, and ductal division eliminates concern about residual ductal patency.

The advent of minimally traumatic transcatheter device closure 25 years ago compelled surgeons to refine their technique. To decrease the chest wall trauma of thoracotomy, incision length was reduced, and muscle-sparing incisions were devised. These maneuvers negate some of the advantages of the open technique by reducing operative exposure and hampering instrument manipulation. Despite these modifications in thoracotomy technique, rib retraction could not be avoided, and chest wall pain and scoliosis remained as significant long-term sequelae.

Transcatheter device development was slow and erratic until the advent of coil occlusion, which is now being used extensively by interventional cardiologists. To avoid chest wall trauma, a different set of complications related to catheterization are introduced: catheter injury to the femoral vessels, device embolization, obstruction of the left pulmonary artery, endarteritis related to an intravascular foreign body, and exposure to fluoroscopic radiation.

VATS for congenital heart disease was a natural evolution of endoscopic techniques gaining favor in adult general and thoracic surgery to minimize surgical trauma. Access to the pleural space is achieved through small thoracostomies, visualization is acquired with a magnifying video camera, and dissection is performed with endoscopic tools. This technique allows ductal closure with minimal chest wall trauma without introducing the uncertainties associated with the intravascular devices. The loss of direct vascular control must be acknowledged, and rapid conversion to thoracotomy constitutes a fallback option during each procedure. Familiarity with the nuances of the open approach, particularly in difficult circumstances, remains essential.

Diagnostic Considerations and Indications for the Procedure

Patent ductus arteriosus (PDA) may present as a murmur in an asymptomatic infant or as congestive heart failure in a premature newborn. Echocardiography confirms ductal patency while ruling out concurrent intracardiac lesions, arch anomalies, left pulmonary artery stenosis, and aortic coarctation. Failure of indomethacin therapy in a premature newborn with a patent ductus constitutes an indication for surgery. Spontaneous closure in term infants is rare after the first few months of life, and the duct should be closed. Patients with large ducts and pulmonary hypertension have an obvious need for closure. The long-term risk of bacterial endocarditis with an audible patent duct mandates closure; however, the risk in patients with a silent, echocardiographically diagnosed ductus is unclear and remains open to individual assessment.

There are no contraindications related to patient size or hemodynamic condition for open or endoscopic ductal closure. This is an important distinction from transcatheter procedures, which are not appropriate in small newborns (<5 kg), where femoral vessel size is prohibitive for catheter placement, or in patients with large ducts (>4 mm in diameter), where devices tend to embolize and larger coils (which can obstruct the left pulmonary artery) must be used. Endoscopic closure is easily performed in premature newborns. Although the overall incision length may not be much less than with an open procedure, rib retraction is avoided. This retraction is usually considerable during an open procedure and may produce significant long-term chest wall effects. Contraindications to the endoscopic approach include calcified ducts, which should not be clipped, given the risk of laceration and bleeding; ducts of >1 cm in diameter, greater than the span of a large vascular clip; and patients with dense pleural adhesions from infection or prior surgery. These patients should be considered for transcatheter occlusion or open division.

Perioperative Patient Management

Term infants are usually admitted the day of surgery. General anesthesia is established with a single-lumen endotracheal tube. Oxygen saturation and end-tidal carbon dioxide levels are monitored.

Premature newborns who are not on an oscillating ventilator are transferred to the operating room for endoscopic patent ductus arteriosus interruption; temperature and oxygen saturation are monitored. End-tidal carbon dioxide assessment is unreliable in small patients, and arterial blood gas monitoring is used selectively. Patients requiring an oscillating ventilator undergo open duct interruption via thoracotomy in the neonatal intensive care unit.

Operative Technique (Exposure)

Video-assisted thoracoscopic PDA ligation is performed with the patient in a right lateral decubitus position (Fig. 73-1). A transesophageal echocardiographic probe is advanced into the esophagus, and the anatomy is confirmed. The left chest is prepared as for a posterolateral thoracotomy, and four thoracostomy incisions are made (Fig. 73-2). The incisions are made with a No. 15 blade and cauterized to prevent bleeding. Blunt dissection with a curved hemostat allows entry into the pleural space, and four trocars are placed to facilitate instrument insertion. The medial port admits the grasping forceps, the next port admits the expanding lung retractor, and the next is for the videoscope

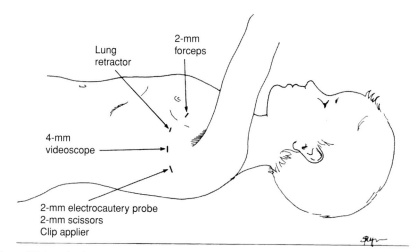

Figure 73-2. The four thoracostomy incisions for endoscopic interruption of a patent ductus.

(4-mm, 30-degree face angle for infants and 2.7-mm, 30-degree angle for premature infants). The posterior incision admits the cautery and the clip applier. The camera is advanced first as the anesthesiologist limits the ventilation to allow the lung to fall away from the chest wall. A cotton swab is advanced through the posterior incision to further push the lung away from the chest wall and to create a space for the lung retractor, which is advanced until it can be seen by the videoscope. The retractor is then opened under direct vision in the chest, and the left upper lobe is retracted medially and inferiorly (Fig. 73-3). The superior segment of the left lower lobe may overlie the duct and can be captured by the lower limb of the retractor to hold it out of the way. The scope is advanced farther into the pleural space using the left subclavian artery as a landmark for the origin of the ductus, which is just distal to it. The left-handed grasper and right-handed cautery probe are used to elevate the pleura over the duct and create a pleural flap (Fig. 73-4). The vagus and recurrent laryngeal nerves are easily seen. Tissue is lifted away from the aorta before the cautery is activated. When the pleural flap is thick with fatty tissue or lymphatics, it can be retracted by inserting a hook retractor through a small puncture wound between the medial two thoracostomies. Carrying the pleural flap up to the take-off of the left subclavian improves exposure (Fig. 73-5). Lymphatics at the upper end of the pleural dissection must be carefully sealed with the cautery. The lower duct angle is dissected with blunt and cautery dissection, with care being taken to avoid the recurrent nerve. The upper angle is opened with sharp dissection to create a plane; development of the plane is then continued with blunt spreading dissection. Once the upper and lower angles are free, the duct is sized by juxtaposing a cotton swab (Fig. 73-6). The appropriate-sized clip applier is advanced through the posterior incision using the grasper to clear first the lower and then the upper angle. The clip applier should fall easily into place (Fig. 73-7). When resistance is felt, usually posteriorly, the back wall of the duct should be further separated from the underlying esophagus with blunt dissection. The clip is

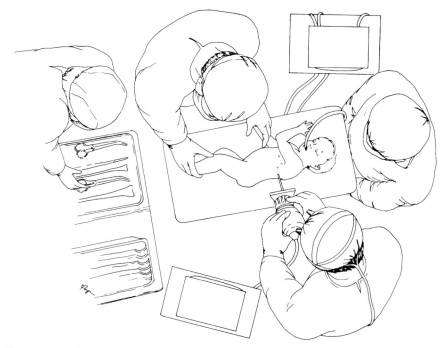

Figure 73-1. The operative setup for video-assisted thoracoscopic interruption of a patent ductus arteriosus.

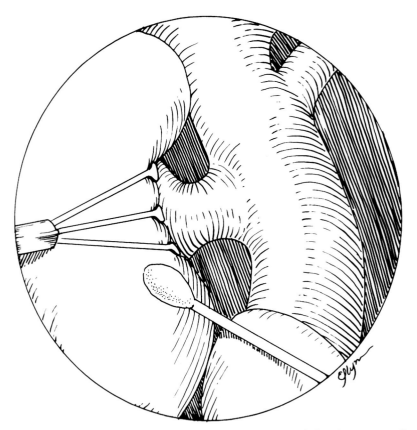

Figure 73-3. Endoscopic view as the left upper lobe is retracted medially using an expanding retractor. A cotton swab is used to manipulate the lung into position.

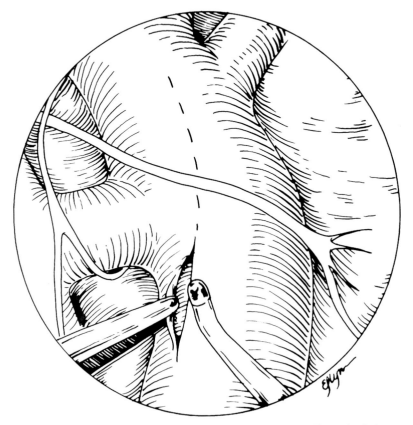

Figure 73-4. The left subclavian artery take-off is used for orientation. The parietal pleura overlying the duct is incised with the cautery. The crossing vein is usually divided.

placed around the duct, and ductal closure is confirmed by simultaneous intraoperative transesophageal echocardiography. Patency of the left pulmonary artery and aorta is ensured. The pleural edges are cauterized to prevent chylous leak, and the instruments are removed, with care being taken to avoid scissoring the lung when closing the retractor. A 12-F thoracostomy tube is advanced through the retractor port, and the individual incisions are closed with subcuticular absorbable sutures. The thoracostomy tube is removed in the operating room. Infants are awakened and extubated in the operating room, and premature newborns are returned to the neonatal intensive care unit.

Conventional exposure is required for duct division in patients with large ducts, calcified ducts, or bleeding during an endoscopic procedure. With the patient in a right lateral decubitus position, a posterolateral thoracotomy incision is made, preserving the latissimus and serratus anterior muscles. During conversion from an endoscopic VATS procedure, the individual thoracostomy incisions are connected to create the thoracotomy. The fourth interspace is entered by detaching the intercostal muscle from the superior rib margin and sharply incising the parietal pleura. The ribs are retracted, and two malleable retractors are used to control the left upper lobe and the superior segment of the left lower lobe (Fig. 73-8). With the take-off of the left subclavian artery used for orientation, the parietal pleura is opened. Pleural retraction sutures are used to expose the duct. The crossing vein is divided when it obscures dissection of the upper duct angle. The upper and lower angles are dissected, with care being taken to avoid cautery near the recurrent nerve as it sweeps under the duct. The posterior margin is freed with a blunt right-angle clamp. Large ducts whose caliber matches the aorta, should be clamped proximally and distally with duct clamps. The duct is then divided; each end is oversewn with running monofilament suture.

Duct division or ligation via median sternotomy requires dissection of the plane between the aorta and main pulmonary artery, which is often vascular in cyanotic patients. The right pulmonary artery origin orients the dissection, and the adventitial plane just superior to this is developed; the dissection is carried under the ductus. The pericardium over the left pulmonary artery is opened to allow dissection in the angle between the duct and the left pulmonary artery. Freeing the ductus posteriorly with a right-angled clamp allows sutures to be passed.

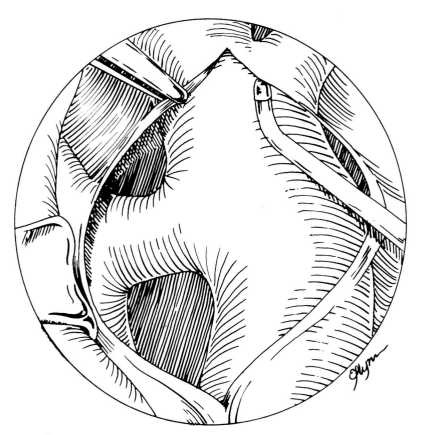

Figure 73-5.   The pleural incision is carried up to the subclavian take-off.

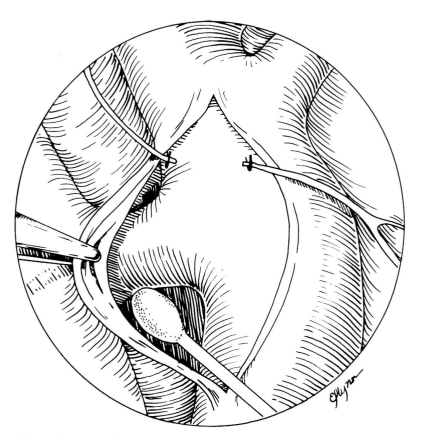

Figure 73-6.   A cotton swab may be used to bluntly dissect the posterior ductal attachments, avoiding injury to the recurrent nerve.

The sutures are secured to the adventitia proximally and distally to maintain separation (Fig. 73-8). Sutures are tied with minimal retraction on the main pulmonary artery to avoid suture cut through, and the duct is divided with tenotomy scissors. Clamping and oversewing the aortic and pulmonary ends may be necessary when the ductus is short. Precise suture placement at the left pulmonary artery origin minimizes the risk of proximal stenosis. Arterial bleeding at the completion of complex intracardiac repairs can often be traced back to the proximal or distal duct division because the ductal tissue is often friable, particularly in cyanotic patients on prostaglandins.

Surgical Complications and Postoperative Care

Remote-access surgery amplifies the risk of bleeding by introducing a delay before direct vascular control can be achieved. Secure intravenous access and prior preparation for rapid thoracotomy are necessary precautions allowing prompt response in the event of hemorrhage. As with open division, the greatest risk exists while the posterior duct wall is being dissected, which should be minimized, and while the vascular clips are being applied. Pediatric patients with esophageal reflux, notably Down syndrome patients, often have dense inflammatory adhesions between the esophagus and aorta in the area of the duct that require precise cautery dissection to avoid bleeding. In the event of hemorrhage, prompt thoracotomy allows entry into the pericardial space to control the left pulmonary artery. Proximal and distal aortic clamping allows time for volume infusion and arterial repair in a clear field.

Open and endoscopic ductal interruptions by sutures or vascular clips introduce the possibility of persistent ductal patency or recanalization. Intraoperative transesophageal echocardiographic confirmation of complete ductal closure can minimize but not eliminate this risk. Persistent flow detected in the operating room during the VATS procedure is usually caused by incomplete duct dissection and failure of the clip to completely encircle the duct wall. Further dissection posteriorly, separating the esophagus from the aortic wall behind the duct, may allow deeper placement of a second clip to complete the closure. Patients with persistent flow detected in the operating room or in the immediate postoperative period should undergo immediate

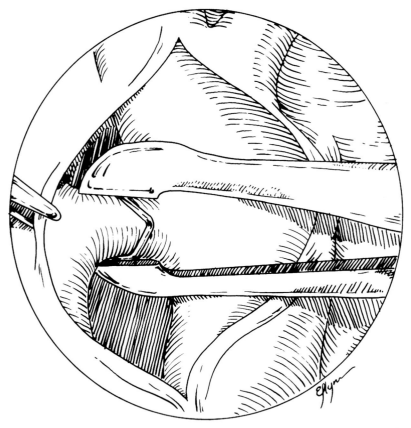

Figure 73-7. The endoscopic clip applier is advanced around the duct while countertraction is maintained with the grasping forceps.

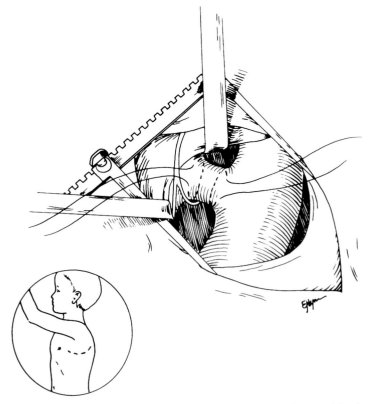

Figure 73-8. To convert to an open procedure, the thoracostomy incisions are joined, and the fourth interspace is entered. Malleable retractors are used for exposure, and proximal and distal sutures are placed.

re-exploration, either endoscopic or open, while the pleural space is clear to complete ductal closure by further ligation or, preferably, division and oversewing.

True ductal aneurysm, related to endocarditis, and false aneurysm, seen with ductal division and oversewing when the pulmonary arterial wall delaminates, are best approached via median sternotomy (when the left pleural space is scarred) or thoracotomy using cardiopulmonary bypass.

Accidental ligation of the aorta or left pulmonary artery has been described in patients with an anatomic optical illusion in which a large ductus overlies, and appears to be, the aortic arch. The recurrent nerve may contribute to the illusion, and in uncertain cases, each element of the aortic arch should be identified and dissected before ductal ligation.

Chylothorax may occur when lymphatics crossing the parietal pleura overlying the duct and in the periaortic adventitia are divided. Several large lymphatics are encountered at the take-off of the left subclavian artery. Risk is increased in patients with recent upper respiratory infections when lymphatics are engorged and more difficult to seal completely with electrocautery. These patients may benefit from pleural reapproximation by continuous suture. When detected early, chylothorax can be directly corrected by returning to the operating room and exploring the left pleural space endoscopically. Leaking lymphatics are readily identified and can be controlled with cautery or vascular clips, obviating the need for prolonged hospitalization and dietary manipulations.

Avoiding recurrent nerve injury is a technical challenge, demanding precise and gentle dissection. Cautery near the nerve is particularly hazardous, making scissors or blunt dissection preferable around the lower ductal angle. Clamp placement during open division and clip placement during open or endoscopic ligation must avoid the nerve, particularly posteriorly. Clip placement parallel to the aorta may minimize the risk of nerve injury.

Elective patients are extubated in the operating room and transferred to the recovery room and then the surgical ward. After a minimally invasive procedure, they advance to regular diet and activity by evening and are prepared for discharge the next morning. A chest film is obtained before discharge to detect pneumothorax and chylothorax, and a follow-up echocardiogram is performed at 1 month to ensure persistent ductal closure.

SUGGESTED READING

Castaneda AR. Patent ductus arteriosus: a commentary. Ann Thorac Surg 1981;31:92.

Fan LL, Campbell DN, Clarke DR, et al. Paralyzed left vocal cord associated with ligation of patent ductus arteriosus. J Thorac Cardiovasc Surg 1989;98:611.

Gray DT, Fyer DC, Walker AM. Clinical outcomes and costs of transcatheter as compared with surgical closure of patent ductus arteriosus. N Engl J Med 1993;329:1515.

Gross RE, Hummard JP. Surgical ligation of a patent ductus arteriosus: report of first successful case. JAMA 1939;112:729.

Laborde F, Noirhomme P, Karam J, et al. A new video-assisted thoracoscopic surgical technique for interruption of patent ductus arteriosus in infants and children. J Thorac Cardiovasc Surg 1993;105:278.

Panagopoulos PG, Tatooles CJ, Aberdeen E, et al. Patent ductus arteriosus in infants and children. Thorax 1971;26:137.

Pontius RG, Danielson GK, Noonan JA, Judson JP. Illusions leading to surgical closure of the distal left pulmonary artery instead of the ductus arteriosus. J Thorac Cardiovasc Surg 1981;82:107.

Wagner HR, Ellison RC, Zierler S, et al. Surgical closure of patent ductus arteriosus in 268 preterm infants. J Thorac Cardiovasc Surg 1984;87:870.

EDITOR'S COMMENTS

Because the ductus arteriosus is a normal fetal structure representing the left sixth aortic arch, persistent patency of the ductus arteriosus is one of the most common congenital heart defects. Ductal patency seems to be more common in girls, and persistent ductal patency occurs in approximately 1 in 2,000 term births. In premature infants, ductal patency is common. By 1 year of age, only about 1% of ducts remain open, and after 1 year of age, <1%/year spontaneously close. Thus, persistent patency of the ductus arteriosus at 6 months to 1 year of age is generally considered an indication for ductal closure. Certainly ducts that are large, producing significant left-to-right shunts with congestive heart failure symptoms, should be closed promptly.

As discussed in this chapter, the approach to ductal closure remains controversial. Although the incidence of endarteritis associated with ductus arteriosus is low, the occurrence of this problem even in clinically silent ducts (D Balzer, TL Spray, CE Cantor, AW Strauss. Endarteritis associated with a clinically silent patent ductus arteriosus. Am Heart J 1993;125:1192) suggests that ductal closure should be effected in all patients including those with a clinically silent duct.

Coil occlusion techniques are being used increasingly for ductal closure and have the advantage of avoiding chest incisions and direct dissection of the ductus with attendant risks of recurrent nerve injury or bleeding; however, these techniques are limited somewhat by vascular access in very small children, and in very large ducts, coils may embolize or be difficult to place without protruding into the pulmonary artery or aorta. In addition, an inadequately closed ductus with a metallic foreign body and the attendant potential risk of late endarteritis remain a concern with this technique. If, however, complete ductal closure can be effected with coil occlusion, there appears to be no disadvantage to this approach. Certainly adults with calcified ducts have a significant enough risk from operative intervention that transcatheter occlusion should be considered primary treatment if at all possible. In older patients, the incisions for thoracoscopy closure or routine thoracotomy closure are relatively large and the morbidity higher, and therefore transcatheter closure should be considered.

Surgical closure of the ductus arteriosus with clips or simple ligatures has been associated with recanalization rates as high as 20% to 25% in some series (KE Sorenson, BO Kristensen, OK Hansen. Frequency of occurrence of residual ductal flow after surgical ligation by color flow mapping. J Am Coll Cardiol 1991;67:653). Therefore, despite documented complete closure after thoracoscopic ductal ligation with clips, recanalization must be considered a relative risk. Certainly the gold standard for ductal occlusion with the lowest incidence of recanalization is ductal division, although the technical aspects of ductal division require larger incisions and far more complete control of the vessel before division. Longer follow-up on the use of transcatheter occluder devices and clip ligation with the thoracoscopic technique should address the issue of late recanalization and residual patency before these techniques completely supplant open division, especially for the significant-sized ductus arteriosus.

Ligation of the ductus arteriosus through a median sternotomy incision is relatively simple, although it is very important to identify the origin of the duct just beyond the take-off of the right pulmonary artery and to adequately dissect the groove between the ductus and the left pulmonary artery before the duct is mobilized for ligation.

T.L.S.

74

Vascular Rings, Slings, and Other Arch Anomalies

Erle H. Austin III and Minoo N. Kavarana

Historical Aspects

Recognition of anomalies of the aortic arch and pulmonary artery began in 1737 when Hommel first described a double aortic arch. Fifty-seven years later, Bayford discovered an aberrant retroesophageal subclavian artery in a patient with a history of dysphagia. He called the anomaly a "lusus naturae," or "prank of nature," and coined the term "dysphagia lusoria" to describe the symptoms. The first surgical correction of a double aortic arch was performed by Gross in 1945 on a 1-year-old boy with chronic wheezing. The pulmonary arterial sling anomaly was described by Glaevecke and Doehle in 1897 and was first repaired by arterial division with reimplantation by Potts in 1954.

Embryology

By 5 weeks of fetal development, the primordial heart tubes have fused and six aortic (branchial) arches have formed between the ventral roots and dorsal aortae (Fig. 74-1). Migration and involution of the arches results in the complex system of the higher mammal. During normal development, persistence of the left fourth aortic arch forms the arch of the aorta and proximal left subclavian artery. The right fourth aortic arch forms the innominate and right subclavian arteries. Involution of the distal right aorta results in an unpaired single aortic arch. Table 74-1 shows the fate of the remaining arches.

Failure of involution or migration of specific segments of the aortic arches results in anomalies that may form partial or complete vascular rings about the trachea and

esophagus. The most common of these are diagrammed in Fig. 74-2.

Pulmonary artery development arises from two separate vascular sources: (1) the lung buds deriving their blood supply from the splanchnic plexus and (2) the proximal left and right sixth aortic arches (Fig. 74-3). Figure 74-4 demonstrates how abnormal migration of the separate blood supplies can result in dislocation of the left pulmonary artery posterior to the trachea, resulting in the pulmonary artery sling anomaly with its associated tracheal compression.

Classification and Incidence

Aortic arch anomalies producing tracheoesophageal constriction account for 1% to 2% of all congenital heart defects. A simple and commonly used system of classifying these vascular anomalies is given in Table 74-2. The relative prevalence of these lesions in surgical series is also indicated.

Group I: Complete Vascular Rings

Anatomy

A double aortic arch (type IA) occurs when the right dorsal aorta fails to involute (Fig. 74-2), resulting in persistence of the right and left fourth aortic arches. The right aortic arch is most commonly dominant. The descending aorta is usually in its normal position on the left, as is the ligamentum arteriosum (or patent ductus arteriosus). Generally, each subclavian and common carotid artery arises independently from its respective aortic arch. The innominate vessels do

not develop. Twenty percent of cases have other cardiac anomalies, with ventricular septal defect and tetralogy of Fallot being most common.

Type IB vascular rings (right aortic arch with retroesophageal ligamentum arteriosum) account for 45% of complete vascular rings. The majority of these defects have left descending aortas. A right aortic arch with retroesophageal left subclavian artery and ligamentum results from abnormal involution of the left fourth arch. A remnant or stump of the left fourth arch (Kommerell's diverticulum) may persist. The left subclavian artery arises aberrantly behind the esophagus from the right-sided arch or from Kommerell's diverticulum. Near this point the left-sided ligamentum emanates and joins the left pulmonary artery to create a complete ring about the trachea and esophagus.

A right aortic arch may occur with mirror image branching with the left innominate artery arising anteriorly and dividing into the left carotid and subclavian arteries. If the ligamentum arteriosum occurs between the left innominate artery and the left pulmonary artery, as is commonly seen in association with tetralogy of Fallot, there is no vascular ring. Therefore, these patients are usually asymptomatic. However, when the ligamentum arises from the aorta behind the esophagus and connects with the left pulmonary artery, a compressive vascular ring is formed.

A rare variant among vascular rings is the cervical aortic arch, in which case the arch exists in the neck above the clavicle, sometimes as high as the C2 vertebral body. There are two main subtypes. The first and the larger group are type IB anomalies with a right-sided arch, an anomalous left subclavian artery, and a retroesophageal

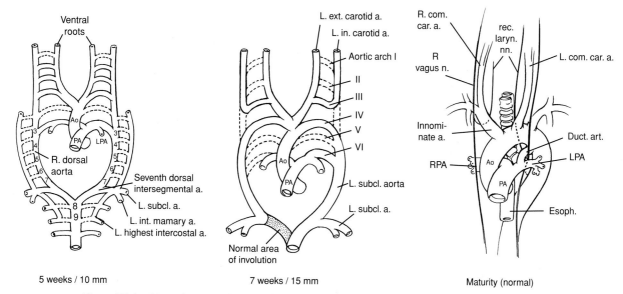

Figure 74-1. Normal aortic arch development. The normal aortic arch arises from the persistence of the left fourth embryologic arch. Note that the recurrent laryngeal nerve recurs about the derivative of the sixth embryologic arch on the left, that is, the ductus arteriosus, and the derivative of the fourth embryologic arch on the right, that is, the right subclavian artery. This occurs because of the normal involution of the right sixth embryologic arch. (a. = artery; Ao = aorta; car. = carotid; com. = common; Duct. art. = ductus arteriosus; Esoph. = esophagus; ext. = external; int. = internal; LPA = left pulmonary artery; L. = left; n. = nerve; PA = pulmonary artery; R. = right; Rec. laryn. nn. = recurrent laryngeal nerves; RPA = right pulmonary artery; subcl. = subclavian.)

ligamentum arteriosum. The second group has a left-sided arch with a normal branching pattern and thus does not form a complete ring. These anomalies are thought to result from a failure of the normal descent of the aortic arch from its cephalic location at 3 weeks to its intrathoracic location at 7 weeks of gestation.

Clinical Presentation

The clinical presentation of vascular rings can vary from mild dyspnea or dysphagia to respiratory distress and apnea. Signs and symptoms often depend on the type of anomaly.

A double aortic arch produces the earliest and most severe symptoms as a result of the presence of a tight ring around the trachea and esophagus. Seventy-five percent of affected patients develop symptoms by 1 year of age, often within the first month of life and rarely after 6 months of age. Stridor, a nonproductive cough, or a hoarse cry may be noted soon after birth. The stridor generally worsens with feedings, especially solid foods. The cough is characterized as a "seal bark" or "brassy cough." Respiratory distress can lead to choking, cyanosis, and apnea. Vomiting may precede or follow choking. Despite the esophageal compression, most infants with double aortic arch tolerate liquids well and appear well fed.

Table 74-1   Outcome of the Embryonic Aortic Arches

Embryonic Vessel	Outcome
1. Truncus arteriosus	Proximal ascending aorta and pulmonary root
2. Aortic sac	Distal ascending aorta, brachiocephalic artery, and arch up to origin of the left common carotid artery
3. First arch	Portions of the maxillary artery
4. Second arch	Portions of the stapedial artery
5. Third arch	Common carotid artery and proximal internal carotid artery
6. Fourth arch	
Right	Proximal right subclavian artery
Left	Aortic arch segment between the left common carotid and left subclavian arteries
7. Fifth arch	No known derivations
8. Sixth arch	
Right	Proximal part becomes proximal segment of the right pulmonary artery; distal portion involutes
Left	Proximal part becomes proximal segment of the left pulmonary artery; distal portion becomes ductus arteriosus
9. Right dorsal aorta	Cranial portion becomes right subclavian artery distal to contribution from right fourth arch; distal portion involutes
10. Left dorsal aorta	Aortic arch distal to left subclavian artery
11. Right seventh intersegmental artery	Distal right subclavian artery
12. Left seventh intersegmental artery	Left subclavian artery

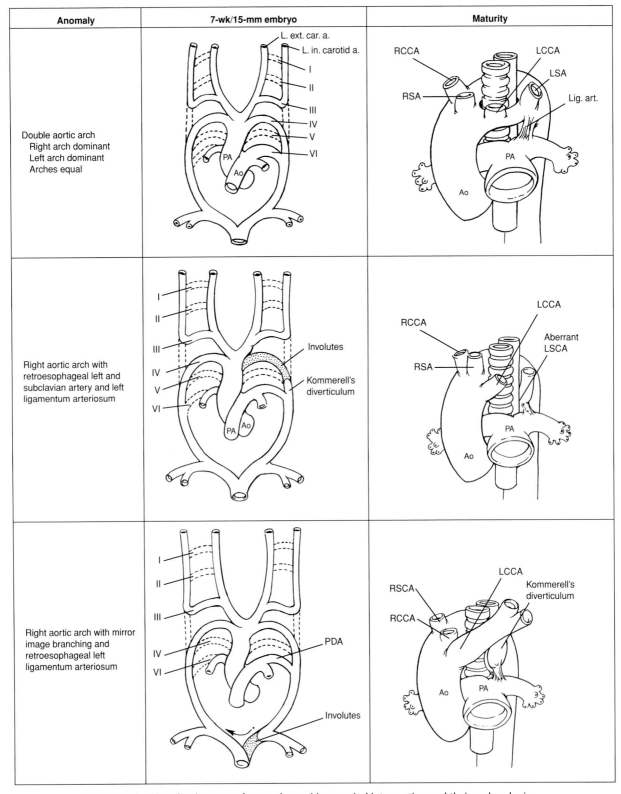

Anomaly	7-wk/15-mm embryo	Maturity

Figure 74-2.   Vascular rings most frequently requiring surgical intervention and their embryologic development. Kommerell's diverticulum is a remnant of the involuted left fourth aortic arch, which may be the origin of the ductus (ligamentum), the left subclavian artery (LSA), or both. (a. = artery; Ao = aorta; L. ext. car. a. = left external carotid artery; L. int. carotid. a. = left internal carotid artery; LCCA = left common carotid artery; Lig. art. = ligamentum arteriosum; LSA, LSCA = left subclavian artery; PA = pulmonary artery; PDA = patent ductus arteriosus; RCCA = right common carotid artery; RSA, RSCA = right subclavian artery; roman numerals refer to embryologic aortic arches.)

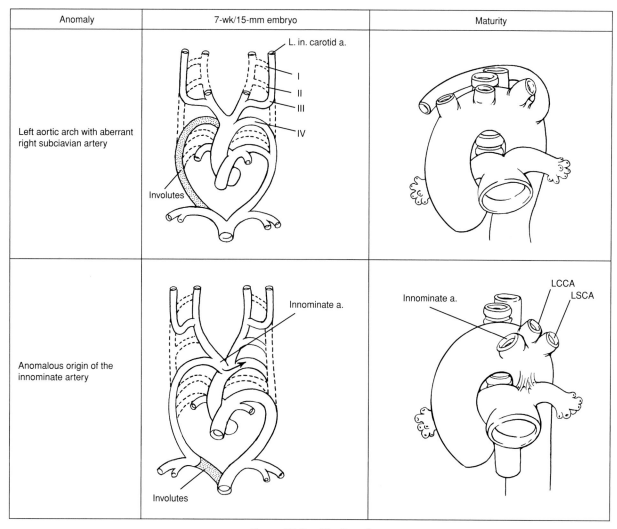

Figure 74-2. (*Continued*)

When tracheoesophageal compression results from a right aortic arch and a retroesophageal ligament, symptoms are similar in nature but are usually less severe and present later in infancy or in early childhood. These rings are generally less stenotic and become notable as the aorta grows.

Patients with cervical arches are usually asymptomatic, but may present with a pulsatile mass in the neck or the supraclavicular fossa. Infants with the type IB anomaly may also exhibit the compressive symptoms of dyspnea and stridor. Adults more commonly present with dysphagia. Some adults have presented with central nervous system symptoms and the subclavian steal syndrome as a result of stenoses of the left subclavian artery and origin of the vertebral artery.

Diagnosis

A vascular ring may be suggested on chest radiography by the presence of a pulmonary infiltrate, atelectasis, or unilateral or bilateral hyperinflation. The presence of a right aortic arch should raise suspicion.

Barium esophagogram remains a useful diagnostic measure. In cases of double aortic arch, the lateral view will reveal a posterior indentation in the esophagus. In the anterior projection, there are dual indentations, higher on the right and lower on the left. An aberrant right subclavian artery from a left aortic arch will also produce posterior esophageal indentation on the lateral view. On the anterior view, however, the aberrant right subclavian artery takes an oblique course descending left to right. The aberrant retroesophageal left subclavian artery from a right aortic arch will show a similar posterior indentation on the lateral view, but the oblique course on the anterior view runs in the opposite direction: from right to left.

Historically, the clinical presentation and barium esophagogram have provided sufficient information to proceed to surgical treatment. The increasing availability and sophistication of magnetic resonance imaging (MRI) and computed tomography (CT), however, have elevated these noninvasive imaging techniques to the preferred diagnostic modality at most institutions. MRI provides the most detailed and complete depiction of the anatomy and compressive effects of a vascular ring. MRI, however, is expensive and requires sedation in the younger patients who are at the greatest risk from airway compression. Without sedation, motion artifacts frequently result in poor image quality. CT scanning with three-dimensional reconstruction can also provide excellent images but is limited by the need for intravenous contrast and exposure to radiation and may also require sedation for adequate imaging. Aortography is the most invasive technique and is rarely used. It can establish the completeness of a double aortic arch and identify areas of luminal irregularity. It cannot, however, distinguish between a double

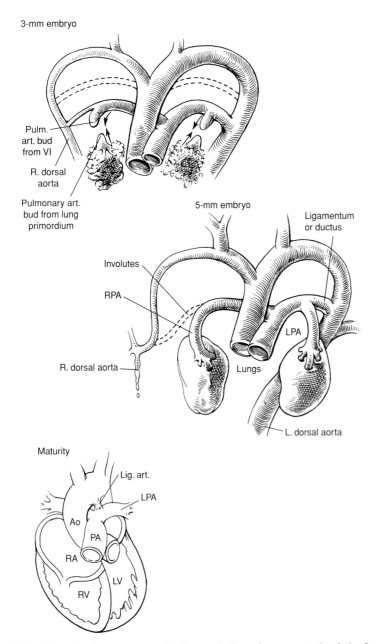

Figure 74-3. Normal pulmonary artery development. The pulmonary arteries derive from two separate vascular buds, the sixth aortic arches (left and right), and the splanchnic plexus. These buds fuse to form the left and right pulmonary arteries. (Ao = aorta; L. = left; Lig. art. = ligamentum arteriosum; LPA = left pulmonary artery; LV = left ventricle; PA, Pulm. art. = pulmonary artery; R. = right; RA = right atrium; RPA = right pulmonary artery; RV = right ventricle.)

aortic arch with an atretic segment and a right aortic arch with a retroesophageal ligament. Transthoracic echocardiography is used to detect associated cardiac anomalies and is reasonably sensitive in evaluating vascular rings but appears deficient in determining atretic and nonluminal segments.

Cervical arches may be suspected by the presence of a wide mediastinum, the absence of the aortic knob, and anterior tracheal deviation on chest radiography. Although angiography has been the standard for diagnosis, CT scanning and MRI now provide a noninvasive technique to confirm the diagnosis.

Indications for Surgery

Surgical correction of complete vascular rings is indicated when symptoms are present. Anomalies identified shortly after birth or within the first 6 months of life require surgical correction much more fre-

quently than those discovered after the age of 6 months. Very mild symptoms presenting in the older infant or young child may resolve as the child grows. A watchful approach may be appropriate in such cases.

Surgical Technique

Ninety percent of vascular ring cases can be corrected through a left posterolateral thoracotomy. Single-lumen general endotracheal anesthesia is applied.

Double Aortic Arch. In cases of double aortic arch, where flow is present in both arches, the dominant arch is preserved. Division is performed at the location on the ring that preserves the greatest brachial and cephalic flow. When an atretic segment of the vascular ring is present, division is performed at the atretic segment. Before vascular division, the carotid and radial pulses are monitored by the anesthesiologist to confirm flow after clamps have been placed.

After induction of general orotracheal anesthesia the infant is placed in a full lateral position with the left side up (Fig. 74-5). Through a posterior lateral muscle-preserving incision, the left chest is entered through the fourth intercostal space. The lung is retracted anteriorly and inferiorly, exposing the posterior mediastinum. This position is retained with malleable retractors secured to the chest retractor with nonpenetrating towel clamps.

The descending aorta, anterior (left) aortic arch, left subclavian artery, and the vagus and phrenic nerves are identified before the pleura is opened (Fig. 74-5). The vagus nerve descends anterior to the left subclavian artery, crossing the left aortic arch, giving off the recurrent laryngeal nerve as it penetrates into the mediastinum medially around the ligamentum arteriosum. The posterior (right) aortic arch may or may not be visualized initially depending on the extent of mediastinal fat.

The pleura is incised from the descending aorta inferiorly to the left subclavian artery, and then elevated from the mediastinum anteriorly and posteriorly with stay sutures (Fig. 74-6). The vagus nerve is elevated off the mediastinum with the anterior pleural flap exposing the branching of the recurrent laryngeal nerve. This is similar to the exposure of a patent ductus arteriosus. The ligamentum arteriosum (or ductus arteriosus) is identified between the distal anterior (left) aortic arch and the left pulmonary artery. The ligamentum is sharply dissected out in its entirety in preparation for ligation and division in standard fashion.

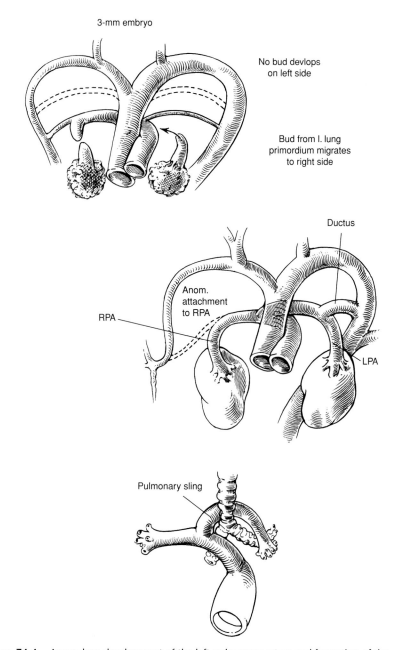

3-mm embryo

No bud devlops
on left side

Bud from l. lung
primordium migrates
to right side

Ductus

Anom.
attachment
to RPA

RPA

LPA

Pulmonary sling

Figure 74-4. Anomalous development of the left pulmonary artery and formation of the pulmonary artery sling. When the splanchnic bud of the left pulmonary artery fails to fuse with the left sixth aortic arch, it migrates posteriorly between the trachea and esophagus to fuse with the right pulmonary artery. This results in a compressive "sling" about the trachea. (Anom. = anomalous; LPA = left pulmonary artery; RPA = right pulmonary artery.)

smaller and should be divided at its junction with the anterior arch (Figs. 74-6 and 74-7). If both arches are of equal size, division is planned for the most accessible point in the ring: usually between the left subclavian artery and the posterior arch.

The ligamentum arteriosum (ductus arteriosus) is divided in standard fashion (Fig. 74-7). Once the appropriate site for ring division is identified, vascular clamps are applied and all radial and carotid pulses confirmed (Fig. 74-8). The vessel is then divided and each end is closed with a running 4-0 polypropylene suture. Clamps are slowly removed to assure hemostasis. Dissection of the posterior arch in its course through the posterior aspect of the mediastinum is performed to allow for retraction of the posterior arch away from the posterior wall of the esophagus (Fig. 74-9). Final inspection for hemostasis is performed and the pleura is closed. A single chest tube is then placed posteriorly along the mediastinum into the apex of the left chest.

Figures 74-10 and 74-11 demonstrate the surgical anatomy and division of the anterior (left) arch using a similar technique. If necessary, the vagus and recurrent laryngeal nerves may be mobilized with the posterior pleural flap to achieve better exposure of the proximal anterior arch and prevent nerve injury.

When MRI or CT scan clearly shows that the right (posterior) arch is smaller than the left, a right thoracotomy is the preferred approach. The smaller posterior arch is easily accessed through the right chest. The divided posterior segment of the arch does not retract behind the spine (as it does through a left thoracotomy) but remains readily controllable should significant bleeding occur.

Right Aortic Arch with Retroesophageal Ligament.
In cases of right aortic arch with a retroesophageal ligament, the surgical approach is through a left thoracotomy. Division of the ring is achieved by division of the ligament. Through a posterolateral muscle-sparing thoracotomy, the vagus nerve is identified in the pleura overlying the mediastinum. The pleura is opened from the proximal descending aorta to the left subclavian artery posterior to the vagus nerve. The anterior flap of pleura is elevated to expose the left pulmonary artery, at which point the ligamentum arteriosum is identified. Several different potential origins of the ligament exist: (1) from a Kommerell's diverticulum off the posterior (right) arch, (2) directly from the right posterior arch, and (3) from the retroesophageal left subclavian artery.

The posterior pleural flap is gently elevated off the mediastinum. With this, the posterior (right) aortic arch becomes visible as it penetrates the mediastinum posterior to the esophagus and joins the left (anterior) aortic arch to form the descending aorta. Opening the pleura extensively in this fashion will provide wide exposure to the mediastinal structures. The anterior arch is dissected to the level of the left common carotid artery. The left subclavian artery is mobilized dis-

tally toward the thoracic outlet. The posterior arch is fully isolated from its mediastinal attachments, and all adhesive bands are sharply divided. At this point, the narrowest portion of the vascular ring is identified. In most cases, the narrowest segment will involve the anterior (left) arch either between the left carotid and left subclavian arteries (Figs. 74-10 and 74-11) or between the left subclavian artery and the posterior (right) arch. In 20% of cases the posterior arch is

Table 74-2   Classification of Vascular Rings and Pulmonary Artery Sling

Classification	Relative Prevalence in Surgical Series (%)
Group I. Complete vascular rings	**75**
IA. Double aortic arch	55
Right arch dominant	80
Left arch dominant	15
Arches equal	5
IB. Right aortic arch/retroesophageal ligament	45
Aberrant left subclavian artery	70
Mirror image branching	30
IC. Left aortic arch/right descending aorta/tight ligament	<1
Group II. Partial vascular rings	**20**
Left aortic arch	100
Aberrant right subclavian artery/left ligament	20
Innominate artery compression	80
Group III. Pulmonary artery sling	**5**

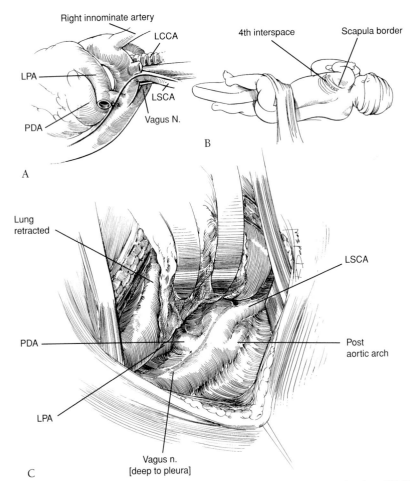

Figure 74-5. Surgical approach, exposure, and anatomy of a complete vascular ring. **(A)** The patient is placed in the right lateral decubitus position with an axillary roll. The right leg is bent at the hip and knee. Legs are separated by pillows, and the left leg is straight. The incision is a gentle S-curve, at the tip of the scapula. With a muscle-sparing technique, the chest is entered through the fourth interspace. **(B)** The chest retractor is placed with the cross bar anteriorly. The lung is retracted anteriorly and inferiorly and is held into position with a moistened sponge secured with malleable retractors that are fixed to the retractor cross bar. **(C)** Before the pleura is incised, note the position of the vagus nerve, aorta, left pulmonary artery, and, if possible, the posterior (right) arch and ligamentum arteriosum. (LCCA = left common carotid artery; LPA = left pulmonary artery; LSCA = left subclavian artery; n = nerve; PDA = patent ductus arteriosus.)

Dissection of the ligamentum is performed to the point of its origin while the recurrent laryngeal nerve is protected. The ligamentum arteriosum is divided in standard fashion. All adhesive bands are released. In most cases it is not necessary to excise the ligament or Kommerell's diverticulum. With adequate mobilization, the structures will retract, releasing impingement on the trachea and esophagus. When Kommerell's diverticulum appears large or dilated it should be resected to prevent subsequent independent compression of the trachea and esophagus. In these cases transfer of the left subclavian artery to the left carotid artery should be considered to relieve any slinglike effect of the posterior arch and left subclavian artery on the trachea.

Vascular Rings Requiring Right Thoracotomy.   A right thoracotomy is indicated in correction of vascular rings in 10% to 20% of cases. As discussed, the most common of these indications is the double aortic arch with dominant left arch. Rarer cases include (1) left aortic arch with a right descending aorta and right ligamentum arteriosum between the right descending aorta to the right pulmonary artery and (2) left aortic arch with aberrant right subclavian artery and right ligamentum arteriosum. The surgeon should be alerted to these rare cases by a distinctive esophagogram demonstrating significant indentation high in the upper left posterior aspect of the esophagus. MRI and CT will also identify these cases. Similar principles apply to correct these anomalies. The recurrent laryngeal nerve recurs around the right-sided ligamentum arteriosum. Division of the ring is achieved by division of the ligamentum arteriosum. Isolation of the ligamentum arteriosum and caution with dissection of the recurrent laryngeal nerve are applied. Dissection of the arch of the aorta through the mediastinum posterior to the esophagus is performed to divide adhesive bands to the posterior wall of the esophagus.

Vascular Rings Requiring Median Sternotomy.   Median sternotomy accounts for approximately 5% of surgical approaches to vascular rings. This approach is used when the vascular ring is associated with correction of another cardiac defect such as tetralogy of Fallot, in which 20% to 25% of cases have an associated right-sided arch. In most cases of tetralogy with right aortic arch, however, there is mirror image branching with the ligamentum arteriosum between the left innominate artery and left pulmonary artery and thus no vascular ring.

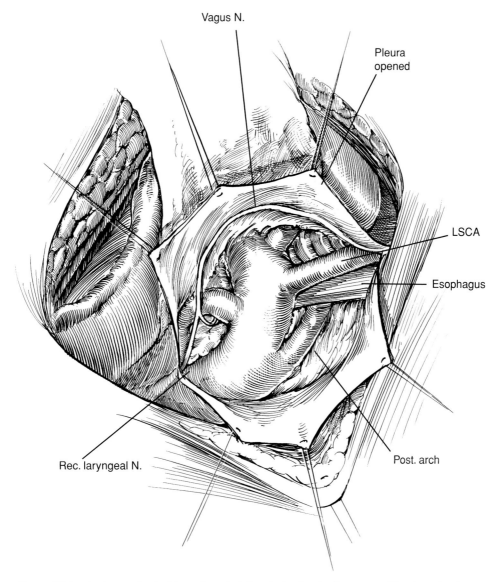

Figure 74-6. Anatomy of a double aortic arch, left arch dominant, pleura open. The pleura has been opened from the proximal descending aorta to the thoracic outlet of the left subclavian artery. The vagus and recurrent laryngeal nerves have been mobilized with the anterior pleural flap. The posterior (right) arch penetrates through the mediastinum deep to the esophagus. (LSCA = left subclavian artery; n = nerve; post. = posterior; Rec. = recurrent.)

Surgical repair for cervical arches is rarely indicated but may be required for complications such as compressive symptoms, arch hypoplasia, and aneurysm of the arch. The surgical approach in these cases is dictated by the anatomy of the complicating feature and may range from division of the ligamentum arteriosum to aneurysm resection with graft interposition.

Group II: Partial Vascular Rings

Partial vascular rings include (1) left aortic arch with retroesophageal right subclavian artery and left ligamentum arteriosum and (2) leftward origin of the innominate artery resulting in anterior tracheal compression.

Left Aortic Arch with Aberrant Right Subclavian Artery

The anomaly of left aortic arch with aberrant right subclavian artery is the most common anomaly of the aortic arch, found in 0.5% to 1.8% of the population. Most patients are asymptomatic. It forms as a result of involution of the entire right dorsal aorta. The right subclavian artery migrates posteriorly behind the esophagus as the left subclavian artery migrates cranially. Coarctation is often associated with this lesion. When symptoms do occur they are most commonly related to difficulty in swallowing. A barium esophagogram is usually sufficient for diagnosis. Surgery is rarely indicated for this anomaly. When symptoms persist, correction consists of left thoracotomy and mobilization and division of the retroesophageal right subclavian artery.

Anomalous Innominate Artery with Tracheal Compression

Anatomy. This entity is described in patients with a normal left aortic arch and left-sided ligamentum arteriosum. In these patients the innominate artery arises either

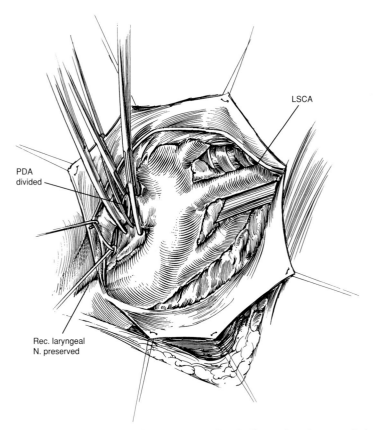

Figure 74-7. Division of the patent ductus arteriosus (PDA). Clamps have been applied to the ductus, using caution to exclude the recurrent laryngeal nerve. The ends of the ductus are closed with 5-0 polypropylene suture. (LSCA = left subclavian artery; n = nerve; Rec. = recurrent.)

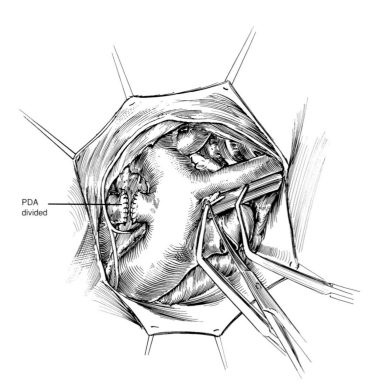

Figure 74-8. Division of the posterior (right) aortic arch. Appropriately sized vascular clamps are applied to the right arch after it has been mobilized. Carotid and subclavian artery pulses are verified by palpation or Doppler ultrasound before division. (PDA = patent ductus arteriosus.)

partially or completely to the left of the trachea and in its course from left to right produces anterior compression on the distal trachea. The degree of tracheal compression varies considerably, with only a small proportion of patients developing symptoms of airway obstruction.

Clinical Presentation. Innominate artery compression occurs most commonly in children younger than 2 years of age. Primary symptoms are respiratory and include repeated bronchopulmonary infections, stridor, and apnea.

Diagnosis. Diagnosis of innominate artery compression is best obtained with bronchoscopy, during which an anterior pulsatile indentation is noted compressing the trachea 1 cm to 2 cm above the carina. The trachea should be narrowed at least 50% to 75% for the symptoms to be attributed to this anomaly. The diagnosis can also be made with MRI.

Indications for Surgery. Surgical therapy is dictated by the severity of symptoms. Patients with mild symptoms are managed conservatively and allowed to improve with growth. Patients with a history of apnea, severe stridor, or respiratory distress or two or more episodes of bronchopneumonia or tracheobronchitis are candidates for surgery if significant tracheal compression is demonstrated.

Surgical Technique. Several techniques for correction of innominate artery compression have been described. Mustard's technique requires division of the artery overlying the trachea. Langlois's technique involves division of the artery and reimplantation on the ascending aorta. We prefer Gross's technique of innominate artery suspension.

Although Gross used a left anterior thoracotomy, we prefer a right anterior thoracotomy through the second intercostal space (Fig. 74-12). The right lobe of the thymus is excised, and the innominate vein is mobilized to expose the innominate artery. The innominate artery should not be dissected from the trachea so that suspension of the artery exerts traction on the compressed segment of trachea restoring the lumen of the airway. Video-assisted rigid bronchoscopy is extremely valuable in assessing the effect of suture placement and tension on the tracheal lumen. Several 3-0 braided sutures are placed in the adventitia of the innominate artery at the level of the pericardium at a point directly beneath

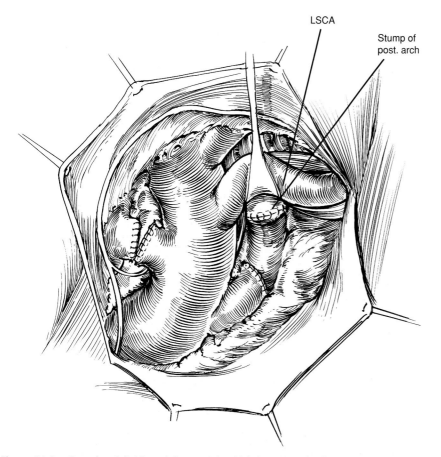

LSCA

Stump of
post. arch

Figure 74-9.   Completed division of the posterior (right) aortic arch. The posterior aortic arch is divided and oversewn in two layers. The proximal and distal stumps of the divided arch are dissected free of adhesive bands, releasing the esophagus and trachea. This allows the proximal stump to retract, relieving esophageal compression. Should bleeding from this stump become problematic, obtaining control can be difficult. For that reason a right thoracotomy approach may be preferable when preoperative imaging clearly demonstrates a smaller posterior (right arch). (LSCA = left subclavian artery; post. = posterior.)

rior membranous portion of the trachea and proximal primary bronchi, replaced by complete tracheal rings. This ring deformity can occur in an isolated segment of the distal trachea or can be much more debilitating when it involves the entire length of the trachea. Predominately, this defect is limited to the area impinged on by the pulmonary arterial sling.

Clinical Presentation

Pulmonary artery slings produce symptoms of tracheal compression due to posterior impingement of the trachea. Infants generally present soon after birth with stridor that is episodic. They are often treated as asthmatics and may have a history of chronic respiratory infections. On examination, stridor, tachypnea, nasal flaring, inspiratory and expiratory wheezing, and intercostal retraction may be noted.

Diagnosis

In cases of pulmonary artery sling, chest radiography may demonstrate anterior bowing of the right mainstem bronchus, deviation of the lower trachea and carina to the left, and unequal aeration of the lung. As with vascular rings, barium esophagography may be diagnostic. The position of the anomalous left pulmonary artery between the trachea and esophagus creates an anterior indentation in the esophagus when viewed in the lateral projection. MRI, however, provides more complete three-dimensional information and is the preferred diagnostic modality for this lesion.

the sternum (Fig. 74-13). These sutures are then placed deeply into the periosteum of the posterior surface of the sternum. Alternatively, the ends of the sutures may be passed through holes bored in the sternum, tying the sutures over the anterior surface of the sternum. It is important to achieve a secure suspension to the sternum in either case. Two to four additional 3-0 sutures are placed more distally in the innominate artery and secured to the periosteum of the adjacent ribs such that the entire extent of the innominate artery producing compression on the anterior wall of the trachea is suspended (Fig. 74-14). Emphasis is placed on bronchoscopic guidance to assure relief of the tracheal obstruction. In the rare case in which innominate artery suspension fails to significantly improve the tracheal compression, reimplantation of the innominate artery via a median sternotomy should be considered.

Group III : Pulmonary Artery Sling

Anatomy

In cases of pulmonary arterial sling the left pulmonary artery originates from the posterior aspect of the right pulmonary artery, proceeds over the right mainstem bronchus, between the trachea and the esophagus, and reaches the hilus of the left lung at a level lower than normal (Fig. 74-15). This lesion does not form a ring, but forms a sling around the distal trachea and right mainstem bronchus, producing compression of these structures. The esophagus is not obstructed, but indentation on the anterior wall of the esophagus can be noted on esophagoscopy or barium esophagogram.

Pulmonary artery sling anomalies are associated with tracheal stenosis in 33% to 50% of cases. In these cases, tracheal stenosis results from absence of the normal poste-

Indications for Surgery

Patients with pulmonary artery sling and signs and symptoms of significant respiratory obstruction are candidates for operative repair. All patients should undergo preoperative bronchoscopic evaluation to assess the position, degree, and extent of any tracheal or bronchial constriction.

When workup demonstrates extrinsic tracheal compression without fixed stenosis, surgical repair entails relocation of the left pulmonary artery anterior to the trachea. This can be done by reimplantation of the left pulmonary artery or by transection of the trachea with reanastomosis behind the undivided left pulmonary artery. When a fixed and localized tracheal stenosis is noted, the affected segment of trachea is resected, the undivided left pulmonary artery is relocated anteriorly, and primary anastomosis of the trachea is performed.

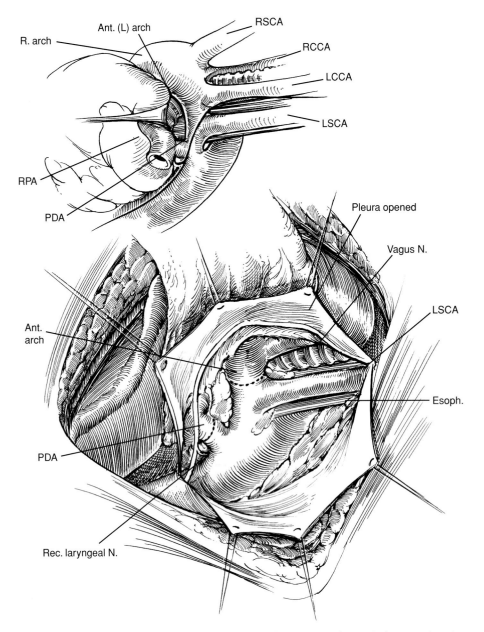

Figure 74-10. Anatomy of a double aortic arch, right arch dominant. The surgical approach and exposure are similar to that in Figs. 74-6 through 74-9. The vagus and recurrent laryngeal nerves are mobilized with the anterior pleural flap in this view. These structures may be mobilized with the posterior pleural flap if division of the anterior (left) arch is expected proximal to the origin of the left common carotid artery. This will allow proximal exposure without undue tension on these nerves. (Ant. = anterior; Esoph. = esophagus; L = left; LCCA = left common carotid artery; LSCA = left subclavian artery; n. = nerve; PDA = patent ductus arteriosus; R. = right; RCCA = right common carotid artery; Rec. = recurrent; RPA = right pulmonary artery; RSCA = right subclavian artery.)

Surgical Technique

Patients not requiring tracheal resection may be approached through an anterolateral left thoracotomy or a median sternotomy. Although cardiopulmonary bypass is not essential for reimplantation of the anomalous left pulmonary artery, its use does replace respiratory function and allows a wide anastomosis on empty and open vessels. The use of cardiopulmonary bypass also provides the option of dividing the trachea without dividing the left pulmonary artery. For this reason we prefer a median sternotomy with cardiopulmonary bypass for all patients with pulmonary artery sling with or without fixed tracheal stenosis.

After standard median sternotomy the pericardium and left pleura are opened. After appropriate heparinization the patient is cannulated via the aorta and right atrium. Cardiopulmonary bypass is instituted, and the patient is cooled to 32°C. The proximal right and left pulmonary arteries are dissected free and the trachea is identified. The ligamentum arteriosum (ductus arteriosus) is divided and oversewn. At this point, options include division of the left pulmonary

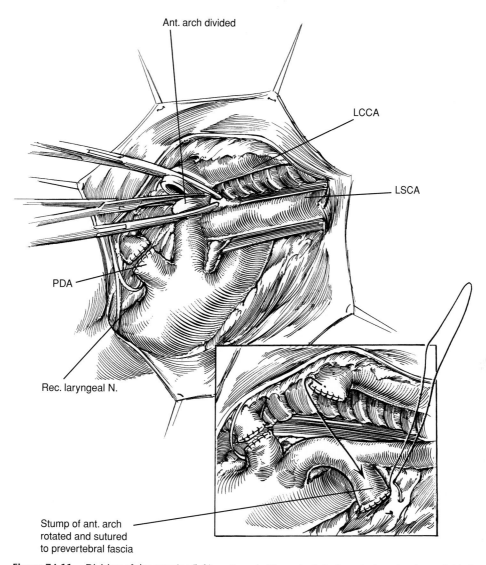

Ant. arch divided

LCCA

LSCA

PDA

Rec. laryngeal N.

Stump of ant. arch
rotated and sutured
to prevertebral fascia

Figure 74-11. Division of the anterior (left) aortic arch. The patent ductus arteriosus has been divided and oversewn. Vascular clamps are applied, with care being taken to make sure that the recurrent laryngeal nerve is not trapped in the clamp on the posterior surface of the left arch. The anterior (left) arch is divided and oversewn in two layers. The distal stump may be rotated and attached to the prevertebral fascia. Adhesive bands about the trachea and esophagus are divided sharply, relieving esophageal and tracheal compression. (Ant., ant. = anterior; LCCA = left common carotid artery; LSCA = left subclavian artery; n = nerve; PDA = patent ductus arteriosus; Rec. = recurrent.)

artery at its origin with reimplantation anterior to the trachea or simple transection of the trachea with anterior relocation of the undivided left pulmonary artery.

When little or no tracheal compromise exists, we prefer to divide the left pulmonary artery and anastomose it to the left lateral aspect of the main pulmonary artery at a site approximating the take-off of a normal LPA.

In patients with localized fixed tracheal stenosis (Fig. 74-16) the stenotic segment is excised (usually four to five rings) and the left pulmonary artery is left intact and mobilized through the tracheal defect. A

primary tracheal anastomosis is then performed with a full-thickness, simple, continuous 5-0 polydioxanone suture (Fig. 74-17). When the length of tracheal stenosis exceeds five rings, patch tracheoplasty with autologous pericardium or rib cartilage may be required. The tracheal repair is then tested under 40 cm H_2O to rule out air leaks.

Once the integrity of the tracheal anastomosis is ensured, ventilation is reinstituted and cardiopulmonary bypass is discontinued. After heparin reversal and satisfactory hemostasis, the sternotomy is closed in the standard fashion.

Postoperative Care

Particular care must be given to respiratory management in all cases. In most vascular ring and pulmonary sling cases, extubation can occur immediately or within 24 hours of surgery. Occasionally, if postobstruction collapse or pneumonia were present preoperatively, prolonged intubation is necessary for tracheal suctioning, positive-pressure breathing, and oxygen administration. Humidified oxygen with bronchodilator therapy should be initiated. After

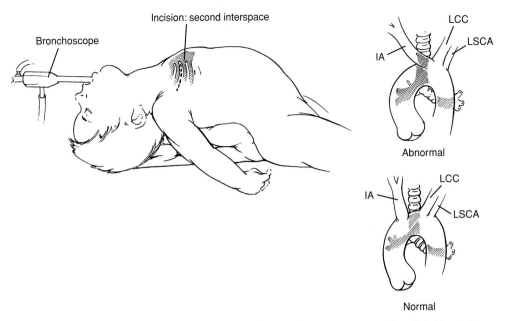

Figure 74-12.   Positioning and approach for relief of innominate artery compression. A right anterior thoracotomy through the second interspace is used. A ventilating fiberoptic rigid bronchoscope with video attachment is placed before the incision is made. (IA = innominate artery; LCC = left common carotid artery; LSCA = left subclavian artery.)

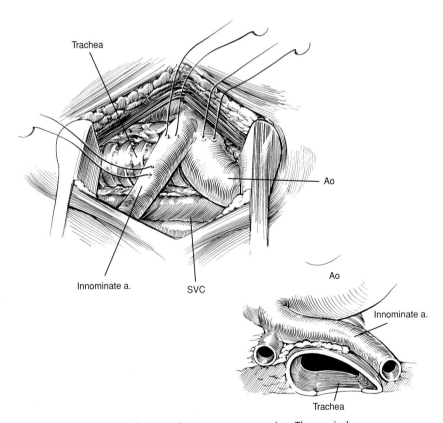

Figure 74-13.   Arteriopexy for innominate artery compression. The surgical exposure demonstrates the leftward origin of the innominate artery. Braided 3-0 sutures are placed in the adventitia of the vessel. The cross-sectional view reveals the mechanism of anterior tracheal compression. The adventitial tissue between the vessel and the trachea must not be dissected if satisfactory retraction of the anterior tracheal wall is to be achieved. (a. = artery; Ao = aorta; SVC = superior vena cava.)

extubation, continued administration of humidified air and bronchodilator therapy are required, as well as aggressive pulmonary toilet. After resectional repair of pulmonary arterial sling with tracheal stenosis, cervical hyperextension is avoided by placement of a heavy suture from the chin to the skin at the sternal notch.

Symptoms frequently are not resolved immediately, and may take days to weeks for edema to resolve. Infrequently, recurring upper respiratory infections and chronic brassy cough may persist for as long as 1 to 2 years. Such prolonged postoperative symptoms are especially prominent in children who had onset of symptoms at age <6 months but were operated on late in their disease process.

Video-Assisted Thoracoscopic Surgery

Video-assisted thoracoscopic surgery (VATS) has been successfully applied to some patients with complete vascular rings. Safe use of this technique requires a significant VATS experience on the part of the operator as well as appropriate patient selection. The most suitable patients are those with a right aortic arch with aberrant left subclavian artery and left ligamentum arteriosum (type IB) and the occasional patient with a double aortic arch with

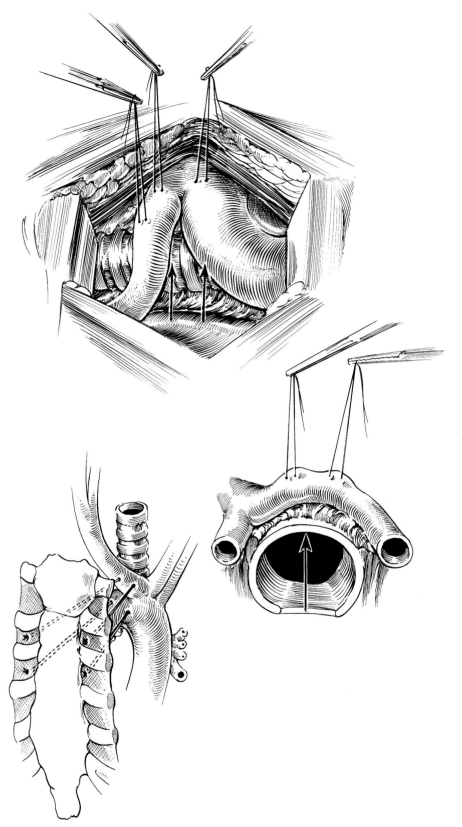

Figure 74-14. Reduction of innominate artery compression. Retraction on the adventitial sutures elevates the innominate artery and the anterior wall of the trachea. Use of video-assisted bronchoscopy assures ideal suture placement for maximal tracheal decompression. Fixation to the sternum is demonstrated in the 30-degree view.

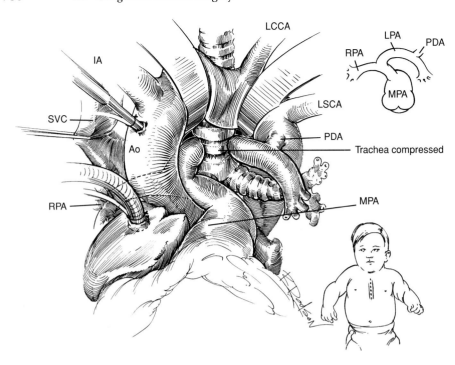

Figure 74-15. Surgical anatomy of the pulmonary artery sling. Exposure via median sternotomy is shown with cardiopulmonary bypass. Localized tracheal stenosis is present in this case. (Ao = aorta; IA = innominate artery; LCCA = left common carotid artery; LPA = left pulmonary artery; LSCA = left subclavian artery; MPA = main pulmonary artery; PDA = patent ductus arteriosus; RPA = right pulmonary artery; SVC = superior vena cava.)

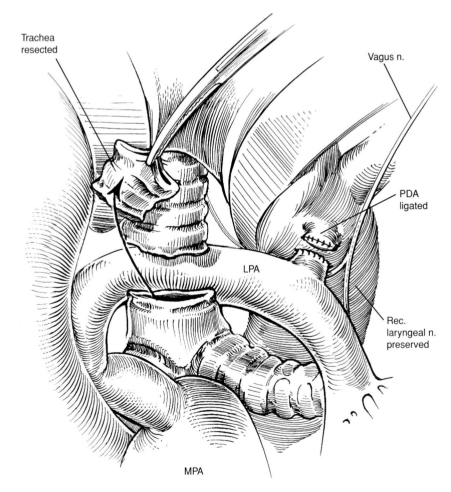

Figure 74-16. Tracheal resection in pulmonary artery sling repair. The stenotic segment of the trachea has been resected. The anomalous left pulmonary artery is mobilized anteriorly through the tracheal defect. This avoids arterial division. (LPA = left pulmonary artery; MPA = main pulmonary artery; n. = nerve; PDA = patent ductus arteriosus; Rec. = recurrent.)

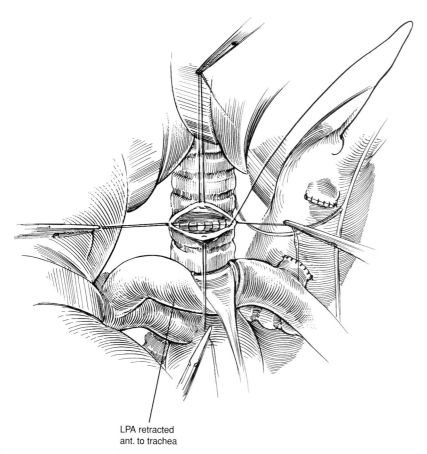

Figure 74-17. Tracheal anastomosis in pulmonary artery sling repair. The trachea undergoes primary anastomosis with a running 5-0 polydioxanone suture. (ant. = anterior; LPA = left pulmonary artery.)

LPA retracted
ant. to trachea

an atretic left arch. In these patients a non-vascular segment of the ring can be approached endoscopically and safely divided. Endoscopic vascular clamps are not reliable enough to recommend this technique for division of a patent vascular segment. MRI can accurately detect segmental patency or atresia and thereby identify those vascular ring patients suitable for the VATS approach.

Results

In cases of true vascular rings, mortality rate ranges from 0.5% to 6.0%. Most deaths are due to postoperative complications secondary to upper respiratory infections, pneumonia, and pulmonary failure in children undergoing delayed operation. Morbidity approximates 30% in children with complete vascular rings and 25% in cases of innominate artery compression. This morbidity most frequently includes chronic wheezing and upper respiratory infections. Infrequent complications include

recurrent laryngeal nerve injuries and chylothorax.

Historically, pulmonary artery sling repair was performed with division and reimplantation of the artery. This repair has been complicated by left pulmonary artery thrombosis in as many as 90% of cases, with death in 50% of cases. More recently, patency rates exceed 75% and mortality rates are less than 5%.

SUGGESTED READING

Backer CL, Mavroudis C. Surgical approach to vascular rings. Adv Card Surg 1997;9:29.

Backer CL, Mavroudis C, Gerber ME, et al. Tracheal surgery in children: An eighteen year review of four techniques. Eur J Cardiothorac Surg 2001;19:777.

Burke RP, Rosenfield HM, Wernovsky T, et al. Video-assisted thoracoscopic vascular ring division in infants and children. J Am Coll Cardiol 1995;24:943.

Dodge-Khatami A, Tulevski II, Hitchcock JF, et al. Vascular rings and pulmonary arterial sling: from respiratory collapse to surgical cure, with

emphasis on judicious imaging in the hi-tech era. Cardiol Young 2002;12:96.

Edwards JE. Anomalies of the derivatives of the aortic arch system. Med Clin North Am 1948(July): 925.

Gross RE. Surgical relief for tracheal obstruction from a vascular ring. N Eng J Med 1945;233:586.

Haramati LB, Glickstein JS, Issenberg HJ, et al. MR imaging and CT of vascular anomalies and connections in patients with congenital heart disease: Significance in surgical planning. Radiographics 2002;22:337.

Hellenbrand WE, Kelley MJ, Talner NS, et al. Cervical aortic arch with retroesophageal aortic obstruction: Report of a case with successful surgical intervention. Ann Thorac Surg 1978;26:86.

Skandalakis JE, Gray SW, Symbas P. Embryology for Surgeons: The Embryological Basis for the Treatment of Congenital Anomalies. Baltimore: Williams and Wilkins, 1994; Chapter 28.

EDITOR'S COMMENTS

As noted in the chapter on imaging modalities, MRI scanning has become perhaps the most useful imaging technique for evaluation of vascular rings and slings. Although barium swallow studies can give a fairly accurate assessment of arch anatomy, the relative size of the anterior and posterior arch in double aortic arch is not readily determined by this type of study.

Rapid multislice helical CT scanning has been very useful for assessment of arch anomalies. The advantage of CT reconstruction is the ability to gain images in a very brief time, which may obviate the need for sedation or intubation with general anesthesia as for MRI scanning. Images are usually quite good and comparable to MRI images. However, the increased amount of radiation and the need for contrast are disadvantages to this technique.

In patients with aberrant left subclavian artery with right aortic arch and Kommerell's diverticulum, it is sometimes valuable to perform a pexy of the diverticulum or the base of the left subclavian artery to the prevertebral fascia to maintain complete opening of the ring and to mobilize the trachea and the esophagus in the middle portion to ensure that there is no adventitial tissue that may result in residual compression. As noted by the authors, resection of Kommerell's diverticulum is rarely necessary, although some centers have routinely done this, believing that greater relief of potential reobstruction is possible with this approach. If a resection of Kommerell's diverticulum is performed, we prefer to reimplant the left subclavian artery to the left carotid or the aorta to maintain flow to the left arm as suggested by the authors.

The situation with innominate artery compressive syndromes is a complex one. In most cases, the innominate artery compresses the trachea because of abnormal location more to the left on the aortic arch than normal. Often this is associated with abnormalities of chest wall symmetry with either pectus excavatum or a decreased anteroposterior diameter. We believe that these abnormalities often predispose patients to innominate artery compression, and simple innominate arteriopexy to the chest wall through a thoracotomy may not completely relieve the compression. In these cases, we believe that it is valuable to relocate the innominate artery on the ascending aorta more to the right, which completely relieves the obstruction even in an abnormal chest geometry. This procedure can easily be undertaken through a sternotomy incision.

Although retroesophageal aberrant right subclavian artery is rarely associated with significant symptoms, we have seen patients who have had true dysphagia or chronic cough from this anatomy. Whereas ligation and division of the subclavian can relieve obstructive symptoms, we prefer to relocate the subclavian vessel from behind the esophagus over to the right side, either to the carotid or directly to the arch of the aorta. This maintains the patency of the subclavian vessel and prevents subclavian steal syndrome. This can generally be done through a right thoracotomy incision

The anatomy of pulmonary artery sling is complex, and the results with repair of this defect are suboptimal. As noted by the authors, patients with pulmonary artery sling have had a very high mortality and a high occlusion rate of the left pulmonary artery when it has been divided and relocated anterior to the trachea. The causes for this are multifactorial; however, often these are small infants, and the pulmonary artery flow may not be adequate to maintain growth of the anastomosed vessel. If reimplantation of the left pulmonary artery to the main pulmonary artery is performed in pulmonary artery sling, it is often advisable to shorten the posterior aspect of the pulmonary artery slightly to prevent kinking and to patch augment the anterior aspect with pericardium or homograft material to decrease the risk of stenosis. In our experience relocation of the pulmonary artery anterior to the trachea, because of the abnormal origin of the left pulmonary artery, can lead to kinking and stenosis of the origin of the left pulmonary vessel due to the elongated nature of the left pulmonary artery, which now sits anterior to the trachea. In some cases, even with simple translocation of the left pulmonary artery anterior to the trachea, it may be necessary to patch augment the origin of the vessel to prevent development of kinking or stenosis.

Much of the mortality in patients with pulmonary artery sling is related to airway complications, and, as noted in this chapter, direct attention to the airway is the primary component of surgical repair for this condition. We have seen several patients who have a tracheal origin of the right upper lobe bronchus with complete tracheal rings of the distal trachea to the bifurcation. Because of the early take-off of the upper lobe bronchus, the distal trachea is quite small and the bifurcation into the mainstem bronchi also is relatively small. In these patients, either extensive resection of the complete rings with slide tracheoplasty or rib cartilage patch tracheoplasty is necessary in addition to division of the trachea and relocation of the pulmonary artery anteriorly. These complex operations can be done with good results, and we prefer to use rib cartilage grafts rather than pericardial patches if sliding tracheoplasty is not feasible in most of these patients because of the rigidity of the tissue and the maintenance of a patent airway without anterior malacia from a pericardial patch. In some cases, however, the diminutive size of the trachea requires the use of a pericardial patch to prevent cartilage bowing into the lumen of the airway. In more typical forms of pulmonary artery sling, simple resection of involved tracheal segments can completely relieve the obstructions.

Although the authors suggest fixation of the chin to the anterior chest wall to relieve potential tension on tracheal reconstruction suture lines, we have rarely found it necessary to perform this procedure in infants or young children. Mobilization of the trachea with hilar releases is often fully sufficient to prevent tension on the anastomosis, even with extensive slide tracheoplasty for long segment tracheal obstruction.

These patients must be diligently managed postoperatively to prevent secretions from pooling in the airway, and repeated bronchoscopic examinations also are necessary to examine the airway to clear secretions and to avoid the development of obstructive granulation tissue at the tracheal anastomosis. Associated cardiac defects such as ventricular septal defect or tetralogy of Fallot may also be present with a pulmonary artery sling complex and can be addressed at the time of the tracheal repair

T.L.S.

75

Atrial Septal Defects

Richard D. Mainwaring and John J. Lamberti

Substantial changes have occurred in the management of atrial septal defects (ASDs) since publication of the first edition of this book. With Food and Drug Administration approval of the Amplatzer ASD occluder device in 2002, the vast majority of ASDs are now closed in the cardiac catheterization laboratory. This has resulted in an overall decrement in the number of open-heart operations performed in most congenital heart surgery programs. In spite of these changes, it is still imperative that surgeons performing pediatric heart operations understand the physiology of these defects, the indications for intervention, and the surgical techniques for their repair. Secundum-type ASDs are frequently a component of more complex congenital heart defects in which the ASD will need to be closed surgically as part of the procedure, and it would appear that the other forms of ASD will remain in the surgical domain at least for the foreseeable future.

Secundum-type atrial septal defects account for approximately 80% to 85% of all ASDs. Sinus venosus defects (both the superior and the inferior type) and incomplete atrioventricular canal defects each constitute between 5% and 10% of all ASDs. Coronary sinus defects are a relatively uncommon form of ASD. The topic of incomplete atrioventricular (AV) canal–type ASDs is reviewed in Chapter 82.

Secundum-type ASDs are three times more frequent in female than in male patients, and there is also a significant incidence of familial inheritance. These observations indicate that genetic factors play an important role in the formation of secundum ASDs. The exact gene locus responsible for this phenomenon has not been identified.

Most ASDs result in a left-to-right shunt (Qp:Qs) of about 2 or 3:1. The amount of flow across an ASD is determined by the relative ratio of diastolic compliance between the right and left ventricles because antegrade flow of the systemic and pulmonary venous return within the heart require the AV valves to be open. The amount of shunt is also influenced by the size of the interatrial communication, the presence or absence of pulmonary valve stenosis, and the pulmonary vascular resistance. Despite the increase in pulmonary blood flow seen with ASDs, most patients will have normal pulmonary artery pressures.

The chronic volume overload associated with an ASD has several adverse effects. The increase in flow through the left atrium, right atrium, and right ventricle (RV) results in enlargement of these structures. It is clear that cardiac enlargement, regardless of its etiology, will eventually translate into decreased quality of life as well as decreased life expectancy. With ASDs, the heart enlargement may take many decades before it leads to ventricular dysfunction or the onset of atrial arrhythmias. Similarly, the increase in pulmonary blood flow is initially well tolerated, but on a long-term basis may result in increased pulmonary vascular resistance.

The natural history of an ASD has been well documented. Studies indicate that patients with unrepaired ASDs and a Qp:Qs of >1.5:1 will have a diminished life expectancy, averaging about 45 years. There is a great deal of variability in the natural history of these patients. Most infants and young children with ASDs are asymptomatic, demonstrating normal growth and absence of cyanosis. Some school-age children will tire a bit more easily than their peers or siblings and occasionally demonstrate perioral or periorbital cyanosis following exertion. As patients with untreated ASDs enter into their teens and 20s, they

may have a gradual decline in their exercise capacity. Also during this time, women enter into their childbearing years. Women with an untreated ASD who become pregnant have a significant incidence of fetal (20% to 30%) and maternal (2%) mortality. As patients enter into their 30s and 40s, most experience a progressive decline in their exercise tolerance coincident with the deterioration in right ventricular function. Atrial arrhythmias are usually a late occurrence and may be the cause of palpitations. The development of arrhythmias may tip a previously well-compensated patient into congestive heart failure because of the loss of atrial contraction. Cyanosis is usually a very late and ominous sign of irreversible pulmonary vascular disease. Patients with a right-to-left shunt or a minimal left-to-right shunt are at risk for paradoxical embolus, although the actual risk is difficult to quantitate. The combination of right heart failure, arrhythmias, and cyanosis generally progresses and eventually leads to the eventual demise of the patient.

Diagnosis

The diagnosis of ASD is usually suspected based on the physical examination. The history may not be particularly helpful in children but is an important part of the assessment in adults. Echocardiography is used to confirm the diagnosis and to delineate the pulmonary venous drainage (Fig. 75-1). Echocardiographic diagnosis is sufficient in most cases because the vast majority of patients identified with ASDs are infants and children. Diagnostic cardiac catheterization is indicated in two specific circumstances. In children, the need for catheterization arises when there remains doubt as to the complete

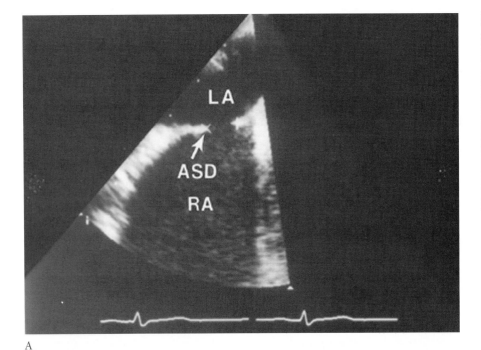

A

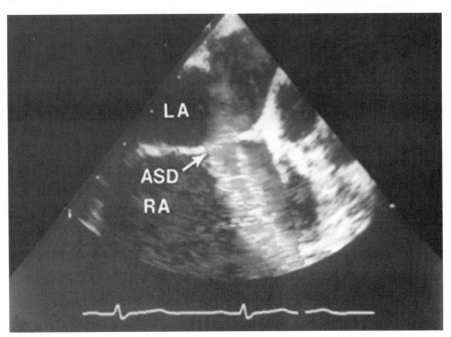

B

Figure 75-1.   **(A)** Echocardiogram demonstrating a secundum-type atrial septal defect (ASD). The positions of the left atrium (LA) and right atrium (RA) are noted. **(B)** The ASD shown in panel A. The flow from the left atrium to the right atrium is shown by color flow (in this case in black and white).

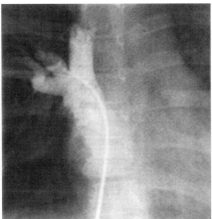

Figure 75-2.   Cardiac catheterization in a patient with a sinus venosus–type atrial septal defect. The entrance of the anomalous right upper lobe pulmonary veins into the superior vena cava is demonstrated.

diagnosis (Fig. 75-2). This can occur with abnormalities of systemic or pulmonary venous drainage or to exclude other associated congenital heart defects. Diagnostic catheterization is indicated in adult patients to assess pulmonary vascular resistance and to exclude the presence of acquired heart disease.

Recommendation for Closure of Atrial Septal Defects

The recommendation for closure of ASDs is based on the premise that the risk of the intervention is substantially lower than

the risk incurred by following the natural history. ASD repair prevents the progression of cardiac and pulmonary changes and in younger patients restores a normal life expectancy. When the diagnosis of ASD is made in infancy or early childhood, closure is generally recommended between 2 and 4 years of age. Regardless of the technique selected (surgical vs. interventional catheterization), these procedures are usually well tolerated and are typically associated with a rapid recovery. The psychosocial aspects of the hospitalization may also be better handled at this age.

Patients with an ASD detected in adulthood will usually benefit from closure of the defect and remain good candidates for whichever technique is selected. Assessment of the adult patient is based on a combination of clinical history, physical findings, echocardiographic information, and cardiac catheterization data. Patients who are fully saturated (i.e., have a left-to-right shunt by echo) and have RV enlargement consistent with a volume load from the shunt will almost certainly derive considerable benefit from closure. Conversely, most patients who have developed cyanosis should not be considered for closure because they rarely benefit from this intervention. Cardiac catheterization may better define those patients in the gray zone. Pulmonary vascular resistance approaching systemic or a shunt ratio barely exceeding 1 suggests that the patient is not a candidate for closure (approximately 10% of patients by the fourth decade will have reached this stage). The conventional teaching has been that surgical intervention is warranted in patients with a Qp:Qs of

>1.5:1, but this criterion can probably be lowered to a Qp:Qs of 1.2 or 1.3:1 with the less invasive septal occluder devices. Closure should also be strongly considered in patients with a history of stroke even if the defect is very small, in order to preclude subsequent events.

Women who are discovered to have an ASD during pregnancy represent a unique clinical situation. During pregnancy, the circulating blood volume expands by about 50%, allowing even more blood to shunt through the ASD. Women who previously were well compensated may develop signs and symptoms of heart failure during the third trimester of their pregnancy. Every attempt should be made to avoid cardiac surgery in this circumstance because the risk to both mother and fetus is quite high. Most pregnant women can be successfully managed using a combination of medical therapy and bed rest. However, on occasion a patient cannot be stabilized and must undergo urgent intervention. This mode of presentation was more common years ago than it is today, presumably because of improved methods of diagnosis.

Surgical Technique

ASDs are usually closed through a sternotomy approach. In boys, this can be performed through a relatively short, low-lying midline incision. Our preference in girls has been to use a curvilinear, transverse (inframammary) skin incision as shown in Fig. 75-3. This technique, once it has been learned, provides a superior cosmetic result without compromising in any way the exposure or versatility. Independent of the orientation of the skin incision, the sternum is divided vertically through the midline. The sternal retractor is then positioned for exposure. The retractor does not need to be opened widely for this operation because visualization of the ASD is relatively straightforward. Excessive retraction can result in sternal fracture.

The thymus is a relatively large structure in younger children and can present an obstacle to cannulation of the aorta. A portion of the thymus can be excised to improve exposure. This maneuver is not necessary in adult patients. The pericardium is then opened according to the intended operation. For repair of a secundum-type ASD, we prefer to open the pericardium slightly to the left of midline with the anticipation that the patch will be cut to the appropriate size and shape once the defect has been

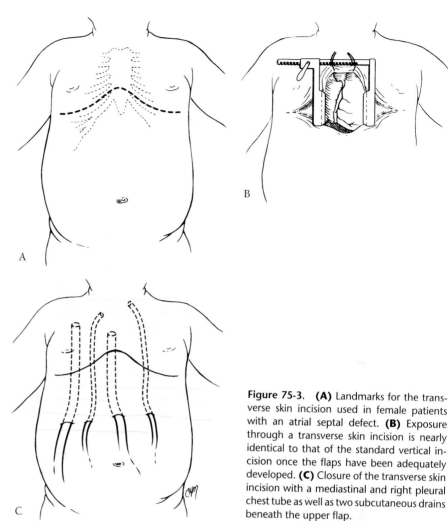

Figure 75-3. (A) Landmarks for the transverse skin incision used in female patients with an atrial septal defect. **(B)** Exposure through a transverse skin incision is nearly identical to that of the standard vertical incision once the flaps have been adequately developed. **(C)** Closure of the transverse skin incision with a mediastinal and right pleural chest tube as well as two subcutaneous drains beneath the upper flap.

visualized. For repair of a sinus venosus–type defect, the anterior pericardium can be harvested and preserved. Some surgeons prefer to treat the pericardium with glutaraldehyde because this both strengthens the patch and makes handling it a bit more straightforward. The remaining pericardial edges are sutured to the drapes to form a pericardial well. Inspection of the anatomy is then conducted with several specific considerations:

1. The heart is inspected with regard to its size and configuration. Often the degree of cardiac enlargement will seem disproportionate to that seen on chest x-ray film.
2. The great vessels are inspected and palpated. The pulmonary artery is usually enlarged consistent with increased flow through this vessel. A thrill at the level of the pulmonary annulus may signify the presence of pulmonary stenosis.
3. The systemic veins are inspected to ensure that there are no abnormalities. A small or absent innominate vein suggests the presence of a left superior vena cava. In the case of a superior sinus venosus defect, the superior vena cava is isolated, and the presence or absence of anomalous pulmonary veins is confirmed. The position of the azygos vein should also be identified.
4. The pulmonary veins on the right are visualized, with the intent of inspecting the left pulmonary veins once on bypass. As indicated, in the case of a sinus venosus defect the anomalous pulmonary veins should be identified at this point.

Cannulation is commenced by placing purse strings in the superior and inferior vena cavae as well as the aorta. If there are anomalous pulmonary veins in association with a sinus venosus defect, the superior vena caval cannulation site should be at the junction of the superior vena cava and innominate vein in order to be well above the entrance of the anomalous veins. Once the patient is cannulated, cardiopulmonary bypass is instituted, and the patient is cooled by decreasing the temperature of the blood. Mild hypothermia (32°C to 34°C) is used in most cases. Deeper levels of hypothermia (28°C to 30°C) may be used when a longer cross-clamp time is anticipated (e.g., sinus venosus ASD with partial veins). Inspection of the heart is completed at this time. Specifically, the position of the left pulmonary veins and the presence of a left superior vena cava can be ascertained by tilting the heart to the right. After inspection, caval tapes are placed around the superior and inferior vena cavae and a cardioplegia needle is inserted into the aortic root. The aortic cross-clamp is applied, and cardioplegia is delivered to achieve electromechanical silence. During this time, the caval tapes are tightened and the right atrium opened to collect the coronary venous effluent.

Surgical Repair of Secundum-Type Atrial Septal Defects

Secundum-type ASDs are approached through a standard right atriotomy (Fig. 75-4). Traction sutures can be placed at the edges of the atriotomy to facilitate exposure. The ASD is identified at its position just beneath the superior limbus. A few moments should be taken to identify the position of the coronary sinus and its relative position with respect to the tricuspid valve. These two structures along with the tendon of Todaro form the triangle of Koch. The AV node should lie at the superior apex of this triangle and may not be too far from the medial border of the ASD. A right-angled clamp can be passed through the ASD into the pulmonary veins to confirm their position. Finally, the position of the inferior vena cava cannula should be inspected along with its relationship to the inferior border of the ASD and the Eustachian valve. Misinterpretation of this anatomy can result in inadvertent baffling of the inferior vena caval flow across the ASD into the left atrium.

After this checklist of anatomic landmarks is completed, repair of the defect is undertaken. The majority of secundum ASDs in young children can be closed primarily, whereas in teenagers and adults the defects are usually large and the tissues less compliant, so that a patch repair is

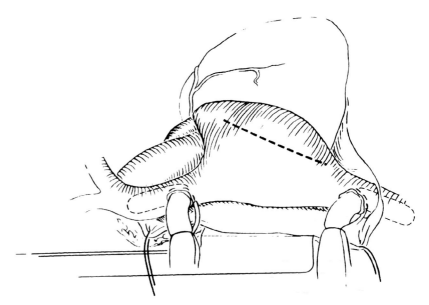

Figure 75-4. View of the right atrium and superior and inferior venae cavae from the surgeon's perspective. Right-angled cannulas have been placed in each vena cava. The dashed line demonstrates the placement of the atrial incision for repair of a secundum atrial septal defect.

almost always indicated under these circumstances. Our preference has been to use autologous pericardium, although synthetic patches also can be used. Pericardial patch repair of an ASD is straightforward, and the technique described here is one of several possible variations. Two separate sutures of 5-0 or 6-0 nonabsorbable vascular suture are placed at the superior and inferior ends of the defect. Each of these sutures is passed through the pericardium at a distance slightly exceeding the length of the

ASD (Fig. 75-5). The pericardial patch is cut and lowered into position with the smooth side towards the left atrium. Each of the sutures is tied, and then each arm of the double-armed suture is run 90 degrees to meet its opposite suture. Just before completing this process, the left side of the heart is filled with blood by ventilating the patient to increase pulmonary venous return and thereby expressing any air remaining in the left atrium (Fig. 75-6). The patient is then positioned in a steeply head-down position

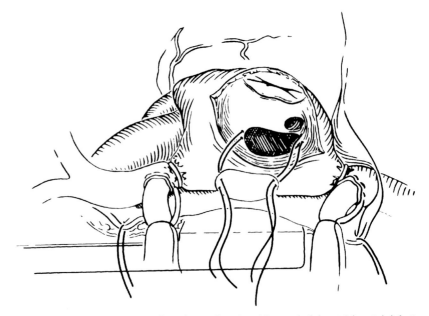

Figure 75-5. Two separate sutures have been placed at either end of the atrial septal defect and then through the pericardium. The pericardial patch has been cut and is now lowered into position. Each of these sutures is then tied and run toward its opposite suture.

of tissue surrounding the ASD, particularly along the inferior aspect of the defect. For these reasons, there still is an occasional secundum defect that is best served through surgical closure.

There are a number of early and late complications that have been reported following Amplatzer insertion that may need surgical intervention. Systemic thromboembolism has been observed following implantation of an Amplatzer; patients who experience this problem should undergo evaluation for hypercoaguable state (e.g., anti-thrombin 3 deficiency, protein C or S deficiency) and be anticoagulated. Repeat thromboembolism is a reasonably strong mandate for removal of the Amplatzer and conventional surgical closure of the ASD. Erosion of the Amplatzer device through the atrial wall has presented as a hemopericardium associated with cardiac tamponade. This complication may be managed by repairing the laceration in the atrial wall with or without removal of the device and closure of the defect with a patch. Erosion has also been reported into the aortic root, resulting in an aortoatrial fistula. In this situation, the device must be removed, the ASD repaired with a patch, and the aorta repaired either primarily or with a patch if the defect is of significant size.

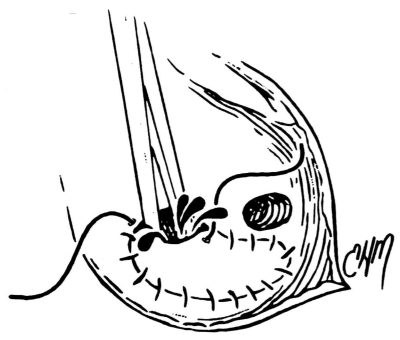

Figure 75-6. Just before completion of the repair, the left heart is de-aired.

and the cross-clamp removed with the aortic root on suction. Rewarming is performed while the right atriotomy is closed with a double running 5-0 or 6-0 nonabsorbable vascular suture. The patient is weaned from cardiopulmonary bypass once rewarming is completed.

Amplatzer Repair of Secundum-Type Atrial Septal Defects

As indicated, the majority of secundum type ASDs are now closed in the catheterization laboratory. The original ASD devices were developed >30 years ago, but were prone to late structural failures. The current design has proven to be both effective and durable (Fig. 75-7). The advantages of device closure are that it is less invasive than surgery and the recovery from the procedure is shorter. The limitations of the device include the fact that it requires a 7-F or 8-F sheath in the femoral vein, so that patients need to be at least 10 kg to 12 kg to accommodate the vascular access. Amplatzer device closure may not be feasible from a technical standpoint in patients with a deficient rim

Repair of the Superior-Type Sinus Venosus Atrial Septal Defect

The superior type of sinus venosus ASD is far more common than the inferior type. The hallmark of this diagnosis is the position of the ASD high in the right atrium above the superior limbus. The majority of the time the right upper and right middle pulmonary veins drain anomalously into the lateral aspect of the superior vena cava (SVC). The distance between the entrance of the pulmonary veins into the cava and the entrance of the cava into the roof of the right atrium can usually be assessed from the outside by dissecting these structures in advance. The azygos vein is also identified in advance so that it is not confused with a pulmonary vein when these structures are inspected from the internal aspect of the cava. When the pulmonary vein entrance is near the cavoatrial junction, a simple patch repair can be performed to channel the pulmonary vein blood flow across the ASD into the left atrium. However, it is not infrequent that the pulmonary vein entrance is a considerable distance from the cavoatrial junction. In this circumstance, we prefer the "double-patch" technique. A lateral atriotomy is performed

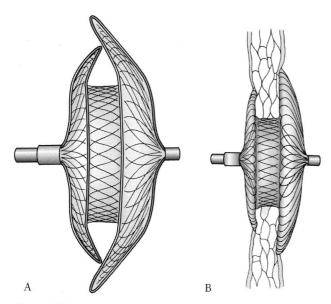

A   B

Figure 75-7. Artist's schematic of the Amplatzer septal occluder.

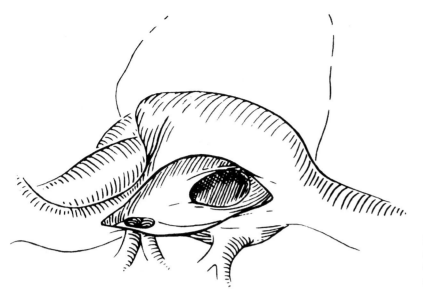

Figure 75-8. A lateral atriotomy is performed extending onto the superior vena cava. The orifice of the anomalous right superior pulmonary vein is seen entering into the cava.

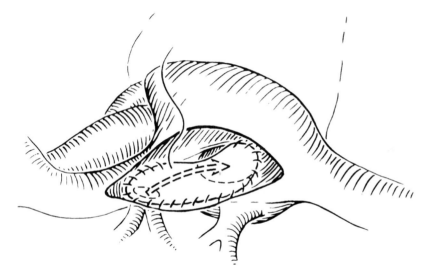

Figure 75-9. A pericardial patch is sutured above the orifice of the anomalous vein and continued inferiorly to encompass the orifice of the sinus venosus atrial septal defect.

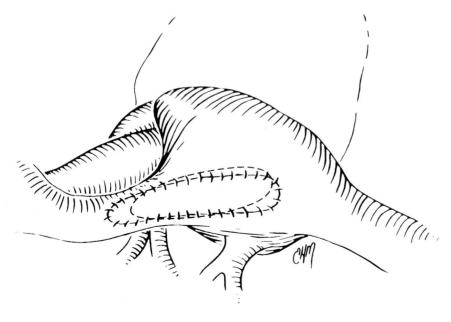

Figure 75-10. The superior vena cava and right atrial junction are augmented with a second pericardial patch to prevent narrowing of the superior vena caval orifice at this point.

and extended cephalad across the cavo-atrial junction onto the superior vena cava (Fig. 75-8). Traction sutures may be helpful to facilitate exposure. A portion of previously harvested pericardium is used to baffle the anomalous veins to the left atrium. The patch is sutured in position with 5-0 or 6-0 nonabsorbable suture, beginning at the superior apex just above the entrance of the superiormost anomalous pulmonary vein (Fig. 75-9). Suturing is continued along the lateral border of the cava and then around the lateral and inferior border of the ASD. De-airing is performed before final completion of the suture line. The repair can be inspected for leaks by having the anesthesiologist ventilate the lungs (Valsalva maneuver). Because the pericardial baffle takes up a portion of the superior vena caval cross-sectional area, primary closure of the cava might result in compromise of the lumen. Therefore, a second pericardial patch is used to augment the cava along its anterior surface (Fig. 75-10).

An alternative approach to sinus venosus defects particularly well suited when the entrance of the anomalous pulmonary veins is high in the cava is to divide the SVC above the level of the pulmonary vein entrance (the top end of the cava still attached to the right atrium is oversewn). A patch is then placed in the roof of the right atrium to divert blood flow from the right upper and middle lobe veins across the ASD into the left atrium. The patch simultaneously closes the superior vena cava from the remainder of the right atrium. The right atrial appendage is then opened and sutured to the distal portion of the SVC. The length of the atrial appendage is usually adequate to permit creation of an anastomosis without tension. Many other variations of these repairs have been described, but it is unclear whether any one technique is superior to the others.

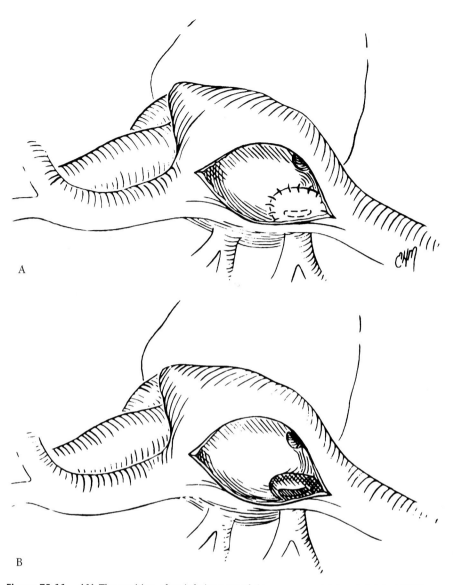

Figure 75-11. **(A)** The position of an inferior type of sinus venosus atrial septal defect (ASD, being inferior and lateral to the fossa ovalis. Through the ASD, one can see the orifice of the anomalously draining right lower lobe pulmonary vein. **(B)** A pericardial patch is used to perform the repair.

Repair of the Inferior-Type Sinus Venosus Atrial Septal Defect

The inferior type of sinus venosus ASD is relatively rare and is often a surprising finding at operation. The hallmark of this defect is the absence of a rim of tissue from the inferior vena cava (IVC) to the left atrium. This defect is positioned just above the inferior cavoatrial junction with the right lower pulmonary vein orifice quite visible through the ASD (Fig. 75-11). Thus, inferior sinus venosus defects are inferior and lateral in position as compared to secundum-type ASDs. It should also be noted that the Eustachian

valve is often quite prominent in these patients, and care must be taken to create a suture line around the inferior vena cava that does not divert the IVC flow into the left by mistaking the Eustachian valve for the inferior rim of the defect.

Repair of the inferior-type sinus venosus ASD is accomplished by closing the atrial defect with a (pericardial) patch, leaving the inferior pulmonary vein on the left atrial side of the patch and the inferior cava on the systemic venous side of the patch. If it is known in advance (by echocardiography) that an ASD is an inferior sinus venosus type, the inferior vena cava cannulation can be performed a bit lower by incising the diaphragmatic pericardium overlying the cava. How-

ever, this differentiation between secundum and inferior sinus venosus defects is difficult to make by echocardiography, and statistically the secundum type is far more common. If the IVC is cannulated in a standard position, it may be discovered after the right atriotomy that the cannula overlies the defect. Repair can still be accomplished by clamping and removing the inferior cannula, placing a cardiotomy sucker through the cannulation site, and completing the inferior aspect of the suture line in this fashion. The cannula can be replaced once the inferior corner has been completed. The pericardial patch is brought above the entrance of the right inferior pulmonary vein to maintain proper pulmonary venous drainage.

Repair of Coronary Sinus Atrial Septal Defects

Coronary sinus ASDs are relatively rare and are usually associated with complex congenital heart disease or anomalies of systemic venous return. Conceptually, these defects can be divided into those with and those without a left superior vena cava (LSVC). In the absence of an LSVC, a coronary sinus ASD exists when the coronary sinus is unroofed into the left atrium. The distal coronary sinus acts as a passageway for blood to shunt from the left atrium to the right atrium. When an LSVC is present, it can be the cause of abnormal shunting either when it enters directly or is unroofed into the left atrium. Coronary sinus ASDs may be associated with a secundum ASD or a common atrium but may also be seen with an intact atrial septum.

The goal in repairing coronary sinus ASDs is to separate systemic and pulmonary return and eliminate shunting at the atrial level. Because these defects are adjacent to the conduction system and the pulmonary veins, care must be taken in planning and performing these repairs in order to minimize morbidity.

Repair of a coronary sinus ASD without an LSVC is accomplished by what is referred to as a "roofing" procedure. The operation is performed using bicaval venous cannulation and a standard right atriotomy. If the atrial septum is intact, the fossa ovalis is incised for exposure. The unroofed coronary sinus is identified medial to the pulmonary veins. A pericardial patch is used to cover the defect (Fig. 75-12). The atrial septum is repaired either primarily or with a second pericardial patch.

Repair of a coronary sinus ASD with an LSVC may be accomplished through one of two principal methods. Selection of the method depends on the anatomy of each particular case. When the LSVC is small, and particularly when there is a bridging vein, the simplest option is usually to ligate the LSVC and perform a roofing procedure as described previously. However, if the LSVC is large, an intra-atrial baffle technique can be considered. The fossa ovalis is incised to allow adequate inspection of the left and right atrial anatomy. A portion of the septum primum is excised under direct visualization to allow placement of the intra-atrial baffle. Autologous pericardium works quite well for this purpose. The suture line begins between the two AV valves along the rim of the ASD. Anteriorly, the suture line dips below the left atrial appendage and the orifice of the LSVC. Laterally, the suture

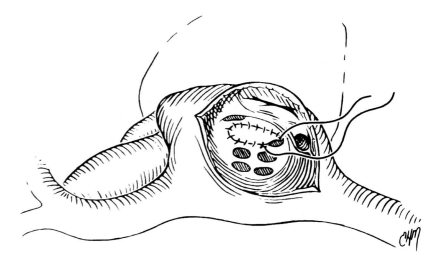

Figure 75-12. The fossa ovalis has been incised to view the left atrial anatomy. The "unroofed" coronary sinus is shown in its position medial to the four pulmonary veins. A pericardial patch is used to repair the defect.

line extends around the right pulmonary veins. Along the inferior border, the suture line follows the rim of the ASD; superficial bites are taken adjacent to the orifice of the coronary sinus (Fig. 75-13). If there is a common atrium, the orifice of the coronary sinus in the right atrium may be absent and thus the landmarks for the conduction system less certain. In this case, the baffle is sutured along the annulus of the tricuspid valve and then is carried out onto the right atrial wall to include the area of the conduction system on the left atrial side (Fig. 75-14).

Raghib syndrome refers to an LSVC to the left atrium with absence of a coronary sinus and a low-lying ASD (near the po-

sition of an inferior sinus venosus ASD). This rare condition is physiologically analogous to a coronary sinus ASD with LSVC and a common atrium (Fig. 75-14). Anatomically, the two are quite distinct because in Raghib syndrome one cannot see the pulmonary veins or left atrial appendage from the right atrium. Simple closure of the ASD results in persistent desaturation because of the LSVC to the left atrium. Raghib syndrome should be suspected whenever there is a low-lying ASD with an LSVC. Correction can be accomplished through ASD repair and ligation of the LSVC (relatively simple) or excision of the septum primum and placement of an intra-atrial baffle (complex).

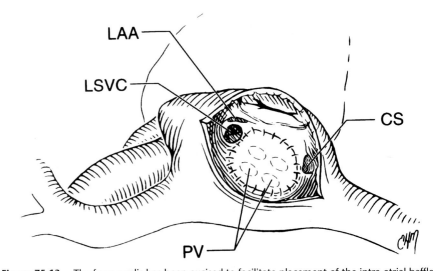

Figure 75-13. The fossa ovalis has been excised to facilitate placement of the intra-atrial baffle. The baffle directs pulmonary venous drainage to the mitral valve while the left superior vena cava (LSVC) and coronary sinus (CS) drain to the right atrium. (PV = pulmonary veins; LAA = left atrial appendage.)

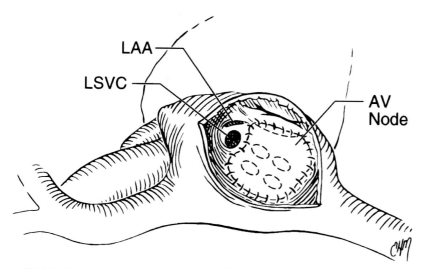

Figure 75-14. Repair of coronary sinus atrial septal defect with a left superior vena cava (LSVC), common atrium, and absence of a coronary sinus in the right atrium. The presumed location of the atrioventricular (AV) node is shown. In this situation, the medial portion of the pericardial patch is sutured to the hinge point of the tricuspid valve to avoid the bundle of His and the AV node. (LAA = left atrial appendage.)

Surgical closure of a secundum ASD in this setting is usually prompted by the poor weight gain in association with a congenital heart defect. The patients are quite frail due to their poor nutritional status and pulmonary hypertension. Thus, they should be approached with caution much like one would approach an infant with failure to thrive associated with a VSD. The operative technique is identical to the standard approach outlined previously. However, we recommend the additional placement of a pulmonary artery catheter to measure PA pressures postoperatively. This measure at first may seem unwarranted, but will serve as an early-warning system for the first time the CO_2 levels increase and the PA pressures rise to systemic or suprasystemic levels. It has been our experience with this entity that many of these patients will continue to demonstrate poor growth after surgical repair of the ASD, but at least the congenital heart defect is removed from the potential list of causes.

Repair of Scimitar Syndrome

Scimitar syndrome is a relatively rare group of findings that may be associated with an ASD. This condition is associated with anomalous venous drainage of the right lung to the inferior vena cava at the level of the diaphragm. This anomalous vein creates a curvilinear density adjacent to the right heart border and was likened to the shape of a Turkish sword (or scimitar). In its full-blown manifestation, scimitar syndrome also includes hypoplasia of the right lung, hypoplasia of the right mainstem bronchus, shift of the mediastinum to the right (dextroposition of the heart), pulmonary sequestration to the right lower lobe, and a secundum-type ASD. Not all of the patients have the complete spectrum of abnormalities, thus accounting for the considerable variability among patients with this syndrome.

Operative techniques for repair of scimitar syndrome have traditionally been (1) baffling of the right pulmonary vein flow through the right atrium across a secundum ASD to the left atrium, (2) reimplantation of the anomalous pulmonary veins higher into the right atrium with baffling across the ASD, and (3) reimplantation of the anomalous pulmonary veins into the left atrium with closure of the ASD. These techniques have all been associated with failures due to kinking and obstruction of the pulmonary veins. A fourth alternative that may be used when it is apparent that the anatomy is not amenable to any of these techniques is to incise the walls of the right atrium and the right common pulmonary vein as they travel in parallel and then sew the edges together in a side-to-side anastomosis. This brings the right pulmonary vein confluence more superiorly in the right atrium and can then be baffled to the left atrium through the ASD without creating any point at which the baffle becomes narrowed or has an acute change in direction.

Atrial Septal Defect with Failure to Thrive

There is the occasional patient who will present in infancy with a secundum-type ASD and failure to thrive. These patients demonstrate poor eating and poor weight gain, and have the clinical appearance that one would normally associate with infants who have a large ventricular septal defect. It is also of note that these patients invariably have significant pulmonary hypertension, with pulmonary artery (PA) pressures typically one-half to three-fourths systemic. The pulmonary vascular resistance tends to be quite elevated, so that the Qp:Qs is usually on the low side (1.5:2.0) for patients with ASDs. The right ventricle is usually noted to be thick due to the increased PA pressures. Some of these patients will have Down syndrome, and others will have a dysmorphic appearance that may be part of an unnamed syndrome. It has been speculated that the primary abnormality in this setting is the pulmonary hypertension and that the ASD is almost an incidental finding.

Conclusion

ASDs are among the more common forms of congenital heart defect. Repair of an ASD is a curative procedure that restores a normal life expectancy. With modern techniques, these procedures can be performed with an extraordinarily low rate of morbidity and mortality.

SUGGESTED READING

Becker RM. Intracardiac surgery in pregnant women. Ann Thorac Surg 1983;36:453.

de Leval MR, Ritter DG, McGoon DC, et al. Anomalous systemic venous connection. Surgical considerations. Mayo Clin Proc 1975;50:599.

Divekar A, Gaamangwe T, Shaikh N, et al. Cardiac perforation after device closure of atrial septal defects with the Amplatzer septal occluder. J Am Coll Cardiol 2005;45:1213.

Gatzoulis MA, Redington AN, Sommerville J, et al. Should atrial septal defects in adults be closed? Ann Thorac Surg 1996;61:657.

Hamilton WT, Haffajee CI, Dalen JE, et al. Atrial Septal Defect Secundum: Clinical Profile with Physiologic Correlates in Children and Adults. In Roberts WC (ed), Congenital Heart Disease in Adults. Philadelphia: FA Davis, 1990;267.

Hoffman JI. Congenital heart disease: incidence and inheritance. Pediatr Clin North Am 1990;37:25.

Mandelik J, Moodie DS, Sterba R, et al. Long-term follow-up of children after repair of atrial septal defects. Cleve Clin J Med 1994;61:29.

Murphy JG, Gersh BJ, McGoon MD, et al. Long-term outcome after surgical repair of isolated atrial septal defect—Follow-up at 27–32 years. N Engl J Med 1990;323:1645.

EDITOR'S COMMENTS

Although ASD usually of the secundum type is one of the most common congenital heart defects seen in any clinical practice, it is not a completely benign lesion. Even small ASDs can be associated with paradoxical embolus late in life, and the association of secundum ASDs and late development of pulmonary hypertension with elevated pulmonary resistance is well known. It appears that there are subsets of patients who in the face of a left-to-right shunt have a predisposition to development of pulmonary vascular disease. Thus, the development of pulmonary vascular disease does not necessarily correlate with the size of the defect or the age of the patient. For these reasons, we believe that even small ASDs should preferentially be closed early in life to prevent late complications. With the advent of occluder devices, it may be possible to close even small ASDs with very little morbidity and eliminate even minor risks of paradoxical emboli or volume overload of the right ventricle with the consequent arrhythmias. As noted by the authors, when an ASD presents in adulthood with only a small shunt, the occurrence of significant pulmonary vascular disease must be suspected and closure might not be indicated if there is any bidirectional or right-to-left shunting.

ASD closure is now commonly being performed for secundum defects with occluder devices such as the Amplatzer device. As noted, there are still complications with these devices, which fortunately are rare, but include erosion into the aorta or through the atrial wall. In addition, as larger devices are being deployed for defects that previously were not amenable to device closure, the incidence of such complications may increase; therefore, continued longitudinal follow-up of patients with occluder devices is necessary. Certainly a small proportion will eventually require removal and standard ASD closure.

The surgical techniques for closure of ASDs are numerous. We prefer a vertical skin incision in both male and female patients, especially when the operation is performed in early childhood. These incisions are quite short and quite low to make them as cosmetic as possible. A sternotomy incision is generally used. We have avoided transverse incisions in young girls because it may be difficult to identify breast tissue, and if the incision cuts across any breast tissue, unsightly scars can occur. In addition, we have abandoned the thoracotomy incision for ASD closure in most cases because if the mammary pedicle is damaged, there may be asymmetric breast development. Thus, we believe that the most cosmetic incision may well be a very small low vertical incision in the midline over the xiphoid (2.5 cm in length), which avoids elevation of major skin flaps and usually heals with excellent cosmetic results.

The minimally invasive approach to secundum ASD repair through a small subxiphoid incision can be done with the use of electrical fibrillation and normothermic bypass, which avoids the need to cross-clamp the aorta. Even in larger secundum defects without a superior rim, where patch closure is necessary, the procedure can be performed through these small incisions without the need for cardioplegic arrest. Operations for atrial septal defects are generally done under normothermia at our institution because bypass and cross-clamp times are generally extremely short.

Some comments are warranted on the multiple techniques for repair of sinus venosus–type ASDs of the superior and inferior types. The authors described a technique for repair of the superior sinus venosus defect that also involves patching of the superior vena cava/right atrial junction. In the majority of cases, sinus venosus defects occur just at the superior vena cava/right atrial junction and the right pulmonary veins enter at that site. In these cases, approach through a right atrial incision as used for secundum defects with gentle retraction on the superior vena cava will expose the defects adequately so that direct patch closure can be performed without narrowing the vena cava as it enters the right atrium. Care must be taken, however, to tailor the patch appropriately so that it does not bulge into the superior vena cava or left atrium. The advantage of this approach is avoidance of an incision across the superior vena cava/right atrial junction, which might interrupt sinus node blood supply. In cases where the right pulmonary veins enter high in the superior vena cava well away from the right atrium we have preferred the use of the Warden-type repair as described in this chapter, in which the superior vena cava is divided and then reconnected to the right atrial appendage and the stump of the superior vena cava, to which the anomalous veins return is baffled across the atrial septal defect to the left atrium. This approach avoids the need for an incision across the caval-atrial junction that may interfere with sinus node blood supply, and there have been many recent reports of excellent consistent results with this technique with a low incidence of late development of superior vena caval stenosis. If superior vena caval stenosis occurs at the suture line, and if the azygos vein is left open, decompression is often to the inferior vena cava, and the SVC can be dilated or stented in the catheterization lab if significant obstruction is present.

The authors described the techniques for repair of scimitar syndrome, which include reimplantation of the anomalous vein or baffling of the vein across an atrial septal defect to the left atrium. They presented a good summary of the various techniques that have been used. Recently there has been a resurgence of interest in reimplantation of the right-sided pulmonary veins directly into the left atrium through a right thoracotomy incision without the use of cardiopulmonary bypass. An advantage of this technique is the fact that the geometry of the vein can be better assessed with the lung slightly inflated through a thoracotomy incision, which may prevent kinking of the vein as it enters the left atrium. This technique is most applicable when there is not a significant atrial septal defect present. Although it is possible to close the atrial septal defect through a right anterior thoracotomy incision and reimplant the anomalous vein, we believe that if bypass is necessary, a standard sternotomy incision is generally the simplest way to get to the areas of interest and avoids struggling with division of the right pulmonary vein entrance at the level of the diaphragm. Although the few reports of direct reimplantation off bypass through a thoracotomy have suggested a very good patency rate, the development of stenosis or occlusion of the reimplanted vein over time needs to continue to be assessed before this technique can be adapted routinely.

It should also be noted that scimitar syndrome presenting in infancy with significant pulmonary hypertension has a very poor prognosis. Because of the high incidence of vein obstruction in scimitar syndrome in adulthood, some authors have recommended that these patients be followed without operative intervention. We still believe, however, that patients with a significant left-to-right shunt and no associated anomalies with no evidence of pulmonary vascular resistance should be considered for surgical therapy with attention to the technical details to prevent vein obstruction.

Drs. Mainwaring and Lamberti also commented on the presence of ASDs with failure to thrive in infancy. Although it is certainly not predictable that closure of a secundum ASD will alter the growth patterns of very young children (because generally these shunts are not large), I have seen several patients over the years who have had marked improvement after a moderate-sized secundum defect was closed in infancy. Care must be taken, however, to ensure that these patients do not have additional left-sided cardiac lesions that exacerbate the left-to-right shunt from a relatively small ASD and that can be unmasked after ASD closure. Nevertheless, in patients with no other cause for failure to thrive and a significant ASD, I believe that the low risk of closing the defect is warranted.

T.L.S.

76

Ventricular Septal Defects

Christopher J. Knott-Craig

Ventricular septal defects (VSDs) are among the most common congenital heart anomalies; isolated VSDs represent about 20% to 30% of all congenital cardiac malformations and have a prevalence of 1 to 2 per 1,000 live births.

The initial description of the clinical signs and symptoms of a VSD is ascribed to Rogier in 1879, and a small, flow-limiting VSD with associated normal pulmonary artery pressures carries the eponym "malady de Rogier ventricular septal defect." At the other end of the clinical spectrum is a large VSD with severe pulmonary hypertension and fixed pulmonary vascular resistance resulting in cyanosis with right-to-left shunting through the VSD; this is known as the "Eisenmenger complex," following the description of such a patient in 1897.

VSDs may be associated with a wide variety of other cardiac defects, including mitral valve disease, atrioventricular (AV) discordance, conotruncal abnormalities such as transposition or double-outlet ventricle, and hypoplasia of either ventricle. In this chapter, I cover isolated VSDs and those associated with patent ductus arteriosus and coarctation of the aorta.

Classification of Ventricular Septal Defects

Of the many classifications of VSDs, the most widely accepted today are those of Soto and van Praagh (Fig. 76-1). The ventricular septum has three main components: (1) an inlet portion beneath the septal leaflet of the tricuspid valve and extending from the tricuspid annulus to the papillary attachments of the tricuspid valve chordae,

(2) a trabecular, or muscular, portion that extends from the chordal attachments of the tricuspid valve to the apex of the ventricles and cephalad to the conal septum, and (3) a smooth-walled conal or outlet septum, which comprises the infundibular septum clasped between the anterior and posterior limbs of the septal band (trabecular septomarginalis) and extends up to the pulmonary and aortic annuli. The inlet and trabecular portions are often referred to collectively as the ventricular septum, in contrast to the conal septum, which is also called the "outlet" or "infundibular" septum.

Conoventricular Defects (Perimembranous Defects)

Conoventricular defects are the most common isolated VSDs, comprising about 70% to 80% in most series. They are situated in the junctional area between the conal and inlet portions of the septum and may extend into the inlet, outlet, or both parts of the septum. They extend up to the tricuspid valve annulus in the region of the anteroseptal commissure of the tricuspid valve. The aortic valve is easily visible through the defect when viewed through the tricuspid valve at operation. Occasionally the noncoronary aortic leaflet may prolapse through the defect, resulting in progressive aortic incompetence.

The bundle of His penetrates the right trigone of the central fibrous body at the anteroseptal commissure of the tricuspid valve. From there it is closely related to the lower half (posteroinferior edge) of the defect, giving off the left fascicles along its course to the medial papillary muscle (also called the muscle of Lancisi or the papillary muscle of the conus). As it passes just inferior to the latter, only the right bundle remains,

and this continues into the trabecula septomarginalis away from the edge of the defect. Conoventricular septal defects are usually repaired through the right atrium.

Conotruncal Defects (Outlet Defects)

Conotruncal defects are also called supracristal, subpulmonary, juxta-arterial, or infundibular. They account for 5% to 10% of isolated defects, except in the Asian population, in whom they are more common. Typically, the defects are oval in shape and extend up to the pulmonary and aortic annuli. Because the normal subpulmonary conus is deficient, the pulmonary and aortic valves are separated only by a very thin rim of fibrous tissue. This results in aortic leaflet prolapse, which occurs in 40% to 50% of conal defects. The right aortic leaflet most commonly is sucked into the defect, resulting in aortic incompetence. The conduction tissue is remote from the borders of this type of VSD, which is most easily repaired through a short transverse incision in the right ventricular outflow tract, or through the main pulmonary artery (Fig. 76-1). If the defect is completely surrounded by muscle, it is referred to as an outlet muscular defect.

Inlet Septal Defects (Atrioventricular Canal–Type Defects)

Inlet septal defects account for about 5% of isolated defects. They are situated beneath the septal leaflet of the tricuspid valve, with the tricuspid valve annulus forming their posterior border. The conduction tissue is closely related to the posteroinferior border of the defect, up to the muscle of Lancisi,

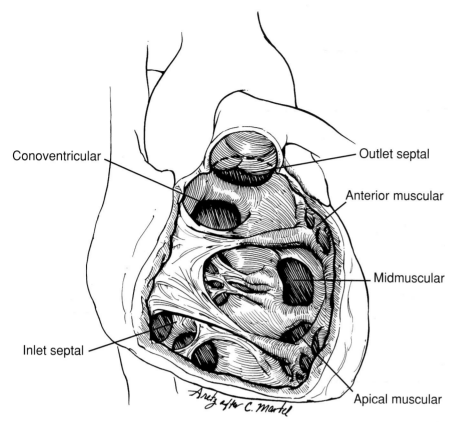

Conoventricular

Outlet septal

Anterior muscular

Midmuscular

Inlet septal

Apical muscular

Aretz after C. Martel

Figure 76-1. The right ventricular free wall has been resected to show the ventricular septal defects: conoventricular = perimembranous; conal septal = outlet septal (subpulmonary); inlet septal = atrioventricular canal type; muscular (trabecular) defects may be midmuscular, anterior, or apical. The penetrating bundle is closely related to the inferior margin of the conoventricular defect and diverges away from this margin into the trabecular septomarginalis beneath the muscle of Lancisi.

at which point the right bundle branch diverges down the trabecula septomarginalis into the moderator band. The AV septum is intact, although occasionally the anterior leaflet of the mitral valve may be partially cleft. Inlet septal defects are best repaired through the tricuspid valve.

Muscular Defects (Trabecular Defects)

Muscular VSDs account for 10% to 15% of isolated VSDs, may be single or multiple, and may occur in any part of the septum. They may be associated with other types of VSDs and are generally divided into midmuscular defects (most common), apical muscular, and anterior muscular defects (Fig. 76-1). Muscular defects may have numerous openings of variable size on the right ventricular side but only a single opening on the left ventricular side of the septum: This is referred to as a "Swiss cheese defect."

The conduction tissue is generally remote from the edges of a muscular defect, with two notable exceptions: (1) When

associated with a conoventricular defect (perimembranous VSD), the penetrating bundle usually runs in the muscle bridge separating the two defects and may easily be injured if they each closed individually, and (2) if a muscular defect is present in the inlet septum (i.e., the defect is separated from the tricuspid valve by a thin rim of muscle), the conduction tissue runs along the defect superior and anterior (leftward) margin—the AV node penetrates the interventricular septum at the anteroseptal commissure of the tricuspid valve and takes the most direct route to the medial papillary muscle along the superior border of the defect.

Indications for Operation

Historically, small infants with a large VSD were initially palliated by placing a constricting band around the main pulmonary artery, suturing this to the adventitia, and

gradually narrowing the band circumference until the systolic pressure in the pulmonary artery distal to the band was reduced by 50%. This decreased the flow through the pulmonary artery, ameliorated congestive cardiac failure, and allowed the patient to grow to a large enough size for the band to be removed and the VSD to be safely repaired. However, as methods of myocardial protection advanced and the surgical skills and the postoperative care of small infants improved, pulmonary artery banding was abandoned in favor of primary closure of the VSD, except in rare instances that will be outlined later.

When reviewing the indications for surgical closure of a VSD, there are four aspects to take into consideration: (1) characteristics of the defect, (2) the patient's age and symptoms, (3) pulmonary vascular resistance, and (4) associated cardiac and noncardiac defects.

Ventricular Septal Defect Characteristics

About 50% to 70% of large VSDs discovered during the neonatal period will close or become small defects spontaneously within 6 to 12 months. This is especially true for conoventricular and muscular defects. Inlet (AV canal) defects and outlet (supracristal) defects do not generally close spontaneously. Defects are considered "large" if they approximate the size of the aortic annulus or result in systemic pulmonary artery pressures. "Medium-sized" defects result in a Qp:Qs ratio of 2:1 to 3:1 and a systolic pulmonary artery pressure that is 40 to 50 mm Hg or about one-half that of the aorta. "Small" defects have essentially normal pulmonary artery pressures and a Qp:Qs ratio of <1.5:1. A simple formula for calculating the Qp:Qs ratio using only oxygen saturations is as follows:

$$Qp:Qs = (Ao\% - RA\%)/(PV\% - PA\%)$$

where Ao% is the . . . , RA% is the . . . , PV% is the . . . , and PA% is the . . . . If a VSD is associated with significant prolapse of the aortic valve leaflet, this should be repaired irrespective of symptoms or the size of the defect. If even mild aortic incompetence is associated with any type of VSD, the defect should be promptly closed and the aortic valve repaired.

Indications for closure of defects in infancy are as follows:

1. All large or symptomatic VSDs.
2. All medium-sized VSDs associated with failure to thrive.

3. All VSDs associated with aortic incompetence.

4. All inlet or outlet VSDs.

5. All residual VSDs >3 mm or those associated with elevated pulmonary artery pressures.

6. All VSDs irrespective of size, if associated with another reason for cardiac surgery.

Patient Characteristics

Infants with large VSDs presenting in the first few months of life with severe congestive heart failure should undergo prompt repair. Delaying surgery until the patient is "bigger" is not beneficial and often results in additional morbidity and mortality. These infants are often too tachypneic to feed orally, experience recurrent chest infections and aspiration of gastric contents, and may have a pulmonary hyperinflation syndrome ("cardiac asthma"). The latter results from systemic pressure in the segmental pulmonary arteries compressing the small bronchi and resulting in chronic air trapping. The exception to early primary closure in a symptomatic infant is the presence of multiple muscular defects, which is still associated with significant mortality when repaired in infancy. This is one of the few remaining indications for pulmonary artery banding. Debanding of the pulmonary artery and repair of the VSDs is done when the patient is about 9 to 18 months of age. Some muscular defects may be suitable for percutaneous catheter device closure by our cardiology colleagues. This can be done either before operation, intraoperatively, or postoperatively. Apical and anterior muscular defects are often difficult to adequately close in the operating room and may be closed percutaneously.

Infants with symptoms controlled with medical therapy and large defects that have not appreciably decreased in size should be electively repaired at between 6 months and 1 year of age. Few of these infants are thriving; most have poor weight gain and failure to thrive, and many may already have developed increased pulmonary vascular resistance. These infants are considered to have "reactive pulmonary hypertension" and are at increased risk of developing pulmonary hypertensive crises during the postoperative period, particularly if their surgery is delayed.

Beyond 12 to 18 months of age, patients with large VSDs should undergo cardiac catheterization and be repaired if (1) their pulmonary vascular resistance is <8 to 10 U/m^2, (2) there is no desaturation with exercise, and (3) the Qp:Qs ratio exceeds 1.3:1 at rest and with exercise.

In the absence of significant symptoms, repair of small or medium-sized VSDs should be delayed until the child is 2 to 3 years of age to allow spontaneous closure of the defect. When small defects are discovered later in childhood, spontaneous closure is unlikely. These defects should be closed if any complications develop; these include endocarditis and psychological trauma (e.g., "I hate this murmur" or "They won't let me take part in school sports with a heart murmur.").

Pulmonary Vascular Resistance

Pulmonary vascular resistance is seldom prohibitive during the first year of life in patients with an isolated VSD, except occasionally in patients with associated Down syndrome; these patients tend to develop pulmonary vascular obstructive disease at an earlier age, sometimes as young as 6 to 9 months of age.

If the VSD is first detected beyond the first 12 to 18 months of age, the patient should be catheterized and the pulmonary vascular resistance (pulmonary arteriolar resistance index, PARI) calculated. If this is >8 U/m^2 or if the Qp:Qs ratio is <1.5:1, the calculations should be repeated with the patient breathing supplemental oxygen (or with an intravenous infusion of a pulmonary vasodilator) to determine whether the increased resistance is reactive or fixed. If the Qp:Qs ratio increases (>1.5:1) and the PARI decreases (<8.0 U/m^2), the defect is repaired. In a patient with high fixed resistance, the defect should not be closed.

Associated Cardiac and Noncardiac Pathologic Conditions

Infants with significant additional left-to-right shunts, such as an atrial septal defect or patent ductus arteriosus, usually have intractable congestive cardiac failure in early infancy. Early primary closure of all defects is thus indicated. There is a slightly increased risk and morbidity associated with repair of these infants, which relates mainly to their poor preoperative condition. In contrast, neonates and young infants with associated coarctation of the aorta should first have the coarctation repaired through a left thoracotomy. If they cannot be weaned from the ventilator or continue to have severe symptoms after the coarctation repair, prompt repair of the VSD is advised during the same hospitalization. This approach has been shown to be superior to simultaneous primary repair of both defects and avoids the unnecessary repair of the VSD in about one half of the patients.

There are a few exceptions to this approach: (1) coarctation and associated multiple muscular septal defects in which pulmonary artery banding may be done at the time of the coarctation repair through the same incision; (2) coarctation and associated large outlet septal (subpulmonary) defect in which simultaneous primary repair is indicated because this type of VSD does not usually undergo spontaneous closure, and (3) VSD and associated aortic interruption, which are best simultaneously repaired through a midline approach.

About 25% of infants undergoing repair of isolated VSD have some noncardiac morphologic syndrome or pathologic condition (e.g., Down syndrome, Vater syndrome, tracheoesophageal fistula, etc.) associated with their VSD. In very symptomatic infants, it is often difficult to quantify the contribution to symptoms of a medium-sized defect. Early closure of the cardiac defect is therefore reasonable.

Technique of Repairing Ventricular Septal Defects

Patients younger than 2 to 3 months of age (or ≤3.5 kg in weight) usually undergo repair with the technique of profound hypothermic (15°C to 18°C) circulatory arrest. The right atrial appendage is cannulated with a single 16-F right-angled venous cannula, and the ascending aorta is cannulated with an 8-F or 10-F cannula. Bypass is commenced at 150 to 200 ml/kg, and the ductus arteriosus is ligated while the patient is being cooled. The ductus should always be ligated before the circulation is arrested to prevent air in the opened right heart from entering the aorta inadvertently through a small undiagnosed patent ductus arteriosus. Once the target temperature has been reached, the aorta is clamped, and a single dose of cold blood is given via a cardioplegia needle in the ascending aorta. The circulation is then stopped, and the venous cannula is removed once the patient has been drained. The defect is then repaired.

For older infants, bicaval cannulation is used and the repair is done using moderate hypothermia (28°C to 32°C) and multidose cold blood cardioplegia. A convenient method for cannulating the venae cavae, especially with very ill or very small infants, small residual defects that may remain after operation.

Repair of Conoventricular Defects

Conoventricular defects are usually repaired through the right atrium, which is opened with an oblique incision parallel to the right AV groove (Fig. 76-2, transatrial approach). A small retractor is used to retract the tricuspid anterior leaflet, and a second, smaller retractor is used to expose the superior margin of the defect in the vicinity of the anteroseptal commissure. Gentle caudal traction on a small right-angled sucker or vascular clamp that has been placed through the VSD brings into view the superior and anterior margins of the defect. The anterosuperior triangle where the aortic valve, tricuspid annulus, and parietoinfundibular fold meet—the "attic" of the VSD—is the most difficult to expose (and therefore the most common site of residual defects). The exposure may be facilitated by the first assistant flexing his or her right index finger, which is positioned at the base of the aortic root between the aorta and the right atrium; this brings into view the "attic."

The VSD is repaired with a Dacron felt patch, which is cut a little larger than the defect, and a continuous suture technique. As viewed by the surgeon through the tricuspid valve, both ends of a 5-0 polypropylene suture, supported by a felt pledget, are passed through the right side of the interventricular septum about 2 mm to 3 mm away from the edge. The suture is begun on the part of the septum farthest away from the surgeon (at 12 o'clock), close to the muscle of Lancisi (Fig. 76-3). The ends are then passed through the patch and tied down; by gently retracting the patch in a caudal (right-hand) direction, the anterior and superior (left-hand) edge of the defect and the "attic" are progressively brought into view and the continuous whipstitch is carried around the superior margin (left-hand half) of the defect until it is passed through the hinge portion of the tricuspid septal leaflet. The other end of the suture is then carried around the posterior and inferior borders (the right-hand half) of the defect, placing the sutures 3 mm to 4 mm from the edge in the vicinity of the conduction tissue (from 2 o'clock to 5 o'clock) until this end is also passed through the tricuspid septal leaflet. The suture line is then completed as a horizontal mattress suture, which allows the patch to lie beneath the septal leaflet. The two ends of the suture are then tied over a pericardial patch, completing the repair (Fig. 76-3, inset). If

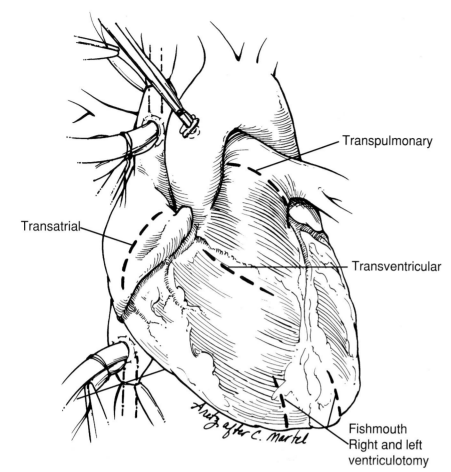

Figure 76-2. The common incisions through which ventricular septal defects are repaired.

is to connect both venous cannulas to the venous line of the bypass machine and then to first cannulate the right atrial appendage with the smaller of the two venous cannulas and commence cardiopulmonary bypass. With the lungs deflated and the heart decompressed on bypass, the next purse-string suture and second venous cannula may then be placed easily in the inferior vena cava. Once this has been done, the first cannula can be clamped, removed from the right atrium, and inserted directly into the superior vena cava through a new purse-string suture. The ductus is then ligated and the patient cooled to the appropriate temperature. No attempt is made to expose or ligate the ductus arteriosus until cardiopulmonary bypass has been established lest the ductus be torn and uncontrollable hemorrhage result. Once the patient is on bypass, the pressure in the aorta and main pulmonary artery is greatly reduced, making dissection of the ductus easy and safe; it may then be obliterated with a 5-0 polypropylene suture or a vascular clip (in neonates).

After the aorta has been clamped and the heart arrested with cardioplegic perfusate, the right atrium is opened with an oblique incision (Fig. 76-2). A pump sump sucker is placed in the left ventricle through a natural defect or stab incision in the interatrial septum to keep the operative field dry. If the repair is done through the right ventricle or pulmonary artery, the sucker is placed in the left ventricle via the right superior pulmonary vein or left atrial appendage.

Occasionally, the defect is small enough for it to be closed using interrupted horizontal mattress sutures of 4-0 or 5-0 polypropylene supported by small felt pledgets. However, usually some sort of patch material is needed for the repair, and polyester (Dacron) velour is the most commonly used patch material. Alternatively, tanned autologous pericardium, glutaraldehyde-treated bovine pericardium, or polytetrafluoroethylene (Gore-Tex) surgical patch may be used. The advantage of using Dacron is the vigorous endocardial reaction that it stimulates; this expedites the spontaneous closure of

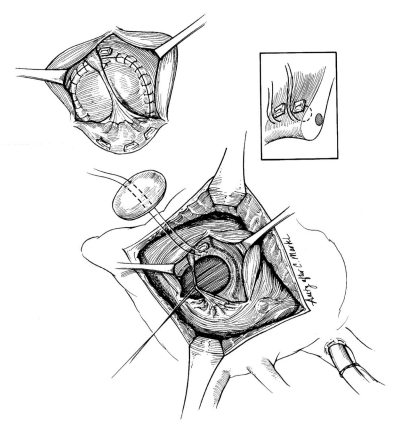

Figure 76-3. Transatrial closure of a ventricular septal defect using a continuous suture technique. The first suture is placed just inferior to the muscle of Lancisi and about 3 mm from the edge of the defect. To the right of this suture the conduction fibers are vulnerable up to the point where the suture is passed through the tricuspid septal leaflet. To the left of the first suture is the "safe" area. **(Inset)** The completed repair.

the septum is very friable or the suture line is unusually long, it is advisable to bolster the continuous suture with a few interrupted pledgeted horizontal mattress sutures to prevent postoperative patch dehiscence.

The sucker is withdrawn from the left atrium, and the cardioplegia line is disconnected from the catheter in the ascending aorta. The left atrium is then filled with enough cold saline so that first air and then saline escapes through the catheter in the ascending aorta. The atrial septal defect or patent foramen ovale is closed, suction is placed on the catheter in the ascending aorta, and the cross-clamp is released. The right atrium is then closed with a running 5-0 monofilament suture while the patient is being rewarmed or while low-flow hypothermic bypass is recommended if the repair was done with circulatory arrest. Spontaneous rhythm usually resumes with rewarming. Temporary atrial and ventricular pacing leads are always placed on the heart before the chest is closed.

Occasionally, the "attic" of the VSD is difficult to visualize either because it extends well into the outlet (infundibular) septum

or because of troublesome tricuspid valve chordae. This part of the VSD may then be better exposed by incising the tricuspid leaflets 1 mm to 2 mm from their hinge point on the annulus and reflecting them caudally (Fig. 76-4). This beautifully exposes that part of the defect, which is then repaired as described. The leaflets are then sutured back to the annulus using a continuous 5-0 polypropylene suture. An alternative technique is to divide the obstructing chordae, complete the repair, then suture the chordae back either to the septum or to the patch with 5-0 polypropylene sutures.

In neonates or very young infants, the tissue is very friable and does not hold sutures well. In these patients it is better to use an interrupted suture technique. Pledgeted horizontal mattress sutures are first placed in the septum around the edge of the defect and individually tagged. Once all the sutures have been placed, they are passed through the patch, which is then lowered and the sutures tied down.

Occasionally, a conoventricular defect is repaired through the right ventricle rather than the right atrium, usually because additional procedures need to be done through the ventriculotomy. An oblique incision is then made in the infundibulum parallel to the right ventricular or conal branches of the

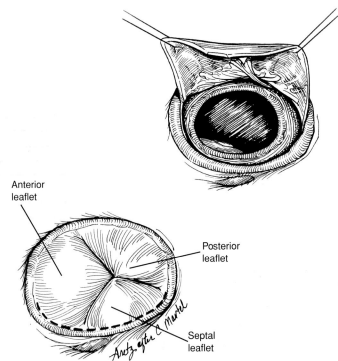

Figure 76-4. The tricuspid leaflets may be detached 1 mm to 2 mm from the annulus to improve exposure in some conoventricular or inlet septal defects. Note that the atrioventricular node penetrates the right trigone of the central fibrous body at the anteroseptal commissure of the tricuspid valve.

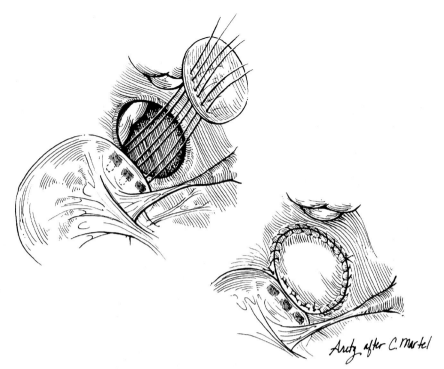

Figure 76-5. Transventricular closure of a conoventricular defect. Initially interrupted pledgeted horizontal mattress sutures are passed from the right atrial side through the tricuspid leaflet, then through the Dacron patch. These are then tied down and the suture line completed with a continuous 5-0 polypropylene suture. The most vulnerable area is the transitional area between the septal leaflet and the muscle of Lancisi (medial papillary muscle). Sutures should be placed 3 mm to 4 mm from the edge of the defect in this area.

may result in significant tricuspid regurgitation. When an interrupted suture technique is used, it is often easier to first position the patch on the septum behind these chordae (the position in which the patch will ultimately lie) before placing any of the sutures through the patch and tying them down.

Repair of Inlet Septal Defects

These defects are generally repaired through the right atrium similar to conoventricular defects. Because the defect is almost entirely beneath the tricuspid septal leaflet, detaching this leaflet from the annulus and retracting it anteriorly makes exposure easy (Fig. 76-4). This is only rarely necessary, though, because inlet (AV canal)-type defects are easily exposed through the tricuspid valve. It is important not to make the patch too wide (from the tricuspid annulus to the crest of the septum), because increased patch bulkiness tends to interfere with the mobility of the septal leaflet. It is important to differentiate an inlet septal defect from a muscular defect in the inlet septum because, in the latter, the bundle of His runs in the thin rim of muscle separating the VSD from the tricuspid valve annulus.

right coronary artery (Fig. 76-2, transventricular). The muscle of Lancisi is again the important landmark, separating the "safe" from the "vulnerable" areas. Usually, two to four interrupted pledgeted horizontal mattress sutures of 5-0 braided material are passed through the hinge portion of the tricuspid leaflet so that the pledgets lie on the right atrial side; the sutures are then passed through the patch, which is then lowered into the ventricle and tied down (Fig. 76-5). A pump sucker placed through the tricuspid valve and retracted inferiorly improves the exposure by separating the tricuspid leaflets. A separate continuous suture of 5-0 polypropylene is then used to complete the repair along the muscular edge (Fig. 76-5). Starting with one end, the suturing advances counterclockwise along the inferior margin of the defect, staying 3 mm to 4 mm away from the vulnerable area. The suture is then tagged, and a new suture is used to complete the repair in a clockwise direction along the superior rim of the defect until the suture line is complete and the two ends are tied (Fig. 76-5). With the continuous suture technique, the needle often needs to be passed back and forth behind important chordae to prevent entrapment, which

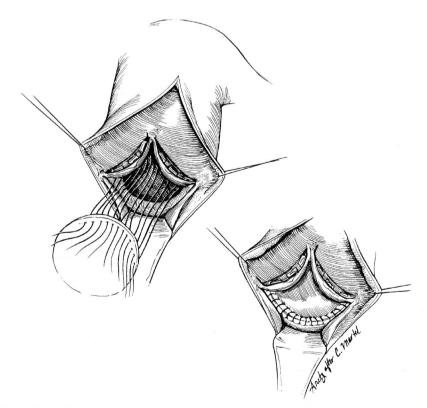

Figure 76-6. Transpulmonary closure of a conal septal (juxta-arterial) defect. The superior margin of the defect is closed by placing interrupted pledgeted sutures through the annulus of the pulmonary valve from within the sinuses. The inferior margin is completed with a running 5-0 polypropylene suture. The conduction fibers are remote from the edge of the defects.

Repair of Conal Septal Defects

Defects in the infundibular septum are approached through the pulmonary valve via a transverse incision in the main pulmonary artery (Fig. 76-2, transpulmonary) or the right ventricular outflow tract just proximal to the pulmonary valve. Conal septal defects are juxta-arterial, the superior margin of the defect being the pulmonary and aortic valves. These are frequently separated by only a thin fibrous rim, which is inadequate to support sutures. In the repair, interrupted pledgeted sutures therefore are placed through the annulus of the pulmonary valve so that the pledgets lie within the pulmonary valve sinuses and are tied below the valve in the right ventricle (Fig. 76-6). The inferior margin of the defect is closed with a continuous suture as for other defects. The conduction tissue is remote from the edges of the VSD. Some of these patients will ultimately come to aortic valve replacement, especially if they have aortic valve prolapse or incompetence at the time of closure of their VSD. Consideration should therefore be given to preserving the pulmonary valve and annulus during the repair lest they need a Ross procedure in the future: If there is a muscular rim below the pulmonary annulus, this should be used rather than the pulmonary annulus, as described previously, to secure the superior sutures.

Repair of Muscular Ventricular Septal Defects

Midmuscular defects are closed in a similar fashion to conoventricular or inlet septal defects through the right atrium. An interrupted horizontal pledgeted mattress suture technique is used, with all of the sutures placed around the perimeter of the defect or defects before the sutures are passed through the patch and tied down. When a midmuscular defect is closely associated with a conoventricular defect, the conduction fibers frequently pass in the muscle bridge between the defects (Fig. 76-7A); for this reason a single large patch is used, and the sutures are placed away from the muscle bridge so that the VSDs are closed as a "single" composite defect (Fig. 76-7B). Anterior muscular defects are repaired via a short vertical incision in the right ventricular outflow tract. The defects usually have multiple small openings on the right ventricular side and are hidden beneath the trabeculations that bind the trabecular septomarginalis to the free wall of the right ventricle. A strip of felt or pericardium is thus used inside

and another outside the right ventricle parallel to the left anterior descending artery (Fig. 76-8A), and the defect is sandwiched between the two strips with interrupted sutures (see Fig. 76-8B). Currently, some of these defects may be closed percutaneously in the catheterization suite.

Apical muscular defects and multiple muscular defects of the "Swiss cheese" variety are the most difficult to repair. Fortunately, many of these defects will close spontaneously after pulmonary artery banding. If congestive heart failure persists or the defects remain despite the band and warrant closure, they should be visualized through the right atrium in the standard fashion. If they cannot be repaired satisfactorily through the tricuspid valve, they may be approached through an apical fish-mouth left ventriculotomy (Fig. 76-1). On the left ventricular aspect of the interventric-

ular septum, there is usually a single defect, and this can be patch closed in the conventional manner. Buttressing the ventriculotomy suture line with a strip of pericardium helps to prevent postoperative hemorrhage. Alternatively, the defects may be closed preoperatively, intraoperatively, or postoperatively with clamshell-type devices in institutions experienced in the deployment of these new devices.

Results of Operation

Hospital mortality associated with the closure of isolated VSDs has steadily improved, from 10% to 15% in the 1970s to 2% to 3% in the 1990s. Incremental risk factors for mortality are (1) multiple defects, particularly those of the "Swiss cheese" variety; (2) associated additional left-to-right shunts such as large atrial septal defects, and (3)

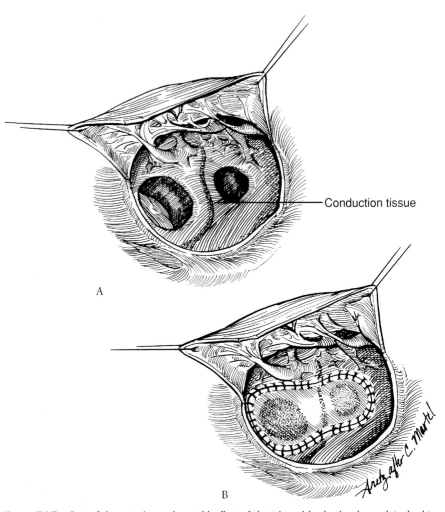

Conduction tissue

A

B

Figure 76-7.   Part of the anterior and septal leaflets of the tricuspid valve has been detached to improve exposure of a conoventricular and midmuscular septal defect. The penetrating bundle lies in the muscle bridge between the two ventricular septal defects. **(A)** The defects are closed using a single composite patch to avoid injury to the conduction tissue. **(B)** Once this has been completed, the tricuspid leaflets are sutured back on the annulus with a continuous 5-0 polypropylene suture.

Park JK, Dell RB, Ellis K, et al. Surgical management of the infant with coarctation of the aorta and ventricular septal defect. J Am Coll Cardiol 1992;20:176.

Rychik J, Norwood WI, Chin AJ. Doppler color flow mapping assessment of residual shunt after closure of large ventricular septal defects. Circulation 1991;84:III-153.

Serraf A, Lacour-Gayet F, Bruniaux J, et al. Surgical management of isolated multiple ventricular septal defects. Logical approach in 130 cases. J Thorac Cardiovasc Surg 1992;103:437.

van Praagh R, Geva T, Kreutzer J. Ventricular septal defects: How shall we describe, name and classify them? J Am Coll Cardiol 1989;14:1298.

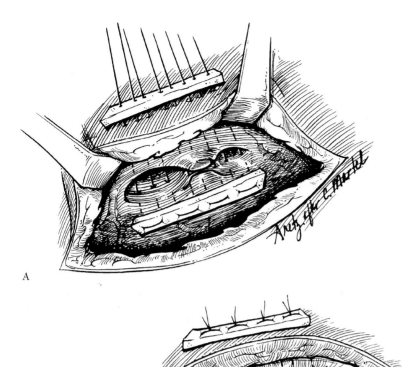

Figure 76-8. Closure of multiple anterior muscular defects through a short vertical right ventriculotomy. **(A)** The defects are sandwiched between two strips of felt or pericardium, one placed inside and the other outside the right ventricle parallel to the left anterior descending coronary artery. **(B)** Interrupted horizontal mattress sutures are used.

EDITOR'S COMMENTS

Knowledge of the anatomy and techniques of closure for the various types of VSDs is critical because VSDs, either isolated or in combination with other defects, are perhaps the most common malformation addressed surgically in congenital heart disease. The approaches to VSDs and techniques for avoiding interfering with the conducting tissue are well outlined in this chapter.

There are several types of VSD that demand specific attention. VSD of either the conoventricular or conoseptal hypoplasia variety associated with prolapse of the right or noncoronary leaflet of the aortic valve is a specific circumstance that can be approached by various operative techniques. It is generally believed that the loss of support for the aortic valve leaflet and commissure causes progressive prolapse of the valve leaflet into the defect and can cause progressive aortic insufficiency. Therefore, the presence of even mild aortic insufficiency in association with a VSD is considered an indication for operative intervention. In most cases, simple closure of the defect either primarily or with a patch can resuspend the aortic valve leaflets and cause either improvement or stabilization of the degree of aortic insufficiency. In unusual cases, more direct repair of the prolapsed aortic valve leaflet is required with techniques that include triangular resection of the central portion of the prolapse in aortic valve leaflet or Truslertype plication of the leaflet at the level of the commissural attachment. In some cases, the defects can be repaired primarily through the aorta with pledgeted sutures placed on the left ventricular side of the ventricular septum through the base of the aortic valve leaflet with plication of the sinus of Valsalva posterior to the aortic valve prolapse, recreating the support for the aortic valve leaflet

severe associated noncardiac pathologic conditions. Small size is no longer a risk factor for mortality, although extreme small size (<2.0 kg) may still be a risk factor for increased morbidity and mortality after surgery.

Small residual defects may be detected by color-flow Doppler studies in about 35% of patients. Small defects (<4 mm) usually close spontaneously and rarely need reoperation. Residual defects of ≥4 mm are less likely to close spontaneously and need reoperation if the Qp:Qs ratio exceeds 1.3 to 1.5:1 or if the pulmonary artery pressures remain significantly elevated. Endocarditis prophylaxis needs to be continued as long as residual defects remain.

Complete heart block occurs in about 1% of patients; right-bundle-branch block develops in about 40% to 60% of patients. The incidence of right-bundle-branch block is slightly higher after a right ventriculotomy compared with a transatrial approach. This is usually not associated with diminished long-term prognosis.

SUGGESTED READING

Barratt-Boyes BG, Neutze JM, Clarkson PM, et al. Repair of ventricular septal defect in the first two years of life using profound hypothermia-circulatory arrest techniques. Ann Surg 1976;184:376.

de Leval MR, Pozzi M, Starnes V, et al. Surgical management of doubly committed subarterial ventricular septal defects. Circulation 1988;78:III-40.

Fishberger SB, Bridges ND, Keane JF, et al. Intraoperative device closure of ventricular septal defects. Circulation 1993;88:II-205.

Hardin JT, Muskett AD, Canter CE, et al. Primary surgical closure of large ventricular septal defects in small infants. Ann Thorac Surg 1992;53:397.

Houyel L, Vaksmann G, Fournier A, et al. Ventricular arrhythmias after correction of ventricular septal defects: importance of surgical approach. J Am Coll Cardiol 1990;16:1224.

Knott-Craig CJ, Elkins RC, Ramakrishnan K, et al. Associated atrial septal defects increase perioperative morbidity after ventricular septal defect repair in infancy. Ann Thorac Surg 1995;59:573.

and dealing with the prolapsed and enlarged sinus of Valsalva simultaneously (Yacoub MH, Khan H, Stavri G, et al. Anatomic correction of the syndrome of prolapsing right coronary aortic cusp, dilatation of the sinus of Valsalva, and septal defect. J Thorac Cardiovasc Surg 1997;113:253). Primary closure with pledgeted sutures can also occasionally be performed through the right atrium.

The approach to closure of conoseptal hypoplasia VSDs through the pulmonary artery is described in the chapter. As noted by Dr. Knott-Craig, it is important when closing these defects to pay attention to suture placement in the base of the leaflets of the pulmonary valve in case later pulmonary autograft valve replacement is necessary. On several occasions, we have been able to use the pulmonary valve for autograft aortic valve replacement in patients who had previous closure of conoseptal hypoplasia defects, either by primary closure or with the use of a patch, if the pledgeted sutures in the base of the pulmonary valve leaflet do not distort the valve unduly. A continuing controversy is the appropriate approach to a symptomatic infant with multiple VSDs. Although pulmonary artery banding and later repair remain a mainstay of therapy in these patients, the progressive right ventricular hypertrophy associated with pulmonary artery banding can often cause additional obscuring of the margins of the ventricular defect from the right ventricular side. In addition, after banding, recatheterization may not identify residual VSDs, which may have little flow in the presence of a tight pulmonary band. After debanding and closure of the identifiable VSDs, with regression of right ventricular hypertrophy, additional muscular defects may reappear. We have therefore advocated a primary approach to multiple VSDs in infancy to close the majority of the defects while ventricular hypertrophy is not severe. In most cases, the defects can be identified. For apical muscular defects, an apical right ventriculotomy may be suitable for closure. Apical left ventriculotomies have the disadvantage of cutting through significant myocardium of the systemic ventricle; however, apical left ventriculotomies have not usually been associated with significant left ventricular dysfunction. In addition, in some cases when multiple anterior muscular defects are associated with a conoventricular defect, it is possible to expose the muscular defects and identify them by passing a right-angled clamp through the conoventricular defect and exploring the ventricular septum. The entrance points in the right ventricle

can then be identified and trabeculae divided to expose the margins of the defect for accurate closure. Most apical midmuscular and conoventricular and conoseptal hypoplasia defects can be closed with a high degree of certainty at primary operation. However, anterior muscular defects remain problematic, because they may be difficult to expose through the atrium. In some cases, these defects can be approached through the aortic valve or a right ventricular outflow tract incision.

In situations where the margins of the muscular defect cannot be readily identified, it may be possible to pass a right-angled clamp through the mitral valve from a transatrial septal approach across the defect into the right ventricle. A large polypropylene suture can then be brought back into the left ventricle and left atrium and a piece of Teflon felt cut larger than the anticipated left ventricular side of the defect. The patch can then be secured with the suture and brought through the mitral valve on to the left side of the septum. The suture is then brought through a similarly shaped Teflon felt patch on the right ventricular side and tied. In this way, the defect is sandwiched between two layers of felt and the actual direct margins of the defect do not have to be identified. This technique can be particularly useful in "Swiss cheese" type ventricular septal defects or occasional anterior muscular defects that are obscure.

The advent of transcatheter closure devices, primarily the umbrella device, has aided surgical intervention for patients with multiple VSDs. In patients in whom residual defects are present or where there are multiple midmuscular defects that can be approached with a transcatheter device, either transcatheter closure before operative closure of remaining defects or after closure of the surgically accessible defects may be associated with a high degree of success

There has been a great deal of interest in use of Amplatzer and clamshell-type VSD closure devices. Although these devices can be deployed in the catheterization laboratory, the approach, across the tricuspid valve, may be difficult. There has been great interest in a hybrid approach in which a standard sternotomy is made, and using a periventricular approach with a needle in the right ventricle, a guide wire is passed across the defect under echocardiographic guidance and then an Amplatzer device deployed with the heart beating off cardiopulmonary bypass under echo guidance. These techniques have the advantage of being able to close even fairly remote api-

cal muscular defects with high degrees of success and avoid the need for cardiopulmonary bypass. As additional experience is gained with these techniques, greater use of hybrid approaches is likely to occur, and even defects that are normally accessible through the right atrium may be closed with a periventricular approach to avoid the need for cardiopulmonary bypass.

Perimembranous VSD devices are being developed and may supplant surgical therapy for many typical conoventricular VSDs. However, the close association of the aortic valve with the superior rim of the VSD may result in some problems with these devices over time, and the incidence of heart block has not completely been identified with the current generation of transcatheter conoventricular closure devices. Nevertheless, the advent of the VSD occluder devices has made pulmonary artery banding for VSDs virtually unnecessary. An additional area of controversy is the approach to patients with coarctation of the aorta and large conoventricular defects. In infants in whom there is a degree of arch hypoplasia in association with a very large conoventricular defect, which is a common association, we have elected to primarily repair both defects through a midline sternotomy with patching of the aortic arch, which relieves the arch obstruction completely. Although in a small percentage of cases these large defects might close spontaneously, the avoidance of pulmonary artery banding and significant shunting early in life controls congestive heart failure immediately and has been associated with good outcomes in our patients

The presence of residual VSD after attempted surgical closure remains a problem. Most commonly with conoventricular defects or malalignment defects, it can be difficult to expose the anterosuperior aspect of the defect, and residual defects can be present in this location. In addition, in patients with tetralogy of Fallot, conal muscle bundles can masquerade as the margin of the defect, and the patch may be attached more on the ventricular muscle than the superior rim of the defect, leaving an abnormal connection from the left ventricle to the right ventricle underneath the aortic valve and obscured by the trabecular muscle. Often these defects are best approached through the aortic valve, where the superior margin of the patch can be readily identified, and either direct primary closure with sutures to the base of the right coronary leaflet of the aortic valve or additional patch closure can be undertaken.

T.L.S.

77

Aortopulmonary Window

James S. Tweddell

Embryology and Anatomy

Aortopulmonary window is a rare defect caused by failure of fusion of the two opposing conotruncal ridges that are responsible for separating the truncus arteriosus into the aorta and pulmonary artery. The aortopulmonary window therefore occurs between the two structures that normally result from septation of the truncus arteriosus, namely the ascending aorta and the main pulmonary artery, and may be found just above the semilunar valves or between the more distal ascending aorta and main pulmonary artery. With increasing size of the defect, aberrations in flow result in abnormal incorporation of the right sixth arch, destined to become the right pulmonary artery, such that the right pulmonary artery arises from the rightward aspect of the ascending aorta. With larger aortopulmonary windows flow patterns can be disturbed such that there is preferential flow through the ductus arteriosus and diminished flow in the developing aortic arch resulting in distal arch hypoplasia including coarctation or interrupted aortic arch (Fig. 77-1). Origin of the right pulmonary artery from the ascending aorta is probably the result of the absence of a large portion of the aortopulmonary septum associated with abnormal incorporation of the right sixth arch and represents a more severe form of aortopulmonary window rather than a distinct anomaly. Similarly, interrupted aortic arch and severe coarctation are likely caused by the flow characteristics of a large aortopulmonary window limiting development of the aortic isthmus rather than representing a distinct anomaly. Support for this concept comes from the observation that interrupted arch associated with aortopul-

monary window is nearly always type A and that aortopulmonary window is not associated with DiGeorge syndrome, suggesting that aortopulmonary window is a distinct malformation not related to abnormalities of the conal septum, such as interrupted aortic arch with ventricular septal defect (VSD), tetralogy of Fallot, and persistent truncus arteriosus. Abnormal origin of the coronary arteries is commonly associated with aortopulmonary window. The coronary arteries may arise from the edge of the defect, or the origin may occur just on the pulmonary artery side of the defect.

Presentation, Diagnostic Considerations, and Indications for Surgery

Antenatal diagnosis of aortopulmonary window has only recently been reported. Simple aortopulmonary window may not be identified by fetal echocardiography because equal pressure in the ascending aorta and pulmonary root in the fetus results in minimal detectable flow through the defect. Although the diagnosis of interrupted aortic arch should be possible, when associated with aortopulmonary window, the patient with an interrupted aortic arch lacks the characteristic posterior deviation of the infundibular septum that may prompt further interrogation of the arch. The antenatal diagnosis of aortopulmonary window with interrupted aortic arch has not been reported.

The presentation of patients with aortopulmonary window is similar to that of other patients with left-to-right shunts, such as patent ductus arteriosus or VSD. Although small, restrictive aortopulmonary

windows do occur; generally, the communication is large, and patients present in the first weeks of life when pulmonary vascular resistance drops and increased pulmonary blood flow with congestive heart failure develops. Signs of congestive heart failure such as tachypnea, diaphoresis, poor feeding, and inadequate weight gain are common. In early infancy, cyanosis is usually not a prominent feature, but with large defects, bidirectional shunting can produce systemic desaturation.

Physical examination demonstrates a tachypneic infant with accessory respiratory muscle use. Cardiac examination reveals an enlarged heart, and as in patients with patent ductus arteriosus, the pulses are bounding. A systolic murmur can be heard along the left sternal border; however, unlike the situation with patients with a patent ductus arteriosus, a diastolic component to the murmur is rare. Chest x-ray films reveal cardiomegaly and increased pulmonary vascular markings consistent with increased pulmonary blood flow. Patients with associated arch abnormalities frequently present with pulmonary edema, low cardiac output, and metabolic acidosis coinciding with closing of the ductus arteriosus.

The diagnosis is routinely made with echocardiography. The location and size of the communication as well as associated anomalies are carefully identified. Cardiac catheterization is occasionally indicated for the patient who presents after early infancy and therefore is at risk for elevated pulmonary vascular resistance or any patient in whom the anatomy cannot be adequately defined by echocardiography. Although using cardiac catheterization to assess the origin of the coronary arteries is theoretically appealing, the large defect occurring just above the sinuses of Valsalva

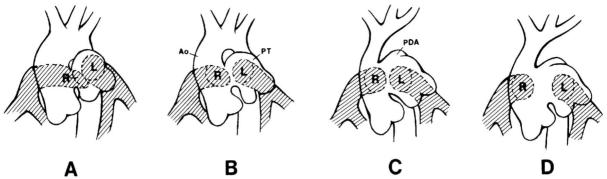

Figure 77-1.   The spectrum of aortopulmonary window. **(A)** Proximal aortopulmonary septal defect with normal origin of the right pulmonary artery from the pulmonary artery trunk. **(B–D)** As the defects extend distally, they are larger and more likely to be associated with abnormal origin of the right pulmonary artery from the aorta (Ao) as well as aortic arch hypoplasia, coarctation, and interruption. **(B)** A mild form of distal aortopulmonary window with the pulmonary artery bifurcation straddling the posterior margins of the defect combined with mild hypoplasia of the aortic arch. **(C)** Aortic origin of the right pulmonary artery and interrupted aortic arch with a patent ductus arteriosus (PDA). **(D)** The most extreme end of the spectrum, with wide separation of the right and left pulmonary arteries associated with absence of the entire aortopulmonary septum combined with an interrupted aortic arch. (R = right; L = left; PT = pulmonary trunk.) (Adapted with permission from T Berry, S Bharati, AJ Muster, et al. Distal aortopulmonary septal defect, aortic origin of the right pulmonary artery, intact ventricular septum, patent ductus arteriosus and hypoplasia of the aortic isthmus: A newly recognized syndrome. Am J Cardiol 1982;49:108.)

combined with the tremendous pulmonary flow makes assessment of coronary artery anatomy with catheterization impractical. Those patients who are found to have an elevated pulmonary vascular resistance should undergo testing with pulmonary vasodilators to determine whether the pulmonary vascular resistance can be reduced. Presence of an aortopulmonary window is an indication for surgery because untreated infants die of intractable heart failure or rapidly develop pulmonary vascular obstructive disease.

Preoperative Management

Initial resuscitative efforts are aimed at improving systemic output by limiting excessive pulmonary blood flow and are similar to those used in the patient with single-ventricle anatomy and unobstructed pulmonary blood flow or patients with truncus arteriosus. For the patient with a large aortopulmonary window, this often requires intubation and mechanical ventilation as well as sedation and sometimes neuromuscular blockade to achieve a balanced circulation. The use of hypercapnea and minimizing the fraction of inspired oxygen (FIO_2) will increase the pulmonary vascular resistance, decrease left-to-right shunting, and

improve systemic oxygen delivery. Inotropic support may be required. Prostaglandin infusion is necessary to maintain ductal patency in patients with aortopulmonary window and interrupted aortic arch or coarctation. These measures should be successful in restoring systemic output, and the patient should go to surgery without a metabolic acidosis.

Operative Technique

A median sternotomy incision is used for aortopulmonary window regardless of associated abnormalities. The anatomy should be carefully assessed (Fig. 77-2). The external extent of the aortopulmonary window and the coronary arteries should be identified. Coronary arteries involved in the defect can be seen arising from the area of the communication and coursing down the proximal aorta before reaching the myocardium. The position of the right pulmonary artery should be noted.

Simple Aortopulmonary Window

The right and left pulmonary arteries should be loosely encircled with snares so that once cardiopulmonary bypass is established, pulmonary flow can be controlled (Fig. 77-3). General anesthesia can produce a drop

in pulmonary vascular resistance, resulting in excessive pulmonary blood flow at the expense of systemic perfusion. It is sometimes helpful to snare one of the branch pulmonary arteries to limit excessive pulmonary blood flow while continuing with preparation for cardiopulmonary bypass. The aorta should be dissected nearly circumferentially distal to the extent of the aortopulmonary window to allow for subsequent placement of the cross-clamp. After the administration of heparin, the aortic cannula is placed in the ascending aorta near the origin of the innominate artery (Fig. 77-3). If there is an associated atrial septal defect or VSD, bicaval cannulation should be undertaken; otherwise, a single venous cannula can be used. Cardiopulmonary bypass is begun and simultaneously the branch pulmonary arteries are snared. A left ventricular vent is placed through the junction of the right superior pulmonary vein and left atrium. A cardioplegia cannula is placed in the ascending aorta. For simple aortopulmonary window, moderate hypothermia to 32°C is adequate. The aorta is cross-clamped distal to the communication. Cardioplegic solution is infused while the pulmonary arteries are snared. The defect can be repaired via an incision in the window itself, through the aorta, or through the pulmonary artery (Fig. 77-4). An approach through the window is preferable

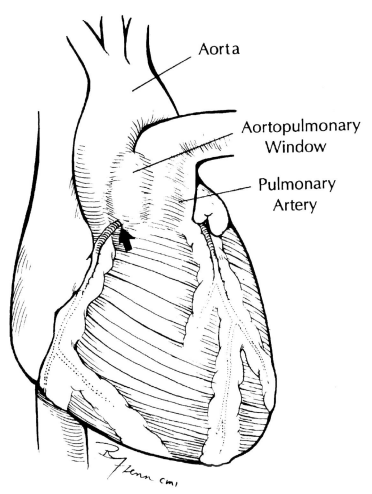

Figure 77-2. External view of aortopulmonary window. The area of communication between the great vessels can be easily identified. The extent of the defect and the origins of the right pulmonary artery and right coronary artery should be identified. As in this figure, the right coronary artery (*arrow*) can be sometimes seen originating near the inferior margin of the defect and coursing proximally on the aorta before taking its normal position in the atrioventricular groove. This finding should prompt careful internal inspection for abnormal origin of the coronary artery from the inferior ridge of the defect or the pulmonary artery.

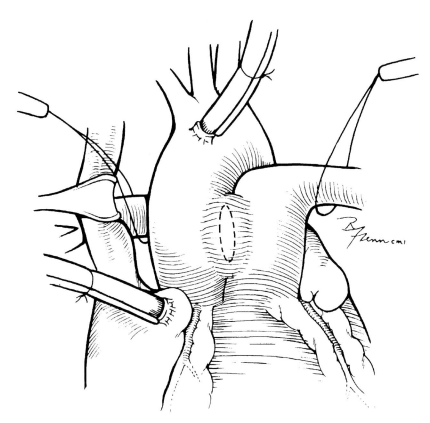

Figure 77-3. Preliminary steps in the repair of a simple aortopulmonary window. The left and right branch pulmonary arteries are loosely encircled. The aorta is cannulated beyond the distal extent of the aortopulmonary window so that there is adequate room for a cross-clamp. Generally, a single venous cannula placed through the right atrial appendage is used for venous drainage. After cardiopulmonary bypass has begun, the branch pulmonary artery snares are tightened. A left ventricular vent (not shown) is placed through the right superior pulmonary vein.

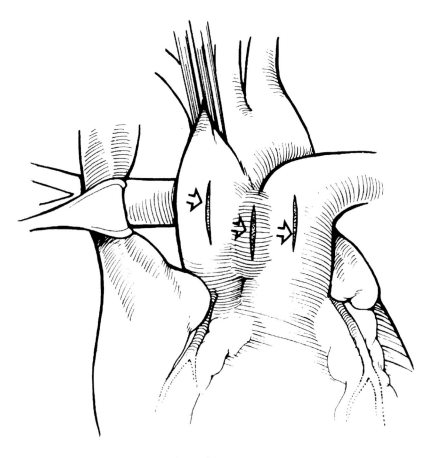

Figure 77-4. Aortopulmonary window can be repaired via an incision in the window itself, through the aorta, or through the pulmonary artery.

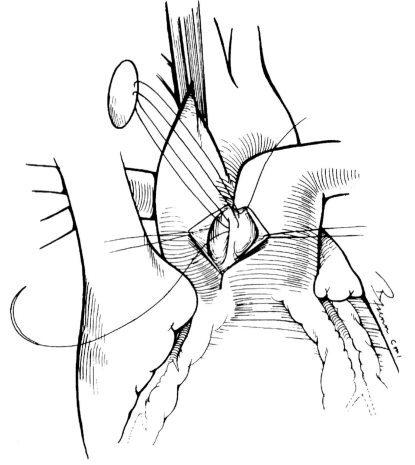

Figure 77-5. Approach through the aortopulmonary window. An incision is initiated in the anterior-superior portion of the window, and after the origin of the right coronary artery is identified, the incision is extended proximally, transecting the anterior half of the window. After the origins of the coronary arteries and the right pulmonary artery are identified, an appropriately sized patch of PTFE or pericardium is secured to the posterior rim of the defect.

because the origin of the coronary arteries can be easily assessed and the patch placed such that an abnormal coronary ostial origin is incorporated into the aorta. In addition, there is less potential for compromise of either of the great vessels or injury of the semilunar valves. The incision is initiated in the anterior-superior portion of the window, and, after the origin of the right coronary artery is identified, the incision is extended proximally, transecting the anterior half of the window. After the origins of the coronary arteries and the right pulmonary artery are identified, an appropriately sized patch of polytetrafluoroethylene (PTFE) or pericardium is secured to the posterior wall of the defect using continuous suture (Fig. 77-5). The anterior incision in the window is then closed, incorporating the patch into the suture line (Fig. 77-6). Rewarming to normothermia is begun as the window is closed. The aortic root is de-aired, and the cross-clamp is removed. Preparation for weaning from cardiopulmonary bypass includes placement of a pulmonary artery line through the right ventricular free wall as well as a left atrial line placed through the vent site. A milrinone infusion is initiated prior to weaning from cardiopulmonary bypass because this provides both inotropy and pulmonary vasodilation. Additional pulmonary vasodilators, such as inhaled nitric oxide, should be available especially in the older infant.

Repair of Aortopulmonary Window with Interrupted Aortic Arch

Aortopulmonary window with interrupted aortic arch is usually a large defect and is more frequently associated with abnormal origin of the right pulmonary artery (Fig. 77-7). A median sternotomy incision is used. Initial preparation is the same as for simple aortopulmonary window; again, the branch pulmonary arteries are loosely encircled with snares. Because of the large aortopulmonary communication, a single arterial cannula can be used. This is placed in the ascending aorta (Fig. 77-8). Flow to the distal half of the body will be through the aortopulmonary window and then via the ductus arteriosus. After cardiopulmonary bypass is established, the branch pulmonary arteries are snared and a left ventricular vent is placed. The patient is cooled over a period of at least 30 minutes to a bladder temperature of 18°C. During the cooling period, the aortic arch, head vessels, ductus arteriosus, and proximal descending thoracic aorta are mobilized. After reaching the target

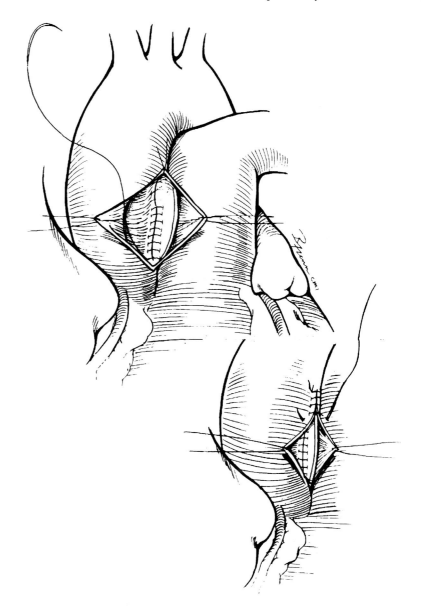

Figure 77-6. Approach through the aortopulmonary window (continued). The patch is secured to the posterior margin of the aortopulmonary window using a continuous suture technique. Anteriorly, closure of the arteriotomy in the aortopulmonary window incorporates the patch.

temperature, circulatory arrest is established, the head vessels are snared, a C-shaped vascular clamp is placed across the descending thoracic aorta at least 1 cm distal to the insertion of the ductus arteriosus, and cardioplegic solution is infused via the arterial cannula. With the branch pulmonary arteries, descending thoracic aorta, and head vessels occluded, cardioplegic solution will be directed into the coronary arteries. The entire procedure can be performed using deep hypothermic circulatory arrest, or alternatively continuous cerebral perfusion can be used by selectively perfusing the innominate artery. The ductus arteriosus is ligated near the pulmonary

artery, and all ductal tissue is excised from the descending thoracic aorta. The undersurface of the proximal aortic arch is incised, and the incision is continued into the ascending aorta. The descending thoracic aorta is then brought up and anastomosed to the undersurface of the aortic arch and distal ascending aorta. Construction of the aortic anastomosis is facilitated by holding the descending thoracic aorta in a C clamp (Fig. 77-9). This provides for close approximation while the anastomosis is performed. After reconstruction of the aortic arch, a cross-clamp is placed between the aortopulmonary window and the reconstructed arch and cardiopulmonary bypass

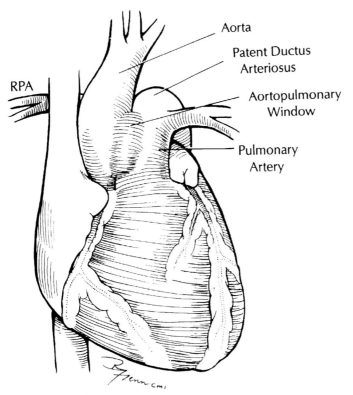

Figure 77-7. External appearance of the aortopulmonary window and interrupted aortic arch. (RPA = right pulmonary artery.)

is re-established. Alternatively, a single period of deep hypothermic circulatory arrest can be used for the entire repair. The window is approached as described. Again, the origins of the right pulmonary artery and coronary arteries are assessed (Fig. 77-10). A patch of PTFE or pericardium is placed to close the window such that the right pulmonary artery is incorporated into the main pulmonary artery trunk and the lumen of the right pulmonary artery is not compromised. The patient is rewarmed, monitoring lines are placed, and weaning from cardiopulmonary bypass is conducted as for simple aortopulmonary window.

An alternative approach to repair of aortopulmonary window with interrupted aortic arch may be necessary in cases in which there is little distal ascending aorta or proximal arch present. In this case additional patch augmentation of the arch anastomosis and proximal great vessels may be necessary to complete reconstruction; this technique is described in Figs. 77-11 through 77-14.

Surgical Complications and Postoperative Care

For simple aortopulmonary window and even aortopulmonary window with

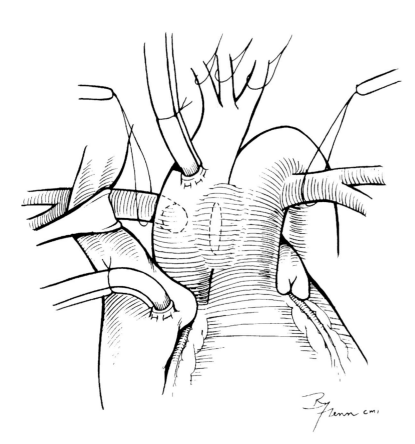

Figure 77-8. Cannulation for repair of aortopulmonary window and interrupted aortic arch. The right and left branch pulmonary arteries are loosely encircled with snares. Unlike interrupted aortic arch with ventricular septal defect, a single aorta cannula is satisfactory because distal perfusion can be carried via the aortopulmonary window and a ductus arteriosus to the lower half of the body. Aortopulmonary window and interrupted aortic arch are rarely associated with ventricular septal defect, and a single venous cannula is usually all that is required. After establishment of cardiopulmonary bypass, the branch pulmonary artery snares are tightened. During the period of cooling, the brachiocephalic vessels are mobilized and loosely encircled with snares.

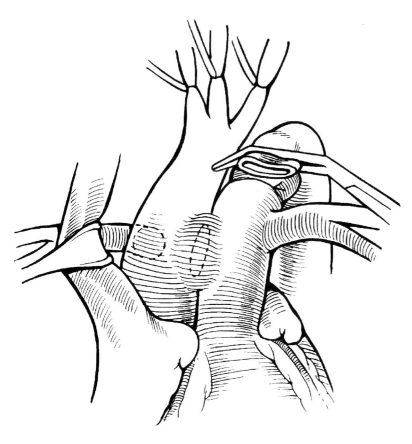

Figure 77-9. Repair of aortopulmonary window and interrupted aortic arch. After the establishment of deep hypothermic circulatory arrest or continuous cerebral perfusion, a C-clamp is placed on the descending thoracic aorta approximately 1 cm distal to the insertion of the ductus arteriosus. The ductus arteriosus is ligated and divided. Residual ductal tissue is excised from the proximal descending thoracic aorta. By placing gentle traction on the C-clamp, the open end at the descending thoracic aorta is brought up to the undersurface of the proximal aortic arch and distal ascending aorta. An anastomosis is constructed between the descending thoracic aorta and distal ascending aorta/proximal arch with continuous suture.

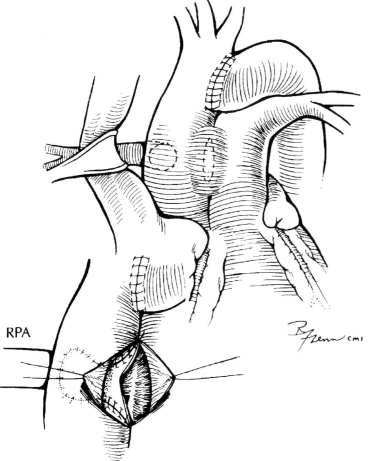

RPA

Figure 77-10. Repair of aortopulmonary window and interrupted aortic arch (continued). After reconstruction of the aortic arch, full cardiopulmonary bypass can be re-established and an aortic cross-clamp placed between the arch reconstruction and the aortopulmonary window. Alternatively, the entire procedure can be carried out using one period of deep hypothermic circulatory arrest. Again, the aortopulmonary window is approached via an incision in the window itself. A patch of polytetrafluoroethylene or pericardium is placed such that the origin of the right pulmonary artery (RPA) is connected to the main pulmonary artery trunk and the lumen of the right pulmonary artery is not compromised. The anterior margin of the patch is incorporated into the arteriotomy closure.

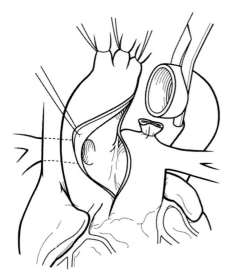

Figure 77-11.   An alternative approach to the repair of an aortopulmonary window with interrupted aortic arch may be necessary in cases in which there is little distal ascending aorta or proximal arch present. In this case there may not be sufficient aorta distal to the aortopulmonary window to permit construction of an unobstructed anastomosis to the descending thoracic aorta. Cannulation is performed as shown in Fig. 78-8, and perfusion techniques can include either continuous cerebral perfusion or deep hypothermic circulatory arrest. The ductus arteriosus is ligated, and all residual ductal tissue is excised from the mobilized descending thoracic aorta. An incision is made in the undersurface of the proximal arch initiated at the origin of the distal brachiocephalic vessel, in this case the left subclavian artery, and extended proximally into the aortopulmonary window.

interrupted aortic arch, postoperative inotropic support should be minimal. As in other patients with large left-to-right shunts there is potential for acute elevation of pulmonary vascular resistance with the development of critically low cardiac output after repair. Patients operated on in the first 2 weeks of life should be at low risk for pulmonary vascular resistance elevation and may be candidates for early extubation. Older patients may require sedation and neuromuscular blockade for the first 12 to 24 hours. In higher-risk patients pulmonary artery pressure should be continuously monitored until extubation. If pulmonary hypertension develops, pulmonary vasodilators (inhaled nitric oxide) should be started promptly. In addition to routine hemodynamic monitoring, the adequacy of systemic oxygen delivery should be assessed by sampling of mixed venous blood from the pulmonary artery.

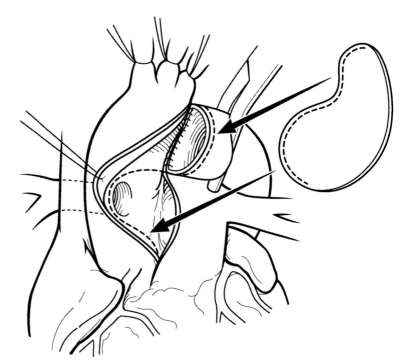

Figure 77-12.   The posterior one half of the circumference of the descending thoracic aorta is sutured to the posterior edge of the arch incision. A patch (either pulmonary homograft or pericardium) is fashioned as shown. The dashed line indicates the initial suture line. Reconstruction begins by suturing the patch to the anterior one half of the proximal descending thoracic aorta and then transitioning the suture line to the posterior wall of the ascending aorta such that the abnormally positioned right pulmonary artery is placed on the left side of the patch. The suture line then continues to the bottom of the aortopulmonary window.

Catheter-Based Approaches

The utility of transcatheter closure is limited by the large size of the defect, the small size of patients with correspondingly small femoral vessels, and the potential for

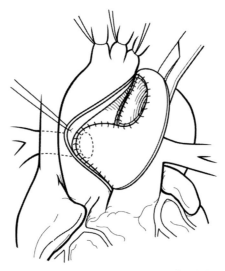

Figure 77-13.   The posterior suture line is in place. The anterior edge of the patch will now be secured to the edge of the ascending aorta.

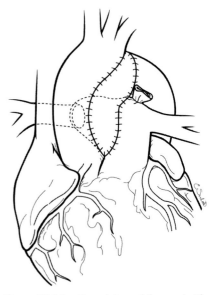

Figure 77-14.   Completion of the repair. The pulmonary artery edge of the aortopulmonary window is sutured to the centerline of the patch to complete closure of the main pulmonary artery. In this way the patch augments both ascending aorta and main pulmonary artery and minimizes the potential for compromise of the caliber of either of these vessels or the right pulmonary artery. In addition, the patch allows augmentation of the arch reconstruction.

complications related to anomalous origin of the coronary arteries that are hard to define prior to intervention. Nevertheless, device closure of aortopulmonary window may be suitable for small defects in which the risk of anomalous origin of the coronary arteries is low, specifically those with a more distal location.

Results of Surgery

Between 1983 and 2004, 18 patients underwent repair of aortopulmonary window at the Children's Hospital of Wisconsin. Patients were divided into two categories based on the presence of important additional lesions. Simple aortopulmonary window ($n = 8$) included those patients with an isolated aortopulmonary window with or without an atrial level communication. Complex aortopulmonary window ($n = 10$) included those patients with important additional lesions including; interrupted aortic arch ($n = 3$), coarctation of the aorta ($n = 2$), ventricular septal defect ($n = 1$), pulmonary atresia with ventricular septal defect and anomalous origin of the right coronary artery ($n = 1$), pulmonary atresia with intact ventricular septum and partial anomalous pulmonary venous return ($n = 1$), aortopulmonary window with d-malposed great vessels ($n = 1$), and congenital absence of the left pulmonary artery with pulmonary artery hypertension ($n = 1$). There were no deaths early or late in the simple aortopulmonary window group. In the complex group there was one early death in the patient with aortopulmonary window, pulmonary atresia, and intact ventricular septum. There was one late death following lung transplantation in the patient with aortopulmonary window, absent left pulmonary artery, and pulmonary hypertension.

In the current era, early mortality following repair of uncomplicated aortopulmonary window approaches zero and long-term outcome should be excellent. Early morbidity includes pulmonary artery stenosis and residual aortopulmonary septal defects. Long-term follow-up is indicated to look for the development of branch pulmonary artery stenosis. For patients with aortopulmonary window and interrupted aortic arch, the outcome should also be very good with extremely low operative mortality. Long-term observation for recurrent coarctation is indicated.

SUGGESTED READING

Backer CL, Mavroudis C. Surgical management of aortopulmonary window: A 40-year experience. Eur J Cardiothorac Surg 2002;21:773.

Bagtharia R, Trivedi KR, Burkhart HM, et al. Outcomes for patients with an aortopulmonary window, and the impact of associated cardiovascular lesions. Cardiol Young 2004;14:473.

Berry TE, Bharati S, Muster AJ, et al. Distal aortopulmonary septal defect, aortic origin of the right pulmonary artery, intact ventricular septum, patent ductus arteriosus and hypoplasia of the aortic isthmus: A newly recognized syndrome. Am J Cardiol 1982;49:108.

Bourlon F, Kreitmann P, Jourdan J, et al. Anomalous origin of left coronary artery with aortopulmonary window: A case report with surgical correction and delayed control. Thorac Cardiovasc Surg 1981;29:91.

Brouwer MH, Beaufort-Krol GC, Talsma MD. Aortopulmonary window associated with an anomalous origin of the right coronary artery. Int J Cardiol 1990;28:384.

Collinet P, Chatelet-Cheront C, Houze de l'Aulnoit D, et al. Prenatal diagnosis of an aorto-pulmonary window by fetal echocardiography. Fetal Diagn Ther 2002;17:302.

Hew CC, Bacha EA, Zurakowski D, et al. Optimal surgical approach for repair of aortopulmonary window. Cardiol Young 2001;11:385.

Johansson L, Michaelsson M, Westerholm CJ, et al. Aortopulmonary window: A new operative approach. Ann Thorac Surg 1978;25:564.

EDITOR'S COMMENTS

As noted by Dr. Tweddell, aortopulmonary window is a rare congenital cardiac condition that presents in infancy with severe congestive failure and pulmonary overcirculation. Preoperative stabilization is imperative for low operative morbidity and mortality. As suggested by Dr. Tweddell, ventilatory maneuvers preoperatively can aid in stabilization of these patients. Because these maneuvers are often temporary, however, prompt resuscitation and early operation are indicated in virtually all infants with this condition.

Many operative techniques have been described for closure of aortopulmonary window. The one most commonly used, however, is the technique described by Dr. Tweddell, in which the window is opened anteriorly, and after careful identification of the edges of the defect, an intra-aortic or intrapulmonary patch is placed to close the defect and septate the great vessels.

In many cases we have elected to divide the aortopulmonary window completely to carefully identify the origins of the coronary arteries and then patch the aortic and pulmonary sides separately. This can be especially useful if there is stenosis of the right pulmonary artery at its origin, which occasionally occurs. In these cases the origin of the right pulmonary artery can be patched with the closure of the pulmonary artery.

In isolated cases of aortopulmonary window, in which the window is distally located and relatively small, it may even be possible to simply divide the defect or ligate the defect as one would a ductus arteriosus. These situations are rare, however, and can avoid the need for cardiopulmonary bypass. In this circumstance, direct identification of the origin of the coronary arteries is very important to avoid leaving a coronary coming from the pulmonary artery side of the defect.

In situations where aortopulmonary window is associated with interrupted aortic arch, we have elected to perform a more radical arch reconstruction than that described by Dr. Tweddell. Because there is often very little distance distal to the aortopulmonary window and the take-off of the innominate artery and carotid vessels, we generally will ligate the ductus arteriosus, excise ductal tissue, and then make an incision into the left subclavian artery (if a type B interruption is present) or widely open the descending aorta (if a type A interruption is present), removing all ductal tissue. The aortopulmonary window is then opened and superiorly the incision is carried up into the origin of the left carotid artery for a short distance. The descending aorta is then anastomosed in a superior aspect of the incision in the ascending aorta and carotid, creating natural tissue approximation in this region. A generous patch of pulmonary homograft is then used to augment the undersurface of the aortic arch to take tension off the suture line and ensure that no kinking or narrowing of the anastomosis creates later arch obstruction. This patch is then fashioned in such a way as to augment the ascending aorta and at its proximal portion to close the aortopulmonary window. With division of the aortopulmonary window the pulmonary arterial side can be separately patched with a small patch of pulmonary homograft material to prevent any distortion or limitation of flow into the branch pulmonary vessels.

T.L.S.

78

Coarctation of the Aorta

Irving Shen and Ross M. Ungerleider

Coarctation of the aorta can present as a severe and emergent problem in a neonate or as a subtle and essentially asymptomatic problem in an older child (or adult). This chapter focuses primarily on coarctation in neonates or infants because it is in that population that many of the important issues of coarctation are highlighted and best appreciated.

Coarctation is a form of left ventricular outflow tract obstruction (LVOTO) and imposes an increase in afterload to the left ventricle. It is often but not necessarily found in association with a variety of other important cardiac defects, and these can have a crucial effect on the physiology of the defect and on the patient's presentation. In its "pure" form, coarctation is simply a constriction, or narrowing, of the aorta that usually occurs near the site of insertion of the ductus arteriosus. Because of this typical location, coarctation is often described as being "juxtaductal," and this term is used to distinguish the more common forms of coarctation from a less common form that can involve the aorta proximal to the ductus arteriosus and extend into the transverse aortic arch. This latter type is sometimes referred to as "preductal" coarctation, and because it will usually present early in infancy, it can also be referred to as "infantile coarctation." In practice, the use of the terms "juxtaductal" and "preductal" is not of critical importance as long as the extent of the coarctation is appreciated by the surgeon (Fig. 78-1).

Because of the obstruction to left ventricular (LV) outflow as well as to distal aortic flow that is created by the coarctation, infants will present in severe LV failure with poor distal perfusion. This is manifested as pulmonary hypertension, and therefore "secondary" right ventricular (RV) hypertrophy is common in newborns with severe aortic coarctation. The LV failure may be reflected by a dilated, hypocontractile left ventricle with reduced output, and for this reason, the gradient across the coarctation site is not an indicator of the severity of the defect. The RV and LV features may be nicely demonstrated by transthoracic echocardiography. Furthermore, a well-performed two-dimensional echocardiogram will demonstrate the anatomy of the aortic arch and the great vessels and the discrete area of aortic narrowing near the ductus. Flow to the distal aorta can be severely restricted, and patency of the ductus arteriosus is often essential in the newborn to preserve perfusion to the lower body (Fig. 78-1). Therefore, neonates with coarctation should be started on an intravenous infusion of prostaglandin E_1 (PGE$_1$). Maintaining ductal patency with PGE$_1$ infusion will also allow decompression of the pulmonary circulation due to downstream obstruction of the LV. In neonatal coarctation, the RV may provide most of the perfusion in the descending aorta, and because the RV pressure may equal systemic pressure (especially if there is an associated ventricular septal defect [VSD]), there can be essentially no difference in the pressure above and below the coarctation. Therefore the pressure gradient between the upper and the lower body will underestimate the severity of the coarctation. If no VSD is present, the descending aorta may be perfused with systemic venous blood from the RV and thereby results in the "differential cyanosis" that has been described for this lesion, with the lower body appearing more cyanotic than the upper body.

It is important to look for other commonly associated defects, which can occur anywhere along the "left heart/aorta complex," and include mitral stenosis (often with mitral anomaly such as single papillary muscle), hypoplastic left ventricle (defined as an LV volume of <20 mL/m^2), endocardial fibroelastosis (a generalized scarring of the LV endothelium that appears as "brightness" on echocardiographic examination and that probably represents LV subendocardial ischemia), VSD (often with posterior malalignment of the infundibular septum that narrows the subaortic area), aortic stenosis (valvar or subvalvar), and atrial septal defect (ASD). All of these defects can be recognized by echocardiography, and it is not usually necessary to perform cardiac catheterization in these critically ill infants. The severity of the problem and the long-term prognosis are related to (1) age (young age, such as newborn, increases the risk), (2) the number and extent of associated defects, and (3) the actual anatomy of the defect (greater risk is incurred in patients whose defect extends proximal to the left subclavian artery).

Initial management of the newborn patient with aortic coarctation requires increasing distal perfusion to the lower body by restoring the patency of the ductus arteriosus with an intravenous PGE$_1$ infusion. Intubation and mechanical ventilation may be necessary due to the 15% to 20% incidence of apnea that occurs with PGE$_1$ infusion. Once the patient has been stabilized, complete diagnostic assessment can be accomplished. This usually can be limited to an echocardiogram, which should demonstrate the anatomy of the aortic arch and isthmus, patency of the ductus arteriosus, the coarctation segment, and any important associated cardiac defects. It is not necessary to perform a cardiac catheterization for diagnostic purposes, but catheterization should be done when there is any question about the arch anatomy, the nature

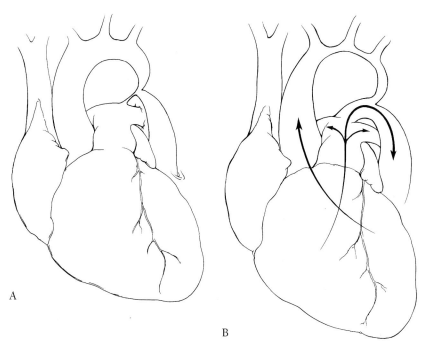

Figure 78-1. **(A)** A juxtaductal coarctation with discrete narrowing at the level of the ligamentum arteriosum. **(B)** An "infantile" or "preductal" coarctation with distal aortic perfusion maintained across a patent ductus arteriosus. In these patients, the aortic arch is usually hypoplastic, as shown.

essary, and less attractive than alternatives. Finally, and importantly, this procedure does not address hypoplasia of the aortic arch that is proximal to the left subclavian artery—a frequent finding in neonatal coarctation.

Patch Aortoplasty

Several groups have advocated repair of discrete coarctation using a large patch of prosthetic material like Dacron, polytetrafluoroethylene (PTFE; Gore-Tex), or cryopreserved homograft (Fig. 78-3). Unlike the subclavian flap procedure, this technique does not require division of the subclavian artery, and the patch can be much larger than the subclavian flap patch. Furthermore, the patch can be extended proximally onto the aortic arch when necessary. Late aneurysm formation opposite the patch has been reported by some, and this has tempered enthusiasm for this technique. More-recent studies have suggested that the occurrence of these aneurysms may be related to easily controlled technical factors such as the type of prosthetic material used and to how the coarctation ridge is managed. Most late aneurysms have been associated with the use of Dacron as compared to PTFE. Avoiding resection of the coarctation shelf has also contributed to reducing the incidence of this complication. Patch aortoplasty has also been described using a technique in which the coarctation tissue is resected and the back wall of the aorta is anastomosed, with a patch then placed over the anterior wall. However, this more complicated technique may not be justified, considering the good results with simpler patch aortoplasty without resection of the coarctation shelf. The recurrence rate after patch aortoplasty is very low, and this remains a very acceptable option for some patients. It is especially useful for recurrent coarctation when mobilization of the aorta is limited.

End-to-End and Extended End-to-End Anastomoses

The original coarctation repair was accomplished by resection of the coarctation region and end-to-end (ETE) anastomosis of the proximal and distal segments. This repair still plays a large role in the surgical treatment (Fig. 78-4). In infants, where the narrowing of the aorta can extend into the aortic arch (Fig. 78-1B), the anastomosis can be fashioned in a manner such that

of the coarctation, or the significance of a related defect that might require concomitant repair. Furthermore, cardiac catheterization has a role when an intervention is desired before coarctation repair (such as a Rashkind atrial septostomy in patients with associated transposition of the great arteries with intact septum who are not candidates for proceeding directly to the operating room). Operative repair should be considered once the diagnosis is confirmed. Coarctation of the aorta is an urgent problem in neonates, and prolonged medical management has a limited role reserved for unusual circumstances. There are several operative techniques in use for repair of aortic coarctation. Each has advantages and disadvantages, and the surgeon should be knowledgeable about each of these options. In most instances, repair is most easily and satisfactorily accomplished through a left thoracotomy, but occasionally median sternotomy is a useful approach and is discussed later.

Subclavian Flap Repair

The technique of subclavian flap repair was once considered by many authorities to be the procedure of choice for neonates and infants. However, we do not favor it and recommend against its routine use. The technique requires division of the subclavian artery and turning it down as a flap to augment the area of coarctation (Fig. 78-2). Those who favor this procedure believe that it is simple and safe, and that the patch of subclavian artery will grow with the patient and therefore will lead to lower incidence of recurrent coarctation or late aneurysm formation. Unfortunately, recurrent coarctation does occur after this procedure with about the same incidence as after other commonly used procedures, and late aneurysm development has been reported after this procedure. The subclavian flap procedure has the disadvantage that it requires permanent division of the left subclavian artery, and although this may be well tolerated in most patients, it can lead to long-term weakness of the left arm. Subclavian steal phenomenon has been described if the vertebral artery is left intact on the distal subclavian segment. Division of the left subclavian artery is problematic in the occasional patient with anomalous origin of the right subclavian artery below the coarctation site because in these patients, permanent loss of the left subclavian artery leaves no way to follow pressures above the coarctation site. Although some have suggested ingenious ways to reimplant the left subclavian as an augmentation patch without division and with relief of more proximal problems, these procedures are cumbersome, unnec-

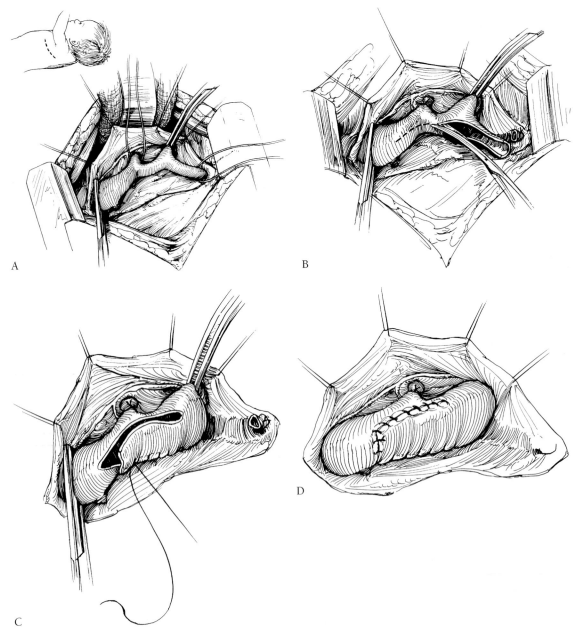

Figure 78-2. **(A)** The coarctation is exposed through a left thoracotomy, and the aortic arch and descending aorta are controlled with clamps. The left subclavian artery and ductus arteriosus are encircled; collateral vessels can be temporarily controlled with hemoclips. **(B)** The ductus arteriosus is ligated, and the subclavian artery is ligated and divided as far distal as possible. It also is important to tie the vertebral artery (first branch off the subclavian artery) to reduce the possibility of late subclavian steal syndrome. An incision is then made through the subclavian artery and extended onto the descending aorta through the area of coarctation. **(C)** The subclavian artery is then sewn as a flap to cover the incision on the descending aorta. **(D)** The finished subclavian flap procedure provides augmentation of the juxtaductal area. The hemoclips previously placed on collateral vessels can be removed.

it uses the underside of the aortic arch to enlarge the anastomotic area (Fig. 78-5). This latter technique has been referred to as extended ETE anastomosis. The major advantage of the ETE techniques is that they do not require division of the subclavian artery nor do they use any prosthetic material. Furthermore, these techniques allow resection and removal of all remnant ductal tissue in the aorta, and this may play a role in limiting restenosis as well as the potential for degeneration of the aortic wall and aneurysm formation. It should be recognized, however, that there is a 10% to 15% recurrence rate of recoarctation after ETE repair, and aneurysms have been reported after balloon dilation of these recurrences. Nevertheless, the attractiveness of ETE techniques in removing the abnormal ductal tissue and in providing an essentially normal thoracic aorta, even in infants with hypoplasia of the transverse arch, has established these as our techniques of first choice in most cases of neonatal and infant coarctation.

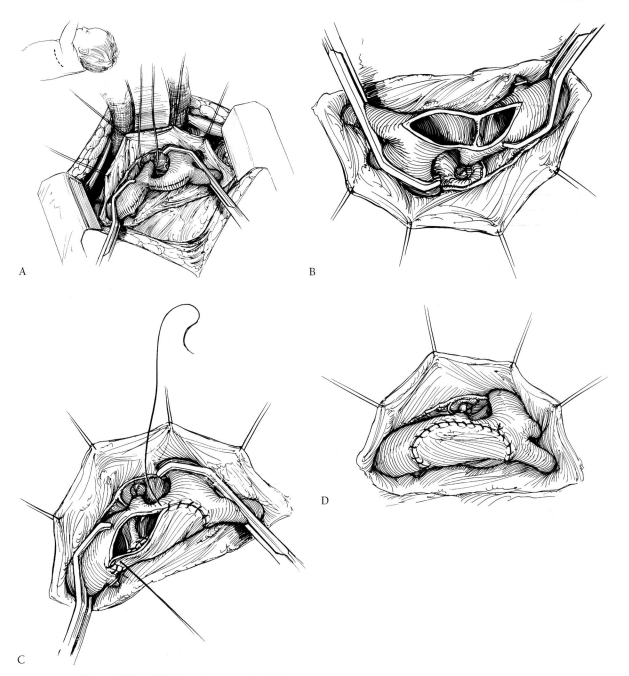

Figure 78-3. **(A)** When the coarctation is discrete and juxtaductal, vascular occlusion clamps can be placed on the aortic arch and descending aorta after the anatomy is exposed through a left thoracotomy. The ductus arteriosus is encircled with a ligature. A Satinsky-type clamp on the descending aorta can be useful in controlling posterior collaterals. An incision is then made across the area of coarctation. **(B)** The coarctation ridge is left intact. This is usually the narrowest part of the aorta and is usually opposite the ligated ductus arteriosus. **(C)** A large patch of either prosthetic or homograft material can then be placed with running monofilament suture. This patch material should be large enough to restore a normal size to the aortic lumen. **(D)** The completed repair provides augmentation of the aorta in the juxtaductal region.

Interposition Graft

Even though ETE repair is now our preferred method of repairing discrete aortic coarctation in neonates and young infants, this technique may not be suitable for repairing aortic coarctation in older children and adults or in recurrent coarctation. In these patients, it may be difficult to adequately mobilize the aorta proximal and distal to the coarctation segment to provide a tension-free ETE anastomosis. A prosthetic interposition graft consisting of Dacron or PTFE can be used for repair in these patients. This technique should be reserved for patients only when it is possible to place an adult-size graft (>18 mm to 20 mm). Extra-anatomic bypass using prosthetic graft for the repair

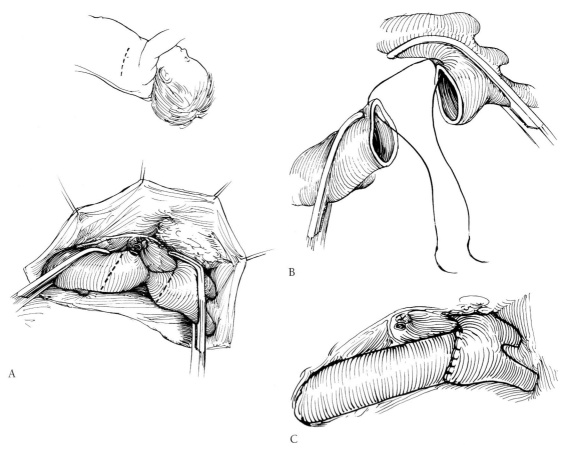

Figure 78-4. End-to-end resection and anastomosis are easily accomplished through a left thoracotomy. **(A)** The proximal ductus arteriosus is securely tied. Vascular clamps control the aortic arch and the descending aorta. When present, collateral vessels can be controlled with hemoclips. The area of coarctation is excised and removed. **(B)** The two ends of the aorta are then anastomosed using a running monofilament suture. **(C)** This provides a normal appearance to the reconstructed aorta, and in most patients there is little difficulty in mobilizing the aorta to be reconstructed in this manner.

of aortic coarctation should be avoided except in unusual circumstances like complex recurrent coarctation.

Surgical Approaches

The majority of coarctations can be exposed and repaired through a left lateral thoracotomy. The ductus arteriosus can be encircled and securely tied just before or after the vascular clamps are placed on the proximal and distal aorta. Most patients, even infants, can have several collateral vessels arising from the aorta near the coarctation site. We prefer to control these with small or medium-sized hemoclips. These hemoclips can be removed easily after coarctation repair. For ETE repair, the aorta can be divided above and below the site of ductal insertion and the excess ductal tissue removed. It is usually only necessary to place a tie on the pulmonary end of the ductus;

this will stay in place quite well after division of the ductus as long as enough tissue remains distal to the tie. The ETE anastomosis can be performed using a fine, running, nonabsorbable monofilament suture. Use of absorbable suture or interrupted rather than running anastomosis has not been shown to decrease the incidence of recurrent coarctation. If a patch technique is chosen, we recommend that the posterior coarctation ridge not be resected. This may decrease the incidence of aneurysm formation in the future. Using a large patch of PTFE will compensate for the intrusion of the posterior ridge into the aortic lumen. Closing the mediastinal pleura after ETE or subclavian flap repair depends on personal preference. Some believe that closing the mediastinal pleura over the repair can cause compression of the repair site and thereby increase the incidence of recurrent coarctation. Others believe that closing the mediastinal pleura after coarctation repair may prevent the lung from

adhering to the repair site, decrease the incidence of postoperative chylothorax, and create a circumferential wrap around the repair site, which will make balloon dilation safer if recurrent coarctation occurs. After patch aortoplasty repair, closing the mediastinal pleura over the repair may not be possible, and it may cause compression of the newly enlarged aorta and produce a suboptimal outcome.

Aortic coarctation can also be approached via a median sternotomy (Fig. 78-6). In these cases, the patient should be placed on cardiopulmonary bypass and cooled to a nasopharyngeal or rectal temperature of 16°C to 18°C. During the cooling period, the entire aortic arch and head vessels can be dissected from surrounding tissue. Once the patient is on cardiopulmonary bypass, the patent ductus arteriosus can be ligated. In cases that approach aortic arch interruption (type A interruption), distal cooling may be limited from the aortic infusion cannula, and

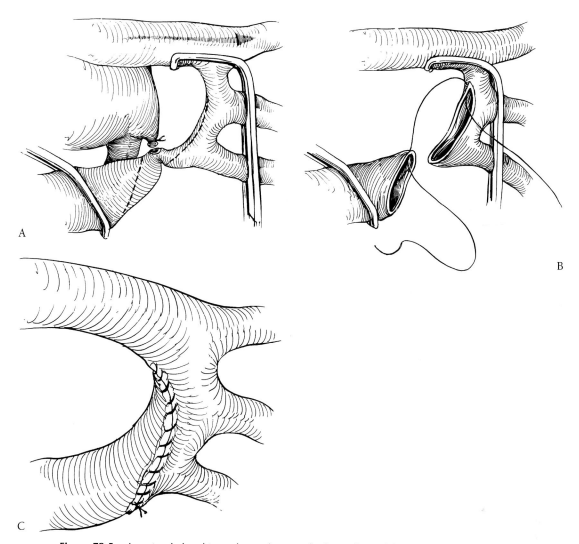

Figure 78-5. An extended end-to-end resection can also be performed through a left thoracotomy. **(A)** It is necessary to place the proximal clamp across the left subclavian and left common carotid artery. This clamp should extend onto the ascending aorta and occlude part of the innominate artery so that the proximal incision on the underside of the aorta can extend proximally as far as the origin of the left common carotid (or farther, if necessary). The ductus arteriosus is ligated, and a distal clamp is placed on the descending aorta. It is important to mobilize the descending aorta as far distally as possible, and hemoclips can be used to control collateral vessels. These hemoclips can be removed at the completion of the procedure. **(B)** The incision on the underside of the aortic arch is carried as far proximal as necessary. The incision on the descending aorta is enlarged so that it will match the size of the proximal incision. **(C)** The two ends of the aorta are then anastomosed using running suture, and this provides augmentation of a hypoplastic aortic arch.

an additional arterial cannula can be placed in the main pulmonary artery and advanced across the ductus arteriosus into the distal aorta. A snare around the ductus, and this cannula, can improve distal perfusion and cooling. After sufficient cooling, the patient's head is packed with ice, cardiopulmonary bypass is stopped, and the arterial cannula is removed. Snares placed around the previously dissected head vessels are occluded. The ductus arteriosus can be divided, and the distal aorta can be elevated by gentle traction on the distal ligature. This maneuver will facilitate dissection of the aorta well

beyond the stenotic segment. In some instances, a vascular clamp placed as far distal as possible on the descending aorta will help to keep it elevated in the surgical field, improving the surgical exposure. All residual ductal tissue in the descending aorta near the ductal insertion should be excised. If the coarctation segment is discrete, a simple ETE repair can be performed (Fig. 78-6). If the coarctation is associated with arch hypoplasia, repair can be achieved by a combination of suturing the back wall together and using a patch to augment the arch and the repair site. Homograft is preferable in

infants, especially if the entire aorta is being augmented, such as in stage 1 palliation for hypoplastic left heart syndrome (HLHS). Gore-Tex works well in older children, especially if the area is a recurrence and is surrounded by scar tissue. The sternotomy approach is convenient when the patient has significant associated cardiac defects that can be repaired at the same time or in patients with recurrent coarctation in whom control of the aorta to enable adequate access to the most proximal extent of the lesion would be challenging from the thoracotomy approach.

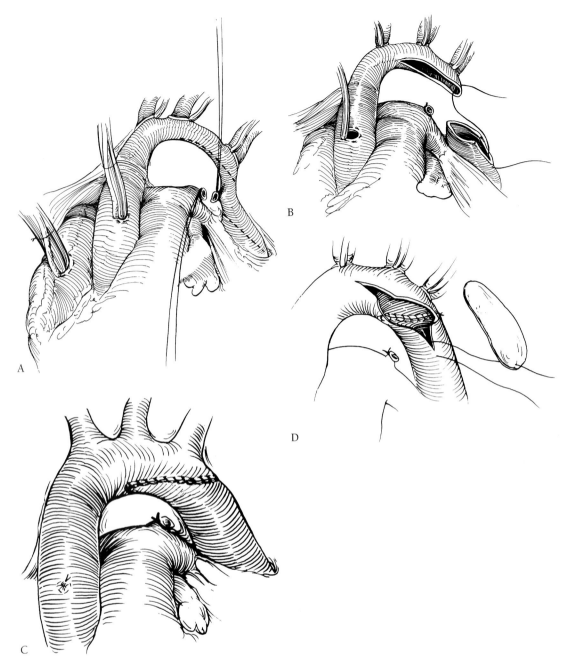

Figure 78-6. Aortic coarctation, especially when it is associated with a hypoplastic aortic arch and other intracardiac defects, can be approached through a median sternotomy. **(A)** With the patient on cardiopulmonary bypass and cannulated through the ascending aorta and the right atrium, the aortic arch, the head vessels, and the descending aorta are aggressively mobilized. The ductus arteriosus can be divided between ligatures, and gentle traction on the ligature attached to the pulmonary arteries will retract the left pulmonary artery away from the area of coarctation. At the same time, gentle upward traction on the distal ligature will help to elevate the descending aorta so that it can be adequately dissected. **(B)** After hypothermic circulatory arrest is instituted, the aortic cannula is removed. Snares on the head vessels are secured, and an incision is then made in the underside of the aortic arch as well as on the descending aorta, as shown. **(C)** These two openings are then connected with fine, running monofilament suture, providing reconstruction of the aorta as well as the hypoplastic aortic arch. **(D)** If the two aortic segments are separated (such as may be present in interrupted aortic arch) such that significant tension is created with the anastomosis, the posterior wall of the aorta can be connected, and the anterior portion of the repair can be augmented with a patch (usually homograft), as shown. **(E)** The completed aortic repair. **(F)** Occasionally (such as in re-do operations for coarctations), a sternotomy approach can be used to enlarge a recurrent coarctation. In this case, the patient is cooled on cardiopulmonary bypass and circulatory arrest is instituted. An incision is then made through the narrowest portion of the aorta. The incised area is then repaired with a patch and the patient is then replaced on bypass and rewarmed. (*Continued*)

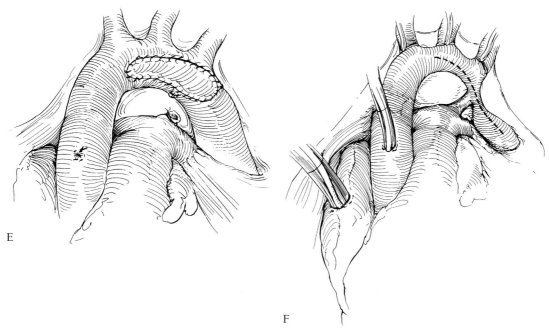

E

F

Figure 78-6. (*Continued*)

Complications

The most dreaded complication of coarctation repair is paraplegia. This has been reported to occur in 0.4% to 0.5% of patients undergoing coarctation repair. Risk factors are difficult to identify, but in some series, an aberrant retroesophageal right subclavian artery or a VSD and patent ductus arteriosus appears to put the patient at higher risk. Absence of adequate collateral vessels has also been implicated as a risk factor, but it is not always possible to delineate the adequacy of collaterals in infants, especially because they are often brought to surgery without preceding angiographic studies. Even with angiography, these tiny collaterals cannot always be delineated. Furthermore, the techniques for coarctation repair in infants are identical regardless of the extent of any collateral vessels. The use of shunts or monitoring of the distal aortic pressure has no role in infant coarctation repair and is of arguable benefit in coarctation repair in older patients. Although it would seem logical that the length of aortic cross-clamp time would relate to the incidence of paraplegia, this has not been supported by published information. Nevertheless, most surgeons attempt to limit the aortic cross-clamp time and generally try to perform the repair with clamp times of <20 to 30 minutes. The presence of hyperthermia during aortic cross-clamping has also been linked to some cases of postcoarctectomy paraplegia. In neonates, rectal or nasopharyngeal temperatures of 34°C to 35°C

can be achieved simply by turning the ambient room temperature down at the beginning of the procedure. Older patients may require active surface cooling with a cooling blanket. Although there has been some investigation into ways to prevent paraplegia (such as by identifying the arterial supply to the anterior spinal cord before surgery), this complication is not preventable by any reliable method, and families should always be informed of its potential. Other complications include postoperative hypertension (especially in older children) and abdominal pain (mesenteric arteritis). Abdominal pain may present in as many as one third of patients who have hypertension after coarctation repair. Treatment for hypertension and for abdominal pain includes beta-blockers and "bowel rest" with intravenous fluids as necessary. An occasional patient may have a postoperative chylothorax, which can present several days after surgery. This is usually caused by transection of small lymphatic vessels during the dissection for repair, and if it does not resolve with conservative management, surgical exploration to ligate the source of the chyle leak may be required.

Results

Despite the seriousness of this defect in neonates, surgical results are excellent. Hospital mortality in neonates after coarctation repair should be between 2% and 9%. Sur-

gical mortality is usually related to other factors such as associated defects, the size of the left ventricle, and the extent of the coarctation. In older patients, hospital mortality should approach zero. Depending on the age and weight of the patient at operation, the technique used, the quality of the initial repair, and factors beyond control such as growth at the repair site, between 5% and 20% of patients may develop a recurrent coarctation (defined as a gradient across the repair site of >20 mm Hg). In most instances, this can be successfully dilated by balloon angioplasty, and surgical intervention is rarely required for recurrent coarctation.

Special Situations

Coarctation and Ventricular Septal Defect

Aortic coarctation can be commonly associated with a VSD. In all cases, the coarctation should be repaired. These infants are usually in fairly significant congestive heart failure because of the left ventricular outflow tract obstruction from the coarctation and the left-to-right shunt from the VSD. At the time of coarctation repair, the VSD can be dealt with by (1) pulmonary artery banding, (2) VSD closure (via a sternotomy with one-stage repair or with separate thoracotomy and sternotomy incisions during one operative setting), or (3) coarctation repair alone with nothing done for the VSD. In the latter instance, the patient can be observed postoperatively and referred for VSD closure as indicated for treatment of that lesion as a separate entity. The Congenital Heart Surgeons Society (CHSS) data suggest that the safest approach is coarctation repair with pulmonary artery banding, but we prefer complete one-stage repair when it is apparent that the VSD will require surgical intervention. In particular, we recommend VSD closure concomitant with coarctation repair when the VSD is large (and especially when the LV outflow tract is small, including patients within the spectrum of interrupted aortic arch) or when the VSD is in a location that is not associated with spontaneous VSD closure (e.g., supracristal). We have done this through a sternotomy as well as through two separate incisions, and both provide excellent results. We do not favor pulmonary artery banding as palliation for a VSD.

Balloon Angioplasty for Native Coarctation

Balloon angioplasty has a limited role in the treatment of native coarctation. Results have been marginal with a high incidence of early recoarctation and development of aortic aneurysms at the coarctation site. Furthermore, there seems to be a disturbingly high incidence of paraplegia in patients who come to surgical coarctation repair after unsuccessful balloon angioplasty, and it is postulated that this may be related to the decreased stimulation for development of collateral circulation once the pressure gradient across the stenotic area has been partially relieved by angioplasty. The excellent results with surgical repair of native coarctation make balloon angioplasty a much less attractive treatment option. Therefore balloon angioplasty of native coarctation only should be reserved for unusual circumstances where operative repair is not possible or desirable.

Coarctation and the Hypoplastic Left Ventricle

Aortic coarctation commonly exists in the spectrum of lesions that constitute hypoplastic left heart syndrome. In the case of unequivocal hypoplasia of the left ventricle, the coarctation is repaired with patch augmentation as part of a standard Norwood procedure. Occasionally the size of the left ventricle is borderline (approximately 20 mL/m^2) with regard to whether it is adequate to support the entire systemic circu-

lation. Instead of staging toward a univentricular physiology, it is possible to repair the aortic coarctation by using a patch technique so that the ductus arteriosus can be left open (on PGE$_1$ infusion) after the procedure. This will serve to decompress the pulmonary hypertension that these patients may have postoperatively and to maintain systemic perfusion while the left ventricle recovers. If the left ventricle is inadequate to support the systemic circulation, right-to-left ductal blood flow will persist and the patient will need to be staged to a univentricular physiology. However, if the left ventricle is adequate to support the entire systemic circulation, blood flow in the ductus will change to left to right after the left ventricle recovers from the coarctation repair. The ductus arteriosus is then allowed to close by stopping the PGE$_1$ infusion. Occasionally, the ductus in these patients is large and will not close after cessation of the PGE$_1$. In these cases, it may be necessary to tie the ductus surgically.

Recurrent Coarctation

The incidence of recurrent coarctation ranges between 5% and 20%, depending on (1) the age of the patient at operation, (2) the extent of the original coarctation lesion, (3) the technique used for coarctation repair, and (4) the length of the follow-up period. Reintervention for these patients should be considered if the peak-to-peak gradient (by cardiac catheterization) across the coarctation site is >20 mm Hg (a peak instantaneous gradient, by echocardiography, of >35 mm Hg). Surgery can be challenging because of the adhesions and scar tissue around the aorta and lung from previous surgery. As a result, it can be very difficult and hazardous to gain proximal control of the aortic arch for placement of a vascular clamp. Repeat ETE reconstruction is nearly impossible in these patients because the aorta cannot be mobilized adequately without placing excessive tension on the suture line. The treatment of choice for recurrent coarctation is balloon angioplasty. If balloon angioplasty is not successful and reoperation is necessary, patch aortoplasty should be considered. This can be done either through a thoracotomy or through a sternotomy on cardiopulmonary bypass with a limited period of hypothermic circulatory arrest. Alternatively, an extra-anatomic bypass graft from the ascending to the descending aorta can be used for complex recurrent coarctation, especially ones with a long segment of arch hypoplasia. Frequently this can be done either through a right thoracotomy

or a median sternotomy without using cardiopulmonary bypass.

SUGGESTED READING

Backer CL, Paape K, Zales VR, et al. Coarctation of the aorta: Repair with polytetrafluoroethylene patch aortoplasty. Circulation 1995;92:II-132.

Brewer LA, Fosburg RG, Mulder GA, et al. Spinal cord complications following surgery for coarctation of the aorta: A study of 66 cases. J Thorac Cardiovasc Surg 1972;64:368.

Castaneda AR, Mayer JEI, Jonas RA, et al. Cardiac Surgery in the Neonate and Infant. St. Louis: Mosby, 1994.

Elliott MJ. Coarctation of the aorta with arch hypoplasia: Improvements on a new technique. Ann Thorac Surg 1987;44:321.

Kirklin JW, Barratt-Boyes BG. Cardiac Surgery (2nd ed). New York: Churchill Livingstone, 1993.

Lerberg DB, Hardesty RL, Siewers RD, et al. Coarctation of the aorta in infants and children: 25 years of experience. Ann Thorac Surg 1982;33:159.

Locher JP Jr, Kron LL. Coarctation of the Aorta. In Mavroudis C, Backer CL (eds), Pediatric Cardiac Surgery. St. Louis: Mosby, 1994.

Quaegebeur JM, Jonas RA, Weinberg AD, et al. Congenital Heart Surgeons Society. Outcomes in seriously ill neonates with coarctation of the aorta: A multi-institutional study. J Thorac Cardiovasc Surg 1994;108:841.

Schwengel DA, Nichols DG, Cameron DE. Coarctation of the Aorta and Interrupted Aortic Arch. In Nichols DG, Cameron DE, Greeley WI, et al. (eds), Critical Heart Disease in Infants and Children. St. Louis: Mosby, 1995.

Ungerleider RM, Ebert PA. Indications and techniques for midline approach to aortic coarctation in infants and children. Ann Thorac Surg 1987;44:517.

EDITOR'S COMMENTS

Although numerous techniques have been used for coarctation repair, all of the accepted techniques have been associated with excellent results with very low morbidity and mortality. The risk of death after coarctation repair now approaches zero for most children even with complex associated defects, except those associated with severe forms of LVOTO. Coarctation of the aorta in isolation, without associated congenital heart defects and of such severity as to not require immediate repair in infancy, is generally repaired in our institution when the patient is younger than 1 year of age. The exact timing of repair of coarctation in asymptomatic individuals remains controversial. Whereas later repair beyond 1 to 2 years of age is associated with a low incidence of late recurrence, the presence of a significant afterload on the ventricle with resulting hypertrophy may alter LV mass and compliance late in life. In addition, some patients, even after successful coarctation repair, continue to have proximal arterial hypertension, possibly related to an abnormal renin–angiotensin system or compliance differences in the aorta above and below the coarctation repair site. Many of these patients have refractory hypertension despite a completely unobstructed anastomosis.

The advent of successful balloon dilation for recurrent coarctation has permitted extension of early coarctation repair to younger than 1 year of age in the majority of patients and may help decrease the pressure load on the left ventricle. The subclavian flap technique for repair of coarctation of the aorta in infants, as popularized by John Waldhausen, has the advantage of being performed rapidly, and can be done with a single Satinsky-type partial occlusion clamp placed across the base of the ductus arteriosus incorporating the descending aorta and the arch of the aorta. The subclavian is ligated distally and divided, and the flap can be rapidly opened and sewn down across the coarctation site. I have not found it possible to resect much coarctation shelf in most of these children because there is often residual ductal tissue and the material is extremely friable. We have elected to utilize absorbable suture for coarctation repair in hopes of aiding growth of the anastomoses, although a fine, nonabsorbable suture has also been associated with growth. We have elected to use the subclavian flap only in situations in which a rapid anastomosis needs to be constructed or in children in whom ductal patency is being maintained until after the coarctation repair is complete. Patch repair as advocated by the authors is another good choice. In patients in whom the ability of the ventricle to withstand coarctation repair is questionable because of LV volume overload, it is possible to perform a subclavian flap repair, leave the ductus open, and then snare the ductus temporarily after repair while observing the effects on ventricular function and cardiac output or to leave the ductus patent and allow spontaneous closure after discontinuation of prostaglandin therapy. If patients with a relatively small LV volume continue to require ventilatory support after coarctation repair and ductal closure, conversion to a Norwood-type operation can be performed through the midline at a separate procedure.

Controversy continues regarding the use of patch material for coarctation repair in infants and older children. Although significant late problems have developed with the use of Dacron patches in the aorta, aneurysm formation has often been opposite the site of the patch, consistent with abnormalities of flow in the region of the coarctation repair. Thus, although Gore-Tex patch has not been associated with late deterioration, the same concerns about late aneurysm formation must be considered. In addition, Gore-Tex may bleed significantly when used proximally in the ascending aorta, and therefore we have not utilized Gore-Tex preferentially for coarctation repair except in exceptional circumstances. Like Dr. Ungerleider, we have preferred to perform one-stage coarctation repair and VSD closure in children in whom the VSD is large and in whom there is associated arch hypoplasia and in those patients in whom the VSD is of a type not likely to spontaneously close. Care must be taken during coarctation repair in these children to tailor the pulmonary homograft patch adequately so that as it is brought down toward the ascending aorta; it is tapered so that a gentle take-off in size of the aorta is created to prevent kinking of the ascending aorta where the size changes abruptly to the patched arch.

In general, we have not elected to perform primary ETE anastomoses through a sternotomy incision because any tension on the anastomosis can result in bleeding that may cause stenosis of the repair site when repair stitches are used to control hemorrhage. In the same fashion as for reconstruction for interrupted aortic arch, we have elected to augment the entire arch with a portion of pulmonary homograft material or to create an ETE anastomosis at the level of the subclavian and carotid vessel and then augment the undersurface with a patch of pulmonary homograft to take tension off the anastomosis. This has resulted in a lower incidence of recurrent coarctation in our patients.

If subclavian flap repair or ETE anastomosis is performed, we have elected to routinely close the mediastinal pleura over the repair site in the hope of decreasing the possibility of late aneurysm formation and to allow better control of any disruption at the time of balloon dilation if recurrent stenosis occurs. Although pseudo-aneurysm formation at coarctation repair has been extremely uncommon, we have seen this occur with primary disruption in at least one older individual. Control of the localized hemorrhage by mediastinal pleural closure can permit salvage of these patients even if aortic disruption occurs. If closure of the pleura will compromise the repair by compression, it is omitted.

The management of recurrent coarctation not amenable to balloon angioplasty remains problematic. In most individuals, it is not possible to create an ETE anastomosis after a previous coarctation repair by any of the usual techniques, and mobilization of the aorta can be difficult and create excessive tension on an ETE suture line. Therefore, recurrent coarctation may best be treated by patch augmentation of the coarctation site. We tend to use patch augmentation with either Gore-Tex or pulmonary homograft in these individuals, usually with cardiopulmonary bypass and a brief period of circulatory arrest to decrease the risk of paraplegia. Because these patients often have inadequate collateral supply, they appear to be at greater risk for development of paraplegia postoperatively.

The use of graft material for bypass of recurrent coarctation segments should be discouraged. Although in exceptional circumstances such grafts may be necessary, we have seen at least two individuals who presented late after graft bypass of recurrent coarctation segments with pseudo-aneurysm formation and aortobronchial fistulae. The extensive scarring in the chest after these operations and the protrusion of the graft to the adjacent lung complicated repair of the pseudo-aneurysm. Thus, if a graft is to be placed, we prefer to place it in the anatomic location with an ETE anastomosis and, if at all possible, to cover the graft with mediastinal pleura to prevent erosion into adjacent structures or to contain pseudo-aneurysm formation.

Unusual circumstances in which recurrent coarctation is present in association with complex arch hypoplasia or previous extensive thoracotomies have been performed occasionally require extra-anatomic bypass. In situations where the aortic arch and coarctation are not readily accessible due to previous surgery or there are other complicating factors, it is simple to create an ascending aorta-to-descending aorta bypass intrapericardially using an adult-size Dacron graft anastomosed to the side of the ascending aorta and then to the descending aorta posteriorly in the intrapericardial space above the level of the diaphragm. These extra-anatomic bypasses appear to have a decreased incidence of pseudo-aneurysm formation compared to extra-anatomic bypass performed in the left chest and can readily relieve any residual gradients.

An area of controversy is the use of balloon dilation and stent implantation in native coarctation in adults. In some cases this approach may be the most desirable because repair of coarctation in older adolescents or adults is associated with difficulty in mobilizing the arteries for direct anastomosis, and large collateral vessels in the chest wall may be associated with significant bleeding. Although the results with the use of stents for native coarctation appear to be good in the short term, long-term follow-up will be necessary to see whether the incidence of pseudo-aneurysm formation or late gradients will limit the use of this technique. Nevertheless, in older patients the relative risk and benefit of catheter-based intervention versus surgical treatment would tend to favor catheter intervention should there be a low incidence of late complications. Paradoxical hypertension, however, can occur with both catheter and surgical approaches.

It has now become common to use stents in recurrent coarctation in older individuals. The advantages of stent implantation are the decreased risk of recurrent obstruction and good relief of any residual gradients. Nevertheless, the long-term potential complications of a stent implanted into the wall of an abnormal aorta with abnormal compliance at the stent site have not been addressed and deserve further study. Nevertheless the use of stents has significantly decreased the recurrence rate even after balloon dilation of recurrent obstruction at the coarctation repair site.

Postoperative complications after coarctation repair are infrequent. The most common complication, as noted, is paradoxical hypertension, which is often treated best by infusion of a short-acting beta-blocking agent such as esmolol. The use of nitroprusside is less effective in controlling hypertension after coarctation repair, and very large doses of nitroprusside may be needed to control the blood pressure. In addition, nitroprusside may increase the force of ventricular ejection and predispose to possible aortic dissection in patients with abnormal aortic tissue. Therefore, we have elected to use esmolol as the primary treatment of significant hypertension postcoarctation repair. In most patients, the beta-blocker can be discontinued within 24 hours after the operation without recurrence of hypertension.

Although enthusiasm has developed for the use of balloon dilation for native coarctation in infants in some centers, we discourage the use of this technique. The results of primary repair of coarctation have become excellent and result in a low incidence of recurrent coarctation or late aneurysm formation. The use of balloon dilation, which does not remove ductal tissue and may result in a primary disruption of the endothelium, seems an unattractive option in patients in whom an operative procedure may be associated with excellent early and late results. This is especially true because most infants who require coarctation repair have associated congenital anomalies that should be addressed promptly.

I.L.K.

79

Interrupted Aortic Arch Complex

Richard G. Ohye, Takaaki Suzuki, Eric J. Devaney, and Edward L. Bove

Interruption of the aortic arch (IAA) is a congenital anomaly characterized by complete discontinuity of blood flow between two portions of the aorta. This malformation may exist as a long-distance physical separation between adjacent segments or in the form of discontinuity between adjacent lumens of vessels that are otherwise connected externally. The latter anomaly is more commonly considered among discussions of coarctation of the aorta and is not discussed further here. IAA occurs uncommonly as an isolated lesion, being frequently associated with a number of complex intracardiac defects. Therefore, the diagnosis and management of IAA complex are best considered in combination with the cardiac anomaly as a whole. Recent advances in the management of IAA and the associated cardiac defects have resulted in a significant improvement in the overall outcome for patients with this complex anomaly. The approach of a single-stage repair of all coexisting defects simultaneously with the IAA has been shown to be a safe and effective management protocol.

Anatomy

The aortic arch is that portion of the aorta between the innominate artery and the ductus arteriosus, and interruption of the arch may occur between any of the arch vessels. According to the classification originally described by Celoria and Patton (Fig. 79-1), type A occurs just distal to the origin of the left subclavian artery, between that vessel and the insertion of the ductus arteriosus itself. In this type, a fibrous cord is frequently found connecting the proximal and distal portions of the arch. The most common variety, type B, occurs between the origins of the left common carotid artery and the left subclavian artery. This type accounts for approximately two thirds of all cases of IAA. In the rarest form, type C, the interruption occurs between the innominate and left common carotid arteries. This type is seen in only 5% of patients.

Associated cardiovascular anomalies are nearly always present in IAA. The most common condition is that of isolated ventricular septal defect (VSD). In a recent multi-institutional study by the Congenital Heart Surgeons Society (CHSS), which analyzed 250 neonates entered into the study over a 5-year period by 29 participating institutions, isolated VSD was present in 183 patients (73%). Other commonly associated lesions included truncus arteriosus, transposition of the great arteries (TGA) with VSD, and various forms of single ventricle. The frequency of associated anomalies, as found in the CHSS report, is shown in Table 79-1.

The VSD in patients with IAA is frequently of the malalignment type and is commonly associated with posterior deviation of the infundibular (outlet) septum. The displacement of the infundibular septum to the left of the posterior limb of the septal band results in narrowing of the left ventricular outflow tract and the potential for subaortic obstruction. Anomalous origin of the right subclavian artery from the descending aorta frequently occurs with IAA and is associated with a greater prevalence of subaortic obstruction secondary to reduced flow in utero through the left ventricular outflow tract and the aortic valve. Additional levels of left heart obstruction may also occur at the aortic valve leaflets, aortic annulus, mitral valve, and the ascending aorta.

Presentation and Diagnosis

In the majority of patients, the diagnosis of IAA is first made on the discovery of signs and symptoms of congestive heart failure within the first few days of life. Lower-extremity pulses may be poorly palpable or not palpable at all. In some cases, the diagnosis is not suspected until ductal closure occurs. While the ductus remains patent, flow to the lower body remains unobstructed, and the elevated pulmonary vascular resistance normally found in the newborn delays the expected increase in pulmonary blood flow through the VSD. This combination effectively delays the development of heart failure. Abrupt ductal closure, however, results in profound acidosis, cardiovascular collapse, and shock as lower-body perfusion is severely reduced. Resuscitation with an infusion of prostaglandin E_1 to maintain ductal patency should be established when the diagnosis is made. If shock has occurred and there is associated renal and hepatic dysfunction, administration of dopamine is generally used as well. A period of a few days may be necessary to allow return of end-organ function before operative repair is performed. During this time, careful control of ventilation is needed to avoid hyperventilation, which serves to increase pulmonary blood flow and may worsen systemic perfusion further. In addition, treatment of associated conditions, including sepsis, necrotizing enterocolitis, and coagulation abnormalities, must be performed. Because DiGeorge syndrome is a commonly associated condition in patients with IAA, occurring in 27% of patients in the CHSS report, careful control of calcium balance will often

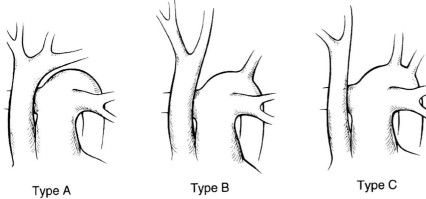

Type A   Type B   Type C

Figure 79-1. The most commonly used classification of the three types of interruption of the aortic arch. In type A, the interruption occurs distal to the left subclavian artery. In type B, the arch is interrupted between the left carotid and the left subclavian arteries. In type C, the rarest form, the aorta is interrupted proximal to the left carotid artery.

be necessary. All transfused blood should be irradiated to avoid graft-versus-host disease until the diagnosis of DiGeorge syndrome is definitively excluded.

The diagnosis of IAA can be accurately made from two-dimensional Doppler/echocardiographic studies. Cardiac catheterization with aortic angiography is rarely needed to define the anatomy. The exact site of the interruption in addition to the location of the branch vessels and the distance between interrupted segments should be determined. The presence of an anomalous origin of the right subclavian artery may be more difficult to diagnose by echocardiography but would not significantly alter the operative approach. In addition to the anatomy of the aortic arch, it is important to define the intracardiac anatomy in anticipation of a complete one-stage repair. The location and boundaries of the VSD, particularly in relation to the left ventricular outflow tract,

aortic valve, and pulmonary valve, must be accurately seen. The majority of VSDs occur in the outlet portion of the septum, but other locations as well as additional defects must be sought. Although measurement of gradients across the left ventricular outflow tract is not possible in the presence of a nonrestrictive VSD and patent ductus arteriosus, some guidelines are helpful in predicting those patients who are likely to develop important left ventricular outflow tract obstruction after repair. When the echocardiographically measured ratio of the smallest diameter of the left ventricular outflow tract normalized to the diameter of the descending thoracic aorta at the level of the diaphragm is 1.0 as measured in diastole or is 0.6 when measured in systole, we have found that the risk of subaortic obstruction after closure of the VSD is high and that efforts to resect or incise that portion of the infundibular septum that is deviated poste-

riorly beneath the aortic annulus are beneficial in avoiding or reducing postoperative obstruction. Other groups have suggested other preoperative echocardiographic measurements, including cross-sectional area of the left ventricular outflow tract indexed to body surface area, subaortic diameter index, and subaortic diameter Z-score. However, the optimal parameter that consistently displays a high degree of sensitivity and specificity remains elusive.

Operative Management of Interrupted Aortic Arch with Isolated Ventricular Septal Defect

The preferred operative management of a newborn with IAA and isolated VSD is a single-stage repair performed through a midline sternotomy approach. Nasopharyngeal and rectal temperature probes are placed. Arterial monitoring is achieved by the placement of a catheter in the umbilical or femoral artery, which has usually been accomplished in the intensive care unit before surgery. Additional noninvasive arterial monitoring should be done with a blood pressure cuff on the right arm to allow measurement of blood pressures above and below the repair site. If the right radial artery has already been cannulated, the cuff is placed on the leg. Venous access is accomplished through an umbilical or femoral venous catheter; internal jugular access is avoided in babies smaller than approximately 5 kg because of the increased risk of superior vena caval thrombosis. A midline sternotomy incision is made, and the presence or absence of thymic tissue is noted. If the thymus is present, it is totally or partially resected for exposure, preserving the cervical extensions. Heparin is administered at this time, and the pericardium is opened. Purse-string sutures for cannulation are placed in the right atrial appendage, the ascending aorta at the base of the innominate artery, and the main pulmonary artery (Fig. 79-2). Alternatively, bicaval venous cannulation may be established at this time. A tourniquet is placed around the right pulmonary artery before bypass, and this vessel may be occluded at this time if significant hypotension exists. A Y-adapter is placed in the arterial line of the pump to allow cannulation of both the ascending aorta and pulmonary artery. Once bypass is initiated, a tourniquet is placed around the left

Table 79-1   Associated Cardiovascular Conditions in Neonates with Interrupted Aortic Arch

Condition	Lesion Number	Percentage
Isolated ventricular septal defect	183	73
Truncus arteriosus	25	10
Transposition of the great arteries/ventricular septal defect[a]	12	5
Aortopulmonary window	10	4
Single ventricle	9	4
Other	7	3
None	4	2

[a]Includes Taussig-Bing anomaly.
Source: Reprinted with permission from RA Jonas, JM Quaegebeur, JW Kirklin, et al. Outcomes in patients with interrupted aortic arch and ventricular septal defect: a multi-institutional study. J Thorac Cardiovasc Surg 1994;107:1099.

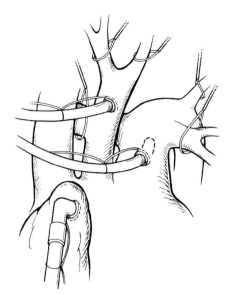

Figure 79-2. Cardiopulmonary bypass and cannulation for repair of type B interruption of the aortic arch. Arterial cannulation is performed through the ascending aorta and proximal main pulmonary artery with the branch pulmonary arteries occluded with tourniquets. Venous return is through the right atrium. Additional tourniquets are placed around the head vessels for occlusion during the period of circulatory arrest.

pulmonary artery and is engaged (as well as the right if not already done) to direct all pump flow through the ductus and to the lower body. This method of cannulation allows for even cooling of the upper and lower body in preparation for circulatory arrest. Bypass is initiated at a blood temperature of approximately 30°C, and progressive cooling to a nasopharyngeal temperature of 18°C or less is accomplished. Ice bags are placed around the head. Systemic vasodilatation with phentolamine (0.1 mg/kg) is given to facilitate even cooling between the nasopharyngeal and rectal temperatures. A minimal cooling period of 20 minutes is allowed, regardless of when the desired temperatures are reached.

During the interval required for cooling, the ascending and descending aorta and the brachiocephalic vessels are mobilized widely. Sufficient intercostal arteries are divided to permit a tension-free anastomosis. After appropriate cooling, the circulation is arrested, and the arch vessels are snared. Blood cardioplegia is delivered through a separate cannula after placement of a cross-clamp or through the arterial cannulation site to induce arrest. The ductus arteriosus is ligated on the pulmonary artery side and excised distally, with care being taken to remove all ductal tissue on the descending

aorta. A vascular clamp on the descending aorta facilitates exposure and avoids the need to place excess tension with forceps on the vessel itself. When there is an anomalous right subclavian artery, ligation and division are usually required to permit an anastomosis without tension or compression of the trachea. In the case of a type B IAA, the descending aorta is sutured to an opening beginning at the base of the left common carotid artery, which is extended proximally along the underside of the ascending aorta (Fig. 79-3). Proper alignment is important, and care must be taken to avoid spiraling this incision. The anastomosis is performed with a continuous technique using 6-0 or 7-0, absorbable or nonabsorbable monofilament suture. In cases of type A IAA, the transverse aortic arch may be hypoplastic, as is frequently seen with coarctation of the aorta. The anastomosis should be spatulated to enlarge the transverse arch using the distal aorta, bringing the suture line proximally to the level of the innominate artery to ensure that there is no residual narrowing.

The total elapsed circulatory arrest time at this point of the procedure is generally no more than 12 to 15 minutes, allowing ample time for VSD closure through an incision in the right atrium. Alternatively, bicaval cannulation can be used rather than single atrial access. If this approach is used, cardiopulmonary bypass may be resumed at this point for the VSD closure to minimize circulatory arrest time. Occasionally, when there is deficiency or absence of the infundibular septum and over-riding of the

VSD by the pulmonary valve, optimal exposure is best achieved through an incision in the main pulmonary artery. Transatrial exposure of the defect usually is accomplished easily with traction sutures placed on the anterior and septal leaflets of the tricuspid valve, and an appropriately trimmed patch of polytetrafluoroethylene material is placed with a continuous 6-0 polypropylene suture. When there is coexisting posterior deviation of the infundibular septum (Fig. 79-4) and important postrepair subaortic obstruction is considered likely, wedge resection of the septum is performed through the VSD itself (Figs. 79-5 to 79-7). On occasion, an incision in the septum alone is performed, which is usually sufficient to enlarge the left ventricular outflow tract. The atriotomy is closed, and the cannulas are reinserted for cardiopulmonary bypass, with air being evacuated through a generous needle hole in the ascending aorta. Rewarming is accomplished, during which time epicardial pacing wires are placed on the right atrium and ventricle. After bypass is discontinued, one or two additional catheters are placed in the right atrium through the cannulation purse string. Left atrial pressure monitoring lines may also be placed. Routine sternal closure over a mediastinal drain is performed; occasionally, sternal closure is delayed if there is hemodynamic compromise or significant edema.

An alternative to deep hypothermic circulatory arrest for the repair of IAA is regional cerebral perfusion. For this technique, a limited amount of flow is delivered

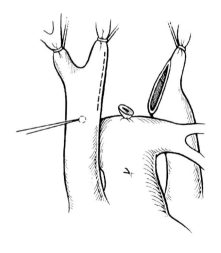
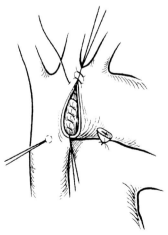

Figure 79-3. Direct anastomosis between the descending thoracic aorta and the ascending aorta is performed with a continuous suture technique after all ductal tissue is resected. The anastomosis is begun at the base of the left carotid artery.

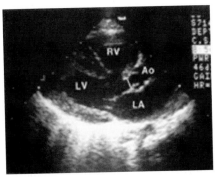

Figure 79-4. An echocardiogram in the long-axis view demonstrating a malalignment ventricular septal defect with posterior deviation of the infundibular septum typically seen with interruption of the aortic arch. (Reprinted with permission from EL Bove, LL Minich, AK Pridjian, et al. The management of severe subaortic stenosis, ventricular septal defect, and aortic arch obstruction in the neonate. J Thorac Cardiovasc Surg 1993;105:289.)

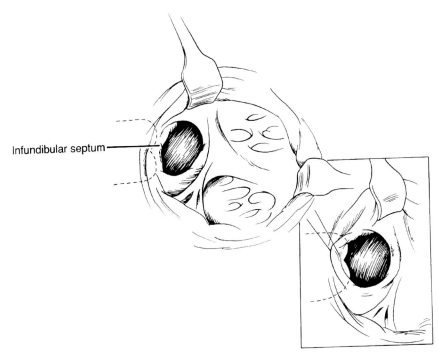

Infundibular septum

Figure 79-5. View of the ventricular septal defect through the tricuspid valve. A traction suture in the infundibular septum facilitates exposure of the aortic valve. (Reprinted with permission from EL Bove, LL Minich, AK Pridjian, et al. The management of severe subaortic stenosis, ventricular septal defect, and aortic arch obstruction in the neonate. J Thorac Cardiovasc Surg 1993;105:289.)

to the brain through the innominate artery. The ascending aorta cannula is placed near the base of the innominate artery. The patient is cooled and otherwise prepared in the same manner as for circulatory arrest. Cerebral oxygen saturation by near-infrared spectroscopy is used to monitor cerebral perfusion, and a right radial arterial line can be inserted to monitor perfusion pressure. At the time that circulatory arrest would be initiated, the aortic cannula is advanced up the innominate artery and snared in place. Flow is started at 5 cc/kg per minute and gradually advanced to 20 cc/kg per minute while monitoring cerebral oxygen saturation for a return to baseline (and pressure if a right radial arterial line is present). The arterial cannula in the pulmonary artery is removed, the venous return is collected by the venous cannula(e), and the remainder of the procedure is identical to that performed during circulatory arrest. Although many centers have adopted this approach in an effort to provide better neurodevelopmental outcome, there are no data to suggest a benefit, particularly when compared to circulatory arrest times less than 20 to 30 minutes.

Special Circumstances

Interrupted Aortic Arch with Aortic Valve Hypoplasia or Atresia

When left ventricular outflow tract obstruction secondary to hypoplasia or atresia of the annulus of the aortic valve is present in conjunction with a VSD, one of two modifications of the Damus-Kaye-Stansel procedure may be used to bypass the aortic valve, depending on the specific anatomy. The approach is tailored to achieve an optimal surgical result with respect to a widely patent, tension-free aortic reconstruction while avoiding compression of adjacent structures, such as the left mainstem bronchus and pulmonary artery. One option is to divide the distal ascending aorta and repair the IAA by direct anastomosis. This reconstructed distal aortic segment, which may be augmented with a patch of allograft material, is then sutured end to end to the divided proximal main pulmonary artery. The ascending aorta is then sewn end to side into the main pulmonary artery. This method of repair can be facilitated by performing a Lecompte maneuver. Alternatively, the ascending aorta may be transected at the level of the divided main pulmonary artery. The IAA is repaired forming the posterior wall for a modified Norwood-type augmentation patch of the aorta, as is described later for IAA with single ventricle. This reconstructed aorta is then sewn end to end to the proximal pulmonary artery, incorporating the proximal ascending aorta, as in a modified Norwood procedure. Following either technique of aortic reconstruction,

the VSD is closed to channel left ventricular blood to the pulmonary valve, and a conduit is interposed between the right ventricle and the pulmonary artery bifurcation. Although we prefer a one-stage approach, the pulmonary artery bifurcation may alternatively be closed with a patch, and pulmonary blood flow is provided through a modified Blalock-Taussig shunt, deferring complete repair until a later date.

The third alternative for patients with IAA and aortic valve hypoplasia, with or without VSD, is a Ross/Konno procedure. The ascending aorta is divided and the proximal ascending aorta and aortic valve are resected. The IAA is repaired, generally by forming a posterior wall at the site of the interruption, with an anterior Norwood-type patch augmentation. The pulmonary autograft is harvested in the usual fashion. and a standard Ross procedure is performed. For the Konno portion of the operation, it is often not necessary to fully divide the ventricular septum and place a patch to enlarge the left ventricular outflow tract. It is generally sufficient to divide the aortic annulus and simply incise the septum up to, but not through, the endocardium of the right ventricular outflow tract (Fig. 79-8). A wedge of muscle can also resected from the septum to further enhance unobstructed left ventricular output.

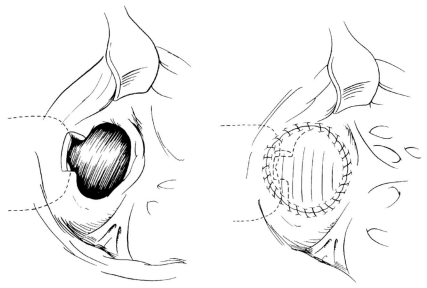

Figure 79-6. Resection of the infundibular septum is performed until the aortic valve is reached. The ventricular septal defect is then closed with a patch. (Reprinted with permission from EL Bove, LL Minich, AK Pridjian, et al. The management of severe subaortic stenosis, ventricular septal defect, and aortic arch obstruction in the neonate. J Thorac Cardiovasc Surg 1993;105:289.)

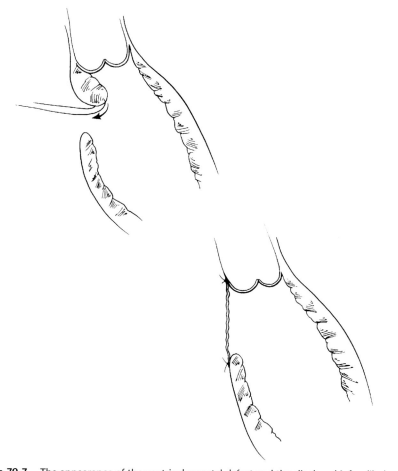

Figure 79-7. The appearance of the ventricular septal defect and the displaced infundibular septum as seen from the lateral view. Note the position of the traction suture in the septum **(upper left)** and the position of the ventricular septal defect patch **(lower right)**. (Reprinted with permission from EL Bove, LL Minich, AK Pridjian, et al. The management of severe subaortic stenosis, ventricular septal defect, and aortic arch obstruction in the neonate. J Thorac Cardiovasc Surg 1993;105:289.)

Interrupted Aortic Arch with Truncus Arteriosus

When interrupted aortic arch is associated with truncus arteriosus, significant modifications in the technique of repair are required. Nearly all interruptions are type B, although a single patient with type A has been seen in our center (Fig. 79-9). The ascending aorta distal to the origin of the ductus arteriosus and the pulmonary arteries is usually quite small in this condition. The arterial cannula is placed into the distal ascending aorta because it will be subsequently augmented, and the branch right and left pulmonary arteries are occluded at the onset of cardiopulmonary bypass. During cooling in preparation for circulatory arrest or regional cerebral perfusion, the innominate, left carotid, and left subclavian arteries are mobilized and encircled with snares for subsequent occlusion, as described in the preceding section. The remaining ascending and proximal descending aorta are also mobilized. Once circulatory arrest or regional perfusion is established, the ductus arteriosus is excised, and the orifices of the right and left pulmonary arteries are excised from the aorta with a button of adjacent arterial tissue that is as large as is feasible. The large opening in the proximal ascending aorta resulting from the excision of both the ductus arteriosus and the pulmonary artery bifurcation is extended superiorly along the medial side of the ascending aorta and into the base of the left carotid artery (Fig. 79-10). Primary end-to-end anastomosis with the descending aorta is then begun, using a running suture technique and placing the descending aorta and left subclavian artery distally to the ascending aorta beginning at the base of the left carotid artery. The large defect remaining below this portion of the anastomosis is then reconstructed and further augmented with a patch of allograft tissue beginning from the sinus of Valsalva and carrying it upward into the lower aspect of the primary arch anastomosis (Fig. 79-11). In this fashion, two potential problems are avoided. First, placing the descending aorta too far proximally onto the ascending aorta may result in obstruction to the left pulmonary artery or compression of the left mainstem bronchus and residual aortic obstruction between the truncal valve and the anastomosis of the aortic arch. Second, this technique also maintains the potential for growth because neither the suture lines nor the prosthetic material are placed circumferentially. After completion of this aspect of the procedure, the VSD is then repaired in the usual fashion

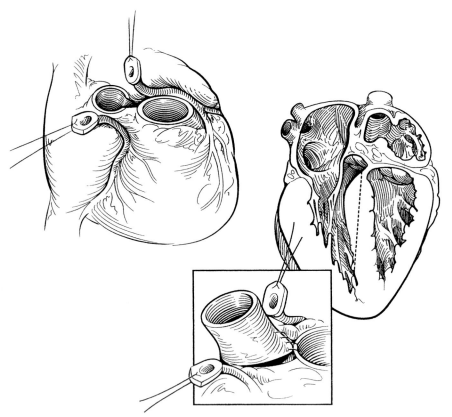

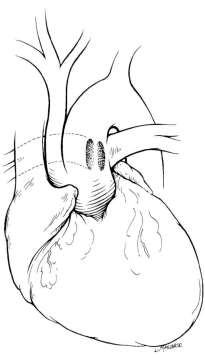

Figure 79-8. After removal of the aortic valve and harvesting of the autograft, a partial thickness septal incision is performed to enlarge the aortic annulus **(left)**. If necessary, a septal myomectomy may be performed for subaortic stenosis **(right)**. In the region of the incision, the autograft is anastomosed directly to the endocardium of the right ventricular outflow tract **(inset)**.

Figure 79-9. A truncus arteriosus associated with type B interruption of the aortic arch. Note the small ascending aorta distal to the origin of the pulmonary arteries and the ductus arteriosus. (Reprinted with permission from AE Baue, AS Geha, GL Hammond, et al. [eds]. Glenn's Thoracic and Cardiovascular Surgery [6th ed]. Norwalk CT: Appleton & Lange, 1994;1216.)

generally on full cardiopulmonary bypass. The right ventricle-to-distal pulmonary artery continuity is established with a cryopreserved allograft conduit.

Interrupted Aortic Arch with Transposition of the Great Arteries

Single-stage arterial switch and IAA repair are performed for TGA with IAA with few modifications. The arch anastomosis is performed first in a fashion identical to that described in the section on IAA with VSD. Because the ascending aorta will be transected for the arterial switch and relocated posterior to the pulmonary artery bifurcation, the division is performed a few millimeters distal to the sinotubular ridge to foreshorten the ascending aorta and avoid kinking.

Interrupted Aortic Arch with Single Ventricle

When IAA coexists with single ventricle, the technique of repair must be individually tailored to the specific anatomy. In the usual situation, IAA is found with TGA and tricuspid atresia or with double-inlet left ventricle (Fig. 79-12). In these conditions, there will be unrestricted pulmonary blood flow and a restrictive or potentially restrictive outlet (bulboventricular) foramen that will result in subaortic obstruction. Therefore, the initial operative procedure must be designed to relieve all levels of systemic outflow tract obstruction and to control pulmonary blood flow. This is best accomplished with a modified Norwood procedure, which augments the entire ascending aorta and aortic arch with a patch of cryopreserved pulmonary allograft material (Fig. 79-13). The ascending and descending portions of the arch are sutured directly only along their posterior walls, and the undersurface is opened distally for at least 1 cm to 2 cm in length. The ascending aorta is divided above the valve and opened posteriorly as well. The allograft patch is then used to augment the entire aorta, which is then sutured end to end to the proximal main pulmonary artery, incorporating the proximal end of the ascending aorta to ensure unobstructed coronary blood flow (Fig. 79-14). A 3.5-mm

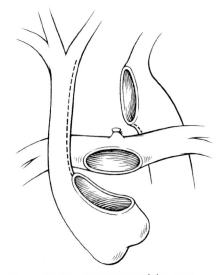

Figure 79-10. Appearance of the great vessels after removal of the pulmonary arteries and ligation of the ductus arteriosus. The distal ductal tissue is excised from the descending aorta, and the ascending aorta is opened from the pulmonary artery excision site to the base of the left carotid artery. (Reprinted with permission from AE Baue, AS Geha, GL Hammond, et al. [eds]. Glenn's Thoracic and Cardiovascular Surgery [6th ed]. Norwalk CT: Appleton & Lange, 1994;1216.)

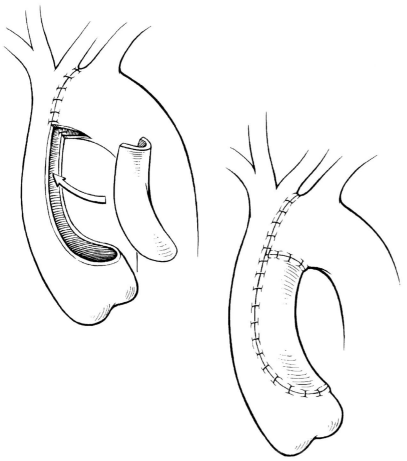

Figure 79-11. A direct anastomosis is made between the descending aorta and the distal ascending aorta-proximal left carotid artery. The proximal ascending aorta is augmented with allograft tissue or prosthetic material. (Reprinted with permission from AE Baue, AS Geha, GL Hammond, et al. [eds]. Glenn's Thoracic and Cardiovascular Surgery [6th ed]. Norwalk CT: Appleton & Lange, 1994;1217.)

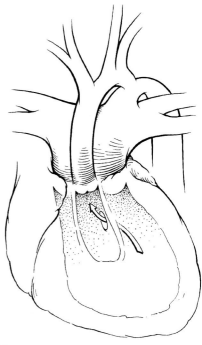

Figure 79-12. The typical appearance of tricuspid atresia with transposition of the great vessels and coarctation of the aorta. The aortic blood flow is dependent on the bulboventricular foramen. Although the illustration shows a coarctation, the approach is similar for patients with arch interruption. (Reprinted with permission from RS Mosca, HA Hennein, TJ Kulik, et al. Modified Norwood operation for single left ventricle and ventriculoarterial discordance: An improved surgical technique. Ann Thorac Surg 1997;64:1127.)

modified Blalock-Taussig shunt is routinely used, with a 4-mm shunt reserved for infants >3.8 kg to 4.0 kg. This technique of aortic reconstruction bypasses the restrictive outlet foramen with the pulmonary valve, allows appropriate size matching of the main pulmonary artery and augmented ascending aorta, and avoids circumferential suture lines or prosthetic grafts in the arch repair.

Postoperative Management and Outcome

Survival

Early and late survival for patients with IAA and VSD treated by single-stage repair has steadily improved over the last decade. The results for 60 consecutive neonates undergoing simultaneous arch and intracardiac repair (excluding single-ventricle patients)

between 1986 and 1994 at the University of Michigan are shown in Table 79-2. Although this series includes patients with coarctation in addition to IAA, the management and outcomes were sufficiently similar, especially considering all were younger than 1 month of age at the time of repair. Early mortality was 11.6% for the entire group; overall mortality (early plus late) was 15%. Not surprisingly, those patients with isolated VSD had a better outcome than those with more complex intracardiac defects. Among 37 neonates with coarctation or IAA and isolated VSD, there were 3 early deaths (8%) and only 1 late (noncardiac) death. For the 23 neonates with coarctation or IAA and more complex anomalies, there were 4 early deaths (17%) and one 1 late death.

The results reported from the multi-institutional study by the CHSS were less optimistic, however. Among 174 neonates with IAA and VSD undergoing repair, survival was 73%, 65%, and 63% at 1 month,

1 year, and 4 years, respectively. In contrast to the series from Michigan, myotomy or myectomy in the presence of narrowing of the subaortic area was found to be a risk factor for death in the CHSS report. Paradoxically, the CHSS data showed that repair without concomitant procedures to address subaortic narrowing (myotomy/myectomy, Damus-Kaye-Stansel) was a risk factor, as was subaortic narrowing itself, leaving no clear solution to that difficult problem.

Intensive Care Unit Management

When single-stage repair of IAA and associated intracardiac defects is performed, the early postoperative management is similar to that for any neonate or young infant undergoing a complex cardiac repair. Mechanical ventilation is generally required for 2 to 4 days, and extubation is carried out after excess edema is mobilized. If weaning from the

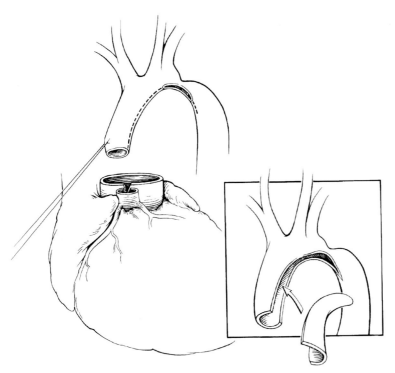

Figure 79-13. Modified Norwood operation for single ventricle with ventriculoarterial discordance. Both great vessels are transected, and the distal tissue is excised. The entire ascending aorta is opened and augmented with a patch of allograft tissue. (Reprinted with permission from RS Mosca, HA Hennein, TJ Kulik, et al. Modified Norwood operation for single left ventricle and ventriculoarterial discordance: an improved surgical technique. Ann Thorac Surg 1997;64:1127.)

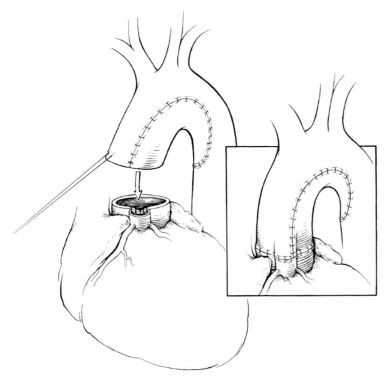

Figure 79-14. The aorta is anastomosed in an end-to-end fashion to the pulmonary artery, incorporating the proximal ascending aorta into the suture line. Pulmonary blood flow is provided through a systemic-to-pulmonary artery shunt or a cavopulmonary connection. (Reprinted with permission from RS Mosca, HA Hennein, TJ Kulik, et al. Modified Norwood operation for single left ventricle and ventriculoarterial discordance: initial management with an improved surgical technique. Ann Thorac Surg 1997;64:1128.)

ventilator is unsuccessful, diaphragm paralysis from phrenic nerve injury, upper airway obstruction secondary to left recurrent laryngeal nerve injury and resultant vocal cord paralysis, and tracheal compression from the reconstructed aortic arch must all be investigated. Inotropic support with low- or intermediate-dose dopamine (5 to 10 μg/kg per minute) is routinely used and should be all that is necessary to maintain hemodynamic stability. When more significant levels of support are required, a detailed search for residual hemodynamic lesions must be carried out. Doppler/echocardiography is useful in diagnosing ventricular dysfunction, residual VSD, left ventricular outflow tract obstruction, tamponade, and atrioventricular or semilunar valve regurgitation. Residual aortic arch obstruction may be diagnosed or highly suspected by simple four-limb blood pressure recordings, although if cardiac output is low, gradients may be underestimated. Cardiac catheterization should be used if any doubt remains as to the cause of low cardiac output.

In patients with single ventricle who have undergone aortic arch repair and a systemic-to-pulmonary artery shunt, systemic output is dependent on the delicate balance between the systemic and pulmonary vascular resistance. Residual arch obstruction is extremely poorly tolerated and usually results in rapid deterioration. Excessive pulmonary blood flow is generally not a problem provided a shunt of correct size is placed. Reduction of systemic vascular resistance with the appropriate medications is of benefit in improving oxygen delivery to the tissues.

Late Problems

Late complications are specific to the type of intracardiac defect repaired or to the expected difficulties that arise after palliation for those patients with single-ventricle lesions. The patient should always be monitored for residual or recurrent arch obstruction, and treatment is usually indicated for resting gradients of >30 mm Hg. Residual gradients of 20 mm Hg occurred in only 2 of 53 late survivors of simultaneous neonatal arch repair for either IAA or coarctation and intracardiac repair of associated defects performed in our institution between 1986 and 1994. No patient has required reoperation for recurrent arch obstruction (mean follow-up, 23 months; range, 1 to 78 months) with the only 2 patients found to have gradients of >20 mm Hg satisfactorily treated with balloon dilation. Both of these patients

Table 79-2 Early and Late Mortality for Single-Stage Repair of Interrupted Aortic Arch and Associated Intracardiac Defects

Group	Number	Early Mortality	Late Mortality	Weight (mean ± SEM; kg)	Age (median; days)
Coarctation/VSD	19	1 (5%)	0	1.4–4.7 (3.1 ± 0.2)	1–29 (11)
Interrupted aortic arch/VSD	18	2 (11%)	1	1.3–4.0 (3.0 ± 0.02)	2–15 (6)
Coarctation/VSD and complex	23	4 (17%)	1	2.1–4.0 (3.1 ± 0.1)	2–24 (8)

SEM = standard error of the mean; VSD = ventricular septal defect.
Source: Reprinted with permission from SK Sandhu, RH Beekman, RS Mosca, et al. Single-stage repair of aortic arch obstruction and associated intracardiac defects in the neonate. Am J Cardiol 1995;75:370.

had coarctation of the aorta and were repaired early in our series, and neither had an extended arch anastomosis, which is now routinely used. Percutaneous balloon dilation is an effective treatment modality for this problem and usually avoids the need for reoperation. If prosthetic tube grafts are used during the arch repair, replacement is inevitable, and reoperation is often technically complex.

As discussed, left ventricular outflow tract obstruction remains a significant source of late postoperative morbidity and mortality. From 1991 to 2001, 27 neonates underwent primary repair for IAA and an isolated malalignment-type VSD at our institution. Fifteen of these patients with the smallest subaortic areas were felt to be at risk for early or late postrepair subaortic obstruction. Consequently, these patients underwent transatrial myectomy or myotomy of the infundibular septum concomitant with the VSD closure and IAA repair, as described previously. Those patients requiring myectomy/myotomy (group I) had significantly smaller subaortic diameters (3.7 ± 0.9 mm) than those who had only IAA with VSD repair (group II, 4.5 ± 0.7 mm; $p = 0.0231$). This remained significant when indexed to body surface area (BSA) (0.83 ± 0.16 vs. 0.99 ± 0.13 cm × $BSA^{0.5}$; $p = 0.012$). There was no difference in the mean aortic Z-value between groups. There were 2 hospital deaths in group I and 1 in group II. No late deaths have occurred. No patient in group II has required reoperation. Six patients required nine reoperations for left ventricular outflow tract obstruction, all of whom were in group I and underwent myectomy/myotomy at the initial operation. Five of those patients underwent resection of a new subaortic membrane. Only 1 patient required myectomy for recurrent muscular subaortic obstruction. The mean interval between initial operation and first reoper-

ation was 3.7 ± 4.1 years (range 0.5 to 9.5 years). Three patients required a second reoperation, primarily related to aortic valvar stenosis. These data reflect the continuing improvement in hospital survival (89%, 24 of 27) for single-stage IAA with VSD repair in the neonatal period. They also support an approach tailored to the degree of subaortic narrowing, with resection or incision of the infundibular septum at the time of primary repair for those patients felt to be at risk for residual or recurrent subaortic stenosis. Although these patients continue to be at risk for other levels of left ventricular outflow tract obstruction, this approach was very effective in preventing or prolonging the interval to recurrent muscular subaortic stenosis when compared to other published series.

SUGGESTED READING

Bove EL, Minich LL, Pridjian AK, et al. The management of severe subaortic stenosis, ventricular septal defect, and aortic arch obstruction in the neonate. J Thorac Cardiovasc Surg 1993;105:289.

Jonas RA, Quaegebeur JM, Kirklin JW, et al. Outcomes in patients with interrupted aortic arch and ventricular septal defect: A multi-institutional study. J Thorac Cardiovasc Surg 1994;107:1099.

Mosca RS, Hennein HA, Kulik TJ, et al. Modified Norwood operation for single left ventricle and ventriculoarterial discordance: improved surgical technique. Ann Thorac Surg 1997;64:1127.

Sandhu SK, Beekman RH, Mosca RS, et al. Single-stage repair of aortic arch obstruction and associated intracardiac defects in the neonate. Am J Cardiol 1995;75:370.

Schreiber C, Mazzitelli D, Haehnel JC, et al. The interrupted aortic arch: An overview after 20 years of surgical treatment. Eur J Cardiothorac Surg 1997;12:466.

Scott WA, Rocchini AP, Bove EL, et al. Repair of interrupted aortic arch in infancy. J Thorac Cardiovasc Surg 1988;96:564.

Sell JE, Jonas RA, Mayer JE, et al. The results of a surgical program for interrupted aortic arch. J Thorac Cardiovasc Surg 1988;96:864.

Serraf A, Lacour-Gayet F, Robotin M, et al. Repair of interrupted aortic arch: A ten-year experience. J Thorac Cardiovasc Surg 1996;112:1150.

EDITOR'S COMMENTS

As noted by the authors, the results with repair of IAA in isolation or in association with other complex congenital heart disease have increasingly improved such that now the majority of infants with these conditions have satisfactory one-stage complete repair. The earlier poor results with neonatal one-stage repair led several surgeons to advocate pulmonary artery banding and arch reconstruction with artificial grafts or with the carotid artery to re-establish arch continuity. However, the late problems with development of subaortic obstruction and the necessity of replacing these conduits during growth have led to universal adoption of one-stage primary repair as the treatment of choice for this condition. Minor variations in operative technique are used in many centers. We have elected in virtually all cases to avoid a direct circumferential primary anastomosis of the descending aorta to the ascending aorta and have used direct anastomosis with absorbable suture over one half of the circumference of the arch in its most superior aspect with incision into the head and neck vessels and then augmentation of the undersurface of the arch with a generous patch of pulmonary homograft material. In this fashion, native aorta is primarily anastomosed to allow for growth, and the arch is additionally enlarged to prevent any tension on the anastomosis. When bleeding is encountered in IAA repair with primary anastomosis, additional sutures to control bleeding may result in narrowing at the area of reconstruction; use of pulmonary homograft to augment the arch prevents this problem. With this technique, we have not found it necessary to divide an aberrant right subclavian artery in type B interruption and have left the right subclavian in place, incising the left subclavian artery at its origin as well as the left common carotid artery and sewing the carotid and subclavian together in their superior extent as part of the arch reconstruction.

The most difficult issue in repair of IAA with associated VSD is the issue of the subaortic infundibular septum, which may cause significant subaortic obstruction.

As noted by the authors, it is not readily possible to identify those patients preoperatively who have significant subaortic obstruction by either echocardiography or catheterization because most flow goes across the VSD to the pulmonary arteries preoperatively. The difficulty in identifying patients with significant outflow tract obstruction may account for the fact that in the CHSS data, the narrowness of the subaortic region as determined by echocardiography did not correlate with outcome, leading the group to advocate primary repair in all circumstances. In spite of this recommendation, we have elected not to perform primary repair in some infants with very small subaortic regions, especially when the aortic valve annulus itself is severely hypoplastic.

A small number of infants have very significant hypoplasia of the aortic valve annulus and associated bicuspid aortic valve with very severe subaortic outflow tract obstruction. In these patients we have elected to perform a Yasui procedure, baffling the VSD to the pulmonary artery and reconstructing the aortic arch as in the Norwood operation with connection of the right ventricle to the pulmonary bifurcation with a homograft conduit.

The incidence of development of subaortic obstruction after complete repair of IAA with associated VSD is significant. Even with resection of some subaortic muscle, recurrent obstruction can occur. The muscle is difficult to excise in very small infants, and the resection, if carried superiorly enough, can damage the aortic valve. In addition, once the resection is performed, the superiormost extent of the VSD patch is difficult to anchor because there is little tissue remaining in this location. Alternate methods of dealing with the subaortic muscle have been described. When possible, we prefer to place the VSD patch on the left ventricular side of the muscle superiorly and then bring the suture line to the right ventricular side on the inferior margin to avoid the conducting tissue. In this fashion, the pressure of the left ventricle pushes the subaortic infundibular muscle away from the outflow tract during systole and seems to cause less stimulus for hypertrophy of this muscle, which can then develop into later outflow tract obstruction. If exposure is good, certainly resection is a reasonable approach. Starnes has recommended closure of the VSD via the pulmonary artery with pulling of the infundibular muscle to the right ventricle to address the subaortic outflow tract obstruction. The follow-up with all of these techniques has been relatively short, and the possibility of late development of residual outflow tract obstruction remains a concern.

Regardless of the technique for dealing with the subaortic infundibular muscle and interrupted aortic arch, a significant incidence of recurrent left ventricular outflow tract obstruction and need for reoperation has been reported in most series. Although patients with even small aortic annulus and subaortic area can successfully undergo single-stage complete repair as a neonate, it is not infrequent for these patients to have a bicuspid aortic valve and recurrent outflow tract obstruction, which requires a Ross-Konno operation as a second procedure often within the first 6 months of life. The results with these repairs, however, have continued to improve such that the overall survival with repair of interrupted aortic arch now approaches 95% in many centers.

T.L.S.

80

Left Ventricular Outflow Tract Obstruction and Aortic Stenosis

Flavian M. Lupinetti and Michael F. Teodori

Valvar Aortic Stenosis in the Neonate and Infant

In the neonate or infant with significant left ventricular outflow tract obstruction, by far the most common pathology is a congenitally stenotic aortic valve. This assumes that an appropriate distinction has been made between left ventricular outflow obstruction with an adequate left ventricle and hypoplastic left heart syndrome in its varying degrees. A congenitally stenotic aortic valve is often quite dysplastic and irregular. Recognition of two or three leaflets with commissural fusion may be possible, but many stenotic valves exhibit an eccentric orifice with no appreciable leaflet formation, the so-called "unicuspid" morphology. Other cardiac anomalies occurring concomitantly with aortic valve stenosis include patent ductus arteriosus, aortic coarctation, ventricular septal defect, and mitral stenosis.

Diagnosis of aortic stenosis is made accurately by echocardiography. Echo examination also allows delineation of most other associated defects and exclusion of left ventricular hypoplasia. Catheterization is now performed most commonly when transcatheter balloon aortic valvotomy is anticipated.

Because many neonates and infants with valvar aortic stenosis present with profound congestive heart failure, cyanosis, and end-organ impairment, treatment must be instituted promptly to prevent catastrophic complications. Endotracheal intubation and mechanical ventilation are usually necessary. Correction of fluid and electrolyte ab-

normalities must be performed prior to operation to enhance the chances of a successful operative outcome. Inotropic support is indicated when ventricular function is diminished, as is usually the case. When the ductus arteriosus can be opened with prostaglandin E_2, cardiac output may be considerably augmented and renal function and acid-base balance markedly improved.

Although balloon dilation has substantially supplanted surgical intervention in many institutions, the risk and results of operative treatment are similar to those of catheter-based therapies. Three major technical approaches to the infant with critical aortic stenosis have been described: open valvotomy with inflow occlusion, open valvotomy during cardiopulmonary bypass, and closed, transventricular dilation. Individual surgeon preference is probably the major determinant of which approach is used.

Open valvotomy with inflow occlusion can be performed quickly and obviates the need for heparinization and bypass. The superior and inferior venae cavae are occluded with snares or clamps for 3 to 4 seconds to allow the heart to empty. The aorta is quickly clamped and opened, and an expeditious valvotomy is performed. In the neonate, the valvotomy is perhaps best accomplished by simple blunt separation with a hemostat. The extremely dysplastic nature of the aortic valve in these patients makes it difficult to identify well-demarcated commissures that lend themselves to precise scalpel division. The aorta and left ventricle are filled with saline to evacuate air, and a side-biting clamp is placed across the aor-

totomy to permit reperfusion while the aorta is sutured closed. The caval tourniquets are released. At this point, the anesthesiologist must vigorously institute resuscitative measures.

Open valvotomy with cardiopulmonary bypass and cardioplegic arrest allows conduct of the operation with a greater margin of safety and reduced time pressure. Once again, the valve is approached via an aortotomy (Fig. 80-1). With bypass support, a more meticulous inspection of the valve is possible, and definite lines of commissural fusion are occasionally identified. A valvotomy is performed with care taken not to create insufficiency of the valve (Fig. 80-2). A third, extremely effective surgical approach to neonatal aortic stenosis is transventricular dilation on cardiopulmonary bypass. Bypass is preferred because of the greater safety during this otherwise risky maneuver but also because of the immediate advantages of bypass itself. In an infant in shock because of aortic stenosis, bypass provides adequate cardiac output, appropriate end-organ perfusion, and correction of acidosis and hypoxia that are beneficial in themselves. After the institution of extracorporeal circulation at normothermia, a purse-string suture of 5-0 polypropylene suture with pledgets is placed in the apex of the left ventricle (Fig. 80-3). A small stab wound is made within the purse string and dilated with a hemostat. Hegar dilators are then introduced through the stab wound and advanced to the aortic valve (Fig. 80-4). The surgeon's index finger of the hand not holding the dilator may be placed on the aorta to obtain feedback regarding positioning of the dilator. The dilator is

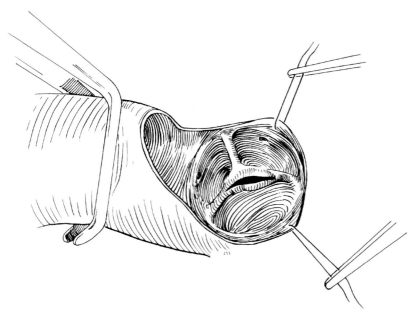

Figure 80-1. Inspection of a stenotic aortic valve approached via an aortotomy.

firmly advanced through the valve into the proximal aorta. A popping sensation is usually appreciated, confirming that the valvotomy has been accomplished. Typically, a 3-mm Hegar dilator is used first, followed by additional dilators in 1-mm increments. The largest dilator used is typically 1 mm larger than the echocardiographically measured diameter of the aortic valve ring, most commonly 5 mm to 6 mm. The patient is

then separated from bypass, and a transvalvar pressure is measured by direct needle puncture of the left ventricle and aorta. A gradient of 25 mm Hg or less is considered adequate. Intraoperative echocardiography can also be helpful in confirming the adequacy of the valvotomy. In some cases, the gradient may not be much different from that measured or calculated preoperatively. It must be remembered, however, that a low cardiac output results in a much lower gradient than would be the case if transvalvar flow was normal. Therefore, if the cardiac function appears to be satisfactory and blood pressure is normal, small to moderate gradients are not a cause for concern.

Operation for neonatal aortic valve stenosis has demonstrated improved results, especially as patients with hypoplastic left ventricle have become more accurately diagnosed and appropriately treated with another procedure. With a normal-size ventricle survival should exceed 90%. Operative survival is not adversely affected by concomitant repair of atrial or ventricular septal defect, coarctation, or patent ductus.

Valvar Aortic Stenosis in the Older Child

In the older child with valvar aortic stenosis, a highly dysplastic morphology is less common than in the neonate. Older children have two distinct leaflets, with fusion of the commissures in >75% of cases. The leaflets are characteristically asymmetric, which probably allows a greater effective orifice area than would a symmetrically bicuspid valve.

Children with aortic valve stenosis may report exercise intolerance, angina, and syncope or near-syncope. Usually the diagnosis is established and the transvalvar gradient estimated by echocardiography. Operation is indicated for a patient with a gradient >40 mm Hg who is symptomatic or who demonstrates hypertrophy or ischemia by electrocardiography. We also suggest intervention for most asymptomatic children with a gradient >50 to 75 mm Hg, although the decision to perform surgical or balloon valvotomy is controversial.

The vast majority of children with congenital valvar aortic stenosis undergoing initial surgical treatment can be adequately palliated with open surgical valvotomy. Valve replacement is seldom necessary except in patients with severe aortic insufficiency or

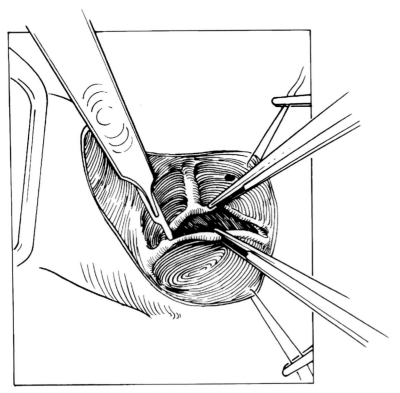

Figure 80-2. A valvotomy is performed by incising the fused commissures. Care is taken to avoid incisions in false raphes, which may result in valve insufficiency.

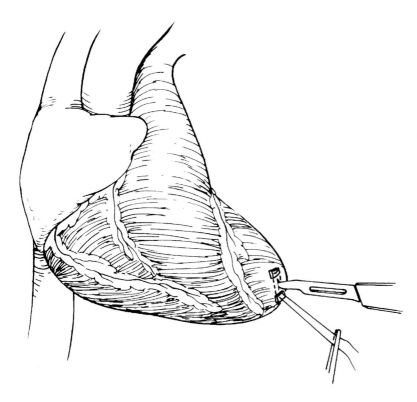

Figure 80-3. Transventricular aortic valvotomy begins with a purse-string suture placed in the apex of the left ventricle.

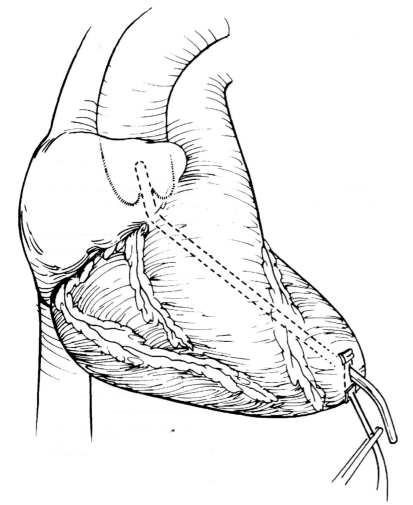

Figure 80-4. Hegar dilators are used to open the stenotic aortic valve and dilate the orifice according to echocardiographic measurements of annular diameter.

in the rare rheumatic heart disease patient in whom reconstructive procedures are not possible. When valve replacement is required, the Ross procedure is the operation of choice.

Aortic valvotomy is performed with moderate hypothermia and cardioplegic arrest. The aortic valve is inspected via an oblique aortotomy extending into the noncoronary sinus. Stay sutures placed on the edges of the proximal and distal aorta facilitate exposure without the need for bulky retractors. As in the infant, care must be taken to achieve a maximum opening of the valvar orifice without creating insufficiency. In the older child, this can usually be accomplished by incising the fused leaflets with a No. 11 scalpel blade to within 1 mm of the aortic wall. Only if this fails to result in an adequate opening is it necessary to further undermine the leaflets. If a satisfactory opening can be achieved with a simple division into a bileaflet valve, it is often unwise more aggressively to attempt further enlargement. In particular, one must guard against making an incision into a false raphe. Aortic valve raphes are distinctive from commissures in that the former do not extend up the aortic wall, whereas the latter do. Incision into a raphe will almost inevitably results in aortic valve incompetence and will likely necessitate valve replacement within a few years.

The mortality of aortic valvotomy in children is <5%. Postoperatively, myocardial performance improves, although hypertrophy is slow to resolve. At least half of all survivors of successful aortic valvotomy ultimately require reoperation. Whether reoperation occurs early or several decades later may depend on the quality of the initial surgical procedure.

Discrete Subaortic Stenosis

Discrete subaortic stenosis is characterized by a diaphragm of muscular and fibrous tissue oriented in a plane parallel and proximal to the aortic valve (Fig. 80-5). The membrane is circular or crescentic in form, attached to the interventricular septum, and often extends to involve the anterior leaflet of the mitral valve. Discrete subaortic stenosis is an acquired condition. There is evidence that an abnormal angulation of the connection between the left ventricle and the aorta may establish a flow pattern that forms the substrate for this lesion.

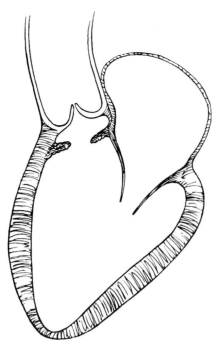

Figure 80-5. Sagittal section of the heart with a discrete subaortic membranous obstruction.

Patients with discrete subaortic stenosis frequently present with an asymptomatic murmur. An important manifestation of subaortic stenosis is aortic valve insufficiency resulting from disordered flow pat-

terns that prevent normal leaflet motion. The presence or progression of aortic valve insufficiency is the most frequent indication for operation. It should be acknowledged that there are few data to support the thesis that repair of subaortic stenosis alters the natural history of aortic valve insufficiency once it becomes manifest.

Complete removal of the subaortic obstruction is best accomplished via an aortotomy. The aortic valve is inspected for any abnormalities at that level. Such abnormalities are uncommon, except perhaps for some tethering of a leaflet by the membrane. If the aortic valve is bicuspid and commissural fusion exists, a valvotomy is necessary to provide relief of obstruction at that level and to achieve adequate access to the subaortic area. The valve leaflets are retracted to expose the subaortic membrane. The first assistant holds a nasal speculum or finger retractors, atraumatically opening the valve and providing visibility of the ventricular outflow tract (Fig. 80-6). A frequent approach to the membrane is to sharply shave it flush with the septum. Such an approach demonstrates a lack of recognition of the depth of the membrane within the ventricular muscle. A more effective measure is to enucleate the membrane. This is accomplished by making a shallow incision in the endocardium at the junction of the membrane and the septal muscle

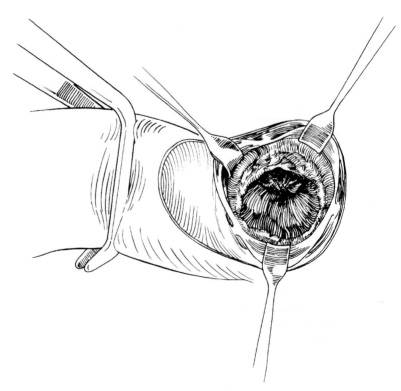

Figure 80-6.   Inspection of a subaortic fibromuscular membrane.

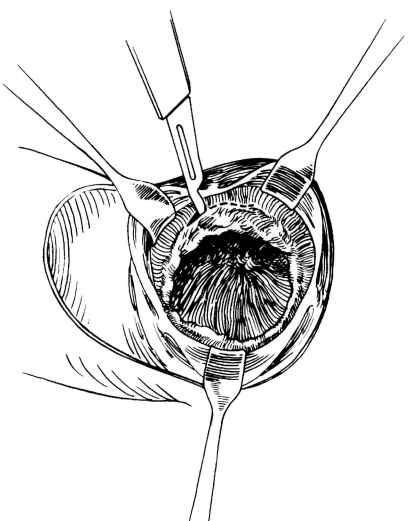

Figure 80-7. The endocardium of the membrane is incised.

(Fig. 80-7). Using a hemostat or right-angled clamp, one dissects the membrane bluntly (Fig. 80-8). In this fashion, the surgeon appreciates that the membrane is a coherent structure that extends within the muscle for 1 mm to 3 mm. This enucleation is initiated to the left side of an imaginary line descending from the right coronary ostium to avoid injury to the conduction system. The dissection is continued in a counterclockwise fashion. With further dissection, the membrane either feathers off neatly or may extend onto the anterior leaflet of the mitral valve. Delicate dissection is required in this area to avoid perforation of the mitral leaflet. The enucleation is then completed by clockwise dissection toward the right. The resulting specimen is then removed and can be seen to have encompassed 180 to 360 degrees of the left ventricular outflow tract

(Fig. 80-9). At this point it is often advantageous to resect some septal muscle to further reduce the risk of recurrence. Either a wedge excision is carried out or a more generous trough is created, again avoiding the conduction system by performing this maneuver to the left of the right coronary ostium.

Reoperations for recurrent subaortic stenosis are performed using the same technique as that for primary repairs. In these cases, which are often associated with a less complete initial operation, the recurrent membrane appears remarkably similar to those operated on for the first time. This suggests that an appropriately aggressive removal of the obstruction may result in a lower incidence of recurrence. A useful way of approaching the removal of the membrane is considering it as one would a benign neoplasm, with a complete

removal of the "capsule" required to avoid its return.

The operative mortality after treatment of discrete subaortic stenosis should approach zero. Left ventricular function should be well preserved, and aortic valve insufficiency should be negligible. Outflow gradients often persist even after appropriately aggressive enucleation. This finding may be attributable to some component of dynamic obstruction due to ventricular hypertrophy, anterior motion of the mitral valve, or other factors. Left-bundle-branch block is quite common after operation. Complete heart block requiring insertion of a permanent pacemaker is less common. There is evidence that a more complete resection is not associated with a higher frequency of complete block.

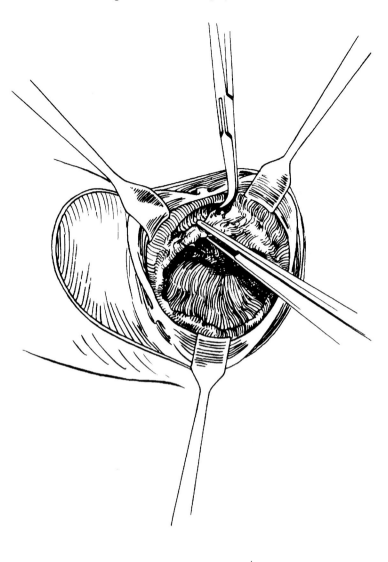

Figure 80-8.   Blunt dissection is initiated. The membrane is enucleated, not excised.

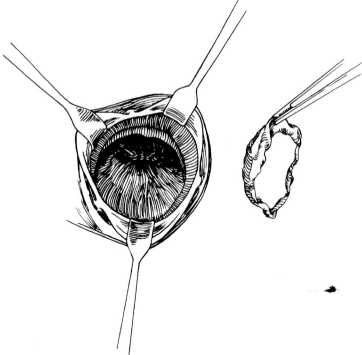

Figure 80-9.   The enucleated membrane is sometimes removed as a complete, circumferential ring.

Diffuse Subaortic Stenosis

Diffuse, or tunnel-type, subaortic stenosis is a much more complicated and morbid condition than the discrete form. Unlike other forms of left ventricular outflow obstruction, in which the obstructive structure is almost always muscular or fibromuscular, diffuse subaortic stenosis is sometimes caused by a rigid, fibrotic formation. The resulting tubular narrowing predictably exhibits a less dynamic appearance and is more likely to retain a constant morphology throughout the cardiac cycle.

Effective treatment of diffuse subaortic stenosis requires aggressive resection of the obstructing tissues. At times, such radical approaches as aortic valve replacement with aorticoventriculoplasty, such as that described by Konno and Rastan, are required. Apicoaortic valved conduits have also been used occasionally with beneficial results. In patients with no intrinsic defects of the native aortic valve, a modified Konno procedure that includes septal myectomy and septoplasty may provide satisfactory relief of obstruction and avoid the adverse consequences of valve prostheses. Cardiopulmonary bypass with bicaval cannulation is established. Under moderate hypothermia and cardioplegic arrest, an aortotomy is performed. The aortic valve is assessed and the subaortic obstruction is examined. An opportunity for excising the subaortic obstruction via the aortotomy is available, but this rarely suffices for the truly diffuse form of obstruction. A better approach to this problem is achieved with a transverse right ventriculotomy performed in the infundibulum well proximal to the pulmonary valve (Fig. 80-10). An incision is made through the interventricular septum (Fig. 80-11). The resulting ventricular septal defect is then extended toward the apex of the heart as well as in the opposite direction toward the aortic valve. Repeated viewing of the enlarging hole from both the aortotomy and the ventriculotomy helps to avoid injury to the aortic and tricuspid valves. The incision is complete when the ventricular communication appears to be adequate for relief of the subaortic narrowing. The ventricular septal defect is then closed with an expanded polytetrafluoroethylene patch (Fig. 80-12). This is secured by a combination of running sutures and interrupted pledgeted sutures of 4-0 or 5-0 polypropylene. The aortotomy and right ventriculotomy are closed, the patient is separated from bypass, in the left ventricle

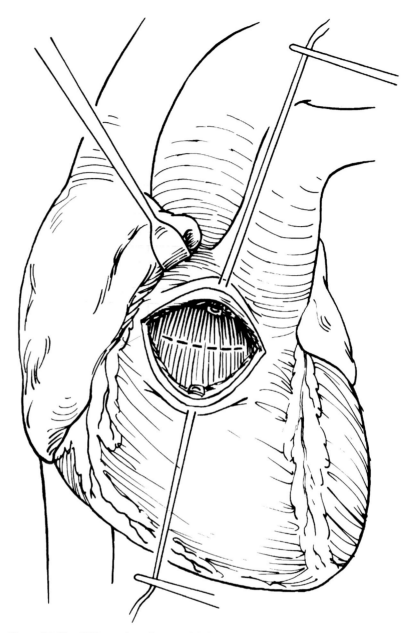

Figure 80-10.   Diffuse subaortic stenosis is best approached via a right ventriculotomy.

and pressures and aorta are measured by direct needle puncture.

In some hearts, a similar septoplasty can be performed via a right atriotomy, which has the advantage of avoiding a right ventricular scar. The right atrial approach may be most successful in the presence of a ventricular septal defect or after a ventricular septal defect has been closed.

Operative mortality is low in both infants and older children. A major risk of septoplasty is complete heart block, which requires insertion of a permanent pacemaker. Another major concern is inadequate relief of obstruction, which may require additional surgical intervention. If an initial

septoplasty fails to relieve the obstruction, a subsequent similar intervention is far less likely to succeed. In such cases, a Ross procedure or a Ross-Konno procedure may be more effective.

Supravalvar Aortic Stenosis

Less than 10% of patients with aortic stenosis have the supravalvar form. Supravalvar aortic stenosis is characterized by a narrowing of the external aortic diameter distal to the commissures of the aortic valve

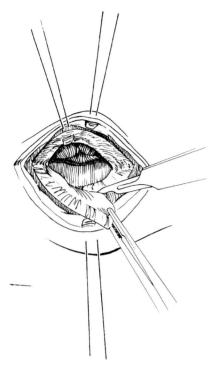

Figure 80-11.   A generous septectomy is required to remove all muscular obstruction. Care must be taken to avoid injury to the nearby aortic valve leaflets.

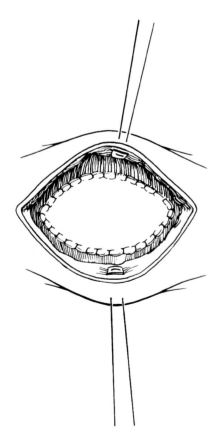

Figure 80-12.   The resulting ventricular defect is closed with a polytetrafluoroethylene patch that enlarges the subaortic area.

accompanied by a thickening of the aortic wall. This may result in profound luminal narrowing. The coronary artery origins may be narrowed as well. The aortic valve leaflets are usually normal, although they may attach to the distal site of narrowing. Supravalvar stenosis may be relatively focal or diffuse, and coarctation of the aorta at the usual site may also be present. In some patients, peripheral pulmonary artery stenosis may coexist.

Manifestations of supravalvar aortic stenosis include poor exercise tolerance, angina, and syncope, although about half of all patients have asymptomatic murmurs as their presenting sign. Echocardiography is useful in suggesting the diagnosis, but cardiac catheterization and angiography are usually necessary to demonstrate the extent of the aortic arch that is involved. This is important because a large external diameter may be consistent with a narrowed lumen that is difficult to appreciate on an initial inspection in the operating room. Operation is performed in the presence of symptoms or in asymptomatic patients with clinically important left ventricular hypertrophy, electrocardiographic changes, or a resting gradient of >50 to 75 mm Hg. Stenosis of the branch pulmonary arteries is seldom an indication for intervention. This is partly because attempts to surgically enlarge the pulmonary arteries are rarely successful and partly because these lesions commonly show spontaneous regression.

A variety of operative approaches to supravalvar aortic stenosis have been devised. The particular approach used must depend on the anatomic nuances in a given individual. All techniques require cardiopulmonary bypass with cardioplegic arrest. Deeper hypothermia with low flow or even circulatory arrest is used for the more extensive forms if reconstruction of the entire aortic arch is required or if a discrete coarct is present.

For all forms of supravalvar stenosis, it is necessary to inspect thoroughly the aortic valve leaflets to make sure that they are freely mobile and to relieve any possible obstruction to the coronary arteries. A meticulous inspection of the sinuses frequently demonstrates some degree of obstruction to coronary artery flow. This obstruction is often a consequence of the reduced diameter at the level of the sinus rim and the reduced excursion of the leaflets. Although the lengths of the free edges of the leaflets are usually normal, there may also be some tethering of the leaflets, again contributing to coronary obstruction. The subaortic region should be inspected as well, and there may be instances

in which some subaortic narrowing requires surgical resection.

For the simplest form of supravalvar stenosis, treatment may require only a vertical incision into the aorta, extending it into the noncoronary sinus of Valsalva, and an endarterectomy. The aorta is enlarged with an elliptical patch of expanded polytetrafluoroethylene or pericardium. A more extensive procedure, first described by Doty, also begins with a longitudinal aortotomy extending into a sinus of Valsalva (Fig. 80-13). The Doty technique then extends a second incision from the first into a second sinus of Valsalva. This inverted Y-shaped incision creates a more spacious opening of the vessel and allows a larger patch to be used (Fig. 80-14).

When the entire aortic arch is hypoplastic, it is necessary to extend the patch to a point well beyond all remaining areas of stenosis. If this is the case, allograft pulmonary artery tissue is quite useful to use as the patch material because of its ability to conform to a complicated curve and because of its hemostatic properties. If there is a discrete coarct, the surgeon may consider a simple extension of the patch to an even more distal extent. Alternatively, the coarct site may be resected, and an elongated end-to-end anastomosis may be performed.

On occasion, the best approach to reconstruction may be excision of the ascending aorta and interposition of a synthetic tube graft. This is obviously less preferable unless the child has reached full growth. A Ross procedure or allograft aortic root replacement may sometimes be a better choice for complex, multilevel disease. Finally, an apicoaortic conduit may be the only option in rare cases. These alternatives are most commonly required in reoperations after failed primary repairs.

The technique of Myers is an extremely effective approach for many patients with supravalvar aortic stenosis. This approach transects the aorta at its narrowest point (Fig. 80-15). Any thickened area on the distal aorta is excised as a horizontal ring to maintain a parallel relationship to the proximal aorta. Three vertical incisions, 120 degrees apart, are made in the sinuses of Valsalva. In the coronary sinuses, care is taken to avoid injury to or distortion of the coronary ostia. This usually necessitates making all three incisions off the center of the sinuses. Three complementary vertical incisions are made in the distal aorta, also 120 degrees apart and out of phase with the proximal incisions (Fig. 80-16). This allows interdigitation of the proximal

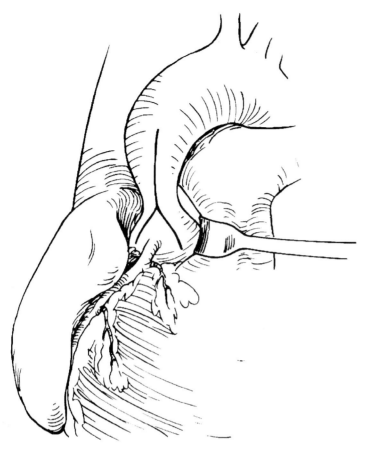

Figure 80-13. Supravalvar aortic stenosis repair as described by Doty begins with an inverted Y-shaped incision.

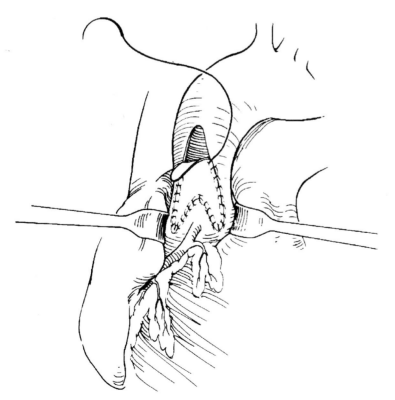

Figure 80-14. The aorta is enlarged with a bifurcated patch.

and distal flaps of aortic tissue to create a maximum enlargement of the aortic root without the use of prosthetic material (Fig. 80-17). A zigzag suture line is then sewn using a fine monofilament absorbable suture (Fig. 80-18). The aorta can be thoroughly mobilized to achieve this repair without the need for removing the aortic cannula, thus allowing this technique to be carried out with moderate hypothermia and continuous cardiopulmonary bypass. Deep hypothermia with circulatory arrest is required only if there are distal arch stenoses as well.

Special mention should be made of the treatment of pulmonary artery stenosis in patients with supravalvar aortic stenosis, a lesion that is most commonly encountered in Williams syndrome patients. It is often unnecessary to attempt repair of these pulmonary arteries. This is because the most severe stenoses are highly refractory to attempts at surgical enlargement and because many such arteries exhibit a remarkable propensity to become less stenotic over time. Although the immediate outcomes after treatment of supravalvar aortic stenosis are good, with an operative mortality of <5%, the late results are less favorable. The more discrete and localized forms of supravalvar stenosis do much better, with a low likelihood of recurrence and good long-term survival. Patients with Williams syndrome and those with more diffuse disease do less well. Such individuals have less complete relief of obstruction, a higher frequency of reoperation, and reduced longevity. The additional burden of pulmonary stenosis, when persistent, is particularly associated with unfavorable long-term results.

Hypertrophic Cardiomyopathy

Hypertrophic cardiomyopathy is characterized by ventricular hypertrophy without apparent cause and a histologic pattern of bizarrely disorganized muscle fibers. The interventricular septum is usually, but not always, disproportionately hypertrophied compared to the left ventricular free wall. This results in obstruction to ventricular ejection and impaired ventricular filling. Frequently, the mitral valve is thickened and may contribute to outflow obstruction by abnormal anterior motion during systole. Although the coronary arteries are usually normal in hypertrophic cardiomyopathy, evidence of ischemic injury is often present on autopsy specimens.

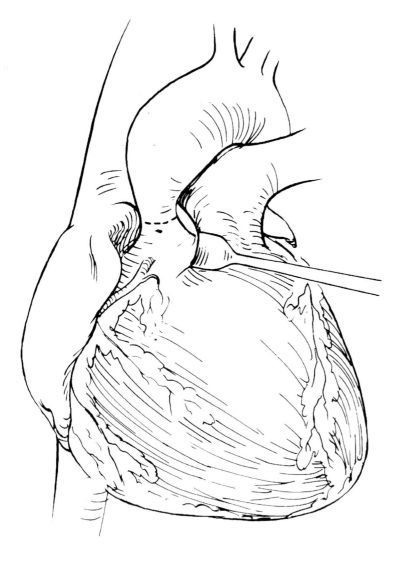

Figure 80-15. Supravalvar aortic stenosis repair as described by Myers starts with transection of the aorta at its narrowest point.

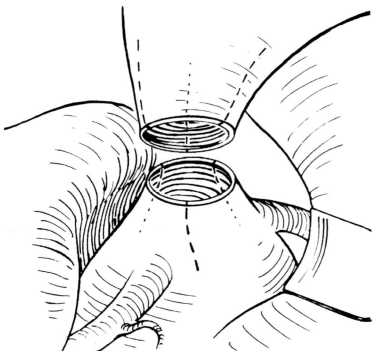

Figure 80-16. Three vertical incisions are made in the proximal and distal aorta.

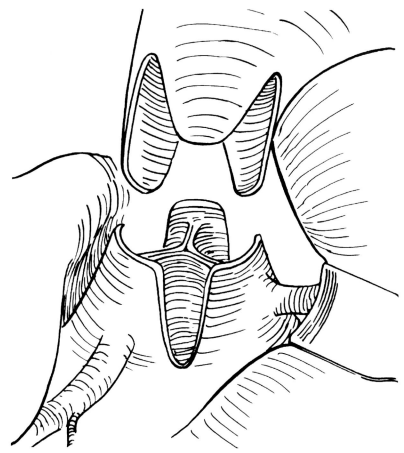

Figure 80-17. The incisions are out of phase, allowing interdigitation of the proximal and distal flaps.

Many patients with hypertrophic cardiomyopathy are asymptomatic. The most common symptoms are exercise-related fatigue and dyspnea. Syncope may occur and is considered a risk factor for sudden death, the most common mode of death among patients who die as a direct consequence of the cardiomyopathy. Other symptoms may result from myocardial ischemia or restriction of ventricular filling, which may limit physical exertion. Mitral insufficiency and bacterial endocarditis are less common manifestations of hypertrophic cardiomyopathy.

Nonoperative treatment of hypertrophic cardiomyopathy has relied on beta-blocking agents and calcium-channel blockers because of their beneficial effects on reducing outflow obstruction. Dual-chamber pacemaker implantation has been used in patients with hypertrophic cardiomyopathy. The rationale of using a pacemaker for treatment of this entity is that delay of septal muscle activation reduces dynamic obstruction. In appropriately selected patients, pacing has resulted in a decreased outflow gradient and symptomatic improvement.

The natural history of hypertrophic cardiomyopathy is unpredictable, and operation is reserved for the patient with symptoms unresponsive to medical management. There are two basic methods for relieving the left ventricular outflow tract obstruction of hypertrophic cardiomyopathy: resection of the subaortic muscle and mitral valve replacement. Septal myectomy as described by Morrow is performed under moderate hypothermia with cardioplegic arrest. An aortotomy is performed, and the aortic valve leaflets are retracted. As for discrete subaortic stenosis, a nasal speculum is an excellent instrument for exposing the region of interest. Additional exposure can be obtained by retracting the anterior leaflet of the mitral valve with a malleable ribbon-type retractor. Another useful maneuver is to press on the anterior surface of the right ventricle with a bulky sponge or laparotomy pad. All of these techniques accentuate the subaortic muscular obstruction and assist the surgeon in recognizing the magnitude of the septal hypertrophy.

Placement of a stay suture within the area of muscle to be resected elevates the hypertrophied septum and provides traction to facilitate the incisions. The septectomy is initiated by making two parallel incisions from the immediate subaortic area down toward the apex of the left ventricle. The initial incision is made immediately beneath the right coronary ostium a few millimeters below the origin of the aortic valve leaflet on the septum. The second incision is further to the left. Placement of these incisions should allow protection of the conduction system. Palpation with the other hand helps the surgeon to appreciate how deeply the incisions may be made without entry into the right ventricle. The length of the incision toward the apex should be to the limits of the surgeon's view and even beyond that. The two parallel incisions are then connected by a third incision perpendicular to the others (Fig. 80-19). Again, palpation is helpful in judging the depth of myectomy that is appropriate. Ideally, the excised specimen is removed as a single, large slab of muscle, and the relief of the outflow obstruction should be obvious. In most cases, this initial excision helps the surgeon to see how much more muscle can be removed, and this is performed in a similar fashion to the initial myectomy. After the myectomy has been completed, it should be obvious that the septal site of mitral valve leaflet contact is now excavated (Fig. 80-20). In a larger child the surgeon's finger may be inserted into the left ventricle so that bimanual palpation can assess how much septum remains. Creation of an interventricular communication should be quite rare if appropriate inspection and palpation are performed periodically during the muscle excision. The left ventricle is carefully flushed with saline to remove any small pieces of muscle that might otherwise embolize. The aortotomy is closed, and the patient is separated from bypass.

Transesophageal echocardiography is useful in assessing the operative repair. A short-axis view of the heart commonly demonstrates a keyhole-like appearance of the ventricular lumen. The mitral valve should be seen as no longer capable of contact with the septum. Echocardiography can also inspect for iatrogenic complications, such as ventricular septal defect or aortic insufficiency. Finally, a left ventricular outflow tract gradient can be calculated. Typically, sufficient relief of the obstruction can be achieved that the outflow tract gradient is <20 mm Hg.

Mitral valve replacement has been advocated by some surgeons, in part based on the view that the dynamic component of the obstructive process is of overwhelming importance. Mitral valve replacement at this

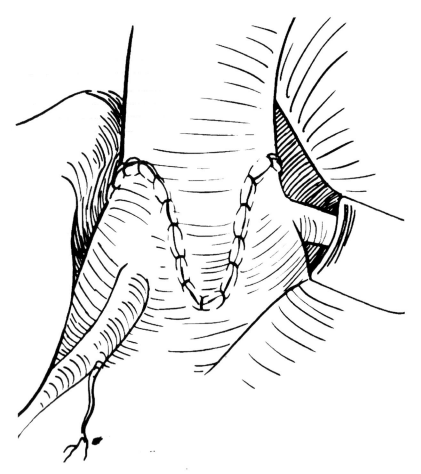

Figure 80-18. Reanastomosis of the aorta in a zigzag fashion achieves maximal enlargement of the aortic root.

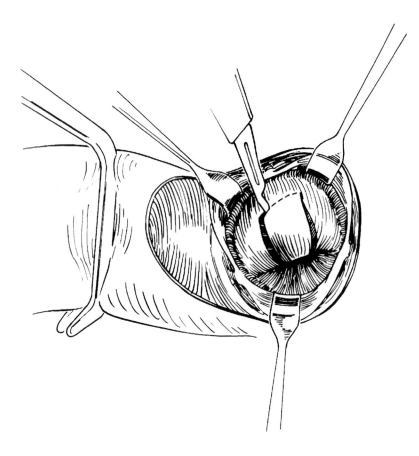

Figure 80-19. Transaortic myectomy for hypertrophic obstructive cardiomyopathy.

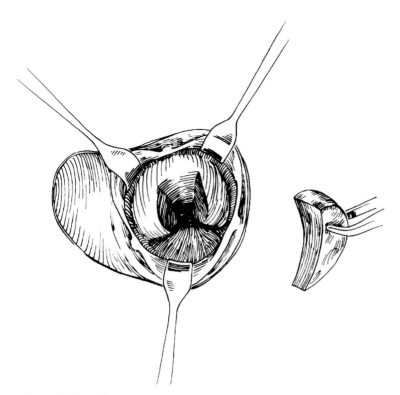

Figure 80-20. After myectomy, the outflow tract should be visibly enlarged.

institution has been recommended only for patients with hypertrophic cardiomyopathy as well as intrinsic mitral valve disease or for those with a poor response to a previous myectomy. Mitral valve replacement for hypertrophic cardiomyopathy is performed in a fashion similar to that for primary mitral disease. Leaflet-sparing techniques, valuable in preserving overall ventricular function in mitral valve repair, are not used in patients with hypertrophic cardiomyopathy. When a mitral valve replacement is performed for this condition, a septal myectomy should usually be done as well to create the maximum improvement in outflow obstruction. Probably the best valve for use in this setting is one with the lowest profile, that is, a bileaflet prosthetic valve.

The results of the Morrow procedure are quite good, with an operative mortality of <5% expected. In the patient with significant symptoms, there is evidence that this procedure both relieves those symptoms and prolongs life. Even after a good operative repair, the patient should probably continue preoperative medical management, beta blockers or calcium-channel blockers, for an indefinite period. The major reason for continuing medication is that hypertrophic cardiomyopathy patients remain at risk for atrial and ventricular arrhythmias irrespective of operative results. Reopera-

tion for recurrent outflow tract obstruction may sometimes be required. The mortality of mitral valve replacement for these patients is similar to that for myectomy, and the reduction in symptoms may be as great. Mitral valve replacement is also similar to myectomy in the degree of reduction in left ventricular outflow gradient and the magnitude of fall in left ventricular end-diastolic pressure. The major reason, though, to prefer myectomy to mitral valve replacement is the risk of valve prostheses with the attendant requirement for anticoagulation.

SUGGESTED READING

Brown JW, Ruzmetov M, Vijay P, et al. Surgery for aortic stenosis in children: A 40-year experience. Ann Thorac Surg 2003;76:1398.

Caldarone CA, Van Natta TL, Frazer JR, Behrendt DM. The modified Konno procedure for complex left ventricular outflow tract obstruction. Ann Thorac Surg 2003;75:147.

Doty DB, Polansky DB, Jenson CB. Supravalvar aortic stenosis. Ann Thorac Surg 1977;74:362.

McElhinney DB, Petrossian E, Tworetzky W, et al. Issues and outcomes in the management of supravalvar aortic stenosis. Ann Thorac Surg 2000;69:526.

Myers JL, Waldhausen JA, Cyran SE, et al. Results of surgical repair of congenital supravalvular aortic stenosis. J Thorac Cardiovasc Surg 1993;105:281.

Rayburn ST, Netherland DE, Heath BJ. Discrete membranous subaortic stenosis: improved results after resection and myectomy. Ann Thorac Surg 1997;64:105.

Stamm C, Li J, Ho SY, et al. The aortic root in supravalvular aortic stenosis: The potential surgical relevance of morphologic findings. J Thorac Cardiovasc Surg 1997;114:16.

Theodoro DA, Danielson GK, Feldt RH, Anderson BJ. Hypertrophic obstructive cardiomyopathy in pediatric patients: results of surgical treatment. J Thorac Cardiovasc Surg 1996;112:1589.

EDITOR'S COMMENTS

Balloon dilation techniques have essentially supplanted surgery as the primary treatment for critical aortic stenosis of newborns and infants. These catheter interventions have a mortality rate that is virtually identical to surgical mortality rates for the same condition. Maintenance of ductal patency during the procedure is useful in aiding distal perfusion and for resuscitation after the procedure. Thus, surgical approaches to valvar aortic stenosis are relegated to cases in which initial balloon attempts have failed or there are other associated conditions. As noted by the authors, in a newborn with critical aortic stenosis, even direct exposure of the aortic valve is difficult, and usually valvotomy is performed in a relatively blind fashion either antegrade with a dilator as described in this chapter or retrograde from above with a clamp or dilator. Thus, there is little benefit to operative dilation in these patients over balloon dilation except for the benefit of supporting the patient on cardiopulmonary bypass. Surprisingly, even though the aortic valve in these infants is a structure that often appears very dysmorphic, late aortic valve development appears quite good in many cases, and the aortic valve can have a long-lasting improvement in orifice area and essentially normal anatomic and physiologic function. In most patients, however, eventual additional valve procedures will be necessary because of either restenosis or progressive calcification of a bicuspid valve.

Patients who have only moderate improvement in valve function with balloon dilation can undergo repeat dilation, and the most common complication is production of aortic regurgitation. Patients can then be stabilized, with aortic regurgitation, often for several months or years before valve replacement with the Ross procedure is necessary. Thus, the need for Ross aortic valve replacement in neonates is extremely unusual. In older infants and children in whom balloon dilation has been unsuccessful in relieving obstruction, direct aortic valvotomy may be valuable. As noted by the authors, incision into a true raphe should be avoided if possible. However, raphes can be debrided to aid mobility of the leaflet and to improve the effective orifice area of the valve. This often can be accomplished without significant development of regurgitation. In patients in whom there is significant fibrotic thickening of the aortic valve leaflet edges, debridement and thinning of the valve leaflets can be undertaken, and the incision in the commissures can be extended back to the annulus and then along the annulus for a short distance to improve effective orifice area and to prevent tethering of the valve leaflets at the commissural attachments.

Discrete subaortic stenosis is a relatively common finding either in isolation or in association with previous cardiac repairs. It is not uncommon for patients with interrupted aortic arch and ventricular septal defect closure to develop acquired subaortic stenosis from the development of a subaortic membrane. In addition, certain patients with atrioventricular canal defects can develop these membranes after repair, and the defect has also been reported after isolated closure of ventricular septal defect. Thus, these subaortic membranes appear to be always an acquired phenomenon related to abnormalities of geometry of the left ventricular outflow tract and turbulent blood flow in this region. An important feature is the fact that these membranes are actually attached to the endocardium of the left ventricular outflow tract, and enucleation can be performed simply by incising the junction of the membrane with the endocardium and identifying the endocardial layer. The membrane often can then be completely removed with blunt dissection with an endarterectomy spatula. On occasion, the membrane can extend up onto the aortic valve leaflets, causing some thickening and valve immobility and can be associated with aortic insufficiency. In these cases, it is valuable to excise the membrane and to debride the membrane from the valve leaflets. Because the membrane is an acquired structure, it is distinct from the endocardial surface of the valve leaflet and often can be peeled off completely without any disruption of the valve's intrinsic structure. The major problem with removal of subaortic membranes is the fact that recurrence is common. The high incidence of recurrence is not surprising considering that these are acquired defects related to the geometry of the outflow tract, and simple removal of the membrane does not alter this anatomic feature. I therefore be-

lieve it is important to perform a myotomy and myectomy of the left ventricular outflow tract wherever possible in association with resection of subaortic membrane to alter the geometry of contraction of the outflow tract, eliminate additional sources of obstruction, and potentially decrease the turbulent flow in the outflow tract, which can cause recurrence.

Tunnel subaortic stenosis is a more diffuse process and often presents a difficult surgical problem. In most cases, there is some hypoplasia of the aortic valve annulus or abnormality of the aortic valve in association with diffuse hypoplasia or tunnel obstruction of the outflow tract. On rare occasions, however, the aortic valve disease may be minor, and a direct approach with septoplasty can provide adequate relief of obstruction. In our experience, however, such patients are unusual. One difficulty with septoplasty is that in true diffuse subaortic obstruction, the obstruction extends all the way to the base of the aortic valve leaflet, and therefore the superior extent of the septoplasty incision has to stop before the aortic annulus level is reached. Thus, there may always be a bridge of muscle tissue beneath the aortic valve leaflet that will become a potential source of obstruction. If there is an area of relatively normal outflow tract below the aortic valve, septoplasty can be very effective. In patients in whom septoplasty alone fails to relieve the obstruction because of the superior extent of the narrowing or associated aortic valve disease, we believe that a Ross-Konno autograft valve replacement supplies the best chance for long-term durability and complete relief of obstruction. Apicoaortic conduits are avoided because of the problems with late valve degeneration and abnormal coronary artery flow patterns. The use of the Ross-Konno operation has virtually eliminated the need for apicoaortic conduits in our experience.

Supravalvar aortic stenosis commonly associated with Williams syndrome represents an unusual condition but one in which good surgical results have been obtained with multiple techniques. We often have found it impossible to perform a simple patch of the ascending aorta with endarterectomy of the thickened supravalvar ridge in these patients because the ridge is often adherent to the commissural attachments of the aortic valve and excision of the ridge may result in damage to the valve commissures. The Doty technique using a Y-shaped patch has been useful, but it does not generally address the narrowing of the orifice into the left coronary ostium that is formed by the commissural attachment to

the supravalvar ring posteriorly and is often associated with thickening of the endothelium and intima around the orifice of the coronary artery. Thus, we have used either a trifurcated patch to enlarge all three coronary sinuses or the technique described by Myers in which the aorta is primarily anastomosed into the base of the aortic sinuses. Although all of the techniques described can result in excellent relief of gradients across the left ventricular outflow tract, we believe that the primary anastomosis with attention to all three of the aortic sinuses permits the most optimal flow in the coronary arteries.

In many patients with Williams syndrome there is significant hypoplasia of the ascending aorta and the aortic arch. In these cases, interdigitation of the distal aorta into the aortic sinuses for repair of supravalvar aortic stenosis is not possible. I have found it quite advantageous to patch the entire arch of the aorta with a triangular patch of pulmonary homograft material and then insert triangular patches into each of the coronary sinuses individually. The opening up of the sinus and sinotubular junction is quite effective with this technique, and then the size match is appropriate for anastomosis to the ascending aortic and arch reconstruction. In addition, if there is ostial stenosis of the left or right coronary or both, the triangular patches of homograft material can be carried down into the origin of the coronary artery itself, creating essentially an arterioplasty of the proximal coronary artery in addition to enlarging the aortic sinus and relieving the supravalvar obstruction. Often these patients have significant pulmonary stenosis and branch pulmonary artery hypoplasia, and transection of the aorta to perform this operation gives good exposure to place a T-shaped patch on the main pulmonary artery and onto the branch pulmonary arteries to the hilum of the lung.

The approach to hypertrophic subaortic stenosis in infants and children is primarily surgical. The early results with surgical resection of the subaortic septal myocardium have been excellent and the long-term results good. Thus, in children with significant gradients remaining despite medical management with calcium-channel blockers or beta blockers, surgical intervention should be considered the primary treatment. We have not found pacing to be particularly beneficial in children, and in fact there is controversy as to the beneficial effects of pacing for this condition. Extensive resection of septal muscle has resulted in virtually complete relief of gradients and good long-term outflow tract obstruction relief in children, and the incidence of significant conduction disturbance has been quite low. When we perform left ventricular myomectomy for subaortic stenosis or for hypertrophic cardiomyopathy, we use the technique described by the authors, although now we more extensively debride all of the muscle to the left of the vertical incision in the ventricular septum all the way to the mitral valve to remove as much muscle as possible from the outflow tract in the area away from the conduction tissue. When associated mitral valve disease is present, valve replacement can be considered; however, the problems of prosthetic valves in children warrant a very conservative approach to valve replacement. We have elected to perform extensive muscle resection of the septum in association with primary mitral valve repair when feasible.

T.L.S.

81

Anomalies of the Sinuses of Valsalva and Aortico-Left Ventricular Tunnel

Luca A. Vricella and Duke E. Cameron

Introduction

Congenital anomalies of the aortic root sinuses typically present as either enlargement or anomalous communication between supravalvular aorta and left ventricular cavity. In the former (sinus of Valsalva aneurysm) the process develops progressively and can be associated with connective tissue disorders that have as phenotypic expression that of diminished tensile strength of the aortic root. The latter is, on the contrary, the result of a perturbation in cardiac development that is almost uniformly clinically evident in the newborn period or in early infancy.

Aortic root dilation is also a late finding in children who have undergone repair of various forms of congenital heart defects, such as common arterial trunk, transposition of the great arteries, or bicommissural aortic valve. With regard to sinus of Valsalva (SoV) aneurysm we will focus,on isolated dilation of one sinus because treatment of uniform aortic root enlargement (seen more commonly in association with other forms of congenital, atherosclerotic or connective tissue disease) is detailed elsewhere in this book.

Aneurysm of the Sinus of Valsalva

Morphologic Considerations

Each coronary sinus is limited inferiorly by the semicircular hinge point of the corresponding aortic valve cusp. The intercommissural triangles are inferior to the festoon-like line of ventriculoaortic continuity (commonly referred to as "annulus"), whereas the sinotubular junction delineates the circular superior margin of the aortic root.

The sinuses of Valsalva are normally thinner than the tubular portion of the aorta, and this macroscopic finding is usually associated with a lesser degree of histologic representation of the tunica media. In patients with SoV aneurysm, this normal characteristic is accentuated. Thinning of the aortic wall with disconnection of the media from the aortoventricular junction is seen histologically and increases over time.

Figure 81-1 schematically demonstrates the anatomic relations of the aortic root with the adjacent cardiac structures when the aortic valve is observed from the operating surgeon's viewpoint. These relations account in turn for the different modes of clinical presentation that are seen with pathologic enlargement of the sinuses of Valsalva. Dilation of the right SoV (most common) will therefore typically progress in the direction of the right ventricular outflow tract or the right atrium, whereas the noncoronary sinus will involve either left or right atrial chambers. Isolated enlargement of the left SoV (with possible rupture into the left atrium) is the rarest form of this pathology. Although typically SoV aneurysms involve one of the three sinuses as a well-defined diverticular outpouching, two or three sinuses can be affected simultaneously by the pathologic process. A ventricular septal defect (VSD) is present in 25% to 50% of cases at presentation.

Aneurysms of the sinuses of Valsalva are rare. They are observed in 0.1% of autopsy series and in 0.14% to 0.96% of large operative cohorts and are five times more common in patients of Asian descent.

Clinical Presentation

Pathologic SoV enlargement is often diagnosed incidentally in asymptomatic patients. Clinical presentation can otherwise either be in the form of aortic catastrophe (free intrapericardial rupture) or acute (rupture within right or left atrium, right ventricle, endocarditis) or assume a more indolent clinical course during childhood. In this last mode of presentation, progressive dilation, distortion, and subsequent loss of cusp coaptation can lead to clinically significant aortic insufficiency.

Rupture or fistulization almost always involves the right coronary sinus, with a minority of patients presenting with involvement of the noncoronary (up to 30%) or left coronary (<2%) sinuses. In perhaps the largest reported surgical series (149 patients with SoV aneurysm), intracardiac rupture was seen at presentation in just less than 50% of cases. Aortic root rupture into a neighboring cardiac chamber is a rare event in the first two decades of life. If we extrapolate from data available in young patients with connective tissue disorders, this is not surprising. In a meta-analysis of 286 patients age <20 years with Marfan syndrome, Knirsh and coworkers reported aortic dissection in only 5 patients (1.7%) and rupture in 3 (1.0%). All but one patient (14 years old) were 19 years of age at the time of the acute event involving the aortic root. When intracardiac rupture of a SoV aneurysm occurs, a mean survival period of 3.9 years has been reported in untreated patients.

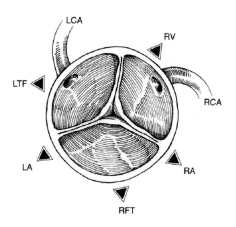

Superior view of Aortic Valve

Figure 81-1. Superior schematic view of the aortic root with adjacent structures (LA = left atrium; LCA = left coronary artery; LFT = left fibrous trigone; RA = right atrium; RCA = right coronary artery; RFT = right fibrous trigone; RV = right ventricle.)

When symptomatic, patients may present with chest discomfort, palpitations, dyspnea on exertion, or florid congestive heart failure, with diastolic hypotension and pulmonary overcirculation from acute left-to-right shunting between aorta and right-sided chambers. Of patients with fistulization, >60% will be symptomatic at presentation. A continuous murmur is usually heard on auscultation of the precordium in cases of fistulization. The clinical picture can be that of sepsis in cases of associated endocarditis (up to 20% of patients). Dyspnea or even cyanosis can rarely result from progressive right ventricular outflow tract obstruction by an enlarging SoV aneurysm that protrudes into the right ventricle. Atrioventricular conduction abnormalities can be observed at presentation in 10% of patients.

The diagnosis is easily confirmed by transthoracic echocardiography, with cardiac catheterization reserved for patients with significant risk factors for coronary artery disease.

Surgical Indications and Technique

Indications for surgery in patients with uniform dilation of the aortic root are fairly well established. Enlargement beyond 5.5 cm, or progression of greater >1.0 cm/ year are well-accepted indications for surgical intervention in asymptomatic patients. Aortic regurgitation from distraction

of the commissural posts with ventricular enlargement is also an accepted indication for surgery, as is aortic dissection. Threshold for intervention can be lowered for young adults with lesser degrees of enlargement and family history of aortic dissection or rupture. In our practice, we have used similar criteria for pediatric patients with root enlargement, although, as mentioned, the risk of rupture in the first decade is quite low.

In case of isolated enlargement of a sinus, indications are not as well defined. Strong consideration to surgical intervention should be given in asymptomatic patients because of the high likelihood of progressive increase in size and the possibility of rupture or endocarditis. The latter is obviously an indication for urgent surgical correction.

A transesophageal echocardiogram is routinely performed after induction of anesthesia to confirm preoperative diagnosis, assess valvular competence, and rule out the possibility of a concomitant septation defect.

The operative approach is via a median sternotomy, with bicaval cannulation and cardiopulmonary bypass and moderate hypothermia (24°C to 28°C). A right superior pulmonary vein vent is inserted, and the heart is arrested with either antegrade administration of cold blood cardioplegia (direct intracoronary delivery is used in case of ruptured aneurysm or significant aortic regurgitation) or with retrograde coronary perfusion. If the tip of the "windsock" is palpable through the right atrium, it can be compressed manually to allow antegrade administration of cardioplegia in spite of runoff secondary to rupture or fistulization. We use continuous topical cooling, as well as carbon dioxide flooding of the surgical field to minimize retention of air within the left-sided chambers.

A transverse aortotomy is performed, and the root anatomy assessed. An oblique right atriotomy is performed next, allowing for identification of both ends of the aneurysm or of the fistulous tract in case of rupture (Fig. 81-2). In case of protrusion or rupture into the right ventricle, exposure can be obtained through a right atriotomy or a limited ventriculotomy (Fig. 81-3). When the fistulous tract or diverticulum is in the right ventricular infundibulum, the lesion can also be exposed through a transverse pulmonary arteriotomy. The defect must be repaired through the aortic root, using a patch of autologous or bovine pericardium to exclude the aortic inlet into the aneurysm. Primary closure predisposes to a higher risk

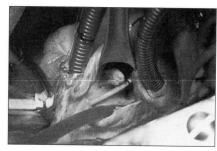

Figure 81-2. Intraoperative photograph of unruptured aneurysm of the right sinus of Valsalva with "windsock" morphology, seen through a right atriotomy. A stay suture is retracting the aneurysm caudally. (Courtesy of Dr. David Yuh, Johns Hopkins Cardiac Surgery.)

of recurrence (as high as 20%) or aortic valve regurgitation from deformation of the root. In ruptures or diverticula, the opening on the atrial or ventricular side should be addressed as well. The ventricular or atrial aspect of the fistula can be closed primarily, but a patch should be used to incorporate closure of a coexisting ventricular septal defect (Fig. 81-3). Great care should be taken in avoiding the atrioventricular conduction system at the time of VSD closure.

In tri-sinus enlargement of the aortic root, we attempt aortic root replacement with valve preservation. The techniques involved in aortic valve-sparing root replacement are detailed elsewhere in this book, and can be successfully applied to pediatric patients as well. Need for aortic valve replacement has been reported in 30% to 50% of patients with significant preoperative aortic valve regurgitation; with fairly reproducible aortic valve repair techniques (such as valve resuspension or shortening of the free margin) this requirement has been significantly lowered in more recent series.

Alternatives to valve preservation in case of diffuse enlargement and unrepairable aortic regurgitation are valve replacement with mechanical, xenograft, or homograft prostheses. The Ross procedure (pulmonary valve autotransplantation) can be considered as a potential option in patients without stigmata of connective tissue disorders or bicuspid aortic valve.

Results

In a large contemporary series, Au and coworkers reported long-term results on 53 patients operated with SoV aneurysms; there

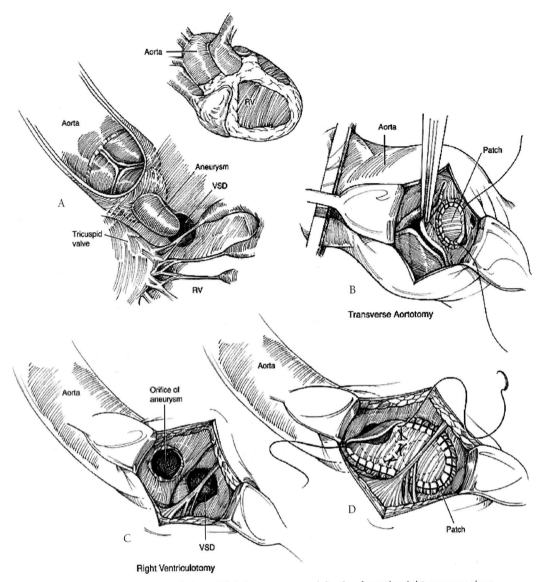

Figure 81-3. **(A)** Unruptured sinus of Valsalva aneurysm originating from the right coronary sinus and associated with a ventricular septal defect (VSD). **(B)** Patch repair of the aneurysm with autologous pericardium through a transverse aortotomy. **(C, D)** Transventricular aneurysm and VSD closure with synthetic patch. (RV = right ventricle.)

was no operative mortality, and overall survival was 83% at 15 years. Over a 32-year period, 22 patients underwent repair of single-sinus SoV aneurysm at the Johns Hopkins Hospital. Nineteen patients presented with intracardiac rupture; congestive heart failure was the most frequently presenting symptom. Operative survival was 95%, with 5- and 10-year survival of 84.9% and 59.4%, respectively. The lower long-term survival in our series might reflect the older age at presentation, associated cardiac conditions, and noncongenital etiology observed more frequently in a Western patient population. Factors such as bacterial endocarditis, aortic valve replacement, and concomitant VSD do not appear to adversely influence operative

and long-term survival. Preoperative VSD and presence of aortic insufficiency appear, however, to have an effect on late reintervention for aortic regurgitation. Especially in cases with progressive dilation without rupture, prolapse of the involved cusp with leaflet fibrosis and insufficiency appears to jeopardize long-term viability of aortic valve repair. Need for late aortic valve replacement has been reported in 25% of patients at 10 years, in particular for patients with VSD on presentation and residual aortic regurgitation at time of discharge. Need for late reintervention for recurrent regurgitation or prosthetic valve dehiscence, endocarditis, and thrombosis has a uniformly negative effect on late survival.

Aortico-Left Ventricular Tunnel

Morphology

Aortico-left ventricular tunnel (ALVT) is an exceedingly rare condition. It represents 0.001% of all congenital cardiac anomalies, with <100 cases reported in the world literature up to 2004.

In this developmental abnormality, an endothelialized paravalvular communication exists between aortic root (typically right coronary sinus) and left ventricle, very rarely leading to the right ventricle by means of a ventricular septal aneurysm. The lesion can often be appreciated as a bulging

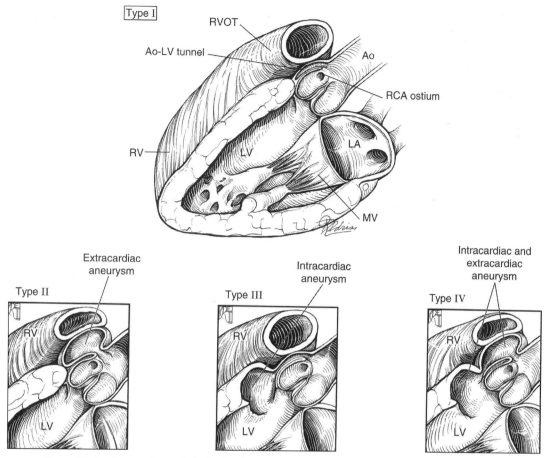

Figure 81-4. Proposed morphologic classification of aortico-left ventricular tunnel. Type I: Simple tunnel with slit-like opening at aortic end, no aortic valve distortion. Type II: Large tunnel with oval aortic opening with or without aortic valve distortion. Type III: Intracardiac aneurysm of the ventricular portion of the tunnel, with or without right ventricular outflow tract obstruction. Type IV: Combination of types II and III. (Ao = aorta; LV = left ventricle; MV = mitral valve, RCA = right coronary artery; RV = right ventricle; RVOT = right ventricular outflow tract.) (Reprinted with permission from D Shum-Tim, CI Tchervenkov. Aortic-Left Ventricular Tunnel. In: Mavroudis C, Backer CL (eds), Pediatric Cardiac Surgery, 3rd ed. Philadelphia: Mosby, 2003;576.)

and pulsatile mass, visible externally between the aorta and pulmonary artery. Although the trajectory of the tunnel has a variable course, the supravalvular inlet is usually located in the right coronary sinus above, below, or at the level of the right coronary ostium. The ventricular opening is readily visible on retraction of the aortic valve cusps and typically located below the right coronary leaflet. The paravalvular tract is directed inferiorly and leftward into the left ventricle. The proximal opening is usually larger, and can be slit-like or oval in appearance. The tunnel can be either aneurysmal or serpiginous and narrow. There are therefore two distinct portions of the tunnel: (1) aortic, located between aortic opening and interventricular septum, and (2) intracardiac, located between the latter and the left ventricular (LV) opening. The latter portion is located within the septum

that forms the posterior wall of the right ventricular outflow tract. The variable morphologic features of ALVT have been summarized as types I to IV of the Hovaguimian classification (Fig. 81-4).

The aortic valve is usually competent or mildly regurgitant. Coronary anomalies can be seen in 30% of patients; otherwise relatively simple associated cardiac defects (VSD, bicommissural aortic valve, aortic stenosis among others) are observed in up to 45% of cases.

Clinical Presentation and Diagnosis

The severity of symptoms clearly depends on the size of the aortico-left ventricular communication and the consequent regurgitant volume. The lesion should be suspected in any neonate or infant with

systolic-diastolic murmurs and congestive heart failure. Differential diagnosis includes patent arterial duct, aortopulmonary window, absent pulmonary valve syndrome, congenital coronary artery fistula, and, in older children, ruptured SoV aneurysm. Tachypnea, poor weight gain, cardiomegaly, and widened pulse pressure with bounding peripheral pulses are other typical signs and symptoms of ALVT. Rarely, cyanosis can be present, secondary to progressive right ventricular outflow tract obstruction from septal bulging beneath the pulmonary valve.

Chest X-ray typically reveals cardiomegaly, plethoric lung fields, and a tortuous ascending aorta. Transthoracic echocardiography is the diagnostic modality of choice, demonstrating the typical septal "drop-out" under the right coronary sinus. Left ventricular hypertrophy, left-axis deviation, and repolarization abnormalities are usually seen on electrocardiography. Cardiac ischemia from diastolic runoff into the fistulous tract can rarely be present. Occasionally, it is very difficult to differentiate between aortic and paravalvular regurgitation. In such cases, aortic root angiography (with or without simultaneous occlusion of the ALVT) readily establishes the diagnosis. Magnetic resonance imaging has also been used as an alternative to angiography to define morphology in unclear cases.

Surgical Indications and Technique

Given the often impressive symptoms at the time of presentation and the risk of progressive aortic valve insufficiency in patients with lesser degrees of clinical acuity, operative intervention is indicated on diagnosis, even in asymptomatic patients. The goal of preventing aortic valve regurgitation from progressive root distortion and secondary valvular changes is particularly relevant in small patients, in whom the alternative to aortic valve repair is homograft aortic root replacement. In case of small ALVT diagnosed in asymptomatic patients, careful medical management and expectant followup can nevertheless be considered because spontaneous closure of small communications has been reported.

Intraoperatively, transesophageal echocardiography is used to assess competence of the valve and adequacy of repair after discontinuation of cardiopulmonary bypass.

In the absence of a septal communication, bypass is established between a single right atrial cannula and the distal ascending aorta. The left atrium is vented through the right superior pulmonary vein after institution of bypass, and systemic cooling to moderate degrees of hypothermia (24°C to 28°C) is started. Because of the paravalvular regurgitation, it is important to avoid left ventricular distension once the heart fibrillates. The aorta is therefore immediately cross-clamped, and an aortotomy is performed above the sinotubular junction. Blood cardioplegia (30 cc/kg in pediatric patients) is then directly infused into the coronary ostia and redosed at 30-minute intervals. Retrograde cardioplegic delivery can be used as an alternative myocardial protection strategy.

As in SoV aneurysm, the defect should be approached both from the aortic root and left ventricle, addressing both inlet and outlet of the ALVT. This is critically important because isolated inlet closure has been associated with AVLT recurrence. Concerns have been raised about the technique of closure of the AVLT inlet, with direct closure resulting in possible distortion of the aortic valve. We favor patch closure (with Gore-Tex or

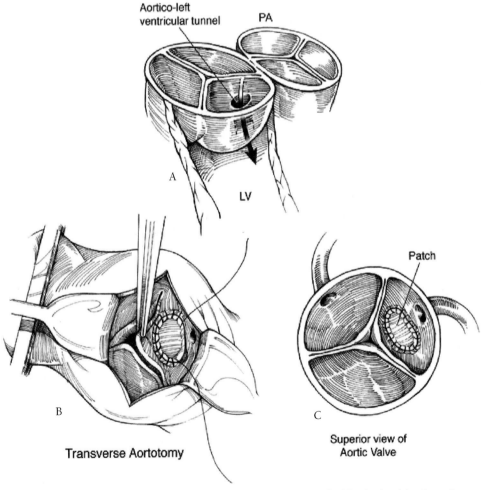

Figure 81-5.   **(A)** Aortico-left ventricular tunnel, as typically observed arising in the right sinus of Valsalva. **(B, C)** Through an aortotomy the inlet orifice to the tunnel is closed with an autologous pericardial patch. The ventricular opening of the tunnel is closed through the aorta separately, either primarily or with a second patch. (LV = left ventricle; PA = pulmonary artery.)

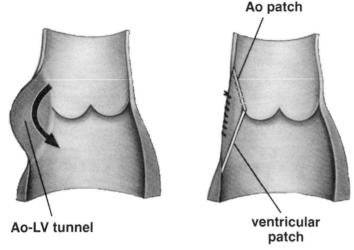

Figure 81-6. Alternative surgical approach to repair of aortico-left ventricular (Ao-LV) tunnel. Inlet and outlet orifices are exposed *through* The tunnel **(left)**. Patch closure of both aortic and ventricular openings is accomplished, followed by closure of the tunnel between aorta and pulmonary artery **(right)**. (Reprinted with permission from J Stark. Congenital Anomalies of the Sinuses of Valsalva and Aortico-Ventricular Tunnel. In: Stark J, deLeval M (eds), Surgery for Congenital Heart Defects, 2nd ed. Philadelphia: Saunders, 1994;633.)

bovine or autologous pericardium) in infants and small children with an oval rather than slit-like aortic opening (Fig. 81-5). In the latter, a pledgeted repair appears to offer a more reliable outcome in case of direct closure. Tunnel plication is now rarely performed. The ventricular outlet of the tunnel can be exposed either through the retracted leaflets of the aortic valve or directly through the tunnel, approached between aorta and pulmonary root (Fig. 81-6).

Results

Reported operative mortality ranges between 0% and 16%, with specific early complications represented by atrioventricular heart block and predischarge aortic valve regurgitation.

The major postoperative concern is need for late reintervention; up to 50% of patients may require late aortic valve replacement either because of valvar deformity (likely the result of postrepair turbulence) or progressive aneurysmal dilation of the aortic root (secondary to poor support of the right aortic cusp). Significant early or late aortic insufficiency is seen more frequently in children undergoing repair at an older age.

Aortico-left ventricular tunnel recurrence is very rare, especially if closure is performed at both ends. If a residual small ALVT is observed, consideration may be given to coil embolization, but proximity to the aortic valve and right coronary artery orifice must be balanced against the benefits of the percutaneous approach.

SUGGESTED READING

Au KW, Chiu SW, Mok CK, et al. Repair of sinus of Valsalva aneurysm: Determinant of long-term survival. Ann Thorac Surg 1998;66:1604.

Azakie A, David TE, Peniston CM, et al. Ruptured of sinus of Valsalva aneurysm: Early recurrence and fate of the aortic valve. Ann Thorac Surg 2000;70:1466.

Cameron DE, Vricella LA. Valve-sparing aortic root replacement in Marfan syndrome. Semin Thorac Cardiovasc Pediatr Card Surg Ann 2005;8:103.

Harkness JR, Fitton TP, Barreiro CJ, et al. A 32 year-experience with surgical repair of sinus of Valsalva aneurysm. J Card Surg 2005;20:198.

Hovaguimian H, Cobanoglu A, Starr A. Aortico-left ventricular tunnel: A clinical review and a new surgical classification. Ann Thorac Surg 1988;45:106.

Martins JD, Sherwood MC, Mayer, JE, et al. Aortico-left ventricular tunnel: 35-year experience. J Am Coll Cardiol 2004;44:446.

Murashita T, Kubota T, Kamikubo Y, et al. Long-term results of aortic valve regurgitation after repair of ruptured sinus of Valsalva aneurysm. Ann Thorac Surg 2002;73:1466.

Naka Y, Kadoba K, Ohtake S, et al. The long-term outcome of a surgical repair of sinus of Valsalva aneurysm. Ann Thorac Surg 2000;70:727.

Takach TJ, Reul GJ, Duncan JM, et al. Sinus of Valsalva aneurysm or fistula: Management and outcome. Ann Thorac Surg 1999;68:1573.

Van Son JAM, Danielson GK, Shaff, HV, et al. Long-term outcome of surgical repair of ruptured sinus of Valsalva aneurysm. Circulation 1994;90:20.

Vricella LA, Williams JA, Ravekes WJ, et al. Early experience with valve-sparing aortic root replacement in children. Ann Thorac Surg 2005.

EDITOR'S COMMENTS

Aneurysms of the sinus of Valsalva are often identified after rupture occurs. As noted by the authors, most sinus of Valsalva aneurysms rupture into the low-pressure right atrial or right ventricular chamber. Left coronary sinus of Valsalva aneurysms, however, can rupture into the left atrium, although even in this location rupture into the right atrium or ventricle is more common. Ventricular septal defect is associated with approximately one third of sinus of Valsalva aneurysms and therefore should be carefully looked for in these patients. Although fistulous communications between the sinuses of Valsalva and cardiac chambers can be approached with a catheter technique and occluder devices, surgery remains the procedure of choice because of the direct approach to each end of the fistula and the ability to either primarily close or patch these defects without significant prosthetic material. One of the more current causes of ruptured sinus of Valsalva into the atrium is related to the use of atrial septal defect occluder devices, which, when excessively large, can erode into the base of the aortic wall and aortic sinus, resulting in an aortic to atrial fistula. Complete removal of the device and surgical closure of the aneurysm would seem to be the most appropriate treatment for these complications of device intervention. The very low morbidity and mortality of operative intervention should continue to lend favor to this approach.

Aortico-left ventricular tunnel is an extremely rare defect; however, it is important to emphasize that when this defect is approached, both the aortic and ventricular ends of the tunnel should be closed. Simple closure of the aortic end of the defect can result in a chamber developing in the septum from systolic inflow, and the pulsatility in this chamber can create an aneurysm of the ventricular septum, which can distort the aortic valve annulus and cause progressive aortic insufficiency.

The optimal technique for dealing with sinus dilation in patients with Marfan syndrome or other degenerative connective tissue diseases of the aortic root remains controversial. As discussed in this chapter, the dilated sinuses of Valsalva can be addressed by graft replacement down to the level of the aortic annulus with preservation of the commissural attachments of the aortic valve and a portion of aortic wall as in the Yacoub operation, or the valve can be resuspended inside a tubular Dacron graft as in the David operation. Both of these procedures have relatively short follow-up, and the incidence of progressive aneurysmal dilation of aortic tissue remaining in the Yacoub operation is unknown. The valve leaflets are also abnormal in these conditions, and progressive aortic insufficiency may occur even with valve-sparing procedures, as in the David operation. Thus, if there is any concern about significant aortic valve disease or aortic insufficiency, complete replacement of the aortic root with a homograft or prosthetic valve and conduit may be the best approach. With these techniques, the operative results have been excellent in the authors' series from Johns Hopkins University, and despite the frequent need for reoperation on other portions of the aorta or the mitral valve in these patients, late morbidity from valve replacement has been low.

T.L.S.

82

Atrioventricular Canal Defects

Martin J. Elliott, Mazyar Kanani, and Jeffrey P. Jacobs

Anatomic Considerations

Atrioventricular canal defects have also been called endocardial cushion defects and atrioventricular septal defects (AVSDs). These defects are characterized by varying degrees of incomplete development of the septal tissue surrounding the atrioventricular (AV) valves along with varying degrees of abnormalities of the AV valves themselves. Consequently, AVSD may include defects in the inferior portion of the atrial septum, defects in the inflow portion of the ventricular septum, and defects in the tissue forming the left and right AV valves. We prefer the term AVSD because the anomaly is primarily caused by the deficiency of normal AV septal structures.

AVSDs represent a spectrum of cardiac anomalies subdivided into partial AVSDs, intermediate AVSDs, and complete AVSDs. *Partial AVSDs* (also known as incomplete AVSDs) have a crescent-shaped atrial septal defect (ASD) in the inferior portion of the atrial septum just above the AV valve. This defect may also be referred to as an ostium primum defect. The partial AVSDs also have varying degrees of malformation of the left AV valve, leading to varying degrees of left AV valve regurgitation. *Complete AVSDs* have both defects in the atrial septum just above the AV valves and defects in the ventricular septum just below the AV valves. In complete AVSD, the AV valve is one valve that bridges both the right and left sides of the heart, creating superior and inferior bridging leaflets. Partial AVSDs and complete AVSDs represent a spectrum of cardiac pathologic conditions. An intermediate form in the middle of this spectrum has been described and termed *intermedi-*

ate AVSD (also known as transitional AVSD). This form of AVSD has two distinct left AV valve and right AV valve orifices but also has both an ASD just above and a ventricular septal defect (VSD) just below the AV valves. The VSD in this intermediate form of AVSD is often restrictive. Although these AV valves in the intermediate form do form two separate orifices, they remain abnormal valves.

The AV valve apparatus in AVSD has been described as having either five or six leaflets. In partial AVSD (Fig. 82-1A), the AV valve apparatus is easily understood as having six leaflets. On the left side, the leaflets have been termed left superior, left lateral, and left inferior. On the right side, the leaflets have similarly been termed right superior, right lateral, and right inferior. In partial AVSD, the right superior and right inferior leaflets both fuse with the ventricular septum to complete the structure of the right AV valve. The left superior and left inferior leaflets similarly fuse with the septum to form the left AV valve. The commissure between the left superior leaflet and left inferior leaflet represents the "cleft" of the left AV valve, which is found in partial AVSD. This cleft is equivalent to the line of abutment of the superior bridging leaflet and inferior bridging leaflet in complete AVSD.

In complete AVSD (Fig. 82-1B,C), it is more difficult to conceive of the common AV valve as a six-leaflet valve. A five-leaflet model is more realistic for complete AVSD. A superior bridging leaflet and an inferior bridging leaflet are always present. These bridging leaflets have very variable morphology in both the amount of leaflet that crosses over the ventricular septum and the degree of chordal attachment to the ventricular septum. Furthermore, scalloping of the bridging leaflets may create the illusion

of extra leaflets. In addition to the superior and inferior bridging leaflets, the five-leaflet model is completed by a left lateral leaflet, a right lateral leaflet, and a right anterosuperior leaflet.

The degree of bridging and chordal attachment by the superior bridging leaflet forms the basis for the Rastelli classification of complete AVSD originally described in 1966. The Rastelli classification does not relate to the anatomy of the inferior bridging leaflet because this leaflet displays greater anatomic variation, and no consistent relationship exists between the morphology of the superior bridging leaflet and the inferior bridging leaflet. In a Rastelli type A defect (Fig. 82-1B), the superior bridging leaflet is effectively limited to the left ventricle, with its right margin being attached to the ventricular crest. The anterosuperior leaflet of the right AV valve is also attached to the ventricular septal crest, giving the appearance that the superior bridging leaflet is split at the interventricular septum. In many cases, chordal attachments pull the plane of the AV valve down into the VSD below the plane of the annulus. In Rastelli type C defects (Fig. 82-1C), there is marked bridging of the ventricular septum by the superior bridging leaflet. The superior bridging leaflet floats freely over the ventricular septum without chordal attachment to the crest of the ventricular septum. Rastelli type B is somewhere between A and C and is very rare in our experience; Rastelli type B involves anomalous papillary muscle attachment from the right side of the ventricular septum to the left side of the common superior (anterior) bridging leaflet.

The other important anatomic consideration when planning the repair of an AVSD is the location of the conduction system because it is very vulnerable during surgical

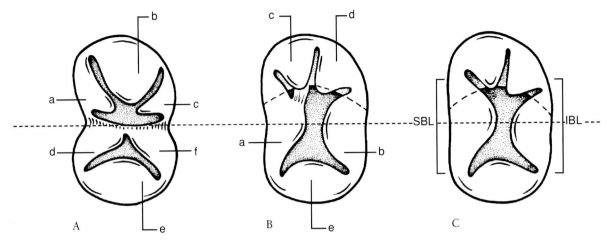

Figure 82-1. **(A)** The atrioventricular valve apparatus in partial atrioventricular septal defect has six leaflets (a = right superior leaflet; b = right lateral leaflet; c = right inferior leaflet; d = left superior leaflet; e = left lateral leaflet; f = left inferior leaflet). The dashed line denotes the plane of the interventricular septum. **(B)** A five-leaflet model demonstrates a Rastelli A atrioventricular septal defect (a = superior bridging leaflet; b = inferior bridging leaflet; c = right anterosuperior leaflet; d = right lateral leaflet; e = left lateral leaflet). Again, the plane of the interventricular septum is demonstrated by the dashed line. **(C)** The anatomy of a Rastelli C defect. The free-floating superior bridging leaflet (SBL) is demonstrated, as is the inferior bridging leaflet (IBL).

repair (Fig. 82-2). The AV node is displaced posteriorly and inferiorly toward the coronary sinus. The AV conduction axis then runs from this node toward the ventricle through the crest of the ventricular septum. Here, the posteriorly displaced bundle of His is usually covered by the inferior bridging leaflet of the AV valve. Thus, the AV node lies in the tissue between the coronary sinus and the margin of the VSD, if present. The location of the AV node is altered in AVSD because the ostium primum ASD often pushes the coronary sinus posteriorly and inferiorly toward the left atrium. This distorts the triangle of Koch and creates a second triangle called the nodal triangle. The nodal triangle is bounded by the coronary sinus, the posterior attachment of the inferior bridging leaflet, and the leading edge of the atrial septum at the septal defect. The ASD pushes the AV node and corresponding conduction tissues posteriorly and inferiorly along with the coronary sinus. The AV node therefore lies at the apex of the nodal triangle in a more posterior and inferior location. The bundle then travels down on the crest of the ventricular septum under the inferior bridging leaflet on the rim of the VSD.

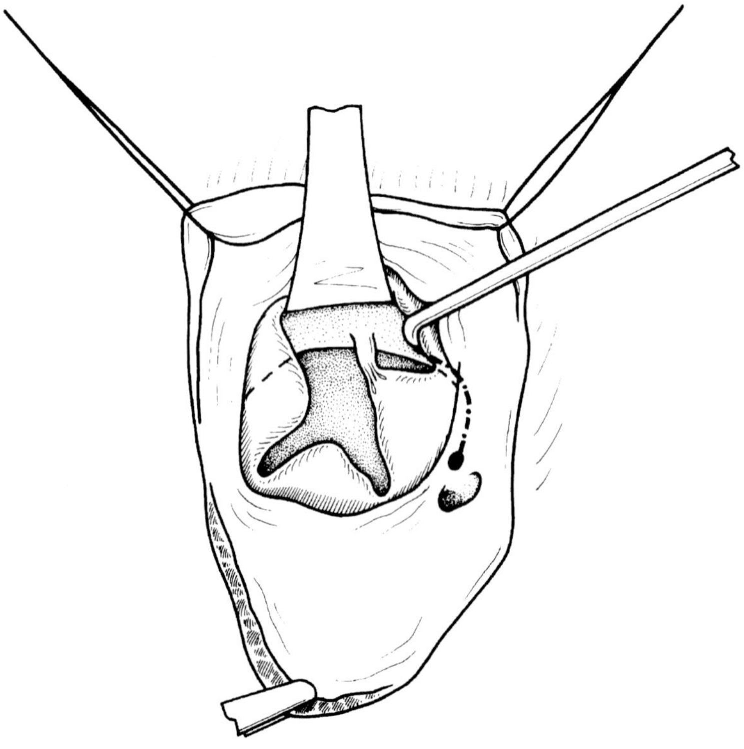

Diagnostic Considerations

Patients with AVSD present in a variety of clinical conditions depending on the size of the septal defects, the direction and magnitude of the associated shunt, and the associated lesions. Patients with partial AVSD may have an asymptomatic cardiac murmur similar to patients with secundum ASDs. However, when left AV valve insufficiency is more pronounced, patients may have symptoms of pulmonary congestion, cardiac failure, and dyspnea. Patients with complete AVSD are more likely to have prominent left-to-right shunting and are similarly more likely to have symptoms of congestive heart

Figure 82-2. A dashed line is used to indicate the location of the atrioventricular node and the bundle of His. The coronary sinus is also demonstrated.

failure, fatigue, and dyspnea. Complete AVSD presents with a more malignant course than partial AVSD. With the complete defect, severe cardiac failure is often present in infancy, and severe pulmonary hypertension will eventually develop, resulting in the death of up to 65% of infants before 1 year of age without surgical intervention. More than one half of the patients with complete AVSD also have Down syndrome.

Physical examination often reveals a variety of cardiac murmurs. A systolic ejection murmur may be found in the pulmonary area because of increased flow across the pulmonary valve. A holosystolic apical murmur is also present when left AV valve regurgitation is significant. The ASD and VSD may also have associated cardiac murmurs.

A chest radiograph often reveals enlargement of the pulmonary artery. The film may also show right ventricular hypertrophy as symptoms of failure progress and left ventricular enlargement with significant left AV valve regurgitation. An electrocardiogram often reveals right ventricular hypertrophy and sometimes left ventricular hypertrophy as well. A vectorcardiogram usually shows a counterclockwise frontal plain loop.

Echocardiography is the modality of choice for establishing a definitive diagnosis in the current era. Two-dimensional echocardiography along with color Doppler studies usually provide complete preoperative information for both partial AVSD and complete AVSD. Three-dimensional echocardiography is undergoing assessment in a number of centers and may ultimately help in the surgeon's understanding of AV valve morphology and in the planning of surgery. Cardiac catheterization is required only when clinical evidence of pulmonary vascular disease exists, making operability questionable, or when additional major cardiac anomalies coexist. A left ventriculogram in the anterior posterior projection shows a typical "goose-neck" deformity caused by the long, narrow left ventricular outflow tract, the lower boundary of which is made up of the superior bridging leaflet. Cardiac catheterization can also be used to measure pressures, flows, and resistances in the pulmonary and systemic circuits as well as the direction and the magnitude of shunting.

Indications for Surgery

The natural history of untreated AVSD depends on the morphology of the lesion and dictates the indications and timing of surgical intervention. Partial AVSD without significant left AV valve regurgitation has a natural history similar to that of ASD. Up to 15% of patients may develop high pulmonary arteriolar resistance in their adult life. The development of symptoms in adulthood often relates to the onset of atrial fibrillation. The natural history of partial AVSD with significant left AV valve regurgitation is much worse. These patients present earlier in life, and without surgical treatment many may die in the first decade of life. Infants with complete AVSD have an even more malignant presentation, and without surgical correction the majority die within the first year of life.

Patients with asymptomatic partial AVSD should be treated similarly to patients with secundum ASD. Elective repair is indicated before school age unless the patient develops symptoms of heart failure or failure to thrive. A minority of patients with partial AVSD and severe left AV valve regurgitation present with severe symptomatology in the first year of life and thus require earlier surgical intervention. Those few infants with severe left AV valve regurgitation who are asymptomatic should be treated surgically.

Infants with complete AVSD should undergo elective correction between 2 and 4 months of life. The management of infants with complete AVSD and trisomy 21 has been somewhat controversial and has depended on the philosophy of the individual cardiologist, cardiac surgeon, and family. In our view, however, they should be treated exactly as those without trisomy 21. The surgical procedure of choice for both partial AVSD and complete AVSD is complete repair of the lesion as will be described. Pulmonary artery banding to palliate symptoms of congestive heart failure plays no role in the management of these lesions except in patients with complex associated cardiac anomalies or those with severely unbalanced hearts or single functional ventricular physiology. Severe pulmonary infection may also be a relative indication for pulmonary artery banding.

Contraindications to surgery are based on fixed severe elevation of pulmonary vascular resistance. Pulmonary vascular resistance >10 units/m² of body surface area (or a pulmonary-to-systemic resistance ratio >0.7) represents a contraindication to repair. Elevated pulmonary vascular resistance of <10 units/m² (or a pulmonary-to-systemic resistance ratio of <0.7) represents an indication for more urgent surgical intervention. The assessment of elevated pulmonary vascular resistance should include cardiac catheterization under conditions of oxygen, nitric oxide, and prostacyclin to assess reversibility.

Operative Technique for Complete Atrioventricular Septal Defects

After routine anesthesia, preparation, and draping, a standard median sternotomy is

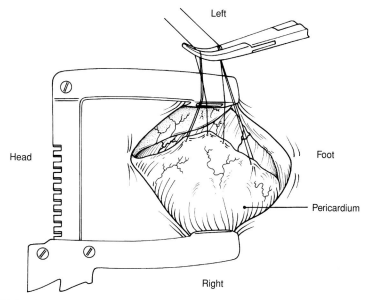

Figure 82-3. An eccentric pericardiotomy to the left is performed leaving a large piece of pericardium attached to the right for later use as a patch. (Note: All operative drawings in this and subsequent figures are viewed from the surgeon's perspective.)

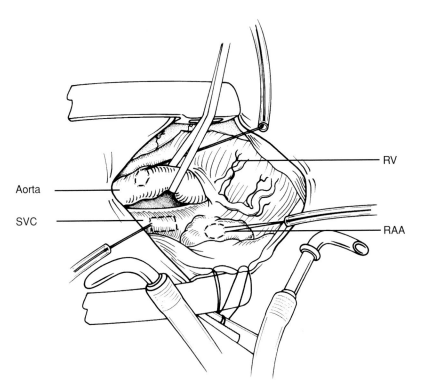

Aorta

SVC

RV

RAA

Figure 82-4. Purse strings are demonstrated in the aorta, the right atrial appendage (RAA), and the superior vena cava (SVC). Note the position of the longitudinally oriented, narrow, rectangular purse string on the SVC about 0.5 cm to 1.0 cm above the junction with the right atrium. (RV = right ventricle.)

The aorta is then cannulated. We prefer the DLP (Medtronic, Grand Rapids, MI) aortic cannula because of its flexibility. Next, the inferior vena cava (IVC) angled metal Pacifico venous cannula (DLP, Grand Rapids, MI) is placed temporarily into the right atrial appendage. Cardiopulmonary bypass is then established (Fig. 82-5), and the ductus arteriosus is ligated with the previously placed silk ligature.

The SVC is then grasped with two mosquito hemostats on each side of the previously placed purse string. The SVC is incised longitudinally with a scalpel, and the SVC is then cannulated with the second angled metal cannula (Fig. 82-6).

A vent is then inserted into the right atrial appendage after the IVC cannula is removed (Fig. 82-7). The pericardial reflection anterior to the IVC is then released, and the subdiaphragmatic IVC is exposed down to the level of the first hepatic vein. A purse string (5-0 polypropylene) is then placed directly into the IVC below the pericardial reflection (Fig. 82-8), and the IVC is cannulated with the IVC angled metal cannula. Nylon caval tapes are passed around the IVC and the SVC.

The patient is cooled to 25°C. The aorta is cross-clamped, the two venae cavae are

performed followed by a subtotal thymectomy. An eccentric pericardiotomy to the left is then performed, leaving a large piece of pericardium attached on the right for later use as a patch (Fig. 82-3). (All operative drawings presented here are viewed from the surgeon's perspective.) The aorta, ductus arteriosus, and superior vena cava (SVC) are then mobilized. Identification of the ductus is best achieved by first finding the "axilla" between the right pulmonary artery and the ductus and then finding the "axilla" between the left pulmonary artery and the ductus using traction on the main pulmonary artery. Once the right and left pulmonary arteries have been formally identified, anything remaining in between must be the ductus. A silk ligature is passed around the ductus but is not yet tied, with care being taken to avoid injuring the ductus.

The lateral aspect of the SVC should be mobilized with scissors to avoid diathermy damage to the right phrenic nerve. A vascular tape is passed around the aorta. Purse strings of 5-0 polypropylene are then placed into the aorta and the right atrial appendage. An additional, longitudinally oriented, narrow, rectangular purse string is placed on the SVC about 0.5 cm to 1.0 cm above the junction with the right atrium (Fig. 82-4).

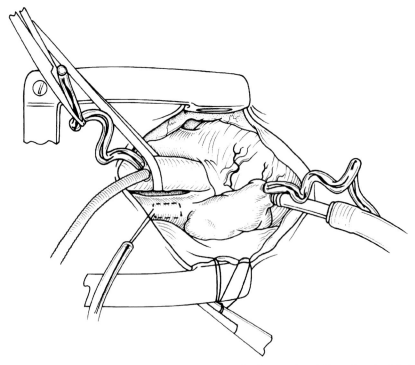

Figure 82-5. The aorta and right atrial appendage are both cannulated. Note that the inferior vena cava angled metal cannula is placed temporarily into the right atrial appendage. Cardiopulmonary bypass may now be established.

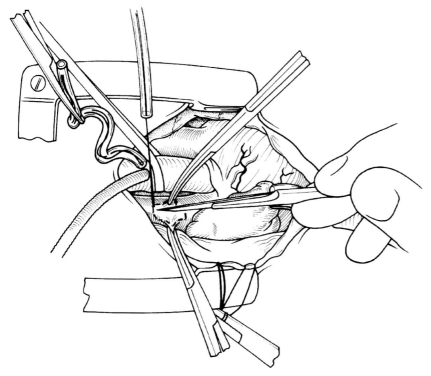

Figure 82-6. The superior vena cava is grasped with two mosquito hemostats on each side of the previously placed purse string. The superior vena cava is incised longitudinally with a scalpel.

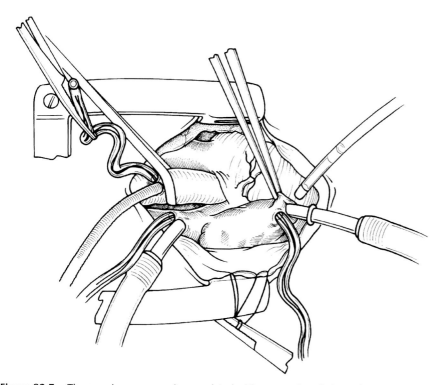

Figure 82-7. The superior vena cava is cannulated with a second angled metal cannula. A vent is then inserted into the right atrial appendage after the inferior vena cava cannula is removed.

snared, the right atrium is opened parallel to the AV groove, and cardioplegic solution is instilled into the aortic root (Fig. 82-9).

A right-angled instrument is then passed through the opening of the right atrium into the left atrium and up into the right superior pulmonary vein. A No. 11 scalpel blade is then used to open the junction of the right superior pulmonary vein and the left atrium between the tips of the right-angled instrument (Fig. 82-10). The vent is then passed into the left atrium and secured into position with a 6-0 polypropylene purse-string suture.

Stay sutures are then applied to the atrial wall, and the anatomy of the AV valve is inspected (Fig. 82-11). Stay sutures of 6-0 polypropylene on an 8-mm needle are then applied to approximate the "kissing points" of the bridging leaflets (Fig. 82-12). The kissing points may be defined as the points of the superior bridging leaflet and inferior bridging leaflet that (1) intuitively come together at the center of the superior and inferior bridging leaflets, (2) usually overlie the interventricular septum, and (3) can be identified as the midpoint between the left and right chordae on each bridging leaflet. Unwanted secondary chordae (which may limit exposure and whose function will partially be replaced by the new interventricular patch) can be divided. This permits elevation of a tethered bridging leaflet from the ventricular crest up to the plane of the annulus.

The size required for the VSD patch is then measured using black silk ligatures. Two pieces of black silk are trimmed. One silk measures the length of the patch by measuring the distance from the superior to the inferior margin of the annulus of the common AV valve in the plane of the interventricular septum (Fig. 82-13A). Inferiorly, extra length must be allowed to permit the patch to extend beyond the predicted position of the bundle. The second silk measures the depth of the patch by measuring the distance from the plane of the annulus of the freed common AV valve to the crest of the interventricular septum beyond the base of the VSD (Fig. 82-13B). The importance of this depth measurement is that it dictates the degree of elevation of the revised AV valve apparatus up to the plane of the annulus. A patch of 0.4-mm polytetrafluoroethylene (Gore-Tex) is then trimmed to size using the previously cut silk sutures as guides (Fig. 82-13C).

This patch of 0.4-mm Gore-Tex is then sutured into position with a 5-0 polypropylene continuous suture. We start this suture inferiorly with the suture being brought

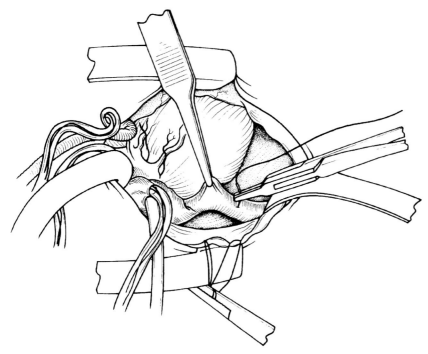

Figure 82-8.   The pericardial reflection anterior to the inferior vena cava (IVC) is released and the subdiaphragmatic IVC is exposed. A purse string (5-0 polypropylene) is then placed directly into the IVC below the pericardial reflection. (The length of the IVC is exaggerated for clarity.)

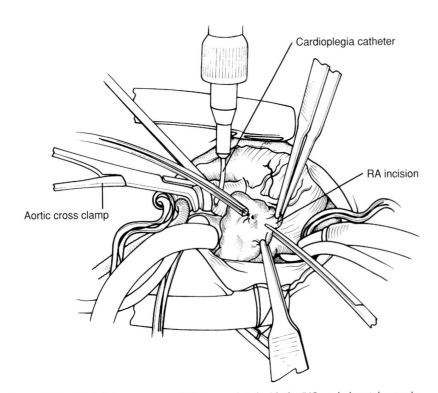

Cardioplegia catheter

RA incision

Aortic cross clamp

Figure 82-9.   The inferior vena cava (IVC) is cannulated with the IVC angled metal cannula. Nylon caval tapes are passed around the IVC and the superior vena cava. The patient is cooled to 25°C. The aorta is cross-clamped, the two venae cavae snared, the right atrium (RA) opened parallel to the atrioventricular groove, and cardioplegic solution instilled into the aortic root.

through the right AV valve close to the annulus, well away from (inferior to) the position of the bundle (Fig. 82-14). It is easiest to place this first suture by going through the inferior bridging leaflet on the right side of the interventricular septum, passing the needle behind the right-sided chordae to the inferior bridging leaflet, and then passing the needle through the corner of the crescentic Gore-Tex patch. The needle is then taken back behind the chordae before positioning the suture deep into the muscle of the septum well away from the position of the bundle but close to the annulus. This will fix the patch in good position before commencing the running suture. This first suture is facilitated by retracting the inferior bridging leaflet inferiorly using a nerve root retractor. The running suture line is then brought superiorly along the right side of the septum, weaving behind chordae as required. The conduction system is avoided inferiorly, and the aortic valve leaflets are carefully visualized and avoided superiorly. The 5-0 polypropylene suture is brought through the superior bridging leaflet at the annular margin and is placed on a rubber-shod clamp once the superior margin is reached (Fig. 82-15).

It is now necessary to septate the valve into a left and a right component, simultaneously preparing the atrial component of the patch. Interrupted horizontal mattress sutures of 6-0 polypropylene double-armed with 8-mm needles are then placed along the crest of the interventricular patch, with the surgeon bringing them out through the superior and inferior bridging leaflets, respectively, and then through a patch of autologous pericardium, not yet detached from the right side of the pericardium (Fig. 82-16). These sutures should start inferiorly, beginning by retracting the inferior bridging leaflet once again with a nerve root retractor. The first of these sutures is placed through the Gore-Tex patch close to the inferior VSD running suture. The needle is then passed through the inferior bridging leaflet next to the inferior VSD running suture, and finally is passed through the attached pericardial patch. The second arm of this first 6-0 polypropylene double-armed suture should then be placed a little bit farther along the crest of the Gore-Tex patch, with the surgeon bringing it in turn through the inferior bridging leaflet in a line between the inferior arm of the VSD running suture and the kissing-point stay suture. This line is important because it will represent the line of demarcation between the left and the right AV valves (Fig. 82-15). The second arm of this first 6-0 polypropylene

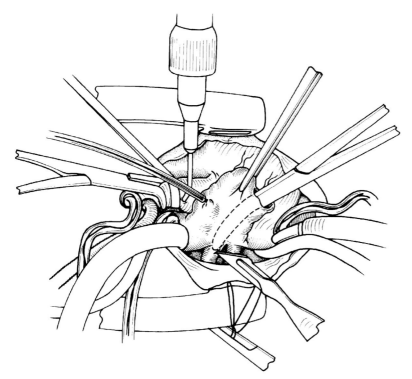

Figure 82-10.   A right-angled instrument is passed through the opening of the right atrium into the left atrium and up into the right superior pulmonary vein. A No. 11 scalpel blade then opens the junction of the right superior pulmonary vein and the left atrium between the tips of the right-angled instrument. The vent can then be passed into the left atrium and secured into position with a 6-0 polypropylene purse-string suture.

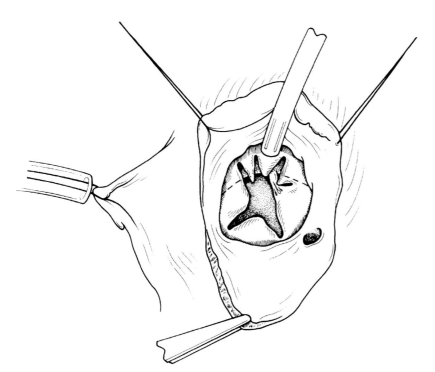

Figure 82-11.   Stay sutures are used to hold the atrial wall open to inspect the anatomy of the atrioventricular valve. The suction tip is useful as a retractor to examine the anatomy of the atrioventricular septal defect.

double-armed suture is then also passed through the attached pericardial patch and held in a rubber-shod clamp. The remaining interrupted horizontal mattress sutures of double-armed 6-0 polypropylene are then placed along the crest of the interventricular patch, with the surgeon bringing them out through the inferior and superior bridging leaflets, respectively, and then through the pericardial patch. We have found it to be a major advantage to keep the pericardium attached because this makes it easier to understand the relationships between the two AV valves and the atrial patch. The horizontal mattress sutures are then tied, and this brings the pericardium down to the ridge of the valve complex (Fig. 82-17). The pericardial patch is detached (Fig. 82-18A) and then swung anteriorly (Fig. 82-18B).

Attaining Left Atrioventricular Valve Competence

1. The first important element in left AV valve repair is the size of the VSD patch. Too big a patch and the valve will not coapt, too small a patch and the valve will become stenotic at annular level.

2. The cleft in the left-sided AV valve (or zone of abutment between the left superior bridging leaflet and the left inferior bridging leaflet) is an unsupported commissure that needs to be closed to create a neoseptal leaflet akin to the aortic leaflet of a normal mitral valve. This is best achieved using one or two horizontal mattress sutures of 6-0 polypropylene reinforced with autologous pericardial pledgets (Fig. 82-19). The valve is then tested for competence by suspending the leaflets with saline (Fig. 82-20). All tension is released from all stay sutures. The autologous pericardial patch is held gently forward, and a 50-ml syringe is used to inject ice-cold saline via a size 10 nasogastric tube through the left AV valve. The valve should float up nicely and demonstrate no regurgitation (Fig. 82-21). If necessary, an additional 6-0 polypropylene suture reinforced with autologous pericardial pledgets is placed in the cleft nearer the central orifice.

3. If the valve continues to leak, the problem should not be ignored. First, the location of the leak is identified: central orifice, separate orifice, or a gap between scalloped components of the bridging leaflets. If a central leak exists and the cleft is already reapproximated to the chordae, an annuloplasty, such as a De-Vega annuloplasty, may be performed at whatever commissures are visible. If the

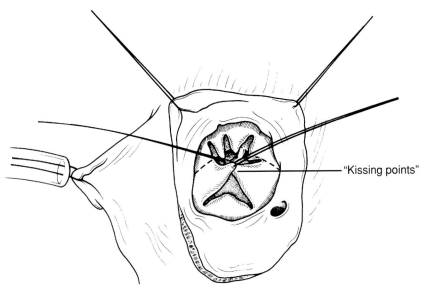

Figure 82-12.   Stay sutures of 6-0 polypropylene on an 8-mm needle are then applied to approximate the "kissing points" of the bridging leaflets.

valve is leaking at the cleft, an annuloplasty will not help. The leaflets and the cleft must be dealt with first. Annuloplasty is supportive and cannot result in primary competence in this morphology.

4. Paradoxically, it may be better in certain circumstances not to close the cleft and to leave the superior and inferior bridging leaflets unapproximated. This is the case when the mural leaflet is tiny or absent as in the parachute arrangement of left AV valve support apparatus. There is always a balance between stenosis and regurgitation in these circumstances, and it is important to size the left AV valve using Hegar dilators to ensure good baseline information for future follow-up, and occasionally to guide removal of an overtight stitch in the cleft, resulting in a degree of "acceptable" regurgitation.

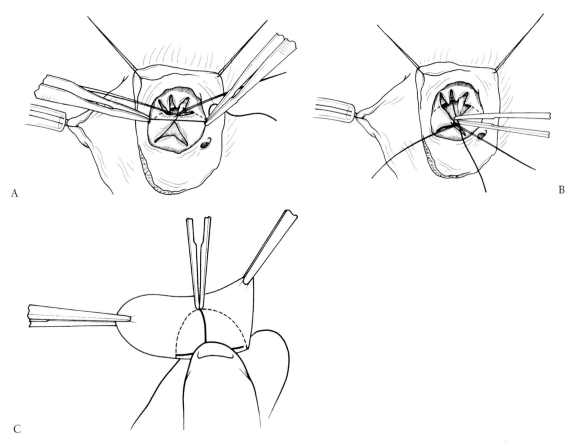

Figure 82-13.   **(A)** A piece of black silk is used to measure the length of the patch by measuring the distance from the superior to the inferior margin of the annulus of the common atrioventricular valve in the plane of the interventricular septum. Inferiorly, extra length must be allowed to permit the patch to extend below the predicted position of the bundle. **(B)** A second piece of silk measures the depth of the patch by measuring the distance from the plane of the annulus of the freed common atrioventricular valve to the crest of the interventricular septum beyond the base of the ventricular septal defect. **(C)** A patch of 0.4-mm polytetrafluoroethylene (Gore-Tex) is then trimmed to size using the previously cut silk sutures as guides.

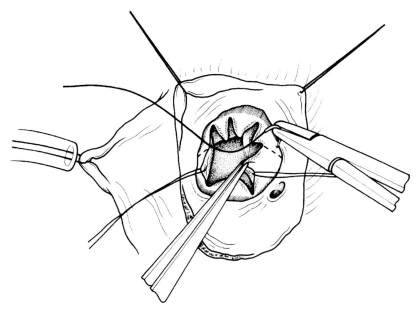

Figure 82-14. The first suture begins inferiorly with the suture being brought through the right atrioventricular valve close to the annulus, well away from and inferior to the position of the bundle.

The ASD patch is then sutured in place with continuous 5-0 polypropylene suture. The coronary sinus may be left on the left or right atrial side. If there is a large ASD or an additional secundum ASD, we keep the coronary sinus on the left side of the heart (Fig. 82-22). However, we try to place the coronary sinus on the right whenever possible. It is essential to place the coronary sinus on the right side when there is a left-sided SVC. We also try to keep the coronary sinus on the right when we are concerned about possible postoperative left AV valve dysfunction because a high left atrial pressure may result in high coronary sinus pressure.

During closure of the ASD, care is taken to ensure that the IVC remains on the right side and that the conduction system is carefully avoided. The first stitch of the continuous 5-0 polypropylene suture used to secure the atrial pericardial patch is placed on the inferior aspect of the ASD next to the previously placed VSD running suture currently held in a rubber-shod clamp. This first stitch is placed in the same way whether the coronary sinus will be placed on the left or the right, and this stitch is used to secure the VSD suture. If the coronary sinus is to go on the left, this continuous 5-0 polypropylene suture is then used to stitch the pericardial ASD patch along the atrial wall well inferior to the bundle and out around the coronary sinus, avoiding the Eustachian valve and keeping the IVC on the right. If the coronary sinus is to go on the right, this continuous 5-0 polypropylene suture is then used to stitch the pericardial ASD patch along the left AV valve itself at its annular margin and then onto the septum beyond the bundle. The continuous 5-0 polypropylene suture is interrupted at the top of the ASD patch to prevent this patch from ever becoming constrictive. The ASD pericardial patch is trimmed as the suture line progresses and often ends up smaller than originally anticipated.

Cardioplegic solution is administered every 20 to 30 minutes throughout the cross-clamp period. After the atrial patch is sewn into position (Fig. 82-23) and all communications between the right heart and the left heart are definitely closed, the aortic cross-clamp is removed and the heart is de-aired through the aortic root and through the right superior pulmonary vein. The right atrium is then closed with a 6-0 polypropylene suture on a 13-mm needle with the cross-clamp off during rewarming. Once the child is warm, ventilation is begun, de-airing is completed, the vent is removed, and a left atrial pressure monitoring line is inserted via the right superior pulmonary vein. The child is then weaned from cardiopulmonary bypass and modified ultrafiltration is carried out. We favor intraoperative echocardiographic assessment to define the functional status of the repair and will redo any part of the procedure as indicated by the study. Protamine is then administered. Two atrial and two ventricular pacing wires are placed and chest drains are placed.

If the left AV valve is potentially regurgitant or dysfunctional or if any other reason exists to increase the likelihood of a redo sternotomy, a 0.1-mm-thick, low-porosity, expanded polytetrafluoroethylene pericardial membrane (Preclude Pericardial Membrane, formerly called the Gore-Tex Surgical Membrane; W. L. Gore and Associates, Flagstaff, AZ) is placed. Routine closure then follows.

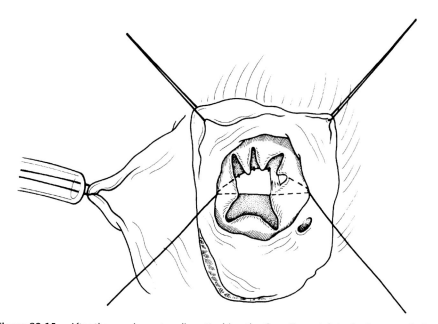

Figure 82-15. After the running suture line attaching the Gore-Tex patch to the interventricular septum is completed, the 5-0 polypropylene suture is placed on a rubber-shod clamp at the superior margin.

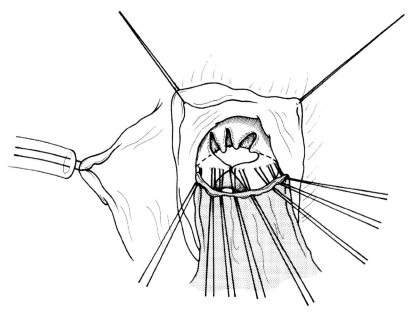

Figure 82-16.   Interrupted horizontal mattress sutures of 6-0 polypropylene double-armed with 8-mm needles are placed along the crest of the interventricular patch, with the surgeon bringing them out through the superior and inferior bridging leaflets, respectively, and then through a patch of autologous pericardium not yet detached from the right side of the pericardium. (The chordae are omitted for clarity.)

Management of Unusual Variants of Complete Atrioventricular Septal Defects

Atrioventricular Septal Defect with Tetralogy of Fallot

Here, the common atrioventricular junction occurs in the setting of deviation of the outlet septum, producing different degrees of aortic override. Necessarily, there will be right ventricular outlet obstruction at variable levels that will have to be dealt with surgically.

The deviation of the outlet septum has consequences for the morphology of the leaflets of the AV junction and the shape of the ventricular septal crest.

The superior bridging leaflet is always free-floating, enabling the left ventricle to access the deviated aorta. Consequently, this combination of defects does not occur in the setting of partial AVSD.

Given that such patients have a protected pulmonary vascular bed, operation is still often deferred to 2 to 3 years of age. Although the valve is larger in these older patients, valvar function and dysplasia may be paradoxically worse in the setting of chronic regurgitation. A competent repair may therefore be more challenging and crucial, especially of the right AV valve, the competence of which is vital for good right ventricular function postoperatively. Right AV valve annuloplasty and/or commissuroplasty are commonly employed as a further, supportive measure for the right AV valve.

The ventricular septal patch must be tear shaped rather than elliptical, taking account of the deviated outlet septum (Fig. 82-24). The aortic margin of the patch may be difficult to access through the right atrium but can be approached through the right ventricular outflow tract that was opened at the time of assessment of the pulmonary valve.

Unbalanced Atrioventricular Septal Defect

This is difficult to define. It could be said that there is ventricular imbalance when the ventricular cavities are of unequal size or when the common atrioventricular junction is committed preferentially to one ventricle over the other. These two problems often coexist. Not only may the overall ventricular cavity be small, but it may also lack one segment of the normal tripartite ventricular morphology, such as the apical trabecular segment.

Severe imbalance of either ventricle is approached with a univentricular, Fontan, strategy, but the cut-off ratio of ventricular size that defines which strategy should be used is undefined. This is compounded by difficulty in measuring ventricular volumes. In our institution, we prefer "eye-balling" ventricular size at two-dimensional echocardiography, but three-dimensional echo and magnetic resonance imaging might have a future role in the decision-making process.

A small left ventricle may coexist with a solitary papillary muscle arrangement (the so-called parachute valve), left ventricular outflow tract obstruction, or coarctation, as in the setting of Shone complex. A small right ventricle may be seen with right ventricular outflow tract obstruction or after previous pulmonary trunk banding.

The approach to the small ventricle must be individualized according to a common morphologic algorithm. Not only must the

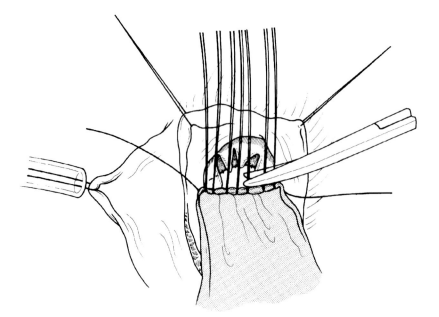

Figure 82-17.   The horizontal mattress sutures are tied, with the surgeon bringing the pericardium down to the ridge of the valve complex.

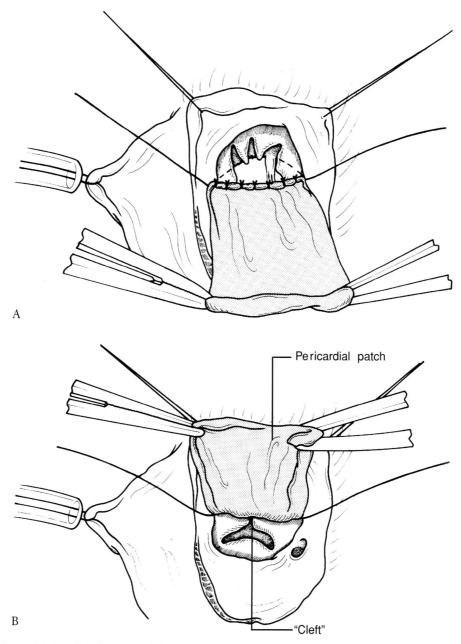

A

B

Pericardial patch

"Cleft"

Figure 82-18. **(A)** The pericardial patch is detached. **(B)** The pericardial patch is then swung anteriorly. This allows visualization of the "cleft" in the left atrioventricular valve. This cleft may be seen as the zone of abutment of the left superior bridging leaflet and the left inferior bridging leaflet.

size of the cavity be assessed at operation, but so must the atrioventricular valve ring size and the state of the papillary muscles. If subjectively little of the common atrioventricular valve is committed to one ventricle, then a biventricular repair will not possible irrespective of the cavity size. Thus, the surgeon must inspect the ventricles at the annular, valvar, and subvalvar levels to determine whether a biventricular approach is feasible. If so, the so-called cleft must almost always be left open to prevent valvar stenosis. Is it possible to "recruit" cavity volume through the division of muscle bundles, in

an manner similar to the ventricular overhaul seen with pulmonary atresia and intact ventricular septum? This is being investigated, and but we advocate close inspection of the ventricular cavity for such bundles with the view of dividing them, so long as the AV valve ring is of good size.

Accessory Left Atrioventricular Valvar Orifice

This unusual variant is commonly cited as a risk factor for postoperative mortality and left AV valve regurgitation.

In these cases, the larger AV valve orifice occurs in association with a smaller orifice that is almost always located at the junction of the inferior bridging leaflet (IBL) and mural leaflet. Developmentally, these two leaflets may have failed to separate or may have fused at their tips, producing a small accessory orifice along their line of closure.

At operation, this orifice must not be closed because it is nearly always supported by cords and therefore is competent. Closure can result in left AV valve stenosis. For similar reasons, the zone of apposition in the main orifice must be closed

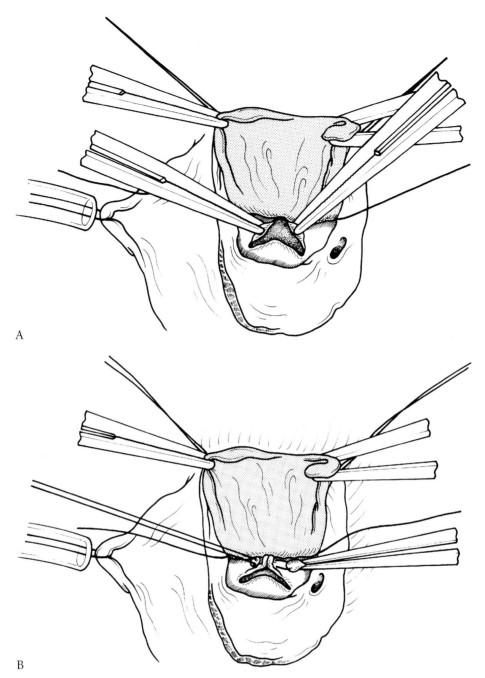

Figure 82-19. **(A)** The cleft in the left atrioventricular valve is demonstrated. **(B)** One or two horizontal mattress sutures of 8-0 polypropylene reinforced with autologous pericardial pledgets are then used to close the cleft in the left atrioventricular valve.

carefully, ensuring that there is no resulting stenosis.

Deficiency of Atrioventricular Valve Tissue

This is a difficult problem and can result in on-table mortality. Although any of the leaflets may be deficient, it almost always results from deficiency of the IBL over the ventricular septum. Thus, the surgical approach must be tailored according to the degree and pattern of this deficiency. Here, annuloplasty may be particularly helpful in improving the degree of central coaptation of the other leaflets. Some degree of resulting valvar stenosis has to be tolerated, given that the unwanted alternative is valvar replacement at a very young age

The Role of Atrial Septal Defect Patch Fenestration

In all of the foregoing instances, the ASD may be closed with fenestration. This technique has the advantage of acting as a "blow-off" (or "pop-off") valve when the ventricle is small, improving the postoperative hemodynamics and salvaging a difficult biventricular repair in this setting. It also gives the

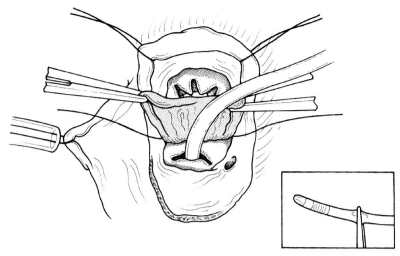

Figure 82-20. The valve is then tested for competence by suspending the leaflets with saline. The inset demonstrates the catheter used to inject the saline to float the valve.

chance for the AVV and ventricle to grow, redressing some of the imbalance and improving left AV valve function over time.

A hole is punched in the middle of a Gore-Tex patch that is sutured to the margins of the atrial septal defect or atrial septectomy. This not only prevents widening of the fenestration that can occur with an incision in autologous pericardium, but also permits transcatheter closure of the hole at the appropriate postoperative time.

Surgical Management of Partial Atrioventricular Septal Defect

The surgical management of partial AVSD has many similarities with that of complete

AVSD, and repetition of the principles is not required. However, there are important differences that need to be highlighted.

Cardiopulmonary Bypass

We prefer to repair partial AVSD at temperatures of >32°C, and recently have begun to perform the procedure at 37°C. Cannulation is as for complete AVSD, and cardioplegia is used.

Repair

We assess the defect carefully using an approach and pericardial patch preparation similar to those described for complete AVSD. Stay sutures are not required, but attention should be paid to the quality of the valve tissue above the crest of the interventricular septum. If the tissue is judged to

be of good quality (strong, thick, holding sutures well), we sometimes use a continuous suture of 5-0 polypropylene to secure the patch along the line of division between right and left components of the AV valve. If the tissue is of poor quality (friable, thin, deficient, or holding sutures poorly), we prefer an interrupted suture technique using an appropriately sized suture as horizontal mattress sutures. If the valve tissue is particularly bad, we often take a strip of autologous pericardium from the left side of the patient and use this as a buttress to the sutures along the valve leaflets at the crest of the septum, creating a very robust sandwich (pericardium-valve-pericardium). At the inferior margin, the bundle is avoided, and the coronary sinus is positioned exactly as for complete AVSD. After the patch has been attached to the crest of the septum, the patch is swung anteriorly and the left AV valve assessed and repaired as for complete AVSD.

Surgical Complications and Postoperative Care

Improved modern surgical techniques and modern intensive care units have drastically reduced the operative mortality for these procedures. Most centers report operative mortality of 1% to 3% for surgical intervention for partial AVSD defects. This mortality decreases to <1% if the partial AVSD is not associated with significant left AV valve regurgitation. Operative mortality for complete AVSD is <5%, and most major centers report operative mortality of <3% for this problem. The operative risk does increase in several subsets of patients, including those with severe AV valve incompetence, those with hypoplasia of one of the ventricles, and those with pulmonary vascular disease.

Potential postoperative complications include pulmonary hypertensive crisis, left AV valve insufficiency, and heart block. Children with significant preoperative left AV valve regurgitation and older children with complete AVSD are at risk of postoperative pulmonary hypertensive crises. The concern for pulmonary hypertension leads to certain fundamental postoperative management principles. Children believed to be at risk for postoperative pulmonary hypertensive problems, including children in the range of 6 to 9 months (or older) undergoing repair of complete AVSD, fall into a late-extubation group. These children are managed with a pulmonary artery line and a left atrial pressure monitoring line in situ and are kept sedated over the first 48 hours after

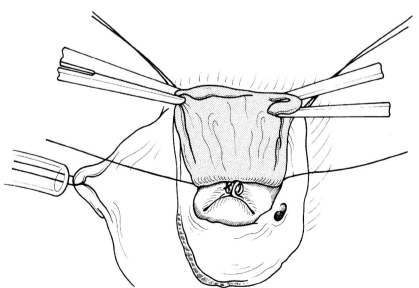

Figure 82-21. The valve should float up nicely, demonstrating no regurgitation.

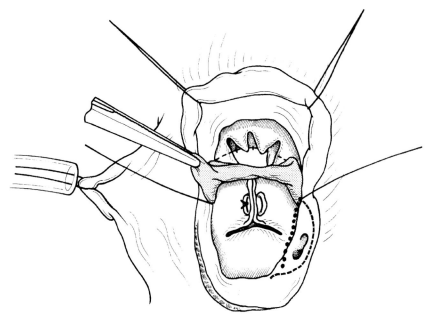

Figure 82-22.   The atrial septal defect pericardial patch is then sutured in place using continuous 5-0 polypropylene suture. The coronary sinus may be left on the left or right atrial side. The dotted line demonstrates the suture line if the coronary sinus is to be placed on the right atrial side. The dashed line demonstrates the suture line if the coronary sinus is to be placed on the left atrial side.

surgery. They are monitored for pulmonary hypertension and are in a position in which pulmonary hypertensive crises can be appropriately managed. Our first-line therapy, after conventional ventilation support, is inhaled nitric oxide (2 ppm to 20 ppm). Phenoxybenzamine, a long-lasting alpha-adrenergic blocking agent, has been used in these patients prophylactically. It is given before cardiopulmonary bypass and during rewarming at doses of 1 mg/kg. It is also given postoperatively at doses of 0.5 mg/kg per dose every 8 to 12 hours until extubation. These children remain sedated and monitored. If a pulmonary hypertensive crisis occurs, appropriate interventions can be initiated. These interventions include increased sedation, increased supplemental oxygen, hyperventilation to a CO_2 pressure of <25 mm Hg or <3.5 kPa, intravenous nitroglycerin or sodium nitroprusside, intravenous aminophylline, possible pharmacologic paralysis, intravenous prostacyclin administration, and inhaled nitric oxide. If a pulmonary hypertensive crisis occurs, a 24-hour period of stability is required before attempts are made to wean the patient from the ventilator. If no pulmonary hypertensive crises occur, children in this group are extubated at approximately 48 hours. Younger infants, in the range of 2 to 4 months, with complete AVSD as well as children with partial AVSD are often not at risk for pulmonary hypertensive crises. Consequently, these children are often extubated sooner, often within the first 24 hours.

Postoperative left AV valve insufficiency is present to some degree in approximately 10% of patients undergoing repair of AVSD. These children are initially managed medically with afterload reduction. This may be done intravenously in the intensive care unit with nitroglycerin or nitroprusside. Long-term afterload reduction can be done orally with angiotensin-converting-enzyme inhibitors such as captopril or with other oral medications such as prazosin (Minipress). A small subgroup of these patients with left AV valve insufficiency require redo operations for either left AV valvuloplasty or left AV valve replacement in the future. Repair should not be delayed if the child is in the intensive care unit.

A third potential complication after repair of AVSD is heart block. In the early days of repair of AVSD, this problem represented a leading cause of operative and postoperative mortality. This complication is not as problematic currently because it occurs with much lower frequency with careful attention to the anatomy of the conduction system and also because, when it does occur, it can be managed appropriately. The incidence of permanent heart block in major centers repairing AVSD is <1%. Most episodes of postoperative heart block in these patients are temporary episodes caused by edema and resolve in the several days after surgery. When permanent heart block does occur, it should be treated by placement of a permanent pacemaker before discharge from the hospital.

Long-term prognosis is excellent after repair of AVSD. Several series have reported long-term survival over 10- to 20-year periods of >90%. Long-term freedom from reoperation is similarly high except in the subgroup of patients requiring intervention for severe left AV valve regurgitation. The short-term and long-term prognoses in

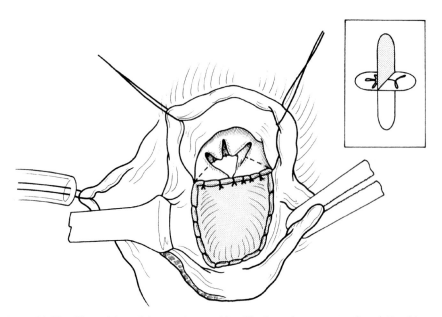

Figure 82-23.   The atrial patch is sewn into position. The inset demonstrates the relationship between the atrial patch, the ventricular patch, the right atrioventricular valve, and the left atrioventricular valve.

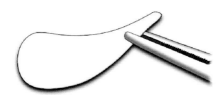

Figure 82-24. In atrioventricular septal defect with tetralogy of Fallot, the shape of the ventricular septal patch must be tear shaped rather than elliptical, taking account of the deviated outlet septum.

children with AVSD and Down syndrome are similar to those for children without Down syndrome.

Controversial Issues

Several issues remain controversial regarding the repair of AVSD. These include whether a single patch or two patches should be used for the repair, which type of material should be used for the patch or patches, whether the cleft in the left AV valve should be closed in partial AVSD, and where to leave the coronary sinus after repair. We prefer to use separate patches because we believe that this allows us greater ease in the reconstruction of the AV valves. By placing two patches, we believe that we are better able to avoid distorting the valves and that we have greater flexibility in creating competent AV valves. Moreover, we believe that we have greater ability to avoid conduction tissue with the use of two patches.

We choose to use Gore-Tex or polyester (Dacron) patches for closure of the VSD. However, we prefer to use autologous pericardial patches for closure of the ASD. We also like to use pericardial pledgets to reinforce this patch closure as previously described. We believe that the pericardial closure of the ASD helps to prevent the small risk of problematic postoperative hemolysis. Otherwise, a jet of regurgitation through the left AV valve can strike a Gore-Tex or Dacron patch and subsequently lead to this hemolytic problem.

It has been proposed that the cleft leaflet in the left AV valve in partial AVSD defect does not need to be completely reapproximated because this valve is actually a trileaflet valve completely different in fundamental structure from a normal mitral valve. In our view, this cleft should be closed because our experience demonstrates that left AV valve cleft closure helps to prevent left AV valve regurgitation.

Finally, several options exist regarding placement of the coronary sinus on the left atrial side or the right atrial side of the patch. We try, whenever possible, to place the coronary sinus on the normal anatomic side (the right atrial side). Placement of the coronary sinus on the right atrial side eliminates an additional element of mixing of saturated and desaturated blood. Furthermore, we believe that placement of the coronary sinus on the right side can be accomplished safely in the majority of instances as long as careful attention is paid to the anatomy of the conduction system. Certainly when a left-sided superior vena cava drains into the coronary sinus, it is extremely important that the coronary sinus be placed on the right side of the atrial septum. It is also important to direct the coronary sinus blood flow to the right side in the setting of an unbalanced AVSD with a small left ventricle. Because the AV node typically lies at the apex of the nodal triangle, the coronary sinus can be directed to the right atrial side of the atrial patch, and the AV node can be safely avoided in the majority of circumstances. In some hearts, a sizable post-Eustachian sinus near the base of the coronary sinus allows for placement sutures that avoid conduction tissue and safely allow the coronary sinus to drain to the right atrium. In other hearts, this post-Eustachian sinus is smaller; in these hearts, it is often necessary to place the suture line within the coronary sinus ostium to keep the coronary sinus draining to the right side of the heart. Using these techniques, we believe that in the majority of circumstances we can allow coronary sinus drainage to remain in its anatomic position of the right side by paying careful attention to the anatomy of the conduction system and the nodal triangle.

SUGGESTED READING

Elliott M. Cannulation for Cardiopulmonary Bypass for Repair of Congenital Heart Disease. In RA Jonas, M Elliott (eds), Cardiopulmonary Bypass in Neonates, Infants, and Young Children. Boston: Butterworth–Heinemann, 1994;127.

Jacobs JP, Burke RP, Quintessenza JA, Mavroudis C. Congenital heart surgery nomenclature and database project: Atrioventricular canal defect. Ann Thorac Surg 2000;69(4 Suppl):S36.

Lillehei CW, Cohen M, Warden HE, Varco RL. The direct-vision intra-cardiac correction of congenital anomalies by controlled cross circulation: results of thirty-two patients with ventricular septal defects, tetralogy of Fallot, and atrioventricular communis defects. Surgery 1958;38:11.

MacCartney FJ, Rees PG, Anderson RH, et al. Angiographic appearances of atrioventricular defects with particular reference to distinction of ostium primum atrial septal defect from common atrioventricular orifice. Br Heart J 1979;42:640.

McMullan MH, Wallace RB, Weidman WH, McGoon DC. Surgical treatment of complete atrioventricular canal surgery. J Thorac Cardiovasc Surg 1972;72:905.

Newfeld EA, Sher M, Paul MH, Nikaidoh H. Pulmonary vascular disease in complete atrioventricular canal defect. Am J Cardiol 1977; 39:721.

Pacifico AD, Ricchi A, Bargeron LM, et al. Corrective repair of complete atrioventricular canal defects and major associated cardiac anomalies. Ann Thorac Surg 1988;46:645.

Pacifico AD. Atrioventricular Septal Defects. In Stark J, de Leval M (eds), Surgery for Congenital Heart Defects (2nd ed). Philadelphia: Saunders, 1994;373.

Rastelli GC, Kirklin JW, Titus JL. Anatomic observations on complete form of persistent common atrioventricular canal with special reference to atrioventricular valves. Mayo Clin Proc 1966;41:296.

Rastelli GC, Ongley PA, Kirklin JW, McGoon DC. Surgical repair of the complete form of persistent common atrioventricular canal. J Thorac Cardiovasc Surg 1968;55:299.

Thiene G, Wenink A, Anderson RH, et al. Surgical anatomy and pathology of the conduction tissues in atrioventricular defects. J Thorac Cardiovasc Surg 1981;82:928.

EDITOR'S COMMENTS

The progressive improvement in results of repair of complete AVSD has permitted primary repair in infancy to become the procedure of choice for this condition. The incidence of the development of pulmonary vascular occlusive disease by 1 year of age has progressively decreased the optimal age at repair to the point that now elective repair can be undertaken at any age when congestive heart failure is not controlled, and optimally between 2 and 4 months of age in most infants. We agree with the authors that pulmonary artery banding is virtually never indicated for complete AVSDs because the banding may cause increased right ventricular hypertrophy, which actually complicates the exposure of the AV valves at the time of complete repair and in our experience has resulted in less optimal exposure for placement of the ventricular patch and reconstruction of the common AV valve. Even very tiny infants can undergo successful complete repair without resorting to banding. One subset of patients who may benefit from banding are the rare infants who have abnormal attachment of the anterior bridging leaflet that is significant enough to create left ventricular outflow tract obstruction. These patients may best be considered to have functionally single ventricle.

Partial AVSD ("ostium primum defect") is generally simple to repair, with good long-term results. However, significant left AV valve regurgitation can occur in this condition despite an adequate primary repair. We agree that closure of the cleft in the anterior mitral leaflet in this condition should be routinely performed to attempt to decrease the incidence of late AV valve regurgitation. In spite of this recommendation, some patients will nevertheless develop AV valve regurgitation despite an adequate closure and require valvuloplasty procedures at a later time. A particularly difficult subgroup of patients are those with a relatively hypoplastic left ventricle in association with primum ASD, who have a high mortality with primary repair.

Technically, our technique for repair of complete AVSDs is similar to the technique described in this chapter. We also favor a two-patch technique, which allows the best exposure of the AV valves for assessment of competence and also permits closure of the VSD without the need to divide a common anterior bridging leaflet except in rare circumstances. If the anterior bridging leaflet is maintained undivided, the chances of dehiscence of the valve attachments to the patch become less and may decrease the need for reoperation. In addition, we have found that securing a ventricular septal patch below the common AV valve leaflets permits a suture line to which the superiorly located pericardial patch can be attached, reinforcing the suture line at the AV valves to minimize the risk of dehiscence. We have generally used Dacron for VSD closure because the patch is more flexible and small residual defects will often close spontaneously. We have elected to place the midportion of the ventricular septal patch first, and then, using gentle traction on each stitch in a running fashion, the suture line can be carried superiorly and inferiorly to complete the repair to the level of the AV valve attachments. The patch can then be trimmed again if nec-

essary to allow the appropriate plane for attachment of the AV valve leaflets to the superior crest of the patch, which we perform in a running fashion. The common AV valve leaflets are then floated with saline solution to assess the coapting surfaces, which are then directly approximated using polytetrafluoroethylene suture, which does not cut through the tissue as readily as polypropylene suture and may avoid the need for pledget material. It is important not to evert the edges of the cleft of the mitral leaflet, which can lead to central regurgitation at the tip of the anterior mitral leaflet. In rare instances in which there is an accessory mitral valve orifice, usually posteriorly and inferiorly, the accessory orifice is not addressed in the repair. We have elected to place the coronary sinus on the right side of the atrial septal patch in essentially all patients and have not found an increased incidence of conduction defects utilizing this technique.

We use intraoperative transesophageal echocardiography at the completion of surgery in every patient who undergoes repair of partial or complete AVSDs to assess the magnitude of mitral valve competence at the end of the procedure. Patients with more than moderate residual mitral regurgitation can then undergo immediate revision of the valve repair to decrease the incidence of late reoperation. With this technique, our experience with complete AVSD repair has resulted in a mortality of 2.9% or less, with a marked reduction in reoperation rate to <10% (CE Canter, TL Spray, CB Huddleston, E Mendeloff. Intraoperative evaluation of atrioventricular septal defect repair by color flow mapping echocardiography. Ann Thorac Surg 1997;63:592).

We have not elected to use pulmonary arterial monitoring lines in most patients with AVSD repairs because with early operative intervention, the incidence of pulmonary hypertensive events has been very low.

Patients who have a restrictive VSD in unbalanced AV canal to the right may have adequate inflow into the left ventricle for a two-ventricle repair even if there is an-

tegrade flow out the aorta and across the aortic arch. Decision making for these patients can be extremely difficult, and careful attention must be given to the attachments of the common AV valve, the inflow patterns into the ventricles, and the relative size of the AV valves and ventricles.

Dr. Elliott and his associates have suggested that leaving an atrial septal defect in patients with a relatively small left ventricle or compromised left AV valve may be beneficial as a "pop-off." Although this has been shown to be effective in some cases, it is not clear how this improves the hemodynamic situation, given that all of the blood decompressing from the left atrium will be represented back to the left atrium. It is thought perhaps that such atrial septal defects simply allow a larger capacitance of the left atrial chamber and may therefore limit pulmonary hypertension at the expense of a lower cardiac output and increased pulmonary blood flow. We generally believe that if an ASD is required to prevent severe left atrial hypertension, then the left-sided structures are probably too small for a two-ventricle repair.

With the advent of nitric oxide, pulmonary hypertensive events have become less of a cause of morbidity and mortality after repair of AVSD, resulting in marked improvement in operative results. Current operative survival after repair of these defects approaches 98%.

In our experience, the indication for reoperation in AVSD repair has generally been left-sided AV valve regurgitation. Rare instances of patch dehiscence have occurred that required reoperation; however, the long-term durability of the left AV valve repair remains the primary determinant of late morbidity. In many cases, the valve can be repaired at a second operative intervention either with more complete closure of the cleft of the anterior mitral leaflet or with additional annuloplasty sutures. Valve replacement should be extremely unusual after AVSD repairs.

T.L.S.

83

Truncus Arteriosus

Thomas L. Spray

Truncus arteriosus represents an unusual congenital heart defect in which a single arterial trunk arises from the heart, providing the origins of the coronary arteries, the true pulmonary arteries, and the brachiocephalic vessels. The defect is usually associated with a ventricular septal defect and a single, large semilunar valve. Typically, the semilunar valve contains up to four separate leaflets, which may be dysmorphic in infancy. In situations in which more than four leaflets are present, incorporation of remnants of the pulmonary valve into the truncal valve is presumed. Very rare instances of absence of ventricular septal defect in truncus arteriosus have been reported, but usually the infundibular septum is virtually absent superiorly. Thus, the ventricular septal defect is similar to that seen in tetralogy of Fallot but with no superior rim of infundibular septum separating the pulmonary and aortic valves. This feature can be used to distinguish truncus arteriosus from pulmonary atresia with ventricular septal defect. Embryologically, the development of truncus arteriosus is related to deficiency of the aorticopulmonary septum, with absence of the subpulmonary infundibulum and partial or complete absence of pulmonary valve tissue. These defects are associated with neural crest abnormalities, and because the neural crest also develops into thymus and parathyroids, DiGeorge syndrome is commonly associated with truncus arteriosus.

The development of aortic arches 4 and 6 varies in truncus arteriosus such that infants with hypoplasia or interruption of the aortic arch have associated large ductal connections between the truncus and the descending aorta, and infants in whom the arch is fully developed usually have absence of the ductus arteriosus.

The primary classification systems for truncus arteriosus have focused on the origins of the pulmonary arteries. The classification scheme of Collett and Edwards defines truncus arteriosus types by the presence of a main pulmonary trunk or the separation of the pulmonary arteries from the arterial trunk. From a surgical standpoint, however, the variations in the origin of the pulmonary arteries are often similar enough among the various types that separation by this classification scheme has not been as useful as the alternate scheme developed by Van Praagh. The Van Praagh classification system is described in Table 83-1. The advantage of the Van Praagh classification is the inclusion of variations of truncus in which interrupted or undeveloped aortic arch is present or in situations in which one pulmonary artery arises from the truncal vessel and the other pulmonary artery arises separately from the ductus arteriosus. These are important surgical differences that are well defined by this classification scheme. Some authors have described as "hemitruncus" a situation in which the right pulmonary artery arises from the ascending aorta and the left pulmonary artery from the right ventricle. This defect is typically not associated with a ventricular septal defect. In our opinion, it is not a variation of truncus arteriosus and is best defined as aortic origin of the right pulmonary artery. Such a description distinguishes this anomaly from the Van Praagh type 3A truncus. The truncal valve typically straddles the ventricular septum with balanced contributions from the left and right ventricles. However, in a few cases the truncal valve straddles the right ventricle, offering the potential for restriction of blood flow from the left ventricle to the truncal valve at repair.

Coronary anomalies seen in truncus are typically a high origin of the left coronary artery from the truncus near the pulmonary origins and an anomalous anterior descending coronary from the right coronary artery crossing the right ventricle to supply the anterior ventricular septum.

Pathophysiology of Truncus Arteriosus

The defect of truncus arteriosus in the absence of arch interruption or severe hypoplasia is one of complete mixing of systemic and pulmonary venous blood with pulmonary overcirculation. As the pulmonary vascular resistance falls in the early neonatal period, the tendency is for unrestricted pulmonary blood flow from the truncus, resulting in severe congestive heart failure. Mild cyanosis may be present because of the complete mixing at the level of the atrium and ventricle. The presence of a large connection between the ascending aorta and the pulmonary arteries above the level of the semilunar valve results in pulmonary blood flow during systole and diastole, increasing the amount of pulmonary overcirculation. It is believed that this situation results in early development of pulmonary vascular obstructive disease in children with truncus arteriosus, which accounts for the high mortality of untreated patients with this condition. Infants born with truncus arteriosus and unrestricted pulmonary blood flow have a mortality of as high as 50% in the first month of life because of congestive heart failure. Pulmonary vascular obstructive disease typically develops to a significant degree by 6 months of age. Other physiologic consequences of truncus arteriosus relate to the

Table 83-1 Van Praagh Classification of Truncus Arteriosus

1. Partially formed aorticopulmonary septum (main pulmonary artery segment present)
2. Absent aorticopulmonary septum (no main pulmonary artery segment)
3. Absence of one branch of the pulmonary artery from the trunk (ductal or aortic origin of one pulmonary artery)
4. Hypoplastic or interrupted aortic arch with a large patent ductus arteriosus

Type A: Ventricular septal defect present
Type B: Ventricular septal defect absent

presence or absence of truncal valve stenosis or insufficiency. Although major truncal valve stenosis is rare, truncal valve insufficiency occurs in a significant proportion of children with this condition. The presence of significant truncal valve insufficiency not only complicates the operative repair of the lesion, but also may have a significant impact on morbidity and mortality after complete repair.

The presence of interrupted aortic arch in association with truncus arteriosus results in cardiovascular instability early after birth. Maintenance of ductal patency by prostaglandin E_1 infusion is critical to provide distal perfusion to the body in this condition but is associated with progressive pulmonary overcirculation, which is not dissimilar to the situation seen in hypoplastic left heart syndrome.

Diagnosis and Indications for Surgical Intervention

The diagnosis of truncus arteriosus can generally be made with accuracy from echocardiograms. Cardiac catheterization is indicated only when the patient presents late after birth and the issue of pulmonary vascular resistance is raised. Some children may have significant pulmonary arterial stenosis, which permits control of congestive heart failure early in life, and catheterization to define the level and degree of obstruction may be beneficial. In addition, abnormalities of coronary arteries and the severity of truncal valve abnormalities may occasionally prompt catheterization for greater characterization of the defects.

We have generally considered the presence of truncus arteriosus an indication for

operation in a relatively urgent fashion. Because hemodynamics may be quite unstable in children with unrestricted pulmonary blood flow and because we have seen patients deteriorate rapidly while awaiting surgical intervention, we have elected to repair truncus arteriosus promptly after the diagnosis is made. This policy reflects the clear advantages of neonatal repair of truncus arteriosus. Review of series of truncus repairs reflects the trend toward earlier intervention. Whereas the first repairs of truncus arteriosus were performed in 1962 by Behrendt and associates, in 1967 McGoon first used a valved allograft for the repair. This operation was a refinement of the procedure described by Rastelli at the Mayo Clinic. The results of early repairs were quite poor, however, because of the development of pulmonary vascular obstructive disease. In most of these early repairs, the operation was undertaken after the patient reached 6 months of age, when pulmonary vascular resistance was already significantly elevated. In 1984, Ebert reported a series of 100 infants who underwent complete repair of truncus arteriosus at 6 months of age with an 11% mortality. This landmark report em-

phasized the improved results in early intervention in children with this lesion. In our experience, repair of truncus arteriosus has gradually improved as surgical techniques have evolved such that operative survivals of >95% are anticipated with neonatal repair in patients without associated valvar lesions. The late results of truncus arteriosus have been favorable, with little late mortality despite the need for reoperation to replace right ventricular outflow tract conduits.

Surgical Techniques

Repair of Truncus Arteriosus

The heart is exposed with a median sternotomy incision. The presence of thymic tissue is confirmed because many of these children have athymia associated with DiGeorge syndrome. The clear presence of thymic tissue therefore may have implications for later management and prognosis. The heart is suspended in a pericardial cradle and the great vessels examined. If the patient is severely overcirculated with congestive heart failure, it may be advisable

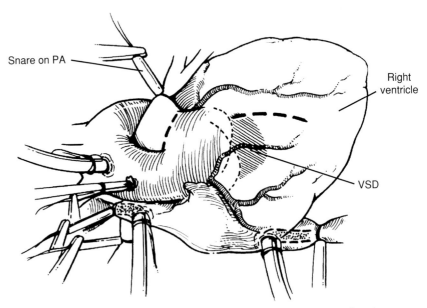

Figure 83-1. Repair of simple truncus arteriosus. The infant is placed on cardiopulmonary bypass with either bicaval cannulation or single venous cannulation in the right atrium for circulatory arrest. The aorta is cannulated as distally as possible to allow cross-clamping proximal to the aortic cannulation site for division of the pulmonary arteries from the truncal vessel. Snares are placed on the right and left pulmonary arteries to prevent pulmonary overcirculation during warming and to allow delivery of cardioplegic solution to the myocardium. After cardioplegia is achieved, the snares are released from the pulmonary arteries and the pulmonary bifurcation is excised from the back of the truncal artery, with care being taken to avoid the origin of the left coronary artery posteriorly, which can originate very close to the pulmonary bifurcation. An incision is made in the right ventricle, with care being taken to avoid major epicardial coronary branches and the base of the truncal valve. (PA = pulmonary artery; VSD = ventricular septal defect.)

to promptly encircle one of the pulmonary arteries with a snare to limit the total pulmonary blood flow. On occasion this can stabilize the patient while dissection is performed around the arch vessels.

The operation can be performed either with the patient on continuous cardiopulmonary bypass or by utilizing circulatory arrest. We have elected to use both of these techniques, and in simple truncus arteriosus, the complete operative repair can be performed during a single period of circulatory arrest of <40 minutes in most cases. The right and left pulmonary arteries are mobilized and encircled with tourniquets for control and the origins of the pulmonary arteries examined. In addition, on opening the pericardium, it is important to determine the location of the anterior descending coronary artery and confirm that it does not cross the right ventricular wall in the area of anticipated ventriculotomy. Heparin is administered and the aorta cannulated as distally as possible. Distal cannulation is particularly important because the pulmonary bifurcation may come off relatively distally and there is little room for cross-clamping of the aorta between the anticipated division of the pulmonary bifurcation and the distal aorta. Either the venae cavae are cannulated if continuous bypass is used, or a single right atrial cannula is used with circulatory arrest. If mobilization of the pulmonary artery confluence behind the aorta is considered to be too close to the anticipated cross-clamp application site, the brachiocephalic vessels are encircled with tourniquets and circulatory arrest is used, with clamping of the aorta more distally on the arch during the reconstruction of the back of the truncus arteriosus after excision of the pulmonary bifurcation. The infant is placed on cardiopulmonary bypass and the snares on the right and left pulmonary arteries tightened as shown in Fig. 83-1 to prevent pulmonary overcirculation during cooling. The child is cooled to 18°C for circulatory arrest or 34°C to 37°C for continuous bypass repair. In the presence of significant truncal valve insufficiency, venting of the left ventricle is important during cooling and may be accomplished by placing a vent through the right superior pulmonary vein across the mitral valve into the ventricle, or if truncal insufficiency is severe, by compressing the heart to maintain emptying of the ventricle during cooling.

The aorta is then cross-clamped and cardioplegic solution administered into the truncal root with the pulmonary artery snares applied to force the cardioplegic solution into the coronary arteries. Alternatively,

cardioplegia can be induced in a retrograde manner or the aorta opened and the coronaries directly cannulated. After cardioplegia is achieved, the snares are removed from the pulmonary arteries, and an incision is made near the take-off of the pulmonary bifurcation anteriorly. Through this initial incision, the truncal valve is examined and the origin of the left coronary artery carefully identified. The left coronary can arise high from above the truncal sinuses and be intimately associated with the origin of the pulmonary bifurcation. Once the coronary arteries are identified, the pulmonary bifurcation is excised from the back of the truncus arteriosus. The aorta is then repaired using a patch of pulmonary homograft. Primary suture closure of the defect in the truncus may be used; however, we believe that placement of a patch allows for less tension on the anastomosis and therefore a decreased risk of bleeding from behind the aorta. This is important after the right ventricular reconstruction has been performed because exposure of the back of the aorta is difficult after the completion of the repair. In addition, suturing bleeding sites in this area may be hazardous because the origin of the left coronary artery may be very close to the

margins of the excision of the pulmonary bifurcation. Although pericardium can also be used for a patch, we have elected to use a portion of the pulmonary or aortic homograft that will be used for right ventricular outflow tract reconstruction because it results in a hemostatic suture line and is easier to work with than nontanned pericardium.

After the repair of the truncus arteriosus is complete and the pulmonary bifurcation is mobilized to bring the bifurcation to the left for reconstruction, additional cardioplegic solution is injected into the aortic root to test the suture line of the truncal patch, and additional sutures are placed if necessary. Next, an incision is made in the right ventricle, avoiding major conal branches of the coronary arteries. This incision is made at the base of the truncal valve, and care must be taken not to carry the incision too far superiorly into the truncal valve annulus. The absence of infundibular septum in this area results in the possibility of damage to the truncal valve if the incision is started too far superiorly. The orientation of the incision is made so that the take-off of the conduit from the right ventricle will be directed toward the pulmonary bifurcation. As shown in Fig. 83-2, the ventricular septal

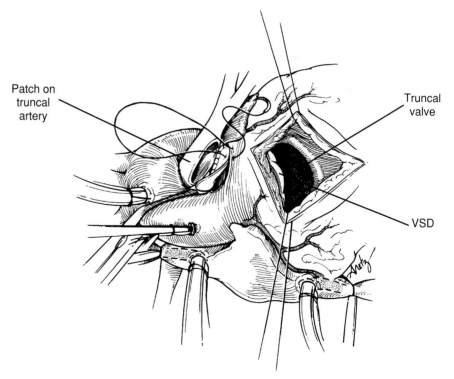

Patch on truncal artery

Truncal valve

VSD

Figure 83-2.   The defect in the main trunk from excision of the pulmonary bifurcation is closed with a patch of pulmonary homograft material or pericardium with meticulous suture technique to ensure hemostasis. Cardioplegic solution is then administered to observe any leaking of the suture line because the area will be difficult to expose after complete repair. The ventricular septal defect (VSD) is exposed through the ventriculotomy incision. There is no muscle rim typically present at the superior margin of the VSD, and therefore the patch is secured to the epicardial portion of the ventriculotomy incision superiorly.

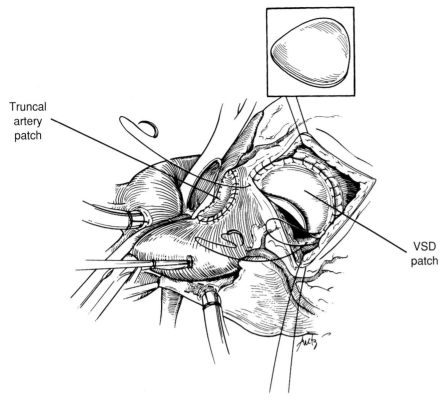

Figure 83-3.   The ventricular septal defect (VSD) is closed with an ovoid patch of polyethylene terephthalate (Dacron) material sewn to the superior margin of the ventriculotomy incision **(inset)**. Typically, a rim of muscle is present inferiorly between the ventricular septal defect and the tricuspid valve septal leaflet, and in these patients a running suture line can be created that avoids the conduction tissue. If the muscle bridge is not present, the inferior margin of the suture line is carried along the base of the septal tricuspid valve leaflet on the right ventricular aspect to avoid the conducting tissue.

defect is exposed through the incision in the right ventricle. The defect is closed with a patch of polyester (Dacron) material using a running technique. Superiorly, the absence of the infundibular septum mandates that the patch be more ovoid in shape, and the patch is secured to the epicardial margin of the ventriculotomy incision superiorly to avoid interference with the truncal valve (Fig. 83-3). In the majority of cases, there is a bridge of muscle between the margin of the ventricular septal defect and the tricuspid valve septal leaflet, and in these patients, suturing in this area can be performed without risk to the conduction tissue. In a minority of cases, there is absence of this muscle tissue, and suturing of the ventricular septal patch to the base of the septal leaflet of the tricuspid valve is necessary to avoid interference with the conduction pathway.

After closure of the ventricular septal defect is complete, the right ventricular outflow tract is reconstructed using a pulmonary or aortic homograft. To allow for the maximum possible growth of the infant before conduit change is necessary, we have

elected to use the largest possible pulmonary homograft that will fit in the chest of the newborn. Typically, this means a homograft of 14 mm to 18 mm. This size is significantly greater than the normal pulmonary valve size for an infant and allows growth to 3 to 4 years of age or greater before the first conduit change.

Occasionally an aortic homograft is a better choice than a pulmonary homograft due to the curved nature of the ascending aorta of the aortic homograft that can be positioned to the left, curving around the enlarged truncal root in patients in whom the truncus is particularly enlarged. The anterior mitral leaflet of the aortic homograft then can create a gusset, creating a gentle take-off from the right ventricular incision. Although pulmonary homografts are preferable due to the ability to dilate and a decreased amount of calcification, it is important not to oversize the pulmonary homograft because even though it is desirable to have a larger homograft to allow for future growth and decrease the need for reoperation early, the capacitance of a large pulmonary homograft may

equal the stroke volume of the right ventricle and limit forward cardiac output in patients when there is severe oversizing of the homograft conduit. The conduit in such cases acts like an aneurysm of the right ventricle, decreasing overall right ventricular performance. To accommodate such a large homograft, the pulmonary bifurcation is incised, with the incision slightly into the origin of the right pulmonary artery but more into the left pulmonary artery so that the conduit will lie toward the left. An anastomosis is then created between the homograft and the pulmonary bifurcation with running monofilament suture (Fig. 83-4). We have elected to use pulmonary homografts in most patients when available because use of aortic homografts has been associated with calcification

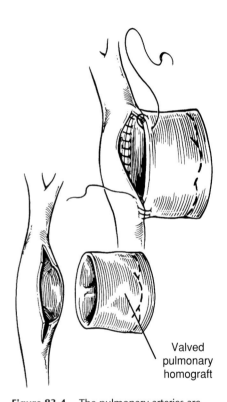

Figure 83-4.   The pulmonary arteries are reconstructed with a pulmonary homograft. To prevent kinking of the homograft with distention, it is trimmed 2 mm to 3 mm distal to the commissural attachments of the pulmonary valve. To provide an adequate anastomosis and size match to the pulmonary bifurcation using a large pulmonary homograft of 12 mm to 18 mm in diameter, an incision is carried into the origin of the right pulmonary artery for a short distance and more significantly into the left pulmonary artery if additional opening is necessary. An anastomosis is then created with a running fine monofilament suture between the pulmonary homograft and the pulmonary bifurcation.

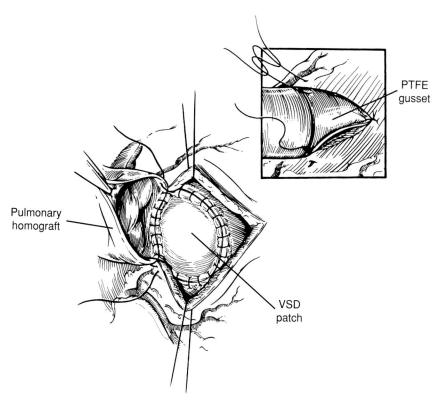

Figure 83-5. The pulmonary homograft is then sewn proximally to the superior aspect of the ventriculotomy incision for approximately one third of its circumference. As noted in the text, if adequate muscle is present on the pulmonary homograft, it can be sewn directly down to the right ventricular outflow tract. However, if inadequate tissue is present, the outflow tract is augmented with a gusset of polytetrafluoroethylene (PTFE) material, as shown in the inset, to create a gentle take-off of the homograft from the right ventricular outflow tract to avoid compression. (VSD = ventricular septal defect.)

of the aortic wall and early conduit stenosis. The pulmonary homograft appears to calcify less readily and to maintain its pliability. As noted in Fig. 83-5, the pulmonary homograft is then anastomosed to the superior margin of the ventricular incision to which the ventricular septal defect patch has been sewn. Approximately one third of the circumference of the ventriculotomy incision is sutured in this fashion. In some cases, the pulmonary homograft will have an adequate amount of right ventricular muscle attached so that it can be trimmed to allow a very small margin of muscle at the suture line to the ventricle but with an adequate amount of muscle remaining anteriorly to create a complete reconstruction without augmentation. In this case, the suture line is continued around the margins of the ventricular incision until the homograft is completely sewn to the right ventricular outflow tract. Care must be taken to trim the homograft appropriately so that it is not compressed as it originates from the right ventricle and also so that the length of the homograft is not excessive, which can result in kinking of the

posterior wall of the homograft and right ventricular outflow tract obstruction.

Typically in a neonate or infant, division of the pulmonary homograft just above the level of the commissural attachments of the

valve results in sufficient length to prevent kinking after completion of the reconstruction. If insufficient right ventricular muscle is available on the pulmonary homograft for a direct anastomosis, a gusset of polytetrafluoroethylene (PTFE) material is used to augment the take-off of the homograft from the right ventricle to prevent compression of its origin as noted in the inset of Fig. 83-5. Whereas pericardium may be used for this gusset, we use PTFE because we have seen aneurysm formation of nonpreserved pericardium when it is used in this position if there is distal stenosis of the homograft or the pulmonary arterial anastomosis.

After the repair is completed, the atrial septum is examined, working either through an atrial purse string or direct atrial incision. In a significant proportion of patients, a secundum-type atrial septal defect is present, and this is closed partially as noted in Fig. 83-6 to allow the capacity for right-to-left shunting at the atrial level if right ventricular dysfunction occurs in the early postoperative period. If a foramen ovale is present without a significant defect, the foramen is left open to permit decompression of the right atrium.

After completion of the repair, the patient is rewarmed and weaned from cardiopulmonary bypass. We have used modified ultrafiltration in our recent series of infants to decrease myocardial edema and improve early postoperative hemodynamics. Because large pulmonary homografts are used for construction of the outflow tract, occasionally the homograft conduit may appear to be compressed by the sternum during closure, and in these cases, opening the left pleural space widely either anterior or posterior to the phrenic nerve may permit rotation of the

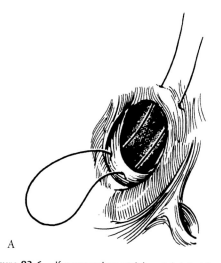

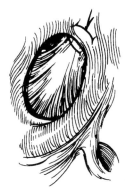

Figure 83-6. If a secundum atrial septal defect is present **(A)**, a partial closure is accomplished **(B)** to allow for the capacity for right-to-left shunting at the atrial level if ventricular dysfunction occurs postoperatively.

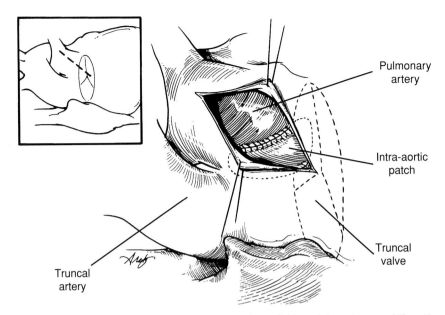

Figure 83-7. Truncal repair can be accomplished without division of the pulmonary bifurcation by incising the truncus anteriorly toward the pulmonary bifurcation **(inset)** and patching the origin of the pulmonary arteries from the inside of the truncus using a piece of pulmonary homograft or autologous pericardium. Care must be taken to avoid suturing near the origin of the left coronary artery and to avoid obstruction to outflow from the truncal valve. Again, meticulous suture technique is imperative to prevent leakage of this patch and resultant left-to-right shunt into the pulmonary artery after complete repair. In addition, the patch cannot be made too redundant or it will bow into the main pulmonary artery, potentially compromising the right ventricular outflow reconstruction. The pulmonary outflow tract is then reconstructed with a conduit or by alternative techniques.

conduit into the left pleural space and allow the chest to be closed without compression.

Alternative Repairs of Truncus Arteriosus

Several variations on repair of truncus arteriosus have been described, primarily to avoid the need for an allograft conduit from the right ventricle to the pulmonary arteries, which will commit most children to eventual conduit replacement. We have used conduit reconstruction in the majority of infants because the early morbidity and mortality after truncus arteriosus repair are commonly related to the occurrence of pulmonary vascular hypertensive crises and right ventricular dysfunction, and in this setting the absence of a truncal valve exacerbates the hemodynamic instability. The presence of a competent valve in the right ventricular outflow tract seems to minimize the early hemodynamic instability in these patients, and replacement of the right ventricular outflow allograft is associated with a low morbidity and mortality.

In the interest of completeness, several alternative techniques are described here. The first alternative repair involves incision

of the truncus arteriosus above the semilunar valve on the pulmonary arterial side of the common trunk (Fig. 83-7). Working through this incision, the surgeon can patch the origin of the pulmonary bifurcation from the arterial trunk with a piece of homologous pericardium or homograft material, with care being taken to avoid interference with the coronary ostium of the left coronary artery and allowing unobstructed flow from the truncal valve to the ascending aorta. An advantage of this technique is the lack of external bleeding with this suture line, which can be troublesome after patching of this area after division of the pulmonary bifurcation. A potential disadvantage, however, is that any dehiscence of this suture line will result in a significant left-to-right shunt. If this type of repair is performed, an incision is made in the right ventricle, and the ventricular septal defect is closed. The pulmonary bifurcation is then mobilized freely and either brought anterior to the ascending aorta or mobilized sufficiently to allow direct anastomosis to the superior margin of the right ventriculotomy. In situations in which the pulmonary bifurcation cannot be anastomosed directly to the right ventriculotomy without compres-

sion of the pulmonary bifurcation by the ascending aorta or if an anomalous anterior descending coronary artery crosses the outflow tract, it is possible to create a floor for the outflow tract reconstruction by use of autologous tissue, such as the left atrial appendage. In Fig. 83-8, the left atrial appendage is opened, creating a flap of tissue that is then brought over the outflow tract and secured to the superior margin of the ventricular incision and the pulmonary bifurcation. The base of the atrial appendage is oversewn. This creates an autologous connection between the right ventricle and pulmonary bifurcation that has the potential for growth. The outflow tract is then augmented by an anteriorly placed patch of homologous pericardium or pulmonary homograft material. In this fashion, a valveless connection is created between the right ventricle and the pulmonary bifurcation.

Another alternative is the use of a monocusp reconstruction of the right ventricular outflow tract, which has the potential advantage of early pulmonary valve competence during the initial period of hemodynamic instability postoperatively and the potential for later growth to decrease the need for conduit reconstruction later in life. In this technique (Fig. 83-9), a piece of homologous pericardium is used to create a single cusp, which is sewn to the wall of an outflow patch of pulmonary homograft, homologous pericardium, or PTFE material. This pericardial monocusp is created in a generous fashion to allow it to close against the right ventricle (Fig. 83-10). The posterior floor of the reconstruction is performed as noted in Fig. 83-8; however, the anterior reconstruction is completed with this monocusp outflow patch. The monocusp valve appears to function adequately for as long as several months and may decrease the incidence of late conduit changes, but it is more difficult to accomplish without at least some early postoperative pulmonary insufficiency.

Repair of Truncus Arteriosus with Interrupted Aortic Arch

When interrupted aortic arch is associated with truncus arteriosus, the operation is performed with the patient under circulatory arrest. Because of the instability of these infants, surgery in the first week of life is typical. After mobilization and snaring of the pulmonary arteries to prevent pulmonary overcirculation on bypass, cannulation of the main trunk and the right atrial appendage is performed. Because perfusion of both the brachiocephalic vessels and the distal aorta across the ductus arteriosus will

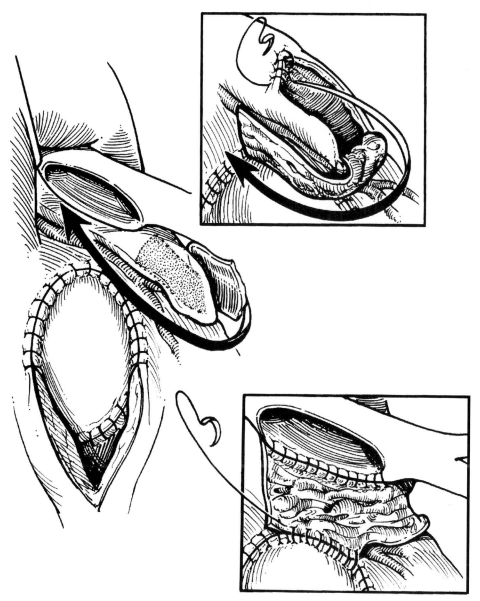

Figure 83-8. In situations in which a pulmonary homograft is not used for outflow reconstruction, autologous tissue may be used. In this alternative technique, the left atrial appendage is incised at its base and a flap of atrial appendage anastomosed to the pulmonary bifurcation superiorly and to the ventriculotomy incision inferiorly to bridge the ventriculotomy incision and the pulmonary bifurcation with autologous tissue. The base of the atrial appendage is then oversewn. It is important if this technique is used to open the atrial appendage to create a long bridge of tissue. Use of the unopened atrial appendage has been suggested; however, in our experience, sufficient tension may be present on this atrial appendage that with cardiac distention and contraction of the atrium the bridge of tissue may compress the left coronary artery and cause myocardial ischemia. The repair is then completed with augmentation of the autologous floor of the outflow tract reconstruction with an anteriorly positioned patch of pericardium or homograft material.

be accomplished by a single cannulation, the arterial cannulation can be placed proximally in the main portion of the truncal vessel. Snares also are placed on the brachiocephalic vessels originating from the ascending aorta. The infant is placed on bypass and cooled to a nasopharyngeal temperature of 18°C while snares on the right and left pulmonary arteries prevent pulmonary

overcirculation and distal perfusion is provided across the ductus arteriosus. During cooling, the descending aorta and left subclavian artery may be mobilized and a snare placed on the left subclavian artery if necessary. In some cases, aberrant origin of the right subclavian artery is present in this condition. In these cases, it may be necessary to divide the right subclavian artery to gain

adequate mobilization for repair, as in repair of interrupted aortic arch. Although several techniques are available for reconstruction of the aortic arch, we prefer to use a technique in which the arch is augmented with pulmonary homograft material to prevent tension on the anastomosis. After circulatory arrest is established and cardioplegia induced, which can be

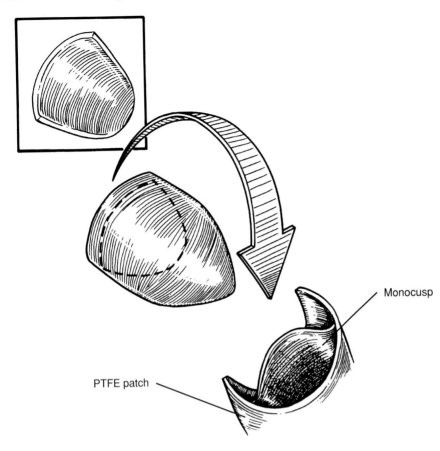

Figure 83-9. An additional variation of outflow reconstruction uses a monocusp of homologous pericardium positioned in a polytetrafluoroethylene (PTFE) or homograft outflow patch, which can provide temporary pulmonary competence in the early postoperative period. We have elected to create a generous cusp of autologous pericardium and secure it to the undersurface of a PTFE patch fashioned to the size of the outflow tract and then suture the PTFE reconstruction with the monocusp already in place. An alternative technique involves sewing a patch of pericardium that contacts the ventricular septum to the right ventricular incision and then placing an onlay PTFE patch over this area.

accomplished by snaring of the ductus arteriosus and the brachiocephalic vessels and infusion of cardioplegic solution through the aortic cannula in the proximal arterial trunk, the cannulae are removed from the heart. With the arch vessels snared, an incision is made on the lateral aspect of the ascending aorta beyond the origins of the pulmonary arteries and then carried inferiorly and across the pulmonary bifurcation (Fig. 83-11). Ductal tissue is excised and the ductus ligated on the pulmonary arterial end. In this fashion, the pulmonary bifurcation is excised from the truncus. The pulmonary arteries are mobilized freely; then all ductal tissue is excised from the descending aorta and an incision made superiorly into the origin of the left subclavian artery. A side-to-side anastomosis is then created from the origin of the left carotid to the origin of the left subclavian artery, providing a

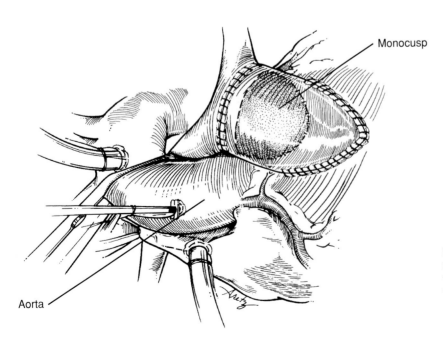

Figure 83-10. After reconstruction with a monocusp, the pericardial patch closes against the superior margin of the ventricular incision or the base of the autologous reconstruction of the right ventricular outflow tract and can limit pulmonary insufficiency

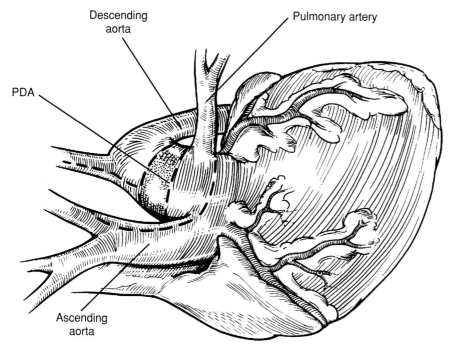

Descending aorta

PDA

Ascending aorta

Pulmonary artery

Figure 83-11.   Repair of interrupted aortic arch with truncus arteriosus. A vertical incision is made in the ascending aorta and brachiocephalic vessels onto the origin of the left carotid artery. This incision is placed medially and then carried transversely across the truncus to the base of the left pulmonary artery origin. The pulmonary bifurcation is then excised from the back of the truncus. The ductus arteriosus is ligated distal to the pulmonary bifurcation, and ductal tissue is excised from the descending aorta. An incision is then made vertically in the left subclavian artery and onto the descending aorta beyond any ductal tissue remnants. (PDA = patent ductus arteriosus.)

length of autologous tissue on the superior surface of the arch to allow for growth of the arch (Fig. 83-12). We perform this anastomosis with absorbable suture in hopes of encouraging growth. The ventriculotomy and closure of the ventricular septal defect are then performed in the usual fashion, and the arch of the aorta is reconstructed with a patch of pulmonary homograft to provide unobstructed flow through the arch of the aorta and to decrease tension on the anastomosis to decrease the risk of bleeding or distal coarctation (Fig. 83-13). The pulmonary artery reconstruction is then performed as in simple truncus arteriosus.

Repair of Truncus Arteriosus with Truncal Valve Repair or Replacement

Newborns who have significant truncal valve stenosis and insufficiency represent a higher-risk subset for neonatal repair. Fortunately, significant truncal valve stenosis is rare, and in only the most severe forms of truncal stenosis is valve replacement necessary at primary operation. Often the elimination of the large left-to-right shunt seen in these patients decreases the flow across

the truncal valve, and what appears to be a significant level of stenosis preoperatively may be acceptable after the ventricular septal defect is closed and the truncal repair has been completed. Thus, primary valve replacement for repair of truncus arteriosus should be extremely rare.

A more common situation is the presence of significant truncal valve insufficiency in association with unrepaired truncus arteriosus with or without interrupted aortic arch. Over the last several years an increasing experience has been reported of valve repair for truncal valve regurgitation at the initial repair of truncus arteriosus or as a secondary procedure. In patients in whom the truncal valve is quadricuspid and there is significant prolapse or abnormality of a single cusp, resection of the cusp and recreation of a trileaflet truncal valve may result in significant improvement in truncal valve insufficiency. In this repair, after division of the truncal root, an incision is made in the aortic wall immediately adjacent to the commissural attachment of the valve leaflet that is to be excised and the incision carried across the valve annulus obliquely. A second incision is made in the more anterior commissural attachment of this same valve cusp, and the cusp is excised with a portion of the truncal wall. Primary repair of the defect then results in a trileaflet valve, which may have less central insufficiency and a more normal distribution of forces

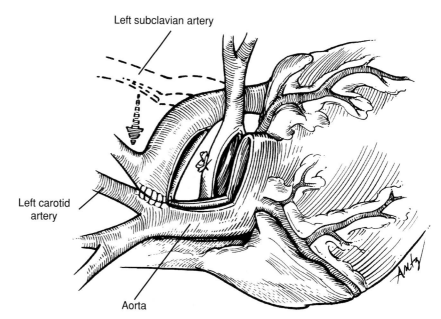

Left subclavian artery

Left carotid artery

Aorta

Figure 83-12.   The arch is reconstructed by direct anastomosis of the origins of the subclavian and carotid vessels with absorbable suture to create an autologous superior aspect to the arch reconstruction.

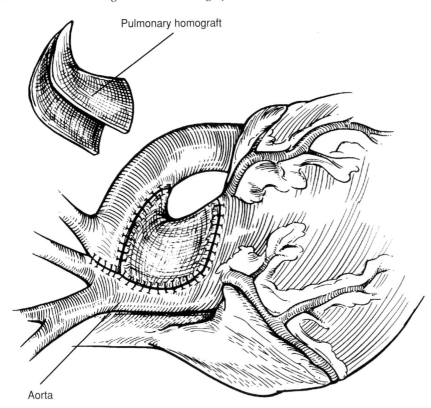

Pulmonary homograft

Aorta

Figure 83-13. A patch of pulmonary homograft material is then used to create arch augmentation beyond all ductal tissue to the proximal trunk. In this fashion, an unobstructed arch is created with the least amount of tension on the suture lines, which prevents compression of the pulmonary bifurcation from the descending aorta and decreases the risk of coarctation of the arch anastomosis.

on the valve sinuses, aiding closure of the valve centrally (Fig. 83-14A,B,C). In other cases, if the truncal valve leaflets are not obviously abnormal, or if there is an obvious area of truncal regurgitation at a commissural attachment, closure of the commissure between adjacent truncal valve leaflets may result in significant improvement in truncal insufficiency. In most cases, however, primary suturing of the valve commissures does not eliminate the truncal regurgitation, which is often centrally located. Thus, this type of repair should be used relatively infrequently (Fig. 83-14D).

Often the valve leaflet that needs to be excised in patients with truncal regurgitation and quadraleaflet truncal valve is the leaflet adjacent to the left coronary ostium. In these cases, excision of the leaflet can be performed as described in Fig. 83-14E,F. However, the left coronary artery needs to be mobilized with a button on the aortic wall prior to excision of the valve leaflet and then reimplanted into a suitable site in the truncal root as is often performed with the arterial switch procedure. With these techniques any of the leaflets of the truncal valve can be excised, although excision of leaflets adjacent to the conduction tissue in the anterolateral aspect of the aorta can be associated with the development of heart block, and therefore, it is preferable to excise noncoronary leaflets or left-sided leaflets if possible.

In the situation of truncus repair with truncal valve replacement, the operation is typically performed with the patient on continuous cardiopulmonary bypass with intermittent circulatory arrest. Bicaval cannulation is used and the aortic cannulation performed as distally as possible. The left heart is vented through the right superior pulmonary vein across the mitral valve to maintain decompression during cooling and rewarming. The aorta is clamped and cardioplegic solution administered directly into the truncal root if there is only modest truncal insufficiency or directly into the coronary arteries after the truncal vessel is opened if severe insufficiency is present. Alternatively, cardioplegia can be induced in a retrograde manner. In our experience, however, direct cannulation of the coronary ostia is possible in even very small neonates, permitting adequate distribution of cardioplegic solution. The truncus is divided transversely at the level of the take-off of the pulmonary bifurcation and the bifurcation mobilized freely. An incision is then made vertically across the truncal valve annulus into the right ventricle, widely opening the right ventricular outflow tract (Fig. 83-15). The right and left coronary ostia are mobilized with a button of aortic wall for anastomosis to the reconstruction. The truncal valve is then excised as in Fig. 83-16. The ventricular septal defect is readily apparent. Although early in our ex-

perience we used aortic allografts for valve replacement and used the anterior mitral leaflet of the allograft valve for closure of the ventricular septal defect, we have more recently elected to use pulmonary allografts in the hope of decreasing the calcification of the allograft wall, allowing greater pliability of the allograft and decreasing the risk of allograft valve stenosis and insufficiency. When a pulmonary allograft is used, the proximal anastomosis of the allograft is performed to the annulus of the truncal valve posteriorly. This suture line is created for approximately one half to two thirds of the circumference of the truncal valve annulus (Fig. 83-17). The ventricular septal defect is then closed with a patch of Dacron or PTFE material, baffling the left ventricular flow to the pulmonary allograft valve. Thus, the superior margin of the ventricular septal defect patch is sewn to the base of the pulmonary valve allograft anteriorly, reconstructing the left ventricular outflow tract. At suitable sites on the pulmonary allograft, buttons of tissue are excised and the coronary arteries reimplanted as for the arterial switch operation for transposition of the great arteries (see Chapter 79). The distal anastomosis of the pulmonary allograft to the ascending aorta is then completed. At this point, additional cardioplegic solution is injected into the aortic root to ensure that the suture lines are hemostatic and that no insufficiency of the allograft valve is present.

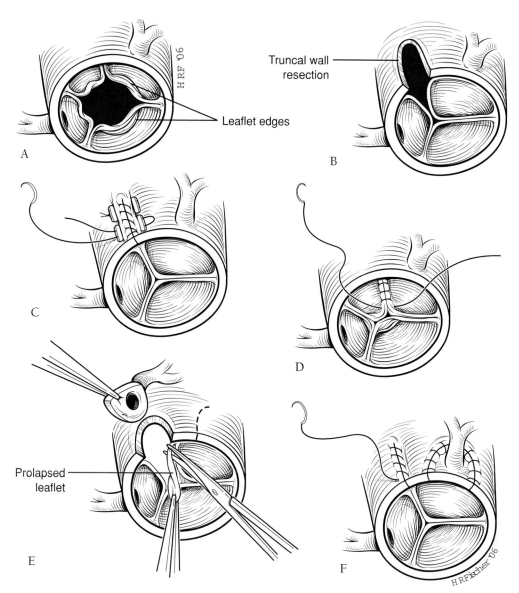

Figure 83-14. Repair of truncal valve insufficiency. **(A)** The truncus is transected, and the leaflet to be excised is identified. Typically, a quadricuspid valve is present, and there may be a significant prolapse of one leaflet. An incision is made adjacent to the commissural attachment of the leaflet to be excised and is carried down across the truncal valve annulus obliquely. **(B)** A second incision is made anteriorly in a similar fashion, and the valve leaflet along with a 1-mm to 2-mm section of the valve annulus is excised. **(C)** Primary closure of the valve annulus and the aortic wall then results in coaptation of the commissural attachments of the remaining truncal leaflets and decreases the magnitude of central insufficiency, improving the central coaptation between the remaining truncal valve leaflets. **(D)** In patients with truncal insufficiency in whom there is prolapse or dysplasia of a truncal valve leaflet resulting in localized regurgitation, closure of the commissural attachments between valve leaflets may be effective. The truncus is divided, and the truncal valve is examined from above. If areas of deficiency between valve leaflets at the commissures are identified, the commissure can be closed with interrupted or running sutures of monofilament PTFE material. We prefer PTFE suture, which seems to cut through the very delicate valve leaflet tissues less than other types of suture material. **(E)** In patients in whom the valve leaflet to be excised is associated with an adjacent coronary ostium, mobilization of the coronary ostium with excision of a button of aortic wall allows the valve leaflet and annulus to be excised as in panel B, permitting primary reconstruction of a trileaflet valve. **(F)** The coronary button can then be reimplanted at a suitable site on the aortic wall either to a punch opening or to a medially based flap incision in the aortic wall.

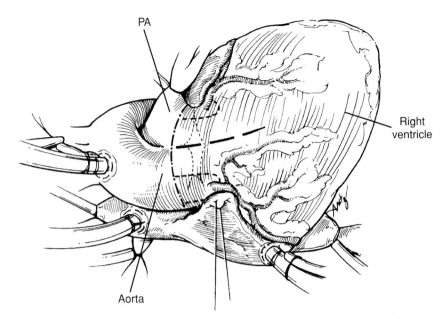

Figure 83-15. Repair of truncus arteriosus with truncal valve replacement. After circulatory arrest or with continuous bypass, the aorta is cross-clamped and cardioplegic solution injected into the truncal root. The pulmonary arteries are snared to allow flow of cardioplegic solution into the coronary arteries if possible. If truncal insufficiency is severe, the truncus is opened superiorly as noted in this diagram and then cardioplegic solution injected into the left and right coronary ostia under direct vision. The right and left coronary ostia are excised with a button of aortic wall, and a vertical incision is made down across the truncal valve annulus into the right ventricle. (PA = pulmonary artery.)

The right ventricular reconstruction is then performed (Fig. 83-18), with an allograft valve from the right ventricular incision to the pulmonary bifurcation augmented with a gusset of PTFE material if necessary or by one of the other alternative techniques described previously. If truncal valve replacement is required later after initial repair, it is performed as in homograft root replacement (see Chapter 92).

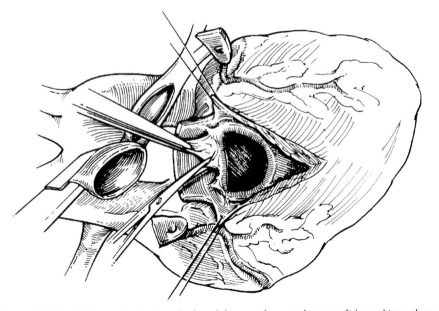

Figure 83-16. The truncal valve is excised, and then a pulmonary homograft is used to replace the truncal valve sewn to the truncal valve annulus over the posterior one half to two thirds of its circumference.

Postoperative Care

The management of infants after repair of truncus arteriosus is primarily directed at minimizing pulmonary vascular resistance and right heart dysfunction. Sedation and occasionally paralysis with hyperventilation are standards of postoperative management. Low-dose inotropic support with phospho-diesterase inhibitors may be necessary to improve right ventricular function in the early postoperative period. With these techniques, pulmonary hypertensive crises and acute right heart dysfunction have been relatively uncommon in our more recent series. However, significant right ventricular dysfunction or unmanageable pulmonary hypertension with low cardiac output may result in severe hemodynamic instability and on rare occasion has been successfully managed with extracorporeal membrane oxygenation support for several days.

Results

Although mortality rates for truncus arteriosus repair were as high as 60% to 70% until the early 1980s, the trend toward earlier repair and improvements in surgical and postoperative management techniques have resulted in a progressive improvement in the operative results such that survival rates of >95% are anticipated in simple truncus arteriosus. The association of severe truncal insufficiency or interrupted aortic arch is a relative risk factor for early mortality; however, good results have been achieved in these subsets of patients also. Patients who survive the perioperative interval have surprisingly good long-term results after repair of truncus arteriosus. Recent evaluation of the long-term results from San Francisco have shown a significant need for reoperation for conduit revision; however, the rates of late morbidity and mortality with this lesion are very low, and the long-term functional results are excellent.

Conclusion

Whereas truncus arteriosus has been associated with a very significant early and late mortality in the past, the repair of truncus arteriosus in the neonatal period has been associated with a progressive improvement in results. Although several innovative techniques of repair have been developed to obviate the need for use of allograft conduits for outflow tract reconstruction of the

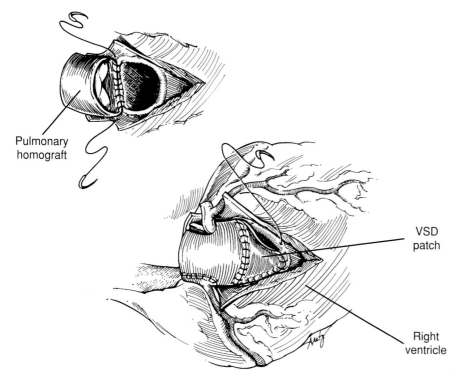

Figure 83-17. The anterior circumference of the pulmonary homograft is secured with a polytetrafluoroethylene (Gore-Tex) or a polyethylene terephthalate (Dacron) patch sewn to the margins of the ventricular septal defect (VSD) up to the pulmonary homograft, reconstructing the left ventricular outflow tract. The coronary ostia are then reimplanted into the pulmonary homograft in the usual fashion and the distal anastomosis to the ascending aorta created.

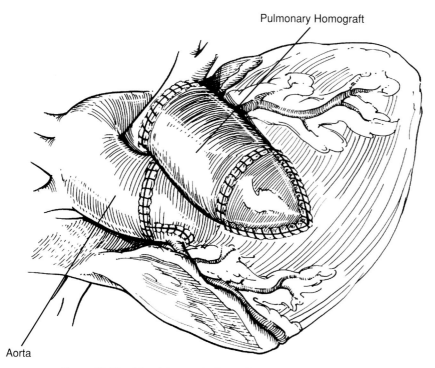

Figure 83-18. The right ventricular outflow tract is reconstructed.

right ventricle, we believe that the presence of a competent pulmonary valve early after repair leads to improved postoperative hemodynamic stability. The low morbidity and mortality from late conduit revision have supported this approach. Nevertheless, the use of an allograft conduit in a neonate will lead to a virtually certain need for operative reintervention for conduit change; therefore, use of autologous tissue in right ventricular outflow tract reconstruction has inherent appeal. Improvements in postoperative management of neonates after complex reconstructive surgery have resulted in significant improvement in the prognosis for children with truncus arteriosus complex, even those with significant additional abnormalities including truncal valve stenosis and regurgitation or interrupted aortic arch.

SUGGESTED READING

Barbero-Marcial M, Riso A, Atik E, et al. A technique for correction of truncus arteriosus type I and II without extracardiac conduits. J Thorac Cardiovasc Surg 1990;99:364.

Bove EL, Beekman RH, Snider AR, et al. Repair of truncus arteriosus in the neonate and young infant. Ann Thorac Surg 1989;47:499.

Ebert PA, Turley K, Stanger P, et al. Surgical treatment of truncus arteriosus in the first six months of life. Ann Surg 1984;200:451.

Rajasinghe HA, McElhinney DB, Reddy BM, et al. Long-term follow-up of truncus arteriosus repaired in infancy: a twenty year experience. J Thorac Cardiovasc Surg 1997;113:869.

Van Praagh S. The anatomy of common aorticopulmonary trunks (truncus arteriosus communis) and its embryonic implications. A study of 57 necropsy cases. Am J Cardiol 1965;16:406.

EDITOR'S COMMENTS

Dr. Spray has clearly described truncus arteriosus. He appropriately gives standard alternative approaches. We agree completely with his approach to using pulmonary homografts for this condition and use these whenever possible. They are prone to less calcification and often avoid early return to the operating room. The use of various interventional techniques has also increased the time period for reoperation to perform the first conduit change. There is now potential, at least, for only one conduit change in these infants with truncus arteriosus.

We have been interested in the best approach for treating the patient with truncal valve insufficiency. We almost never replace the truncal valve at the time of the initial operation. Dr. Spray states that merely closing the commissures often does not solve the problem. However, the use of transesophageal echocardiography can at least give the surgeon a physiologic approach to the truncal valve insufficiency. Although regurgitation is often central, prolapse does occur in most situations.

Correcting the valve prolapse can be helpful. Although this approach may not be permanent, it will allow for at least some temporizing to either avoid or to put off valve replacement in these children.

Finally, Dr. Spray states that it is important to consider reoperations in these patients. Appropriate placement of the pulmonary homograft out of the way of the previous sternotomy will allow for much easier re-entry without catastrophic results. Opening the left pleura and careful placement are critical for the overall long-term benefits to these children.

I.L.K.

84

Double-Outlet Ventricles

Kirk R. Kanter

Double-Outlet Right Ventricle

Definition

Double-outlet right ventricle (DORV) refers to a heterogeneous group of cardiac malformations characterized by an abnormal ventriculoarterial connection in which both great arteries are related to the right ventricle. Although the term *double-outlet right ventricle* can be correctly applied to hearts with atrioventricular discordance (e.g., congenitally corrected transposition of the great arteries) or to hearts with univentricular atrioventricular connections (e.g., double-inlet left ventricle), for simplicity of discussion, only hearts with atrioventricular concordance and two adequate ventricles are discussed in this chapter.

The definition of what constitutes a DORV has been the source of controversy. Although some have required the presence of bilateral infundibula or atrioventricular valve–semilunar valve discontinuity (most commonly mitral–aortic discontinuity), these criteria are not essential in establishing the diagnosis of DORV. From a surgical perspective, it is most useful to adopt the "50% rule" in defining DORV. With this rule, a heart is termed DORV if >50% of both great arteries arise from the right ventricle. Usually, all of one great artery and 50% or more of the other great artery arise from the right ventricle in DORV.

Classification

A ventricular septal defect (VSD) is almost always present with DORV. Based on the work of Lev and his colleagues, DORV is classified into four groups based on the relationship of the VSD to the great arteries (Table 84-1): subaortic, subpulmonary, doubly committed, and noncommitted (remote).

Subaortic Ventricular Septal Defect

DORV with subaortic VSD (Fig. 84-1A) is the most common group of DORV. It may or may not be associated with pulmonary stenosis. The presentation without pulmonary stenosis is similar to that of a child with a large VSD (heart failure). If there is pulmonary stenosis, it is usually infundibular, so the clinical presentation in this subgroup is similar to that of tetralogy of Fallot (cyanosis, hypercyanotic episodes). Accordingly, if a patient is not a candidate for complete repair at the time of presentation because of size, clinical condition, or other variables, a palliative procedure in DORV with subaortic VSD without pulmonary stenosis is pulmonary artery banding; in children with pulmonary stenosis, a systemic-to-pulmonary artery shunt is appropriate.

Subpulmonary Ventricular Septal Defect

DORV with subpulmonary VSD (the Taussig-Bing heart) is the second-most-common group of DORV (Fig. 84-1B). Because of the location of the VSD, oxygenated left ventricular blood preferentially streams through the VSD into the pulmonary artery and desaturated right ventricular blood streams into the aorta as in transposition of the great arteries with VSD. These children present with cyanosis and heart failure. Associated coarctation of the aorta occurs commonly. Because DORV with subpulmonary VSD is prone to early development of pulmonary vascular obstructive disease, intervention in infancy is usually

necessary. In addition to repair of the aortic coarctation, if present, balloon atrial septostomy is commonly needed to improve mixing of oxygenated blood at the atrial level as in transposition of the great arteries. Although palliation can be accomplished with pulmonary artery banding, it is preferable to proceed with complete repair in infancy.

Doubly Committed Ventricular Septal Defect

In DORV with doubly committed VSD, the VSD is immediately beneath both the pulmonary artery and the aorta (Fig. 84-1C). Usually, the infundibular septum is absent or hypoplastic. As in DORV with subaortic VSD, there may be associated pulmonary stenosis. Thus, clinical presentation and surgical approach would be similar to those for DORV with subaortic VSD with or without pulmonary stenosis.

Noncommitted Ventricular Septal Defect

In the final group of DORV, the VSD is committed neither to the aorta nor to the pulmonary artery (Fig. 84-1D). The remote location of the VSD may be in the inlet septum as with atrioventricular septal defects or a muscular VSD in the trabecular septum. Pulmonary stenosis may be present. The presentation and surgical palliation of DORV with noncommitted VSD are similar to those for DORV with subaortic VSD with or without pulmonary stenosis.

Surgical Techniques

The goal of surgical repair in DORV is to achieve a biventricular repair using the left

Table 84-1 Classification of Double-Outlet Right Ventricle		
VSD Relationship	**Pulmonary Stenosis**	**Clinical Mimicry**
Subaortic	Absent	VSD
Subaortic	Present	TOF
Subpulmonary	Absent	TGA/VSD
Doubly committed	Absent	VSD
Doubly committed	Present	TOF
Noncommitted	Absent	VSD
Noncommitted	Present	TOF

TGA = transposition of the great arteries; TOF = tetralogy of Fallot; VSD = ventricular septal defect.

ventricle as the systemic ventricle with unobstructed right and left ventricular outflow tracts. Usually this can be accomplished within the first 6 to 12 months of life, thus obviating the need for palliative procedures. If it is anticipated that the final repair will require an extracardiac valved conduit or a complicated intraventricular tunnel, it is reasonable to delay correction to allow for growth by palliating, if necessary, with a pulmonary artery band or a systemic-to-pulmonary artery shunt. In addition, in children who eventually will need a Fontan procedure, it is critical to protect the pulmonary vascular bed early on with appropriate palliation.

Roughly 10% of children with DORV have a restrictive VSD. By definition, this means that outflow from the left ventricle is obstructed, and therefore early repair with enlargement of the VSD is mandated because spontaneous closure of the VSD, rather than being curative as in isolated VSD, would be fatal in DORV. Pulmonary artery banding is certainly not appropriate in patients with DORV and a restrictive VSD.

Tunnel Repair of Double-Outlet Right Ventricle with Subaortic Ventricular Septal Defect without Pulmonary Stenosis

Repair of DORV with a subaortic VSD is accomplished by creating an intraventricular tunnel channeling left ventricular blood through the VSD to the aorta

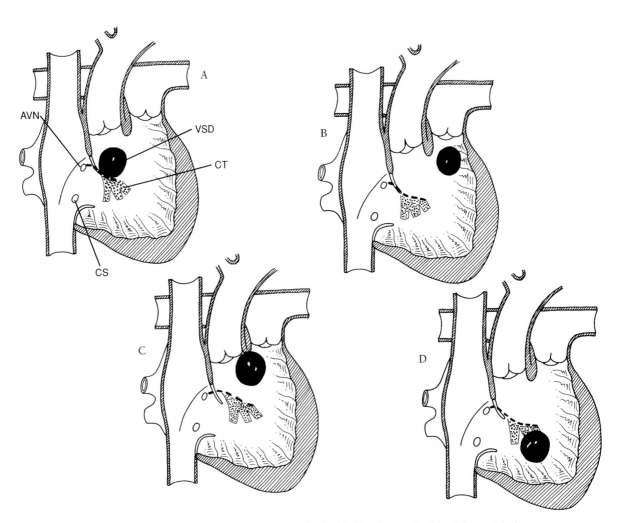

Figure 84-1. Types of double-outlet right ventricle classified by the relationship of the ventricular septal defect (VSD) to the great arteries. The locations of the atrioventricular node and conduction tissue are depicted. **(A)** Subaortic VSD. **(B)** Subpulmonary VSD. **(C)** Doubly committed VSD. **(D)** Noncommitted VSD. (AVN = atrioventricular node; CS = coronary sinus; CT = conduction tissue.)

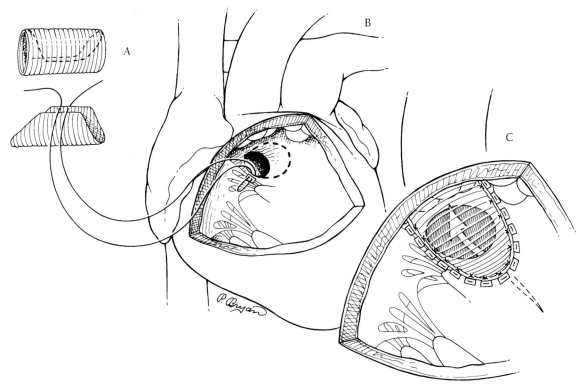

Figure 84-2. Intraventricular tunnel repair of double-outlet right ventricle with subaortic ventricular septal defect (VSD) without pulmonary stenosis. **(A)** A (polyester) Dacron or Hemashield tube graft the size of the aorta is opened longitudinally for use as the patch. Suturing is started through the midportion of the graft and the base of the anteroseptal commissure of the tricuspid valve. **(B)** The VSD is exposed through a right ventriculotomy. The safe area for enlargement of the VSD is shown with a dashed line. **(C)** The intraventricular tunnel is completed with pledgeted or continuous sutures. Care is taken to maintain orientation of the tube graft so that one end is at the anterior-inferior margin of the VSD and the other end is anterior to the aortic valve. The arrow indicates flow of blood from the left ventricle through the enlarged VSD and tunnel to the aorta.

(Fig. 84-2). This is facilitated by the use of a polyester (Dacron)- or collagen-impregnated polyester tube graft corresponding to the size of the aorta. This is opened longitudinally so that about two thirds of its circumference is available (Fig. 84-2A). The advantage of using a tube graft for the intraventricular tunnel is that the corrugations keep the required curve in the baffle to allow unobstructed left ventricular outflow. A flat Dacron or polytetrafluoroethylene (Gore-Tex) patch that one would use to close a simple VSD would be prone to kinking and would create obstruction unless the geometry and size of the patch were exactly perfect.

After routine establishment of cardiopulmonary bypass with bicaval cannulation and cardioplegic arrest, the intracardiac anatomy is carefully inspected through a right atriotomy. The VSD is visualized through the tricuspid valve and its relationship to the aorta is confirmed. If there is any suspicion preoperatively or intraoperatively that the VSD is

smaller than the aorta, it should be enlarged. This can be accomplished through the tricuspid valve or through the right ventricle with either a transverse or a longitudinal right ventriculotomy. The VSD is enlarged superiorly and anteriorly (Fig. 84-2B), thus resecting some of the infundibular septum. Enlarging the VSD posteriorly and superiorly through the ventriculoinfundibular fold runs the risk of going outside the heart. The conduction tissue runs inferiorly and of course should be avoided (Fig. 84-1A).

Once the VSD is enlarged (if necessary), the Dacron tube graft is oriented so that the longitudinal axis of the graft corresponds to an imaginary line from the anteriormost portion of the aorta to the anterior-inferior limit of the VSD (Fig. 84-2C). It is helpful to place the first suture through the base of the tricuspid valve leaflet at the anteroseptal commissure, then through the midportion of the tube graft (Fig. 84-2B). About one third of the VSD sutures are placed along

the posterior and inferior rim of the defect through the tricuspid valve, with care taken to avoid the conduction tissue, with several of these pledgeted sutures on the atrial side of the septal leaflet of the tricuspid valve. These sutures are passed through the Dacron tube graft, which is seated down and the sutures tied. The remainder of the circumference of the VSD is closed through the right ventriculotomy, with being care taken to maintain proper orientation of the patch (Fig. 84-2C). Anteriorly and superiorly, it may be advantageous to anchor some of the pledgeted sutures through the anterior wall of the right ventricle above the aortic valve, as is done in a Rastelli procedure. Rather than using interrupted pledgeted sutures, the VSD can be closed with a continuous suture technique completely through the right ventriculotomy.

If it appears that the intraventricular tunnel is bulging into the right ventricular outflow tract, the right ventriculotomy is closed with a patch of autologous pericardium to avoid right ventricular outflow tract obstruction.

Repair of Double-Outlet Right Ventricle with Subaortic Ventricular Septal Defect and Pulmonary Stenosis

In the group of patients with DORV with subaortic VSD and pulmonary stenosis, it is useful to mark the planned right ventriculotomy incision with stay sutures before cardioplegic arrest after carefully identifying the course of the epicardial coronary arteries (Fig. 84-3A). The intraventricular tunnel repair of the VSD is identical to that used for patients with DORV and subaortic VSD without pulmonary stenosis (Fig. 84-3B). If a major coronary artery crosses the right ventricular outflow tract, if the pulmonary vascular resistance is elevated, or if there is distal pulmonary arterial obstruction, a valved conduit should be used to establish right ventricle–pulmonary artery continuity. The pulmonary trunk is divided, with the proximal main pulmonary artery oversewn (Fig. 84-3B). The proximal portion of a valved homograft is sewn to the superior aspect of the right ventriculotomy. The homograft is trimmed to the proper length, and an end-to-end anastomosis between the distal homograft and the distal main pulmonary artery (or pulmonary bifurcation if the main pulmonary artery is small) is performed. Finally, the gap between the proximal right ventriculotomy and the proximal homograft is roofed with leftover homograft material or autologous pericardium (Fig. 84-3C). Alternatively, the native pulmonary trunk can be left intact and the distal homograft conduit sewn end to side to the junction of the native pulmonary trunk and pulmonary bifurcation, allowing blood flow through both the stenotic native pulmonary valve and the new conduit.

Sometimes it is possible to establish an adequate right ventricular outflow tract without a valved conduit as is done with

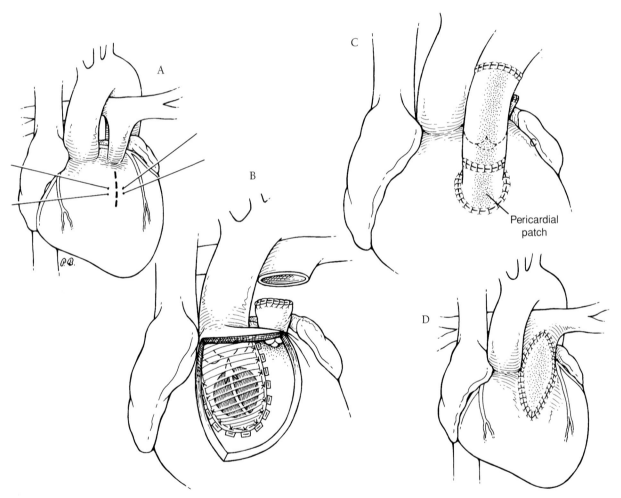

Figure 84-3. Repair of double-outlet right ventricle with subaortic ventricular septal defect and pulmonary stenosis. **(A)** The site of the proposed right ventriculotomy is shown by a dashed line. Marking sutures are placed before cardioplegic arrest to aid with retraction and to properly orient the ventricular incision. **(B)** An intraventricular tunnel is fashioned as in Fig. 84-2. The main pulmonary artery is divided and the cardiac end oversewn. **(C)** Right ventricle-to-pulmonary artery continuity is reestablished with a valved homograft conduit. About one half of the circumference of the proximal homograft is sutured to the superior aspect of the right ventriculotomy. A piece of pericardium or homograft material is used to roof the gap between the right ventricle and the homograft. **(D)** Alternatively, a nonvalved transannular right ventricular outflow tract patch can be used to relieve the pulmonary stenosis.

repair of tetralogy of Fallot. In this case, after division of obstructing right ventricular muscle bundles, a transannular outflow tract patch is created using autologous pericardium (Fig. 84-3D). If the pulmonary valve annulus is of good size, a non-transannular patch is adequate after a pulmonary valvotomy is performed. Otherwise, a transannular patch is necessary.

Sakamoto and colleagues described an interesting transaortic approach for enlarging the VSD and tunneling left ventricular outflow through the VSD to the aorta in two patients with DORV with subaortic VSD and pulmonary stenosis.

Anatomic Repair of Double-Outlet Right Ventricle with Subpulmonary Ventricular Septal Defect

The preferred surgical repair of DORV with subpulmonary VSD (the Taussig-Bing heart) is anatomic repair (the arterial switch operation). Because coarctation of the aorta is commonly seen in this group, these patients may have had prior coarctation repair with a pulmonary artery band, although simultaneous repair of the coarctation at the time of anatomic repair is now the accepted standard.

The VSD is closed either through a right atriotomy or a right ventriculotomy channeling left ventricular blood into the pulmonary artery (Fig. 84-4A). The aorta is transected slightly higher than the pulmonary trunk (Fig. 84-4A). If present, the coarctation and associated aortic arch hypoplasia can be corrected at this time with a patch of homograft material using a brief period of profound hypothermia with circulatory arrest or regional low-flow perfusion.

Particularly with side-by-side great arterial relationships, the circumflex coronary artery often arises with the right coronary artery from the right posterior-facing sinus, whereas the anterior descending coronary artery originates from the left posterior-facing sinus. In this situation, the anterior descending coronary artery is excised as a button and transferred to a defect created in the left anterior-facing sinus of the proximal pulmonary trunk (neoaorta, Fig. 84-4B). The right and circumflex coronary ostium is excised as a large U-shaped button. It is transferred above the right anterior-facing sinus of the proximal pulmonary trunk (neoaorta) and incorporated into the suture line between the proximal pulmonary trunk (neoaorta) and the distal ascending aorta (Fig. 84-4B). Positioning this coronary button more superiorly as it is transferred to the

left avoids potential kinking of the circumflex coronary artery.

Reconstruction of the right ventricular outflow tract when the great arteries are side by side can cause compression of one of the coronary arteries or predispose to right ventricular outflow tract obstruction if performed exactly as one would with typical transposition of the great arteries because there is so much offset between the "old" proximal ascending aorta (neopulmonary artery) and the distal pulmonary trunk. This potential problem can be addressed by opening the right lateral aspect of the distal pulmonary trunk onto the undersurface of the right pulmonary artery (Fig. 84-4B) after performing the Lecompte maneuver (bringing the pulmonary bifurcation anterior to the distal ascending aorta). The U-shaped defect in the "old" proximal ascending aorta at the site of the right and circumflex coronary ostial button is repaired with a patch of autologous pericardium that is much wider distally. This increases the circumference of the proximal neopulmonary artery to accommodate for the typical size discrepancy between the smaller proximal aorta and the larger distal pulmonary trunk. This same patch is incorporated into the incision on the undersurface of the right pulmonary artery (Fig. 84-4C) to allow for a generous tension-free pulmonary arterial anastomosis and has the benefit of pulling the new pulmonary trunk to the right away from the right coronary artery. Both the old site of the anterior descending coronary artery button and the slight overhang on the left lateral aspect of the distal pulmonary trunk are closed with small pericardial patches. If the U-shaped patch filling the defect in the right posterior facing sinus is broad enough distally, it accomplishes the same effect as a pantaloon patch for repairing both coronary button defects and is somewhat easier to do.

Alternatively, with side-by-side arteries, pulmonary artery reconstruction can be performed using the same techniques outlined previously without incorporating the Lecompte maneuver (Fig. 84-4D). To do this, it is very important to transect the aorta higher than the pulmonary trunk at the beginning of the repair (Fig. 84-4A).

Intraventricular Repair of Double-Outlet Right Ventricle with Subpulmonary Ventricular Septal Defect

In patients with DORV and subpulmonary VSD with side-by-side great arteries, an intraventricular tunnel repair is feasible.

The subpulmonary VSD is exposed through a transverse right ventriculotomy (Fig. 84-5A). Often it is necessary to enlarge the VSD anteriorly and superiorly. The infundibular septum between the aorta and pulmonary artery is usually quite prominent and in fact can cause subaortic obstruction preoperatively. This is excised to provide an unimpeded channel from the left ventricle through the VSD to the aorta (Fig. 84-5B). Usual care must be taken to avoid injury to the conduction tissue (Fig. 84-1B). The intraventricular tunnel is now created using an opened Dacron or Hemashield tube graft as employed with DORV and subaortic VSD (Fig. 84-5C). Although the illustration in Fig. 84-5C depicts interrupted pledgeted sutures, a continuous suture technique can also be used.

If the relationship of the great arteries is more anteroposterior than side by side, there is inadequate distance between the tricuspid valve and the pulmonary valve. The intraventricular tunnel will obstruct the subpulmonary region. Therefore, patients with DORV and subpulmonary VSD with anteroposterior great arteries should not undergo an intraventricular tunnel repair; anatomic repair with closure of the VSD to the pulmonary artery and an arterial switch operation is preferable.

Damus-Kaye-Stansel Repair of Double-Outlet Right Ventricle with Subpulmonary Ventricular Septal Defect

There is a subset of patients with DORV and subpulmonary VSD who have significant subaortic stenosis that may not lend itself to adequately successful resection. This would preclude an arterial switch operation because postoperative right ventricular outflow tract obstruction would result. There is also a small number of patients with coronary artery anatomy that makes it too risky to perform an arterial switch operation depending on the experience of the individual surgeon (e.g., intramural coronary artery or single coronary artery), although these situations have become less common as techniques dealing with these more challenging coronary abnormalities have evolved. In these situations, an arterial switch operation without coronary translocation (Damus-Kaye-Stansel procedure) is a feasible alternative.

With the Damus-Kaye-Stansel procedure, the subpulmonary VSD is closed either through the right atrium or through a right ventriculotomy incision to direct left ventricular blood through the pulmonary

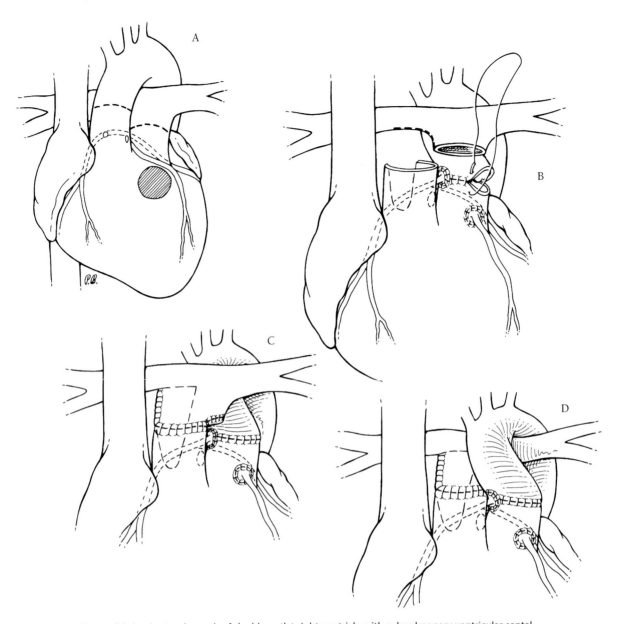

Figure 84-4.   Anatomic repair of double-outlet right ventricle with subpulmonary ventricular septal defect (arterial switch operation). **(A)** The level of transection of the great arteries is shown with a dashed line. With a side-by-side relationship of the great arteries, the aorta should be divided higher than the main pulmonary artery. The ventricular septal defect is closed through a right ventriculotomy or right atriotomy, directing blood to the pulmonary artery. **(B)** The anterior descending coronary ostial button is transferred to an oval defect in the neoaorta. The right coronary–circumflex coronary ostial patch extends to the level of aortic transection as a U-shaped button. It is incorporated into the aortic suture line. The pulmonary bifurcation has been brought anterior to the distal aorta (the Lecompte maneuver). The incision along the undersurface of the right pulmonary artery (RPA) is indicated with a dashed line. **(C)** A large pericardial patch closes the U-shaped defect in the proximal neopulmonary artery and extends onto the undersurface of the RPA. Separate patches close the harvest site of the anterior descending coronary ostial button and the left lateral aspect of the pulmonary trunk. **(D)** With the same technique as in panel C, the Lecompte maneuver can be avoided, leaving the pulmonary bifurcation posterior to the ascending aorta.

valve (Fig. 84-6A). The pulmonary trunk is transected just proximal to the pulmonary bifurcation. It is critical to avoid distortion of the proximal pulmonary trunk or ascending aorta, which may result in semilunar valve insufficiency. Before cardioplegic arrest, it is helpful to place a marking suture on the right medial aspect of the proximal pulmonary trunk at the planned site of transection. A corresponding marking suture is placed on the left medial aspect of the ascending aorta to define the proximal extent of the aortic incision and to ensure proper orientation of both great arteries. The aorta is opened along its left medial aspect

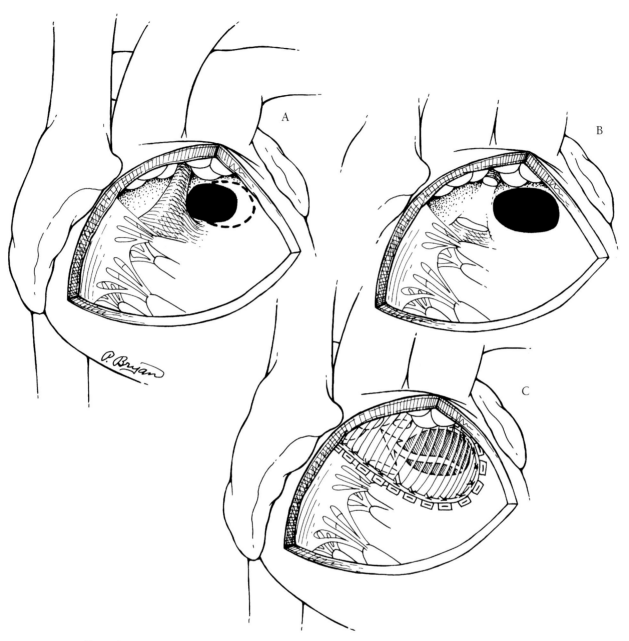

Figure 84-5. Intraventricular repair of double-outlet right ventricle with subpulmonary ventricular septal defect (VSD). **(A)** The VSD is exposed through a transverse right ventriculotomy. The safe area for enlargement of the VSD is marked with a dashed line. The prominent infundibular septum is well seen. **(B)** The infundibular septum is partially excised and the VSD is enlarged. **(C)** The intraventricular tunnel is created with an opened polyester (Dacron) tube graft, channeling left ventricular blood through the enlarged VSD to the aorta (*arrow*).

from the previously placed marking suture distally for a length corresponding to the diameter of the pulmonary trunk. The incision on the aorta should start just above the commissural posts of the aortic valve. Attention should be given to carefully identifying the coronary arteries and avoiding any distortion. An end-to-side anastomosis between the proximal pulmonary trunk and the left medial aspect of the ascending

aorta is performed using a continuous suture technique. It is surprising how often this anastomosis can be performed primarily without additional patch augmentation (Fig. 84-6A). However, in children with previous pulmonary artery banding, the level of transection of the pulmonary trunk is at the level of the band. After the scar tissue is excised from the band site, it is usually necessary to augment the end-to-side

pulmonary–aortic anastomosis with autologous pericardium or homograft material. Right ventricle-to-pulmonary artery continuity is now established with a homograft valved conduit (Fig. 84-6B).

Alternatively, the ascending aorta can be transected at the same level as the pulmonary trunk. A partial side-to-side anastomosis is constructed between the proximal ascending aorta and the proximal

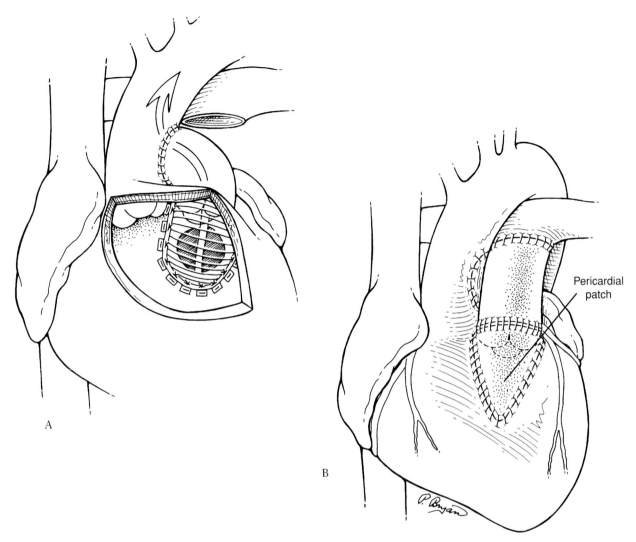

Figure 84-6.   Damus-Kaye-Stansel repair of double-outlet right ventricle with subpulmonary ventricular septal defect (VSD). **(A)** The VSD is closed, channeling left ventricular blood to the pulmonary artery (*arrow*). The main pulmonary artery is transected, and an end-to-side anastomosis is created with the proximal ascending aorta. The aortic valve remains connected to the right ventricle. **(B)** Right ventricle-to-pulmonary artery continuity is reestablished with a valved homograft; about one half of the circumference of the proximal homograft is sutured to the superior aspect of the right ventricle. A piece of pericardium or homograft material is used to roof the gap between the right ventricle and the homograft.

pulmonary trunk. The distal ascending aorta is anastomosed to this double-barreled arterial connection, commonly after patch enlargement of the ascending aorta and arch. The advantage of this double-barreled technique compared with the end-to-side anastomosis depicted in Figure 84-6 is less risk of semilunar valve distortion with subsequent insufficiency as well as the ease of enlarging the distal aorta.

With the Damus-Kaye-Stansel procedure, the aortic valve is still connected to the right ventricle. Because aortic pressure is always higher than right ventricular pressure throughout the cardiac cycle,

the aortic valve remains closed. Right ventricular output is through the valved conduit into the lower-pressure pulmonary arteries rather than through the aortic valve into the higher-pressure systemic circulation. Obviously, any significant aortic valve insufficiency would be poorly tolerated because the regurgitant blood would flow into the right ventricle, causing a left-to-right shunt that could be misdiagnosed as a residual VSD. In the case of significant aortic valve insufficiency, the aortic valve itself can be oversewn primarily without much difficulty. With advances in the arterial switch procedure and the creation of

intraventricular tunnels, it is uncommon to resort to a classical Damus-Kaye-Stansel procedure.

Repair of Double-Outlet Right Ventricle with Doubly Committed Ventricular Septal Defect

Surgical repair of the uncommon variant of DORV with doubly committed VSD is managed in much the same fashion as described for DORV with subaortic VSD. The VSD is usually large, so channeling left ventricular blood to the aorta with an intraventricular tunnel does not present much difficulty. If there is pulmonary stenosis or if the VSD patch obstructs flow into the pulmonary artery, it may be necessary to perform a right ventricular outflow tract patch or to use a right ventricle-to-pulmonary artery valved conduit.

Repair of Double-Outlet Right Ventricle with Noncommitted Ventricular Septal Defect

A satisfactory biventricular repair of DORV with noncommitted VSD is more difficult because the remoteness of the VSD necessitates a complex intraventricular tunnel to direct blood from the left ventricle through the VSD to the aorta. If the VSD is in the inlet perimembranous location, the VSD must be carefully inspected for straddling tricuspid valve or even mitral valve tissue, which would preclude biventricular repair. If the VSD is small, it can be safely enlarged superiorly and anteriorly (Fig. 84-7A) because the conduction tissue in a perimembranous inlet VSD courses along the posterior and inferior rim of the defect on the left ventricular side of the septum similar to DORV with subaortic VSD (Fig. 84-1A). The intraventricular tunnel is then fashioned with a patch tailored from a Dacron or Hemashield tube graft (Figs. 84-7B and 84-2A). The techniques and precautions described in the section on intraventricular tunnel repair of DORV with subaortic VSD are very much applicable to this repair of DORV with noncommitted perimembranous inlet VSD. Usually, even if there is no preexisting pulmonary stenosis, the large and bulky intraventricular patch creates some obstruction to the pulmonary valve so that a right ventricular outflow tract patch or a right ventricle-to-pulmonary artery valved conduit is necessary.

Sometimes the noncommitted VSD is a muscular defect in the trabecular septum. If the VSD is small, it is enlarged anteriorly and inferiorly (Fig. 84-8A) because the conduction tissue courses on the superior posterior aspect of the defect (Fig. 84-1D). A suture line with the intraventricular tunnel repair as described previously not only would place the conduction tissue at jeopardy as the patch is brought up to the aorta, but would also risk distortion of the tricuspid valve apparatus. For these reasons,

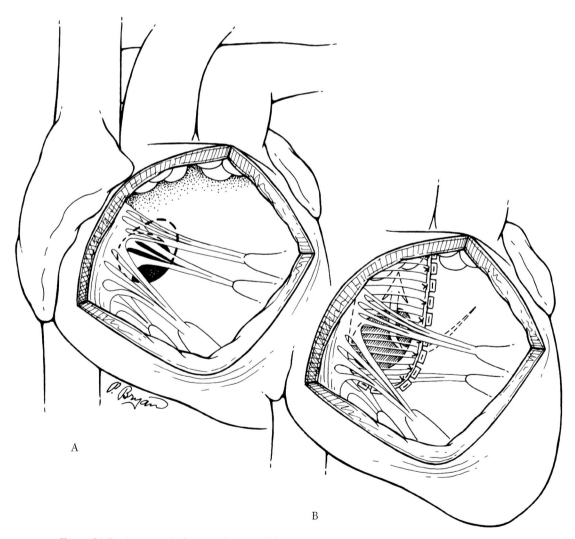

Figure 84-7. Intraventricular tunnel repair of double-outlet right ventricle with noncommitted perimembranous inlet ventricular septal defect (VSD). **(A)** The VSD is exposed through a right ventriculotomy. The safe area for superior and anterior enlargement of the VSD is marked with a dashed line. **(B)** The intraventricular tunnel is created with an opened polyester (Dacron) tube graft, channeling left ventricular blood through the VSD to the aorta (*arrow*).

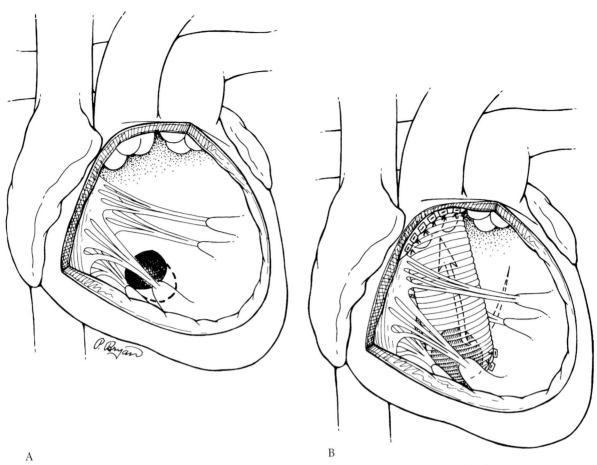

A   B

Figure 84-8.   Repair of double-outlet right ventricle with noncommitted muscular trabecular ventricular septal defect (VSD). **(A)** The VSD is exposed through a right ventriculotomy. The safe area for inferior and anterior enlargement of the VSD is marked with a dashed line. **(B)** An intact polyester (Dacron) tube graft is used with one end sutured around the VSD and the other end up to the aortic valve, creating an intraventricular conduit for blood from the left ventricle through the VSD to the aorta (*arrow*).

in this situation the Dacron or Hemashield tube graft is left intact, with one end sutured around the VSD and the other end around the aortic valve (Fig. 84-8B). This large intraventricular tube is quite bulky and may obstruct right ventricular outflow, mandating the use of a right ventricular outflow tract patch or right ventricle-to-pulmonary artery valved conduit. An obvious disadvantage to this intraventricular tube graft repair is the lack of potential for growth in the channel from the VSD to the aorta. Therefore, the tube graft must be of adult size at the time of the original repair, or one must be resigned to reoperation to enlarge the tube as the child outgrows it.

An alternative approach to correction of DORV with noncommitted VSD was described by Lacour-Gayet and colleagues wherein an intraventricular baffle is constructed to route the left ventricular outflow through the VSD (after surgical enlargement) to the pulmonary artery and then an arterial switch procedure is performed. An even more complex biventricular repair strategy is the use of multiple intraventricular patches to direct left ventricular outflow through the noncommitted VSD to the aorta.

There are situations in which a satisfactory biventricular repair cannot be safely accomplished with DORV and noncommitted VSD. Examples are multiple muscular VSDs, an inability to reliably channel the remote VSD to the aorta, or straddling atrioventricular valve tissue (although Serraf described innovative techniques for establishing a biventricular repair with straddling atrioventricular valves). In these patients unsuitable for a biventricular repair, a modified Fontan procedure can be used effectively. Even though this will result in a physiologic univentricular repair, it is reasonable to enlarge a restrictive VSD when

present to allow unobstructed left ventricular contribution to the systemic output. In these children whose eventual repair will be a Fontan procedure, careful consideration must be given to protecting the pulmonary vascular band with a pulmonary artery band early, particularly if there is no associated pulmonary stenosis.

Complications and Postoperative Considerations

Many of the important complications after surgical repair of DORV are mechanical in nature and should be routinely sought out in the operating room after the patient is separated from cardiopulmonary bypass and addressed at that time if possible. With the routine use of intraoperative transesophageal echocardiography, many of these problems are recognized early, allowing expeditious correction.

The same possible complications seen with closure of straightforward VSDs can occur during repair of DORV with VSD, particularly if it is necessary to enlarge the VSD during the correction. Surgically induced heart block can occur, and this underscores the importance of assiduously avoiding the area of the conduction tissue during repair (Fig. 84-1). Residual left-to-right shunting across the VSD patch or intraventricular baffle can severely compromise the patient's hemodynamic status. In addition to intraoperative transesophageal echocardiography, which will help precisely locate any residual leak, measurements of oxygen saturations across the right heart will help to quantify the magnitude of the shunt. Certainly, any residual calculated ratio of pulmonary to systemic blood flow (Qp/Qs) of 2:1 should be addressed in the operating room, and probably a ratio of >1.5:1 should also be corrected.

The use of an intraventricular tunnel in the repair of most forms of DORV raises the possibility of left ventricular outflow tract obstruction either from inadequate enlargement of a restrictive VSD or poor configuration of the intraventricular tunnel patch with resultant obstruction. Again, intraoperative echocardiography is helpful in identifying and localizing any narrowings. Careful simultaneous measurements in the operating room of left ventricular and aortic pressures will identify any residual left ventricular outflow tract gradient. If there is a significant residual gradient, it is helpful to inspect the left ventricular outflow tract through an aortotomy. Residual obstructing muscle often can be resected through the aortic valve. If the patch is the cause of obstruction, rather than replacing the entire intraventricular tunnel patch, it is possible to visualize the narrowed area through the aorta and relieve the obstruction through the right ventricle by incising the intraventricular tunnel patch at the site of narrowing and enlarging it with a separate patch of Dacron or pericardium. Although perhaps not aesthetically pleasing, this technique can be an easy solution to a potentially life-threatening complication.

Similarly, significant right ventricular outflow tract obstruction can occur after repair as a result of inadequate relief of preexisting pulmonary stenosis, obstructing muscle bundles, or obstruction from the intraventricular tunnel patch. Again, intraoperative pressure measurements and echocardiography help to identify and locate the site of obstruction, which should be dealt with at the time of recognition if it is significant.

Myocardial dysfunction can be a significant problem postoperatively because of the complex and sometimes lengthy intraoperative repairs as well as the uniform presence of significant right ventricular hypertrophy and possibly even left ventricular hypertrophy in patients with a restrictive VSD. Naturally, diligent intraoperative myocardial protection is crucial. Postoperatively, in addition to inotropic support, fairly high right-sided filling pressures are often necessary to maintain adequate cardiac output because of the stiff, poorly compliant, hypertrophied right ventricle. In patients in whom it is anticipated that there will be postoperative right ventricular dysfunction due to existing right ventricular hypertrophy, extensive right ventricular incisions, or residual right ventricular outflow tract obstruction, it can be helpful to leave an interatrial communication (typically by not closing the patent foramen ovale) to allow right-to-left shunting. This strategy maintains systemic ventricular output at the expense of usually well-tolerated systemic arterial desaturation.

Particularly in children without pulmonary stenosis, pulmonary hypertension can be problematic in the early postoperative period and should be identified and treated with the usual measures of sedation, paralysis, pulmonary vasodilation, and hyperventilation. In the past, when complete repair was delayed until later in life, pulmonary vascular obstructive disease was an important cause of postoperative mortality. Occasionally, delaying sternal closure until after improvement of myocardial dysfunction and reduction of tissue edema can be life-saving.

Finally, children undergoing the arterial switch repair of DORV with subpulmonary VSD can develop coronary ischemia even with technically adequate coronary transfer. Avoidance of ventricular distention and systemic hypertension in this situation are key.

Double-Outlet Left Ventricle

Definition

Double-outlet left ventricle (DOLV) is a rare form of congenital heart disease in which >50% of both great arteries arise from the left ventricle. As with DORV, DOLV can be associated with atrioventricular discordance or with univentricular atrioventricular connections. For the purposes of this chapter, only DOLV with concordant atrioventricu-

lar connections and two adequate ventricles is discussed.

Anatomy and Presentation

A VSD is almost always present with DOLV and is usually subaortic in location, although it can be subpulmonic. There are no reports of DOLV with two well-developed ventricles in which the VSD is remote or absent. Pulmonary stenosis is present in most cases of DOLV and can be either valvular or subvalvular.

Children with DOLV with pulmonary stenosis present with a clinical picture similar to that for tetralogy of Fallot with cyanosis. Palliation with a systemic-to-pulmonary shunt is very satisfactory. The uncommon patient with DOLV without pulmonary stenosis presents with symptoms of excessive pulmonary blood flow with heart failure, much like a patient with an unrestricted VSD. There may be some systemic desaturation due to the mixing of systemic and pulmonary venous return in the left ventricle. These children may be palliated early in life with a pulmonary artery band.

Surgical Technique

Complete surgical repair of DOLV is usually simpler than repair of DORV because the aorta arises completely from the left ventricle, thus eliminating the need for a complex intraventricular tunnel. Furthermore, the VSD is unrestrictive, so there is no need to enlarge the VSD.

In patients with DOLV with pulmonary stenosis, the VSD is exposed through a right ventriculotomy (Fig. 84-9A). It is closed with a Dacron patch, with standard precautions taken to avoid injury to the conduction tissue, which lies in the usual location on the left ventricular side of the posterior-inferior portion of the defect (Fig. 84-9B). The proximal main pulmonary artery is divided and the cardiac end oversewn (Fig. 84-9A). Right ventricle-to-pulmonary artery continuity is established using a homograft valved conduit (Fig. 84-9C).

There are reports of total intracardiac repairs of DOLV without pulmonary stenosis in which the VSD is patched to direct right ventricular outflow through the VSD into the pulmonary artery. However, except in the most ideal situations, it is still probably easier to repair DOLV without pulmonary stenosis in the same fashion as DOLV with pulmonary stenosis (i.e., perform simple patch closure of the VSD, oversew the proximal pulmonary artery, and establish right ventricle-to-pulmonary artery continuity with a homograft valved conduit;

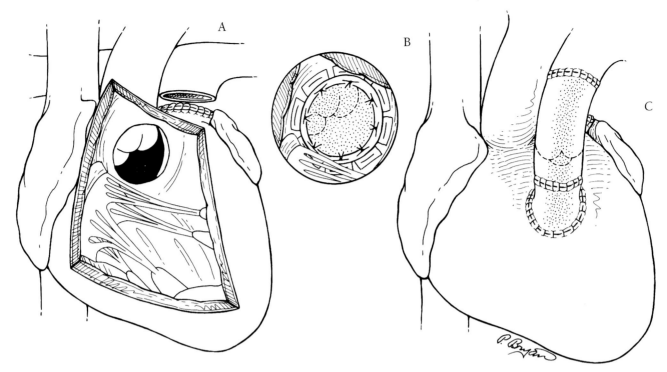

Figure 84-9.   Repair of double-outlet left ventricle. **(A)** The ventricular septal defect (VSD) is exposed through a right ventriculotomy. The aortic valve can be visualized through the subaortic VSD. The main pulmonary artery is divided and the cardiac end oversewn. **(B)** The VSD is closed with a polyester (Dacron) patch using interrupted pledgeted sutures or a continuous suture technique, with care taken to avoid the conduction tissue. **(C)** Right ventricle-to-pulmonary artery continuity is established with a valved homograft; about one half of the circumference of the proximal homograft is sutured to the superior aspect of the right ventricle. A piece of pericardium or homograft material is used to roof the gap between the right ventricle and the homograft.

Fig. 84-9). In many cases with subaortic VSD and pulmonary outflow tract obstruction, the anatomic substrate for the pulmonary obstruction is typically subvalvular with only mild or no pulmonary valve stenosis. In these cases, after closing the subaortic VSD channeling left ventricular outflow to the aorta, the pulmonary root can be harvested with the valve intact (similar to the technique for a Ross procedure) and then translocated to the right ventricle. This obviates the need for a homograft valved conduit with its attendant requirement for eventual replacement.

Complications and Postoperative Considerations

As with surgical closure of a routine VSD, in repair of DOLV the risks of surgically induced heart block or residual left-to-right shunts exist, but there is nothing about DOLV that makes these complications more or less likely when the usual precautions and careful surgical techniques are used.

Because all patients with DOLV have hypertrophied right ventricles, postoperative right ventricular dysfunction with a stiff, poorly compliant right ventricle can occur but is usually not problematic. Finally, as with any extracardiac valved conduit, improper technique can result in right ventricular outflow tract obstruction, which should be identified and corrected in the operating room.

SUGGESTED READING

Barbero-Marcial M, Tanamati C, Atik E, Ebaid M. Intraventricular repair of double-outlet right ventricle with noncommitted ventricular septal defect: advantages of multiple patches. J Thorac Cardiovasc Surg 1999;118: 1056.

Belli E, Serraf A, Lacour-Gayet F, et al. Double-outlet right ventricle with non-committed ventricular septal defect. Eur J Cardiothorac Surg 1999;15:747.

Ceithaml EL, Puga FJ, Danielson GK, et al. Results of the Damus-Stansel-Kaye procedure for transposition of the great arteries and

for double-outlet right ventricle with subpulmonary ventricular septal defect. Ann Thorac Surg 1984;38:433.

Chiavarelli M, Boucek MM, Bailey LL. Arterial correction of double-outlet left ventricle by pulmonary artery translocation. Ann Thorac Surg 1992;53:1098.

DeLeon SY, Ow EP, Chiemmongkoltip P, et al. Alternatives in biventricular repair of double-outlet left ventricle. Ann Thorac Surg 1995; 60:213.

Kawahira Y, Yagihara T, Uemura H, et al. Ventricular outflow tracts after Kawashima intraventricular rerouting for double outlet right ventricle with subpulmonary ventricular septal defect. Eur J Cardiothorac Surg 1999;16: 26.

Kawashima Y, Fujita T, Miyamoto T, Manabe H. Intraventricular rerouting of blood for the correction of Taussig-Bing malformation. J Thorac Cardiovasc Surg 1971;62:825.

Kleinert S, Sano T, Weintraub RG, et al. Anatomic features and surgical strategies in double-outlet right ventricle. Circulation 1997;96:1233.

Lacour-Gayet F, Haun C, Ntalakoura K, et al. Biventricular repair of double outlet right ventricle with non-committed ventricular septal defect (VSD) by VSD rerouting to the pulmonary artery and arterial switch. Eur J Cardiothorac Surg 2002;21:1042.

Lev M, Bharati S, Meng CC, et al. A concept of double-outlet right ventricle. J Thorac Cardiovasc Surg 1972;64:271.

Lui RC, Williams WG, Trusler GA, et al. Experience with the Damus-Kaye-Stansel procedure for children with Taussig-Bing hearts or univentricular hearts with subaortic stenosis. Circulation 1993;88(Pt 2):II170.

Masuda M, Kado H, Shiokawa Y, et al. Clinical results of arterial switch operation for double-outlet right ventricle with subpulmonary VSD. Eur J Cardiothorac Surg 1999;15:283.

Mavroudis C, Backer CL, Muster AJ, et al. Taussig-Bing anomaly: arterial switch versus Kawashima intraventricular repair. Ann Thorac Surg 1996;61:1330.

McElhinney DB, Reddy VM, Hanley FL. Pulmonary root translocation for biventricular repair of double-outlet left ventricle with absent subpulmonic conus. J Thorac Cardiovasc Surg 1997;114:501.

Sakamoto K, Charpentier A, Popescu S, et al. Transaortic approach in double-outlet right ventricle with subaortic ventricular septal defect. Ann Thorac Surg 1997;64:856.

Serraf A, Nakamura T, Lacour-Gayet F, et al. Surgical approaches for double-outlet right ventricle or transposition of the great arteries associated with straddling atrioventricular valves. J Thorac Cardiovasc Surg 1996;111:527.

Tchervenkov CI, Marelli D, Beland MJ, et al. Institutional experience with a protocol of early primary repair of double-outlet right ventricle. Ann Thorac Surg 1995;60(Suppl):S610.

Tchervenkov CI, Walters III HL, Chu VF. Congenital Heart Surgery Nomenclature and Database Project: Double outlet left ventricle. Ann Thorac Surg 2000;69(Suppl):S264.

Walters III HL, Mavroudis C, Tchervenkov CI. Congenital Heart Surgery Nomenclature and Database Project: Double outlet right ventricle. Ann Thorac Surg 2000;69(Suppl):S249.

Wetter J, Sinzobahamvya N, Blaschczok HC, et al. Results of arterial switch operation for primary total correction of the Taussig-Bing anomaly. Ann Thorac Surg 2004;77:41.

Yacoub MH, Radley-Smith R. Anatomic correction of the Taussig-Bing anomaly. J Thorac Cardiovasc Surg 1984;88:380.

EDITOR'S COMMENTS

The anatomic spectrum of DORV continues to require multiple operative approaches. In complex forms of these defects, surgical decision-making can be difficult. The use of intraventricular tunnel repairs, often with the need for right ventricular outflow tract reconstruction with valved conduits, has led to a significant incidence of reoperation in these patients for conduit exchange. In addition, inadequate resection of septal muscle and enlargement of the VSD can result in progressive obstruction of the intraventricular tunnel and subaortic stenosis. The problems with these late defects have led some authors to suggest that in complex forms of DORV, conversion to a single-ventricle type of repair is preferable and may actually decrease the risk of late reoperation and complications.

A patient with subpulmonary VSD and DORV (the Taussig-Bing heart) commonly has associated coarctation of the aorta. Although repair of the coarctation and pulmonary artery banding can be performed for this condition, we perform primary complete repair in these infants. The division of the aorta at the time of the arterial switch procedure allows reconstruction of the arch by patch enlargement without difficulty and a low risk of recurrence of stenosis.

Even when complete correction requires the use of an extracardiac conduit, we primarily repair most patients with nonrestrictive pulmonary outflow tracts to prevent the complications of pulmonary artery banding, which may exacerbate myocardial hypertrophy and, in some cases with relatively restrictive VSDs, cause progressive subaortic obstruction. The progression of subaortic obstruction then drives more blood through the pulmonary artery band. These patients represent a very difficult subgroup at second-stage operation. Often they have been followed with a pulmonary artery band with good oxygen saturations and yet have had progressive subaortic obstruction. Thus, the actual Qp/Qs ratio may not be restricted, and a significant left-to-right shunt may predispose the patient to development of pulmonary vascular disease. This is a particularly difficult situation in those patients who are being staged to single-ventricle correction. Bidirectional Glenn shunting or hemi-Fontan procedures should be performed early even if pulmonary artery banding is undertaken in infancy. Subjecting these patients to significant left-to-right shunts as subaortic stenosis develops in the face of a pulmonary band results in a very high risk of inadequate pulmonary circulation at the time of reoperation for Damus-Kaye-Stansel connection and bidirectional Glenn shunting. Therefore, close follow-up is necessary after pulmonary artery banding to avoid this complication.

When a Damus-Kaye-Stansel operation is necessary because of subaortic obstruction, we augment the arch of the aorta as in the Norwood operation in most cases. Patients with significant subaortic obstruction in infancy often have hypoplasia of the ascending aorta, and there is a significant size discrepancy between the ascending aorta and the proximal pulmonary artery. Therefore, direct connection of the pulmonary artery to the aorta, either primarily or with an augmentation hood, can result in kinking of the distalmost portion of the superior anastomosis with obstruction of the aorta, requiring additional augmentation or stenting. Creation of a long patch underneath the arch of the aorta prevents this kinking and augments the entire ascending aorta. A brief period of circulatory arrest is used for this portion of the operation.

Late restriction of the VSD when an intracardiac conduit is used is common enough that one should consider enlargement of virtually all VSDs in DORV at the time of complete repair. The exception may be isolated subaortic defects where there is a 50% override of the aorta and where the VSD is clearly as large as or larger than the aortic annulus.

Although intracardiac conduits can obstruct right ventricular outflow, it is also possible that the conduit attachments to the septal tricuspid leaflet can limit leaflet mobility and cause functional tricuspid stenosis.

Patients with DORV and uncommitted VSDs remain a difficult surgical challenge. Although resection of the anterior septum with inlet defects can occasionally permit an adequate left ventricular outflow without interfering with tricuspid valve function, in many cases complex intraventricular tunnels may be necessary, creating a virtual right-angled tunnel along the ventricular septum to the aorta.

In some cases with noncommitted VSD, the VSD is more directly related to the pulmonary artery than it is to the aorta. In these cases, in the absence of significant pulmonary stenosis, closure of the VSD to the pulmonary artery and arterial switch procedure is the best approach as is done in Taussig-Bing anomaly. In each case with noncommitted VSD, it is imperative to identify the relationship of the VSD to the great arteries and to conceptually craft a pathway from the VSD to the great vessels to decide when a two ventricle repair can be accomplished. Very complex baffles with significant angulation are most likely to result in late stenosis; in such cases the potential for obstruction is significant, and therefore in many cases a single-ventricle-type repair might be the best approach.

DOLV remains an unusual condition. Although patch closure of the VSD is simple, oversewing of the pulmonary outflow and creation of a right ventricle-to-pulmonary artery conduit exposes the child to recurrent operation for conduit changes. As noted by Dr. Kanter, in some cases with unrestricted right ventricular outflow, the entire pulmonary valve and annulus can be excised from the ventricle and relocated onto the right ventricle with patch closure of the defect in the left ventricle. In this fashion, a native valve can be reconstructed to the right ventricular outflow tract and potentially decrease the risk of late reoperation. Patients with significant pulmonary stenosis, however, are best treated with outflow reconstruction, either with a valved conduit or by direct reconstruction of the pulmonary confluence onto the right ventricle with the Lecompte maneuver and an anterior patch of pericardium or homograft material to create a nonvalved reconstruction. Coronary location often precludes primary outflow tract reconstruction with a transannular patch.

T.L.S.

85

Transposition of the Great Arteries

Thomas L. Spray

Complete transposition of the great arteries (TGA) is a congenital cardiac defect in which there is anatomic reversal of the relationship of the great arteries: The aorta arises entirely or largely from the right ventricle, and the pulmonary artery arises entirely or largely from the left ventricle (ventriculoarterial discordant connection). The lesion is incompatible with life without surgical intervention because in the resulting physiologic abnormality the pulmonary and systemic circulations exist in parallel instead of in series. Survival therefore depends on mixing between the pulmonary and systemic circulations. In spite of the severity of this cardiac defect, surgical therapy has become standardized such that anatomic and physiologic repair can be accomplished in the first few weeks of life in the majority of affected children.

TGA may coexist with other cardiac lesions, including coarctation of the aorta and patent ductus arteriosus. Transposition is associated with intact ventricular septum in approximately 50% of patients, with ventricular septal defect (VSD) in 25%, and with VSD and functional or anatomic left ventricular outflow tract obstruction (pulmonary stenosis) in 25%. Transposition with interruption of the aortic arch is a rare association.

Anatomy

Complete TGA is characterized by atrioventricular concordance and ventriculoarterial discordance ({S,D,D} according to the Van Praagh classification system). Although some have used the term *transposition* to describe a discordant ventriculoarterial connection, other authors have used *transpo-*

sition to describe any heart in which the aorta is anterior to the pulmonary artery. Use of the term "transposition of the great arteries" is confused by the use of this definition in some patients with double-inlet ventricle or absent atrioventricular connection and in patients with nonlateralized atrial arrangements (some heterotaxy syndromes). The term "D-transposition of the great arteries" has also been used to describe a concordant atrioventricular and discordant ventriculoarterial arrangement, but this nomenclature does not adequately describe patients in whom the aorta is anterior and to the *left* of the pulmonary artery. Thus, in this chapter, *complete TGA* is defined as atrial situs solitus, atrioventricular concordance, and ventriculoarterial discordance, {S,D,D}.

The morphogenesis of the abnormal relationship between the great arteries and the ventricles in TGA is controversial. Van Praagh suggested that the subaortic conus persists during normal looping of the ventricles, whereas the subpulmonary conus undergoes absorption, thus establishing fibrous continuity between the mitral and pulmonary valves. In normal cardiac development, the subaortic conus is static, and dominant growth of the pulmonary conus forces the pulmonary valve anterior, superior, and to the left. Differential growth of the subaortic conus in transposition therefore pushes the aorta anteriorly and disrupts the aortic valve continuity. If the subpulmonary conus fails to develop, the pulmonary artery will maintain a posterior location and pulmonary-to-mitral valve continuity will occur. As a consequence of this relationship, the aortic valve becomes anterior to the pulmonary valve, permitting both semilunar valves to con-

nect with the distal great vessels without the rotation that is hypothesized to occur in normal cardiac development. Because conal development determines rotation of the truncus arteriosus, the great arteries are similar in relationship at the semilunar valves as they are at the arch. Anatomic variations are often encountered, although the heart is left-sided with atrial situs solitus in 95% of patients. Left-to-right juxtaposition of the atrial appendages is a sign of other intracardiac anomalies. A true ostium secundum atrial septal defect is present in 10% to 20% of cases; however, the majority of atrial communications are via a patent foramen ovale. Right aortic arch is present in 4% of patients with intact ventricular septum and up to 16% of those with VSD. Up to 50% of patients with TGA will have an associated VSD, many of which will spontaneously close. The VSDs are commonly perimembranous (conoventricular) in location, although they may be found anywhere in the ventricular septum. Pulmonary stenosis or atresia, overriding or straddling atrioventricular valves, coarctation of the aorta, and interruption of the aortic arch have all been noted in association with transposition and VSD.

The spatial relationship of the great vessels is quite variable; however, the aorta is most frequently to the right and anterior to the pulmonary artery. In most cases, the sinuses of Valsalva and coronary artery ostia face the corresponding pulmonary arterial sinuses of Valsalva, although direct alignment of the commissures is universal. This situation permits transfer of the coronary arteries in the arterial switch operation. Only a small number of patients who have a coronary artery that originates from a nonfacing coronary sinus pose a problem for arterial switch reconstruction.

The most common coronary pattern in D-TGA (68%) consists of the left main coronary arising from the leftward coronary sinus, giving rise to the left anterior descending and circumflex coronary arteries. The right coronary arises as a separate ostium from the rightward posterior-facing sinus. Occasionally there is no true circumflex coronary artery, but separate branches arise from the left coronary to supply the corresponding portion of the left ventricle. In up to 20% of cases, the circumflex coronary arises from the right coronary artery off the rightward posterior-facing sinus and passes behind the posterior great vessel. The left anterior descending then arises from a separate ostium off the left coronary sinus. More rare coronary patterns involve a single right coronary artery from the rightward posterior sinus (4.5%) or a single left coronary artery from the leftward coronary sinus (1.5%). Intramural coronary arteries, which proceed in the aortic wall for a distance before exiting to the epicardial surface, have been described and commonly occur at the commissural attachment of the atrioventricular valve. Single coronary ostium or separate ostia close together arising from a single sinus have also been described. Abnormal coronary anatomies are more commonly seen in transposition with associated VSD than when an intact ventricular septum is present.

Important left ventricular outflow tract obstruction is unusual in association with TGA but has significant implications for management strategies. The most common type of left ventricular outflow tract obstruction is dynamic as a result of leftward displacement of the muscular ventricular septum secondary to the development of higher right systemic ventricular pressure. The septum may then narrow the outflow tract, resulting in abnormal systolic anterior mitral leaflet motion and a situation similar to that noted in hypertrophic obstructive cardiomyopathy. Occasionally, obstruction may be produced by a subvalvular fibrous ridge. Posterior malalignment of the ventricular septum may create a tunnel-like obstruction, and fibrous tags arising from the mitral apparatus or membranous septum can result in significant subvalvar obstruction, most commonly when a VSD is present. Valvar stenosis is uncommon, but nonobstructive bicuspid pulmonary valve is not infrequently present. In rare cases, aortic arch obstruction with coarctation or true interruption of the aortic arch has been observed in patients with TGA, left ventricular outflow tract obstruction, and VSD.

Pathophysiology

TGA {S,D,D} is a relatively common form of congenital heart disease, accounting for 9.9% of infants with congenital heart disease in a New England study and representing a frequency of 0.206 per 1,000 live births. A distinct male predominance is noted, with a male-to-female ratio of 2 to 1, which increases to 3.3 to 1 when the ventricular septum is intact. In complex forms of transposition, a sexual predominance has not been noted. Untreated, 90% of children with D-TGA and an intact septum will die by 1 year of age.

The parallel relationship of the pulmonary and systemic circulations in TGA results in nonoxygenated venous blood passing through the right ventricle to the aorta, whereas the oxygenated pulmonary venous blood passes through the left ventricle back to the pulmonary arterial circulation. Mixing between the pulmonary and systemic circulations at the atrial, ventricular, or great vessel level through a patent foramen ovale or atrial septal defect, a VSD, or a patent ductus arteriosus, respectively, is mandatory for survival. Patients with TGA and an intact ventricular septum survive initially because of aortopulmonary flow through a patent ductus arteriosus. After birth, both ventricles are relatively noncompliant, and infants with transposition often have an increased pulmonary blood flow, which causes enlargement of the left atrium and functional incompetence of the foramen ovale, resulting in atrial level mixing of oxygenated and nonoxygenated blood. Inadequacy of this mixing, however, may result in only marginal tissue oxygenation that does not improve with oxygen administration. Atrial balloon septostomy results in improved admixture and an improved tissue oxygen delivery in these patients.

Patients with TGA and significant VSD often have higher oxygen saturations by virtue of greater pulmonary blood flow and greater mixing at both the atrial and ventricular levels. In children with high pulmonary blood flow, pulmonary resistance may progressively increase throughout infancy. The early development of severe pulmonary vascular disease in children with TGA is exacerbated in patients with associated VSD. The rapidity of development of pulmonary obstructive disease has been suggested to be related to hypoxemia associated with increased sympathetic activity and in association with excessive pulmonary blood flow.

Although neonatal pulmonary vascular resistance is elevated in infants with TGA, the resistance falls progressively during the neonatal period with associated changes in the pulmonary and systemic ventricular compliance. In a normal infant, there is an increase in the left ventricular volume load and pressure load and a decrease in right ventricular volume and pressure load shortly after birth, resulting in a rapid

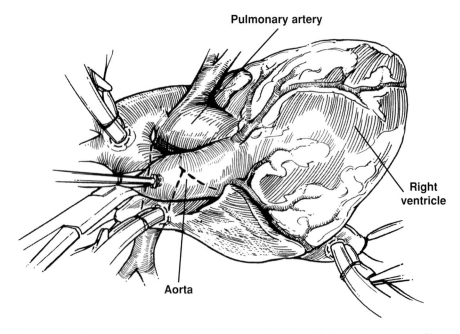

Figure 85-1. The anatomy in transposition of the great arteries with the aorta anterior and to the right of the pulmonary artery. The aorta is cannulated distally, and bicaval cannulation with snares is placed.

increase in the left ventricular myocardial mass. This normal development of the left ventricle is lost in infants with D-TGA, in which the left ventricle ejects to the low-resistance pulmonary vascular bed. Thus, the left ventricle does not increase muscle mass relative to the right ventricle and within a few weeks loses the ability to maintain adequate cardiac output against significant afterload. This change occurs despite the fact that the left ventricle maintains a volume load in patients with transposition and intact ventricular septum. However, when a VSD or large patent ductus arteriosus is present, both volume and pressure overload of the left ventricle is maintained. In D-transposition with left ventricular outflow tract obstruction without a VSD, a ventricular pressure load is imposed without a significant volume load. These physiologic changes in the neonatal heart are important for the consideration of surgical approaches because after a few weeks of postuterine life, the left ventricle in D-transposition with intact ventricular septum takes on the characteristics and wall thickness of a pulmonary ventricle and may not be adequate to support the systemic circulation.

Clinical Features

The most common clinical finding in an infant with TGA is cyanosis (arterial partial pressure of oxygen 25 to 40 mm Hg), which varies in degree depending on associated anomalies. Typically, the cyanosis is more pronounced when the ventricular septum is intact and is often present at birth. The development of cyanosis later in infancy is usually associated with the presence of a significant VSD or left ventricular outflow tract obstruction. Congestive heart failure may be the predominant clinical finding in patients with a large VSD or patent ductus arteriosus. Symptoms of cardiac failure, however, are rarely present in the first week of life but commonly appear by 1 month of age as pulmonary vascular resistance decreases and pulmonary blood flow becomes excessive, even in a patient with an intact ventricular septum.

Management

The widespread use of fetal ultrasound techniques has resulted in the common antenatal diagnosis of TGA. This fact and the fact that the majority of children with TGA are cyanotic in the first week of life have led to the

initiation of treatment at a very early age in these patients. Although in the past cardiac catheterization was generally necessary to confirm the position of the cardiac chambers and the associated lesions, echocardiography has now generally supplanted cardiac catheterization in the majority of patients with simple complete transposition. Cardiac catheterization is now often indicated only in infants in whom inadequate shunting is noted or if associated intracardiac or extracardiac abnormalities require clarification. Echocardiographic views confirming a posterior great vessel that divides into right and left pulmonary arteries and arises from the left ventricle in association with an anterior aorta arising from a right ventricle confirm the diagnosis of TGA. The intracavitary shunts can be determined by Doppler echocardiography techniques, and several echocardiographic views can determine the size and location of VSDs with reference to the infundibular septum, the nature and size of atrial communications, the anatomy of the atrioventricular valves, and the presence and location of significant degrees of subpulmonary stenosis. In addition, in the majority of cases the origins and anatomic distributions of the coronary arteries can be adequately visualized by echocardiogra-

phy. Because the majority of coronary arterial variations can be successfully addressed at surgery, identification of the origins of the coronary arteries is usually sufficient by echocardiography to permit operation without catheterization.

Cardiac catheterization is reserved for patients with significant clinical instability to improve the degree of intracavitary shunting by enlarging the interatrial septal communication. At catheterization, the left atrial pressure is usually greater than the right atrial pressure, and the pressure in the pulmonary (left) ventricle depends on the presence or absence of a VSD, valvar or subvalvar stenosis, the age of the patient, and the magnitude of elevation of pulmonary vascular resistance.

If inadequate interatrial shunting is noted and results in clinical instability (acidemia, severe hypoxemia), the mainstay of management has been a Rashkind balloon atrial septostomy. A balloon-tipped catheter is passed through the systemic veins, through the right atrium and foramen ovale, and into the left atrium. The balloon is inflated and pulled vigorously across the atrial septum to tear the foramen ovale, improving admixture of pulmonary and systemic venous blood. This procedure

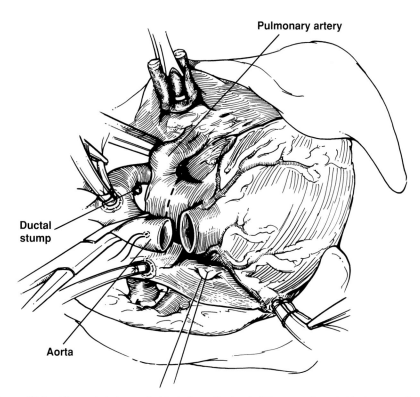

Figure 85-2. The aorta is transected just above the level of the commissural attachments of aortic valve, and the pulmonary artery bifurcation is transected at the dashed line at the bifurcation. Care must be taken not to cut into the origin of the right pulmonary artery. The pulmonary bifurcation is mobilized freely bilaterally out to the hilar branches to allow for translocation anteriorly.

may be performed in the intensive care unit with echocardiographic guidance in children who are clinically unstable. The atrial septostomy results in decompression of the left ventricle and therefore may result in poor left ventricular performance if a subsequent arterial switch procedure is delayed. Therefore, patients who are good anatomic candidates for an arterial switch procedure who have acceptable arterial oxygen saturations are generally referred for early arterial switch without intervening atrial septostomy if the clinical condition permits. Prostaglandin E_1, however, is usually administered to maintain ductal patency and increase pulmonary blood flow to improve stabilization of patients before early operative repair. In addition, relative dehydration may decrease the degree of interatrial shunting, and volume infusions may improve hemodynamics.

History of Surgical Repair

Initial surgical therapy for TGA involved creation of an atrial septal defect using a closed technique to increase the mixing between the systemic venous and pulmonary venous circulations. This was first performed by Blalock and Hanlon in 1950. Although early mortality was high with this operative approach, successful creation of an atrial septal defect resulted in significant palliation in many of these children. Initial attempts to reverse the transposed vessels by both Mustard and Bailey were frustrated by an inability to maintain coronary perfusion and the poor function of the anatomic left ventricle. Thus, initial surgical therapy was directed toward atrial transposition of the pulmonary and systemic venous returns. In 1952, Lillehei and Varco transferred the right-sided pulmonary veins to the right atrium and connected the inferior vena cava to the left atrium. A successful modification of this technique using an allograft to connect the inferior vena cava to the left atrium was described by Baffes in 1956.

Multiple attempts were made at both atrial and arterial repairs of TGA during the 1950s, and in 1954 Albert suggested the concept of switching the atrial septum so that caval return was directed to the left ventricle and the pulmonary venous return to the right ventricle at the atrial level. This atrial switch concept was first successfully accomplished by Senning in 1959 using an ingenious technique for relocating the walls of the right atrium and the atrial septum.

Many of the early attempts at atrial repair were frustrated by the fact that the operation was performed on patients between 1 and 2 years of age, and significant pulmonary vascular obstructive disease had already developed in many of these children. In 1964, Mustard described an alternate procedure for intra-atrial repair: excising the atrial septum and creating a large interatrial baffle of pericardium to redirect pulmonary and systemic venous blood. This repair resulted in larger atrial size than the Senning operation. Early results with the Mustard operation were markedly improved over the previously reported Senning repairs and reflected the significant population of patients in Toronto who had undergone successful Blalock-Hanlon atrial septectomies early in life.

A major development in the surgical treatment of TGA occurred in 1966 when Rashkind and Miller reported the use of a balloon catheter technique to enlarge the atrial septal defect in patients with TGA, resulting in improved early physiologic stability and decreasing the need for operative atrial septectomy. During the 1960s, the Mustard operation became the most commonly performed procedure for transposition, and it became clear that repair in the first few months of life could be accomplished with a low operative mortality and

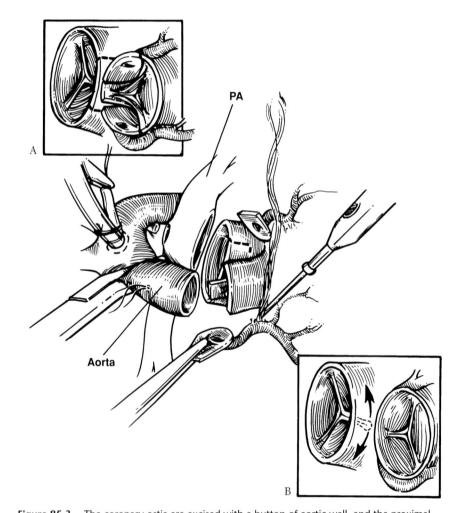

Figure 85-3.   The coronary ostia are excised with a button of aortic wall, and the proximal coronary arteries are mobilized with the cautery, sacrificing small conal branches if necessary to allow unrestricted translocation to the posterior great vessel. Medially based flap incisions are made posteriorly for reimplantation of the coronary arteries as noted by the dashed lines. **(Inset A)** The excision of the coronary ostia down to the sinuses of the aorta is noted, and the relationship of the vertical incisions in the posterior great artery is shown. **(Inset B)** The fact that the commissural attachment of the pulmonary valve may vary in location and relationship to the anterior great artery is shown. Division of the pulmonary artery at the bifurcation allows a 5-mm or 6-mm distance of pulmonary artery (PA) above the commissural attachments so that the coronary arteries can be reimplanted above the sinuses if necessary.

improved results compared with repair at a later age as techniques of cardiovascular surgery became improved over this decade. In 1970, the Senning procedure re-emerged as the persistent problems of baffle obstruction and arrhythmias after the Mustard operation became well defined and the ability to use autologous tissue for the atrial reconstruction became a preferred approach.

The success with the atrial switch operations for TGA with intact septum did not translate to repair of transposition with a large VSD. Disappointing results with VSD closure and atrial repair in this group of patients continued to be a stimulus for development of an arterial switch procedure, which was first successfully performed by Jatene and colleagues in 1975. Yacoub shortly thereafter reported additional successful cases. The success of the arterial switch procedure with reimplantation of the coronary arteries in some patients with transposition and VSD led to reintroduction of this technique for patients with intact ventricular septum. Yacoub's initial attempts in patients with TGA and an intact ventricular septum were unsuccessful in 1972; however, additional reports by 1976 suggested that such repair was possible in infancy. Early mortality with the arterial switch in infancy was related to the fact that the pulmonary left ventricle was not prepared to sustain systemic pressure. Therefore, initial approaches included pulmonary arterial banding (with or without a systemic-to-pulmonary shunt) as a first stage followed by a later arterial switch. However, Yacoub, Quaegebeur, Brawn, and Castaneda subsequently demonstrated the ability to repair simple transposition in the first few days of life by an arterial switch operation while the pulmonary ventricle has relatively high pressure. The rapidly decreasing mortality for arterial switch operations has resulted in this surgical approach becoming the standard corrective surgical procedure, which results in both an anatomic and physiologic reconstruction of this cardiac defect.

Operative approaches to TGA, VSD, and significant left ventricular outflow tract obstruction were less successful in the early period of cardiac surgery. In 1969, Rastelli suggested the combination of an intraventricular tunnel repair: closing the VSD and baffling the pulmonary venous blood from the left ventricle to the aorta, closing the pulmonary artery exit from the left ventricle, and creating an extracardiac conduit from the anatomic right ventricle to the pulmonary bifurcation, resulting in an anatomic repair for TGA/VSD and left ventricular outflow tract obstruction. Obstruction of the reconstructed left ventricular outflow tract remains a common complication of the Rastelli-type repair and has led to recommendation of a variation of intraventricular repair by Lecompte (the "réparation à l'étage ventriculaire" [REV] procedure).

Operative Intervention: Palliative Operations

The advent of the balloon atrial septostomy by Rashkind and Miller has essentially eliminated the need for the Blalock-Hanlon atrial septectomy. Infants with associated cardiac abnormalities and a thick atrial septum who are considered for later atrial baffle repair may benefit from the Blalock-Hanlon technique, although the safety of cardiopulmonary bypass has resulted in the common use of open atrial septectomy in such patients. Pulmonary arterial banding has been used for palliation with TGA and VSD in young infants who have intractable congestive heart failure until operative repair at 3 to 6 months of age. As the results with the arterial switch procedure and VSD closure in infancy have improved, banding in most instances is unnecessary because complete repair can be affected in infancy. Therefore, banding of the pulmonary artery has now been limited to very small neonates who might benefit from a delay in

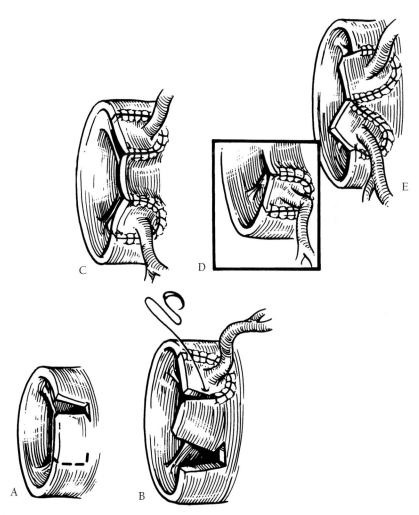

Figure 85-4. **(A)** The medially based flap incisions in the posterior great artery are shown. **(B)** The coronary arteries are translocated to these incisions and anastomosed with absorbable running suture. **(C)** The transfer of the coronary arteries is complete and the takeoff of the vessels noted. **(D)** If the coronary artery is implanted vertically, in some cases the vessel is too low in the posterior great artery, and the origin of the vessel can kink during distention of the neoaorta. **(E)** In these cases, translocation of the coronary artery at an angle that is more superior can result in an unobstructed takeoff of the coronary artery from the aorta.

corrective surgery and those patients with transposition and an intact ventricular septum who present late for arterial switch repair and require "training" of the left ventricle to work at a higher pressure to become the systemic ventricle. For similar reasons, pulmonary arterial banding is used in patients with TGA who develop right ventricular dysfunction and failure after atrial baffle operations as a component of staged conversion to an arterial switch repair. Pulmonary arterial banding in TGA is a delicate procedure because limitation of pulmonary blood flow results in significant hypoxia and metabolic acidosis, and loose banding results in inadequate protection of the pulmonary vascular bed and poor development of the left (pulmonary) ventricle. Thus, in most situations in which preparation of the left ventricle is undertaken for conversion to an arterial switch procedure, banding must be associated with creation of an aortopulmonary shunt to maintain adequate pulmonary blood flow and prevent hypoxemia and ventricular dysfunction.

Surgical Correction

Satisfactory correction of TGA results in rerouting of systemic venous blood to the pulmonary circulation and the pulmonary venous blood into the systemic arterial circulation. This may be accomplished at the atrial, the ventricular, or the great arterial level. The earliest repairs of TGA involve rerouting of the systemic and pulmonary venous returns at the atrial level, resulting in an adequate physiologic repair but not an anatomic repair because the morphologic right ventricle continues to be the systemic ventricle. Both ventricular (Rastelli) and great arterial (arterial switch) repairs are more anatomic corrections resulting in a morphologic left ventricle as the systemic ventricle.

Atrial Repair

Despite the excellent results with atrial switch operations for TGA, anatomic correction by the arterial switch procedure has resulted in the arterial switch procedure becoming the standard surgical correction for TGA. Therefore, the Senning and Mustard operations will not be described in detail in this chapter.

Arterial Repair

The technique of the arterial switch operation involves transection of the great arteries, transfer of the coronary arterial origins,

and repositioning of the great vessels. The procedure is performed with a median sternotomy incision and the use of cardiopulmonary bypass with hypothermia, although in some cases the entire operation can be performed with a single period of circulatory arrest, or circulatory arrest can be used for a brief period for atrial septal defect exposure and coronary transfer. After the sternotomy incision is made, a portion of the anterior pericardium is excised for use as an autologous patch for reconstruction of the anterior great vessel. The patch can be used either fresh or fixed in a glutaraldehyde solution to make handling easier. In addition, we have used pulmonary homograft patch material for pulmonary artery reconstruction. The ligamentum arteriosum or patent

ductus arteriosus is dissected out and the branches of the right and left pulmonary arteries mobilized well out to the hilum of the lung bilaterally. It is important to freely mobilize the pulmonary arterial branches out beyond the bifurcation to the lobar branches so as to permit anterior relocation of the pulmonary artery in the Lecompte maneuver without compression of the pulmonary arteries by the aorta. As noted in Fig. 85-1, the aorta is cannulated as distally as possible to allow room for manipulation of the proximal aorta during the reconstruction. A cardioplegia needle is inserted into the aortic root, and bicaval cannulation is performed in most cases. In D-TGA, the aorta is anterior and to the right of the pulmonary artery, and the pulmonary artery is typically larger than

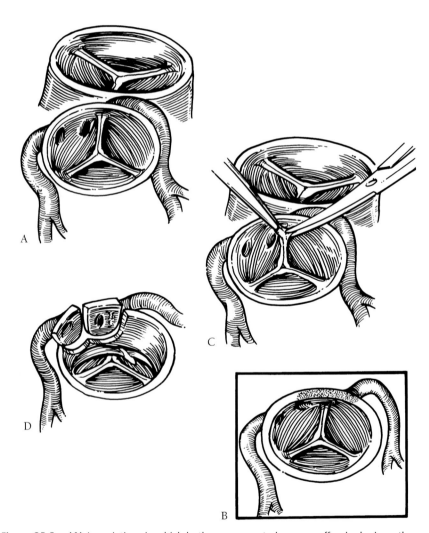

Figure 85-5. **(A)** In variations in which both coronary arteries come off a single sinus, the coronary ostia may have an intramural course. **(B)** Care must be taken not to transect the coronary artery during excision of the coronary button from the aortic wall (*stippled area*). **(C)** The aortic valve leaflet may need to be detached from the commissure to allow access to the coronary ostia for excision. **(D)** Separate excision of the two coronary ostia can be effective in most cases.

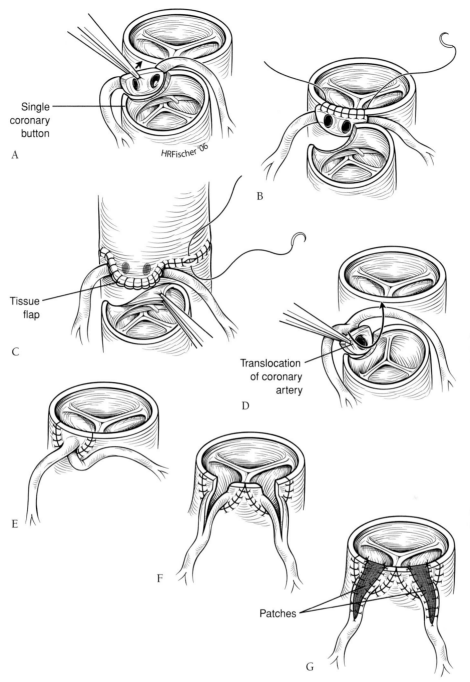

Figure 85-6. **(A)** In some cases, excision of the single coronary ostium supplying both right and left circulations or side-by-side ostia from the same sinus are best translocated with a single coronary button excised from the sinus of the aortic valve. **(B)** The superior margin of the coronary button is anastomosed to the superior margin of the posterior great vessel. In this fashion, there is no translocation of the coronary ostia posteriorly, but they are left in their normal anatomic relationships to prevent kinking of the arteries. **(C)** The aorta is then mobilized to create a flap of tissue sewn down over the coronary ostia, allowing unobstructed flow into the coronary vessels. **(D)** Translocation of a single coronary artery to the posterior great vessel can be effective in most cases. Care must be taken, however, to orient the artery such that kinking of the left coronary branch does not occur. **(E)** A more superior location of the coronary artery on the posterior great vessel generally relieves such kinking. **(F)** In situations with intramural coronaries with ostia that arise adjacent posteriorly from the aorta, the coronary buttons can be excised and the intramural course opened inside the aortic wall. The coronaries are then rotated and then reimplanted into the posterior great artery in the usual fashion. **(G)** The narrow nature of the coronary arteries despite opening of the intramural course still often leaves stenosis, and therefore incision of the coronary with patch augmentation with a small triangular patch of pulmonary homograft or pericardium material can ensure that there is no coronary inflow problem. This patch coronary ostioplasty must be done in a meticulous fashion to prevent distortion and kinking of coronary flow.

the ascending aorta. After bypass is established, the ductus arteriosus is ligated but not divided. The aorta is then clamped as close to the aortic cannula as possible, and cardioplegic solution is administered into the aortic root.

If a VSD is present, we have found it valuable to approach it either through the right atrium across the tricuspid valve or occasionally through the anterior great vessel or pulmonary artery. In the majority of cases, however, we have chosen to approach the VSD across the tricuspid valve and have had adequate exposure. We prefer to address the VSD and atrial septal defect after the initial cross-clamping of the aorta and administration of cardioplegic solution so that additional doses of cardioplegic solution can be administered before aortic reconstruction. The VSD is closed in the usual fashion across the tricuspid valve as described in Chapter 76. Anterior muscular or conoseptal hypoplasia defects are approached through the aorta or pulmonary artery. If an atrial septal defect is present, it is closed partially to allow for right-to-left shunting if necessary in the early postoperative period; if a patent foramen ovale is present, it is left unclosed. After the VSD is closed, if present, additional cardioplegic solution is injected into the aortic root, and then the aorta is transected above the level of the commissural attachments of the aortic valve and the pulmonary artery transected at the level of the bifurcation as noted in Fig. 85-2. The ductus arteriosus is divided on the pulmonary arterial end, and the pulmonary arteries are freely mobilized from adjacent tissue. At this point, we have found it valuable to relocate the pulmonary bifurcation anterior to the aorta and then re–cross-clamp the aorta, keeping the pulmonary bifurcation cephalad and out of the operative field while coronary reconstruction is performed. The coronary ostia are then examined carefully and excised from the anterior great vessel with a button of aortic wall extending down to the base of the sinuses of Valsalva, as noted in Fig. 85-3 (inset A). The epicardial courses of the coronary arteries are then mobilized adequately to permit translocation of the coronary ostia to the posterior great vessel without kinking of the epicardial course of the vessels, as noted in Fig. 85-3. On occasion, small conal branches of the coronary arteries may need to be sacrificed to permit adequate mobilization. At a suitable site on the posterior great artery, a vertical incision is made and a medially based flap incision created to allow takeoff of the coronary ostia without tension or kinking. Whereas generally the sinuses of the aortic and pulmonary valves

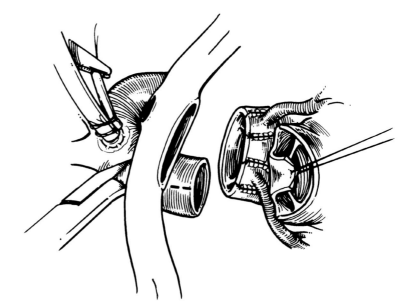

Figure 85-7. The pulmonary bifurcation is translocated anterior to the great artery in the Lecompte maneuver. To obtain an adequate size match between the distal ascending aorta and the proximal great artery to which the coronaries have been transferred, a vertical incision is used.

face each other, the commissural attachment of the pulmonary valve may be dislocated superiorly or inferiorly and does not necessarily align directly with the commissural attachment of the aortic valve, as noted in Fig. 85-3 (inset B). This fact must be taken into account in decisions regarding relocation of the coronary ostia. It is not uncommon for both coronary ostia to end up arising superior to the commissural attachments of the pulmonary valve or for both coronary ostia to be reimplanted to the same sinus of the pulmonary valve because of the variations in anatomy of the commissural

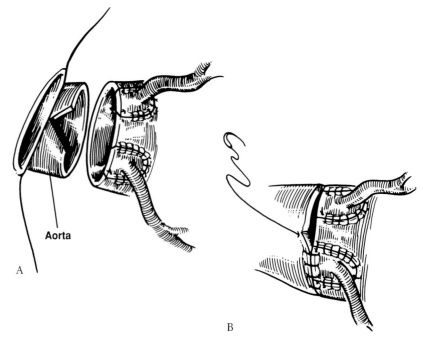

Figure 85-8. The vertical incision in the distal aorta is shown, creating an adequate size match for the anastomosis **(A)**, which is completed with a running absorbable suture **(B)**.

attachments. It is generally preferable to reimplant the coronary arteries somewhat higher in the pulmonary artery than down into the sinuses of the pulmonary valve. This permits the coronary to come off of the neoaorta with less risk of kinking at the origin during distention of the aorta. As shown in Fig. 85-4, the coronary ostia are then reimplanted into the medially based flap incisions. We prefer to use absorbable suture for these anastomoses in the hope of encouraging growth at the suture lines. On occasion, the placement of a vertically oriented suture line can result in kinking of the origin of the coronary artery, as noted in Fig. 85-4D; in these cases, rotation of the coronary medially (Fig. 85-4E) can resolve the distortion.

Common variations in coronary translocation techniques are illustrated in Figs. 85-5 and 85-6. As noted in Fig. 85-5, when both coronaries come off a single sinus with the origin of the left coronary artery from an orifice near the commissural attachment of the aortic valve, it is possible to mobilize the commissure and excise the coronary arteries in the usual fashion before translocation to the posterior great vessel. It is particularly important to note that the coronary artery may run intramurally in the aortic wall before exiting to the epicardial surface, and care must be taken not to cut across the coronary course (Fig. 85-5B). An alternative technique for translocation that does not require separate coronary transfer is noted in Fig. 85-6. The common coronary orifice or adjacent coronary orifices can be excised from the aortic wall as a single patch and then sewn side-to-side to the posterior great artery. The distal aorta can then be fashioned to create a flap over the origin of the coronary arteries, allowing unobstructed flow into the vessels (Fig. 85-6C). In the majority of cases, however, it is possible to transfer the coronary arteries directly to the posterior great vessel even when there is a single coronary from the right posterior-facing sinus, as noted in Fig. 85-6D,E. Care must be taken, however, to position the coronary artery in such a fashion that it does not kink one of the branches (Fig. 85-6E). Rotation of the coronary flap or translocation to a higher level on the pulmonary artery can adjust for many of the variations and possible kinking of the origins of the coronary arteries and allow coronary transfer in virtually all anatomic variations of TGA. In situations of single coronary ostium or side-by-side origin of the coronaries from the same sinus with very little distance between the orifices and intramural course, take-down of the commissure, division of the coronary

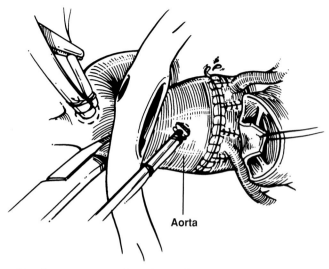

Figure 85-9. After the coronary transfer and ascending aortic reconstruction are completed, cardioplegic solution is injected into the aortic root to ensure free flow into the coronary arteries and hemostasis at the suture lines.

arteries, and rotation and reimplantation into the posterior great vessel may still leave an intramural course of the coronary that is prone to kinking and occlusion. The flap technique described earlier leaving the coronaries in situ may sometimes solve this potential problem; however, the Lecompte maneuver, bringing the pulmonary bifurcation anterior to the aorta, may create compression on the anteriorly located flap and limit inflow into the coronaries, causing ischemia and potential late arrhythmias during exercise. One technique that has worked well for us in this situation is dividing the coronary arteries with reimplantation to the posterior great vessel and then performing an ostial

coronary arterioplasty, cutting into the orifice of the intramural course of the coronary vessel and augmenting the origin with a small triangular patch of pulmonary homograft material or pericardium. This widely opens the orifice to the coronary artery and prevents kinking at the end proximal portion of the intramural course of the vessel (Figure 85-6F,G).

Once coronary artery transfer has been completed, the distal aorta is then anastomosed to the posterior great vessel to which the coronaries have been transferred. Because of the frequently present size discrepancy between the neoaorta (to which the coronaries have been transferred) and the

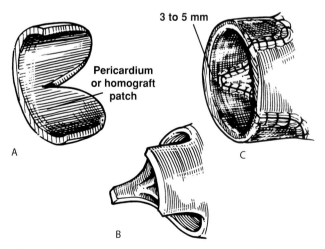

Figure 85-10. The anterior pulmonary artery is then reconstructed with a pantaloon-shaped patch of pulmonary homograft or autologous pericardium with an extension approximately 3 mm to 5 mm above the posterior commissure to elongate the pulmonary artery before the bifurcation.

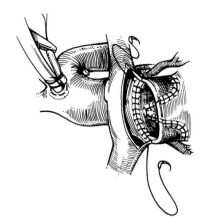

Figure 85-11. The pulmonary bifurcation is then reconstructed onto the anterior great artery using running nonabsorbable suture. Incisions onto the right and left pulmonary arteries are made as necessary to create an adequate size match.

distal aorta, a vertical incision is used to make up the size discrepancy (Fig. 85-7). As noted in Fig. 85-8, this incision can allow for adequate primary anastomosis in most circumstances even if there is a significant size discrepancy. The suture line is performed with absorbable suture, again in the hope of maximizing growth potential. The anteriorly placed vertical incision in the aorta has the additional advantage of pulling the aorta posteriorly, which helps to prevent compression of the pulmonary bifurcation that has now been anteriorly translocated. At this point in the procedure, additional cardioplegic solution is injected into the aortic root (Fig. 85-9) to check for hemostasis of the suture lines and to ensure that free perfusion of the coronary ostia without kinking is present. Next, the defects in the anterior great vessel from which the coronaries

have been excised are repaired with a generous portion of glutaraldehyde-fixed pericardium or pulmonary homograft material (Fig. 85-10). The patch is fashioned in a pantaloon shape and posteriorly is extended for 3 mm to 5 mm to allow for some extension and length of the pulmonary artery to the bifurcation. Anteriorly, native tissue is left in place and the patch trimmed appropriately to allow for an anterior portion of native tissue to be anastomosed to the pulmonary bifurcation in the hope of encouraging growth at this portion of the suture line. As noted in Fig. 85-11, the anterior great vessel is then sutured to the pulmonary artery bifurcation with care being taken to avoid tension on the pulmonary arteries, which may interfere with symmetric pulmonary blood flow. If necessary, an incision is carried out onto the origin of the pulmonary arteries to allow for an adequate size match and to prevent distortion of the origins of the pulmonary arteries. This anastomosis is occasionally completed with the aortic cross-clamp released and the heart reperfusing. After completion of the pulmonary artery reconstruction, the right atrium is closed, and then finally the pulmonary origin of the ductus oversewn with an absorbable suture, with care being taken not to interfere with the flow into the origin of the left pulmonary artery (Fig. 85-12).

In situations in which the great vessels are side to side rather than anteroposterior in relationship, it is occasionally advisable to leave the pulmonary confluence posterior to the aorta and incise onto the right pulmonary artery, closing the pulmonary bifurcation on the left to transpose the opening in the pulmonary artery more to the right. This may facilitate reconstruction to the right ventricle after the arterial switch has been performed.

After completion of the repair, right atrial lines are placed for postoperative monitoring and volume infusions and temporary pacemaker wires applied to the right atrium and right ventricle. After the patient is weaned from cardiopulmonary bypass, a systemic pressure of no more than 60 to 70 mm Hg is preferable to prevent distention of the newly systemic left ventricle.

The Rastelli Operation

Infants with significant left ventricular outflow tract obstruction represent a small proportion of children with TGA. Left ventricular outflow tract obstruction in TGA is often dynamic in nature; therefore, the relative contributions of the dynamic components of obstruction and the fixed components such as subvalvar fibrous rings and mitral valve leaflet tags are difficult to

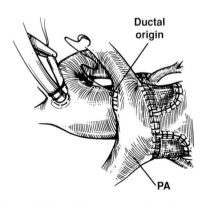

Figure 85-12. After reconstruction, the origin of the ductus arteriosus is oversewn with absorbable suture, with care being taken not to narrow the takeoff of the left pulmonary artery (PA).

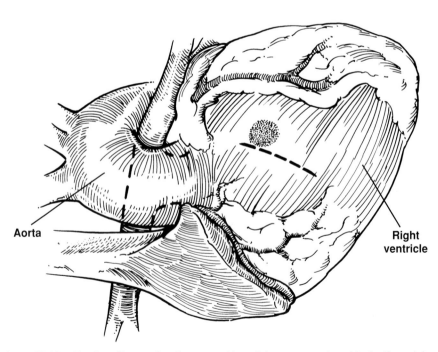

Figure 85-13. The Rastelli operation. In transposition of the great arteries with significant left ventricular outflow tract obstruction, the aorta is larger than the posteriorly located pulmonary artery. The dashed lines show the direction for the ventriculotomy incision in the right ventricle avoiding major epicardial coronaries, and the location of the ventricular septal defect is noted.

determine. Although fixed forms of left ventricular outflow tract obstruction occasionally may be resected with exposure across the pulmonary valve at the time of arterial switch operation, complete relief of obstruction often is not possible. In the majority of cases, however, moderate relief of left ventricular outflow tract obstruction can be well tolerated because the pulmonary ventricle

has been preconditioned to elevated intracavitary pressure.

When significant left ventricular outflow tract obstruction in association with TGA presents in infancy, creation of an interatrial communication and a systemic-to-pulmonary arterial shunt is often the best early approach followed by later complete repair by the Rastelli operation. In some

institutions, early complete repair is preferred, and we have generally elected to complete the operative procedure by the time the patient is 6 months of age even if a systemic-to-pulmonary artery shunt is initially selected.

In the Rastelli operation (Figs. 85-13 to 85-18), pulmonary venous blood is directed by a patch across the VSD to the aorta and

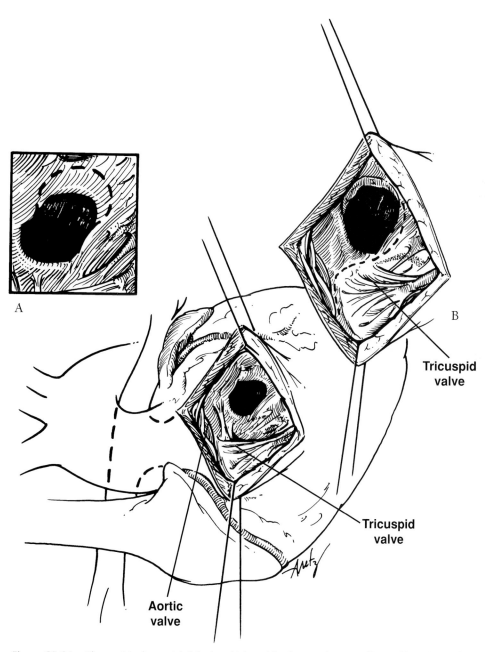

Figure 85-14. The ventricular septal defect and tricuspid valve attachments. **(Inset A)** Excision of the anterior superior margin of the ventricular septal defect away from the conducting tissue allows an unobstructed connection from the left ventricle to the aorta. **(Inset B)** In the "réparation à l'étage ventriculaire" (REV) procedure, the conal muscle beneath the aorta separating the aorta and pulmonary valves is also resected at the anterior left lateral margin of the ventricular septal defect away from the conducting tissue (*stippled lines*). The direction of the suture line for the ventricular septal defect patch to the aorta is shown by the dashed lines, avoiding the conduction tissue.

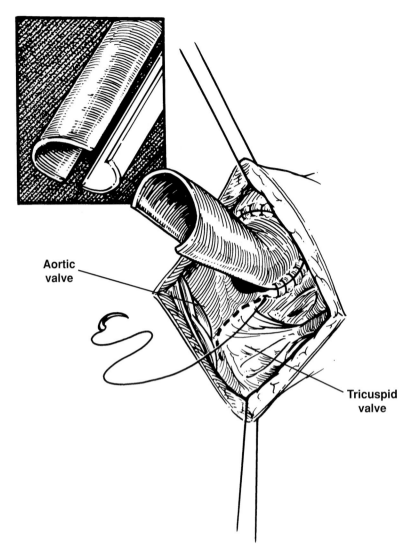

Figure 85-15. A baffle created from a polytetrafluoroethylene (Gore-Tex) tube graft **(inset)** is used to create the connection from the left ventricle to the aorta.

a valved conduit is used to reconstruct the right ventricular outflow tract to the distal pulmonary arteries. Figure 85-13 shows the transposed great arteries with the ascending aorta larger than the posteriorly located pulmonary artery because significant pulmonary stenosis is a feature of this condition. The incision in the right ventricle for placement of the conduit is directed toward the pulmonary bifurcation to the left, and the VSD is exposed through this ventriculotomy incision. As noted in Fig. 85-14, the VSD is often somewhat smaller than the ascending aorta, and enlargement of the VSD is recommended to prevent late development of obstruction from the left ventricle across the VSD, which becomes the outlet to the ascending aorta. Restriction of the VSD is one of the most common late problems after the Rastelli operation. In Fig. 85-14 (inset A), the enlargement of

the VSD is shown anteriorly and superiorly away from the area of the conducting tissue. The pathway of the conducting tissue along the right ventricular septum is noted in Fig. 85-14B (stippled line), and the suture line for placement of the baffle from the left ventricle to the aorta is noted by the dashed line. In Fig. 85-15, the creation of a conduit-like patch from either a polyester (Dacron) tube graft or a polytetrafluoroethylene (Gore-Tex) tube graft is described. Alternately, a patulous rectangular patch of Dacron material can be used, allowing for a large amount of the material to bow into the right ventricle to permit an unobstructed connection from the VSD at the ascending aorta. We prefer to use Gore-Tex material for these connections because the rough surface of the Dacron patch material may cause hemolysis early postoperatively.

After the baffle is completed, the left ventricular output is directed across to the ascending aorta anteriorly (Fig. 85-16). The pulmonary artery is then divided and the pulmonary bifurcation incised for connection to a pulmonary homograft conduit of the largest size that will satisfactorily fit into the chest cavity (Fig. 85-17). Homograft material is preferred for re-creation of the right ventricular outflow tract because it is compressible and therefore will allow the conduit to sit in the left chest underneath the sternum without significant distortion in the majority of cases. The pulmonary valve is oversewn, and the stump of the pulmonary artery also is oversewn to prevent antegrade flow out of the ventricle into a blind pouch, which could be a source of potential thrombi and thromboembolism. The right ventricular outflow tract is then reconstructed with a pulmonary valved homograft with a polytetrafluoroethylene gusset, allowing a gentle takeoff from the right ventricle to the pulmonary outflow tract (Fig. 85-18).

Unusual cases of children with transposition and intact ventricular septum with significant left ventricular outflow tract obstruction may be treated by atrial baffle repair and connection of a conduit from the left ventricular cavity to the pulmonary bifurcation on the left.

Lecompte modified the Rastelli operation to decrease the risk of obstruction of the conduit from the left ventricle to the aorta by creation of the REV procedure. In this operation, the resection of the subaortic conus is more extensive than in the Rastelli operation, and resection of muscle is carried to just below the pulmonary valve annulus superiorly (Fig. 85-19A,B). In addition, when tricuspid valve attachments to the ventricular septum are abnormal, a septal flap containing the important tricuspid valve attachments can be created and repositioned onto the ventricular septal patch after it is sewn in place. These more extensive resections of the ventricular septum create a more direct pathway from the left ventricle to the ascending aorta with a lower risk of recurrent stenosis. In addition, Lecompte suggested translocation of the pulmonary bifurcation anteriorly in these patients with resection of a short portion of the ascending aorta to reposition the aorta more posteriorly and allow direct connection of the pulmonary bifurcation to the right ventricular outflow tract with a monocusp patch or nonvalved direct connection. In this fashion, complete repair can be effected in patients with TGA, VSD, and left ventricular outflow tract obstruction

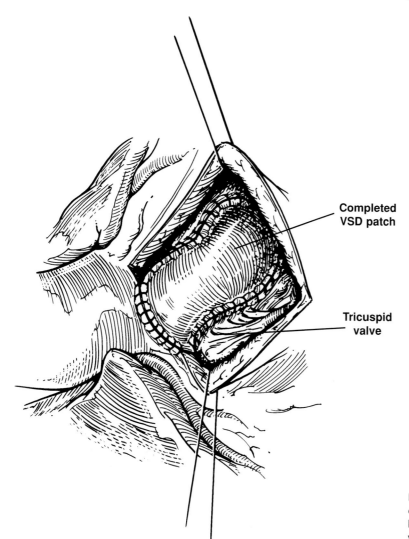

Figure 85-16. Completion of the baffle creates a conduit from the left ventricle to the aorta sewn to the base of the septal tricuspid valve leaflet inferiorly. (VSD = ventricular septal defect.)

without the need for a homograft conduit, which would require later revision. A modification of the approach described by Lecompte resects a short segment of the aorta decreasing the length of the aorta and bringing it into a more posterior position. This short segment of aorta that is excised can then be used to reconstruct the pulmonary outflow tract using autologous tissue to allow for potential growth.

A variation on the REV procedure has been described by Nikaidoh and is useful for patients who have transposition-like forms of double-outlet right ventricle with ventricular septal defect and small pulmonary valve annulus. In this approach the pulmonary annulus can be incised across the conal muscle into the ventricular septal defect and the aorta excised with mobilization of the coronary arteries as in the pulmonary autograft procedure for aortic valve replacement. The entire aortic root with the coronaries attached can then be positioned more posteriorly into the left ventricular outflow tract and secured to the pulmonary valve annulus posteriorly (Fig. 85-20A,B,C). The VSD is then closed anteriorly with a patch secured to the inferior margin of the translocated aorta (Fig. 85-20D). In this fashion the outflow from the left ventricle becomes more directly related to the aorta without a complex intracardiac baffle and often without requiring enlargement of the ventricular septal defect. The right ventricular outflow tract can then be reconstructed either with direct connection to the pulmonary bifurcation or with use of a homograft valve conduit (Fig. 85-20E). In some cases it is simpler to excise the coronary artery buttons and mobilize them to gain access to the subaortic area for excision of the aortic root before translocation of the aortic root more posteriorly. The coronary buttons can then be reimplanted in a suitable orientation to the mobilized aorta, decreasing the potential risk of kinking of the epicardial course of the vessels. Only limited series of the Nikaidoh operation have been reported; however, the operation has several advantages in suitable patients when there is moderate hypoplasia of the pulmonary valve annulus and associated ventricular septal defect.

Surgical Results of Repairs of Transposition of the Great Arteries

The results of either a Mustard or a Senning surgical atrial switch procedure have generally been good, with survival rates of 80% to 95% reported for complete repair in infancy in patients with intact ventricular septum. Complications of the atrial operation, however, have been a high incidence of sinus node dysfunction or other atrial dysrhythmias and the development of dynamic left

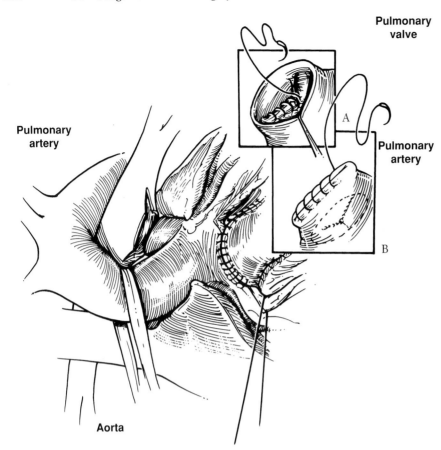

Pulmonary valve

Pulmonary artery

Pulmonary artery

A

B

Pulmonary artery

Aorta

Figure 85-17. After the intracardiac portion of the repair is completed, the pulmonary artery is transected and the pulmonary valve **(inset A)** and main pulmonary artery **(inset B)** are oversewn to prevent stasis and bleeding. Alternatively, the pulmonary valve can be excised. The distal pulmonary artery is opened adequately for reconstruction with a pulmonary homograft.

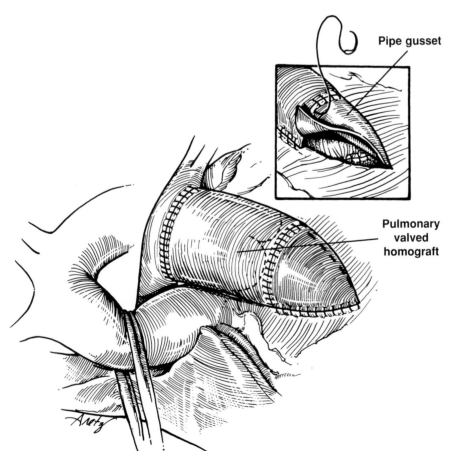

Pipe gusset

Pulmonary valved homograft

Figure 85-18. The right ventricular outflow tract is reconstructed using a pulmonary valved homograft to the pulmonary bifurcation augmented by a polytetrafluoroethylene (PTFE) gusset from the right ventricle **(inset).**

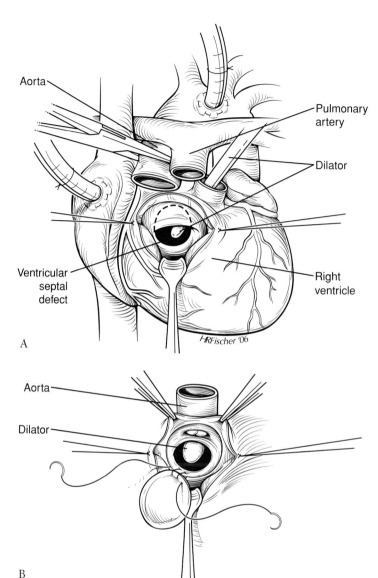

Aorta

Pulmonary
artery

Dilator

Ventricular
septal
defect

Right
ventricle

HRFischer '06

A

Aorta

Dilator

B

Figure 85-19. **(A)** In the "réparation à l'étage ventriculaire" (REV) procedure the aorta and pulmonary artery are transected, and through an incision in the right ventricular outflow tract the infundibulum is widely excised to create an unobstructed pathway from the ventricular septal defect (VSD) to the aorta. A dilator can be passed across the outflow to guide resection of the VSD to avoid damage to the semilunar valve. **(B)** A generous patch of Dacron is used to close the VSD, directing flow to the aorta. The resection of conal muscle provides a more direct connection of the ventricle to the aorta than in the standard Rastelli operation. The pulmonary artery is then reconnected to the right ventricular outflow tract after a Lecompte maneuver is performed, bringing the pulmonary arteries anterior to the aorta.

ventricular outflow tract obstruction from systemic right ventricular pressure loading. The Senning operation has been associated with improved rates of sinus rhythm compared with the Mustard operation, although atrial arrhythmias are not uncommon with this approach. The incidence of late deterioration in systemic right ventricular function is unknown but may approach 10% of patients. Results with atrial correction appear to be improved with early repair before the development of significant pulmonary vascular obstructive disease, and age alone does not appear to be a significant independent predictor of operative risk.

Arterial switch operations have been associated with progressive improvement in mortality rates such that hospital survival

approaches 95% to 100% in the current era. Perhaps the largest series of arterial repairs for transposition of the great vessels has been reported by the group at Boston Children's Hospital, in which the 1-, 5-, and 8-year survival rates were 93%, 92%, and 91%, respectively. Significant risk factors for death after repair included abnormal coronary artery patterns and longer duration of circulatory arrest during the operation, and approximately 5% of the patients required some reintervention to relieve right ventricular or pulmonary arterial stenosis. The same group has shown that left ventricular size, mass, functional status, and contractility are normal on followup with no evidence of late deterioration. In addition, follow-up studies of atrial and

ventricular arrhythmias after the arterial switch operation have shown a 96% incidence of sinus rhythm on electrocardiographic and 99% during Holter monitoring studies at a mean of 2.1 years after the procedure, which represent a marked improvement over the results with the atrial operations. The results of these careful studies have confirmed the superiority of the anatomic arterial switch procedure over atrial repairs, and therefore, despite evolution in the management of patients with TGA, current surgical techniques have resulted in favorable long-term outcomes for these children. In spite of the excellent intermediate-term results with the arterial switch operation, late problems occur in some of these children. Dilation of

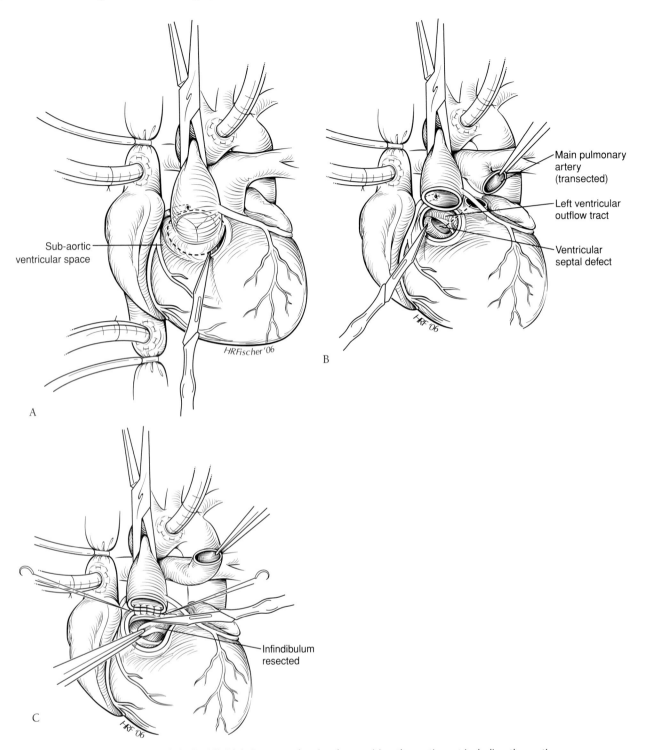

Figure 85-20. **(A)** The Nikaidoh-Bex procedure involves excising the aortic root including the aortic valve from the ventricle by making an incision below the aortic valve annulus and mobilizing the entire root along with the attached coronary arteries. If exposure is difficult, the coronaries can be excised for reimplantation, much as in an arterial switch operation. **(B)** Once the aortic root has been mobilized, the muscle between the pulmonary annulus and the ventricular septal defect (VSD) is divided, widely opening up the outflow from the left ventricle to the pulmonary valve annulus, and additional muscle resected if necessary. **(C)** After infundibular muscle is resected, the aortic root is reimplanted into the left ventricular outflow tract at what was the previous pulmonary valve annulus. (*Continued*)

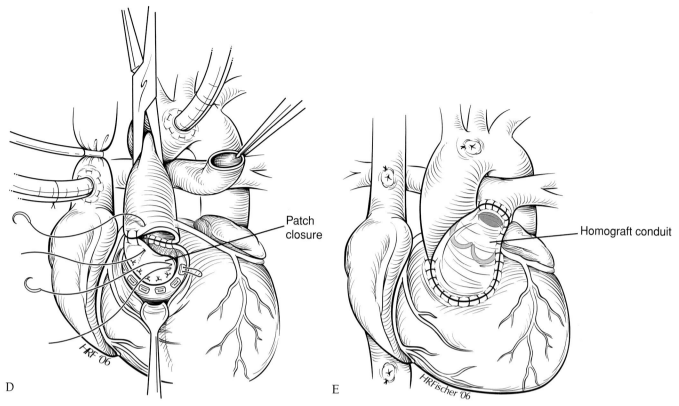

D   E

Figure 85-20. (*Continued*) **(D)** After the aortic root is translocated posteriorly, the anterior VSD is closed with a patch of Dacron or polytetrafluoroethylene material, which is secured anteriorly to the anterior portion of the aortic root, thus baffling the blood from the left ventricle to the aorta. **(E)** The right ventricular outflow tract reconstruction is created with an aortic or pulmonary homograft conduit.

Patch closure

Homograft conduit

the aortic root with aneurysmal dilation of the aorta and progressive aortic insufficiency has been seen in increasing frequency in older patients after the arterial switch operation, perhaps reflecting the abnormal pulmonary arterial wall of the aortic root in these patients. There is also an incidence of asymptomatic occlusion of the coronary artery, which is not completely known, but may have potential implications for these patients as they get into adulthood and middle age.

SUGGESTED READING

Castaneda AR, Trusler GA, Paul MH, et al. Congenital Heart Surgeons Society: The early results of treatment of simple transposition in the current era. J Thorac Cardiovasc Surg 1988;95:14.

Colan SD, Boutin C, Castaneda AR, Wernovsky G. Status of the left ventricle after arterial switch operation for transposition of the great arteries: hemodynamic and echocardiographic evaluation. J Thorac Cardiovasc Surg 1995;109,2:311.

Lecompte Y. Réparation à l'étage ventriculaire— The REV procedure: technique and clinical results. J Cardiol Young 1991;1:63.

Rhodes LA, Wernovsky G, Keane JF, et al. Arrhythmias and intracardiac conduction after the arterial switch operation. J Thorac Cardiovasc Surg 1995;109:303.

Trusler GA, Williams WG, Duncan KF, et al. Results with the Mustard operation in simple transposition of the great arteries. Ann Surg 1987;206:251.

Wernovsky G, Mayer Jr JE, Jonas RA, et al. Factors influencing early and late outcome of the arterial switch operation for transposition of the great arteries. J Thorac Cardiovasc Surg 1995;109:289.

EDITOR'S COMMENTS

Dr. Spray has described, in detail, surgery for transposition of the great arteries. The chapter is complete and the technical detail excellent.

This operation has become the index operation for most surgical programs. Excellent survival is mandatory because survival is essentially based on the technical aspects of the operation. These children should do extremely well; if they do not, mortality relates to coronary ischemia. Dr. Spray is entirely correct in stating that the point of coronary transfer into the aorta is definitely a little bit higher that what would normally seem to be the site in order to avoid kinking. We spend some time with the heart full marking the point of coronary transfer. The only difference in our practice from Dr. Spray's is that we try to avoid circulatory arrest. We use two vena cava cannulas, which seems cumbersome but, in fact, makes the operation a little bit easier. This is particularly helpful when a VSD repair is required.

The major concern of this operation is the late outcome. We too are concerned with dilation of neoaortas. This seems to be particularly true in patients who have had a VSD repair as well. We are concerned that these sinuses will continue to enlarge, but,we have not had any neoaortic roots that had to be repaired. I am certain that this will be a part of our practice in the future.

The arterial switch operation is a huge addition to the care of infants with transposition. The results have been superb, but the procedure requires attention to detail.

I.L.K.

Congenitally Corrected Transposition of the Great Arteries

Victor Bautista-Hernandez and Pedro J. del Nido

Introduction

Congenitally corrected transposition of the great arteries (ccTGA) is a complex cardiac defect, first reported in 1875 by von Rokitansky and representing approximately 1% of all congenital cardiac anomalies. In ccTGA there are discordant connections between the atria and ventricles and between the ventricles and the great arteries. The systemic veins usually connect normally with the right atrium, which then connects to a right-sided, morphologically left ventricle (LV). The morphologic LV connects to the pulmonary artery and is frequently referred to as the "pulmonary" ventricle. On the left side, the pulmonary veins connect normally to the left atrium, which is connected to a left-sided, morphologically right ventricle (RV). The left-sided RV, frequently referred to as the "systemic" ventricle, is connected to the aorta. The atrioventricular (AV) valve morphology corresponds with the ventricle, that is, the mitral valve is the inlet valve for the right-sided, morphologically left ventricle, and the tricuspid valve is the inlet valve for the left-sided right ventricle. The circulatory pathway is therefore in series and normal because systemic venous blood from the right atrium enters the pulmonary circulation, and the pulmonary venous blood is ejected into the systemic circulation via the aorta. Thus, the term "corrected" transposition has been used extensively to describe this lesion, even though anatomically the connections are discordant.

The terminology used to describe this entity has varied and has contributed to the confusion relating to the anatomic connections. In addition, there is a high association with other cardiac defects such as ventricular septal defects (VSDs), subpulmonary obstruction, and abnormal tricuspid valve with septal leaflet attachments. Less frequent is the association of ccTGA with aortic arch abnormalities, particularly in situs inversus. The Van Praagh convention describes the situs, ventricular loop, and relation of the aorta to the pulmonary artery. Thus, the most common form of ccTGA has situs solitus (S), L-loop (L), and the aorta to the left of the pulmonary artery (L), or {S, L, L}. In situs inversus with mirror image anatomy, the defect is classified as {I, D, D}. Alternatively, description of segmental connections had been used to depict ccTGA. The term "atrioventricular discordance" is used to describe the atrioventricular (AV) connection, and "ventriculoarterial discordance" is used to describe the ventriculoarterial (VA) connections. In this convention, the situs must also be described. Regardless of the convention used, it is important to note that the anatomy of the ventricle determines the type of AV valve (mitral or tricuspid), the morphologic RV connects to the aorta and is supporting the systemic circulation, and the AV node and bundle of His are located anteriorly, adjacent to the right AV valve orifice, next to the orifice of the atrial appendage. The elongated and tethered connection between the AV node and His bundle makes these patients more susceptible to conduction defects, including AV block.

Embryology and Anatomy

Early in embryonic development, the primitive heart tube begins to acquire several curvatures that give it an S shape. This transformation, also called looping, does not appear to be so much determined by blood flow characteristics within the developing cardiac segments as be predetermined by the shape and position of the fetal myocardium. Evidence for this comes from experiments in which the cardiac tube was isolated from flow or its attachments and curvature still developed. More recently, genetic manipulations in chick embryos have resulted in mutants that have abnormal development of the cardiac loop. In the human embryo, the normal looping process causes a curvature to the right, and these are referred to as having a "D-loop." Curvature to the left, or L-loop, eventually leads to abnormal connection among the atrial, ventricular, and arterial segments of the developing heart. Furthermore, the normal process of septation and valve formation is also affected so that ventricular morphology is maintained consistent within the ventricular chamber. That is, the AV valve and conduction tissue correspond to the overall morphology of each ventricle. If there is also malseptation of the conotruncus, the aorta will be supported by a complete muscular infundibulum and will arise from the morphologic RV and the pulmonary artery from the morphologic LV. This process of malseptation frequently leads to the existence of a VSD. In fact, a VSD is the most frequent associated anomaly, presenting in approximately 80% of patients with ccTGA. Although the defect can be located at any position, it is usually membranous and large, extending either anteriorly toward the aorta or inferiorly toward the atrioventricular canal. Malposition of the heart is also common. Dextrocardia is present in approximately 25% of cases, and mesocardia is seen in occasional patients.

The abnormal looping process also leads to malalignment of the atrial and ventricular septa and the presence of two AV nodes. One node is at the apex of the triangle of Koch and does not penetrate to the ventricular tissue. A secondary node is located beneath the opening of the atrial appendage in the area of pulmonary valve-to-mitral valve fibrous continuity. This secondary node, first described by Monckeberg in 1913, has a long, penetrating bundle that courses on the anterior segment of the septum below the pulmonary outflow tract for some distance before branching. The anterior and superior position of the conduction bundle is of particular importance when there is a VSD in the membranous septum. When compared with a similar defect in a heart with D-loop, the conduction bundle courses on the opposite or anterior superior edge of the septum as opposed to the posterior inferior edge in a D-looped heart. The exception to this rule is the ccTGA heart with situs inversus, or {I, D, D}, in which the posterior AV node penetrates to connect with the conduction bundle that courses on the posteroinferior rim of the VSD, similar to that in AV concordant hearts.

In the {S, L, L} relationship, the outflow tracts of the two ventricles are most often in a parallel position rather than crossing, as in the normal {S, D, D} heart. Thus, the two ventricles are often in a side-by-side position, although other relationships do exist, such as criss-cross or inferosuperior position. The subpulmonary outflow tract is wedged between the mitral and tricuspid valves, and the pulmonary valve annulus can override the ventricular septum. Thus, hemodynamically significant obstruction of the outflow tract of the morphologic LV is a common finding, occurring in about 40% of patients, particularly in the presence of a VSD. Subaortic obstruction or obstruction of the morphologic RV outflow, however, rarely occurs.

Tricuspid valve anomalies are frequent, occurring in as many as 90% of {S, L, L} hearts when examined at autopsy. Most defects, however, do not cause dysfunction of the valve. The abnormality most frequently described is an Ebstein-like deformity with short, thick chordae arising from the septum tethering the valve. Unlike the Ebstein anomaly, however, apical displacement of the valve annulus, enlargement of the anterior leaflet, and stenosis are rare. Clinically important insufficiency of the tricuspid valve is uncommon in younger children but appears to increase in incidence with age,

being seen an as many as 40% of adults with this deformity. Incompetence of the tricuspid valve is probably the most important adverse prognostic factor. Overriding or straddling of the AV valves can occur but is more commonly seen with hypoplasia of one of the ventricles, mainly RV underdevelopment, or with unusual position of the ventricles (criss-cross or superoinferior).

The coronary arteries in ccTGA are inverted and follow the course appropriate for the ventricle. In {S, L, L}, the right-sided coronary artery arises from the right posterior sinus and gives rise to the anterior descending and circumflex branches. The circumflex coronary courses over the outflow of the pulmonary ventricle and travels in the AV groove around the right-sided mitral valve. The left-sided coronary travels in the AV groove of the morphologic RV around the left-sided tricuspid valve. The origin and distribution of the coronary arteries is quite constant in ccTGA. The most common variation is the existence of a single coronary artery that arises from the right-facing sinus and divides into right and left main branches. In ccTGA there is also a tendency toward early branching of the left main.

Diagnosis

Patients with ccTGA usually present as older infants or children, and the clinical findings are often subtle. Congestive heart failure from excessive pulmonary flow is uncommon, even in the presence of a large VSD, in the first year of life. This is due to the high incidence of pulmonary valvar or, most commonly, subvalvar obstruction restricting pulmonary blood flow. The degree of pulmonary outflow obstruction, however, is infrequently severe enough to warrant surgery early in infancy. Thus, most often the defect manifests itself in older childhood or in the second decade, most commonly with symptoms of exercise intolerance or cyanosis. Tricuspid valve regurgitation and RV dysfunction can appear spontaneously during the second decade of life, exacerbating the symptoms in children. Tricuspid regurgitation is a significant risk factor for death. Some patients with no associated lesions (1% to 2%) can remain asymptomatic during decades and present later in life or at postmortem examination. However, a high late mortality is expected

Bradycardia can be the initial presenting sign, most often caused by complete heart block. AV block can present as intermittent episodes, although usually it will become

permanent in these children. Approximately 5% of infants with ccTGA are born with rhythm disturbances. Conduction tissue is prone to fibrosis of the junction between the AV node and the AV bundle, and complete heart block can develop at any time during the natural history of the disease. This connection can also be congenitally absent. The proportion of patients with complete heart block increases 2%/year to reach 30% by adult life. Conduction defects can also be induced by cardiac surgery, especially when VSD closure is attempted.

The physical findings generally do not provide sufficient information to confirm the diagnosis of ccTGA. The chest radiograph, with a leftward aorta and rightward posterior pulmonary artery placing the hilar vessels more medially and producing a straight left upper heart border, often suggest the diagnosis. An electrocardiogram may demonstrate the presence of AV block, and a Q wave may be present in the right precordial leads.

The diagnosis is most often established by echocardiography, including the ventricular and septal morphology and the position of the two ventricles and their respective outflow tracts. Pulse Doppler and color-flow mapping are used to demonstrate the presence and severity of outflow obstruction and confirm the presence of AV valve regurgitation. Detailed information regarding the size, location, and relationship of VSDs to AV valves can also be obtained from the echocardiogram. Particularly useful is the information the echocardiogram provides regarding the size, function, and chordal attachments of the AV valves.

Cardiac catheterization and cineangiography confirm the ventricular morphology and associated defects such as outflow obstruction, septal defects, and AV valve regurgitation. However, because of the accuracy and sensitivity of the echocardiogram, cardiac catheterization is more often indicated to assess the degree of pulmonary hypertension and to visualize the peripheral pulmonary arteries after previous operations.

Surgical Treatment

Palliative Operations

Palliative procedures are rarely required in infants with ccTGA unless there is severe hypoplasia of one ventricle precluding reparative surgery or if there is severe cyanosis in the neonatal period. Congestive heart failure in children with two adequate-size ventricles and a large VSD is unlikely to present in infancy and can usually be treated by corrective surgery. Severe cyanosis in the neonatal period caused by pulmonary vale or subvalve obstruction is usually treated with a palliative shunt. We prefer to construct a modified Blalock-Taussig shunt from the subclavian to the pulmonary artery using a polytetrafluoroethylene graft 3.5 mm to 4.0 mm in diameter for newborns and young infants, respectively. Subsequent procedures are determined by the ventricular anatomy.

Because of the frequent existence of subvalvar, valvar, and/or supravalvar pulmonary obstruction, banding is rarely required. Furthermore, pulmonary artery banding has been identified as a risk factor for the development of aortic root dilation and aortic regurgitation in patients who subsequently underwent an arterial switch procedure. However, when a double-switch procedure is planned, particularly in an older infant, and the left ventricular pressure has been less than approximately two thirds of the right ventricular pressure, a pulmonary artery banding may be necessary to prepare the left ventricle, that is, increase left ventricular muscle mass.

If a single-ventricle approach is planned, a bidirectional Glenn shunt can be performed followed by a total cavopulmonary connection. The univentricular strategy should be reserved for patients in whom an anatomic repair is not feasible. In patients with severe ventricular hypoplasia and/or associated straddling AV valves, a univentricular repair is usually advocated. The existence of multiple VSDs or the unsuitability for baffling the VSD to the aorta may also preclude a biventricular repair. For the Fontan operation we usually perform a lateral tunnel constructed of polytetrafluoroethylene. The prosthesis is usually fenestrated to permit some right-to-left shunting early after surgery, which has been shown to shorten the period of recovery. The anastomosis between the right atrium and the right pulmonary artery is usually supplemented in the anterior surface with a rhomboidal patch to avoid stenosis of the anastomosis. No ventricular incisions are made.

Another option in patients with ccTGA and small or poorly functioning pulmonary ventricle is the 1 1/2 ventricular repair. Introduced by Billingsley et al., this approach combines a bidirectional Glenn shunt with intracardiac correction. Although some authors have reported good results with this strategy, an anatomic repair is preferred unless there is severe hypoplasia of the morphologic right ventricle, in which case a Fontan procedure may be preferable.

Intracardiac Repair

Repair of ccTGA has been possible since the late 1950s. The so-called "classic" or "physiologic" approach addresses only the associated defects such as VSD or subpulmonary obstruction but leaves the morphologic RV connected to the systemic circulation. The potential drawbacks of this approach are the risk of injury of the conduction system from the VSD closure and late tricuspid valve regurgitation and RV dysfunction. For these reasons, this approach has fallen into disfavor.

Closure of Ventricular Septal Defects

The most common location for VSD in ccTGA is in the conoventricular or membranous septum. The defect is often a malalignment type, with the pulmonary valve overriding the septum. AV canal (inlet) defects and conal septal defects (single or multiple) can also occur in association with ccTGA.

Because of the unusual course of the specialized conduction tissue and the difficulty often encountered in visualizing the VSD, several techniques have been developed to close the VSD in children with ccTGA. The usual approach to the defect is through the right atrium, with the right-sided mitral valve retracted. As recommended by de Leval and associates, the stitches should be placed on the morphologic right ventricular side of the septum, particularly in the danger area of the conduction tissue (anterosuperior). If the VSD cannot be seen well through the mitral valve, the valve can be partially taken down by incising the leaflets near the base of the anterior commissure into the mural leaflet, exposing the subpulmonary area of the VSD. Alternatively, the VSD can be approached through the aortic valve or, if a conduit between the right-sided ventricle and pulmonary artery is required, through a ventriculotomy in the right-sided LV. Although the VSD can be seen through the pulmonary valve, we do not recommend closing the VSD through it because the traction often required to expose the defect can cause injury to the conduction tissue running in the subpulmonary infundibulum.

In the {S, L, L} type of ccTGA, the conduction tissue runs in the subpulmonary infundibulum and along the anterior border of the VSD. To avoid injury to the conduction tissue, the sutures must be placed on the left (systemic) side of the defect anteriorly 3 mm to 4 mm away from the edge of the defect (Fig. 86-1). Posteriorly, left-sided tricuspid valve frequently has attachments to the edge of the VSD, and therefore the

sutures need to be placed on the morphologic left ventricular side of the VSD. Commonly, the mitral and tricuspid valves are in fibrous continuity, and the VSD patch is attached to this fibrous structure.

If the aortic root is sufficiently large, the VSD can be closed through the aortic valve. In this case, all the sutures are placed on the left (systemic) side of the VSD. Care must be taken, however, not to interfere with the chordae or leaflets of the tricuspid valve because this may cause systemic AV valve insufficiency.

In patients with situs inversus {I, D, D} and ccTGA, the conduction tissue runs posteriorly on the edge of the septal defect. In this case the entire VSD patch can be placed on the left (pulmonary) side of the VSD with the posterior suture line staying 3 mm to 4 mm away from the edge of the defect.

Repair of Subpulmonary Obstruction

Pulmonary or subpulmonary obstruction is found in 30% to 50% of patients with ccTGA and is most often caused by a narrowed outflow tract that is wedged posteriorly between the two AV valves and accessory mitral valve chordae attaching to the subpulmonary area. In cases in which the obstruction is primarily valvar with an adequate pulmonary valve annulus, simple valvotomy may be sufficient to relieve the obstruction. On occasion, a subvalvar fibrous membrane, accessory mitral valve tissue, or an aneurysm of the membranous septum may be the major source of obstruction. In those cases, resection of the extra tissue may be all that is necessary. Resection of subpulmonary myocardium should not be done because this is likely to lead to AV block as a result of the presence of the conduction bundle in the subpulmonary area.

If a "physiologic" repair of ccTGA and LV outflow obstruction is contemplated, an extracardiac conduit is often required to adequately relieve subpulmonary obstruction. A site for the ventriculotomy to accommodate the conduit connection must be chosen carefully. Usually the anterior surface inferiorly on the morphologic LV is chosen, away from the papillary muscles. This maneuver usually requires direct inspection of the papillary muscles from an atriotomy or digital palpation of the papillaries through the mitral valve to prevent direct injury or damage to their blood supply. Allograft valved conduits are most frequently used, although a nonvalved synthetic tube graft can also be used when pulmonary resistance is low and the distal pulmonary arteries are of adequate size. Because of the distance

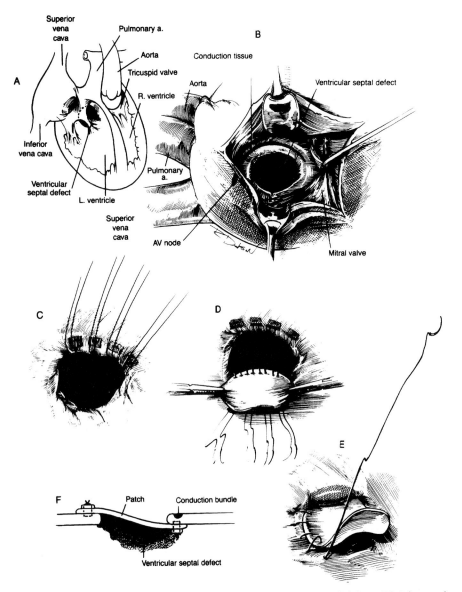

Figure 86-1. Congenitally corrected transposition and ventricular septal defect. **(A)** Schema of the anatomic relationship {S, L, L}. **(B)** Transatrial exposure of the ventricular septal defect (VSD). Note the anterior location of the atrioventricular (AV) node between the right AV valve and the stoma of the right atrial appendage. **(C)** To avoid damage to the conduction tissue, interrupted horizontal mattress sutures reinforced with polytetrafluoroethylene (Teflon) pledgets are guided through the defect and anchored approximately 4 mm from the edge of the VSD within the left-sided ventricular surface, particularly along the anterior and superior rim of the defect. **(D)** Interrupted sutures are passed through the polyester (Dacron) patch. **(E)** The remainder of the patch is sewn to the rim of the VSD with a continuous suture. **(F)** Schematic representation of anchoring of the patch within the right ventricular surface anteriorly and on the left ventricular surface posteriorly. (a. = artery; L. = left; R = right.) (Reprinted with permission from AR Castaneda, RA Jonas, JE Mayer, et al. Cardiac Surgery of the Neonate and Infant. Philadelphia: Saunders, 1994;440.)

between the ventriculotomy and the distal main pulmonary artery, a tube graft extension is frequently needed to extend the allograft valved conduits. The tube graft is most often sewn to the valve annulus of the homograft and should be of sufficient length to place the allograft valve away from

the posterior surface of the heart to prevent compression by the sternum. However, compression of the conduit is not uncommon and may be avoided by opening the right pleura and positioning the conduit to the right over the right atrium and by delaying sternal closure.

Repair of Left Atrioventricular Valve

Left-sided tricuspid valve insufficiency is usually seen late, even though anomalies of the leaflets are a common finding. Exposure of the tricuspid valve can be difficult because of its more anterior location. Incision of the interatrial septum may be required. A left thoracotomy approach exposing the valve through the left atrium has also been advocated. This approach also facilitates closure of a VSD by placing the VSD patch on the left side of the defect and away from conduction tissue.

Repair of the regurgitant tricuspid valve is rarely successful but may be attempted if annular dilation or inadequate leaflet coaptation at a commissure is the underlying cause of the insufficiency. Valve replacement is most often required, and the same considerations regarding the choice of the type and size of prosthesis apply to patients with ccTGA as to patients with normal ventricular connections.

Anatomic Repair

Double-Switch Operation. This approach should be used in the rare cases in which there is no subpulmonary obstruction or the subpulmonary obstruction is due to accessory mitral or tricuspid valve tissue that can be resected without affecting valve function. An arterial switch procedure is performed, transposing the great vessels and the coronary arteries to achieve an anatomic repair without the need for a conduit.

The operation is performed through a standard median sternotomy. The thymus is partially resected, and a large section of anterior pericardium is harvested and treated with 0.6% glutaraldehyde for 10 minutes approximately. The ascending aorta and the branch pulmonary arteries are dissected free for later mobilization. The patient is then cannulated through the aorta and vena caves. Care must be taken in placing the cannulas as far from the surgical field as possible. Moderate hypothermic cardiopulmonary bypass is then established, and the patient is cooled to 25°C to 28°C. At this point, control should be obtained of any systemic-to-pulmonary shunts, which should then be divided. The main pulmonary artery is transected with the heart fibrillating or arrested, and the pulmonary valve is carefully inspected. Valvotomy or resection of the subpulmonary extra tissue is performed when necessary. As previously described, excision of subpulmonary myocardium should not be done.

Subsequently, a right atriotomy is carried out parallel to the AV groove, and the interatrial septum is exposed. The septum primum as well as the roof of the atrial septum is widely resected to facilitate baffling of the systemic venous return to the posterior tricuspid valve. Either the Senning procedure or the Mustard baffling operation can be performed with similar results. However, in patients with atrial adhesions from previous palliative procedures or in those with dextrocardia and small right atrium the Senning procedure may be technically quite difficult, and therefore a Mustard operation is preferred. In some cases of dextrocardia, opening the left pleural space and displacing the heart into the left pleural cavity may improve exposure to the atrium and therefore may allow performance of a Senning procedure. For the Mustard operation, glutaraldehyde-treated pericardium is used to baffle the inferior and superior vena cavae to the posterior pulmonary ventricle and, by exclusion, the pulmonary veins to the anterior systemic ventricle. Supplementation of the right atrium with a patch of pericardium or prosthetic material is advised to provide an unobstructed pulmonary venous pathway in the Senning procedure, particularly in cases of dextrocardia.

Because the double-switch procedure is technically demanding and usually requires a long cross-clamp time, the atrial switch procedure can be performed with the heart cold fibrillating, taking care to maintain adequate coronary perfusion pressure and the ventricles adequately vented. For the arterial switch part of the procedure, the aorta is cross-clamped and the heart arrested with cold blood cardioplegia. The aorta is transected and the VSD closed, as previously described. Although the VSD can be closed through the right atrium, we usually prefer to transect the aorta as needed for the arterial switch procedure and inspect the VSD through the neo-pulmonary valve once the coronary buttons have been removed because this usually affords more direct access to the VSD away from conduction tissue. Subsequently, an arterial switch procedure is undertaken. Coronary translocation may be difficult in cases of side-by-side vessel orientation. Often there is a relatively short left main, and extensive mobilization is usually needed. This is also the case when a single coronary artery is present. The Lecompte maneuver is also undertaken, except in the rare cases of posterior aorta. For reconstruction of the coronary button areas in the neo-pulmonary artery a trouser-shaped patch of autologous treated pericardium works best. Transesophageal echocardiography is performed to exclude baffle pathway obstruction and to determine the status of the LV and RV outflow tracts. It is also useful to place a central venous catheter for measuring the gradient across the superior vena cava.

If during rewarming or before the surgery there is evidence of complete AV block, placement of permanent dual-chamber epicardial leads should be considered. In patients with AV valve regurgitation, a DDD-mode atrioventricular sequential pacemaker improves cardiac output and AV valve function.

Senning (or Mustard) plus Rastelli Operation. An alternative approach in children with a VSD and subpulmonary obstruction is to divert the morphologic LV outflow through the VSD to the aorta in combination with an atrial level switch procedure (Senning or Mustard). Incision, cannulation, and cardiopulmonary bypass are performed as previously described. The approach to the VSD is through the infundibulum of the left-sided RV via an infundibular incision, and an intracardiac baffle is then constructed to divert the VSD to the aorta (Fig. 86-2). The VSD may be enlarged to assure an unobstructed connection between the LV and the aorta; however, this carries a very high risk of inducing complete heart block and should only be considered if the defect appears restrictive. The baffle is sutured to the septum away from the edge of the VSD anteriorly to avoid injury to the conduction tissue. Posteriorly, the baffle is attached to the fibrous continuity between the tricuspid and mitral valve. The site for the ventriculotomy is carefully selected as described earlier, and the Senning or Mustard procedure is subsequently undertaken.

Establishment of RV-to-pulmonary artery continuity may be performed with a *réparation à l'étage ventriculaire* as described by Lecompte in 1982, or, most commonly, with an extracardiac valved conduit. In the first case, an anteriorly placed patch is usually needed to supplement the anastomosis. The technique for placing the extracardiac conduit was described earlier. The RV-to-pulmonary artery conduit is usually a homograft and is best placed to the left of the aorta to avoid compression by the sternum.

Results

"Classic" Repair and Univentricular Repair
In 1957 Anderson and Lillehei reported their initial experience with ccTGA at the University of Minnesota. This approach was directed at treating the associated lesions, and the RV remained in the systemic circuit. Although that therapy resulted in improved outcomes, the operative risk remained relatively high (14% to 15%), and the actuarial survival at 10 years was low (55% to 85%). These disappointing results were related to late tricuspid regurgitation and RV dysfunction. The suboptimal results obtained with the so-called "classic" approach has moved surgeons since the mid-1990s to place the LV supporting the systemic circulation with the hope of improving surgical results and long-term outcomes.

In experience at Children's Hospital Boston with classic and univentricular repair for ccTGA between 1963 and 1996, 123 patients underwent a "classic" approach or a Fontan procedure. Actuarial survival was 84% at 1 year, 75% at 5 years, 68% at 10 years, and 61% at 20 years. Risk factors for death by multivariable analysis were RV end-diastolic pressure of >17 mm Hg before operation, complete heart block after operation, subvalvular pulmonary stenosis, Ebstein-like malformation of the tricuspid valve, and preoperative systemic RV dysfunction. The best outcomes were seen in patients undergoing the Fontan procedure, whereas the poorest outlook was seen in patients who required tricuspid valve replacement.

Anatomic Repair
In 1990, Ilbawi and coworkers first reported successful anatomic correction in two patients, aged 31 and 38 months, respectively, with {S, L, L} ccTGA by means of a Mustard plus Rastelli procedure. One of the children had pulmonary atresia, and the other had dextrocardia with severe subpulmonic infundibular stenosis. Both patients had a large, nonrestrictive VSD. No postoperative heart block was seen. Two years later, Di Donato and colleagues adopted the principle of anatomic repair and repaired two cases of {I, D, D} ccTGA and nonrestrictive malalignment VSDs. Previous palliative systemic-to-pulmonary shunting had been placed in both children. Their ages were 3 1/3 and 9 years, respectively. Both patients were discharged home in good condition.

In 1993 Yamagishi, Imai, and others reported a series of 11 patients with a median age of 6.7 years, 5 with ccTGA and 6 with double-outlet right ventricle, in whom anatomic repair was undertaken. Three patients with situs solitus and ccTGA received a double-switch procedure. The Senning plus arterial switch operation was performed in 2 patients, and the Mustard plus arterial switch in 1. This last patient had dextrocardia and grade III tricuspid regurgitation and

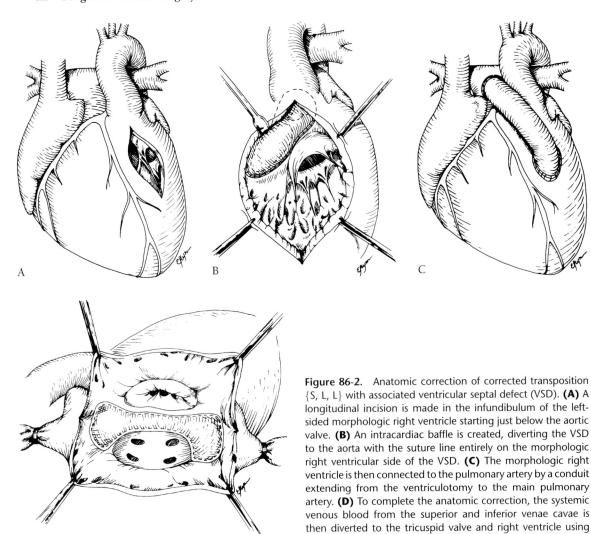

A

B

C

D

Figure 86-2. Anatomic correction of corrected transposition {S, L, L} with associated ventricular septal defect (VSD). **(A)** A longitudinal incision is made in the infundibulum of the left-sided morphologic right ventricle starting just below the aortic valve. **(B)** An intracardiac baffle is created, diverting the VSD to the aorta with the suture line entirely on the morphologic right ventricular side of the VSD. **(C)** The morphologic right ventricle is then connected to the pulmonary artery by a conduit extending from the ventriculotomy to the main pulmonary artery. **(D)** To complete the anatomic correction, the systemic venous blood from the superior and inferior venae cavae is then diverted to the tricuspid valve and right ventricle using a pericardial or polytetrafluoroethylene baffle.

was the only hospital death in the series. One year later, Yagihara and coworkers published excellent results of anatomic repair in 10 patients with ccTGA, 2 of them undergoing the Mustard plus arterial switch operation. The largest series of anatomic repair for ccTGA was presented by Imai et al. in 2001. Between 1989 and 2000, 76 patients underwent anatomic repair for ccTGA. Surgery at the atrial level consisted of 47 Mustard and 29 Senning procedures. Arterial switch operation was performed in 14 patients, external conduit in 40, direct anastomosis between the RV and the pulmonary artery in 21, and intraventricular rerouting in 1 patient. Mean age at operation was 6.6 years (range 3 months to 15 years). In-hospital mortality was 7.9% with 4 late deaths. At a mean follow-up of 5 years, 64 patients were in New York Heart Association class I and 2 patients were in class II.

In a series of 27 patients with ccTGA published by Imamura et colleagues, 22 under-

went anatomic repair at Cleveland Clinic. Senning plus arterial switch was performed in 10 patients and Senning plus Rastelli in 12. LV retraining by means of pulmonary artery banding was performed in 6 patients. At a median follow-up of 27.8 months, there were no early or late mortality, and tricuspid valve function improved in all patients but 1. Two patients required pacemaker implantation. In a previous study of the same institution, Poirier and Mee reported 84 patients, 45 with ccTGA, who underwent LV reconditioning in preparation for an arterial switch procedure. The overall mortality was 15.4%, with all deaths occurring in patients with D-transposition. Ninety-one percent of survivors presented normal LV function at follow-up.

In 2002, Ilbawi and associates updated their results and reported intermediate follow-up of a series of 12 patients with ccTGA. Palliative systemic-to-pulmonary artery shunts were performed in 10 patients.

Two patients received a double-switch operation and 10 a Mustard plus Rastelli. The mean age at operation was 9 months. In-hospital mortality was 9% (1 patient). At a median follow-up of 7.1 years, all hospital survivors were asymptomatic. Five patients required RV-to-pulmonary artery conduit replacement after a mean interval of 5.3 years.

Results reported by Devaney et al. from the University of Michigan achieved successful double-switch operation in 17 patients with ccTGA with no early or late mortality. Seven patients underwent pulmonary artery banding for left ventricular retraining, and 1 patient required heart transplantation. Mean follow-up was 36 months.

From March 1992 to January 2002, 28 patients with a median age of 1.7 years underwent anatomic correction at Children's Hospital Boston for {S, L, L} (24 patients) or {I, D, D} (4 patients) ccTGA. Associated cardiac anomalies were VSD and pulmonary stenosis in 12 patients, VSD in 8 patients, and VSD and pulmonary atresia in 7 patients. Preoperative palliative systemic-to-pulmonary shunt was performed in 10 children. Two patients required pulmonary banding for LV preparation. At the atrial level 20 Senning and 8 Mustard procedures were done. Ventriculoarterial concordance was reestablished by a Rastelli approach in 17 patients and by arterial switch in 11. There were 2 early deaths (7%), and 1 patient required heart transplantation. Six patients underwent pacemaker implantation for complete heart block. At a median follow-up of 1.2 years (range 5 days to 7.6 years), 88% of patients had preserved ventricular function and 11 patients required reinterventions, including homograft angioplasty (4), systemic venous obstruction (3), device closure of baffle leak (2), revision of pulmonary venous obstruction (2), pacemaker replacement (1), and conduit change (1).

Recently, Langley and coworkers reported their experience with a large series of 54 patients, 51 with ccTGA and 3 with double-outlet right ventricle. In the group of patients with ccTGA, 29 underwent a double-switch procedure and 22 a Senning plus Rastelli. Median age at operation and follow-up was 3.2 and 4.4 years, respectively. Early mortality was 5.6%, and 2 late deaths occurred. There were no statistically significant differences between groups in terms of survival or freedom from reoperation. The most frequent early morbidity was complete heart block. Interestingly, 4 patients with previous pulmonary artery banding developed postoperative aortic regurgitation in the double-switch group.

Despite excellent results for anatomic repair of ccTGA with respect to RV and tricuspid valve function, postoperative LV dysfunction late, after repair has been reported and remains a concern. We have recently updated our experience on anatomic repair for ccTGA, especially focusing on late LV performance. From August 1992 to July 2005, 44 patients (median age at surgery 1.6 years; range from 0.6 to 39.6 years) with ccTGA had anatomic repair. Twenty-three patients had a Rastelli procedure while 21 underwent an arterial switch. Twelve patients (27%) were pacemaker dependent at latest follow-up. Early mortality was 4.5% (n = 2) with one late death from leukemia. Median follow-up was 3 years (range from 7 days to 12.4 years). LV function deteriorated in 8 patients (18%). Development of LV dysfunction was significantly associated with pacemaker implantation and a widened QRS (>20%, >98% percentile of normal).

Resynchronization may be of value in patients requiring a pacemaker.

SUGGESTED READING

Victor Bautista-Hemandez, Gerald R. Marx, Kilmberlee Gauvreau, et al. Maxwell Chamberiain memorial paper for congenital heart surgery: determinants of left ventricular dysfunction after anatomic repair of congenitally corrected transposition of the great arteries. Ann Thorac Surg 2006, In press.

Bove EL. Congenitally corrected transposition of the great arteries: ventricle to pulmonary artery connection strategies. Semin Thorac Cardiovasc Surg 1995;7:139.

Connelly MS, Liu PP, Williams WG, et al. Congenitally corrected transposition of the great arteries in the adult: functional status and complications. J Am Coll Cardiol 1996;27:1238.

Devaney EJ, Charpie JR, Ohye RG, Bobe EL. Combined arterial switch procedure and Senning operation for congenitally corrected transposition of the great arteries: Patient selection and intermediate results. J Thorac Cardiovasc Surg 2003;125:500.

Di Donato R, Troconis C, Marino B, et al. Combined Mustard and Rastelli operations: an alternative approach for repair of associated anomalies in congenitally corrected transposition in situs inversus (IDD). J Thorac Cardovasc Surg 1992;104:1246.

Feingold B, O'Sullivan B, del Nido P, Pollack P. Situs inversus totalis and corrected transposition of the great arteries {I,D,D} in association with a previously unreported vascular ring. Pediatr Cardiol 2001;22:338.

Fyler DC. Corrected transposition of the great arteries. In: *Nadas' Pediatric Cardiology.* Philadelphia, Hanley and Belfus, 1992.

Graham Jr TP, Bernard YD, Mellen BG, et al. Long-term outcome in congenitally corrected transposition of the great arteries: a multi-institutional study. J Am Coll Cardiol 2000;36:255.

Hancock Friesen CL, Jonas RA, Del Nido PJ, et al. Anatomic repair of corrected transposition of the great arteries. Circulation 2002;106(Suppl II):395.

Hraska V, Duncan BW, Mayer Jr JE, et al. Long-term outcome of surgically treated patients with corrected transposition of the great arteries. J Thorac Cardiovasc Surg 2005;129:182.

Ilbawi MN, DeLeon SY, Backer CL, et al. An alternative approach to the surgical management for physiologically corrected transposition with ventricular septal defect and pulmonary stenosis or atresia. J Thorac Cardiovasc Surg 1990;100:410.

Ilbawi MN, Ocampo CB, Allen BS, et al. Intermediate results of the anatomic repair for congenitally corrected transposition. Ann Thorac Surg 2002;73:594.

Imai Y, Seo K, Aoki M, et al. Double-switch operation for congenitally corrected transposition. Semin Thorac Cardiovasc Surg Pediatr Card

Surg Annu 2001;4:16.

Imamura M, Drummond-Web JJ, Murphy DJ, et al. Results of double switch operation in the current era. Ann Thorac Surg 2000;70:100.

Kirklin JW, Barratt-Boyes BG. Congenitally Corrected Transposition of the Great Arteries. In: *Cardiac Surgery.* New York: Churchill Livingstone, 2003:1549.

Langley SM, Winlaw DS, Stumper O, et al. Midterm results after restoration of the morphologically LV to the systemic circulation in patients with congenitally corrected transposition of the great arteries. J Thorac Cardiovasc Surg 2003;125:1229.

Mauvroudis C, Backer C. Physiologic versus anatomic repair of congenitally corrected transposition of the great arteries. Semin Thorac Cardiovasc Surg Pediatr Card Surg Annu 2003;6:16.

McKay R, Anderson RH, Smith A. The coronary arteries in hearts with discordant atrioventricular connections. J Thorac Cardiovasc Surg 1996;11:988.

Moons P, Gewilling M, Sluysmans T, et al. Long-term outcome up to 30 years after the Mustard or Senning operation: A nationwide multicentre study in Belgium. Heart 2004;90:307.

Poirier NC, Mee RB. Left ventricular reconditioning and anatomical correction for systemic right ventricular dysfunction. Semin Thorac Cardiovasc Surg Pediatr Card Surg Annu 2003;3:198.

Presbitero P, Somerville J, Rabajoli F, et al. Corrected transposition of the great arteries without associated defects in adult patients: clinical profile and follow-up. Br Heart J 1995;74:57.

Prieto LR, Hordof AJ, Secic M, et al. Progressive tricuspid valve disease in patients with congenitally corrected transposition of the great arteries. Circulation 1998;98:997.

Sano T, Riesenfeld T, Karl TR, et al. Intermediate-term outcome after intracardiac repair of associated cardiac defects in patients with atrioventricular and ventriculoarterial discordance. Circulation 1995;92(9 Suppl):II-272.

Sarkar D, Bull C, Yates R, et al. Comparison of long-term outcomes of atrial repair of simple transposition with implications for a late arterial switch strategy. Circulation 1999;100(19 Suppl):II-176.

Schwartz ML, Gauvreau K, del Nido P, et al. Long-term predictors of aortic root dilatation and aortic regurgitation after arterial switch operation. Circulation 2004;110(11 Suppl 1):II-128.

Voskuil M, Hazekamp MG, Kroft LJ, et al. Post-surgical course of patients with congenitally corrected transposition of the great arteries. Am J Cardiol 1999;83:558.

Yagihara T, Kishimoto H, Isobe F, et al. Double switch operation in cardiac anomalies with atrioventricular and ventriculoarterial discordance. J Thorac Cardiovasc Surg 1994;107:351.

Yamagishi Y, Imai Y, Hoshino S, et al. Anatomic

correction of atrioventricular discordance. J Thorac Cardiovasc Surg 1993;105:1067.

EDITOR'S COMMENTS

ccTGA, or {S,L,L} transposition, continues to present a challenge for surgical intervention. The tenuous nature of the conducting tissue in this condition has resulted in a significant incidence of late complete AV block with or without surgical intervention. Despite attention to the surgical details of VSD closure, AV block continues to be a late problem requiring pacemaker insertion in up to one third of cases. In addition, even with direct intracardiac repair, patients are left with a systemic morphologic right ventricle with often an abnormal AV valve and, in addition, frequently a conduit from the morphologic left ventricle to the pulmonary arteries that will require replacement. Thus, the incidence of late reoperation is high and the problem of late systemic ventricular dysfunction significant. Valve reparative procedures on the left side of the heart to the abnormal anatomic tricuspid valve have not been particularly successful, and valve replacement has been associated with late ventricular function deterioration and the complications of prosthetic heart valve insertion. Even conversion to the single-ventricle type of morphology in patients with significant pulmonary stenosis has not been associated with improved long-term results because left AV valve regurgitation may compromise ventricular performance after conversion to single-ventricle physiology. The suboptimal late results have led some authors to suggest the use of a double-switch procedure for selected patients with {S,L,L} anatomy. As described by Dr. del Nido and associates, the double-switch procedure creates a Senning or Mustard baffle at the atrial level associated with closure of the VSD to the pulmonary artery and an arterial switch procedure at the level of the great vessels. In this case, the anatomic left ventricle becomes the systemic ventricle, and ventricular inflow is switched at the atrial level. The abnormal tricuspid valve then is associated with the pulmonary ventricle, which is presumably at a lower pressure, and therefore the regurgitation is better tolerated. The use of this technique has been relatively rare, and the long-term follow-up results for these patients are unknown, although the number of series reported in the literature is increasing every few years. As nicely summarized by the authors of this chapter, there are now several series with significant numbers of patients being reported with intermediate short-term follow-ups of up to 5 years with a low incidence of atrial arrhythmias but with the need for reoperation in a significant number of the patients. Overall mortality, however, has been quite low. The known problems of atrial arrhythmias from atrial baffles and the need for conduit revision with these repairs may very well limit the long-term durability of the operation even though ventricular function may be preserved. The operation may also be used for patients with right ventricular dysfunction and tricuspid regurgitation who present later in life either without prior palliative procedures or with prior palliative shunts or bands. Some patients who have had late ventricular deterioration after complete intracardiac repairs despite good anatomic results have had sufficient cardiac dysfunction to require cardiac transplantation for corrected transposition.

T.L.S.

87

Pulmonary Stenosis and Pulmonary Atresia with Intact Septum

Mark D. Plunkett and Hillel Laks

Pulmonary Stenosis

Pulmonary stenosis at the valvar level has been reported to account for 8% to 10% of all congenital heart defects. Although critical pulmonary stenosis may present in the newborn period and may require immediate intervention, most of these lesions are less severe and present after the neonatal period. The pulmonary valve is usually stenotic and dome shaped with a small central orifice. The right ventricle is usually normal in size, but secondary hypertrophy of the ventricle and infundibulum may occur. The etiology is not known and is probably multifactorial. There is a reported increased incidence of 2% to 4% in siblings of patients with this defect. Treatment of this congenital defect with either balloon valvotomy or surgical valvotomy is associated with low morbidity and mortality and excellent long-term outcomes.

Diagnostic Considerations

Infants with critical pulmonary stenosis may present in the newborn period with severe cyanosis and heart failure. The clinical manifestations are relative to the severity of the stenosis and the patency of a foramen ovale or an atrial septal defect. In most children with pulmonary valve stenosis and intact ventricular septum, symptoms develop more slowly. Most patients are initially identified by a harsh systolic ejection murmur and a thrill over the pulmonic region on physical examination. An electrocardiogram usually reveals right-axis deviation, prominent P waves, and right ventricular (RV) hypertrophy. A chest radiograph may show

prominent pulmonary artery shadows secondary to poststenotic dilation. The heart shadow is normal except in severe cases with congestive failure. Subsequent studies should include echocardiography to establish the severity of the lesion and identify associated abnormalities. Doppler evaluation allows estimation of the gradient across the valve and right ventricular outflow tract. Finally, cardiac catheterization may be performed for additional diagnostic information and for therapeutic intervention with balloon valvotomy.

Surgical Treatment and Techniques

Patients with pulmonary valve stenosis and intact ventricular septum require intervention for symptomatic lesions and for significant transvalvular pressure gradients. Historically, surgery was the mainstay of therapy for isolated pulmonary valvar stenosis. Currently, however, catheterization with balloon valvotomy has replaced surgery as the cornerstone of initial treatment. In cases of recurrent stenosis, repeat balloon valvotomy may be attempted before surgical therapy. The incidence of pulmonary insufficiency after balloon valvotomy is high (80%), but it is clinically mild and tolerated well in most patients. Failed balloon valvotomy can be an indication for urgent surgical intervention. Surgical pulmonary valvotomy may be performed as an open technique using cardiopulmonary bypass or through a closed transventricular approach. Operative mortality is minimal except in cases of critical stenosis with associated RV hypoplasia and congestive heart failure. The

results of treatment are directly related to the size of the RV chamber and the age of the patient at presentation.

Open Pulmonary Valvotomy Using Cardiopulmonary Bypass

Exposure for open pulmonary valvotomy is obtained through a median sternotomy. After heparinization, an aortic cannula is placed in the ascending aorta, and bicaval cannulation is performed. Snares are placed around the inferior and superior venae cavae. A catheter is placed in the ascending aorta for the antegrade delivery of cold blood cardioplegia. A patent ductus arteriosus must be ligated or snared at the initiation of cardiopulmonary bypass. An aortic cross-clamp is applied, and cardioplegia is delivered antegrade to achieve myocardial arrest.

A longitudinal pulmonary arteriotomy is performed above the level of the valve commissures. The stenotic valve is inspected, and the fused commissures are identified and carefully incised with a No. 11 scalpel blade. The incisions should extend to the annulus. Any valvar adhesions to the pulmonary arterial wall are sharply incised. A partial valvectomy may be performed to remove thickened valve tissue or dense scarring on the leaflets. Dysplastic portions of the valve may require excision. The infundibulum is then inspected through the valve for any residual subvalvular stenosis. Sharp infundibular resection through the valve should be performed if necessary. Rarely, a ventriculotomy is required with an infundibular or transannular patch closure. If a small annulus is present, a Hegar dilator may be used to size the valve annulus.

The need for a transannular patch can be determined based on this measurement. If there is supravalvular hypoplasia, a pericardial patch is used to close the incision in the pulmonary artery from the annulus to the base of the left pulmonary artery. The arteriotomy is otherwise closed with a running polypropylene (Prolene) suture.

If there is evidence of an atrial septal defect or patent foramen ovale, a right atriotomy is performed and the atrial septum is inspected. Closure of a patent foramen ovale or atrial septal defect is performed using primary closure or pericardial patch closure with a running Prolene suture technique. The tricuspid valve leaflets are retracted to expose the infundibular outflow tract. Infundibular resection may be performed through the tricuspid valve to relieve any remaining stenosis. The tricuspid valve is tested for competence before closure. The atriotomy is then closed in a two-layer fashion with a running Prolene suture.

The patient is weaned from cardiopulmonary bypass. If the right ventricle is hypoplastic, a patent foramen ovale is left open or controlled with an adjustable snare. Measurements of pressure in the right ventricle and the main pulmonary artery will document any residual gradient and should be performed before decannulation. Intraoperative transesophageal echocardiography may be used to assess any residual gradient or pulmonary valve insufficiency. There is often a small residual gradient across the valve postoperatively, which may regress with time.

Off-Pump Transventricular Pulmonary Valvotomy

If a restrictive patent foramen ovale is present or the atrial septum is intact, pulmonary valvotomy may be performed using a closed technique that avoids the use of cardiopulmonary bypass. A wet pump should be available on standby for possible use if necessary. A median sternotomy is used, and a purse string of 4-0 Prolene suture is placed on the anterior aspect of the right ventricle just below the infundibulum. A 14-gauge angiocatheter with a pressure transducer is first introduced through the right ventricle into the pulmonary artery. Hegar dilators of progressively larger sizes (up to 7 mm or 8 mm) are then introduced across the valve. If the membrane does not dilate easily, a long vascular clamp can be passed through the purse string and right ventricle to disrupt the valve membrane. We now prefer the use of a balloon dilation catheter with a balloon,

1 mm larger in diameter than the annulus of the pulmonary artery. The balloon can be positioned by measurement and by palpation. A needle pressure transducer is then used to assess the remaining gradient across the valve. After adequate dilation is achieved, the purse string is tied and an additional reinforcing suture is placed in the ventricular epicardium.

Perioperative Management

Most patients with pulmonary stenosis are operated on electively with routine preoperative and postoperative care. Neonates with critical stenosis should be stabilized in the intensive care unit and operated on as soon as possible. Acidosis, electrolyte abnormalities, and congestive heart failure are corrected preoperatively.

These patients may also have stenosis in the infundibular region secondary to RV myocardial hypertrophy. Inotropes must be used with caution in the preoperative and postoperative periods because increased contractility may cause increased dynamic obstruction across the pulmonary outflow tract and further compromise pulmonary blood flow.

Postoperative Care and Surgical Complications

Postoperative care for patients after surgical pulmonary valvotomy should focus on adequate RV filling pressures and reduced pulmonary artery pressures. Pulmonary vasodilators may be used in the early postoperative period to increase pulmonary flow and reduce RV afterload. Inotropic support may be useful for the first few days.

Transthoracic monitoring catheters may be placed in the right atrium or through the right ventricle into the pulmonary artery to continuously monitor hemodynamics postoperatively. These are generally discontinued within the first 48 hours.

Pulmonary insufficiency may result from either open or closed valvotomy. Most patients will tolerate this residual valve incompetence with little difficulty. RV dysfunction may be present in the early postoperative period. This is usually transient, but may require moderate inotropic support during the early postoperative recovery.

If the obstruction is adequately relieved, any residual infundibular hypertrophy will regress over time. Most patients recover without complications, and long-term outcomes are excellent for both balloon valvotomy and surgical valvotomy.

Pulmonary Atresia with Intact Septum

Pulmonary atresia with intact septum (PA/IVS) represents between 1% and 3% of all congenital heart defects. The exact cause or event that leads to pulmonary atresia is unknown. The lesion is sporadic, and no significant familial pattern has been identified. By definition, there is no communication between the right ventricle and the pulmonary arteries. Consequently, a patent ductus arteriosus is essential for early survival with this defect. There are usually varying degrees of hypoplasia of the right ventricle and hypoplasia of the tricuspid valve, and RV-to-coronary artery fistulas may be present. Morphologically and functionally, the hypoplasia of the tricuspid valve usually varies directly with the hypoplasia of the right ventricle. Coronary artery fistulas are present in 45% of cases and are more common in patients with severely hypoplastic right ventricles and small competent tricuspid valves. Without early surgical intervention, children with PA/IVS have an extremely high mortality rate. The natural history is associated with 50% mortality at 2 weeks and 85% mortality at 6 months.

Diagnostic Considerations

Diagnosis of this lesion is usually made in neonates and is prompted by the presence of hypoxia in varying degrees. Physical examination findings are often remarkable for prominent cervical venous pulsations and hepatic enlargement. A significant murmur is indicative of tricuspid regurgitation or may be related to the patent ductus arteriosus. An electrocardiogram shows progressive evidence of right atrial enlargement with peaked right atrial P waves. A chest radiograph is unremarkable at birth, but may later reveal an increased cardiac shadow secondary to right atrial and left ventricular enlargement. The diagnosis of pulmonary atresia with intact ventricular septum is easily made by two-dimensional echocardiography. Ventricular cavity sizes, valve dimensions and function, and the nature of the pulmonary artery obstruction can be determined by echocardiography. Cardiac catheterization is used for a definitive diagnosis and further evaluation. Information determined during right and left heart catheterization should include the size and competency of the tricuspid valve, the functional status of the ventricles, the degree of RV hypoplasia, the degree of infundibular hypoplasia, the presence or absence of coronary sinusoids and their communications, with the anatomy of the coronary arteries, and the size of the pulmonary arteries. In addition to an injection of contrast medium into the right ventricle, selective coronary angiograms are required to assess the native coronary anatomy, particularly in the severely hypoplastic group. Newborns with hypoxemia and poor perfusion in spite of medical management should be assessed for the presence of a restrictive atrial septal defect, which can be enlarged by balloon septostomy at the time of catheterization. If the ductus arteriosus is closed or restrictive, prostaglandin E_1 (PGE_1) is infused to open the ductus.

Anatomic Considerations

Our initial management of patients with pulmonary atresia and intact septum is based largely on an anatomic classification, which specifically defines the RV morphology and degree of RV hypoplasia. This classification not only allows initial management strategies, but also has predictive value for the possible use of the right ventricle in subsequent definitive repair. An alternate approach is to base therapy on a quantitative Z-score assessment of the tricuspid valve diameter. The Z-score is determined by comparing the diameter of the tricuspid valve (as measured by echocardiography) to the "expected" size and calculating the difference in standard deviations. This allows for a quantitative assessment of the degree of hypoplasia of the tricuspid valve, which in most patients varies directly with the degree of hypoplasia of the RV. We and others have found the degree of RV hypoplasia to correlate with short- and long-term outcomes of surgical management. In this classification, neonates with PA/IVS are initially separated into three groups of mild, moderate, and severe RV hypoplasia. In neonates, the degree of RV hypoplasia correlates closely with the degree of tricuspid hypoplasia. In patients with mild RV hypoplasia, the tricuspid valve and RV cavity are approximately two thirds or greater of calculated normal size and the RV outflow tract is well developed. This usually correlates with a Z-score for the tricuspid valve of 0 to 2. In patients with moderate RV hypoplasia, the tricuspid valve and the RV cavity are approximately one half of calculated normal size (with a range of one-third to two-thirds normal) and the outflow tract is developed enough to allow an effective pulmonary valvotomy. This usually correlates with a Z-score for the tricuspid

valve of −2 to −4. In patients with severe RV hypoplasia, the tricuspid valve and RV cavity are one third or less of calculated normal size and the outflow tract is severely hypoplastic or obliterated and is not amenable to an effective pulmonary valvotomy. This usually correlates with a Z-score for the tricuspid valve of −4 to −6. Our approach is not based on a single anatomic finding, but instead assesses the overall RV morphology and the degree of both tricuspid valve and RV hypoplasia.

The tricuspid valve is often anatomically and functionally abnormal in patients with PA/IVS. Therefore, a tricuspid valve Z-score or valve diameter may not be enough to assess the likelihood of a biventricular repair. Some patients with moderate RV hypoplasia may have a severe tricuspid malformation and may ultimately undergo a Glenn or Fontan procedure as a single-ventricle approach.

A fourth subgroup of patients may present with marked cardiomegaly caused by right atrial enlargement, severe tricuspid regurgitation, and an Ebstein's anomaly of the tricuspid valve. Dilation and dysfunction of the RA, RV, and ventricular septal wall in these patients often compromises left ventricular function and leads to biventricular failure. Surgical intervention in these patients is associated with >50% mortality.

During the initial evaluation of patients with PA/IVS, particular attention must be paid to the anatomy of the coronary circulation. Abnormalities of the coronary circulation are often found in the severely hypoplastic group and may dictate which surgical management option is indicated. During fetal development, RV hypertension may cause intramyocardial sinusoids to develop. These sinusoids often communicate by fistulas with the coronary artery circulation. The morphology of these sinusoids and their specific communications are extremely variable. Proximal coronary artery stenosis or obstruction may develop in a coronary artery supplied by these intramyocardial sinusoids. If the distal coronary artery flow is dependent on these sinusoids for adequate myocardial perfusion, they are termed RV-dependent coronary circulations (RVD-CCs). Decompression of the right ventricle in these patients is contraindicated because it may lead to myocardial ischemia and death. Our limited experience has shown that a shunt from the aorta to the right ventricle may be beneficial in these patients to augment myocardial perfusion and coronary blood flow.

Initial Surgical Treatment and Techniques

Most infants with PA/IVS will require surgical management early in life to survive. Treatment with PGE_1 will maintain pulmonary flow through the patent ductus arteriosus and allows time for evaluation and interventional decision making. Recently, some neonates have been successfully palliated with stenting of the ductus arteriosus at the time of catheterization. This has allowed delay of surgical intervention in those neonates who would otherwise be treated with a central shunt as an initial palliation. The efficacy of this catheter-based therapy appears promising for some neonates with PA/IVS, but the indications remain to be defined. Once the anatomy and morphology of these lesions have been identified at cardiac catheterization, classification is determined and an appropriate operative strategy is planned. Delay in surgical treatment is often hazardous and may reduce survival. The choice of surgical approach is based on the anatomic classification (Table 87-1).

Initial Procedures for Neonates with Mild Right Ventricular Hypoplasia

Neonates with mild RV hypoplasia (the right ventricle approximates two thirds of normal or greater) are best treated with pulmonary valvotomy, ligation of the patent ductus arteriosus, and creation of a central systemic-to-pulmonary shunt. Occasionally, there are cases in which a valvotomy alone will be adequate to restore pulmonary blood flow. These are rare and should be performed with caution. Most patients will require a shunt as an additional source of pulmonary blood flow. Neonates with moderate RV hypoplasia are treated with a pulmonary valvotomy, patch augmentation of the pulmonary outflow tract, insertion of a central shunt, and ligation of the patent ductus arteriosus. Pulmonary valvotomy with patch augmentation of the pulmonary outflow tract relieves RV hypertension, reduces tricuspid regurgitation, and promotes growth of the RV cavity and tricuspid valve. Neonates with severe RV hypoplasia are treated with a shunt only. If there is no RV-dependent coronary circulation and no pulmonary valvotomy is performed, the tricuspid valve can be made incompetent and the RV decompressed with a closed tricuspid valvotomy.

Off-Pump Transventricular Pulmonary Valvotomy. Closed pulmonary valvotomy is performed on patients with mild to

Table 87-1   Initial Surgical Management of Pulmonary Atresia with Intact Septum According to the Degree of Right Ventricular (RV) Hypoplasia

Classification of RV Hypoplasia	Classification	Treatment
Mild	Tricuspid valve and RV cavity more than two thirds of normal size, well-developed RV outflow tract	Valvotomy with shunt or occasionally valvotomy
Moderate	Tricuspid valve and RV cavity one third to two thirds of normal size, moderately hypoplastic RV outflow tract	Valvotomy with shunt
Severe	Tricuspid valve and RV cavity less than one third of normal size, severely hypo-plastic or absent RV outflow tract	Shunt only; possible closed tricuspid valvotomy

moderate RV hypoplasia who have an adequately developed RV outflow tract below the obstructed pulmonary valve. We have wet-pump standby in case there is hemodynamic instability during the procedure. The procedure is performed as previously described. Many of these patients can now be treated with perforation of the membrane and balloon dilation by transcatheter techniques.

Aorta-to-Pulmonary Artery Shunt.   A median sternotomy is used in performing a central shunt. The shunt insertion is performed by connecting either the innominate artery to the right pulmonary artery or the ascending aorta to the main pulmonary artery using a polytetrafluoroethylene (Gore-Tex) graft. A 3.0-mm shunt is used for neonates $\leq$3.0 kg, a 3.5-mm shunt in those >3.0 kg, and 4.0-mm shunt in those >4.0 kg. Cardiopulmonary bypass is usually not necessary. Partial occluding thin-bladed vascular C-clamps of appropriate sizes are applied to either the innominate artery or the aorta and to the pulmonary artery. Care must be taken to avoid occluding the patent ductus. The arteriotomies are performed with a No. 11 scalpel blade and fine vascular scissors. The proximal anastomosis is performed on the anterior aspect of the aorta or the innominate artery in an end-to-side manner using a running 7-0 Prolene suture technique. A similar anastomosis is performed to the anterior aspect of the main pulmonary artery or the right pulmonary artery. The clamps are released slowly to de-air the graft, and flow is established through the shunt. The ductus arteriosus is ligated after completion of the central shunt procedure.

Initial Procedures for Neonates with Moderate Right Ventricular Hypoplasia

Neonates with moderate RV hypoplasia are best treated with ligation of the patent ductus arteriosus, insertion of a central shunt, pulmonary valvotomy, and patch augmentation of the pulmonary outflow tract. We have used a closed technique to perform a pulmonary valvotomy and place a transannular outflow tract patch of pericardium without using cardiopulmonary bypass. We prefer to avoid the use of cardiopulmonary bypass in neonates in whom a shunt-dependent circulation will persist postoperatively.

Off-Pump Pulmonary Valvotomy with Transannular Right Ventricular Outflow Tract Patch.   In neonates with moderate RV hypoplasia, the infundibulum may be long and narrow, but reaches the pulmonary valve membrane. In these patients, a pulmonary valvotomy and a pericardial transannular patch may be performed without using cardiopulmonary bypass.

A median sternotomy incision is used. Wet-pump bypass is available with the lines on the field in case bypass is necessary. A pediatric cross-clamp is placed immediately beneath the bifurcation of the pulmonary artery. The ductus is kept patent to provide pulmonary blood flow. A vertical incision is made in the main pulmonary artery down to the atretic valve and RV junction. A partial-thickness myocardial incision is made over the right ventricle to bring the incision over the RV cavity. Part of the muscle is resected to a depth of 1 mm to 2 mm to thin out the right ventricle. An elliptical pericardial patch is now sutured to the pulmonary artery incision with a running

5-0 or 6-0 Prolene suture down to the RV junction. The suture line is continued onto the myocardium to the edges of the RV incision, leaving the sutures loose inferiorly. A No. 12 blade scalpel is then used to incise the pulmonary valve membrane and to cut through the remaining myocardium into the RV cavity under the pericardial patch. The sutures are pulled up to control bleeding and the cross-clamp on the pulmonary artery is removed. If the RV pressure is not adequately reduced to between one half and one third of systemic pressure, a rhizotomy knife is introduced through a purse string in the pericardial patch and the RV muscle is further incised until an adequate outflow tract has been created to adequately reduce the RV pressure (Fig. 87-1).

Initial Procedures for Neonates with Severe Right Ventricular Hypoplasia

Neonates with severe RV hypoplasia (less than one-third normal) are difficult to manage. If there is a restrictive atrial communication, then balloon atrial septostomy may be performed at the time of catheterization. The ductus is kept patent with PGE_1 and may be stented at the time of initial catheterization. At the time of surgery, simple pulmonary valvotomy is usually not effective in relieving RV hypertension. An extensive myomectomy and pericardial outflow tract patch may be performed using cardiopulmonary bypass. A Gore-Tex central shunt is inserted from the aorta to the main pulmonary artery, and the ductus arteriosus is ligated. If there are no sinusoids or if the sinusoids are tortuous and narrow and the native coronary circulation is normal, the right ventricle may be decompressed by incising the tricuspid valve using the closed technique as described later. Repeat cardiac catheterization in 3 months is performed in this group of patients.

Closed Tricuspid Valvotomy.   Closed tricuspid valvotomy is used in patients with severe RV hypoplasia where the possibility of a subsequent biventricular repair is minimal. Preoperative catheterization must determine the absence of sinusoids or an RV-dependent coronary circulation before decompression of the right ventricle. An RV-dependent coronary circulation is defined as one in which the native coronary circulation has stenoses and the sinusoids have broad-based communications with the RV cavity and the coronary circulation.

The closed tricuspid valvotomy is performed through a median sternotomy. The pericardium is opened, and a purse-string

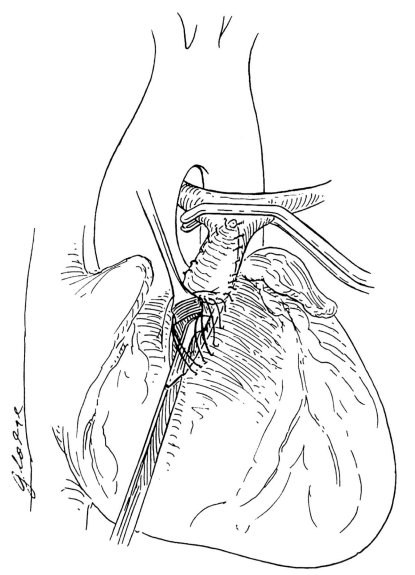

Figure 87-1. A transannular pulmonary outflow tract pericardial patch inserted without the use of cardiopulmonary bypass. The cross-clamp is placed on the main pulmonary artery just proximal to the bifurcation. The suture is left loose along the inferior edge of the patch until the annulus is divide anteriorly and right ventricular myocardium is completely incised.

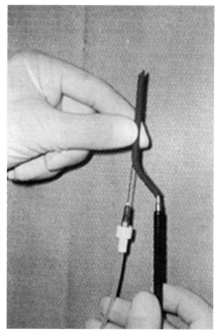

Figure 87-2. The device used to perform closed tricuspid valvotomy via the right atrium. A rhizotomy knife is inserted in rubber tubing of appropriate size and connected to a needle pressure transducer. The knife may be advanced or withdrawn in the rubber tubing, avoiding damage to structures on insertion or withdrawal.

suture is placed around the right atrial appendage. An instrument is made using a rhizotomy knife with a small, curved blade passed through a segment of red rubber tubing (Fig. 87-2). A pressure-measuring needle is placed into the tubing and connected to a transducer monitor. The tubing is then introduced into the right atrium via the right atrial appendage and passed into the right ventricle while the pressure is monitored. The knife blade is then exposed in the right ventricle and the tricuspid valve is cut anteriorly. Care is taken to avoid incising the area of the conduction system. When the RV pressure has fallen to one-half systemic pressure or less, the knife is retracted into the tubing, which is then removed from

the right atrium. The purse-string suture is tied to achieve hemostasis. We have found in patients without a pulmonary valvotomy that decompression of the right ventricle with a tricuspid valvotomy results in regression of the narrow tortuous types of sinusoids and has not resulted in myocardial ischemia if the native coronary circulation is intact.

Definitive Surgical Treatment and Techniques

Cardiac catheterization is repeated when the patient is 3 to 6 months of age, depending on the anatomy and echocardiographic findings. Further procedures will be based on the anatomic findings at catheterization. Our patients are again divided into those with mild, moderate, or severe RV hypoplasia (Table 87-2).

Definitive Procedures for Patients with Mild Right Ventricular Hypoplasia

Some patients with mild hypoplasia treated by pulmonary valvotomy may not require subsequent surgery unless the obstruction to the outflow tract has recurred. Relief of obstruction with pulmonary regurgitation and an open atrial communication can produce a large right-to-left shunt resulting in hypoplasia of the tricuspid valve annulus while the right ventricle develops well due to the regurgitation. This may lead to a discrepancy in the size of the tricuspid valve and the right ventricle cavity. In a patient with mild RV hypoplasia, definitive repair consists of primary or patch closure of the atrial septal defect with an adjustable snare, enlargement of the RV cavity and RV outflow tract by myocardial resection, and pericardial patch augmentation of the RV outflow tract. A monocusp or bicuspid autologous pericardial valve or a tissue valve is inserted in the pulmonary outflow tract, depending on the size of the child.

Table 87-2 Approaches for Definitive Repair of Patients with Pulmonary Atresia and Intact Septum

Classification of RV Hypoplasia	Treatment Options
Mild	Closure of ASD (adjustable snare), enlargement of RV and RVOT, and transannular patch. Ligation of previous shunt.
	Closure of ASD (adjustable snare), enlargement of RV and RVOT, and pulmonary homograft. Ligation of previous shunt.
Moderate	Closure of ASD (adjustable snare), modified Glenn shunt, enlargement of RV and RVOT, and transannular patch. Ligation of previous shunt.
	Closure of ASD (adjustable snare), modified Glenn shunt, enlargement of RV, and pulmonary homograft. Ligation of previous shunt.
Severe	Fontan procedure with ligation of previous shunt.
	Right atrium-to-right ventricle communication.
	Right atrium-to-pulmonary artery communication.

ASD = atrial septal defect; RV = right ventricular; RVOT = right ventricular outflow tract.

Enlargement of the Right Ventricular Cavity and Right Ventricular Outflow Tract.

The RV cavity is enlarged by sharp resection of trabecular myocardium. The procedure is performed using cardiopulmonary bypass with bicaval cannulation and both antegrade and retrograde blood cardioplegia. The right atrium is opened obliquely and the tricuspid valve is inspected. The annulus is measured and compared with normal values, and its competence is tested with cold saline. An incision is made longitudinally from the main pulmonary artery, through the annulus. If the outflow tract is hypoplastic, the incision is extended to the right ventricular cavity. Obstructive hypertrophied muscle in the outflow tract is resected. Care is taken to work between the papillary muscles, which must be preserved. A glutaraldehyde-treated pericardial outflow patch is then placed on the transannular incision. If the RV cavity is adequate and the tricuspid valve is competent, a valve may not be required. In infants, we generally prefer a pericardial monocusp valve. In older children, we have used a pulmonary homograft or porcine valve within the RV outflow tract.

Adjustable Atrial Septal Defect.

If the atrial septal defect is large, it is closed with a pericardial patch, leaving an open defect adjacent to the right superior pulmonary vein for the adjustable snare. If the defect is small with firm edges, it may be closed with the purse string of the "adjustable atrial septal defect." The adjustable atrial septal defect is performed by placing a No. 1 Prolene suture as a purse string around the tissue edges of the existing septal defect. A pericardial

pledget is used to avoid tearing of the tissue edges. The No. 1 Prolene is secured to the edges of the defect with 5-0 Prolene interrupted sutures. Both ends of the No. 1 Prolene are then brought out through the interatrial groove. An 8-F polyethylene tube is measured so that the end will lie under the

linea alba closure. The Prolene sutures are passed through this tube to create a snare to control the size of the atrial communication. The end of the tubing is sutured to the atrial wall with a single chromic catgut suture. The size of the atrial septal defect is adjusted by tightening or loosening the snare. Retracting the Prolene snare results in closure of the ASD, and pushing on the Prolene, opens the communication. The Prolene is then fixed to the tube with medium hemoclips. The end of the snare is left under the linea alba, where it can be retrieved under local anesthesia postoperatively for subsequent adjustment. The same technique can be used to create an adjustable defect in a patch repair using pericardium. The defect in the suture line is left on the right side adjacent to the right superior pulmonary vein, where it is encircled by the No. 1 Prolene snare as described. The ASD is left open until the patient is weaned from bypass. The atrial septal defect is then slowly closed using the snare while the right atrial pressure and the arterial oxygen saturations are monitored. A right atrial pressure of about 10 to 12 mm Hg with an oxygen saturation of $\geq 88\%$ on 100% fraction of inspired oxygen (FIO_2) is the goal (Fig. 87-3).

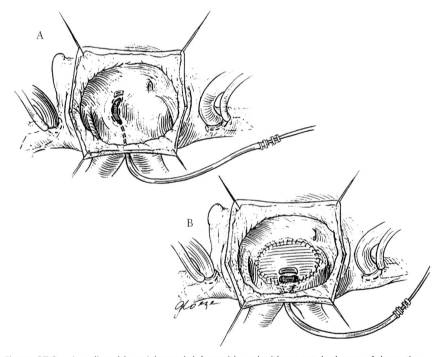

Figure 87-3. An adjustable atrial septal defect with and without patch closure of the native atrial septal defect. **(A)** A purse string is sewn around the border of the atrial septal defect. Pledgets may be used to reinforce the purse string. The snare is constructed using an 8-F polyethylene tubing placed over the No. 1 polypropylene (Prolene) and measured to reach the linea alba. **(B)** If a large secundum atrial septal defect is present, it is closed with a pericardial patch and a defect is left in the lateral wall. The No. 1 Prolene is brought through the interatrial septum and placed as a horizontal mattress stitch through the edge of the patch. The No. 1 Prolene is then anchored to the patch with a 5-0 Prolene suture.

Definitive Procedures for Patients with Moderate Right Ventricular Hypoplasia

In a patient with moderate RV hypoplasia, definitive repair is dictated by the previous growth and development of the right ventricle and the tricuspid valve. If the RV and tricuspid valve diameter are one half to two thirds of normal size, repair consists of partial closure of the atrial septal defect with an adjustable snare, enlargement of the RV cavity by myocardial resection, and insertion of a valved connection between the right ventricle and pulmonary artery. A monocusp transannular patch from native pericardium may be used in younger patients. If the RV and tricuspid valve diameter is one third to one half of normal, repair consists of partial closure of the atrial septal defect with an adjustable snare, enlargement of the RV cavity, creation of a bidirectional cavopulmonary Glenn shunt, and insertion of a valved connection between the right ventricle and pulmonary artery. The Glenn shunt reduces the volume load on the small right ventricle and provides an obligatory source of pulmonary blood flow from approximately one third of the systemic venous return. This has been termed the "one and one-half ventricle" or "partial biventricular" repair. The atrial septal defect is adjustable to create a gradient between the right atrium and left atrium to encourage forward flow through the RV, which will enhance development of the of the tricuspid valve and the right ventricle. Either a two-ventricle repair (with takedown of the Glenn shunt) or a completion of the Fontan reconstruction will follow based on the subsequent growth of the right ventricle and tricuspid valve.

Tissue Valve Insertion. A transannular incision is made vertically across the pulmonary outflow tract and extended onto the left pulmonary artery and down into the right ventricle. Any residual membrane in the region of the annulus is resected, as well as obstructive muscle in the outflow tract. The distance between the RV outflow tract and the pulmonary artery bifurcation is assessed. If it is short, an outsized porcine valve can be placed under a pericardial or Gore-Tex patch within the RV outflow tract as shown in Fig. 87-4. A running 3-0 Prolene suture is used to insert the valve, which is also sutured to the patch anteriorly. The pericardium is treated with glutaraldehyde for 3 minutes and rinsed with saline. If the distance between the RV outflow tract and the pulmonary artery bifurcation is adequate, an appropriately sized pulmonary

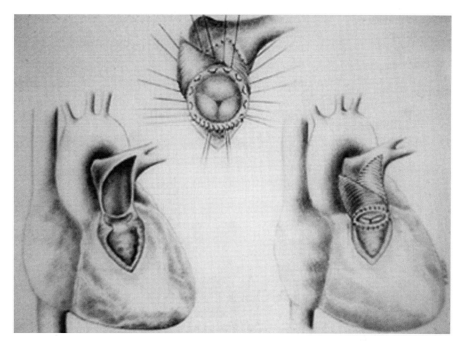

Figure 87-4. Insertion of a porcine valve under a transannular patch for enlargement of the right ventricular outflow tract. A large valve is chosen and is sutured to the annulus posteriorly and to the patch anteriorly.

homograft is chosen. A running suture of 4-0 Prolene is used distally just below the pulmonary artery bifurcation. Proximally, the homograft is sutured to the RV outflow tract just below the pulmonary valve annulus with a running suture of 3-0 Prolene (Fig. 87-5). A hood of pericardium or Gore-Tex may be used to complete the reconstruction.

Transannular Pericardial Patch with Monocusp Valve. The technique of a transannular pericardial patch with a monocusp valve is usually used for neonates and infants but can also be used for older children. It is best used for patients with mild or moderate RV hypoplasia with normal pulmonary artery size, because the valve will remain competent for a shorter period of

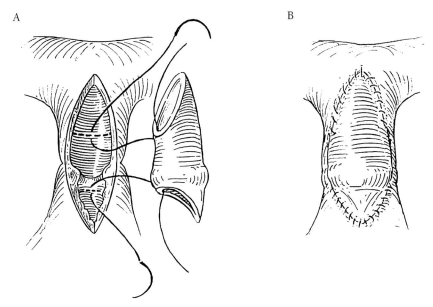

Figure 87-5. A pulmonary homograft used to enlarge the right ventricular outflow tract. The size of the homograft is carefully selected, and the graft is fashioned on both ends. The homograft is inserted as shown using a running polypropylene (Prolene) suture for the proximal and distal anastomoses.

time than a tissue valve. It has the advantage, however, of not causing obstruction even when the valve has become incompetent. Insertion of a transannular patch with a monocusp valve is performed through median sternotomy using cardiopulmonary bypass and bicaval cannulation. After harvesting, the pericardium is treated with glutaraldehyde for 5 minutes and then rinsed in saline. Both the transannular patch and the monocusp valve leaflet are outlined on the harvested pericardium using a sterile marking pen. Sizing of the monocusp valve is made using a metal dilator approximately 20% larger than the "normal" diameter for the pulmonary annulus. The width of the monocusp leaflet at its base should be approximately one half of the circumference of the dilator. It should also correspond with the width and shape of the inferior end of the transannular patch. The superior edge of the monocusp valve leaflet should be attached to the edges of the incised pulmonary artery 5 mm to 10 mm distal to the area of the true valve annulus. The monocusp valve is attached to the edges of the pulmonary artery and the right ventricle using the same suture that attaches the edges of the transannular patch.

Definitive Procedures for Patients with Severe Right Ventricular Hypoplasia

In a patient with severe RV hypoplasia (one third of normal size or less), a biventricular repair is usually not possible. Most patients will undergo insertion of a central shunt in the neonatal period with or without decompression of the right ventricle depending on whether or not there is an RV-dependent coronary circulation.

An RV-dependent coronary circulation is one in which there are sinusoidal connections between the RV cavity and the coronary circulation either with obstruction in the native coronary circulation or with broad sinusoidal connections that would result in runoff from the coronary circulation into the low-pressure right ventricle. Tortuous sinusoidal connections without coronary stenoses do not usually denote an RV-dependent coronary circulation. Decompression of the right ventricle at the time of the bidirectional Glenn shunt will usually result in closure of these sinusoids as opposed to the broad-based fistulous connections. In some cases, the large fistulous connections can be identified on the surface of the heart and can be suture ligated at the time of the bidirectional Glenn shunt, allow-

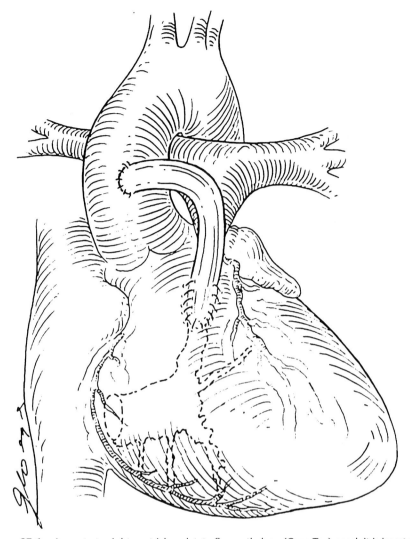

Figure 87-6.   An aorta-to-right ventricle polytetrafluoroethylene (Gore-Tex) conduit is inserted to augment coronary flow in cases where ischemia develops secondary to the presence of a right ventricle–dependent coronary circulation.

ing RV decompression at that time. RV decompression can be performed via the right atrium using the closed technique described previously to incise the anterior leaflet of the tricuspid valve.

If there is an RV-dependent coronary circulation, a bidirectional Glenn shunt is performed at 3 to 4 months of age without RV decompression and without bypass. Any additional source of pulmonary blood flow such as a previously placed central shunt is reduced to give an estimated combined Qp:Qs ratio of 1.2:1 from the Glenn shunt and the systemic-to-pulmonary artery shunt.

At 2 to 4 years of age, the Fontan procedure is completed. To bring oxygenated blood to the tricuspid valve, the septum is excised and the coronary sinus is unroofed.

If there are signs of myocardial ischemia, either preoperatively or intraoperatively, the

RV-dependent coronary circulation can be improved by creating an aorta-to-right ventricle shunt at the time of the Glenn shunt or at the time of the Fontan procedure (Fig. 87-6).

Bidirectional Cavopulmonary Glenn Shunt.   A median sternotomy incision is usually used for the Glenn shunt. Care should be taken in dissecting out the superior vena cava (SVC) and the right pulmonary artery to stay in the perivascular plane and avoid disrupting lymphatic tissue, which could result in a chylothorax. Injury to the phrenic nerve as it courses along the pericardium on the lateral aspect of the superior vena cava must also be avoided. The pulmonary artery pressure is measured on both sides. The azygos vein is ligated and divided.

A left SVC may be present and is usually found anterior to the left pulmonary artery. Care must be taken not to mistake a left upper-lobe pulmonary vein for a systemic vein. The SVC is then clamped just above the right atrium, and the proximal pressure is monitored. If the pressure does not rise above a mean of 30 mm Hg, then a left SVC should be suspected. If there is a left SVC with a venous communication to the right SVC, the pressure will usually not rise above 30 mm Hg and bypass or a temporary shunt is not necessary.

If the proximal pressure in the clamped SVC is ≥30 mm Hg, a temporary shunt should be used. The use of bypass is avoided if at all possible, particularly if there are sinusoids. The SVC is dissected from surrounding tissue starting at its right atrial junction and extending to the confluence of the innominate vein. The right pulmonary artery is identified and dissected circumferentially from surrounding tissue both medially and laterally to the site of primary branching. A purse-string suture of 5-0 Prolene is placed in the SVC at the junction of the innominate vein. A second purse string is placed in the right atrial appendage. The patient is heparinized, and a temporary bypass shunt is created using two modified aortic cannulas and a Y-connector with a chapeau attachment. The SVC is cannulated with one modified aortic cannula at the junction of the innominate vein. The distal end of this cannula should be beveled so that the opening is as large as possible relative to the venous cannulation site and should face superiorly toward the right internal jugular vein. The second cannula is placed in the right atrial appendage. The circuit is connected after air is completely evacuated from the cannulas and the clamps are removed. Flow should be visualized in the shunt after removal of the clamps. The cannulas are then supported by towels in a medial position that allows exposure of the SVC and right pulmonary artery.

The SVC is then clamped at its junction with the right atrium and at its junction with the innominate vein. The pressure may be measured in the proximal SVC with the first clamp in place to ensure proper functioning of the shunt. Methylene blue is used to mark the anterior aspect of the SVC and the superior aspect of the PA to ensure proper alignment of the subsequent cavopulmonary anastomosis. The azygos vein is ligated and divided. The SVC is divided at the atrial junction, with care being taken to leave an adequate cuff of tissue with the clamp to allow subsequent closure of this SVC stump. Attention to the rhythm

at this point helps to avoid clamp injury to the sinoatrial node. The open end of the SVC is enlarged by an incision in the posterior wall of the vessel. This enlargement ensures a widely patent anastomosis. The right pulmonary artery is clamped with a C-clamp, and a V-shaped incision is made on its superior aspect with the apex pointing anteriorly. The anastomosis is performed with 6-0 or 7-0 Prolene. The cannula in the SVC is removed, followed by removal of the right atrial cannula. If the SVC is narrowed at the site of the purse string, a vascular C-clamp is applied, the purse string is removed, and the incision in the SVC is closed with a running 7-0 Prolene suture. Any previously placed systemic-to-pulmonary artery shunt is now reduced in size to give an estimated combined Qp:Qs ratio of 1.2:1 from the systemic-to-pulmonary artery shunt and the Glenn shunt. The change in arterial systolic blood pressure, with the shunt open versus closed, should be no more than 5 to 7 mm Hg.

The SVC and pulmonary artery pressures are measured, as well as the arterial oxygen saturations on 100% oxygen. The heparinization is not reversed. If a jugular vein line has been inserted, it is used for measuring the pulmonary artery pressure and for the infusion of pulmonary vasodilators, if necessary. The line is removed within 24 hours to avoid venous thrombosis. A Gore-Tex membrane is left as a pericardial substitute to facilitate reoperation for the Fontan procedure (Fig. 87-7).

Lateral Tunnel Fontan with Adjustable Atrial Septal Defect.
A Fontan procedure is usually performed as a second-stage operation after the creation of a cavopulmonary Glenn shunt. A median sternotomy is performed, and bicaval venous cannulation is used for total cardiopulmonary bypass. Note that the SVC cannula is placed above the previous Glenn shunt anastomosis. Systemic hypothermia to 24°C is used in addition to cold blood cardioplegia.

A right atriotomy is performed just anterior to the linea terminalis, and the edges are retracted with stay sutures. The coronary sinus is identified and cannulated with a retrograde cardioplegia catheter. A Prolene purse string is placed at the opening of the coronary sinus to secure the catheter and achieve more efficient delivery of the cardioplegia. The atrial septum is excised. The SVC orifice is identified from within the right atrium. It is important that this orifice be widely open and not restrictive. The right pulmonary artery is incised adjacent to the opening in the SVC stump. The posterior

wall of the anastomosis is achieved by suturing the adjacent pulmonary artery and right atrium together with 5-0 Prolene. Anteriorly, the connection is bridged with a pericardial patch.

After the right atrium-to-pulmonary artery anastomosis has been completed, the lateral tunnel is constructed. A rectangular Gore-Tex patch is cut from 0.8-mm-thick Gore-Tex vascular patch material. The length is carefully measured from the orifice of the inferior vena cava (IVC) to the SVC orifice. The width is left about two thirds of the length to be trimmed after completion of the posterior suture line.

A running 4-0 Prolene suture with an RB1 needle is used for the posterior suture line, which is begun posteriorly at the IVC orifice. The suture line is carried superiorly to the site of the adjustable atrial septal defect orifice, where it ends. This site is chosen because there is a natural recess close to the right superior pulmonary vein at the superior and lateral end of the fossa ovalis. A second 4-0 Prolene suture line is begun at the superior end of the atrial septal defect and carried superiorly around the SVC orifice. The atrial septal defect is sized according to the age of the patient and made large in diameter so that it may be reduced in size if necessary after the patient is taken off bypass. As a rule of thumb, the defect size is 4 mm for 2-year-olds, 6 mm for 4-year-olds, and 8 mm for 6year-olds and older. The patch is trimmed appropriately as the suture line advances. Before the anterior suture line is completed, the snare control is placed for the adjustable atrial septal defect. A No. 1 Prolene suture is brought through a pericardial pledget, through the interatrial septum at the lower border of the atrial septal defect, and through the edge of the Gore-Tex patch as shown in Fig. 87-8. It is then brought back through the upper edge of the Gore-Tex patch and out through the interatrial septum and through the pericardial pledget. An 8-F polyethylene tube is cut to the appropriate length to reach the linea alba, and the Prolene sutures are brought through this snare. The No. 1 Prolene is sutured to the edge of the Gore-Tex patch with a 5-0 Prolene suture, the polyethylene tubing is sutured to the lateral wall with 2-0 chromic catgut, and the Prolene is fixed to the tubing with a medium hemoclip. These three points of fixation prevent inadvertent closure of the atrial septal defect by tension on the Prolene. The patch is now trimmed to create a wide-open connection and to reach just anterior to the linea terminalis. The anterior part of the suture line is completed using full-thickness sutures to avoid a suture line

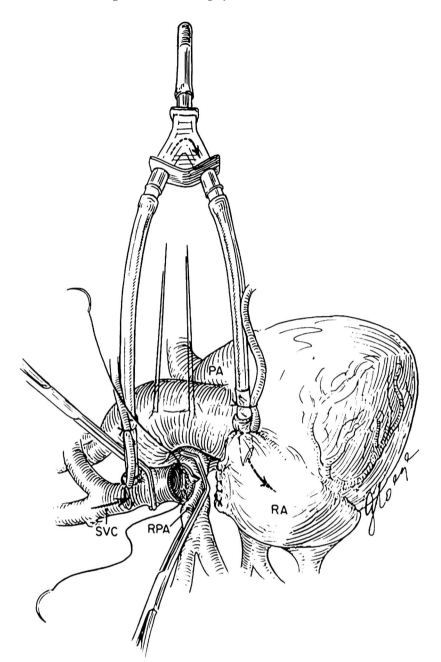

Figure 87-7.   A bidirectional Glenn shunt is performed using a superior vena cava-to-right atrial shunt. This technique avoids the use of cardiopulmonary bypass. The cannulas are placed in the superior vena cava and the right atrium (as shown), allowing continuous flow of venous return to the right atrium during creation of the cavopulmonary anastomosis. (RA = right atrium; RPA = right pulmonary artery; SVC = superior vena cava.)

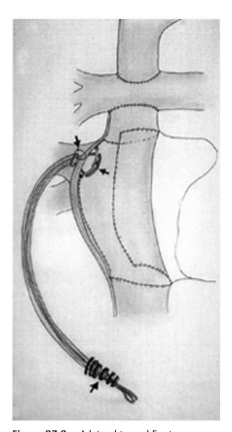

Figure 87-8.   A lateral tunnel Fontan procedure with an adjustable atrial septal defect. A tunnel of uniform caliber is created by suturing a piece of polytetrafluoroethylene (Gore-Tex) vascular patch to the orifice of the inferior vena cava and the superior vena cava and to the sinus venosus portion of the lateral wall. A defect is left in the lateral tunnel. The adjustable atrial septal defect is created by passing the No. 1 polypropylene (Prolene) through the lateral portion of the interatrial septum and through the edge of the Gore-Tex tunnel. The No. 1 Prolene is then secured to the edge of the Gore-Tex with a 5-0 Prolene suture. The suture is brought back out the interatrial septum and through a pericardial pledget. The snare is constructed with 8-F polyethylene tubing and anchored to the heart through the pledget and through the atrial wall. Medium hemoclips are used at the end of the snare to fix the atrial septal defect.

leak. The right atrial incision is then closed with 4-0 Prolene (Fig. 87-9).

The coronary sinus cannula and the purse-string suture are removed, and the right atrium is closed in a two-layer fashion with a running Prolene suture. Transthoracic lines are generally placed in the left and right atria. If an internal jugular line is not inserted, then the right atrial line can be inserted to measure the pressure in the pulmonary system via the Fontan tunnel or the Glenn shunt. Air is evacuated from all structures. The patient is warmed to normothermia and subsequently weaned from cardiopulmonary bypass. The adjustable atrial septal defect snare is adjusted to achieve arterial saturations of 80% to 85% while an attempt is made to maintain pressure in the lateral tunnel Fontan at or below 15 mm Hg.

Extracardiac Fontan with Adjustable Fenestration.   The extracardiac Fontan is performed through a median sternotomy using cardiopulmonary bypass and bicaval cannulation. The procedure can be completed in most patients without the need for cardioplegic arrest of the heart. A clamp is placed on the inferior vena cava near its junction to the right atrium. The inferior vena cava is then divided between the snared venous cannula and the clamp. The atrium is repaired and the clamp is removed. The open right ventricle, and the distal end of the graft is anastomosed to this site using a running polypropylene suture (Fig. 87-6).

Postoperative Care and Surgical Complications after the Fontan Procedure.

Early management after the Fontan procedure is focused on optimizing cardiac output and reducing the systemic venous pressure. The adjustable atrial septal defect or fenestration is useful because it allows as much as one third of the systemic venous return to traverse the atrial septal defect to the left atrium, thus lowering the systemic venous pressure while increasing the cardiac output. A Fontan pressure of ≤15 mm Hg is ideally achieved by adjustment of the fenestration.

The pulmonary vascular resistance may be reduced with the use of inhaled nitric oxide. This drug has an advantage over other pulmonary vasodilators, because its effect is confined to the pulmonary vascular bed and the systemic vascular resistance is not reduced. Methemoglobin levels should be monitored carefully with the use of nitric oxide.

Inotropes are routinely used, starting with 5 μg/kg per minute of dopamine and dobutamine. If the systemic vascular resistance is low, dopamine or epinephrine in higher doses is infused via the left atrial line. If these medications are not effective, milrinone or isoproterenol (Isuprel) may be added.

If the hemodynamics is optimal with minimal support, early extubation is attempted. In more critical cases, the patients are sedated and paralyzed for 12 hours before being weaned from the ventilator. If the systemic venous pressure has been high early in the postoperative course, the patient is diuresed before extubation. The patient must be actively monitored for the development of pleural and pericardial effusions, which must be drained immediately. If the venous pressure or the left atrial pressure is high, echocardiography is performed to assess ventricular and valvular function and to exclude the presence of any obstruction within the systemic venous pathway or pulmonary arteries. Rarely, recatheterization may be necessary for postoperative assessment.

The atrial septal defect may require adjustment early postoperatively. In most cases, it is left partially open. In some patients, as the left ventricular function improves, the right-to-left shunt increases, resulting in a decrease in the arterial oxygen saturation. The snare can be exposed under local anesthesia behind the linea alba and is

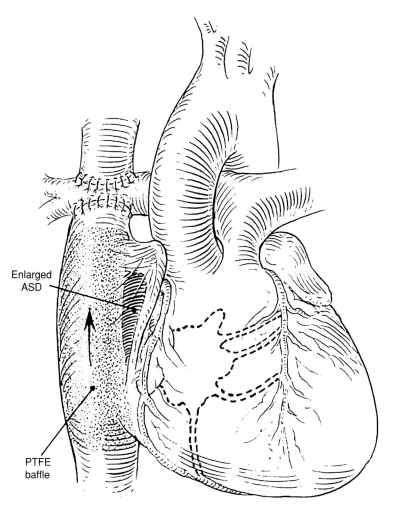

Figure 87-9. The completed lateral tunnel Fontan with adjustable atrial septal defect (ASD) (snare not shown). The atrial septal defect is left open at the completion of the procedure and adjusted postoperatively to achieve the desired hemodynamic measurements and oxygen saturations. (PTFE = polytetrafluoroethylene.)

end of the inferior vena cava is anastomosed end to end to a Gore-Tex conduit (16 mm to 20 mm in diameter) using a running Gore-Tex suture. The proximal anastomosis is performed end to side between the Gore-Tex conduit and the inferior aspect of the right pulmonary artery. The clamps are released and flow is established between the inferior vena cava and the pulmonary arteries.

To insert the adjustable atrial septal defect, a partial occluding vascular C-clamp is placed on the Gore-Tex graft. A direct anastomosis is performed between the extracardiac conduit and the right atrium. A snare is inserted to control the opening and closing of this "atrial septal defect." An alternate method uses a conduit for the defect. With this technique, an 8.0-mm Gore-Tex graft is anastomosed end to side to the middle of the larger conduit. A similar technique is used to create an opening in the right atrium, and the other end of the 8.0-mm graft is anasto-

mosed to this site. A snare is inserted around the smaller conduit. A distinct drawback to the extracardiac Fontan is the need for anticoagulation with warfarin postoperatively for 6 months to 1 year, with subsequent conversion to aspirin therapy.

Aorta-to-Right Ventricle Shunt.

The aorta-to-right ventricle shunt is performed through a median sternotomy using cardiopulmonary bypass and bicaval cannulation. Cardioplegic arrest of the heart may or may not be necessary. The shunt is created using a 5.0-mm ringed Gore-Tex graft. A partial occluding clamp is placed on the anterior wall of the ascending aorta. An aortotomy is created, and an end-to-side anastomosis is performed between the graft and the ascending aorta using a running polypropylene suture. A ventriculotomy is made in the infundibular portion of the further tightened using medium hemoclips. Betadine is used to irrigate the wound and is injected into the polyethylene snare. The atrial septal defect can also be opened further by pushing on the Prolene sutures, but this is not as reliable as the ability to close the atrial septal defect. At 6 to 12 weeks, an echocardiogram and arterial oxygen saturation measurement are used to assess the size of the defect. If it is small, it is left to close spontaneously. If it is still large, the defect is closed in the catheterization laboratory with a balloon, and if the venous pressures are acceptable, the snare is exposed behind the linea alba and the defect is closed completely.

Summary

In neonates with pulmonary atresia and intact septum, we have found that the surgical classification of RV and tricuspid hypoplasia into mild (more than two thirds of normal), moderate (one third to two thirds of normal), and severe (less than one third of normal) has been useful in selecting a surgical approach.

A similar classification is used in older children, and patients are stratified into those who will benefit from an attempt to achieve a biventricular repair and those who are best suited to a Fontan procedure. With this approach, the surgical mortality and morbidity can be reduced.

Results of Surgical Treatment

At the UCLA School of Medicine, our surgical approach to patients with PA/IVS has been based on classification of the degree of right ventricular hypoplasia. Between 1982 and 2001, 111 patients with a diagnosis of PA/IVS underwent surgical interventions at our institution. Six patients had Ebstein's anomaly of the tricuspid valve and were excluded from analysis.

Sixty-three patients with PA/IVS underwent palliative procedures at UCLA as neonates. Twenty patients were classified as severe right ventricular hypoplasia and/or demonstrated severe coronary abnormalities with RVDCC. There were 3 early deaths in this group. Forty-three patients were classified as mild to moderate right ventricular hypoplasia without significant right ventricle sinusoids or fistulae. These patients all underwent procedures to open the right ven-

tricular outflow tract with or without a central shunt. There were 3 early deaths and 2 late deaths in this group. Early survival in this total group is 90% and late survival is 87%.

Eighty-two patients surviving palliative procedures from UCLA and referring institutions underwent later interventions at UCLA based on our classification system. Fifty-seven patients underwent complete or partial biventricular repair. Nineteen of these patients underwent partial biventricular repair with a bidirectional cavopulmonary shunt and an adjustable ASD. There were 3 deaths in this group. Twenty-three of these patients underwent Fontan operations as a later intervention. Two patients underwent cardiac transplantation after initial palliation. There were 2 early deaths and 1 late death after discharge. Actuarial survival in this total group is 96% at 1 year, 89% at 5 years, and 86.3% at 10 years. As evidenced by our experience, the prognosis for children with this PA/IVS continues to improve as a more structured and methodical surgical approach is used. The role of catheter-based interventions in these patients, including balloon valvotomy and stenting of the ductus arteriosus, is evolving and remains to be defined.

SUGGESTED READING

Ashburn DA, Blackstone EH, Well WJ, et al. Determinants of mortality and type of repair in neonates with pulmonary atresia with intact ventricular septum. J Thorac Cardiovasc Surg 2004;127:1000.

Daubeney P, Delany D, Anderson R, et al. Pulmonary atresia with intact ventricular septum: Range of morphology in a population-based study. J Am Coll Cardiol 2002;39:1670.

Dyamenahalli U, McCrindle BW, McDonald C, et al. Pulmonary atresia with intact ventricular septum: Management of, and outcomes for a cohort of 210 consecutive patients. Cardiol Young 2004;14:299.

Hanley FL, Sade RM, Freedom RM, et al. Outcomes in critically ill neonates with pulmonary stenosis and intact ventricular septum: A multi-institutional study. J Am Coll Cardiol 1993;22:183.

Laks H, Gates RN, Grant PW, et al. Aortic to right ventricular shunt for pulmonary atresia and intact ventricular septum. Ann Thorac Surg 1995;59:342.

Laks H, Pearl JM, Drinkwater DC, et al. Partial biventricular repair of pulmonary atresia with intact ventricular septum. Use of an adjustable atrial septal defect. Circulation 1992;86(Suppl II):159.

Laks H, Pearl JM, Haas GS, et al. Partial Fontan: Advantages of an adjustable interatrial communication. Ann Thorac Surg 1991;52:1084.

McCrindle BW, Kan JS. Long-term results after balloon pulmonary valvuloplasty. Circulation 1991;83:1915.

Mi YP, Chiu CS, Yung TC, et al. Evolution of the management approach for pulmonary atresia with intact ventricular septum. Heart 2005;91:657.

Odim J, Laks H, Plunkett M, et al. Successful management of patients with pulmonary atresia with intact ventricular septum using a three tier grading system for right ventricular hypoplasia. Ann Thorac Surg 2006;81:678–84.

Polansky DB, Clark EB, Doty DB. Pulmonary stenosis in infants and young children. Ann Thorac Surg 1985;39:159.

Rychik J, Levy H, Gaynor JW, et al. Outcome after operations for pulmonary atresia with intact ventricular septum. Cardiovasc Surg 1998;116:924.

Weber HS. Initial and late results after catheter intervention for neonatal critical pulmonary valve stenosis and atresia with intact ventricular septum: A technique in continual evolution. Catheter Cardiovasc Interv 2002;56:394.

Yoshimura N, Yamaguchi M, Ohashi H, et al. Pulmonary atresia with intact ventricular septum: Strategy based on right ventricular morphology. J Thorac Cardiovasc Surg 2003;126:1417.

EDITOR'S COMMENTS

Infants with critical pulmonary stenosis and an adequate-sized pulmonary valve annulus are now treated with balloon valvuloplasty rather than surgical intervention. However, patients with severely dysplastic pulmonary valves or significant RV outflow tract obstruction with dynamic infundibular obstruction may still come to surgical intervention and require valvectomy or outflow patching as recommended by Drs. Laks and Plunkett. Transventricular dilation of a stenotic pulmonary valve is rarely necessary, but may be applied to certain patients with pulmonary valve atresia.

The multiple creative techniques pioneered by Dr. Laks have permitted surgical intervention in the majority of patients with pulmonary atresia and intact ventricular septum. The classification scheme described in this chapter relating the relative size of the right ventricle to the surgical approach taken has several advantages. A more classic technique used by the Congenital Heart Surgeons Society has related tricuspid valve diameter (or Z-value) to the optimal technique of repair. Because the tricuspid valve size depends on RV size, these two approaches would seem to be similar. It should also be noted, however, that the tricuspid valve is often abnormal in pulmonary atresia, and therefore, tricuspid valve diameter alone may not accurately reflect tricuspid valve function. Thus, some patients with a moderate-sized right ventricle may be limited in long-term repair by abnormal tricuspid valve inflow and require a Glenn shunt and outflow reconstruction or the Fontan operation. In addition, the compliance of abnormal right ventricles with significant ventricular hypertrophy and small size may limit the utility of complete two-ventricle repair in those with moderate hypoplasia. The use of an adjustable atrial septal defect at complete repair as pioneered by Dr. Laks has permitted right-to-left shunting in those cases in which early ventricular compliance limits forward flow into the pulmonary vascular bed and may help to stabilize these patients in the critical early postoperative period.

Decompression of the right ventricle by tricuspid valve incision remains somewhat controversial. Although in the majority of patients tricuspid valve incision/avulsion is well tolerated, patients who have had valvotomies with associated pulmonary insufficiency may not tolerate decompression of the right ventricle well, because the shunt flow may be directed retrograde across the outflow tract to the right ventricle and then into the right atrium, resulting in a steal of blood away from the pulmonary vascular bed. Whereas decompression of the ventricle may result in resolution of some sinusoidal connections to the coronary arteries, in many cases it is not necessary to decompress the ventricle, and late results have not yet shown a significant effect of decompression on arrhythmias or ventricular dysfunction. As noted in this chapter, decompression of a ventricle that has RV-dependent coronary circulation to greater than one coronary system is contraindicated, and these patients have a significant risk of morbidity and mortality from coronary ischemia regardless of the operative approach taken. Thus, in some cases, early bidirectional Glenn shunting or augmentation of RV flow with an aorta-to-right ventricle connection and an early Fontan procedure may result in improved oxygenation of the coronary flow from in the right ventricle. However, these patients continue to have problems with ventricular dysfunction and may have acute myocardial infarction early in life, causing ventricular dysfunction or early death. Thus, in patients with significant ventricular dysfunction in association with RV-dependent coronary circulation, early shunting for stabilization followed by orthotopic cardiac transplantation has been advocated by some centers, and we have performed this procedure in several infants.

A major area of controversy regarding pulmonary atresia and intact ventricular septum is the use of radiofrequency ablation and perforation of the right ventricular outflow tract with balloon dilation in preference to surgical intervention in these neonates. Although the experience of the Toronto Hospital for Sick Children is relatively good with radiofrequency ablation and perforation of the right ventricular outflow tract with balloon dilation (followed by ductal stenting if necessary to maintain pulmonary blood flow), the disadvantage of this technique is the fact that in patients with severely hypoplastic right ventricular outflow tract, there is not complete relief of the gradient. Residual obstruction may limit right ventricular growth, and a more radical relief of RV outflow tract obstruction and even division of hypertrophied muscle bundles in the cavity of the right ventricle may permit better growth. The technique can be very effective, however, in patients who have a platelike pulmonary valve atresia with a reasonable-sized pulmonary annulus and relatively well developed right ventricle. In these cases, balloon dilation while maintaining the patient on prostaglandin and then gradually letting the ductus arteriosus close can permit total interventional repair with closure of the atrial septal defect with an occluder device at a later time. Hybrid therapies, including a Blalock-Taussig shunt and RV outflow reconstruction with later occlusion of the Blalock-Taussig shunt and atrial septum in the catheterization lab, have also been used with good success in selected patients. A comparison of these relatively noninvasive approaches with surgical approaches in all patients with pulmonary atresia and intact septum has not been performed, and therefore the selection criteria for these various interventions are controversial.

When outflow tract patches are required, we have elected to use cardiopulmonary bypass in most cases, because it makes the operation simpler. Incision of the RV outflow tract in pulmonary atresia must be done carefully, because even a slight deviation of the incision can cut into the base of the aortic valve leaflet. Thus, the use of cardioplegia and cardiopulmonary bypass has resulted in more accurate placement of the incision. In addition, we have elected to place the shunts through a median sternotomy incision rather than a thoracotomy in the majority of patients so that the ductus arteriosus can be ligated at the time of shunt placement. If ductal patency remains, pulmonary overcirculation can occur; therefore, closure of the ductus in the operating room with maintenance of distal saturations is a good sign that the shunt is adequate in size. In addition, competitive flow from the ductus, which may compromise shunt patency in the early postoperative period, is eliminated.

A particularly difficult group of patients are those with pulmonary atresia and Ebstein's malformation of the tricuspid valve with severe tricuspid insufficiency. These patients may have significant compromise of the left ventricle by the dilated right ventricle, and the inefficient flow of blood in and out of the right ventricle compromises overall systemic blood flow. The creation of an aortopulmonary shunt may stabilize pulmonary blood flow in these patients, but the effect of the dilated right ventricle on systemic output remains problematic. Patch closure of the tricuspid valve is not suitable for these patients, because there will be no outflow of the coronary sinus return, and often sinusoidal connections and Thebesian vessels into the ventricle cannot then be decompressed. In these rare instances, the best approach would appear to be early cardiac transplantation. Sano and his colleagues in Okayama, Japan, have suggested either radical plication or complete excision of the right ventricular free wall (with closure of the tricuspid valve orifice) in patients with Ebstein's malformation and pulmonary atresia to eliminate the effect of the right ventricle on left ventricular function. These very radical approaches seem to have been successful in a small number of cases and should be considered in patients with pulmonary atresia with severe Ebstein's malformation because patch closure of the tricuspid valve will, as mentioned, often not relieve the dilation of the right ventricle and the secondary effects on left ventricular function.

When valve insertion is required, homograft valves can often be used. If the homograft valve is too long from the pulmonary bifurcation to the normal annulus level, it is possible in most circumstances to use a pulmonary homograft and cut the valve just at the commissural attachments, sewing the distal end of the homograft to the pulmonary bifurcation and sewing the proximal homograft in the RV outflow tract to the infundibular septum. In this situation, the pulmonary valve is positioned more inferiorly in the right ventricle but maintains a normal anatomic outflow tract.

When monocusp outflow tract reconstruction is used, we have elected to use either a Gore-Tex patch with a pericardial monocusp fashioned in the operating room or homograft tissue with a contained monocusp, Gore-Tex pericardial membrane, or native pericardium. The aortic homograft monocusps used by Dr. Laks can develop calcification of the wall and also are ex-

pensive. Nevertheless, they have the distinct advantage of having a gusset of anterior mitral leaflet that is readily available to create a gentle take-off from the RV outflow tract. For Fontan operations, we have preferred use of the fenestrated lateral tunnel or extracardiac conduit Fontan with a fixed 4-mm

fenestration rather than an adjustable defect as used by Dr. Laks. In most cases, the defect will close spontaneously. The approach to the Fontan operation and hemi-Fontan versus bidirectional Glenn shunt will be commented on in a later chapter.

T.L.S.

88

Pulmonary Atresia with Ventricular Septal Defect and Major Aortopulmonary Collaterals

Malcolm J. MacDonald, V. Mohan Reddy, and Frank L. Hanley

Pulmonary atresia with ventricular septal defect (VSD) and major aortopulmonary collaterals is a complex lesion in which great morphologic variability exists regarding the sources of pulmonary blood flow. The situation with regard to the true central pulmonary arteries ranges from normal size to complete absence. Major aortopulmonary collateral arteries (MAPCAs), probably derived embryologically from the splanchnic vascular plexus, are also highly variable in their size, number, course, origin, arborization, and histopathologic makeup. A given segment of the lung may be supplied solely from the true pulmonary arteries, solely from the aortopulmonary collaterals, or from both, sometimes with connections between the two sources occurring at central or peripheral points and at single or multiple sites. In contrast, the intracardiac morphology of this lesion is relatively straightforward, often with a single anteriorly malaligned VSD, well-developed right and left ventricles, and normal atrioventricular and ventriculoarterial connections.

The ultimate goal of surgical therapy in this lesion is to construct completely separated, in-series pulmonary and systemic circulations. The traditional surgical management strategy for achieving this goal is to embark on a staged reconstruction to centralize the multifocal pulmonary blood supply, recruiting as many lung segments as possible, then close the VSD and provide egress from the right ventricle to the "unifocalized" pulmonary arterial system. In the past, this generally has required multiple operations.

The most important physiologic factor signifying a favorable outcome for these pa-

tients after complete repair is the postrepair peak right ventricular pressure. This should be as low as possible. The peak right ventricular pressure depends greatly on the number of lung segments that are unifocalized and on the status of the pulmonary microvasculature in those segments. Another important factor is that the reconstruction must achieve unobstructed delivery of blood from the right ventricle to the pulmonary microvasculature. A number of impediments to achieving this ideal outcome exist. Lung segments can be lost for several reasons. The natural history of these MAPCAs often follows a course of progressive stenosis and occlusion, sometimes making the segment of lung supplied by that collateral inaccessible at the time of unifocalization. Even if accessible, a long-standing severe stenosis of the collateral can lead to distal arterial hypoplasia and underdevelopment of preacinar and acinar vessels and alveoli. In addition, iatrogenic occlusion can occur when these collaterals are unifocalized in stages using nonviable conduits, sometimes resulting in loss of these segments. Finally, MAPCAs without obstruction can lead rapidly to pulmonary vascular obstructive disease in their supplied segments. Similarly, staged unifocalization necessitating the use of modified Blalock-Taussig or central shunts may result in pulmonary vascular obstructive disease.

Therapeutic Goals and Patient Selection

It seems logical that the longer the microvasculature of a given lung segment

is left to the hemodynamic vagaries of a MAPCA, the more likely it is that it will either develop pulmonary vascular obstructive disease or involute. Only the "perfectly stenosed" MAPCA may allow normal distal development. Furthermore, stenoses in MAPCAs are well known to progress with time, suggesting that even a "perfectly stenosed" vessel is not likely to remain that way. Extending this logic, it seems clear that the sooner these hemodynamic vagaries can be removed, the greater is the likelihood that the largest number of healthy lung segments can be incorporated into the unifocalized pulmonary circuit. The pulmonary microvasculature taken in aggregate is healthiest at birth and declines thereafter. From these arguments, it seems logical that one-stage complete unifocalization and repair early in life gives the greatest chance of achieving a healthy and complete pulmonary vascular bed.

We have prospectively applied a complex surgical management protocol that reflects these goals and principles. The first priority is to completely unifocalize the pulmonary arterial and MAPCA complex via a median sternotomy incision. This removes the MAPCAs from the abnormal physiologic milieu as early as possible. Whenever possible we also perform intracardiac repair at the first operation. If simultaneous intracardiac repair is not considered advisable because of concern about pulmonary hypertension, a polytetrafluoroethylene (PTFE) shunt is constructed between the ascending aorta and the fully reconstructed single-compartment pulmonary arterial system. Based on experience with more than 300 patients, this approach of one-stage complete bilateral unifocalization was performed in

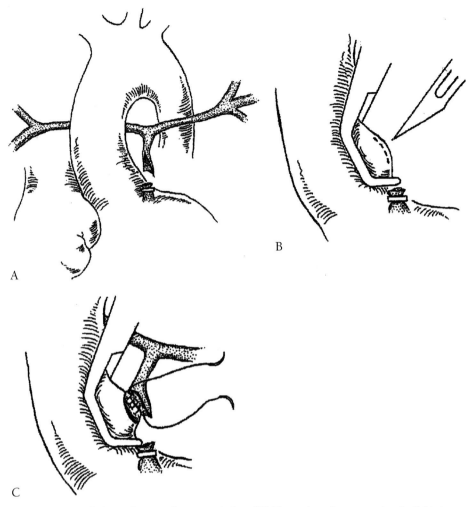

Figure 88-1.   Technique of aortopulmonary window. **(A)** The main pulmonary artery is divided as proximally as possible and spatulated with a longitudinal incision. **(B)** It is important to carefully apply the clamp such that the sequestered portion of the aorta is somewhat posterior to the direct lateral aspect of the aortic circumference. **(C)** Aortotomy is made, and the anastomotic site is enlarged by excising an aortic wall button. Anastomosis is performed with continuous 7-0 monofilament absorbable suture.

about 85% of all patients. In 56%, intracardiac repair was also performed. In 29%, a central shunt was created; intracardiac repair was achieved within 2 years in the great majority of patients in whom shunts were created. The remaining 15% of patients typically fall into two general categories. In one group centrally confluent true pulmonary arteries were present in association with a relatively complete arborization pattern to most or all lung segments. The source of pulmonary blood flow is via MAPCAs that share dual-supply vascular distribution with the true pulmonary arteries. In this anatomic variant we construct a neonatal aortopulmonary window by removing the blind end of the main pulmonary artery from the infundibulum and connect it to the ascending aorta, and we concurrently ligate important MAPCAs (Fig. 88-1). If patients are selected

properly, the central source of pulmonary blood flow will distribute to all lung segments. Patients are then evaluated for intracardiac repair at 3 to 6 months of age. In the second group true pulmonary arteries may or may not be present. The important factor is that the majority of MAPCAs have multiple stenoses at the segmental and subsegmental branches. In our opinion these patients are best managed by sequential staged thoracotomies.

Regardless of which approach is taken, creative surgical techniques are used to achieve native tissue-to-tissue continuity. If use of allograft patch material is necessary, we use it non-circumferentially so that the growth potential of the native tissue is preserved. We limit the use of circumferential nonviable conduits to the central mediastinum.

Ideal age of repair of this lesion is unknown. Our current approach involves the following. If the patient is well balanced physiologically, we prefer to perform this procedure when the patient is between 3 and 6 months of age. However, if the patient is severely cyanotic or overshunted, repair is feasible at an even earlier age. The advantages of early one-stage repair are numerous. Early normalization of cardiovascular physiology and correction of cyanosis is achieved. Protection against pulmonary hypertension, related either to high flow through collaterals or through systemic shunts, is accomplished. The number of operations is reduced. The use of nonviable material in the periphery of the lung is completely eliminated in the great majority of cases. The number of patients who can be completely repaired is likely to be enhanced.

Technique: One-Stage Complete Unifocalization and Intracardiac Repair

Surgical access to the mediastinum is via a generous midline incision and a median sternotomy (Fig. 88-2). A subtotal thymectomy is performed. The right pleura is widely opened anterior to the phrenic nerve, the right lung is lifted out of the pleural cavity, and the right-sided collaterals are identified and dissected. Similarly, the left pleura is opened and the left-sided collaterals are

identified and dissected. Avenues for collateral rerouting are developed by opening the pleura on both sides posterior to the phrenic nerves in the hilar regions (Fig. 88-3). The descending aorta is exposed in the posterior mediastinum and all the collaterals from it are identified, dissected, and controlled. After this, the pericardium is opened, and a large piece is harvested and fixed in glutaraldehyde. Attention is then directed to the central mediastinum, and the native pulmonary arteries, if present, are dissected out (Fig. 88-4A). Any further collaterals from the upper descending aorta are identified and dissected in the subcarinal space (between the tracheobronchial angle and the

roof of the left atrium) by an approach between the right superior vena cava and the aorta (Fig. 88-4B). The floor of the pericardial reflection in the transverse sinus is opened, and the posterior mediastinal soft tissues are dissected to expose the aortic segment and the collaterals in this region. This is an important maneuver for gaining access to collaterals, which typically can arise from this location. Opening this space also provides the most direct avenue for collateral rerouting for direct tissue-to-tissue anastomosis, which would otherwise be impossible. In addition, in some cases collaterals arising from the aortic arch or the neck vessels are exposed and dissected. All

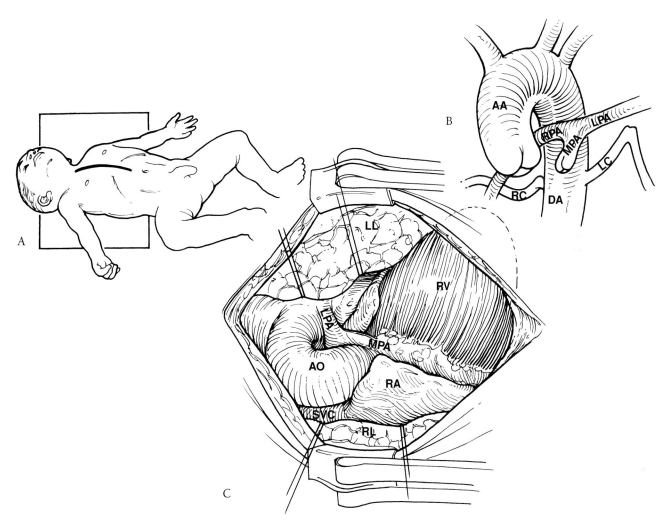

Figure 88-2. **(A)** An extended midline incision and sternotomy are performed to facilitate generous sternal retraction. **(B)** The pulmonary blood supply. The pulmonary arteries are small: The right pulmonary artery (RPA) supplies only the right lower lobe, and the left pulmonary artery (LPA) supplies only the upper lobe. The collaterals supply the remainder of the lung segments. **(C)** View from the surgeon's side after harvest of the pericardial patch. The pericardial edges are suspended with silk stay sutures and held with hemostats to facilitate hilar dissection. (AA = ascending aorta; AO = aorta; DA = descending aorta; LC = left collateral; LL = left lung; MPA = main pulmonary artery; RA = right atrium; RC = right collateral; RL = right lung; RV = right ventricle; SVC = superior vena cava.)

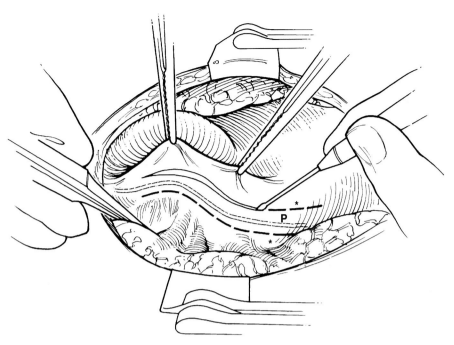

Figure 88-3. The pericardium and parietal pleura on both sides are incised longitudinally above and below the pericardium (the phrenic nerve is left on a strip of tissue with careful attention not to injure the nerve during the entire procedure). This facilitates hilar dissection for isolating, rerouting, and unifocalizing the collaterals. (P = phrenic nerve.)

collaterals are snared to achieve control before cardiopulmonary bypass is instituted.

As many collaterals as possible are permanently ligated at their origin, mobilized, and unifocalized without cardiopulmonary bypass (Fig. 88-4C, D). When the patient's oxygenation reaches a compromising level, cardiopulmonary bypass is instituted, and the remainder of the collaterals are unifocalized at mild to moderate hypothermia with the heart beating. A calcium-supplemented blood prime is used in the cardiopulmonary bypass pump circuit to maintain normal cardiac function. During the unifocalization process, the emphasis is on avoiding

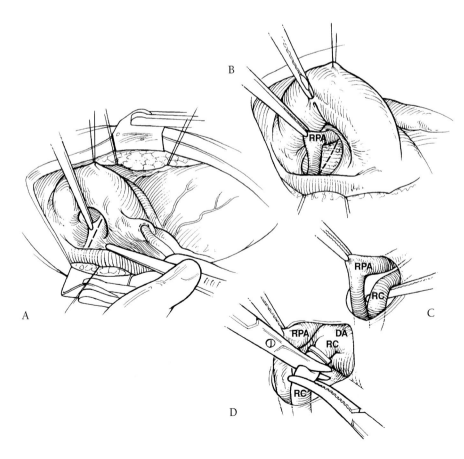

Figure 88-4. **(A)** The pericardium is incised over the right pulmonary artery. **(B)** The right pulmonary artery (RPA) is mobilized extensively all the way into the hilum. Transverse sinus dissection is performed in the area shown by the dashed line. **(C)** The right collateral (RC) is identified and mobilized. **(D)** The aortic end is occluded with a large hemoclip, and the collateral is transected. As much length of the collateral as possible is taken to facilitate tissue-to-tissue reconstruction of the neopulmonary arteries. (DA = descending aorta.)

synthetic or allograft conduits in the periphery and on achieving unifocalization by native tissue-to-tissue anastomosis. One or more of the following techniques of unifocalization are generally used in these patients:

1. Side-to-side anastomosis of the collateral to the central pulmonary arteries, thereby augmenting the hypoplastic central pulmonary arteries.
2. Side-to-side anastomosis of collateral to collateral or of collateral to peripheral native pulmonary artery.
3. End-to-side anastomosis of collateral to collateral or of collateral to native pulmonary artery.
4. Anastomosis of button of aorta (giving rise to multiple unobstructed collaterals) to the native pulmonary arteries.
5. End-to-end or end-to-side anastomosis of collateral to central conduit.
6. Allograft patch plasty of stenotic distal segments of the collaterals.
7. Allograft patch augmentation of the reconstructed neo-central pulmonary arteries.

These anastomoses are achieved directly by bringing collaterals through the transverse sinus or below the lung hilum or occasionally above the hilum, using as much of the collateral length as possible. Collateral length is given the highest priority to achieve tissue-to-tissue anastomosis. For example, if a discrete stenosis is present in the midportion of a collateral, the entire collateral would still be used. The stenosis is managed by side-to-side reconstruction at the necessary level or, if that is not possible, by patching. Even collaterals that had a dual supply to a lung segment along with true pulmonary artery supply are unifocalized to build up the size of the reconstructed pulmonary arteries. However, particularly difficult aspects of unifocalization occasionally are completed after cardioplegia is induced and aortic cross-clamping at moderate hypothermia. The important concepts necessary to achieve this type of unifocalization are flexibility regarding reconstruction, aggressive mobilization, maximizing the length of the MAPCAs, and creative rerouting (Figs. 88-5 through 88-8).

After unifocalization is completed the new single-compartment pulmonary arterial system is assessed for suitability for VSD closure (see next section for criteria for VSD closure). If VSD closure is indicated, a longitudinal ventriculotomy is made in the right ventricular infundibulum and the hypertrophied muscle bundles are resected (Figs. 88-9 through 88-12). The VSD is closed with a glutaraldehyde-fixed autologous pericardial patch or a polyester (Dacron) patch using interrupted mattress pledgeted, braided polyester sutures. The right atrium is opened to inspect the atrial septum. An atrial septal defect or patent foramen ovale, if present, is partially closed to leave a small unidirectional interatrial communication as a "pop-off" valve for venous blood in case of postoperative right ventricular dysfunction. In some cases with intact atrial septum, a small one-way interatrial communication is created. At this stage rewarming is started.

An allograft valved conduit is tailored and used in all cases to connect the right ventricle to the reconstructed neopulmonary arterial system (Fig. 88-10). The distal conduit is anastomosed to the reconstructed pulmonary arteries. If needed, a distal tongue of tissue is shaped to augment the reconstructed central branch pulmonary arteries.

In a total of >1,100 unifocalized collaterals, only a small number have been reconstructed with circumferential nonviable conduit (expanded polytetrafluoroethylene) (Fig. 88-13). In patients with absent or stringlike true pulmonary arteries, sometimes a second, nonvalved allograft conduit may be necessary to reconstruct the central left and right pulmonary arteries. In such patients, in whom growth potential is an issue, the hilar regions are reconstructed only with native tissue using the techniques described, and this second conduit serves as the main left and right pulmonary artery only with the conduit

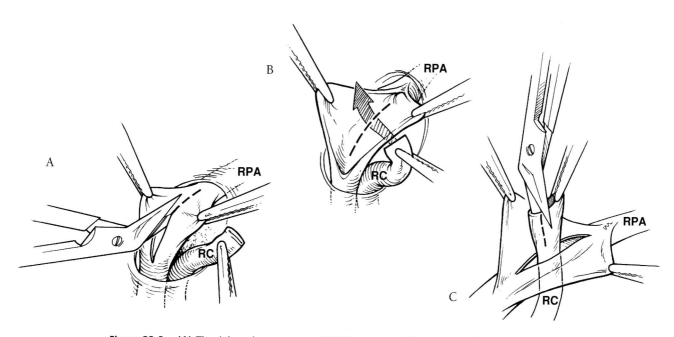

Figure 88-5.   **(A)** The right pulmonary artery (RPA) is opened. This arteriotomy is later extended to augment the right pulmonary artery. **(B)** An arteriotomy is then made in the posterior wall of the right pulmonary artery. **(C)** The end of the collateral vessel is splayed open. (LPA, left pulmonary artery; MPA, main pulmonary artery; RC = right collateral.)

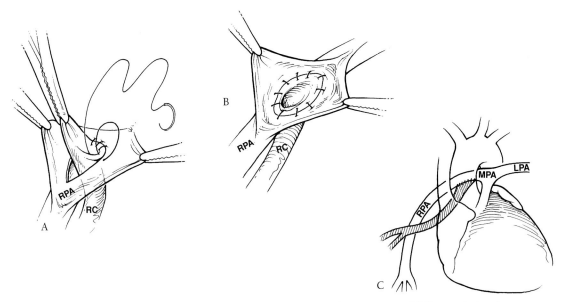

Figure 88-6. **(A)** The collateral is anastomosed to the right pulmonary artery (RPA) posteriorly using 7-0 absorbable monofilament suture. The site of the anastomosis varies depending on the position and course of the collateral. **(B)** The unifocalized collateral through the right pulmonary artery. The opening should be unobstructed, wide, and without any kinks. **(C)** The appearance of the right-sided pulmonary arteries after unifocalization. (LPA = left pulmonary artery; MPA = main pulmonary artery; RC = right collateral.)

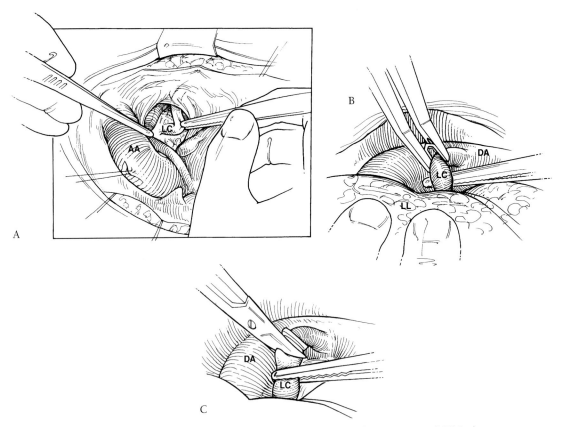

Figure 88-7. **(A)** The aorta is retracted to the right side. The left pulmonary artery (LPA) is shown being held by the forceps on the left, and the left collateral is shown being held by the forceps on the right. The left collateral (LC) is dissected and mobilized as much as possible in the mediastinum through the transverse sinus. **(B)** The left lung (LL) is retracted out of the pleural cavity and the descending aorta (DA) is exposed. The LC is dissected at its origin, mobilized, and occluded with hemoclips close to the origin from the aorta. **(C)** The collateral is further mobilized and transected. (AA = ascending aorta; MPA = main pulmonary artery.)

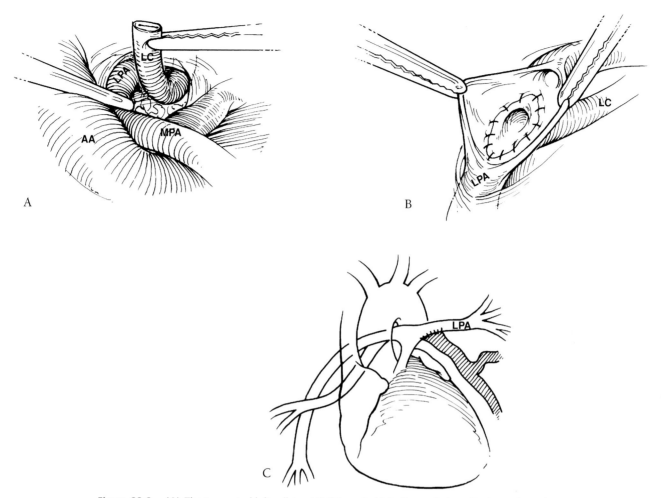

Figure 88-8. **(A)** The transected left collateral (LC) is routed into the central mediastinum through the transverse sinus. **(B)** The collateral is then unifocalized to the left pulmonary artery (LPA) using the technique described for the right side. **(C)** The appearance of the pulmonary arteries after the unifocalization is completed. (AA = ascending aorta; MPA = main pulmonary artery.)

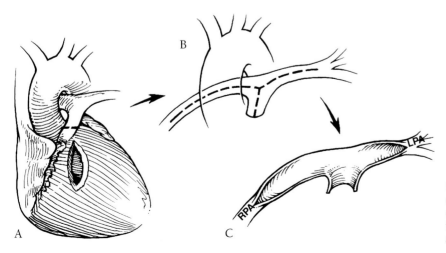

Figure 88-9. The hypoplastic main pulmonary artery is disconnected from the heart and opened into both branch pulmonary arteries all the way into the hilum. (LPA = left pulmonary artery; RPA = right pulmonary artery.)

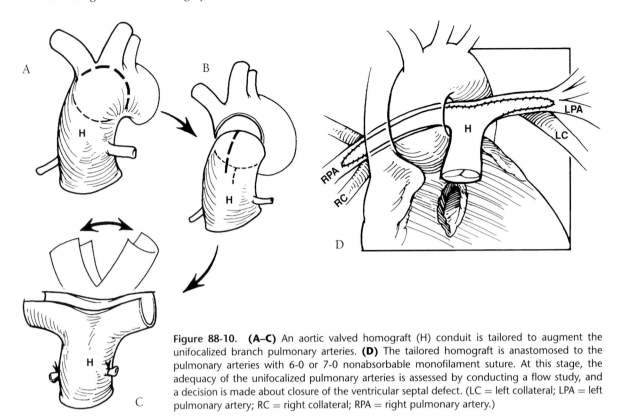

Figure 88-10. **(A–C)** An aortic valved homograft (H) conduit is tailored to augment the unifocalized branch pulmonary arteries. **(D)** The tailored homograft is anastomosed to the pulmonary arteries with 6-0 or 7-0 nonabsorbable monofilament suture. At this stage, the adequacy of the unifocalized pulmonary arteries is assessed by conducting a flow study, and a decision is made about closure of the ventricular septal defect. (LC = left collateral; LPA = left pulmonary artery; RC = right collateral; RPA = right pulmonary artery.)

limited to the pericardial cavity (Fig. 88-14). In patients with adequate collateral length, the collaterals alone are used to reconstruct the central main, right, and left pulmonary arteries, without the need for a second conduit (Fig. 88-13). The proximal right ventricle-to-conduit anastomosis is performed with a running nonabsorbable monofilament suture. A pressure-monitoring catheter is placed through the right ventricular free wall into the pulmonary arteries across the right ventricular outflow tract. The right ventriculotomy is then closed with a pericardial or an allograft patch shaped like a hood, extending from the proximal conduit onto the right ventricle.

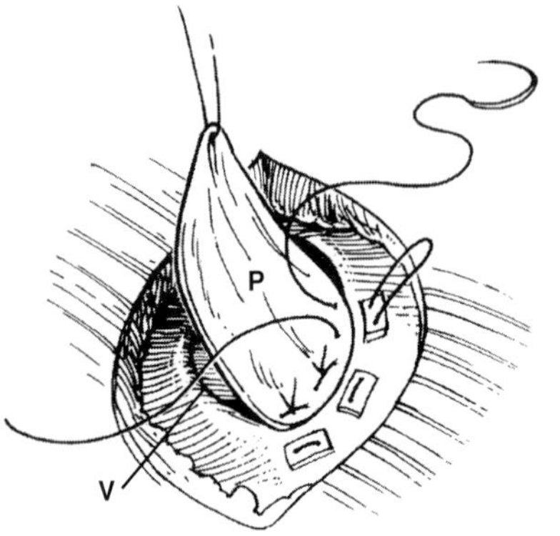

After separation from cardiopulmonary bypass, aortic, pulmonary arterial, and atrial pressures are measured continuously. A transesophageal echocardiogram is performed to ensure that there are no significant residual defects.

Bilateral pleural and mediastinal tube drains are placed and the sternum is closed. If bleeding or ventilation is an issue, we electively leave the sternum open and close the chest wound with a silicone rubber (Silastic) patch. Secondary sternal closure is performed on the second or third postoperative day.

Criteria for Closure of the Ventricular Septal Defect

Once the complete unifocalization has been performed, while the patient is still on cardiopulmonary bypass, the total resistance of the pulmonary vascular bed is assessed by an intraoperative pulmonary flow study. The pulmonary vascular bed is cannulated and perfused using a calibrated pump head from the cardiopulmonary bypass machine, with gradually increasing flow leading up to the equivalent of at least one cardiac output. At the same time a pressure catheter is placed in the pulmonary artery system, and the left atrium is vigorously vented. If the mean pulmonary artery pressure is <25 mm Hg, the decision is made to close the VSD. If the mean pulmonary pressure is >25 mmHg a central shunt is created.

Postoperative Care

The significant postoperative events are phrenic nerve palsy, severe episodic bronchospasm, pulmonary parenchymal reperfusion injury, and pulmonary hemorrhage. In an occasional patient, splanchnic end-organ injury has occurred.

With proper attention to the phrenic nerve, we have minimized this complication. Severe bronchospasm is probably caused by the extensive dissection and disruption of lymphatics and blood vessels around the tracheobronchial tree. It is also possible that the autonomic nerve balance is affected because of the dissection. We

Figure 88-11. The ventricular septal defect is closed with a glutaraldehyde-fixed pericardial patch (or a polyethylene terephthalate [Dacron] patch) (P) and interrupted pledgeted 5-0 or 4-0 braided polyester sutures. (V = ventricular septal defect.)

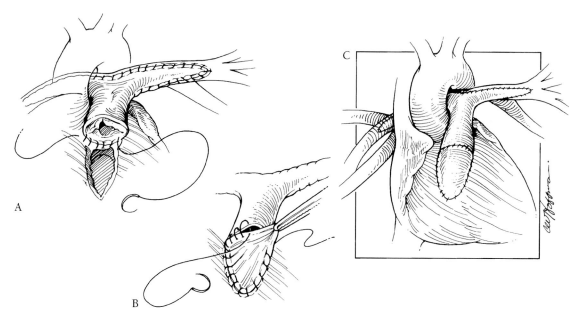

Figure 88-12.   (A) The homograft conduit is anastomosed to the right ventricle with 4-0 or 3-0 nonabsorbable monofilament suture. **(B)** The ventriculotomy is closed with a hood of homograft or glutaraldehyde-fixed pericardial patch and 4-0 or 3-0 nonabsorbable monofilament suture. **(C)** The final appearance after complete repair.

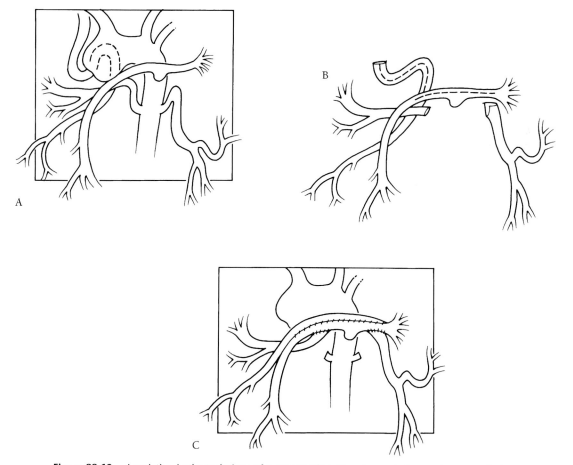

Figure 88-13.   A variation in the technique of reconstruction. Here the central neopulmonary arteries are created using only the collaterals and without any homograft patches. In cases in which there are no true pulmonary arteries and the collaterals are of adequate length and size, we reconstruct the central pulmonary arteries with similar techniques using the collateral tissue only.

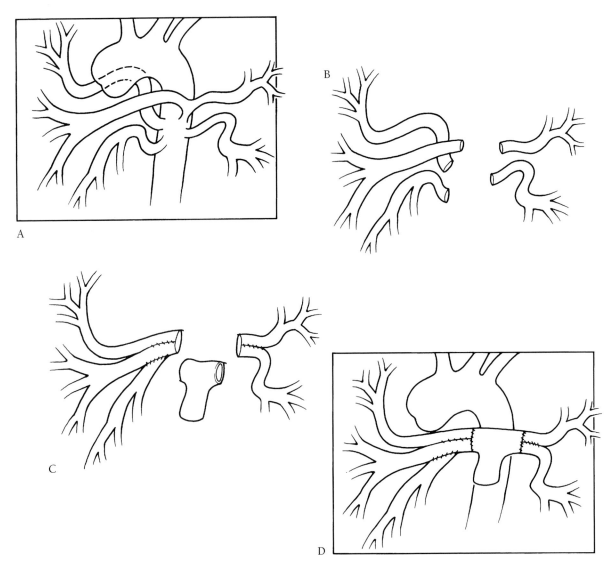

Figure 88-14. Another technical variation. In this instance there are no true pulmonary arteries. After the collaterals are unifocalized, part of the central pulmonary arteries is reconstructed entirely with pulmonary homograft (or sometimes with a second homograft conduit).

now routinely perform bronchoscopy before and after repair. The findings from this approach may reveal the cause of such episodes. Another important observation is the development of reperfusion injury of the lung. This is generally limited to the segments that are severely underperfused before unifocalization. The splanchnic end-organ injury is manifested in the form of acute hepatic insufficiency and rarely bowel necrosis. Aggressive monitoring of serum potassium, serum glucose, and hepatic enzyme profiles is strongly recommended. Hyperkalemia and hypoglycemia should be promptly detected and aggressively treated in such cases. The cause of this phenomenon is not completely known, although in the latter half of our series this complication has been rare. We believe that maintaining perfusion pressure >40 mm Hg on cardiopulmonary bypass has been an important factor in the elimination of this complication.

Follow-Up Management

All completely repaired patients are followed clinically, and a cardiac catheterization is performed at about 1 year postoperatively or earlier if necessary. In addition, during the first year the patients are followed every 3 months by echocardiography and nuclear pulmonary flow scan to promptly detect and manage alterations in pulmonary blood flow distribution or pulmonary hypertension. In patients where the VSD is left open after one-stage complete unifocalization a follow-up cardiac catheterization is performed electively at 3 months postoperatively and assessed for possible VSD closure. Some patients require one or more balloon angioplasty interventions before VSD closure. If the ratio of pulmonary to systemic blood flow (Qp/Qs) at catheterization is >2:1, the VSD is closed. If the Qp/Qs ratio is <2:1, the pulmonary artery stenosis assessment is made intraoperatively. In all patients with a second-stage closure of the VSD, an intraoperative pulmonary flow study is performed to assess the feasibility of VSD closure.

SUGGESTED READING

DeRuiter MC, Gittenberger-de Groot AC, Poelmann RE, et al. Development of the pharyngeal arch system related to the pulmonary and bronchial vessels in the avian embryo. With a concept on systemic-pulmonary collateral artery formation. Circulation 1993;87:1306.

Haworth SG. Collateral arteries in pulmonary atresia with ventricular septal defect. A precarious blood supply. Br Heart J 1980;44:5.

Iyer KS, Mee RBB. Staged repair of pulmonary atresia with ventricular septal defect and major systemic to pulmonary artery collaterals. Ann Thorac Surg 1991;51:65.

Marelli AJ, Perloff JK, Child JS, Laks H. Pulmonary atresia with ventricular septal defect in adults. Circulation 1994;89:243.

Pacifico AD, Allen RH, Colvin EV. Direct reconstruction of pulmonary artery arborization anomaly and intracardiac repair of pulmonary atresia with ventricular septal defect. Am J Cardiol 1985;55:1647.

Puga FJ, Leoni FE, Julsrud PR, Mair DD. Complete repair of pulmonary atresia, ventricular septal defect, and severe peripheral arborization abnormalities of the central pulmonary arteries. J Thorac Cardiovasc Surg 1989;98:1018.

Rabinovitch M, Herrera-DeLeon V, Castaneda AR, Reid L. Growth and development of the pulmonary vascular bed in patients with tetralogy of Fallot with or without pulmonary atresia. Circulation 1981;64:1234.

Reddy VM, Liddicoat JR, Hanley FL. Midline one stage complete unifocalization and repair of pulmonary atresia with ventricular septal defect and major aortopulmonary collaterals. J Thorac Cardiovasc Surg 1995;109:832.

Reddy VM, McElhinney D, Amin Z, et al. Early and intermediate outcomes after repair of pulmonary atresia with ventricular septal defect and major aortopulmonary collateral arteries. Experience with 85 patients. Circulation 2000;101:1826.

Rodefeld M, Reddy VM, Thompson LD, et al. Surgical creation of aortopulmonary window in selected patients with pulmonary atresia with poorly developed collaterals and hypoplastic pulmonary arteries. J Thorac Cardiovasc Surg 2002;123:1147.

Rome JJ, Mayer JE, Castaneda AR, Lock JE. Tetralogy of Fallot with pulmonary atresia. Rehabilitation of diminutive pulmonary arteries. Circulation 1993;88:1691.

Sawatari K, Imai Y, Kurosawa H, et al. Staged operation for pulmonary atresia and ventricular septal defect with major systemic collateral arteries. J Thorac Cardiovasc Surg 1989;98:738.

EDITOR'S COMMENTS

Surgical repair of pulmonary atresia with ventricular septal defect and aortopulmonary collateral sources of blood flow is a technical challenge. The aortopulmonary collaterals may supply only a relatively small portion of the total parenchymal volume of the lung or may supply the majority of the pulmonary vascular bed. In addition, some collaterals may be unobstructed, leading to rapid development of pulmonary vascular disease, and others may develop peripheral or proximal stenoses. In the most severe cases, no central pulmonary arteries are present; however, in the majority of cases there is a very small central pulmonary confluence that may not supply much of the distal parenchyma. Multiple surgical approaches have been applied to this complex congenital heart defect, including staged unifocalizations of the collateral vessels to the lungs by bilateral thoracotomies with either pericardial tube reconstruction and unifocalization of the vessels with bilateral shunting and then a repeat operation for central unifocalization and connection to the right ventricular outflow tract, or in cases with diminutive central pulmonary arteries with distal reasonable arborization, connection of the central pulmonary arteries directly to the aorta posteriorly as advocated by Roger Mee.

All of these approaches suffer from the problems of development of distal stenoses and the inability to centrally unifocalize all of the collateral segments at a single setting. In addition, patients who have had bilateral thoracotomies for unifocalization who ultimately fail unifocalization procedures represent a very difficult subset of patients for lung transplantation and cardiac repair at a later time. The severe cyanosis in these patients and the development of significant chest wall collateral vessels has resulted in severe hemorrhage at the time of lung transplant and cardiac repair in our experience and has limited the applicability of lung transplantation in these patients. Therefore, the approach recommended by the authors has appeal because direct intervention to unifocalize all major aortopulmonary collaterals is performed at an early age through a median sternotomy incision, which will, it is hoped, limit development of aortopulmonary collaterals from the chest wall to the pulmonary parenchyma. Thus, if failure of unifocalization occurs, it may be possible in these patients to undertake lung transplantation with cardiac repair at a later time without the problem of severe hemorrhage from the pleural spaces.

Although one-stage unifocalization as advocated in this chapter has become increasingly popular, there are some patients in whom staged unifocalization may be associated with excellent long-term results as described by Dr. Laks and associates from the University of California at Los Angeles. The advantage of peripheral unifocalization by thoracotomy is the relative accessibility of the collateral vessels. The use, however, of pericardial tube grafts for unifocalization leads to difficulty in centralizing these pericardial tube grafts and then reconstructing the vessels to the right ventricle. We have found that non–glutaraldehyde-fixed pericardium has been associated with significant dilation and aneurysm formation if used for central unifocalization, and, in addition, the central pulmonary arteries often need to be placed anterior to the aorta to prevent compression by the generally large aorta in these patients. There is often very little room behind the aorta for creation of a central pulmonary artery confluence. Thus, patient selection and tailoring of the specific operation to the individual anatomy are paramount in this particular cardiac lesion.

The extensive nature of operations to provide complete unifocalization in infancy is well described in this chapter. The problems with organ system dysfunction from long bypass times for these complex operations and the difficulties in preventing steal from the collateral vessels with initiation of bypass will require additional development of these procedures for wider use. Nevertheless, in most cases, central unifocalization can be performed with reconstruction to the right ventricular outflow tract, which has the advantage of providing access to the distal pulmonary vasculature for catheter interventional procedures to deal with distal stenoses.

The primary difficulty in one-stage unifocalization is deciding when VSD closure can be performed. Complete reconstruction with a Dacron patch of the ventricular septal defect and right ventricular outflow tract reconstruction can be performed with creation of a superiorly located defect in the VSD patch, which can be encircled with a purse-string suture of polypropylene that is brought out superiorly on the right ventricle. In this fashion, a VSD can be left after reconstruction, and after the patient is weaned from cardiopulmonary bypass with pressure monitoring in the main pulmonary artery, decisions can be made regarding snaring of the residual VSD. If the VSD can be closed with maintenance of right ventricular pressures of half systemic or less, then complete occlusion of the VSD may be undertaken. In other cases, the VSD may be left open to allow for right-to-left shunting in the early postoperative period, and later snaring of the residual defect can be performed by leaving the VSD tourniquet snare in the subcutaneous tissue near the linea alba for exposure under local anesthesia. In this fashion, decisions regarding VSD closure can be made at a period after the operation when hemodynamic stability and recovery of organ system dysfunction from the operative procedure have occurred.

Recently, if there is concern that the complete VSD closure is not possible, we place a VSD patch with a central opening that can create an unrestricted flow, but we leave a rim of Dacron material for potential anchoring of a VSD closure device in the future. This adds the possibility of avoiding reoperation when distal dilations of the pulmonary vascular bed result in adequate pulmonary flow to permit VSD closure.

Despite the outstanding results with surgical treatment of pulmonary atresia, VSD, and MAPCAS presented by Dr. Hanley's group, these continue to be very difficult patients. Even when excellent pulmonary flow can be achieved with VSD closure and a relatively low ventricular pressure in the operating room, development of distal stenosis and distortions of the pulmonary vascular bed can result in gradual and progressive elevation of pulmonary resistance with right ventricular failure. The long-term outlook of patients who have VSD closure and unifocalization remains to be completely elucidated. Nevertheless, the approaches described by Dr. Hanley and his associates have resulted in a VSD closure rate that is higher than has been traditionally seen with other staged surgical approaches, suggesting that early intervention with extensive patching of any areas of stenosis may result in better overall long-term outcomes. Nevertheless, these patients require a great deal of attention and observation for development of distal stenosis that will require catheter or surgical intervention.

In patients with inadequate collateral vessels to the lungs, severe progressive cyanosis, and a distal pulmonary vascular bed that is not amenable to unifocalization and reconstruction, we use bilateral lung transplantation and cardiac repair. This procedure is best performed in patients who have not had extensive previous pleural surgery because of the severe adhesions and hemorrhage at reoperation. Hemorrhage has been the primary cause of operative mortality with transplantation in this setting. Thus, avoidance of thoracotomy incisions if at all possible at reconstruction in these patients is preferable if later lung transplantation or heart-lung transplantation is contemplated.

T.L.S.

89

Tetralogy of Fallot

Robert D. B. Jaquiss

With an incidence of approximately 3 to 5 per 10,000 live births, tetralogy of Fallot is the most common of the cyanotic "T" lesions (tetralogy of Fallot, transposition of the great arteries, total anomalous pulmonary venous return, and tricuspid atresia) that require operation during the first year of life. Beginning with successful palliation by means of the Blalock-Taussig shunt, through the development of "complete" repair by Lillehei and Kirklin, to the present early one-stage approach, the surgical management of tetralogy has exemplified the evolution of pediatric cardiac surgery. The guiding principles in tetralogy surgery have been the minimization of early and late mortality, together with a recent focus on reduction of long-term morbidity, particularly as concerns the consequences of pulmonary insufficiency and chronic right ventricular volume overload.

Initial palliative operations are less commonly employed in simple tetralogy and are well described in Chapter 71. The subset of tetralogy with pulmonary valvar atresia and major aortopulmonary collaterals is discussed fully in Chapter 88. In this chapter, discussion will focus on the group of patients with an anterior malalignment ventricular septal defect in association with varying degrees of infundibular, valvar, and supravalvar right ventricular outflow tract obstruction.

Operative Strategy and Timing of Intervention

As expertise and experience with the use of cardiopulmonary bypass in neonates and small infants has accumulated, the management of children with tetralogy has evolved from a two-stage approach (initial palliation with a systemic-to-pulmonary shunt with definitive repair delayed for months or years) to an approach of early one-stage repair. Considerations favoring one-stage management include the avoidance of palliation-related morbidity (pulmonary artery distortion, phrenic nerve injury, seroma formation, shunt thrombosis) and palliation-related mortality. Other theoretical advantages of early complete repair are rescue of the right ventricle from grossly abnormal pressure- and volume-loading conditions as well as the avoidance of prolonged exposure of the developing brain to cyanosis. In the past, relative contraindications to early repair have included major coronary artery anomalies (anterior descending originating from the right coronary and crossing the distal infundibulum), multiple muscular septal defects, extreme pulmonary arterial hypoplasia, and pulmonary arterial discontinuity. The excess risk associated with these factors for the most part has now been overcome with modern techniques. It is generally agreed that these conditions can be managed well without initial palliation, although some controversy remains. The major indication for initial palliation is probably the coexistence of illnesses or conditions (recent intracranial hemorrhage, severe renal or hepatic dysfunction, or complicated infectious illness) that would greatly increase the risks inherent in the use of cardiopulmonary bypass. In such circumstances initial palliation with a small systemic to pulmonary shunt (3.5- or 4-mm polytetrafluoroethylene [PTFE]) is reasonable. Alternatively, palliation of severe cyanosis by means of balloon angioplasty may be accomplished in cases with predominantly valvar obstruction of the right ventricular outflow tract, although such cases are rare.

The timing of intervention is influenced both by patient characteristics and institutional preference. Absent the occurrence of hypercyanotic "spells," elective repair should probably be undertaken if the level of baseline oxygen saturation is <75% to 80%. If hypoxemic spells occur, standard management includes the administration of volume, sedation, and supplemental oxygen. Beta-adrenergic blockade may be added, but should probably not be used as justification to delay surgery significantly. The creation of an institutional policy for the timing of elective operation for asymptomatic patients with only minimal or moderate cyanosis is also desirable. Without such a policy, such patients may become "lost," and in any case there seem to be little data to support "watchful waiting," particularly beyond 3 to 6 months of age.

After the timing of surgery has been set, an operative plan is created with two primary goals in mind: maximal relief of right ventricular outflow obstruction and complete separation of the pulmonary and systemic circulations by closure of the ventricular septal defect. Preservation of right ventricular function is also of paramount importance, and is accomplished by minimizing right ventricular incisions and minimizing pulmonary valvar incompetence. To tailor the surgical strategy to the patient, complete anatomic information is necessary, and can generally be obtained from detailed echocardiography. If the information gleaned from echocardiography is incomplete, cardiac catheterization may be required, particularly to assess pulmonary artery distortion if a palliative shunt has been employed and to assess the coronary branching pattern if this has not been well seen. As an alternative to cardiac catheterization, cardiac magnetic resonance imaging has recently shown increasing promise and is attractive because of its noninvasive nature. In the preoperative evaluation of anatomy, specific features to be considered include the size and arborization of the pulmonary arteries, presence of a ductus arteriosus, details of the origin and course of the major coronary arteries, levels and severity of right ventricular outflow tract obstruction (infundibular, valvar, supravalvar), presence of additional ventricular septal defects, and presence of other significant anomalies such as a persistent left superior vena cava. Palliative shunts as well as any consequent pulmonary artery distortion must also be identified.

Operative Technique

After sternotomy (which may be a resternotomy if a palliative shunt is in place) preliminary dissection is accomplished. This consists in separating the ascending aorta from the main pulmonary artery, mobilizing any systemic-to-pulmonary connections (ductus arteriosus or palliative shunt), and encircling the vena cavae for subsequent tourniquet placement. The anterior surface of the right ventricle is inspected for the presence of major coronary artery branches.

After administration of heparin, the patient is cannulated for cardiopulmonary bypass employing direct bicaval venous cannulation with right-angled, metal-tipped cannulas (Fig. 89-1). The conduct of cardiopulmonary bypass generally requires only mild or moderate hypothermia (28°C to 32°C) and limited hemodilution (hematocrit on bypass ≥30%). In the past, deep hypothermic circulatory arrest was routinely employed for complete repairs in neonates and small infants, although there seems little justification for this unless the patient is extraordinarily small (<2.0 kg). With the initiation of bypass, palliative shunts are occluded and should be divided. If shunt-associated pulmonary artery distortion has been identified, reconstruction of the pulmonary artery is accomplished at this point, generally by means of a small patch to augment the diameter of the artery. A catheter is inserted through a purse-string suture at the junction of the right upper pulmonary vein and the left atrium and then advanced across the mitral valve to serve as a left heart vent. (Fig. 89-2). Even on total cardiopulmonary bypass, children who have been cyanotic

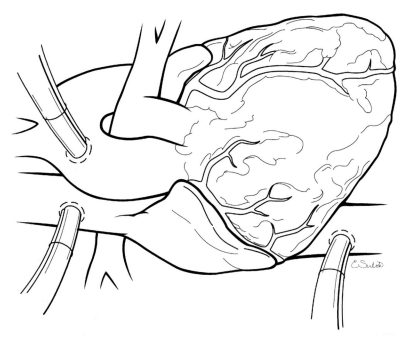

Figure 89-1.   Cannulation for repair of tetralogy of Fallot.

often have such well-developed collateral sources of pulmonary blood flow that the amount of pulmonary venous return may be prodigious. A well-functioning left heart vent is therefore absolutely essential to permit the visualization and closure of the ventricular septal defect.

Next, the aortic is cross-clamped and cardioplegia administered, with redosing at 20- to 30-minute intervals. A longitudinal right atriotomy is performed, and the interatrial septum is inspected. In older infants and children, a patent foramen ovale or atrial septal defect is closed. In neonates and young infants, a patent foramen is left open; if an atrial septal defect is present in younger children, it is reduced in size to approximately 4 mm.

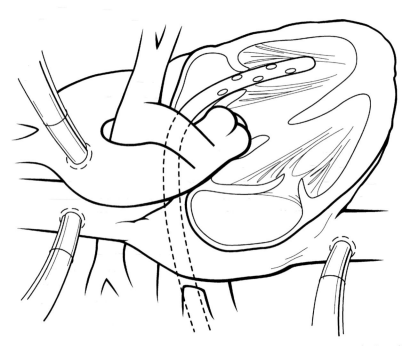

Figure 89-2.   A left-sided vent catheter is placed through a purse-string suture at the junction of the left upper pulmonary vein and the left atrium, and then advanced across the mitral valve.

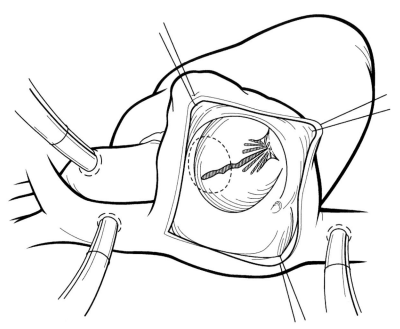

Figure 89-3. Traction sutures on the edges of the right atriotomy allow visualization of the tricuspid valve. The approximate location of the ventricular septal defect is indicated by the dashed circle beneath the anteroseptal commissure of the tricuspid valve.

Traction sutures on the posterior aspect of the atriotomy and the right atrial wall immediately anterior to the anterior leaflet of the tricuspid valve allow excellent visualization of the ventricular septum (Figs. 89-3 and 89-4). Additional ventricular septal defects that may not have been visible on preoperative echocardiography because of equalization of pressures should be sought at this time and closed if present.

The right ventricular outflow tract is inspected from below through the tricuspid valve. Except in the very rare instance of pure subvalvar obstruction (normal pulmonary artery and valve diameter), the pulmonary artery is also opened longitudinally at this point. With visualization from above and below, relief of right ventricular obstruction is then accomplished. From below, obstructing muscle bundles are incised and resected if necessary, taking care to avoid injury to the anterior papillary muscle and the moderator band. In older children the fibrous rim of an os infundibulum must be completely resected. From above, the pulmonary valve is inspected, with sharp division of any fused commissures. The adequacy of the pulmonary valve annulus is assessed by calibrated dilators (Fig. 89-5). If the annulus is judged to be inadequate, that is, <1 or 2 mm larger than the predicted normal pulmonary annulus for the patient, the pulmonary arterial incision is extended across the annulus for a distance of a few millimeters, respecting the presence of any larger coronary arterial branches. The proximal extent of this incision is then determined by the perceived adequacy of the infundibular gradient relief accomplished by the previously described muscle resection and division. Additional muscle resection is easily accomplished at this point, but may not be adequate if the infundibulum is diffusely hypoplastic, in which case the transannular incision should be extended more proximally.

Closure of the ventricular septal defect is then accomplished via an atrial approach. Exposure is generally excellent from this vantage point, particularly with retraction of the septal and anterior tricuspid leaflets, either with a hand-held retractor or traction sutures. Occasionally difficulty may be encountered in visualizing the upper margin of the ventricular septal defect just beneath the junction of the septal and anterior leaflets. In such cases, exposure may be improved by gentle external pressure on the anterior portion of the aortic root that, in effect, pushes the upper margin of the defect into view allowing accurate suture placement. Alternatively, a limited incision can be made in the tricuspid valve, parallel to the annulus, through which visualization is simple. After placement of the ventricular septal defect (VSD) sutures, the incision in the valve leaflet is closed with a fine Prolene suture.

The septal defect is typically closed with a Dacron patch, although PTFE and glutaraldehyde-tanned autologous pericardium are reasonable alternatives. Generally, an interrupted suture technique is preferred, except in neonates and small infants, in whom repeated tying of multiple sutures in friable ventricular muscle may be more

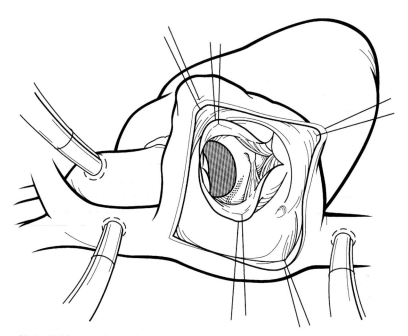

Figure 89-4. With retraction of the septal and anterior leaflets of the tricuspid valve the ventricular septal defect is exposed. Also seen are the aortic valve leaflets in proximity to the upper margin of the defect. The stippled area along the crest of the muscular septum denotes the area of the conduction system.

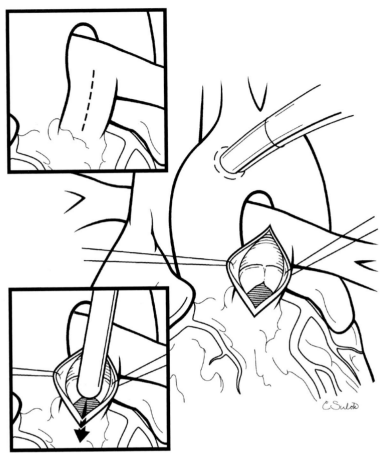

Figure 89-5.   A longitudinal incision in the main pulmonary artery allows inspection of the right ventricular outflow tract from above. A calibrated dilator is introduced from above to size the pulmonary valve annulus and infundibular region.

likely to cause sutures to tear out. Regardless of suture choice, attention to the depth and location of suture placement is crucial in the posterior-inferior aspect of the ventricular septal defect to avoid surgical heart block. As the sutures are placed along the inferior rim of the defect, they should be placed on the right ventricular aspect of the rim approximately 3 mm to 5 mm away from the crest of the septum. At the posteroinferior corner, a transition is made in suturing from the right ventricular aspect of the septum up onto the septal leaflet of the tricuspid valve itself (Fig. 89-6). A similar transition in made superiorly from the ventriculo-infundibular fold onto the tricuspid annulus. With both transition sutures two pledgets are used, one located on the atrial aspect of the septal leaflet annulus and one below the valve level against the right ventricular aspect of the septum. With all the sutures tied, the margins of the patch are gently probed to detect any "between-stitch" residual defects (Fig. 89-7).

With the ventricular septal defect closed, a final evaluation of the right ventricular outflow tract must be made, with the aortic root pressurized. This may be accomplished by means of the administration of a dose of antegrade cardioplegia or by simply removing the aortic cross-clamp. The point of this examination is to evaluate the right ventricular outflow tract under physiologic conditions with the aortic root in its normal state and position, which is quite different from its location in an arrested, vented heart. Any significantly obstructive outflow tract muscle should be resected at this time, or if no further muscle resection is possible, the proximal extent of the right ventricular outflow tract incision may be extended. After removal of the aortic cross-clamp, reconstruction of the right ventricular outflow tract is then completed using a gusset of PTFE, Dacron, or glutaraldehyde-tanned pericardium, the distal extent of which will serve to enlarge the main pulmonary artery and even the proximal left pulmonary artery if necessary. Alternatively, if the main pulmonary artery is of adequate size, a separate incision and patch may be used to address isolated branch pulmonary artery stenosis

or hypoplasia. Last, the right atriotomy is closed with a two-layer running monofilament suture.

After closure of the cardiac incisions, pacing wires are placed on the right atrium and right ventricle. Mediastinal and pleural drains are placed as well, and a left atrial pressure-monitoring catheter is brought through the chest wall. After reperfusion for an appropriate interval, attainment of normothermia, and the institution of inotropic infusions, transesophageal echocardiography is performed to confirm the completion of cardiac de-airing. The left ventricular vent is then removed and replaced with a left atrial pressure-monitoring line. Separation from cardiopulmonary bypass is then accomplished, and a complete transesophageal echocardiogram is performed. The evaluation should include assessments of residual right ventricular outflow obstruction, pulmonary valve competence, residual septal defects, tricuspid valve function, and biventricular systolic function. A simultaneous hemodynamic assessment may be accomplished by direct needle puncture of the right ventricle and distal pulmonary artery. If the right ventricular pressure is >70% to 80% of systemic pressure, a remediable cause must be sought and addressed by means of additional muscle resection, proximal extension of the pulmonary artery or transannular patch, or revision of the distal aspect of the patch. If right ventricular hypertension is caused by distal pulmonary artery hypertension, then the pulmonary bed must be presumed to be diffusely hypoplastic. In such cases, consideration should be given to creating a fenestration in the ventricular septal defect patch.

Once a satisfactory surgical result has been achieved, modified ultrafiltration is performed, after which routine decannulation and chest closure is accomplished. Every attempt is then made to accomplish immediate postoperative extubation, provided hemodynamic stability is assured.

Special Circumstances

Severe Pulmonary Insufficiency

If placement of a transannular patch is necessary, some degree of pulmonary insufficiency is the inevitable consequence. The magnitude of this insufficiency will depend on several factors including the width of the patch relative to the native annulus, the adequacy of the pulmonary vascular bed,

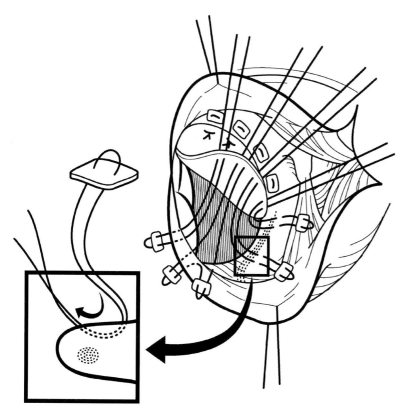

Figure 89-6. A series of interrupted horizontal mattress sutures with pledgets is placed around the margin of the defect. A transition suture with two pledges is shown at the 7-o'clock position. One pledget is below the valve and another is above the tricuspid annulus. A similar transition stitch (not shown) is used at the inferoposterior margin. The inset shows safe placement of sutures on the right ventricular aspect of the septum in the region of the conduction system, which is denoted by stippling.

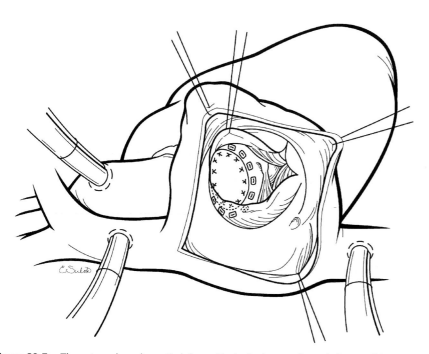

Figure 89-7. The sutures have been tied down. Typically three or four pledgets will be above the annulus (two transition sutures plus one or two sutures between them).

the functionality of any residual native pulmonary valve tissue, and the diastolic function of the right ventricle. In addition, the impact of the insufficiency will also be influenced by the competence (or lack thereof) of the tricuspid valve. In circumstances in which it is felt that pulmonary insufficiency will be poorly tolerated, the placement of a so-called monocusp valve may be helpful. The valve is fashioned as a generously proportioned hemioval attached over the proximal half of the transannular patch (Figs. 89-8 and 89-9) so as to allow coaptation with the right ventricular outflow tract rather than with the residual native pulmonary valve. (Figs. 89-10 and 89-11). The long-term fate of such valves has been disappointing, particularly when they have been constructed of native pericardium (although the importance of such valves is probably greatest in the immediate postoperative phase). Encouraging short- and intermediate-term data have recently been reported with monocusps created of thin (0.1 mm) PTFE.

Anomalous Coronary Artery Course

The traditional management of such patients has often involved the creation of a right ventriculotomy proximal to the anomalous coronary artery with the placement of an allograft valved conduit between the right ventricle and the pulmonary artery confluence. More recently reports have appeared describing successful transatrial, transpulmonary repair without conduit in the vast majority of cases of anomalous coronary arteries, limiting conduit implantation to only patients with severe hypoplasia of the right ventricular outflow tract. Transection of the native main pulmonary artery with reimplantation of the distal artery down to the proximal ventriculotomy has also been described as an alternative to conduit placement.

Tetralogy of Fallot with Absent Pulmonary Valve

Patients with this anomaly typically present shortly after birth with severe ventilatory compromise from massively dilated central pulmonary arteries that in turn have caused severe tracheobronchomalacia or as older, mildly cyanotic infants with much less airway malacia. The former group must be approached at the time of diagnosis and require the implantation of a competent pulmonary valve. Simultaneous reduction arterioplasty of the central pulmonary arteries is also performed. Recently, very encouraging

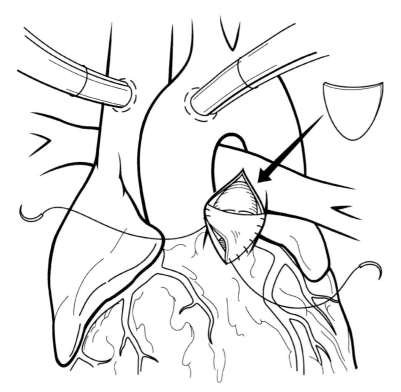

Figure 89-8. A monocusp valve in the form of a hemioval constructed of 0.1-mm polytetrafluoroethylene is used if a transannular incision will result in significant pulmonary insufficiency.

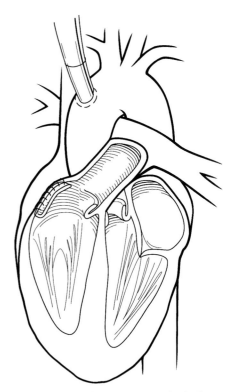

Figure 89-10. The monocusp valve in the open position.

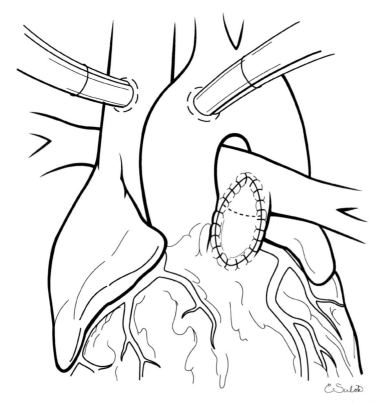

Figure 89-9. The completed transannular patch is in place, with the monocusp valve size denoted by the dashed line.

results have been described with the addition of the Lecompte maneuver, bringing the pulmonary bifurcation anterior to the aorta and very effectively minimizing airway compression. In the minimally symptomatic infant coming to elective repair, pulmonary valve competence is probably less important, and neither valve implantation nor Lecompte maneuver may be necessary, although downsizing of the central pulmonary arteries is reasonable.

Surgical Complications and Postoperative Care

Pitfalls to avoid in the repair of tetralogy of Fallot relate to either injudicious suture placement during ventricular septal defect repair or unfortunately placed incisions in the right ventricular outflow tract. The consequences of poor suture placement include injury to the aortic or tricuspid valve with resultant valvar insufficiency, incomplete closure of the ventricular septal defect, and surgically induced heart block requiring implantation of a permanent pacemaker. All of these are avoidable complications and require thorough understanding of the location of the conduction system of the heart

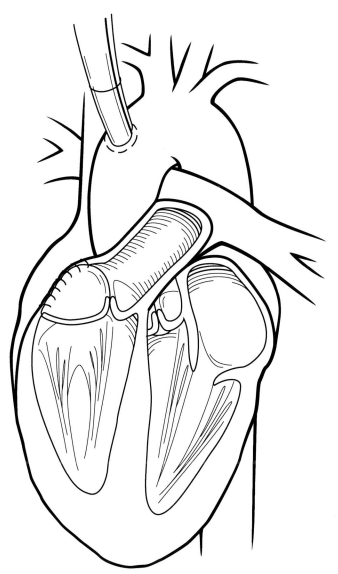

Figure 89-11. The monocusp valve in the closed position, with apposition against residual pulmonary valvar tissue or outflow tract muscle.

as well as optimum visualization of the margins of the septal defect and adjacent valve leaflets.

Complications related to poorly placed muscular incisions include injury to the papillary muscles of the tricuspid valve or the more ominous transection of a major coronary branch. The former problem is generally the result of overly enthusiastic "muscle bundle" division performed with incomplete visualization and should be entirely preventable. Likewise, injury to an anomalous anterior descending coronary artery is preventable if the surgeon has anticipated its existence based on preoperative imaging studies, confirmed by intraoperative visualization of the artery. In extremely rare cases the anomalous coronary artery is entirely intramyocardial for a portion of

its course, but this should be suspected based on echocardiography and examination. Other coronary arteries, particularly septal perforator branches of the anterior descending artery, may be transected during intracavitary right ventricular muscle resection with the subsequent development of coronary-cameral fistulae. These fistulae are rarely hemodynamically significant and generally do not require intervention.

Other postoperative complications observed immediately after tetralogy of Fallot repair include low-cardiac-output syndrome, junctional ectopic tachycardia, and pleural effusions. Low cardiac output is virtually always related to right ventricular dysfunction, which may be systolic failure, diastolic failure, or more commonly both. The etiology of right ventricular failure is

likely multifactorial but includes such factors as imperfect myocardial protection of the hypertrophied right ventricle during the cross-clamp interval, extensive right ventricular incisions, residual pulmonary valve dysfunction (obstruction, insufficiency, or both), and tricuspid valve insufficiency. The best approach to right ventricular dysfunction in tetralogy of Fallot patients is obviously prevention, but failing that ideal solution, treatment generally consists in optimizing filling with adequate volume resuscitation, minimizing mean airway pressure to reduce right ventricular afterload, and supporting the systemic blood pressure with appropriate inotropic medication to maximize coronary perfusion pressure to the right ventricle. If significant right ventricular dysfunction is anticipated, the provision of a small atrial septal communication will allow preservation of left-sided filling and systemic cardiac output, albeit at the expense of mild or even moderate systemic arterial oxygen desaturation.

Right-sided pleural effusions are frequently seen after repair of tetralogy of Fallot, and are likely related to the increased right atrial pressure often noted after surgery in the setting of right ventricular diastolic dysfunction. In anticipation of these effusions, it is reasonable to place a right pleural drain at the time of surgery to avoid the need for postoperative thoracentesis or tube thoracostomy. If the effusions are small, they often respond to aggressive diuresis in the event that a pleural drain has not been left.

Junctional ectopic tachycardia is an infrequent complication of tetralogy repair, particularly if there has been extensive right ventricular muscle resection and division. The tachycardia may be well tolerated if it is relatively slow, but at heart rates >180 to 200 beats/min may significantly impair biventricular filling and cardiac output. The traditional approaches to postoperative junctional tachycardia have included induced hypothermia and a variety of antiarrhythmic medications, with avoidance of beta-adrenergic medications if possible. More recently, amiodarone has emerged as the drug of choice for this arrhythmia, the appearance of which is generally confined to the first few days after surgery.

Late Complications

The majority of late issues facing patients with repaired tetralogy of Fallot arise from dysfunction of the pulmonary valve, with consequent impairment of right ventricular function. Clinical manifestations include varying degrees of right heart failure, ranging from exercise intolerance to peripheral edema and anasarca in extreme cases. Other late problems include the development of ventricular arrhythmias and the development of progressive aortic valvar insufficiency. The optimal timing of intervention to prevent irreversible right ventricular damage remains unclear and is the subject of a great deal of investigation. When such intervention is undertaken, typically in the form of implantation of a pulmonary valve, cryoablation and/or implantation of an antitachycardia device is often performed at the same time.

SUGGESTED READING

Brizard CP, Mas C, Sohn YS, et al. Transatrial-transpulmonary tetralogy of Fallot repair is effective in the presence of anomalous coronary arteries. J Thorac Cardiovasc Surg 1998;116:770.

Castaneda AR, Freed MD, Williams RG, et al. Repair of tetralogy of Fallot in infancy. Early and late results. J Thorac Cardiovasc Surg 1977;74:372.

Chen Q, Monro JL. Division of modified Blalock-Taussig shunt at correction avoids distortion of the pulmonary artery. Ann Thorac Surg 2001;71:1265.

Cheung MM, Konstantinov IE, Redington AN. Late complications of repair of tetralogy of Fallot and indications for pulmonary valve replacement. Semin Thorac Cardiovasc Surg 2005;17:155.

Davlouros PA, Karatza AA, Gatzoulis MA, et al. Timing and type of surgery for severe pulmonary regurgitation after repair of tetralogy of Fallot. Int J Cardiol 2004;97(Suppl 1):91.

Dodge-Khatami A, Miller OI, Anderson RH, et al. Surgical substrates of postoperative junctional ectopic tachycardia in congenital heart defects. J Thorac Cardiovasc Surg 2002;123:624.

Fraser CD Jr, McKenzie ED, Cooley DA. Tetralogy of Fallot: surgical management individualized to the patient. Ann Thorac Surg 2001;71:1556; discussion, 1561.

Fyler DC. Report of the 1980 New England Regional Infant Cardiac Program. Pediatrics 1980;65(Suppl):375.

Geva T, Greil GF, Marshall AC, et al. Gadolinium-enhanced 3-dimensional magnetic resonance angiography of pulmonary blood supply in patients with complex pulmonary stenosis or atresia: comparison with x-ray angiography. Circulation 2002;106:473.

Hraska V. A new approach to correction of tetralogy of Fallot with absent pulmonary valve. Ann Thorac Surg. 2000;69:1601; discussion, 1603.

Kolcz J, Pizarro C. Neonatal repair of tetralogy of Fallot results in improved pulmonary artery development without increased need for reintervention. Eur J Cardiothorac Surg 2005;28:394.

Laird WP, Snyder CS, Kertesz NJ, et al. Use of intravenous amiodarone for postoperative junctional ectopic tachycardia in children. Pediatr Cardiol 2003;24:133.

Marshall AC, Love BA, Lang P, et al. Staged repair of tetralogy of Fallot and diminutive pulmonary arteries with a fenestrated ventricular septal defect patch. J Thorac Cardiovasc Surg 2003;126:1427.

Pigula FA, Khalil PN, Mayer JE, et al. Repair of tetralogy of Fallot in neonates and young infants. Circulation 1999;100(19 Suppl):II157.

Rhodes J, O'Brien S, Patel H, et al. Palliative balloon pulmonary valvuloplasty in tetralogy of Fallot: Echocardiographic predictors of successful outcome. J Invasive Cardiol 2000;12:448.

Starnes VA, Luciani GB, Latter DA, et al. Current surgical management of tetralogy of Fallot. Ann Thorac Surg 1994;58:211.

Tchervenkov CI, Pelletier MP, Shum-Tim D, et al. Primary repair minimizing the use of conduits in neonates and infants with tetralogy or double-outlet right ventricle and anomalous coronary arteries. J Thorac Cardiovasc Surg 2000;119:314.

Turrentine MW, McCarthy RP, Vijay P, et al. Polytetrafluoroethylene monocusp valve technique for right ventricular outflow tract reconstruction. Ann Thorac Surg 2002;74:2202.

Van Arsdell G, Yun TJ. An apology for primary repair of tetralogy of Fallot. Semin Thorac Cardiovasc Surg Pediatr Card Surg Annu 2005;128.

EDITOR'S COMMENTS

The optimal approach to tetralogy of Fallot remains somewhat controversial. Although the number of operative deaths has decreased with tetralogy of Fallot repair and approaches zero in many series, the optimal age at repair is unknown. In centers where neonatal repair is commonplace, operative intervention for complete repair of tetralogy of Fallot can be undertaken at any age. We have elected to perform tetralogy repair at the age of presentation when patients have significant cyanosis. If this approach is used, there is a small subset of patients who present early in neonatal life with significant cyanosis and ductal dependence of pulmonary blood flow. These patients often have the most severe forms of tetralogy of Fallot with significant outflow tract obstruction, small pulmonary arteries, and significant risk for left branch pulmonary artery stenosis after repair. Nevertheless, direct primary repair in these patients may have better results than staged reconstruction with palliative shunting because involution of ductal tissue in these patients often results in pulmonary artery discontinuity when a shunt

is placed, and then the advantages of forward flow in the pulmonary arteries may be lost.

Anomalous origin of the left coronary artery has not generally been a contraindication to complete repair in our experience. Short transannular incisions are now the rule, and often are able to avoid anomalous coronaries in the right ventricular outflow tract (RVOT). Sometimes a flap of left atrial appendage can be used to cover the coronary artery on the RVOT to maintain an autologous tissue connection to the pulmonary arteries, or in unusual cases the pulmonary artery can be divided and brought down to the ventriculotomy incision directly, bridging the anomalous coronary vessel. It therefore is not generally necessary to use a valved conduit in reconstruction in these patients. When neonatal repair is undertaken, we have generally left the foramen ovale open or partially closed the secundum atrial septal defect to allow a pop-off of pressure in the right atrium, which may result from elevation of pulmonary resistance in the newborn. In older patients, we agree with Dr. Jaquiss that closure of the atrial septal defect should be performed to prevent right-to-left shunting and cyanosis in the early postoperative period due to right ventricular compliance decrease.

The primary controversy in repair of tetralogy of Fallot is the age of the patient at primary repair and the use of transatrial/transpulmonary approaches to complete reconstruction with avoidance of transannular patching. Patients with extensive transannular patches may develop progressive late right ventricular dilation because of progressive pulmonary insufficiency, and these patients have a significant late morbidity and mortality from ventricular arrhythmias and right ventricular dysfunction. Pulmonary valve replacement may be necessary. It is unclear, however, whether pulmonary regurgitation is a result of extensive right ventricular muscle resection or extensive patching as a result of tubular hypoplasia of the RVOT. The exact cause of right ventricular dysfunction and pulmonary insufficiency is not clear. It seems logical, however, to limit the extent of right ventriculotomy and transannular patching to the minimal amount possible to prevent late right ventricular dysfunction. In most cases, even with transannular patching, pulmonary regurgitation is only modest, and right ventricular dilation does not occur. Although it is important to relieve RVOT obstruction if at all possible even at the cost of more extensive transannular patching, the extensive studies of late ventricular function performed by Dr Andrew Reddington and his associates suggests that the characteristics of the right ventricle are more important than the pulmonary insufficiency alone in late function of the right ventricle. These studies suggest that residual stenosis is well tolerated and can limit the magnitude of pulmonary insufficiency with resultant ventricular dilation and late RV failure. Thus, the trend is to leave more residual RV outflow tract obstruction than has typically been the case in the past with anticipation that there will be a gradual decrease in the ventricular systolic pressure over time and that mild degrees of obstruction (20 mm to 30 mm) are well tolerated over a lifetime. Thus, minimal transannular patches are becoming more standard and attempts to preserve pulmonary valve function are becoming increasingly desirable.

Nevertheless, the relative advantages of leaving residual obstruction that may in fact progress over time and require reoperation and the problems of placing monocusps or other valve-bearing or valve-creating procedures in the RV outflow tract with the potential need for reoperation make continued follow-up of these patients mandatory. If postoperative residual pulmonary hypertension is anticipated, we have also used monocusp valves in the RVOT to aid in the postoperative hemodynamic stability of these patients. Primary repair in the neonatal or infant period without previous palliative procedures such as systemic-to-pulmonary shunts has resulted in the ability to perform primary repair without extensive right ventricular muscle resection in the majority of cases.

Transatrial and transventricular approaches to the ventricular septal defect are both suitable; however, transatrial repair allows the greatest exposure to avoid the conduction tissue. Closure of the ventricular septal defect before muscle resection allows adequate endocardium for anchoring the patch and avoids having to sew the patch for the ventricular septal defect to raw divided muscle, which may not hold sutures well. We have elected to use pulmonary homograft material or Gore-Tex for RVOT reconstruction when necessary. Although nonfixed homologous pericardium can be used, if a small residual ventricular septal defect is present, a jet directed toward the outflow patch can result in aneurysmal dilation and require reoperation. Therefore, if outflow tract reconstruction is necessary, we have generally preferred to use either glutaraldehyde-fixed autologous pericardium or homograft or Gore-Tex material, which has less tendency to stretch.

Patients with particularly difficult situations are those with tetralogy of Fallot and absent pulmonary valve. In these patients, the ductus arteriosus is typically absent and the to-and-fro blood flow in the main pulmonary arteries causes severe central pulmonary artery dilation and bronchial compression. Ventricular septal defect closure and extensive posterior and anterior internal plication of the pulmonary arteries to a normal diameter with placement of a valved homograft from the right ventricle to the pulmonary arteries may result in the most optimal repair of this defect. The use of a valved conduit decreases the pulsatility in the central pulmonary arteries and therefore decreases the tendency for bronchial compression. Extensive posterior internal plication of the pulmonary arteries results in a more normal anatomic diameter of the pulmonary arteries and adds substance to the pulmonary artery, which can support the underlying bronchial wall. In spite of these technical modifications, some patients will require long-term ventilatory support because of distal arborization abnormalities and distal tracheomalacia with significant developmental abnormalities of the lung. Nevertheless we believe that obtaining the most normal hemodynamic and physiologic conditions of the RVOT at the initial operation will maximize early recovery and the ability to wean the patient from ventilatory support. It is not uncommon in these patients to require reoperation for additional pulmonary artery plication in the first 2 to 3 months after initial repair because pulmonary artery size can continue to enlarge even with adequate initial plication and can compromise lung function late after the procedure. There has been increasing interest in the use of a Lecompte maneuver to bring the dilated central pulmonary arteries anterior to the aorta in tetralogy of Fallot with absent pulmonary valve syndrome to avoid bronchial compression. It is not clear how this technique affects the malacia that has been assumed to be present in the bronchi because this would not be addressed by this technique. Nevertheless, the results with this approach seem to be good and can avoid the need for placing a competent valve in the right ventricular outflow tract in patients with respiratory compromise. Presumably also progressive dilation of the pulmonary arteries will not result in increased airway symptoms as has been seen in the more traditional plication approaches. The exact physiology of tetralogy of Fallot with absent pulmonary valve syndrome and dilated pulmonary arteries and the effect of the pulmonary pulsatility on the airways have not been extensively studied. Prone positioning in these patients seems to result in some improvement, even when the VSD is open, suggesting that rather than specific airway compression by the dilated pulmonary arteries, distribution of blood flow in the lungs may be a more important factor.

Repair of tetralogy of Fallot now is associated with mortality approaching zero in many large series from several pediatric cardiovascular surgical centers. The optimal age at repair is unknown; however, we have generally elected to repair these patients early in infancy in the majority of cases. Because symptoms generally occur early in neonates with the most complex forms of tetralogy of Fallot, operative intervention therefore must be initiated early in these patients. Asymptomatic neonates with tetralogy of Fallot in our center generally are followed until they are 2 to 4 months of age, at which time elective complete repair can be undertaken with very low morbidity and mortality.

T.L.S.

90

Cavopulmonary Shunts and the Hemi-Fontan Operation

W. Steves Ring

Cavopulmonary shunts were first developed in the early 1950s as an alternative to systemic-to-pulmonary artery shunts for patients with cyanotic congenital heart disease. Experimental work in dogs was carried out independently by Carlon at the University of Padua in Italy; Glenn at Yale University in the United States; and Galankin, Darbinian, and Meshalkin in Russia. After the first unsuccessful clinical application of a cavopulmonary shunt in a patient with truncus arteriosus by Shumacker in 1955, Meshalkin performed and reported the first successful end-to-end cavopulmonary anastomosis for tetralogy of Fallot. However, because it was published in the Russian literature and there was very little intellectual communication between the East and West at the time, this advance went unrecognized in the English-language literature. In 1958, Glenn reported the first successful cavopulmonary shunt (superior vena cava to distal right pulmonary artery) in a 7-year-old child with a univentricular heart, transposition, and pulmonary stenosis. In 1984, Glenn reported that the patient was working full time 25 years later at the age of 32.

In 1948, Rodbard and Wagner first demonstrated the feasibility of completely bypassing the right ventricle in dogs by anastomosing the right atrial appendage to the pulmonary artery and ligating the main pulmonary artery proximally. Fontan performed the first successful complete bypass of the right ventricle in 1968 on a patient with tricuspid atresia and a previous cavopulmonary (Glenn) shunt. The right atrium was connected directly to the proximal stump of the right pulmonary artery, and a pulmonary homograft was placed at

the junction of the inferior vena cava to the right atrium. Later modifications by Fontan and others demonstrated that direct connections without interposed valves were superior, permitting unrestricted flow of blood from the systemic venous system into the pulmonary arterial system. The success of the Fontan procedure with its modifications and the late complications associated with the cavopulmonary (Glenn) shunt led Robiscek to write an article entitled An Epitaph for Cavopulmonary Anastomosis in 1982. In 1981, however, Pennington reported that patients who had an established cavopulmonary (Glenn) shunt at the time of the Fontan procedure experienced a more hemodynamically stable postoperative course with fewer complications of pleural effusion, ascites, and renal dysfunction.

Haller developed the technique of bidirectional cavopulmonary anastomosis in dogs in 1966. The first successful clinical application of this technique was reported by Azzolina, Eufrate, and Pensa in 1972. Since the mid 1980s, this technique has been widely used as an intermediate-stage procedure in higher-risk Fontan candidates. It has also been used as a definitive procedure for some patients with a univentricular heart and interrupted inferior vena cava with azygos or hemiazygos continuation, as reported by Kawashima in 1984. Because most bidirectional cavopulmonary shunts are performed as preparation for a Fontan-type procedure, Norwood and Jacobs developed the hemi-Fontan procedure in 1989. It is a more advanced staging procedure than the bidirectional cavopulmonary shunt and is designed to make the completion of the Fontan operation easier. In the hemi-Fontan

procedure, the connection between the right atrium and pulmonary artery is completed and temporarily closed off with a patch at the junction of the superior vena cava and right atrium. This permits later completion of the Fontan connection by simply creating an intracardiac baffle from the inferior vena cava to the superior vena cava after the patch is removed, without further pulmonary reconstruction.

Indications and Preoperative Assessment

A cavopulmonary shunt should be considered as a preparatory stage for any patient older than 2 months of age in which a univentricular repair is anticipated, particularly in those patients with risk factors for a Fontan-type procedure (Table 90-1). In these situations, a cavopulmonary shunt may be combined with a procedure to alleviate a Fontan risk factor (e.g., relief of subaortic obstruction, correction of atrioventricular [AV] valve insufficiency, removal of ventricular volume loads such as systemic-to-pulmonary artery shunts or bands, enlargement of a restrictive atrial septal defect, or repair of pulmonary artery distortion or stenosis). It may also be beneficial in selected patients in whom a two-ventricle repair is anticipated when the right ventricle is believed to have inadequate size or function.

The cavopulmonary shunt has several advantages as a first- or second-stage procedure in preparation for a Fontan-type

Table 90-1   Risk Factors for Fontan-Type Procedure
Young age (<18–24 months)
Anatomic pulmonary artery distortion, hypoplasia, or stenosis
Elevated pulmonary artery pressure (>18–20 mm Hg) or resistance (>2 Wood units)
Systemic ventricular systolic (ejection fraction of <60%) or diastolic (end-diastolic pressure >12 mm Hg) dysfunction
Systemic atrioventricular valve insufficiency or unfavorable anatomy (tricuspid or common atrioventricular valve)
Systemic ventricular outflow obstruction (gradient of >10 mm Hg)
Anatomy other than tricuspid atresia

Table 90-2   Essentials of Preoperative Assessment
1. Anatomic evaluation by angiography
Pulmonary artery size and anatomy: hypoplasia, distortion, stenosis
Systemic-to-pulmonary artery shunt anatomy and patency
Pulmonary artery band anatomy
Systemic venous anatomy: superior vena cava size, contralateral superior vena cava, inferior vena caval drainage
Systemic ventricular outflow tract anatomy
2. Functional evaluation by echocardiography and/or ventriculography
Systemic ventricular function (ejection fraction, dimensions, end-diastolic pressure)
Systemic atrioventricular valve function (insufficiency)
3. Hemodynamic evaluation by catheterization
Pulmonary artery pressures (direct or pulmonary venous wedge) and resistance
Mean atrial and end-diastolic ventricular pressures
Cardiac output and pulmonary-to-systemic flow ratios (Qp/Qs)
Systemic arterial and mixed venous oxygen saturations
Systemic ventricular outflow tract gradient

operation. First, it can be performed with a lower mortality and morbidity than a Fontan procedure or a total cavopulmonary connection, particularly in infants from 3 to 12 months of age. Second, in contrast to a systemic-to-pulmonary artery shunt, a cavopulmonary shunt increases effective pulmonary blood flow by directing fully desaturated blood into the pulmonary circulation. Third, the risk of developing pulmonary vascular disease is reduced by lowering the pressure and reducing the flow through the pulmonary vascular bed. Fourth, the risk of pulmonary artery distortion is less than with a systemic-to-pulmonary artery shunt. Finally, and perhaps most important, the cavopulmonary shunt, when combined with removing systemic-to-pulmonary artery shunts or antegrade pulmonary blood flow, reduces ventricular work by reducing the volume load on the single ventricle. This often improves ventricular function and reduces systemic AV valve regurgitation, which would compromise candidacy for a Fontan-type procedure.

Careful assessment of anatomic, functional, and hemodynamic variables by echocardiography and catheterization is essential before creation of a cavopulmonary shunt (Table 90-2). This information is necessary to determine the risk and feasibility of performing the cavopulmonary shunt, the suitability for a later Fontan-type procedure or total cavopulmonary connection, the need for additional procedures at the time of cavopulmonary shunt, and the optimal technique for conducting the cavopulmonary shunt (e.g., the need for cardiopulmonary bypass).

Adequate pulmonary artery anatomy is critical to the success of a cavopulmonary anastomosis. Significant pulmonary artery distortion or stenosis should be identified during preoperative evaluation and corrected at the time of cavopulmonary shunt because it is associated with increased morbidity and mortality after both the cavopulmonary shunt and the Fontan procedure. A determination of pulmonary artery size using the Nakata index may be useful in predicting morbidity after cavopulmonary shunt and suitability for the Fontan procedure in patients with marginal pulmonary artery beds. The Nakata index is the sum of the cross-sectional areas of the right and left pulmonary arteries normalized for body surface area in square millimeters per square meter. Pulmonary artery hypoplasia, defined as a Nakata index of <200 mm^2/m^2, is associated with increased morbidity after cavopulmonary shunt, although success has been achieved with indices as low as 70 mm^2/m^2.

The patency of systemic-to-pulmonary artery shunts, the extent of systemic-to-pulmonary artery collaterals, and the anatomy of pulmonary artery band sites should be evaluated preoperatively along with the pulmonary-to-systemic flow ratio (Qp/Qs) to determine whether accessory sources of pulmonary blood flow should remain or be interrupted. In general, alternative sources of pulmonary blood flow may be left if Qp/Qs is <1.0 preoperatively or if the systemic oxygen saturation is $<70\%$ after completion of the cavopulmonary shunt. However, leaving alternative sources of pulmonary blood flow when the preoperative Qp/Qs is >1.0 will cause an excessive

volume load on the systemic ventricle, which might otherwise compromise later completion of the Fontan-type procedure.

Systemic venous anatomy is carefully evaluated angiographically during preoperative catheterization to determine the size of the ipsilateral superior vena cava, the presence of a contralateral superior vena cava (e.g., a persistent left superior vena cava), and the presence of azygos or hemiazygos continuation of the inferior vena cava. The presence of normal-sized bilateral superior venae cavae usually permits sequential performance of bilateral, bidirectional cavopulmonary anastomoses off cardiopulmonary bypass and without a temporary decompressing shunt if additional intracardiac or major pulmonary reconstruction is not required. A small contralateral superior vena cava or any other venous communication between the superior vena cava and the coronary sinus, pulmonary veins, or inferior vena cava should be surgically ligated and divided to prevent collateralization and reduced efficiency of the cavopulmonary shunt. If azygos or hemiazygos continuation of an interrupted inferior vena cava is found, a modified total cavopulmonary connection such as described by Kawashima can be performed by dividing the superior vena cava below the azygos or hemiazygos connection and directly anastomosing it to the pulmonary artery, thus directing all systemic venous return except the hepatic and splanchnic venous return into the pulmonary circulation.

Accurate assessment of ventricular function and AV valve competence are essential before cavopulmonary anastomosis is attempted. This should include measurement of systemic ventricular ejection fraction, ventricular end-diastolic pressure, extent of AV valve insufficiency, and Qp/Qs to determine whether ventricular dysfunction might be the result of excessive volume loading of the systemic ventricle. Although a depressed ejection fraction (<50%) and moderate elevations of filling pressures (end-diastolic pressure of 10 to 15 mm Hg) may not absolutely preclude a cavopulmonary shunt, they are associated with higher risk for both the shunt and later Fontan procedure. Any anatomic or functional factor that contributes to excessive hemodynamic pressure or volume loads on the systemic ventricle should be corrected at the time of cavopulmonary shunt. This may include removal of alternative sources of inefficient pulmonary blood flow (systemic-to-pulmonary artery shunts or native pulmonary outflow tracts) and correction of any significant AV valve insufficiency that might contribute to excessive volume loading. Any significant (>10 to 15 mm Hg) systemic ventricular outflow tract obstruction should also be corrected because it will contribute to both systolic and diastolic ventricular dysfunction.

Measurement of the pulmonary artery pressure and transpulmonary gradient should be accomplished at catheterization directly across the pulmonary outflow tract or very carefully across a systemic-to-pulmonary artery shunt because this can occasionally result in intimal dissection and occlusion of the prosthetic shunt with disastrous consequences. Pulmonary artery pressure may also be measured indirectly from a pulmonary venous wedge pressure or directly at the time of surgery. A mean pulmonary artery pressure of >18 mm Hg or a transpulmonary gradient of >10 mm Hg is considered to be a risk factor for morbidity and mortality after either a Fontan-type procedure or a cavopulmonary shunt. A pulmonary vascular resistance of >2 Wood units/m² is also associated with increased risk for a Fontan procedure and warrants consideration for prior staging with a cavopulmonary shunt. This should be performed along with removal of any alternative sources of pulmonary blood flow (if systemic oxygen saturation permits) to permit the resistance to fall before a Fontan-type procedure. However, if the pulmonary vascular resistance exceeds 4 Wood units/m², a cavopulmonary anastomosis may also result in excessive morbidity or mortality.

Operative Technique

Appropriate invasive and noninvasive monitoring is essential for successful operative management and postoperative evaluation after cavopulmonary connections. A peripheral pulse oximeter and a cerebral near-infrared spectroscopic (NIRS) monitor are used to continuously monitor systemic oxygen saturation and cerebral perfusion both during and after surgery. An arterial line is placed in a vessel that is not supplying a systemic-to-pulmonary artery shunt for continuous pressure monitoring and arterial blood gas determination. Central venous access is obtained through the contralateral (usually left) internal jugular or subclavian vein to avoid interfering with cannulation of the superior vena cava. An atrial pressure line is inserted intraoperatively to monitor ventricular filling pressures and transpulmonary gradients if the superior vena caval pressure is elevated after completion of the cavopulmonary connection. Both the central venous and atrial pressure lines are removed as quickly as possible postoperatively to minimize the risk of thrombosis and thromboembolism. External defibrillator patches are placed before induction for any patient with a prior intrapericardial surgical procedure.

Unidirectional Cavopulmonary Shunt

The "unidirectional" or "classic Glenn" cavopulmonary shunt is largely of his-
torical interest. It has been replaced by the "bidirectional" Glenn cavopulmonary shunt, which maintains pulmonary artery continuity and better prepares patients for a Fontan-type procedure. The "unidirectional" cavopulmonary shunt is reserved for unusual palliative situations in which separation of the two pulmonary beds is needed or when a Fontan procedure is unlikely or contraindicated.

The "classic" Glenn shunt was originally performed off cardiopulmonary bypass using a posterolateral muscle-sparing thoracotomy incision through the fourth intercostal space. Today, it is more commonly performed through a median sternotomy to avoid pleural entry and the subsequent development of systemic-to-pulmonary collaterals. In the thoracotomy approach, the pleura and pericardium are incised posterior to the phrenic nerve from the thoracic inlet superiorly to the pulmonary veins inferiorly (Fig. 90-1). The phrenic nerve is left attached to the widely mobilized anterior pleuropericardium to avoid excessive traction directly on the nerve. The superior vena cava is dissected free from the level of the innominate vein to the right atrium. Lymphatic tissue located medial and posterior to the cava is carefully avoided to minimize the risk of postoperative chylothorax. The azygos vein is suture ligated and divided to provide better mobility of the superior

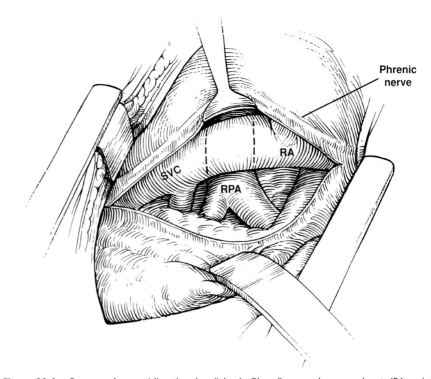

Figure 90-1. Exposure for a unidirectional or "classic Glenn" cavopulmonary shunt. (RA = right atrium; RPA = right pulmonary artery; SVC = superior vena cava.)

vena cava and to prevent collateral venous connection with the lower-pressure inferior vena cava. The right pulmonary artery is dissected from the pulmonary bifurcation to beyond the first hilar branches. After partial heparinization, a trial occlusion of the proximal right pulmonary artery with an angled pediatric vascular clamp is performed to determine whether pulmonary blood flow to the contralateral lung is sufficient to maintain systemic saturations, which may fall into the 50% to 60% range. Raising the systemic blood pressure temporarily with pressor agents may improve systemic saturation by augmenting flow across the pulmonary valve or through a contralateral systemic-to-pulmonary artery shunt during the 10 to 15 minutes needed to complete the cavopulmonary anastomosis. However, these agents should be avoided when significant dynamic subpulmonary obstruction is present. When a stable systemic saturation of >50% is achieved, the distal right pulmonary artery branches are controlled with microvascular occluders. The right pulmonary artery is then divided along the medial border of the superior vena cava, the proximal end is oversewn with 6-0 or 7-0 polypropylene suture, and the clamp is removed. The inferior margin of the distal right pulmonary artery is incised approximately two-thirds the width of the vena cava, and the ends are gently rounded to enlarge the effective width of the cavopulmonary anastomosis (Fig. 90-2). A partially occluding pediatric Satinsky clamp is placed on the superior vena cava from above the divided azygos vein to just above the right atrium, providing a long segment of vena cava (double the width of the pulmonary artery) for construction of the anastomosis. The clamp should leave approximately half of the superior vena cava patent, with a caval pressure of <30 mm Hg above the clamp. The lateral aspect of the superior vena cava is incised beginning where the inferior margin of the right pulmonary artery crosses the vena cava and extending superiorly through the orifice of the divided azygos vein for a distance 50% greater than the width of the right pulmonary artery. The anastomosis is completed with absorbable 7-0 or 6-0 monofilament running suture from cephalad to caudad; often a second traction suture is placed at the inferior aspect of the anastomosis to prevent purse stringing. After the anastomosis is de-aired by releasing the distal vessel loops, the caval clamp is removed. The right lung is inflated and ventilated to permit the pulmonary vasculature to dilate before the superior vena cava is temporarily occluded above the right atrial junction.

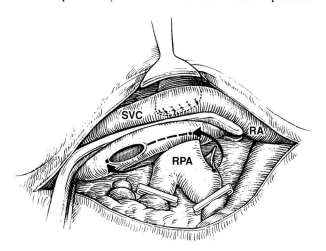

Figure 90-2. Technique for enlarging the width of the "classic Glenn" cavopulmonary shunt.

The upper superior vena cava pressure and systemic saturation are monitored, with the lower superior vena cava occluded. Pressures of 10 to 15 mm Hg are considered ideal, with pressures up to 20 mm Hg being acceptable, because the pressure will usually fall with spontaneous ventilation and resolution of perioperative atelectasis. If satisfactory pressures are obtained, the superior vena cava is ligated just inferior to the anastomosis (Fig 90-3). Superior vena cava pressures >20 mm Hg are of concern and should prompt a determination of the transpulmonary gradient by placing a right atrial pressure-monitoring line and a measurement of any anastomotic gradient obtained either directly or by pullback across the anastomosis.

Bidirectional Cavopulmonary Shunt

The bidirectional cavopulmonary shunt is the preferred procedure when a future extracardiac conduit Fontan is planned. It is usually performed through a median sternotomy approach, and cardiopulmonary bypass is used for bidirectional cavopulmonary anastomoses by most surgeons. However, cardiopulmonary bypass has several adverse effects, including a systemic inflammatory response, altered pulmonary vascular reactivity, hemodilution requiring transfusion, and increased need for postoperative mechanical ventilation. These adverse effects of cardiopulmonary bypass can be reduced by employing modified ultrafiltration

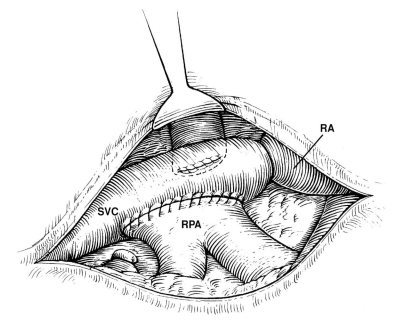

Figure 90-3. A completed "classic Glenn" cavopulmonary shunt with ligation of the lower superior vena cava. (RA = right atrium; RPA = right pulmonary artery; SVC = superior vena cava.)

techniques. Cardiopulmonary bypass can be avoided when no intracardiac procedures are required if the contralateral lung receives pulmonary blood flow sufficient to maintain adequate systemic arterial saturation during clamping of the ipsilateral branch pulmonary artery and if adequate cerebral blood flow is maintained. This is accomplished by constructing a temporary shunt circuit that decompresses the superior vena caval circulation directly into the right atrium. After full systemic heparinization, a right-angled, metal-tipped cannula is inserted through a purse string at the junction of the innominate vein with the superior vena cava and oriented cephalad. A second cannula is inserted into the right atrium and connected directly to the superior vena cava cannula, with the surgeon carefully avoiding any air within the cannulae. Cardiopulmonary bypass is required when additional cardiac procedures are needed, if total occlusion of the ipsilateral proximal pulmonary artery causes excessive systemic desaturation, if an ipsilateral aortopulmonary shunt is present, if superior vena caval pressure exceeds 25 mm Hg, or if the cerebral NIRS monitor falls below 40%.

After either isolated superior caval bypass or partial cardiopulmonary bypass is initiated, the azygos vein is suture ligated and divided. If an ipsilateral aortopulmonary shunt is present, it is occluded and divided. The superior vena cava is occluded with a tourniquet placed around the right-angled cannula superiorly just below the innominate vein, and a vascular clamp is placed inferiorly just above the right atrial junction. The superior cava is transected just above the inferior border of the right pulmonary artery and the lower end oversewn with 6-0 polypropylene (Prolene). The upper end of the superior vena cava is opened along the lateral margin to a point below the superior border of the right pulmonary artery, and the corners are gently rounded to create an opening for an anastomosis that will be wider than the cava itself (Fig. 90-4). This also leaves some redundancy of the cava to move it medially where the anastomosis can be accomplished to the superior margin of the right pulmonary artery closer to the pulmonary bifurcation. A vascular clamp is placed horizontally across the origin of the right pulmonary artery for proximal control. The distal branches are controlled with microvascular occluders. A longitudinal pulmonary arteriotomy is created along the superior margin of the right pulmonary artery, usually incorporating the distal aortopulmonary shunt anastomotic site medially. Traction sutures are

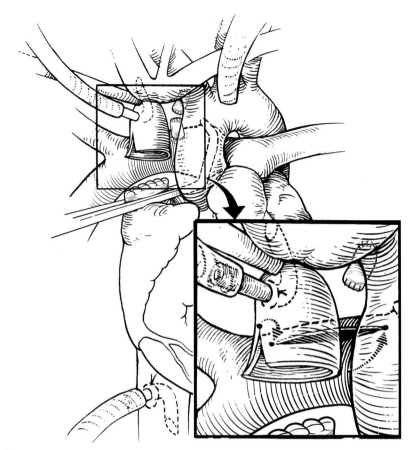

Figure 90-4. Exposure and cannulation for a bidirectional cavopulmonary anastomosis with the technique for medial displacement and augmentation of the caval anastomosis (inset).

placed in the corners of the arteriotomy and passed through the medial and lateral borders of the superior vena cava to prevent purse stringing of the anastomosis. An additional traction suture through the anterior wall of the pulmonary arteriotomy also facilitates exposure for the anastomosis. Twisting of the superior vena cava can be prevented by placing marking sutures on the cava before transection, by correctly orienting the upper corner of the lateral enlarging incision in the cava toward the lateral corner of the pulmonary arteriotomy, and by using the stump of the azygos vein as a posterior landmark. The anastomosis is accomplished with running 7-0 or 6-0 monofilament absorbable suture with meticulous attention to achieving smooth intimal apposition. If systemic oxygen saturation is <70%, alternative sources of pulmonary blood flow are best left patent. However, if saturation is >80%, some or all of the alternative sources of pulmonary blood flow should be occluded. If the main pulmonary artery is to be divided, the pulmonary valve should be oversewn directly to prevent a blind pouch of proximal pulmonary artery, which can

lead to stasis, thrombus, and systemic embolization (Fig. 90-5).

Hemi-Fontan Procedure

The hemi-Fontan procedure is preferred if a later intracardiac lateral tunnel Fontan procedure is planned. It is performed through a median sternotomy, generally using cardiopulmonary bypass, although deep hypothermic total circulatory arrest may also be used. Standard arterial cannulation of the aorta and bicaval venous cannulation are used for cardiopulmonary bypass. Single venous atrial cannulation is used if circulatory arrest is anticipated. The superior vena cava is cannulated near the junction with the innominate vein using a right-angled, metal-tipped cannula oriented superiorly as for a bidirectional cavopulmonary shunt. The inferior vena cava is cannulated with a right-angled, metal-tipped cannula placed at the right atrial-caval junction. Both venae cavae are looped with tourniquets. Cardiopulmonary bypass is initiated, with cooling to 32°C or lower if extensive intracardiac repair is planned. All other

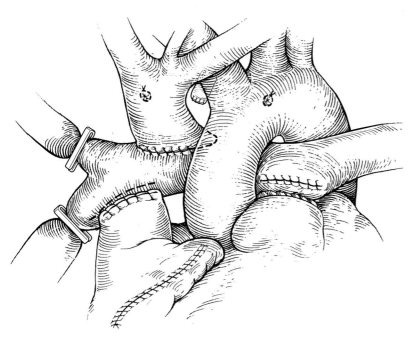

Figure 90-5. A completed bidirectional cavopulmonary anastomosis with division of accessory sources of pulmonary blood flow and orientation for a hemi-Fontan procedure.

intracardiac procedures (e.g., AV valve repair, enlargement of the bulboventricular foramen, Damus-Kay-Stansel procedure, division of the main pulmonary artery with oversewing of the pulmonary valve, etc.) and pulmonary artery reconstruction should be accomplished during the hemi-Fontan procedure, along with occlusion of all other sources of pulmonary blood flow. The aorta is cross-clamped, and cardioplegia is obtained with cold blood perfusate. A right atriotomy is made parallel and anterior to the crista terminalis to minimize the risk of compromising atrial conduction, as recommended by the group from Washington University in St. Louis. If necessary, the atrial septal defect may be enlarged within the confines of the limbus. Other intracardiac procedures are accomplished at this point. The superior atrial-caval junction is closed by suturing a patch of polytetrafluoroethylene (Gore-Tex) obliquely to the right atrial side of the orifice with 6-0 or 5-0 Prolene running suture is placed superficially through the endocardium to avoid injuring the sinoatrial node (Fig. 90-6). The right atriotomy is closed and the heart extensively de-aired before the aorta is unclamped. With a brief period of cardioplegia, the heart will usually return spontaneously to a sinus rhythm and not require cardioversion. However, ventricular fibrillation and asystole must be corrected promptly with cardioversion or pacing to prevent distention of the single ventricle. Once the heart

resumes a regular rhythm, the superior vena cava is transected at the level of the inferior right pulmonary artery. The bidirectional cavopulmonary anastomosis is performed as outlined in the previous section, angling the upper superior vena cava

slightly medially toward the pulmonary bifurcation (Figs. 90-4 and 90-5). A second pulmonary arteriotomy is made along the inferior margin of the right pulmonary artery, offset laterally from the incision made for the superior anastomosis. This creates better flow dynamics for both cavopulmonary anastomoses, ultimately directing the inferior caval blood to the right lung and the superior caval blood to the left lung once the direct cavopulmonary connection is completed (Fig. 90-7). The lower superior vena cava is opened along the lateral margin and anastomosed to the inferior aspect of the right pulmonary artery, either directly or augmented laterally with a diamond-shaped patch of pericardium. Alternatively, the hemi-Fontan as originally described by Norwood and Jacobs in 1993 can be performed in which the superior vena cava is anastomosed crosswise to the right pulmonary artery posteriorly. Anteriorly, a patch of homograft is used to augment the anastomosis and close the superior vena cava-to-right atrial connection. Disadvantages of this technique include application only to an intracardiac lateral tunnel repair, and it usually requires hypothermic circulatory arrest. It does have the advantage of simplifying the later lateral tunnel Fontan procedure and may decrease energy loss in the region of the connection due to the caval offset created.

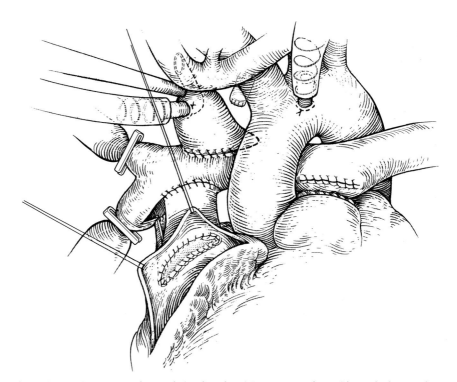

Figure 90-6. Exposure and cannulation for a hemi-Fontan procedure with patch closure of superior vena caval–atrial junction and enlargement of the lower superior vena cava-to-right pulmonary artery anastomosis.

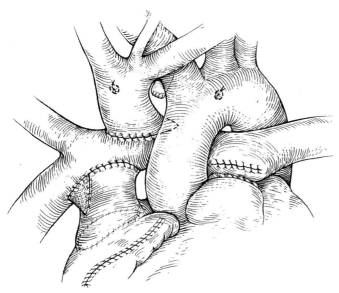

Figure 90-7. A completed hemi-Fontan procedure with division of accessory sources of pulmonary blood flow.

Postoperative Care

Postoperatively, hemodynamics (cardiac rhythm, arterial blood pressure, superior vena cava pressure, atrial pressure) and pulmonary status (chest x-ray film, arterial blood gas analysis, pulse oximetry, ventilator mechanics) are monitored closely. Most patients, particularly those with any evidence for ventricular dysfunction, are maintained on inotropic support to optimize cardiac output and minimize atrial filling pressures. The administration of maintenance fluids and blood products is minimized to prevent pulmonary edema and pleural effusion. Early extubation is anticipated if the arterial and mixed venous (superior vena cava) blood gases are satisfactory and the superior vena cava pressure is <18 mm Hg with good blood pressure and perfusion. The head and upper body are elevated to reduce the risk of superior vena cava syndrome by providing a hemodynamic advantage for upper-body blood return. Low-dose heparin (10 units/kg/hr) and aspirin (5 mg/kg) therapy is started as soon as bleeding is controlled to reduce the risk of caval thrombosis. Central lines are removed as soon as possible after extubation. Because most univentricular hearts have some degree of volume overload, we prefer to manage most patients with digoxin and diuretics. Those with hypertension, significant ventricular dysfunction, or systemic AV valve insufficiency are also managed with an angiotensin-converting-enzyme (ACE) inhibitor.

Early Postoperative Complications

With appropriate patient selection, significant early morbidity and mortality after isolated cavopulmonary anastomosis is unusual. Most complications are seen when cavopulmonary anastomosis is combined with other cardiac procedures. Careful attention to patient selection and attention to technical details at the time of surgery will minimize the risk of most complications. Superior vena cava syndrome, transient systemic hypertension, sinoatrial node dysfunction, supraventricular arrhythmias, and pleuropericardial effusions are the most common early complications after cavopulmonary shunt. Excessive superior vena cava pressure or hypoxemia with a high transpulmonary gradient and no evidence for pulmonary dysfunction warrants early study by echocardiography and angiography of the superior vena cava to rule out anatomic obstruction caused by anastomotic stricture, kinking, or branch pulmonary artery stenosis. Pleural effusions can be reduced by minimizing superior vena cava pressures without compromising cardiac output, optimizing plasma oncotic pressure, and avoiding fluid overload. Chylothoraces can be minimized by limiting dissection of the lymphatic tissue between the aorta and the superior vena cava posterior to the right pulmonary artery. Phrenic nerve injury is very uncommon except in reoperations but may result in significant morbidity, particularly after a "classic" cavopulmonary shunt. Hypertension is usually only transient and resolves without treatment before discharge. Persistent hypertension is treated with ACE inhibitors and diuretics.

Late Postoperative Complications

Progressive cyanosis is the most common late complication after cavopulmonary anastomosis. Cyanosis may result from normal growth with proportionately less of the cardiac output supplying the upper body. However, more commonly, the disproportionate venous pressure in the superior vena cava relative to the inferior vena cava causes systemic venous collaterals to develop that decompress the superior vena cava into the inferior vena cava or hepatic veins. Pulmonary arteriovenous connections also result in progressive late cyanosis. These have been noted to develop late after the "classic" Glenn anastomosis but have also been noted within the first year after a bidirectional cavopulmonary shunt, most notably following the Kawashima modification. The absence of a humoral factor from the hepatic venous circulation has been implicated in the development of pulmonary AV connections by the group at Boston Children's Hospital. When conversion to a modified Fontan or total cavopulmonary connection occurs within several years, pulmonary arteriovenous fistulas are only rarely a problem.

Acute thrombosis of the superior vena cava has been reported and remains a potential late complication after cavopulmonary connection. Most often this is associated with mechanical obstruction to flow through the anastomosis caused by kinking or stenosis of the anastomosis or distal branch pulmonary arteries. Thrombolytic therapy may reopen the shunt acutely, but angiography is needed to anatomically evaluate the shunt and the pulmonary arteries. Late stenosis of the anastomosis is unusual and is most often caused by technical problems at the time of surgery.

SUGGESTED READING

Bove EL, de Leval MR, Migliavacca F, et al. Computational fluid dynamics in the evaluation of hemodynamic performance of cavopulmonary connections after the Norwood procedure for hypoplastic left heart syndrome. J Thorac Cardiovasc Surg 2003;126:1040.

Bradley SM, Mosca RS, Hennein HA, et al. Bidirectional superior cavopulmonary connection in young infants. Circulation 1996;94(Suppl II):II-5.

Castaneda AR. From Glenn to Fontan: a continuing evolution. Circulation 1992;86:II-80.

Chang AC, Hanley FL, Wernovsky G, et al. Early bidirectional cavopulmonary shunt in young infants: Postoperative course and early results. Circulation 1993;88:II-149.

de Leval MR, Dubini G, Migliavacca F, et al. Use of computational fluid dynamics in the design of surgical procedures: Application to the study of competitive flows in cavopulmonary connections. J Thorac Cardiovasc Surg 1996;111:502.

Duncan BW, Desai S. Pulmonary arteriovenous malformations after cavopulmonary anastomosis. Ann Thorac Surg 2003;76:1759.

Gandhi SK, Bromberg BI, Rodefeld MD, et al. Lateral tunnel suture line variation reduces atrial flutter after the modified Fontan operation. Ann Thorac Surg 1996;61:1299.

Kawashima Y, Kitamura S, Matsuda H, et al. Total cavopulmonary shunt operation in complex cardiac anomalies. J Thorac Cardiovasc Surg 1984;87:74.

Liu J, Lu Y, Chen H, et al. Bidirectional Glenn procedure without cardiopulmonary bypass. Ann Thorac Surg 2004;77:1349.

Norwood WI, Jacobs ML. Fontan's procedure in two stages. Am J Surg 1993;166:548.

Pridjian AK, Mendelsohn AM, Lupinetti FM, et al. Usefulness of the bidirectional Glenn procedure as staged reconstruction for the functional single ventricle. Am J Cardiol 1993;71:959.

Robiscek F. An epitaph for cavopulmonary anastomosis. Ann Thorac Surg 1982;34:208.

Srivastava D, Preminger T, Lock JE, et al. Hepatic venous blood and the development of pulmonary arteriovenous malformations in congenital heart disease. Circulation 1995;92:1217.

Trusler GA, Williams WG, Cohen AJ, et al. The cavopulmonary shunt: evolution of a concept. Circulation 1990;82:IV-131.

Webber SA, Horvath P, LeBlanc JG, et al. Influence of competitive pulmonary blood flow on the bidirectional superior cavopulmonary shunt—A multi-institutional study. Circulation 1995;92:II-279.

EDITOR'S COMMENTS

The use of early cavopulmonary shunts and the hemi-Fontan operation in staged reconstruction for single-ventricle physiology has resulted in marked improvement in late outcomes after the Fontan procedure. The primary reason for this salient benefit in late outcome after the Fontan procedure is the ability to address pulmonary artery distortions and minimize excessive pulmonary blood flow early to prevent problems with pulmonary vascular resistance. Thus, in many cases, staged reconstruction with an initial cavopulmonary shunt is the preferable approach to a one-stage complete Fontan procedure. In very favorable patients with optimal ventricular anatomy and protected pulmonary vascular beds, a one-stage Fontan procedure can be contemplated; however, the staged reconstruction has particular benefit in patients with hypoplastic left heart syndrome in whom a high incidence of left pulmonary artery hypoplasia is noted. In addition, decreasing volume loading of the functional right single ventricle early may improve late ventricular function and minimize the significance of tricuspid valve regurgitation in these patients.

Although the unilateral cavopulmonary anastomosis as advocated by Glenn can be accomplished technically without the use of cardiopulmonary bypass, there is little use for this technique at present. The bilateral cavopulmonary connection has supplanted the standard Glenn anastomosis in virtually all circumstances. The use of a unilateral cavopulmonary connection has been associated with significant development of late arteriovenous malformations of the lung. Even with bilateral cavopulmonary connections and certainly with the Kawashima operation (in which the majority of inferior vena caval flow is directed to the lungs without contributions from hepatic venous return), development of arteriovenous malformations of the lung is commonplace and results in progressive cyanosis. Early conversion of these patients to the completed Fontan procedure with fenestration is advocated to maintain some hepatic flow to the lung to diminish or resolve the development of arteriovenous malformations.

Although the bidirectional cavopulmonary anastomosis can be accomplished simply with the use of either decompressing shunts from the superior vena cava to the right atrium or with the use of cardiopulmonary bypass (as is preferred in our institution), we continue to use the hemi-Fontan procedure for some patients with single-ventricle physiology. This operation uses a homograft patch to widely enlarge the pulmonary bifurcation and create a dam between the superior vena cava and right atrium without actual disconnection of the superior vena cava from the atrium at operation. Although this operation is extensive and is often done under a brief period of circulatory arrest, the reconstruction of the pulmonary bifurcation eliminates causes of maldistribution of pulmonary blood flow and permits a very simple completion Fontan procedure, which is generally done when the patient is 1 1/2 to 2 years of age. More complex types of hemi-Fontan reconstruction with a Gore-Tex dam in the superior vena caval orifice in the right atrium followed by division of the superior vena cava with anastomosis to the right pulmonary artery superiorly and inferiorly results in additional multiple suture lines and a longer operative procedure. In addition, the superior vena cava at the right atrial junction is often augmented with additional pericardium to create a larger opening into the pulmonary artery. It is unclear that this technique offers any distinct advantage over the hemi-Fontan procedure. The only relative advantage is the lack of an incision crossing the superior vena cava-to-right atrial junction, which can interfere with the blood supply to the sinus node and potentially increase the risk of late development of atrial arrhythmias.

Whereas the azygos vein is usually ligated or divided with creation of bidirectional Glenn shunts or the hemi-Fontan operation, it has been left open in many patients in our center and has not resulted in significant decompression of the superior vena cava. Most decompression of superior vena cava-to-pulmonary anastomoses occurs when there is a left-sided vena cava, which can decompress to a low-pressure chamber such as the right atrium through the coronary sinus. Although the Nakata index has been useful for defining the extent of the pulmonary vascular bed for completion Fontan operation, we have not used this index in our center. In most cases, patients with an adequate oxygen saturation with an aortopulmonary shunt and a pulmonary venous wedge pressure that is low can undergo a cavopulmonary anastomosis with satisfactory results, even with a low Nakata index number. It is not uncommon for patients with even a single pulmonary arterial supply to have satisfactory results with a cavopulmonary anastomosis in the presence of discontinuous pulmonary arteries if pulmonary vascular resistance is low in the remaining vascular bed.

In our operative techniques, no monitoring lines are placed in the superior vena cava or jugular veins. Such monitoring lines can result in thrombosis and have catastrophic consequences if pulmonary embolization occurs after a cavopulmonary anastomosis. We have used transthoracic lines positioned through the hemi-Fontan reconstruction into the pulmonary artery directly and into the pulmonary venous atrium by placing these catheters on either side of the homograft baffle at the superior vena cava-to-right atrium anastomosis. These lines are generally left in place for <24 hours. In all cases, operations are performed through a median sternotomy incision because there is little benefit to the thoracotomy incision for construction of the cavopulmonary anastomosis. The majority of these patients require a later completion Fontan procedure, and therefore the ease of creation of the anastomosis by sternotomy is not a disadvantage. In addition, we use right-sided systemic-to-pulmonary artery shunts at initial palliation and take down the shunt and place the cavopulmonary anastomosis at the shunt insertion site at reoperation through the same sternotomy incision. This eliminates the need for left-sided aortopulmonary shunts and the difficulty in take-down of these shunts with its potential risk to the left phrenic nerve.

A significant addition to the creation of cavopulmonary shunts or hemi-Fontan procedures is the use of modified ultrafiltration postoperatively. In our experience, use of modified ultrafiltration markedly decreases the risk of pleural effusions after these operations and is associated with a mortality rate that approaches zero.

Currently almost all patients undergoing Fontan procedure have had intermediate staging with a cavopulmonary shunt. As the results with surgery for hypoplastic left heart syndrome have improved, the cavopulmonary shunts have been done at a younger age to decrease the risk of interstage mortality between the first-stage reconstruction and the second stage. It is unclear what age is the minimum at which one can complete a cavopulmonary shunt with low morbidity. Many centers routinely perform the cavopulmonary shunt at 3 to 4 months of age rather than 6 months of age, which was our practice in the past. In rare cases and with documented low pulmonary resistance, even earlier cavopulmonary shunt can be contemplated in some cases. Although the mortality does not appear to be higher with early cavopulmonary shunt, the morbidity does appear to be slightly greater, with a longer hospital stay and possibly more venous congestion early after the procedure. Nevertheless, early conversion to a cavopulmonary connection may decrease the morbidity of shunt thrombosis from aortopulmonary shunts and improve oxygen saturations in patients who have shunt stenosis and limited pulmonary blood flow.

T.L.S.

91

Tricuspid Atresia/Single Ventricle and the Fontan Operation

John E. Mayer, Jr.

Patients who are born with a single functional ventricle (including those with tricuspid atresia) have a dismal prognosis without surgical intervention, and the results of the Fontan operation, which is the "definitive" procedure for these patients, are now quite good. This chapter focuses on the Fontan operation and its modifications, but it is critically important that the management of these patients begin at birth, well before they are physiologically ready for a Fontan operation. This management frequently involves one or more palliative interventions during the first few years of life, and these early interventions can have an important effect on the suitability of the patient for the subsequent Fontan operation. The goal of these initial interventions is to avoid either life-threatening cyanosis due to inadequate pulmonary blood flow or congestive heart failure due to excessive pulmonary blood flow. A variety of surgical procedures may be necessary to fulfill short-term goals, such as banding the pulmonary artery to relieve heart failure or creating a systemic-to-pulmonary artery shunt to improve cyanosis. However, these interventions must not only achieve these short-term goals, but they also must be carefully designed to achieve the additional goal of creating a suitable candidate for a "repair" based on the Fontan principle (unless the supply of heart transplant donors and the therapeutic index of immunosuppressive agents both markedly improve). In simplest terms, candidates for Fontan operations should have undistorted pulmonary arteries, good systolic and diastolic ventricular function, competent atrioventricular valves, and low pulmonary vascular

resistance. Although this chapter discusses the selection of patients for the Fontan operation and various modifications of this procedure, the pre-Fontan management of these patients is the source of much of their mortality and is clearly related to the subsequent suitability of patients for the operation.

Anatomy

A variety of anatomic defects exist that should be considered as a single ventricle from the standpoint of surgical interventions. The classic defect for which the Fontan operation was first performed is *tricuspid atresia*. In this defect, there is no identifiable tricuspid valve tissue or valve remnant. Instead, the floor of the right atrium is completely muscular, and the floor is separated from the ventricular mass by the fibrofatty tissue of the atrioventricular (AV) sulcus. Generally in association with the atretic right atrioventricular valve, there is a total absence of the inlet and varying portions of the trabecular portion of the right ventricle. There is almost always an associated ventricular septal defect (VSD), which is frequently restrictive. The great vessels may be transposed (aorta arising from the infundibular chamber) or normally related (aorta arising from left ventricle [LV]). The VSD (also referred to as a bulboventricular foramen [BVF]) is frequently restrictive, which results in restriction to pulmonary blood flow when the great vessels are normally related but results in subaortic stenosis when there is transposition of the great arteries (TGA). When transposition is present, even if the BVF is initially large and unrestrictive, with

time it can be expected to become smaller, resulting in subaortic stenosis later in life. If there is a coarctation present, then it is very likely that the BVF will be restrictive in the newborn period.

The most common form of single ventricle is a *single left ventricle*. Single LV exists in two forms, one in which the morphologic left ventricle is left sided (ventricular D-loop), and the second (more common) form in which the morphologic LV is right sided (ventricular L-loop). In L-loop single LV, the aorta most commonly arises from a left-sided infundibular chamber (L-TGA), and the pulmonary artery arises from the right-sided morphologic LV. However, both great vessels may arise from the outlet chamber (double outlet right ventricle [DORV]). In this situation, similar to tricuspid atresia with transposition, the pathway from the LV to the aorta involves a BVF that may become restrictive (resulting in subaortic stenosis from a functional standpoint). In both forms of single LV there is almost always obstruction to either pulmonary or systemic blood flow. If there is an associated coarctation of the aorta, then it is likely that there will be subaortic obstruction as well (usually at the level of the BVF). There may be one or two atrioventricular valves leading into the single left ventricle, but by definition, neither will connect into the infundibular or outlet chamber.

Another form of single ventricle is *single right ventricle*. In this anatomic subtype, the single ventricle is more heavily trabeculated, and typically there are insertions of the tricuspid valve into the septal surface. The great vessels most commonly both arise from the right ventricle, but there may be stenosis or atresia of either the aorta or, more commonly, the pulmonary artery. One variant of single right ventricle is the *hypoplastic left heart syndrome*, in which there is functionally a single right ventricle in association with mitral stenosis or atresia, aortic stenosis or atresia, a severely hypoplastic left ventricle, and coarctation of the aorta.

Finally, there is a series of disorders known as the *heterotaxy syndromes*, which are associated with either asplenia or polysplenia, and many of these patients have a single ventricle, most commonly with right ventricular morphology. There is a high incidence of "right-left" abnormalities in these patients resulting in abnormalities of systemic (bilateral superior vena cava [SVC]) and pulmonary venous connections, a common atrium, and a common AV valve. Patients with asplenia frequently have total anomalous pulmonary venous connection to a systemic vein and separate connections of right and left hepatic veins to the floor of the common atrium, whereas patients with polysplenia frequently have interruption of the infrahepatic portion of the inferior vena cava (IVC) with connection of lower body venous drainage to the azygous vein. Polysplenia patients are more likely to have ipsilateral pulmonary venous connections (right pulmonary veins to the right side of the atrium and left pulmonary veins to the left side of the atrium). There is a high incidence of obstruction to pulmonary blood flow in heterotaxy patients, with asplenia patients commonly having pulmonary atresia, and polysplenia patients more likely to have pulmonary stenosis.

From the standpoint of planning the Fontan operation, regardless of the precise anatomic diagnosis, the critical *anatomic* details are the locations of the connections of the systemic and pulmonary venous return to the atrium, the size and anatomy of the pulmonary arteries, and the specific anatomy of the atrioventricular valves and their relationships to the systemic and pulmonary venous connections.

Pre-Fontan Management

The initial management of the single-ventricle patient is the subject of other discussions in this book. The major focus of attention in the medical management of the patient with single ventricle after the initial diagnosis, with or without palliative surgical interventions, should be directed at attempting to ensure that the patient will be a candidate for a Fontan type of operation in the future. The identification of residual or newly developing anatomic or physiologic problems is a critical aspect of management during this pre-Fontan interval. The most commonly encountered problems are recurrent obstruction in the aortic arch, progression or new development of subaortic stenosis at the infundibular or bulboventricular foramen levels, anatomic narrowing or distortion of the pulmonary arteries, deterioration of ventricular or atrioventricular valve function, and the development of elevated pulmonary vascular resistance. In particular, continuing difficulties with congestive heart failure should alert the clinician to the potential development of subaortic or aortic arch obstruction or the deterioration of ventricular or AV valve function. The development of obstruction in the aortic arch and/or at the level of the BVF occurs most frequently in those patients who present with excessive pulmonary blood flow initially and require procedures to reduce pulmonary blood flow. This observation has led us to carry out pulmonary artery-to-aortic anastomoses and systemic-to-pulmonary artery shunts much more frequently than a pulmonary artery banding operation for single-ventricle patients with excessive pulmonary blood flow, especially when there is associated aortic arch obstruction. If the patient has previously undergone a pulmonary artery banding operation, the pulmonary valve may have become distorted and will be more likely to be insufficient if a pulmonary artery-to-aortic anastomosis is required because of the development of subaortic stenosis.

Echocardiography may identify some of these problems, but routine cardiac catheterization has generally been carried out in essentially all single-ventricle patients by the age of 6 months. We are engaged in a study to determine whether echocardiography and magnetic resonance imaging in combination may be able to reduce the need for catheterization, but the results of this study are not final. In addition to the measurements of pressures and flows and the calculation of pulmonary vascular resistance at catheterization, the presence of significant aortopulmonary collaterals should be aggressively sought at catheterization. We have attempted to occlude all significant connections in the catheterization laboratory using coils and other devices because it has seemed that the presence of these collaterals would provide retrograde flow in the pulmonary arteries, which would then retard the forward flow into the pulmonary arteries after a systemic venous-to-pulmonary artery connection in a Fontan or bidirectional cavopulmonary shunt operation. If significant residual anatomic problems are identified, they should be addressed at the time of Fontan or bidirectional cavopulmonary artery shunt operations or, if necessary, at a separate operation.

After the first few months of life, pulmonary vascular resistance generally falls, and then the goals of subsequent surgical interventions should be to reduce the volume load on the single ventricle. This goal is met by eliminating systemic arterial-to-pulmonary artery shunts or eliminating connections between the single ventricle and the pulmonary circulation. Once these systemic-to-pulmonary artery connections are removed, pulmonary blood flow is re-established by creating direct connections between the venous system and the pulmonary arteries (generally by means of a bidirectional cavopulmonary artery shunt). Any residual anatomic problems such as pulmonary artery distortion, obstruction to systemic blood flow, atrioventricular valvar regurgitation, or a restrictive atrial septal defect should be dealt with at the same procedure to simplify the "definitive" management (Fontan operation).

Indications for the Bidirectional Cavopulmonary Shunt Operation

The physiologic advantage of the bidirectional cavopulmonary artery shunt (BDCPS) operation is that it allows the elimination of systemic-to-pulmonary artery shunts and of connections between the systemic ventricle and the pulmonary arteries, thereby eliminating the volume load on the single ventricle and maintaining a viable level of oxygenation. We prefer to carry out this operation within the first 4 to 6 months of life in the hope of reducing the volume load on the single ventricle and thereby preserving ventricular function for a subsequent Fontan operation. In addition, the BDCPS circulation seems to be inherently more stable than a "shunted" or "banded" single-ventricle circulation, and sudden death after a BDCPS is much less common than in patients with single ventricle and a pulmonary artery band or a systemic-to-pulmonary artery shunt. Calculated pulmonary vascular resistance as high as 3 to 4 Wood units (indexed to body surface area) or pulmonary artery pressures as high as 20 mm Hg are compatible with a successful bidirectional cavopulmonary artery shunt operation.

An important question is how to choose between a BDCPS and a Fontan operation in the young patient (usually between 9 and 18 months of age) who requires an intervention because of increasing cyanosis. Typically, this is a patient who has undergone a neonatal shunting or banding operation and develops increasing cyanosis. In our initial review of the Fontan operation, young age (<4 years) was not found to be an independent risk factor for failure of the operation, but our subsequent analysis of a larger experience suggested that age <3 years is a risk factor by multivariant analysis. Based on this experience I have adopted the approach that the younger patient is not excluded from consideration for a Fontan operation based on age alone, but must be an "ideal" candidate as outlined later. It is my impression that younger patients tolerate elevated venous pressures less well than older patients, and therefore the criteria for carrying out a Fontan operation for these patients should be more strict. Otherwise, the young patient should undergo a BDCPS as an interval step. Conversely, we have also observed that the older patient is likely to have a lower arterial oxygen saturation after a BDCPS, and therefore may be better considered as a candidate for a "fenestrated" Fontan operation.

A second question centers around whether any systemic-to-pulmonary artery sources of pulmonary blood flow (e.g., a systemic-to-pulmonary artery shunt or a patent ventricle-to-pulmonary artery pathway) should be allowed to persist along with the superior vena cava. If these systemic arterial sources of blood flow remain, then one advantage of the BDCPS procedure in reducing the volume load on the single ventricle is lost. There are multiple opinions on this question, and the definitive answers are unknown. My inclination is to remove these systemic sources of pulmonary blood flow unless the arterial oxygen saturations are inadequate after the BDCPS. Assuming that sources of SVC decompression into either the IVC or atrium are not present, opening systemic-to-pulmonary artery connections will provide additional pulmonary blood flow, which will likely improve oxygenation.

Operative Technique for the Bidirectional Cavopulmonary Shunt

The concept for the BDCPS is to create a functional end-to-side connection between the cranial end of the superior vena cava and both pulmonary arteries. This operation is generally carried out using cardiopulmonary bypass with an ascending aortic cannula for arterial inflow and two venous cannulas in the innominate vein and in the right atrium. All systemic-to-pulmonary artery shunts should be looped before the start of bypass to prevent systemic pump flow from being "stolen" into the pulmonary circulation via the shunt, which would thereby compromise systemic flow. Most commonly, this cavopulmonary connection is created by dividing the SVC at the level of the right pulmonary artery and then sewing the cranial end of the SVC into an incision in the superior aspect of the right pulmonary artery (Fig. 91-1). I have found it useful to dissect out the entire SVC up to the level of the innominate vein entrance site and to divide the azygous vein as an initial step before bypass. Care must be taken to remain close to the SVC during this dissection, particularly on the lateral aspect of the SVC to avoid injury to the phrenic nerve. Once bypass is initiated and systemic-to-pulmonary artery shunts are divided, the SVC is divided between angled vascular clamps that are placed above and below the level of subsequent transection of the SVC. Then an incision is made in the superior aspect of the right pulmonary artery, and the cranial end of the SVC is sewn into this incision with running absorbable monofilament suture material. It is often convenient to make the anastomosis in the region of a previous right-sided Blalock-Taussig shunt by excising all shunt material and then extending the incision proximally and/or distally. The cardiac end of the SVC can then be oversewn with running nonabsorbable monofilament suture. I have recently begun to suture this oversewn cardiac end of the SVC to the undersurface of the right pulmonary artery to preserve SVC length on the cardiac end, which may reduce the

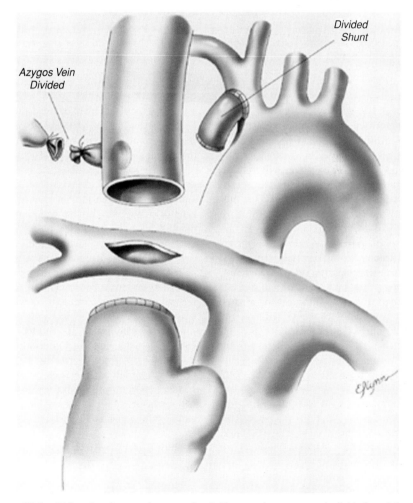

Figure 91-1. Bidirectional cavopulmonary shunt. The superior vena cava is divided, and the cardiac end is oversewn. The azygos vein is divided. A previous modified Blalock-Taussig shunt is shown after division and oversewing.

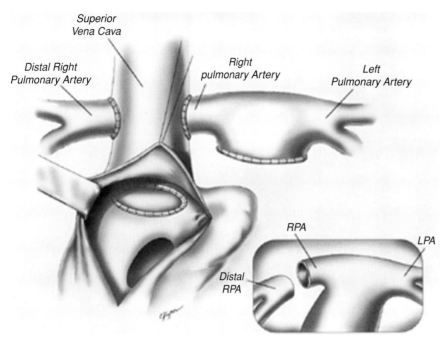

Figure 91-2. The hemi-Fontan variation of bidirectional cavopulmonary shunt. The superior vena cava entrance site into the right atrium is occluded with a polytetrafluoroethylene patch. The cavopulmonary connections are shown, with the right pulmonary artery (RPA) divided and sewn into the sides of the superior vena cava and the main pulmonary artery divided. Alternatively, the superior vena cava can be divided as shown in Fig. 91-1, and the cranial and cardiac ends of the superior vena cava can be sewn into incisions in the superior and inferior surfaces of the right pulmonary artery. (LPA = left pulmonary artery.)

likelihood of sinus node injury when the patient returns for the Fontan operation.

An alternative approach, which we have termed a "hemi-Fontan" procedure, is to create anastomoses between both the cranial and cardiac ends of the SVC and the pulmonary artery using arteriotomies in both the superior and inferior surfaces of the right pulmonary artery. To prevent SVC blood from reaching the right atrium and bypassing the lungs, the SVC-right atrial orifice must then be occluded, and I prefer to effect this occlusion by sewing a patch of polytetrafluoroethylene (PTFE) into the right atrium at the entrance site of the SVC (Fig. 91-2). I have tried both homograft patch material and pericardium, but I believe that it is easiest to remove the PTFE patch when carrying out the subsequent Fontan operation. To place the intra-atrial patch in carrying out the "hemi-Fontan" operation, the heart must either by fibrillating or arrested and total bypass must have been established by looping the inferior vena cava. The advantage of the "hemi-Fontan" approach is that it simplifies the subsequent Fontan operation into a procedure in which the SVC–right atrial junction patch is removed and the intra-atrial baffle

is placed. This approach thereby avoids dissection around the sinus node at the time of the Fontan operation.

As an alternative to dividing the SVC, the right pulmonary artery can be divided and sewn into the sides of the superior vena cava (Fig. 92-2). This technique can be particularly useful if there is a localized right pulmonary artery stenosis at the site of a previous Blalock-Taussig shunt.

In the presence of both left and right superior vena cavae, both should be anastomosed to their respective pulmonary arteries, unless one is clearly much smaller and can therefore be ligated. If one SVC is not connected to the pulmonary arterial system, then this SVC will decompress the contralateral SVC into either the inferior vena caval system or into the atrium directly and there will be inadequate pulmonary blood flow with resulting greater cyanosis.

Results of the Bidirectional Cavopulmonary Shunt Operation

The results of the initial experience with the bidirectional cavopulmonary artery shunt operation are, in general, quite favorable.

In one group of 28 patients undergoing this procedure as a second-stage operation in the management of their single-ventricle anatomy in our institution, 27 survived. The major sources of difficulty have been primarily related to either markedly elevated pulmonary vascular resistance or unrecognized venous collaterals from the superior vena cava system to either the inferior vena cava or to the atrium, which leads to decreased oxygen saturation.

Fontan Operation

Indications

We believe that most patients with single ventricle will be best served over the long term by undergoing a Fontan type of operation. However, the true long-term (lifetime) outcome of the Fontan operation is unknown, and the wisdom of directing all single-ventricle patients toward a Fontan procedure as the "definitive" treatment is unproven. However, if one accepts this treatment strategy as a preferred approach, the issue is not the indication for the operation, but the definition of the contraindications to this approach. Several studies have been undertaken to identify risk factors for this operation, and the relative importance of the various risk factors has evolved. We view pulmonary vascular resistance >2 Wood units (indexed to body surface area), significant pulmonary artery narrowings that cannot be repaired surgically, and pulmonary artery pressures >15 mm Hg as indicators of greater risk, although none of these variables should be viewed as absolute contraindications. Each piece of data should be carefully evaluated for potential measurement errors, calculation errors, and physiologic conditions that might temporarily alter the patient's physiology and thereby convey an erroneous impression of the patient's ability to tolerate a Fontan operation. For example, calculation of pulmonary vascular resistance requires knowledge of both pulmonary artery mean pressure and calculation of pulmonary blood flow (PBF). Calculation of PBF by the Fick method depends on measurement of oxygen uptake and on accurate measurement of pulmonary artery and pulmonary venous oxygen content. If there is more than one source of pulmonary blood flow, and if the two sources do not have the same oxygen content, then calculation of pulmonary blood flow and resistance is not likely to be accurate. Similarly, if the patient is hypoventilating with an elevated CO_2 tension and low pH during the catheterization, then pulmonary resistance will be artificially elevated. When pulmonary resistance is measured in a nonpulsatile system, such as will be present after a bidirectional cavopulmonary shunt, the calculated pulmonary vascular resistance (PVR) tends to be higher (presumably due to the nonpulsatile nature of the pulmonary blood flow), and we do not view a PVR of up to 2.5 to 3 Wood units in this type of circulation as acceptable for a Fontan operation. Ventricular function can be difficult to precisely quantify because of the variable geometry of many single ventricles. Magnetic resonance imaging allows accurate measurement of ventricular volumes and ejection and regurgitant fractions, but the usefulness of these volume determinations as predictors of outcome after Fontan operations is not clear. The presence of atrioventricular valvar regurgitation may occur as a consequence of volume loading of the single ventricle if the patient has a systemic-to-pulmonary artery shunt or a persistent anatomic connection between the ventricle and the pulmonary circulation, and the regurgitation may improve when the volume load is removed. In addition, we have at least a few patients who have AV valve regurgitation post-Fontan and who tolerate this quite well. However, our practice is aggressively to attempt to correct or reduce atrioventricular valve regurgitation whenever possible. Finally, it must be emphasized that our loosening of the criteria for a Fontan operation is based on the fact that almost all of our patients now undergo a fenestrated Fontan operation, which we believe allows less "ideal" patients to tolerate this operation.

Operative Technique

The technique of the *Fontan operation* has become fairly standardized, and I routinely use the "lateral tunnel" technique with direct cavopulmonary anastomoses. The operation is carried out using hypothermic cardiopulmonary bypass (24°C) with venous cannulas placed in either the SVC or innominate vein and the inferior vena cava–right atrial junction. All systemic-to-pulmonary artery shunts must be controlled before the institution of cardiopulmonary bypass for the reasons outlined previously. Both superior and inferior vena cavae are surrounded with tourniquets, and a cardioplegia catheter is introduced into the ascending aorta. It is important to avoid ventricular distention once the heart has stopped having effective contractions, and a vent catheter is generally placed either in the right superior pulmonary vein or in

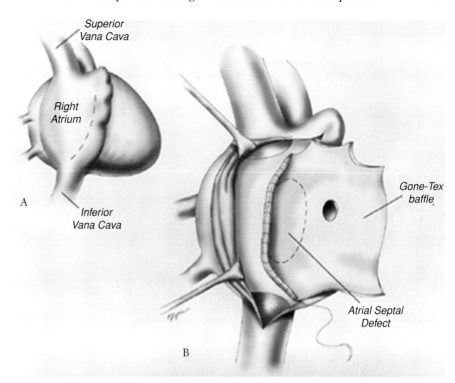

Figure 91-3. Fontan operation (lateral tunnel technique). The incision in the atrium is shown **(A)**. The suture line begins medial to the inferior vena cava and proceeds posterior to the inferior vena caval orifice and then superiorly along the lateral wall of the atrium (anterior to the atrial septal remnant).

the left atrial appendage. Once the aorta is clamped and cardioplegia is given, the right atrium is opened with an incision parallel to the atrioventricular groove (Fig. 91-3). The atrial septum should be inspected, and a large defect should be created to prevent any restriction to flow between the atria. The creation of a large ASD is particularly important when there is left atrioventricular valve atresia or stenosis because a restrictive ASD will cause pulmonary venous obstruction, which will virtually guarantee the failure of the Fontan operation. The location of all pulmonary and systemic venous connections must be confirmed. The "lateral tunnel" technique involves placement of a baffle along the lateral aspect of the right atrium that conveys inferior vena cava blood to the superior vena caval orifice. This baffle is cut in the form of a half cylinder. We use PTFE patch material and do not use PTFE vascular graft material to form the baffle because the vascular graft material has a "wrap" that may be more thrombogenic. The two ends of the hemicylindrical patch are beveled with the medial end being longer than the part of the baffle that will run along the lateral wall of the atrium (Fig. 91-3). I generally sew this baffle in with running nonabsorbable monofilament suture begin-

ning medial to the inferior vena cava orifice and then sewing posterior to the IVC and then along the lateral wall of the atrium. I try to stay anterior to the atrial septum to minimize the risk of creating obstruction to the right pulmonary venous return. When the superior vena cava orifice is reached, the baffle length can be adjusted. The suture line is then carried around the SVC orifice. Because this area of the right atrium can be very trabeculated, I tend to sew the baffle into the smooth inner wall at the origin of the superior vena cava (crista terminalis). The sinus node is in this region, and therefore sutures must be placed superficially. After about three fourths of the superior vena cava circumference has been completed, the anterior portion of the baffle-to-inferior vena cava orifice suture line is constructed with the other end of the original suture. The fenestration is then made in the medial aspect of the baffle opposite the ASD so that there will be ample room for a device to be placed in the fenestration at later catheterization without creating pulmonary venous obstruction (Fig. 91-4). The diameter of the baffle can be altered to keep the baffle from protruding into the pulmonary venous pathway at this point as well. Then the anterior lip of the baffle is sewn to the lateral right atrial

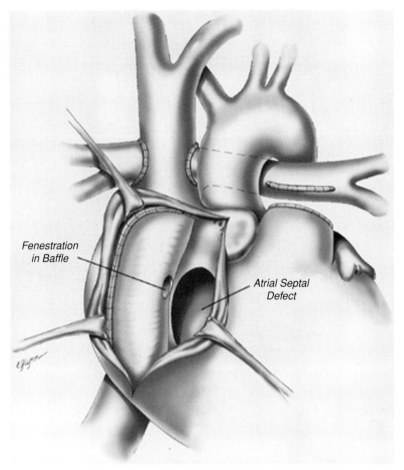

Figure 91-4. Fontan operation (lateral tunnel technique). The intra-atrial baffle is shown completed along with a fenestration in the baffle. A variation of the technique of cavopulmonary anastomosis is shown in which the right pulmonary artery is divided and sewn to the medial and posterolateral aspects of the superior vena cava.

wall, completing the inferior vena cava-to-superior vena caval pathway.

If the patient has not had a "hemi-Fontan" procedure previously, the cardiac end of the superior vena cava is connected to the inferior aspect of the right pulmonary artery using an end-to-side technique as described previously *prior to the construction of the lateral tunnel.* This sequence is used because the right atrium may have to be pulled up to reach the right pulmonary artery, and it can be difficult to gauge the appropriate length of the lateral tunnel to account for this stretching unless the SVC-to-right pulmonary artery anastomosis is constructed first. I have not made a major point of offsetting the cranial and caudal cavopulmonary anastomoses, believing that the kinetic energy losses due to turbulence must be quite small because the blood flow velocity is low. All connections between the systemic arterial system or systemic ventricle and the pulmonary arteries must be obliterated to

prevent competitive flow, which will elevate systemic venous pressures.

Generally it is preferable to divide the pulmonary artery and to resect any remaining pulmonary valve tissue (unless there is pulmonary valvar atresia) rather than simply ligating the pulmonary artery (Fig. 91-4). I try to divide the main pulmonary artery relatively close to the semilunar valve, and in closing the proximal orifice, I also incorporate any residual pulmonary valve leaflets into the closure so that there will not be any residual sinuses of Valsalva where there could be stasis. We have observed thrombus formation in the "stump" of the main pulmonary artery that has been divided above the valve, and on at least a few occasions, this "stump" seems to have been the source of systemic arterial emboli.

After completing the Fontan baffle and the closure of the main pulmonary artery and the cavopulmonary connections, the heart is de-aired, and the aortic cross-clamp

is removed. The heart is kept decompressed with the vent catheter until effective cardiac contractions have been restored during rewarming.

The clearest advantage of the lateral tunnel technique is that it minimizes the likelihood of obstruction of the pulmonary venous return when the pulmonary venous return must reach the right atrioventricular valve (as in cases with mitral atresia or hypoplastic left heart syndrome). This problem of the systemic venous pathway causing pulmonary venous obstruction was a common cause of the mortality in our early experience with Fontan operations for hypoplastic left heart syndrome. A second advantage of the lateral tunnel technique is that it avoids the marked right atrial enlargement that frequently occurs when the entire right atrium is exposed to elevated venous pressure. This "giant" right atrium can lead to turbulence and consequent energy losses in the systemic venous return reaching the right atrium, although the magnitude of these energy losses is difficult to evaluate. The distended right atrium can also cause compression of the right pulmonary veins, which lie immediately behind the right atrium. Either of these consequences of a giant right atrium will be disadvantageous for the patient with a Fontan circulation.

We use a "fenestration" in the lateral tunnel baffle in virtually all patients because there is reasonably good evidence to suggest that both mortality and morbidity are reduced. We use a 4-mm coronary punch to create the fenestration. Many fenestrations spontaneously close with time, and those that do not close can be closed in the catheterization laboratory with ASD devices. We believe that cavopulmonary anastomoses are preferable to atriopulmonary connections because there is less likelihood of kinking or obstruction at these anastomoses.

Less common anatomic situations may require different approaches to achieve the goals of an unobstructed systemic venous pathway from the superior and inferior vena cavae to the pulmonary arteries and an unobstructed pathway for pulmonary venous blood to reach the atrioventricular valves and systemic ventricle. In the patients with a left superior vena cava, the operation is modified by adding a left superior vena cava (LVSC)-to-left pulmonary artery anastomosis using the same technique as for a right superior vena cava. We generally place a third venous cannula in the LSVC when there are bilateral superior vena cavae. In patients with the heterotaxy syndromes, there are frequently anomalies of systemic and pulmonary venous connections as outlined in the section on anatomy. In these situations, it may be difficult to construct a standard lateral tunnel without creating pulmonary venous obstruction. It may seem necessary to construct the baffle across the posterior wall of the atrium with the open part of the baffle sewn to the posterior wall of the atrium rather than the lateral wall. However, I have found that this technique may lead to pulmonary venous obstruction because the posterior wall of the atrium also may form the anterior wall of the some or all of the pulmonary veins. In this situation, it seems preferable to use a complete tube (conduit) to convey IVC blood to the pulmonary arteries, and this conduit may lie either within or outside the atrium. If this situation is anticipated, I generally try to defer the Fontan operation until the patients are older (>5 to 6 years) so that the IVC and the atrium will be large enough to accommodate a 14- to 16-mm internal PTFE conduit. If the conduit is placed outside the atrium, then the inferior vena cava is divided from its junction with the atrium, and the atrial defect is closed. A PTFE conduit (which may be of larger diameter) is sewn end to end to the IVC, and the other end of the conduit is sewn to the underside of the ipsilateral pulmonary artery. A fenestration may be created by sewing a 4-mm defect created in the external conduit to a similar defect in the atrial free wall (side to side).

Another anatomic situation worthy of mention is the presence of total anomalous pulmonary venous connection to the superior vena cava (almost always in asplenia patients). In this situation the pulmonary veins usually enter the SVC in the position of an azygous vein (Fig. 91-5). In this situation, one is tempted to leave the pulmonary venous blood to drain into the superior vena cava to reach the atrium and to divide the SVC above the pulmonary vein entrance site into the SVC. The cranial end of the SVC can then be sewn into the pulmonary artery directly. However, the pulmonary venous drainage then is "draped" over the pulmonary artery (because the azygous vein enters the SVC superior to the pulmonary artery), and we have found that pulmonary venous obstruction will be present when this technique is used. I believe that it is preferable in this situation to construct a direct connection between the pulmonary veins and the atrium if possible. If not, then the pulmonary artery should be divided and reanastomosed anterior to the pulmonary vein–SVC junction to prevent the pulmonary venous obstruction caused as the pulmonary veins course posteriorly

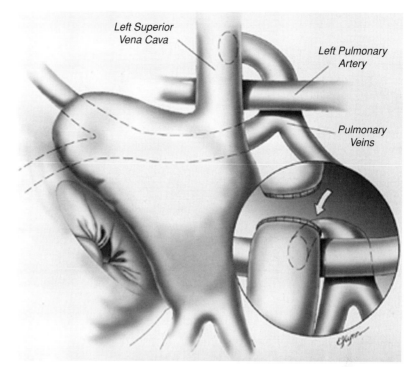

Figure 91-5. Total anomalous pulmonary venous connection to the superior vena cava in asplenia. This figure depicts a total anomalous pulmonary venous connection to a left superior vena cava in an asplenia patient. Shown in the inset is the effect of simply dividing the superior vena cava. The native elasticity of the superior vena cava inferiorly and "bowstringing" of the pulmonary veins over the top of the pulmonary artery lead to pulmonary venous obstruction.

to reach the more anteriorly positioned SVC.

Postoperative Management after Fontan and Bidirectional Cavopulmonary Shunt Operations

After either of these operations, pulmonary blood flow will be driven by the difference between systemic venous pressure and the pulmonary venous pressure. Therefore, it is important to monitor these pressures, and measures to minimize pulmonary vascular resistance are important. In general, poor hemodynamics should prompt a through investigation for any residual anatomic problems with the operation, including a cardiac catheterization. In the patient with a bidirectional cavopulmonary artery shunt, the arterial saturation will generally be >80%, although older patients will be more likely to have lower saturations because superior vena caval return is a smaller percentage of the total systemic venous return. More severe cyanosis may imply the presence of a

vein that decompresses the superior vena cava into either the inferior vena cava (such as an azygous vein) or into the atrium. We have frequently observed systemic arterial hypertension after the BDCPS operation, which we believe is a reflex response to cerebral venous hypertension. It is generally treated acutely with systemic afterload reduction.

After the Fontan operation it is again important to monitor systemic and pulmonary venous pressures and indicators of cardiac output such as strength of pulses, arterial blood pressure, urine output, and capillary refill time. An unfavorable hemodynamic course should result in prompt investigations such as echocardiogram and catheterization to determine whether there are residual anatomic problems with the operation. Systemic venous hypertension, which is obligatory after a Fontan operation, seems to cause reflex arterial vasoconstriction, which may impair ventricular output. We liberally employ vasodilator agents in the postoperative period (e.g., amrinone, nitroprusside) to offset this vasoconstriction. In the absence of a correctable cause for a failing Fontan circulation, early takedown to a bidirectional cavopulmonary shunt offers the best hope for patient survival. Because it is relatively uncommon for there to be severe low cardiac output after a fenestrated Fontan operation, we regard low cardiac output that does not respond to low- to moderate-dose pharmacologic intervention and for which there is no correctable anatomic cause as an indication for this takedown operation.

Atrial pacing wires are an essentially obligatory adjunct to postoperative management as well. There may be sinus node dysfunction due to surgical manipulation in this area, and patients after both Fontan and bidirectional cavopulmonary artery shunt operations seem to be quite sensitive to the loss of sinus rhythm. Atrial pacing in these situations may be life-saving. In addition, the atrial pacing wires allow the accurate diagnosis of arrhythmias in the postoperative patient, which allows accurate therapy for the arrhythmia.

Pleural effusions are the most common problem after a Fontan operation, and they have not been totally eliminated by the use of the fenestration. There is reasonably good evidence that the liver and/or mesenteric circulation are the source of the fluid that collects in the pleural or pericardial spaces. Complete drainage of effusions is generally advisable because a large fluid collection will compress the lung and can therefore raise the pulmonary vascular resistance. It is important to maintain adequate fluid replacement and nutrition for the patient who is having large chest tube losses for more than a few days after the operation. Fortunately, most patients with effusions will stop draining within 1 to 3 weeks after the operation. For patients with persistent drainage, cardiac catheterization is advisable to rule out residual anatomic problems.

Results of Fontan Operations

The results of the entire Fontan experience from 1973 through 1991 at the Children's Hospital Boston are shown in Table 91-1. This experience involved a number of techniques for carrying out the Fontan operation, and over this period of time involved a significant "learning curve." The results clearly improved over time (Table 91-2). The results with the lateral tunnel technique and with cavopulmonary anastomoses (rather than atriopulmonary anastomoses or atriopulmonary conduits) were better (86.6% success vs. 80.9%) although it was difficult to separate the effect of technique from the effect of year of operation. The effects of fenestration of the lateral

Table 91-1 Overall Outcome of Fontan Operations 1973 to 1991

Diagnosis	Success[a]	Failure[b]	Percentage Success
Single LV-NRGA	131	20	86.8
Single LV-TGA	168	28	85.7
Heterotaxy	32	9	78.1
Single RV	46	14	76.7
HLHS	16	11	59.3
Other	23	2	92.3
Total	500	84	83.2

HLHS = hypoplastic left heart syndrome; LV = left ventricle; RV = right ventricle; NRGA = normally related great arteries; TGA = transposed great arteries.
[a]Survived Fontan operation.
[b]Death or takedown of Fontan operation.

Table 91-2 Effect of Date of Operation

Years of Operation	n	Success	Failure	Percentage Success
1973–1984	133	98	35	73.7
1985–1989	233	195	38	83.7
1990–1991	134	125	9	93.3
2001–2004	196	194	2	98.9

Table 91-3 Effect of Fenestration 1973 to 1991 (n = 498)

	n	Success	Failure	Percentage Success
Fenestrated	136	127	9	93.4
Nonfenestrated	361	289	72	80.0

tunnel during this earlier era are shown in Table 91-3. In more recent years, the mortality results have continued to improve. In the years 2001 to 2004, 196 fenestrated Fontan procedures were carried out with an operative mortality rate of 1% (Table 91-2).

When all variables from the earlier era are considered in a multivariant analysis excluding date of operation as a variable, the important risk factors for the entire series of 500 patients are as shown in Table 91-4. Although a similar analysis for risk of mortality is no longer feasible because of the marked reduction in mortality with this procedure, the lessons from the earlier era analyses are appropriate for the lessons about case selection that were learned during that interval. The actuarial late survival at 10 years using the lateral tunnel technique was 91%.

Atrial arrhythmias have emerged as an important late outcome problem. The late results of patients operated on in the period 1987 to 1991 using the lateral tunnel technique at Children's Hospital Boston were reported in 2001 by Stamm et al. The overall rates of freedom from tachyarrhythmias and bradyarrhythmias at 10 years are

91% and 79%, respectively (Table 91-5). The major risk factors for the development of tachyarrhythmias include heterotaxy syndrome, atrioventricular valve abnormalities, and preoperative bradyarrhythmia. The major risk factor for bradyarrhythmias is the presence of systemic venous anomalies, a

Table 91-4 Multivariant Analysis (1973 to 1991): Early Outcome[a]

Risk Factor	p value
Heterotaxy diagnosed	.029
Age <4 years	.001
Prior atrial septectomy	.003
Pulmonary artery pressure >18 mm Hg	<.001
Pulmonary artery distortion	.011
Use of conduit	.015
Cardiopulmonary bypass time	.001
Fenestration (lower risk)	<.001

[a]Without operative date considered in analysis.

Table 91-5 Incidence of Arrhythmias

Arrhythmia	Percentage Free at 5 Years	Percentage Free at 10 Years
Supraventricular tachycardia	94	90
New-onset supraventricular tachycardia	96	91
Bradyarrhythmia	83	73
New-onset bradyarrhythmia	88	79

Mean follow-up = 8.7 years.

factor that is highly associated with heterotaxy syndrome. Although some have advocated the use of the extracardiac conduit technique for the Fontan procedure, our limited experience with this technique for selected diagnoses suggests that early postoperative atrial arrhythmias still occur.

Summary

The management of single-ventricle patients clearly remains a challenge for both surgeons and cardiologists involved in their care. The continuing mortality and morbidity after neonatal palliative operations suggest that earlier reinterventions to establish a pulmonary circulation that is in series with the systemic circulation rather than in parallel (i.e., bidirectional cavopulmonary shunt or Fontan procedure rather than systemic-to-pulmonary artery shunt) may have the potential for reducing some of this interval mortality. The technical refinements to the Fontan operation outlined here have contributed to significant improvements in early patient outcome after this operation, but long-term follow-up is clearly necessary to determine whether this approach is optimal for all single-ventricle patients or for certain (as yet to be defined) physiologic and/or anatomic subsets of patients. Continued follow-up and reassessment of the "unnatural" history of the surgically treated patient with single ventricle beginning with neonatal and infant interventions and continuing through Fontan operations will be essential to refine the treatment of this difficult group of patients.

SUGGESTED READING

Bridges ND, Mayer JE, Lock JE, Castaneda AR. Effect of fenestration on outcome of Fontan repair. Circulation 1991;84(Suppl II):II-120.

Edwards JE. Congenital Malformations of the Heart and Great Vessels: C. Malformations of the Valves. In: Gould SE (ed), Pathology of the Heart and Blood Vessels (3rd ed). Springfield, IL: Charles C Thomas,1968: 312.

Fontan F, Baudet E. Surgical repair of tricuspid atresia. Thorax 1971;26:240.

Franklin RCG, Spiegelhalter DJ, Anderson RH, et al. Double-inlet ventricle presenting in infancy. J Thorac Cardiovasc Surg 1991;101:767.

Matitiau A, Geva T, Colan SD, et al. Bulboventricular foramen size in infants with double-inlet left ventricle or tricuspid atresia with transposed great arteries: Influence on initial palliative operation and rate of growth. J Am Coll Cardiol 1992;19:142.

Mayer Jr JE, Bridges ND, Lock JE, et al. Factors associated with marked reduction in mortality for Fontan operations in patients with single ventricle. J Thorac Cardiovasc Surg 1992;103:444.

Mayer Jr JE, Helgason H, Jonas RA, et al. Extending the limits for modified Fontan procedures. J Thorac Cardiovasc Surg 1986;92:1021.

Moodie DS, Ritter DG, Tajik AJ, O'Fallon WM. Long-term follow-up in the unoperated univentricular heart. Am J Cardiol 1984;53:1124.

Stamm C, Friehs I, Mayer JE, et al. Long-term results of the lateral tunnel Fontan operation. J Thorac Cardiovasc Surg 2001;121:28.

Van Praagh R, Ongley PA, Swan HJC. Anatomic types of single or common ventricle in man. Am J Cardiol 1964;13:367.

EDITOR'S COMMENTS

The Fontan operation has been a major advance in the treatment of complex congenital heart disease. It is applicable to multiple forms of complex defects, including all forms of single ventricle and situations in which biventricular repair is either not feasible or is associated with long-term complications and late reoperation. Multiple modifications of the Fontan procedure have permitted a marked improvement in late morbidity and mortality, such that the Fontan operation is associated with a mortality of <5% in most centers and long-term results remain quite good despite the lack of a ventricle pumping blood through the pulmonary circulation.

In spite of these very salient features of the Fontan operation, multiple modifications have been recommended to decrease late morbidity. Perhaps the most significant advance in the Fontan operation has been the advent of a fenestration in the intra-atrial baffle, which has been shown to maintain ventricular preload in situations of elevated pulmonary vascular resistance and improve cardiac output. Initial use of the fenestration in high-risk Fontan procedures at Children's Hospital Boston was associated with a marked improvement in the incidence of pleural effusions and a decreased incidence of takedown of the Fontan operation even in "high-risk" Fontan candidates. Although initial approaches were directed at closure of the fenestration at a later catheterization procedure, it is interesting that in all patients with temporary occlusion of the fenestration, cardiac output dropped, suggesting that there is a potential benefit of maintaining ventricular preload with a fenestration. For these reasons, we use fenestrations in all Fontan operations, and although spontaneous closure occurs in at least 30% of patients with a 4.0-mm fenestration of an intra-atrial baffle, it is unclear whether closure of the fenestration is necessarily beneficial in all patients. This controversy is heightened by the fact that patients who have developed protein-losing enteropathy after the Fontan operation or who have persistent effusions that are not resolving with medical management may have complete resolution of the problems by creation of a fenestration in a previously nonfenestrated atriopulmonary connection. This fact would suggest that the optimal hemodynamics with fenestration of the atrial baffle may be very beneficial in the long term for Fontan patients. Arterial desaturation may be an acceptable price to pay for adequate oxygen delivery with improvement in cardiac output in these patients if late morbidity is in fact improved.

As noted in the commentary to Chapter 90, we use a hemi-Fontan procedure in most patients for staging to a completion fenestrated Fontan procedure. The hemi-Fontan procedure is generally done between 3 and 6 months of age, and the completion Fontan operation is performed by 1.5 to 2.0 years of age. In a consecutive series of 120 such patients with the hemi-Fontan and Fontan procedures in our institution, the operative mortality was <1%, and morbidity from pleural effusions was very low. We found that use of modified ultrafiltration after the operation results in a marked decrease in volume load and improved hemodynamics and shortened hospital stay and a marked decrease in morbidity from pericardial and pleural effusions. Prolonged pleural effusions lasting > 1 week are now extremely unusual after Fontan operations in our institution.

A major issue for long-term function after the Fontan operation is the incidence of atrial flutter and fibrillation, which can compromise ventricular function and cardiac output. Much attention has been directed to the contribution of atrial suture lines to the development of atrial arrhythmias. The creation of extensive atrial sutures lines has resulted in areas of conduction block that may contribute to atrial flutter. For this reason, some centers have advocated use of extracardiac connections from the inferior vena cava to the pulmonary artery to completely eliminate pressure loading of the right atrium and to eliminate suture lines in the right atrium. Long-term follow-up of these extracardiac connections is not available, however, and longitudinal growth may result in constriction of the conduits and require late conduit replacement in some cases. In addition, it is difficult to fenestrate extracardiac Fontan connections with a satisfactory degree of long-term patency. Direct anastomosis to the right atrial wall results in rapid spontaneous closure, and a graft from the extracardiac conduit to the right atrium may also thrombose rapidly. If a hemi-Fontan procedure done with a homograft baffle from the SVC to the right atrium is used as an initial-stage procedure, extracardiac Fontan connection can be performed with creation of a fenestration through the "dam" between the SVC and right atrium at the hemi-Fontan connection and results in adequate fenestration patency over the intermediate term in most cases.

As emphasized by Dr. Mayer, it is particularly important to avoid development of subaortic obstruction in patients who have had procedures to reduce PBF with single-ventricle physiology. Therefore, creation of Norwood-type operations or Damus-Kaye-Stansel procedures with systemic-to-pulmonary shunts is preferable to pulmonary banding in most cases to protect the pulmonary vascular bed for later Fontan reconstruction. An additional emphasis should be placed on the need to oversew pulmonary artery stumps if the pulmonary arteries are disconnected from the ventricles at the time of bidirectional Glenn or Fontan operations to prevent stasis thrombosis in the stump of the pulmonary artery and potential embolization. In situations in which the pulmonary valve cannot be readily oversewn, excision of the pulmonary valve and oversewing of the pulmonary stump to eliminate an area of stasis is recommended. We have seen several cases in which thrombus formation in the pulmonary artery stump has been associated with late embolization and cerebrovascular accidents.

We use a hemi-Fontan procedure with circulatory arrest to avoid caval cannulation and potential caval distortion at second-stage reconstruction. With this approach, a completion fenestrated Fontan procedure can be accomplished in an additional brief period of circulatory arrest, generally averaging <20 minutes. In this operation, an incision is made in the right atrium on a line from the SVC to the inferior vena cava. The dam of homograft material in the superior margin of the right atrium is then excised, and a baffle (using a PTFE [Impra, Inc., Tempe, AZ] graft, which is incised longitudinally and in which a 4.0-mm fenestration is created) is trimmed and sewn in the lateral tunnel technique. Inferiorly, the suture line is carried around the Eustachian valve, which creates a good size match to the inferior vena cava. Superiorly, the suture line is carried around the homograft suture line to the superior aspect of the right atrium, which avoids any trabecular muscle of the right atrium that can result in additional patch leaks and creates a secure suture line avoiding the sinus node. The atriotomy incision is then closed, with the baffle sandwiched between the two edges of the atrial incision to complete the lateral tunnel. The ease of this operation and use of modified ultrafiltration have been associated with very low morbidity. Atrial monitoring lines are brought through the chest wall and positioned on either side of the atrial suture line in which the baffle is sandwiched, creating a pressure-monitoring line on the pulmonary venous and pulmonary arterial side of the baffle. Patients are generally extubated shortly after the operation, and the average hospital stay has decreased to 5 to 7 days after the Fontan operation, with very low morbidity from pleural effusions with this technique.

The long-term benefits from Fontan reconstruction remain to be determined; however, it is apparent that the late results with single-ventricle repairs have been markedly better than most surgeons would have anticipated. Although a certain population of patients will develop protein-losing enteropathy late after the operative procedure, the incidence of this condition at intermediate follow-up is relatively low. Thus, the Fontan operation has become a mainstay of repair for complex congenital heart disease, and continued refinement is being undertaken to optimize late hemodynamic results. Modification of atrial suture lines and division of potential conduction zones for atrial flutter may be added to the Fontan operation in the future to prevent late arrhythmias. In addition, diversion of inferior vena caval flow preferentially to the right lung with superior vena caval flow directed to the left lung may optimize flow distribution in the pulmonary arteries after the operation. The use of lateral tunnel techniques has decreased the incidence of significant stasis in the right atrium, and giant right atrium after the operation, although rare, must be taken down to create the lateral baffle superior to the right pulmonary vein entrances to prevent compression of the pulmonary veins and late stenosis. Failure of Fontan operations requiring takedown is now extremely unusual with attention to staging of the operations and addressing of significant sources of pulmonary artery distortion before a complete Fontan procedure.

T.L.S.

92

Hypoplastic Left Heart Syndrome

Peter J. Gruber and Thomas L. Spray

Introduction

Hypoplastic left heart syndrome (HLHS) comprises a wide spectrum of anatomic abnormalities with the common feature of left ventricular hypoplasia and hypoplasia of the ascending aorta. At one end of the spectrum there may be some mild left ventricle hypoplasia, mild aortic stenosis, and aortic coarctation. At the other end of the spectrum, however, there is complete absence of the left ventricle, aortic atresia, and aortic arch hypoplasia or even interrupted aortic arch.

HLHS is a uniformly fatal disease if untreated. It represents 5% of all congenital heart disease and is responsible for nearly 25% of cardiac deaths in the first week of life. Of 10,000 live births, approximately 1.8 will be born with HLHS, with a slight male predominance. Of these, 25% will also have a noncardiac anomaly and 5% a chromosomal abnormality (trisomies 13, 18, and 21). Syndromic lesions are rare, with Turner syndrome (monosomy X) the most common. The recurrence risk is 2.2% for one affected sibling and 6% for two affected siblings, suggesting some genetic predisposition but arguing against a simple effect.

Surgery for HLHS has been one of the great successes in the management of congenital heart disease. Before the 1980s, HLHS was a uniformly lethal condition. Over the last 25 years, the repair of HLHS has become a standard operation in nearly all institutions. In 1952, Lev first described maldevelopment of the left-sided cardiac structures in combination with a small ascending aorta and transverse arch. By 1958, Noonan and Nadas had further defined the syndrome to describe a variety of cardiac malformations of left heart structures. The

first report of any attempt to palliate a patient with mitral atresia was by Redo in 1961, who performed an atrial septectomy using inflow occlusion through a right thoracotomy; the patient died soon after the operation. In 1968, Sinha outlined management principles still in use today that include creation of an unobstructed atrial communication, unrestricted ductal flow, and control of pulmonary blood flow. Cayler described an anastomosis between the right pulmonary artery (PA) and ascending aorta with banding of both right and left pulmonary arteries. It is of interest that 35 years later, PA banding is being used in certain centers for selected children who present with a medical or anatomic situation unsuitable for stage-one Norwood reconstruction; this first-stage hybrid procedure involves stenting the ductus arteriosus and atrial septal defect and using bilateral PA bands. Litwin, Mohri, and others performed operations that were variations of the principles of palliation that were unsuccessful but contributed to the development of the knowledge of the disease and its repair. In 1977, Doty described primary reconstruction that included atrial septation and an right atrium (RA)-to-PA Fontan circuit. Again, although no patients survived, this experience established the principle that one-stage reconstruction with a Fontan repair would not be successful due to high neonatal pulmonary vascular resistance. Levitsky, Behrendt, and others described multiple variations of surgical procedures that, although they demonstrated no long-term success, established the principle of staged reconstruction with initial palliation followed by later separation of the systemic and pulmonary circulations. However, it was Norwood who in 1980 first achieved successful palliation in infants. In 1983, he described the first successful staged

approach culminating in a Fontan repair. The Norwood procedure remains the primary reconstructive approach.

Anatomy

Patients with HLHS can be categorized on the basis of atrioventricular (AV) and semilunar valvular morphology into three primary subsets: (1) aortic atresia with mitral atresia (40%), (2) aortic stenosis with mitral stenosis (30%), and aortic atresia with mitral stenosis (30%) (Fig. 92-1). Aortic stenosis with mitral atresia is rare. HLHS variants include malaligned AV canal, double-outlet right ventricle with mitral atresia, tricuspid atresia with transposed great arteries, and univentricular heart with aortic stenosis. There is frequent leftward and posterior deviation of the septal attachment of the septum primum, but this feature is unlikely to be a shared developmental mechanism because it is commonly seen in other congenital heart disease patients. Usually, the superior vena cava (SVC) and inferior vena cava (IVC) are normally connected to the right atrium, although in about 15% of patients a left SVC-to-coronary sinus is present. Other structural abnormalities of the heart are rare, with <5% of patients demonstrating AV valvular dysplasia. Also rare (<5%) are abnormalities of pulmonary venous return or an interrupted aortic arch. Abnormalities in brain development are being increasingly associated with children with severe congenital heart disease, who may be a high-risk group for operative repair. The pulmonary vascular tree is also abnormal, with an increase in number of vessels as well as muscularity.

The developmental mechanisms that underlie HLHS are obscure from a molecular

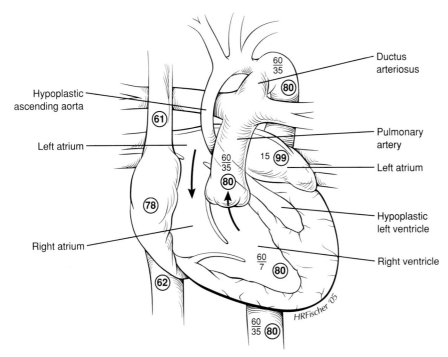

Figure 92-1. Anatomic features and representative hemodynamic parameters for unrepaired hypoplastic left heart syndrome. Oxygen saturations are enclosed in circles, and blood pressures are indicated by standard nomenclature.

standpoint because there are no mutations that have been robustly associated with this condition. Despite the existence of rare family clustering of HLHS, linkage analysis has been unproductive; however, embryologically, there are clues. The severe hypoplasia of left heart structures is probably a consequence of limited flow during development secondary to a primary abnormality of either left ventricular inflow or left ventricular outflow. Primary defects of myocardial growth are unlikely to be a mechanism for this disease because the myocardium appears normal. In addition, in approximately 5% of patients with aortic atresia there exists an unrestrictive ventricular septal defect, and in such cases there is nearly always normal development of the left ventricle and mitral valve.

Presentation and Initial Management

The normal fetus has a parallel circulation that adequately supports single-ventricle physiology before birth. Three communications (the ductus venosus, foramen ovale, and ductus arteriosus) shunt oxygenated placental blood largely past the hepatic and pulmonary beds to supply the splanchnic circulation. HLHS is well supported in this

situation, and, as a result, HLHS is rarely a cause of fetal demise. HLHS is likely a secondary result of early obstructive lesions of either mitral or aortic valvular development. This has been supported in animal models of either mitral or aortic stenosis with resulting left ventricular hypoplasia. However, the primary cause of the obstructive flow lesion leading secondarily to HLHS is unknown. There are no known genetic animal models that recapitulate HLHS despite the existence of a large number of mutations that affect valvular development. This argues either for a complex early event that is the result of multiple factors or, more likely, a transient early insult.

The presentation of infants with congenital heart disease has changed dramatically over the last 10 years. In most large centers the majority of patients are identified through prenatal echocardiography, although this early identification has not consistently correlated with better outcome. Although some tachypnea and mild cyanosis may be present, it is not until the ductus arteriosus begins to close that the children exhibit impaired systemic perfusion with pallor, lethargy, and diminished femoral pulses. Cardiac examination reveals a dominant right ventricular impulse, a single-second heart sound, and often a nonspecific soft systolic murmur. Electrocardiogram examination reveals right atrial enlargement and

right ventricular hypertrophy. Chest x-ray occasionally shows mild cardiomegaly and increased pulmonary vascular markings.

Physical examination of children with HLHS usually appears normal. The examination is determined by the underlying anatomy as well as the duration of the disease. Poor perfusion, weak distal pulses (that may or may not be present, depending on the size of the ductus), acidosis, and a sepsis-like picture may all confound the diagnosis. In the absence of risk factors or laboratory findings consistent with sepsis, one should search for left-sided obstructive lesions. There are no specific laboratory indicators of HLHS, and most patients usually exhibit normal values. With ductal closure and malperfusion, end-organ compromise may be reflected by altered hepatic and renal function tests.

Many mothers of fetuses with HLHS will have had a fetal echocardiogram at 20 weeks with reasonable visualization of cardiac structures. It is neither feasible nor cost effective to screen all pregnancies; therefore a selective approach is taken in which only those mothers at high risk are screened. Frequently, a ventricular size discrepancy is the first hint of impending problems. Certainly, the presence of intact or restrictive atrial septum with HLHS should prompt term high-risk delivery in an institution in which an urgent postdelivery atrial septectomy can be performed safely and rapidly. The use of prenatal screening improves the prenatal condition of the child but may not improve outcome (at least in cases of transposition of the great arteries or HLHS). After delivery, the infant should undergo two-dimensional and Doppler echocardiography, which can define the anatomy sufficiently for medical and surgical decision-making. It is important to distinguish HLHS from other diseases that may mimic certain of its features. Chest radiography often demonstrates mild cardiomegaly and excessive pulmonary blood flow. Head ultrasound should be obtained in all patients to rule out intracranial hemorrhage and minimize the risks of heparinization and circulatory arrest. Patients with medical necrotizing enterocolitis should ideally have a 7-day course of intravenous antibiotics before repair if they are hemodynamically stable.

Preoperative stabilization is critical to the ultimate outcome of patients with HLHS regardless of anatomic subtype. Nearly all patients with suspected HLHS are transported to our center on prostaglandin E$_1$ at a dose of 0.01 to 0.025 μg/kg/minute. Two clinically important dose-dependent side effects of prostaglandin E$_1$ are hypotension and apnea, although these are infrequent. Umbilical arterial and umbilical venous lines are used for central access in most patients. Most patients can ventilate with a natural airway and indeed often have more favorable hemodynamics while extubated. Supplemental oxygen should generally be avoided because this will act as a pulmonary vasodilator, decreasing pulmonary vascular resistance, increasing the ratio of pulmonary-to-systemic blood flow, and thus decreasing systemic perfusion. Inotropic support is required in patients who have suffered a perinatal insult but rarely is necessary otherwise. The goal of these maneuvers is to get the patient to the operating room in as stable condition as is possible.

Surgical Therapy

There are two primary therapies for hypoplastic left heart syndrome: (1) staged-reconstructive surgery leading to a modified Fontan-Kreutzer procedure and (2) heart transplantation. Heart transplantation is discussed in detail in other sections of this text, and therefore we will concentrate in the remainder of this section on staged reconstructive surgery.

Over the last 20 years, the Norwood procedure has evolved and by now is a standard operation in nearly all institutions for hypoplastic left heart syndrome. There are three primary goals of stage I palliation: (1) establishment of unrestricted interatrial communication to provide complete mixing and avoid pulmonary venous hypertension, (2) establishment of a reliable source of pulmonary blood flow, allowing pulmonary vasculature development and minimizing the volume load on the single ventricle, and (3) providing unobstructed outflow from the ventricle to the systemic circulation.

We offer surgical palliation to nearly all patients with hypoplastic left heart syndrome, including very low birth weight infants and those with nonlethal genetic syndromes. In certain complicating situations primary transplantation should be considered, including severe aortic regurgitation, dilated cardiomyopathy, and severe atrioventricular valve regurgitation.

Stage I Reconstructive Surgery

The child is brought to the operating room and ventilated on room air, with care taken to avoid hyperventilation. A full midline sternotomy is performed and a sternal retractor placed. The thymus is removed in its entirety, with care being taken to avoid the phrenic nerves. The pericardium is opened, and an obligatory mediastinal inspection is performed to confirm the echocardiography, especially to identify abnormalities of the aortic arch and coronary arteries. The ascending and descending aorta, head vessels, ductus arteriosus, and pulmonary arteries are extensively mobilized, with care taken to avoid damage to the recurrent laryngeal nerve. No attempt is made to dissect the systemic veins. Purse-string sutures are placed in the proximal main pulmonary artery and generously around the right atrial appendage, through which heparin is administered. A previously thawed pulmonary homograft hemipatch is then trimmed in an extended arrowhead shape and set aside (Fig. 92-2A). Two perfusion techniques can be used for operative repair: deep hypothermic circulatory arrest (DHCA) and selective antegrade continuous cerebral perfusion. There is no consensus regarding the superior approach, although DHCA is more common. After the activated clotting time reaches 300 seconds, the patient is cannulated with the arterial cannula at the base of the main pulmonary artery and a single venous cannula in the right atrium. Cardiopulmonary bypass is initiated and tapes brought down around the branch pulmonary arteries. The patient is cooled to 18°C over 15 minutes, during which time any remaining dissection is performed. A side-biting clamp is placed on the innominate artery, and a polytetrafluoroethylene (PTFE) graft (usually 4.0 mm for patients >3.2 kg and 3.5 mm in all smaller infants) is anastomosed in an end-to-side fashion. The clamp is removed and flow assessed. If blood does not easily flow out of the open shunt, the anastomosis should be revised. A hemoclip is gently placed to temporarily occlude the shunt. On initiation of circulatory arrest, tapes are brought down around the head vessels, and a vascular clamp is placed on the descending aorta distal to the ductal insertion site. Cardioplegia is administered retrograde through a side port on the arterial cannula. After draining the patient of blood, all cannulas and PA tapes are removed. The ductus arteriosus is ligated on the PA side and divided on the aortic side. The atrial septum is completely excised working through the atrial purse string (Fig. 92-2B). Visualization can be improved through a right atriotomy, although this is seldom necessary. Next, the main pulmonary artery (MPA) is divided close to the branch pulmonary arteries, and the defect in the distal MPA segment is closed either with an oval homograft patch or primarily in a vertical fashion.

At a point beginning immediately adjacent to the divided MPA the diminutive aorta is incised medially and the incision carried superiorly along the underside of the transverse arch through the ductal insertion site to a point approximately 1 cm distant. It is important that all redundant ductal tissue be excised from the previous insertion site and the coarctation shelf be debrided (or the segment excised and the remaining vessel reanastomosed.) The proximal aortic-to-proximal PA connection is now performed using interrupted, fine polypropylene sutures (Fig. 92-2C). Next, the arch is reconstructed using the homograft patch, carrying this suture line down to complete the Damus-Kaye-Stansel proximally (Fig. 92-2D). The distal Blalock-Taussig shunt–PA anastomosis is now performed to the origin of the right pulmonary artery (RPA), although some surgeons prefer to do this with the cross-clamp off during warming (Fig. 92-2E). The arch is infused with cold saline to assess the geometry and to rule out kinking or residual obstruction, the atrium is infused with cold saline to de-air, and the cannulas are replaced. Cardiopulmonary bypass is begun and the patient warmed to 37°C over 22 minutes. It is important at this point to assess prompt and equivalent filling of coronary distributions, and any perfusion defect should be addressed immediately with revision of the aortic-to-PA anastomosis. During warming, obvious bleeding should be controlled. After the patient has been rewarmed to 37°C the clip is removed from the shunt and atrial lines are brought through the chest wall and positioned in the right atrium and the patient begun on low-dose dopamine and milrinone support. The patient is then weaned off cardiopulmonary bypass, and modified ultrafiltration is routinely performed. Oxygen saturations at this point should be in the mid to 80% range, which is indicative of adequate pulmonary blood flow. Any base deficit is corrected completely with sodium bicarbonate, and continued persistent acidosis is a relative indication of poor cardiac function and requires examination of the repair. After protamine is administered to adverse the affects of heparin, hemostasis is meticulously obtained. If there are no issues with bleeding, the chest is routinely closed. In approximately 20% of cases either hemodynamic or respiratory instability or continued potential bleeding results in the potential for cardiac compromise with chest closure, and in these cases a PTFE patch is cut to an appropriate size and approximated to the skin edges, leaving the sternum open for 12 to 24 hours.

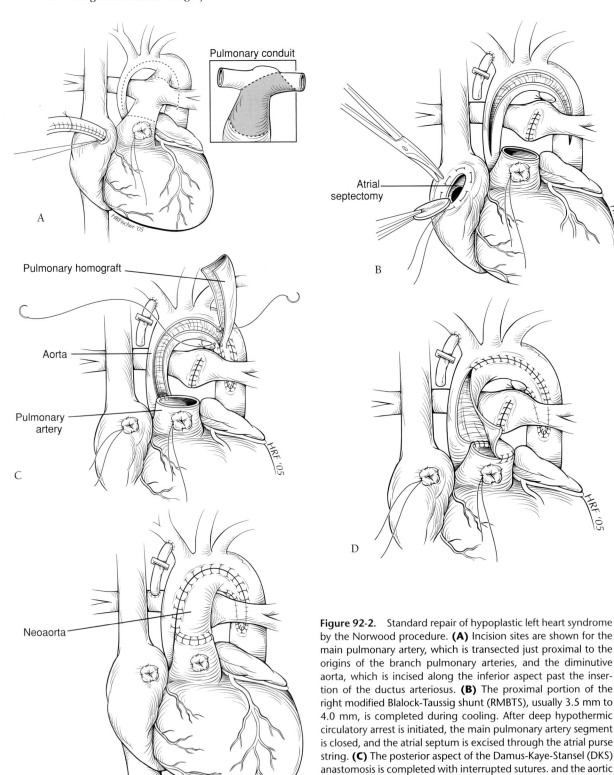

Pulmonary conduit

Pulmonary homograft

Aorta

Pulmonary artery

Neoaorta

Figure 92-2.   Standard repair of hypoplastic left heart syndrome by the Norwood procedure. **(A)** Incision sites are shown for the main pulmonary artery, which is transected just proximal to the origins of the branch pulmonary arteries, and the diminutive aorta, which is incised along the inferior aspect past the insertion of the ductus arteriosus. **(B)** The proximal portion of the right modified Blalock-Taussig shunt (RMBTS), usually 3.5 mm to 4.0 mm, is completed during cooling. After deep hypothermic circulatory arrest is initiated, the main pulmonary artery segment is closed, and the atrial septum is excised through the atrial purse string. **(C)** The posterior aspect of the Damus-Kaye-Stansel (DKS) anastomosis is completed with interrupted sutures. and the aortic arch is augmented with a homograft patch. **(D)** The remainder of the DKS is completed with the homograft patch. (E) The distal end of the RMBTS is completed to the right pulmonary artery.

Postoperative management of these patients includes low-dose dopamine and milrinone, although some centers use phenoxybenzamine as an afterload-reducing agent. The use of milrinone has resulted in good vasodilation with right ventricular inotropic support and generally removes the need for any greater inotropic support. In rare cases, low-dose epinephrine is used if there is significant hypotension. Patients are lightly sedated and given either a low dose of fentanyl analgesic as a continuous drip or intermittent morphine doses. The patient is not routinely paralyzed with pancuronium unless the sternum is left open and an

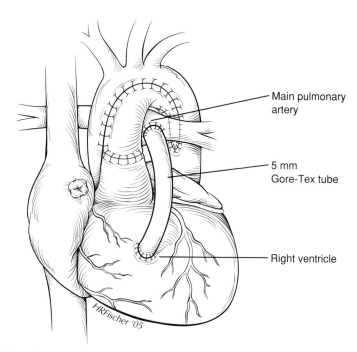

Figure 92-3. Alternative approach to stage I palliation using the Sano modification. Instead of a right modified Blalock-Taussig shunt, pulmonary blood flow is supplied by a 5.0-mm polytetrafluoroethylene (Gore-Tex) shunt from a right ventriculotomy to the main pulmonary artery.

attempt is made to allow the patient to awaken and to wean the ventilator support such that extubation can be performed on the first to second postoperative day. If the chest is left open, the chest is closed the day after surgery and then the patient allowed to waken, and weaning from the ventilator is performed over the next 24 to 48 hours. Rapid deintensification with initiation of nasogastric feedings and removal of central lines is preferred. Aspirin is usually administered after the first night when heparin is used at a low dose to decrease the potential risk of shunt thrombosis. When oral intake is established, low-dose aspirin is administered enterly. Patients are usually extubated between postoperative days 1 and 3. Average duration of hospitalization is between 7 and 21 days, the limiting factor often being establishment of adequate oral caloric intake. Recent reports suggest that a right ventricular-to-pulmonary artery (RV-PA) shunt as popularized by Sano may improve outcome after the stage I reconstruction (Fig. 92-3). However, further studies indicate the need for caution before broad adoption of the RV-PA conduit, with an increased incidence of shunt reinterventions, an earlier return for stage II reconstruction, and no difference in overall mortality.

For high-risk infants, some have advocated catheter-based hybrid approaches (stage I, ductal stenting, PA banding; stage

II, septectomy, arch augmentation, cavopulmonary anastomosis; stage III, catheter-based Fontan completion). Although there have been some early promising results, these techniques may be limited in certain anatomic subsets such as aortic atresia in which preductal, retrograde coarctation is a significant problem (Fig. 92-4). Palliative catheter-based hybrid approaches may be the most useful in identifiable subsets of patients with HLHS who have very low birth weight or associated cardiac anomalies. These patients are still a high-risk group for stage I reconstruction in most series.

Stage II Reconstructive Surgery

Two important observations by Norwood and colleagues early in the reconstructive experience prompted the institution of an intermediate stage. The first was that there was a time-related interstage mortality. The second was that the chronic volume load of a systemic-to-pulmonary shunt could create diastolic ventricular dysfunction. Thus, an intermediate stage was initiated as either a bidirectional cavopulmonary (Glenn) shunt or a hemi-Fontan procedure. A bidirectional cavopulmonary anastomosis sets the patient up for an extracardiac conduit, whereas a hemi-Fontan sets the stage for a lateral tunnel completion Fontan. There is

no long-term data that prove the efficacy of one approach over another. In general, at approximately 4 to 6 months of age the stage I survivors are catheterized to evaluate both pressures throughout the heart and the anatomy of pulmonary arteries. Use of a cavopulmonary anastomosis before approximately 3 months of age is sometimes associated with increased hypoxia and upper-body venous congestion, although bidirectional Glenn shunts have been done in children at even 6 weeks to 2 months of age with good results when there is clearly demonstrable low pulmonary vascular resistance. The technique for a bidirectional cavopulmonary anastomosis is fairly standard (Fig. 92-5).

An alternative operative approach is the hemi-Fontan procedure, which we perform under deep hypothermic circulatory arrest. The approach is through a reoperative median sternotomy, during which time care is taken around the dissection of the neo-aorta, which is often adherent to the left side of the sternum and somewhat fragile. The patient is cannulated in a standard fashion with an arterial cannula in the neo-aorta and a single straight cannula in the body of the right atrium. Cardiopulmonary bypass is begun, and the patient is cooled to 18°C. The previous shunt is divided and ligated near the innominate artery and the azygous vein ligated. After cardioplegic arrest, the PAs are opened on the anterior aspect and the pulmonary insertion of the shunt excised. If preoperative catheterization revealed pulmonary arterial stenosis, the incisions are carried beyond this point well onto the left PA and onto the right lower lobar branch. Next, the right atrium is incised superiorly and medially from 12 to 6 o'clock beginning just superior to the cannulation site and ending at the level of the right upper pulmonary artery (Fig. 92-6). The SVC and right aspect of the pulmonary arteriotomy are anastomosed with fine monofilament suture. Next, an extended triangular pulmonary homograft patch is used to augment the pulmonary arteries and create a roof over the anastomosis of the SVC to the RPA, as well as simultaneously create a dam to prevent blood flow between the SVC and right atrium. The patch-augmented PAs are infused with saline to examine anatomy and de-air. The venous cannula is replaced, cardiopulmonary bypass is reinitiated, cross-clamp is removed, and warming to 37°C is completed over 22 minutes. Occasionally, additional procedures such as atrial septectomy or arch augmentation may need to be completed in the same setting. One or two right atrial lines are inserted into

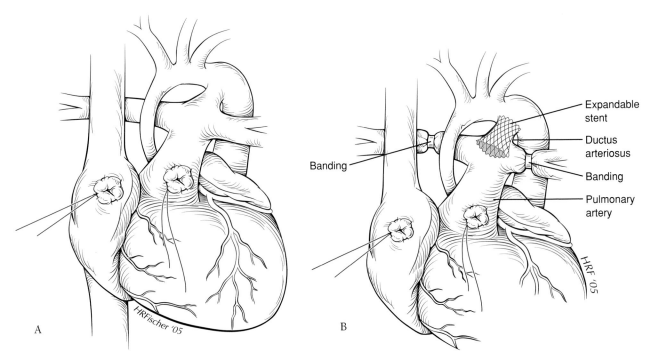

Figure 92-4. Alternative approach to stage I palliation using ductal stenting and pulmonary artery bands. **(A)** Unrestricted, stable systemic and pulmonary blood flow is created by insertion of an expandable stent in the ductus arteriosus. **(B)** Next, pulmonary blood flow is restricted by placement of bilateral pulmonary artery 3.0-mm bands.

the body of the right atrium or into the PA through the suture line. The patient is weaned from cardiopulmonary bypass, and modified ultrafiltration is performed, during which time all suture lines are checked for hemostasis. All cannulas are removed, and protamine is administered. The chest is then closed in a standard fashion and the patient returned to the intensive care unit (ICU). In general, these patients can be extubated soon after return to the ICU. With reduction of the volume load provided by this procedure, inotropic support is usually brief. Blood-oxygen saturations are generally 80% to 90%, and patients are generally discharged within 5 to 7 days after surgery.

Stage III Reconstructive Surgery

Between ages 1.5 and 5 years (usually determined by a combination of the patient's weight, growth characteristics, and arterial saturations) the patient is reimaged by echocardiography or magnetic resonance imaging and, if necessary, catheterization. If there are no anatomic issues to be addressed via catheterization (e.g., distal arch coarctation,) the patient is referred for Fontan reconstruction via either an extracardiac conduit or lateral tunnel completion Fontan. For the extracardiac

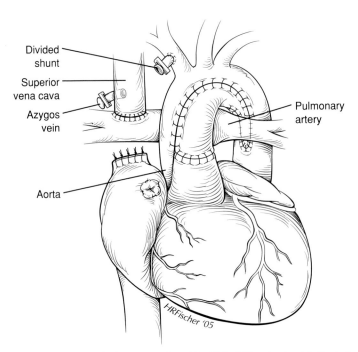

Figure 92-5. The bidirectional Glenn procedure. The Blalock-Taussig shunt is ligated proximally and removed distally from the right pulmonary artery. The azygous vein is ligated and the superior vena cava (SVC) is detached from the right atrium, oversewing the atrial portion. Finally, the SVC is anastomosed to the right pulmonary artery.

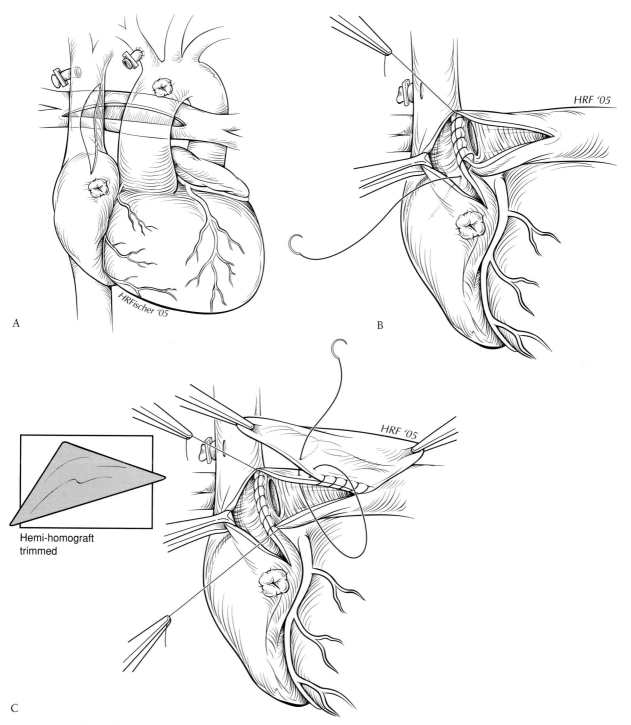

Figure 92-6. The hemi-Fontan procedure. **(A)** The pulmonary artery is incised widely from the left lower pulmonary artery to the left pulmonary artery. The right atrium is incised vertically in a spiral clockwise fashion from the superior portion of the right atrial (RA) appendage into the superior vena cava (SVC) to the superior aspect of the right pulmonary artery. The azygous vein is ligated. **(B)** The posterior aspect of the incision in the SVC is anastomosed to the rightward aspect of the pulmonary arteriotomy. **(C)** An extended triangular homograft patch is trimmed and sewn to augment the pulmonary arteries. **(D)** The homograft patch suture line continues along the SVC-RA junction to create the bottom of the dam. **(E)** The patch is folded on itself to create a triangular-shaped dam. **(F)** The suture line is continued to complete the dam. **(G)** The same homograft patch is used to simultaneously complete the pulmonary artery augmentation and SVC-PA anastomosis. (*Continued*)

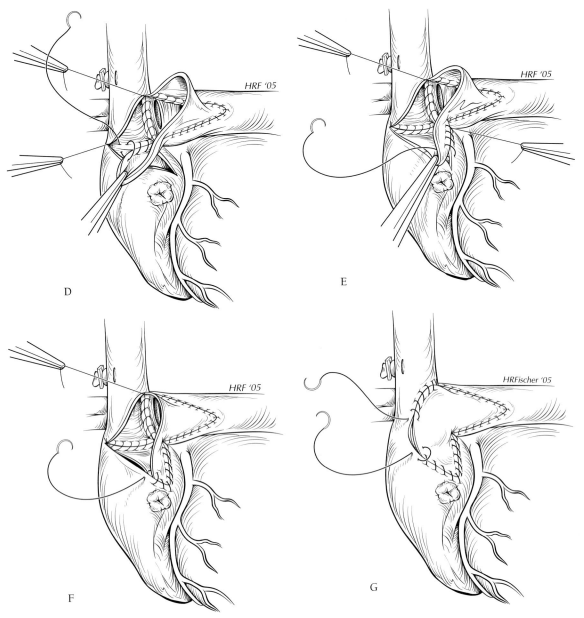

Figure 92-6. (*Continued*)

conduit, DHCA or continuous bypass with or without aortic cross-clamp is employed, and DHCA is used for the lateral tunnel. The approach is again through a reoperative median sternotomy.

For the extracardiac Fontan procedure, the patient is bicavally cannulated in a standard fashion and an arterial cannula placed high in the aortic reconstruction. Cardiopulmonary bypass is begun and tourniquets are applied around the caval cannulas. A vascular clamp is placed at the IVC-RA junction and the IVC divided (Fig. 92-7). The atrial portion is partially closed in two layers with fine monofilament suture. The conduit (18-mm to 22-mm PTFE) is trimmed

to the appropriate length to avoid compression of the right pulmonary vein (shorter than one might expect), and a 4-mm fenestration is punched in the medial aspect near the IVC portion. The IVC-conduit anastomosis is completed with monofilament suture followed by a side-to-side anastomosis of the remaining cardiac portion of the IVC opening with the exterior conduit, leaving a rim of conduit around the fenestration. Next, the PAs are opened along the inferior margin and inspected directly. If preoperative studies revealed any pulmonary arterial stenosis and the beveled end of the PTFE conduit will not span the area of stenosis, this is addressed with

pulmonary homograft patch augmentation. The conduit is then anastomosed to the inferior aspect of the pulmonary arteries angled slightly medial to the SVC. Practically, the angled nature of the superior portion of the conduit augments the PAs from left pulmonary artery (LPA) to the RPA. The conduit is infused with saline to de-air, and the patient is weaned off of cardiopulmonary bypass. The SVC cannula is removed, and a period of modified ultrafiltration is begun. All suture lines are checked for hemostasis. At the completion of modified ultrafiltration, the SVC pressure is measured directly with a transthoracic line. An additional monitoring line is placed in the right atrium. All

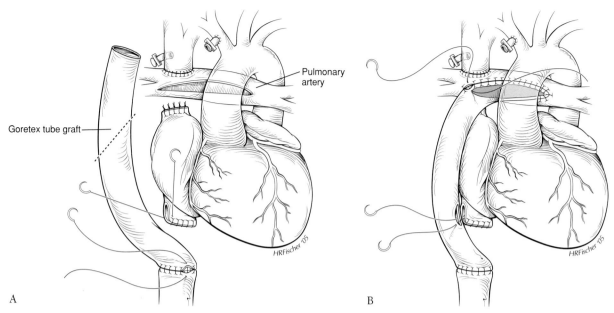

Figure 92-7. The extracardiac Fontan procedure. **(A)** The inferior vena cava is detached from the right atrium, and the right atrial portion is partially closed. An 18-mm to 22-mm polytetrafluoroethylene (PTFE; Gore-Tex) conduit is anastomosed to the inferior vena cava (IVC), and a 4.0-mm fenestration is created next to the partially closed IVC. **(B)** A side-to-side anastomosis is fashioned between the fenestration and IVC opening in the right atrium. The distal end of the PTFE conduit is beveled to create a large opening that augments the pulmonary arteries, and the conduit-PA anastomosis is completed.

cannulas are removed, and protamine is administered. The chest is then closed in a standard fashion and the patient returned to the ICU. In general, these patients can be extubated soon after return to the ICU.

An alternative operative approach is the lateral-tunnel Fontan procedure, which we perform under deep hypothermic circulatory arrest using a piece of fenestrated PTFE patch to baffle blood from the IVC to the PAs (Fig. 92-8). The patient is cannulated in a standard fashion with an arterial cannula in the neo-aorta and a single straight cannula in the body of the right atrium. Cardiopulmonary bypass is begun, and the patient is cooled to 18°C. An aortic cross-clamp is applied and cardioplegic arrest achieved. The patient is drained of blood and the venous cannula removed. A vertically based incision is made in the body of the right atrium parallel to Waterson's groove. The previously constructed PA-RA homograft dam is excised, and the Eustachian valve is removed. A 10-mm PTFE tube graft is split longitudinally and trimmed to length, and a 4-mm fenestration is created. Inferiorly, the graft is sewn around the IVC orifice and the suture line carried superiorly along the line of the interatrial communication. Superiorly, the baffle is sewn around the edge of the newly created opening between the atrium and PAs. Care must be exercised here to assure that the trabecular portion of the atrium contains no leaks. The free, superior edge of the PTFE baffle is then closed in a single sandwich between the two free edges of the right atrium. Thus the medial aspect of the lateral tunnel is PTFE, whereas the lateral aspect is native right atrial tissue. The heart is infused with saline to de-air and the venous cannula replaced. Cardiopulmonary bypass is reinitiated, and the patient is warmed to 37°C over 22 minutes. Atrial lines are brought into the atrium on either side of the baffle through the suture line. The patient is weaned from bypass and undergoes modified ultrafiltration. Inotropic support is rarely necessary.

Results

Despite continued developments, patients with HLHS continue to present formidable challenges. Since its institution in 1984, results from staged reconstruction have improved significantly. This has been the case across multiple institutions, and many centers report excellent outcomes, approaching 90% hospital survival. Some of the variability in outcome may be influenced by anatomy, although it now appears that the diagnosis of HLHS is not a predictor of mortality compared to stage I palliation for other HLHS variants. However, risk factors such as low birth weight, associated cardiac anomalies, longer total support time, and extracorporeal membrane oxygenation (ECMO) or ventricular assist device (VAD) support are predictors of operative mortality. Additional perioperative or operative treatment strategies may improve morbidity and mortality such as use of anti-inflammatory treatment strategies, continuous mixed venous oxygen saturation monitoring, and use of systemic vasodilators. Another approach has been the development of home surveillance programs. Interstage mortality in monitored patients when compared to historical controls is significantly reduced, suggesting that monitoring programs may provide significant benefit toward the reduction of interstage mortality.

Our group compared the outcomes of all neonates who underwent a stage I reconstruction between 2002 and 2004 with use of the RV-PA conduit and modified Blalock-Taussig shunt. In all, 149 infants underwent a stage I reconstruction for hypoplastic left heart syndrome or variants. There was no difference in surgical mortality, time to extubation, or length of hospital stay. However, there was an increased incidence of shunt reinterventions in the patients with the RV-PA conduit. Patients with RV-PA

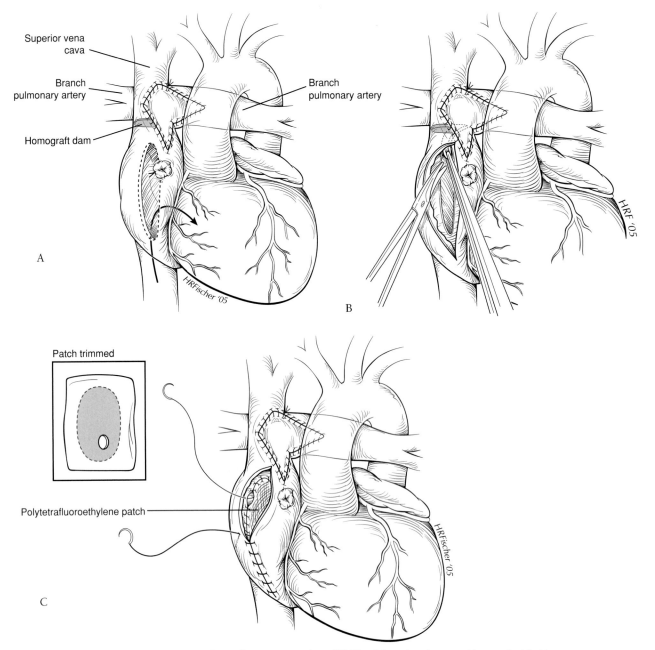

Figure 92-8. The lateral tunnel Fontan procedure. **(A)** The right atrium is opened in a vertical fashion medial to Waterson's groove. **(B)** The homograft dam is excised, creating an unobstructed opening from right atrium to pulmonary artery. **(C)** A polytetrafluoroethylene (PTFE) baffle is sewn along the posterior rim of the remnant atrial septum, on the medial aspect of the inferior vena cava (IVC), and to the medial aspect of the superior vena cava–pulmonary artery (PA) junction. The free edge of the PTFE dam is sewn in a sandwich to close the right atrium, baffling blood from the IVC to the PA.

conduit returned earlier for stage II reconstruction but there was no difference in overall mortality.

Although they are promising for certain high-risk populations, catheter-based hybrid approaches are in an experimental phase. These techniques may be inadvisable in certain anatomic subsets such as aortic atresia in which preductal retrograde coarctation is a significant problem.

Results for the final palliation to the Fontan circulation and for the second- and third-stage reconstruction for HLHS continue to improve. Survival rates for the bidirectional Glenn or Hemi-Fontan are well above 95% in most centers, and similarly the survival rates for Fontan completion are >95% to 98% in most recent reports. These excellent results confirm the utility of staged reconstructive surgery to the

Fontan circulation as the preferred strategy for patients with HLHS, saving transplantation for patients who fail at any stage of the reconstruction sequence. Our experience with the Fontan procedure for HLHS shows a >95% survival with a median hospital stay of 5 to 6 days. Effusions, although not uncommon, rarely last more than a few days, and prolonged effusions (>2 weeks) occur in <15% of patients with current strategies. This improvement in overall Fontan survival has been reflected in series from many institutions, suggesting that there has been a marked improvement in cardiac function in survivors of single-ventricle staged reconstruction over the last 15 years. Hospital survival of >90% is common, with guardians reporting their child's overall health as excellent or good. Physical activity is normal in one third of patients, with $\frac{1}{2}$ reporting only slight physical limitations. School performance varies widely, with about one third of patients above average, one third average, and one third below average.

When comparing outcomes of extracardiac conduit and lateral tunnel Fontan connections, results are conflicting. Some have reported that the lateral tunnel Fontan procedure has a significantly higher incidence of postoperative sinoatrial node dysfunction, supraventricular tachycardia, duration of intensive care unit stay, and ventilatory support. However, others have found contrasting data with a lower incidence of sinus node dysfunction in the lateral tunnel versus extracardiac Fontan reconstruction. The potential advantages of extracardiac Fontan reconstruction include the lack of complicated atrial suture lines, although most patients with HLHS will have atrial septectomy as part of their initial procedure. The incidence of late development of atrial arrhythmias is unknown in this population of patients, and it is not clear whether the extra cardiac conduit Fontan will have significant advantages over the lateral tunnel operation. There have been studies suggesting that the hemodynamic flow characteristics of the extracardiac Fontan may be superior to a lateral tunnel connection; however the offset created by a hemi-Fontan procedure may be beneficial. These conflicting results have not been correlated with clinical findings and late outcomes.

With the progression of improvement in surgical techniques and pre- and postoperative management, current survival to the Fontan procedure for all patients with HLHS as a group is approximately 75% in centers with the greatest experience. Survival rates of >80% to 90% are common in low-risk patients who have normal birth weight and no associated cardiac or noncardiac anomalies. However, the frequent coexistence of low birth weight or tricuspid regurgitation or other noncardiac anomalies continues to create a high-risk group that lowers overall survival in centers who see a large proportion of patients with these comorbidities. Selective application of the variations in the Norwood procedure and hybrid strategies for these subsets of high-risk patients may improve overall survival with greater experience.

Developments in preoperative evaluation, operative techniques, and postoperative management based on rigorous controlled trials and rational application of these results will provide continued progress with this challenging disease.

SUGGESTED READING

Bacha EA, Daves S, Hardin J, et al. Single-ventricle palliation for high-risk neonates: The emergence of an alternative hybrid stage I strategy. J Thorac Cardiovasc Surg 2006;131:163.

Fontan F, Baudet E. Surgical repair of tricuspid atresia. Thorax 1971;26:240.

Gaynor JW, Bridges ND, Cohen MI, et al. Predictors of outcome after the Fontan operation: Is hypoplastic left heart syndrome still a risk factor? J Thorac Cardiovasc Surg 2002;123:237.

Gaynor JW, Mahle WT, Cohen MI, et al. Risk factors for mortality after the Norwood procedure. Eur J Cardiothorac Surg 2002;22:82.

Kreutzer G, Galindez E, Bono H, et al. An operation for the correction of tricuspid atresia. J Thorac Cardiovasc Surg 1973;66:613.

Kumar SP, Rubinstein CS, Simsic JM, et al. Lateral tunnel versus extracardiac conduit Fontan procedure: A concurrent comparison. Ann Thorac Surg 2003;76:1389.

Lev M. Pathologic anatomy and interrelationship of hypoplasia of the aortic tract complexes. Lab Invest 1952;1:61.

Mahle WT, Spray TL, Wernovsky G, et al. Survival after reconstructive surgery for hypoplastic left heart syndrome: A 15-year experience from a single institution. Circulation 2000;102:III136.

Mitchell ME, Ittenbach RF, Gaynor JW, et al. Intermediate outcomes after the Fontan procedure in the current era. J Thorac Cardiovasc Surg 2006;131:172.

Norwood WI, Kirklin JK, Sanders SP. Hypoplastic left heart syndrome: Experience with palliative surgery. Am J Cardiol 1980;45:87.

Norwood WI, Lang P, Hansen DD. Physiologic repair of aortic atresia-hypoplastic left heart syndrome. N Engl J Med 1983;308:23.

Pizarro C, Norwood WI. Pulmonary artery banding before Norwood procedure. Ann Thorac Surg 2003;75:1008.

Sano S, Ishino K, Kawada M, et al. Right ventricle-pulmonary artery shunt in first-stage palliation of hypoplastic left heart syndrome. Semin Thorac Cardiovasc Surg Pediatr Card Surg Annu 2004;7:22.

Sinha SN, Rusnak SL, Sommers HM, et al. Hypoplastic left ventricle syndrome. Analysis of thirty autopsy cases in infants with surgical considerations. Am J Cardiol 1968;21:166.

Tabbutt S, Dominguez TE, Ravishankar C, et al. Outcomes after the stage I reconstruction comparing the right ventricular to pulmonary artery conduit with the modified Blalock Taussig shunt. Ann Thorac Surg 2005:80:1582.

EDITOR'S COMMENTS

Although patients with hypoplastic left heart syndrome (HLHS) represent some of the highest-risk groups of patients, the results of treatment have improved dramatically over the last 20 years. Dr. Gruber and his colleagues at Children's Hospital of Philadelphia give an excellent summary of their approach to the management of the HLHS population based on their extensive and excellent experience. Probably the most significant and controversial change in the management of these children over the last 5 years has been the reintroduction and widespread adoption of the right ventricular-to-pulmonary artery conduit in substitution for the traditional modified Blalock-Taussig shunt as part of stage I reconstruction. Although this version of the stage I reconstruction was described by Norwood in his initial publications, the use of the modified Blalock-Taussig shunt became the uniformly adopted version of the operation. It was not until Sano and his colleagues reintroduced the RV-to-PA conduit concept in the literature that its practical and theoretical appeal led to its widespread reintroduction. The RV-to-PA conduit version of the Norwood procedure seems to address at least two of the difficult features of the care of patients after stage I reconstruction using the modified Blalock-Taussig shunt: perioperative hemodynamic lability and interstage death. Many institutions have introduced effective strategies in dealing with hemodynamic instability in stage I Norwood procedures, but these concerns still exist at many centers. In addition, the reported rates of interstage death after the Norwood procedure using a modified Blalock-Taussig shunt continue to run in the 10% to 15% range. The experience of most surgeons with the Sano modification shows dramatic reductions in interstage death. In our institution, the interstage death rate is <4% after the Sano procedure. Indeed, with the adoption of the Sano modification of the Norwood procedure, a great number of surgeons throughout the world have seen decreased surgical mortality rates and significant reductions in interstage mortality. The tradeoff with the Sano procedure is the need for a right ventriculotomy for the proximal takeoff of the right ventricular-to-pulmonary artery conduit. The long-term effects of the ventriculotomy in terms of right ventricular function and arrhythmia generation are largely unknown given the relatively recent reintroduction of the procedure. Other concerns raised about the Sano procedure are even less clear in their importance. Concerns raised regarding increased need for shunt reinterventions and earlier stage II reconstruction have been completely absent in our experience at the University of Virginia.

Many surgeons feel that the use of regional perfusion strategies as an adjunct to complex aortic reconstruction to avoid long periods of deep hypothermic circulatory arrest is a valuable advance. This concept, however, is not uniformly accepted by all surgeons, especially those accustomed to using DHCA. I think it is fair to say that the use of regional perfusion may at least add a safety factor for many surgeons during these complex reconstructions. In our experience it is rare to need more than 4 to 5 minutes of DHCA (during transection of the ductus and atrial septectomy) using regional perfusion techniques.

Despite the considerable improvements in the overall result of stage I reconstruction for HLHS, the treatment of patients in the highest-risk categories remains a great challenge at all centers. The availability of donor hearts continues to be scarce, and thus the search for novel therapies has continued. Although the exact criteria by which patients are deemed to be higher risk vary among institutions, the patients that raise the most concern are those with the lowest birth weights, ascending aortic size <2 mm, significant atrioventricular valve regurgitation, and significant extracardiac abnormalities and those that present in profound shock. The novel strategy that has garnered the most attention recently has been so-called "hybrid palliation." This involves bilateral pulmonary artery banding, stenting of the ductus arteriosus, and atrial septostomy. The hope for this procedure is to allow a more stable hemodynamic situation while the patient is listed for transplantation or to allow the child to grow before undergoing a later, larger reconstructive procedure. Several institutions have reasonably good early data regarding this procedure. Our early data with a group of patients have also been good, although our intermediate-term experience with this procedure has been dismal. This is concurrent with near-uniform survival of our HLHS patients who undergo the Norwood (Sano) procedure. In our HLHS patients, we are significantly restricting our use of the hybrid procedure. It will be some time before the true place for this procedure in the care of these patients is truly known.

Most centers now have excellent results with both stage II (Glenn/hemi-Fontan) and stage III (Fontan) procedures. Success rates are well above 90% as techniques and timing of the operations have improved. We use the bidirectional Glenn procedure for stage II reconstruction, which in some cases can be performed without the use of cardiopulmonary bypass by leaving the RV-PA conduit open to the left lung while the Glenn anastomosis is performed. The extracardiac (fenestrated) Fontan procedure is used for stage III reconstruction in our institution. Although this also can be done off-pump in some cases, we have found that the procedure proceeds much more simply and efficiently and takes less time with a short run of cardiopulmonary bypass.

B.B.P., I.L.K.

93

Anomalies of Pulmonary Venous Return

Benjamin B. Peeler, V. Seenu Reddy, and Irving L. Kron

Anomalies of pulmonary venous return form a spectrum of embryologically related congenital heart defects that have in common the failure of the pulmonary veins to unite normally with the left atrium. The lesion may involve anomalous connection of all four pulmonary veins with the right atrium, which is referred to as total anomalous pulmonary venous return (TAPVR). Conversely, there may exist abnormal drainage of at least one but not all pulmonary veins into the systemic venous circulation, referred to as partial anomalous pulmonary venous return (PAPVR).

Total Anomalous Pulmonary Venous Return

Historical Aspects

The earliest description of TAPVR was by Wilson in 1798. The first series of patients with this anomaly was an autopsy series presented by Brody in 1942. Muller in 1951 at UCLA is credited with the initial attempt at surgical treatment of TAPVR. He described a closed operation consisting of a side-to-side anastomosis between the common pulmonary vein trunk and the left atrial appendage. In 1956, Lewis, Varco, and associates at the University of Minnesota reported the first successful total correction of TAPVR using hypothermia and inflow occlusion. The same year Burroughs and Kirklin described their experiences with surgical correction using cardiopulmonary bypass (CPB). The introduction of deep hypothermic circulatory arrest by Barratt-Boyes and colleagues in the early 1970s was a major advance toward accomplishing

surgical repair because this technique provides a bloodless operative field. Further advances in early diagnostic modalities, neonatal intensive care, including the availability of extracorporeal membrane oxygenation (ECMO), and pediatric cardiac surgical anesthesia, as well as an awareness of the merits of early surgical intervention, have contributed to the excellent results with TAPVR repair reported recently by many centers.

Embryology

The respiratory system develops as an evagination from the foregut at 26 days. The venous plexus surrounding the early lung buds drains into the anterior cardinal and umbilico-vitelline veins, both of which are part of the splanchnic (systemic) venous system. The anterior cardinal veins give rise to the superior vena cava, the coronary sinus, and the azygos vein, and the umbilico-vitelline veins later form the portal venous system. In normal circumstances, the common pulmonary vein develops as an outpouching from the dorsal left atrial wall, eventually fusing with the pulmonary venous plexus at 27 days' gestation. Shortly thereafter, the anterior cardinal and umbilico-vitelline venous channels normally undergo involution (Fig. 93-1). However, failure of the common pulmonary vein to unite with the pulmonary venous plexus is associated with persistence of these embryonic pulmonary venous-to-systemic venous anastomoses, yielding total anomalous pulmonary venous drainage into right atrial tributaries. In some instances, abnormal leftward displacement of the developing atrial septum results in anomalous connection of all four pulmonary venous ostia directly with the right atrium.

Anatomic Defects and Classification

The common underlying anatomic defect in all cases of TAPVR involves anomalous drainage of the entire pulmonary venous circulation directly into the right atrium or via systemic vein or sinus connecting with the right atrium via the superior vena cava (SVC), inferior vena cava (IVC), or coronary sinus. The pulmonary venous blood may drain into the systemic venous circulation through a single common channel or by multiple portals of entry. An interatrial communication, usually manifested as a patent foramen ovale (PFO) or secundum atrial septal defect (ASD), is mandatory for shunting of oxygenated blood to the left heart.

In 1957, Darling and associates proposed a four-part classification system to describe the various routes of pulmonary venous drainage in TAPVR. They described supracardiac, or type I TAPVR, as an anomalous connection with a persistent left SVC, also referred to as an ascending left vertical vein or a persistent left anterior cardinal vein (Fig. 93-2). In addition, pulmonary venous connection with the right superior vena cava is a less frequently encountered supracardiac variant. The more common anatomic subtype of supracardiac TAPVR has blood from all four pulmonary veins draining into a horizontal common pulmonary venous confluence (a left vertical vein) immediately posterior to the left atrium, which then drains into either the innominate vein, azygos vein, right SVC, or right atrium. Type II, or cardiac-type TAPVR, is characterized by total pulmonary venous drainage into a markedly dilated coronary sinus (Fig. 93-3) or, less commonly, directly into the right atrium (Type III) or the infracardiac variant, involves descent of a vertical vein

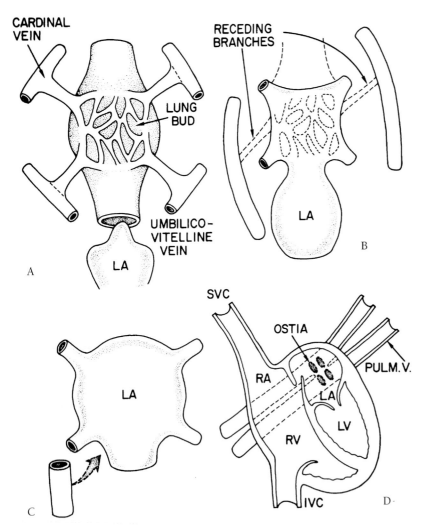

Figure 93-1.   Normal embryonic development of the pulmonary veins. **(A)** Common pulmonary vein evagination from the dorsal left atrial wall growing toward the pulmonary venous plexus surrounding the lung buds. Embryonic pulmonary-to-systemic venous anastomoses still exist. **(B)** The common pulmonary vein fuses with the pulmonary venous plexus as pulmonary-to-systemic communications begin to involute. **(C, D)** Complete incorporation of the pulmonary veins into the dorsal left atrial wall with disappearance of embryonic pulmonary-to-systemic venous communications. (IVC = inferior vena cava; LA = left atrium; LV = left ventricle; PULM V. = pulmonary vein; RA = right atrium; RV = right ventricle; SVC = superior vena cava.)

includes visceral heterotaxy, isomerism, dextrocardia, and splenic abnormalities (asplenia, polysplenia, hyposplenia).

Alternate classification systems have been based on the length and degree of obstruction between the pulmonary venous and systemic venous pathways. In general, the supracardiac and cardiac level defects initially have minimal symptoms of obstruction, whereas the infracardiac variants have significant obstruction due to the length of the venous channel and resistance created in the hepatic portal system. The most complete system proposed by Herlong describes the anatomic variant, the degree of obstruction, and the type of obstruction (extrinsic or intrinsic compression).

Pathophysiology

In those cases with nonobstructed anatomy, TAPVR functions as a large left-to-right shunt. Pulmonary blood flow is greatly increased, and right ventricular overload occurs as a result of both the pulmonary venous and systemic circulations returning to the right atrium. Consequently, pulmonary hypertension, pulmonary edema, right ventricular enlargement, and congestive heart failure supervene. The physiologic consequences of TAPVR depend largely on the presence and magnitude of pulmonary venous obstruction. Cyanosis results from the mixing of fully oxygenated pulmonary venous blood with desaturated systemic venous blood. A compensatory right-to-left shunt through a patent foramen ovale or, less commonly, via an ASD is mandatory for survival because this allows shunting of partially oxygenated blood to the left atrium for systemic distribution. Although left atrial and left ventricular volumes are generally small due to shunting, these chambers are rarely hypoplastic.

Obstruction to pulmonary venous blood flow in TAPVR may occur as a result of extrinsic compression, intrinsic luminal narrowing of the vein, or a combination of both. The infracardiac TAPVR is most often associated with obstruction, occurring in 80% to 100% of patients. Usually the descending vertical vein is obstructed at its junction with the portal vein or ductus venosus. In addition, resistance to blood flow through the hepatic sinusoids in the setting of a closed ductus venosus produces a functional obstruction. Obstruction in the supracardiac subtype is characterized by a "viselike" compression of the vertical vein between the left pulmonary artery anteriorly and the left mainstem bronchus posteriorly. Another site of potential impediment to pulmonary

from the common pulmonary venous trunk through the esophageal hiatus to below the diaphragm, where it most often makes an anomalous connection with the portal vein, one of its branches (Fig. 93-4), or the ductus venosus. In such cases, pulmonary venous blood returns to the right atrium by way of the IVC. Type IV TAPVR comprises all mixed defects with connections at multiple levels.

Most series report that supracardiac connection is the most common TAPVR variant (45%), whereas the cardiac and infracardiac types are encountered somewhat less frequently (25% each) and the mixed type is the rarest (5%). A recent review of the authors' series at the University of Virginia

corroborates this frequency distribution (Table 93-1).

Whereas the majority of TAPVR cases are isolated anomalies, the lesion occasionally coexists with other cardiac and extracardiac congenital malformations. TAPVR, especially in autopsy series, has been diagnosed concomitantly with a variety of other acyanotic and cyanotic heart defects, including patent ductus arteriosus, valvular atresia and stenosis, ventricular septal defect, transposition of the great arteries, tetralogy of Fallot, double-outlet right ventricle, and common atrioventricular canal. In addition, there is a well-known association between TAPVR and the heterotaxy syndrome, which

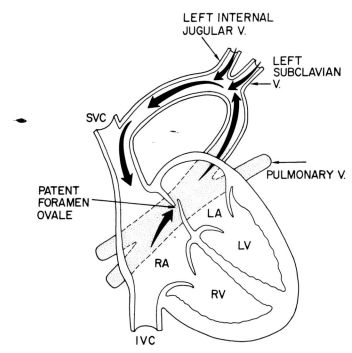

Figure 93-2. The pathologic anatomy of supracardiac-type total anomalous pulmonary venous return via the ascending left vertical vein. (IVC = inferior vena cava; LA = left atrium; LV = left ventricle; RA = right atrium; RV = right ventricle; SVC = superior vena cava; V. = vein.)

venous flow may be attributed to a restrictive communication at the atrial level (e.g., a small PFO), which is suggested by the presence of a transatrial pressure gradient.

The sequelae of pulmonary venous obstruction are striking, particularly in obstructed patients. Profound pulmonary edema results from the increased hydro-static pressure in the pulmonary capillaries bed proximal to the obstruction. In addition, cyanosis is apparent because of the impeded return of oxygenated blood to the heart. Pulmonary hypertension is usually present and most severe in patients with significant obstruction. In those patients, pulmonary artery pressures approach or exceed

systemic pressures. Conversely, pulmonary venous obstruction also has the effect of unloading the right ventricle, thereby circumventing the right ventricular dilation and hypertrophy that are constant features in nonobstructed TAPVR.

Diagnosis

Signs and Symptoms

The condition of infants with TAPVR is determined largely by the presence and degree of obstruction to pulmonary venous return. Nonobstructed TAPVR often eludes diagnosis at birth and in the early neonatal period. Months later, patients may present with the gradual onset of tachypnea, dyspnea, congestive heart failure, and mild cyanosis. Often, subtle complaints of feeding difficulties and failure to thrive may be the only clues of congenital heart disease in these children. Liver congestion with hepatomegaly and cardiomegaly along with a prominent right ventricular impulse are consistent features.

Cardiac examination may be unimpressive. There may exist either a gallop or a faint systolic murmur, most often a result of increased flow across the tricuspid valve. Other findings are the hallmarks of increased pulmonary blood flow, such as a systolic ejection murmur over the left second interspace and a prominent fixed S2 component.

In contrast, infants with obstructed TAPVR present in extremis within hours to days after birth. These infants are profoundly cyanotic and in severe congestive heart failure. Hypotension and metabolic acidosis are frequently present. Findings on cardiac examination are inconsistent, but the right-sided cardiac chambers may be of normal size. The liver may also be of normal span and free of congestion if the ductus venosus remains patent and thus is able to divert pulmonary venous blood directly into the inferior vena cava.

Chest X-Ray

Chest roentgenographic features of TAPVR are again dependent on the presence or absence of pulmonary venous obstruction. No-obstructed TAPVR is characterized by a normal-sized heart with increased pulmonary vascularity, possibly a distinct pulmonary artery silhouette, and occasional enlargement of the right cardiac silhouette. The classic roentgenographic images of a "snowman" or "figure-of-eight" in supracardiac connection are rarely appreciated before 6 months of life. In cases of obstructed TAPVR, the cardiac silhouette is usually of

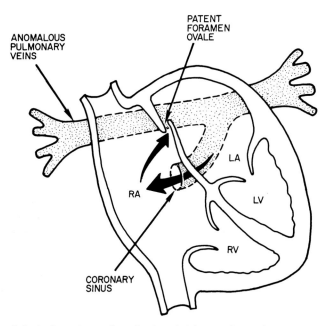

Figure 93-3. Pathologic anatomy of cardiac-type total anomalous pulmonary venous return via the coronary sinus. (LA = left atrium; LV = left ventricle; RA = right atrium; RV = right ventricle =.)

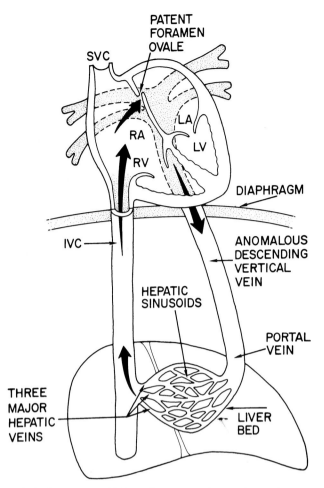

Figure 93-4. Pathologic anatomy of infracardiac-type total anomalous pulmonary venous return via the descending vertical vein to the portal vein. (IVC = inferior vena cava; LA = left atrium; LV = left ventricle; RA = right atrium; RV = right ventricle; SVC = superior vena cava.)

catheterization and angiography in these ill infants may have the untoward effects of a hyperosmotic contrast load, including precipitation of potentially fatal pulmonary edema or acute renal failure. Since the 1980s, echocardiography has become the mainstay for preoperative diagnosis and classification of TAPVR. Two-dimensional echocardiography with Doppler color-flow mapping is extremely accurate and reliable in diagnosing TAPVR, delineating the exact drainage pattern of each individual pulmonary vein, detecting the presence and degree of obstruction, and identifying any concomitant cardiac malformations.

Cardiac Catheterization and Angiocardiography

In the current era, cardiac catheterization is reserved for patients in whom more precise examination of the individual pulmonary veins or elucidation of the presence of obstruction is required, for cases in which echocardiographic findings are inconsistent with the clinical course, or in the presence of associated complex cardiac anomalies. The precise site of anomalous pulmonary venous connection is identified by a "step-up" in oxygen saturation in a systemic vein, whereas the exact course of pulmonary venous drainage is delineated during the levophase of selective pulmonary arteriography.

It is common for the blood in all four cardiac chambers to have equal or similar oxygen saturations, which reflects the mixing of pulmonary and systemic venous circulations. TAPVR and transposition of the great arteries are the only two conditions in which the oxygen saturation of blood in the main pulmonary artery is equal to or greater than that in the aorta. Right ventricular and pulmonary artery pressures are frequently elevated in TAPVR but are virtually always so in the presence of obstruction. It is estimated that in 75% of cases in which the pulmonary artery pressure exceeds that of the systemic circulation there is underlying pulmonary venous obstruction. The adequacy of the patent foramen ovale in terms of its ability to shunt partially oxygenated blood to the left side of the heart may be estimated by the difference between right atrial pressure and pulmonary capillary wedge or left atrial pressure. The detection of a transatrial pressure gradient suggests a restrictive foramen ovale or obstructed pulmonary venous return.

In neonates, umbilical vein catheterization allows direct injection of contrast into the anomalous connection in the

normal size, but there is marked engorgement of the pulmonary vasculature and diffuse interstitial infiltrates indicative of severe pulmonary edema. Furthermore, as opposed to nonobstructed TAPVR, the main pulmonary artery silhouette is not unusually prominent.

Echocardiography

Modern two-dimensional echocardiographic technology and techniques have revolutionized the noninvasive diagnosis of TAPVR. In unstable, critically ill neonates, echo prevents any undue delay in diagnosis and surgical therapy. Cardiac

Table 93-1 Frequency Distribution of Types of Total Anomalous Pulmonary Venous Return (TAPVR) at the University of Virginia			
Type of TAPVR	**Number**	**Percentage**	**Number (Percentage) Obstructed**
Supracardiac	23	60.5	10/23 (43.5)
Ascending vertical vein	16		
Right superior vena cava	7		
Cardiac	5	13.2	0/5 (0)
Coronary sinus	2		
Right atrium	3		
Infracardiac	6	15.8	5/6 (83.3)
Portal vein	6		
Mixed	4	10.5	1/4 (25)
Total	38	100	16/38 (42.1)

infradiaphragmatic subtype of TAPVR. If the connection is of the supracardiac type, the vertical vein and common pulmonary venous sinus can be demonstrated. In the cardiac subtype, the coronary sinus is seen as a large opacified structure to the left of the spine but within the right atrial contour.

Preoperative Management and Timing of Surgical Intervention

Infants presenting with obstructed TAPVR represent a surgical emergency. An intensive resuscitation period should be followed by expeditious surgical intervention. Immediate interventions include endotracheal intubation and hyperventilation with 100% oxygen to a partial arterial pressure of carbon dioxide ($PaCO_2$) of <30 mm Hg and a systemic pH of >7.6. Induced respiratory alkalosis decreases pulmonary vascular resistance and improves oxygenation. Metabolic acidosis should be treated with sodium bicarbonate or tromethamine (THAM) infusions. Function of the failing heart is augmented with the administration of inotropic and diuretic agents. Isoproterenol has special merit for inotropic support in obstructed TAPVR because it also possesses pulmonary vasodilatory properties. Maintenance of ductal patency with a prostaglandin E_1 infusion may also be of some physiologic benefit.

ECMO has been employed in those infants with severe pulmonary hypertension or cardiac failure refractory to conventional medical measures, although prompt surgical intervention is the mainstay of definitive therapy. A brief period of ECMO may assist in stabilizing these critically ill infants and prevent end-organ dysfunction before operative correction.

Nonobstructed TAPVR patients with a nonrestrictive ASD are usually in stable condition. Therefore, these infants rarely need significant preoperative intervention or pharmacologic support. Nonetheless, the current practice in most centers is to perform elective corrective surgery within a few days of diagnosis irrespective of the patient's age or weight. The impetus for early surgery has been a heightened awareness of the extremely high mortality associated with uncorrected TAPVR as well as the substantial risk of progression to irreversible cardiac and pulmonary vascular disease while awaiting delayed repair.

Surgical Technique

Preparation for and Management of Extracorporeal Circulation

The following descriptions apply specifically to TAPVR repair in neonates and young infants, with the understanding that older children and even adults also infrequently undergo corrective surgery for TAPVR. Central venous and umbilical arterial pressure catheters are usually placed during the preoperative resuscitation period. High-dose fentanyl is an ideal agent for induction of anesthesia because it reduces stress-induced increases in pulmonary vascular resistance. Access to the heart and mediastinal structures is gained via a median sternotomy. After partial thymectomy, creation of a pericardial well, and systemic heparinization, an arterial cannula is placed in the ascending aorta. A single venous cannula is then positioned in the right atrial appendage. Care is taken to avoid any undue manipulation of the heart until the institution of CPB because the myocardium of hypoxic, acidotic neonates with obstructed TAPVR is especially irritable and prone to ventricular fibrillation. Immediately after commencement of CPB, the patent ductus arteriosus is dissected and ligated. During core cooling to a nasopharyngeal temperature of 18°C, the posterior pericardium is incised where it directly overlies the common pulmonary venous trunk. Once a core temperature of 18°C is achieved, the aorta is cross-clamped and antegrade cold blood potassium cardioplegic solution is infused into the aortic root. Topical cold is also applied to the heart. Blood is then drained from the patient into the oxygenator to initiate the period of deep hypothermic circulatory arrest. At this point, the venous cannula may be removed to facilitate repair. The technique of circulatory arrest is a valuable adjunct to surgical repair of supracardiac, infracardiac, and mixed types of TAPVR because it provides a completely bloodless and quiescent operative field for fashioning of as large a pulmonary venous-to-left atrial anastomosis as possible. However, for repair of TAPVR to the coronary sinus, standard CPB with two venous cannulas and moderate hypothermia (28°C) often suffices.

Supracardiac Type. Ligation of the vertical vein may be accomplished just after commencement of CPB or after completion of the repair. It is best to ligate the vein in its extrapericardial portion to avoid narrowing the ostium of the left upper lobe pulmonary vein. Because the condition of TAPVR renders the heart untethered by the pulmonary veins, excellent exposure of the posteriorly-lying common pulmonary venous trunk is afforded by retraction of the heart to the left; we use such an approach exclusively. Alternatively, a superior approach between the aorta and superior vena cava may be used. However, an inferior approach with retraction of the apex anteriorly is inadvisable because this maneuver may distort the cardiac and pulmonary venous anatomy and result in kinking of the anastomosis when the heart is replaced to its natural position. A transverse biatrial incision is made starting inferior to the right atrial appendage and carrying it posteriorly through the foramen ovale and into the posterior wall of the left atrium (Fig. 93-5). It may be necessary in some cases to extend this incision superiorly into the left atrial appendage for construction of a wider anastomosis. A generous corresponding transverse incision is made in the common pulmonary venous trunk where it lies in direct apposition to the posterior wall of the left atrium. For as wide an anastomosis as possible, this incision is usually carried up to but not including the individual pulmonary venous ostia. A continuous 6-0 polydioxanone suture is used for the pulmonary venous-to-left atrial anastomosis. The application of this continuous technique with absorbable suture material yields a low incidence of delayed anastomotic stenosis, presumably by allowing growth of the anastomosis. Using a bovine pericardial patch with continuous 6-0 polypropylene suture, one closes the foramen ovale through the right atrium; direct suture closure of the foramen may jeopardize the patency of the common pulmonary vein-to-left atrium anastomosis. The right atriotomy is then closed with a continuous 6-0 polypropylene suture.

After completion of the repair, the heart is filled with saline, air is vented through the cardioplegia catheter site, and the venous cannula is reinserted into the right atrium. CPB is resumed, with systemic rewarming to a core temperature of 34°C to 35°C. During rewarming, atrial and ventricular pacing wires are placed, as is a right atrial catheter.

Cardiac Type. Repair of TAPVR to the coronary sinus is approached through a longitudinal right atriotomy (Fig. 93-6). After performance of a median sternotomy and institution of CPB as described for supracardiac repair, the patient is cooled to 28°C. A segment of atrial septal tissue is excised between the dilated coronary sinus ostium and the patent foramen ovale; the valve of the foramen ovale is removed in the process. An unroofing incision is then made in the superior wall of the coronary sinus such that drainage of pulmonary venous and coronary sinus blood is redirected to the left atrium. A bovine pericardial patch is sutured with continuous 6-0 polypropylene to the perimeters

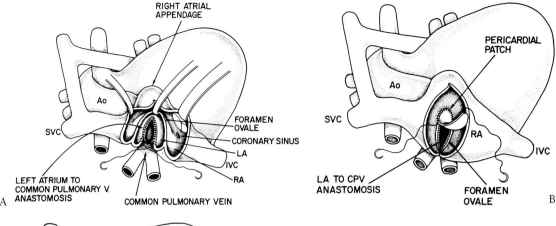

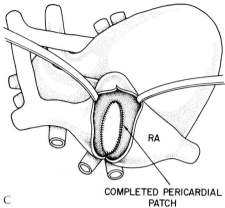

Figure 93-5. Technique for repair of supracardiac-type total anomalous pulmonary venous return via the ascending left vertical vein. **(A)** A transverse incision is made in the right atrium, through the foramen ovale, into the left atrium. The heart is retracted to the left. A corresponding transverse incision is made in the anterior wall of the common pulmonary venous trunk for fashioning of an anastomosis to the dorsal left atrium. Note that the right atrial cannula is removed during circulatory arrest to facilitate exposure. **(B)** Left atrium-to-common pulmonary vein anastomosis is completed. A pericardial patch is used to close the patent foramen ovale. **(C)** The completed repair, yielding total pulmonary venous blood flow to the left atrium and closure of the interatrial communication. (Ao = aorta; CPV = common pulmonary vein; IVC = inferior vena cava; LA = left atrium; RA = right atrium; SVC = superior vena cava; V = vein.)

of the foramen ovale and the coronary sinus ostium to close the resultant interatrial communication.

TAPVR directly to the right atrium is also approached through a transverse right atriotomy. The pulmonary venous ostia are visualized as they open into the posterior aspect of the right atrium, usually by way of a single venous hunk from each lung. A large ASD is created by excision of a portion of atrial septum surrounding the foramen ovale. An autologous or bovine pericardial patch is then sutured over the resultant defect to include the pulmonary venous ostia. The functional results of such a repair are that the interatrial communication is closed and pulmonary venous drainage is tunneled to the left atrium.

Infracardiac Type. TAPVR below the diaphragm is obstructed in the vast majority of patients; thus, patients diagnosed with this anomaly usually undergo an emergency operation in the neonatal period. A midline sternotomy CPB and deep hypothermic circulatory arrest are used as described earlier. During the period of systemic cooling, the apex of the heart is retracted anteriorly to facilitate dissection and long mobilization of the descending vertical vein. As in

the case involving repair of supracardiac TAPVR, routine ligation of the anomalous vertical vein in the infracardiac type is controversial; our bias is to never ligate the descending vertical vein. There have been anecdotal reports describing hepatic necrosis after ligation of the descending vertical vein. Furthermore, some surgeons maintain that the unligated anomalous vein serves as a useful postoperative reservoir until the small left-sided cardiac chambers are able to grow to a normal capacity. As opposed to the supracardiac variant, the common pulmonary venous trunk in infradiaphragmatic TAPVR lies predominantly in a vertical orientation. Hence, a lengthy vertical incision in the vein is often required, extending from the origin of the left upper lobe vein into the descending vertical vein. The heart is then retracted to the left as in supracardiac repair. A longitudinal right atriotomy is performed, with extension through the foramen ovale and into the posterior left atrial wall. The left atrial incision is then continued inferiorly such that it parallels the venous incision. Superior extension into the left atrial appendage may be required for a wider anastomosis. The common pulmonary venous-to-left atrial anastomosis is fashioned in a manner similar to that used for the repair of

supracardiac lesions, using a continuous 6-0 absorbable monofilament suture. Pericardial patch closure of the foramen ovale and continuous suture closure of the right atriotomy are performed in an identical fashion to that described for supracardiac repair.

Mixed Type. Mixed patterns of pulmonary venous drainage, in which one or more pulmonary veins do not enter into the common pulmonary venous confluence but instead connect with the systemic venous circulation independently, are treated by a combination of techniques described in the preceding paragraphs. In addition, pulmonary veins with separate anomalous routes of drainage may be individually anastomosed to the left atrium. In the event that only a single pulmonary vein from one lobe drains separately, it may be left uncorrected with minimal adverse physiologic sequelae.

Postoperative Management

In those infants who present initially with an obstructed subtype of TAPVR, pulmonary pressures are elevated due to high pulmonary vascular resistance secondary to preoperative injury and the inflammatory

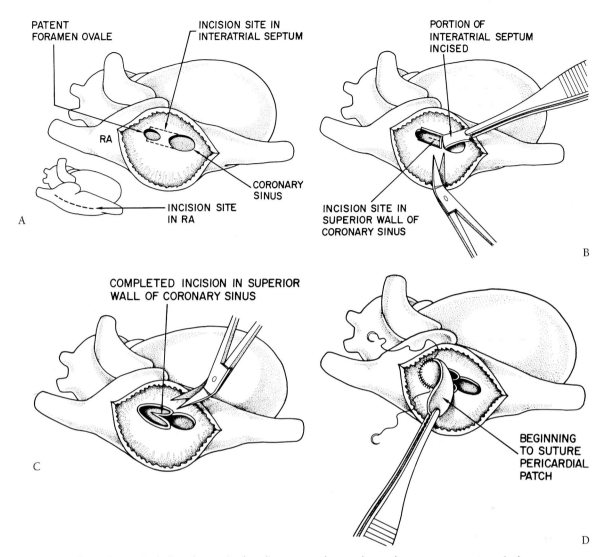

Figure 93-6. Technique for repair of cardiac-type total anomalous pulmonary venous return via the coronary sinus. **(A)** Inset shows the site of the longitudinal incision in the right atrium. A portion of atrial septum is excised between the coronary sinus and foramen ovale, removing the valve of the latter. **(B)** Site of the incision in the superior wall of the coronary sinus. **(C)** An unroofing incision is made in the coronary sinus, allowing redirection of coronary sinus blood flow into the left atrium. **(D)** A pericardial patch is sutured around the perimeters of the coronary sinus and foramen ovale such that pulmonary venous blood returning to the former is diverted underneath the patch, through the patent foramen ovale, and into the left atrium. (RA = right atrium.)

effects of CPB. Persistent pulmonary hypertension is a major cause of early morbidity and mortality after repair of obstructed TAPVR. It is not uncommon to see significant pulmonary hemodynamic lability and pulmonary hypertensive crises in the postoperative period in these patients. Although pulmonary artery–monitoring catheters are not a standard requirement for management during the first 24 to 48 postoperative hours, it is essential to institute prophylactic measures to maintain an acceptably low pulmonary vascular resistance. Such strategies include hyperventilation-induced respiratory alkalosis and careful titration

of the inspired oxygen concentration to minimize pulmonary vasoconstriction. If pulmonary pressures remain elevated beyond two thirds or more of systemic pressure, right ventricle end-diastolic pressures may rise higher than left atrium pressure, thereby reducing stroke volume. In these cases, acidemia may ensue and should be vigorously treated pharmacologically as well as with ventilator management.

In addition, a continuous narcotic infusion (usually fentanyl) is useful for sedation, providing postoperative analgesia and blunting stress-induced increases in pulmonary vascular resistance. A paralytic

agent to inhibit skeletal muscle activity with the intent of obtaining complete control of ventilation and minimizing oxygen consumption is similarly useful in the acute postoperative period. Milrinone is an ideal agent when inotropic support is required because it also produces pulmonary artery vasodilation. Rarely a sodium nitroprusside infusion may be required for management of difficult cases of pulmonary hypertension. Nitric oxide is often a useful agent in cases of difficult-to-manage pulmonary hypertension. ECMO has been infrequently used when maximal combinations of the foregoing noninvasive measures fail to improve pulmonary vasospasm and right heart function. Before ECMO is initiated, mechanical causes of refractory pulmonary hypertension, such as pulmonary venous obstruction or anastomotic stricture, should be ruled out with echocardiography.

Usually a progressive decrease in pulmonary vascular tone permits weaning of ventilation, inotropes, and pulmonary vasodilators within 24 to 48 hours after surgery. Pulmonary edema is a frequent complication after TAPVR repair, especially in nonobstructed cases in which there is long-standing preoperative right ventricular volume overload and in the presence of a diminutive left ventricle. Postoperative fluid management is critical, as is the judicious administration of diuretic agents such as furosemide. If there is deviation from the expected postoperative course or the patient is refractory to the usual interventions, an echocardiogram should promptly be obtained to investigate the possibility of pulmonary venous obstruction or anastomotic stricture.

Results

Historically, the surgical mortality for TAPVR repair has been extremely high, as evidenced by a 65% to 85% rate of early death for infants undergoing repair in the 1960s. With the advent of deep hypothermic circulatory arrest in the 1970s, the 30-day operative mortality decreased markedly to 12% to 18%. Further advances in noninvasive diagnosis, surgical technique, cardiac anesthesia, and perioperative cardiopulmonary support, as well as adoption of the routine practice of early surgical intervention, have resulted in mortality rates of <5% in our institution and in many recently reported series. Although young age at operation, preoperative pulmonary venous obstruction, infracardiac type of TAPVR, and emergent operation have all been previously indicted as risk factors for early death after isolated TAPVR repair, management practices of this lesion have virtually eliminated any identifiable preoperative risk factors for adverse outcome in the current era. Refractory pulmonary hypertension and cardiac failure continue to constitute the majority of intraoperative and early postoperative deaths in most series.

The most significant cause of late morbidity and mortality after corrective surgery for TAPVR remains recurrent pulmonary venous obstruction, which develops in 5% to 15% of patients within the first 6 to 12 postoperative months. The predominant pathologic manifestations of this compli-cation are anastomotic fibrotic stricture, discrete stenoses of the individual pulmonary venous ostia, and a poorly understood diffuse fibrotic process that may involve the entire length of a pulmonary vein. Although the use of absorbable polydioxanone suture has reportedly decreased the incidence of anastomotic stricture in recent years, there have been no technical factors that have reliably predicted or prevented the more insidious occurrence of diffuse, fibrotic stenosis of one or more pulmonary veins. This process accounts for a large proportion of the 5% to 10% late mortality rate after TAPVR repair. Various surgical techniques for managing postoperative pulmonary venous obstruction have been proposed, including revision of the common pulmonary vein-to-left atrium anastomosis, patch angioplasty of stenotic pulmonary veins, creation of a sutureless pericardial well, and suturing of individual pulmonary veins directly to the left atrium. Lung transplantation recently has been proposed for treating patients who have no other surgical alternatives. Junctional rhythms and various degrees of heart block are relatively common sequelae of TAPVR repair of the cardiac type. The internodal tracts and the atrioventricular node itself may be disrupted during suturing around the coronary sinus, particularly around its anterior margin. Although some patients do sustain spontaneous conversion to a normal sinus rhythm after a few days of external pacing in the early postoperative period, others require implantation of a permanent pacemaker as a result of a persistent postsurgical rhythm disturbance.

Partial Anomalous Pulmonary Venous Return

PAPVR is a congenital cardiac anomaly in which one or more, but not all, of the pulmonary veins connect with the right atrium or one of its systemic tributaries. By definition, at least one pulmonary vein must drain normally into the left atrium. Whereas the lesion is reported to occur in up to 0.7% of autopsy specimens, the frequency of antemortem diagnoses is somewhat lower as a result of a relatively high number of asymptomatic cases. The initial pathologic description was presented by Winslow in 1739, but it was not until 1949 that the first antemortem diagnosis was reported by Dotter and colleagues using angiocardiography.

Pathologic Anatomy

PAPVR results from involution of the right or left portion of the common pulmonary vein at a stage in embryonic development when primitive pulmonary-to-systemic venous anastomoses still exist. In approximately 80% of cases the anomalous vein or veins arise from the right lung, whereas in only 10% of cases does the left lung represent the sole source of PAPVR. Most commonly the pulmonary veins from the right upper and middle lobes drain anomalously into the right superior vena cava or, less frequently, connect directly with the right atrium. The innominate vein, coronary sinus, azygos vein, portal vein, and inferior vena cava represent uncommon sites of systemic venous connection. The anomalous pulmonary veins may enter the systemic circulation as a common trunk or as multiple individual connections. An associated ASD is identified in at least 80% of patients with PAPVR. Although a high-lying sinus venosus defect is the most frequent coexisting cardiac malformation, secundum ASD is also seen. In addition, a host of associated complex cardiac anomalies has been described in patients with PAPVR; in such cases, these complex defects dominate the clinical picture.

Scimitar Syndrome

By definition, the scimitar syndrome involves PAPVR from the right lung to the inferior vena cava. Some or all of the pulmonary veins unite in a common trunk to descend in a gentle curve alongside the right heart border en route to the inferior vena cava, giving the radiographic appearance of a scimitar (Turkish sword). The conjoined anomalous veins may enter the inferior vena cava near the cavoatrial junction or in its subdiaphragmatic portion. The right pulmonary artery and lung are hypoplastic in more than one-half of cases. Other associated anomalies include systemic arterial supply to the right lung (especially the right lower lobe) from aortopulmonary collaterals, abnormal lobation and bronchial distribution, secundum ASD, pulmonary vein stenosis, and a variety of other complex cardiac malformations.

Pathophysiology

The hemodynamic consequences of PAPVR are very similar to those of a large, isolated ASD. Pulmonary blood flow is substantially increased, but pulmonary vascular disease per se usually does not supervene for several decades with the lesion. The chronic right ventricular volume overload eventually yields right ventricular hypertrophy, dilation, and failure. The onset of pulmonary hypertension heralds an end-stage manifestation of a long-standing, uncorrected left-to-right atrial shunt. For unclear reasons, the scimitar syndrome is associated with pulmonary hypertension at a younger age and more frequently than other types of PAPVR.

Diagnosis

The majority of patients with PAPVR remain asymptomatic throughout early childhood. Those who eventually develop symptoms usually do so in the third or fourth decade of life, with the most common complaints being easy fatigability and mild exercise intolerance. Younger patients come to medical attention as a result of an incidentally discovered cardiac murmur, abnormalities on a chest roentgenogram, or recurrent pulmonary infections. Patients with associated major cardiac anomalies present in infancy with hemodynamic features referable to these complex lesions; in most such cases PAPVR is an incidental finding.

The mainstay in the diagnosis of PAPVR has become two-dimensional echocardiography with Doppler color-flow mapping. As in TAPVR, this modality is highly accurate in delineating the anomalous pulmonary veins and ASD. Cardiac catheterization is reserved for cases in which there are associated complex lesions or pulmonary hypertension is believed to exist. The pulmonary-to-systemic blood flow ratio (Qp/Qs) is usually discovered to be >1.5:1.

Surgical Management

To avert onset of the potentially irreversible complications of right heart failure and pulmonary hypertension, elective surgical repair should be undertaken in all patients diagnosed with PAPVR. In general, the surgical principles of PAPVR repair include separation of the systemic and pulmonary venous circulations, avoidance of creating obstruction to superior vena cava or pulmonary venous blood flow, complete closure of the ASD, and preservation of sinoatrial (SA) node function.

Partial Anomalous Pulmonary Venous Return to the Low Superior Vena Cava or Right Atrium

We use a technique very similar to the simple pericardial baffle procedure originally described by Kirklin and associates in 1956 (Fig. 93-7). The heart and mediastinal structures are approached through a median sternotomy. The right pleural space may be entered to verify the origin of the anomalous veins from the right lung. The superior vena cava is dissected from the cavoatrial junction to the level of the innominate vein. The azygos vein is usually ligated and divided to allow greater mobilization of the superior vena cava. With care taken to avoid obstructing access to the anomalous pulmonary venous ostia, the superior vena cava is cannulated with an angulated venous cannula placed through the right atrial appendage or, occasionally, directly into the superior vena cava above the anomalous pulmonary veins. More commonly, direct cannulation of the innominate vein can be used. A standard venous cannula is used for inferior vena caval drainage. CPB is initiated with cooling to moderate systemic hypothermia (28°C to 32°C). Occasionally, in our experience, cooler temperatures have been used, allowing temporary low flow or complete circulatory arrest to provide a bloodless field. The aorta is then cross-clamped, and cold blood potassium cardioplegic solution is infused in the aortic root.

A vertical incision is made in the right atrium lateral to the right atrial appendage extending upward to a level above the entrance of the highest anomalous pulmonary vein. Such an incision affords excellent exposure to all pulmonary venous ostia and the ASD and avoids injury to the SA node. If the ASD is narrow or the atrial septum is intact, a surgical atrial septostomy is created. A baffle of bovine pericardium is sutured into the lumen of the superior vena cava and the right atrium such that blood flow from the anomalous pulmonary veins is redirected from the superior vena cava, across the ASD, and into the left atrium. Care is taken to avoid narrowing the lumen of the superior vena cava or obstructing the pulmonary venous ostia with the pericardial baffle. The incision in the right atrium and superior vena cava is most safely closed with a bovine pericardial patch, thus eliminating the possibility of superior vena caval stenosis.

Partial Anomalous Pulmonary Venous Return to the High Superior Vena Cava

For repair of PAPVR to the superior vena cava 1 cm or higher above the cavoatrial junction, we again prefer the simple pericardial baffle technique just described. Historically, this has been regarded as the standard technique for repair of PAPVR to the superior vena cava at all levels. The only technical difference between low and high superior vena cava repairs using this technique is that in the latter it is usually necessary to place the upper venous cannula in the superior vena cava or innominate vein. In our experience as well as that reported recently in several large series, the intracardiac baffle technique provides excellent total correction of PAPVR with low morbidity.

However, concerns arising from the development of the postoperative complications of superior vena caval obstruction, pulmonary venous obstruction, residual atrial shunts, and SA node dysfunction at other centers have led to a host of proposed alternative yet complex procedures for repair of PAPVR to the high superior vena cava. Perhaps the most commonly used alternative procedure is that proposed by Warden et al. in 1984. This technique involves transection and oversewing of the cardiac end of the superior vena cava, followed by fashioning of an anastomosis between the cephalad end of the transected superior vena cava and the right atrial appendage. Redirection of pulmonary venous flow to the left atrium is then achieved by coaptation of the ASD to the anterior border of the intracardiac orifice of the superior vena cava. Although this and other complex procedures for high superior vena cava repair were developed in the interest of reducing the postoperative complications just described, there are no clear advantages of these more complicated procedures over the simpler and more expedient pericardial baffle technique.

Scimitar Syndrome

In general, pulmonary resection rather than vascular reconstruction is recommended for treatment of PAPVR in the scimitar syndrome if the right lung has been destroyed by recurrent infections, when it does not contribute appreciably to gas exchange, or in patients in whom an anomalous pulmonary vein arises from only a single lobe. Conversely, a variety of vascular reconstructive procedures have been proposed to reroute the pulmonary venous drainage to the left atrium in patients with sufficient right lung function and adequate pulmonary arterial blood supply. The anomalous pulmonary venous trunk is often too short for direct reimplantation into the left atrium; therefore, most procedures involve redirecting the anomalous drainage from the right atrium, across an ASD, and into the left atrial cavity via a pericardial tunnel. Aberrant aortopulmonary collaterals may be successfully treated by either surgical ligation or transarterial embolization.

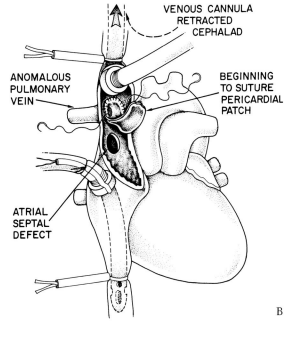

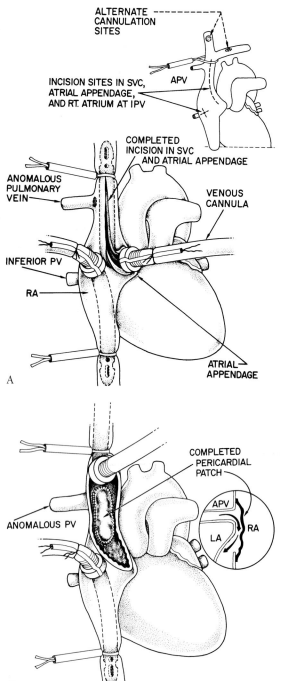

Figure 93-7. Technique for repair of partial anomalous pulmonary venous return (PAPVR) to the superior vena cava. **(A)** Inset demonstrates potential venous cannulation sites for PAPVR repair. The site of superior cannula placement is dictated by the level of connection of the highest anomalous pulmonary vein with the systemic venous circulation. Distal superior vena cava or innominate vein cannulation is used for PAPVR to the high superior vena cava. A cannula is placed in the inferior vena cava. Cardiopulmonary bypass is initiated. A vertical incision is made in the right atrial appendage and extended through the anterior wall of the superior vena cava to just above the ostium of the anomalous pulmonary vein. **(B)** The superior vena cava cannula is retracted in a cephalad direction to facilitate exposure. A pericardial patch is sutured to the margins of the anomalous pulmonary venous ostium and atrial septal defect. **(C)** Pericardial patch repair is completed. Inset shows the direction of blood flow after repair of partial anomalous pulmonary venous return. (APV = anomalous pulmonary vein; IPV = inferior pulmonary vein; LA = left atrium; RA = right atrium; RT. = right; PV = pulmonary vein; SVC = superior vena cava.)

Results

The surgical mortality for PAPVR repair is <1%. However, the higher mortality after repair of PAPVR in patients with the scimitar syndrome is a reflection of the frequently associated pulmonary hypertension and multiple complex cardiovascular anomalies. Although the reported incidences of late superior vena caval obstruction, pulmonary venous obstruction, residual atrial shunts, and rhythm disturbances is low after PAPVR repair, no single surgical technique has demonstrated a distinct advantage in further reducing these complications.

SUGGESTED READING

Cooley DA, Hallman GL, Leachman RD. Total anomalous pulmonary venous drainage: correction with the use of cardiopulmonary bypass in 62 cases. J Thorac Cardiovasc Surg 1966;51:88.

Darling RC, Rothney WB, Craig JM. Total pulmonary venous drainage into the right side of the heart. Lab Invest 1957;6:44.

Katz NM, Kirklin JW, Pacifico AD. Concepts and practices in surgery for total anomalous pulmonary venous connection. Ann Thorac Surg 1978;25:479.

Kirklin JW, Ellis FH, Wood EH. Treatment of anomalous pulmonary venous connections in association with interatrial communications. Surgery 1956;39:389.

Neill CA. Development of the pulmonary veins:

with reference to the embryology of anomalies of pulmonary venous return. Pediatrics 1956;18:880.

Van Praagh R, Corsini I. Cor triatriatum: pathologic anatomy and a consideration of morphogenesis based on 13 postmortem cases and a study of normal development of the pulmonary vein and atrial septum in 83 human embryos. Am Heart J 1969;78:379.

Warden HE, Gustafson RA, Tarnay TJ, Neal WA. An alternative method for repair of partial anomalous pulmonary venous connection to the superior vena cava. Ann Thorac Surg 1984;38:601.

EDITOR'S COMMENTS

The surgical results of complete repair of TAPVR have dramatically improved over the last two decades. Currently, with the techniques described in this chapter, operative mortality for these defects is <5% in most major centers. Isolated patients still do not survive operation primarily because of severe obstruction of the pulmonary venous confluence or restrictive ASD. These infants often present in extremis with multisystem organ failure before operative intervention. Thus, early recognition of this congenital lesion with prompt medical stabilization and urgent surgical therapy may result in a marked improvement in overall survival.

We use the same approaches to supracardiac and intracardiac forms of TAPVR as described by the authors. The biatrial transverse incision allows a very wide exposure of the back of the left atrium and the widest possible anastomosis between the common pulmonary venous confluence and the left atrium. In most cases, we incise into the individual pulmonary veins to create the widest possible anastomosis and open beyond potential constrictive tissue, which may occur at the entrance points of the pulmonary veins to the common pulmonary venous confluence. We use absorbable suture for this anastomosis. In some cases, the pulmonary venous confluence is sutured to the back of the atrium such that the confluence extends beyond the atrial septum, and in this case, the atrial septum is recreated with a pericardial or homograft patch. In some cases, the right atrium is also enlarged during closure with a patch.

Because of the difficulties with development of late obstruction in patients with single ventricle and total anomalous pulmonary venous return we have more recently used "sutureless" techniques for primary repair of total anomalous pulmonary venous return in these patients and are extending this technique to patients with more standard isolated total anomalous pulmonary venous return. The advantages of a sutureless repair technique are that the venous confluence can be widely excised out into each of the branch veins and then the pericardium or perivascular adventitial tissue can be sewn to a wide opening in the back of the left atrium. With this technique in a primary repair situation there is no need to suture at any point to the actual pulmonary vein wall, which may decrease the risk of scarring and late development of stenosis.

The mixed types of TAPVR may represent technical problems in very small infants because anastomotic techniques for individual pulmonary veins may lead to significant late stenosis. In addition, patients who have all four pulmonary veins entering separately into the right atrium (although simple to repair by excising the atrial septum and baffling the veins to the left atrium) have a very high incidence of late development of pulmonary venous obstruction of the individual veins and severe pulmonary hypertension. These patients must have continued surveillance postoperatively, and if pulmonary venous obstruction occurs, prompt lung transplantation is the optimal therapy.

Controversy continues regarding the relative contributions of anastomotic strictures to the late development of pulmonary venous obstruction in TAPVR. It is our impression that most pulmonary venous obstruction is not related to an inadequate anastomosis, but instead to involution of tissue of the common pulmonary vein or the individual pulmonary venous entrances into the common pulmonary venous channel, which occurs in the first 2 months after birth. Thus, a widely patent anastomosis may become restrictive with time. In situations in which the common pulmonary venous channel and individual veins are dilated with a restriction at the level of the entrance into the heart, surgical revision can be undertaken using sutureless techniques with good success rates. This appears to be most common in patients who have cardiac forms of TAPVR, in whom a wide anastomosis to the left atrium is created by unroofing the coronary sinus. In some of these patients, continued involution of the common pulmonary venous tissue can cause restriction of this anastomosis and require revision. Where individual pulmonary veins are stenotic and the proximal vein not dilated, operative intervention has virtually no role in resolving severe pulmonary hypertension. These patients appear to have a diffuse process in the pulmonary vein extending back into the hilum of the lung, and even sutureless techniques of vein repair do not result in a significant drop in the pulmonary resistance in most cases. If there is mixed dilation of some veins and not others, then sutureless repair techniques may be attempted before consideration for lung transplantation. Nevertheless, these patients have not responded to interventional catheterization techniques or surgical therapy in most cases and should be referred early for consideration for lung transplantation. Very high mortality with conservative measures in these patients and the inability to stent veins to relieve obstruction in the more proximal vessels have been noted. Even with consideration of lung transplantation, these patients develop severe pulmonary hypertension and often have a progressive downhill course before a lung donor becomes available.

An additional problematic group comprises patients with scimitar syndrome. Although the authors recommend that all patients with PAPVR and significant left-to-right shunts undergo operative repair, scimitar syndrome repair has been associated with a high incidence of pulmonary venous obstruction despite an initial successful baffling of the venous return to the left atrium. These patients then develop pulmonary venous obstruction and often hemoptysis from the right lung, which has little pulmonary blood flow other than bronchial supply. In addition, the aberrant aortopulmonary collaterals that enter the lung through the diaphragm and inferior pulmonary ligament may cause sources of bleeding; recurrent infection is not uncommon. In these patients, pneumonectomy of the affected lung can often resolve the hemoptysis and improve overall ventilation perfusion match.

Patients with scimitar syndrome presenting in infancy are a very difficult subgroup of patients with this anatomy. Often these children have hypoplasia of the right lung with a significant shunt from the aortopulmonary collateral vessels. In addition, associated congenital heart lesions are common. Even with complete correction of the cardiac defects, persistent pulmonary hypertension is common, and the mortality for operative intervention in these infants is significant. For these reasons, some authors advocate lung removal in these patients or medical management alone if possible.

The significant incidence of pulmonary venous obstruction after cardiac repair in isolated scimitar syndrome has led other authors to suggest that these patients not undergo operative therapy. Reimplantation of the pulmonary veins into the back of the right atrium with baffling to the left atrium or direct anastomosis into the left atrium may be complicated by kinking of the pulmonary veins when the lung expands. Dr. John Brown and his colleagues have shown good success with direct anastomosis of the scimitar vein into the left atrium using a right thoracotomy approach with a low incidence of any turbulence or potential obstruction at intermediate follow-up. The encouraging results with this technique have led many centers, including ours, to preferentially use reimplantation through a thoracotomy approach if the patient does not have a significant additional intracardiac defect that would require cardiopulmonary bypass or a sternotomy approach. Long baffles created from the entrance of the pulmonary veins at the level of the diaphragm along the right atrium into the left atrium have been associated with progressive stenosis. This is primarily because the veins take a right-angle course as they enter the inferior vena cava, and a baffle vertically into the atrium creates an obstructive junction at this site that can progressively occlude. We therefore incise the right atrial wall between the pulmonary veins and right atrium and suture the opening in the vein and atrium together, enlarging the pulmonary venous entrance

point into the inferior vena cava up into the right atrium. In this fashion, the veins enter in a wider orifice, which therefore can be baffled to the left atrium without creating a right-angle juncture. In a short follow-up, this approach has resulted in good patency of the pulmonary venous confluence.

Repair of partial anomalous pulmonary venous return remains a surgical challenge because of the potential for pulmonary venous anastomoses in the atrium to develop obstruction. Vigilance in assessing the results of operative intervention and catheter intervention to maintain patency of the anastomoses may be necessary in some forms of anomalous venous return to ensure good long-term outcomes. For PAPVR associated with a sinus venosus ASD, we make incisions in the right atrium without extending the incision across the junction of the superior vena cava and right atrium. In this way, the sinus node artery is generally preserved. In most cases, with a cannula placed very high in the superior vena cava, one can examine the pulmonary venous entrance into the superior vena cava from below, and with gentle retraction on the superior vena cava, the suture line of the pericardial baffle can be accurately placed in the superior vena cava without actually

opening the vena cava directly. This technique is useful if there is significant dilation of the superior vena cava-to-right atrial junction due to the anomalous venous return. In these cases the floor of the superior vena cava can be patched closed, baffling the veins to the left atrium without creation of significant SVC obstruction. However, if there is only modest dilation of the vena cava then a more elaborate approach may be necessary, including the use of the Warden procedure (dividing the superior vena cava above the entrance of the anomalous pulmonary veins, baffling the orifice of the superior vena cava and right atrium across the atrial septum into the left atrium, and then reconnecting the remaining superior vena cava to the right atrial appendage to reestablish flow to the right atrium). These techniques have resulted in very low complication rates with excellent results. It may be advantageous to leave the azygous vein open if possible, rather than ligation and division of the azygous vein routinely, because if any stenosis of the superior vena cava-to-right atrial anastomosis occurs, some decompression through the azygous system can be permitted with this technique.

T.L.S.

94

Coronary Artery Anomalies in Children

J. William Gaynor

This chapter discusses the management of coronary artery anomalies in patients without other congenital heart defects. Most variations in the number, origin, and distribution of the coronary arteries are of intellectual interest only; however, a few are clinically important. Clinically significant coronary artery anomalies may result in myocardial ischemia, left ventricular dysfunction, and sudden death. Anomalies discussed in this chapter include anomalous origin of a coronary artery from the pulmonary artery, coronary artery fistula, and anomalous course of a coronary artery between the pulmonary artery and aorta.

Normally, two coronary arteries arise from separate ostia in the right and left aortic sinuses of Valsalva. The left main coronary artery (LMCA) originates from the left aortic sinus. The LMCA usually bifurcates into the left anterior descending coronary artery (LAD), which traverses the anterior interventricular groove, and the left circumflex coronary artery, which courses in the left atrioventricular groove. The right coronary artery (RCA) originates anteriorly from the right aortic sinus, courses along the right atrioventricular groove, and commonly gives rise to the posterior descending artery at the crux.

The coronary ostia are usually located near the center of the sinuses of Valsalva. The ostium may be eccentrically located, however, and in some patients a coronary artery will arise very near a valve commissure. One or both coronary ostia may arise from the tubular aorta above the sinotubular junction, which is usually a benign finding. This anomaly becomes important if an aortotomy is necessary for aortic valve replacement or another reason. If the abnormal course is not recognized, the coronary artery could be transected. Both coronary arteries

may arise from the same aortic sinus with either a single ostium or two separate ostia (Table 94-1). If either the LMCA or RCA arises from the opposite sinus and courses between the aorta and pulmonary artery, myocardial ischemia and even sudden death may occur.

Anomalous Origin of a Coronary Artery from the Pulmonary Artery

The most important congenital coronary artery anomaly is anomalous origin of the LMCA from the pulmonary artery. This is a very rare lesion, and before the advent of surgical correction, it was often lethal in infancy. Anomalous origin of the LMCA from the pulmonary artery occurs more frequently than anomalous origin of the RCA. Anomalous origin of both the LMCA and the RCA from the pulmonary artery is very rare and almost uniformly fatal. Occasionally, the LAD alone arises from the pulmonary artery. Associated anomalies are uncommon. Without surgical correction, anomalous origin of the LMCA from the pulmonary artery is usually lethal in infancy, with a mortality of 90% by 1 year of age.

Children with anomalous origin of the LMCA from the pulmonary artery usually develop symptoms after ductal closure and the resultant fall in the pulmonary vascular resistance. Before ductal closure, the pulmonary artery pressure is elevated, and perfusion of the anomalous coronary artery is maintained. The clinical course after ductal closure is largely determined by the presence or absence of collaterals from the RCA to the left coronary system. If collaterals are inadequate, myocardial ischemia and ven-

tricular dysfunction result from inadequate perfusion. Death usually occurs if there is no surgical intervention. If collaterals are adequate, perfusion of the left coronary system is maintained. As the pulmonary vascular resistance falls, however, a left-to-right shunt develops from the RCA to the pulmonary artery. There is progressive dilation of the RCA and left coronary artery systems, with reversal of flow in the left coronary leading to a steal of blood from the myocardium. Children with significant collaterals may survive past infancy; however, there is usually progressive left ventricular dysfunction. Severe mitral regurgitation may be present secondary to papillary muscle dysfunction and ventricular dilation. Myocardial infarction may lead to formation of a left ventricular aneurysm. Infants frequently present at a few weeks of age with evidence of congestive heart failure and symptoms of distress and discomfort during feeding that likely represent myocardial ischemia.

Left ventricular dysfunction secondary to anomalous origin of the LMCA from the pulmonary artery can be difficult to distinguish from a dilated cardiomyopathy. Any infant with dilated cardiomyopathy must be extensively evaluated to rule out anomalous origin of the LMCA. Anomalous origin of the left coronary artery from the pulmonary artery must also be considered in older children and adolescents with a dilated cardiomyopathy because occasional patients survive past infancy. The symptoms associated with anomalous origin of the RCA from the pulmonary artery are less severe; however, myocardial ischemia and death can still occur. The electrocardiogram may show evidence of myocardial ischemia but is not diagnostic. Echocardiographic examination often demonstrates left ventricular dilatation and dysfunction with significant

Table 94-1   Origin of Both Coronary Arteries from One Sinus

1. Left main coronary artery originates from the right sinus of Valsalva (either from the right coronary artery or separate ostia).
   Left main coronary artery courses anterior to pulmonary artery.
   Left main coronary artery courses through interventricular septum.
   Left main coronary artery courses between aorta and pulmonary artery.
   Left main coronary artery courses posterior to aorta.
   Rarely the left anterior descending coronary or the left circumflex coronary artery alone may originate from the right sinus.
2. Single left main coronary artery arises from the left sinus and bifurcates into the left anterior descending coronary and the left circumflex coronary arteries. The left circumflex coronary artery crosses the crux and continues as the right coronary artery.
3. Single right coronary artery from the right sinus, which crosses the crux, continues as the left anterior descending coronary artery and the left circumflex coronary artery.
4. Right coronary artery originates from the left sinus of Valsalva (either from the left main coronary artery or as separate ostium).
   Right coronary artery courses posterior to aorta.
   Right coronary artery courses anterior to pulmonary artery.
   Right coronary artery courses between aorta and pulmonary artery.

mitral regurgitation. Visualization of the coronary ostium by either two-dimensional or color-flow Doppler echocardiography may be difficult. If the origins of both coronary arteries cannot be clearly visualized by echocardiography, cardiac catheterization is mandatory to rule out an anomalous origin of the LMCA. The anomalous LMCA ostium may be located almost anywhere on the main pulmonary artery or the branch pulmonary arteries. Most commonly, an anomalous LMCA originates from the rightward posterior sinus (facing) of the pulmonary artery (Figs. 94-1 and 94-2). The anomalous LMCA may originate from the leftward posterior (nonfacing) and rarely from the anterior (facing) sinus of the main pulmonary artery (Fig. 94-2). An anomalous RCA most commonly originates from the anterior portion of the pulmonary artery.

The first successful operation for correction of anomalous origin of the LMCA from the pulmonary artery was simple ligation of the anomalous artery at the pulmonary artery. Ligation prevents the left-to-right shunt, allowing perfusion of the left ventricle through collaterals from the RCA. Because of concern over early mortality and an increased risk of late sudden death with simple ligation, a variety of techniques were developed to create a dual coronary artery system, including bypass grafting using the left subclavian artery, the internal mammary artery (IMA), and saphenous vein. Meyer and colleagues reported the first successful left subclavian artery-to-left coronary bypass in 1968. The results of bypass grafting especially with saphenous vein have been

disappointing. Takeuchi and associates described creation of an aortopulmonary window and intrapulmonary artery baffle using a flap of pulmonary artery to direct blood from the aorta to the anomalous coronary artery. As experience with the arterial switch operation for transposition of the great vessels has increased, direct reimplantation of the anomalous coronary into the aorta has become the procedure of choice in many centers.

Because of the high mortality associated with medical therapy in these children, surgical intervention is indicated at the time of initial diagnosis in children with anomalous origin of the LMCA or RCA from the pulmonary artery. The goal of surgery is restoration of a two-coronary system; therefore, simple ligation of the anomalous coronary should not be performed. Severe left

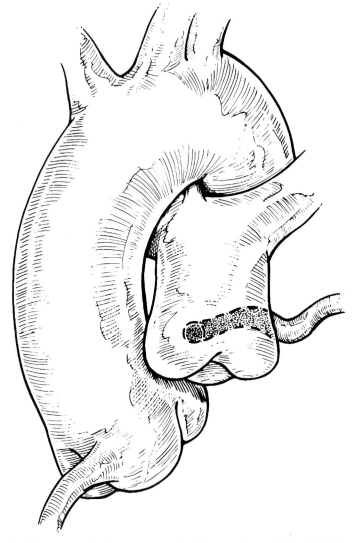

Figure 94-1.   The aorta and pulmonary artery showing anomalous origin of the left main coronary artery from the posterior-facing sinus of the pulmonary artery with the anomalous artery coursing behind the pulmonary artery.

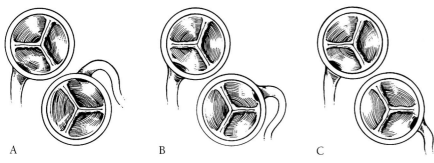

Figure 94-2. **(A)** Anomalous origin of left main coronary artery from the rightward aspect of the posterior-facing sinus of the pulmonary artery. **(B)** Anomalous origin of the left main coronary artery from the leftward aspect of the posterior-facing sinus. **(C)** Anomalous origin of the left main coronary artery from the nonfacing sinus of the pulmonary artery.

ventricular dysfunction and mitral insufficiency are not contraindications to revascularization in infants because significant recovery usually occurs. Left ventricular aneurysmectomy and mitral valve repair are rarely indicated at the time of initial procedure even if severe mitral regurgitation is present because the severity of mitral regurgitation almost always decreases after revascularization. Mitral valve repair or replacement is rarely necessary. Because of the increased risk of late death after ligation of the anomalous coronary, establishment of a dual coronary artery system should be considered in children who survive initial ligation.

Method of Operation

Aortic Reimplantation

Direct reimplantation of the anomalous coronary artery onto the aorta can be performed in most patients with anomalous origin of the LMCA from the pulmonary artery. The procedure is straightforward when the ostium is located in the posterior-facing sinus. If the ostium is located in the nonfacing sinus, excision of a generous button of pulmonary artery allows extension of the coronary artery, making direct implantation possible.

After induction of anesthesia and placement of monitoring lines, the chest is prepared and draped. A median sternotomy is performed and the thymus resected. The pericardium is opened and suspended in stay sutures. Myocardial ischemia and left ventricular dysfunction are usually present, and the left ventricle may be very dilated. Contact with the myocardium should be minimized until the patient is placed on cardiopulmonary bypass to avoid ventricular fibrillation. The aortic purse-string suture is placed distally near the innominate artery

and a purse-string suture is placed in the right atrial appendage for a single venous cannula. Heparin is administered, the aortic and right atrial cannulas are inserted, and cardiopulmonary bypass is instituted. The operation may be performed using either continuous low-flow bypass with moderate hypothermia (25°C to 28°C) or deep hypothermic circulatory arrest (18°C) in very small infants. A left ventricular vent should be placed via the right superior pulmonary vein to decompress the left ventricle. The pulmonary artery and epicardial course of the left coronary artery are carefully inspected. If the anomalous left coronary orig-

inates far to the left or anteriorly on the pulmonary artery, direct reimplantation may not be possible. The aorta is fully mobilized, as are the right and left pulmonary arteries. The ductus (or ligamentum) arteriosus is ligated and divided to improve mobility of the pulmonary artery. Tourniquets are placed around both the right and left branch pulmonary arteries. A cannula is placed in the ascending aorta for administration of cardioplegia solution. The aorta is cross-clamped, and cold cardioplegia solution is administered via the aortic root. Occlusion of the branch pulmonary arteries with tourniquets prevents runoff of cardioplegic solution into the lungs. Alternatively, the origin of the coronary artery from the pulmonary artery may be compressed during administration of cardioplegic solution to prevent runoff. If circulatory arrest is used, the head vessels are occluded with tourniquets, the circulation is arrested, venous blood is drained into the reservoir, and the cannulae are removed. After adequate arrest, the pulmonary artery is opened transversely immediately above the sinotubular junction (Fig. 94-3). The orifice of the anomalous coronary is identified, and the pulmonary artery is divided. The coronary ostium is excised from the pulmonary artery, as in the arterial switch operation, with a generous button of arterial wall. The excised pulmonary artery wall extends the

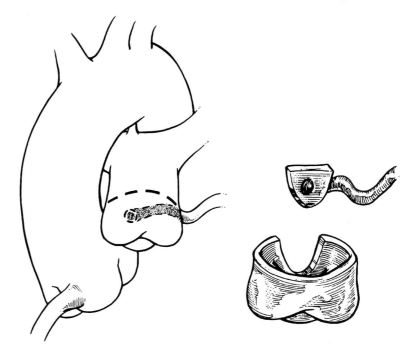

Figure 94-3. After institution of cardiopulmonary bypass and induction of cardioplegia, the pulmonary artery is transected above the sinotubular junction and the anomalous coronary ostium excised with a generous button of pulmonary artery wall.

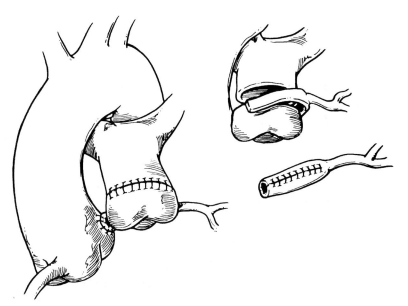

Figure 94-4. Occasionally when the coronary artery arises from the leftward or anterior aspect of the pulmonary artery, direct reimplantation may not be possible. In these situations, a tube can be constructed from a segment of pulmonary artery to lengthen the coronary and allow reimplantation on the aorta.

proximal end of the coronary artery, allowing the anastomosis to the aorta to be constructed without tension. If the coronary ostium is located near a commissure, it may be necessary to take down the commissure to excise the coronary button. If the coronary arises anteriorly on the pulmonary artery or from a branch pulmonary artery, the coronary artery can be extended using a tube constructed from pulmonary artery wall to allow reimplantation (Fig. 94-4). The proximal portion of the coronary artery is mobilized using cautery, with care being taken to avoid any small branches. The aorta is opened transversely just above the sinotubular junction, as in the arterial switch operation, and the incision is carried posteriorly above the left posterior sinus (Fig. 94-5). The sinus is incised vertically to accept the coronary button. The coronary button is carefully aligned with the incision in the aorta to avoid twisting or kinking. The anastomosis is begun at the most inferior aspect of the coronary button, which is attached to the most inferior portion of the incision in the sinus with a continuous suture of 7-0 polypropylene (Prolene). The suture line is carried to the top of the incision anteriorly and posteriorly. The aorta is closed with a continuous suture of 7-0 Prolene, which is tied to the coronary button suture as the anastomosis is completed (Fig. 94-5). After completion of the aortic closure, cardioplegia solution is administered and the anastomosis inspected to ensure adequate filling of the coronary and to assess

hemostasis. The pulmonary artery may be repaired primarily with a continuous suture of 7-0 Prolene in most cases (Fig. 94-6). Division of the ductus improves mobility of the pulmonary artery confluence, allowing re-

construction without tension. If there is any tension or narrowing, however, the defect in the pulmonary artery should be repaired with a patch of autologous pericardium (Fig. 94-6). If a commissure was taken down during excision of the coronary buttons, the pulmonary artery should be reconstructed with pericardium and the commissure resuspended. The patient is rewarmed, and the aorta cross-clamp is removed. If preferred, the cross-clamp may be removed before pulmonary artery reconstruction to decrease the ischemic time. The left ventricle is inspected to assess perfusion and function. The suture lines are inspected for hemostasis. Right and left atrial lines are inserted for pressure monitoring and drug administration. Atrial and ventricular pacing wires are also placed. After full rewarming, the patient is separated from cardiopulmonary bypass. The electrocardiogram should be monitored during reperfusion and after separation from bypass for evidence of ischemia. Because of the preoperative left ventricular dysfunction, temporary inotropic support may be necessary. In infants or children with very severe preoperative dysfunction, support with a ventricular assist device or extracorporeal membrane oxygenation occasionally may be necessary in the postoperative period.

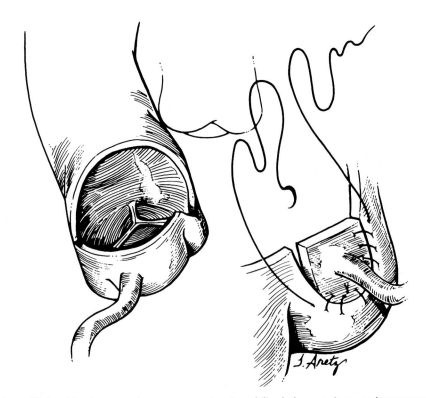

Figure 94-5. After the anomalous coronary artery is mobilized, the aorta is opened transversely above the sinotubular junction and a vertical incision is made in the left posterior sinus to accept the reimplanted coronary.

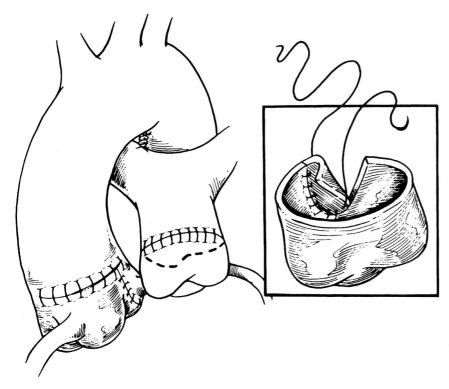

Figure 94-6. After the coronary is reimplanted, the aorta is closed primarily. The pulmonary artery may frequently be closed primarily. Ligation and division of the ligamentum arteriosus improves mobility of pulmonary artery. Occasionally, patch repair of the defect in the pulmonary artery with autologous pericardium may be necessary **(inset)**.

Modified Takeuchi Repair

An alternative method for repair of anomalous origin of the left coronary artery from the pulmonary artery is the Takeuchi repair, or intrapulmonary artery tunnel. In the original Takeuchi repair, an aortopulmonary window was created and a portion of anterior pulmonary artery wall used to create a baffle that directed blood from the aorta to the ostium of the anomalous coronary. In the modified repair, the baffle is constructed with a polytetrafluoroethylene (PTFE) (Gore-Tex) patch. Creation of a baffle may not be possible if the ostium is located near a commissure or arises from a branch pulmonary artery. The procedure may be performed with either continuous low-flow cardiopulmonary bypass (25°C to 28°C) or deep hypothermic circulatory arrest (18°C). Cannulation is performed as for direct reimplantation. After cardioplegic arrest of the heart, an anterior longitudinal pulmonary arteriotomy is performed (Fig. 94-7). The ostium of the aberrant coronary is identified. Using a punch, a 5-mm-diameter opening is made in the aorta above the sinotubular junction on the leftward aspect (Fig. 94-8). If there is any question concerning placement of the aortic opening, an anterior aortotomy should be performed and the incision performed under direct vision to avoid damage to the aortic valve.

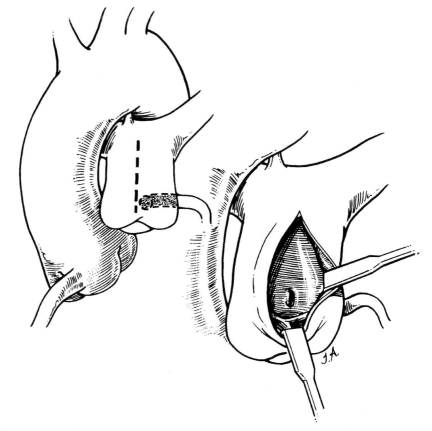

Figure 94-7. After institution of cardiopulmonary bypass and induction of cardioplegia, a longitudinal incision is made in the main pulmonary artery, and the ostium of the abnormal coronary is identified.

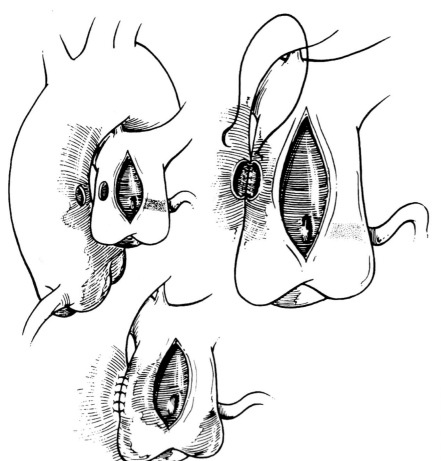

Figure 94-8. Using a punch, a 5-mm opening is made in the aorta on the leftward aspect above the sinotubular junction. A similar opening is made in the pulmonary artery at the same level, and these are anastomosed to create an aortopulmonary window.

Placement of the aortopulmonary window above the sinotubular junction allows the baffle to angle downward into the sinus if the ostium is located deep within a sinus. A similar incision is made in the pulmonary artery directly opposite the opening in the aorta, and an aortopulmonary window is created with a continuous suture of 7-0 Prolene (Fig. 94-8). A 4-mm PTFE tube graft is split longitudinally and tailored to an appropriate length (Fig. 94-9). This graft is used to create an intrapulmonary artery tunnel, baffling blood from the aortopulmonary window to the coronary ostium. The suture line begins at the coronary artery and is continued inferiorly along the pulmonary artery wall to the aortopulmonary window. The suture line is completed by starting again at the coronary artery and completing the superior portion of the baffle. After creation of the baffle, the pulmonary artery should be repaired with a prosthetic patch or autologous pericardium to avoid supravalvar right ventricular outflow tract obstruction (Fig. 94-10). Complications of the modified Takeuchi procedure include baffle leak, baffle occlusion, and supravalvar right ventricular outflow tract obstruction.

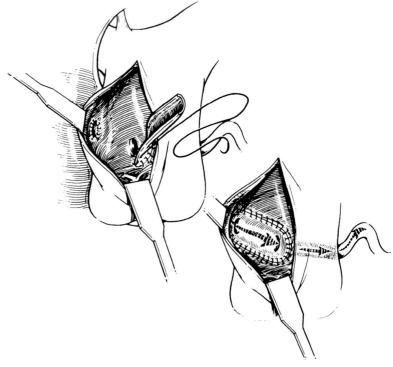

Figure 94-9. A segment of 4-mm polytetrafluoroethylene (Gore-Tex) graft is opened longitudinally and used to fashion a baffle that directs blood flow from the aortopulmonary window to the anomalous coronary ostium.

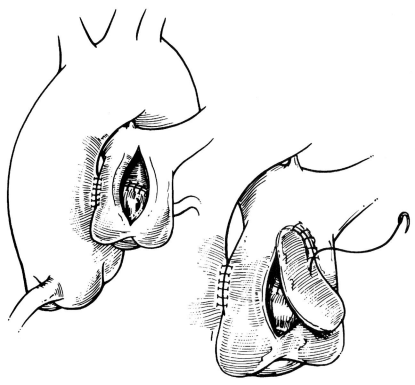

Figure 94-10. After the baffle is completed, the pulmonary arteriotomy is repaired with a patch to avoid creation of supravalvar right ventricular outflow tract obstruction.

Coronary Artery Bypass Grafting

Left Subclavian-to-Left Coronary Artery Anastomosis. Left subclavian-to-coronary artery anastomosis may be performed via a median sternotomy using cardiopulmonary bypass or via a left posterolateral thoracotomy without cardiopulmonary bypass. Cardiopulmonary bypass is useful for stabilization of critically ill infants and allows the anastomosis to be performed under optimal conditions. However, mobilization of the subclavian artery may be difficult through a median sternotomy. If a left thoracotomy is used, the subclavian artery is fully mobilized and divided distally after heparin administration. The pericardium is opened and the anomalous coronary mobilized. After a partial occlusion clamp is placed, the ostium of the anomalous coronary is excised with a small button of pulmonary artery. An end-to-end anastomosis is created between the subclavian and coronary arteries with 7-0 Prolene. The pulmonary artery may be repaired primarily or with a patch of autologous pericardium. Alternatively, the anomalous coronary is ligated at the take-off from the pulmonary artery, and an end-to-side anastomosis is created between the subclavian and coronary arteries. The major com-plication of left subclavian-to-left coronary artery anastomosis is anastomotic stenosis or occlusion.

Left Internal Mammary Artery Grafting. Coronary artery bypass grafting is rarely necessary in patients with anomalous origin of a coronary artery from the pulmonary artery. The most common indications are creation of a dual coronary artery system after previous ligation or because of stenosis or occlusion after a previous attempt at repair. The internal mammary artery (IMA) is the preferred conduit. Because of the risk of occlusion and poor long-term results, saphenous vein should be used only if no other conduit is available. The IMA can be successfully used for bypass grafting even in neonates and infants. There is also evidence for growth of the IMA after bypass grafting in children.

Results

Simple ligation of an anomalous left coronary artery has been shown to have unacceptable early and late mortality. In general, survival after creation of a dual coronary system is excellent. Burton and coworkers reported 11 cases of coronary ligation or ostial closure with a 27% early mortality and a 25% late mortality over a 10.5-year follow-up period. In the same report there were no early or late deaths in 11 children undergoing a Takeuchi procedure with an 18.5-month follow-up. After Takeuchi repair, 2 of 11 patients developed right ventricular outflow tract obstruction (1 also had a baffle leak), and 1 additional patient was found to have baffle occlusion. Backer and associates reported the follow-up results of 20 patients with anomalous left coronary artery. Nine patients underwent ligation, 10 patients underwent creation of a dual coronary artery system, and 1 underwent cardiac transplantation. Three of the 9 patients who underwent ligation died. There were no deaths among the patients undergoing creation of a dual coronary artery system. Five patients in this series underwent left subclavian-to-left coronary anastomosis and 2 developed significant anastomotic stenosis. Vouhé and associates reported isolated reimplantation of the anomalous coronary in 31 consecutive children. There were 3 hospital deaths and 2 additional deaths within the first 3 months. There were no late deaths. The only risk factor identified for early mortality was a shortening fraction of <20%. Twenty-three survivors were studied >1 year after repair. Left ventricular function had normalized in all patients, and in 5 of 7 patients who had severe mitral regurgitation preoperatively, the severity had decreased to mild or no regurgitation. The reimplanted coronary artery was patent in all patients. Cardiac transplantation is occasionally indicated if left ventricular function does not improve after revascularization.

Coronary Artery Fistula

A congenital coronary artery fistula is a communication between a coronary artery and a cardiac chamber, the coronary sinus, the vena cavae, the pulmonary artery, or a pulmonary vein. Coronary fistulas that terminate in right-sided structures, including the right atrium, right ventricle, and pulmonary artery, are called coronary arteriovenous fistulas. Fistulas that terminate in left heart chambers are arterioarterial fistulas. Coronary artery fistulas may arise from either the right or the left coronary artery. The most common sites of termination are the right ventricle and the right atrium. Most fistulas arise from a coronary artery with an otherwise normal distribution. The fistulous connection may arise either in the midportion of the vessel with a normal vessel continuing past the origin of the fistula or at the most distal part of the vessel as an end artery. Coronary fistulas result in a "left-to-right" or "left-to-left" shunt, and the involved vessel is usually dilated proximally. Fernandez and colleagues described 93 patients with coronary artery fistulas. A single fistula was present in 83 patients, and the remainder had multiple fistulas. The RCA was the most common site of origin and the right ventricle the most common drainage site. Isolated coronary fistulas were present in 56 patients, and the remainder had associated cardiac lesions. A review of 286 patients by Lowe and coworkers found the RCA was the site of origin in 56% and the left coronary artery system in 36%. The site of drainage was the right ventricle in 39%, the right atrium (including the coronary sinus and superior vena cava) in 33%, and the pulmonary artery in 20%. The remainder (8%) drained to the left atrium or left ventricle.

Patients with coronary artery fistula rarely present in infancy and are often older than 20 years of age at the time of diagnosis. Many patients are asymptomatic, and the fistula is discovered during evaluation for a murmur. The fistula may "steal" flow from the coronary circulation; however, angina is uncommon. Ventricular dysfunction and congestive heart failure may occasionally be present. The electrocardiogram may show normal results or may show evidence of ventricular volume overload. Chest x-ray films are usually normal unless congestive heart failure has developed. Giant aneurysms of the involved coronary artery can occasionally be present. Two-dimensional echocardiography can demonstrate enlarged coronary arteries, and the actual fistula may be demonstrated by color-flow echocardiography. Coronary catheterization with selective coronary angiography is necessary to accurately delineate the anatomy and plan the surgical repair.

The natural history of coronary artery fistulas has not been fully delineated. It is likely that the fistulas are present early in life and gradually increase in size. All patients with symptomatic fistulas should undergo closure. Patients with very small fistulas may not require surgical closure; however, they should be followed because progressive enlargement may occur. Patients who are asymptomatic but have moderate to large fistulas should undergo elective surgical closure. Despite progressive enlargement of the coronary arteries, spontaneous rupture is rare. Bacterial endocarditis may occur secondary to turbulent flow. Spontaneous closure of small fistulas has been reported. Successful transcatheter coil embolization of coronary artery fistula has been reported. The indications for coil embolization have not been defined, and for most

patients surgical closure is the preferred therapy.

Method of Operation

The coronary artery anatomy must be clearly defined by coronary angiography before surgical closure and the operation individualized based on the anatomy. The fistula frequently can be ligated or oversewn at its origin or termination. Many fistulas can be closed without the use of cardiopulmonary bypass; however, cardiopulmonary bypass must always be available. After median sternotomy, the thymus is resected and the pericardium opened. The coronary anatomy is carefully inspected and the distribution of the coronary arteries and the site of the enlarged vessel noted. When the fistula is located at the distal end of a coronary artery and there is no viable myocardium distal to the fistula, the fistula may be closed by ligation without the use of cardiopulmonary bypass (Fig. 94-11). A ligature is placed around the coronary artery immediately proximal to the fistula, and the fistula is temporarily occluded. The heart is observed for signs of ischemia, and the electrocardiogram is monitored. If there are no signs of ischemia and myocardium perfusion remains adequate, the ligature is tied. A second suture ligature should also be placed to ensure obliteration. Intraoperative echocardiography may be used to document closure of the fistula.

If the fistula arises from the midportion of a coronary artery or if the course cannot be fully defined, cardiopulmonary bypass should be used. An aortic cannula is placed in the ascending aorta, and both vena cavae are cannulated and bypass initiated. If it is necessary to open a coronary artery or cardiac chamber, cardioplegic arrest should be induced. The aorta is cross-clamped, and cardioplegia solution is administered. The fistula should be compressed during administration of the cardioplegia solution to prevent runoff into the heart. If an adequate arrest is not obtained because of runoff through the fistula, retrograde administration of cardioplegia solution may be useful. A variety of techniques may be used to close the fistula. If the fistula arises from the midportion of a dilated aneurysmal coronary artery, the fistulous communication may be obliterated by placing multiple pledgeted sutures beneath the coronary, with care being taken to avoid compromising the distal perfusion (Fig. 94-11). If distal perfusion of the coronary bed is compromised when the fistula is closed, coronary bypass grafting may be necessary. Alternatively, the artery may be opened and the fistula identified and oversewn from within the coronary artery (Fig. 94-12). The coronary artery is closed primarily. If the fistula terminates in the right atrium or right ventricle, the fistula may be closed directly from within the chamber (Fig. 94-13). A right atriotomy is

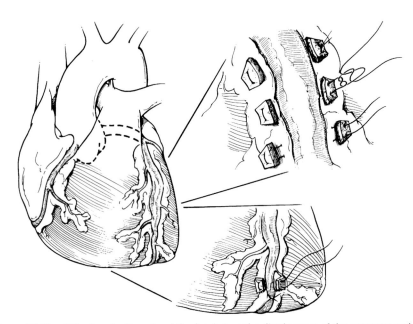

Figure 94-11. If the termination site of the fistula is at the distal aspect of the coronary and no significant myocardium is in jeopardy, the coronary may be ligated proximal to the termination site. If the fistula terminates in the midportion of the left anterior descending coronary artery, the fistulous communication may be closed with multiple pledgeted sutures placed underneath the coronary artery so as not to impair distal perfusion.

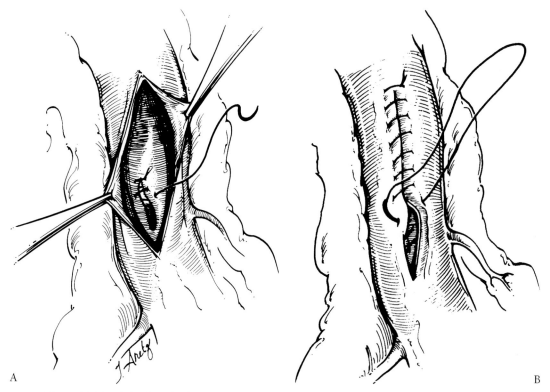

Figure 94-12. **(A)** When the fistulous communication arises from the midportion of the dilated coronary, the coronary may be opened longitudinally and the origin of the fistula oversewn from within the coronary. **(B)** The coronary artery is closed primarily.

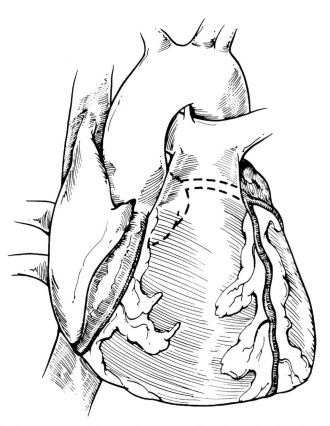

Figure 94-13. A coronary arterial venous fistula arising from the midportion of the right coronary artery and terminating in the right atrium.

performed and the termination site of the fistula identified. Administration of cardioplegic solution may be helpful for localization. The termination site fistula may be closed primarily or with a pericardial patch (Fig. 94-14).

Results

The operative mortality for repair of coronary artery fistula should be very low. The late results of repair are excellent, and very few patients have recurrence. Lowe and colleagues reported 22 patients undergoing surgical closure of coronary artery fistulas. In 14 patients, the fistula was obliterated with sutures without cardiopulmonary bypass. Six patients underwent closure of the termination of a fistula within a cardiac chamber while under cardiopulmonary bypass. In the remaining 2 patients, saphenous vein grafts were used to maintain distal perfusion after obliteration of the fistula. There were no operative or late deaths with a mean follow-up of 10 years. One patient had a small residual fistula, but there were no recurrent fistulas. Fernandez and colleagues reported closure of isolated coronary artery fistula in 56 patients with no early or late mortality. Two patients had perioperative myocardial infarctions.

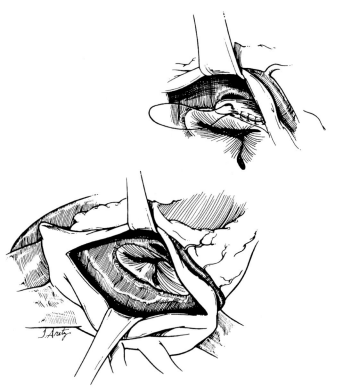

Figure 94-14. After institution of cardiopulmonary bypass and induction of cardioplegia, the right atrium is opened and the termination site of the fistula identified from within the right atrium. This may be closed primarily or with a patch of pericardium.

Anomalous Course of a Coronary Artery between the Aorta and Pulmonary Artery

An anomalous course of a coronary artery between the aorta and pulmonary artery trunk may result in myocardial ischemia and sudden death. This situation may be found when there is a single coronary arising from the right aortic sinus and the LMCA or LAD passes between the great vessels or when a single coronary arises from the left aortic sinus and the RCA courses between the great vessels (Fig. 94-15). Similarly, if either the RCA or LMCA arises from a separate ostium in the opposite sinus and courses between the great vessels, myocardial ischemia may occur. When there are two ostia in the same sinus, the ostium of the anomalously arising coronary artery is frequently abnormal and slitlike. The anomalous course of a coronary artery between the aorta and pulmonary trunk is associated with a high incidence of sudden death particularly associated with exercise. These lesions are often asymptomatic until an episode of syncope or sudden cardiac death. If the RCA arises from the left aortic sinus and is nondominant, however, this appears to be a benign lesion. In all other patients in whom a coronary artery arises anomalously and courses between the aorta and pulmonary trunk, surgical intervention should be considered. A variety of techniques have been used to repair these lesions, including aortocoronary bypass grafting with either the IMA or a saphenous vein graft, and direct reimplantation of the anomalous coronary. If the ostium of the anomalous coronary is slitlike and abnormal, direct reimplantation alone may not relieve the obstruction. An alternative technique has been described for use both in anomalous origin of either the LMCA from the right sinus or the RCA from the left sinus in which there is an abnormal slitlike ostium of the coronary. This repair consists in enlarging and remodeling the ostium to prevent compression between the great vessels and to relieve the ostial obstruction. When there is a single coronary artery and

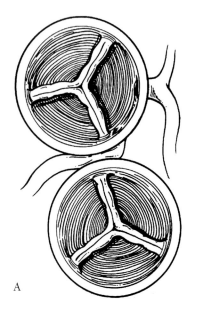

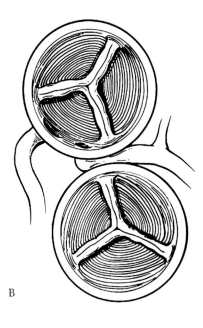

Figure 94-15. **(A)** Anomalous origin of the right coronary artery from the left aortic sinus with abnormal coursing of the right coronary artery between the aorta and pulmonary artery. **(B)** Abnormal origin of the left main coronary artery from the right aortic sinus with abnormal coursing of the left main coronary artery between the aorta and pulmonary artery.

A

B

the LMCA or RCA courses between the great vessels, relief of the obstruction by reimplantation or remodeling of the ostia is not possible. In these patients, bypass grafting may be necessary.

There are no characteristic physical findings in patients with an anomalously coursing coronary. The diagnosis must be considered in any patient with exercise-induced myocardial ischemia or sudden death. Noninvasive imaging techniques such as echocardiography and magnetic resonance imaging may visualize the anomalous course of the coronary. Before surgical repair, however, coronary artery angiography may be necessary to accurately delineate the anatomy and rule out other associated coronary disease.

The incidence and natural history of anomalous course of a coronary artery between the great vessels are not known. A recent review of 242 patients with either an anomalous course of the coronary artery or an abnormal ostium (slitlike, acute angle of origin, or valvelike ridges) found an incidence of cardiac death of 59% (142 patients). Sudden cardiac death occurred in 78 patients and was often exercise related. Origin of the LMCA from the right aortic sinus and origin of the RCA from the left aortic sinus were associated with the highest risk of sudden death. Surgical intervention is indicated in any patient with angina, syncope, or risk of sudden death who is found to have an anomalous course of a coronary between the great vessels. The indications for surgery in asymptomatic patients have not been defined. Because the defect can only be diagnosed by angiography, however, it is unlikely to be discovered in truly asymptomatic patients.

Method of Operation

Remodeling of Abnormal Ostium.   A median sternotomy is performed, the pericardium is opened, and the anatomy is inspected. The aorta is cannulated near the innominate artery, and a two-stage venous cannula is inserted via the right atrial appendage. Cardiopulmonary bypass with moderate hypothermia is instituted, and a left ventricular vent is placed via the right superior pulmonary vein. A cannula for administration of cardioplegic solution is placed in the ascending aorta, the aorta is cross-clamped, and cardioplegic solution is administered. After adequate arrest is achieved, a transverse aortotomy is performed, and the coronary ostia are identified. When the anomalous coronary arises from the opposite sinus, it is necessary to

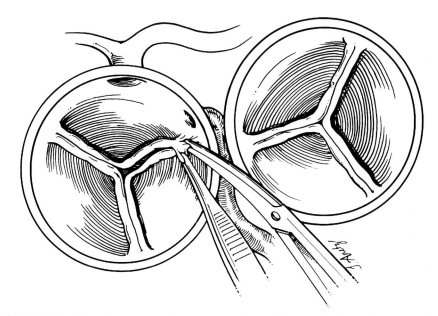

Figure 94-16.   When the coronary arises anomalously from the opposite sinus of Valsalva and courses between the pulmonary artery, the ostium is frequently abnormal. Repair may be undertaken by remodeling of the ostium. The abnormal ostium is usually located near a commissure, and this commissure must be initially taken down to allow remodeling of the ostium.

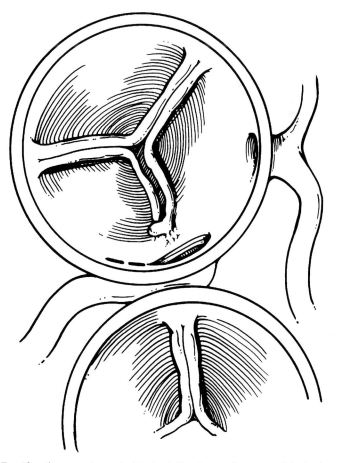

Figure 94-17.   After the commissure is detached, the abnormal coronary is incised longitudinally beginning at the abnormal ostium, and this incision is carried into the right aortic sinus. A portion of the common wall between the aorta and coronary is excised.

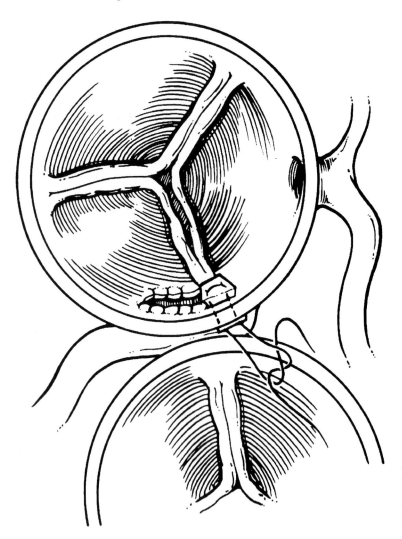

Figure 94-18. The walls of the coronary artery and aorta are anastomosed with interrupted sutures of 8-0 polypropylene (Prolene), enlarging the ostium and preventing compression by the great vessels. The commissure of the aortic valve is resuspended with a pledgeted suture.

detach the aortic valve commissure (Fig. 94-16). The slitlike ostium is opened along the longitudinal axis of the anomalous coronary. A portion of the common wall between the aorta and coronary is excised, and the intimal surfaces are approximated with interrupted sutures (Fig. 94-17). The aortic valve commissure is resuspended with a pledgeted suture (Fig. 94-18). The aortotomy is repaired, and the cross-clamp is removed after de-airing. The patient is rewarmed, the electrocardiogram is monitored for signs of myocardial ischemia, and the patient separated from cardiopulmonary bypass in the usual fashion.

Alternative surgical techniques have been described. A technique that is useful when the anomalous coronary passes below the commissure is creation of a neo-ostium in the correct sinus (Figure 94-19). A probe is passed through the intramural segment into the correct sinus. At the point the artery

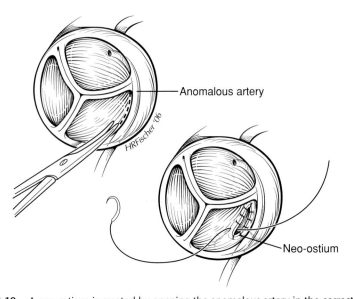

Figure 94-19. A neo-ostium is created by opening the anomalous artery in the correct sinus as it exits the aortic wall. The intima is sewn to the aortic wall with interrupted sutures.

leaves the aorta, the artery is opened to create a neo-ostium. The intima is sewn to the aortic wall with interrupted sutures. This technique avoids the need to take down the commissure. It has also been suggested that compression of the coronary artery can be prevented by translocating the main pulmonary artery to the left pulmonary artery or by translocating the right pulmonary artery and bifurcation anterior to the aorta. The long-term success of pulmonary artery translocation procedures is not known.

SUGGESTED READINGS

Backer CL, Stout MJ, Zales VR, et al. Anomalous origin of the left coronary artery. A twenty-year review of surgical management. J Thorac Cardiovasc Surg 1992;103:1049.

Barth CW, Robert WC. Left main coronary artery originating from the right sinus of Valsalva and coursing between the aorta and pulmonary trunk. J Am Coll Cardiol 1986;7:366.

Berdjis F, Takahashi M, Wells WJ, et al. Anomalous left coronary artery from the pulmonary artery. Significance of intercoronary collaterals. J Thorac Cardiovasc Surg 1994;108:17.

Blanche C, Chaux A. Long-term results of surgery for coronary artery fistulas. Int Surg 1990;75:238.

Bunton R, Jonas RA, Lang P, et al. Anomalous origin of left coronary artery from pulmonary artery. J Thorac Cardiovasc Surg 1987;93:103.

Davis JT, Allen HD, Wheller JJ, et al. Coronary artery fistula in the pediatric age group: a 19-year institutional experience. Ann Thorac Surg 1994;58:760.

Dua R, Smith JA, Wilkinson JL, et al. Long-term follow-up after two coronary repairs of anomalous left coronary artery from the pulmonary artery. J Card Surg 1993;8:384.

El-Said GM, Ruzyllo W, Williams RL, et al. Early and late result of saphenous vein graft for anomalous origin of left coronary artery from pulmonary artery. Circulation 1973;47 (Suppl III):III-2.

Farooki ZQ, Nowlen T, Hakimi M, et al. Congenital coronary artery fistulae: a review of 18 cases with special emphasis on spontaneous closure. Pediatr Cardiol 1993;14:208.

Fernandes ED, Kadivar H, Hallman GL, et al. Congenital malformations of the coronary arteries: the Texas Heart Institute experience. Ann Thorac Surg 1992;54:732.

Kesler KA, Pennington DG, Nouri S, et al. Left subclavian–left coronary artery anastomosis for anomalous origin of the left coronary artery. J Thorac Cardiovasc Surg 1989;98:25.

Kitamura S, Kawachi K, Nishii T, et al. Internal thoracic artery grafting for congenital coronary malformations. Ann Thorac Surg 1992;53:513.

Kitamura S, Seki T, Kawachi K, et al. Excellent patency and growth potential of internal mammary artery grafts in pediatric coronary artery

bypass surgery: new evidence for a "live" conduit. Circulation 1988;78(Suppl I):I-129.

Kragel AH, Roberts WC. Anomalous origin of either the right or left main coronary artery from the aorta with subsequent coursing between aorta and pulmonary trunk: Analysis of 32 necropsy cases. Am J Cardiol 1988;62:771.

Laks H, Ardehali A, Grant PW, et al. Aortic implantation of anomalous left coronary artery. Improved surgical approach. J Thorac Cardiovasc Surg 1995;109:519.

Lowe JE, Oldham HN, Sabiston DC. Surgical management of congenital coronary artery fistulas. Ann Surg 1981;194:373.

Montigny M, Stanley P, Chartrand C, et al. Postoperative evaluation after end-to-end subclavian–left coronary artery anastomosis in anomalous left coronary artery. J Thorac Cardiovasc Surg 1990;100:270.

Mustafa I, Gula G, Radley-Smith R, et al. Anomalous origin of the left coronary artery from the anterior aortic sinus: a potential cause of sudden death. J Thorac Cardiovasc Surg 1981;82:297.

Reidy JF, Anjos RT, Qureshi SA, et al. Transcatheter embolization in the treatment of coronary artery fistulas. J Am Coll Cardiol 1991;18:187.

Rinaldi RG, Carballido J, Giles R, et al. Right coronary artery with anomalous origin and slit ostium. Ann Thorac Surg 1994;58:828.

Roberts WC. Major anomalies of coronary arterial origin seen in adulthood. Am Heart J 1986;III:941.

Roberts WC, Kragel AH. Anomalous origin of either the right or left main coronary artery from the aorta without coursing of the anomalously arising artery between aorta and pulmonary trunk: Analysis of 32 necropsy cases. Am J Cardiol 1988;62:1263.

Roberts WC, Shirani J. The four subtypes of anomalous origin of the left main coronary artery from the right aortic sinus (or from the right coronary artery). Am J Cardiol 1992;70:119.

Rodefeld MD, Casey B, Culbertson CB, et al. Pulmonary artery translocation: A surgical option for complex anomalous coronary artery anatomy. Ann Thorac Surg 2001;72:2150.

Romp RL, Herlong R, Landolfo CK, et al. Ann Thorac Surg 2003;76:589.

Roynard JL, Cattan S, Artigou JY, et al. Anomalous course of the left anterior descending coronary artery between the aorta and pulmonary trunk: a rare cause of myocardial ischaemia at rest. Br Heart J 1994;72:397.

Sauer U, Stern H, Meisner H, et al. Risk factors for perioperative mortality in children with anomalous origin of the left coronary artery from the pulmonary artery. J Thorac Cardiovasc Surg 1992;104:696.

Shirani K, Roberts WC. Solitary coronary ostium in the aorta in the absence of other major congenital cardiovascular anomalies. J Am Coll Cardiol 1993;21:137.

Shivalkar B, Borgers M, Daenen W, et al. ALCAPA syndrome: An example of chronic

myocardial hypoperfusion J Am Coll Cardiol 1994;23:772.

Smith A, Arnold R, Anderson RH, et al. Anomalous origin of the left coronary artery from the pulmonary trunk. J Thorac Cardiovasc Surg 1989;98:16.

Takeuchi S, Imamura H, Katsumoto K, et al. New surgical method for repair of anomalous left coronary artery from pulmonary artery. J Thorac Cardiovasc Surg 1979;78:7.

Taylor AJ, Rogan KM, Virmani R. Sudden cardiac death associated with isolated congenital coronary artery anomalies. J Am Coll Cardiol 1992;20:640.

Turley K, Szarnick RJ, Flachsbart KD, et al. Aortic implantation is possible in all cases of anomalous origin of the left coronary artery from the pulmonary artery. Ann Thorac Surg 1995;60:84.

Virmani R, Chun PKC, Goldstein RE, et al. Acute takeoffs of the coronary arteries along the aortic wall and congenital coronary ostial valve-like ridges: Association with sudden death. J Am Coll Cardiol 1984;3:766.

Vouhé PR, Tamisier D, Sidi D, et al. Anomalous left coronary artery from the pulmonary artery: Results of isolated aortic reimplantation. Ann Thorac Surg 1992;54:621.

Wesselhoeft H, Fawcett JS, Johnson AL. Anomalous origin of the left coronary artery from the pulmonary trunk. Its clinical spectrum, pathology, and pathophysiology, based on a review of 140 cases with seven further cases. Circulation 1968;68:403.

Yamanaka O, Hobbs RE. Coronary artery anomalies in 126,595 patients undergoing coronary arteriography. Cathet Cardiovasc Diagn 1990;21:28.

EDITOR'S COMMENTS

Multiple operations have been devised for treatment of anomalous left coronary artery in children and are well outlined by Dr. Gaynor in this chapter. Although each technique may be applicable in certain circumstances, we believe that reimplantation of the coronary is the most ideal technique and establishes a two-coronary system with the least risk of late stenosis or occlusion. Past experience with the Takeuchi operation has also been favorable; however, we have seen cases in which the baffle dehisced in the pulmonary artery and created a left-to-right shunt, which in addition allowed decompression of the coronary artery. Thus, the reimplantation technique prevents the possibility of any left-to-right shunt through the coronary, and in the worst-case scenario, if the coronary occludes, the patient would have a situation similar to coronary ligation but at least would not have an additional volume load on the ventricle.

As described by Dr. Gaynor, we have taken the approach of reimplanting the coronary ostium in the left coronary sinus of Valsalva in a more anatomic location. Other authors have used a punch to create an opening in the aorta for reimplantation of the coronary. However, when this is used, the opening must be made more distally on the aorta to avoid blind damage to the commissural attachments of the aortic valve. Thus, we believe that it is simplest to open the aorta transversely, make an incision down into the left coronary sinus, and use the same suture line to close the aortotomy incision. In this way, damage to the aortic valve can be avoided and excellent exposure is obtained. We have used absorbable suture for the suture lines in young infants to encourage growth.

An additional controversy with anomalous left coronary artery is the management of significant mitral valve regurgitation in these patients. As noted by Dr. Gaynor, in the majority of cases, mitral regurgitation resolves when a two-coronary system is reestablished with resolution of distal myocardial ischemia and ventricular dysfunction. However, there are very rare cases of infants who have significant myocardial damage at the time of presentation and situations in which the papillary muscles themselves have undergone infarction with progressive elongation and fibrosis. In these patients, mitral valve repair can be undertaken with good results, often with papillary muscle shortening. Valve replacement for this condition should be extremely rare. One technical note at the time of operation in patients with anomalous left coronary artery is the fact that there is often a thin-walled venous plexus in the area between the aorta and pulmonary artery that has to be mobilized for exposure to the coronary for reimplantation. This troublesome area of venous collaterals may require meticulous cauterization to avoid significant bleeding after the reimplantation is performed.

Coronary arterial fistulas are rare, but the majority of fistulas should be closed. The transcatheter coil embolization or occlusion device techniques have become increasingly popular, and these fistulas can be closed in the catheterization laboratory. However, in patients with a broad-based fistula proximal in the coronary artery, occluder devices will potentially compromise coronary flow, and therefore surgical treatment is the procedure of choice. As noted by Dr. Gaynor, in the majority of cases, either direct ligation in the epicardial course of the fistula or suture obliteration beneath the coronary artery as the fistula dives into the myocardium can be performed with the patient off cardiopulmonary bypass, with excellent closure rates. More distal end artery fistulas at the distal ends of coronary arteries can often be difficult to close because the exact distal extent of the origin of the fistula is sometimes difficult to determine from the epicardial surface. Ligation and even suture obliteration of these distal coronary arteries may be the most satisfactory technique for ensuring that there is no recurrence of the fistula or residual flow. Even when from an epicardial inspection the fistula appears to be completely closed, intraoperative echocardiography is valuable because minor amounts of flow may still be present and complete obliteration is the goal in all cases. Not uncommonly, we have seen residual flow that requires additional sutures or ligatures for complete obliteration. The situation of anomalous origin of the left coronary from the right or the right coronary from the left passing between the great vessels is becoming an increasingly recognized entity. Although in the past these coronary anomalies were most commonly seen at catheterization, more recently the techniques of echocardiography and ultrafast computed tomography have identified these coronary anomalies more frequently. They are especially frequently identified in children who are undergoing echocardiography for participation in sports or for some other nonassociated vague symptomatology. This has led to a situation in which many of these patients are being identified who are totally asymptomatic and brings up the question of whether all patients with these anatomies should undergo surgical treatment. The overall incidence in the general population is not completely known. These lesions have been associated with sudden death in athletes, especially when there is a slitlike origin of the anomalous coronary. We have therefore found it difficult not to recommend surgical intervention in patients with a slitlike orifice of these anomalous coronaries because it is unclear which patients will have sudden cardiac symptoms and potentially even death from coronary compression.

T.L.S.

95

Pediatric Heart Transplantation

Charles B. Huddleston

Indications

Although cardiac transplantation in children had been performed in the 1960s and 1970s, it was not until the 1980s that this mode of therapy became established as an appropriate tool for those children with heart failure or unreconstructable congenital heart disease. The development of cyclosporine and the work of Bailey and associates at Loma Linda University were two important events contributing to this. Since then, many modifications of techniques and indications for transplantation have occurred, with a general shift away from transplantation for hypoplastic left heart syndrome in neonates to an increasing number of procedures in which young adults and children in their teenage years undergo transplantation after single-ventricle palliation. Survival after heart transplantation in infants and in children with complex congenital heart disease as the indication lags behind that after transplantation in children with cardiomyopathy. This is likely related to three factors. Many children with congenital cardiac lesions have had one or more palliative procedures so that the transplant takes place in the setting of a reoperation, increasing the risk of bleeding and increasing the technical difficulty of the operation. In many instances some sort of reconstructive surgery is required with the transplant procedure. Many children will have preformed antibodies due to exposure to multiple blood products and/or homograft material used during prior operations. These factors can lead to higher operative risk and higher risk of rejection or complications of enhanced immunosuppression that might be required. Many of the technical challenges related to transplantation in this setting have been worked out. This chapter presents some of these advances.

In general, the indications for transplantation in children include refractory heart failure, life-threatening arrhythmias refractory to medical therapy, and unreconstructable congenital heart disease. There are few cases in which arrhythmias cannot be controlled with medications, implantable defibrillators, or ablation techniques. Although hypoplastic left heart syndrome was at one time considered a lesion in which reconstructive surgery posed too high a risk, this is no longer the case. Most centers now report survival in the range of 80% or better for first-stage palliation. "Unreconstructable" congenital cardiac lesions are, in fact, quite unusual. Most transplants for an underlying congenital cardiac lesion are performed because of poor ventricular function, usually late after corrective or palliative procedures. Overall, approximately 50% of all transplants performed in children are due to idiopathic cardiomyopathies and 50% are in the setting of an underlying congenital heart disease.

Patients with single-ventricle anatomy represent a group requiring special consideration. Transplantation may be necessary in the setting of hemodynamics unfavorable for palliative procedures, poor ventricular function, poor ventricular compliance, valve regurgitation or stenosis, elevations of pulmonary vascular resistance resulting in failure of the Fontan circulation, arrhythmias, or other late complications of the Fontan procedure. It is clear that early palliation results in an increase in the number of children with acceptable anatomy and hemodynamics for ultimate Fontan reconstruction. It is also clear that the survival curves for patients after the Fontan procedure show a steady decline that significantly exceeds that of the general population. Many children born with single-ventricle anatomy have the anatomic right ventricle as the systemic ventricle, hypoplastic left heart syndrome being the most common anatomic diagnosis for patients born with this category of congenital heart disease This is substantially different from the late 1970s and 1980s, when most patients undergoing palliation for single-ventricle anatomy had tricuspid atresia with the anatomic left ventricle serving as the systemic ventricle; those with hypoplastic left heart syndrome either were not treated at all or died during attempted palliation. Thus, over the next several years we will have the opportunity to evaluate the durability of the anatomic right ventricle in this setting. If permitted to use the analogy of patients after the atrial repair of transposition of the great arteries or those with congenitally corrected transposition of the great arteries, the right ventricle may not stand up to the demands of systemic circulation over the long term. It is certainly possible, if not likely, that a large percentage of these patients will ultimately come to transplantation and become the predominant indication not only in children, but also in adults.

Contraindications

The contraindications to heart transplantation include multisystem organ failure, "uncured" malignancy, HIV infection, uncontrolled infection, and significant psychosocial issues. Severe renal and hepatic dysfunction failing to respond to medical therapy of the heart failure is a relative contraindication. In some cases renal dysfunction will be improved by the improved cardiac output produced by the transplanted heart, but immunosuppressants (cyclosporine and tacrolimus) critical to the survival of the organ have significant nephrotoxic effects. Dialysis post-transplant may be necessary and certainly allows time for the presumed recovery of renal function. Thus, one must be cautious about accepting a patient for transplantation with significant reduction in creatinine clearance.

The classic guidelines regarding pulmonary vascular disease and its impact on risk for heart transplantation are that the indexed pulmonary vascular resistance should be <6 to 8 Woods units and the transpulmonary gradient should be <15 mm Hg. These are only guidelines. These hemodynamic values may be difficult to measure or calculate in a patient with congenital heart disease in whom intra- or extracardiac shunts significantly complicate the computations necessary to derive the pulmonary vascular resistance value. The patients identified as high risk on the basis of elevated pulmonary vascular resistance should be evaluated extensively in the cardiac catheterization laboratory to examine their response to vasodilators such as nifedipine, oxygen, nitric oxide, prostacyclin, and so on. Patients with significant elevation of pulmonary vascular resistance failing to respond to any of these agents may be treated with prostacyclin or inotropic agents for an extended period of time and restudied. On occasion, there will be a favorable response related to either a reduction in the end-diastolic pressure of the systemic ventricle and/or remodeling of the pulmonary vasculature, so that some patients might become suitable candidates. The alternative for these patients would be heart-lung transplant, a procedure associated with much worse prognosis than isolated heart transplant alone.

Anatomic Considerations General Comments

The number of different combinations of congenital defects and their anatomic nuances preclude an encyclopedic description of each method of implanting the donor heart. However, the described procedures to meet the individual needs can be modified accordingly. This is particularly true for complex single-ventricle anatomy after palliation. These patients often have anomalies of both systemic and pulmonary venous return in addition to the obligatory abnormalities in the pulmonary artery anatomy.

It is important to obtain appropriate tissue from the donor at the time of retrieval so that necessary anatomic modifications are possible. This may involve a particularly long length of superior vena cava with the innominate vein, additional length of aorta, or all of the mediastinal branch pulmonary arteries. If the lungs are being harvested for another recipient, there will be limitations on the pulmonary artery available. Likewise, there may be a need to use some of the native tissue that might otherwise be discarded in order to patch pulmonary arteries or other areas where deficient tissue is a problem. In short, advanced planning based on knowledge of the specific anatomy from imaging studies and prior operative reports is of critical importance in the conduct of transplant procedures for these complex patients. In addition to these complex anatomic issues, most of these patients will have robust aortopulmonary collaterals, resulting in a large volume of pulmonary venous blood returning to the left side of the heart. One must account for this by either increasing the cardiopulmonary bypass flow or reducing the perfusate temperature.

Some controversy exists regarding the venous anastomotic technique—whether it should be directly to the major veins or at the level of the atria. Evidence supporting caval anastomoses over right atrial anastomosis is accumulating. There appears to be a better hemodynamic result in addition to allowing greater flexibility for the anatomic needs. However, in small infants the superior vena cava (SVC) is correspondingly small and delicate. The risk of anastomotic stricture is fairly high, so that right atrial connection is probably a better approach in children younger than the age of 1 year. There does not appear to be as much support for pulmonary venous over left atrial anastomoses. Technically right and left isolated pulmonary venous anastomoses are a bit more difficult than isolated left atrial anastomosis and may be more complicated due to wider separation of the pulmonary venous orifices in a patient with significant left atrial dilatation.

Donor Assessment/ Management

Once a donor has met the usual criteria for general acceptance for organ procurement on the basis of blood type compatibility and absence of transmissible disease, size match and organ function become the issues to be evaluated. The degree of size discrepancy

allowable depends upon the size of the recipient. For neonates, donors may approach as much as three times the weight of the recipient. For older children, the range by weight is usually on the order of 20% above or below. It is generally felt (without much objective data) that a heart from a larger donor will tolerate higher pulmonary vascular resistance in the recipient. Whereas this may be preferable in this circumstance, the luxury of such selectivity in this era of limited donor availability with an ever-increasing recipient pool is often not feasible. Although blood type compatibility has generally been a barrier that could not be crossed, it has been demonstrated that this is not necessarily the case for infant recipients.

Donor heart function evaluation includes a careful review of the past history of the donor, a review of the process that led to brain death, including whether or not there was prolonged cardiopulmonary resuscitation, the inotropic and vasotonic support the donor is currently receiving, an echocardiogram, an electrocardiogram, and direct examination. Laboratory testing for the myocardial fraction of creatine phosphokinase and cardiac troponin I is also part of the routine donor evaluation, particularly in the setting of possible cardiac contusion from blunt trauma. Donor hearts that might be considered borderline may be "resuscitated" using hormonal therapy. Brain death is associated with reduction in cortisol and thyroid hormone production. There are conflicting reports regarding the efficacy of replacement therapy using triiodothyronine and cortisol in improving myocardial function. The use of vasopressin for diabetes insipidus results in elevation of the blood pressure and often the reduction in overall inotropic support. There are no clear guidelines for the upper limit of inotropic support for donor hearts, but one should avoid those requiring high doses of two or more agents.

Post-Transplant Complications

Graft Failure

This is the most common cause of early deaths, particularly in the neonatal age group. Mechanical support for infants is generally limited to extracorporeal membrane oxygenation (ECMO). Intra-aortic balloon counterpulsation is generally not effective in small children because of relatively small size, high heart rates, and the distensibility of the aorta preventing effective counterpulsation. Small size is also the limiting factor for the use of ventricular assist devices. ECMO is clearly the simplest form of mechanical support for these small children because it requires only right atrial and aortic cannulation and provides "biventricular" support, albeit with the use of an oxygenator. As with other nontransplant cardiac procedures, it usually requires 5 to 7 days for recovery of the heart to be able to wean from support.

Right heart failure with tricuspid valve regurgitation may be treated in a number of ways. However, before initiating treatment, one must ensure that there is no technical problem leading to obstruction at the level of the pulmonary arterial or venous anastomoses. This is particularly true in the setting of prior Fontan or other palliative procedures in which the transplant has involved reconstruction of the pulmonary arteries. In the setting of elevated pulmonary vascular resistance, nitric oxide, prostacyclin (either inhaled or intravenous), as well as inotropic support and sedation with neuromuscular paralysis may effectively stabilize the patient until some recovery of the right ventricle has occurred. As mentioned, pretransplant pulmonary vascular resistance of >6 Woods units or a transpulmonary gradient of >15 mm Hg has generally been considered a contraindication to isolated heart transplantation. However, these newer pulmonary vasodilators have clearly extended these limitations. It is often assumed that patients in heart failure secondary to failed Fontan should have acceptable pulmonary vascular resistance by virtue of the fact that they are surviving with venous connections to the pulmonary arterial tree absent the force generated by a ventricle. However, this is not necessarily the case.

Bleeding

This is an issue in patients coming to transplantation in the setting of multiple prior corrective or palliative procedures. The use of aprotinin is relatively routine and has had a significant benefit at least on a subjective level. The number of prior cardiac procedures should not affect candidacy for transplantation.

Rejection

The rate of rejection in neonates appears to be lower than that seen in older children and adults. This is presumably a product of an immature immune system. Reduction in the immunosuppression used in these patients is typical, and many patients come

off steroids altogether. The diagnosis of rejection depends on endomyocardial biopsy with histologic examination. Noninvasive tests are not 100% reliable for this diagnosis. Treatment is generally with high-dose steroids (10 mg/kg methylprednisolone intravenous) daily for 3 days. Repeated bouts of rejection may require cytolytic therapy and change of baseline immunosuppression.

Other Complications

A complete cataloging of the complications after cardiac transplantation is beyond the scope of this chapter. The immunosuppressant drugs are responsible for a number of these including neurologic events, renal insufficiency, infections, hypertension, and hirsutism. Gastrointestinal complications include gastric and duodenal ulcers, acalculous cholecystitis, and pancreatitis. Phrenic nerve injury can occur from direct surgical trauma particularly in patients requiring extensive dissection of right superior vena cava or of the branch pulmonary arteries. This is generally well tolerated except in young infants, who depend almost exclusively on the diaphragm for inspiration; they will likely require diaphragm plication for weaning from the ventilator. Post-transplant coronary vasculopathy and lymphoproliferative disease are long-term complications that occur in children as well as adults.

Operative Techniques

Hypoplastic Left Heart Syndrome

As mentioned, transplantation for this entity is used much less frequently now than in the early 1990s. Mortality for first-stage reconstruction in most centers is now about 20% and occurs primarily in infants with additional risk factors such as small size or poor right ventricular function. The waiting time for small infants may range from 6 weeks to 3 months, and the procedure is notable for a mortality of 15% to 20%. Therefore, transplantation is generally reserved for those infants with poor right ventricular function, severe tricuspid valve regurgitation, or pulmonary valve stenosis or regurgitation. These patients are poor candidates for single-ventricle palliation even if they survive the Norwood procedure.

Donor Procurement

The key issue here is to acquire sufficient donor aorta to allow for reconstruction of

the recipient aorta as part of the transplant procedure. The ascending aorta, aortic arch including the head vessels, and proximal descending thoracic aorta are all dissected out (Fig. 95-1A). To enhance exposure, the innominate vein may be ligated and divided. After aortic clamping, cardioplegia administration, and cooling with topical cold saline and ice, the innominate, left common carotid, and left subclavian arteries are divided just beyond their origin. The proximal descending aorta is divided just beyond the origin of the ligamentum arteriosum. The remainder of the organ harvest proceeds as for any other cardiac procurement. The aorta is prepared by taking off the superior portion of the aortic arch beginning just proximal to the origin of the innominate artery and going all the way to the ligamentum arteriosum. I prefer to begin this preparation of the arch by incising into the mouth of the innominate and taking the rest of the superior aspect of the aortic arch. This leaves a small piece of the right lateral proximal wall of the innominate artery as a convenient way to increase the length available for the arch reconstruction. It also provides a convenient fit for the native arch and head vessels. The remainder of the donor preparation is similar to that for any transplant.

Recipient Operation

The ductus arteriosus, branch pulmonary arteries, and aortic arch with its branches are dissected out extensively (Fig. 95-1). When dissecting out the ductus arteriosus and during the distal arch reconstruction, care must be taken to avoid injury to the recurrent laryngeal nerve. Cannulation for arterial inflow may be performed by one of three methods: via the main pulmonary artery with control of the branch pulmonary arteries, directly into the ductus arteriosus with ligation of the pulmonary artery end of the ductus arteriosus, or via the innominate artery usually through a small graft sewn to the innominate artery. The last method provides the greatest flexibility in arch reconstruction with a minimal amount of time subjecting the patient to circulatory arrest. Bicaval venous cannulation is performed also to limit the circulatory arrest time. Once cardiopulmonary bypass has commenced, the patient is cooled to 18°C. While the cooling is going on, the donor heart is prepared as described. If cannulation is either via the ductus arteriosus or via the graft sewn to the innominate artery, the heart can be excised without circulatory arrest. There are techniques for arch reconstruction without complete circulatory arrest. This requires

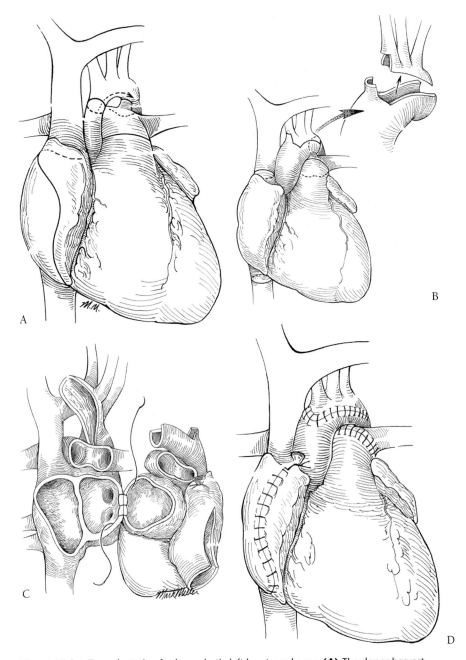

Figure 95-1. Transplantation for hypoplastic left heart syndrome. **(A)** The donor harvest procedure involves removing the heart as with any donor harvest. In addition, a long segment of aorta—from the arch distal to the ligamentum arteriosum—is removed. Preparation of the donor aorta for arch reconstruction is shown in the inset. The top of the arch is removed beginning with the midportion of the innominate artery. The right lateral wall of the innominate artery is left to extend the length of the donor arch available for the reconstruction. **(B)** The anatomy of hypoplastic left heart syndrome and the incisions necessary for the recipient cardiectomy. **(C)** The recipient cardiectomy has been performed, and appropriate cuffs have been left for the left and right atrial anastomoses. Most of the small ascending aorta has been removed. The underside of the aortic arch is opened all the way through the insertion of the ductus and 1 cm distally into the descending thoracic aorta. The left atrial anastomosis is performed first and then the arch reconstruction. **(D)** The completed transplant with the newly created aortic arch. (IVC = inferior vena cava; LA = left atrium; PA = pulmonary artery; RA = right atrium; SVC = superior vena cava.)

cannulation of the innominate artery with occlusion of the arch branches and proximal descending thoracic aorta. The arch reconstruction can usually be performed in a fairly short period of time, however, using circulatory arrest. The potential benefit of eliminating circulatory arrest must be weighed against the potential benefit of a quicker, less cumbersome procedure.

After recipient cardiectomy the left atrial anastomosis is performed in the usual fashion. The posterior aspect of the right atrial anastomosis is performed sewing the lateral free edge of the donor right atrium to the right lateral suture line of the left atrial anastomosis. Once the suture line comes around the recipient right atrial free wall, this is left to be completed later. The circulation is shut down at this point, and the patient is exsanguinated into the cardiopulmonary bypass circuit. The arch reconstruction is then performed. The residual ductal tissue is excised in its entirety from the aorta. The underside of the recipient aortic arch is opened to the insertion point of the ductus arteriosus and then beyond approximately 1 cm. The donor heart with the attached aorta is brought up onto the field. The donor aortic arch is then attached to reconstruct the recipient aorta. The circulation may be recommenced at this point and the patient rewarmed. The pulmonary artery anastomosis is performed as an end-to-end anastomosis, and the anterior portion of the right atrial anastomosis is completed. The usual de-airing maneuvers are performed, and the patient is weaned from cardiopulmonary bypass.

Approximately 15% of all patients with hypoplastic left heart syndrome have a bilateral superior venae cavae. As mentioned, a very simple method of handling this is to alter the recipient cardiectomy such that the left SVC continues to drain via the recipient coronary sinus into the new right atrium (Fig. 95-2). The right atrial anastomosis is slightly more complicated to accommodate this, and one must be careful to include the cut edge of the recipient left atrial free wall in the left atrial anastomosis to avoid bleeding from the divided coronary veins.

Frequently the donors used for these young infants are considerably larger, often twice by weight. This may present problems with chest closure immediately. The chest may be left open with either a Silastic or some other synthetic patch material sewn to the skin edges to prevent compression. With resolution of edema over the ensuing first few post-transplant days the chest may be closed. Some maneuvers that might allow for closure of the chest include resecting the pericardium and opening the left

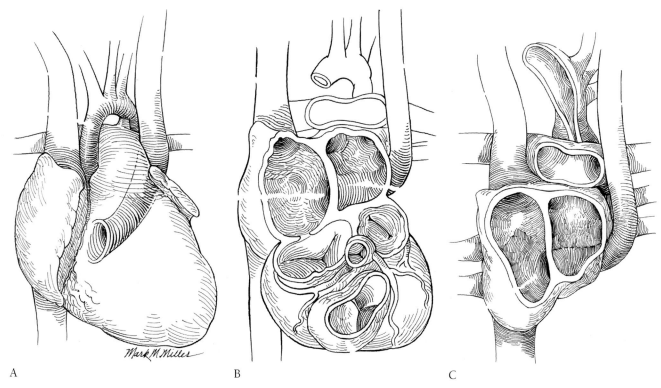

Figure 95-2. Transplantation for hypoplastic left heart syndrome with a left superior vena cava. **(A)** The same view as in Fig. 95-1B except that there is a left superior vena cava that drains into an enlarged coronary sinus. The innominate vein is absent. **(B)** The recipient cardiectomy is altered so that the coronary sinus remains intact along its course in the posterior left atrioventricular groove. The incision in the inferolateral portion of the left atrial free wall is moved into the atrioventricular groove. **(C)** The recipient cardiectomy is completed, and the left superior vena cava and coronary sinus are intact. The donor heart is sewn in place just as it would be otherwise. (LSVC = left superior vena cava; RSVC = right superior vena cava.)

pleural space to allow the heart to "fall" into the left chest to some degree. Using smaller tidal volumes and lower positive end-expiratory pressure may also be of some benefit.

The postoperative management of these infants is similar to that for any neonate undergoing major cardiac reconstructive surgery with the possible exception that the risk of pulmonary hypertension may be higher than in most other cases. This is related to the length of waiting time before transplant and the large left-to-right shunt imposed by the native circulation of hypoplastic left heart syndrome with the ductus arteriosus patency maintained by prostaglandin E1 infusion. Patients waiting for >1 month under these circumstances should be prophylactically managed with neuromuscular paralysis, sedation, and mild hyperventilation in the first 24 hours post-transplant. Other measures, such as use of inhaled nitric oxide, may be necessary as well.

"Congenitally Corrected" Transposition of the Great Arteries (S,L,L)

This congenital cardiac anomaly involves discordant connections on both the ventriculoarterial level and the atrioventricular level—the systemic venous blood returns to the right atrium, which connects to the anatomic left ventricle, which gives rise to the pulmonary artery, and the pulmonary venous return drains to the left atrium, which connects to the anatomic right ventricle, which gives rise to the aorta. Typically, right (systemic) ventricular function begins to deteriorate by the second or third decade of life. Left atrioventricular valve (tricuspid valve) regurgitation accompanies this. The basis for heart failure in these patients is presumably related to the fact that the anatomic right ventricle is not well suited to support the demands of the systemic circulation on a chronic basis. Patients with a history of prior repair of another anomaly (ventricular

septal defect with pulmonary stenosis) who also develop heart block seem to be at greater risk for right ventricular dysfunction.

Donor Operation

Procurement for transplantation in patients with this anomaly is not particularly different than that for any other transplant with the exception that a longer segment of aorta and main pulmonary artery may be necessary.

Recipient Operation

The aorta is generally to the left and slightly anterior to the pulmonary artery (Fig. 95-3). Arterial cannulation should be as high on the ascending aorta as possible. All aspects of the transplant procedure are just as they are for hearts with normal anatomy except for the handling of the great arteries. The recipient aorta is transected relatively high, where it is closer to the midline. The main pulmonary artery is taken at about the level

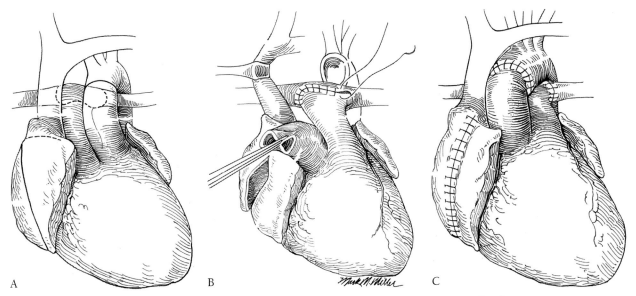

Figure 95-3.   Transplant for congenitally corrected transposition of the great arteries (S,L,L). **(A)** Congenitally corrected transposition of the great arteries results in the aorta positioned to the left and anterior; it is occasionally displaced far off into the left chest. The main pulmonary artery is to the right and posterior to the aorta. **(B)** The recipient cardiectomy has been performed, with the aorta excised in a sufficiently distal position so that the open end for the anastomosis is more to the patient's right. The venous or atrial anastomoses are performed as they would be otherwise. The pulmonary artery anastomosis is performed before the aortic anastomosis because it will come to lie almost directly posterior to the aorta when that anastomosis is completed. A long segment of main pulmonary artery from the donor will assist in this part of the procedure. **(C)** The completed transplant demonstrating the aorta now in a more normal position to the right of the pulmonary artery bifurcation. (SVC = superior vena cava.)

of the bifurcation, which is located generally further to the right of the patient than normal. The arteriotomy may be extended out onto the proximal left pulmonary artery, and the right side of the cuff of main pulmonary artery is closed, moving the pulmonary artery opening leftward a short distance to get it out from behind the aorta and avoiding the potential of kinking of the main pulmonary artery. The left atrial anastomosis is performed first. The pulmonary artery anastomosis should be done before the aortic anastomosis to avoid an obstructed view of this connection. The aortic anastomosis may be constructed in a relatively normal position near the midline as opposed to the left side of the patient by using this relatively long length of donor aorta to connect to the distal ascending aorta. The anastomoses of the venae cavae are performed in the usual fashion.

Status Post Fontan Procedure
Donor Operation
Pulmonary artery reconstruction and correction of systemic venous anomalies are the most common problems requiring modification of the standard technique in these patients. Thus, the harvest should include

as much of the venae cavae and pulmonary arteries as possible, with the caveat that other organ procurement teams have their own needs for the same vascular structures. A segment of donor descending thoracic aorta provides a conduit allowing for more flexibility in the recipient reconstruction that inevitably accompanies the transplant procedure. The innominate vein in continuity with the SVC may also be very useful.

Recipient Operation
The illustrations demonstrate a patient with bilateral SVCs, each anastomosed to the pulmonary artery directly, who has had an intra-atrial lateral tunnel type of Fontan procedure (Fig. 95-4). The blood from the inferior vena cava (IVC) reaches the pulmonary artery via a lateral intra-atrial baffle (cavopulmonary connection) and anastomosis of the cardiac end of the SVC and pulmonary artery. Venous cannulation needs to be high in both SVCs and low in the IVC. Both SVCs do not necessarily have to be cannulated. Often one SVC (usually the right) can be cannulated and one (usually the left) can be snared without cannulation owing to the venous collateral network through facial and intracranial venous

connections. The pressure in the snared SVC above the snare should be measured to ensure that venous hypertension will not be an issue. This is done simply to limit the tubing and equipment in the operative field. The recipient cardiectomy is performed removing most of the right atrium and the entire cavopulmonary baffle. This is often difficult owing to the stiffness of the baffle (usually polytetrafluoroethylene [PTFE]) and the growth of the tissue into this. A small cuff of right atrial tissue may be left on the orifice of the IVC to provide a bit more length for this anastomosis. The SVCs may be handled in a couple of ways. Each of these will be presented separately.

The first method involves removing each SVC from its site of connection to the pulmonary artery with a plan of attachment to the donor innominate vein and right SVC. In most cases the pulmonary artery defects left will require patching with appropriate material rather than directly oversewn. The transplant procedure is modified to allow for an anastomosis between the innominate vein and the left SVC. This donor innominate vein is usually best positioned behind the ascending aorta rather than draped across the top of the aorta. The left SVC is in a somewhat posterior position as well. The

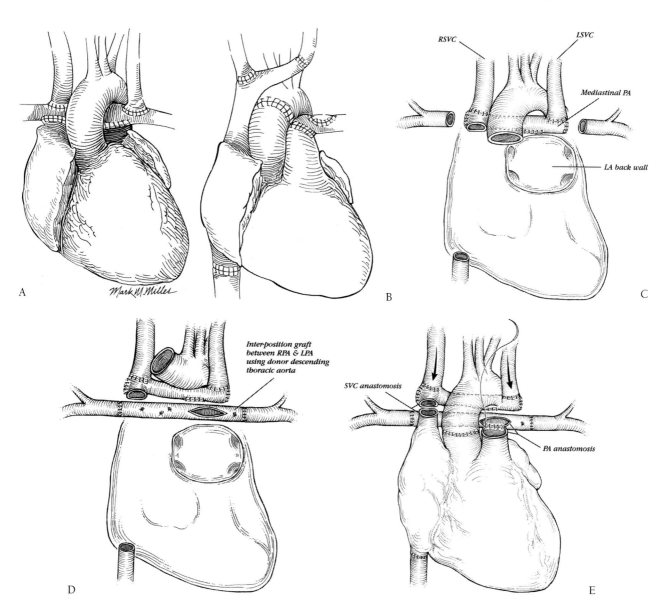

Figure 95-4.   Transplant for a failed Fontan procedure. **(A)** A patient after a total cavopulmonary connection in which there are bilateral superior venae cavae. Both superior venae cavae are anastomosed directly to the pulmonary artery, and the blood returning from the inferior vena cava is directed via an intra-atrial baffle to the cardiac end of the right superior vena cava, which is anastomosed to the underside of the right pulmonary artery. **(B)** By obtaining a long segment of the innominate vein from the donor, one can perform direct caval anastomoses to both the right and left superior venae cavae. Direct caval anastomosis is also performed to the inferior vena cava. The sites of the superior vena caval anastomoses to the pulmonary artery usually need to be patched with pericardium or other tissue obtained from the donor at the time of the harvest, such as additional aorta. **(C–E)** Another method of handling bilateral superior venae cavae after caval anastomoses to the pulmonary artery as either part of the Glenn procedure or Fontan procedure. The branch pulmonary arteries are divided just distal to the caval connections and the medial ends oversewn or patched. This intervening segment of pulmonary artery between the superior venae cavae in effect becomes the innominate vein. **(D)** The distal branch pulmonary arteries are connected with either a synthetic tube graft or the descending thoracic aorta harvested from the donor. This is sewn end to end to both distal pulmonary arteries in the hilar regions. An opening in this interposition graft is placed appropriate for the anastomosis of the donor main pulmonary artery. **(E)** The donor heart is then sewn in place with the donor superior vena cava sewn to the underside of what was the right pulmonary artery, the donor pulmonary artery is sewn to the appropriate location on the graft connecting the distal branch pulmonary arteries, the donor and recipient inferior vena cava is connected, and the left atrial anastomosis is performed as it usually would be (La = left atrium; LPA = left pulmonary artery; LSVC = left superior vena cava; PA = pulmonary artery; RPA = right pulmonary artery; RSVC = right superior vena cava; SVC = superior vena cava.)

right SVC is anastomosed directly to the donor SVC, and the recipient IVC is attached to the donor IVC end to end. The donor main pulmonary artery is connected to the mediastinal pulmonary artery using a relatively long segment of donor pulmonary artery.

Alternatively, the SVCs may be left attached to the recipient pulmonary artery, and this intervening segment of mediastinal pulmonary artery can become the "innominate vein." This then requires reconstruction of the mediastinal pulmonary arteries with donor pulmonary artery, donor descending thoracic aorta, or synthetic tube graft. The advantage of leaving the SVCs connected to the recipient pulmonary artery is that it avoids the tedious nature of an anastomosis of a very thin-walled, fragile vein to another, risking suture line anastomotic stenosis and possibly occlusion. The disadvantage is that the reconstruction involves anastomoses to both branch pulmonary arteries in the hilar regions. If the donor aortic segment or synthetic tube graft is used for the pulmonary artery reconstruction, however, this can be performed with the recipient heart out of the field and before the donor heart being inserted into the field. This simplifies the connections considerably and makes the remainder of the transplant procedure more straightforward.

In the presence of a "classic" Glenn shunt (where the pulmonary arteries are rendered discontinuous), the pulmonary artery reconstruction will nearly always require an additional segment of donor vascular tissue for an interposition graft. Again, either a long segment of donor right pulmonary artery or a segment of the donor descending aorta will frequently be available and relatively simple to harvest. Generally speaking, the pulmonary artery reconstruction/anastomoses should be performed before the aortic anastomoses for optimal visualization.

Situs Inversus

Patients with situs inversus may present for transplantation because of associated severe congenital cardiac defects such as single-ventricle physiology with failed Fontan or occasionally with an isolated cardiomyopathy and no other anomalies. In either instance, this entity is a significant technical challenge primarily related to handling of the systemic venous return. Certainly the expectation of finding a donor with situs inversus and an otherwise normal heart is extremely low, given that it is estimated to occur at a rate of only 2 per 10,000 population. Thus, techniques designed to modify the recipient so that a heart with normal situs may be implanted are necessary.

Donor Operation

Donor procurement depends on how the surgeon specifically plans to handle the systemic and pulmonary venous connections as well as the needs based on associated anomalies and prior palliative procedures. To allow for greatest flexibility, the harvest should include all of the SVC and a long segment of innominate vein. If the recipient has had a prior Fontan or Glenn procedure, harvest of as much mediastinal pulmonary artery or descending thoracic aorta should be performed.

Recipient Operation

Cannulation directly into the SVC and IVC at points as far distant from the right atrium is advised (Fig. 95-5). The aorta should be cannulated in a distal location as well. The incision in the right atrium is near the atrioventricular groove, leaving sufficient amount of tissue for the modifications necessary for implantation of the donor heart. The incision in the left atrium is also near the atrioventricular groove. As much of the atrial septum as possible should be left behind. The pulmonary artery is transected close to the bifurcation. The aorta is transected distally to move the anastomosis closer to the midline.

One acceptable technique for implantation of the donor heart is reminiscent of the Senning procedure for transposition of the great arteries. The atrial septum of the donor is mobilized by dividing it at its caudad and cephalad portions. It is then reattached to the free wall of the left atrium anterior to the right-sided pulmonary veins. When an atrial septal defect is present, pericardium or prosthetic patch material may be used in addition to or in place of the atrial septal tissue. This directs the pulmonary venous return from the right lung to the left across the midline. The interatrial groove is then mobilized extensively. An atriotomy is placed anterior to the left-sided pulmonary veins. The left atrial anastomosis is thus placed on the left side of the mediastinum. It is usually necessary to perform the right atrial anastomosis next. A portion of the left superior aspect of the new right atriotomy can be closed primarily to move more of this anastomosis to the right and to better match the size of the donor right atrial cuff. The recipient pulmonary artery is usually positioned to the patient's right. This can be effectively moved to the left by mobilizing the branches or by extending the arteriotomy out onto the left pulmonary artery while partially closing the right side. The pulmonary artery anastomosis should be performed before the aortic anastomosis so that the pulmonary artery can be accurately seen. The aortic anastomosis is performed in the usual fashion.

There are other techniques (not illustrated) that may be applied and may serve as better options, depending on the associated anomalies. The first of these is a modification of that described previously in which the atrial groove is dissected extensively and split so that two separate atria result. Frequently the anterior portion of the atrial septum is too thin to precisely split; in that case the septum should be devoted to the pulmonary venous atrium. These two atrial orifices are then transposed, moving the systemic (left-sided) atrium anterior and to the right and moving the pulmonary (right-sided) atrium posterior and to the left. The SVC and IVC need to be extensively mobilized—dividing the azygous vein above and mobilizing subdiaphragmatic veins below. The atrial and arterial connections are then performed as described previously.

The next modification is based on the principle of devoting the atrial mass to the pulmonary venous connection and reestablishing systemic venous flow with bicaval anastomoses. This may be the preferred technique when the patient has undergone palliation for associated single-ventricle physiology or other major intracardiac anomalies, particularly one of the heterotaxy syndromes. Cannulation in the SVC must be at or above the entry of the innominate vein and in the inferior vena cava below the diaphragm. The left-sided SVC is removed by transecting it at its junction with the heart and just below the entry of the innominate vein. The short segment is then anastomosed to the innominate vein on the patient's right side. The donor SVC can then be anastomosed to the newly constructed right-sided SVC; alternatively, a long segment of donor SVC may be anastomosed directly to the innominate vein on the right side. The IVC is effectively moved across the midline to the right by using a flap of right atrial tissue. The inferolateral portion of the right atrium is separated from the left atrium, and the septum is resected. The incision in the right atrium is carried down into the IVC orifice medially to the level of the junction of the pericardium with the diaphragm. From there the IVC is then sewn to the pericardium to create a tunnel, which continues across the midline using the flap of right atrium to continue on to the right, where the donor IVC can be sewn to this

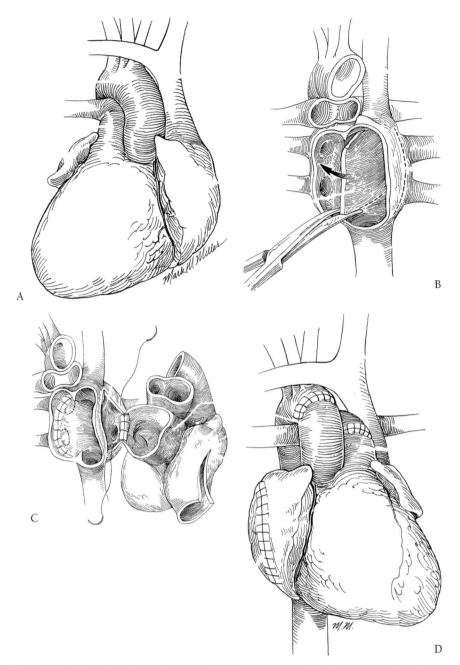

Figure 95-5. Transplant for situs inversus. **(A)** The appearance of the heart in a patient with situs inversus. The superior vena cava and inferior vena cava enter the right atrium on the left side, and the left atrium is on the right side of the patient. **(B)** The recipient cardiectomy has been performed, leaving as much of the atrial wall and septum as possible. The atrial septum is mobilized by incising it at its cephalad and caudad attachments. The dashed line in the atrial groove is the site of the left atriotomy for the left atrial anastomosis. **(C)** The cut edge of the atrial septum is sewn to the left atrial free wall anterior to the entrance of the pulmonary veins on the right. The atrial groove is extensively dissected out, and an atriotomy is placed anterior to the pulmonary veins on the left. The donor heart is then sewn in place beginning with the left atrial anastomosis to the new atriotomy anterior to the pulmonary veins on the left. The right atrial anastomosis is placed to the newly created right atrium. This may be made easier by partially closing the new right atrial orifice by sewing up the left superior corner near the entry of the superior vena cava. **(D)** The great artery anastomoses are performed in a fashion similar to that for congenitally corrected transposition of the great arteries. The pulmonary artery anastomosis may need to be performed before the aortic anastomosis so that it can be adequately seen. (IVC = inferior vena cava; LA = left atrium; RA = right atrium; SVC = superior vena cava.)

tunnel; some of the IVC is sewn to the pericardial portion of the newly created "tunnel." The left atrial anastomosis is carried out by using the lateral portion of the recipient right atrium as the left side of the anastomosis, and the rest is carried out in the usual fashion.

Heterotaxy Syndromes

Patients with heterotaxy syndromes (or splenic syndromes) have ambiguous visceral and atrial situs associated with anomalies of systemic and pulmonary venous drainage. Virtually all these patients have single-ventricle physiology and most have undergone prior palliative procedures. In addition, an endocardial cushion defect with its associated single common atrioventricular valve and large atrial septal defect is often present. This valve frequently becomes insufficient, resulting in either failed Fontan procedures or lack of candidacy for them, thus leading to transplantation as a treatment option. The key issue once again pertains to the venous drainage—either systemic or pulmonary. Anomalies of the pulmonary venous drainage are associated with both polysplenia and asplenia syndromes, although the extracardiac forms occur almost exclusively with the asplenia syndrome. Anomalies of the systemic venous drainage occur with both also, but they are more common with polysplenia, for which the vast majority of patients have bilateral SVCs with or without an interrupted IVC with azygous continuation. The hepatic veins may enter the atrium separately as well. It is crucial that both systemic and pulmonary venous drainage be carefully defined by cardiac catheterization, echocardiography, or other imaging studies such as computed tomography or magnetic resonance.

Donor Operation

This is performed much like that for situs inversus. Sufficient length of SVC is necessary to allow for flexibility in the transplant operation. Other considerations for the harvest of the great arteries depend on the associated anatomic defects and prior palliative procedures. The left atrial portion of the harvest does not need to be altered significantly. Although it may be more convenient to obtain the entire left atrium including the orifices of the pulmonary veins, this would preclude lung harvest for transplantation of this organ into another recipient. It is entirely possible to perform isolated heart transplantation in these patients with only a small left atrial cuff from the donor.

Recipient Operation

The transplant procedure should in general be based on the principle of devoting the atrial mass to the pulmonary atrial anastomosis and connecting the venae cavae by direct anastomoses. The illustrations provided are for a patient with total anomalous pulmonary venous connection to the right SVC and a midline IVC (Fig. 95-6). The SVC is of necessity very large just as it enters a large common atrium, which these patients frequently have. Cannulation is high in the SVC (well above the entry for the pulmonary veins) and very low in the IVC. The heart is excised with an atrial incision that proceeds around the heart near the atrioventricular groove. The SVC is divided below the cannula and above the entry of the pulmonary veins, and the cardiac end is then oversewn. The IVC is separated from the atrium, leaving a short cuff of atrium attached for added length. This leaves only the pulmonary venous drainage to empty into the atrial mass. This very large atrial orifice frequently needs to be reduced in size by sewing up the corners or by any other method deemed suitable as long as it puts the "left atrial" opening generally to the left of the midline. The transplant is then performed beginning with the left atrial anastomosis. The connections for the pulmonary artery and aorta depend on the associated anomalies but are generally not difficult to accomplish. Finally, the systemic venous connections are made with caval anastomoses.

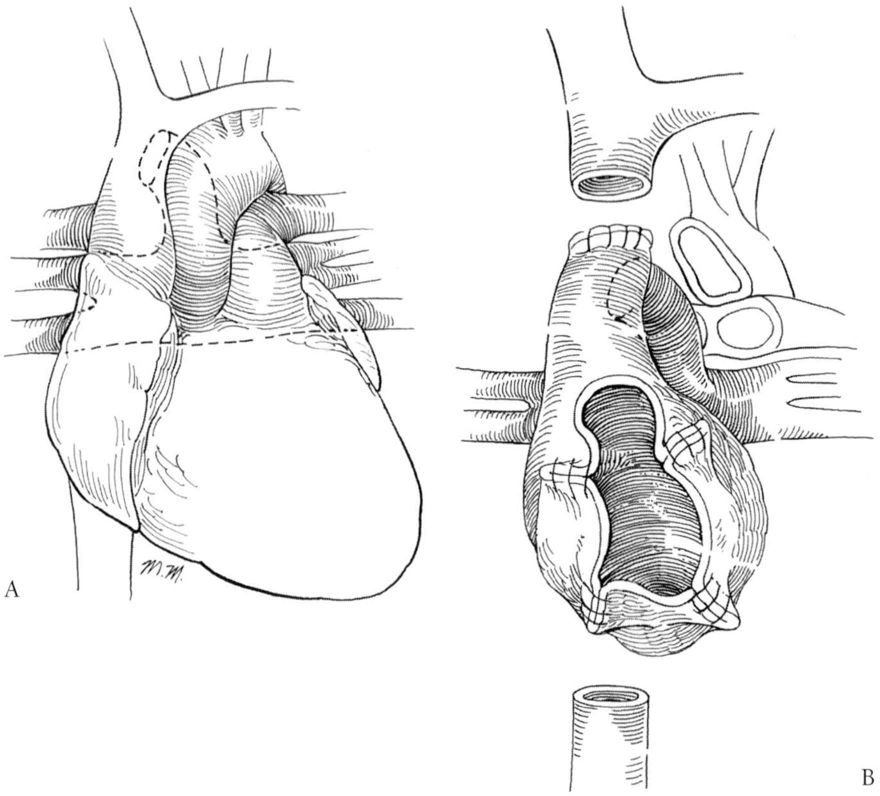

Summary

There are no anatomic contraindications to heart transplantation. Any anomaly has a suitable means of implantation of the donor heart, although it may be necessary to alter the recipient anatomy and donor procurement to meet the individual needs. In addition, heart transplantation can be successfully performed in the presence of situs inversus totalis. It is essential that a full anatomic evaluation of the recipient be performed in addition to a careful review of prior operative reports so that appropriate plans can be made for donor procurement as well as the transplant procedure itself. The surgeon should have thorough understanding of congenital heart disease and experience in the various palliative and corrective procedures employed therein.

SUGGESTED READING

Allard M, Assaad A, Bailey L, et al. Surgical techniques in pediatric heart transplantation. J Heart Lung Transplant 1991;10(Part 2): 808.

Bailey LL, Concepcion W, Shattuck H, et al. Method of heart transplantation for treatment of hypoplastic left heart syndrome. J Thorac Cardiovasc Surg 1986;92:1.

Doty DB, Renlund DG, Caputo GR, et al. Cardiac transplantation in situs inversus. J Thorac Cardiovasc Surg 1990;99:493.

Kawaguchi A, Gandjbakhch I, Pavie A, et al. Cardiac transplant recipients with preoperative pulmonary hypertension. Circulation 1989;80(Suppl III):90.

Michler RE, Rose EA. Pediatric heart and heart-lung transplantation. Ann Thorac Surg 1991;52:708.

Mitchell MB, Campbell DN, Boucek MM. Heart transplantation for the failing Fontan circulation. Semin Thorac Cardiovasc Surg Pediatr Card Surg Annu 2004;7:56.

Razzouk AJ, Gundry SR, Chinnock RE, et al. Orthotopic transplantation for total anomalous pulmonary venous connection associated with complex congenital heart disease. J Heart Lung Transplant 1995;14:713.

Vouhe PR, Tamisier D, Le Bidois J, et al. Pediatric cardiac transplantation for congenital heart defects: surgical considerations and results. Ann Thorac Surg 1993;56:1239.

Figure 95-6. Transplant for heterotaxy syndrome with anomalous pulmonary venous drainage. **(A)** Total anomalous pulmonary venous drainage to the right superior vena cava. The course of the pulmonary veins behind the heart is shown by a series of dashed lines. The superior vena cava is enlarged. The inferior vena cava is in the midline. **(B)** The recipient cardiectomy has been performed, dividing the superior vena cava above the entry of the pulmonary veins and oversewing the cardiac end. The corners of the huge common atrial orifice are sewn up to diminish the size of the orifice and to move the orifice to the left. The inferior vena cava is separated from the atrial mass, leaving a small cuff of atrial tissue attached for added length.

EDITOR'S COMMENTS

As greater experience has been gained in transplantation of the heart in pediatric patients, especially those with congenital heart disease, it is apparent that virtually all anatomic malformations are amenable to orthotopic implantation of a donor heart. Abnormalities of systemic and pulmonary venous return can generally be addressed either by relocating the vessels or adding additional length from donor tissues. In addition, experienced congenital heart surgeons can use prosthetic materials to reconstruct most venous connections so that orthotopic implantation of the heart can be performed. One remaining concern exists in patients who have dextrocardia associated with either normal situs or situs inversus. Although successful orthotopic cardiac transplantation has been performed in patients with situs inversus, patients with dextrocardia and normal situs represent a situation in which the implantation of the heart in the pericardial space may produce rotation of the apex toward the right and can distort the septal position and tricuspid valve. This is less of an issue if there is cardiac enlargement and the pericardial space is large enough that the apex can assume a more normal location after transplantation. However, in children with a relatively normal heart size in whom transplantation is performed with situs inversus or dextrocardia, it may be necessary to excise a portion of anterior pericardium on the left to allow the apex of the heart to sit in the left chest.

As cardiac transplantation becomes more commonly applied in children with congenital heart disease, the need for donor organs increases. The success of reconstructive procedures for congenital heart disease has created a fairly large population of children and young adults with complex cardiac reconstructions, a significant proportion of whom may ultimately require cardiac replacement. Thus, children, particularly those in the early teenage group, often present for cardiac replacement at a time when donor organs of suitable size for adult recipients are becoming increasingly infrequent. The use of assist devices such as implantable left ventricular or right ventricular assist pumps and total cardiac replacements needs to be extended to the pediatric population to permit survival while these patients are awaiting a donor organ. In most pediatric heart transplant centers, the average waiting time for donor organs has progressively increased, and many patients coming to transplant are on some form of assist.

ECMO has been the primary method of ventricular assistance in patients awaiting organ transplantation in the pediatric population until recently. Now, various pulsatile cardiac assist devices are becoming available for the pediatric population. Although the Thoratec and Heart Mate devices can be used in older children and adolescents, there is still a limitation on available devices in the Untied States for small infants and children. The new DeBakey Child Heart may permit fully implantable devices in smaller children, but it is not currently useful for infants and neonates. The availability of the Berlin Heart assist device in the United States has made it possible to bridge even neonates and small infants to heart transplantation over waiting times of several months. These devices have the advantage of multiple different sizes for the potential population of recipients. Nevertheless, all assist devices still have significant complication rates, with thrombosis, thromboembolism, and problems of anticoagulation being the primary issues.

Whereas 1-year survival after heart transplantation in children is approximately 80%, the results of the international heart and lung transplant registries suggest that 10-year survival of adult recipients will be approximately 30% to 40%. Thus, the long-term survival of patients after heart transplantation is still significantly lower than that of an age-matched population. It is therefore logical to attempt to preserve the native heart as long as possible if an adequate functional result is obtained in any patient with congenital heart disease. Cardiac transplantation can then be used as an additional palliative therapy after earlier palliative interventions have failed.

The approach to cardiac transplantation in infancy for children with hypoplastic left heart syndrome remains controversial. As more centers have achieved excellent results with staged palliative reconstructive operations, such as the Norwood procedure and ultimately Fontan reconstruction, it becomes increasingly difficult to justify the use of scarce donor organs for patients who have other surgical options. For these reasons, most centers, including ours, have abandoned cardiac transplantation as primary therapy for hypoplastic left heart syndrome. Reconstructive surgery with the Norwood operation has been extended to even infants of very low birth weight, and there has been no incremental increase in mortality with patients who have aortic and mitral atresia and an extremely diminutive ascending aorta. The early mortality of approximately 20% is comparable with the mortality on the waiting list for most centers that do primary transplantation for patients with hypoplastic left heart syndrome. Although the percentage of patients who will ultimately require transplantation after Fontan reconstruction is unknown, it is anticipated that the majority of transplants will not be re-quired until patients reach the teenage years at which time better availability of organs may occur. A particular concern in centers doing high-volume infant cardiac surgery is the need for cardiac transplantation in patients who failed an early reconstructive operation and require ECMO support for postoperative survival. These patients may be salvageable if a donor heart were to become available within a reasonably short time frame. Because of the limited availability of infant organs, such salvage of these critically ill patients is not currently likely. It is perhaps in these patients that the limited available infant organs should be preferentially used. Several centers have shown satisfactory results if transplantation can be performed in a timely fashion even in patients on ECMO support before transplant.

Because of the concerns of increasing waiting times for infants and neonates who may be unstable, there is increasing interest in the use of ABO-incompatible transplantation for these patients. The ability to use a non–ABO-compatible donor heart in infants extends the potential donors available and can potentially decrease the waiting time for some of the sickest patients. The early results with these techniques have been quite acceptable, with no increase in rejection episodes or early morbidity and mortality. The exact age at which ABO-incompatible transplantation can no longer be accomplished is not clearly delineated, but after 1 year of age, measurement of antibodies titer to other blood groups would appear to be appropriate.

One difficulty with transplantation of patients who have undergone staged reconstructive surgery for hypoplastic left heart syndrome and have developed contraindications to continuing down the single-ventricle repair pathway is that often allograft tissue is necessary for reconstruction of the aortic arch and pulmonary arteries. It has been demonstrated that implantation of allograft tissue can result in significant elevations of panel reactive antibodies (PRA), which can increase the difficulty in cross-matching donor heart to a recipient and increase the risk of early rejection or chronic rejection episodes. Complex strategies including plasmapheresis, and exchange transfusions may be necessary to permit transplantation with elevated PRA; clearly an increased incidence of rejection is a potential complication. Use of decellularized allograft material may decrease the risk of this complication; however the routine use of the decellularized allografts has not been advocated for staged reconstruction due to the friability of this tissue at second- and third-stage reconstruction, making the surgery more difficult at the time of reoperation.

The optimal implantation technique for orthotopic heart transplantation remains controversial. Caval anastomotic techniques have been associated with a lower incidence of tricuspid regurgitation and better atrial function after transplant and therefore may be preferred in most cases. The late incidence of caval stenosis in children has not been identified but potentially can be treated with balloon dilation or stenting if it occurs. The use of separate pulmonary venous anastomoses has been raised in adult cardiac transplantation in the hope of improving left atrial and mitral valve function; however, the use of separate pulmonary venous cuff anastomoses may be associated with greater risk of arrhythmia.

The immunosuppression regimen after pediatric cardiac transplantation is variable from one institution to another. There is no clearly accepted superior technique for immunosuppression. The majority of centers use a triple-drug technique of azathioprine or mycophenolate mofetil, cyclosporine or tacrolimus, and steroids. Steroid-free regimens have been promoted in the hope of increasing late linear growth. In most centers, attempts are made to wean infant patients from steroids 6 months after the transplant, beyond the period when most early rejection and infection episodes occur. Use of tacrolimus for primary immunosuppressive therapy rather than cyclosporine in infants and very young children decreases the risk of hirsutism and gingival hyperplasia, which can impede feeding.

Controversy remains regarding the level of pulmonary hypertension at which ortho-topic cardiac transplantation cannot succeed. Patients with significant transpulmonary gradients and elevations of pulmonary vascular resistance may have satisfactory results from orthotopic cardiac transplantation if the pulmonary resistance is reversible. Hemodynamic evaluation is important to assess in each patient before listing for heart transplantation. In some patients with an elevated transpulmonary gradient but in whom primary left heart dysfunction is present, heterotopic heart transplantation can permit use of a heart transplant rather than a heart and lung transplant with acceptable outcome. The number of heterotopic heart transplants performed in children, however, is so few as to preclude any evaluation of long-term effectiveness of this therapy.

T.L.S.

96

Lung and Heart-Lung Transplantation in Children

Thomas L. Spray

Clinical heart-lung transplantation began in the late 1960s when the first heart-lung transplant was performed in an infant with an atrioventricular canal defect and pulmonary hypertension; the child died of pulmonary insufficiency 14 hours after the operation. The first clinical success was not achieved until 1981 when Reitz performed a heart-lung transplant in a 45-year-old patient with pulmonary hypertension. As success was achieved in adult patients, heart-lung transplantations were performed in an increasing number of pediatric patients, from only a few in 1984 to as many as 40 in 1988. Successful clinical use of isolated lung transplantation by Cooper in 1984 established the possibility of lung transplantation alone for certain forms of cardiopulmonary disease. These techniques were ultimately extended to the pediatric population, such that the use of heart-lung transplantation in children has gradually been restricted to children with irreparable cardiac defects associated with pulmonary disease, and isolated lung transplantation (either single or bilateral) has become an accepted modality of therapy for children with pulmonary vascular disease or primary pulmonary disease with reparable cardiac defects. By 1996, as many as 200 children younger than age 16 years had undergone single-lung or bilateral lung transplantation, approaching the total number of heart-lung transplantations that have been performed in the pediatric population.

Indications for Transplant

General indications for heart-lung or lung transplantation in pediatric recipients are similar to the indications in adults. End-stage restrictive or obstructive pulmonary disease or primary or secondary end-stage pulmonary vascular disease is the major indication. Some forms of secondary pulmonary vascular disease associated with correctable congenital heart defects can be considered for cardiac repair and lung transplantation if the cardiac repair is durable and not associated with significant inherent mortality. The presence of significant left ventricular dysfunction or cardiopulmonary defects that are uncorrectable or correctable only with a high likelihood of need for future surgical repair may best be treated by heart-lung transplantation.

Although general indications for lung transplantation are similar in adults and children, the types of pulmonary disease seen in children are different from those noted in adults. It is particularly important to note that obstructive pulmonary disease is extremely unusual in children. In addition, pulmonary fibrotic diseases (except for cystic fibrosis) are very unusual in children and often associated with previous therapy of underlying malignancies such as leukemia and lymphomas. This fact accounts for radiation fibrosis as a significant indication for lung transplantation in children.

Infectious complications are more common after cardiopulmonary and pulmonary transplantation than after solid-organ transplants. Of particular importance in pediatric recipients is the common occurrence of viral infections of the transplanted lungs. Children continue to be exposed to a wide range of viruses, including adenovirus and respiratory syncytial virus in addition to the influenza viruses. In addition, cytomegalovirus (CMV) infection is very common after pediatric lung transplantation because many children have not yet been exposed to CMV infection and active immunity is not present. An additional concern in children is the presence of Epstein-Barr virus (EBV). There is a higher incidence of seronegativity for this viral pathogen in children than in adults, and EBV infection can be quite subtle in early childhood, making diagnosis difficult. A significantly increased risk of associated lymphoproliferative disease in patients who have sustained an EBV infection after transplant has been reported, and lymphoproliferative disease may progress despite decreased immunosuppression in these children.

Children with cystic fibrosis represent the single largest group of pediatric patients who require lung or heart-lung transplantation. Most of these children are teenagers because the majority of cystic fibrosis patients survive to adulthood with intensive medical management. Indications for consideration of pulmonary or cardiopulmonary transplantation in cystic fibrosis include increasing hospitalization for antibiotic therapy, progressive weight loss in older patients or persistent lack of weight gain in younger patients despite nutritional supplementation, and an increase in oxygen dependence or hypercarbia with gradual deterioration of pulmonary function. In general, a forced expiratory volume in 1 second (FEV_1) of <30% of predicted values is a relative indication for transplantation.

Cardiopulmonary diseases requiring transplantation in infancy are rare but include congenital diaphragmatic hernia, surfactant protein deficiencies, pulmonary vein stenosis or veno-occlusive diseases, and primary pulmonary hypoplasia.

The indications for transplantation in children with pulmonary hypertension are somewhat subjective because of the poorly defined natural history of pulmonary hypertension, either primary or secondary, in this age group. Generally, indications for consideration for transplantation include progressive exercise intolerance, the onset of syncope, hemoptysis, angina pectoris, and significant right ventricular failure. These symptoms often are correlated with hemodynamic abnormalities, with elevations of right atrial pressure to >8 mm Hg with a decreased cardiac index and a total pulmonary vascular resistance of >20 Woods units/m². When the product of right atrial mean pressure and pulmonary vascular resistance index is >360, poor survival is expected, and transplantation is considered. Some children with significant pulmonary vascular disease may respond to vasodilators, including prostacyclin, and the use of chronic prostacyclin infusion may improve the stability of patients while they await suitable donor organs. In patients with Eisenmenger syndrome and a right-to-left cardiac shunt, the onset of severe polycythemia in association with hemoptysis, right ventricular failure, or progressive exercise intolerance may be considered a relative indication for transplantation.

A particularly difficult subgroup of patients who are considered for lung or heart-lung transplantation comprises those with pulmonary vein stenosis and pulmonary veno-occlusive disease. These children are often extremely unstable and the pulmonary hypertension severe. Because delivery of blood to the left ventricle is limited in these patients, there has been a high incidence of death while awaiting organs, and therefore these children should be listed early in the course of their disease after diagnosis. Although it is possible to use chronic ventilation, nitric oxide therapy, and even extracorporeal membrane oxygenation as bridges to lung transplantation or cardiopulmonary transplantation in children, patients with pulmonary vein stenosis are often unable to be adequately resuscitated with chest compressions while extracorporeal membrane support is initiated because of the inability to get adequate blood flow to the left ventricle to provide cerebral blood flow during the arrest.

Contraindications to Transplantation

Contraindications to transplantation are primarily mechanical. Patients with severe scoliosis or restrictive chest wall mechanics may have chronic hypoventilation even if normal lungs are implanted. Significant as-

sociated metabolic diseases including renal insufficiency or uncontrolled diabetes are relative contraindications to transplantation, and patients with portal hypertension and biliary cirrhosis may also be considered poor candidates for cardiopulmonary transplantation alone. Patients who have had multiple prior surgical procedures involving the pleural spaces require more complicated operations for implantation of donor organs. This is a particular problem in patients with chronic cyanosis, who may have multiple and extensive collateral vessels in the adhesions from previous surgeries that may be difficult or impossible to control at the time of transplant. Severe and even fatal bleeding complications have been noted in these patients in our series. High-dose steroid dependence is a relative contraindication to transplantation because of poor healing or sepsis. However, moderate doses of steroids have not been considered a contraindication in our experience. A long-standing history of noncompliance with medical interventions by the patient or the family may be considered a relative contraindication to undertaking a procedure of such magnitude. Uncontrolled collagen vascular disease and ongoing malignancy also are contraindications to consideration for transplantation.

Selection of Operative Procedure

The majority of transplantations performed in children have been by the heart lung en bloc technique. Whereas it is apparent that comparable results can be obtained with heart-lung or lung transplantation in many children, the need to maximize the availability of scarce donor organs and use the heart for other patients has produced a gradual decrease in the use of combined heart-lung transplantation for primary pulmonary diseases. Most heart-lung transplantation is now reserved for patients with uncorrectable congenital heart defects associated with severe pulmonary vascular disease in patients with elevated pulmonary resistance alone. Heterotopic heart transplantation may be used in some children with elevated pulmonary resistance in whom improvement in pulmonary resistance can be anticipated with improvement in cardiac output. We use heart-lung transplantation for only those children with congenital heart disease who have poor chance of long-term correction or those children with severe left or biventricular dys-

function. Pulmonary transplantation with preservation of the native heart is preferred in children with cystic fibrosis or other septic lung diseases, patients with pulmonary fibrosis, or children with primary or secondary pulmonary vascular disease associated with normal ventricular function and a relatively simple or correctable congenital heart defect. Even children with severe right ventricular dysfunction are considered candidates for pulmonary transplantation alone if the right ventricular ejection fraction is >10% and tricuspid valve insufficiency is graded less than severe. Patients with repairable cardiac defects can receive cardiac repair and lung transplantation alone, and our experience includes children with atrial septal defect, ventricular septal defect, patent ductus arteriosus, vascular rings, atrioventricular canal defects, pulmonary vein stenosis, peripheral pulmonary arterial stenosis, and pulmonary atresia with nonconfluent pulmonary arteries in addition to children with anomalies of pulmonary venous return.

An additional consideration in pediatric patients is the preference of single-lung or bilateral sequential lung transplantation. In children with cystic fibrosis, bilateral lung transplantation is preferred to remove the infected lungs and decrease the sources of potential sepsis. A similar consideration is given to patients with chronic bronchiectasis who may be best served by bilateral sequential transplantation and removal of infection sources in the lungs. Single-lung transplantation is a possibility in patients with pulmonary fibrosis and pulmonary vascular disease. Although there have been successful series of single-lung transplantations for primary and secondary pulmonary hypertension, these reports have suggested that the postoperative course is more complicated in such patients. The entire cardiac output is delivered to the transplanted lung if single-lung transplantation is used in the presence of severe pulmonary vascular disease. Thus, patients may be unstable in the postoperative period and have additional instability when infection, rejection, or bronchiolitis obliterans occurs in the transplanted lung. We therefore prefer bilateral sequential lung transplantation in most children with pulmonary vascular disease to improve postoperative stability and the distribution of pulmonary blood flow. In addition, the use of bilateral sequential transplantation in younger children and infants allows for maximum possible growth and development of the lungs. Single-lung transplantation is still considered in children with primary pulmonary hypertension in whom there is a relative contraindication to entering one pleural space, such as those children who have had multiple previous thoracotomies with cyanosis.

Donor Selection

Donors for cardiopulmonary or pulmonary transplantation are uncommon compared with donors for other organs. Only 10% to 15% of cardiac donors may be suitable for donation of a heart-lung block or lungs. This rarity reflects the damage often done to the lungs during gastric aspiration, at trauma, or with a sudden neurologic event. In addition, severe pulmonary edema from either neurogenic or cardiac cause can affect oxygen exchange of the potential donor lungs. General criteria for pulmonary donors includes normal gas exchange with an arterial partial pressure of oxygen (PaO_2) of >100 mm Hg on 40% oxygen and 5-cm positive end-expiratory pressure. A clear chest x-ray film, age younger than 45 years, and normal findings on electrocardiograms and echocardiograms are criteria for cardiopulmonary and pulmonary donors. A history of pulmonary disease or prolonged smoking or asthma is a relative contraindication for donation. In addition, demonstrated aspiration of gastric contents, contamination of the tracheobronchial tree, or severe lung contusion are considered contraindications to donor use. In some cardiopulmonary donors, the requirement of very high dose inotropic drugs in the face of suitable fluid management or significant ventricular hypertrophy or dysfunction on an echocardiogram is considered a contraindication to using the combined heart-lung block.

As in all organ donation, the presence of human immunodeficiency virus or hepatitis A or B is a contraindication for use of donor organs. Hepatitis C organs may be used in a hepatitis C–positive recipient and in some cases may be used if the severity of the condition of the recipient warrants the risk of hepatitis C transmission. Although it is generally advisable to match CMV-seropositive donors with CMV-positive recipients, successful transplantation is not precluded with CMV mismatching. CMV prophylaxis is routinely used after transplantation, and CMV infection usually is adequately treated if it occurs. Although donor criteria may be unsuitable, with aggressive donor management many unsuitable organs may be rendered usable. Careful evaluation of each potential donor is therefore important to maximize the availability of suitable donor organs. Size matching between donor and recipient is important in pediatric lung and heart-lung transplantation. For heart-lung transplantation, it is desirable to have the donor weight within 20% to 30% of the weight of the recipient. Although it is possible in cardiac transplantation to use hearts of donors several times the body weight of the recipient, the fact that excessive lung size may compress the heart limits the size discrepancy that is acceptable for combined heart-lung transplantation in children. Donor–recipient size matching is more liberal when double-lung or single-lung transplant is contemplated. Because the lungs have the capacity to expand to fill chest cavities of significantly larger recipients, it is possible to use smaller donor lungs than the recipient's. In addition, it is possible to use large donor lungs and use lobes or trim portions of the parenchyma of the lungs to allow them to fill the chest cavity without impinging on cardiac function. Bronchial size match between donor and recipient is better correlated with height and age than with weight. Thus, most patients are listed for lung transplantation with a size range of 3 in. to 4 in. above and below the size of the recipient. However, heights of twice the size of the recipient can be considered if lobes are to be used from larger donors.

Organ Procurement

Bronchoscopy is preferable at the time of lung procurement. The presence of direct trauma to the lungs or pulmonary contusions should be evaluated before the heart-lung or lung block is removed. The donor receives methylprednisolone and antibiotics and is heparinized before organ procurement. The technique of organ procurement from pediatric donors is similar to that in adults except that the volumes of cardioplegic and pulmonoplegic solutions are adjusted for the weight of the donor. Cardioplegic solution is given for a total dose of approximately 20 mL/kg of donor weight and pulmonoplegic solution from 25 to 40 mL/kg of donor weight. Crystalloid cardioplegic solution and Euro-Collins or University of Wisconsin pulmonoplegic solution has been used in most centers for organ preservation.

When a heart-lung block is harvested for a single recipient, the cardioplegic solution is administered into the aorta and pulmonoplegic solution administered directly into the pulmonary artery with venting of the heart by division of the left atrial appendage. Division of the inferior vena cava at the diaphragm permits evacuation of cardioplegic solution without ventricular distention. The trachea is mobilized above the level of the carina, and minimal dissection of the carina is done. The lungs are then gently inflated and the trachea stapled. The superior vena cava is ligated and divided and the esophagus mobilized in the superior mediastinum and stapled and divided. The aorta is transected at the level of the innominate artery, and the distal aorta in the posterior pericardial space is mobilized and ligated and divided also. If additional aortic length is necessary, the aorta is not transected, but the arch vessels are divided individually. With incision of the pleura at the paraspinal region bilaterally, the entire heart-lung block is then excised in toto and the esophagus then removed from the specimen away from the operative field. If the heart and lung are to be harvested separately, cardioplegic and pulmonoplegic solutions are administered as in the combined heart-lung technique; however, the interatrial groove is developed, and then the heart is excised by division of the aorta and pulmonary artery, leaving the bifurcation of the pulmonary artery for the lung. The left atrium is then excised with a limited left atrial cuff, leaving as much as possible of the pulmonary venous confluence bilaterally for the lung implantation. The superior and inferior venae cavae are divided at the pericardial reflection, and the lung block is excised as in the heart-lung block by division of the trachea with the lungs and gentle inflation after the esophagus is stapled proximally and distally. The heart-lung block or lung blocks are then placed in iced saline solution in sterile bags and transported to the recipient center in ice. Although some groups have used cardiopulmonary bypass for cooling of the entire heart-lung block, this technique is not widely used in the United States. Preservation times of >9 hours for lung transplantation have satisfactorily been achieved with the use of these techniques.

Recipient Operation

It is particularly important to take care in the removal of the recipient organs for heart-lung or lung transplantation to obtain absolute hemostasis in the mediastinum and pleural spaces and to avoid injury to the thoracic nerves including the phrenic, recurrent laryngeal, and vagus nerves. The bilateral thoracosternotomy (clamshell incision) (Fig. 96-1, inset) allows excellent access to the pleural spaces for takedown

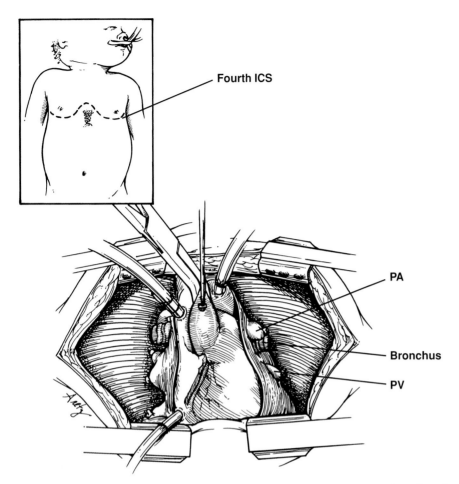

Fourth ICS

PA

Bronchus

PV

Figure 96-1. The right and left lungs are removed sequentially with ligation of the branches of the pulmonary arteries and veins and stapling and division of the bronchus. The bronchial stump is left stapled, the bronchus is divided distal to the staple line, and the lungs are excised. The patient is on cardiopulmonary bypass, allowing removal of both lungs with support of the circulation. As is illustrated, a cross-clamp can be applied, cardioplegia induced, and the cardiac repair performed before lung implantation. **(Inset)** The clamshell thoracosternotomy incision. The incision is carried transversely in the midline as high as possible to allow adequate sternum for sternal stability after rewiring with chest closure. The fourth intercostal space (ICS) is opened bilaterally and the incision carried out into the axillae. The incision in the chest can be carried more inferiorly because the trap door–like opening of the clamshell incision allows greater superior mobility than inferior mobility. It is therefore imperative not to enter the chest too high or dissection of the lungs will be impeded near the pulmonary veins and inferior pulmonary ligaments. (PA = pulmonary artery; PV = pulmonary vein.)

of adhesions and aids in obtaining hemostasis before implantation of the donor organs. When the clamshell incision is made, the incision needs to be carried as superiorly as possible in the midline so as to transect the sternum above the xiphoid to add stability of the sternal fragments when they are rewired after the procedure. Entrance in the fourth intercostal space is preferred; however, it is generally better to enter the chest more inferior than superior because the opening of the clamshell incision allows greater exposure in the superior mediastinum than it does inferiorly.

Heart-Lung Transplantation

The technical aspects of heart-lung implantation in children are similar to those used in adults. Cardiopulmonary bypass is used while the lungs are excised bilaterally. The phrenic nerves are carefully protected on a pedicle of pericardium, which is mobilized before the organs are removed. The lungs are excised individually with division of the mainstem bronchus, pulmonary artery, and pulmonary veins after ligation

and division of the vessels. After the lungs have been removed, the heart is excised, leaving a cuff of right atrium and distal aorta for implantation of the new organs. A portion of the wall of the left pulmonary artery can be left in situ to avoid dissection around the recurrent laryngeal nerve on the left. After excision of the heart and each lung, the trachea is mobilized in the mediastinum behind the stump of aorta and divided approximately two rings above the carina. After meticulous hemostasis is obtained, the donor heart-lung block is placed in the mediastinum and the lungs passed behind the pedicles of pericardium containing the phrenic nerves. Anastomoses between the donor and recipient trachea, aorta, and right atrium are then accomplished with the patient on cardiopulmonary bypass and cannula placed in the superior and inferior venae cavae and caval tapes placed to eliminate venous return to the right atrium. In older children, the tracheal anastomosis can be accomplished with a running suture; however, our preference is to perform a running anastomosis of the membranous portion of the trachea and interrupted anastomosis of the cartilaginous portion anteriorly. We have used absorbable sutures in children in hopes of permitting better growth of the anastomoses. The aorta is then anastomosed with an absorbable running suture and the right atrium anastomosed between the donor and recipient. In most cases, separate superior vena caval and inferior vena caval anastomoses are used and the right atrium of the recipient is excised with the heart at the time of recipient preparation. Use of separate caval anastomoses tends to maintain better geometry of the right atrium and decrease the incidence of tricuspid regurgitation after transplantation. In very small children, however, caval anastomoses may lead to purse stringing of the suture line and obstruction, and therefore atrial anastomoses are used in very small infants. To prevent distention of the heart during reperfusion while rewarming before weaning from cardiopulmonary bypass, a vent is inserted through the amputated left atrial appendage into the heart.

Bilateral Sequential Lung Transplantation

The child is positioned supine and the shoulders elevated on a rolled towel. With this positioning, the entire chest can be prepared down to the axillae and draped as a sterile field (Fig. 96-1, inset). The transverse thoracosternotomy (clamshell incision) is made in the fourth intercostal space. The internal mammary pedicles are divided bilaterally. Chest retractors are placed in each thoracotomy incision, and the thymus is divided in the midline or resected completely if exposure of the superior mediastinum is poor. The pericardium is opened, and the heart is suspended with pericardial stay sutures. After heparinization, the aorta and right atrium are cannulated for bypass. We prefer to use cardiopulmonary bypass in all lung transplant procedures in children because of the ease with which bypass permits removal of the recipient lungs and the fact that after removal of both lungs the airway can be irrigated with antibiotic solution if necessary to decrease septic secretions. In addition, removal of both lungs before implantation decreases the ischemia time on the second implanted lung. In most pediatric patients, we use aprotinin to decrease bleeding complications.

Separate caval cannulation is used if heart-lung transplantation or cardiac repair is contemplated in addition to lung implantation. With the child on cardiopulmonary bypass and cooled to approximately 30°C, the lungs are removed bilaterally by ligation of the pulmonary artery branches, pulmonary venous drainage, and stapling of the right and left mainstem bronchi (Fig. 96-1). Care is taken to dissect around the bronchial stumps as minimally as possible to aid in revascularization of the bronchial anastomosis. The donor lung block is then brought to the field, and the right and left lungs are separated from the combined lung block by division of the bronchus approximately two rings from the take-off of the upper lobe orifices bilaterally. The pulmonary arteries are trimmed to appropriate length for suturing to the recipient, and the pulmonary venous confluence is divided by dividing the remnant of left atrium between the right and left pulmonary veins. The left lung is usually implanted first because traction on the heart may be necessary to aid in exposure, and, once the lung is implanted, the heart can then recover from any injury while the right lung is implanted. The bronchial stump on the left is cut as short as practical; however, generally the length of the left mainstem bronchus at implantation is longer than the right mainstem bronchus because it extends for a longer distance in the mediastinum. The bronchial anastomosis between donor and recipient is then created with running absorbable suture for the membranous bronchus and interrupted simple absorbable sutures for the cartilaginous bronchus (Fig. 96-2, inset B). An end-to-end

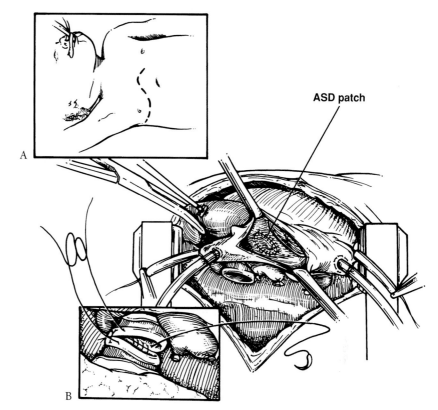

Figure 96-2. The aorta is cross-clamped and bicaval cannulation with caval tapes is used. With cardioplegia or fibrillatory arrest, the right atrium can be opened and an atrial septal defect (ASD) closed primarily or patched. Ventricular septal defects can be approached across the tricuspid valve through this incision and closed with a polyester (Dacron) patch. The atrium is then closed, and the heart is allowed to reperfuse during implantation of the lung. **(Inset A)** For single-lung transplantation and repair of intracardiac defects of the atrial or ventricular septum, a right anterior thoracotomy crossing the sternum can be used. Again, the sternum is transected as high as possible to aid in sternal stability postoperatively. The fourth intercostal space or fifth intercostal space is then opened and the pleura entered. **(Inset B)** The bronchial anastomosis is created using a running absorbable suture for the membranous portion of the bronchus and interrupted simple sutures for the cartilaginous bronchus without telescoping. In this way, an end-to-end anastomosis is created that allows the least chance for stenosis and granulation tissue at the suture line. No bronchial wrap is used, but peribronchial tissues may be tacked over the anastomosis if they are available.

anastomosis of the bronchus without telescoping of one bronchus into the other is used to prevent stenosis or malacia of the anastomosis. If a significant size discrepancy between donor and recipient bronchus is present, then minor telescoping of the bronchial anastomosis is accepted. The pulmonary arterial anastomosis is then created with a partial occlusion clamp on the pulmonary artery of the recipient, and a running absorbable suture is used to complete the anastomosis. The arterial clamp is left in place while the venous anastomosis is completed. A partial occlusion clamp is placed on the pulmonary vein confluence, the pulmonary vein confluence is opened widely between the stumps of the individually ligated upper and lower veins, and then a wide anastomosis is created with absorbable su-

ture. Just before completion of the venous anastomosis, venous return is permitted to the heart, the arterial clamp is released, and air is aspirated from the veins before opening of the lungs for reperfusion. The same technique is then used for implantation of the right lung. On the right, the stump of the right mainstem bronchus is generally cut within two to three rings of the carina to have the shortest distance for revascularization of the anastomosis. Protection of the bronchial suture lines is accomplished with peribronchial tissues tacked over the anastomosis with absorbable suture if such tissue is available. However, with suitable trimming of the recipient bronchus, the suture line will be retracted into the mediastinal tissues such that good revascularization and protection of the anastomosis is available. We have abandoned the use of pericardial pedicle wraps or omentum for bronchial wraps in children, and the incidence of bronchial complications has not increased by using an unprotected anastomotic technique.

If cardiac repair is to be performed in association with bilateral sequential lung transplantation, the patient is cannulated for bypass, the lungs are removed as noted earlier, and the aorta is cross-clamped and cardioplegic solution administered (Fig. 96-1). Closure of intracardiac defects is performed through the right atrium if possible to prevent ventricular incisions in patients with significant pulmonary hypertension in whom right ventricular function may be depressed. After completion of the cardiac repair, reperfusion of the myocardium is permitted while the sequential lung implantation is performed.

Single-Lung Transplantation

In children in whom only a single lung is required, the operation is performed either through a posterolateral thoracotomy on the transplant side or, more commonly, with the patient in a supine position and via a partial thoracosternotomy (Fig. 96-2, inset A). An anterior thoracotomy can be used, or the sternum can be crossed partially in the midline, allowing better access to the heart for cannulation and cardiopulmonary bypass. Closure of atrial septal and ventricular septal defects can be readily accomplished with this technique. The patient is placed on cardiopulmonary bypass with caval cannulation through the right chest and direct aortic cannulation. With cardioplegia, the right atrium can be opened and the atrial septum patched or primarily closed and ventricular septal defects approached across the tricuspid valve (Fig. 96-2). Explantation of the lung and implantation of the donor lung then proceeds as in bilateral sequential lung implantation.

Special Situations

Congenital pulmonary vein stenosis is an extremely rare condition in children but is associated with high mortality and is usually not amenable to direct surgical repair. These children often present with severe pulmonary hypertension, and it is not uncommon for transcatheter attempts at stabilization, including balloon dilation and stent implantation of the pulmonary veins,

to have been performed before referral of the children for lung transplantation. In addition, interventional techniques have been used to stabilize patients while they are awaiting donor organs because this subgroup of children has the highest mortality under such circumstances. Because these children have often had stents implanted in the pulmonary veins, the implantation of the donor lungs is altered. At the time of lung implantation on cardiopulmonary bypass, it is necessary to excise the pulmonary venous confluence bilaterally including the excision of the stents, which often extend into the left atrium. This can be accomplished in either of two ways: (1) by implanting the right and left lungs with bronchial and pulmonary arterial anastomoses and then subjecting the patient to a period of aortic cross-clamping and cardioplegia while the pulmonary venous confluence is excised bilaterally and the pulmonary venous confluence of the donor lung is implanted directly into the left atrium with a running suture line bilaterally or (2) if possible by implanting both lungs and completing all anastomoses under a single period of cardioplegia. The anastomoses in lung transplantation in very small children are simple and often require only 15 to 20 minutes per lung implant, and therefore a total period of cardioplegia may not exceed 40 to 50 minutes for the entire procedure. We have used both of these techniques for implantation in patients with pulmonary vein stenosis with equal success.

In children in whom a patent ductus arteriosus is associated with severe pulmonary hypertension, it is advisable to place the patient on cardiopulmonary bypass and to divide and oversew the ends of the ductus arteriosus rather than ligate the ductus in situ. The elevation in pressure during ligation may result in enough pressure on the suture line to allow recanalization, and division of the ductus ensures that recanalization will not occur.

A particular concern after cardiac repair at lung transplantation is the development of dynamic right ventricular outflow tract obstruction after the procedure. Many patients with elevated right ventricular pressure in the presence of shunt lesions such as ventricular septal defect or a large patent ductus arteriosus may have severe right ventricular hypertrophy that creates dynamic outflow tract obstruction when the right ventricular pressure drops after successful lung implantation. In severe cases, these patients may best be treated by patch augmentation of the right ventricular outflow tract, but in the majority of patients the avoidance of inotropic drugs postoperatively or use of

beta-blocking agents may be sufficient to relieve the dynamic obstruction in the early postoperative period. In the majority of patients, this dynamic obstruction will resolve spontaneously after several days.

An unusual subgroup of children who may require lung transplantation comprises those with pulmonary atresia with ventricular septal defect and nonconfluent pulmonary arteries. These children often have undergone multiple previous attempts at unifocalization operations to recreate a distal pulmonary vascular bed. Thus, many children will have had previous thoracotomies or median sternotomy incisions. In these children, typically the ascending aorta is markedly dilated and somewhat posteriorly located. Thus, the space available in the mediastinum for placement of the pulmonary arteries is limited, and placement behind the ascending aorta can result in compression of the right pulmonary artery by the dilated ascending aortic root. The operation is performed through the thoracosternotomy incision, as in bilateral sequential lung transplantation described earlier. The aorta is cross-clamped with the patient on bypass, and cardioplegia is induced. In this case, an incision is made in the right ventricular outflow tract to gain exposure to the ventricular septal defect, which is closed with a polyester (Dacron) patch (Fig. 96-3). A pulmonary homograft conduit is then sutured to the superior margin of the ventriculotomy incision and augmented with a gusset of polytetrafluoroethylene (PTFE) to allow a gentle take-off of the newly reconstructed right ventricular outflow tract from the right ventricle (Fig. 96-4). The remainder of the operation can then be performed with the heart reperfused and fibrillating at 18°C to 20°C or under continued cardioplegia. The lungs are then implanted sequentially as described earlier; however, the pulmonary artery anastomoses are performed last. After the bronchial and pulmonary venous anastomoses are completed, the pulmonary arteries are brought to the midline, either anterior or posterior to the ascending aorta. When brought anterior to the aorta, the pulmonary confluence is recreated in the midline with an absorbable suture posteriorly (Fig. 96-5). The reconstructed right ventricular outflow tract is then connected to the recreated pulmonary bifurcation with nonabsorbable suture because the homograft tissue is nonviable and growth is therefore not an issue (Fig. 96-6). After reconstruction, venous flow is returned to the lungs and air is evacuated through a vent in the left ventricle and from the ascending aorta to fully

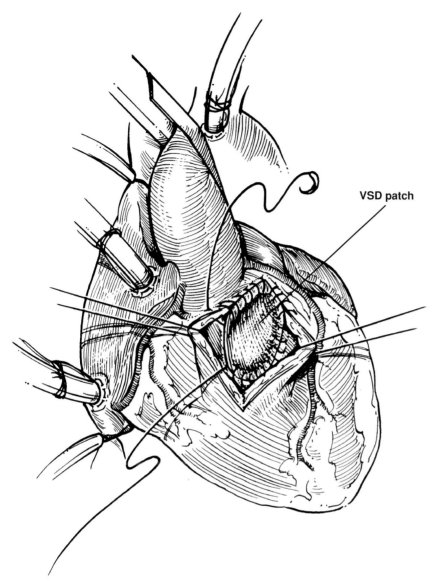

VSD patch

Figure 96-3. Technique for cardiac repair and lung transplantation for pulmonary atresia with ventricular septal defect (VSD) and nonconfluent pulmonary arteries. With the heart on cardiopulmonary bypass and under diastolic cardioplegia, a right ventriculotomy incision is made vertically, avoiding major epicardial coronary branches. Through this defect, the VSD is exposed and patched with a polyester (Dacron) patch. Running or interrupted mattress sutures can be used for placement of the patch, and in the posteroinferior aspect, care must be taken to avoid the conducting tissue if the defect is in the usual conoventricular location. Superiorly, the patch can be secured to the free margin of the ventriculotomy incision or to the conal septum. Care must be taken to ensure complete closure of the defect because reoperation for residual cardiac defects will be difficult in a patient on chronic immunosuppression.

de-air the heart before the patient is weaned from cardiopulmonary bypass.

Lobar Lung Transplantation

Because suitably sized donor lungs are often not readily available, techniques have been devised to use lung grafts of reduced size (lobes) for selected children. Cadaveric and living donor lobar transplants have now been performed with satisfactory results. The use of living donors for lobar lung transplantation has made donor organs available rapidly for children with very unstable conditions who might not survive waiting for suitable cadaveric organs to become available. In addition, the use of cadaveric lobes from larger donors has expanded the donor pool for infants and very young

children for whom identical-size donors are rare. Because lung growth can continue to late childhood, we generally prefer to use lobes from pediatric cadaveric donors for infants and very small children in the hope that additional lung growth of the donor lobe will continue. In older children, lobar transplants from adults may provide quite adequate alveolar volume even for continued growth despite the theoretical disadvantage of lack of additional donor lung alveolar growth. The indications for lobar lung transplantation and donor evaluation are similar to those for whole-lung transplant. Living donors, however, add additional concerns of donor evaluation. Both psychosocial and physiologic factors must be considered in these patients because the harvest of the lobe must result in the least possible morbidity to the donor. If bilateral lung implantation is contemplated, the larger donor generally is preferred for donation of the right lower lobe because the total lung volume is lower in this lobe than the left lower lobe.

Technique of Donor Lobectomy

If lobes are used from larger cadaveric lungs, variations in lobar anatomy can be addressed at the time of dissection away from the operative field and the most suitable lobes identified for implantation into the recipient. In general, we prefer to use lower lobes for implantation because of the geometric advantages of the shape of the lower lobes bilaterally and the relatively consistent bronchial and vascular anatomy. Often the right upper lobe has multiple lobar arterial branches that require reconstruction to create a single pulmonary artery for anastomosis to the recipient.

The right middle lobe is a relatively small amount of lung tissue for implantation and has variable venous drainage, which may complicate venous anastomosis and dissection. Use of a middle lobe from an adult to a young child or infant might be associated with poor lung growth because addition of alveolar number is unlikely to occur from an adult lung. For these reasons, we prefer to use lower lobes in most patients.

The technique of donor right lower lobectomy is shown in Fig. 96-7. A posterolateral thoracotomy is performed and the inferior pulmonary ligament taken down with electrocautery. Dissection in the fissure between the upper and lower lobes is created to identify the branches of the pulmonary artery to the right lower lobe and to define the take-off of the right middle lobe pulmonary artery branch. The pericardium is

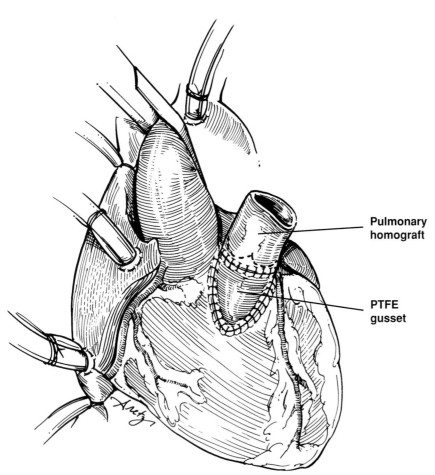

Pulmonary
homograft

PTFE
gusset

Figure 96-4.   After closure of the ventricular septal defect, a pulmonary homograft of the largest size that will fit in the chest cavity to allow for adequate growth of the recipient is selected and secured to the superior margin of the ventriculotomy incision with nonabsorbable suture. A gusset of polytetrafluoroethylene (PTFE) is used to create a gentle take-off of the conduit from the right ventricle. Care must be taken to obtain adequate hemostasis of this suture line to avoid late pseudoaneurysm formation.

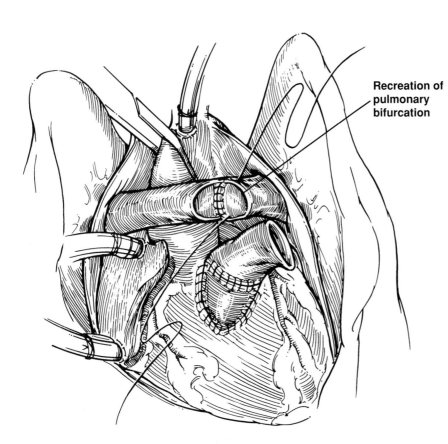

Recreation of
pulmonary
bifurcation

Figure 96-5.   If the aorta is large and posteriorly located, the pulmonary arteries are brought anterior to the aorta for reconstruction. The lungs are implanted bilaterally with bronchial and venous anastomoses and then the pulmonary arteries are brought anterior or posterior to the phrenic nerves to the ascending aorta and reapproximated in the midline.

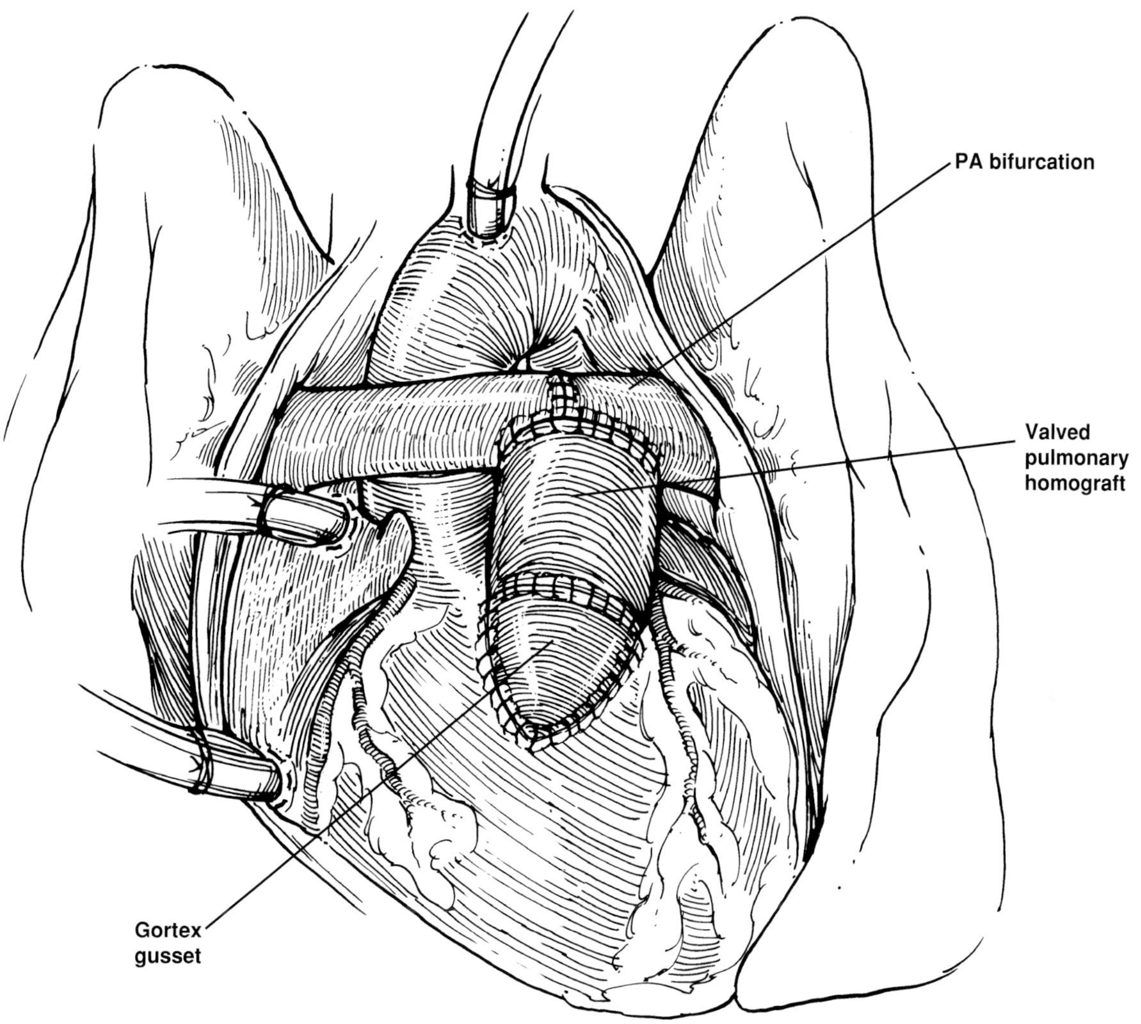

Figure 96-6. The reconstruction is completed by anastomosis of the pulmonary homograft reconstruction of the right ventricular outflow tract to the newly reconstructed pulmonary confluence anterior to the aorta. (PA = pulmonary artery.)

opened around the inferior pulmonary vein and the venous drainage from the middle lobe identified to ensure that it does not enter the inferior pulmonary vein directly. After heparinization, a vascular clamp can be placed below the take-off of the right middle lobe pulmonary artery, leaving a stump of pulmonary artery adequate for anastomosis to the recipient. A vascular clamp can then also be placed on the lower lobe pulmonary vein at its entrance to the left atrium with dissection in the interatrial groove to allow a suitable stump of tissue for oversewing of the venous entrance in the donor and leaving an adequate stump of pulmonary venous confluence for anastomosis to the recipient. The vessels are then divided, and the remaining fissures are divided with the stapler. After division of the pulmonary artery, the bronchus to the right lower lobe is dis-

sected as minimally as possible to preserve blood supply to the lobe. The middle lobe bronchus is identified, and the bronchus is divided with a scalpel. The donor lobe is then removed and taken away from the operative field for preparation and preservation. The pulmonary artery and left atrium are closed with running nonabsorbable suture, and the bronchus is closed with a stapler if adequate length is available or with simple nonabsorbable sutures. A pleural flap can be used to cover the bronchial stump if necessary.

The technique of donor left lower lobectomy is illustrated in Fig. 96-8. Again, the inferior pulmonary ligament is divided, and the pulmonary artery is dissected within the fissure to identify the lingular and lower lobe branches. The pericardium is opened around the inferior pulmonary vein, and fis-

sures are completed with a stapler. With the patient heparinized, a clamp is placed on the pulmonary artery proximal to the take-off of the superior segment of the lower lobe. Either lingular pulmonary arterial branches are preserved after removal of the donor lobe or small branches are ligated and divided, sacrificing some blood supply to segmental lingular vessels. The pulmonary vein is clamped and divided, and then the bronchus to the left lower lobe is exposed behind the pulmonary artery. Once the lingular bronchus is identified, the main bronchus is transected obliquely with care taken to include the superior segmental bronchus in the donor lobe, leaving a 2-mm to 3-mm rim of bronchus above the take-off of the superior segmental lobar branch. The pulmonary artery is then oversewn with nonabsorbable suture, or a pericardial patch is used if

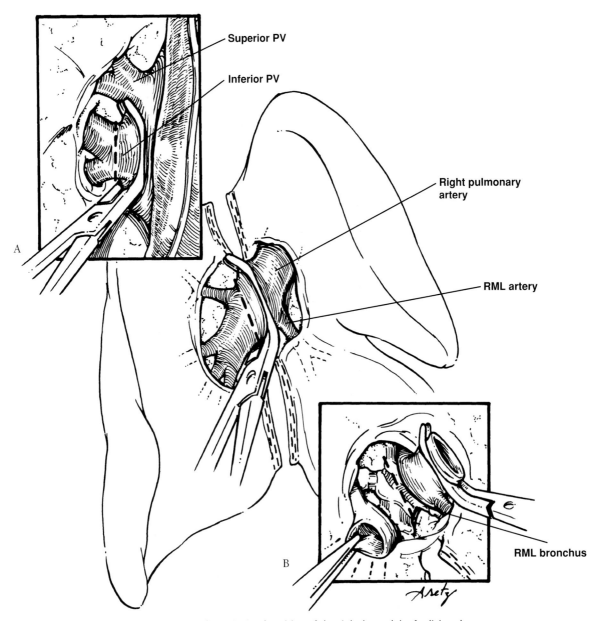

Superior PV

Inferior PV

Right pulmonary artery

RML artery

A

B

RML bronchus

Figure 96-7.   Technique for dissection and excision of the right lower lobe for living donor lobectomy. The pulmonary artery is exposed in the fissure, and dissection is completed to allow identification of the right middle lobe (RML) pulmonary artery. Mobilization of the pulmonary artery is then performed so that a vascular clamp can be applied just distal to the takeoff of the middle lobe vessel. The fissures are completed with staplers and before placement of clamps. **(Inset A)** The pulmonary venous dissection is created by takedown of the pericardial reflection and isolation of the right lower lobe pulmonary venous confluence. Care must be taken to identify the middle lobe vein entrance into the upper lobe bifurcation or the superior aspect of the lower lobe and to protect this venous drainage if at all possible. Heparinization of the donor is then performed, a clamp is placed on the pulmonary artery and pulmonary venous confluence, and the artery and vein are divided. **(Inset B)** With retraction of the stumps of the pulmonary artery, the bronchus is identified and the bronchus divided just distal to the take-off of the middle lobe bronchus. The donor lobe is then removed for preservation, and the vessels and bronchus are oversewn. (PV = pulmonary vein.)

necessary to maintain patency of the lingular segment. The left atrium is closed with nonabsorbable suture, and the bronchial stump is closed with interrupted nonabsorbable suture and covered as in the right donor lobectomy.

Preservation of the living donor lobes is performed by infusion of pulmonoplegic solution in the pulmonary artery until the venous effluent is clear. Gentle inflation can be used during flushing to aid in evacuation of any residual blood. Prostaglandin E_1 may ei-

ther be added to the pulmonoplegic solution or infused in the donor before lobectomy. Because of the anticipated short ischemia time on donor lobes, gentle inflation and clamping of the bronchus during transport can be used, or the lungs can be left uninflated

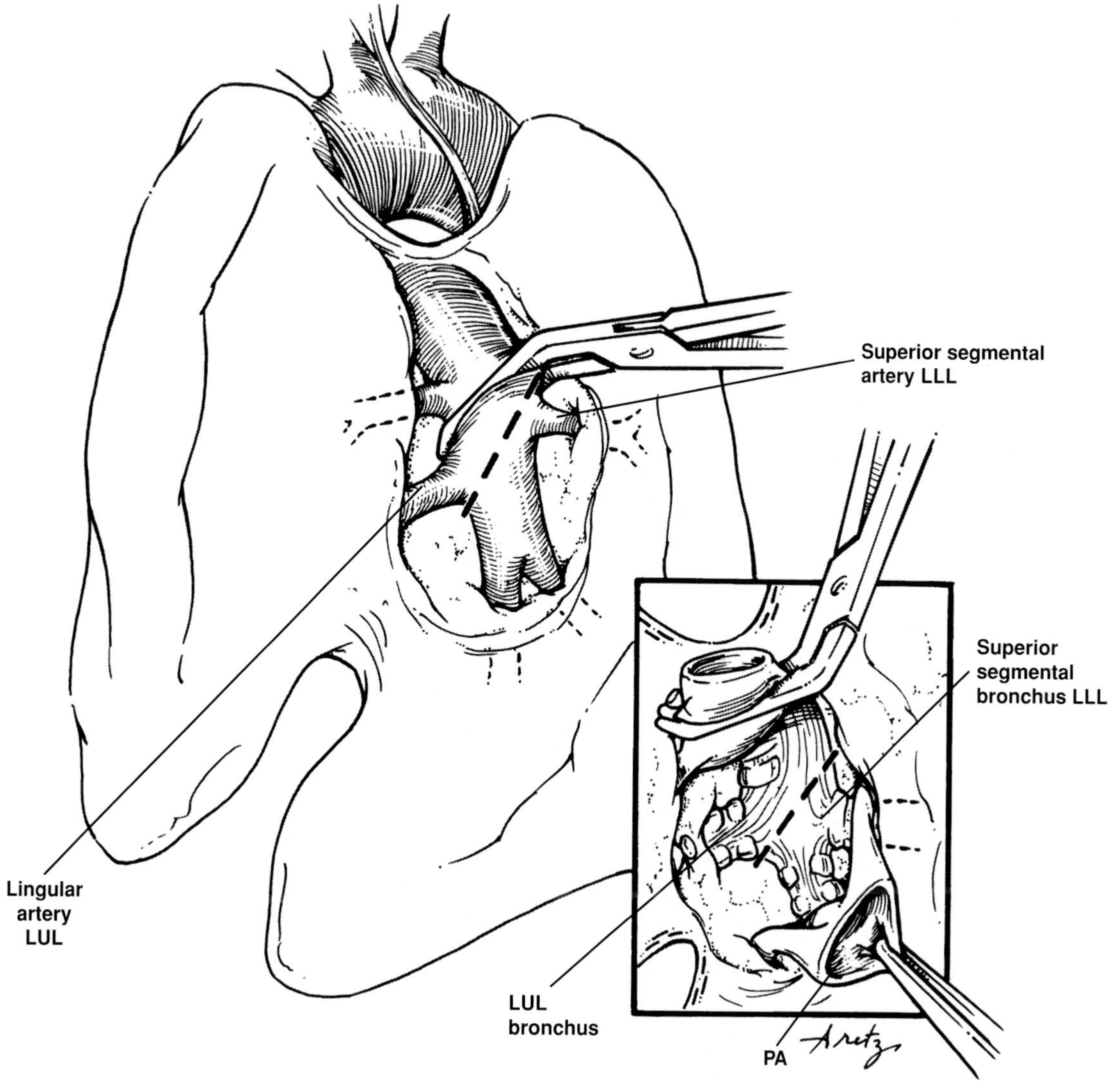

Figure 96-8. Technique for preparation of left lower lobe (LLL) living donor lobectomy. The left pulmonary artery (PA) is identified in the fissure and mobilized, and the take-offs of the superior segmental branch of the lower lobe and the lingular branches are identified. After completion of the fissures with staplers and dissection of the pulmonary veins, the patient is heparinized, and a vascular clamp is placed on the PA above the take-off of the superior segmental branch of the lower lobe. Small lingular branches may be ligated or, as illustrated, left in situ and an oblique incision made just distal to the take-off of the lingular branch and obliquely carried superior to the take-off of the superior segmental branch. The PA then can be patched or oversewn with care taken to maintain perfusion to the lingular branch of the PA. The bronchus is then exposed behind the PA and an oblique incision made, keeping the origin of the superior segmental bronchus with the donor lobe and the lingular bronchus with the upper lobe. (LUL = left upper lobe.)

during the short period of transportation to the recipient.

Recipient Operation

The recipient operation for implantation of donor lobes is similar to the complete lung implantation technique. The short length of the pulmonary venous confluence from single lobes makes it valuable to leave longer stumps of pulmonary veins in the recipient to gain length for the anastomosis. If proper organization and timing of donor and recipient operations is performed, it is possible to limit the ischemia time on each donor lobe to <45 minutes.

Postoperative Management

Postoperative management and restriction of postoperative fluid administration are important after heart-lung and lung transplantation to decrease the magnitude of reperfusion edema of the transplanted organs. In addition, the effects of immunosuppression agents such as cyclosporine and tacrolimus on renal function may be minimized by use of diuretics and low-dose dopamine. Isoproterenol is often used in heart-lung transplant recipients to maintain the cardiac rate from 110 to 150 beats per minute. The isoproterenol may also lower pulmonary vascular resistance early post-transplant. Weaning of the fraction of inspired oxygen (FIO_2) is performed to maintain a PaO_2 of >70 mm Hg and low amounts of positive end-expiratory pressure used to prevent water accumulation in the lungs and atelectasis. We generally perform a fiberoptic bronchoscopic examination of the anastomosis 12 to 24 hours after lung transplantation to assess the blood supply and to suction any residual airway secretions before extubation of the patient.

It is generally advisable to keep children with severe pulmonary hypertension and congenital heart disease sedated and paralyzed for 12 to 24 hours after transplant to minimize hemodynamic instability. Patients who are chronically debilitated or who have been chronically ventilated pretransplant may require prolonged weaning after successful transplant procedures. Early reperfusion damage of the transplanted lungs, which is generally manifested by a diffuse pulmonary infiltrate on chest x-ray films, usually resolves after 5 to 7 days posttransplant. Often, copious serous drainage from the chest cavities may occur, representing transudative fluid loss across the visceral pleura or exudative fluid loss from takedown of extensive intrapleural adhesions. Early mobilization is encouraged to aid in re-expansion of the transplanted lungs, and surveillance cultures of sputum, urine, and blood routinely are performed along with bronchoalveolar lavage cultures for viruses. Immunologic staining of donor and recipient lung samples for common viruses has been performed to identify early potential viral infections of the transplanted lung. In our experience, most of the early graft dysfunction after lung transplantation is associated with positive viral cultures of the donor organs, which are particularly common in pediatric donors.

The immunosuppressive regimen used for heart-lung and lung transplantation is similar to that used for pediatric heart transplants. No standardized regimen has been devised; however, we have used primarily tacrolimus and mycophenolate mofetil with steroids in our most recent pediatric experience. For heart-lung and lung transplants, ganciclovir for a 6-week period posttransplant is used to prevent early CMV infection. It is unclear that there is any significant superiority of one immunosuppression protocol; however, we have used tacrolimus to make dosing and administration easier in children, who may often require multiple doses of cyclosporine to maintain adequate drug levels, and for cystic fibrosis patients, who may have difficulty with gastrointestinal cyclosporine absorption. Common

complications of cyclosporine include hirsutism, seizures, and gum hyperplasia in addition to renal dysfunction, and these complications are diminished somewhat with the use of tacrolimus. Steroids have been associated with the onset of diabetes, but we have not noted an increased incidence of infection with steroid use. Although weight gain has been appropriate in small children who have undergone lung or heart-lung transplantation, bone growth may be somewhat decreased by the use of immunosuppressive regimens that include steroids.

Rejection Surveillance and Management

Bronchoscopy is used even in small infants and children for rejection and infection surveillance. Bronchoalveolar lavage for cultures is routinely performed, and biopsy specimens are obtained either through a fiberoptic bronchoscope or through a suction catheter positioned in the distal airways under fluoroscopic guidance if the airways are too small to allow an adequate-sized fiberoptic bronchoscope to pass into the distal airways. Significant documented rejection is treated by pulse steroids and increases in dosage of tacrolimus or cyclosporine as necessary.

Refractory rejection can be treated with cytolytic agents such as OKT3 if the patient does not rapidly respond to an increase in steroid dose. Echocardiography is used to evaluate cardiac function in children after heart-lung transplantation. Differential rejection of heart and lungs is well documented; however, cardiac rejection appears to be rare in the absence of associated pulmonary rejection. In addition, the incidence of cardiac rejection in cardiopulmonary transplantation appears to be lower than in cardiac transplantation alone. Thus, in the absence of evidence for pulmonary rejection, cardiac biopsies are not routinely performed.

Results

Relatively few results of cardiopulmonary or pulmonary transplantation have been reported in children. The overall reported results to the Registry of the International Society of Heart and Lung Transplantation show approximately a 45% survival of heart-lung transplant recipients at 3 years in patients older than 6 years at the time of transplantation and 25% to 30% at 3 years in

patients younger than 5 years of age at the time of transplantation. Lung transplantation has virtually identical survival statistics in pediatric populations, with an actuarial survival in the 16- to 18-year range of 40% at 3 years. As might be expected, the initial operative mortality is higher in children requiring pulmonary transplantation and cardiac repair and in patients with pulmonary hypertension. Nevertheless, the long-term results are similar after initial operative mortality is excluded from analysis. The major obstacle to long-term survival after lung transplantation in children is the development of bronchiolitis obliterans, which may be a manifestation of chronic rejection. The onset of bronchiolitis obliterans is associated with progressive dyspnea and reduction of oxygen saturation on room air plus a documented decrease in FEV_1 or in forced expiratory flow over midexpiration (FEF_{25-75}). The clinical diagnosis of bronchiolitis obliterans may be considered if there is a sudden decrease in FEV_1 of 20% or greater from the maximum post-transplant baseline level, unassociated with infection, acute rejection, or bronchial complication. Although some patients have had stabilization of the level of bronchiolitis obliterans with increased immunosuppression, in other children a progressive decline in lung function has occurred that required retransplantation or resulted in late mortality. In heart-lung transplant recipients, the onset of bronchiolitis obliterans may occur independent of the development of coronary graft atherosclerosis or chronic rejection of the transplanted heart.

Conclusion

Long-term follow-up data are not available on a significant number of children after cardiopulmonary or pulmonary transplantation. The medium- and intermediate-term results appear to be similar to results noted in adults, for whom there is a somewhat longer follow-up. Although results are encouraging, obliterative bronchiolitis remains a serious late concern that must be addressed for the future success of cardiopulmonary transplantation in children. As increasing experience has been gained in cardiac repair and lung transplantation and the use of reduced-size donor grafts, the technical limitations to cardiopulmonary and pulmonary transplantation have been largely eliminated. The immunologic issues related to late development of chronic rejection and bronchiolitis obliterans, however, make cardiopulmonary and pulmonary transplantation a palliative procedure for the majority of recipients.

SUGGESTED READING

Conte JV, Robbins RC, Reichenspurner H, et al. Pediatric heart lung transplantation: Intermediate term results. J Heart Lung Transplant 1996;15:692.

Spray TL. Lung transplantation in children with pulmonary hypertension and congenital heart disease. Semin Thorac Cardiovasc Surg 1996;8:286.

Spray TL, Mallory GB, Canter CE, Huddleston CB. Pediatric lung transplantation: Indications, technique, and early results. J Thorac Cardiovasc Surg 1994;107:990.

Spray TL, Mallory GB, Canter CE, et al. Pediatric lung transplantation for pulmonary hypertension and congenital heart disease. Ann Thorac Surg 1992;54:216.

Starnes VA, Marshall SE, Lewiston NJ, et al. Heart lung transplantation in infants, children and adolescents. J Pediatr Surg 1991;26: 434.

Watson TJ, Starnes VA. Pediatric lobar lung transplantation. Semin Thorac Cardiovasc Surg 1996;8:313.

EDITOR'S COMMENTS

Dr. Spray describes the management and operative care of children requiring lung and heart-lung transplantation. I agree completely with the vast majority of his comments. I believe that he has the largest series of patients with pulmonary venous issues that lead to lung transplantation, and he describes the techniques in a thorough and easily understandable fashion.

Spray discusses the techniques of bronchial anastomosis, including the importance of not telescoping the individual bronchi during anastomosis. I think this needs to be emphasized. We went through a phase early in our program during which telescoping was performed and did lead to airway complications. These have disappeared with the techniques that Spray describes.

A more important issue is reperfusion injury. Reperfusion injury still occurs in between 5% and 20% of recipients. They often can be managed medically using pharmacologic techniques as well as appropriate ventilating care. However, in some circumstances, the injury is much more severe. We are true believers in early extracorporeal membrane oxygenation intervention after severe reperfusion injury. It turns out that the injury tends to last no more than 48 hours and, once they are supported, most patients survive. However, one episode of reperfusion injury does increase the chances for late bronchiolitis obliterans. These high-risk patients are always at risk for this late complication and must be closely monitored.

I.L.K.

97

Ebstein's Malformation of the Tricuspid Valve in Children

Brian L. Reemtsen and Vaughn A. Starnes

Introduction

Ebstein's malformation is a syndrome that may involve malformation of the tricuspid valve, the right ventricle, and the right atrium. Symptoms range from none to life-threatening instability. This anomaly is rare, occurring in 1 in 200,000 live births, accounting for <1% of all congenital heart disease cases. Due to the varied anatomy and presentation, the surgical therapy is different for selective groups.

In 1866, Wilhelm Ebstein described the first known case of malformation of the tricuspid valve, in a paper entitled, "Concerning a very rare case of insufficiency of the tricuspid valve caused by a congenital malformation." He very thoughtfully discussed the pathophysiology of the malformed valve, which he described as an enlarged and fenestrated anterior leaflet with hypoplastic adherent remaining leaflets. He proposed that the valve malfunction was responsible for the patient's marked cyanosis with marked jugular venous distension.

Since the first clinical case reported in the 1950s, the medical and surgical management of this anomaly has not been particularly effective, and the survival of patients with severe malformation has been dismal. Recently, advances in valve repair and replacement in older individuals and univentricular strategies in neonates have revolutionized the treatment of symptomatic patients with Ebstein's malformation.

Embryology

The embryology of Ebstein's malformation is not clearly defined. It is known that the substance of the tricuspid valve is derived from both the endocardial cushions and the atrioventricular myocardium. One of the major contributors to leaflet genesis is the delamination of the atrioventricular myocardium. Hearts with Ebstein's malformation do not demonstrate normal delamination and have resultant valve morphology. The mechanism of the failure of delamination is not well understood.

Anatomy

Ebstein's malformation occurs when the posterior and septal leaflets are downwardly displaced into the right ventricular cavity away from the normally positioned tricuspid valve annulus (Fig. 97-1). The degree of displacement is variable. The leaflets are also abnormal. The septal and posterior leaflets are usually hypoplastic and can be tethered to the ventricular wall. The anterior leaflet, however, which is normally attached at the annulus, is enlarged and "sail-like." It too can have abnormal chordal tethering to the ventricular wall even to the point of complete fusion. These leaflet abnormalities of position, size, and attachment affect the ventricular and atrial anatomy. The portion of the right ventricle between the tricuspid annulus and the displaced septal and posterior leaflets becomes "atrialized." The wall is usually thinned out and dilated. The remainder of the right ventricle is usually reduced in size with lack of an inlet chamber and a small trabecular component. Incompetence of the valve results in right atrial enlargement. The degree of leaflet abnormality directly affects the degree of ventricular and atrial abnormality. The tethering of the anterior leaflet can cause right ventricular outflow obstruction. In some cases, the anterior leaflet totally obstructs the infundibulum except for a small perforation or cleft in the leaflet. The atrium becomes massively enlarged in cases of severe regurgitation and significant right ventricular outflow tract obstruction.

Carpentier et al. developed a grading system based on ventricular morphology, leaflet movement, and right ventricular outflow tract (RVOT) obstruction (Fig. 97-2):

Type A: The volume of the right ventricle is adequate

Type B: There is a large atrialized component of the right ventricle, but the anterior leaflet moves freely

Type C: The anterior leaflet is severely restricted in its movement and may cause significant obstruction of the RVOT

Type D: There is almost complete atrialization of the ventricle with the exception of a small infundibular component. The only communication between the atrialized ventricle and the infundibulum is through the anteroseptal commissure of the tricuspid valve.

Associated Anomalies

The most common associated cardiac anomaly is an atrial septal communication. In most series 80% to 95% of patients have a significant interatrial defect, with the next most common being ventricular septal defects. Frequently associated defects can be found on the left side of the heart, including mitral valve prolapse, left ventricular noncompaction, and bicuspid aortic valve.

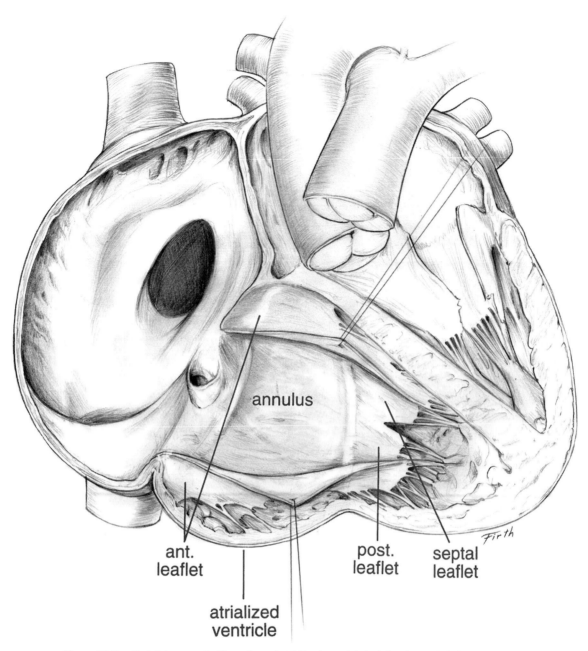

Figure 97-1.   Ebstein's anomaly. The enlarged atrialized ventricle is defined superiorly by the tricuspid valve annulus and inferiorly by the septal and posterior leaflets. The greatly enlarged anterior leaflet is divided for visualization. (Ant. = anterior; Post. = posterior.)

Familial cases of Ebstein's have been described but are exceedingly rare. There is a correlation of maternal lithium exposure and the development of Ebstein's malformation. Environmental exposure to viruses in utero is thought to cause sporadic cases of this anomaly. No specific cause or genetic factor has been elucidated.

Pathophysiology and Clinical Course

The clinical course of a child with Ebstein's malformation is determined largely by the degree of displacement of the tricuspid valve leaflets, the relationship of the anterior leaflet to the right ventricular outflow tract, and the presence of certain associated cardiac anomalies.

At birth, the pulmonary vascular resistance is elevated to near systemic levels. Depending on the degree of malformation and the presence of an atrial septal defect, right-to-left shunting occurs with resulting

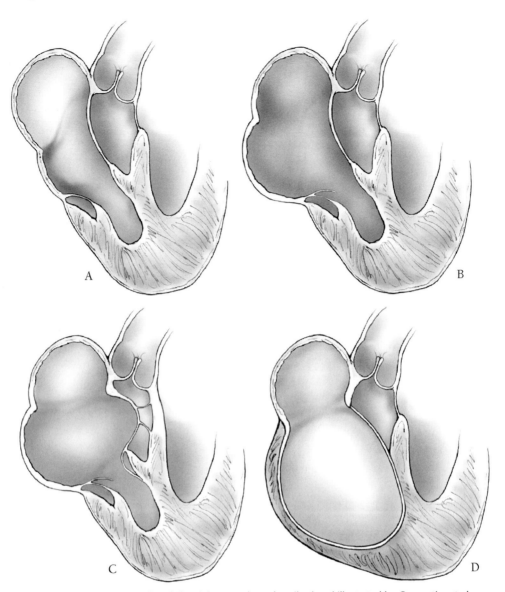

Figure 97-2.   The four grades of Ebstein's anomaly as described and illustrated by Carpentier et al. See the text for the description of types A through D.

cyanosis. In patients with relatively mild tricuspid valve displacement and no right ventricular outflow tract obstruction, the shunting of blood across the atrial defect decreases as the pulmonary vascular resistance falls over the ensuing 7 to 10 days. As this occurs, the cyanosis decreases. In those individuals with significant atrialized ventricles and/or obstruction of the right ventricular outflow tract by the anterior leaflet of the tricuspid valve, cyanosis will persist and the severity of congestive heart failure will increase. Individuals with massive cardiomegaly and cardiac-to-thoracic cavity ratios of ≥ 0.65 generally do not tolerate medical management alone. The factors that have been associated with a failure of medical management in infants are listed in Table 97-1.

In the fetus severe malformations can lead to presentation in utero. Fetal echocardiography can demonstrate hydrops, cardiomegaly, and tachyarrhythmias, as well as features of the malformation to be described later. Greater than 50% of the cases diagnosed in utero do not survive to live birth due to spontaneous or elective termination of pregnancy.

Neonates presenting with Ebstein's malformation 1 have a varied course depending on the severity of their anomaly. Patients diagnosed post-partum usually have a survival advantage over those diagnosed by fetal echocardiogram because the severity of their malformation is usually less. Neonates presenting early generally have severe cyanosis and cardiovascular instability.

Severe tricuspid valve regurgitation results in cardiomegaly and cardiovascular embarrassment requiring urgent surgical management. Until recently the survival of these children with or without intervention was dismal. From 20% to 40% of all presenting neonates do not survive 1 month, with an overall mortality of nearly 50% at 5 years. More important to survival is the timing of symptoms. Those patients presenting in the neonatal period have a dismal outlook, with a survival of only 47%. Predictors of neonatal death are well described. Tables 97-2 and 97-3 show independent risk factors for death and reduced time to death, respectively.

After the neonatal period, presentation is more variable, with most patients reaching adolescence or adulthood when symptoms

Table 97-1 Presenting Features in the Different Age Groups

	Fetuses 21 Pts	Neonates 88 Pts	Children 73 Pts	Adolescents 15 Pts	Adults 23 Pts	Total (%) 220 Pts
Cyanosis	0	65	15	2	1	83 (38)
Heart failure	0	9	14	2	6	31 (14)
Incidental murmur	0	8	36	5	3	52 (24)
Arrhythmia	1	5	7	6	10	29 (13)
Abnormal fetal scan	18	0	0	0	0	18 (8)
Other	2	1	1	0	3	7 (3)

Pts = patients.
Neonates, 0–1 month; children, >1 month to 10 years; adolescents, >10 to 18 years; adults, >18 years at time of presentation.
Adapted from Celermajer DS, Bull C, Till JA, et al. Ebstein's anomaly: Presentation and outcome from fetus to adult. J Am Coll Cardiol 1994;23:170.

arise. Some present with progressive right heart failure, but more present with dysrhythmias. In patients >10 years of age the most common presenting symptom is an electrophysiologic one. Presenting features of certain age groups are given in Table 97-3. If untreated, nearly 50% of patients develop signs of heart failure as an adult.

Diagnosis

The clinical presentation of Ebstein's anomaly is determined by the degree of tricuspid regurgitation and right ventricular outflow tract obstruction and the size of the atrialized portion of right ventricle. Regurgitation manifests itself as massive right atrial enlargement. A systolic murmur and a prominent jugular venous "v" wave can be seen. Outflow tract obstruction in combination with an atrial septal defect results in significant right-to-left shunting and cyanosis. A similar situation occurs at birth, and the pulmonary vascular resistance is elevated. As the resistance drops, forward flow of blood is restored in the absence of outflow tract obstruction. When the portion of atrialized right ventricle is extensive, poor cardiac output occurs with accompanying symptoms of congestive heart failure.

Diagnostic studies include chest x-ray films, echocardiography, cardiac catheterization, magnetic resonance imaging, and angiography. The chest x-ray film can vary from appearing normal in slightly affected patients to exhibiting massive cardiomegaly from an enlarged right atrium and atrialized ventricle. The pulmonary vascular markings can vary from normal to decreased. An echocardiogram is the diagnostic test of choice. This modality can demonstrate the degree of leaflet malformation, displacement, and attachment as well as the extent of ventricular atrialization. Doppler signals can be used to estimate the severity of regurgitation and outflow tract obstruction. Celermajer et al. devised an echo grading scale for neonates with Ebstein's anomaly. The Great Ormond Street (GOS) score grades severity from 1 to 4. The score is the ratio of the combined area of the right atrium and atrialized ventricle over the area of the functional right ventricle added to the area of the left heart chambers in diastole on a four-chamber view. Grade 1 is characterized as a ratio <0.5; grade 2 as a ratio of 0.5 to 0.99; grade 3 as a ratio of 1.0 to 1.49; and grade 4 as a ratio of ≥1.5. Studies have demonstrated that ratios >1.0 can predict 100% mortality. Cardiac catheterization is rarely necessary, although exceptions occur when noninvasive tests and the expected clinical course do not agree or if other lesions need examination. During catheter examination the key sign of Ebstein's malformation is the occurrence of a ventricular electrocardiographic pattern at the same point as an atrial pressure pattern. Finally, magnetic resonance imaging has come into vogue, and this noninvasive examination may more accurately measure chamber sizes.

Medical Management

The spectrum of the presentation of Ebstein's anomaly dictates the medical management. Aggressive management is required for patients who present in the neonatal period to prepare them for surgery. The main problems are severe cyanosis with progressive heart failure and malperfusion. Intubation and mechanical ventilation are a starting point. Efforts to decrease pulmonary vascular resistance and maintain ductal patency are necessary until the resistance falls or the patient is stabilized for an operative procedure. Hyperventilation, alkalosis, supplemental oxygen, and nitric oxide may be used. Prostaglandin E_1 may be necessary. Congestive heart failure can be treated with inotropic agents such as dopamine, dobutamine, milrinone, and amrinone. If symptoms resolve, support can be withdrawn slowly, but if they persist, operative treatment is indicated.

Asymptomatic or mild forms of Ebstein's anomaly can be managed conservatively, with routine cardiology follow-up to assess

Table 97-2 Predictors of Death in Neonates with Ebstein's Anomaly

1. Cardiothoracic ratio >0.85 (100% fatal)
2. Echocardiography score grade 4/4 (>1.5:1, 100% fatal)
3. Echocardiography score grade 3/4 (>1.1:1) and cyanosis (100% fatal)
4. Severe tricuspid regurgitation (mostly fatal)
5. Echocardiography score grade 3/4 (>1.1:1, 45% fatal in infancy)

Adapted from Knott-Craig CJ, Overholt ED, Ward KE, et al. Repair of Ebstein's anomaly in the symptomatic neonate: An evolution of technique with 7-year follow up. Ann Thorac Surg 2002;73:1786.

Table 97-3 Independent Association of Clinical Characteristics with Reduced Time to Death

Variable	Relative Risk (95% CI)
Reduced left ventricular function	4.10 (1.70–9.91)
Presence of moderate to large atrial septal defect	2.39 (1.05–5.45)
Pulmonary atresia	
Absent	1.00
Functional	2.44 (1.34–4.44)
Anatomic	5.97 (3.28–10.8)

From Cox's proportional hazard regression modeling of survival; n = 43.
CI = confidence interval.
Adapted from Yetman AT, Freedom RM, McCrindle BW. Outcome in cyanotic neonates with Ebstein's anomaly. Am J Cardiol 1998;81:749.

ventricular function and valve competence. Standard endocarditis prophylaxis is recommended. Patients who are being actively treated for heart failure should be evaluated for surgical intervention.

Surgical Indications

Operative intervention is guided by symptoms. Operative technique depends on anatomy and age at presentation. Neonates who present in the postnatal period are generally in extremis and require prompt surgical attention. The right heart is severely dilated and causes poor systemic perfusion. This is coupled with severe cyanosis and arrhythmias, causing difficulty in medical management. It is sometimes difficult to discern the need for medical "tuning up" or the need for emergent operation.

Patients who are asymptomatic can generally be followed until symptoms arise. Children who make it through infancy usually have many years until symptoms become apparent. The most frequent late presentation is with arrhythmias. Surgery must be considered when atrial or ventricular arrhythmias occur, objective dilation and malfunction of the right ventricle are documented, and/or cyanosis becomes apparent. Once the patient is in overt heart failure with a New York Heart Association class of III or IV, medical management has little to offer. The determination of what procedure to be performed depends on anatomy and age.

A special subset of patients are those with significant pulmonary stenosis, pulmonary atresia, or absent pulmonary valve. Attempts at combining right ventricular outflow tract reconstruction with either single- or double-ventricle repair have been uniformly fatal in most studies. An option for these patients may be heart-lung transplantation. In addition, severely affected patients diagnosed in utero have been shown to have dismal outcomes and may benefit from heart transplant listing with the hopes of transplantation. Many ethical issues come to bear when the need for extracorporeal membrane oxygenation support arises when on the waiting list for a transplant as a neonate, and this needs to be weighed by the surgeon and family.

Operative Technique

Two-Ventricle Repair

The two-ventricle repair attempts to transpose the tricuspid leaflets to the tricuspid annulus. In doing so, the atrialized ventricle is

obliterated. Tricuspid regurgitation is minimized, and right ventricular outflow tract obstruction is relieved.

The procedure is done through a median sternotomy incision with bicaval venous cannulation and aortic arterial perfusion. After initiation of cardiopulmonary bypass, a vent is placed through the right superior pulmonary vein into the left ventricle. The patient is cooled to 25°C, the aorta is cross-clamped, and cardioplegic solution is administered in an antegrade fashion. Caval tourniquets are applied, and the right atrium is opened obliquely. The tricuspid valve leaflets and annulus are inspected. The sizes of the functional and atrialized ventricles are assessed. The presence of an atrial septal defect is investigated.

Danielson et al. described using pledgeted sutures to pull the papillary muscles to the septum, thereby displacing the anterior leaflet toward the annulus. The posterior and septal leaflets are then brought up to the level of the annulus by a series of pledgeted mattress sutures placed through the base of the leaflets. The same sutures are then passed through the atrialized ventricle in a plicating fashion and then through the anatomically adjusted annulus (Fig. 97-3). Care must be taken to not injure the posterior descending coronary artery, which can be evaluated by direct vision. The spacing between each mattress suture is wider at the

annulus than at the leaflet (Fig. 97-4). This has the effect of narrowing the annulus. No attempt is made to plicate leaflet tissue that overlies the septum. The annulus may be further narrowed by plicating the free wall portion of the annulus to the septal portion using pledgeted mattress sutures (Fig. 97-5). This maneuver can potentially cause distortion of the coronary sinus or right coronary artery. A posterior annuloplasty is then performed to once again decrease the size of the dilated annulus (Fig. 97-6). The annuloplasty sutures should remain lateral of the coronary sinus to avoid heart block. Any perforations or clefts in the leaflets may be closed with fine, simple interrupted sutures. These techniques create a functional monocusp valve in a patient with a large anterior leaflet. In patients with a normal-sized anterior leaflet, a bicuspid or tricuspid leaflet valve may be constructed depending on the individual anatomy. The competency of the reconstructed valve is tested by injecting saline into the ventricle and observing the valve for leaks. The atrial septal defect is then closed with a patch (Fig. 97-7). A portion of the right atrial wall is resected to reduce cardiomegaly and the incidence of atrial arrhythmia. The atriotomy is closed, and the cross-clamp is removed. The patient is then rewarmed and weaned from cardiopulmonary bypass. Dopamine and dobutamine are used to augment ventricular

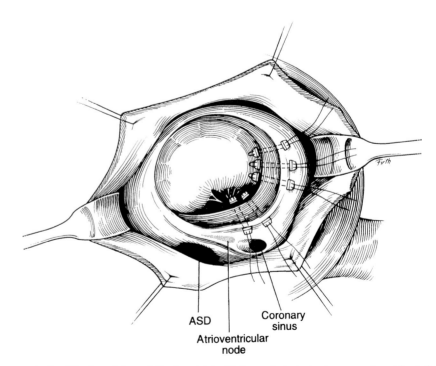

Figure 97-3.   Plication of the atrialized ventricle. Mattress pledgeted sutures are placed from the free wall of the right ventricle around to the coronary sinus, avoiding the sinus node. (ASD = atrial septal defect.)

ASD

Coronary sinus

Atrioventricular node

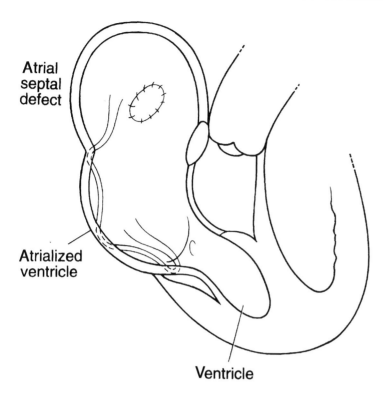

Figure 97-4. Schematic depiction of plication of the atrialized ventricle. Mattress sutures are passed from the level of the septal and posterior leaflets through the ventricular wall and then to the anatomic level of the tricuspid annulus.

Atrial septal defect

Atrialized ventricle

Ventricle

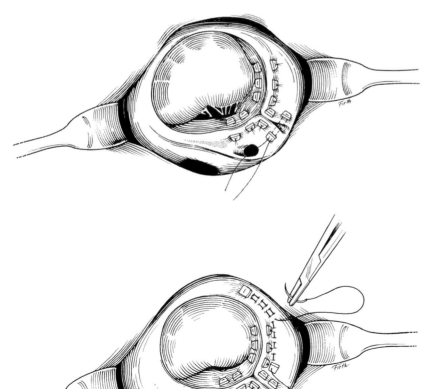

Figure 97-5. Lateral tricuspid annuloplasty is performed by placing mattress sutures in the dilated annulus laterally.

Figure 97-6. Semicircular annuloplasty. Further reduction of the tricuspid annulus can be achieved by a circular annuloplasty of the lateral free wall.

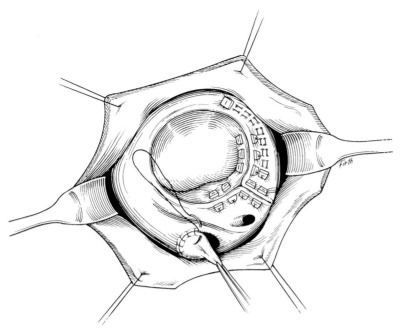

Figure 97-7. Patch closure of the atrial septal defect.

atrial septal defect is not present or is small, the atrial septum is excised to ensure complete right-to-left shunting. The orifice of the tricuspid valve is then closed with a pericardial patch (Fig. 97-8). The patch is positioned on the valve annulus and travels inferior to the coronary sinus so only Thebesian veins drain into the excluded right ventricle. A portion of the enlarged atrial wall is then resected (Fig. 97-9), and the atriotomy is closed. The right atrium is downsized, and, depending on the size of the atrialized portion of the RV, plication is performed. This univentricular strategy evolved to include a fenestration in the patch for RV decompression. The patch is incised in the center, and a 4-mm punch is used to make a uniform opening.(Fig. 97-10). This opening serves to decompress the RV. Pulmonary blood flow is provided by a modified Blalock-Taussig shunt of 3.5- to 4.0-mm polytetrafluoroethylene (PTFE) constructed from the innominate artery to the right pulmonary. The patient is rewarmed and weaned from cardiopulmonary bypass.

performance. Prostaglandin, hyperventilation, and, potentially, nitric oxide are used to reduce right ventricular afterload.

Variations of this repair have been described and have excellent results. Carpentier's group described a monocusp creation by mobilization of the anterior leaflet in combination with a full annuloplasty ring. This method has similar results to the repair just described.

This group also showed that the addition of a bidirectional cavopulmonary shunt is useful in patients at high risk (i.e., massive tricuspid regurgitation, extensive atrialized ventricle, poor ventricular function, and long-standing atrial fibrillation). A randomized study demonstrated that addition of a Glenn shunt significantly decreased operative mortality and reoperation.

Single-Ventricle Repair (Starnes Procedure)

The procedure is performed through a median sternotomy. The anterior pericardium is harvested and treated with glutaraldehyde. The inferior and superior venae cavae are dissected for bicaval cannulation. After institution of bypass, the patient is cooled to 20°C. A ventricular vent catheter is placed through the right superior pulmonary vein, and an intrapericardial cooling system is placed to bathe the heart in continuous cold saline. The septal temperature is monitored. The ascending aorta is clamped, and

cold blood cardioplegic perfusate is administered. A septal temperature of 8°C is desired. Caval tourniquets are applied, and the right atrium is opened obliquely. The anatomy is carefully inspected, and the position and size of the leaflets and the degree of atrialized right ventricle (RV) are noted. If an

Postoperative Care and Complications

The most common difficulty facing a neonate after single-ventricle repair for

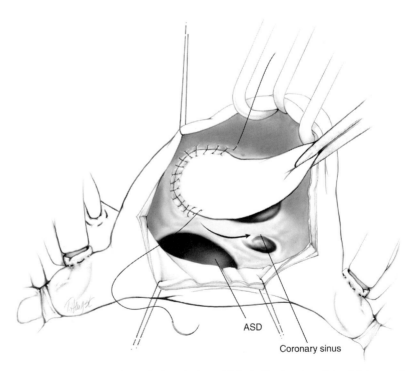

Figure 97-8. Right ventricular exclusion. A glutaraldehyde-fixed pericardial patch is used to cover the inlet to the right ventricle. (ASD = atrial septal defect.)

ASD

Coronary sinus

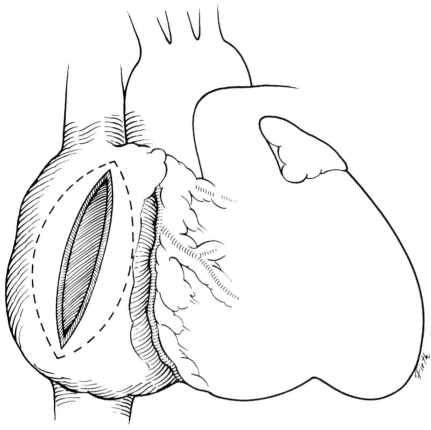

Figure 97-9. Downsizing atriotomy. The excess atrial wall is excised before the atriotomy is closed.

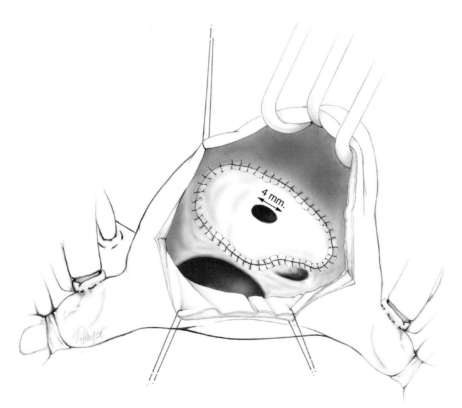

Figure 97-10. Completed patch with 4-mm fenestration.

Ebstein's malformation is low cardiac output. Postoperatively, the coronary sinus and Thebesian veins drain into the right ventricle. Inotropic support of the right ventricle with dopamine and dobutamine is necessary to prevent distention. These inotropes also support the left ventricle, which may function poorly as a result of preoperative congestive failure. Right ventricular distention is also avoided by decreasing the pulmonary vascular resistance with hyperventilation (pH of >7.45, partial pressure of carbon dioxide of <35 mm Hg), prostaglandin E_1 (0.05 to 0.20 μg/kg per minute), and inhaled nitric oxide (1 to 40 ppm). These agents have the additive effect of reducing resistance to flow from the systemic-to-pulmonary shunt. These efforts at hemodynamic manipulation should be continued for the first 24 hours postoperatively in addition to sedation with midazolam (1 μg/kg per minute), analgesia with continuous fentanyl (1 μg/kg per hour), and neuromuscular paralysis. Pulmonary vascular pressure may be monitored by transventricular pulmonary artery catheter placed at the time of operation.

In extreme cases of ventricular dysfunction, leaving the sternum open and covered with a silicone rubber (Silastic) patch can improve diastolic function and prevent cardiac compression due to myocardial edema. The open sternum also allows the lungs to be ventilated at lower pressures, thereby decreasing pulmonary vascular resistance. Usually after 3 to 4 days, the sternum can be closed after inotropes have been minimized and oxygen saturations in the 80s are maintained on low inspired oxygen.

After 24 hours or when the sternum is closed, the patient is allowed to awaken. The pulmonary artery pressures are monitored carefully, and the doses of inotropes and pulmonary vasodilators are tapered. Patients with single-ventricle physiology are treated with digoxin and furosemide. Maintenance of shunt patency is improved by the administration of aspirin in the early postoperative period after significant bleeding has stopped.

Palliated patients typically require construction of a superior cavopulmonary shunt at 6 months to 1 year of age. Eventually, at age 2 to 3 years a complete cavopulmonary connection is constructed. Alternatively, patients who exhibit poor ventricular function or have other criteria that would preclude completion of the total cavopulmonary connection may be evaluated and listed for cardiac transplantation.

In addition, patients with Ebstein's malformation are subject to supraventricular arrhythmias because of accessory atrioventricular conduction pathways. Use of antiarrhythmic agents in the postoperative period and for 6 months after discharge is recommended. If arrhythmias have not been a problem, the antiarrhythmic may be tapered off. Arrhythmias that do not respond to pharmacologic agents may require ablation. Arrhythmias present at the time of surgery should undergo operative ablation. The specific technique of ablation is described elsewhere.

Results

The historical results with neonatal valve repair were uniformly dismal until recently, when some progress was demonstrated with improved outcomes in one small series. Our institutional experience with neonatal Ebstein's anomaly has been significant. From 1992 to 2005, 16 neonates underwent univentricular surgical intervention for Ebstein's anomaly at our institution. Two patients received the Starnes procedure after attempted valve repair. Overall actuarial survival for patients with RV exclusion was 70% at 1 month, 1 year, and 5 years. Survival with the fenestration improved to 80% at 1 month, 1 year, and 5 years. Of 10 RV exclusion survivors, 7 went on to cavopulmonary shunts and 3 to completion Fontan.

For older children and adults, the results with Ebstein's anomaly are good. Although a study of 294 patients revealed no significant difference between valve repair versus replacement, we continue to advocate for valve repair and feel it is a more potentially durable alternative, especially for younger patients.

SUGGESTED READING

Anderson KR, Zuberbuhler JR, Anderson RH, et al. Morphologic spectrum of Ebstein's anomaly of the heart: A review. Mayo Clin Proc 1979;54:174.

Attenhofer Jost CH, Connolly HM, Edwards WD, et al. Ebstein's anomaly—Review of a multifaceted congenital cardiac condition. Swiss Med Wkly 2005(May 14);135(19-20): 269.

Carpentier A, Chauvaud S, Mace L, et al. A new reconstructive operation of Ebstein's anomaly of the tricuspid valve. J Thorac Cardiovasc Surg 1988;96:92.

Celermajer DS, Cullen S, Sullivan ID, et al. Outcomes in neonates with Ebstein's anomaly. J Am Coll Cardiol 1992;191:41.

Chauvaud S, Fuzellier JF, Berrebi A, et al. Bidirectional cavopulmonary shunt associated with ventriculo and valvuloplasty in Ebstein's anomaly; benefits in high risk patients. Eur J Cardiothorac Surg 1998;13:514.

Ebstein W. Uber einen sehr seltenen Fall von Insufficienz der Valvula tricuspicalis, bedingt durch eine angeborene haochgradige Missbildung derselben. Arch Anat Physiol 1866;238.

Eustace S, Kruskal JB, Hartnell GG. Ebstein's anomaly presenting in adulthood: the role of cine magnetic resonance imaging in diagnosis. Clin Radiol 1944;49:690.

Khositseth A, Danielson GK, Dearani JA, et al. Superventricular tachyarrhythmias in Ebstein anomaly: Management and outcome. J Thorac Cardiovasc Surg 2004;128:826.

Kiziltan HT, Theodoro DA, Warnes CA, et al. Late results of bioprosthetic tricuspid valve replacement in Ebstein's anomaly. Ann Thorac Surg 1998;66:1539.

Knott-Craig CJ, Overholt ED, Ward KE, et al. Repair of Ebstein's anomaly in the symptomatic neonate: An evolution of technique with 7-year follow-up. Ann Thorac Surg 2002; 73:1786.

McElhinney DB, Salvin JW, Colan SD, et al. Improving outcomes in fetuses and neonates with congenital displacement (Ebstein's malformation) or dysplasia of the tricuspid valve. Am J Cardiol 2005;96(4):582.

Watson H. Natural history of Ebstein's anomaly of the tricuspid valve in childhood and adolescence. Br. Heart J 1974;36:417.

Yetman AT, Freedom RM, McCrindle BW. Outcome in cyanotic neonates with Ebstein's anomaly. Am J Cardiol 1998;81:749.

EDITOR'S COMMENTS

Until relatively recently, patients with Ebstein's malformation of the tricuspid valve with atrial septal defect who survived infancy were managed medically for many years before any surgical intervention was recommended. The primary reason for delay in operative intervention was the fact that these patients remained relatively stable despite severe cardiomegaly on chest x-ray films and cyanosis from right-to-left shunting at the atrial level. It was believed that the only operative intervention would be valve replacement, and a high incidence of heart block was associated with valve replacement in the earlier surgical eras. Thus, operative intervention was delayed until the patient became old enough to accept a satisfactorily-sized adult prosthesis with probable epicardial pacemaker placement.

The markedly improving results with valve repair for Ebstein's malformation as pioneered by Danielson at the Mayo Clinic has changed the approach to patients with Ebstein's malformation significantly. Because most valves can be repaired (approximately 70% in most series), earlier intervention may be recommended for patients with severe cardiomegaly and cyanosis. With earlier repair and with valve repair rather than replacement, the biventricular function can be maintained, and elimination of atrial level shunting decreases the chronic effects of cyanosis and markedly improves exercise tolerance in these patients. With current techniques, a low incidence of complete heart block has been noted. Nevertheless, as emphasized by the authors, arrhythmias are common after repair of Ebstein's malformation of the tricuspid valve. Many of these patients may have accessory conduction pathways, and long-term antiarrhythmic therapy or ablation, either before valve repair or at the time of operation, may be necessary to control arrhythmias. Direct surgical approaches for controlling atrial arrhythmias at the time of valve repair have been advocated, and the results have been quite excellent.

The optimal valve replacement for patients who require replacement rather than repair is somewhat controversial. Mechanical valves in the right side of the heart require anticoagulation, and thrombosis may be more frequent than on the left side of the heart despite adequate warfarin (Coumadin) therapy. Therefore, tissue valves have preferentially been used on the right side of the heart and have the additional advantage of permitting access for catheterization if necessary. Tissue valves, however, in young children have a significant incidence of degeneration even on the right side of the heart, and therefore valve repair should be undertaken if at all possible in all cases.

Multiple technical modifications of valve repair have been described; however, the most commonly used repair, as described in this chapter, is that pioneered by Danielson. Other approaches have plicated the atrialized portion of the ventricle in a more vertical fashion with valve annular reconstruction, as advocated by Carpentier. Several variations of repair for Ebstein's malformation have been described and have basically used the principle of creation of a unileaflet valve. Many of these repairs do not involve plication or resection of the atrialized right ventricle. Repairs by Quaguebeur and Hetzer represent variations on Carpentier's techniques. An infant with significant congestive heart failure with Ebstein's malformation represents a continuing therapeutic dilemma. These patients often have abnormal ventricular function or obstruction to the right ventricular outflow tract, which accounts for the severity of the hemodynamic instability early in life. Thus, simple valve repair may not be possible in most of these infants, and the operative mortality with surgical intervention has been high. If infants do not respond to medical management, then the optimal operative approach remains controversial. As described in this chapter, in some patients who have only mild right ventricular outflow tract obstruction from leaflet tissue rather than at the valvar level, it is occasionally possible to close the entrance into the right ventricle with a patch to control the magnitude of tricuspid regurgitation and convert the patient to single-ventricle physiology. In these patients, coronary sinus flow and Thebesian flow must still be ejected from the right ventricle, and therefore an unobstructed outflow tract to the pulmonary artery is necessary. Recognition of the distention of the small ventricle has led Starnes to modify his original procedure, creating a punch opening or fenestration in the center of the patch to allow decompression of the right ventricle. Even with these approaches, operative mortality is significant. As noted in this chapter, the most significant problem occurs in infants with Ebstein's malformation and pulmonary atresia or significant pulmonary stenosis. These patients often are ill immediately after birth, and the right ventricle is markedly dilated and can cause abnormal ventricular function on the left side of the heart. If such patients can be identified in utero, then in utero listing for heart or heart-lung transplantation may be the most appropriate therapy. Operative intervention after birth in these rare children has been often unsuccessful, and in our experience heart transplantation may be the best option. As reparative techniques improve, however, some of these infants may be suitable for operative intervention if the right ventricle has adequate volume and function.

An increasing experience with repair of Ebstein's malformation in neonates and infants has been reported by Knott-Craig. In his small series of patients who were unstable in the neonatal and infant period and did not respond to medical management, valve reparative techniques were successful in the majority of cases. Thus, it may be reasonable to attempt valve repair in the majority of these patients before converting them to single-ventricle physiology.

Attempts to ablate the right ventricle have been unsuccessful because of the amount of inflow into the ventricle from Thebesian veins, and therefore occlusion of the inflow into the ventricle without adequate outflow has not been successful. Attempts to reconstruct the right ventricular outflow tract and eliminate inflow into the ventricle have also not been successful because of the inability of the right ventricle to adequately decompress. Ventricular dysfunction is common in these patients with a thin-walled, poorly contractile right ventricle, probably secondary to in utero severe tricuspid regurgitation. Sano and his associates have been successful in complete excision of the right ventricular free wall in rare cases with pulmonary atresia and Ebstein's malformation with patch closure or oversewing of the tricuspid valve inlet. These radical approaches of RV exclusion have been successful in isolated cases and may represent a reasonable alterative in patients who have significant RV dilation and RV dysfunction and abnormal ventricular septum that can bulge into the left ventricular outflow tract and cause left ventricular outflow tract obstruction. In these cases, removal of the free wall of the right ventricle may allow septal repositioning and improvement in left ventricular outflow tract diameter.

Overall, the surgical approach to Ebstein's malformation remains a technical challenge. Although repair techniques are evolving and use of the bidirectional Glenn or cavopulmonary shunt permits more drastic reduction of the tricuspid annulus to achieve better competence, the wide variation in ventricular function, valve morphology, and age at presentation make this patient population medically challenging.

T.L.S.

98

Mitral Valve Repair in Children

Christian Brizard

Introduction and Background

Mitral valve repair in children is guided by the same surgical rules as in adults, but the anatomic substrate differs greatly. The rules were set out by Carpentier more than two decades ago. The technical difficulties vary according to the anatomy and the size and age of the patient. The indications for surgery and the timing of the surgery have to take into account a large range of issues and are therefore less straightforward than in adults.

This chapter covers mitral valve repair in children, congenital and acquired, excluding the mitral valve in atrioventricular discordance, the mitral valve in univentricular hearts, the mitral valve of the hypoplastic left heart syndrome, and the left atrioventricular valve in atrioventricular septal defects.

Anatomy and Embryology

Anatomy

The normal anatomy of the mitral valve in children does not differ from that in adults and has been described in the adult section of this and other books. Precise knowledge of the normal anatomy is essential for reading the echocardiographic study, understanding the pathologic anatomy, and planning the repair.

Embryology

The leaflet and chordal tissue derive from the endocardial cushion tissue lying on the inner surface of the atrioventricular junction. As the cushion tissue elongates and grows toward the ventricular cavity, the leaflets shape progressively into a funnel-like structure totally attached to the myocardium while perforations appear in the valve leaflet edges. The perforations grow and form the chordae tendineae. The ventricular layer of the cushions generates the fibrous part of the mitral valve and the chordae. Simultaneously, the development of the papillary muscle takes place: the anterior and posterior parts of a horseshoe ridge within the left ventricle lose contact progressively with the ventricular wall. They form the papillary muscles, increasing their size while keeping contact with the cushion tissue at their tip.

Pathology

Congenital Anomalies of the Mitral Valve

Congenital valve stenosis and congenital mitral valve insufficiency are presented together because they have identical pathology and associated lesions. They are frequently associated in the same patient and require similar surgical techniques for treatment.

Cleft Mitral Valve

Very often isolated, the cleft mitral valve can be easily differentiated from a left atrioventricular valve in a partial atrioventricular septal defect. The cleft is centered on the aortic commissure between the noncoronary cusp and the left coronary cusp, and there is no suspension apparatus on the edges of the defect. The papillary muscles are normal. Lack of valvular tissue can be seen and is secondary to the regurgitation through the cleft. The defect is not stenotic and may generate only little regurgitation for a long time.

Accessory Valve Tissue and Valvular Tags

In these anomalies, which are often found in association with other valvar anomalies, the spaces between the chordae are filled with a network of myxoid, valve-like tissue. When there is continuity between the anterior and the posterior leaflet the accessory tissue may generate a gradient directly related to the size of the perforations in the accessory tissue. When the accessory valve tissue is entrapped in the left ventricular outflow tract, the mitral valve may become regurgitant due to the traction exerted by the accessory valvular tissue on the anterior leaflet, opening the valve in midsystole; however, in such cases, the left ventricular outflow tract obstruction is the predominant hemodynamic lesion and is the most frequent mode of diagnosis. The accessory mitral valve tissue in isolation often does not generate significant gradient or insufficiency.

Lesions Associated with Lack of Valvular Tissue

Three major anatomic types have been identified, although there is a continuum among them. Their recognition is useful for the planning of the repair. The functional lesion can be either predominantly regurgitant or predominantly stenotic, it can be both stenotic and regurgitant, or the valve can have a normal function.

Parachute Mitral Valve. The parachute mitral valve can be found in isolation. It is, however, often integrated in Shone syndrome. There is a dominant papillary muscle with the orifice of the mitral valve overriding the tip of the papillary muscle. There is a spectrum of lesions for the chordae ranging from complete absence and fusion of the tip of the papillary muscle to the free leaflet edge to relatively normal looking chordae with good mobility of the leaflet. An accessory papillary muscle, usually very small, is devoted to a short segment of the free edge, or even to the under surface of the leaflet tissue with or without a second orifice (double-orifice mitral valve). The functional anatomy depends on the interaction between the amount and mobility of leaflet tissue, the size of the fenestrations, and the presence, length, and quality of the chordae. The parachute mitral valve almost always has a stenotic component.

Papillary Muscle-to-Commissure Fusion.
This syndrome is a spectrum that ranges from papillary muscle tip fused to the commissural area of the free edge to short, almost normal-looking chordae. This anomaly can be limited to one papillary muscle only. The valve is generally more regurgitant than stenotic. When the papillary muscles are hypertrophied, the bulk of their mass is responsible for a valve that is predominantly stenotic.

Hammock Valve (Arcade Valve).
The suspension apparatus may have lost all resemblance to the normal anatomy. There is either no papillary muscle identifiable or multiple very small ones behind the posterior leaflet. The leaflets are suspended directly by a network of chordae directly attached to the posterior wall of the ventricle. This attachment is generally displaced toward the base of the heart with an excess of tension on the anterior leaflet and extreme limitation of posterior leaflet motion. The valve is most often predominantly regurgitant.

Regurgitant Mitral Valves with Normal Anatomy Associated with Congenital Cardiac Lesions
These conditions are associated with isolated annular dilation and isolated elongation of the chordae and/or the papillary muscle. There is no evidence of the congenital origin of these lesions. They are not found at birth, unlike the anomalies described earlier. They are usually associated with significant volume loading of the left ventricle, that is, large ventricular septal defect or large patent ductus arteriosus. Sometimes minor anomalies of the

valvular tissue or the papillary muscles can give an indication of a true congenital origin. Sometimes the papillary muscle has an ischemic aspect, which is mostly seen in neonates.

Anomalous Coronary Artery from the Pulmonary Artery.
The mitral regurgitation in patients with anomalous coronary artery from the pulmonary artery is of ischemic origin. The anatomy is normal. The functional classification is of systolic restriction of one of the segments of the posterior leaflet.

Supravalvar Mitral Ring.
Noted as a common cause of congenital mitral valve stenosis, the supravalvar mitral ring is in fact an acquired fibrous construction attached to the posterior annulus of the mitral valve and from both commissures to the mid-height of the anterior leaflet. The supravalvar mitral ring is secondary to turbulent flow through the mitral orifice. The primary lesion of the mitral valve responsible for the turbulent flow can be obvious, stenotic or regurgitant, or can be very discrete and difficult to identify. The supravalvar mitral ring is prone to reoccur after surgical resection unless the underlying anatomic anomaly has been identified and corrected. The supravalvular ring can be encountered very early in life. It has to be suspected every time the transvalvular gradient increases during follow-up or when the Doppler gradient is greater than what the anatomy depicted with the echocardiographic study would suggest; sometimes, it is only found at operation.

Mitral Valve Disease with Excess Leaflet Tissue, Mitral Valve Prolapse, and Connective Tissue Disorder
These conditions are associated with mitral valve prolapse, Marfan syndrome, Barlow disease, Ehler-Danlos syndrome, and mucopolysaccharidosis type I. All include elastic fiber alteration and myxomatous tissue proliferation of various degrees. Most are well associated with chromosomal mutations.

Acquired Mitral Valve Disease
Rheumatic Heart Disease
Acute rheumatic fever (ARF) is an autoimmune disorder. The immune response to group A streptococcal (GAS) M protein generates T cells and antibodies that cross-react with cardiac antigens. In some patients, the acute damage to the valves induces chronic and evolving lesions secondary to the scarring process and/or the hemodynamic mod-

ifications. This is known as rheumatic heart disease (RHD).

Acute Lesions.
Acute lesions are exclusively regurgitant. On inspection, the valvar tissue and the chordae are swollen but supple. Prolapse predominantly affects the anterior leaflet. This prolapse is usually related to large elongation of the marginal chordae that appear stretched; chordal ruptures are rare. Multiple small nodules (2 mm to 3 mm in diameter) can be seen on the free edge of either mitral leaflet. The annular dilation is secondary to the myocarditis.

Chronic Lesions.
The healing of the spongiosa induces fusion of chordae as demonstrated by reduction in their number and increase in their thickness. The physiology of the regurgitation is always a combination of prolapse of the anterior leaflet, retraction of the posterior leaflet, and annular dilation. In the pediatric age group, the mitral valve is exclusively or predominantly regurgitant. The stenosis appears later, and the age of appearance of the mitral stenosis varies greatly with the geographic origin of the population affected, suggesting a different pattern of infection (i.e., age of first ARF episode) and influence of other factors (alimentation and genetic).

Infective Endocarditis
Bacterial endocarditis of the mitral valve is rare. It is always a regurgitant lesion. At the Royal Children's Hospital, Melbourne, Australia, in the last decade most patients had normal native mitral valve. It is very important for the surgeon to be able to differentiate intact valvar tissue, which is supple, thin, and resistant, from infected tissue, which is thickened, edematous, and friable.

Indication and Planning of the Repair

Echocardiography
The long-axis view obtained from the apex or from the subcostal view of the transthoracic study is best for grading the regurgitation, providing an accurate estimate of transvalvular gradient, and defining the precise amplitude of any prolapse or restriction. The short-axis view gives a direct evaluation of the area of the mitral orifice and a precise localization of the regurgitant jet. It allows an analysis of the papillary muscles (presence, size, location, and symmetry). The transesophageal echo is

superior for visualizing the anatomic details of the suspension apparatus and evaluating the functional classification in relation to the anatomy (how much prolapse/restriction and where?), but it is less useful in grading the severity of the regurgitation. The transgastric position allows for a short-axis cut with precise measurement of the shortening fraction and an en face view of the mitral valve.

For mitral stenoses, the peak instantaneous and mean gradients across the valve have to be interpreted according to the diastolic performance of the heart and the associated lesions (mainly ratio of pulmonary to systemic blood flow [Qp/Qs], presence of an intra-atrial shunting, and gradient across the foramen ovale/atrial septal defect). The overall effect of the gradient on the surgical indication has to be weighted with the pulmonary artery pressure but mostly the clinical tolerance.

Functional Classification

Through the use of transthoracic and transesophageal echocardiography, we can classify the malformations according to the motion of the leaflets into one of the three following types:

Type I: Normal leaflet motion. The regurgitation results from a lack of coaptation between the leaflets.
Type II: Leaflet prolapse. The free edge of one or both leaflets overrides the plane of the orifice during systole.
Type III: Restricted leaflet motion. The motion of one or both leaflets is limited.

This can be secondary to short or stiff leaflet tissue or suspension apparatus (type IIIa), or the leaflet can be pulled away from the coaptation area by a paradoxical motion of the ventricular wall (type IIIb or systolic).

Other Investigations

Catheter study and angiography generate no additional information to the echocardiography and should not be performed.

Three-dimensional echocardiography, magnetic resonance imaging, and electron-beam computed tomography are of limited use in pediatric patients for the analysis of the leaflet tissue and the subvalvar apparatus because of the limited spatial resolution.

Indications

The indications for surgical intervention have to weigh several considerations.

Size of Mitral Valve Annulus

Large Mitral Valve Annulus (Greater Than 30 mm in Female Patients and 32 mm in Male Patients). With a wide range of mitral valve repair techniques, the probability of a successful repair of the valve is very high. A remodeling annuloplasty will not be outgrown and will not generate stenosis with the growth of the patient. The surgical indications are similar to those in the adult population: Patients should be operated on as soon as the regurgitation is severe, irrespective of the severity of other symptoms. The probability of repair is directly related to the experience of the surgical team, but the repair of virtually all valves is an accessible goal.

Mitral Valve Annulus Less Than 18 mm. Biventricular repair should be considered only if the mitral valve annulus is *not* hypoplastic (Z value greater than −1.5). The repair is technically very challenging, and the replacement is only possible with the use of surgical artifacts associated with significantly increased mortality. In these patients the surgery should be deferred as long as the patient can be managed with intense medical therapy, including transfusion. Aggressive medical therapy allows delaying the surgery for several months in some instances and can generate significantly more favorable operating conditions.

Intermediate Mitral Valve Annulus (Greater Than 19 mm and Smaller Than Adult Size). In these patients, the mitral valve replacement can be safely performed in anatomic position. Therefore, the mitral valve repair does not need to be delayed by fear of replacement in supra-annular position; it is generally safe to wait for a long time (up to several years) with a severe regurgitation, provided that adequate monitoring of the pulmonary artery pressure and ventricular function is achieved. Contrary to adult patients, in children, long-term ventricular function returns to normal in patients with decreased systolic function preoperatively.

Associated Lesions

Large Left-to-Right Shunts. These shunts can generate severe functional regurgitation that subsides with the treatment of the shunt. The mitral regurgitation should be addressed separately only if a prolapse of the anterior leaflet or a congenital valve can be identified. Similarly, modest mitral valve anomaly can generate severe gradient in this context. No or only minimal intervention on the valve may be required.

Aortic Valve Stenosis and Shone Syndrome. Whether to embark on a biventricular repair or a univentricular pathway in neonates with combined aortic and mitral valve anomalies is one of the most difficult problems in pediatric cardiology. The minimal size of the left ventricle required to survive a biventricular repair in isolated critical aortic stenosis is not a satisfactory criterion. The aim of a biventricular repair should be an excellent long-term functional result, which supposes normal ventricular function and normal pulmonary resistances. At the Royal Children's Hospital, Melbourne, we limit this surgery to patients who have (1) no endocardial fibroelastosis (EFE) on the echocardiographic study *and* intraoperatively, (2) a left ventricle of normal or very close to normal size, (3) a normal-size mitral valve annulus, and (4) the possibility of having the mitral *and* aortic valves satisfactorily repaired. In the early postoperative period, any difficulty in weaning from the ventilator or an absence or minimal pulmonary pressure decrease with persisting reactivity should indicate a revision of the surgical strategy.

Surgical Technique

Bypass Technique

At our institution cardiopulmonary bypass is conducted with moderate hypothermia (32°C), hemoglobin of 10 to 12 g/dL, and pump flow of 150 mL/min per kg or 1 liter/min per m². Myocardial protection is provided with intermittent cold blood cardioplegia administered every 20 to 30 minutes. Venous cannulation should allow ample access to the inter-atrial groove. Limited dissection of the groove is performed. The left atrium is entered through the interatrial groove. The exposure is enhanced with mattress sutures inserted into the posterior annulus pulling the valve upward and toward the operator. The snugger on the inferior vena cava is pulling upward and to the left. A self-retaining retractor for mitral surgery adapted to the size of the patient has to be used in all cases. Once satisfactory exposure of the mitral valve is gained, the valve is systematically analyzed, confronting the observation with the preoperative echocardiographic study. The functional classification is confirmed, but the extension of mitral valve prolapse or restriction is based on echocardiographic study on the beating heart. Then the analysis of the anatomy takes place. The operator must evaluate the texture, aspect, and size of the mitral valve leaflets, the presence and location of jet lesions, the number, aspect, and distribution of the chordae, the presence of commissural tissue and dedicated suspension apparatus, and the presence, size, location, and morphology of the papillary muscles. The examination finishes with a careful check for accessory mitral valve tissue in the interchordal spaces. A supravalvular ring is confirmed or eliminated. The diameter of the annulus and of the opening of the mitral valve is compared to the reference value for the patient's body surface area. At our institution we use a modification of the sizes provided by Kirklin.

Mitral Valve Repair According to the Functional Classification

Correction of Type I Malformation

An annuloplasty is mandatory in all mitral valve repairs for regurgitation with the exception of some isolated type I malformations without annular dilation, mostly cleft mitral valve. Attempts to perform mitral valve repair without annuloplasty have resulted in recurrence. To accommodate an adult-size device or a larger annulus than what would be indicated from the area of the anterior leaflet, leaflet enlargement with glutaraldehyde-treated pericardium of the posterior leaflet, the anterior leaflet, or both is used. When no annuloplasty device is available for the size of the patient or when the device is too small, an annuloplasty limited to the posterior annulus is indicated. The annuloplasty has to incorporate both trigones and can be divided in the middle to allow for further growth. For that purpose, we use expanded polytetrafluoroethylene sheet folded to provide rigidity. The mattress sutures should not be tied too tightly to avoid a corrugating effect (Fig. 98-1).

Correction of Type II Malformation

Correction of type II malformation is rarely necessary in mitral valves with abnormal anatomy but is common in other types of valves. Multiple techniques are available, and are used in isolation or in combination depending on the width of the prolapsus (evaluated intraoperatively), the height of the prolapse (based on the echocardiographic study), and the aspect of the chordae. All techniques are efficient and reliable, provided that the repair is adequate (restores a large surface of apposition between anterior and posterior leaflet) and avoids overcorrection.

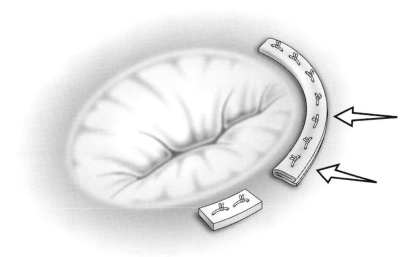

Figure 98-1. Annuloplasty limited to the posterior annulus in patients with annulus less than adult size. A band of polytetrafluoroethylene (PTFE) or pericardium can be used and divided in two or three to allow for growth, or short strips of PTFE can be used.

Chordal shortening requires thin and flexible chordae. The correction generates significant shortening of the chordae and is only adopted when a significant degree of shortening is necessary (Fig. 98-2).

Chordal transfer, mostly between secondary chordae and the free edge, corrects a localized prolapse (Fig. 98-3).

Wedge resection (Fig. 98-4) and *sliding plasty* (Fig. 98-5) generate different degrees of correction of prolapsus to multiple chordae. They are very well adapted to prolapsus extended to a large segment of the anterior leaflet.

The use of *artificial chordae* should be restricted to cases of absence of available chordae of appropriate strength and quality in the area of prolapse. The insertion requires a rigorous technique to avoid overcorrection and large knots at the free edge (Fig. 98-6).

Correction of Type III Malformation

Successful correction of restricted leaflet motion and insufficient leaflet tissue is the essence of treating congenital mitral anomalies, especially in the first year of life.

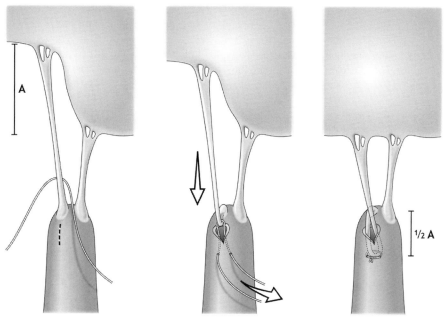

Figure 98-2. Chordal shortening. Note the extent of the shortening achieved. (A = the height of the prolapse to be corrected.)

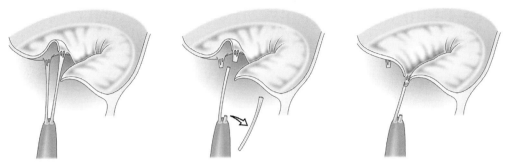

Figure 98-3. Chordal transfer. Only secondary chordae should be used but not the basal chordae.

Access to the suspension apparatus is the key to adequate mobilization of the latter. It can be done through the mitral valve orifice when it is sufficient. In very small patients, the mitral orifice is very small and does not allow for good access to the suspension apparatus. In these situations, the detachment of the posterior leaflet generates a good view of the papillary muscles. Adequate thinning, mobilization from the posterior wall, splitting, and fenestration of the papillary muscles can then be performed safely with good exposure (Figs. 98-7 and 98-8). The posterior leaflet is afterward reconstructed with enlargement of the valvar tissue (Fig. 98-7) when necessary.

The augmentation of the valvular leaflet tissue can be limited to the posterior leaflet or to the anterior leaflet (Fig. 98-9) or used in both. The extension of the posterior leaflet should be less than one half of the height of the leaflet. It can be limited to the area of the middle scallop; alternatively, when the detachment is extended from one commissure to another, to allow for a large opening in diastole, the extension should either be a band or emulate the shape of the posterior leaflet with three scallops and two commissures but should *not* have a crescent shape. The extension of the anterior leaflet should be done in the body of the leaflet, leaving a strip of valvar tissue close to the hinge point to avoid mechanical stress at this level. The height of the extension should not be greater than two fifths of the height of the leaflet, and should leave the area close to the free edge intact to allow for supple and efficient surface of coaptation. It should be symmetric from trigone to trigone.

Resection of Supravalvular Rings and Accessory Mitral Valve Tissue

Resection of supravalvar tissue requires an excellent exposure of the leaflet tissue. The supravalvar tissue can sometimes be peeled off the valvular tissue. More often, there will be a need for a careful cleavage with blunt dissection. Perforation to the anterior leaflet may occur and should be closed with a simple figure-of-eight suture.

The resection of accessory mitral valve tissue requires similar rigorous surgical technique to delineate perfectly the mitral valve chordae from what can be resected without compromising the integrity of the suspension apparatus (Fig. 98-8). Various approaches to the suspension apparatus may have to be combined.

Results

The results have to be presented for two groups: patients ≤1 year of age and patients >1 year of age, or alternatively patients with mitral annulus ≤18 mm and those with

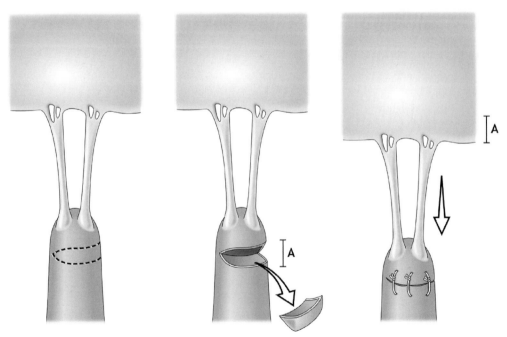

Figure 98-4. Wedge resection. This achieves limited shortening distributed to several chordae. (A = the height of the prolapse to be corrected.)

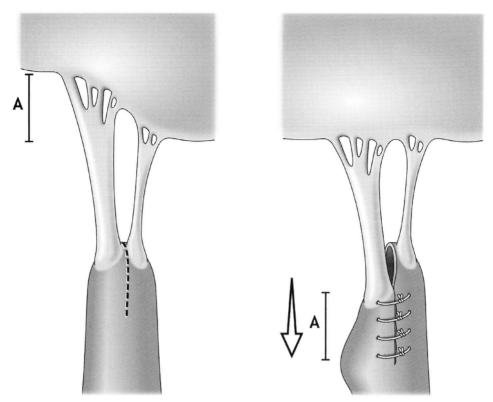

Figure 98-5. Sliding plasty. This achieves controlled shortening for thickened chordae. (A = the height of the prolapse to be corrected.)

mitral annulus >18 mm. In the first group the survival of the patient is the primary goal, which is best achieved through repair. After 1 year of age the technical conditions approach those for adults, the repair of all valves is an achievable goal, and replacement of mitral valves is exceptional. Replacement does not influence long-term survival significantly with current anticoagulation protocols and mechanical prosthesis.

Congenital Mitral Valves in Neonates and Infants

At the Royal Children's Hospital, Melbourne, 10 patients <1 year of age had 13

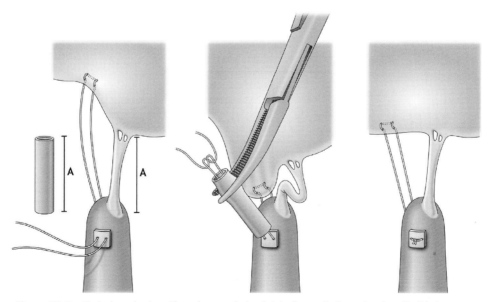

Figure 98-6. Technique for insertion of expanded polytetrafluoroethylene chordae. **(Left)** A template is made from a short plastic tube cut at the required length and slid over the distal part of the stitch. **(Middle)** The free edge of the leaflet is lowered to the contact of the papillary muscle. The artificial chordae is tied while the template is clamped. **(Right)** The template is removed, and the mattress suture is pulled to bring the knot in contact with the papillary muscle. (A = the height of the prolapse to be corrected.)

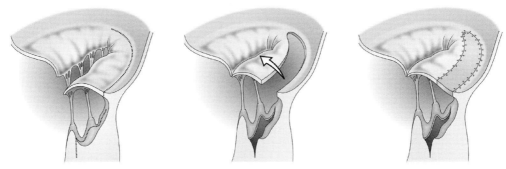

Figure 98-7. Detachment of the posterior leaflet allows access to the suspension apparatus for mobilization (here in a hammock valve). The patch enlargement of the posterior leaflet treats the type III malformation and allows for a larger annuloplasty.

mitral valve procedures for mitral valve regurgitation between 1996 and the end of 2005. All underwent initial valve repair. Two reoperations required valve replacement. There was 1 early death and 1 late hospital death related to inappropriate orientation to biventricular repair for a patient with Shone syndrome.

During the same time span, 7 patients <10 months of age were operated on for congenital mitral stenosis. The median age was 5 months (range 1 week to 10 months). All had severe failure to thrive and severe pulmonary hypertension. The mean preoperative gradient was 13 ± 2.3 mm Hg. The malformations included papillary muscle-to-commissure fusion (n = 3), parachute mitral valve (n = 2), excess tissue (n = 1), and supravalvular ring (n = 1), and 1 of these patients had Shone syndrome. Two patients underwent late reoperations, and

1 required mitral valve replacement. There were no deaths.

Congenital Mitral Valves in Patients Older Than One Year of Age

Mitral Regurgitation

According to the recent series, repair should be expected in more than 90% of the patients, with a hospital mortality rate <10%. Result in the current era should be significantly improved compared to previous series stretching over a long time span. The expected reoperation rate should be <15% at 15 years.

Mitral Stenosis

The hospital mortality should be very low when the mitral stenosis is isolated. Mitral

stenoses with associated cardiac lesions generate high mortality and reoperation rate but are rare in this age group. After mitral valve repair for mitral stenosis, residual gradients are frequent but often well tolerated and reoperations are indicated according to the level of pulmonary hypertension. Supravalvar mitral ring has a high recurrence rate.

Rheumatic Mitral Valves

Mitral valve repair in the pediatric age group in units with significant experience with this surgery is achieved in >90% of the patients, with hospital mortality <2%. Large variations in the reoperation rate are reported (45% to <10% at 5 years). These variations could be attributed to the quality of the follow-up, regional and national specificities, including whether access to surgery is free or not, and, most important, compliance

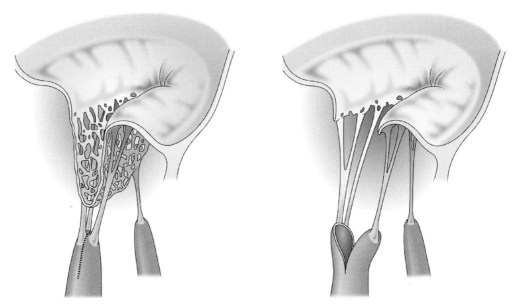

Figure 98-8. Excision of extravalvular tissue, here within a parachute mitral valve. Great care must be taken to preserve the suspension apparatus

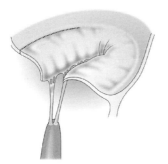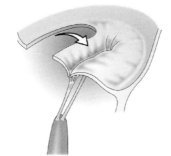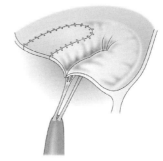

Figure 98-9. Patch enlargement of the anterior leaflet to treat the lack of tissue in congenital valve or the retraction of the rheumatic leaflet.

with secondary antibioprophylaxis. At the Royal Children's Hospital, Melbourne, between 1996 and 2005, 88 patients aged 6 to 24 years of age had surgery for rheumatic mitral valve insufficiency. All had mitral valve repair initially. Freedom from reoperation at 70 months with 32 patients at risk is 78%. There were 15 reoperations in 13 patients, of which 7 were replacements and 8 were further repairs. There was 1 early death and 1 late death.

Conclusion

Mitral valve repair is the objective in all children with significant mitral valve disease. If the mitral valve replacement is unavoidable, it should be delayed until it can be done at low risk. In that context an imperfect repair represents a satisfactory palliation if the surgical indication cannot be delayed altogether.

SUGGESTED READING

Acar C, de Ibarra JS, Lansac E. Anterior leaflet augmentation with autologous pericardium for mitral repair in rheumatic valve insufficiency. J Heart Valve Dis 2004;13:741.

Caldarone CA, Raghuveer G, Hills CB, et al. Long-term survival after mitral valve replacement in children aged <5 years: A multi-institutional study. Circulation 2001;104:1143.

Chauvaud S, Fuzellier JF, Houel R, et al. Reconstructive surgery in congenital mitral valve insufficiency (Carpentier's techniques): Long-term results. J Thorac Cardiovasc Surg 1998;115:84.

Chauvaud S, Mihaileanu S, Gaer J, Carpentier A. Surgical treatment of congenital mitral stenosis: "The Hôpital Broussais" experience. Cardiol Young 1997;7:15.

Disse S, Abergel E, Berrebi A, et al. Mapping of a first locus for autosomal dominant myxomatous mitral-valve prolapse to chromosome 16p11.2-p12.1. Am J Hum Genet 1999;65:1242.

Fann JI, Ingels Jr NB, Miller DC. Pathophysiology of mitral valve disease. Card Surg Adult 2003;2:901.

Guilherme L, Dulphy N, Douay C, et al. Molecular evidence for antigen-driven immune responses in cardiac lesions of rheumatic heart disease patients. Int Immunol 2000;12:1063.

Kohl T, Silverman NH. Comparison of cleft and papillary muscle position in cleft mitral valve and atrioventricular septal defect. Am J Cardiol 1996;77(2):164.

Krishnan US, Gersony WM, Berman-Rosenzweig E, Apfel HD. Late left ventricular function after surgery for children with chronic symptomatic mitral regurgitation. Circulation 1997;96:4280.

Lymbury RS, Olive C, Powell KA, et al. Induction of autoimmune valvulitis in Lewis rats following immunization with peptides from the conserved region of group A streptococcal M protein. J Autoimmun 2003;20:211.

McCarthy JF, Neligan MC, Wood AE. Ten years' experience of an aggressive reparative approach to congenital mitral valve anomalies. Eur J Cardiothorac Surg 1996;10(7):534.

Oosthoek PW, Wenink AC, Vrolijk BC, et al. Development of the atrioventricular valve tension apparatus in the human heart. Anat Embryol (Berl) 1998;198:317.

Oosthoek PW, Wenink AC, Wisse LJ, Gittenberger-de Groot AC. Development of the papillary muscles of the mitral valve: Morphogenetic background of parachute-like asymmetric mitral valves and other mitral valve anomalies. J Thorac Cardiovasc Surg 1998;116:36.

Pomerantzeff PM, Brandao CM, Faber CM, et al. Mitral valve repair in rheumatic patients. Heart Surg Forum 3(4):2000;273.

Pope FM, Burrows NP. Ehlers-Danlos syndrome has varied molecular mechanisms. J Med Genet 1997;34(5):400.

Prifti E, Frati G, Bonacchi M, et al. Accessory mitral valve tissue causing left ventricular outflow tract obstruction: Case reports and literature review. J Heart Valve Dis 2001;10:774.

Schmid AC, Zund G, Vogt P, Turina M. Congenital subaortic stenosis by accessory mitral valve tissue, recognition and management. Eur J Cardiothorac Surg 1999;15:542.

Streif W, Andrew M, Marzinotto V, et al. Analysis of warfarin therapy in pediatric patients: A prospective cohort study of 319 patients. Blood 1999;94:3007.

Tamura M, Menahem S, Brizard C. Clinical features and management of isolated cleft mitral valve in childhood. J Am Coll Cardiol 2000;35:764.

van Karnebeek CD, Naeff MS, Mulder BJ, et al. Natural history of cardiovascular manifestations in Marfan syndrome. Arch Dis Child 2001;84:129.

Wood AE, Healy DG, Nolke L, et al. Mitral valve reconstruction in a pediatric population: Late clinical results and predictors of long-term outcome. J Thorac Cardiovasc Surg 2005;130:66.

EDITOR'S COMMENTS

Mitral valve repair continues to be a surgical challenge in pediatric cardiac surgery. The wide range of anatomic abnormalities and the often palliative nature of valve repair in association with the extreme rarity of congenital valvular abnormalities results in only relatively small reported series of operations for these abnormalities. The results of valve repair in the pediatric population for more common adult diseases (such as rheumatic heart disease) are much more reproducible, and significant series of valve repairs with good results have been published. Patients with mitral regurgitation from either a congenital or acquired cause may respond to valve reparative operations as eloquently described by Dr. Brizard; however, the surgical technique has to be individually tailored to each anatomy. The effect of newer technology, such as three-dimensional echocardiography, on the preoperative assessment of valvular function and anatomy for guiding surgical repair is unknown; however with development of these techniques and more real-time imaging, better assessment of valve function may lead to improved outcomes in the future.

Dr. Brizard and his colleagues have had excellent results with valve leaflet augmentation extension procedures of both the posterior and anterior leaflets. Although we have had very limited experience with these techniques at the Children's Hospital of Philadelphia, the results have not been quite as good as those presented by Dr. Brizard and his group. In situations in which a restricted leaflet motion is present it is not clear that augmenting the leaflet surface in its superior margin with these extensions will always result in better coaptation because the free margin is still tethered by the restricted motion. In augmentation of the anterior leaflet again the chordal attachments at the free margin may be as important as the overall surface area in creating accurate valve function. Nevertheless, Dr. Brizard makes a very good point that these leaflet augmentation methods need to be accurately tailored to the valve anatomy, and excessive patching may actually cause problems.

An area of controversy concerns the supravalvar mitral ring. There is often confusion in the reported series of repair of supravalvar mitral ring between the anatomic entity described by Dr. Brizard and the patient with cor triatriatum sinister. Membrane-like structures dividing the left atrium with a stenotic central orifice can be completely excised with a very low recurrence rate. The acquired form of supravalvar mitral ring such as described by Dr. Brizard is distinguishable from cor triatriatum by the attachment of the supravalvar ring to the mid-portion of the anterior mitral leaflet. This may well be an acquired structure as noted; however, the pathophysiology of development of the lesions is not known. Although recurrence is a possibility due to abnormal flow characteristics across the mitral valve, there have been only a few reported cases of recurrence of supravalvar mitral rings in the literature. Perhaps this is related to the extreme rarity of the condi-

tion or the fact that the underlying stenotic or regurgitant process, which leads to the development of the ring, is addressed at the time of the resection of the ring itself. There appears to be a slightly greater incidence of supravalvar mitral obstruction when there is a left superior vena cava entering the coronary sinus, perhaps creating abnormal flow characteristics across the mitral valve.

Although infective endocarditis of the mitral valve is usually associated with mitral regurgitation, large vegetations on the mitral valve can lead to primary mitral stenosis. The most common situation is a combination of regurgitation and stenosis. If the vegetation is obstructive, resection of the vegetation and valve repair can be performed; however, regurgitation can develop as additional healing of the valve occurs. In most cases, if there has not been extensive destruction of leaflet tissue, valve reparative techniques are preferable to valve replacement in infective endocarditis with the goal of maintaining the native valve for as long possible.

Cardiac catheterization is rarely necessary in the current era for evaluation of valvular lesions on the left side of the heart. Nevertheless, catheterization to measure right ventricular pressure and pulmonary pressure and resistance may be necessary in some cases to determine optimal timing for valve intervention. Interventional catheterization with balloon valvuloplasty of even significant congenital mitral stenosis may be an effective palliative measure in some children. There are small reported series of balloon dilation of congenital mitral stenosis that resulted in adequate relief of valvular obstruction with only modest regurgitation and permitted palliation for sometimes many years prior to the need for surgical intervention.

As noted in Chapter 99 on aortic valve repair, valve reparative procedures are certainly preferable to valve replacement in

all children and young adults if a reasonably durable repair can be achieved. In the mitral position even only modest improvement in stenosis can result in significant palliation. When valve reparative techniques have failed and there is significant pulmonary hypertension or increasing congestive heart failure, valve replacement may be warranted. It is not uncommon to perform multiple valve reparative procedures for mitral regurgitation or stenosis if necessary to avoid valve replacement until an older age when a prosthetic valve can be implanted without increased morbidity and mortality.

The situation of the Shone complex of aortic and mitral valve disease remains difficult. Many patients with this complex anatomy have significant aortic disease as newborns that require balloon dilation. The balloon dilation can then result in only temporary relief of stenosis or can cause significant aortic regurgitation. These patients may then require an autograft aortic valve replacement as a newborn or young infant. Often the nature of the mitral valve disease is not readily apparent until the relief of the distal aortic obstruction is achieved. In situations in which the mitral valve is abnormal in structure, it may be best to consider single-ventricle reconstruction for these patients. Nevertheless, decision-making continues to be difficult, and many patients have an intervention on the aortic valve before consideration is given to the single-ventricle pathway. If aortic regurgitation becomes significant, then it may preclude a single-ventricle reconstruction approach such as the Norwood operation.

Mitral valve procedures in children should be considered palliative. In experienced centers such as the Royal Children's Hospital, Melbourne, the success of mitral valve reparative operations is enviable and a standard to which other pediatric cardiac programs should aspire.

T.L.S.

99

Aortic Valve Repair in Children

Mary Jane Barth, Chawki el-Zein, and Michel N. Ilbawi

Surgical management of aortic valve disease in children presents a difficult dilemma. On one hand, early surgery protects the myocardium from volume and pressure overload, decreases the chance of fibrosis and remodeling, and is consistent with current surgical philosophy of early complete repair of all congenital heart defects. On the other hand, early valve replacement in children is suboptimal because of the lack of an ideal valve substitute that allows growth and does not need anticoagulation or frequent replacement.

The dichotomy created by the absence of the ideal valve substitute and the mounting evidence of deleterious effects of long-standing volume and/or pressure overload have renewed interest in aortic valvuloplasty. Although several techniques, such as annular reduction, commissural resuspension, and cusp extension, were used in the past, valvuloplasty remained an evolving approach rather than a definitive treatment, due in part to lack of complete understanding of the functional anatomy and the precise geometry of the aortic valve. More recently, the successful repair of the atrioventricular valves, the significant progress made in myocardial protection, and the detailed analysis of valve anatomy and function have led to improved results of aortic valve reconstruction.

Anatomy and Function of the Aortic Valve

The three leaflets of the aortic valve are attached to the aortoventricular junction. The collagenous condensation at the point of attachment of each leaflet has been termed the annulus fibrosis. There is, however, no true "ring" of annular tissue supporting the leaflets in a straight circular plane. The hemodynamic stresses on the leaflets, therefore, is counteracted at several structural levels. The margin of coaptation of a competent valve is more than a finite point of contact. It extends along the whole margin of the leaflet in length and several millimeters in depth. Beneath the apices formed by leaflet attachment, the so-called commissures, there are subcommissural or interleaflet triangles (Fig. 99-1) The wide base of these triangles follows the ventricular contraction pattern and allows optimal retraction of leaflets during systole. The sinotubular bar marks the junction with the ascending aorta. It is thicker than the adjacent sinuses. It is circular with areas of increased collagen. It acts as a suspension post that supports the peripheral attachments (the commissures) of the valve leaflets. The parabolic shape of the leaflets resembles a suspension bridge. Their attachments to the sinotubular bar are several millimeters above the level of coaptation. As these support poles stretch outward by as much as 16% during systole, the leaflet edges (the cables) become straighter, aiding in the opening of the valve.

The aortic root is also a complex hemodynamic system. Its component parts change in size and shape during the cardiac cycle. Its upper portion is exposed to the aortic pressure. It expands during systole to allow leaflet retraction. The base of the valve is exposed to ventricular dynamics. It contracts during peak of systole to decrease the distance the leaflets have to close and may reduce the stress forces applied to leaflets during diastole. Moreover, the leaflet—sinus assembly behaves as an independent unit to store the diastolic pressure within. It allows the aortic valve to remain competent even if the interleaflet triangles are partly incised.

The instantaneous changes in aortic valve orifice have been shown to precede movement of blood in the ventricle. The transformation of the aortic orifice from a closed position to a triangle and then to a circle without causing flexion deformity of cusp tissue is related to aortic root distensibility and the mechanism of leaflet suspension.

Pathology and Function of the Abnormal Aortic Valve

Aortic Valve Stenosis
The Bicuspid Aortic Valve
In contrast to the normal tricuspid valve, the leaflet edges are excessive and sagging. As a result, there is increased folding and crossing and a compensatory extension of the area of leaflet approximation from their edges (doming). The opening of the valve is eccentric due to discrepancy in leaflet sizes. The orifice also has an elliptical rather than a circular opening. The resultant distortion in blood flow pattern exaggerates turbulence and predisposes to degenerative changes. Frequently, there is commissural fusion that limits the leaflet movement and further exaggerates eccentricity of the valve opening and effective orifice. The narrowed opening, in combination with annular hypoplasia, impairs the ability of the leaflets to escape systolic or diastolic pressure load, further exaggerating the stress on the valve. The subcommissural triangle is severely attenuated. It limits the leaflet movement in early systole and the change in orifice configuration necessary for appropriate leaflet coaptation at the end of systole. The leaflet edges are suspended below

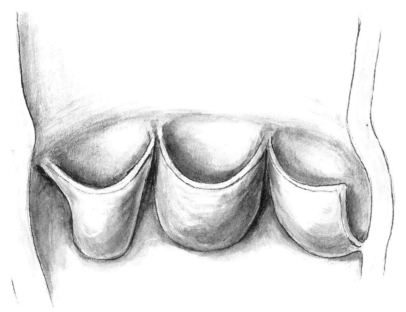

Figure 99-1.   Anatomy of normal aortic valve opened longitudinally. The relationship of the sinotubular bar to commissures is shown. The subcommissural triangle is wide and deep.

the sinotubular bar. This, combined with redundant leaflet edges, results in shallow sinuses, decreases coaptation area, and exaggerates leaflet-deforming dynamic forces (Fig 99-2).

The Rheumatic Aortic Valve

The continued inflammatory process causes progressive scarring and thickening of the leaflets and fusion of the commissures. The valve becomes progressively stenotic.

Valve Regurgitation

Regurgitation Associated with Ventricular Septal Defect

There is discontinuity between the aortic media and the crest of the ventricular septum that results in a decreased support of the sinus wall and progressive prolapse and deformity of the involved cusp. The sagging leaflet edge loses coaptation contact with the other two leaflets and central regurgitation ensues. The noncoronary cusp is usually affected with perimembranous ventricular septal defects, whereas the right coronary cusp is involved with the subarterial, more anterior, ventricular septal defect.

Regurgitation in Patients with Congenital Valvar Stenosis

The continued trauma to the leaflet edges produced by hemodynamic stress and abnormal flow patterns results in progressive scarring, thickening, deformity, and retraction of the leaflet edges and subsequent lack of coaptation.

Aortic Regurgitation Secondary to Subaortic Fibromuscular Stenosis

The abnormal jet pattern produced by the stenosis and the tethering of the leaflet by subvalvar fibrous tissue result in progressive deformity of the leaflet and consequent regurgitation.

Regurgitation in Marfan Syndrome

This condition results from progressive dilation of the weakened aortic root due to fragmentation of its elastic support. The dilated sinotubular bar and valve sinuses stretch apart the commissural suspension and leaflet edges. The increase in hemodynamic stress due to changes in the leaflet suspension mechanism combined with enlarged aortoventricular junction lead to poor leaflet coaptation and central regurgitation.

Post-Balloon Regurgitation

This condition is usually caused by leaflet(s) that tear close to the fused commissure. The leaflet becomes flail and eccentric regurgitation results.

Regurgitation after Arterial Switch Operation

This condition is most likely related to disruption of the sinotubular mechanism and undue dilation of the aortic sinuses caused by the implantation of the coronary artery buttons.

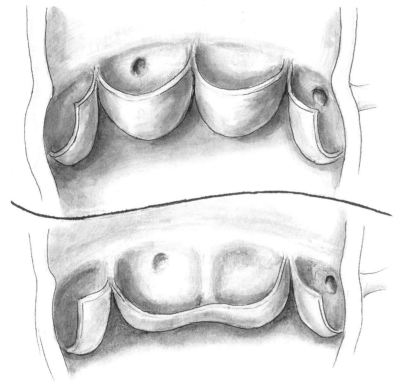

Figure 99-2.   Comparison of normal and bicuspid stenotic valves. The sinuses are shallower and the edges of the leaflets are sagging. The sinotubular bar is superior to the commissures.

Aortic Regurgitation Secondary to Rheumatic Disease

There is cusp retraction secondary to inflammation and scarring. The hemodynamic sequelae result in progressive annular dilation and worsening of the regurgitation.

Timing of Surgical Intervention

To achieve optimal short- and long-term results, surgical intervention should be timed appropriately. The decision relies on achieving the goals of valve surgery, which include relief of symptoms, restoration of exercise capacity, improved quality of life, and, most important, protection of the myocardium from chronic pressure and/or volume overload. Most of the reported guidelines for valve surgery are based on studies in the adult population and on the premise that valve replacement is the only option. These studies use mortality rates as a follow-up endpoint but fail to analyze myocardial performance and reserve several years postoperatively. They use as their database several single-center observational studies and very few prospective, randomized trials.

The introduction of and refinement in valvuloplasty technique have prompted critical evaluation of these older guidelines. The availability of a surgical alternative that avoids valve replacement or anticoagulation has liberalized the old rigid criteria. Although large-scale, long-term data on repaired valves are not available, there is unquestionable evidence that valvuloplasty extends the functional longevity of the native aortic valve in children and may safely delay the need for replacement, thus justifying earlier surgical intervention. Waiting for symptoms to appear or for ejection fraction to decrease might put extra load on the ventricle and lead to long-term ventricular dysfunction.

Assessment of the severity of valve dysfunction and timing of valvuloplasty involves several echocardiographic and Doppler-derived indices. For isolated aortic valvar stenosis, pressure gradients of 40- to 50 torr associated with progressive left ventricular hypertrophy or impaired exercise tolerance are indications for intervention. Measurement of effective valve orifice and the extent of valve pathology are also helpful in deciding the timing of surgery. In isolated aortic valvar regurgitation, a ratio of regurgitant jet to annulus diameter of >40% and the progressive increase in indexed end-diastolic left ventricular dimensions for two consecutive measurements, especially if they exceed a Z score of 3, have been found to correlate with early ventricular dysfunction before onset of symptoms and therefore constitute valid and rather objective indications for intervention.

Techniques of Surgical Valvuloplasty

Most of the surgical techniques used for aortic valve repair were devised many years ago or have been used for a long time. Thorough understanding of the pathology and improvement in cardiopulmonary bypass and myocardial protection have made their successful application possible. In addition, several principles have evolved that helped in improving outcome. These include the following: (1) detailed pre- and intraoperative analysis of pathology is essential. This is best achieved by two- and three-dimensional echocardiography; (2) more than one technique needs to be performed to achieve both competence and relief of obstruction; (3) reconstructive steps should be preceded by as complete as possible relief of obstruction; (4) repair of only one leaflet or cusp is inadequate and leads to early failure; (5) fresh autologous tissues such as pericardium or fascia lata cannot withstand dynamic stress when used for repair; (6) "overcorrection" in cases of aortic valve incompetence might be needed, but excessive correction may lead to crowding and distortion of the repaired valve; and (7) centralizing blood flow through the valve decreases turbulence and extends the longevity of the repair.

Techniques for Restrictive or Stenosis Valve

Unrolling and Thinning of Leaflets

Patients with chronic stenosis, turbulence, and abnormal blood flow patterns have progressive leaflet thickening and distortion. As a result, nodules of scar tissue are formed and edges are rolled away from the center, further restricting leaflet mobility. Thinning of leaflet edges with unrolling may improve valve function but has to be combined with other techniques to yield long-lasting benefits.

Commissurotomy

Harkens et al. introduced the concept of commissurotomy in 1958. The technique involves cutting along the edges of the fused leaflets to allow improved mobility. Classically, the incision is extended up to the commissure. Although this technique results in larger valve orifice, it fails to address many pathologic features of congenital aortic valve stenosis and therefore has had poor long-term outcome.

Extended Commissurotomy

This approach was introduced in 1985 in an attempt to improve on the results of simple commissurotomy. The incision along the edge of the fused leaflets is extended into the aortic wall in curvilinear fashion, splitting inner media at the leaflet junction with the wall. The added extension results in a longer free edge, mobilizes the subcommissural triangle, and centralizes blood flow across the orifice (Fig 99-3). However, it decreases leaflet support and may result in long-term progressive regurgitation if it is

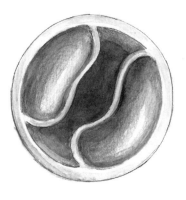
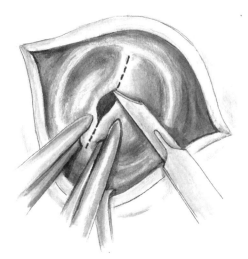

Figure 99-3. Technique of extended commissurotomy. The incision is extended into the aortic wall on both sides to increase the mobility of leaflets.

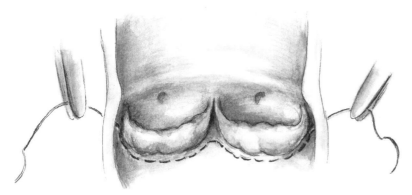

Figure 99-4. Reduction annuloplasty technique. The suture is passed in and out at the base of the aortoventricular junction in a circular fashion.

not combined with leaflet augmentation and suspension.

Techniques for Dilated Annulus

1. In *commissural annuloplasty*, U-shaped pledgeted sutures are placed at each commissure to plicate the aortic wall and reduce its total circumference. It is primarily applicable to valves with normal cusp mobility and moderately dilated annulus. Severe annular dilation cannot be repaired using this technique.
2. *Annular reduction using a circumferential suture around the base of the valve leaflets* may reduce annular dilation. Its use in small children and young adults may limit growth and result in future stenosis (Fig. 99-4).
3. *Patch closure of discrete leaflet perforation* due to infective endocarditis or catheter intervention involves the use of a small patch of autologous or bovine pericardium secured in place with multiple sutures.
4. *Triangular resection and repair of redundant leaflet edge* is rarely successful when performed as an isolated step. Additional leaflet augmentation with a thin strip of pericardium and resuspension of the reconstructed leaflet at the commissures(see next technique) are needed to support the repair (Fig. 99-5).
5. *Leaflet augmentation and resuspension* is the most commonly used technique. After thorough mobilization of all aortic valve leaflets (see techniques for reduced mobility) a piece of autologous or bovine pericardium is fashioned (Fig. 99-6A). The curvilinear longitudinal dimension GHI should equal the length of the leaflet free edge plus two 0.5-cm extensions on both sides (FA and EJ). It is tailored to fit the deficiencies and irregularities of

the leaflet edge. The longitudinal dimension BCD should be slightly straighter and shorter than GHI (Fig. 99-6A). The width CH should provide enough additional depth to the leaflet so that the reconstructed leaflet free edge is level with the sinotubular bar at the commissures but deeper (more caudad) at the center (C). The pericardial patch is sutured to the free edge of the leaflet using 5-0/6-0 running suture from its center toward the commissures. The patch ends (or wings) are then sutured to the aortic wall with pledgeted suture, resulting in a rounded leaflet edge suspended at the sinotubular bar (Fig. 99-6B). The suspending sutures

are placed in such a way as to enhance the bar. The step is repeated for at least one additional leaflet, with special attention such that the heights (width) of the augmenting patches equalize the depth of all sinuses.(Fig. 99-6C,D) This allows effective leaflet enlargement and surface for coaptation. In bicuspid valves with fused but well-developed rudimentary commissure, the commissure is opened and the valve is converted into a tricuspid valve. The three leaflets are then augmented. Centralization of the valve orifice by appropriate mobilization of the leaflets or conversion of the valve into trileaflet should be attempted whenever possible to reduce postrepair turbulence and long-term leaflet scarring and restenosis. An alternative augmentation technique is to release the leaflet-annular attachment and close the created defect in the bottom of the sinus by a patch of pericardium.

The choice of patch material for valve augmentation has evolved through the years. As mentioned earlier, fresh autologous pericardium does not withstand the hemodynamic stress. Treating the pericardium with a high concentration of glutaraldehyde (2%) resulted in a very stiff patch and predisposed to early calcification and stenosis. The use of low concentration

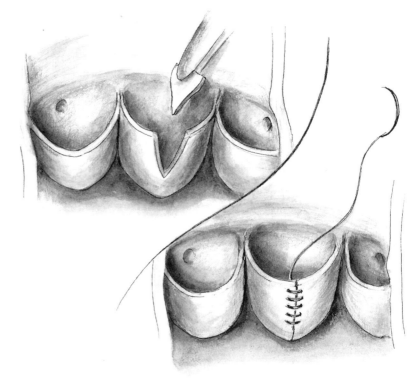

Figure 99-5. Triangular resection and repair of redundant leaflet.

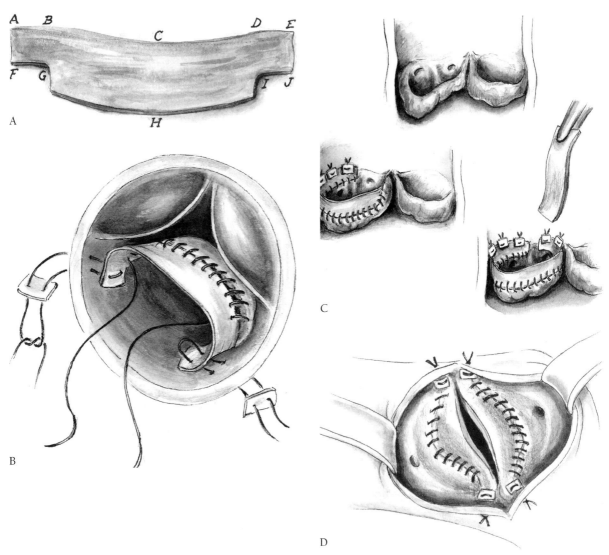

Figure 99-6. Technique of augmentation valvuloplasty. **(A)** The harvested pericardial patch; **(B)** augmentation of the leaflet with the patch and resuspension at the sinotubular bar; **(C)** the end result from the side; **(D)** the appearance of reconstructed valve from above.

of glutaraldehyde (0.6%) with a short fixation time (5 minutes) results in a more pliable patch material and decreases the incidence of restenosis. Thin bovine pericardium processed using infrared wave technology provides a good alternative with minimal calcification or stenosis on follow-up.

Results

The techniques of aortic valvuloplasty are in evolution. Several series have reported results using one or more of the techniques mentioned here. None of these results, however, reflects the present knowledge of the surgical anatomy nor the outcome of the synchronized combination of these technical steps as currently used.

Review of our total experience with these different approaches in 78 patients revealed a significant drop in pressure gradient across the valve, a decrease in aortic regurgitation as judged by grade and by ratio of the ratio of regurgitant jet to aortic annulus diameter, and a decrease in indexed left ventricular end-diastolic dimensions.

Postoperative follow-up from 6 months to 8 years (mean 5.6 ± 1.9 years) revealed a progressive increase in pressure gradient in 42% of patients, associated with stiffening or calcification of the patch used for leaflet augmentation. When restenosis was analyzed further, it was apparent that patients who had valvar stenosis and annular hypoplasia had the highest incidence of restenosis (Fig. 99-7). This might reflect the crowding of these hypoplastic aortic roots

when aggressive overcorrection was used early in the experience. Recurrence of regurgitation was not a problem on follow-up, and most patients maintained competent valves (Fig. 99-8).

Conclusions

Aortic valvuloplasty as currently used has very low operative mortality. It provides an excellent alternative to valve replacement, especially in children and young adults, in whom anticoagulation and repeated valve replacements are serious drawbacks. It maintains the patient's own valve and does not preclude other alternatives when deemed necessary. It is probably superior to the Ross procedure in patients who

Freedom from Reintervention

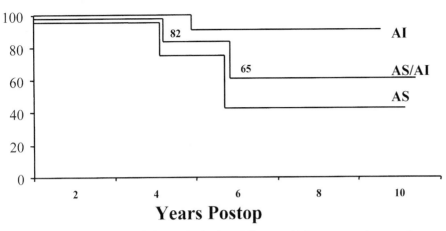

Figure 99-7. Functional life of the repaired valves. Failure was highest among the stenosis group (AS). (AI = aortic insufficiency.)

Regurgitant Jet/Annulus Ratio

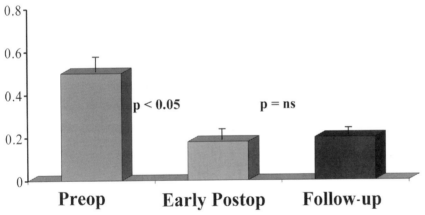

Figure 99-8. Incidence of regurgitation in repaired valves on follow-up.

are very young or have significant annular dilation, due to regurgitation or other causes. Its use in patients with aortic annular hypoplasia should be reduced and limited to avoid recurrent stenosis. The use of patch material not fixed with glutaraldehyde might provide a decrease in the incidence of restenosis because calcification is less likely to happen.

SUGGESTED READING

Becker A. Surgical and Pathological Anatomy of the Aortic Valve and Root. In Cox JL, Sund T (eds), Operative Techniques in Cardiac and Thoracic Surgery. Philadelphia: WB Saunders, 1996;1:3.

Bonow R, Picone A, McIntoch C. Survival and functional results after valve replacement for aortic regurgitation from 1971 to 1983: Influences of preoperative left ventricular function. Circulation 1985;72:1244.

Borer J, Hochreiter C, Herrold EMCM, et al. Prediction of indications for valve replacement among asymptomatic or minimally symptomatic patients with chronic aortic regurgitation and normal left ventricular performance. Circulation 1998;97:525.

Borer J, Truter S, Herrold E, et al. Myocardial fibrosis in chronic aortic regurgitation. Circulation 2002;105:1837.

Bozbuga N, Erentug V, Kirali K, et al. Midterm results of aortic valve repair with the pericardial cusp extension technique in rheumatic valve disease. Ann Thorac Surg 2004;77:1272.

Chartrand C, Saro-Seervvando E, Vobecky J. Long term results of surgical valvuloplasty for congenital valve aortic stenosis in children. Ann Thorac Surg 1999;68:1356.

Cheung M, deLeval M, Tsang V, Redington A. Optimal timing of the Ross procedure in the management of chronic aortic incompetence in the young. Cardiol Young 2003;13:253.

Duran C: Present status of reconstructive surgery for aortic valve disease. J Card Surg 1993;8:443.

Grande-Allen K, Cochran R, Reinhall P, Kunzelman K. Mechanisms of aortic valve incompetence: Finite-element modeling of Marfan syndrome. J Thorac Cardiovasc Surg 2001;122:946.

Guidelines for the management of patients with valvular heart disease. A report of the American College of Cardiology/American Heart Association Task Force on Practice Guidelines. Circulation 1998;98:1949.

Hasaniya N, Grundy S, Razzouk A, et al. Outcome of aortic valve repair in children with congenital aortic valve insufficiency. J Thorac Cardiovasc Surg 2004;127:970.

Hawkins J, Minich L, Shaddy R, et al. Aortic valve repair and replacement after balloon aortic valvuloplasty in children. Ann Thorac Surg 1996;61:1355.

Ilbawi MN, DeLeon SY, Wilson WR, et al. Extended aortic valvuloplasty. A new approach for the management of congenital valve aortic stenosis. Ann Thorac Surg 1991;52:663.

Kiodas E, Enriquez-Sarano M, Tajik AJ, et al. Optimizing timing of surgical correction in patients with severe aortic regurgitation. J Am Coll Cardiol 1997;30:746.

Lambert V, Obreja D, Losay J, et al. Long-term results after valvotomy for congenital aortic valvar stenosis in children. Cardiol Young 2000;10:590.

Okura H, Yoshida K, Hozumi T, et al. Planimetry and transthoracic two dimensional echocardiography in noninvasive assessment of aortic valve area in patients with valvular aortic stenosis. J Am Coll Cardiol 1997;30:753.

Robicsek F, Thubrikar M, Cook J, Fowler B. The congenitally bicuspid aortic valve: How does it function? Why does it fail? Ann Thorac Surg 2004;77:177.

Smith P, Barth M, Ilbawi M. Pericardial leaflet extension for aortic valve repair: Techniques and late results. Semin Thorac Cardiovasc Surg Pediatr Card Surg Annu 1999;2:83.

Sutton J, Ho Yen S, Anderson R: The forgotten interleaflet triangles: A review of the surgical anatomy of the aortic valve. Ann Thorac Surg 1995;94:419.

Thubrrikar M, Piepgrass W, Shaner T, Nolan SP. The design of the normal aortic valve. Am J Physiol 1981;241:H795.

Vandervoort P, Rivera J, Mele D, et al. Application of color Doppler flow mapping to calculate effective regurgitant orifice area: An in vitro study and initial clinical observation. Circulation 1993;88:1150.

Yacoub M, Cohn L. Novel approaches to cardiac valve repair: From structure to function: Part I. Circulation 2004;109:942.

Yacoub M, Cohn L. Novel approaches to cardiac valve repair: From structure to function: Part II. Circulation 2004;109:1064.

Yacoub MH, Gehie P, Chandrasekavan V, et al. Late results of a valve-preserving operation in patients with aneurysm of ascending aorta and root. J Thorac Cardiovasc Surg 1998;115:1080.

Yacoub M, Kilner P, Birks E,et a!. The aortic outflow and root: A tale of dynamism and cross talk. Ann Thorac Surg 1999;68(3 Suppl):537.

EDITOR'S COMMENTS

There has been a resurgence of interest in aortic valve repair based on the pioneering work of Dr. Ilbawi and his associates. As very nicely summarized in this chapter, the complex geometry of the aortic valve requires multiple approaches to achieve a competent repair, and the procedure must be tailored to the individual patient's anatomy and pathophysiology. The use of valve extension techniques as pioneered by Dr. Ilbawi has permitted the creation of trileaflet valves even in patients with bicuspid valves to achieve a more central orifice and improve the long-term outcome.

Valve reparative techniques may offer the option for earlier surgical intervention in patients with significant aortic stenosis and insufficiency. The indications for intervention, however, remain somewhat vague. In most cases, stenosis with a measured peak-to-peak gradient of greater than 40 to 50 mm Hg is a relative indication for surgical or balloon intervention, especially when there is associated left ventricular hypertrophy or strain pattern on electrocardiogram. Exercise testing with evidence for ventricular dysfunction is another relative indication. Symptoms are a late finding in aortic stenosis and should not be the indication for surgical intervention. Aortic insufficiency of a severe degree causing diastolic flow reversal in the descending aorta and significant progressive ventricular volume overload are indications for surgical intervention. Documented increase in left ventricular end-diastolic dimension on serial measurements that are greater than three standard deviations above normal despite use of afterload reduction therapy is a relative indication for surgery, as is a decrease in systolic performance on exercise. Exercise intolerance is another relative indication for intervention.

An increasing number of patients are coming to aortic valve repair or replacement after balloon dilation of aortic valve stenosis in infancy. In many cases these valves can be repaired by the techniques described by Dr. Ilbawi's group. However, many of these patients have relative hypoplasia of the aortic annulus, and the reparative techniques to alleviate the regurgitation may result in varying degrees of stenosis. Therefore, these valves may be best suited to a valve replacement rather than valve repair. Concerns about longevity and aortic root dilation over time of the autograft aortic valve replacement have led to an increasing use of valve reparative techniques as a temporizing measure. We use valve repair whenever possible if we believe a relatively durable (>5 year) good result can be anticipated. If the valve is significantly distorted or if valve reparative techniques will result in relative stenosis, we believe that the Ross operation may be a better choice. Nevertheless, patients with predominant aortic insufficiency can often have a quite durable valve repair, which may allow children to grow and provide more options for valve replacement in the future.

We consider valve repair a palliative procedure that will ultimately require reoperation and valve replacement; however, in small and growing children, female patients, and young adults it may be advisable to perform a valve repair of limited durability to allow the patient to grow into adulthood, when mechanical valve replacement may be a better option. In addition, the increasing interest in development of tissue-engineered valves lends hope that in the future viable valves can be developed that will alleviate many of the concerns with bioprosthetic or mechanical valve replacement.

The tissue used for valve leaflet extension is controversial. As noted, glutaraldehyde-fixed tissue tends to calcify and stiffen over time and may lead to valve degeneration and recurrent regurgitation or stenosis, requiring reoperation. Fresh pericardium tends to shrink and may lead to a relatively unstable early repair. The use of any nonautologous tissue such as homograft material or bovine pericardium has not been examined at long enough follow-up to determine whether these tissues might provide a more reliable alternative. Nevertheless, the use of nonviable tissue for reconstruction is likely to result in degeneration over time.

The complex geometry of the aortic valve and the difficulty in assessing the valve function in the operating room make the use of newer imaging modalities for pre- and postoperative assessment important. Three-dimensional echocardiography is a new modality that may preoperatively identify the mechanism of valve dysfunction and guide the surgical intervention for valve repair. When three-dimensional reconstruction can be done in real time, it may significantly improve our ability to perform accurate valve repairs.

The complications of valve replacement as noted in Chapter 100 have led most pediatric centers to begin more aggressive repair of valves in all positions in the heart in the hope of providing reasonably durable palliation before anticipated later valve replacement.

T.L.S.

Valve Replacement in Children/Ross Procedure

Ronald C. Elkins

Operative repair or replacement of a cardiac valve is relatively uncommon in children, and delays in operative care in children with significant hemodynamic valvular disease are frequent, because the options for valve replacement are not satisfactory for many of these young, growing patients. The cardiac surgeon involved in the clinical management of an infant or child with valvular heart disease must constantly be aware of the unique characteristics and requirements of such a patient. Growth, activity level, lifestyle, and difficulty of medical compliance produce a unique set of requirements that must be considered when consulting on or planning the operative care of a child. In most situations, valvular heart disease should be managed with these concepts in mind so that the child's cardiac growth will not be compromised by prosthetic materials and lifestyle will not be altered unnecessarily. Valve repair by a well-conceived and well-executed surgical procedure is frequently the best alternative for a young child. Many of the operative procedures that allow valve conservation in an adult are not applicable to children because of the requirement of growth. The need for innovative techniques with maintenance of viability of transplanted or transposed tissue is paramount (see Chapters 97 to 99).

A detailed discussion of anatomic and pathologic valve abnormalities is not presented in this chapter, because they have been discussed previously. This chapter presents operative techniques and indications in young patients with aortic valve disease, mitral valve disease, tricuspid valve disease, and pulmonary valve disease requiring valve replacement.

Aortic Valve Disease

The most common congenital abnormality of the heart is a bicuspid aortic valve. It has been estimated that one third of the patients with this abnormality are born with or develop significant aortic stenosis (AS) during their lifetime. A significant number of patients with AS and a bicuspid aortic valve also have a component of subvalvular obstruction that may be a limited subvalvular membrane, whereas others have diffuse narrowing of the left ventricular outflow tract. One third of the patients with a bicuspid aortic valve have aortic valve insufficiency (AI), and this is frequently noted during adolescence or young adulthood. One third of the patients do not develop significant aortic valve dysfunction unless they develop endocarditis of their bicuspid aortic valve.

Children born with significant aortic valve obstruction may present with congestive heart failure in the first few hours of life and require early intervention as a lifesaving measure. If the left ventricle is of adequate size, an urgent aortic valvotomy in the form of a balloon valvuloplasty by the interventional cardiologist, a surgical aortic valvotomy using the transventricular approach, or an open valvotomy with the use of cardiopulmonary bypass is indicated (see Chapter 80). In situations in which a successful valvotomy cannot be accomplished or in which severe AI is created by the valvotomy, an aortic valve replacement with a pulmonary autograft (Ross operation) has been performed in a number of patients with excellent short-term results. This operation is accomplished as a root replacement, and when done with absorbable sutures, the potential for growth is excellent. Long-term results of this operation are not available, but the early success and the results with a significant number of patients having a Ross operation during the first year of life are encouraging. The techniques used in this operation are discussed later in this chapter.

With the increased use of aortic balloon valvuloplasty for primary aortic stenosis or recurrent aortic stenosis, an increased number of children require surgical intervention for severe aortic insufficiency after balloon valvuloplasty. Some centers advocate an aortic valve repair using techniques of surgical repair of leaflet tears, patch repairs of perforations, leaflet augmentation with glutaraldehyde-fixed autologous pericardium, and surgical repair of commissures. Early results with these types of repair have shown good results with a freedom from valve reoperation (valve repair or replacement) of 100% at 3 years and freedom from increased aortic insufficiency of 75% at 3 years. Whether this approach will equal the results obtained with a similar group of patients having a primary Ross operation is unknown.

Patients with a normal-sized ventricle and reduced ventricular function, even if associated with significant endocardial fibroelastosis (increased echogenicity of the left ventricular endocardium) and severe obstruction at the aortic annulus or subvalvular level, can have successful surgical management with an extended Ross operation (Ross operation using the Konno procedure to enlarge the aortic outflow tract with a septal myotomy and myectomy).

Successful aortic valvotomy or resection of subvalvular obstruction should be viewed as a palliative procedure. The development of recurrent left ventricular obstruction or the development of significant AI is related to the underlying pathologic abnormality and to the surgeon's ability to correct the abnormality. In our experience with 237 patients surviving after aortic valvotomy or resection of subvalvular obstruction, slightly >50% of children required reoperation within 10 years. In those patients requiring aortic valve surgery before age 5 years, almost 80% required reoperation before age 15 years. In children who develop recurrent stenosis without AI or only mild insufficiency that can be treated with a repeat aortic valvotomy, either as a balloon valvuloplasty or as a second surgical procedure, serious consideration should be given to the pathologic abnormality of the valve and the ability to restore valve function, which will provide significant duration (>15 years) of near-normal valve function. A decision to replace the aortic valve with a pulmonary autograft may be a more conservative approach than doing a limited aortic valvotomy and having a patient that requires a third median sternotomy and aortic valve replacement in a few years. Even though the patient remains at risk for additional surgery because of the presence of the pulmonary homograft used for reconstruction of the right ventricular outflow tract (actuarial freedom from reoperation on the pulmonary homograft is 86 ± 5% at 14 years in our series of 201 patients), this reoperation has significantly less risk than a third operation for aortic valve replacement.

Children who develop significant AI after aortic valvotomy should be treated medically and followed closely with clinical assessment and echocardiographic evaluation of valve function and left ventricular function and size. When the patient becomes functionally limited or shows signs of increasing left ventricular size or decreasing left ventricular function, aortic valve replacement should be considered. The early and late results with replacement of the aortic valve in the Ross operation support its use as the operation of choice in children and young adults.

AI may be associated with a ventricular septal defect (VSD). The VSD may be in the outlet septum or located in the perimembranous portion of the septum. Usually, the right coronary leaflet prolapses through a subconal VSD and the noncoronary leaflet if the VSD is perimembranous. With time, the leaflet becomes elongated and redundant. In about one half of patients, the aortic valve is tricuspid, and in the remaining patients there may be fusion at the right and noncoronary commissure. Use of patch closure of the VSD and a valvuloplasty consisting of decreasing the length of the elongated leaflet has been the traditional approach to management of this lesion. Recently, Carpentier identified the increased diameter of the aortic annulus caused by the presence of the VSD and proposed the use of a circumferential purse-string suture placed at the annulus in the base of the coronary sinuses and extending below the annulus in the interleaflet triangle. In the area of the VSD patch, this suture line will be at or near the attachment of the patch. This suture is brought external to the aorta in the noncoronary sinus and is tied over a pledget. The redundant portion of the free margin of the prolapsed leaflet is then resected as a triangular resection in the mid-portion of the leaflet. This restores a more normal anatomy of the three leaflets, and with the reduction annuloplasty, more appropriate leaflet coaptation is obtained. In those patients in whom a bicuspid aortic valve is associated with a VSD, I have used the Ross operation as a root replacement and have closed the VSD by increasing the length of the right ventricular free wall on the autograft at the time of mobilization of the autograft and have used this extension of the autograft root to close the VSD.

Operative Technique

In the performance of aortic valve surgery in children, I prefer to have optimal exposure with a "quiet" operative field. I have found that mild systemic hypothermia with cold blood cardioplegic perfusate provides excellent myocardial protection that allows time to accomplish the necessary procedure in a very careful and deliberate fashion. I routinely use bicaval cannulation, with one cannula placed high in the superior vena cava (SVC). This allows the retrograde infusion of cardioplegic solution in almost all patients, even in very small ones, in whom cannulation of the coronary sinus may require direct vision. Placement of the superior vena caval cannula high in the SVC ensures that it will not obstruct the view of the aortic valve. I use a left ventricular vent in all patients, and place this vent through the right superior pulmonary vein, across the mitral valve, into the left ventricle. The aorta should be cannulated high, either at the origin of the innominate artery or more distally if significant disease of the ascending aorta is identified. I always dissect the aortic fat pad and expose the origin of the right coronary artery so that the aortotomy can be properly positioned depending on the planned operative procedure. I prefer a transverse aortotomy about 1 cm to 2 cm above the origin of the right coronary artery with a vertical extension into the noncoronary sinus at its midpoint. With properly placed stay sutures, this allows excellent exposure of the aortic valve and subvalvular outflow tract.

Several anatomic relationships must be kept in mind, because the outcome of an operation to restore valve function or to replace the aortic valve with a nonstented tissue valve depends on the successful recreation of these normal anatomic relationships. Aortic valve competence depends on aortic valve leaflet coaptation, and it is this coaptation that allows the very thin, delicate normal aortic valve leaflet or pulmonary valve leaflet to withstand the stress associated with systemic resistance and also to provide essentially zero impedance to forward flow. Proper coaptation depends on aortic annulus dimensions (size and configuration), sinotubular dimensions, and the height and position of each commissure in relation to the other two commissures (Fig. 100-1). Lack of appreciation for these principles and the inability to reproduce these relationships delayed the widespread use of nonstented tissue valves for many years. The evolution of experience with replacement of the ascending aorta and aortic valve as a Bentall procedure, the experience developed with the arterial switch procedure, the use of homograft valves as a root replacement, and the introduction of the

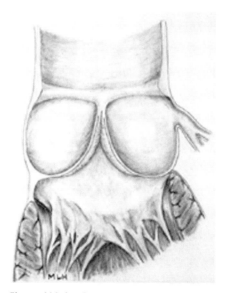

Figure 100-1. Proper coaptation depends on aortic annulus dimensions (size and configuration), sinotubular dimensions, and the height and position of each commissure in relation to the other two commissures.

root replacement technique for the Ross operation have led many surgeons to use this operation in the management of young patients with aortic valve disease (see Chapter 46 for a description of the Ross operation). After excision of the abnormal aortic valve, the aortic annulus should be carefully sized with a Hegar dilator or an appropriate valve sizer. This diameter is compared to a nomogram of the expected size based on the patient's body surface area. In patients with a Z-value of −2 or smaller, the annulus should be enlarged by careful removal of all obstructing fibrous tissue and a portion of the aortic annulus in the noncoronary sinus. In most patients, this will be adequate; however some patients may require resection of a subvalvar membrane and a left ventricular myomectomy or they may require a Ross-Konno to relieve their obstruction. In those patients with an aortic annulus Z-value of +2 or greater, an annular reduction should be performed. In children in whom significant somatic growth is anticipated and in whom at the time of Ross operation the aortic annulus is normal in size, I use absorbable sutures for the suture lines in inserting the autograft valve. This enhances the likelihood of growth of the autograft valve. All other technical aspects of the Ross operation are similar to those used in adults.

Aortic Valve Replacement

When the pathologic state of the aortic valve is not amenable to a valvuloplasty, replacement with a pulmonary autograft is the procedure of choice if the pulmonary valve is normal. In 1% to 2% of patients with a bicuspid aortic valve, the pulmonary valve is bicuspid, and in these patients we replace the aortic valve with an aortic homograft as a root replacement. The pulmonary autograft may be used as an intra-aortic implant or as a root replacement. When using the autograft as an intra-aortic implant, the inclusion technique allows the autograft to be inserted as an anatomic unit and reduces the risk of altering the intercommissural dimensions. In adult-sized patients with an annulus size between 20 mm and 25 mm and relatively normal anatomy, we initially preferred the intra-aortic insertion of the pulmonary autograft. The long-term results of this operation have been reported by Ross with an actuarial survival of 80% at 20 years and a freedom from replacement of the autograft of 85% at 20 years. The root replacement, first used

in 1986, has become the most frequently used technique for insertion of the autograft. This technique allows the surgeon to use the pulmonary autograft for a wide variety of pathologic lesions involving the aortic valve and the left ventricular outflow tract. The valve is translocated as an anatomic unit, and intraoperative distortion cannot occur if significant mismatch between the pulmonary annulus and the aortic annulus is avoided or an appropriate annulus reduction is performed when aortic annular dilation is a component of the patient's disease. In 201 patients (age 1 day to <18 years of age, median 9.9 years) having a Ross procedure between August 1986 and June 2002, actuarial survival for operative survivors was 97% ± 2% at 14 years. Operative mortality was 5%, and there have been 4 late deaths, 1 of them valve related. One hundred and sixty-one patients had a root replacement, 13 had a Ross-Konno procedure, and 40 had an intra-aortic implant (17 scalloped subcoronary and 23 inclusion cylinder implants). Actuarial freedom from autograft degeneration (autograft reoperation or severe autograft insufficiency not related to infection, or valve-related death) in the 190 operative survivors was 83% ± 8% at 14 years. In the 148 root replacements, excluding 2 patients with bicuspid pulmonary valves that had relatively early degeneration, actuarial freedom from autograft degeneration was 95% ± 3% at 13 years (Fig. 100-2). Autograft reoperation in all patients was for technical error in 2 patients, an abnormal pulmonary autograft valve in 2, aortic annulus dilation in

4, and autograft sinus dilation in 3. Actuarial freedom from explant of the autograft valves was 88% ± 7% at 14 years. Actuarial freedom from allograft degeneration (allograft intervention [replacement, balloon valvuloplasty, stent placement, or allograft reoperation], peak gradient 50 mm Hg, or more or severe valve insufficiency) was 67% ± 6% at 14 years. Twenty-five patients had a valve-related event. There were no valve-related embolic or bleeding events, 2 patients developed endocarditis (1 allograft valve and 1 autograft valve), 1 valve-related death, 11 autograft valve reoperations (1 autograft reoperation was for recurrent subvalvar obstruction), and 11 pulmonary allograft reoperations. Actuarial freedom from all valve-related events was 67% ± 9% at 14 years.

In patients with an abnormal pulmonary valve, either a bicuspid pulmonary valve or significant structural abnormality of one or more leaflets, we have used an aortic homograft to replace the aortic valve. A homograft that is slightly larger than the patient's aortic annulus and obtained from a donor of relatively young age is selected. The homograft is inserted as a root replacement and is inserted in a normal anatomic orientation. The left coronary is implanted to an opening in the left coronary sinus of the homograft after excision of the ostium of the homograft left coronary. The coronary is implanted with a large cuff of aorta so that re-replacement will be simplified. The right coronary is implanted after the homograft has been inserted and the distal suture line has been completed. The ho-

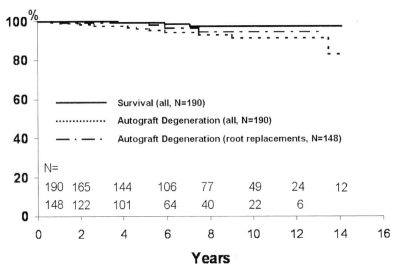

Figure 100-2. Actuarial survival and freedom from autograft degeneration in 190 operative survivors over 14 years and actuarial freedom from autograft degeneration in 148 root replacement patients (excludes 2 patients in whom bicuspid pulmonary valves were used as autografts, which showed early degeneration).

mograft is then distended with cardioplegic solution, and the site for implantation of the right coronary is selected so that distortion of the right coronary attachment will not occur. Frequently, the site of attachment of the right coronary is cephalad to the origin of the homograft right coronary artery origin. The early results of aortic valve replacement with a homograft valve as a root replacement are excellent. The late results depend on the recipient's immunologic reaction to the homograft and to the degeneration of the nonviable leaflets. In very young patients, accelerated deterioration of the valve and dysfunction that requires valve replacement has been seen. The long-term results of allograft replacement of the aortic valve with a cryopreserved allograft have recently been reported, and the actuarial freedom from reoperation from structural degeneration in a patient <20 years of age is 47% at 10 years, with most of the reoperations occurring between 5 and 10 years.

Annulus Enlargement

To completely relieve left ventricular outflow tract obstruction, it may be necessary to significantly enlarge the aortic annulus and widen the outflow tract with an aortoventriculoplasty. The pulmonary autograft replacement of the aortic valve lends itself to this operation and simplifies it. After the pulmonary artery and its contained valve are mobilized, the right ventriculotomy

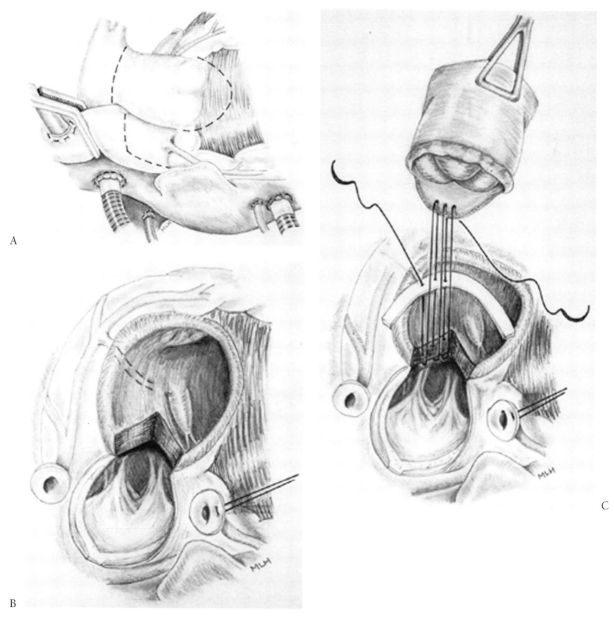

Figure 100-3. **(A)** After the pulmonary artery and its contained valve are mobilized, the right ventriculotomy is positioned so that 1.0 cm to 1.5 cm of the anterior free wall of the right ventricle, proximal to the pulmonary valve annulus, is enucleated with the pulmonary autograft. **(B)** This ventriculotomy is extended toward the conal papillary muscle, which is readily visualized. **(C)** The pulmonary autograft is positioned in an anatomic position, with the anterior free wall of the right ventricle being used to close the ventriculotomy, and the pulmonary root is attached to the aortic annulus in the normal fashion.

is positioned so that 1.0 cm to 1.5 cm of the anterior free wall of the right ventricle, proximal to the pulmonary valve annulus, is enucleated with the pulmonary autograft (Fig. 100-3A). The aortic valve is resected, the coronary arteries are mobilized for implantation of the autograft as a root replacement, and the aortic root is resected. A septal ventriculotomy is then made near the commissure between the left and right coronary sinuses. This ventriculotomy is extended toward the conal papillary muscle, which is readily visualized (Fig. 100-3B). If a septal myectomy is required, it can be accomplished before insertion of the autograft. The pulmonary autograft is positioned in an anatomic position with the anterior free wall of the right ventricle being used to close the ventriculotomy, and the pulmonary root is attached to the aortic annulus in the normal fashion (Fig. 100-3C). I use a polytetrafluoroethylene (Teflon) felt buttress when attaching the autograft to the septal myocardium along the ventriculotomy, but absorbable sutures are used along the aortic annulus. The right ventricular muscle should revascularize, and this technique should allow "growth" of the autograft. The remainder of the Ross operation is as previously described. Once the autograft has been inserted, the cross-clamp can be removed and the integrity of the coronary and annular anastomoses can be inspected. Homograft reconstruction of the right ventricular outflow tract is then accomplished in the usual fashion. A pulmonary homograft that is slightly larger than the size of the distal pulmonary artery confluence should be selected. The homograft is attached as usual to the cut edge of the right ventricle, except where the septal closure has occurred. In this area, the homograft will be sutured to the autograft for a short distance. The use of this technique should allow correction of almost any left ventricular outflow tract obstructive lesion and has the potential to provide normal aortic valve function for the patient's lifetime. We have used this extension of the Ross operation in very young patients with complex left ventricular outflow tract problems, in young adults, and in patients with previous atrioventriculoplasty and a prosthetic valve who have desired or required discontinuation of their anticoagulation.

Annuloaortic Dilation or Ectasia

Patients with significant aortic annulus dilation, AI, and a bicuspid aortic valve are candidates for aortic valve replacement when symptoms of left ventricular dysfunction occur or when significant and progressive ventricular dilation is identified on echocardiographic examination. These patients are frequently teenagers or young adults, and use of a prosthetic valve and the long-term risk and complications of anticoagulation in this group of patients, who have difficulty with medical compliance, has been associated with poor long-term results. The Ross operation provides an opportunity to restore valve function with the least disruption of the patient's lifestyle. However, an uncorrected significant discrepancy between the aortic annulus and pulmonary annulus has been associated with early autograft valve failure. We have recently modified our technique of autograft insertion in these patients in the hope of improving the intermediate-term and long-term results. A pulmonary autograft is inserted as a root replacement in combination with a reduction annuloplasty of the aortic annulus and fixation of the size of the aortic annulus with an external reinforcement. The reduction annuloplasty is accomplished with two purse-string sutures of 2-0 polypropylene placed in the aortic annulus beginning in the noncoronary sinus and extending along the annulus in the depths of the coronary sinus and below the annulus in the interleaflet triangle. The suture is brought through the aorta in the noncoronary sinus and tied over a pledget, and the annulus size is reduced to the determined size based on body surface area (Figs. 100-4 to 100-6). The pulmonary autograft is performed as a root replacement. The proximal suture line is completed with interrupted 4-0 polypropylene sutures placed to include the annular reduction sutures, and, after the autograft is seated, the sutures are tied over a reinforcing cuff of woven Dacron. This cuff is used to "fix" the size of the aortic annulus (Fig. 100-7). In a young child with significant expected somatic growth, the annulus reduction can be accomplished using a Z-value of the aortic annulus that is between +2 and 0, recognizing that the pulmonary autograft valve may be associated with mild autograft insufficiency, but with a "fixed" aortic annulus,

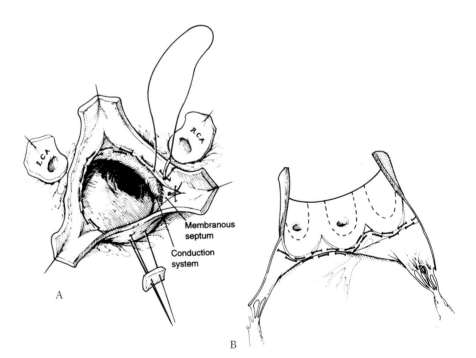

Figure 100-4. **(A)** Two purse-string sutures of 2-0 polypropylene are placed at the aortic annulus in the nadir of the coronary sinuses, in the lateral fibrous trigone in the interleaflet triangle between the left and noncoronary sinus, in the muscle of the ventricular septum at the commissure between the left and right coronary sinuses, and in the membranous septum between the right and noncoronary sinus. The sutures are brought through the aortic annulus external to the aorta in the midpoint of the noncoronary sinus and passed through a felt pledget. **(B)** An opened view of the aortic annulus showing the exact placement of the sutures. Notice the placement of the sutures in the membranous septum to avoid the conduction system. (With permission from RC Elkins. The Ross Operation in Patients with Dilation of the Aortic Annulus and of the Ascending Aorta. In Cox JL, Sundt III TM (eds), Operative Techniques in Cardiac and Thoracic Surgery, Vol. 2. Philadelphia: WB Saunders, p. 333, 1997.)

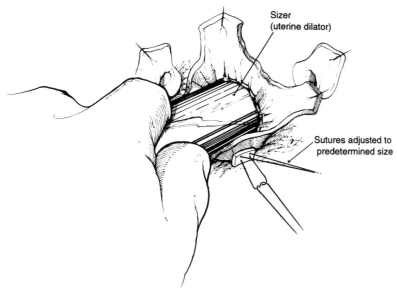

Figure 100-5.   The two sutures are tied over the felt pledget with a graduated dilator in the aortic annulus of appropriate size for the patient. (With permission from RC Elkins. The Ross Operation in Patients with Dilation of the Aortic Annulus and of the Ascending Aorta. In Cox JL, Sundt III TM (eds), Operative Techniques in Cardiac and Thoracic Surgery, Vol. 2. Philadelphia: WB Saunders, p. 334, 1997.)

the autograft insufficiency should not increase.

Our early results have been very encouraging, and we are using this technique in an increasing number of older children and young adults. We have been able to use this technique to decrease the aortic annulus from between 34 mm and 35 mm to between 23 mm and 24 mm without difficulty. In some of these patients, the aortic annular di-

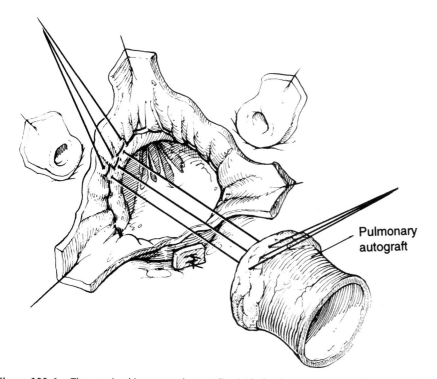

Figure 100-6.   The proximal interrupted suture line includes the annulus reduction sutures at the level of the aortic valve annulus. (With permission from RC Elkins. The Ross Operation in Patients with Dilation of the Aortic Annulus and of the Ascending Aorta. In Cox JL, Sundt III TM (eds), Operative Techniques in Cardiac and Thoracic Surgery, Vol. 2. Philadelphia: WB Saunders, p. 335, 1997.)

lation has been associated with an ascending aortic aneurysm or with significant dilation of the ascending aorta. In patients with an ascending aortic aneurysm, the aneurysm was resected and replaced with a Dacron graft of appropriate size (Fig. 100-8). We use a size similar to the selected size of the aortic annulus reduction and suture the graft to the pulmonary autograft just distal to the sinotubular junction. In patients with dilation of the ascending aorta, an aortoplasty with excision of a semi-ellipse of the aorta and reduction of its diameter to that of the aortic annulus is accomplished before the distal suture line is completed (Fig. 100-9).

Mitral Valve Replacement

In a child requiring a mitral valve replacement, valve selection is limited to a mechanical valve because of the lack of durability of bioprosthetic xenografts or of allograft valves. The newer, low-profile tilting–disc valves have a favorable orifice-to-annulus ratio and have demonstrated early excellent hemodynamics. They all require anticoagulation with warfarin and, particularly in very young children, are subject to pannus ingrowth that will obstruct the valve leaflets or cause a significant reduction in the valve orifice. In adult-sized older children, mitral valve replacement is similar to that in adults and appears to have similar early and intermediate-term results. There appears to be an increased risk of thromboembolic complications, especially valve thrombosis in older children and young adults. In a small child, mitral valve replacement can be difficult because of the small mitral annulus, small left atrium, and small left ventricle. In these patients, a median sternotomy provides excellent exposure. In patients with a small left atrium, it may be helpful to use hypothermic circulatory arrest to avoid the presence of atrial cannulas that may hamper exposure. Either an atriotomy in the interatrial groove or a right atriotomy extending into the atrial septum provides good exposure. The largest prosthetic mitral valve that can be inserted should be used in the hope that the requirement for repeat mitral valve replacement can be minimized. In a neonate, it is usually possible to insert a 19-mm or larger valve. In situations in which the mitral annulus is extremely small or the left ventricular outflow is narrow, the mitral valve can be inserted in a supra-annular position, 0.5 cm to 1.0 cm above the annulus, anchoring the prosthetic valve ring to the

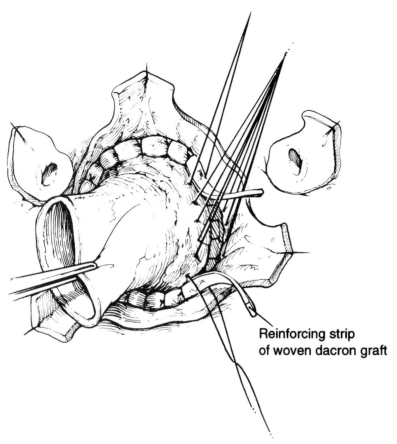

Reinforcing strip
of woven dacron graft

Figure 100-7. The proximal suture line is tied over a thin strip of woven Dacron graft, with care taken to keep the Dacron material external to the autograft and not between the apposition line of the aortic annulus and the autograft. The two ends of the Dacron graft are tied together with the last two sutures to complete the "fixation" of the aortic annulus. (With permission from RC Elkins. The Ross Operation in Patients with Dilation of the Aortic Annulus and of the Ascending Aorta. In Cox JL, Sundt III TM (eds), Operative Techniques in Cardiac and Thoracic Surgery, Vol. 2. Philadelphia: WB Saunders, p. 335, 1997.)

left atrial wall. The early results have been successful in a small number of neonates, and this procedure has allowed successful replacement of the mitral valve in a very difficult situation. When inserting a prosthetic mitral valve, the surgeon should avoid the use of additional prosthetic material, such as felt pledgets, to reinforce the valve suture line. These pledgets enhance local scar formation, make the repeat mitral valve replacement more difficult, and may limit the ability to utilize a significantly larger prosthesis at the repeat operation. The surgeon and the patient's cardiologist should anticipate that a successful mitral valve replacement in a neonate has an 80% likelihood of requiring reoperation within 5 years.

Recently, there has been renewed interest in pulmonary autograft replacement of the mitral valve in children and young adults. This operation was originally described by Ross in 1967 and has been revived by Kabbani and Ross with modifications of the

"top hat" replacement of the mitral valve with an allograft valve as described by Yacoub. They reported very good intermediate–term results in 80 patients with a mean age of 39 years. The pulmonary autograft is inserted into a tube of woven Dacron with the annulus of the pulmonary autograft being sewn to the proximal end of the Dacron tube, which provides support for the autograft valve. The distal pulmonary artery is sewn to the distal end of the Dacron graft, and then the Dacron graft with its contained autograft valve is sutured to the mitral annulus. The Dacron graft is then covered externally with autologous pericardium to avoid thrombus formation in the left atrium. I used the "top hat" technique of pulmonary autograft replacement of the mitral valve in a patient (age 7 years) in 1991. Normal echocardiographic function of the valve was maintained for 10 years. The patient had more than tripled his size by the time of his death from reactive airway disease. At

autopsy, the autograft valve appeared normal with excellent revascularization of the autograft. Initial experience with the use of pulmonary autograft replacement of the mitral valve is now occurring in this country and, if continued favorable results are seen, a mitral valve replacement that does not require long-term anticoagulation may be available for children and young adults.

Pulmonary Valve Replacement

Pulmonary valve replacement as an isolated valve replacement or as a conduit for reconstruction of the right ventricular outflow tract has become an increasing part of the congenital heart surgeon's practice. As our ability to palliate and correct complicated congenital cardiac abnormalities has increased and as these children have grown and reached adulthood, the consequences of residual pulmonary stenosis and pulmonary insufficiency are being recognized with increasing frequency. Many congenital lesions require conduit reconstruction of the right ventricular outflow tract for their original "corrective" procedure. The original conduit used was a Dacron conduit with a contained bioprosthetic valve. The unfavorable performance of these conduits, however, with intimal peel obstruction of the conduit or structural degeneration of the valve in a relatively short time after implantation in young children, led to discontinuation of their use. The pulmonary allograft rapidly became the conduit of choice for right ventricular reconstruction and pulmonary valve replacement in children and young adults. However, the limited supply of allograft conduits, especially in small sizes, and their early failure from calcification and loss of valve function from valve or conduit obstruction has led to a continuing search for an appropriate valved conduit for reconstruction of the right ventricular outflow tract. The cryopreserved allograft pulmonary valve remains the gold standard for right ventricular outflow tract reconstruction. In patients having a Ross operation, the pulmonary allograft performance is more favorable than when used for reconstruction of other congenital abnormalities. In our experience with 190 Ross operation survivors, actuarial freedom from allograft explant is 81% ± 8% at 16 years. However, the actuarial freedom from allograft degeneration (allograft reoperation, balloon valvuloplasty with or without stent placement, peak gradient of 50 mm Hg or more, and/or severe pulmonary

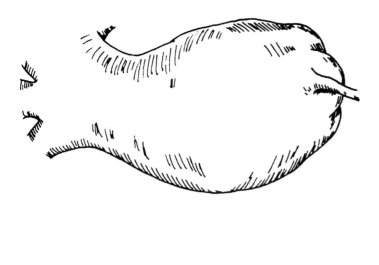

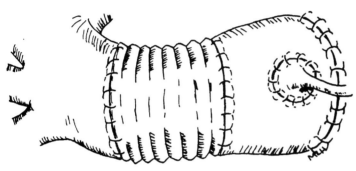

Figure 100-8. In patients with an ascending aortic aneurysm, the aneurysm is resected and replaced with a polyester (Dacron) graft of appropriate size.

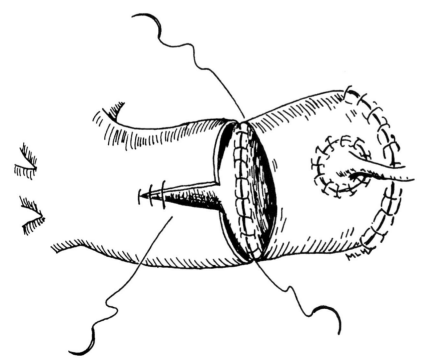

Figure 100-9. In patients with dilatation of the ascending aorta, an aortoplasty with excision of a semi-ellipse of the aorta and reduction of its diameter to that of the aortic annulus is accomplished before the distal suture line is completed.

insufficiency) is 67% ± 6% at 16 years. In a previous study of 72 children requiring allograft reconstruction of the right ventricular outflow tract for other congenital abnormalities, the freedom from allograft failure (reoperation, peak gradient of 40 mm Hg or more, and/or severe pulmonary insufficiency) was 53% ± 10% at 8 years. In a multivariable analysis of these data comparing all allografts implanted in the right ventricular outflow tract through January 1997, donor age <5 years, later year of operation, and non-Ross operation were identified as risk factors for allograft dysfunction.

The demonstration that young patient age, small size of the allograft, pulmonary hypertension, and distal pulmonary artery disease have been associated with allograft failure by other investigators and the decreasing availability of allografts of an appropriate size have led to the search for alternate valved conduits for right ventricular reconstruction. The most promising of the recent generation of valved conduits introduced is the Contegra conduit (Medtronic Inc., Minneapolis, MN). This conduit is a glutaraldehyde-fixed jugular bovine vein with the contained trileaflet venous valve presently marketed in Europe and under investigation in clinical trials in the United States. Early experience has been very good, with limited early complications. In older patients, especially those who require replacement of a prior conduit reconstruction of the right ventricular outflow tract, the Medtronic Freestyle valve has been used with good short-term results. In patients of adequate size, pulmonary valve replacement with a bioprosthesis has been used by a number of investigators. Depending on available right ventricular outflow tract tissue, this type of implantation may require an on-lay patch of pericardium or prosthetic material. The use of mechanical valves for pulmonary valve replacement has been avoided by most surgeons due to the tendency of valve thrombosis on the right side of the heart.

The pulmonary allograft valve continues to be the valve of choice for pulmonary valve replacement in older children and young adults. Whenever possible, the pulmonary allograft conduit should not be implanted with a distal Dacron extension to extend the allograft pulmonary artery or proximal as a Dacron hood, because these techniques appear to be associated with an increased incidence of early failure. If necessary, a piece of pericardium or prosthetic graft material may be used as an anterior gusset to allow implantation of the allograft without distortion or kinking.

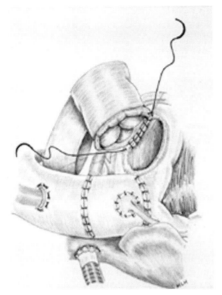

Figure 100-10. Proximal suture line of the pulmonary homograft insertion during the Ross operation. Sutures in the right ventricular septum are superficial to avoid septal coronary arteries.

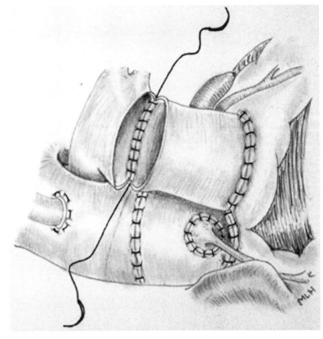

Figure 100-11. Distal suture line of the pulmonary homograft insertion after adjusting the length of the homograft. Fine polypropylene sutures without pledgets.

In reconstruction of the right ventricular outflow tract, it is important to avoid distortion of the allograft conduit during implantation and to attempt to compensate for the normal elongation of the conduit that will occur with distention. It is essential that neither the distal nor the proximal anastomosis be associated with residual obstruction. I have found that performance of the proximal anastomosis first allows me to adjust the conduit length and, if necessary, to perform the distal anastomosis to the distal main pulmonary artery, to the bifurcation of the distal pulmonary artery, or to the right and left pulmonary arteries as necessary to avoid distal obstruction. These anastomoses are performed with fine polypropylene sutures and do not need reinforcement with felt pledgets (Figs. 100-10 and 100-11).

Tricuspid Valve Replacement

Tricuspid valve replacement is a relatively rare occurrence. Its indications are tricuspid stenosis, endocarditis, and severe tricuspid insufficiency not amenable to valvuloplasty. Although there is concern for the use of prosthetic valves on the right side of the heart, most surgeons feel that a prosthetic valve is the valve of choice. Long-term anticoagulation will be required with these valves. They can be inserted in the usual

fashion with pledgeted sutures, but attention must be given to the avoidance of the conduction system. Along the ventricular septum, I place the sutures on the atrial aspect of the tricuspid annulus and use the septal leaflet of the tricuspid valve for anchoring the valve. Attention to this detail is very important as one approaches the junction of the septal leaflet and the anterosuperior leaflet. This is the area where the conduction system is most likely to be injured, and the most common operative complication of tricuspid valve replacement is complete heart block. In patients with Ebstein malformation, the tricuspid valve leaflets, particularly the septal and mural leaflets, are displayed toward the junction of inlet and apical trabecular components of the right ventricle. Frequently, these leaflets are quite large and redundant and may require some resection to avoid obstruction of the replacement valve or of right ventricular outflow. The conduction system can be located in the triangle of Koch, and sutures can be placed in the ventricular muscle between the atrioventricular junction and the septal leaflet attachment. These sutures should be placed carefully to avoid the right coronary artery, which runs below the atrioventricular junction.

Mechanical valve replacement in a very young or small child presents several distinct disadvantages. The mechanical valve will require anticoagulation with its attendant difficulty and limitations of lifestyle.

The valves are obstructive, and the patient will likely have an elevated right atrial pressure that will increase as the child grows, and this may impact the child's growth and development. In this group of patients, some surgeons use allograft pulmonary valves to replace the tricuspid valve. These are inserted as a top hat procedure or unstented, with the proximal anastomosis being completed with pericardium between the allograft annulus and the right atrial floor. Early results with these approaches have been good; however no long-term data about the fate of the allografts are available. One would anticipate that the fate of an allograft in the tricuspid would parallel the experience of allografts used in Ross operation patients of similar age.

Tricuspid valve replacement can be accomplished, but it should be utilized only after careful consideration of surgical repair.

SUGGESTED READING

Aharon AS, Laks H, Milgalter E. Congenital Malformations of the Mitral Valve. In Sabiston D Jr, Spencer FC (eds), Surgery of the Chest. Philadelphia: Saunders, 1995;1544.

Bando K, Danielson GK, Schaff HV, et al. Outcome of pulmonary and aortic homografts for right ventricular outflow tract reconstruction. J Thorac Cardiovasc Surg 1995;109:509.

Capps SB, Elkins RC, Fronk DM. Body surface area as a predictor of aortic and pulmonary valve diameter. J Thorac Cardiovasc Surg 2000;119:975.

Clarke DR, Bishop DA. Ten year experience with pulmonary allografts in children. J Heart Valve Dis 1995;4:384.

Clarke DR, Campbell DN, Hayward AR, Bishop DA. Degeneration of aortic valve allografts in young recipients. J Thorac Cardiovasc Surg 1993;105:934.

Elkins RC, Knott-Craig CJ, Howell CE. Pulmonary autografts in patients with aortic annulus dysplasia. Ann Thorac Surg 1996;61: 1141.

Elkins RC, Knott-Craig CJ, Ward KE, et al. Pulmonary autograft in children: Realized growth potential. Ann Thorac Surg 1994;57:1387.

Gerosa G, McKay R, Ross DN. Replacement of the aortic valve or root with a pulmonary autograft in children. Ann Thorac Surg 1991;51:424.

Kabbani SS, Jamil H, Hammoud A, et al. The mitral pulmonary autograft: Assessment at midterm. Ann Thorac Surg 2004;78:60.

Niwaya K, Knott-Craig CJ, Lane MM, et al. Cryopreserved homograft valves in the pulmonary position: Risk analysis for intermediate-term failure. J Thorac Cardiovasc Surg 1999; 117:141.

O'Brien MF, Harrocks S, Stafford EG, et al. The homograft aortic valve: A 19-year, 99.3% follow up of 1,022 valve replacements. J Heart Valve Dis 2001;10:334.

Editor's Comments

The advent of balloon valvuloplasty for valvar AS and the development of the pulmonary autograft procedure for replacement of the aortic valve and root (Ross operation) have dramatically changed the approach to children with congenital aortic valve disease. As noted in Chapter 80, early surgical intervention by aortic valvotomy has become unusual, and balloon valvuloplasty is the primary procedure of choice for aortic valve stenosis in newborns or infants.

Pulmonary autograft valve replacement has permitted replacement of stenotic or regurgitant aortic valves earlier in life. In the past, as noted by Dr. Elkins, patients with significant valvar disease often were managed medically for prolonged periods at the expense of ventricular function, because the options for valve replacement were limited in children and suboptimal. Mechanical valve replacement in children is associated with need for reoperation as the child outgrows the valve size, and the difficulties of anticoagulating young children are significant, with the added inconvenience of multiple blood drawings for monitoring. Other alternatives for valve replacement are also unappealing, including tissue valves, which degenerate rapidly in children, and

homograft valves, which do not have the growth potential of autografts and also have a reasonably high incidence of late degeneration. However, the Ross pulmonary autograft valve replacement as described in this chapter and as extensively performed by Dr. Elkins and others in many children with complex forms of left ventricular outflow tract obstruction has proved to be a quite durable and satisfactory procedure. Dr. Elkins has shown conclusively that the autograft valves can grow in young children, and the natural endothelial surface and viability of the autograft seems to be ideal for aortic valve replacement. Thus, the favorable characteristics of the autograft valve replacement may actually permit earlier replacement of the aortic valve rather than repeated valvotomies or other procedures, which may provide only short-term palliation and potentially exacerbate ventricular dysfunction by maintaining chronic volume and pressure loads on the ventricle. The pulmonary homograft valve used to replace the right ventricular outflow tract in the Ross operation may not grow with the child; however, in most cases a much larger pulmonary homograft can be inserted than the size of the autograft valve, which in most children >3 or 4 years of age permits the use of an almost adult-sized valve. Although stenosis of the homograft valve has rarely occurred, in most cases the valves become insufficient with time, which is well tolerated hemodynamically on the right side of the heart.

On rare occasions, the pulmonary valve is abnormal, and Dr. Elkins has suggested that he does not use bicuspid pulmonary valves for the Ross operation. However, in young children in whom other valve replacements are unappealing or a homograft replacement of the aortic valve would likely be associated with a significant risk of reoperation because of the patient's growth, we use the bicuspid pulmonary autograft, because it may have satisfactory function over the intermediate term. However, other abnormalities of the pulmonary valve, including any pulmonary valvar insufficiency related to leaflet abnormalities such as quadricuspid valves have been associated with autograft regurgitation when used in the aortic position. Therefore, if significant pulmonary valve abnormalities are noted, even in the presence of delicate valve leaflets, we now believe that the autograft should not be used.

Dr. Elkins has described nicely the Konno modification of the Ross operation for patients in whom enlargement of the left ventricular outflow tract is necessary.

We have also used the technique of excising a portion of right ventricular outflow tract muscle with the autograft as a way of closing the incision in the ventricular septum; however, in patients in whom a larger septal incision is necessary, we have used a Gore-Tex patch to fill in the septal defect and have sewn the autograft to the superior margin of the patch. In these patients, when the pulmonary autograft is much larger than the native aortic root after reconstruction, the pulmonary homograft used to replace the right ventricular outflow tract is relatively large and must swing around the new aortic root, which is larger than the original. Thus, it is important to be sure that there is adequate length of the homograft used for right ventricular outflow reconstruction, and, as the suture line is brought toward the right side of the incision in the right ventricular outflow tract, that it does not become compressed by the autograft aortic root. The homograft has a tendency to be draped across the autograft root. The natural curvature of an aortic homograft may provide a better option for right ventricular outflow reconstruction than a pulmonary homograft in some cases.

Dr. Elkins has also described the technique for decreasing the size of the aorta for the distal anastomosis when the ascending aorta is somewhat dilated with the autograft root replacement procedure. We have used a similar technique; however, we have found that the pulsatility of the autograft in the aortic root caused by the elasticity of the pulmonary artery can cause significant bleeding when there is a diameter discrepancy at the distal suture line, and we therefore tailor the distal aorta as described by Dr. Elkins, but also reinforce the suture line with a strip of Teflon felt or pericardium to decrease the pulsatility at the suture line and decrease the risk of bleeding.

The greatest long-term concern after Ross pulmonary autograft aortic root replacement is the development of progressive dilation of the autograft and AI. Although there does appear to be an incidence of progressive aortic regurgitation in these patients from dilation of the proximal autograft pulmonary artery wall and distortion of the sinuses, the incidence appears to be relatively low and the progression slow. Nevertheless, reoperations will likely be necessary in some of these patients. However, a valve replacement procedure that can be done in young children with a likely reoperation-free rate at 5 years of 80% to 90% or greater, as has been noted for the autograft, is a significant advance for the management of valvular disease in children.

With longer follow-up of the use of the Ross pulmonary autograft as a root replacement in children and young adults, there has been an increasing incidence of autograft root dilation. The sinuses and aortic wall appear to dilate, and even with annular fixation techniques that preserve valve function, significant aneurysms of the proximal aorta can develop. It is unclear at what size intervention is justified, because there is a distal suture line that potentially could prevent distal dissection as seen in Marfan syndrome; however, there has been an isolated case report of dissection of the autograft wall in association with root dilation. Therefore, most centers expect that when root dilation progresses to 5 cm, root replacement should be performed. There is an increasing experience of use of the valve-sparing root replacement in this condition to preserve the autograft valve for as long as possible. In most cases the autograft valve leaflets remain delicate and can coapt well when the autograft wall is replaced with a Dacron graft. There has also been increasing interest in supporting the autograft wall at the time of implantation in older children and young adults, when growth is not an issue, in the hope of preventing the complication of late aortic root dilation. The effect of a rigid prosthetic stenting of the autograft root on overall late autograft function is not known.

Mitral valve replacement in very small children continues to have a significant morbidity and mortality because of the inability to place a small prosthesis in or near the mitral annulus without interference with disk motion. In most very small infants, supra-annular mitral prosthetic valve replacement must be performed, and this procedure ventricularizes a portion of the left atrium below the valve. In patients in whom pre-vious atrioventricular canal defect repairs have been performed, this places a portion of the atrial septal patch and its attachments to the common atrioventricular valve at high pressure, which can be associated with significant risk of dehiscence. Thus, attention must be paid to a secure closure of the atrium below the valve insertion site in these patients. In addition, the valve may partition the left atrium such that a very small chamber is present where the common pulmonary veins enter the atrium above the mitral prosthesis. This has been associated with pulmonary venous hypertension as a result of the lack of compliance in this chamber. On occasion, we have placed a patch on the superior aspect of the left atrium to enlarge the atrial chamber above the prosthetic valve and used this patch to enlarge the atrial septum and the superior aspect of the right atrium as well. This has resulted in improved flow characteristics across the mitral valve. In addition, the technique allows placement of a prosthetic valve in even a newborn infant with enlargement of the right atrium so that the superior vena caval entrance into the right atrium is not compressed by the sewing ring of the prosthetic valve in the left atrium as it is pushed to the right.

As noted by Dr. Elkins, there has been an increasing interest in the use of the pulmonary autograft valve as a mitral prosthesis (the Ross II operation). Various modifications of the technique for implantation have been described with both the "top hat" method described by Dr. Elkins and by placing the valve in a more anatomic position at the mid-portion of the mitral annulus. Some authors have even suggested reinforcing the autograft valve with a graft that is slit to allow for potential growth. The effects of these modifications on long-term valve function are unknown. It does appear, however, that use of the autograft mitral valve in very small infants and newborns is associated with development of stenosis, and obviously the need to support the autograft valve prevents growth. Nevertheless, this technique may be valuable in difficult situations when mitral valve replacement is absolutely required in a very small child. Unfortunately, many children who have significant mitral valve disease as infants and neonates also have significant aortic disease in which the autograft valve may be more necessary for the aortic valve replacement.

We have found it possible to place allograft pulmonary valves in the pulmonary outflow tract in most cases without kinking, even if a short distance is present from the right ventricle to the pulmonary bifurcation, by placing the proximal suture line down into the right ventricle and sewing to the infundibular septum proximally. In this situation, if the allograft valve is cut distally at the level of the commissural attachments, a very short prosthetic conduit can be created and in most cases can be implanted without any kinking. Nonviable prosthetic material extensions of allografts are avoided if at all possible.

Valve replacement in children remains a surgical challenge; however, the autograft valve has markedly improved the results with aortic valve replacement in infants and children. Mitral valve repair and replacement continue to be problematic, and the long-term durability of allograft valves in the pulmonary position and aortic position remains suboptimal. Thus, there continues to be room for improvement in developing viable prosthetic valves for cardiac valve replacement in growing children.

T.L.S.

101

Fontan Conversion/Arrhythmia Surgery

Constantine Mavroudis, Barbara J. Deal, and Carl L. Backer

Catheter ablation of atrial reentry tachycardia after surgical repair of congenital heart disease has immediate success rates of 30% to 80%, with short-term recurrence rates of >50% for certain types of heart disease. The catheter technique is more likely to fail in hearts with residual hemodynamic problems or markedly thickened atria. The Fontan population is particularly problematic; significant atrial arrhythmias occur in as many as 50% of patients with long-term follow-up, and there is limited success after catheter ablation, with high recurrence of tachycardia (Table 101-1). The disappointing results of the catheter approach have been attributed to many factors, including chronic atrial hypertension and dilation, distorted anatomy, multiple reentrant circuits, and limitations of catheter access and delivery. Particularly after lateral tunnel–type repairs, catheter access may be restricted. Markedly thickened atria contribute to an inability to deliver radiofrequency lesions of sufficient depth to create a line of block. The ability to perform three-dimensional mapping of multiple reentrant circuits and to track the continuity of the ablation lines of block, coupled with newer types of energy delivery enabling deeper lesions, may improve the results of catheter ablation in the future.

The majority of Fontan patients with disabling atrial arrhythmias have significant hemodynamic abnormalities, including obstruction of the right atrium-to-pulmonary artery connection, pulmonary venous obstruction, and massively dilated right atria with sluggish venous flow, predisposing to atrial thrombosis. In some patients, atrial reentry tachycardia may degenerate into atrial fibrillation, which is not currently amenable to catheter ablation in this population. The loss of atrial contractility is particularly debilitating in patients with

single-ventricle anatomy. In the early experience of Fontan revision, surgical revision of the Fontan anastomosis, without direct intervention for the arrhythmia substrate, was performed with the expectation that disabling arrhythmias would be ameliorated. This approach resulted in improved hemodynamics, but almost uniform recurrence of the atrial tachycardia (Table 101-2). In postoperative Fontan patients with refractory atrial tachycardia, the association of hemodynamic abnormalities and recurrent tachycardia after surgical repair has led to a combined surgical approach to arrhythmia therapy with revision of the Fontan hemodynamics.

Arrhythmia Substrate

The incidence of atrial arrhythmias after Fontan-type surgery increases steadily with the postoperative interval, with at least 50% of patients experiencing problematic atrial tachycardia by 20 years of follow-up. Although the arrhythmias are generally believed to be a consequence of surgical interventions, electron microscopy has demonstrated that the atria of patients with tricuspid atresia show a distinctly abnormal atrial fiber array compared with normal hearts; the atypical fiber orientation may predispose the atria to the slowing of conduction necessary for reentrant rhythms. Natural history studies of unoperated adults with tricuspid atresia have also shown that at least 40% of patients experienced tachycardia by the fourth decade. In postoperative Fontan patients, supraventricular tachycardia is usually a macro-reentrant rhythm involving the right atrium, although in lateral tunnel–type repairs the reentrant rhythm may be localized to the pulmonary venous

atrium. Slowed conduction with reentry is facilitated by anatomic barriers, such as the orifices of the inferior and superior venae cavae, the os of the coronary sinus, and the atrial septal defect, further confounded by extensive atrial suture lines of either the atriopulmonary anastomosis or the lateral tunnel repair. Residual hemodynamic abnormalities (or simply the dissipation of energy forces within the atria) result in marked distention with fibrosis, complicated by sinus node dysfunction with an irregular atrial rhythm serving as triggers for the onset of tachycardia.

Surgical variables identified as risk factors for the development of tachycardia include an older age at the time of initial repair, early postoperative arrhythmias, sinus node dysfunction, and double-inlet left ventricle. Modifications of the atriopulmonary anastomosis to the lateral tunnel repair were developed in an effort to improve hemodynamics and limit late arrhythmias. Although initial reports suggested a decreased incidence of arrhythmias after the lateral tunnel technique, this difference has become less significant with longer periods of follow-up. The extracardiac total cavopulmonary anastomosis, by limiting atrial suture lines, has a theoretical advantage in limiting the development of tachycardia; this is supported by Amodeo's early follow-up report showing a 5-year arrhythmia-free rate of 92%.

Surgical Management

Surgical treatment of tachycardia localized to the atria may involve resection or cryoablation of atrial tissue in addition to isolation procedures. Some authors had good results with simple cryoablation and

Table 101-1   Ablation Results in Fontan Patients

Authors	Patients	Acute success (%)	Mean follow-up (months)	Recurrence (%)
Triedman et al., 1995[1]	6	33	—	(50)
Kalman et al., 1996[2]	4	50	17	(50)
Chinitz et al., 1996[3]	3	33	12	100
Lesh et al., 1997[4]	3	33	—	—
Betts et al., 2000[5]	5	60	6	66
Chan et al., 2000[6]	1	100	—	100
Collins et al., 2000[7]	43	72	—	32
Nakagawa et al., 2001[8]	6	100	10	33
Triedman et al., 2002[9]	63	43	25	52
Kannankeril et al., 2003[10]	15	—	38	53
Weipert et al., 2004[11]	30	83	18	76[a]

[a]Arrhythmia recurrence not specifically stated; 76% of patients were receiving antiarrhythmic medications at follow-up.

[1]Triedman JK, Saul JP, Weindling SN, Walsh EP. Radiofrequency ablation of intra-atrial reentrant tachycardia after surgical palliation of congenital heart disease. *Circulation* 1995;91:707.

[2]Kalman JM, Van Hare GF, Olgin JE, et al. Ablation of "incisional" reentrant atrial tachycardia complicating surgery for congenital heart disease. Use of entrainment to define a critical isthmus of conduction. Circulation 1996;93:502.

[3]Chinitz LA, Bernstein NE, O'Connor B, et al. Mapping reentry around atriotomy scars using double potentials. Pacing Clin Electrophysiol 1996;19:1978.

[4]Lesh MD, Kalman JM, Saxon LA, Dorostkar PC. Electrophysiology of "incisional" reentrant atrial tachycardia complicating surgery for congenital heart disease. *Pacing Clin Electrophysiol* 1997;20:2107.

[5]Betts TR, Roberts PR, Allen SA, et al. Electrophysiological mapping and ablation of intra-atrial reentry tachycardia after Fontan surgery with the use of noncontact mapping system. *Circulation* 2000;102:419.

[6]Chan DP, Van Hare GF, Mackall JA, et al. Importance of atrial flutter isthmus in postoperative intra-atrial reentrant tachycardia. Circulation 2000;102:1283.

[7]Collins KK, Love BA, Walsh EP, et al. Location of acutely successful radiofrequency catheter ablation of intraatrial reentrant tachycardia in patients with congenital heart disease. Am J Cardiol 2000;86:969.

[8]Nakagawa H, Shah N, Matsudaira K, et al. Characterization of reentrant circuit in macroreentrant right atrial tachycardia after surgical repair of congenital heart disease: Isolated channels between scars allow "focal" ablation. Circulation 2001;103:699.

[9]Triedman JK, Alexander ME, Love BA, et al. Influence of patient factors and ablative technologies on outcomes of radiofrequency ablation of intra-atrial re-entrant tachycardia in patients with congenital heart disease. J Am Coll Cardiol 2002;39:1827.

[10]Kannankeril PJ, Anderson ME, Rottman JN, et al. Frequency of late recurrence of intra-atrial reentry tachycardia after radiofrequency catheter ablation in patients with congenital heart disease. Am J Cardiol 2003;92:879.

[11]Weipert J, Noebauer C, Schreiber C, et al. Occurrence and management of atrial arrhythmia after long-term Fontan circulation. J Thorac Cardiovasc Surg 2004;127:457.

excision of automatic foci when found. Multiple ectopic foci arrhythmia recurrence led surgeons to apply more extensive techniques such as pulmonary vein isolation, left atrial isolation, right atrial isolation, and His bundle cryoablation with pacemaker insertion in difficult cases. In general, refractory cases are rare and require an individualized treatment plan for accurate diagnosis and ablation.

Multiple reports introduced slight modifications to the extant surgical atrial ablative techniques; these modifications include alternative energy delivery systems for ablation and differing anatomic ablative sites. In patients with congenital heart disease, anomalies in embryologic development can result in varying types of anatomic and physiologic atrioventricular (AV) conduction systems. In addition to the congenital lesions are the acquired problems of cavitary dilation and increased atrial wall thickness. In particular, atrial wall thickness, sometimes up to 1.5 cm, represents a significant challenge in achieving adequate transmural ablation, especially for alternative forms of energy delivery systems such as radiofrequency ablation. To ensure transmural lesions in the thickened atrial wall, incision and cryoablative techniques are used. Large atria resulting from abnormal hemodynamics are surgically reduced (Fig. 101-1) and previous atrial scars are resected, especially if pre- or intraoperative electrophysiologic study shows corresponding areas of slow conduction. However, patients with heterotaxy syndrome (occasional absence of the coronary sinus), tricuspid atresia (absence of the tricuspid annulus), anomalous venous drainage (both systemic and pulmonary), gross anatomic thickening of the atrial wall, and endocardial fibrous anatomic jet lesions require alterations of standard techniques based on the preoperative and intraoperative electrophysiologic study.

Specifically, patients with heterotaxy syndrome and absence of the coronary sinus are treated without the obligatory cryoablation lesions that connect the coronary sinus with the inferior vena cava and the tricuspid valve. These patients can be approached by (1) isolation of the superior and inferior venae cavae, (2) linear lesions that connect the orifice of the inferior vena cava with the medial and proximate AV valve (often a common AV valve), (3) a linear lesion that connects the atrial septal area with the base of the resected right atrial appendage, and (4) a linear lesion that connects the atrial septal area with the posterior incised atrial wall across the crista terminalis.

Patients with tricuspid atresia have a tricuspid "dimple" in about one third of cases. Some authors treat this dimple as a diminutive valve and apply cryoablation lesions to connect the coronary sinus with the dimple. However, anatomic dissections by Orie, Anderson, and associates showed the AV node in very close proximity to the proposed cryoablation area. Our approach to patients with atrial reentry tachycardia and tricuspid atresia is to omit the cryoablation lesion that connects the coronary sinus with the presumed annulus of the diminutive tricuspid annulus.

Anomalous systemic and pulmonary venous drainage to the atria are approached as additional anatomic barriers in much the same way as the pulmonary vein orifices. They are, therefore, treated using isolation techniques (either by transection and reanastomosis or by orifice cryoablation) as the case dictates. The other therapeutic cryoablation lesions are added to these ablations as indicated.

The basic tenets of surgical atrial arrhythmia ablation in congenital heart patients are a thorough understanding of the anatomic features referable to the specific congenital anomaly, resection of excess atrial tissue including previous atrial incisions, establishment of lines of block in areas that have been previously shown to be critical parts of a reentrant circuit, and establishment of atrial pacing, especially when sinus node dysfunction exists. Operative strategies for minimizing cross-clamp times can be planned to apply right-sided lesions before cross-clamp placement (assuming no communication between the right and left sides of the heart), to apply lesions during exposure for other left-sided problems (e.g., mitral valve surgery), and to use newly adapted cryoablation probes (Cryocath Technologies, Inc.,

Table 101-2   Results of Fontan Revision without Arrhythmia Surgery

Authors	Patients	Mortality (%)	Transplant (%)	Arrhythmia recurrence (%)
Balaji et al., 1994[1]	3	33	—	0
Kao et al., 1994[2]	3	0	—	67
Vitullo et al., 1996[3]	9	11	—	100
McElhinney et al., 1996[4]	7	14	14	67[a]
Kreutzer et al., 1996[5]	8	12.5	12.5	67
Scholl et al., 1997[6]	12	8.3	—	100
Van Son et al., 1999[7]	18	11	11	69
Petko et al., 2003[8]	13[b]	7.7	—	—
Sheikh et al., 2004[9]	4	0	0	75
Total	77	9	6	76

[a]Two of three patients with preoperative indication of atrial tachyarrhythmias had continued need for arrhythmia medications for improved or stabilized arrhythmias; at follow-up an additional three patients had postoperative arrhythmias treated with medication

[b]Five of 13 patients underwent arrhythmia surgery; arrhythmia recurrence was not stated.

[1]Balaji S, Johnson TB, Sade RM, et al. Management of atrial flutter after the Fontan operation. J Am Coll Cardiol 1994; 23:1209.

[2]Kao JM, Alejos JC, Grant PW, et al. Conversion of atriopulmonary to cavopulmonary anastomosis in management of late arrhythmias and atrial thrombosis. Ann Thorac Surg 1994;58:1510.

[3]Vitullo DA, DeLeon SY, Berry TE, et al. Clinical improvement after revision in Fontan patients. Ann Thorac Surg 1996;61:1797.

[4]McElhinney DB, Reddy VM, Moore P, Hanley FL. Revision of previous Fontan connections to extracardiac or intraatrial conduit cavopulmonary anastomosis. Ann Thorac Surg 1996;62:1276.

[5]Kreutzer J, Keane JF, Lock JE, et al. Conversion of modified Fontan procedure to lateral atrial tunnel cavopulmonary anastomosis. J Thorac Cardiovasc Surg 1996;111:1169.

[6]Scholl FG, Alejos JC, Laks H. Revision of the traditional atriopulmonary Fontan connection. Adv Cardiac Surg 1997;9:217.

[7]van Son JA, Mohr FW, Hambsch J, et al. Conversion of atriopulmonary or lateral atrial tunnel cavopulmonary anastomosis to extracardiac conduit Fontan modification. Eur J Cardiothorac Surg 1999;15:150.

[8]Petko M, Myung RJ, Wernovsky G, et al. Surgical reinterventions following the Fontan procedure. Eur J Cardiothorac Surg 2003;24:255.

[9]Sheikh AM, Tang ATM, Roman K, et al. The failing Fontan circulation: Successful conversion of atriopulmonary connections. J Thorac Cardiovasc Surg 2004;128:60.

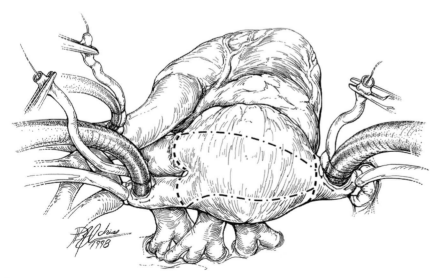

Figure 101-1. Atriopulmonary Fontan connection. Lines of excision (dashed lines) represent the area of atrial excision. After the pulmonary artery is disconnected, the superior and inferior venae cavae are transected and connected by the wide atrial excision, which in most cases includes the cardiac portion of the superior vena cava, the sinoatrial node, and the crista terminalis. (Reproduced with permission from the artist from Mavroudis C, Deal BJ, Backer CL, Johnsrude CL. The favorable impact of arrhythmia surgery on total cavopulmonary artery Fontan conversion. Semin Thorac Cardiovasc Surg Pediatr Card Surg Annu 1999;2:143.)

Montreal, Quebec) that can deliver longer lines of block with each application.

Results

At our center, we have performed 108 Fontan revisions in combination with arrhythmia surgery over the last 10 years. The operation that we first introduced in 1994 for Fontan patients with anatomic hemodynamic problems and debilitating arrhythmias has undergone a significant metamorphosis based on the analysis of our extensive electrophysiologic findings. Three common sites within the right atrium important to these reentrant circuits were found: (1) the area between the coronary sinus os and the inferior vena cava os/right-sided atrioventricular annulus, (2) the region of the atrial septal defect patch, and (3) the lateral right atrial wall. These areas of reentry were addressed by the modified right-sided maze procedure.

Different anatomic diagnoses required different approaches to the cryoablation lesion at the isthmus (area between the coronary sinus os, when present, and the right-sided atrioventricular valve, when present). In general, cryoablation lesions are placed to connect the coronary sinus os with the associated atrioventricular valve to achieve isthmus block and avoid complete heart block. Patients with single ventricle who have a defined right atrium, coronary sinus, and right ventricle have the same predictive location of the atrioventricular node in the triangle of Koch as do patients with normal anatomy. The relationship of the coronary sinus to the atrioventricular node in patients with double-inlet left ventricle, unbalanced atrioventricular canal, and other complex forms of single ventricle are less predictive and cannot be relied on to identify the AV node. Nor can the distance between the coronary sinus and the annulus in these patients be interpreted as the isthmus, even though in our practice we have treated it as such. In many cases, the distance between the coronary sinus and the atrioventricular valve is long and quite distinct from the normal anatomy. Future studies should focus on more detailed electrophysiologic mapping in these complex forms of single ventricle. This will determine whether the area between the coronary sinus os and the atrioventricular valve participates in atrial reentry tachycardia for these complex forms of single ventricle.

Patients with right atrial macro-reentry tachycardia after the Fontan procedure undergo a modified right atrial maze

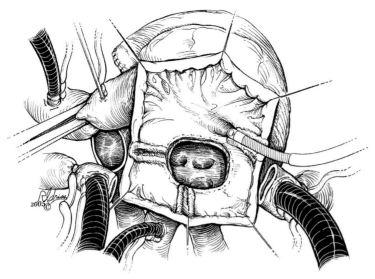

Figure 101-2.   Atrial view of an atriopulmonary Fontan patient after aortic cross-clamping and cardioplegic arrest. The inferior and superior venae cavae have been transected, atrial wall excision has been performed, and the atrial septal patch has been removed. No measures are taken to preserve the sinoatrial node, which is nonfunctional in a significant number of patients. Cryoablation lesions (−60°C for 90 seconds) are placed in three areas to complete the modified right-sided maze procedure. The first two cryoablation lesions are standard for all anatomic substrates and are performed by connecting (1) the superior portion of the atrial septal ridge with the incised area of the right atrial appendage and (2) the posterior portion of the atrial septal ridge with the posterior cut edge of the atrial wall, which extends through the crista terminalis. Third is the isthmus cryoablation. These lines of block depend on the anatomic substrate. In patients with tricuspid atresia, depicted here, the cryoablation lesion is placed to connect (3) the posteroinferior portion of the coronary sinus os with the transected inferior vena cava. (Adapted from Mavroudis C, Backer CL, Deal BJ, et al. Total cavopulmonary conversion and maze procedure for patients with failure of the Fontan operation. J Thorac Cardiovasc Surg 2001;122:863.)

involving the right (Figs. 101-2 –to 101-4) and left (Fig. 101-5) atria. The Cox maze III procedure is designed to limit the ability of the micro-reentrant circuits of atrial fibrillation to propagate while allowing normal conduction of an atrial impulse to the AV node and preserving atrial contractility. The modified right atrial maze procedure can be completed in <10 minutes, whereas the Cox maze III procedure requires an additional 35 to 55 minutes of surgery. The use of linear ablation probes or radiofrequency catheters can considerably shorten the procedure.

At our center, of the initial 13 patients undergoing arrhythmia surgery and Fontan revision, atrial antitachycardia pacemakers were implanted in 12 (Intertach II, Sulzer Intermedics, Angleton, TX). When this pacemaker became unavailable, atrial rate-responsive pacemakers (Kappa SR, Medtronic, Inc., Minneapolis, MN) were implanted in the subsequent 31 patients. The change to the rate-responsive pacemaker was partly due to the decreased incidence of tachycardia seen with use of the more extensive right atrial maze (versus early isthmus block procedure) as well as the need for rate responsiveness. More recently, dual-chamber antitachycardia pacemakers (AT 500, Medtronic) have been implanted due to the potential need for ventricular pacing during late follow-up and to avoid the risk

procedure. The modified right atrial maze is intended to interrupt critical areas of reentry specific to the Fontan patient: the atriotomy scar, the rim of the atrial septal defect and the lateral right atrial wall, and the prior atriopulmonary connection. In addition, the area of "typical" atrial flutter is addressed with cryoablation lesions between the inferior vena cava and the os of the coronary sinus, and between the inferior vena cava and the region of the tricuspid valve or AV groove. Specific lesions and incisions are modified to account for the individual's anatomy and diagnosis (Figs. 101-2 to 101-4).

Atrial fibrillation typically occurs in the presence of markedly dilated left atria, usually in the setting of significant mitral regurgitation, either due to ventricular dysfunction or valve abnormalities. The Cox maze III procedure is designed to eliminate atrial fibrillation while preserving intact AV nodal conduction and atrial contractility. Use of the cryoablation probe or radiofrequency catheter intraoperatively instead of atrial incisions considerably shortens surgical time. Patients with atrial fibrillation after the Fontan procedure undergo a complete Cox maze III procedure

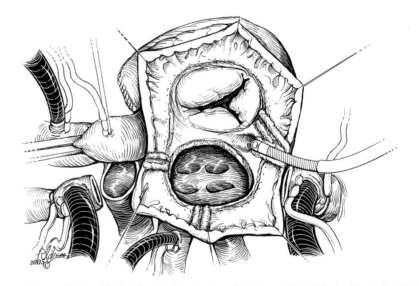

Figure 101-3.   The modified right-sided maze procedure in a patient with double-outlet right ventricle and mitral atresia. As noted in Fig. 101-2, the two standard cryoablation lesions are shown connecting the atrial septal ridge to (1) the incised area of the right atrial appendage and (2) the posterior cut edge of the atrial wall. The isthmus block is accomplished by placing cryoablation lesions to connect the transected inferior vena cava os (3) with the posteroinferior portion of the coronary sinus os and (4) with the tricuspid valve annulus. These isthmus block lesions are usually placed across the ridge of the resected atrial compartmentalization patch. (Adapted from Mavroudis C, Backer CL, Deal BJ, et al. Total cavopulmonary conversion and maze procedure for patients with failure of the Fontan operation. J Thorac Cardiovasc Surg 2001; 122:863.)

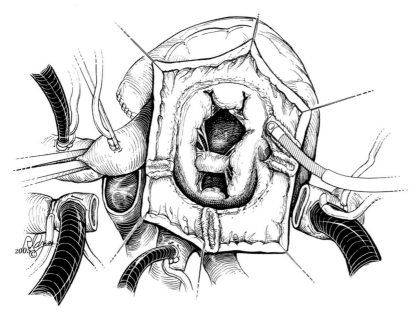

Figure 101-4. The modified right-sided maze procedure in a patient with single ventricle and unbalanced atrioventricular canal. As noted in Fig. 101-2, the two standard cryoablation lesions are shown connecting the atrial septal ridge to (1) the incised area of the right atrial appendage and (2) the posterior cut edge of the atrial wall. The isthmus block is accomplished by placing cryoablation lesions to connect the transected inferior vena cava os (3) with the posteroinferior portion of the coronary sinus os and (4) with the common atrioventricular valve annulus. These isthmus block lesions are usually placed across the ridge of the resected atrial compartmentalization patch. (Adapted from Mavroudis C, Backer CL, Deal BJ, et al. Total cavopulmonary conversion and maze procedure for patients with failure of the Fontan operation. J Thorac Cardiovasc Surg 2001;122:863.)

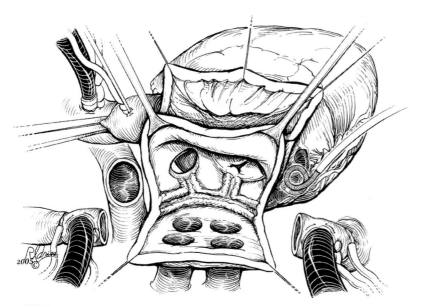

Figure 101-5. Left atrial view of a univentricular heart showing the standard incisions, excisions, and cryoablation lesions that, when combined with the right atrial component (Figs. 101-2 to 101-4), complete the Cox maze III procedure. The incisions include a partial encircling pulmonary vein isolation and a left atrial appendage resection. Standard cryoablation lesions (−60°C for 90 seconds) are placed to complete the pulmonary vein isolation, to create a cryoablation lesion from the isolated pulmonary veins toward the posterior mitral or tricuspid valve annulus, and to extend the pulmonary vein isolation to the cut edge of the left atrial appendage base. A large cryoablation probe (15 mm) is used to place a lesion on the coronary sinus (−60°C for 180 seconds). (Adapted from Mavroudis C, Backer CL, Deal BJ, et al. Total cavopulmonary conversion and maze procedure for patients with failure of the Fontan operation. J Thorac Cardiovasc Surg 2001;122:863.)

of reoperation; most of these pacemakers are programmed for atrial pacing only (Fig. 101-6). Atrial pacing rates are programmed to consistently maintain a regular atrial rhythm faster than the intrinsic rhythm, usually at 70 to 80 beats per minute during late follow-up. One patient received an epicardial defibrillator in addition to multisite ventricular pacing due to a prior cardiac arrest with ventricular tachycardia and ventricular dysfunction with left-bundle-branch block.

Fontan conversion to total cavopulmonary connections in association with arrhythmia surgery is highly effective and safe. Arrhythmias are controlled, functional class is improved, and exercise tolerance is increased. Our center's selection criteria were liberal and included patients with severe ventricular dysfunction, cyanosis-causing pulmonary arteriovenous fistulas, significant associated cardiac lesions, and protein-losing enteropathy. During this period, 11 patients were evaluated for cardiac transplantation. Six of these who eventually underwent Fontan conversion and arrhythmia surgery had anatomic and arrhythmogenic substrates amenable to surgery. The other 5 (not included in our original cohort of 108 patients) had severe ventricular dysfunction that could not be ascribed to atrial arrhythmias or anatomic lesions; 3 of these patients had cardiac transplantation, and the other 2 died on the waiting list. Cardiac transplantation after Fontan conversion was performed in 4 of our patients from the original cohort, similar to the incidence reported in long-term follow-up studies.

Arrhythmia recurrence for the entire Fontan conversion series is 14% (14 of 108); 4 of these patients were among the first 8 patients in our series. Since our conversion to the more extensive modified right-sided maze procedure for atrial reentry tachycardia, recurrence of atrial tachycardia has markedly decreased. Similarly, isthmus cryoablation was ineffective for atrial fibrillation, which has been eliminated with the use of the Cox maze III procedure. The Cox maze III procedure represents a combination of the right-sided maze procedure, appropriate for anatomic substrate (Figs. 101-2 to 101-4), combined with the left-sided series of incisions, excisions, and cryoablation lesions as described by Cox and associates (Fig. 101-5).

Alternatively, intraoperative radiofrequency ablation and microwave energy have been reported as treatment for atrial arrhythmias. However, these methods have been associated with higher recurrence rates. Others report that a right-sided procedure will

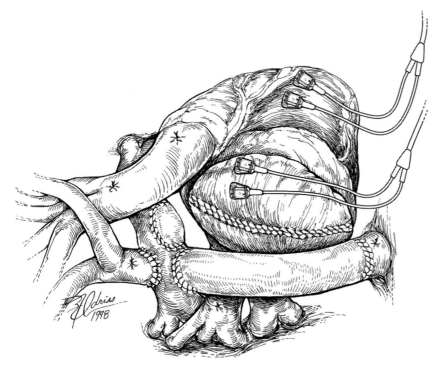

Figure 101-6. Completion of total cavopulmonary connection, showing placement of pacemaker electrodes. (Adapted from Mavroudis C, Backer CL, Deal BJ, Johnsrude CL. The favorable impact of arrhythmia surgery on total cavopulmonary artery Fontan conversion. Semin Thorac Cardiovasc Surg Pediatr Card Surg Annu 1999;2:143.)

effectively treat congenital heart patients with atrial fibrillation; long-term data are not available in that population. In contrast, our experience, which is supported by other studies, shows recurrence of atrial fibrillation with lesions limited to the right atrium. Recurrent atrial fibrillation in our single-ventricle population causes unfavorable hemodynamic consequences that are less well tolerated than in the two-ventricle population. Because of this, we prefer to perform the Cox maze III procedure, which is associated with the lowest recurrence rate.

Most of the complications in our series occurred in the atrial fibrillation group in patients who had the Cox maze III procedure. These patients had significant risk factors when compared to the group that had right-sided procedures. They were older at Fontan conversion, experienced atrial arrhythmias for a longer time, had a longer aortic cross-clamp time, and sustained a higher incidence of perioperative renal insufficiency. These data show important trends. We believe that earlier referral should occur before the onset of atrial fibrillation, at a time when the less invasive and more expedient modified right-sided maze procedure can be performed. Other beneficial effects of early operation include prevention of progressive myocardial dysfunction due to atrial

arrhythmias, cessation of potentially toxic antiarrhythmic agents, and improved functional class that is associated with Fontan conversion and arrhythmia surgery.

Our experience with protein-losing enteropathy is limited to two patients who underwent Fontan conversion with arrhythmia surgery. One patient developed recurrent protein-losing enteropathy with progressive ventricular dysfunction and underwent cardiac transplantation 11 months later. The second, an adult female with chronic atrial fibrillation, cyanosis, and protein-losing enteropathy, developed renal failure after Fontan conversion and underwent cardiac transplantation 6 months later. She died of multi-organ failure following cardiac transplantation. Some authors documented clinical improvement with steroid administration and heparin therapy. Rychik and colleagues believed that although protein-losing enteropathy has a multifactorial etiology, the main component is decreased cardiac output. They reasoned that the increased cardiac output that can be achieved by atrial pacing and/or an atrial fenestration will favorably impact hemodynamics. This, in turn, can lead to cessation of protein-losing enteropathy in a significant percentage of cases. Based on our limited experience, patients with protein-losing en-

teropathy are not suitable candidates for Fontan conversion. Cardiac transplantation has been recommended in the setting of protein-losing enteropathy and decreased ventricular function.

Fontan conversion with arrhythmia surgery is a safe and efficacious operation. Adherence to standard reoperative techniques and patient selection should optimize outcome. Debilitating arrhythmias are cured, functional class is increased, and exercise tolerance is improved. We recommend that patients with atriopulmonary Fontan connections be closely monitored for the development of obstructive pathways, valvular dysfunction, and atrial arrhythmias. Fontan conversion should be seriously considered under these circumstances, even if the only indication is debilitating atrial arrhythmias. Surgical intervention before the development of atrial fibrillation results in less surgical morbidity. Cardiac transplantation may be required in the short or long term in some of these patients.

SUGGESTED READING

Amodeo A, Galletti L, Marianeschi S, et al. Extracardiac Fontan operation for complex cardiac anomalies: Seven years' experience. J Thorac Cardiovasc Surg 1997;114:1020.

Balaji S, Gewillig M, Bull C, et al. Arrhythmias after the Fontan procedure. Comparison of total cavopulmonary connection and atriopulmonary connection. Circulation 1991;84:111–162.

Cohen MI, Rhodes LA, Wernovsky G, et al. Atrial pacing: An alternative treatment for protein-losing enteropathy after the Fontan operation. J Thorac Cardiovasc Surg 2001;121:582.

Cox JL, Boineau JP, Schuessler RB, et al. Modification of the maze procedure for atrial flutter and atrial fibrillation. I. Rationale and surgical results. J Thorac Cardiovasc Surg 1995;110:473.

Cox JL, Jaquiss RD, Schuessler RB, Boineau JP. Modification of the maze procedure for atrial flutter and atrial fibrillation. II. Surgical technique of the maze III procedure. J Thorac Cardiovasc Surg 1995;110:485.

Deal BJ, Mavroudis C, Backer CL, et al. Comparison of anatomic isthmic block with modified right atrial maze procedure for late atrial tachycardia in Fontan patients. Circulation 2002;106:575.

Gelatt M, Hamilton RM, McCrindle BW, et al. Risk factors for atrial tachyarrhythmias after the Fontan operation. J Am Coll Cardiol 1994;24:1735.

Harada A, D'Agostino Jr HJ, Schuessler RB, et al. Right atrial isolation: A new surgical treatment for supraventricular tachycardia. I. Surgical technique and electrophysiologic effects. J Thorac Cardiovasc Surg 1988;95:643.

Mavroudis C, Backer CL, Deal BJ, et al. Total cavopulmonary conversion and maze procedure for patients with failure of the Fontan operation. J Thorac Cardiovasc Surgery 2001; 122:863.

Mavroudis C, Backer CL, Deal BJ, Johnsrude CL. Fontan conversion to cavopulmonary connection and arrhythmia circuit cryoablation. J Thorac Cardiovasc Surg 1998;115:547.

McElhinney DB, Reddy VM, Moore P, Hanley FL. Revision of previous Fontan connections to extracardiac or intraatrial conduit cavopulmonary anastomosis. Ann Thorac Surg 1996; 62:1276.

Orie JD, Anderson RH, Ettedgui JA, et al. Echocardiographic-morphologic correlations in tricuspid atresia. J Am Coll Cardiol 1995; 26:750.

Peters NS, Somerville J. Arrhythmias after the Fontan procedure. Br Heart J 1992;68:199.

Sanchez-Quintana D, Climent V, Ho SY, Anderson RH. Myoarchitecture and connective tissue in hearts with tricuspid atresia. Heart 1999;81:182.

Triedman JK, Bergau DM, Saul JP, et al. Efficacy of radiofrequency ablation for control of intraatrial reentrant tachycardia in patients with congenital heart disease. J Am Coll Cardiol 1997;30:1032.

EDITOR'S COMMENTS

Dr. Mavroudis and his associates have clearly demonstrated that patients with the Fontan circulation who have inefficient venous pathways with areas of stasis and associated arrhythmias and ventricular dysfunction can be effectively treated with Fontan conversion and arrhythmia surgery with a marked improvement in exercise performance and clinical status. These results confirm the concept that the Fontan circulation should be made as hemodynamically efficient as possible, which lends support to the total cavopulmonary connection and extracardiac conduit Fontan modifications that are now the most popular techniques for Fontan completion. The single-ventricle Fontan physiology creates a situation of relatively low cardiac output, and therefore, anything that can be done to maximize the cardiac output and maintain ventricular performance should result in improved long-term outcomes.

It is unknown whether the newest modifications to the Fontan operation (such as the extracardiac conduit), which have the potential of decreasing the number of atrial suture lines, will in fact decrease the risk of late arrhythmias. The follow-up for the extracardiac conduit modification is not yet long enough on average to determine whether the incidence of late arrhythmias will be significantly decreased with this technique. There are encouraging early reports of a lower incidence of arrhythmias at 5 to 8 years of follow-up; however, because the majority of atrial arrhythmias do not occur until 10 years or later after the Fontan operation, the overall effect is still unknown. There may well be anatomic substrates for arrhythmias in the single-ventricle population that will make patients at risk for late arrhythmias regardless of the type of Fontan connection performed. In many cases, the need for atrial septectomy as a first-stage operation in association with other reconstructive procedures means that many patients will have atrial suture lines regardless of the type of completion Fontan.

The majority of Fontan revision procedures that have been performed in most centers have converted an old-style atriopulmonary Fontan connection with very dilated atrial chambers and thick atrial walls to the more hemodynamic extracardiac Fontan. There will probably be an increasing number of lateral tunnel Fontan operations that develop enough dilation of the atrial pathway to require conversion in the future, although the incidence of this phenomenon is not yet clearly determined. It is likely, however, that an increasing number of patients will be referred for arrhythmia modification and conversion as the very large population of children and young adults with the Fontan circulation age. The majority of those Fontan patients who have had the procedure for hypoplastic left heart syndrome are now just entering their preteenage years. These patients may represent an increasing challenge for pediatric cardiac surgeons as they develop potential complications of Fontan physiology as they age into adulthood. Surprisingly, even after many years of follow-up, only a relatively small percentage of Fontan patients have required cardiac transplantation, as nicely demonstrated by Dr. Mavroudis and his colleagues. The primary goal with staged surgical reconstruction in single-ventricle physiology is to maintain ventricular function as much as possible to delay the need for cardiac replacement.

The increasing need for surgical arrhythmia ablation in adults with congenital heart disease has made it imperative that congenital heart surgeons learn these techniques. Our own lesser experience with ablative surgery for arrhythmias and Fontan conversion mirrors Dr. Mavroudis' results. Despite the complexity of the operations, which are often quite prolonged and difficult, the results have been gratifying. Most patients achieve a significant improvement in exercise performance and control of arrhythmias, which dramatically improves their quality of life.

T.L.S.

Index

Page numbers followed by *t* indicate table; those followed by *f* indicate figure.

A

Abdominal phase, of transhiatal esophagectomy, 131–132

Aberrant right subclavian artery, left aortic arch with, 729

Abnormal ostium remodeling, for anomalous coronary artery course, between aorta/pulmonary artery, 969–970, 969*f*, 970*f*

Absent pulmonary valve, tetralogy of Fallot with, 911–912

Accessory left atrioventricular valvar orifice, AVSDs and, 821–822

Accessory valve tissue, pediatric mitral valve repair and, 1008

ACCP. *See* American College of Chest Physicians

Acetylcholine (ACh) receptors, 107

ACh receptors. *See* Acetylcholine receptors

Achalasia
    definition of, 163
    diagnosis of, 163
    etiology of, 163
    incidence of, 163
    laparoscopic esophagomyotomy for, 164–165, 164*f*, 165*f*
    non-surgical treatment options for, 164
    patient with end-stage esophagus with, 168*f*
    surgical indications for, 164
    surgical technique for, 164–168, 165*f*, 166*f*, 167*f*
    symptoms of, 163
    treatment for, 163–170
    treatment principles for, 163–164
    vigorous, 170

Acid-base management, neurologic injury prevention and, 334–335

ACOSOG. *See* American College of Surgeons Oncology Group

Acquired mitral valve disease, pediatric mitral valve repair and, 1009

Acquired shortening of the esophagus, 148–149
    barium esophagram of, 149*f*

Acquired valvular heart disease, 378–389

ACT. *See* Activated clotting time

Activated clotting time (ACT), for lung implantation, 199

Acute ischemic mitral regurgitation
    clinical presentation of, 516–518
    diagnosis of, 516–518
    incidence of, 515–516
    myocardial infarction complications and, 515–519
    natural history of, 518
    operative technique for, 519, 519*f*
    operative timing for, 518–519
    pathogenesis of, 515–516
    preoperative therapy for, 518–519
    survival for, 519

Acute pulmonary embolus, 621–625
    anatomic considerations for, 622
    background on, 621
    diagnosis of, 621
    operative procedure for, 622–625, 623*f*, 624*f*, 625*f*
    postoperative considerations for, 622–625, 623*f*, 624*f*, 625*f*
    surgery indications for, 622

Acute respiratory distress syndrome (ARDS), 59

Acute traumatic aortic transection, 568–576
    background on, 568
    diagnosis of, 568–569
    endovascular aortic stents and, 575–576
    incidence of, 568
    medical therapy for, 569
    natural history of, 568
    patient position for, 570*f*
    surgical management of, 569–574, 570*f*, 571*f*, 572*f*, 573*f*, 574*f*, 575*f*
    surgical outcome for, 574–575

Acute type A aortic dissection, 536–541
    aortic valve repair and, 538*f*
    aortic valve resuspension and, 537*f*
    distal false lumen obliteration and, 538*f*
    surgical technique for, 538–541, 539*f*

Acute type B aortic dissection, 541–543
    intramural hematomas and, retrograde extensions of, 543

malperfusion syndrome and, 542*f*
pseudo-coarctation and, 542*f*

Adrenal adenomas, 12

Adult preoperative risk factors, New York State database, 329*t*

Aerodigestive anatomy, 3

AESOP. *See* Automated Endoscopic System for Optimal Positioning

AF. *See* Atrial fibrillation

Air removal, from heart, in CPB, 313–314. *See also* De-airing, left ventricle

Airway complications, with heart-lung transplantation, 594

Airway reconstruction, carinal resection and, 85*f*

American College of Chest Physicians (ACCP), 621

American College of Surgeons Oncology Group (ACOSOG), 12, 33

Amplatzer repair, of secundum-type atrial septal defects, 743, 743*f*

Anastomosis, pericardial fat wrapped around, 66*f*

Anastomotic technique, interrupted, 66*f*

Anesthesia
    for bronchoplastic procedures, 64
    for carinal resection, 82–83
    for MVST, CABG, 468–469
    for OPCAB, 457
    for robotic mitral valve surgery, 355
    for thoracic/thoracoabdominal aneurysms, 547

Aneurysmal dilation, of superior caval system, 711

Annuloaortic dilation/ectasia, pediatric, operative technique for, 1028–1029, 1028*f*, 1029*f*, 1030*f*

Annuloaortic ectasia, 527–532
    aortic annuloplasty for, 528*f*
    background on, 527

Annuloplasty ring removal, reoperative mitral valve replacement and, 396*f*

Annulus enlargement, pediatric, operative technique for, 1027–1028, 1027*f*

Annulus patch repair, reoperative mitral valve replacement and, 398*f*

Annulus primary repair, reoperative mitral valve replacement and, 398*f*

Anomalous coronary artery course
between aorta/pulmonary artery, 968–969, 968*f*, 969*f*, 970*f*
abnormal ostium remodeling for, 969–970, 969*f*, 970*f*
operation method for, 969–970, 969*f*, 970*f*
tetralogy of Fallot and, 911

Anomalous innominate artery, with tracheal compression, 729–731
anatomy of, 729–730
clinical presentation of, 730
diagnosis of, 730
surgical indications for, 730
surgical technique for, 730–731, 734*f*, 735*f*

Anomalous pulmonary venous return, 947–956

Antegrade cannulas, for cardioplegia, 318, 320*f*

Antegrade pressure, of cardioplegia, 320–321

Antegrade/retrograde cardioplegic perfusion, delivery/monitoring of, 322

Antegrade/retrograde perfusion, for myocardial protection, 316–317

Anterior cervicothoracic approach, 30–31, 31*f*

Anterior leaflet commissuroplasty, for mitral valve repair, 346*f*

Anterior leaflet pathology, 345–347

Anterior leaflet prolapse, 361–364, 362*f*, 363*f*, 364*f*

Anterior left aortic arch, division of, 733*f*

Anterior mediastinotomy, 20–25
alternative procedures of, 23
complications of, 22, 22*t*
contraindications for, 20–21
indications for, 20
sternotomy and, 20
surgical technique for, 21–22, 22*f*
transcarinal aspiration and, 22*f*

Anterior mitral leaflet, triangular resection of, 349*f*

Anterior retrosternal diaphragmatic hernia of Morgagni, 230–231
repair of, 235*f*

Anterior scalene muscle
bone wedge excision, 215*f*
insertion of, superior sulcus tumor resection and, 292*f*
off first rib, 214*f*

Anterior segmental branch, of pulmonary artery, 48*f*

Anterior thoracotomy, 28, 28*f*
patient position for, 27

Anterior ventricular restoration, 483*f*, 484*f*, 485*f*, 486*f*, 487*f* 488–491

Anterolateral thoracotomy
pericardiectomy via, 260*f*
for reoperative mitral valve replacement, 391–392, 392*f*

Anteroseptal infarction, left ventricular reconstruction and, 480*f*

Anticoagulation management protocol, 307*t*

Antireflux procedures, 121–129
complications of, 128–129
patient preparation for, 122
postoperative care for, 127–128
results of, 129
surgical principles of, 122

Aorta, 648
cardiac magnetic resonance imaging of, 665–667, 667*f*

Aorta-to-aorta artery shunt, for neonates, 884

Aorta-to-right ventricle shunt, PA/IS with, definitive surgical treatment for, 891

Aortic anastomoses, fashioning of, 551, 551*f*

Aortic annular dilation, pulmonary autograft replacement in, 431, 431*f*

Aortic annuloplasty, for annuloaortic ectasia, 528*f*

Aortic annulus
enlargement, operative technique for, 422*f*
small, 421–422, 422*f*

Aortic arch
aneurysms, 556–566
cerebral protection and, 563–565
diagnosis of, 556–557
elephant trunk technique for, 560–563, 561*f*, 562*f*
etiology of, 556
hemi-arch technique for, 557–559, 558*f*, 559*f*
indications for, 557
pathology of, 556
perioperative techniques for, 557
postoperative care for, 565–566
preoperative techniques for, 557
reverse elephant trunk technique for, 563, 564*f*
surgical results for, 565*t*
surgical techniques for, 557–565, 558*f*, 559*f*, 560*f*, 561*f*, 562*f*, 564*f*
total arch technique for, 559–560, 560*f*, 561*f*
anomalies
classification of, 722
embryology of, 722
historical aspects of, 722
incidence of, 722
anterior left, division of, 733*f*
double
anatomy of, 729, 732*f*
surgical technique for, 726–727, 728*f*, 730*f*, 731*f*, 732*f*, 733*f*, 930*f*

embryonic, outcome of, 723*t*
interrupted, 779–787
normal development of, 723*f*
obstructions, congenital heart disease and, 686–687
posterior, division of, 730*f*
postoperative care for, 733–734
right, with retroesophageal ligament, 727–728

Aortic cannula/obturator, wire-wound pediatric, 309*f*

Aortic clamping, single period of, 317–318

Aortic coarctation, 768–776
end-to-end anastomosis and, 769–771, 772*f*, 773*f*
extended end-to-end anastomosis and, 769–771, 772*f*, 773*f*
hypoplastic left ventricle and, 776
interposition graft and, 771–772
juxtaductal, 769*f*
patch aortoplasty and, 769, 771*f*
recurrent, 776
special situations for, 775–776
subclavian flap repair for, 769, 770*f*
surgical approaches to, 772–774, 773*f*, 774*f*, 775*f*
surgical complications to, 775
surgical results for, 775
VSDs and, 775–776

Aortic cross-clamping
extracorporeal circulation and, 548–549, 549*f*, 550*f*
for hemodynamic instability control, thoracic/thoracoabdominal aneurysms, 548–551
pharmacologic manipulation and, 548
slow clamp application/release and, 548

Aortic cusp prolapse, repair of, 531, 531*f*

Aortic dissection, 534–544
background on, 534
chronic dissections and, 543–544
classification of, 534–535, 535*f*
clinical presentation of, 535–536
diagnostic evaluation for, 535–536
follow-up on, 543–544
incidence of, 534

Aortic flow velocity, 417*f*

Aortic graft selection, thoracic/thoracoabdominal aneurysms and, 551–553, 551*f*, 552*f*, 553*f*, 554*f*

Aortic pressure, measurement comparisons of, 322*f*

Aortic regurgitation
asymptomatic, 418
diagnosis of, 413
etiology of, 412–413
natural history of, 413
pathophysiology of, 413

Aortic reimplantation, for coronary artery anomalies, 961–962, 962*f*

Aortic root
aneurysm, 527, 528*f*
dilation, 804
remodeling of, 528–529, 528*f*, 529*f*
replacement of, 531–532, 532*f*
sinuses, congenital anomalies of,
804–809
surgical complications of, 532
surgical late outcomes of, 532
Aortic stenosis
asymptomatic patient of, 416–418
congenital heart disease and, 683–685
diagnosis of, 411
low-gradient, 418–420
LVOTO and, 789–801
natural history of treated, 412, 412*f*
pathophysiology of, 411, 411*f*
projected patient outcomes for, 420*f*
symptoms of, 411
Aortic valve, 648
area determination of, 412*f*
calcification, 418*f*
cusp entrapment, MVR and, 388–389
disease, 1024–1025
hypoplasia/atresia, interrupted aortic
arch with, 782
reimplantation of, 528, 529–531, 529*f*,
530*f*, 531*f*
repair
acute type A aortic dissection and,
538*f*
pediatric, 1017–1022
resuspension, acute type A aortic
dissection and, 537*f*
stenosis, pediatric aortic valve repair
and, 1017
surgical anatomy of, 410
Aortic valve replacement (AVR)
actuarial analysis of, 416*f*
with bovine pericardial bioprosthesis,
417*f*
historical perspective of, 410
operative technique for, 413–415, 414*f*
with patent internal mammary artery,
421
pediatric, operative technique for,
1026–1027
Ross procedure for, 424–433
surgical outcomes for, 415
survival improvement for, 419*f*
Aortic valve-related deaths, 416*f*
Aortic valve-sparing operations, 527–531
Aortico-left ventricular tunnel, 806–809
clinical presentation of, 807–808
diagnosis of, 807–808
morphology of, 806–807, 807*f*
surgical indications for, 808–809
surgical technique for, 808–809, 808*f*,
809*f*
Aortopulmonary region, bidigital palpation
of, cervical mediastinotomy
and, 23*f*

Aortopulmonary shunts
anatomy of, 693–704
for congenital heart disease, 693–704,
694*t*
Aortopulmonary window, 759–767
anatomy of, 759
approach through, 763*f*
cannulation for repair of, 764*f*
catheter-based approaches for, 766–767
clinical presentation of, 759–760
diagnostic considerations of, 759–760
embryology of, 759
external appearance of, 764*f*
interrupted aortic arch repair of,
763–764, 764*f*, 765*f*
operative technique for, 760–764, 761*f*,
762*f*, 763*f*, 764*f*, 765*f*, 766*f*
postoperative care for, 764–767
preoperative management of, 760
for pulmonary atresia with ventricular
septal defect, MAPCAs and, 896*f*
repair of, 765*f*
simple, operative technique for,
760–763, 761*f*, 762*f*, 763*f*
spectrum of, 760*f*
surgical complications of, 764–767
surgical indications for, 759–760
surgical results of, 767
Apical blebs, wedge resection of, 98*f*
Apical resection, for subpleural bleb, of
recurrent primary spontaneous
pneumothoraces, 95*f*
Apical subpleural blebs, 94
Apical venous branch, apical-anterior
arterial trunk and, 37*f*
Apical-anterior arterial trunk, apical
venous branch and, 37*f*
ARDS. *See* Acute respiratory distress
syndrome
Arrhythmia. *See also specific* arrhythmia
after pneumonectomy, 59–62
substrate, 1035
surgery, 1035–1040
background on, 1035
Fontan revision results without,
1037*t*
results of, 1037–1040, 1037*t*, 1038*f*,
1039*f*, 1040*f*
Arterial repair, TGA and, 857*f*, 858*f*,
859*f*, 860–864, 860*f*, 861*f*,
862*f*, 863*f*
Arteriopexy, for innominate artery
compression, 734*f*
ASDs. *See* Atrial septal defects
Asymptomatic aortic regurgitation, 418
Asymptomatic aortic stenosis, 416–418
risks without operation, 416
unmasking symptoms of, 417
Atherosclerotic heart disease, 437
Atrial arrhythmias
in congenital heart disease, 603–604
incidence of, 1035

surgical management of, 1035–1037,
1037*f*
Atrial fibrillation (AF), 59
alternatives to surgical ablation for,
608–609, 608*f*
AV nodal ablation for, 599
current clinical algorithm for, 610, 611*t*
epidemic of, 606
future directions for, 610
hypertrophic cardiomyopathy, 604
maze procedure for, 599–605
pathophysiology of, 606
postablative care for, 609–610
pulmonary vein isolation for, 608–609,
608*f*
with connecting lesions, 608*f*, 609
surgical treatment of, 606–611
Atrial lesions, alternate energy sources for,
600–601
Atrial repair, TGA and, 860
Atrial septal defects (ASDs), 739–747
background on, 739
closure recommendations for, 740–741
congenital heart disease and, imaging
children with, 653–655, 654*f*, 655*f*,
656*f*
diagnosis of, 739–740, 740*f*
echocardiogram of, 740*f*
with failure to survive, 747
patch fenestration, deficiency of,
822–823
skin incision landmarks for, 741*f*
surgical technique for, 741–747
Atrial septectomy, for congenital heart
disease, 705*t*
Atrial septum, 645, 646*f*
Atrioventricular alignments, 643*f*, 644*f*
Atrioventricular canal defects, 811–825
anatomic considerations for, 811–812
Atrioventricular canal-type defects,
750–751
Atrioventricular conduction pathway, MVR
and, 388–389
Atrioventricular disruption, in MVR, 388
Atrioventricular nodal ablation, for AF, 599
Atrioventricular septal defects (AVSDs),
811–825
accessory left atrioventricular valvar
orifice and, 821–822
anatomic considerations for, 811–812,
812*f*
attaining left atrioventricular valve
competence and, 817–820
congenital heart disease and, imaging
children with, 653–655, 654*f*, 655*f*,
656*f*
controversial issues with, 825
diagnostic considerations for, 812–813
eccentric pericardiotomy for, 813*f*
operative technique for, 813–820, 814*f*,
815*f*, 816*f*, 817*f*, 818*f*, 819*f*, 820*f*,
821*f*, 822*f*, 823*f*, 824*f*

Atrioventricular septal defects (AVSDs)
     (*Contd.*)
  partial, surgical management of, 823
  postoperative care for, 823–825
  surgical complications for, 823–825
  surgical indications for, 813
  with tetralogy of Fallot, 820
  unbalanced, 820–821
  unusual variants of, management of,
     820–823
Atrioventricular valve stenosis, or
     insufficiency, hemodynamic
     assessment of, 681
Atrioventricular valve tissue, deficiency of,
     822
Automated Endoscopic System for Optimal
     Positioning (AESOP), 353
  procedures for, 356*t*
  video-assisted mitral valve repairs with,
     366
AVR. *See* Aortic valve replacement
AVSDs. *See* Atrioventricular septal defects
Axillary thoracotomy, 26, 28*f*
  advantages of, 27
  incisions, 28*f*
  positioning for, 27
Azygos continuation, to right SVC,
     711–712, 712*f*
Azygous vein, 56

B

BAC. *See* Bronchioloalveolar carcinoma
Balloon angioplasty
  congenital heart disease and, 685–686
  for native coarctation, 776
Balloon valvuloplasty, for congenital heart
     disease, 682–685, 684*f*, 685*f*
Barium swallow study
  for interposed stomach, 143*f*
  for recurrent aspiration/dysphagia, 142*f*
BDCPS. *See* Bidirectional cavopulmonary
     shunts
Beating heart totally endoscopic coronary
     artery bypass grafting (BH-TECB),
     472, 473*f*
Belsey fundoplication, 127*f*
Bernoulli theorem, modified, ultrasound
     physics/applications and, 652
BH-TECB. *See* Beating heart totally
     endoscopic coronary artery bypass
     grafting
Bidigital palpation, of aortopulmonary
     region, cervical mediastinotomy
     and, 23*f*
Bidirectional cavopulmonary shunts
     (BDCPS), 919–920, 919*f*, 920*f*, 921*f*
  indications for, 926–927
  operative results of, 928
  operative technique for, 927–928, 927*f*,
     928*f*
  PA/IS with, definitive surgical treatment
     for, 888–889, 890*f*

postoperative management after,
     931–932
Bilateral lung transplants (BLT), 194
Bilateral lung volume reduction, through
     video-assisted thoracoscopic
     approach, 209*f*
Bilateral sequential lung transplantation,
     pediatric, 988–990, 989*f*
Bilateral superior caval veins
  anatomy of, 709*f*
  drainage to systemic venous atrium,
     708–709
Bilateral thoracosternotomy, 29, 29*f*
Bilateral thoracotomy, pericardiectomy via,
     260–261
Bilobectomy, 44–45, 45*f*
  sleeve resection, 67
  view of, 67*f*
BioGlue application, to outflow graft-aortic
     anastomosis suture line, 507*f*
BIVADs. *See* Biventricular assist devices
Biventricular assist devices (BIVADs), 500
Blalock-Taussig shunt
  for congenital heart disease, 693–694,
     694*f*, 694*t*, 695*f*, 696*f*, 697*f*
  takedown of, with double ligation, 695*f*
Blalock-Taussig shunts, modified, for
     congenital heart disease, 694–697,
     695*t*, 696*f*, 697*f*
Bleeding
  from CABG, 446
  mediastinal biopsy and, 18
  as post-transplant complications for,
     pediatric heart transplantation, 975
Blind/blunt mobilization, in transhiatal
     esophagectomy, 134*f*
BLT. *See* Bilateral lung transplants
Body surface area (BSA), 421*f*
Bougie position, in laparoscopic Collis
     gastroplasty, 151*f*
Bovine pericardial bioprosthesis, AVR with,
     417*f*
BPF. *See* Postpneumonectomy
     bronchopleural fistula
Brachial plexus dissection
  for superior sulcus tumor resection, 289,
     290*f*
  superior sulcus tumor resection and, 292
Brachytherapy, for esophageal cancer, 182
Branch pulmonary artery stenosis,
     congenital heart disease and,
     686–687, 686*f*, 687*f*
Bronchial anastomosis, lung
     transplantation and, 200*f*
Bronchioloalveolar carcinoma (BAC), 71
Bronchoplastic procedures, 64–69
  anesthesia for, 64
  history of, 64
  justification for, 64
  operations, 64–69
  outcome for, 69
  postoperative care and, 69

preoperative assessment for, 64
  preparation for, 64
  principles of, 64
  right-sided resections and, 65–66
Bronchopleural fistula, pneumonectomy
     and, 61–62
Bronchoscopy, 3, 5–6
  flexible, 5*f*
  Jackson rigid ventilating laser, 6
  patient positioning for, 8*f*
  procedure for, 6–9
Bronchus. *See also specific* bronchus
  bronchoscopic view of, 4*f*
  division, 49*f*
     in lung transplantation, 199*f*
BSA. *See* Body surface area
Bugge retractor, sternum elevation using,
     207*f*
Bullous disease, 98
  classification of, 98*t*

C

CAB. *See* Coronary artery bypass
CABG. *See* Coronary artery bypass grafting
CAH. *See* Central alveolar hypoventilation
Calcified mitral annulus, management of,
     385–386
Cannula
  antegrade, 318–319
  retrograde, 318–319
  thin-walled venous, for infants/children,
     311*f*
  tip, non-deep palpation of, 321*f*
Cannulation
  adult preparation for, 306*f*
  aorta incision for, 308*f*
  for CPB, 306–309, 306*f*, 307*f*, 308*f*, 309*f*
  double, 310*f*
  final aorta position for, 308*f*
  infant preparation for, 307*f*
  single venous, 310*f*
  for tetralogy of Fallot, 907*f*
Carcinoid heart disease, tricuspid valve
     and, 404
Cardiac anatomy, 400*f*
Cardiac displacement, for OPCAB, 459,
     460*f*, 461*f*, 462*f*
Cardiac magnetic resonance imaging,
     660–678
  anatomical uses, 665–675
  anatomy, 662*f*
  of aorta, 665–667, 667*f*
  approach to, 662–665
  complex spatial relationships and,
     670–671, 671*f*, 672*f*
  extracardiac conduits/baffles and,
     669–670, 669*f*, 670*f*
  of general morphology, 674–675, 674*f*
  great artery anatomy, preoperative/
     postoperative, 665–669
  of miscellaneous diseases, 674–675
  myocardial perfusion with, 677

myocardial tissue/blood tagging with, 676–677

perfusion/viability/coronary imaging with, 665*f*

physiology/function, 663*f*

for physiology/function, 675–677

of pulmonary arteries, 667–669, 668*f*

of pulmonary veins, 673–674

of systemic veins, 673

tissue/blood-tagging imaging with, 666*f*

types of, 662*f*

venous connections and, preoperative/postoperative, 671–674, 673*f*

Cardiac malpositions, 649

Cardiac neoplasms

benign, 616*t*

malignant primary, 616*t*

metastatic, 616*t*, 618–619

primary malignant, 618, 618*f*

Cardiac pheochromocytomas, 617

Cardiac repair/lung transplantation, for pulmonary atresia, pediatric, 990, 991*f*

Cardiac stress test, 54

Cardiac Surgery Consultants Committee (CSCC), 326

Cardiac surgery databases

background on, 326

challenges/future directions for, 331

construction of, 327–328

current adult, 327–328

data collection for, 327–328

historical considerations on, 326–327

Cardiac surgery, repeat, 324

Cardiac tamponade, diagnosis of, 254–255

Cardiac tumors, 615–619

classification of, 615

epidemiology of, 615

historical background on, 615

myxomas and, 615–616, 616*f*

Cardiac/noncardiac pathologic conditions, associated with VSDs, 752

Cardiology Patient Database, of CHP, 708, 710, 711

Cardioplegia

antegrade cannulas for, 318, 320*f*

antegrade pressure of, 320–321

clinical applications of, 318–322

cold blood, 315

cold multidose blood, solution contents for, 318*t*

components, 315

for coronary grafting/valve replacement, 320*f*

coronary sinus injury and, 320–321

delivery devices for, 318, 319*f*

modified cold blood maintenance solution, 319*t*

monitoring devices for, 318, 319*f*

monitoring pressure of, 320

multidose, 315–316

retrograde cannulas for, 318–319, 320*f*

warm blood, 315

solution contents for, 318*t*

Cardioplegic delivery system, pressure measurement of, 322

Cardioplegic perfusion

antegrade/retrograde, 316–317

delivery of, 323*t*

intermittent/continuous, 317

Cardioplegic solutions, 322–323

Cardioplegic vascular system, pressure measurement of, 322

Cardiopulmonary bypass (CPB), 305–314, 332

air removal from heart in, 313–314

alternate arterial cannulation for, 309–310, 310*f*

CABG using, 437–448

cannulation for, 306–309, 306*f*, 307*f*, 308*f*, 309*f*

completed cannulation, 311*f*

decompressing left heart in, 312–313

draping and, 306

hemacrit management for, for neurologic injury prevention, 335

incisions for, 306

indications for, 439

institution of, 312–313, 443–444

ischemic mitral regurgitation and, 372

lung transplantation and, 199

patient blood volume in, 313*t*

patient management after, 452

patient positioning for, 305–306

plan development for, 305

preparation for, 305

priming volume per tube length/diameter in, 313*t*

for pulmonary stenosis, open pulmonary valvotomy using, 881–882

required tubing diameter, for different patient weights, 313*t*

skin preparation for, 306

weaning from, 387–388, 444

Cardiopulmonary bypass circuit, 310–312, 311*f*, 312*f*

example of, 312*f*

Cardiopulmonary bypass institution, for reoperative mitral valve replacement, 393

Cardiopulmonary bypass machine, effects of, 439–441, 440*f*, 441*f*

Carina, bronchoscopic view of, 4*f*

Carinal resection, 82–86

airway reconstruction and, 84–85, 85*f*

anesthesia for, 82–83

intraoperative evaluation for, 83

introduction to, 82

operative technique for, 83–86

patient evaluation for, 82

postoperative care for, 85–86

release maneuvers for, 83, 84*f*

surgical approaches to, 83, 83*f*

Carpentier transatrial approach, 396*f*

Carpentier-McCarthy-Adams IMR etlogix ring, for ischemic mitral regurgitation, 374–375, 375*f*

Carpentier's functional classification, of ischemic mitral regurgitation, 369

Catamenial pneumothorax, 98–99

Catheter placement, with polyethylene terephthalate cuffs, 251*f*

Cavitary disease, of right upper lobe, chest radiograph of, 296*f*

Cavopulmonary shunts

bidirectional and, 919–920, 919*f*, 920*f*, 921*f*

early postoperative complications for, 922

hemi-Fontan operation and, 916–922

hemi-Fontan procedure and, 920–921, 921*f*, 922*f*

history of, 916

indications for, 916–918

late postoperative complications for, 922

operative technique for, 918–921, 918*f*, 919*f*, 920*f*, 921*f*, 922*f*

postoperative care for, 922

preoperative assessment for, 916–918, 917*t*

risk factors for, 917*t*

unidirectional, 918–919, 918*f*, 919*f*

CBF. *See* Cerebral blood flow

ccTGA. *See* Congenitally corrected transposition of great arteries

Celiac/mesenteric/renal arteries, reimplantation of, 552–553, 553*f*, 554*f*

Central alveolar hypoventilation (CAH), diaphragmatic pacing and, 238

Cephalad movement, transhiatal esophagectomy, umbilical tape pulling in, 135*f*

Cerebral blood flow (CBF), 333

Cerebral perfusion maintenance, neurologic injury prevention and, 333

Cerebral protection

arch aneurysms and, 563–565

techniques, 332–336

Cerebral venous oxygen saturation (CVOS), 335

Cervical dissection, 16*f*

in mediastinoscopy, 16*f*

Cervical incision, 143–144

Cervical mediastinotomy, bidigital palpation of, aortopulmonary region and, 23*f*

Cervical phase, of transhiatal esophagectomy, 132–135

CF. *See* Cystic fibrosis

Chemotherapy, for esophageal cancer, 182

Chest lobe resections, en bloc removal, 291*f*

Chest radiographs (CXR), for
    pneumothorax, 96
Chest roentgenogram
    of empyema
        with pleura effusion, 281*f*
        with pleura space collection, 282*f*
    of multiloculated empyema, 283*f*
Chest tubes
    for empyema, 280–281, 281*f*
    modification of, 27*f*
Chest wall closure, superior sulcus tumor
    resection and, 293
Chest wall resections, 222–227
    en bloc lateral, 223*f*
    en bloc removal, 291*f*
    indications for, 222
    operative planning for, 222–223
    pedicle muscle flaps and, for
        reconstruction, 226*f*
    preoperative evaluation for, 222
    prosthesis inset for, 225*f*
    sternal resections and, 225–227, 226*f*,
        227*f*
    superior sulcus tumor resection and,
        288–289, 289*f*, 293
    surgical technique for, 223–225, 223*f*
    synthetic material choices for, 225
    tissue transfer options for, 225, 225*t*
CHF. *See* Congestive heart failure
Children's Hospital of Pittsburgh (CHP),
    708
    Cardiology Patient Database of, 708,
        710, 711
Chitwood extracorporeal knot-tier, 366*f*
Chordal replacement, technique of, 348*f*
Chordal shortening, technique of, 347*f*
Chordal-sparing mitral valve replacement,
    381–384
    Khonsari I technique, 385*f*
    Khonsari II technique, 385*f*
    technique for, 384*f*
CHP. *See* Children's Hospital of Pittsburgh
Chronic obstructive pulmonary disorders
    (COPD), 194
    diaphragmatic pacing and, 238
Chronic pulmonary thromboembolism,
    626–630
Chronic thromboembolic pulmonary
    hypertension (CTEPH), 626–630
    alternative treatments for, 629
    anesthetic considerations for, 630
    clinical presentation of, 627
    diagnostic modalities for, 627–629, 628*f*
    incidence of, 626–627
    indications for, 629–630
    operative preparation for, 630
    operative principles for, 630, 631*f*
    operative techniques for, 630–633, 631*f*,
        632*f*, 633*f*, 634*f*
    pathology of, 627
    pathophysiology of, 627
    postoperative care for, 633–635

    pulmonary thromboendarterectomy for,
        629–630
    reperfusion response management and,
        635
    surgical complications of, 634–635
Chronic thromboendarterectomy (PTE),
    626
Chyle, composition of, 246*t*
Chylothorax
    definition of, 244
    diagnosis of, 245–246
    etiology of, 245*t*
    internal shunt system for, 248*f*
    management of, 247–252
    octreotide for, 246, 247*t*
    pleuroperitoneal shunt for, 248*f*
    pneumonectomy and, 60–61
    somatostatin for, 246, 247*t*
    thoracoscopic management of, 248*f*
    thoracotomy for, 247*f*
Cine magnetic resonance imaging uses,
    675–676
Circumflex artery injury, in MVR, 388
Citrate phosphate dextrose (CPD), 315
Clamshell. *See* Bilateral thoracosternotomy
Cleft mitral valve, pediatric mitral valve
    repair and, 1008
Closed tricuspid valvotomy, for neonates,
    884–885
Coarctation. *See* Aortic coarctation
Cold blood cardioplegia, for myocardial
    protection, 315
Cold multidose blood cardioplegia,
    solution contents for, 318*t*
Collis gastroplasty, 126–127, 128*f*, 129*f*
Collis procedure, 234
Colon interposition, 176–178
    mobilized left, 177*f*
    preparation for, 176–177
    procedure for, 177–178
    surgical results for, 178
    vagal-sparing esophagectomy with, 175*f*
Complete vascular rings
    anatomy of, 722–729
    clinical presentation of, 723–725
    diagnosis of, 723–725
    surgical indications for, 726
    surgical technique for, 726–727, 728*f*,
        730*f*, 731*f*, 732*f*, 733*f*, 930*f*
Complex spatial relationships, cardiac
    magnetic resonance imaging and,
    670–671, 671*f*
Computed tomography (CT), 54
    tumor staging and, 11, 12*t*
Conal septal defect
    repair of, 755*f*, 756
    transpulmonary closure of, 755*f*
Conduits/shunts, congenital heart disease
    and, 687, 688*f*
Cone resection, with electrocautery, 74*f*
Congenital anomalies, of aortic root
    sinuses, 804–809

Congenital heart disease
    anatomy of, 644–649
    aortic arch obstructions and, 686–687
    aortopulmonary shunts for, 693–704,
        694*t*
    atrial arrhythmias in, 603–604
    atrial septectomy for, 705*t*
    balloon angioplasty and, 685–686
    balloon valvuloplasty for, 682–685,
        684*f*, 685*f*
    Blalock-Taussig shunt for, 693–694,
        694*f*, 694*t*, 695*f*, 696*f*, 697*f*
    branch pulmonary artery stenosis and,
        686–687, 686*f*, 687*f*
    chamber/valve/vessel abnormalities and,
        644–649
    classification of, 639–644
        accuracy in, 640
        aims/principles of, 639–640
        atrioventricular alignments and,
            642–643, 642*f*, 643*f*, 644*f*
        cardiac segment and, 640–641
        economy in, 639
        intersegmental alignments and,
            642–644, 642*f*, 643*f*, 644*f*
        organization of, 639
        precision in, 640
        quantification, 640
        segmental approach to, 640
        segmental notation and, 641–642,
            642*f*
        ventricular loop and, 640–641, 641*f*
        ventriculoarterial alignments and,
            643–644
        visceroatrial situs and, 640
    conduits/shunts and, 687, 688*f*
    device closures and, 690
    echocardiographic evaluation of,
        651–658
    embolizations and, 688–689
    endovascular stenting and, 685–686
    imaging children with, 652–658, 653*t*
        abdomen view of, 652
        atrial/ventricularseptal defects and,
            653–655, 654*f*, 655*f*, 656*f*
        atria/ventricles and, 652–653
        atrioventricular connection and,
            652–653
        conotruncal anomalies and, 656–657,
            657*f*
        extracardiac vessels and, 657–658
        sinus venous ASD and, 654–655, 655*f*,
            656*f*, 657*f*, 658*f*
        situs and, 652
        venous connections and, 657–658
    intraoperative transesophageal
        echocardiography/postoperative
        imaging and, 658
    miscellaneous palliative procedures for,
        704–705, 705*t*
    modified Blalock-Taussig shunts for,
        694–697, 695*t*, 696*f*, 697*f*

palliative operations for, 693–705
Potts shunt for, 698–700, 700f, 700t, 701f
pulmonary artery band for, 700–704, 701t
pulmonic valve stenosis/atresia and, 682–683
retrievals and, 690
septostomy procedures for, 682, 682f
syntax for diagnosis, 649
systemic pulmonary veins and, 687
transcatheter therapy for, 681–690
hemodynamic assessment and, 679–691
Waterston/Cooley shunt for, 697–698, 698f, 698t, 699f
Congenital mitral valves, pediatric mitral valve repair and, 1013–1014
Congenital pulmonary vein stenosis, pediatric, 990
Congenitally corrected transposition of great arteries (ccTGA), 873–879
anatomic repair for, 876–879
anatomy of, 873–874
background on, 873
classical repair of, 877
diagnosis for, 874
embryology of, 873–874
intracardiac repair for, 875–877
left atrioventricular valve repair for, 876
palliative operations for, 874–875
Senning plus Rastelli operation for, 877
subpulmonary obstruction repair for, 875–876, 876f
surgical results of, 877–879
surgical treatment for, 874–879, 876f, 878f
terminology for, 873
univentricular repair of, 877, 878f
ventricular septal defects closure for, 875
Congestive heart failure (CHF), 379, 494
background on, 494
Conical ventricular chamber, in left ventricular reconstruction, 485f
Conotruncal anomalies, 648–649, 649f
congenital heart disease and, imaging children with, 656–657, 657f
Conotruncal defects, 750, 751f
Conoventricular defects, 750
repair of, 753–755, 754f, 755f
transventricular closure of, 755f
Conscious sedation, 7t
Constrictive pericarditis, etiology of, 258t
Continuous positive airway pressure (CPAP), 89
COPD. See Chronic obstructive pulmonary disorders
Coronary artery, 648
fistula
definition of, 965

operation method for, 966–967, 967, 968f
results for, 967
Coronary artery anomalies
aortic reimplantation for, 961–962, 962f
CABG for, 965
left internal mammary artery grafting and, 965
left subclavian-to-left coronary artery anastomosis and, 965
in children, 959–971
modified Takeuchi repair for, 963–964, 963f, 964f, 965f
operation method for, 961–965, 962f, 963f, 964f, 965f
origin from pulmonary artery, 959–961, 960f, 960t, 961f
results of, 965
Coronary artery bypass (CAB), 332
on bypass, conduct of, 441–445
graft-only risk model, 330t
interoperative management for, 441–442, 442f
neurologic injury prevention after, 332–337
operative mortality, risk-adjusted isolated, 438f
preoperative assessment for, 441
procedure, 323
surgical techniques for, 442–443
Coronary artery bypass grafting (CABG), 324, 466
bleeding from, 446
complications from, 445–446
for coronary artery anomalies, 965
evolution of, 437–438
future considerations and, 448
infection from, 446
mortality model, 329t
neurologic complications of, 445
outcomes from, 446–447, 448t
postoperative physiology/management of, 444–445
renal dysfunction and, 446
timeline for, 439t
using CPB, 437–448
Coronary grafting/valve replacement, cardioplegia for, 320f
Coronary sinus (CoS), 644
anomalies of, 713
atrial septal defect, surgical repair of, 745f, 746, 747f
cannula, palpation for position of, 321f
compression of, 321f
injury, cardioplegia and, 320–321
Coronary stabilization, for OPCAB, 459
Coronary targets, for OPCAB, 459, 460f, 461f, 462f
Corticosteroids, for pyridostigmine, 107
CoS. See Coronary sinus

Costotransversectomy, posterior mediastinal neurogenic dumbbell tumor and, 118f
Cox Maze III modifications, 600, 600f, 601f
Cox Maze procedure
mitral valve surgery and, 602–603
recurrent atrial fibrillation after, 604–605
results of, 607–608, 607f, 608f
surgical technique of, 607–608, 607f, 608f
CPAP. See Continuous positive airway pressure
CPB. See Cardiopulmonary bypass
CPD. See Citrate phosphate dextrose
Crawford classification, of thoracic/thoracoabdominal aneurysms, 546f
CSCC. See Cardiac Surgery Consultants Committee
CT. See Computed tomography
CTEPH. See Chronic thromboembolic pulmonary hypertension
Curative debulking, for MPM, 264–265
CVOS. See Cerebral venous oxygen saturation
CXR. See Chest radiographs
Cystic fibrosis (CF), 98, 194

D
da Vinci robotic telemanipulation system, 353, 354f
mitral valve repairs with, 366–367
Damus-Kaye-Stansel repair, of DORV, with subpulmonary ventricular septal defect, 845–848, 848f
Databases. See Society of Thoracic Surgeons (STS) database; Veterans Affairs database
DCT. See Double-clamp technique
De-airing
left ventricle, reoperative mitral replacement and, 401f
during lung transplantation, 200f
for type IIIb, ischemic mitral regurgitation, 374
Debakey forceps, 90
Decompressing left heart, in CPB, 312–313
Deep vein thrombosis (DVT), 626
Degenerative mitral disease, 356–357
DES. See Diffuse esophageal spasm
Diaphragm, 228–243
abdominal view of, 232f
anatomy of, 228–229, 229f, 230f, 231f
embryological development of, 228
eventration of, 237–238
incisions in, 229
phrenic nerve and, 230f
plication of, 239f, 240f, 241f
repair, 229–230

Diaphragm (*Contd.*)
  polypropylene mesh for, 230
  PTFE patch for, 230
  suturing techniques for, 233*f*
  thoracic view of, incisions in, 232*f*
  trauma to, 240–242
  tumors of, 242
Diaphragmatic flap, 243
  harvesting technique for, 242*f*
Diaphragmatic pacing, 238–240
  CAH and, 238
  COPD and, 238
Diaphragmatic paralysis, 236–237
Diaphragmatic surface, transdiaphragmatic
    fenestration and, 95*f*
Diffuse esophageal spasm (DES), 163
  definition of, 170
  diagnosis of, 171
  esophagomyotomy results for, 171
  etiology of, 170–171
  incidence of, 170–171
  laparoscopy for, 171
  long myotomy alone for, 171
  lower esophageal sphincter/partial
      fundoplication, long myotomy
      with, 171
  surgical results for, 171
  surgical technique for, 171
  thoracoscopic long myotomy for, 171
  treatment of, 171
Diffuse subaortic stenosis, 795, 795*f*,
    796*f*
Dilators, flexible, 7*f*
Discrete subaortic stenosis, 792–793, 792*f*,
    793*f*, 794*f*
Distal false lumen obliteration, acute type
    A aortic dissection and, 538*f*
Distal segmental esophagectomy, 180–181
  advantages/disadvantages of, 180–181
  procedure of, 180
Distant metastases, diagnosis of, 11–12
Diverticula. *See specific* diverticula
Domino-donor procedures, with heart-lung
    transplantation, 594
Donor heart procurement, for heart
    transplantation, 580–581, 581*f*
Donor lung retrieval, 194–197
Doppler principle, ultrasound
    physics/applications and, 651–652
Dor fundoplication, in laparoscopic
    esophagomyotomy, 165*f*
Dorsal sympathectomy
  posterior thoracotomy first-rib resection
      with, for recurrent thoracic outlet
      syndrome, 215–217, 217*f*
  transaxillary first-rib resection with,
      214–215, 214*f*, 215*f*, 216*f*
Dorsal sympathetic chain
  division of, 219*f*
  exposure of, 219*f*
  stellate ganglion and, in transaxillary
      approach, 216*f*

Double aortic arch
  anatomy, 729, 732*f*
  surgical technique for, 726–727, 728*f*,
      730*f*, 731*f*, 732*f*, 733*f*, 931*f*
Double cannulation, final position for,
    310*f*
Double venous cannulation, 309*f*
Double-clamp technique (DCT), 334
Double-outlet left ventricle (DOLV),
    851–852
  anatomy of, 851
  clinical presentation of, 851
  complications of, 852
  definition of, 851
  postoperative considerations of, 852
  surgical technique for, 851–852, 852*f*
Double-outlet right ventricle (DORV),
    841–851
  anatomic repair of, with subpulmonary
      ventricular septal defect, 845, 846*f*
  classification of, 841, 842*t*
  complications of, 850–851
  Damus-Kaye-Stansel repair, with
      subpulmonary ventricular septal
      defect, 845–848, 848*f*
  definition of, 841
  doubly committed ventricular septal
      defect with, 841, 849
  noncommitted ventricular septal defect
      with, 841, 849–850, 850*f*
  postoperative considerations of, 850–851
  with subaortic ventricular septal defect
      with pulmonary stenosis, 844–845,
      844*f*
    tunnel repair of, 842–844, 842*f*, 843*f*
  subaortic ventricular septal defect and,
      841
  subpulmonary ventricular septal defect
      and, 841
  surgical techniques for, 841–850, 842*f*,
      843*f*, 844*f*, 846*f*, 847*f*, 848*f*, 849*f*,
      850*f*
Doubly committed ventricular septal
    defect, with DORV, 841, 849
Duke Lung Transplant Program, 194
Duke University immunosuppression
    protocol, for lung transplantation,
    201*t*
Duke University infection prophylaxis, for
    lung transplantation, 202*t*
Dumbbell tumor. *See* Posterior mediastinal
    neurogenic dumbbell tumor
Duodenum migration, paraesophageal
    hernia with, 237*f*, 238*f*
DVT. *See* Deep vein thrombosis

E
Ebstein's anomaly
  anatomy of, 404, 405*f*, 998–999, 999*f*
  associated anomalies of, 998–999
  background on, 998
  complications of, 1004–1006

  diagnosis of, 1001
  embryology of, 998
  grades of, 1000*f*
  medical management of, 1001–1002
  operative technique for, 1002–1004,
      1003*f*, 1004*f*
  pathophysiology of, 999–1001, 1001*t*
  pediatric, 998–1006
  postoperative care for, 1004–1006
  results of, 1006
  single-ventricle repair for, 1004, 1004*f*,
      1005*f*
  surgical indications for, 1002, 1002*f*
  tricuspid valve, repair for, 407*f*, 408, 408*f*
  two-ventricle repair for, 1002–1004,
      1003*f*, 1004*f*
Eccentric pericardiotomy, for AVSDs, 813*f*
ECG. *See* Electrocardiogram
Echocardiographic evaluation, of
    congenital heart disease, 651–658
ECMO. *See* Extracorporeal membrane
    oxygenation
Electrocardiogram (ECG), 660
Electrocautery incision, of periosteum,
    217*f*
Elephant trunk technique, for arch
    aneurysms, 560–563, 561*f*, 562*f*
EM. *See* Environmental Mycobacterium
Embolization
  congenital heart disease and, 688–689
  reduction, neurologic injury prevention
      and, 333–334
Emphysema
  definition of, 204
  giant bullectomy for, 204
  history of, 204
  laser bullectomy for, 204
  LVRS for, 205, 205*t*, 206
  pathophysiology of, 204–205
  surgery for, 204–211
    indications for, 205–206, 205*t*
    preoperative evaluation for, 205–206,
        205*t*
    preoperative preparation for, 206
Empyema
  chest tubes for, 280–281, 281*f*
  history of, 280
  incidence of, 280
  open drainage procedure for, 284*f*
  pneumonectomy and, 61–62
  streptokinase for, 281–284
  treatment for, 280
Endo-ACAB. *See* Endoscope-assisted
    coronary artery bypass
Endocarditis
  of mitral valve, 349–350
  tricuspid valve and, 404
Endoscope-assisted coronary artery bypass
    (Endo-ACAB), 467
Endoscopic endoluminal palliative
    procedures, for esophageal cancer,
    182–183

Endoscopic heart positioner, 471*f*, 472*f*
Endoscopy, 3
    advantages of, 4*t*
    anatomic considerations for, 3–5
    equipment, 5–6, 5*f*
    rigid v. flexible, 4*t*
Endovascular aortic stents
    acute traumatic aortic transection and, 575–576
    congenital heart disease and, 685–686
Endovascular thoracic aortic aneurysm repair, 554
End-to-end anastomosis
    aortic coarctation and, 769–771, 772*f*, 773*f*
    technique of, 84*f*, 85*f*
Environmental Mycobacterium (EM), 295, 296
Erdheim's cystic medial necrosis, 527
Esophageal cancer
    ablative therapies for, 183–184
    brachytherapy for, 182
    chemotherapy for, 182
    endoscopic endoluminal palliative procedures for, 182–183
    incidence of, 139
    laser ablation for, 183–184
    palliation for, 182
    photodynamic therapy for, 183
    radiation for, 182
    stents for, 184, 184*f*, 185*f*
    surgical treatment for, 182
Esophageal diverticula
    definition of, 187
    excision of, 187–193
Esophageal mobilization, for thoracic diverticula, 192*f*
Esophageal motility disorders, 163–173
Esophageal replacement conduits, 174–186
    position of, 181–182
Esophageal replacement, indications for, 168, 168*f*
Esophageal resection, 168
Esophageal rotation, for thoracic diverticula, 192*f*
Esophagectomy
    left thoracoabdominal approach to, 145–146, 145*f*
    minimally invasive approaches to, 146
    postoperative management for, 146–147
    preoperative evaluation for, 139–140
    surgical results of, 168–170
    thoracic approaches to, 139–147
        indications for, 140
        surgical principles of, 140–142
        surgical technique for, 142–146, 144*f*, 145*f*
    three-incision technique, 169*f*
Esophagogastric anastomosis, suturing of, 136*f*
Esophagogastric fat pad, mobilization of, 155*f*

Esophagogastrostomy
    hand-sewn, 144*f*
    mechanical stapler for, 144*f*
Esophagomyotomy
    main techniques of, 167*f*
    videothoracoscopic, 166*f*
Esophagoscope, dilating, 7*f*
Esophagoscopy, 6
    procedure for, 6–9
Esophagus, 4–5
    acquired shortening of, 148–149
Eventration of diaphragm, 237–238
Evolving myocardial infarction, 323–324
Excitotoxicity mechanism, of neural cell injury, 333*f*
Excitotoxin, glutamate as, 332
Extended cervical mediastinoscopy, 21*f*
Extended end-to-end anastomosis, aortic coarctation and, 769–771, 772*f*, 773*f*
Extended vertical trans-septal biatriotomy approach, to MVR, 381*f*
Externalized pleuroperitoneal shunt
    patency of, 252*f*
    placement of, 250*f*
Extracardiac conduits/baffles, cardiac magnetic resonance imaging and, 669–670, 669*f*, 670*f*
Extracardiac Fontan with adjustable fenestration, PA/IS with, definitive surgical treatment for, 890–891
Extracardiac vessels, congenital heart disease and, imaging children with, 657–658
Extracorporeal membrane oxygenation (ECMO), 197, 232, 947, 954
Extrapleural pneumonectomy, eligibility criteria for, 263*t*

F

FDG. *See* Fluorodeoxyglucose
FEV. *See* Forced expiratory volume
Fibromas, heart, 617
First rib removal
    posterior approach incision for, 217*f*
    with Urschel rongeur, 216*f*
First thoracic nerve root, from intervertebral foramen, 290*f*
Flip over technique, for mitral valve repair, 348*f*
Floppy Collis-Nissen wrap creation, in laparoscopic Collis gastroplasty, 152*f*
Flow gradients, 680
Fluorodeoxyglucose (FDG), 55
FMR. *See* Functional mitral regurgitation
Folding plasty technique, for mitral valve repair, 347*f*
Fontan conversion, 1035–1040
Fontan operation, 925–933
    arrhythmias incidence for, 933*t*
    early outcome for, 932*t*

fenestration effect for, 932*t*
    indications for, 928–929
    late outcome for, 932*t*
    operative technique for, 929–931, 929*f*, 930*f*, 931*f*
    overall outcomes for, 932*t*
    postoperative management after, 931–932
    results of, 932–933
Fontan patients, ablation results in, 1036*t*
Fontan revision results, without arrhythmia surgery, 1037*t*
Fontan suture, in left ventricular reconstruction, 481*f*
Foraminectomy, hemilaminectomy and, 118*f*
Forced expiratory volume (FEV), 34, 54
Forced vital capacity (FVC), 34, 108
Fossa ovalis
    excision of, 746*f*
    incision of, 746*f*
Free ventricular wall rupture
    clinical presentation of, 510
    diagnosis of, 510
    incidence of, 510
    myocardial infarction complications, 510–512
    natural history of, 510
    operative technique of, 510–512, 511*f*
    operative timing of, 510
    pathogenesis of, 510
    preoperative treatment of, 510
    survival of, 512
Full blood flow rates, calculation methods for, 312*t*
Full median sternotomy incision, for thymectomy, 103, 105*f*
Full median sternotomy, thymectomy via, 105*f*
Functional mitral regurgitation (FMR), 378
Functional tricuspid regurgitation, 403–404
Fundoplication
    Belsey, 127*f*
    completed view of, 128*f*
    complications of, 128–129
    gastroplasty and, 126–127, 128*f*, 129*f*
    indications for, 121–122
    laparoscopic, 122–123, 122*f*, 123*f*
        access port placement for, 122*f*
    operative techniques for, 122–127, 122*f*, 123*f*, 124*f*, 125*f*, 126*f*, 127*f*
    patient preparation for, 122
    postoperative care for, 127–128
    results of, 129
    surgical principles of, 122
    Toupet, suture rows for, 125*f*
    transabdominal partial, 124–125, 125*f*
    transabdominal total, 123–125, 124*f*
        crural stitches for, 124*f*
        suture placement for, 124*f*

Fundoplication (*Contd.*)
transthoracic partial, 126, 127*f*, 128*f*
transthoracic total, 125–126
crural stitches for, 126*f*
FVC. *See* Forced vital capacity

G

Gastric interposition, 175*f*
Gastric mobilization, 174
Gastric pull-up, completed, 170*f*
Gastric pull-up procedures, 174–176
Gastric staple line, for laparoscopic Collis gastroplasty, 151*f*
Gastric tube
construction of, 143*f*
creation, MIE and, 159*f*
suturing, for MIE, 160*f*
Gastroesophageal migration, paraesophageal hernia with, 237*f*, 238*f*
Gastroesophageal reflux disease (GERD), 121, 125, 127, 129
medications for, 121
surgical candidates for, 121
Gastroesophageal reflux related motility disorders, 172–173
Gastrointestinal anastomosis (GIA), 234
Gastroplasty
after fundoplication, 129*f*
Collis, 126–127, 128*f*, 129*f*
fundoplication and, 126–127, 128*f*, 129*f*
staple line of, 129*f*
GCOs. *See* Ground glass opacities
GERD. *See* Gastroesophageal reflux disease
GIA. *See* Gastrointestinal anastomosis
Giant bullectomy, for emphysema, 204
Giant paraesophageal hernia (GPEH) repair, 153–156
results of, 155–156
technique for, 154–155, 154*f*, 155*f*
Glenn shunts. *See* Bidirectional cavopulmonary shunts
Glucose control, neurologic injury prevention and, 335
Glutamate, as excitotoxin, 332
GPEH repair. *See* Giant paraesophageal hernia (GPEH) repair
Graft failure, as post-transplant complications for, pediatric heart transplantation, 974–975
Graft surveillance, for heart-lung transplantation, 592
Graft-coronary anastomosis, MVST CABG, 470–471, 470*f*, 471*f*
Grafting sequence, for OPCAB, 459
Ground glass opacities (GCOs), 71

H

Hammock valve, pediatric mitral valve repair and, 1007
HCA. *See* Hypothermic circulatory arrest

HCFA. *See* Health Care Financing Administration
Health Care Financing Administration (HCFA), 326
Heart transplantation, 579–586
after ventricular assist device, 585
background on, 579
donor availability/allocation for, 579–580
donor heart procurement for, 580–581, 581*f*
donor selection for, 580
heterotopic, 585, 585*f*, 586*f*
organ preservation for, 581, 582*f*
orthotopic, 581–584
pediatric, 973–982
postoperative management for, 585–586
preoperative evaluation for, 579
recipient selection for, 579
results for, 586
Heart-lung transplantation, 587–595
airway complications with, 594
background on, 587
chronic rejection/late complications with, 593
domino-donor procedures with, 594
early postoperative clinical management for, 591
graft surveillance for, 592
immunosuppressive management for, 591–592
infection prophylaxis for, 592
long-term results of, 595
organ procurement preservation for, 587–588, 588*f*, 588*t*
pediatric, 988
postoperative complications with, 592–593
recipient operation for, 588–591, 589*f*, 590*f*, 591*f*, 592*f*, 593*f*, 594*f*, 595*f*
recipient selection for, 587, 588*t*
retransplantation and, 593–594
HeartMate left ventricular assist device, in situ, 508*f*
Heart-single-lung transplant, 594–595
Heller myotomy, modified, 165–167, 166*f*, 167*f*
Hemacrit management, on CPB, for neurologic injury prevention, 335
Hemi-arch technique, for arch aneurysms, 557–559, 558*f*, 559*f*
Hemiclamshell incision, superior sulcus tumor resection and, 293, 293*f*
Hemi-Fontan procedure, cavopulmonary shunts and, 916–922, 920–921, 921*f*, 922*f*
Hemilaminectomy, foraminectomy and, 118*f*
Hemodynamic assessment
of atrioventricular valve stenosis, or insufficiency, 681

of mitral valve, 681
of patients
with complete mixing lesions, 680–681
with functional single ventricle, 680–681
with left-to-right shunt lesion, 680
with right-to-left shunt lesion, 680
principles of, 679–680
of pulmonary valve, 681
of semilunar valve stenosis, or insufficiency, 681
transcatheter therapy and, for congenital heart disease, 679–691
of tricuspid valve, 681
Hemorrhage, tracheal resection and, 80
Hemostasis, thymectomy and, 105*f*
Hepatic segment, of IVC, absence of, 711, 712*f*
Hernia
of Bochdalek, posterolateral diaphragmatic, 231–233
repair of, 235*f*
hiatal, 153, 234–236, 234*f*
of Morgagni, anterior retrosternal diaphragmatic, 231–233
repair of, 235*f*
paraesophageal
with duodenum migration, 237*f*, 238*f*
with gastroesophageal migration, 237*f*, 238*f*
incidence of, 153
laparoscopic reduction of, 154*f*
symptoms of, 153
treatment for, 153
view of, 236*f*–237*f*
Heterotaxy syndromes, pediatric heart transplantation and, 981–982, 982*f*
Heterotopic heart transplantation, 585, 585*f*, 586*f*
Hiatal hernia, 153, 234–236
abdominal view of, 234*f*
Hiccups, intractable, 238
High superior vena cava, PAPVR to, 955
High-amplitude peristaltic contraction, 171–172
definition of, 171
diagnosis of, 171–172
etiology of, 171
incidence of, 171
therapy of, 172
Hilum
left pulmonary, view of, 47*f*
right pulmonary, view of, 35*f*
HLHS. *See* Hypoplastic left heart syndrome
Hypertrophic cardiomyopathy, 797–801, 800*f*, 801*f*
AF and, 604
Hypoplastic left heart syndrome (HLHS), 935–945
anatomy of, 935–936, 936*f*
initial management of, 936–937, 938*f*

pediatric heart transplantation and, 975–977, 976*f*, 977*f*
donor procurement for, 975, 976*f*
recipient operation for, 975–977, 977*f*
presentation of, 936–937
results for, 942–945
stage I reconstructive surgery for, 937–939, 938*f*, 939*f*
stage II reconstructive surgery for, 939–940, 940*f*, 941*f*, 942*f*
stage III reconstructive surgery for, 940–942, 943*f*, 944*f*
surgical therapy for, 937–942, 939*f*, 940*f*, 941*f*, 942*f*, 943, 944*f*
Hypoplastic left ventricle, aortic coarctation and, 776
Hypothermia level, safe circulatory arrest times and, 314*t*
Hypothermic circulatory arrest (HCA), 332
Hypothermic ventricular fibrillation, 449–453
advantages/disadvantages of, 452–453
clinical results review for, 453
contraindications for, 449
indications for, 449
operative principles of, 449–450
operative technique for, 450–452
preoperative preparation for, 449
primary revascularization for, 450–452
reoperative revascularization for, 452

I

ICM. *See* Intercostal muscle
ICS. *See* Intercostal space
Idiopathic pulmonary fibrosis (IPF), 194
IMLC. *See* Incomplete mitral leaflet coaptation
IMR. *See* Ischemic mitral regurgitation
Inclusion cylinder, Ross procedure and, 425–429
Incomplete mitral leaflet coaptation (IMLC), 379
Infant/pediatric aortic cannulas, 311*f*
insertion/final positioning for, 309*f*
Infection
from CABG, 446
prophylaxis, for heart-lung transplantation, 592
tracheal resection and, 80
Infective endocarditis, pediatric mitral valve repair and, 1009
Inferior caval vein (IVC)
anomalies of, 711–712
hepatic segment of, absence of, 711, 712*f*
interruption of, in visceral heterotaxy, 712
miscellaneous abnormalities of, 712
Inferior pulmonary ligament, 48
view of, 51*f*
Inferior ventricular restoration, 488*f*, 489*f*, 490*f*, 491–492, 491*f*, 492*f*

Inferior/superior horns, of thymus gland, 104*f*
Inferior-type sinus venous atrial septal defect, surgical repair of, 745, 745*f*
Inflow valve conduit, preclotting the, 503*f*
Infundibular septum
resection of, 783*f*
VSDs and, 783*f*
Inlet septal defects, 750–751
repair of, 755*f*, 756
Innominate artery compression
arteriopexy for, 734*f*
positioning/approach for, 734*f*
reduction of, 735*f*
Intercostal arteries, reimplantation of, 552
Intercostal muscle (ICM)
harvesting of, 55*f*
on right mainstem bronchi, 55*f*
Intercostal space (ICS), 89
Internal shunt system
for chylothorax, 248*f*
in position, 250*f*
Internal thoracic artery (ITA)
anatomic considerations, 467–468, 468*f*
graft of, 473*f*
harvesting of, 466, 467, 470*f*
sutures in, 474*f*, 475*f*
Interposed stomach, barium swallow study for, 143*f*
Interposition graft, aortic coarctation and, 771–772
Interrupted aortic arch, 779–787
anatomy of, 779, 780*f*
with aortic valve hypoplasia/atresia, 782
classification of, 780*f*
clinical presentation of, 779
diagnosis of, 779–780
early/late mortality with, 787*t*
intensive care unit management for, 785–786
late problems with, 786–787
neonatal cardiovascular conditions with, 780*t*
operative management of, 780–782, 781*f*, 782*f*
postoperative management for, 785–787
repair of aortopulmonary window, 763–764, 764*f*, 765*f*
with single ventricle, 784–785, 785*f*, 786*f*
special circumstances of, 782–785
survival for, 785–787
with TGA, 784, 786*f*
with truncus arteriosus, 783–784, 784*f*, 785*f*
repair of, 832–838, 835*f*, 836*f*, 838*f*, 839*f*
Intertrigonal area, stabilization of, 346*f*

Intervertebral foramen, first thoracic nerve root from, 290*f*
Intracardiac defects, closure procedures for, 687–690, 689*f*, 690*f*
Intractable hiccups, 238
Intramural hematomas, retrograde extensions of, acute type B aortic dissections, 543
Intraoperative cerebral monitoring, neurologic injury prevention and, 335–336
Intraoperative transesophageal echocardiography/postoperative imaging, congenital heart disease and, 658
Intrathoracic lymphatics
anatomy of, 271
drainage of, 272*f*
graphic representation of, 272*f*
metastases patterns of, 271–273, 273*t*
IPF. *See* Idiopathic pulmonary fibrosis
Ischemic mitral regurgitation (IMR), 369, 378
Carpentier-McCarthy-Adams IMR etlogix ring for, 374–375, 375*f*
Carpentier's functional classification of, 369, 370*f*
CPB and, 372
late outcomes for, 375–376
mild/moderate, 371–372
mitral valve exposure and, 372
mitral valve repair and, 372–375
myocardial protection and, 372
new developments in, 374–375
operative mortality for, 375
perioperative considerations for, 372
residual, 374
severe, 371
surgical approaches to, 372, 373*f*
surgical indications, 371–372
surgical results on, 375–376
type II
clinical presentation of, 376
diagnosis of, 376
medical/surgical treatment for, 376
pathophysiology of, 376
surgical results for, 376
type IIIb
clinical presentation of, 369–370
de-airing process for, 374
diagnosis of, 371
pathophysiology of, 369, 371*t*
segmental valve analysis for, 372
undersized remodeling ring annuloplasty for, 374
Ischemic mitral valve repair, 347–349, 369–377
Isolated atrial fibrillation, minimally invasive epicardial ablation and, 609, 610*f*

Isolated left superior caval veins, 709–710
ITA. *See* Internal thoracic artery
IVC. *See* Inferior caval vein

J

Jackson esophagoscopes, 6*f*
Jackson rigid ventilating laser
    bronchoscope, 6
Jejunal branching pattern, jejunal
    interposition and, 180*f*
Jejunal interposition, 178–181
    jejunal branching pattern and, 180*f*
    long-segment, 181*f*
    long-segment reconstruction and,
        178–179
    mesentery straightening and, 180*f*
    postoperative barium swallow status
        after, 181*f*
Jejunal mesentery, transillumination
    branching within, 179*f*
Juxtaductal coarctation, 769*f*

K

Khonsari I technique, of chordal-sparing
    MVR, 385*f*
Khonsari II technique, of chordal-sparing
    MVR, 385*f*
Khonsari oblique biatriotomy incision, for
    mitral valve replacement (MVR),
    382*f*

L

LAD. *See* Left anterior descending artery
LAO. *See* Left anterior oblique view
Lap Sac, 90
Laparoscopic Collis gastroplasty, 148–153
    bougie position in, 151*f*
    floppy Collis-Nissen wrap creation in,
        152*f*
    gastric staple line for, 151*f*
    neo-esophagus completion in, 152*f*
    results of, 151–153
    technique of, 149–151
Laparoscopic esophagomyotomy
    for achalasia, 164–165, 164*f*, 165*f*
    Dor fundoplication in, 165*f*
    downward retraction in, 165*f*
    trocar port positions for, 164*f*
Laparoscopic fundoplication, 122–123,
    122*f*, 123*f*
Laparoscopic Nissen fundoplication, port
    placement for, 150*f*
Laparoscopic pyloroplasty, MIE and,
    159*f*
Laparoscopic reduction, of paraesophageal
    hernia, 154*f*
Laparoscopy, for DES, 171
Laparotomy, 143–144
Laryngeal dysfunction, tracheal resection
    and, 80
Laser ablation, for esophageal cancer,
    183–184

Laser bullectomy, for emphysema, 204
Lateral chest wall resection, polypropylene
    mesh/methylmethacrylate
    prosthesis for, 224*f*
Lateral decubitus position, for
    posterolateral thoracotomy, 27*f*
Lateral tunnel Fontan with adjustable atrial
    septal defect, PA/IS, definitive
    surgical treatment for, 889–890,
    890*f*, 891*f*
Latissimus dorsi muscle
    outline of, 297*f*
    passed into chest, 298*f*
    sutured to right mainstem bronchus,
        299*f*
LCSG. *See* Lung Cancer Study Group
Leaflet advancement technique, for mitral
    valve repair, 345*f*
Left anterior descending artery (LAD), 466
Left anterior oblique view (LAO), 479
Left anterior thoracotomy, pericardiectomy
    via, 260
Left aortic arch, with aberrant right
    subclavian artery, 729
Left atrial anastomosis, lung
    transplantation and, 200*f*
Left atrioventricular valve competence,
    AVSDs and, 817–820
Left atrioventricular valve repair, for
    ccTGA, 876
Left atrium, left superior caval veins
    drainage into, 710
Left hemithorax, mediastinal lymph node
    dissection and, 275–276, 278*f*, 279*f*
Left inferior pulmonary vein, view of, 58*f*
Left internal mammary artery (LIMA), 323
Left internal mammary artery grafting,
    coronary artery anomalies and,
    CABG for, 965
Left lower lobectomy, 50–52
    sleeve resection, 68–69
Left lower sleeve, view of, 68*f*
Left main bronchial resection, exposure for,
    83*f*
Left main bronchus, left main pulmonary
    artery and, 48*f*
Left main pulmonary artery, left main
    bronchus and, 48*f*
Left pulmonary artery
    anomalous development of, 727*f*
    superior pulmonary artery and, 199*f*
    view of, 50*f*
Left pulmonary atrium, right superior caval
    veins to, 711, 711*f*
Left pulmonary hilum, view of, 47*f*
Left subclavian-to-left coronary artery
    anastomosis, coronary artery
    anomalies and, CABG for, 965
Left superior caval veins
    anatomy of, 708
    drainage to left atrium, 710
    occlusion of, 708

Left superior pulmonary vein, view of, 58*f*
Left thoracoabdominal approach, to
    esophagectomy, 145–146, 145*f*
Left thoracotomy, 144–145
    esophageal mobilization in, 145*f*
    esophagectomy incisions for, 145*f*
Left upper lobe sleeve
    resection, 67–68
    view of, 68*f*
Left upper lobectomy, surgical technique
    of, 46–50
Left ventricular assist devices (LVADs),
    500
    contraindications for, 502*t*
    economic considerations for, 502–503
    indications for, 501*t*
    preoperative evaluation for, 501*t*
Left ventricular end-systolic volume index
    (LVESVI), 479
Left ventricular function, in normal hearts,
    316*f*
Left ventricular outflow tract obstruction
    (LVOTO), 768
    aortic stenosis and, 789–801
    MVR and, 389
Left ventricular oxygen requirements, of
    beating nonworking, fibrillating
    arrested hearts, 316*f*
Left ventricular reconstruction, 479–492
    anteroseptal infarction and, 480*f*
    beating heart myocardial protection and,
        488*f*
    conical ventricular chamber in, 485*f*
    dilated chamber in, 486*f*
    distal inferior wall scar in, 483*f*
    final ventricular running suture and,
        487*f*
    Fontan suture in, 481*f*
    inbrication of inferior wall in, 484*f*,
        485*f*
    inferior infarction area and, 487*f*
    introduction to, 479
    lateral segment sliding in, 486*f*
    narrowing inferior wall scar in, 484*f*
    operative technique for, 479–488, 480*f*,
        481*f*, 482*f*, 483*f*, 484*f*, 485*f*, 486*f*,
        487*f*
    palpation in, 481*f*
    patch size in, 482*f*
    postoperative care for, 492
    preoperative evaluation for, 479
    rim suture for, 483*f*
    suture placement in, 482*f*
    ventricular thinning/necrosis and,
        480*f*
Left ventricular rupture, in MVR, 388
Left-side intrapericardial hilar, release
    technique, 84*f*
Left-sided endotracheal tube, for right
    upper lobe sleeve, 65*f*
Left-sided pneumonectomy, surgical
    procedure for, 57–58

Left-sided pulmonary resections, 46–52
Left-sided resections, 67–69
Left-to-right shunt lesion, hemodynamic assessment, of patients, 680
LES. *See* Lower esophageal sphincter
Lesions
    with lack of valvular tissue, pediatric mitral valve repair and, 1008
    sets, for AV, 600–601
Levoatrial cardinal vein
    anatomy of, 710*f*
    presence of, 710
LIMA. *See* Left internal mammary artery
Limited resections, 71–75
Linear stapler, wedge resection by, 74*f*
Lipomas, within pericardium, 616–617
Lobar lung transplantation, pediatric, 991–995, 994*f*, 995*f*
Lobectomy, 33. *See also specific* lobectomy
    with VATS, 90–91
Long esophagomyotomy, technique of, 170*f*, 171
Long myotomy
    alone, for DES, 171
    with lower esophageal sphincter/partial fundoplication, for DES, 171
Long-segment jejunal interposition, 181*f*
Long-segment reconstruction
    advantages of, 179
    jejunal interposition and, 178–179
    operation course for, 178–179
Low superior vena cava/right atrium, PAPVR to, 955
Lower esophageal sphincter (LES), 163
Lower esophageal sphincter/partial fundoplication, long myotomy with, for DES, 171
Lower lobe bronchus, pulmonary artery and, retraction of, 51*f*
Lower lobe pulmonary artery, stump of, 43*f*
Low-gradient aortic stenosis, 418–420
Lung cancer
    mediastinoscopic radiologic studies in, pathologic nodal stagir, 15*t*
    preoperative evaluation for, 34
    revised TNM staging system, 13*t*
    survival rate, 15*f*
    thoracotomy for, morbidity/mortality reduction for, 34*t*
    TNM staging system for, 12*t*
Lung Cancer Study Group (LCSG), 33
    lobectomy study of, 71
Lung implantation
    ACT for, 199
    preparation for, 197*f*
    procedure for, 199–200, 199*f*, 200*f*
Lung transplantation, 194–203
    anesthetic considerations in, 197–198
    bronchial anastomosis and, 200*f*
    bronchus division in, 199*f*
    clamshell incision for, 198*f*

CPB and, 199
    donor requirements for, 195
    Duke University immunosuppression protocol, 201*t*
    Duke University infection prophylaxis for, 202*t*
    indications for, 194
    left atrial anastomosis and, 200*f*
    lung de-airing during, 200*f*
    patient positioning for, 197
    PGD and, 201–203
    postoperative care for, 202–203
    pulmonary artery anastomosis during, 200*f*
    recipient procedure for, 195–201, 198*f*, 199*f*, 200*f*
    reperfusion in, 200–201
    skin incision for, 197–198
    survival rates for, 195*f*
Lung volume reduction surgery (LVRS), 204
    contraindications for, 205*t*
    for emphysema, 205, 205*t*, 206
    future directions for, 211
    median sternotomy for, 207*f*
    postoperative care for, 208–209
    resection during, 208*f*, 210*f*
    results of, 209–211
    sternum elevation, using Bugge retractor, 207*f*
    thoracoscope insertion during, 209*f*
    tissue grasping during, 208*f*
    unilateral procedures for, 208
    video-assisted bilateral thoracoscopic, 208
Lung/heart-lung transplantation, pediatric, 985–996
    postoperative management of, 995–996
    rejection surveillance/management of, 996
    results of, 996
LVADs. *See* Left ventricular assist devices
LVESVI. *See* Left ventricular end-systolic volume index
LVOTO. *See* Left ventricular outflow tract obstruction
LVRS. *See* Lung volume reduction surgery
Lymph node(s)
    dissection of, 21*f*, 273–274
    identification of, 17, 21*f*
    interoperative assessment of, 274*t*
    map of, for TNM staging, 14*f*
    mediastinal dissection of
        accuracy of, 273–274
        techniques of, 274–277
    mediastinoscopy of, 13–25
Lymphatics, intrathoracic
    anatomy of, 271
    drainage of, 272*f*
    graphic representation of, 272*f*
    metastases patterns of, 271–273, 273*t*

M
MAC. *See* Mycobacterium avian complex
Magnetic resonance imaging (MRI), 34
    advantages/disadvantages of, 661*t*
    for neurologic injury, 336
    role of, 660
    tumor staging and, 11
Major aortopulmonary collaterals (MAPCAs), pulmonary atresia with ventricular septal defect and, 894–903
Malignant pleural mesothelioma (MPM)
    curative debulking for, 264–265
    diagnosis of, 262
    incidence of, 262
    invasive staging studies for, 264
    multimodal approach to, 264–268
        incision for, 265, 266*f*
        introduction to, 264–265
        lung-sparing procedure for, 265–268, 267*f*
        parietal pleurectomy and, 267*f*
        positioning for, 265
        visceral pleural debulking and, 267*f*
    operative techniques for, 263–269, 263*f*, 266*f*, 267*f*
    PDT for, 262
    pericardial reconstruction for, 268–269
    pleural biopsy for, 263*f*
    with pleural effusion
        diagnosis for, 263–264
        palliation for, 263–264
    with pleural rind, diagnosis for, 264
    surgical management of, 262–269
    treatment options for, 262–263
Malperfusion syndrome, acute type B aortic dissection and, 542*f*
MAPCAs. *See* Major aortopulmonary collaterals
Marfan syndrome, 527
Masaoka incision, superior sulcus tumor resection and, 293, 293*f*
Maximal voluntary ventilation (MVV), 34
Maximum intensity projection (MIP), 661, 662*f*
Maze I procedure, 599
Maze II procedure, 599
Maze procedure
    for AF, 599–605
    Cox Maze III modifications and, 600, 600*f*, 601*f*
    future perspectives on, 605
    indications for, 599–600
    outcomes for, 601–602
    postoperative management for, 602
    technique of, 600–601, 600*f*, 601*f*
MDRTB. *See* Multidrug-resistant tuberculosis
Median sternotomy, 28–29
    for LVRS, 207*f*
    patient positioning for, 29*f*

Median sternotomy (*Contd.*)
    pericardiectomy via, 259–260, 259*f*
    vascular rings requiring, 728–729
Mediastinal biopsy
    bleeding and, 18
    complications with, 18–19
    contraindications for, 14–15
    indications for, 13–14
    postoperative care of, 18
    surgical technique for, 15–18, 16*f*
    variations of, 17
Mediastinal lymph node dissection,
        271–279
    left hemithorax and, 275–276, 278*f*, 279*f*
    morbidity of, 277
    right hemithorax and, 274–275, 274*f*,
        275*f*, 276*f*, 277*f*
    survival of, 277–279
    techniques of, 274–277
Mediastinoscopic radiologic studies,
        pathologic nodal stagir, in lung
        cancer, 15*t*
Mediastinoscopy, 11–25
    alternative procedures of, 19
    cervical dissection in, 16*f*
    extended cervical, 21*f*
    of lymph nodes, 13–25
    passive angle of, 19*f*
    patient position for, 16*f*
    staging non-small cell lung cancer,
        algorithm for, 24*f*
    technique of, 13
Mediastinotomy, anterior, 20–25
Merendino. *See* Distal segmental
        esophagectomy
Mesentery straightening, jejunal
        interposition and, 180*f*
Metaiodobenzylguanidine (MIBG), 115
Metastases
    diagnosis of, 12
    distance, 11–12
Methylmethacrylate reconstruction,
        multilevel thoracic
        vertebrectomy/laminectomy and,
        291*f*
Metzenbaum scissors, 90
MG. *See* Myasthenia gravis
MIBG. *See* Metaiodobenzylguanidine
Microvascular reconstruction, proximal
        jejunal branches in, 179*f*
MIDCAB. *See* Minimally invasive direct
        coronary artery bypass
Middle lobe
    bronchus, division of, 42*f*
    sleeve resection, 66–67
    sleeve, view of, 67*f*
MIE. *See* Minimally invasive
        esophagectomy
Mild right ventricular hypoplasia, initial
        neonatal procedures for, 883–884
Minimally invasive coronary artery bypass
        surgery, 466–475

concept of, 466
    technological evolution of, 466–467
    types of, 467
Minimally invasive direct coronary artery
        bypass (MIDCAB), 467
    robot-assisted
        clinical outcomes for, 472–473
        suture directions for, 472–473
Minimally invasive epicardial ablation,
        isolated atrial fibrillation and, 609,
        610*f*
Minimally invasive esophageal procedures,
        148–161
Minimally invasive esophagectomy (MIE),
        156–161
    completed cervical anastomosis, 161*f*
    gastric tube creation and, 159*f*
    gastric tube suturing for, 160*f*
    laparoscopic pyloroplasty and, 159*f*
    proximal esophageal isolation for, 160*f*
    results of, 159–161
    technique of, 157–159
    thoracic esophageal mobilization and,
        158*f*
    thoracoscopic port placement for, 157*f*
    through low transverse cervical incision,
        160*f*
Minimally invasive mitral valve surgery,
        354–355
    patient selection for, 355
MIP. *See* Maximum intensity projection
Mitochondria, neural cell injury and,
        333*f*
Mitral regurgitation (MR), 369, 379, 380
    annuloplasty for, 496, 496*f*
    cardiac catheterization for, 497
    chest X ray for, 497
    clinical presentations of, 496–497
    diagnostic techniques for, 497
    electrocardiogram for, 497, 497*f*
    management of, 497–498
    pathology of, 494–495, 495*f*
    pathophysiology of, 495–496, 496*f*
    prognosis for, 498
Mitral stenosis, 379
Mitral valve, 648
    anatomy of, 378, 494–495
    annuloplasty, 364–366, 365*f*
    anterior/posterior segments of, 343*f*
    disease, repair techniques and, 356–357
    endocarditis of, 349–350
    exposure, ischemic mitral regurgitation
        and, 372
    hemodynamic assessment of, 681
    repair, 341–351
        anterior leaflet commissuroplasty for,
            346*f*
        for cardiomyopathy, 494–498
        with da Vinci robotic telemanipulation
            system, 366–367
        development of techniques for,
            341–342

double-orifice technique for, 349*f*
        flip over technique for, 348*f*
        introduction to, 341
        ischemic mitral regurgitation and,
            372–375
        by leaflet advancement technique,
            345*f*
        pediatric, 1008–1015
        principles of, 342–351
        rheumatic, 350
        robotic technology for, 353–368
        variations on, 344–345
    re-repair, 350–351
    surgery, Cox Maze procedure and,
        602–603
Mitral valve replacement (MVR), 378–389
    anatomic preservation of anterior
        chordae, 386*f*
    anterior leaflet preservation in, 383*f*
        Nara technique for, 383*f*
    aortic valve cusp entrapment and,
        388–389
    atrioventricular conduction pathway
        and, 388–389
    atrioventricular disruption in, 388
    chordal-sparing, 381–384
        technique for, 384*f*
    circumflex artery injury and, 388
    conventional, 381, 382*f*
    diagnostic considerations for, 379
    extended vertical trans-septal
        biatriotomy approach, 381*f*
    Khonsari oblique biatriotomy incision
        for, 382*f*
    left ventricular outflow tract obstruction
        and, 389
    left ventricular rupture in, 388
    operation indicators for, 379
    operative technique for, 380–388, 380*f*,
        381*f*, 382*f*, 383*f*, 384*f*, 385*f*, 386*f*,
        387*f*, 388*f*
    papillary-annular continuity in, 387*f*
    pediatric, operative technique for,
        1029–1030, 1031*f*
    pericardial patch reconstruction in, 387*f*
    perioperative management, 379–380
    perivalvular leak and, 389
    posterior leaflet preservation of, 382*f*
    postoperative management for, 389
    preservation of anterior/posterior
        leaflets, 386*f*
    surgical complications of, 388–389
    vertical left atriotomy incision for, 381*f*
Mobilized gastric conduit, 175*f*
Mobilized latissimus dorsi muscle, with
        resection of third rib, 298*f*
Mobilized left colon interposition, 177*f*
Modified Bernoulli theorem, ultrasound
        physics/applications and, 652
Modified Blalock-Taussig shunts
    for congenital heart disease, 694–697,
        695*t*, 696*f*, 697*f*

takedown of, with hemoclip/division technique, 697f
using PTFE graft, 696f
Modified cold blood cardioplegia maintenance solution, 319t
Modified Dartevelle. *See* Transclavicular approach
Modified Heller myotomy, 165–167
completed view of, 167f
Penrose drains for, 166f
two-stitch fundal wrap for, 167f
Modified Takeuchi repair, for coronary artery anomalies, 963–964, 963f, 964f, 965f
Modified thoracosternotomy. *See* Anterior cervicothoracic approach
Molecular markers, for neurologic injury, 336
Monitoring pressure, of cardioplegia, 320
Morphologic left atrium, 648
Morphologic left ventricle, 648
Morphologic right atrium, 644
Morphologic right ventricle, 645
MOTT. *See* Mycobacterium other than tuberculosis
Mountain lymph node map, 271
MPM. *See* Malignant pleural mesothelioma
MR. *See* Mitral regurgitation
MRI. *See* Magnetic resonance imaging
MTB. *See* Mycobacterium tuberculosis
Multidose cardioplegia, for myocardial protection, 315–316
Multidrug-resistant organism, 295, 296
Multidrug-resistant tuberculosis (MDRTB), chest radiograph of, 296f
Multilevel thoracic vertebrectomy/laminectomy, methylmethacrylate reconstruction and, 291f
Multivessel revascularization, MVST, conduit options for, 468
Multivessel small thoracotomy (MVST), 467
CABG, 467–472
anesthesia/monitoring for, 468–469
graft-coronary anastomosis, 470–471, 470f, 471f
instrument-port sites for, 469f
ITA anatomic considerations, 467–468
ITA harvesting and, 469–470
operating room preparation for, 468
patient positioning for, 469f
patient selection for, 468
pericardial suspensory ligaments in, 470f
postoperative care for‘, 471–472
target vessel exposure in, 470
conduit options for, multivessel revascularization, 468
Muscle sparing. *See* Axillary thoracotomy

Muscular ventricular septal defects, 751
repair of, 756, 756f, 757f
MVR. *See* Mitral valve replacement
MVST. *See* Multivessel small thoracotomy
MVV. *See* Maximal voluntary ventilation
Myasthenia gravis (MG), thymectomy and, 100
Mycobacterium avian complex (MAC), 295
Mycobacterium other than tuberculosis (MOTT), 295
Mycobacterium tuberculosis (MTB), 295, 296
Myocardial infarction complications
acute ischemic mitral regurgitation and, 515–519
free ventricular wall rupture and, 510–512
pump failure and, 519–522
surgery for, 510–522
ventricular septal defect and, 512–515
Myocardial infarction, evolving, 323–324
Myocardial metabolic changes, with cardioplegic solution, 317f
Myocardial perfusion, cardiac magnetic resonance imaging of, 677
Myocardial protection, 315–325
antegrade/retrograde perfusion for, 316–317
during aortic root replacement, 324
beating heart, during systemic vascular resistance, 325f
cold blood cardioplegia for, 315
ischemic mitral regurgitation and, 372
multidose cardioplegia for, 315–316
during OPCAB, 460–462
for reoperative mitral valve replacement, 393
strategies for, 315
ventricular restoration and, 324–325
warm blood cardioplegia for, 315
Myocardial tissue/blood tagging, with cardiac magnetic resonance imaging, 676–677
Myxomas, 615–616, 616t
operative approach to, 616, 617f
Myxomatous floppy mitral valve repair, principles/techniques for, 342–347, 343f, 344f

N

Nara technique, for anterior leaflet preservation, in MVR, 383f
National Emphysema Treatment Trial (NETT), 204, 206
primary results of, 210t
Neo-esophagus completion, in laparoscopic Collis gastroplasty, 152f
Nerve root identification, 218f
NETT. *See* National Emphysema Treatment Trial

Neural cell injury
excitotoxicity mechanism of, 333f
mitochondria and, 333f
Neurogenic dumbbell tumor, resection of, single-stage approach to, 117f, 118f, 119
Neurologic complications, of CABG, 445
Neurologic injuries
assessing, 336
mechanism of, 332
molecular markers for, 336
MRI for, 336
neuropsychologic testing for, 336
spectrum of, 332
Neurologic injury, prevention
acid-base management and, 334–335
after CAB surgery, 332–337
cerebral perfusion maintenance and, 333
embolization reduction and, 333–334
glucose control and, 335
hemacrit management, 335
intraoperative cerebral monitoring and, 335–336
off-pump coronary artery bypass and, 336
pharmacologic intervention for, 335
temperature management and, 334
Neuronal nitric oxide synthase (nNOS), 332
Neuropsychologic testing, for neurologic injury, 336
Neurotoxin, NO as, 332
Neurovascular bundle, tumor dissection and, 116f
New York State database, 327, 328–329
adult preoperative risk factors, 329t
Nissen fundoplication, suture placement for, 126f
Nitric oxide (NO), as neurotoxin, 332
NMDA receptor. *See* N-methyl -D-aspartate receptor
N-methyl -D-aspartate (NMDA) receptor, 332
activation of, 333f
NNE database. *See* Northern New England Cardiovascular Study Group database
nNOS. *See* Neuronal nitric oxide synthase
NO. *See* Nitric oxide (NO)
Noncommitted ventricular septal defect, 841
DORV with, 841, 849–850, 850f
Nonseptic lung disease, 194
Non-small cell lung cancer (NSCLC), 53
Non-tuberculosis Mycobacterium (NTM), 295
Northern New England Cardiovascular Study Group (NNE) database, 327, 328, 329
NSCLC. *See* Non-small cell lung cancer
NTM. *See* Non-tuberculosis Mycobacterium

O

Oblique osteotomy, through clavicle head, 31*f*
Octreotide, for chylothorax, 246, 247*t*
Off-pump coronary artery bypass surgery (OPCAB), 454–464
 anesthesia for, 457
 benefits of, 455*t*
 cardiac displacement for, 459, 460*f*, 461*f*, 462*f*
 clinical outcome after, 454–456
 contraindications for, 456*t*
 coronary stabilization of, 459
 coronary targets for, 459, 460*f*, 461*f*, 462*f*
 future directions for, 463–464
 grafting for, 459–460
 grafting sequence for, 459
 intraoperative management of, 457
 myocardial protection during, 460–462
 neurologic injury prevention and, 336
 operative plan for, 458–463
 patient considerations in, 456
 postoperative care for, 463
 preoperative considerations, 456–457
 prospective randomized studies on, 454–455, 455*t*
 proximal anastomoses and, 462–463
 risk-adjusted retrospective studies on, 455–456
 surgeon considerations in, 456
 surgical preparation for, 458–459
Off-pump pulmonary valvotomy, with transannular right ventricular outflow tract patch, for neonates, 884
Off-pump transventricular pulmonary valvotomy
 for neonates, 883–884
 for pulmonary stenosis, 882
Ondine's curse. *See* Central alveolar hypoventilation
One-stage complete unifocalization/intracardiac repair, for pulmonary atresia with ventricular septal defect, MAPCAs and, 897–902, 897*f*, 898*f*, 899*f*, 900*f*, 901*f*, 902*f*, 903*f*
OPCAB. *See* Off-pump coronary artery bypass surgery
Open drainage procedure, for empyema, 284*f*
Open mitral commissurotomy, 351*f*
Open pulmonary valvotomy, for pulmonary stenosis, using cardiopulmonary bypass, 881–882
OPTN. *See* Organ Procurement and Transplantation Network
Organ preservation
 for heart transplantation, 581, 582*f*
 for heart-lung transplantation, 587–588, 588*f*, 588*t*

Organ procurement
 for heart-lung transplantation, 587–588, 588*f*, 588*t*
 for pediatric lung/heart-lung transplantation, 987
Organ Procurement and Transplantation Network (OPTN), 194
Orthotopic heart transplantation, 581–584
 alternative techniques for, 584, 584*f*
 implantation, 582–584, 583*f*
 operative preparation for recipient, 582
 for recipients with congenital anomalies, 584, 584*f*
 re-do sternotomy and, 584–585
Outflow graft-aortic anastomosis, sewing of, 507*f*
Outlet defects, 750, 751*f*

P

Paget-Schroetter syndrome. *See* Venous thrombosis of axillary-subclavian vein
PA/IS. *See* Pulmonary atresia with intact septum
Papillary fibroelastomas, 61
Papillary muscle-to-commissure fusion, pediatric mitral valve repair and, 1009
Papillary-annular continuity, in MVR, 387*f*
PAPVR. *See* Partial anomalous pulmonary venous return
Parachute mitral valve, pediatric mitral valve repair and, 1008–1009
Paraesophageal hernia
 with duodenum migration, 237*f*, 238*f*
 with gastroesophageal migration, 237*f*, 238*f*
 incidence of, 153
 laparoscopic reduction of, 154*f*
 symptoms of, 153
 treatment for, 153
 view of, 236*f*–237*f*
Paraesophageal hernia sac, excision of, 155*f*
Paravertebral fascia, tumor on, 290*f*
Parietal pleura, 93
Parietal pleurectomy, MPM and, multimodal approach to, 267*f*
Partial anomalous pulmonary venous return (PAPVR)
 definition of, 954
 diagnosis of, 955
 to high superior vena cava, 955, 956*f*
 to low superior vena cava/right atrium, 955
 pathologic anatomy of, 954
 pathophysiology of, 954–955
 results of, 956
 scimitar syndrome and, 954
 surgical management of, 955
Partial sternal-splitting incision, for thymectomy, 101–103, 102*f*, 103*f*
Partial vascular rings, 729–731

Patch aortoplasty, aortic coarctation and, 769, 771*f*
Patent ductus arteriosus (PDA), 716–720
 anatomic considerations of, 716
 diagnosis considerations for, 716
 division of, 730*f*
 operative technique for, 717–719, 717*f*, 719*f*, 720*f*
 perioperative patient management for, 716–717
 postoperative care for, 719–720
 procedure indications for, 716
 surgical complications for, 719–720
 thoracostomy incisions for, 717*f*
 VATS for, 716, 717*f*
Patient blood volume, in CPB, 313*t*
Patient evaluation, for carinal resection, 82
PDA. *See* Patent ductus arteriosus
PDT. *See* Photodynamic therapy
PE. *See* Pulmonary embolism
Pediatric abnormal aortic valve, pathology of, 1017–1021, 1018*f*
Pediatric annuloaortic dilation/ectasia, operative technique for, 1028–1029, 1028*f*, 1029*f*, 1030*f*
Pediatric annulus enlargement, operative technique for, 1027–1028, 1027*f*
Pediatric aortic valve repair, 1017–1022
 anatomy/function of, 1017, 1018*f*
 aortic valve stenosis and, 1017
 background on, 1017
 commissurotomy for, 1019
 dilated annulus techniques for, 1020–1021, 1020*f*, 1021*f*
 extended commissurotomy for, 1019–1020, 1019*f*
 restrictive/stenosis valve techniques for, 1019
 results for, 1021, 1022*f*
 surgical intervention timing for, 1019
 surgical valvuloplasty techniques for, 1019
 valve regurgitation and, 1018–1019
Pediatric aortic valve replacement, operative technique for, 1026–1027
Pediatric bilateral sequential lung transplantation, 988–990, 989*f*
Pediatric cardiac repair/lung transplantation, for pulmonary atresia, 990, 991*f*
Pediatric congenital pulmonary vein stenosis, 990
Pediatric heart transplantation, 973–982
 anatomic considerations for, 974
 background on, 973
 contraindications for, 973–974
 donor assessment/management for, 974
 heterotaxy syndromes and, 981–982, 982*f*
 hypoplastic left heart syndrome and, 975–977, 976*f*, 977*f*
 indications for, 973

operative techniques for, 975–982, 976*f*, 977*f*, 978*f*, 979*f*, 980*f*, 981*f*, 982*f*

post-transplant complications for, 974–975

bleeding as, 975

graft failure as, 974–975

rejection as, 975

situs inversus and, 980–981 , 981*f*

status post Fontan procedure and, 978–980 , 979*f*

transplant for congenitally corrected transposition of great arteries, 977–978, 978*f*

Pediatric heart-lung transplantation, 988

Pediatric lobar lung transplantation

donor lobectomy technique of, 991–995, 994*f*, 995*f*

recipient operation of, 994*f*, 995, 995*f*

Pediatric lung/heart-lung transplantation, 985–996

contraindications for, 986

donor selection for, 987

indications for, 985–986

operative procedure selection for, 986–987

organ procurement for, 987

postoperative management of, 995–996

recipient operation for, 987–988, 988*f*

rejection surveillance/management of, 996

results of, 996

Pediatric mitral valve repair, 1008–1015

accessory valve tissue and, 1008

according to functional classification, 1011–1012, 1011*f*, 1012*f*, 1013*f*, 1014*f*, 1015*f*

acquired mitral valve disease and, 1009

anatomy of, 1008

background on, 1008

bypass technique for, 1010–1011

cleft mitral valve and, 1008

congenital anomalies and, 1008

congenital mitral valves and, 1013–1014

echocardiography for, 1009–1010

embryology of, 1008

hammock valve and, 1009

indications for, 1009–1010

infective endocarditis and, 1009

introduction to, 1008

late outcomes for, 1014–1015

lesions with lack of valvular tissue and, 1008

papillary muscle-to-commissure fusion and, 1009

parachute mitral valve and, 1008–1009

pathology of, 1008

planning for, 1009–1010

regurgitant mitral valves, with congenital cardiac lesions and, 1009

results of, 1012–1015

rheumatic heart disease and, 1009

rheumatic mitral valves and, 1014–1015

supravalvular rings resection and, accessory mitral valve tissue, 1012

surgical technique for, 1010–1012, 1011*f*, 1012*f*, 1013*f*, 1014*f*, 1015*f*

type I malformation correction and, 1011, 1011*f*

type II malformation correction and, 1011, 1011*f*, 1012*f*, 1013*f*

type III malformation correction and, 1011–1012, 1014*f*, 1015*f*

valvular tags and, 1008

Pediatric mitral valve replacement, operative technique for, 1029–1030, 1031*f*

Pediatric pulmonary valve replacement, operative technique for, 1030–1032, 1032*f*

Pediatric single-lung transplantation, 989*f*, 990

Pediatric tricuspid valve replacement, operative technique for, 1032

Pediatric valve replacement, 1024–1032

background on, 1024

incidence of, 1024

operative technique for, 1025–1026, 1025*f*

Pedicle muscle flaps, chest wall resections and, for reconstruction, 226*f*

Penrose drains, for modified Heller myotomy, 166*f*

Peptic esophageal injury, 121

Percent postoperative predicted (popEV$_1$%), 54

Percent postoperative predicted diffusion capacity of lung for carbon monoxide (popDLCO%), 54

Pericardial effusions

diagnosis of, 258

etiology of, 254

pericardial procedures for, 255–258

Pericardial fat

pericardial patch and, 268

wrapped around anastomosis, 66*f*

Pericardial patch, pericardial fat and, 268

Pericardial patch reconstruction, in MVR, 387*f*

Pericardial procedures

introduction to, 254

for pericardial effusions, 255–258

Pericardial reconstruction, for MPM, 268–269

Pericardial suspensory ligaments in, MVST CABG, 470*f*

Pericardial tamponade, physiology of, 254

Pericardiectomy, 258–261

technique of, 258–259

via anterolateral thoracotomy, 260*f*

via bilateral thoracotomy, 260–261

via left anterior thoracotomy, 260

via median sternotomy, 259–260, 259*f*

pitfalls of, 261*t*

via thoracosternotomy, 260–261

Pericardiocentesis, 255

Pericardium, anatomy of, 254

Perimembranous defects, 750

Periosteum, electrocautery incision of, 217*f*

Perivalvular anatomic structures

left atrial appendage and, 402*f*

rendering prosthesis incompetent and, 402*f*

reoperative mitral replacement and, 401*f*

Perivalvular leak, MVR and, 389

PET scans. *See* Positron emission tomographic scans

PGD. *See* Primary graft dysfunction

Pharmacologic intervention, for neurologic injury prevention, 335

Phase-encoded velocity mapping, 676

Photodynamic therapy (PDT)

for esophageal cancer, 183

for MPM, 262

Phrenic nerve, diaphragm and, 230*f*

Pleura grasp, by endoscopic scissors, of posterior mediastinal tumor, 116*f*

Pleural effusion, MPM with

diagnosis for, 263–264

palliation for, 263–264

Pleural gases, 93

Pleural rind, MPM with, diagnosis for, 264

Pleural space, 93

anatomy, 93

physiology, 93

Pleural surfaces, anatomy of, 94*f*

Pleuroperitoneal shunt, for chylothorax, 248*f*

Pneumectomy, VATS and, 91

Pneumonectomy, 53–62. *See also specific* pneumonectomy

arrhythmias after, 59–62

bronchopleural fistula and, 61–62

chest closure after, 57*f*

chylothorax and, 60–61

complication management for, 58–59

empyema and, 61–62

history of, 53

indications for, 53–54

pulmonary embolism and, 61

surgical technique for, 54–58

types of, 53

vocal cord dysfunction and, 58–59

Pneumothorax

catamenial, 98–99

CXR for, 96

diagnosis of, 96

etiology of, 93–95, 95*t*

management of, 93–98

operative intervention for, 97*t*

operative management for, 97–98

pathophysiology of, 93–95, 95*t*

spontaneous, 94

treatment algorithm for, 96*f*

treatment for, 96–97, 96*t*

Polyethylene terephthalate cuffs, catheter placement with, 251*f*

Polypropylene mesh
   for diaphragm repair, 230
   for lateral chest wall resection, 225

Polypropylene mesh/methylmethacrylate prosthesis, for lateral chest wall resection, 224*f*

Polytetrafluoroethylene (PTFE), 225, 230
   for diaphragm repair, 230

popDLCO%. *See* Percent postoperative predicted diffusion capacity of lung for carbon monoxide

popEV₁%. *See* Percent postoperative predicted

Porous-diaphragm syndromes, 242–243

Port placement
   for laparoscopic Nissen fundoplication, 150*f*
   for posterior mediastinal tumor, resection of, 115*f*

Positron emission tomographic (PET) scans, 33, 54
   tumor staging and, 12

Posterior aortic arch, division of, 730*f*

Posterior leaflet
   preservation, of MVR, 382*f*
   prolapse, 357–361, 357*f*, 358*f*, 359*f*, 360*f*, 361*f*

Posterior mediastinal lesions
   postoperative considerations for, 120
   resection of, 113–120
      surgical principles of, 115
      surgical technique for, 115–118
   thoracoscopic resection of, 115–117

Posterior mediastinal neurogenic dumbbell tumor
   costotransversectomy and, 118*f*
   resection of, 118–120
   showing spinal cord compression, 114*f*
   single-stage approach, 119, 119*f*
   single-stage resection incision for, 117*f*
   surgical considerations for, 119–120

Posterior mediastinal neurogenic tumors, 113–115

Posterior mediastinal tumor
   pleura grasp by endoscopic scissors of, 116*f*
   resection of, port placement for, 115*f*

Posterior mediastinum, anatomy, 114*f*

Posterior rib aspect, grasping /freeing of, 215*f*

Posterior right aortic arch, completed division of, 731*f*

Posterior thoracotomy first-rib resection, with dorsal sympathectomy, for recurrent thoracic outlet syndrome, 215–217, 217*f*

Posterolateral approach, for superior sulcus tumor resection, 288

Posterolateral diaphragmatic hernia of Bochdalek, 231–233
   repair of, 235*f*

Posterolateral thoracotomy, 26, 27*f*
   landmarks for, 26
   lateral decubitus position for, 27*f*

Postoperative barium swallow status, after jejunal interposition, 181*f*

Postpneumonectomy bronchopleural fistula (BPF), 61

Postpneumonectomy empyema, 61–62

Postpneumonectomy pulmonary edema (PPE), 59–60

Postpneumonectomy syndrome, 62

Potts anastomosis
   takedown of, with PTFE patch, 701*f*
   view of, 700*f*

Potts shunt
   for congenital heart disease, 698–700, 700*f*, 700*t*, 701*f*
   takedown of, with digital occlusion, 701*f*

PPE. *See* Postpneumonectomy pulmonary edema

Preexisting aortic prosthesis
   annulus reconstruction and, 395–396
   removal of old prosthesis, 395
   reoperative mitral valve replacement and, 394–396, 395*f*, 396*f*

Pre-Fontan management, for single ventricle, 926

Pretracheal fascia
   incision of, 16*f*
   oblique view of, 18*f*

Pretracheal tunnel, identification of, 17*f*

Primary graft dysfunction (PGD), 194
   in lung transplantation, 201–203

Primary malignant cardiac neoplasms, 618, 618*f*

Primary revascularization, hypothermic ventricular fibrillation for, 450–452

Primary sternal tumor, with intended resection lines, 226*f*

Priming volume per tube length/diameter, in CPB, 313*t*

Primum ASD, congenital heart disease and, imaging children with, 653, 654*f*, 655*f*

"Prophylactic" aortic valve replacement, 420

Prosthesis removal, reoperative mitral valve replacement and, 397*f*

Prosthetic aortic valve, choice of, 415–416

Proximal anastomoses, OPCAB and, 462–463

Proximal esophageal isolation, for MIE, 160*f*

Proximal jejunal branches, in microvascular reconstruction, 179*f*

Pseudo-coarctation, acute type B aortic dissection and, 542*f*

PTE. *See* Chronic thromboendarterectomy; Pulmonary thromboembolism

PTFE. *See* Polytetrafluoroethylene

Pulmonary arteries, 647–648. *See also specific* pulmonary arteries
   anterior aspect of fissure, 49*f*
   anterior segmental branch of, 48*f*
   cardiac magnetic resonance imaging of, 667–669, 668*f*
   coronary artery anomalies from, 959–961, 960*f*, 960*t*, 961*f*
   identification of, 43*f*
   normal development of, 726*f*
   retraction of, 49*f*
      lower love bronchus and, 51*f*
   view of, 39*f*

Pulmonary artery anastomosis, 200*f*
   during lung transplantation, 200*f*

Pulmonary artery band
   for congenital heart disease, 700–704, 701*t*
   intraluminal technique of, 705*f*
   placement of, 702*f*
   sequential tightening of, 703*f*
   takedown of
      with PTFE patch, 703*f*
      with pulmonary artery transaction, 704*f*

Pulmonary artery sling, 731–733
   anatomy of, 731
   classification of, 728*t*
   clinical presentation of, 731
   diagnosis of, 731
   surgical anatomy of, 736*f*
   surgical indications for, 731
   surgical technique for, 732–733, 736*f*, 737*f*
   tracheal anastomosis for, 737*f*
   tracheal resection for, 736*f*

Pulmonary atresia with intact septum (PA/IS), 882–892
   anatomic considerations for, 883
   definitive surgical treatment for, 885–892, 886*f*, 886*t*, 887*f*, 888*f*, 890*f*, 891*f*
      adjustable atrial septal defect and, 886, 886*f*
      aorta-to-right ventricle shunt, 891
      bidirectional cavopulmonary Glenn shunt, 888–889
      enlargement of right ventricular cavity and, 886
      extracardiac Fontan with adjustable fenestration, 890–891
      lateral tunnel Fontan with adjustable atrial septal defect, 889–890, 890*f*, 891*f*
      with mild right ventricular hypoplasia, 885–886
      moderate right ventricular hypoplasia, 887

severe right ventricular hypoplasia, 888–892, 888f, 890f, 891f
tissue valve insertion and, 887
transannular pericardial patch with monocusp valve, 887–888, 887f
diagnostic considerations for, 882–883
Fontan procedure
postoperative care for, 891–892
surgical complications after, 891–892
incidence of, 882
initial surgical treatment for, 883–885, 884t, 885f
for neonates, 883–885
surgical results after, 892
Pulmonary atresia with ventricular septal defect, MAPCAs and, 895–904
aortopulmonary window for, 896f
closure criteria of ventricular septal defect of, 902
follow-up management for, 902–904
one-stage complete unifocalization/intracardiac repair for, 897–902, 897f, 898f, 899f, 900f, 901f, 902f, 903f
postoperative care for, 902–904
therapeutic goals of, 895–896
Pulmonary autograft replacement, 424
in aortic annular dilation, 431, 431f
proximal sutures of, 432f
Pulmonary embolism (PE), 626
pneumonectomy and, 61
Pulmonary mycobacterium disease
CT for, 295
diagnostic considerations for, 295–296
operative technique for, 297–299
perioperative management for, 296
postoperative care for, 299
surgery of, 295–300
surgical complications for, 299
surgical indications for, 295–296
Pulmonary rehabilitation, 206
Pulmonary resections, 71–75. See also specific pulmonary resections
history of, 33
introduction to, 33–36
postoperative mortality/morbidity of, 44–45
right-sided, 33–45
of superior sulcus tumor, 290
superior sulcus tumor resection and, 293
Pulmonary stenosis, 881–882
diagnostic considerations for, 881
incidence of, 881
off-pump transventricular pulmonary valvotomy for, 882
open pulmonary valvotomy, using cardiopulmonary bypass for, 881–882
perioperative management for, 882

postoperative care for, 882
subaortic ventricular septal defect with, DORV repair, 844–845, 844f
surgical complications for, 882
surgical techniques for, 881–882
surgical treatment for, 881
Pulmonary thromboembolism (PTE), 61
Pulmonary valve, 647
hemodynamic assessment of, 681
Pulmonary valve replacement, pediatric, operative technique for, 1030–1032, 1032f
Pulmonary vascular resistance, VSDs and, 752
Pulmonary veins
cardiac magnetic resonance imaging of, 673–674
systemic venous connection to, 713
Pulmonic valve stenosis/atresia, congenital heart disease and, 682–683
Pump failure
clinical presentation of, 520
diagnosis of, 520
incidence of, 519–520
myocardial infarction complications and, 519–522
natural history of, 520
operative technique of, 521–522, 521f, 522f
operative timing of, 520
pathogenesis of, 519–520
preoperative treatment of, 520
survival of, 521–522
Pyloric drainage, procedure for, 181
Pyridostigmine, corticosteroids for, 107

R
Radiation, for esophageal cancer, 182
RAO. See Right anterior oblique view
Rastelli operation, on TGA, 864–867, 864f, 865f, 866f, 867f, 868f, 869f, 870f, 871f
Receiver operating characteristic (ROC) curve, 328
Recurrent aspiration/dysphagia, barium swallow study for, 142f
Recurrent atrial fibrillation, after Cox Maze procedure, 604–605
Recurrent laryngeal nerve injury, 59
Recurrent primary spontaneous pneumothoraces, apical resection for, of subpleural bleb, 95f
Recurrent thoracic outlet syndrome, dorsal sympathectomy, posterior thoracotomy first-rib resection with, 215–217, 217f
Re-do median sternotomy technique, for reoperative mitral valve replacement, 392
Re-do sternotomy, orthotopic heart transplantation and, 584–585

Regurgitant mitral valves, with congenital cardiac lesions, pediatric mitral valve repair and, 1009
Renal cell carcinomas, 619, 619f
Renal dysfunction, from CABG, 446
Reoperative mitral valve replacement, 391–402
annuloplasty ring removal and, 397f
annulus patch repair and, 398f
annulus primary repair and, 398f
anterolateral thoracotomy technique for, 391–392, 392f
atriotomy choice for, 393–394, 394f
cardiopulmonary bypass institution for, 393
choice of approach for, 391
closure for, 401–402
de-airing left ventricle and, 401f
incision site for, 392f
myocardial protection for, 393
perivalvular anatomic structures and, 401f
preexisting aortic prosthesis and, 394–396, 395f, 396f
prosthesis removal and, 397f
re-do median sternotomy technique for, 392
transatrial oblique atriotomy and, 395f
trans-septal atriotomy and, 395f
valve implantation and, 396–401, 399f
Reoperative revascularization, hypothermic ventricular fibrillation for, 452
Reperfusion, in lung transplantation, 200–201
Resection of third rib, mobilized latissimus dorsi muscle with, 298f
Residual ischemic mitral regurgitation, 374
Residual volume (RV), 34
Resistance calculation, 680
Retransplantation, heart-lung transplantation and, 593–594
Retroaortic innominate vein, 711
Retrograde cannulas
for cardioplegia, 318–319, 320f
introduction method for, 321f
Reverse elephant trunk technique, for arch aneurysms, 563, 564f
Rhabdomyoma, 617
Rheumatic heart disease, pediatric mitral valve repair and, 1009
Rheumatic mitral valve repair, 350
pediatric, 1014–1015
Right anterior oblique view (RAO), 479
Right aortic arch, with retroesophageal ligament, 727–728
Right hemithorax, mediastinal lymph node dissection and, 274–275, 274f, 275f, 276f, 277f
Right inferior pulmonary vein, view of, 56f
Right lower lobectomy, 42–44, 42f, 43f, 44f
Right mainstem bronchi, intercostal muscle on, 55f

Right mainstem bronchus intermedius, during right upper lobe sleeve, 66f

Right middle lobectomy, 40–41, 41f, 42f

Right pulmonary hilum, view of, 35f

Right superior caval veins
    azygos continuation of, 711–712, 712f
    to left pulmonary atrium, 711, 711f

Right thoracotomy, 143–144
    esophagectomy incisions for, 145f
    vascular rings requiring, 728

Right transcervical incision, superior sulcus tumor resection and, 292f

Right upper lobe bronchus
    division of, 40f
    tumor in, 65

Right upper lobe sleeve, for left-sided endotracheal tube, 65f

Right upper lobectomy, 36–40, 37f, 38f, 39f, 40f
    sleeve resection, 65–66

Right ventricular assist devices (RVADs), 500

Right-sided pneumonectomy, surgical technique for, 54–57

Right-sided pulmonary resections, 33–45
    introduction to, 36
    surgical technique for, 36–45, 37f, 38f, 39f, 40f, 41f, 42f, 43f, 44f, 45f

Right-to-left shunt lesion, hemodynamic assessment, of patients, 680

Robotic arms, 367f

Robotic coronary artery bypass surgery, 466–475
    robotic technology for, 467

Robotic mitral valve surgery, 355–356
    anesthesia for, 355
    clinical outcomes of, 366–367
    exclusion criteria for, 355t
    future directions for, 367
    intraoperative times for, 368f
    limitations of, 367
    monitoring for, 355
    operative field for, 356f
    operative techniques for, 355–356
    procedures for, 356t

Robotic posterior leaflet resection, 357f

Robotic technology, for mitral valve repair, 353–368

ROC curve. See Receiver operating characteristic curve

Root replacement, Ross procedure and, 429–430, 430f, 431f

Ross procedure, 1024–1032
    actuarial freedom from late death, 433f
    for aortic valve replacement, 424–433
    contraindications for, 424
    current thoughts on, 431–433
    inclusion cylinder and, 425–429
    indications for, 424
    operative technique for, 424–430, 425f, 426f, 427f, 428f, 429f, 430f

root replacement, 429–430, 430f, 431f
    surgical results of, 431–433

RV. See Residual volume

RVADs. See Right ventricular assist devices

S

Safe circulatory arrest times, hypothermia level and, 314t

SAM. See Systolic anterior motion

SARS. See Severe acute respiratory syndrome

Scalene biopsy, 23–24
    complications of, 24
    indications for, 23
    surgical technique for, 23–24, 24f

Scimitar syndrome
    PAPVR and, 953, 954
    surgical repair of, 747

Scleroderma
    definition of, 172
    diagnosis of, 172
    etiology of, 172
    surgical options for, 172f
    surgical results for, 172
    treatment for, 172

SCT. See Single-clamp technique

Secundum ASD, congenital heart disease and, imaging children with, 653

Secundum-type atrial septal defects
    Amplatzer repair of, 743, 743f
    surgical repair of, 742–743, 742f, 743f

Sedation, conscious, 7t

Segmental valve analysis, for type IIIb, ischemic mitral regurgitation, 372

Segmentectomy, 72–74
    view of, 73f

Semidorsal/semiventral incision view, of superior sulcus tumor resection, 291f

Semilunar valve stenosis, hemodynamic assessment of, or insufficiency, 681

Senning plus Rastelli operation, for ccTGA, 876

Septostomy procedures, for congenital heart disease, 682, 682f

Severe acute respiratory syndrome (SARS), 95

Severe right ventricular hypoplasia, initial neonatal procedures for, 883–884

Shaded surface display (SSD), 660–661

Short-segment small bowel transposition, 181

Shunt calculation, 680

Silastic occluders, in TECAB, 473f

Simple aortopulmonary window, operative technique for, 760–763, 761f, 762f, 763f

Simultaneous antegrade/retrograde cardioplegic perfusion, delivery/monitoring of, 322

Single venous cannulation, 310f

Single ventricle

anatomy of, 925–926
    interrupted aortic arch with, 784–785, 785f, 786f
    pre-Fontan management for, 926
    tricuspid atresia and, 925–933

Single-clamp technique (SCT), 334

Single-lung transplants (SLT), 194
    pediatric, 989f, 990

Single-stage approach, to neurogenic dumbbell tumor resection, 117f, 118f, 119

Single-ventricle repair, for Ebstein's anomaly, 1004, 1004f, 1005f

Sinus venous ASD, congenital heart disease and, imaging children with, 654–655, 655f, 656f, 657f, 658f

Situs inversus, pediatric heart transplantation and, 980–981, 981f

Sleeve lobectomy, 64

Sleeve resection, 53. See also specific sleeve resection

SLT. See Single-lung transplants

Small aortic annulus, 421–422, 422f

Small bowel transposition, short-segment, 181

Society of Thoracic Surgeons (STS) database
    Adult Cardiac Surgery database, 330
    Congenital Cardiac Surgery database, 330
    database, 326, 330, 330t
    General Thoracic Surgery database, 330–331

Somatostatin, for chylothorax, 246, 247t

Spinal cord compression, neurogenic dumbbell tumor showing, 114f

Spinal cord preservation, thoracic/thoracoabdominal aneurysms and, 549–551

Spontaneous pneumothorax, 94

SSD. See Shaded surface display

SSFP. See Steady-state free-precession

Staging. See Tumor staging

Stapler placement, incisions for, 90t

Starnes procedure. See Single-ventricle repair

Status post Fontan procedure, pediatric heart transplantation and, 978–980, 979f

Steady-state free-precession (SSFP), 660

Stellate ganglion, dorsal sympathetic chain and, in transaxillary approach, 216f

Sternal resections
    for chest wall resections, 225–227, 226f, 227f
    reconstruction of, 227f
    technique for, 226–227

Sternotomy. See also Thymectomy
    anterior mediastinotomy and, 20
    median, 28–29, 28f
    thymectomy via, 100–106

Sternum
    elevation, using Bugge retractor, 207*f*
    retraction of, 103*f*
Streptokinase, for empyema, 281–284
Structural valve deterioration (SVD), 417*f*
STS database. *See* Society of Thoracic
        Surgeons (STS) database
Subaortic ventricular septal defect
    DORV repair, with pulmonary stenosis,
        844–845, 844*f*
    double-outlet right ventricles and, 841
    tunnel repair of, DORV, 842–844, 842*f*,
        843*f*
Subclavian artery dissection
    superior sulcus tumor resection and, 291
    from tumor, 290*f*
Subclavian artery division, superior sulcus
        tumor resection and, 292*f*
Subclavian flap repair, for aortic
        coarctation, 769, 770*f*
Subclavian vein dissection, superior sulcus
        tumor resection and, 291
Subclavian vessel dissection, for superior
        sulcus tumor resection, 289– 290,
        289*f*, 290*f*
Sublobar pulmonary resections, 71
Subpleural bleb, of recurrent primary
        spontaneous pneumothoraces,
        apical resection for, 95*f*
Subpulmonary obstruction repair, for
        ccTGA, 875–876, 876*f*
Subpulmonary ventricular septal defect
    DORV with, anatomic repair of, 845,
        846*f*
    double-outlet right ventricles and,
        841
Subxiphoid pericardial window, 255–256,
        256*f*
    pitfalls of, 256*t*
Superior caval system, aneurysmal dilation
        of, 711
Superior caval veins (SVCs)
    anomalies of, 708–711
    isolated left, 709–710
    left, 708
Superior mediastinum, 17
Superior pulmonary arterial branch,
        dissection of, 73*f*
Superior pulmonary artery, left pulmonary
        artery and, 199*f*
Superior sulcus tumor
    perinduction MRI of, 287*f*
    pulmonary resection of, 290
    resection, 286–294
        anatomical considerations for, 286,
            287*f*
        anterior approaches for, 290–293
        anterior scalene muscle insertion and,
            292*f*
        brachial plexus dissection for, 289,
            290*f*, 292
        chest wall closure and, 293

chest wall resections for, 288–289,
            289*f*, 293
        clinical considerations for, 286
        diagnostic considerations for, 286–287
        hemiclamshell incision and, 293,
            293*f*
        indications for, 287
        investigations for, 287–288
        Masaoka incision and, 293, 293*f*
        operative technique for, 288–293,
            288*f*, 289*f*, 290*f*, 291, 292*f*, 293
        perioperative patient management for,
            288
        posterolateral approach of, 288, 288*f*
        postoperative care and, 293
        postoperative complications and, 293
        pulmonary resection and, 293
        right transcervical incision and, 292*f*
        semidorsal/semiventral incision view
            of, 291*f*
        subclavian artery dissection and, 291
        subclavian artery division and, 292*f*
        subclavian vein dissection and, 291
        subclavian vessel dissection for,
            289–290, 289*f*, 290*f*
        transclavicular approach to, 290–293
        vertebral body resection for, 290, 291*f*
Superior-type sinus venous atrial septal
        defect, surgical repair of, 743–745,
        744*f*, 745*f*
Supravalvar aortic stenosis, 795–796, 797*f*,
        798*f*, 799*f*
Supraventricular tachycardia (SVT), 59
Surgical ventricular reconstruction (SVR),
        479
SVCs. *See* Superior caval veins
SVD. *See* Structural valve deterioration
SVR. *See* Surgical ventricular
        reconstruction
SVT. *See* Supraventricular tachycardia
Sympathetic chain
    division of, 216*f*
    exposure of, 218*f*
Synthetic material choices, for chest wall
        resections, 225
Systemic inflammatory state, minimizing,
        332–333
Systemic pulmonary veins, congenital
        heart disease and, 687
Systemic vascular resistance, myocardial
        protection during, beating heart,
        325*f*
Systemic veins, cardiac magnetic resonance
        imaging of, 673
Systemic venous atrium, bilateral superior
        caval veins drainage to, 708–709
Systemic venous connection
    to pulmonary veins, 713
    total anomalous, 713
Systemic venous drainage
    anomalies of, 708–714
    background on, 708

Systolic anterior motion (SAM), 345

T
Table-mounted retractor, for transhiatal
        esophagectomy, 133*f*
Tachycardia-induced cardiomyopathy, 603,
        603*t*
Takeuchi repair, modified, for coronary
        artery anomalies, 963–964, 963*f*,
        964*f*, 965*f*
Tangential grafting, method of, 324*f*
TAPVR. *See* Total anomalous pulmonary
        venous return
Target vessel exposure in, MVST CABG,
        470
TB. *See* Tuberculosis
TCD. *See* Transcranial Doppler
TCT. *See* Transcervical thymectomy
TECAB. *See* Totally endoscopic coronary
        artery bypass
TEE. *See* Transesophageal
        echocardiography
Temperature management, neurologic
        injury prevention and, 334
Tetralogy of Fallot, 907–914
    with absent pulmonary valve,
        911–912
    anomalous coronary artery course and,
        911
    AVSDs with, 820
    background on, 907
    cannulation for, 908*f*
    incidence of, 907
    intervention timing for, 907–908
    late complications for, 913–914
    operative strategy for, 907–908
    operative technique for, 908–910, 908*f*,
        909*f*, 910*f*, 911*f*
    postoperative care for, 912–913
    severe pulmonary insufficiency and,
        910–911, 912*f*, 913*f*
    special circumstances of, 908, 909*f*, 910,
        910*f*, 911*f*
    surgical complications for, 912–913
TGA. *See* Transposition of great arteries
Thoracic diverticula, 190–193
    clinical presentation of, 190
    diagnosis of, 190–191
    esophageal mobilization for, 192*f*
    esophageal rotation for, 192*f*
    postoperative care for, 192–193, 193*f*
    surgical complications for, 192
    surgical indications for, 191, 191*f*
    surgical procedure for, 191–192, 192*f*
Thoracic duct
    anatomy of, 244–245, 245*f*
    mediastinal structures and, 246*f*
    physiology of, 245
    thoracoscopic approach to, 248*f*
Thoracic esophageal mobilization, MIE
        and, 158*f*
Thoracic incisions, 26–32

Thoracic outlet syndromes, 213–219
  surgical complications for, 218–219
  surgical principles for, 213–214
  surgical results for, 218–219
  surgical technique for, 214–217, 214*f*,
    215*f*, 216*f*, 217*f*
  surgical therapy indications for, 213
Thoracic/thoracoabdominal aneurysms,
    545–555
  anatomic considerations, 545
  anesthesia/monitoring for, 547
  aortic graft selection and, 551–553, 551*f*,
    552*f*, 553*f*, 554*f*
  Crawford classification of, 546*f*
  diagnostic considerations of, 545–547
  hemodynamic instability control, during
    aortic cross-clamping, 548–551
  incision/operative exposure in, 547–548
  operation completion for, 553
  operative procedure for, 547–553, 549*f*,
    550*f*, 551*f*, 552*f*, 553*f*
  spinal cord preservation and, 549–551
  surgical results for, 553–554
Thoracoabdominal incision, 31–32, 31*f*
Thoracoscopic esophagomyotomy, 165
Thoracoscopic long myotomy, for DES, 171
Thoracoscopic pericardial window,
    256–258, 257*f*
  pitfalls of, 258*t*
Thoracoscopic port placement, for MIE,
    157*f*
Thoracosternotomy, 29–30
  incision for, 30*f*
  pericardiectomy via, 260–261
Thoracostomy, incision for, patent ductus
    arteriosus, 717*f*
Thoracotomy
  anterior, 28, 28*f*
  for chylothorax, 247*f*
  left, 144–145
    esophagectomy incisions for, 145*f*
  for lung cancer, morbidity/mortality
    reduction for, 34*t*
  posterolateral, 26, 27*f*
  right, 143–144
    esophagectomy incisions for, 145*f*
Thymectomy, 100–106
  dissection in, 103*f*
  full median sternotomy incision for, 103,
    105*f*
  hemostasis and, 105*f*
  introduction to, 107–108
  MG and, 100
  operative technique for, 101–103, 102*f*,
    103*f*
  partial sternal-splitting incision for,
    101–103, 102*f*, 103*f*
  postoperative recovery of, 103–104
  preoperative preparation for, 101
  surgical approaches to, 100
  surgical results of, 104–105, 104–106
  transcervical, 107–111

via full median sternotomy, 105*f*
  via sternotomy, 100–106
  walking technique in, 102
Thymoma, survival of, 105
Thymus gland
  inferior/superior horns of, 104*f*
  view of, 101*f*
Thymus horns, retraction of, 104*f*
Tissue transfer options, for chest wall
    resections, 225, 225*t*
Tissue/blood-tagging imaging, with cardiac
    magnetic resonance imaging, 666*f*
TLC. *See* Total lung capacity
TNM groups, postoperative survival by, 36*t*
TNM staging system, 11
  for lung cancer, 12*t*
  revisions to, for lung cancer, 13*t*
Total anomalous pulmonary venous return
    (TAPVR)
  anatomic defects of, 947–948, 949*f*, 950*t*
  angiocardiography for, 950–951
  cardiac catheterization for, 950–951
  chest X-ray for, 949–950
  classification of, 947–948
  diagnosis of, 949–950
  echocardiography for, 950
  embryology of, 947, 948*f*
  extracorporeal circulation management
    for, 951–952
    cardiac type, 951–952, 953*f*
    infracardiac type, 952, 953*f*
    mixed type, 952, 953*f*
    supracardiac type, 951, 952*f*
  frequency distribution of types, 950*t*
  historical aspects of, 947
  pathophysiology of, 948–949, 949*f*, 950*f*
  postoperative management for, 952–954,
    953*f*
  preoperative management for, 951
  results for, 954
  signs/symptoms of, 949
  surgical intervention timing for, 951
  surgical technique for, 951–952, 952*f*,
    953*f*
Total anomalous systemic venous
    connection, 713
Total arch technique, for arch aneurysms,
    559–560, 560*f*, 561*f*
Total lung capacity (TLC), 34
Totally endoscopic coronary artery bypass
    (TECAB), 467
  silastic occluders in, 473*f*
Toupet fundoplication, suture rows for,
    125*f*
Trabecular defects, 751
Trachea
  anatomy of, 76
  bronchoscopic view of, 4*f*
Tracheal anastomosis, for pulmonary artery
    sling, 737*f*
Tracheal compression, anomalous
    innominate artery with, 729–731

Tracheal lesions
  clinical presentation of, 77
  diagnostic studies of, 77
  etiology of, 76–77
  surgical indications for, 77
  surgical technique for, 77–79, 78*f*
  treatment options for, 77
Tracheal reconstruction
  anastomotic complications of, 80, 80*t*
  operative procedures for, 79*t*
  patient characteristics, 79*t*
  postoperative management of, 79
  procedure for, 78*f*
  resection and, 76–80
  results of, 79, 80*t*
Tracheal resection
  anastomotic complications of, 80, 80*t*
  deaths and, 80
  hemorrhage and, 80
  infection and, 80
  laryngeal dysfunction and, 80
  operative procedures for, 79*t*
  patient characteristics, 79*t*
  postoperative management for, 79
  for pulmonary artery sling, 736*f*
  reconstruction and, 76–80
  results of, 79, 80*t*
Tracheobronchial angle, exposure of, 50*f*
Tracheobronchial tree, 3–4, 5*f*
Transabdominal partial fundoplication,
    124–125, 125*f*
Transabdominal total fundoplication,
    123–125, 124*f*
Transatrial closure, of VSDs, 754*f*
Transatrial oblique atriotomy, reoperative
    mitral valve replacement and,
    395*f*
Transaxillary approach, dorsal sympathetic
    chain, stellate ganglion and, 216*f*
Transaxillary first-rib resection, with dorsal
    sympathectomy, 214–215, 214*f*,
    215*f*, 216*f*
Transcarinal aspiration, anterior
    mediastinotomy and, 22*f*
Transcatheter therapy
  for congenital heart disease, 681–690
  hemodynamic assessment and, for
    congenital heart disease, 679–691
Transcervical thymectomy (TCT),
    107–111
  clamp placement in, 111*f*
  ligature placement in, 110*f*
  preoperative preparation for, 108
  sternum separation in, 110*f*
  surgical results of, 111
  surgical technique for, 108–111, 109*f*,
    110*f*, 111*f*
  tie on gland in, 109*f*
  view of, 109*f*
Transclavicular approach, 31, 31*f*
Transcranial Doppler (TCD), 335
Transcuspid leaflets, 754*f*

Transdiaphragmatic fenestration, diaphragmatic surface and, 95*f*

Transesophageal echocardiography (TEE), 197, 334, 682*f*

Transhiatal esophagectomy, 131–137
    abdominal phase of, 131–132
    blind/blunt mobilization in, 134*f*
    cervical phase of, 132–135
    introduction to, 131
    operative technique for, 131–135
    patient position for, 132*f*
    postoperative care for, 135–136
    postoperative complications for, 136–137, 136*t*
    preoperative assessment for, 131
    preparation for, 131
    results of, 137
    table-mounted retractor for, 133*f*
    umbilical tape pulling, for cephalad movement in, 135*f*

Transillumination branching, within jejunal mesentery, 179*f*

Transplant for congenitally corrected transposition of great arteries, pediatric heart transplantation and, 977–978, 978*f*

Transposition of great arteries (TGA), 779, 855–871
    anatomy of, 855–856, 856*f*
    arterial repair and, 857*f*, 858*f*, 859*f*, 860–864, 860*f*, 861*f*, 862*f*, 863*f*
    atrial repair, 860
    background on, 855
    clinical features of, 857
    interrupted aortic arch with, 784, 786*f*
    management of, 857–858
    operative intervention of, 857*f*, 859–860
    palliative operations of, 859–860
    pathophysiology of, 856–857
    Rastelli operation on, 864–867, 864*f*, 865*f*, 866*f*, 867*f*, 868*f*, 869*f*, 870*f*, 871*f*
    surgical correction for, 857*f*, 858*f*, 859*f*, 860–867, 860*f*, 861*f*, 862*f*, 863*f*, 864*f*
    surgical repair history of, 858–859
    surgical repair results of, 867–871

Transpulmonary closure, of conal septal defect, 755*f*

Trans-septal atriotomy, reoperative mitral valve replacement and, 395*f*

Transthoracic coronary stabilizer, positioning of, 472*f*

Transthoracic dorsal sympathectomy, 217

Transthoracic esophageal resection/reconstruction
    principles of, 140–142, 144*f*, 145*f*
    surgical technique for, 142–146, 144*f*, 145*f*

Transthoracic partial fundoplication, 126, 127*f*, 128*f*

Transthoracic total fundoplication, 125–126, 126*f*

Transventricular closure, of conoventricular defect, 755*f*

Tricuspid atresia, single ventricle and, 925–933

Tricuspid regurgitation
    evaluation/operative indications for, 403–406
    functional, 403–404

Tricuspid valve, 403–409, 645, 646*f*
    anatomy of, 404– 405, 405*f*
    annuloplasty, 407*f*
    carcinoid heart disease and, 404
    Ebstein's anomaly of, 404, 405*f*
    endocarditis and, 404
    hemodynamic assessment of, 681
    introduction to, 403
    operative setup for, 405– 406, 406*f*
    repair, for Ebstein's anomaly, 407*f*, 408, 408*f*
    replacement, 406–408, 407*f*

Tricuspid valve replacement, pediatric, operative technique for, 1032

Trocar port positions, for laparoscopic esophagomyotomy, 164*f*

Truncal valve repair/replacement, truncus arteriosus with, 835–838, 837*f*, 838*f*, 839*f*

Truncus arteriosus, 827–839
    alternative repair of, 832, 833*f*, 834*f*
    background on, 827
    classification for, 827, 828*t*
    diagnosis of, 828
    interrupted aortic arch with, 783–784, 784*f*, 785*f*
    pathophysiology of, 827–828
    postoperative care for, 838
    repair of, with interrupted aortic arch, 832–838, 835*f*, 836*f*
    surgical indications for, 828
    surgical repair of, 828–832, 828*f*, 829*f*, 830*f*, 831*f*, 832*f*
    surgical results for, 838
    surgical technique for, 828–838, 828*f*, 829*f*, 830*f*, 831*f*, 832*f*, 833*f*, 834*f*, 835*f*, 836*f*, 838*f*, 839*f*
    truncal valve repair/replacement with, 835–838, 837*f*, 838*f*, 839*f*
    van Praagh classification, 828*t*

Tube graft placement, 551–552, 552*f*

Tuberculosis (TB), incidence of, 295

Tumor(s). *See also specific* cancers; *specific* neoplasms; *specific* tumors
    cardiac, 615–619
    of diaphragm, 242
    on paravertebral fascia, 290*f*
    primary, 11–12
    subclavian artery dissection from, 290*f*

Tumor staging
    CT and, 11, 12*t*
    MRI and, 11

PET scans and, 12
    process of, 11
    system, 11

Tunnel repair, of DORV, with subaortic ventricular septal defect, 842–844, 842*f*, 843*f*

Two-ventricle repair, for Ebstein's anomaly, 1002–1004, 1003*f*, 1004*f*

U

Ultrasound frequencies, ultrasound physics/applications and, 651

Ultrasound physics/applications
    Doppler principle and, 651–652
    modified Bernoulli theorem and, 652
    principles of, 651–652
    ultrasound frequencies and, 651

Undersized remodeling ring annuloplasty, for type IIIb, ischemic mitral regurgitation, 374

Unidirectional cavopulmonary shunts, 918–919, 918*f*, 919*f*

Urschel rongeur, first rib removal with, 216*f*

V

VA database. *See* Veterans Affairs database

VADs. *See* Ventricular assist devices

Vagal-sparing esophagectomy, with colon interposition, 175*f*

Vagal-sparing gastric mobilization, 176*f*

Vagal-sparing gastric pull-up, 174–176, 175*f*, 176*f*
    advantages/disadvantages, 176

Valsalva sinus aneurysm, 804–806
    clinical presentation of, 804–805, 805*f*
    morphologic considerations of, 804
    surgical indications for, 805, 806*f*
    surgical results for, 805–806
    surgical technique for, 805, 806*f*

Valvar aortic stenosis
    in neonate/infant, 789–790, 790*f*
    in older child, 790–792, 791*f*

Valve implantation, reoperative mitral valve replacement and, 396–401, 398*f*, 399*f*, 400*f*

Valve regurgitation, pediatric aortic valve repair and, 1018–1019

Valve replacement, pediatric, 1024–1032

Valvular tags, pediatric mitral valve repair and, 1008

Van Praagh classification, for truncus arteriosus, 828*t*

Vascular connections, closure procedures for, 687–690, 689*f*, 690*f*

Vascular rings
    classification of, 728*t*
    complete, 722–729
        anatomy of, 722–729
        embryonic development of, 724*f*–725*f*
    partial, 729–731

Vascular rings (*Contd.*)
   requiring median sternotomy, 728–729
   requiring right thoracotomy, 728
   requiring surgery, 724f–725f
VATS. *See* Video-assisted thoracic surgery
Velocity mapping, with cardiac magnetic
   resonance imaging, 664f
Venae cavae, 644
Venous connections
   cardiac magnetic resonance imaging and,
     preoperative/postoperative,
     671–674, 673f
   congenital heart disease and, imaging
     children with, 657–658
Venous embryology, schematic of, 709f
Venous sinus valves, anomalies of,
   713–714, 713f
Venous thrombosis of axillary-subclavian
   vein, 217–219
Ventricular assist devices (VADs), 500–509
   background on, 500–501
   economic considerations for, 502–503
   heart transplantation after, 585
   patient selection for, 501–502
   perioperative period for, 508t
   postoperative care for, 507–509, 508t
   potential complications for, 507–508
   preoperative evaluation for, 501–502
   surgical procedure for, 503–507, 503f,
     504f, 505f, 506f, 507f
   types of, 501t
Ventricular septal defects (VSDs), 750–757
   aortic coarctation and, 775–776
   background on, 750
   cardiac/noncardiac pathologic
     conditions associated with, 752
   characteristics of, 751–752
   classification of, 750–751
   clinical presentation of, 512
   closure, for ccTGA, 875
   common incisions for, 754f
   diagnosis of, 512
   incidence of, 512
   Infundibular septum and, 784f
   myocardial infarction complications,
     512–515

natural history of, 512
operative technique for, 513–515, 513f,
   514f, 515f, 516f, 517, 518f
operative timing of, 512–513
pathogenesis of, 512
patient characteristics of, 752
preoperative therapy of, 512–513
pulmonary vascular resistance and, 752
repair technique for, 752–756, 753f,
   754f, 755f
surgical indications for, 751–752
surgical results for, 756–757
survival of, 515
transatrial closure of, 754f
view of, 782f
Ventricular septum, 645–647, 647f
Ventricular tachycardia (VT), 59
Ventricular thinning/necrosis, left
   ventricular reconstruction and, 480f
Ventriculoarterial alignments, 645f
Vertebral body resection
   of superior sulcus tumor, 290
   for superior sulcus tumor resection, 290,
     291f
Veterans Affairs (VA) database, 326, 327,
   329–330, 329t
Vicryl suture, 79
Video-assisted bilateral thoracoscopic lung
   volume reduction surgery, 208
Video-assisted mitral valve repairs, with
   AESOP, 366
Video-assisted thoracic surgery (VATS), 27,
   54
   advantages of, 88
   bleeding risk during, 88
   history of, 88
   incisions for, 89–90
   lobectomy, 88
   lobectomy with, 90–91
   oncologic issues with, 88
   for patent ductus arteriosus, 716, 717f
   pneumectomy and, 91
   wedge resection with, 75
Video-assisted thoracoscopic pulmonary
   resections, 88–91
   contraindications for, 88–89, 89t

indications for, 88–89
morbidity/mortality after, 91
operative technique for, 89–91
outcomes of, 91
preoperative evaluation for, 89
survival from, 91
wedge resection with, 90
Videothoracoscopic esophagomyotomy,
   166f
Vigorous achalasia, 170
Vocal cord dysfunction, pneumonectomy
   and, 58–59
Volume-rendered object (VRT), 661, 662f
VRT. *See* Volume-rendered object
VSDs. *See* Ventricular septal defects
VT. *See* Ventricular tachycardia

W

Walking technique, in thymectomy, 102
Warm blood cardioplegia
   for myocardial protection, 315
   solution contents for, 318t
Waterston anastomosis
   construction of, 699f
   preparation for, 698f
   takedown of, with cardiopulmonary
     bypass/PTFE patch, 699f
Waterston/Cooley shunt, for congenital
   heart disease, 697–698, 698f, 698t,
   699f
Wedge resection
   of apical blebs, 98f
   using linear stapler, 74f
   with VATS, 75
   with video-assisted thoracoscopic
     pulmonary resections, 90
Weitlander retractor, 90

Z

Zenker's diverticulum, 187–190
   barium esophagram of, 188f
   clinical presentation of, 187
   diagnosis of, 187
   endoscopic surgical technique for, 188
   preoperative management of, 188
   surgical results for, 189f, 190, 190f